D1294617

Pulmonary
and Critical Care
Pharmacology
and Therapeutics

NOTICE

Medicine is an ever-changing science. As new research and clinical experience broaden our knowledge, changes in treatment and drug therapy are required. The editor and the publisher of this work have checked with sources believed to be reliable in their efforts to provide information that is complete and generally in accord with the standards accepted at the time of publication. However, in view of the possibility of human error or changes in medical sciences, neither the editor nor the publisher nor any other party who has been involved in the preparation or publication of this work warrants that the information contained herein is in every respect accurate or complete, and they are not responsible for any errors or omissions or for the results obtained from use of such information. Readers are encouraged to confirm the information contained herein with other sources. For example and in particular, readers are advised to check the product information sheet included in the package of each drug they plan to administer to be certain that the information contained in this book is accurate and that changes have not been made in the recommended dose or in the contraindications for administration. This recommendation is of particular importance in connection with new or infrequently used drugs.

Samford University Library

Pulmonary and Critical Care Pharmacology and Therapeutics

Editor

Alan R. Leff, M.D.

Professor of Medicine, Pediatrics, Pharmacological and Physiological Sciences, Anesthesia and Critical Care, and on the Committees of Cell Physiology and Clinical Pharmacology
Head, Section of Pulmonary and Critical Care Medicine
Division of the Biological Sciences
The University of Chicago
Chicago, Illinois

Released From
Samford University Library
Howard College

McGraw-Hill
Health Professions Division

New York   St. Louis   San Francisco   Auckland   Bogotá
Caracas   Lisbon   London   Madrid   Mexico City   Milan   Montreal
New Delhi   San Juan   Singapore   Sydney   Tokyo   Toronto

McGraw-Hill

A Division of The McGraw·Hill Companies

PULMONARY AND CRITICAL CARE PHARMACOLOGY AND THERAPEUTICS

Copyright © 1996 by The McGraw-Hill Companies, Inc. All rights reserved. Printed in the United States of America. Except as permitted under the United States Copyright Act of 1976, no part of this publication may be reproduced or distributed in any form or by any means, or stored in a data base or retrieval system, without the prior written permission of the publisher.

1234567890 DOW DOW 98765

ISBN 0-07-037096-6

This book was set in Palatino by Better Graphics, Inc.
The editors were Joseph Hefta and Pamela Touboul;
the production supervisor was Clare Stanley;
the cover designer was Diane Andrews.
R. R. Donnelley & Sons was printer and binder.

This book is printed on acid-free paper.

Library of Congress Cataloging-in-Publication Data

Pulmonary pharmacology and therapeutics / Alan R. Leff, editor.
    p. cm.
   Includes bibliographical references and index.
   ISBN 0-07-037096-6 (alk. paper)
   1. Pulmonary pharmacology.   I. Leff, Alan R.
   [DNLM: 1. Lung Diseases—drug therapy. 2. Respiratory System
Agents—pharmacology, 3. Lung—drug effects. 4. Lung—
physiopathology.   WF 600 P9855 1996]
RM388.P85   1996
616.2'4061—dc20
DNLM/DLC   98-12852
for Library of Congress   CIP

RM
388
.P85
1996

CONTENTS

v

This book is dedicated to Donna

CONTRIBUTORS

Andrew G. Alexander, M.D.
Department of Thoracic Medicine
London Chest Hospital
London, England [80]

Ralph J. Altiere, Ph.D.
Professor, School of Pharmacy
University of Colorado Health Sciences Center
Denver, Colorado [5, 9]

M. D. Altose, M.D.
Professor of Medicine
Case Western Reserve University
Cleveland, Ohio [83]

Gary P. Anderson, Ph.D.
Asthma and Allergy Research
CIBA Geigy
Basel, Switzerland [79]

Alejandro C. Arroglia, M.D.
Director, Fellowship Program
Department of Pulmonary and Critical Care Medicine
The Cleveland Clinic Foundation
Cleveland, Ohio [86]

Arthur S. Banner, M.D.
Adjunct Associate, Professor of Medicine
Dartmouth Medical Center
Lecturer on Medicine, Harvard Medical Center
Department of Veterans Affairs
Medical Center
Manchester, New Hampshire [68]

James N. Baraniuk, M.D.
Assistant Professor of Medicine
Division of Rheumatology, Immunology, and Allergy
Co-director, Adult Asthma and Allergy Service
Georgetown University
Washington, D.C. [7]

Neil C. Barnes, Ph.D.
Royal Brompton Hospital, National Heart & Lung Institute
London, England [80]

Peter J. Barnes, M.A., D.M., DSc., F.R.C.P.
Chairman, Department of Thoracic Medicine, and
    Honorary Consultant Physician
Royal Brompton Hospital
National Heart & Lung Institute
London, England [60, 80]

Robert C. Basner, M.D.
Associate Professor of Medicine
Section of Respiratory and Critical Care Medicine
University of Illinois
College of Medicine at Chicago
Chicago, Illinois [109]

Malcolm N. Blumenthal, M.D.
Director, Section of Allergy and Assistant Professor
Department of Medicine
University of Minnesota
Minneapolis, Minnesota [74]

Rebecca Blumenthal, M.D.
Assistant Professor, The University of Chicago
Chicago, Illinois [11]

Volker Brinkman, M.D. [79]
Asthma and Allergy Research
CIBA Geigy
Basel, Switzerland

Stuart M. Brooks, M.D.
Professor and Chairman, Department of Environmental
    and Occupational Health
University of South Florida
College of Public Health
Tampa, Florida [38]

William W. Busse, M.D.
Professor of Medicine
Head, Allergy / Clinical Immunology
University of Wisconsin Medical School
Madison, Wisconsin [34, 35]

Shannon S. Carson, M.D.
Assistant Professor of Clinical Medicine,
    Department of Medicine
The University of Chicago
Chicago, Illinois [8, 17]

Larry C. Casey, M.D., Ph.D.
Associate Professor of Medicine and Associate Director,
    Department of Pulmonary and Critical Care Medicine
Rush-Presbyterian St. Luke's Medical Center
Chicago, Illinois [25]

David M. Center, M.D.
Professor of Medicine, Research Professor of Biochemistry
Boston University School of Medicine
Boston, Massachusetts [30, 31]

Anoop J. Chauhan, MRCP [57]
Research Fellow
Southampton General Hospital
Southampton, United Kingdom

Neil S. Cherniak, M.D.
Dean, School of Medicine
Case Western Reserve University
Cleveland, Ohio [83]

Kian Fan Chung, M.D., FRCP
Reader in Thoracic Medicine, University of London,
    and Honorary Consultant
Royal Brompton Hospital
National Heart & Lung Institute
London, England [27]

Thomas Corbridge, M.D.
Assistant Professor of Medicine, Physical Medicine
    and Rehabilitation
Northwestern University Medical School
Director, Pulmonary Program
Rehab Institute of Chicago
Chicago, Illinois [78, 111A, 111B]

Alberto de Hoyos, M.D. FCCP [118]
Resident in General Surgery
Department of Surgery
Medical College of Virginia—Virginia Commonwealth
    University
Richmond, Virginia

Gordon Dent, M.D.
Krankenhaus Grosshansdorf
Center for Pharmacology
Grosshansdorf, Germany [16, 49]

Louis Diamond, Ph.D
Professor and Dean, University of Colorado at Boulder
School of Pharmacy
Boulder, Colorado [9]

Jeffrey M. Drazen, M.D.
Parker B. Francis Professor of Medicine
Harvard Medical School
Chief, Respiratory Division
Brigham & Women's Hospital
Boston, Massachusetts [10, 13]

Jack A. Elias, M.D.
Professor and Chief, Pulmonary and Critical Care Medicine
Department of Internal Medicine
Yale University School of Medicine
New Haven, Connecticut [26]

Alan M. Fein, M.D.
Professor of Medicine
Director, Pulmonary and Critical Care Medicine
Winthrop University Hospital
Mineola, New York [117]

Allison D. Fryer, Ph.D.
Assistant Professor of Physiology
School of Hygiene and Public Health
Johns Hopkins University
Baltimore, Maryland [6]

Allan Garland, MD
Assistant Professor of Clinical Medicine
University of Medicine and Dentistry of New Jersey
Robert Wood Johnson Medical School
New Brunswick, New Jersey [81]

Eugene F. Geppert, M.D.
Professor of Clinical Medicine
The University of Chicago
Chicago, Illinois [75, 90, 115, 116]

Leslie C. Grammer III, M.D.
Professor of Medicine
Northwestern University Medical School
Division of Allergy-Immunology
Chicago, Illinois [36]

Nicholas J. Gross, M.D., Ph.D.
Professor, Department of Medicine and Molecular
    Biochemistry
Department of Veterans Affairs
Edward Hines, Jr. Hospital
Hines, Illinois [10, 52, 53, 54]

Ronald F. Grossman, M.D.
Associate Professor of Medicine, University of Toronto
Head, Division of Respiratory Medicine
Mount Sinai Hospital
Toronto, Ontario [118]

Michael M. Grunstein, M.D., Ph.D.
Professor of Pediatrics
Chief, Division of Respiratory Medicine
Department of Pediatrics
Children's Hospital of Philadelphia
University of Pennsylvania School of Medicine
Philadelphia, Pennsylvania [1, 2, 3]

Jesse Hall, M.D.
Director, Critical Care and Professor of Medicine
The University of Chicago
Chicago, Illinois [67, 78, 87, 100, 101, 102]

Kimm J. Hamann, Ph.D.
Research Associate (Assistant Professor)
Department of Medicine
The University of Chicago
Chicago, Illinois [24, 32]

Rana Hejal, M.D.
Assistant Professor of Medicine
Case Western Reserve University
Cleveland, Ohio [73]

Marc B. Hershenson, M.D.
Assistant Professor
Department of Pediatrics
The University of Chicago
Chicago, Illinois [4, 106]

Carol A. Hirshman, M.D.
Professor of Anesthesiology, Critical Care Medicine,
    Environmental Health, Science, and Medicine
Johns Hopkins School of Hygiene
Baltimore, Maryland [119]

Stephen T. Holgate, M.D., DSC, FRCP
MRC Clinical Professor of Immunopharmacology
Southampton General Hospital
Southampton, United Kingdom [57, 58, 59]

Jonathan S. Ilowite
Director, Pulmonary Rehabilitation & Respiratory Care
Winthrop-University Hospital
Mineola, New York [117]

Elliot Israel, M.D.
Assistant Professor of Medicine
Brigham & Women's Hospital
Boston, Massachusetts [70]

David B. Jacoby, M.D.
Associate Professor
Division of Pulmonary and Critical Care
Johns Hopkins University
Baltimore, Maryland [6]

John W. Jenne, M.D.
Professor Emeritus
Loyola University, Stritch School of Medicine
Edward Hines, Jr. Veterans Administration Hospital
Hines, Illinois
Sandia Park, New Mexico [41–48]

Rudolf Jörres, M.D.
Krankenhaus Grosshansdorf
Center for Pharmacology
Grosshansdorf, Germany [37]

Bina Joseph
Allergy/Immunology Fellow
University of Wisconsin Medical School
Madison, WI [35]

Jan-Anders Karlsson, Ph.D.
Program Director, Biology
Rhone-Poulenc Rorer
Central Research
Dagenham Research Center
United Kingdom [61, 62]

Talmadge E. King, Jr., M.D., FACP, FCCP
Executive Vice President for Clinical Affairs
National Jewish Center for Immunology
    and Respiratory Medicine
Denver, Colorado [110]

Aparna Kumar, M.D.
Allergy Fellow
University of Wisconsin Medical School
Madison, Wisconsin [34]

Sophie Laberge, M.D.
Meakins-Christie Laboratories
McGill University
Ontario, Canada [31]

Stephen J. Lane, M.D.
United Medical and Dental Schools of Guys
    and St. Thomas Hospitals
London, England [55]

Tak H. Lee, M.D.
Professor, University of London
United Medical and Dental Schools of Guys
    and St. Thomas Hospitals
Division of Medicine
London, England [55]

Alan R. Leff, M.D.
Professor and Head
Section of Pulmonary and Critical Care Medicine
Department of Medicine
Chief, Pulmonary and Critical Care Medicine
The University of Chicago
Chicago, Illinois [77]

Lucille A. Lester, M.D.
Associate Professor, Department of Pediatrics
The University of Chicago
Chicago, Illinois [69]

Theodore H. Lewis, Jr., M.D.
Assistant Professor of Medicine
Section of Pulmonary and Critical Care Medicine
The University of Chicago
Chicago, IL [71, 103, 104, 105]

Greg Lindsay, M.D.
Research Associate
University of Colorado Health Sciences Center
School of Pharmacy
Denver, Colorado [5, 9]

Melvin Lopata, M.D.
Vice Chairman and Chief
Section of Respiratory and Critical Care Medicine
University of Illinois College of Medicine
Chicago, Illinois [107, 108]

Joseph P. Lynch, III, M.D.
Professor of Internal Medicine
University of Michigan Medical Center
Ann Arbor, Michigan [29]

Helgo Magnussen, M.D.
Krankenhaus Grosshansdorf
Center for Pharmacology
Grosshansdorf, Germany [37, 51]

Bernard Marsh, M.D. [82]
Professor, Otolaryngology
Head and Neck Surgery
Johns Hopkins University Medical Center
Baltimore, Maryland

William J. Martin, II, M.D.
Floyd and Reba Smith Professor of Medicine
Director, Division of Pulmonary, Critical Care
   and Occupational Medicine
Indiana University Medical Center
Indianapolis, Indiana [40]

Richard A. Matthay, M.D.
Boehringer Ingelheim Professor of Medicine
Associate Director, Department of Internal Medicine
Yale University School of Medicine
New Haven, Connecticut [86]

Hernalini Mehta, M.D.
Allergy Fellow
University of Wisconsin Medical School
Madison, Wisconsin [34]

E. Regis McFadden, Jr., M.D.
Argyl J. Barnes, Professor of Medicine
Case Western University School of Medicine
Department of Medicine
University Hospital
Cleveland, Ohio [41, 73]

Richard W. Mitchell, Ph.D.
Research Associate (Associate Professor)
Department of Medicine
The University of Chicago
Chicago, Illinois [18, 19, 20]

William Keith C. Morgan, M.D.
Professor of Medicine
The University of Western Ontario
Ontario, Canada [39]

Rebecca L. Mortenson, M.D. [111A, 111B]
Assistant Professor of Medicine
Department of Medicine, University of Colorado
Denver, Colorado

Jonathan Moss, M.D., Ph.D.
Professor and Vice Chairman for Research and
   Professor of Clinical Pharmacology
Department of Anesthesia and Critical Care
The University of Chicago
Chicago, Illinois [11]

Nilda Maria Muñoz, M.S.
Research Associate (Assistant Professor) of Medicine
The University of Chicago
Chicago, Illinois [12]

Thomas M. Murphy, M.D.
Associate Professor of Pediatrics
Chief, Division of Pediatric Pulmonary
Duke University Medical Center
Durham, North Carolina [91, 92, 93, 94, 95]

Patrick Murray, M.D.
Instructor in Medicine
The University of Chicago
Chicago, Illinois [23]

Jeffrey L. Myers, M.D. [114]
Associate Professor of Pathology
Division of Anatomic Pathology
Mayo Clinic
Rochester, Minnesota

Robert M. Naclerio, M.D.
Professor and Chief
Otolaryngology - Head and Neck Surgery
The University of Chicago
Chicago, Illinois [82]

Lewis W. Neese, M.D. [114]
Fellow, Division of Pulmonary and Critical Care Medicine,
   Department of Internal Medicine
Mayo Graduate School of Medicine

Michael S. Niederman, M.D.
Associate Professor of Medicine
SUNY at Stony Brook
Health Sciences Center
Director, Medical & Respiratory Intensive Care Unit
Pulmonary and Critical Care Medicine
Winthrop-University Hospital
Mineola, New York [89]

Paul O'Byrne, MB, FRCPI, FRCP(C)
Professor, Department of Medicine
Head, Division of Respirology
McMaster University
Hamilton, Ontario, Canada **[56]**

Michael O'Conner, M.D.
Assistant Professor
Department of Anesthesia and Critical Care
The University of Chicago
Chicago, Illinois **[71]**

Philip Padrid, D.V.M.
Assistant Professor of Medicine
Section of Pulmonary and Critical Care Medicine
The University of Chicago
Chicago, Illinois **[63, 64]**

Harold I. Palevsky, M.D.
Associate Professor of Medicine
Pulmonary and Critical Care Division
University of Pennsylvania Medical Center
Philadelphia, Pennsylvania **[113]**

Jonathon D. Plitman, M.D.
Division of Pulmonary and Critical Care Medicine
Vanderbilt University
Nashville, Tennessee **[14]**

Klaus F. Rabe, M.D.
Krankenhaus Grosshansdorf
Center of Pharmacology
Grosshansdorf, Germany **[16, 49, 50, 51]**

Daniel W. Ray, M.D.
Assistant Professor of Clinical Medicine
Northwestern University
Chicago, Illinois **[8]**

Stanley Rehm, M.D. [40]
Clinical Associate Professor
Pulmonary and Critical Division
Indiana University, Medical Center
Indianapolis, Indiana

Cheryl L. Renz, M.D.
Assistant Professor of Medicine
The University of Chicago
Chicago, Illinois **[72]**

Michael H. Ries, M.D., F.C.C.P.
Assistant Professor of Medicine,
Rush Medical College
Director, Medical Intensive Care Unit
Co-Director, Internal Medicine Residency Program
Co-Director, Pulmonary Rehabilitation Program
Rush North Shore Medical Center

Director, Pulmonary Rehabilitation Program
Director, Medical Intensive Care Unit
Director, Pulmonary and Critical Care Division
St. Joseph Health Centers and Hospital
Medical Director, THC-North Side Ventilator Unit
Chicago, Illinois **[88]**

Edward C. Rosenow, III, M.D.
Professor of Medicine
Thoracic Diseases and Internal Medicine
Mayo Clinic
Rochester, Minnesota **[114]**

Chris Rudd, M.D. [91, 92, 93, 94, 95]
Assistant Clinical Professor,
Duke University Medical Center
Durham, North Carolina

Wayne M. Samuelson, M.D. [91, 92, 93, 94, 95]
Associate Professor of Medicine
Division of Respiratory, Critical Care, and Occupational
    Pulmonary Medicine
University of Utah
Salt Lake City, Utah

Jussi J. Saukkonen, M.D.
Assistant Professor of Medicine
Boston University School of Medicine
Boston, Massachusetts **[30]**

Gregory A. Schmidt, M.D.
Associate Professor of Clinical Medicine and Director,
    Critical Care Fellowship
The University of Chicago
Chicago, Illinois **[96–102]**

Craig M. Schramm, M.D.
Assistant Professor of Pediatrics
Pediatric Pulmonary Division
University of Connecticut Health Center
Farmington, Connecticut **[1, 2, 3]**

Paul Schumacker, Ph.D.
Professor of Medicine and Chairman, Committee on
    Comparative Medicine
The University of Chicago
Chicago, Illinois

James R. Snapper, M.D.
Professor of Medicine
Director of Pulmonary and Critical Care Medicine
Department of Medicine
Vanderbilt University Hospital
Nashville, Tennessee **[14, 15]**

Gordon L. Snider, M.D.
Maurice B. Strauss, Professor of Medicine
Chief–Medical Service
Boston Medical Center
Boston, Massachusetts [84, 85]

Julian Solway, M.D.
Associate Professor of Medicine and Pediatrics
Section of Pulmonary and Critical Care Medicine and
    Director, Pulmonary Medicine
The University of Chicago
Chicago, Illinois [8, 17, 81]

Mary E. Strek, M.D.
Assistant Professor of Medicine
Section of Pulmonary and Critical Care Medicine
The University of Chicago
Chicago, Illinois [65, 66]

Eugene J. Sullivan, M.D.
Pulmonary Specialist
Department of Pulmonary and Critical Care Medicine
Cleveland Clinic Foundation
Cleveland, Ohio [110]

Lynn T. Tanoue, M.D.
Assistant Professor of Medicine
Pulmonary and Critical Care Section
Yale University, School of Medicine
New Haven, Connecticut [26]

Galen B. Toews, M.D.
Professor and Chief, Division of Pulmonary
    and Critical Care Medicine
The University of Michigan Medical Center
Ann Arbor, Michigan [29, 33]

Paula L. Watson, M.D.
Fellow, Department of Pulmonary Medicine
Vanderbilt University
Nashville, Tennessee [15]

Craig D. Wegner, Ph.D.
Abbott Laboratories
Abbott Park, Illinois [28]

Steven R. White, M.D.
Associate Professor of Medicine and Section of Pulmonary
    and Critical Care Medicine
The University of Chicago
Chicago, Illinois [76]

Richard H. Winterbauer, M.D.
Head, Section of Chest and Infectious Diseases
Virginia Mason Clinic
Seattle, Washington [112]

Nicholas J. Withers, Ph.D., M.R.C.P.
Research Fellow
University of Southampton
Southampton General Hospital
United Kingdom [58]

Lawrence D. H. Wood, M.D.
Professor of Medicine and Faculty Dean for Education
The University of Chicago
Chicago, Illinois [87]

Mark E. Wylam, M.D.
Assistant Professor of Pediatrics and Medicine
Department of Pediatrics
The University of Chicago
Chicago, Illinois [21, 22, 23]

FOREWORD

There has been an explosion of information in pharmacology, and recently much of this information has been applied to the lung and to respiratory diseases. These advances have been made possible by the development of many new drugs that have a great degree of specificity and by rapid advances in molecular and cell biology. Application of these novel pharmacologic tools and approaches has revealed much new information about the basic mechanisms involved in lung diseases. Pharmacology has greatly broadened its scope in recent years and has become integrated with molecular biology, immunology, and biochemistry. The use of increasingly sophisticated drugs has provided an opportunity to study the mechanisms of lung disease in detail. The development of specific receptor antagonists and enzyme inhibitors has provided new insights into the mechanisms of lung disease, particularly in asthma, where multiple inflammatory mediators are involved.

This book brings together a wealth of talent in the field of pulmonary pharmacology. Until recently the application of pharmacology to lung disease often lagged behind its role in other areas, such as cardiovascular disease and gastroenterology, but this has now been more than compensated for by a rapid increase in interest in pulmonary pharmacology. The respiratory tract is accessible to pharmacologic intervention by administration of inhaled drugs; it also allows sampling of cells and tissue via fiberoptic bronchoscopy, induced sputum, and more recently, exhaled gases such as nitric oxide.

The lung is highly complex, with multiple interacting cell types, and this provides enormous opportunities to examine a great diversity of physiologic and biochemical mechanisms, using pharmacologic techniques. In the past, most emphasis in asthma research was placed on airway smooth muscle; it was believed that abnormal bronchoconstriction was the fundamental problem. It is now apparent that asthma is a complicated inflammatory disease involving many cell types. Much attention has been directed to many of these cell types including inflammatory cells (e.g., eosinophils, T lymphocytes, macrophages, and mast cells) and structural cells, such as epithelial cells, endothelial cells, and fibroblasts. Indeed, it is now emerging that these so-called structural cells actively participate in inflammatory and immune responses in the lung by releasing mediators and growth factors.

Asthma has attracted considerable attention and remains a major clinical problem in industrialized and developing countries alike. This has provided a powerful impetus to research. Pharmacologic approaches have been invaluable in elucidating the underlying inflammatory mechanisms involved. It is clear that immunologic mechanisms are also involved in the pathophysiology of asthma, but as the mediators of these immune mechanisms become better defined, the distinction between pharmacology and immunology becomes blurred. Thus as a cytokine, such as interleukin-5, is identified, it is possible to then study its receptors and their transduction mechanisms, and this comes into the province of pharmacology. Ultimately this will lead to specific drugs that will block the synthesis of or response to IL-5.

However, asthma is not the only disease where pharmacologic approaches have been used to clarify mechanisms. Chronic obstructive pulmonary disease (COPD), cystic fibrosis, interstitial lung diseases, and adult respiratory distress syndrome all involve inflammation with the release of many mediators that may be elucidated by pharmacologic means.

Another important aspect of pharmacology that is amply covered in this book is an understanding of the mechanisms of drug action. Enormous insights recently have been obtained into the molecular mechanisms involved in the action of bronchodilators and anti-inflammatory drugs. This knowledge is important in understanding how best to use these drugs in treating any particular lung disease. Understanding the basic pharmacology of drug action sheds light on the underlying disease mechanisms. The comprehension of molecular mechanisms makes it possible to study and predict the interaction (beneficial and harmful) between different drugs; this will be of increasing importance in the treatment of the future.

Alan Leff, in editing this book, has chosen a careful balance between basic pharmacology and its clinical application to the treatment of lung disease. The first section highlights some of the important recent advances in understanding receptor structure and function. Many of these advances were only made possible through developments in molecular biology and the consequences of all this new knowledge have still to be fully exploited.

Autonomic control is an area where classical pharmacology has been particularly useful in defining neurotransmitters and their receptors that play such a key role in airway diseases. There have been important new advances in our understanding of innervation of the respiratory tract. Novel neurotransmitters, such as multiple neuropeptides and nitric oxide, have been identified in the lung; this may have important implications for understanding disease mechanisms and for the development of new drugs. Over a hundred mediators of inflammation have been associated with inflammatory lung diseases. Enormous advances have been made by the development of specific inhibitors (e.g., leukotriene and thromboxane receptor antagonists) and enzyme inhibitors (e.g., 5-lipoxygenase and nitric oxide synthase inhibitors). Many of these drugs are now in clinical studies. Only with the development of specific drugs can the role of a particular inflammatory mediator be properly evaluated in a disease. For example, cysteinyl-leukotrienes and platelet-activating factor both have potent effects on pulmonary function; therefore, there was reason to believe that both might be involved in asthma. However, leukotriene, and not PAF antagonists, has been found to have useful clinical effects in asthma. An explosion of interest in cytokines has occurred as molecular cloning has revealed more and more of these important and complex signaling molecules. The complexities of the inflammatory response, including the individual inflammatory cells, adhesion molecules, and the role of structural cells, are all covered in detail. This information is important in trying to understand the mechanism of action of the different drugs used in the treatment of lung disease.

A wide range of drugs used to treat lung diseases is now available and many more drugs are currently in development. These drugs are dealt with in detail, both from the point of view of their mechanisms of action and in terms of how they are used in management. All types of pulmonary disease are covered in this book and a wealth of information concerning therapy is also provided.

Pulmonary pharmacology has come of age and is a key component of pulmonary medicine and an important part of pulmonary research. In the future it is likely that the boundaries between the different disciplines will become ever more indistinct as molecular and cell biology blend into biochemistry and pharmacology. Pulmonary pharmacology is in a good position to take advantage of these new developments and apply them to elucidating the underlying mechanisms of pulmonary disease and effective therapy. Undoubtedly this approach will lead to new therapeutic avenues in the future. This book ably sets the stage.

Peter Barnes, M.D.
Chairman, Department of Thoracic Medicine
Royal Brompton Hospital
National Heart and Lung Institute
London, England

PREFACE

The decision to assemble a textbook of pulmonary and critical care pharmacology derives from the recognition that no comprehensive new work has been written on this subject in more than 20 years. The more difficult decision was how to organize the material and what to include. Since 1975, there has been a vast array of scientific discoveries. What were concepts of molecular biology are now preclinical developments that are ready for translation into clinical therapies.

It seems reasonable that a comprehensive text must begin with some sections that relate specifically to the basic science of pharmacology (and immunology) per se, with special emphasis upon those of interest to pulmonologists and intensivists. The text is organized accordingly, and there follows a section relating specifically to the clinical pharmacology of the therapeutic agents. In the title *Pulmonary and Critical Care Pharmacology and Therapeutics*, I meant to consider the broad range of treatments available for diseases of the lung and critical systemic illness. Therapeutics thus relates not only to pharmaceuticals but also, for example, to administration of agents by nebulization, airway management during anesthesia, oxygen therapy, and pulmonary exercise regimens. Indeed, since 1975, the entire field of critical care medicine has been defined as a subspecialty. By nature, critical care medicine is a multidisciplinary specialty involving critical illness of various organ systems, often simultaneously. Because such patients frequently are managed by pulmonologists who are also certified specialists in critical care medicine, it seemed appropriate to consider in detail the critical care aspects of pulmonary diseases and the art and science of management of the critically ill patient. In this endeavor, the emphasis has been upon the management of immune-compromised host (with special emphasis on HIV infection) and on the patient with noncardiogenic pulmonary edema. There has been no attempt to consider systematically the antibiosis per se of pulmonary diseases beyond this context. That would require extensive elaboration beyond the scope of this textbook. Likewise, aspects of lung oncology have been excluded from the text, as they rightfully belong in the literature of that subspecialty to receive the detailed treatment that is required.

All contributions have been referenced extensively, and contributors have been asked to write at the state-of-the-art level in the three basic areas of the book, that is, the basic science, clinical pharmacology, and disease-related therapies. Thus, this book should be of value to all students and practitioners of pulmonary and critical care science and medicine.

I would like to thank my contributors for their generous and selfless efforts. In my view, they have uniformly produced works of outstanding quality, and I am personally honored that they all agreed to deliver contributions of such fine quality. I also wish to thank the editors of McGraw-Hill, who conceived this project. It has been a particular pleasure to work with them, and their tolerance of a text that is twice its estimated size is much appreciated. Special thanks also to Nancy Trojan, Project Manager of the Pulmonary and Critical Care Section at the University of Chicago, for her help in the numerous correspondences necessary to assemble this text. The greatest measure of thanks goes to my family. The work on this textbook involved long nights and times away that cannot be regained, and their continued support of such challenging endeavors is the single most important factor in the production of this text.

Alan R. Leff
The University of Chicago
Chicago, Illinois

Pulmonary
and Critical Care
Pharmacology
and Therapeutics

PART 1

PRINCIPLES OF PULMONARY PHARMACOLOGY

RECEPTORS AND TARGET CELLS

Chapter 1
RECEPTORS 1: G-PROTEIN–LINKED RECEPTORS

MICHAEL M. GRUNSTEIN AND CRAIG M. SCHRAMM

Cellular activation in the lung involves all known forms of transmembrane signaling including those induced by endocrine, paracrine, synaptic, and autocrine processes. The host of mediators, neurotransmitters, and hormones mediating these signaling modalities act through a variety of target-cell surface and intracellular receptors. The cell surface receptors include the guanine nucleotide-binding protein (G protein)–linked receptors, ion channel–linked receptors, and enzyme-linked receptors. In contrast, the family of intracellular receptors encompasses those that respond to water-insoluble hormones that diffuse across the target-cell plasma membrane; these include the steroid hormones, thyroid hormones, retinoids, and vitamin D. The following three chapters highlight much of the information gained to date on the above principal classes of receptors, including their classification, molecular characteristics, regulation, and key signal-transduction mechanisms. This first chapter focuses on the G-protein-linked receptors, beginning with a general overview of the structural and functional characteristics of this receptor class. This is followed by a description of the role of G proteins and their transmembrane signaling processes and concludes with a description of mechanisms regulating G-protein-linked receptor function.

The receptors whose signal transduction involves coupling of heterotrimeric G proteins constitute a superfamily of integral membrane proteins characterized by amino acid sequences containing seven hydrophobic transmembrane-spanning regions. More than 150 G-protein-coupled receptors have been cloned and sequenced. Through their interaction with G proteins, these receptors transduce a myriad of signals, including those represented by lipid analog (e.g., eicosanoids), peptide hormones and neurotransmitters, and other specialized stimuli. In recent years, extensive research using molecular biologic, biochemical, and pharmacodynamic techniques has elucidated certain fundamental structural and functional features of this superfamily of receptors, which are discussed below. For additional in-depth literature in this area, extending beyond the scope of this chapter, the reader is referred to a number of recent comprehensive reviews.[1–5]

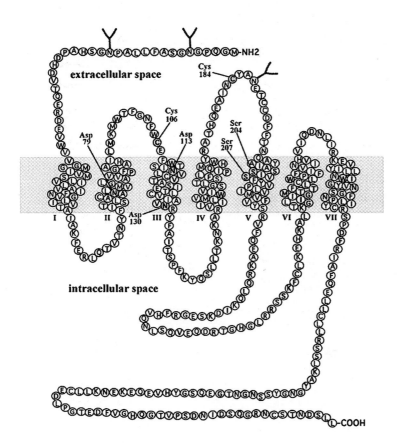

FIGURE 1-1 Primary structure of the β_2-adrenergic receptor depicting topology of the seven-pass transmembrane helical domains, and highlighted key amino acid residues examined using mutational analysis. The amino acid sequence of the receptor is represented by the single-letter code. (*From Savarese and Fraser,*[110] *with permission.*)

G-Protein–Linked Receptors: Structural Characteristics

Cloning of G-protein–coupled receptors has revealed the conservation of a primary structure among G-protein receptor families. Accordingly, G-protein–coupled receptors were found to represent single polypeptides, ranging in size from ~ 400 to over 1000 amino acids, each possessing seven hydrophobic domains of 20 to 25 amino acids, which span the membrane lipid bilayer, as exemplified by the schematic model of the β_2-adrenergic receptor in Fig. 1-1. The overall structure of G-protein receptors resembles a barrel oriented perpendicular to the plane of the cell membrane, with the staves represented by the seven membrane-spanning domains. Analysis of the amino acid composition of these receptors has identified that the membrane-spanning domains depict the largest degree of sequence homology between unrelated receptors and that up to 90 percent of sequence homology exists between various receptor subtypes. Apart from this structural similarity, the membrane-spanning domains were predicted to be α helices and to contain a ligand-binding region.[6,7] Moreover, immunologic mapping studies have demonstrated the presence of a hydrophilic extracellular N-terminal sequence and an intracellular C-terminal sequence[8,9,10] associated with three sets of alternate intra- and extracellular loops of variable length.

The tertiary structure of the transmembrane regions of the G-protein–linked receptor establishes the ligand-binding domain within the core of the barrel. The ligand-binding domain is fairly highly conserved among members of a given receptor family. Studies on the structure of the adrenoceptor family using mutagenesis techniques and synthetic adrenergic ligands have elucidated that the endogenous ligand-binding pocket of the receptor contains acidic amino acid residues on the third transmembrane loop (e.g., Asp 113) that act as counter-ions for the catecholamine nitrogen, whereas conserved serines (Ser 204 and Ser 207) contained within the fifth transmembrane domain interact with the meta- and parahydroxy groups on the catechol ring.[7,11] The latter serine residues are conserved in G-protein–linked receptors having catechol ring ligands (e.g., adrenergic and dopaminergic receptors) but are not contained in receptors lacking catechol ring ligands (e.g., muscarinic and peptide hormone receptors). Four additional serines (Ser 106, Ser 184, Ser 190, and Ser 191) in the first and second intracellular loops have been shown to affect both agonist and antagonist binding to the β-adrenoceptor and are believed to contribute disulfide bridges to the tertiary structure of the receptor. Mutational analysis of the β-adrenergic receptor has also elucidated a number of other structure/function characteristics of this G-protein–linked receptor, several of which are summarized in Table 1-1 in relation to the mutational sites identified in Fig. 1-1.

The binding sites for antagonists have been found to be different from those of naturally occurring ligands. In this regard, construction of chimeric receptors has provided some important clues as to the regions that are crucial for binding. Chimeric receptors are formed using portions of two related G-protein–linked receptors by splicing together

TABLE 1-1   Mutational Effects of the β_2-Adrenergic Receptor Corresponding to the Sites Identified in Fig. 1-1.

Site	Mutation		Effect	Reference
Asp^{113}	Asn^{113}		Reduced antagonist affinity	103,104
			Reduced adenylate cyclase activation	
Asp^{113}	Glu^{113}		Reduced antagonist affinity	103,104
			Reduced agonist potency	
Asp^{79}	Ala^{79}		Decreased agonist affinity	103,104
			Reduced adenylate cyclase activation	
			Normal antagonist binding	
Asp^{79}	Asn^{79}		Normal antagonist binding	105
			Reduced agonist affinity	
			No agonist-mediated cAMP increase	
Asp^{130}	Asn^{130}		Normal antagonist binding	106
			Increased agonist affinity but uncoupled cAMP response	
Ser^{204}	Ala^{204}		Reduced agonist affinity	107
			Unaltered antagonist binding	
Ser^{207}	Ala^{207}		Reduced agonist affinity	107
			Unaltered antagonist binding	
Cys^{106}	or	Cys^{184}	Disrupted disulfide linkage with altered receptor tertiary structure	108,109
			Altered agonist and antagonist binding	

complementary helical regions from the two receptors. In this manner, the junction for splicing of the two receptors can be varied to different sites in the receptor sequence; hence, it is possible to determine which helical domain(s) may be the most crucial for binding of a specific ligand. While this technique is useful for the localization of general sites involved in ligand binding, when coupled to analysis of the effects of specific point mutations in these general regions, the ligand binding characteristics of the receptor can be defined more closely. Accordingly, using chimeric receptors constructed from α_2- and β_2-adrenergic receptors, the seventh transmembrane domain was identified as a key determinant of antagonist binding.[2] Similarly, the amino acid sequence contained within the transmembrane region of the tachykinin NK_1 receptor associated with binding of the antagonist CP 96345 was identified as different from the domain(s) associated with binding of endogenous neurokinin peptide ligands.[12] Moreover, construction of chimeric receptors was useful in identifying the G-protein activation sites for the muscarinic and β-adrenergic receptors. On the other hand, it should be noted that interpretation of the structural determinants for G-protein–linked receptors using the chimeric receptor approach has the limitation that all the interhelical sites of contact responsible for the tertiary structure of the receptor must be maintained. This limitation is often reflected by a reduced binding affinity of the chimeric receptor.

Posttranscriptional Modification of G-Protein–Linked Receptors

Most G-protein–linked receptors undergo posttranscriptional modifications, which alter their structural and functional characteristics, primarily including glycosylation and palmitoylation. The findings that these receptors have molecular weights greater than those predicted from their amino acid sequences and that endoglycosidase treatment results in decreases in the receptors' molecular weights provide evidence that the receptors undergo posttranscriptional glycosylation. Moreover, G-protein–linked receptors have asparagine residues in their extracellular domain, primarily associated with the N-terminus, which confer the glycosylation consensus sequence, Asn-X-Ser/Thr, in the extracellular domain. While believed to play an insignificant role in agonist binding, glycosylation of the receptors has been implicated in determining the cellular distribution of the receptors and some of their functional characteristics.[2,7,13] Palmitoylation, on the other hand, is a posttranscriptional modification associated with the intracellular C-terminus, involving cysteine residues which covalently bind palmitic acid through a thioester bond.[2,7,13,14] With this interaction, the palmitate residues become incorporated into the membrane bilayer, conferring a fourth intracellular loop configuration to the receptor. It has been demonstrated, for the β_2-adrenergic receptor, that disruption of this configuration by mutagenesis of the cysteine residues involved with palmitoylation destabilizes the tertiary structure of the receptor and results in alterations in its binding characteristics and coupling of the receptor to its associated G_s protein.[13] Moreover, the state of palmitoylation of the β_2-adrenergic receptor was found to be influenced by ligand occupancy.[15] Palmitoylation has been implicated in modulating phosphorylation of the receptor by specific receptor kinases (i.e., GRKs), which act on ligand-bound receptors at sites near the C-terminus.[17] Thus, it appears that palmitoylation of G-protein–linked receptors represents an important dynamic feature for modulating receptor/G-protein interac-

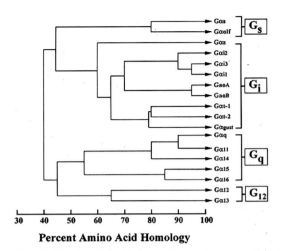

FIGURE 1-2 Classification of G-protein α subunits and their structural relationships. Members of the four principal G-protein classes are grouped in relation to their amino acid homology with branch junctions corresponding to comparative values for the α subunits indicated. *(From Watson and Arkinstall,[111] with permission.)*

tion as well attenuating the receptor activity by altering its anchoring to the cell membrane.[15]

There is also convincing evidence that receptor–G-protein coupling specificity is primarily determined by amino acid sequences in the third intracellular (i3) loop. Synthetic peptides corresponding to the amino- and carboxyl-terminal portions of the i3 loop of the β-adrenoceptor can directly activate G_s.[112] Moreover, chimeric muscarinic receptors, formed by switching the i3 loops between M_2 and M_3 receptors, demonstrate G-protein selectivity of the i3 loop donor.[113] Other receptor hybrids (e.g., M_1-muscarinic/β-adrenergic) with exchanged i3 loops also couple to the G protein associated with the i3 donor, but these chimeras retain the ability to couple to the G protein associated with the i3 recipient as well.[114] Studies with the latter receptor hybrids suggest that the i2 loop may also influence receptor–G-protein interactions.

G Proteins: Structural and Functional Characteristics

The G proteins are heterotrimeric structures containing α, β, and γ subunits, which are encoded by different genes. The diversity in G-protein structure and function is largely given by the heterogeneity of the proteins' α subunits. More than 20 different Gα gene products have been identified, some of which represent alternative RNA-spliced isoforms.[18,19] Based on homology of their primary amino acid sequences, the G-protein α subunits have been classified into four principal classes, including $G\alpha_s$, $G\alpha_i$, $G\alpha_q$, and $G\alpha_{12}$, each class contains various α-subunit members (Fig. 1-2).

The conserved domains of the α subunits are schematically depicted in a linearized model in Fig. 1-3, which highlights certain important Gα-subunit functions. In general, the C-terminal sequence of the α subunit is critical for the interaction of the receptor with its effector. At this site, pertussis toxin acts to ADP-ribosylate certain α subunits, blocking their interaction with the receptor.[20–22] Moreover, certain key amino acid residues within the C-terminal sequence (i.e., sites G_3–G_5) have been identified as sites of Gα-mediated effector activation (e.g., adenylate cyclase,[23,24] whereas adjacent sequences serve as the guanine nucleotide binding pocket contained within the GTPase domain (G_1–G_5), the site of ADP-ribosylation by cholera toxin. In contrast, components of the N-terminal sequence have been identified as crucial for α-subunit anchorage to the membrane, myristoylation, and coupling to the β-γ subunit.

Whereas the α subunit binds and hydrolyzes GTP, the β-γ subunit dimer does not dissociate and functionally represents a monomer. Both the α subunit and β-γ dimer play important roles as mediators of signal transduction. The cycle of receptor-coupled G-protein activation that transduces the extracellular signal to effector activation is depicted schematically in Fig. 1-4. In the absence of receptor activation by its ligand, GDP is bound to the α subunit and the latter is associated with the β-γ dimer, constituting an inactive heterotrimer that is bound to the unstimulated receptor (Fig. 1-4A). Upon activation of the receptor by its ligand, the receptor undergoes a conformational change,

FIGURE 1-3 Linear schematic representation of the generalized G protein α subunit. Domains depicted include those proposed for interaction with receptor, effector, and β-γ dimer. Also indicated are sites for myristolation and ADP ribosylation by cholera toxin and pertussis toxin as well as conserved domains for binding guanine nucleotides and intrinsic GTPase activity (regions G_1-G_5). *(From Watson and Arkinstall,[111] with permission.)*

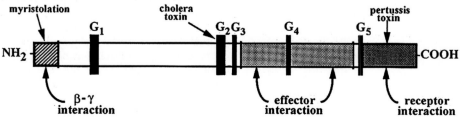

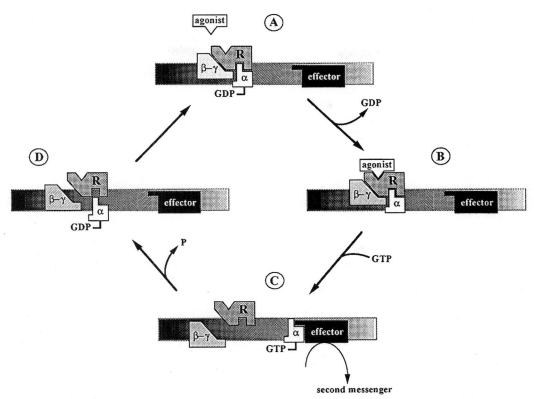

FIGURE 1-4 The cycle of receptor/G-protein interaction in transmembrane signaling. The components include receptor (R), α subunit, β-γ dimer, agonist, and effector. *A:* The receptor bound to G protein has a greater affinity for the agonist. *B:* The binding of agonist to the receptor produces a conformational change in the receptor, which results in the release of GDP and binding of GTP to the α subunit. *C:* The binding of GTP to the α subunit results in dissociation of the α subunit from both the receptor and the β-γ dimer and association of the α subunit with the effector to stimulate the generation of a second messenger. *D:* The α subunit–bound GTP is hydrolyzed to GDP by an intrinsic GTPase, and the α subunit becomes dissociated from the effector and reassociates with the β-γ dimer/receptor complex to repeat the agonist-coupled cycle.

which is associated with a corresponding change in the α subunit. This results in a reduced affinity of the α subunit for GDP and, because the cellular concentration of GTP markedly exceeds that of GDP, the latter becomes dissociated from the active site of the α subunit and is replaced by GTP (Fig. 1-4*B*). When placed in this GTP-bound activated state, the α subunit becomes dissociated from both the receptor and the β-γ dimer. In this activated GTP-bound state (Fig. 1-4*C*), the free α and β-γ subunits activate specific intracellular effectors (e.g., phospholipase C, adenylate cyclase, ion channels, βARK, etc.). The activated state of the GTP-bound α subunit, however, is transient, since the bound GDP is hydrolyzed to GDP by an intrinsic GTPase contained within the α subunit. Accordingly, when replaced by GDP, the α and β-γ subunits reassociate, and the reconstituted heterotrimer also becomes reassociated with the receptor (Fig. 1-4*D*), thereby priming the receptor-coupled G-protein mechanism to respond again to receptor stimulation.

In the above scheme of G-protein activation, it is important to note that while receptors are typically highly selective in interacting with their specific ligands, the specificity with which receptors interact with their G proteins can vary in relation to the range of responses of a particular cell. Thus, whereas a given receptor interacts with only one G-protein subtype to activate a single effector, another type of receptor (or the same receptor in a different cell) may interact with several G proteins, resulting in the activation of several effectors through different signaling pathways. This produces a diversity of cellular responses, which is regulated further by other mechanisms. Among these, the finding that different α subunits possess different intrinsic rates of GTPase activity[25,26] implies that a given receptor coupled to different α subunits may mediate both a relatively transient, short-lived response as well as a more sustained intracellular signal. Also, it has been demonstrated that certain effectors may regulate α-subunit activity reciprocally. For example, phospholipase C and retinal CGMP phosphodiesterase were found to enhance the intrinsic GTPase activity of their activating G proteins,[27,28] thereby facilitating the deactivation of the α subunits. Additional mechanisms potentially regulating G-protein function are covalent modification by phosphorylation of α subunits on serine or threonine residues, lipid modifications including palmitoylation of cysteine residues within the N-terminal sequence of the α subunits, myristoylation of the α subunits at the N-terminal glycine, and isoprenylation of the C-terminal cysteine of the γ subunit.[29]

Apart from the above considerations of receptor-mediated modulation of G-protein function, it has been established that G proteins exert a reciprocal modulatory action on the function of their corresponding receptors. Accordingly, when coupled to an inactive G protein, the receptor exists in a state of high affinity for the agonist. Agonist binding elicits the above conformational change in the G protein, resulting in its activation. In response to the latter event, the α subunit of the G protein is released, and the receptor reverts to a lower-affinity state for the agonist. This sequence of events, wherein the G protein feeds back a modulatory action on the receptor, is referred to as the "guanine nucleotide shift" of the receptor to an altered affinity state and represents a highly sensitive indicator of receptor/G protein coupling. To date, the molecular mechanism underlying this G-protein–induced conformational change in the affinity state of its corresponding receptor remains to be identified.

G-Protein–Linked Effector Systems

G-protein–linked receptors are coupled to several functionally diverse effector and second-messenger systems. A detailed account of each of these known systems is beyond the scope of this chapter; however, consideration is given here to certain principal signal transduction mechanisms associated with G-protein–linked receptors, including activation of the phospholipase C, phospholipase A$_2$, and adenylate cyclase systems, as well as regulation of ion channel activity.

PHOSPHOLIPASE C-COUPLED SIGNALING

Stimulation of specific G-protein–linked receptors by a variety of hormones, neurotransmitters, and certain growth factors leads to activation of phospholipase C (PLC). The latter elicits hydrolysis of membrane phosphatidyl inositol 4,5-bisphosphate (PIP$_2$), which results in the generation of the two key second messengers, inositol 1,4,5-triphosphate (Ins(1,4,5)P$_3$) and diacylglycerol (DAG). Whereas the former acts on its intracellular receptor located in the endoplasmic reticulum to mobilize intracellular Ca^{2+}, DAG elicits activation of a group of protein kinase C (PKC) isozymes which exert a host of cellular regulatory actions.[30–32]

Apart from the diversity of G-protein–linked receptors activating PLC, the latter effector is also structurally and functionally diverse in mammalian cells. Accordingly, PLC isozymes have been classified into the three principal classes—PLC-β, PLC-γ, and PLC-δ—with each class further categorized into different sub-classes based on cloned sequences demonstrating amino acid homology, including PLC-β1, PLC-β2, PLC-β3, PLC-γ1, PLC-γ2, PLC-δ1, and PLC-δ2.[33–35] Collectively, these PLC subtypes depict an overall amino acid sequence homology ranging between 21 and 56 percent and contain an even higher degree of sequenced homology within two domains (X and Y domains) constituting critical sites for catalytic activity of the PLC isozymes (Fig. 1-5). Additionally, the PLC-γ isoforms also contain two *Src* homology 2 (SH2) regions[36] and one SH3 region[37] interposed between the X and Y domains (Fig. 1-5), which display sequence similarities with the regulatory regions of the *Src* protooncogene and are coupled to activation of certain growth-modulatory enzyme-linked receptors having intrinsic tyrosine kinase activity (see Chap. 2).

Activation of the PLC subtypes is accompanied by Ca^{2+}-sensitive hydrolysis of the phospholipids, phosphatidylinositol (PI), phosphatidylinositol 4-monophosphate (PIP), and phosphatidylinositol 4, 5-bisphosphate (PIP$_2$).[38–41] Members of the PLC-β and -γ subtypes are activated by certain pertussis toxin–insensitive G protein α subunits, including αq and α11, α14, α15 and α16, whereas the pertussis toxin–sensitive G$_i$α subunits are ineffective.[42–44] In contrast, the PLC-β isoforms can be activated by the β-γ dimers of certain G proteins (i.e., Gα$_i$ and Gα$_o$), conferring pertussis toxin sensi-

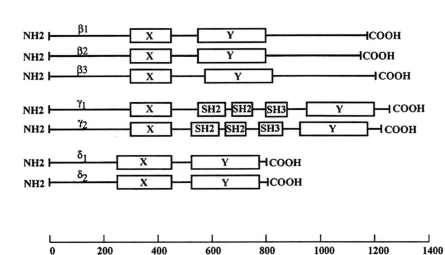

FIGURE 1-5 Linear schematic representation of the structural arrangement of the phospholipase C isoforms. The homologous domains, X and Y, are proposed as containing the catalytic activities of the isoenzymes. These domains are separated in PLCγ$_1$ and PLCγ$_2$ to contain sequences with Src protooncogene homology (SH), including SH2 and SH3, which are involved in transmembrane signaling associated with cellular proliferation. (*From Watson and Arkinstall,*[111] *with permission.*)

Amino Acid Residue Number

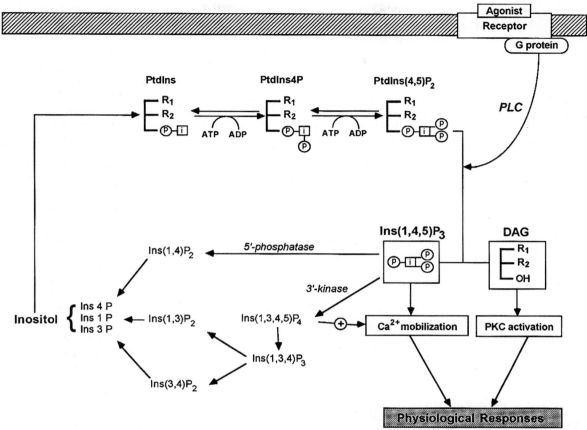

FIGURE 1-6 Schematic representation of G-protein–linked receptor activation of phosphoinositide hydrolysis by phospholipase C (PLC). Note: activation of PLC results in hydrolysis of PtdIns (4,5)P$_2$ to generate the second messengers, Ins(1,4,5)P$_3$ and diacylglyceral (DAG). Ins(1,4,5)P$_3$ elicits mobilization of intracellular Ca^{2+} and DAG activates protein kinase C, both of which induce various cellular responses. Ins(1,4,5)P$_3$ is metabolized via two routes, including phosphorylation to the active Ca^{2+}-regulating isomer, Ins(1,3,4,5)P$_4$, and dephosphorylation to the inactive isomer, Ins(1,4)P$_2$. Further metabolism of these Ins(1,4,5)P$_3$ products ultimately results in the formation of inositol, which becomes reincorporated into the membrane phospholipids.

tivity to phosphoinositol hydrolysis by these PLC isoforms.[45–49] The typical sequence of events associated with receptor/G-protein–coupled activation of PLC is schematically depicted in Fig. 1-6, wherein hydrolysis of PIP$_2$ results in the formation of Ins (1,4,5) P$_3$ and DAG, leading to intracellular Ca^{2+} mobilization and PKC activation, respectively.

PHOSPHOLIPASE A$_2$–COUPLED SIGNALING

Phospholipase A$_2$ (PLA$_2$) catalyzes the hydrolysis of membrane phospholipids to generate free arachidonic acid and lysophospholipid. The liberated arachidonate is subsequently converted to a number of bioactive eicosanoids, which exert significant paracrine and autocrine actions in different cell types. These include the prostaglandins, thromboxane, leukotrienes, and hydroxyeicosatetraeinoic acids (HETEs). The co-liberated lysophospholipids possess detergent-like properties and, therefore, are membrane-lytic and are rapidly reacylated within the plasma membrane, although certain biologic functions have been also attributed to these agents including chemotaxis, mitogenesis, and the

synthesis of platelet activating factor.[31,50–52] Thus, collectively, the products of PLA$_2$ activation exert a host of both acute and long-term cellular responses (e.g., smooth muscle contraction, cellular proliferation, etc.).

While evidence for direct activation of PLA$_2$ by G proteins has not been identified, the demonstration of both pertussis toxin–sensitive and –insensitive activation of PLA$_2$ suggests that multiple G proteins may be involved.[53] One of the PLA$_2$ isoforms, termed cytosolic phospholipase A$_2$ (cPLA$_2$), having a molecular mass of 85 kDa, has been proposed as a key effector in transmembrane signaling coupled to G-protein–linked receptors involving the Ca^{2+}-sensitive release of arachidonic acid.[54,55] Indeed, recombinantly expressed cPLA$_2$ was found to mediate arachidonic acid release by G-protein–linked receptors and demonstrated phosphorylation by MAP kinase.[56–58] Notwithstanding this implicated role for cPLA$_2$, it is likely that other PLA$_2$ isotypes may also be coupled to G-protein–linked receptors, as recently exemplified by the demonstration of carbachol-mediated induction of secretory (s)PLA$_2$ expression in gastric mucosa.[59]

ADENYLATE CYCLASE–COUPLED SIGNALING

A variety of G-protein–linked receptors are associated with activation of adenylate cyclase activity. The latter is represented by a group of related enzyme subtypes that possess distinct molecular structures and are regulated by many different hormones, neurotransmitters, and growth factors. Whereas stimulation of adenylate cyclase activity resulting in cAMP generation from ATP occurs as a result of receptor-coupled activation of the $G\alpha_s$ subtypes, inhibition of adenylate cyclase is mediated by receptor-coupled activation of the $G\alpha_i$ subtypes. Moreover, the β-γ subunits of certain G proteins can also regulate some subtypes of adenylate cyclase.[3,60–64] Finally, certain subtypes of adenylate cyclase are regulated by calcium/calmodulin.[63,65–69]

To date, at least eight molecularly distinct subtypes of adenylate cyclase are believed to exist which, among each other, display an amino acid homology ranging between 35 and 67 percent. Their primary molecular structure consists of two similar transmembrane sequences, each consisting of a cytoplasmic N-terminal segment followed by six membrane-spanning domains and then a large (~40 kDa) C-terminal cytoplasmic segment. The first C-terminal segment forms a large intracellular loop between the two halves of the molecule. This cytoplasmic loop and the C-terminal intracellular sequence as highly homologous, both within a given enzyme and between enzyme subtypes. It is felt that both these intracellular domains are essential for conferring the catalytic properties to the enzyme.[70–74]

Apart from the well-established roles of $G\alpha_s$, $G\alpha_i$, and Ca^{2+}/calmodulin in modulating adenylate cyclase activity, relatively little is known regarding the regulation of the adenylate cyclases by phosphorylation. Recent evidence, however, supports the notion that protein kinase C stimulation can lead to phosphorylation of adenylate cyclase, typically resulting in increased activity of certain isoforms of the enzyme.[75–77] In this regard, treatment of certain cells with phorbol ester to activate protein kinase C has been shown to stimulate the Ca^{2+}-calmodulin–dependent adenylate cyclases types 1, 2, and 3, whereas the subtypes 4, 5, and 6 were relatively unaffected.[76] Thus, intracellular regulatory "cross-talk" between transmembrane signaling pathways, as exemplified by protein kinase C activation, may exert a significant modulatory action on adenylate cyclase activity and its resultant cellular actions.

ION-CHANNEL–COUPLED SIGNALING

G proteins have the capacity not only of coupling membrane receptors to enzyme effectors and intracellular second messengers but also of coupling membrane receptors to ion channels by a cytoplasmic-independent, membrane-limited mechanism. Examples of such direct G-protein–mediated regulation of ion channel activity include muscarinic K^+ channels, voltage-gated dihydropyridine-sensitive Ca^{2+} channels, and rapid tetrodotoxin-sensitive Na^+ channels.[78] The direct G-protein–linked pathway leading to modulation of cardiac muscarinic K^+ channel activity has been most extensively studied; it has been demonstrated that the G_i isoforms 1, 2, and 3 regulate K^+ channel activity in the atria.

Direct G_o-protein–coupled gating of neuronal K^+ channels has also been demonstrated in response to either muscarinic M_2-, adrenergic α_2-, serotonin (5HT-1A)-, dopamine $(D)_2$-, adenosine $(A)_1$-, or $GABA_\beta$-receptor stimulation.[79–82] In contrast to K^+ channels, where G-protein gating is obligatory, G-protein gating is primarily modulatory for Ca^{2+} channels and membrane depolarization represents the obligatory process. In this regard, it has been demonstrated that both G_s and G_i can modulate Ca^{2+} channel activity in different cell types.[78] Moreover, it has been demonstrated that a given G protein may exert dual effector actions coupled to altered Ca^{2+} channel activity, with one action represented by direct modulation of the Ca^{2+} channel and the other given by indirect second-messenger–mediated regulation of the ion channel's activity (e.g., PKA-mediated phosphorylation). This duality of direct and indirect regulation of K^+ channel activity has been recently documented with respect to the effects of β-adrenoceptor stimulation in airway smooth muscle.[83,84]

Regulation of G-Protein–Linked Receptor Function

The ability of most G-protein–linked receptors to sustain a cellular response in the presence of agonist is limited by the phenomenon of desensitization. This phenomenon is attributed to certain key, largely independent processes including phosphorylation of the receptor, its sequestration or cellular internalization, and its downregulation. The process of phosphorylation reflects functional uncoupling of the receptor from its G protein and has been attributed to the actions of different kinases (see below). Sequestration of the receptor is given by its removal from the cell surface and internalization or compartmentalization within intracellular sites. Finally, downregulation represents the process of reduction in total number of receptors either within the cell or on its surface.

RECEPTOR PHOSPHORYLATION

The process of receptor desensitization caused by phosphorylation has been extensively investigated with respect to the β-adrenergic receptor subtypes. Accordingly, it has been shown that the β_2-adrenoceptor can undergo rapid phosphorylation within seconds to minutes, resulting in heterologous and/or homologous desensitization. The former type of desensitization has been attributed to the action of cAMP-dependent protein kinase A (PKA) and involves uncoupling of G_s from its phosphorylated receptor, which normally is associated with cAMP generation (e.g., β_2-adrenergic receptor, PGE_2 receptor, etc.). This process has been found to occur independent of the occupancy of the receptor by its agonist, given that the phenomenon can be elicited in response to exogenous administration of a cell-permeable cAMP analog, such as dibutyryl cAMP.[85] In contrast, the phenomenon of homologous desensitization involves phosphorylation of the receptor only in the presence of agonist occupancy. Accordingly, for the β-adrenergic receptor, uncoupling of the agonist-bound receptor from G_s has been attributed to the action of β-adrenoceptor kinase (βARK).[86,87] Following dissociation of the α subunit, G_s β-γ subunits interact with βARK, binding the kinase and bringing it into contact with its receptor substrate. This process further involves the action of another protein, β-arrestin, which interacts with the βARK phosphorylated receptor to facilitate its uncoupling from G_s.[88,89]

The principal molecular determinants of phosphorylation of the β_2-adrenoceptor by PKA and βARK have been largely identified using mutational analyses, construction of chimeric receptors, and biochemical techniques. In this regard, it has been demonstrated that the consensus sequence, R-R-X-S, at residues 259–262 within the third intracellular loop of the receptor (see Fig. 1-7) serves as a phosphorylation site for PKA, as does the consensus sequence located in the intracellular C-terminal domain at residues 343–346.[90] Similarly, βARK-mediated phosphorylation of the β_2-adrenoceptor involves the serine-and threonine-rich region of the C-terminal limb of the receptor.[91,92] Mutated receptors at either or both of the above determinant sites have been found to display depressed phosphorylation, with resultant relatively enhanced cAMP accumulation in response to agonist when compared to the wild-type receptor.[93]

RECEPTOR SEQUESTRATION

As for phosphorylation, the process of receptor sequestration also occurs along a comparably short time course (i.e., within seconds to minutes). Moreover, similar to the required action of βARK, the process of receptor sequestration also necessitates the presence of agonist occupancy of the receptor; however, the process does not appear to be independent of phosphorylation of the receptor per se.[94] Given the recent findings that agonist-promoted sequestered receptors are less phosphorylated than receptors on the cell surface and that intracellular vesicles containing the sequestered receptors have associated high concentrations of phosphatases,[95] it has been proposed that receptor sequestration may represent a mechanism for dephosphorylating the receptor. For the α_2-adrenoceptor, it has been suggested that sequestration of the receptor may be required for its

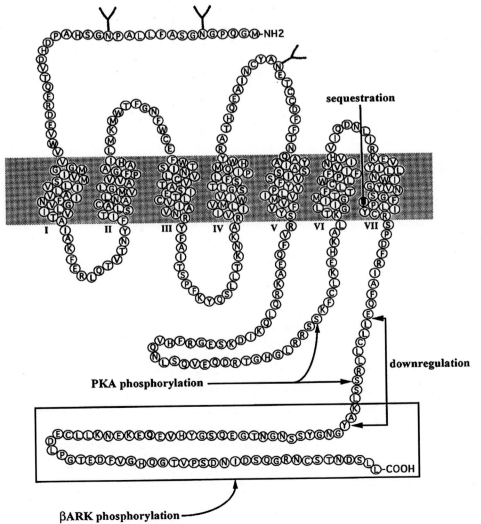

FIGURE 1-7 Schematic representation of the β_2-adrenergic receptor and its presumed residues and sequences required for receptor desensitization, including phosphorylation, sequestration, and downregulation.

agonist-induced downregulation.[96] Although the molecular determinant(s) for sequestration of G-protein–linked receptors remains to be identified, recent evidence pertaining to the β_2-adrenergic receptor supports the view that the proximal portion of the C-terminal domain (see Fig. 1-7) of the receptor is important for conferring its sequestration properties.[97]

RECEPTOR DOWNREGULATION

In contrast to the acute effects of agonist exposure on receptor phosphorylation and sequestration, prolonged agonist exposure typically results in a decrease in the number of G-protein–linked receptors, reflecting the process of agonist-induced receptor downregulation. Potential mechanisms accounting for this phenomenon include a reduction in transcription of the receptor's mRNA, altered stability of the receptor's mRNA, or increased degradation of the receptor protein.

In examining the processes leading to G-protein–linked receptor downregulation, it has recently been demonstrated that the degree of coupling of the receptor to its G protein directly correlates with the extent of its downregulation.[98,99] In contrast, sequestration of the receptor has not been clearly demonstrated as a prerequisite for its downregulation. Rather, apart from the presence of receptor/G-protein coupling, the requirements for downregulation possibly include the presence of tyrosine residues on the C-terminal component of the receptor (see Fig. 1-7) as well as phosphorylation of the receptor.[100] Finally, while transcriptional regulation may play a part, the overall process of receptor downregulation appears largely dependent upon enhanced degradation of the receptor's mRNA.[101,102]

Conclusion

Pulmonary cells contain an array of receptors for many types of chemical and/or physical stimuli. In response to these signals, a host of different types of receptors are coupled to their correspondingly varied selection of G proteins, which, in turn, modulate many intracellular effectors and their second messengers. While any given cell can respond only to those signals for which it has receptors, the specificity with which any given receptor interacts with its coupled G proteins defines the range of responsiveness of the cell. In recent years, remarkable progress has been made in elucidating the molecular structure and functional characteristics of G-protein–linked receptors and the transmembrane signal transduction processes mediating their cellular actions. Cloning and sequence analysis of the family of G-protein–linked receptors have identified a high degree of structural homology between the members of this family, including their ligand and G-protein–binding domains, that reflects their largely common mechanisms of action. Notwithstanding the latter, the naturally occurring ligands for these receptors, as well as their intracellular effector systems, vary widely in both structure and function. Thus, while the G-protein–linked receptors represent a structurally and

functionally similar collection of receptors, the individual members of this family of receptors distinctively contribute to the overall array of cellular responses. As highlighted in the present chapter, much of the complex molecular and biochemical machinery underlying the varied actions and regulation of the G-protein–linked receptors as well as their coupling proteins has been unraveled. Given the rapid progress in this area of research, one can look forward to significant further new insights in the near future.

References

1. Strader CD, Fong TM, Tota MR, Underwood D: Structure and function of G protein-coupled receptors. *Ann Rev Biochem* 1994; 63:101–132.
2. Kobilka B. Adrenergic receptors as models for G protein-coupled receptors. *Annu Rev Neurosci* 1992; 15:87–114.
3. Gilman AG: G proteins: Transducers of receptor-generated signals. *Annu Rev Biochem* 1987; 56:615–649.
4. Jackson TR: Structure and function of G protein coupled receptors. *Pharmacol Ther* 1991; 50:425–442.
5. Hargrave PA, McDowell JH: Rhodopsin and phototransduction: A model system for G protein-linked receptors. *FASEB J* 1992; 6:2323–2331.
6. Findley J, Eliopoulos, E: Three-dimensional modeling of G protein-linked receptors. *Trends Pharmacol Sci* 1990; 11:492–499.
7. Strader CD, Fong TM, Graziano MP, Tota MR: The family of G protein-coupled receptors. *FASEB J* 1995; 9:745–754.
8. Wang H: Site-directed and anti-peptide antibodies define the topography of the beta-adrenergic receptor. *J Biol Chem* 1989; 264:14424–14431.
9. Dohlman HG, Bouvier M, Benovic J: The multiple membrane spanning topography of the beta$_2$-adrenergic receptor: Localization of the sites of binding, glycosylation, and regulatory phosphorylation by limited proteolysis. *J Biol Chem* 1987; 262:14282–14288.
10. Dohlman HG, Thorner J, Caron MG, Lefkowitz RL: Model systems for the study of seven-transmembrane-segment receptors. *Ann Rev Biochem* 1991; 60:653–688.
11. Strader CD, Sigal IS, Dixon RAF: Structural basis of β-adrenergic receptor function. *FASEB J* 1989; 3:1825–1832.
12. Fong TM, MaCascieri H Yu, Bonsal A, et al.: Amino-aromatic interaction between histidine 197 of the neurokinin-1 receptor and CP 96345. *Nature* 1993; 362:350–353.
13. O'Dowd BF, Hnatowich M, Caron MG, et al.: Palmitoylation of the human beta-2-adrenergic receptor: Mutation of Cys341 in the carboxyl tail leads to an uncoupled nonpalmitoylated form of the receptor. *J Biol Chem* 1989; 264:7564–7569.
14. Casey PJ: Lipid modifications of G proteins. *Curr Opin Cell Biol* 1994; 6:219–225.
15. Mouillac B, Caron M, Bonin H, et al.: Agonist-modulated palmitoylation of beta$_2$-adrenergic receptor in Sf9 cells. *J Biol Chem* 1992; 267:21733–21737.
16. Kawate N, Menon KMJ: Palmitoylation of luteinizing hormone/human choriogonadotropin receptors in transfected cells: Abolition of palmitoylation by mutation of Cys-621 and Cys-622 residues in the cytoplasmic tail increases ligand-induced internalization of the receptor. *J Biol Chem* 1994; 269:30651–30658.
17. Inglese J, Freedman NJ, Koch WJ, Lefkowitz RJ: Structure of mechanism of the G protein-coupled receptor kinases. *J Biol Chem* 1993; 268:23735–23738.
18. Kaziro Y, Itoh H, Kozassa T, et al.: Structure and function of sig-

nal-transducing GTP-binding proteins. *Am Rev Biochem* 1991; 60:349–400.

19. Simon MI, Strathmann MP, Gautam N: Diversity of G proteins in signal transduction. *Science* 1991; 252:802–808.

20. Huff RM, Neer EJ: Subunit interactions of native and ADP-ribosylated alpha 39 and alpha 41, two guanine nucleotide-binding proteins from bovine cerebral cortex. *J Biol Chem* 1986; 261:1105–1110.

21. Watkins PA, Burns DL, Kanaho Y, et al.: ADP-ribosylation of transduction by pertussis toxin. *J Biol Chem* 1985; 260:13478–13482.

22. Navon SE, Fung BKK: Characterization of transduction from bovine retinal rod outer segments: Participation of the amino and terminal region of T alpha in subunit interaction. *J Biol Chem* 1987; 262:15746–15751.

23. Berlot CH, Bourne HR: Identification of effector-activating residues of G_s alpha. *Cell* 1992; 68:911–922.

24. Itoh H, Gilman AG: Expression and analysis of Gs alpha mutants with decreased ability to activate adenyl-cyclase. *J Biol Chem* 1991; 266:16226–16231.

25. Carty DJ, Padrell E, Codina J, et al.: Distinct guanine nucleotide binding and release properties of the three G_i proteins. *J Biol Chem* 1990; 265:6268–6273.

26. Linder ME, Ewald DA, Miller RJ, Gilman AG: Purification and characterization of $G_o\alpha$ and three types of $G_i\alpha$ after expression in *Escherichia coli. J Biol Chem* 1990; 265:8243–8251.

27. Arshovsky VY, Bownds MD: Regulation of deactivation of photoreceptor G protein by its target enzyme and cGMP. *Nature* 1992; 357:416–417.

28. Berstein G, Blank JL, Jhon DY, et al.: Phospholipase C-β1 is a GTPase-activating protein for Gq11, its physiologic regulator. *Cell* 1992; 70:411–418.

29. Casey PJ: Protein lipidation in cell signaling. *Science* 1995; 268:221–225.

30. Berridge MJ: Inositol triphosphate and diacylgliceral: Two interacting second messengers. *Annu Rev Biochem* 1987; 56:159–193.

31. Nishizuka Y: Intracellular signalling by hydrolysis of phospholipids and activation of protein kinase C. *Science* 1992; 258:607–614.

32. Berridge MJ, Irvine RF: Inositol phosphates and cell signaling. *Nature* 1989; 341:197–206.

33. Rhee SG: Inositol phospholipids-specific phospholipase C: Interaction of the gamma 1 isoform with tyrosine kinase. *Trends Biochem Sci* 1991; 16:297–301.

34. Rhee SG, Choi KD: Regulation of inositol phospholipid-specific phospholipase C isozymes. *J Biol Chem* 1992; 267:12393–12396.

35. Cockcroft S, Thomas GMH: Inositol-lipid-specific phospholipase C isoenzymes and their differential regulation by receptors. *Biochem J* 1992; 288:1–14.

36. Koch CA, Anderson D, Moran MF, et al.: SH2 and SH3 domains: Elements that control interactions of cytoplasmic signaling proteins. *Science* 1991; 252:668–674.

37. Musacchio A, Gibson T, Lehto VP: SH3—An abundant protein domain in search for a function. *FEBS Lett* 1992; 307:55–61.

38. Rana RS, Hokin LE: Role of phosphoinositides in transmembrane signalling. *Physiol Rev* 1990; 70:115–164.

39. Katan M, Parker PJ: Purification of phosphoinositide-specific phospholipase C from a particulate fraction of bovine brain. *Eur J Biochem* 1987; 168:413–418.

40. Rhee SG, Suh PG, Ryu SH, Lee SY: Studies of inositol phospholipid-specific phospholipase C. *Science* 1989; 244:546–550.

41. Ginger RS, Parker PJ: Expression, purification and characterization of a functional phosphatidylinositol-specific phospholipase C delta 1 protein in *Escherichia coli. Eur J Biochem* 1992; 210:155–160.

42. Taylor SJ, Chae HZ, Rhee SG, Exton VA: Activation of the beta 1 isozyme of phospholypase C by alpha subunits of the Gq class of G proteins. *Nature* 1991; 350:516–518.

43. Smrcka AV, Hepler JR, Brown KO, Sternweiss PC: Regulation of polyphosphoinositide specific phospholipase C activity by purified Gq. *Science* 1991; 251:804–807.

44. Wu D, Katz A, Lee CH, Simon MI: Activation of phospholipase C by alpha 1-adrenergic receptors is mediated by the alpha subunits of Gq family. *J Biol Chem* 1992; 267:1811–1817.

45. Camps M, Carozzi A, Schnabel P, Scheer A, Parker PJ, Gierschik P: Isozyme-selective stimulation of phospholipase C-beta 2 by G protein beta gamma-subunits. *Nature* 1992; 360:684–686.

46. Katz A, Wu D, Simon MI: Subunits beta-gamma of heterotrimeric G protein activate beta2 isoform of phospholipase C. *Nature* 1992; 360:686–689.

47. Blank JL, Brattain KA, Exton VH: Activation of cytosolic phosphoinositide phospholipase C by G-protein beta-gamma subunits. *J Biol Chem* 1992; 267:23069–23075.

48. Carozzi A, Camps M, Gierschik P, Parker PV: Activation of phosphatidylinositol lipid-specific phospholipase beta 3 by G-protein beta-gamma subunits. *FEBS Lett* 1993; 315:340–342.

49. Park D, Jhon DY, Lee CW, et al.: Activation of phospholipase C isozymes by G protein beta-gamma subunits. *J Biol Chem* 1993; 268:4573–4576.

50. Miller B, Sarantis M, Traynelis SF, Attwell D: Potentiation of NMDA receptor current by arachidonic acid. *Nature* 1992; 355:722–725.

51. Piomelli D, Greengard P: Lipoxygenase metabolites of arachidonic acid in neuronal transmembrane signalling. *Trends Pharmacol Sci* 1990; 11:367–373.

52. Hanahan DJ: Platelet activating factor: A biologically active phosphoglyceride. *Annu Rev Biochem* 1986; 55:483–509.

53. Axelrod J: Receptor-mediated activation of phospholipase A_2 and arachidonic acid release in signal transduction. *Biochem Soc Trans* 1990; 18:503–507.

54. Sharp JD, White DL, Chiou XG, et al.: Molecular cloning and expression of human calcium sensitive cytosolic phospholipase A_2. *J Biol Chem* 1991; 266:14850–14853.

55. Clark JD, Lin LL, Kriz RW, et al.: A novel arachidonic acid-selective cytosolic PLA_2 contains a calcium-dependent translocation domain with homology to PKC and GAP. *Cell* 1991; 65:1043–1051.

56. Lin AY, Knopf JL: Cytosolic phospholipase A_2 is coupled to hormonally regulated release of arachidonic acid. *Proc Natl Acad Sci USA* 1992; 89:6147–6151.

57. Wharton M, Lin AY, Knopf VL, et al.: cPLA2 is phosphorylated and activated by MAP kinase. *Cell* 1993; 72:269–278.

58. Nemenoff RA, Winitz S, Qian NX, et al.: Phosphorylation and activation of a high molecular weight form of phospholipase A2 by p42 microtubule-associated protein 2 kinase and protein kinase C. *J Biol Chem* 1993; 268:1960–1964.

59. Ying Z, Tojo H, Nonaka Y, Okamoto M: Cloning and expression of phospholipase A_2 from guinea pig mucosa, its induction by carbachol and secretion in vivo. *Eur J Biochem* 1993; 215:91–97.

60. Birnbaumer L, Abramowitz J, Brown AM: Receptor-effector coupling by G proteins. *Biochem Biophys Acta* 1990; 1031:163–224.

61. Levitzki A, Bar-Sinai A: The regulation of adenylyl cyclase by receptor-operated G-protein. *Pharmacol* 1991; 50:271–283.

62. Tang WJ, Gilman AG: Type-specific regulation of adenyl cyclase by G protein beta-gamma subunits. *Science* 1991; 254:1500–1503.

63. Tang WJ, Gilman AG: Adenylyl cyclases. *Cell* 1992; 70:869–872.

64. Federman AD, Conklin BR, Schrader KA, et al.: Hormonal stimulation of adenylyl cyclase through Gi-protein beta-gamma subunits. *Nature* 1992; 356:159–161.

65. Harrison JK, Hewlett GH, Gnery ME: Regulation of calmod-

ulin-sensitive adenylate cyclase by the stimulatory G-protein, Gs. *J Biol Chem* 1989; 264:15880–15885.

66. Choi EJ, Wong ST, Hinde TR, Storm DR: Calcium and muscarinic agonist stimulation of type I adenylyl cyclase in whole cells. *J Biol Chem* 1992; 267:12440–12442.

67. Tang WJ, Krupinski J, Gilman AG: Expression and characterization of calmodulin-activated (type I) adenylyl cyclase. *J Biol Chem* 1991; 266:8595–8603.

68. Caldwell KK, Boyajian CL, Cooper DM: The effects of Ca^{2+} and calmodulin on adenylyl cyclase activity in plasma membranes derived from neural and non-neural cells. *Cell Calcium* 1992; 13:107–121.

69. Yoshimura M, Cooper DMF: Cloning an expression of a $Ca^{(2+)}$-inhibitable adenylyl cyclase from NCB-20 cells. *Proc Natl Acad Sci USA* 1992; 89:6716–6720.

70. Katsushika S, Chen L, Kawabe J, et al.: Cloning and characterization of a sixth adenylyl cyclase isoform: Types V and VI constitute a subgroup within the mammalian adenylyl cyclase family. *Proc Natl Acad Sci USA* 1992; 89:8774–8778.

71. Chinkers M, Garbers DL: Signal transduction by guanylyl cyclases. *Rev Biochem* 1991; 60:553–576.

72. Singh S, Lowe DG, Thorpe DS, et al.: Membrane guanylate cyclase is a cell-surface receptor with homology to protein kinases. *Nature* 1988; 334:708–712.

73. Bender JL, Wolf LG, Neer EJ: Interaction of forskolin with resolved adenylate cyclase components. *Adv Cyclic Nucleotide Protein Phosphor Res* 1984; 17:101–109.

74. Gao B, Gilman AG: Cloning and expression of a widely distributed (type IV) adenylyl cyclase. *Proc Natl Acad Sci USA* 1991; 88:10178–19182.

75. Yoshimasa T, Sibley DR, Bouvier M, et al.: Cross-talk between cellular signalling pathways suggested by phorbol-ester-induced adenylate cyclase phosphorylation. *Nature* 1987; 327:67–70.

76. Jacobowitz O, Chen J, Premont RT, Iyengar R: Stimulation of specific types of Gs-stimulated adenylyl cyclases by phorbol ester treatment. *J Biol Chem* 1993; 268:3829–3832.

77. Yoshimasa T, Bouvier M, Benovik JL, et al.: In: McKerns KW, Chretien M, eds. *Molecular Biology of Brain and Endocrine Peptidergic Systems.* New York: Plenum Press, 1988; 123–139.

78. Brown AM, Birnbaumer L: Ionic channels and their regulation by G protein subunits. *Annu Rev Physiol* 1990; 52:197–213.

79. Andvade R, Malenka R, Nicoll R: A G protein couples serotonin and $GABA_B$ receptors to the same channels in hippocampus. *Science* 1986; 234:1261–1265.

80. Mihara S, North RA, Suprenant A: Somatostatin increases an inwardly rectifying potassium conductance in guinea pig submucous plexus neurons. *J Physiol* 1987; 390:335–355.

81. North RA, Williams JT, Surprenant A, Christie MJ: μ and δ receptors belong to a family of receptors that are coupled to potassium channels. *Proc Natl Acad Sci USA* 1997; 84:5487–5491.

82. Sasaki K, Sato M: A single GTP-binding protein regulates K+-channels coupled with dopamine, histamine and acetylcholine receptors. *Nature* 1987; 325:259–262.

83. Kume H, Hall IP, Washabau RJ, et al.: β-adrenergic agonists regulate Kca channels in airway smooth muscle by cAMP-dependent and -independent mechanisms. *J Clin Invest* 1994; 93:371–379.

84. Kume H, Graziano MP, Kotlikoff MI: Stimulatory and inhibitory regulation of calcium-activated potassium channels by guanine nucleotide-binding proteins. *Proc Natl Acad Sci USA* 1992; 89:11051–11055.

85. Sibley DR, Peters JR, Nambi P, et al.: Desensitization of turkey erythrocyte adenylate cyclase: Beta-adrenergic receptor phosphorylation is corrected with attenuation of adenylate cyclase activity. *J Biol Chem* 1984; 259:9742–9749.

86. Benovic JL, Strasser RH, Caron MG, Lefkowitz RJ: Beta-adrenergic receptor kinase: Identification of a novel protein kinase that phosphorylates the agonist-occupied form of the receptor. *Proc Natl Acad Sci USA* 1986; 83:2797–2801.

87. Benovic JL, Major F Jr, Staniszewski C, et al.: Purification and characterization of the beta-adrenergic receptor kinase. *J Biol Chem* 1987; 262:9026–9032.

88. Palczewski K, McDowell JH, Jakes S, et al.: Regulation of rhodopsin dephosphorylation by arrestin. *J Biol Chem* 1990; 264:15770–15773.

89. Lohse MJ, Benovic JJ, Codina J, et al.: Beta-arrestin: A protein that regulates beta-adrenergic receptor function. *Science* 1990; 248:1547–1550.

90. O'Dowd BF, Hnatowich M, Regan JW, et al.: Site-directed mutagenesis of the cytoplasmic domains of the human $beta_2$-adrenergic receptor: Localization of regions involved in G protein-receptor coupling. *J Biol Chem* 1988; 263:15985–15992.

91. Lefkowitz RJ, Hausdorff WP, Caron MG: Role of phosphorylation in desensitization of the β-adrenoceptor. *Trends Pharmacol Sci* 1990; 11:190–194.

92. Bouvier M, Hausdorff WP, DeBlasi A, et al.:Removal of phosphorylation sites from the beta 2-adrenergic receptor delays onset of agonist-promoted desensitization. *Nature* 1988; 333:370–373.

93. Liggett SB, Bouvier M, Hausdorff WP, et al.: Altered patterns of agonist-stimulated cAMP accumulation in cells expressing mutant $beta_2$-adrenergic receptors lacking phosphorylation. *Mol Pharmacol* 1989; 36:641–646.

94. Yu SS, Lefkowitz RJ, Hausdorff WP: Beta-adrenergic receptor sequestration. A potential mechanism of receptor resensitization. *J Biol Chem* 1993; 268:337–341.

95. Stadel JM, Nambi P, Shorr RG, et al.: Catecholamine-induced desensitization of turkey erythrocyte adenylate cyclase is associated with phosphorylation of the beta-adrenergic receptor. *Proc Natl Acad Sci USA* 1983; 80:3173–3177.

96. Eason MG, Liggett SB: Subtype-selective desensitization of alpha 2-adrenergic receptors: Different mechanisms control short and long term agonist-promoted desensitization of alpha 2C10, alpha 2C4, and alpha 2C2. *J Biol Chem* 1992; 267:25473–25479.

97. Hausdorff WP, Campbell PT, Ostrowski J, et al.: A small region of the beta-adrenergic receptor is selectively involved in its rapid regulation. *Proc Natl Acad Sci USA* 1991; 88:2979–2983.

98. Cheung AH, Sigal IS, Dixon RAF, Strader CD: Agonist-promoted sequestration of the $beta_2$-adrenergic receptor requires regions involved in functional coupling with Gs. *Mol Pharmacol* 1989; 34:132–138.

99. Campbell PT, Hnatowich M, O'Dowd BF, et al.: Mutations of the human $β_2$-adrenergic receptors that impair coupling to G_s interfere with receptor down-regulation but not sequestration. *Mol Pharmacol* 1991; 39:192–198.

100. Valiquette M, Bonin H, Hnatowich M, et al.: Involvement of tyrosine residues located in the carboxyl tail of the human $β_2$-adrenergic receptor in agonist-induced down-regulation of the receptor. *Proc Natl Acad Sci USA* 1990; 87:5089–5093.

101. Hadcock JR, Wang H, Malbon CC: Agonist-induced destabilization of beta-adrenergic receptor mRNA: Attenuation of glucocorticoid-induced up-regulation of beta-adrenergic receptors. *J Biol Chem* 1989; 264:19928–19933.

102. Hadcock JR, Malbon CC: Downregulation of beta-adrenergic receptors: Agonist-induced reduction in receptor mRNA levels. *Proc Natl Acad Sci USA* 1988; 85:5021–5025.

103. Strader CD, Sigal IS, Register RB, et al.: Identification of residues required for ligand binding to the β-adrenergic receptor. *Proc Natl Acad Sci USA* 1987; 84:4384–4388.

104. Strader CD, Sigal IS, Candelore MR, et al.: Conserved aspartic

acid residues 79 and 113 of the β-adrenergic receptor have different roles in receptor function. *J Biol Chem* 1988; 263:10267–10271.

105. Chung FZ, Wang C-D, Potter PC, et al.: Site-directed mutagenesis and continuous expression of the human β-adrenergic receptor. *J Biol Chem* 1988; 263:4052–4055.

106. Fraser CM, Chung FZ, Wang CD, et al.: Site-directed mutagenesis of human β-adrenergic receptors: Substitution of aspartic acid-130 by asparagine produces a receptor with high-affinity agonist binding that is uncoupled from adenylate cyclase. *Proc Natl Acad Sci USA* 1988; 85:5478–5482.

107. Strader CD, Candelor MR, Hill WS, et al.: Identification of two serine residues involved in agonist activation of the β-adrenergic receptor. *J Biol Chem* 1989; 264:13572–13578.

108. Dixon RAF, Sigal IS, Candelore MR, et al.: Structural features required for ligand binding to the β-adrenergic receptor. *EMBO J* 1987; 6:3269–3275.

109. Dohlman HG, Caron MG, DeBlasi A, et al.: Role of extracellular disulfide-bonded cysteines in the ligand binding function of the β₂-adrenergic receptor. *Biochemistry* 1990; 29:2335–2342.

110. Savarese TM, Fraser CM: In vitro mutagenesis and the search for structure-function relationships among G protein-coupled receptors. *Biochem J* 1992; 283:1–19.

111. Watson S, Arkinstall S: *The G-Protein Linked Receptor: Facts Book.* San Diego, CA: Academic Press, 1994.

112. Cheung AH, Huang R-RC, Graziano MP, Strader CD: Specific activation of G$_s$ by synthetic peptides corresponding to an intracellular loop of the β-adrenergic receptor. *FEBS Lett* 1991; 279:277–280.

113. Wess J: Mutational analysis of muscarinic acetylcholine receptors: Structural basis for ligand/receptor/G protein interactions. *Life Sci* 1993; 53:1447–1463.

114. Wong SK, Parker EM, Ross EM: Chimeric muscarinic cholinergic: Beta-adrenergic receptors that activate G$_s$ in response to muscarinic agonists. *J Biol Chem* 1990; 265:6219–6224.

Chapter 2

RECEPTORS 2: ENZYME-LINKED RECEPTORS

CRAIG M. SCHRAMM AND MICHAEL M. GRUNSTEIN

The serpentine G protein-associated receptors discussed in the previous chapter lack intrinsic enzymatic activity and are coupled to their effector enzymes via specific regulatory G proteins. There also exist other classes of cell surface receptors which, in contrast to the G-protein receptors, contain an enzymatic moiety directly within the receptor molecule. The best characterized of these enzyme-linked receptors are those that demonstrate protein tyrosine kinase activity and are aptly termed receptor tyrosine kinases (RTKs). Two more recently identified and to date less well characterized types of enzyme-linked receptors are receptors demonstrating protein serine/threonine kinase activity (the receptor serine/threonine kinases, or RSTKs) and those having intrinsic protein tyrosine phosphatase activity (the receptor protein tyrosine phosphatases, or RPTPs). The characterization of such receptors known or suspected to be present in lung cells, along with the identification of their ligands and signal transduction pathways, is the focus of this chapter.

Receptor Tyrosine Kinases

The RTKs are a group of structurally related transmembrane molecules that demonstrate tyrosine kinase activity in response to stimulation by the polypeptide cytokines commonly referred to as growth factors. To date, more than 50 vertebrate RTKs belonging to at least 14 different receptor families have been identified. The principal RTKs identified in lung cells include those depicted in Fig. 2-1. Additional RTK classes not considered in this review include the sub-

families of nerve growth factor receptors, EPH receptors, and AXL receptors as well as the recently identified TIE, DDR, and ROR "orphan" subfamilies for which no ligands have yet been identified.[1] Activation of tyrosine kinase receptors by their ligands leads to important physiologic consequences influencing cellular metabolism, proliferation, shape and differentiation, and migration.

All RTKs share a similar general structure consisting of a large extracellular amino-terminal portion, which contains the ligand-recognition domain; a single, short membrane-spanning region; and a cytoplasmic carboxy-terminal portion that contains the receptor's tyrosine kinase activity and autophosphorylation sites. The external domains of RTKs typically contain cysteine-rich regions and/or immunoglobulinlike motifs, with a large number of disulfide bonds forming the highly specific tertiary structure that is needed to establish ligand binding specificity.[2] The transmembrane domain of RTKs markedly differs from the seven membrane-spanning regions of the G protein-linked receptors, in that it consists of a single α-helical region of around 24 amino acids that is not conserved between or even within RTK families. Its main function is to anchor the RTK in the plane of the plasma membrane, and it appears to have only a passive role in signal transduction.[3] On the other hand, the RTK cytoplasmic domain is the most highly conserved region within the RTK classes, and it shares sequence homology with the cytoplasmic protein tyrosine kinases. The cytoplasmic region contains ~250 amino acids (excluding inserts) that determine the protein's tyrosine kinase activity as well as autophosphorylation and ATP binding sites.

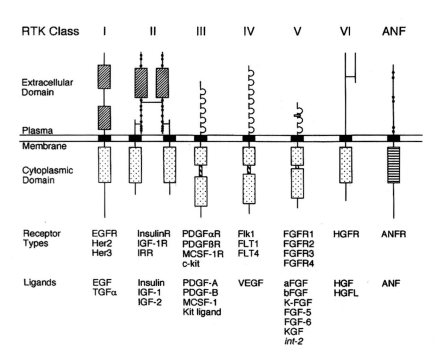

RTK Class	I	II	III	IV	V	VI	ANF
Receptor Types	EGFR Her2 Her3	InsulinR IGF-1R IRR	PDGFαR PDGFβR MCSF-1R c-kit	Flk1 FLT1 FLT4	FGFR1 FGFR2 FGFR3 FGFR4	HGFR	ANFR
Ligands	EGF TGFα	Insulin IGF-1 IGF-2	PDGF-A PDGF-B MCSF-1 Kit ligand	VEGF	aFGF bFGF K-FGF FGF-5 FGF-6 KGF int-2	HGF HGFL	ANF

FIGURE 2-1 Pulmonary receptor tyrosine kinases (RTKs). Representative receptors and specific ligands for each RTK class are listed below the schematized receptors. Stippled boxes symbolize the *tyrosine kinase domain(s)*, separated by slashed *kinase insert regions* in Class III, IV, and V receptors; slashed extra-cellular boxes symbolize *cysteine-rich regions* and dots represent conserved *cysteine residues*; semicircles symbolize *immunoglobulin-like domains*, with an interspersed *acid box domain* depicted by the open box in the Class V receptors; the striped cytoplasmic box of the ANF receptor symbolizes its *guanylyl cyclase domain*. Principal abbreviations: epidermal growth factor and receptor (EGF, EGFR); transforming growth factor-α (TGF-α); insulin-like growth factor types 1 and 2 and receptor (IGF-1, IGF-2, IGF-1R); insulin related receptor (IRR); platelet-derived growth factors and receptor (PDGF, PDGFR); macrophage colony-stimulating growth factor-1 and receptor (MCSF-1, MCSF-1R); vascular endothelial growth factor (VEGF); acidic and basic fibroblast growth factors and receptor (aFGF, bFGF, FGFR); keratinocyte growth factor (KGF); hepatocyte growth factor and receptor (HGF, HGFR); atrial natriuretic factor and receptor (ANF, ANFR).

With the exception of the insulin receptor family, all known RTKs undergo a transition from a monomeric to a dimeric state following binding of their specific ligand(s). Such dimerization may be homodimeric, between two identical receptors, or heterodimeric, between different members of the same receptor family or between a receptor and an accessory protein.[3] It is felt that inactive monomeric receptors exist in equilibrium with active dimeric receptors and that ligand binding stabilizes the active dimeric form of the RTK.[4] Ligand-induced dimerization may occur through several mechanisms, including the following:

1. Monovalent binding of a dimeric ligand to single sites on two receptor molecules, leading to cross-linking and subsequent activation of the receptor (as for platelet-derived growth factor and macrophage colony-stimulating factor 1)
2. Bivalent binding of a monomeric ligand to two or more sites on two receptor molecules (as for epidermal growth factor and human growth hormone)
3. Monovalent binding of a monomeric ligand to its receptor, with concomitant multivalent binding of the ligand to an accessory molecule that promotes dimerization of the ligand-receptor complex (as for fibroblast-derived growth factor and its accessory molecules, heparan sulfates on the cell surface).[4]

The potential for heterodimerization increases the spectrum of ligands that can bind to a given RTK type. Since they may also differ in the pattern of autophosphorylation sites, different heterodimers could recruit different sets of substrate proteins and hence elicit different cellular responses.

CLASSES OF RECEPTOR TYROSINE KINASES

Based on conserved amino acid sequences and overall molecular structure, RTKs have been divided into 14 subclasses,[1,2,4–6] with an additional fifteenth class of RTK-like proteins accounted for by atrial natriuretic peptide (ANP) receptors.[7] A full description of each subclass of RTK is beyond the scope of this chapter. Those RTKs implicated in lung growth, repair, and function are depicted in Fig. 2-1 and discussed briefly below.

EPIDERMAL GROWTH FACTOR RECEPTORS

Receptors for epidermal growth factor (EGF) have been demonstrated in fetal mouse,[8,9] ovine,[10] and human lungs.[11] The EGF receptor (EGFR; also termed *HER-1* or *c-erbB-1* due to its homology to the transforming protein encoded by the *erbB* oncogene of the avian erythroblastosis virus) is a 170-kDa transmembrane protein that serves as the prototype for class I RTKs. In addition to airway epithelium, EGF receptors are expressed on a wide variety of cell types and demonstrate high-affinity, competitive binding to EGF, transforming growth factor-α (TGF-α), vaccinia virus growth factors, amphiregulin, and heparin-binding EGF-like growth factor.[5,12–14] Other members of the EGF receptor family include p185[neu] tyrosine kinase (alternately termed erbB-2 or HER-2) and erbB-3.[6] Two endogenous ligands for p185[neu] have recently been identified and have been termed neu differentiation factor (NDF)[15] and neu/erbB ligand growth factor (NEL-GF),[16] based on their ability to induce phenotypic differentiation in certain cells.

The mature EGFR is a ~170-kDa glycoprotein composed of 1186 amino acids. Like all class I RTKs, the EGFR is a monomeric, transmembrane protein that is divided into a

621-amino acid extracellular portion, a 23-residue hydrophobic membrane-spanning region, and a 542-amino acid cytoplasmic portion. The extracellular region contains a single EGF binding site (domain III) flanked by two clusters of cysteine-rich regions (domains II and IV), as well as an amino-terminal sequence (domain I) that is somewhat homologous to the EGF binding domain and may facilitate ligand binding.[17] The extracellular sequence also contains 10 or 11 *N*-linked oligosaccharides, which appear essential for receptor translocation to the cell surface, EGF binding, and receptor phosphorylation.[18] The cytoplasmic portion of the receptor is made up of a juxtamembrane region (domain VI), a tyrosine kinase domain (VII), an internalization domain (VIII), and an a carboxy-terminal inhibitory domain (IX). Studies with site-directed mutagenesis have shown that lysine-721 within domain VII is necessary for kinase activity of the EGFR.[6] Receptors containing alanine or methionine for lys-721, while expressed on the cell surface and having normal binding for EGF, fail to elicit EGF-stimulated responses and to undergo EGF-induced autophosphorylation.

Wild-type EGF and related receptors dimerize in response to EGF and related ligands and become autophosphorylated. Although EGF is a monomeric protein, it is capable of binding simultaneously to two receptor molecules.[4] EGF binding results in the formation of homodimeric EGF receptors or, preferentially if both RTKs are expressed in the tissue, heterodimeric EGF-p185^{neu} receptors.[19] Once ligand-bound and dimerized, the EGFR is autophosphorylated at tyrosine-992 in the internalization domain[20] and tyrosines 1068, 1148, 1173 within the inhibitory domain.[6,12] Autophosphorylation of the tyrosine residues within the inhibitory domain enhances the tyrosine kinase activity of the EGFR, presumably through a conformational change that removes the carboxy-tail region from competing with cellular substrates for the active kinase site.[21] At least two types of EGF receptors have been characterized based on binding affinities to EGF. The majority of total EGF receptors are of relatively lower affinity, with an apparent K_d of 2 to 15 nM, whereas the remaining 5 to 10 percent of receptors are of high affinity, with K_d values for EGF ranging from 0.1 to 0.3 nM.[22] The structural correlates with these differing affinities are not established, but it has been shown that EGF-stimulated responses are mediated by the high-affinity receptors.[23]

EGF receptors, along with EGF and TGF-α, are expressed in the epithelium and smooth muscle of bronchi and bronchioles and in the epithelium of saccules in late-gestation fetal rat lung.[24] Moreover, the pharmacologic treatment of fetal mouse, rabbit, sheep, and monkey lungs with EGF or TGF-α at various gestational ages results in accelerated airway branching and tracheal and bronchial epithelial hyperplasia.[9,25–27] In contrast, the inhibition of endogenous EGF production with an antisense oligonucleotide in fetal mouse lung explants reduced airway branching.[28] Thus, EGF appears to be a critical factor in airway morphogenesis. In the fetal human lung, EGF immunoreactivity is present in nonciliated tracheal epithelial lining cells from 12 to 24 weeks of gestation.[29] EGF receptors can be identified on epithelial cells of the conducting airways and developing bronchial ducts early in the second trimester and are found

in bronchial epithelial cells by 23 weeks gestation.[11,30] Expression of EGF and TGF-α persists in airway epithelium and alveolar septal cells in adult rat lung, and emerging evidence suggests that these growth factors are important modulators of acute lung injury throughout life.[31,32]

In light of their potent mitogenic and morphogenic properties, it is not surprising that EGF and TGF-α have also been implicated in a number of pulmonary neoplasias. Up to 80 percent of non-small-cell lung carcinomas contain twice the amount of TGF-α as normal lung,[33] and approximately 50 percent of lung adenocarcinomas stain strongly for EGF.[34] Similarly, most non-small-cell lung carcinomas express the high-affinity EGF receptor, often at levels as high as five times that seen in normal lung.[34–36] Of interest, among 131 patients with primary lung adenocarcinoma, those whose tumors expressed the EGF receptor and either EGF or TGF-α showed a 5-year survival only 30 to 50 percent that of patients whose tumors did not express the EGF receptor.[34]

INSULINLIKE GROWTH FACTOR-I RECEPTORS

Receptors for another class of growth factor, insulinlike growth factor-1 (IGF-1), have also been demonstrated in canine tracheal epithelial cells[37] and rabbit tracheal smooth muscle cells.[38] The IGF-I receptor (IGF-IR) is one of three class II RTKs, which are unique among RTKs in that the receptors exist as heterotetrameric proteins in which two α subunits and two β subunits are linked by disulfide bonds. The other RTKs form dimers for activation, but the molecular association is noncovalent in the other subclasses. The $\alpha_2\beta_2$ structure accounts for, in addition to IGF-IR, the insulin receptor (IR), the insulin-related receptor (IRR, a receptor whose sequence is homologous to the sequences of the IR and IGF-IR but whose ligand is unknown), and probably the relaxin receptor.[6] Considerably more is known about the insulin receptor and its signal transduction processes than the IGF-1 receptor.[39,40] The IR and IGF-1R molecules are synthesized as single precursor polypeptides that are cleaved posttranslationally to yield the mature α and β subunits. The α subunits (135-kDa for the IR) are completely extracellular and contain a single cysteine-rich region that stabilizes the ligand binding domain. In the absence of ligand, the α subunit is felt to inhibit the intrinsic tyrosine kinase activity of the β subunit (~95-kDa), which also contains the short membrane spanning region of the receptor.

It has been proposed that the α subunits of the $\alpha_2\beta_2$ receptor contain two primary ligand contact sites, and that the ligand contacts different sites on each half of the receptor.[40] Accordingly, at physiologically relevant hormone concentrations, insulin interacts with high affinity to both binding sites 1 and 2, each on separate halves of the receptor. At greater concentrations, two insulin molecules may bind with lower affinity to a site 1 on each α chain. The proximity of the 1 and 2 contact sites on each α subunit may account for the negative cooperativity exerted by one insulin on the binding of a second insulin molecule to the receptor. The insulin and IGF-1 receptors bind both insulin and IGF-1 but with opposite affinities, such that the IR binds insulin with higher affinity and the IGF-1R preferentially binds IGF-1.

Insulin binding to its receptor rapidly induces receptor autophosphorylation which, in contrast to the class I RTKs, appears essential for activation of the exogenous tyrosine kinase activity of the receptor.[40] In some systems, ligand binding induces each β subunit to phosphorylate itself by an intramolecular *cis* reaction,[41] while in others, β subunit phosphorylation occurs through an intermolecular trans-phosphorylation mechanism.[42]

Class II RTKs also differ from the other RTK subtypes in that most of their effects are mediated through an intermediary, "docking protein" termed insulin receptor substrate 1 (IRS-1, pp185).[43] The IGF-IR, like the IR, phosphorylates IRS-1,[44] and the phosphorylated tyrosine domains of IRS-1 couple the protein to downstream effector enzymes that are involved in the RTK action cascade (as reviewed in Ref. 40).

While IGF-I production is localized to mesenchymal cells, most cell types absolutely require IGF-I for growth in in vitro conditions.[45] More specifically, IGF-I has been shown to be mitogenic for canine tracheal epithelial cells[37] and rabbit tracheal smooth muscle.[38] Furthermore, both IGF-I and IGF-II appear to play important roles in the development of mesodermally derived pulmonary tissues, which determine the ultrastructure of the fetal lung, as well as in the multiplication and differentiation of the respiratory epithelium.[46] Type I IGF receptors are more abundant in growing tissues and proliferating cells than in more quiescent tissue. Hybrid receptors containing subunits of the insulin and IGF-I receptor have been described and have been implicated in some of the growth effects attributed to insulin.[47] IGF-I and insulin also influence the differentiation of tracheal smooth muscle cells grown in culture and, in particular, the expression of muscarinic cholinergic receptors in that cell type.[48] IGF-I is expressed in the lung throughout life, with high relative abundance of IGF-I mRNA compared to most other tissues.[49] Small-cell lung carcinomas elaborate IGF-I at even higher levels, and evidence suggests that IGF-I acts as an autocrine factor to stimulate such carcinoma cell proliferation.[50]

PLATELET-DERIVED GROWTH FACTOR RECEPTORS
Class III TRKs comprise receptors for platelet-derived growth factor (PDGF), macrophage colony-stimulating growth factor (MCSF-1), and the *c-kit* protein (or the steel receptor, important in the development of melanocytes and germ cells and in hematopoiesis).[6] These receptors are monomeric proteins but differ from class I TRKs in the following features: (1) their 10 highly conserved cysteine residues are not contained within a cluster but are distributed throughout the extracellular domain; (2) the extracellular domain contains 5 immunoglobulinlike sequences; and (3) the intracellular domain contains an insert sequence (termed the *kinase insert*) of about 120 amino acids located in the middle of the conserved kinase domain, separating the putative ATP-binding region from the autophosphorylation site.[2,51,52] Although dispensable for kinase activity, because of its several autophosphorylation sites, the kinase insert has an important role in substrate recognition. PDGF receptors are synthesized as 140- to 160-kDa precursor proteins, which undergo extensive posttranslational modification and glycosylation to produce the 170- to 180-kDa mature receptors.[53]

Of the known classes of RTK ligands, only PDGF and related cytokines are covalently dimeric. PDGF exists in three forms, with disulfide-linked A chains and B chains forming either homodimeric (AA or BB) or heterodimeric (AB) combinations. Analogously, there are two known types of PDGF receptor, termed PDGFαR and PDGFβR, that are similar in sequence but differ in tissue distribution and regulation. The receptor subunits also differ in ligand-binding specificity, such that PDGFβR binds only the B-chain PDGF ligand, whereas the PDGFαR binds both the A- and B-chain ligands. Accordingly, PDGF-AA can induce both homo- and heterodimerization of the PDGF receptor to form all PDGFR types (i.e., αα, αβ, or ββ); PDGF-AB can induce formation of the αβ or ββ PDGFR; and PDGF-BB can induce only homodimerization of the ββ receptor. Thus, the type of receptor dimer that is formed (i.e., αα, αβ, or ββ) depends on the type of PDGF dimer (AA, BB, or AB) used to stimulate a given cell type, as well as the type of receptor(s) expressed by the cell.[6] If autophosphorylation patterns vary between the PDGFR dimer types, this multiplicity of interaction could provide a means of selective substrate recruitment following PDGF stimulation in differing cell types and conditions, as discussed below.

PDGF receptors are found on most mesenchymal connective tissue, including fibroblasts, chondroblasts, smooth muscle cells, and capillary endothelial cells.[54–56] Although PDGFR usually is not expressed in epithelial cells, there is emerging evidence that PDGF is involved in distal fetal lung growth and development. The latter consideration is based on observations that:

1. PDGF immunoreactivity is present in distal airway epithelial cells as well as interstitial and smooth muscle cells during late fetal rat lung development.[57]
2. Distal fetal lung epithelial cells express PDGFαR and PDGFβR[58] and respond functionally to exogenous PDGF-AA[58] and PDGF-BB.[59]
3. PDGFαR and PDGFβR gene expression are differentially regulated at the transcriptional and posttranscriptional levels, respectively, during fetal lung development.[60]
4. Antisense PDGF-A oligonucleotide reduces the number of terminal buds formed during branching morphogenesis in embryonic rat lung explants.[61]

PDGF acts to initiate cell cycle events leading to DNA synthesis and proliferation and is, hence, a type of cytokine termed a *competence factor*. Through induction of a group of competence genes (e.g., c-myc, c-fos, and c-jun), competence factors cause cells to enter the $G_0 \rightarrow G_1$ transition but, by themselves, competence factors are incapable of inducing mitosis. Progression through the G_1 phase requires stimulation by complementary cytokines termed *progression factors*, of which EGF and IGF-I are examples.[62]

PDGF has also been implicated in the development of fibrosing lung diseases. Nonactivated human alveolar macrophages constitutively transcribe both PDGF-A and PDGF-B genes but release little PDGF. In contrast, macrophages from patients with fibrosing lung diseases demonstrate increased transcription of the PDGF-B gene[63] and release of PDGF.[64] Secretion of PDGF has also been observed in alveolar macrophages isolated from patients with Hermansky-Pudlak syndrome.[65] An additional source of PDGF in subjects with idiopathic pulmonary fibrosis may be their alveolar epithelial cells which, unlike in normal lungs, express PDGF-B mRNA.[66]

VASCULAR ENDOTHELIAL GROWTH FACTOR

A class IV group of receptors for vascular endothelial cell growth factor (VEGF) has been identified exclusively in endothelial cells. Members of this family include the receptors termed Flk1, FLT1, and FLT4. Because of similarities with the PDGF subfamily of receptors, these RTKs are sometimes included in the class III group. Like the class III receptors, VEGF receptors contain extracellular immunoglobulinlike motifs (although they have seven IG repeats instead of five) and a cytosolic tyrosine kinase domain that is interrupted by a large kinase insert region.[6] Little is known about VEGF receptor-mediated signaling systems, although VEGF has been identified as a mitogen for endothelial cells and an inducer of enhanced vascular permeability.[67] Whether such a role for VGEF exists in pulmonary endothelium remains to be established.

FIBROBLAST GROWTH FACTOR RECEPTORS

Fibroblast growth factor receptors (FGFR), the prototypes for class V RTKs, have features similar to the class III PDGFRs, including a monomeric transmembrane structure, the presence of three consensus Ig-like domains within the extracellular region, and a 14-amino acid kinase inset sequence in the intracellular region that splits the tyrosine kinase domain into two nearly equal halves.[6] Between Ig domains I and II is a short region comprised of eight acidic amino acids and referred to as the acid box domain. Four distinct genes (FGFR1, FGFR2, FGFR3, FGFR4) have been found to be differentially expressed in a variety of mouse tissues during embryogenesis. Further diversity is generated by alternative splicing within the FGFR1 and FGFR2 genes to create FGFR1 and FGFR2 forms with or without the Ig I domain, FGFR2 forms with or without the acid box domain, FGFR1 and FGFR2 forms with three alternative exons coding for the second half of Ig domain III (FGFR1-IIIa, FGFR1-IIIb, FGFR-IIIc, FGFR2-IIIb, and FGFR2-IIIc), and FGFR2 forms with three distinct carboxy-terminal domains.[68–70]

The alternate splicing within Ig III appears to be particularly important in determining binding specificities for the following members of the FGF family: acidic FGF (aFGF), basic FGF (bFGF, encoded by at least seven mRNAs of varying length), the product of the *int-2* oncogene, the product of the *hst* oncogene, FGF 5, FGF 6, and keratinocyte growth factor (KGF).[6] For example, aFGF binds with high affinity to all four gene products and to FGFR1 and FGFR2 forms containing IIIb- or IIIc-type sequences. In contrast, bFGF binds with high affinity only to FGFR1 and FGFR2 forms containing the IIIc-type sequence, with much lower affinity to FGFR3 and to FGFR1 and FGFR2 forms with the IIIb-sequence, and does not bind to FGFR4.[6] Thus, it is believed that tissues can achieve selective responsiveness to individual fibroblast growth factors through tissue-specific FGFR gene expression and/or tissue-specific alternative splicing in the third Ig domain. FGF binding induces receptor dimerization, with both homodimeric and heterodimeric receptor species being formed between FGFR1, FGFR2, and FGFR3 receptor proteins.[71,72] Receptor dimerization is followed by autophosphorylation, which occurs by an intermolecular transphosphorylation mechanism,[6] and activation of the intrinsic tyrosine kinase activity.

FGFs are potent angiogenic factors, stimulating proliferation and chemotaxis of cells of mesodermal origin and inducing an invasive phenotype in endothelial cells. Accordingly, through effects on neovascularization and granulation tissue formation, FGFs play a major role in wound healing. Perhaps to this end, the adult lung expresses an acidic FGF (mRNA 4.6 kb) and seven known basic FGFs (mRNAs 6.0, 3.7, 2.5, 1.8, 1.6, 1.4, and 1.0 kb), as well as types 1 to 3 of the FGF receptor.[73] FGFs also appear to modulate developmental processes, such that INT-2, KGF, and FGF-5 are expressed at precise stages of embryonic and fetal development,[74] and basic FGF is present in epithelial basement membranes and endothelial cells of fetal rat lung.[75] Moreover, preliminary data suggests that mRNAs for FGF receptor types 1, 2, and 3 are also expressed in late-gestational fetal lung, with FGFR2 predominating.[73] The latter is localized to the epithelium and is increased during periods of alveolar septal development.[73]

HEPATOCYTE GROWTH FACTOR

Hepatocyte growth factor (HGF) recently has been identified as a mitogen for rat alveolar type II cells, although not as potent as acidic FGF.[76] HGF acts by binding to a specific type of RTK (class VI) that is expressed in type II pneumocytes[76] and that is structurally identical to the *c-met* gene product. The HGF receptor is composed of an extracellular 50-kDa α-subunit that is disulfide-linked to a membrane spanning 145-kDa β-subunit. HGF binding activates the tyrosine kinase activity of the receptors, allowing association with several signaling molecules and causing biologic responses in epithelial cells, including mitogenesis and stimulation of cell motility.[6]

ATRIAL NATRIURETIC PEPTIDE RECEPTOR

Last, it should be noted that the atrial natriuretic peptide (ANP) receptor shares several structural and sequence similarities with the RTKs, including (1) the presence of 6 conserved cysteine residues distributed throughout the extracellular domain; (2) a single membrane-spanning region; and (3) a cytoplasmic carboxy-terminal portion containing a sequence similar to the tyrosine kinase domain of the PDGFR and the serine protein kinase family but which lacks any tyrosine kinase activity.[7,77] Rather, binding of ANP to its receptor activates membranous forms of guanylyl cyclase and increases cGMP in target tissues. Both the ANP ligand binding site and guanylyl cyclase activity have been shown to exist on a single protein, encoded by the cDNA of rat brain membranous guanylyl cyclase.[77] Thus, the ANP receptor represents a unique receptor type, in which ligand binding induces activation of an intrinsic guanylyl cyclase catalytic domain and the subsequent generation of a second messenger, cGMP.

REGULATION OF PROTEIN TYROSINE KINASE ACTIVITY BY AUTOPHOSPHORYLATION AND HETEROLOGOUS PHOSPHORYLATION

The tyrosine kinase domain is the most highly conserved portion of all RTK classes. Within this domain, all tyrosine kinases contain an ATP binding motif located approximately 50 amino acids downstream from the transmembrane domain and encoded by the consensus amino acid sequence Gly-Xxx-Gly-Xxx-Xxx-Gly-(Xxx)$_{15-20}$-Lys.[2] The lysyl residue is absolutely required for kinase activity, such that its replacement completely abolishes kinase activity and signal transduction in all RTKs.[2,3] A second distinctive motif, found about 140 amino acids beyond the ATP binding site, is delineated by the amino acid sequences Asp-Phe-Gly on the amino-terminal side and Ala-Pro-Glu on the carboxy side. This region contains one or more tyrosyl residues that are surrounded by acidic amino acids and are sites of ligand-induced autophosphorylation.[2] Most RTKs contain 1 tyrosyl residue in this region, and the effect of autophosphorylation on kinase activation is unclear.

For the insulin receptor (IR), however, the above sequence is referred to as the *regulatory region*, since autophosphorylation of the three tyrosyl residues found there (Tyr$_{1146}$, Tyr$_{1150}$, and Tyr$_{1151}$) is necessary for activation of the insulin receptor kinase.[2] Analysis of a mutant insulin receptor in which Tyr$_{1146}$ was replaced with phenylalanine (IR$_{F1146}$) demonstrated normal insulin binding but a 60 to 80 percent reduction in autophosphorylation,[2] suggesting that Tyr$_{1146}$ may have a central role in stimulating autophosphorylation at the other sites. Moreover, IR$_{F1146}$ does not internalize insulin rapidly or stimulate DNA synthesis in the presence of insulin, although insulin-induced glycogen synthesis is not affected.[2] In contrast, substitution of Tyr$_{1150}$ and Tyr$_{1151}$ with phenylalanine, leaving Tyr$_{1146}$ intact, results in a mutant IR with defective insulin stimulation of glucose uptake and glycogen formation, but with normal insulin-induced DNA synthesis.[78] Such demonstrations suggest that the relationship between autophosphorylation and RTK biologic functions is more complicated than the regulation of tyrosine kinase activity. Autophosphorylation likely is involved in the regulation of substrate binding and, hence, the selection of specific signal transduction pathways activated by receptor binding.

The tyrosine kinase domains of class III, IV, and V RTKs are interrupted by insertions of up to 100 mostly hydrophilic amino acid residues. These kinase insert regions vary in length and composition between RTKs but are highly conserved between species for a given receptor. The latter observations suggest that these kinase inserts also play an important role in receptor function, possibly again in modulating receptor interactions with specific cellular effector proteins.[3] Such a function has been reported in the PDGF receptor. Although most of the kinase insert region appears dispensable for kinase activity and mitogenic signaling of the PDGFR, the kinase insert of the receptor contains an autophosphorylation site (Tyr$_{751}$) that appears necessary for receptor interaction with phosphatidylinositol 3-kinase[79] and p21^{ras}-GTPase-activating protein (GAP).[80] That the Tyr$_{751}$ residue is not required for interaction with other PDGFR signal transducing molecules, such as phospholipase C-γ and c-Raf-1,[80] demonstrates how the kinase insert may regulate selectively RTK interactions with cytoplasmic substrate proteins.

Several additional autophosphorylation sites have been mapped to the carboxy-terminal tails of most RTKs. The carboxy-terminus is the most divergent region between RTKs, and the role of this tail region in receptor function largely is undetermined. For the EGF receptor, however, the carboxy-tail has been found to exert negative control on EGF-induced responses, proportedly through an allosteric mechanism. The tail region is believed to be long and flexible enough to interact as a pseudosubstrate with binding sites of the kinase region.[3] Accordingly, autophosphorylation or, alternately, amino acid substitution at autophosphorylation sites[81] or deletions within the tail region[82] removes the competitive potential of these intrinsic sequences and enhances the binding of cellular substrates to the tyrosine kinase site.

In addition to determining substrate specificity, phosphorylation at other tyrosine as well as serine and threonine residues provides a mechanism for heterologous regulation of RTK function. Threonine phosphorylation of the EGFR by PDGFR activation or by protein kinase C abolishes EGF tyrosine kinase activity, decreases high-affinity EGF binding, and may enhance receptor downregulation.[12,13,83] Protein kinase C-mediated phosphorylation of Thr$_{654}$, located just after the transmembrane domain, inhibits EGF-stimulated tyrosyl autophosphorylation and tyrosine kinase activity, but phosphorylation of other serine/threonine residues appears to be responsible for the PKC-induced attenuation of EGF binding affinity.[13,83,84] To the extent that EGF binding to its receptor results in the tyrosyl phosphorylation and likely stimulation of phospholipase C-γ, the subsequent activation of protein kinase C in the PLC-γ signaling pathway may provide a critical negative feedback loop, regulating EGFR tyrosine kinase activity by heterologous phosphorylation of Thr$_{654}$. The exact mechanism of this inhibition is unknown, but it is speculated that the insertion of a negatively charged phosphate near the inner surface of the plasma membrane may interfere with dimerization of occupied EGF receptors.[2] On the other hand, similar findings have been reported for the insulin receptor, wherein serine/threonine phosphorylation by cyclic adenosine monophosphate (cAMP)-dependent protein kinase[85] or by protein kinase C[86,87] results in decreased receptor tyrosine kinase activity. Since the IR already exists in a dimerized state, threonine phosphorylation must also inhibit receptor tyrosine kinase activity by mechanisms other than interference with receptor dimerization.

INTERNALIZATION OF RECEPTOR TYROSINE KINASES

In addition to autophosphorylation, ligand binding to RTKs induces receptor internalization into two types of intracellular vesicles: "pitted" or "coated" vesicles coated with the protein clathrin, and smooth vesicles lacking clathrin. RTKs are believed to undergo spontaneous internalization and recycling even in the absence of ligand, but ligand binding accelerates the process, resulting in a downregulation of cell-surface receptors and a desensitization of the ligand-RTK response. Accordingly, in the absence of EGF, the half-life of the EGFR is 10 to 12 h; in the presence of EGF, the half-life is reduced to approximately 1 h.[13] Once internalized, the ligand-RTK complex dissociates, and the ligand and receptors are degraded. For the EGF receptor, bound EGF-EGFR complexes are incorporated into coated vesicles and transported through endosomes to multivesicular bodies, where the EGF and some of the EGFR are degraded. The remainder of unbound EGF receptors are then recycled back to the plasma membrane.[13] It has been shown that tyrosine kinase activity is indispensable for EGF degradation, in that a kinase-negative EGFR mutant was internalized at nearly the same rate as the wild-type receptor but was rapidly recycled back to the cell surface for reutilization.[88] Only the wild-type, kinase-containing receptors were degraded following EGF-stimulated internalization.[89]

In contrast to the EGF receptor, insulin-IR complexes are internalized through smooth vesicles and transported to the smooth endoplasmic reticulum. Degradation of insulin and the IR occurs with this internalization, but it has also been proposed that nondegraded, active insulin-IR complexes may be transported by this process to cell sites otherwise not accessible to the cell surface RTK (e.g., the nuclear membrane) in order to mediate some of the biologic effects of insulin.[90] As with the EGFR, tyrosine kinase-negative IR mutants fail to undergo ligand-induced down regulation.[91]

RECEPTOR TYROSINE KINASE SIGNAL TRANSDUCTION—SH2 AND SH3 DOMAINS

Whereas the requirement of tyrosine kinase activity for signal transduction clearly has been demonstrated for nearly all classes of RTKs, the molecular link between kinase activity and the subsequent RTK messenger system is just beginning to be understood. It is now known that RTKs, like other tyrosine-phosphorylated proteins, interact with molecules containing Src homology 2 and 3 (SH2 and SH3) domains. These SH2 and SH3 domains are short sequences of about 100 and 50 to 60 amino acid residues, respectively, that function to specify the interaction of a molecule with target proteins.[92,93] Together with Pleckstrin homology (PH) domains, SH2 and SH3 domains share the following properties:

1. They are true domains, such that each forms a compact unit that maintains its structure in isolation from the rest of the protein.
2. Each has its amino and carboxy termini in close apposition so that the domain can be "plugged in" to the surface of a protein.
3. There is no pattern to the number or location of these domains within proteins.
4. They are not restricted to specific types of signal transduction proteins, but occur in protein kinases, lipid kinases, protein phosphatases, phospholipases, Ras-controlling proteins, transcription factors, and certain adaptor proteins that have no enzymatic function.[94]

The SH2 motifs recognize phosphotyrosine residues and are responsible for interactions with autophosphorylated

RTKs, the specificity of which depends upon the amino acid sequences surrounding both the tyrosine autophosphorylation site on the RTK and the substrate's SH2 domain.[95–97] Group I SH2 domains prefer to interact with the following amino acid sequence:

phosphotyrosine—hydrophilic—hydrophilic—hydrophobic

whereas group II SH2s select the sequence:

phosphotyrosine—hydrophobic—xxx—hydrophobic

Conversely, SH3 motifs are not necessary for the interaction of SH2-containing substrates with the phosphotyrosine residue of an RTK. Rather, because of many conserved hydrophobic residues, the SH3 domains recognize sequences of 9 to 12 amino acids containing proline and hydrophobic residues[93] and are thought to interact with cytoskeletal proteins in the localization of the molecule to the cytoplasmic membrane.[92]

RTK substrate proteins containing SH2 and SH3 motifs may contain enzymatic activity or may function solely as adaptor proteins.[93] The best characterized enzymatic RTK substrates are the various cytoplasmic protein tyrosine kinases (e.g., Src, Abl, Csk, Syk), p21^{ras}-GTPase-activating protein (GAP), phospholipase C-γ1 (PLC-γ1), protein tyrosine phosphatases (e.g., PTP1C, Syp/PTP1D), and p91 transcriptional factor. Adaptor protein RTK substrates, on the other hand, are composed almost completely of SH2 and SH3 domains and include Grb2 (one SH2 flanked by two SH3 motifs), c-Crk (one SH2 and two SH3 motifs), Nck (one SH2 and three SH3 motifs), and the p85 subunit of phosphatidylinositol 3 kinase (PI3-K) (two SH2 motifs and one SH3 motif). The p85 subunit is an adaptor protein whose primary function is to carry the associated p110 PI3-K catalytic subunit to the cytoplasmic membrane; however, its Brc homology domain could also allow p85 to function as a GTPase-activating protein (GAP).[93] Due to the ability of their SH2 and SH3 domains to recognize particular amino acid sequences, both adaptor and enzymatic RTK substrate proteins have a pivotal role in directing the specific cellular response to RTK-ligand binding. Schlessinger[93] has proposed three different paradigms for RTK activation of SH2/SH3-containing proteins, although the latter are not necessarily mutually exclusive mechanisms.

PHOSPHOLIPASE C-γ1

The first paradigm is activation by tyrosine phosphorylation, as exemplified by the substrate phospholipase C-γ1 (Fig. 2-2A). There are four families of PLC isoenzymes, PLC-α, -β (formerly PLC-I), -γ (PLC-II) and -δ (PLC-III), based on cDNA sequencing. Of the four types, only PLC-γ has SH2 domains and is an RTK substrate. In contrast, PLC-β and -δ isoenzymes are activated by non-tyrosine kinase receptors via certain G proteins (e.g., Gq is the intermediary in receptor-stimulated activation of PLC-β1).[98] The role of PLC-α in signal transduction has yet to be determined. PLC-γ exists in two isoforms, the first of which (PLC-γ1) being widely expressed and the second (PLC-γ2) being largely restricted to thymus, spleen, and lung.[1] The SH2 motifs of PLC-γ are attracted to autophosphorylation sites on the carboxy-termi-

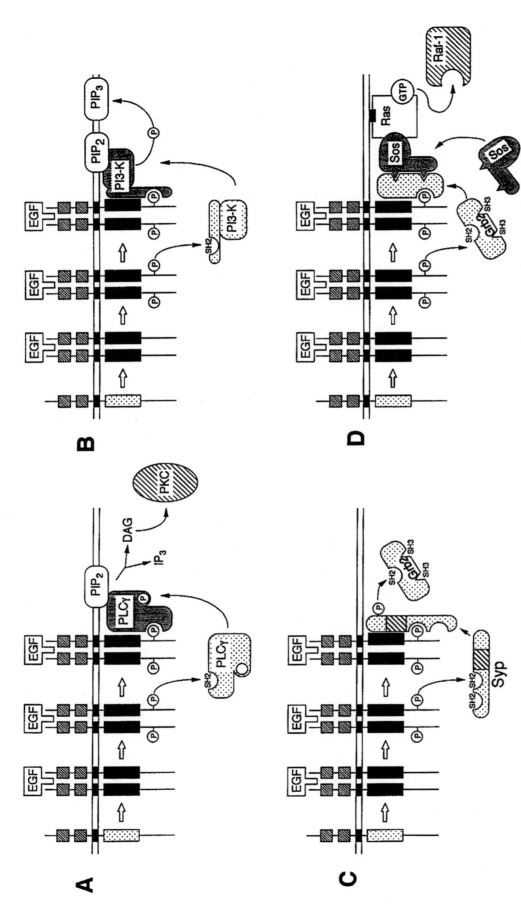

FIGURE 2-2 Paradigms of signal transduction through receptor tyrosine kinases. Panel A: Activation by tyrosine phosphorylation, as shown for epidermal growth factor (EGF) activation of phospholipase Cγ (PLCγ). EGF induces dimerization and autophosphorylation of the epidermal growth factor receptor (EGFR). The SH2 domain of inactive PCLγ interacts with the autophosphorylated (P) EGFR, resulting in phosphorylation and activation of PLCγ, which then hydrolyses membrane phosphatidylinositol 4,5-bisphosphate (PIP₂) to form inositol 1,4,5-trisphosphate (IP₃) and diacylglycerol (DAG). DAG in turn can activate protein kinase C (PKC). Panel B: Activation by conformational change, as shown for EGF-induced activation of phosphatidylinositol 3-kinase (PI3-K). The SH2 domain of the autophosphorylated EGFR, interacts with the autophosphorylated EGFR, resulting in a transformational change in and consequent activation of in the p110 subunit of PI3-K, which can then phosphorylate PIP₂ to form phosphatidylinositol 3,4,5-trisphos-

phate (PIP₃). Panel C: Activation by association and possible phosphorylation, as shown for EGF-induced activation of the cytoplasmic protein tyrosine phosphatase Syp. One of two SH2 domains of Syp interacts with the autophosphorylated EGFR, bringing its protein tyrosine phosphatase domain (striped area) into contact with the RTK. Activated Syp is capable of interacting with the SH2 domain of the Ras-associated adaptor protein, Grb2. Panel D: Activation by localization, as shown for EGF-activation of Ras. The SH2 domain of Grb2 interacts with the autophosphorylated EGFR, and the SH3 domains of Grb2 interact with Ras guanine nucleotide releasing factor, Sos. The translocation of Sos to the inner surface of the cell membrane brings it into contact with the membrane-associated GTPase, Ras. The activated (GTP-bound) Ras can then associate with the regulatory domain of the serine/threonine kinase Raf-1.

nal tail of the RTK, and the binding of PLC-γ to the receptor promotes the tyrosine phosphorylation of PLC-γ by the receptor's tyrosine kinase domain. Tyrosine phosphorylation of PLC-γ1 has been documented in response to the activation of several RTKs, including receptors for EGF,[99–102] PDGF,[103–105] VEGF,[106] FGF,[107,108] and HGF.[109] In contrast, PLC-γ1 phosphorylation does not occur following activation of insulin receptors,[110] MCSF-1 receptors,[111] or the Src cytoplasmic tyrosine kinases.[99] Sequencing studies have demonstrated the presence of three tyrosine phosphorylation sites (Tyr_{771}, Tyr_{783}, and Tyr_{1254}) and one RTK-induced serine phosphorylation site (Ser_{1248}) on the PLC-γ molecule.[92]

Phosphorylation of Tyr_{783} and, to a lesser extent, Tyr_{1254} activates the PLC-γ enzyme[92] and induces the rapid hydrolysis of the plasma membrane phospholipid, phosphatidylinositol 4,5-biphosphate ($PtdIns(4,5)P_2$). Hydrolysis of $PtdIns(4,5)P_2$ generates two second messengers, inositol 1,4,5-trisphosphate ($Ins(1,4,5)P_3$), which binds to a specific receptor and releases calcium from intracellular stores, and diacylglycerol (DAG), which is an activator of protein kinase C (PKC). At least some PKC isoforms are capable of eliciting a mitogenic response, in part via phosphorylation of key signaling molecules such as Raf-1 (Ref. 112, see below).

PHOSPHATIDYLINOSITOL 3-KINASE

The second paradigm is activation by conformational change (Fig. 2-2*B*), as demonstrated by phosphatidylinositol 3-kinase (PI3-K), an enzyme capable of phosphorylating the D-3 position on phosphatidylinositol, phosphatidylinositol-4-phosphate, and phosphatidylinositol-4,5-bis-phosphate ($PtdIns(4,5)P_2$, the substrate for PLC). PI-3 kinase is a heterodimeric complex of an 85-kDa protein and a 110-kDa protein that has several different potential isoforms, in that three distinct p85 cDNAs and two distinct p110 cDNAs have been identified.[113,114] The p85 protein contains two SH2 domains but lacks a typical ATP binding site and does not demonstrate any PI-3 kinase activity. The current view is that the p85 subunit serves as a chaperon or regulatory protein for the p110 subunit, which houses the enzyme's catalytic activity.[92] Interaction of the p85 protein with phosphorylated tyrosine residues on a RTK results in a conformational change in p85 that is transmitted to the p110 subunit, thereby inducing its catalytic activity.[93] Moreover, the translocation of the activated p110 molecule to the plasma membrane, shepherded by the p85 subunit, brings the enzymatic component of PI3-K into contact with its substrate phosphoinositides. The SH2 domains of p85 are attracted to phosphorylated kinase residues on receptors for EGF,[115] PDGF,[105,116] c-kit,[117] VEGF,[106] and HGF[109] as well as the cytoplasmic protein tyrosine kinases, Src, Fyn, and Lyn.[118,119] PI3-K has also been shown to coprecipitate with IRS-1,[120] which contains six tyrosine residues with the YMXM sequence that appears important for binding the p85 SH2 domain.[43,121,122] Thus, PI3-K is activated by insulin in a variety of cell types, including adipose cells,[123] CHO cells,[120,124] and human vascular smooth muscle cells.[125] The potential role of PI3-K in mediating the effects of insulin and/or IGF-1 in pulmonary tissues has yet to be identified.

Indeed, the specific signaling pathways utilized by PI3-K remain unidentified, since the functions of D-3 phosphory-lated phosphoinositides are largely unknown. The latter phospholipids do not appear to be hydrolyzed by any known phospholipase C. Accordingly, PI3-K-stimulated production of $PtdIns(3,4,5)P_3$ from $PtdIns(4,5)P_2$ may serve to inhibit the PLC-signaling pathway, by limiting availability of the $PtdIns(4,5)P_2$ substrate for PLC. Alternately, $PtdIns(3,4,5)P_3$ has recently been shown to activate PKCζ[126] a calcium- and phorbol acid-insensitive isoform of protein kinase C that has mitogenic properties.[127] Additional cellular processes regulated by PI3-K may include activation of p70[S6K], a serine/threonine kinase involved mitogenesis,[128] cellular trafficking,[116] and membrane ruffling and chemotaxis.[129] The latter responses are consistent with the observation that p85 has GAP activity toward Rac, a small molecular weight G protein involved in membrane ruffling.[130]

PROTEIN TYROSINE PHOSPHATASES

Also activated through binding to a RTK and possibly as a result of tyrosine phosphorylation (Fig. 2-2*C*) are the cytoplasmic protein tyrosine phosphatases (PTPs) SH-PTP1 (also known as *SHP*, *PTP1C*, and *HCP*) and SH-PTP2 (alternately termed *Syp*, *PTP1D*, *PTP2C*, and *SH-PTP3*).[1] The latter are SH2 containing enzymes that catalyze the dephosphorylation of phosphotyrosine residues in RTKs and their substrates. Expression of SH-PTP1 is confined to hematopoietic cells and some epithelial cell lines, but SH-PTP2 probably is ubiquitously expressed. Both enzymes have a similar structure consisting of two SH2 domains in the amino-terminal half and a catalytic domain in the carboxy half of the molecule. That SH-PTP1 has been shown to dephosphorylate cytoplasmic phosphotyrosyl residues in PDGFα and PDGFβ receptors, as well as in receptors for MCSF-1, EGF, insulin, and IGF-1,[131,132] suggests that this PTP may be involved in attenuating mitogenic or other responses to these cytokines. The binding sites for SH-PTP1's SH2 domain on these receptors remain to be identified, however.

Conversely, SH-PTP2 is known to bind to a phosphotyrosine at residue 1009 of the PDGF receptor,[133] and SH-PTP2 is phosphorylated in vivo by activated PDGF and EGF receptors.[134,135] Nevertheless, SH-PTP2 does not dephosphorylate the cytoplasmic domains of PDGFα or β receptors, EGF or HER3 receptors, or insulin or IGF-1 receptors.[1] Instead, SH-PTP2 appears to mediate the binding of the PDGF receptor with the Ras-associated adaptor protein, Grb2,[136] as noted below.

RAS—MAP KINASE CASCADE

The third paradigm is activation by localization (Fig. 2-2*D*). Most RTKs stimulate the mitogen-activated kinase (MAP kinase) pathway through a multistep signaling cascade, initiated by translocation of an adaptor protein, Grb2, to the cytoplasmic membrane.[93] Grb2 is a 217 amino acid, 24-kDa protein consisting entirely of a single SH2 domain sandwiched between two SH3 domains. Grb2 is structurally similar to the *C. elegans* protein Sem-5 and the *Drosophila* protein Drk (for *downstream of receptor kinases*). The Grb2 SH2 motif recognizes a phosphotyrosine two amino acids upstream from an asparagine residue on the EGF receptor,[137] IRS-1 protein,[138] and the Shc adaptor protein,[138] which may act as a bridge between tyrosine-phosphorylated T-cell receptors and Grb2/Sos.[97] As noted above, Grb2 also does not appear to interact directly with PDGF receptors but is linked to them via SH-PTP2.

The Grb2 SH3 domains interact with short proline-rich regions in the carboxy-tail of a ubiquitously expressed Ras guanine nucleotide releasing factor termed Sos (the mammalian homolog of the product of the *Son of sevenless* gene in *Drosophila*). In response to EGF binding, the Grb2/Sos complex binds to the autophosphorylated EGFR[137] and thereby is translocated to the plasma membrane, where the 21-kDa Ras protein is located. The three closely related p21 Ras proteins found in most mammalian cells (termed *Ha*, *Ki*, and *N*) are posttranslationally modified at their carboxy ends to allow anchorage to the inner surface of the plasma membrane.[6]

Ras proteins are small molecular weight GTPases that cycle between conformations that are active (GTP-bound) and inactive (GDP-bound). In resting, nontransformed cells, most of the Ras protein is in the inactive form, due to its high binding affinity for GDP and its low intrinsic GTPase activity. Sos activates Ras by promoting the release of Ras-associated GDP and enabling the subsequent binding of GTP to the Ras molecule. GTP binding to Ras displaces the Sos exchange protein, leaving free activated Ras-GTP. Only Ras-GTP (not Ras-GDP) can associate with the amino-terminal regulatory domain of Raf-1 serine/threonine kinases.[139] The latter are a family of isoenzymes (the three mammalian forms being designated *c-Raf-1*, *A-Raf*, and *B-Raf*) that are known activators of the MAP kinase pathway. Ras-GTP also interacts with a protein that activates its intrinsic GTPase activity (i.e., GTPase-activating protein, *GAP*) and converts Ras back to the inactive, GDP-bound state. Of interest, p120-GAP has been shown to interact through its own two SH2 domains with tyrosyl phosphorylated PDGF and VEGF receptors.[106,140,141] The recruitment of p-120 GAP to the plasma membrane would be expected to counter the effects of Sos; however, if RTK-associated GAP is somehow inactivated or sequestered from Ras, then PDGF receptor activation could enhance Ras activity by removing an inhibitory regulator from the Ras protein.

By itself, Ras-GTP is insufficient to activate Raf-1,[142] and artificial fusion of c-Raf-1 to the plasma membrane circumvents the need for Ras in the activation of Raf-1 kinase activity.[143,144] Accordingly, the current model suggests that the principal if not sole function of Ras-GTP is to position Raf-1 at the plasma membrane in the vicinity of additional activator(s) or cofactor(s).[145] One such membrane-associated factor is protein kinase C-α (PKC-α), which also is translocated to the membrane upon activation and which has been shown to phosphorylate and activate c-Raf-1 in 3T3 fibroblasts.[112] Near its Ras binding site, Raf-1 also contains a highly conserved zinc-finger motif of the type Cys-(Xxx)$_2$-Cys-(Xxx)$_9$-Cys-(Xxx)$_2$-Cys.[146] The hydrophobic portion of this zinc finger is believed to be buried within the molecule when the Raf kinase is localized within the cytoplasm of the cell. It has been proposed that interaction with Ras-GTP results in a conformational change in the Raf kinase, and the translocation of Raf to the cell membrane allows the hydrophobic

zinc-finger region to be stabilized within the lipid bilayer and possibly interact with a membrane lipid cofactor.[146] The conformational change in translocated Raf-1 exposes the catalytic domain and results in partial activation of the kinase.

As noted, however, full stimulation of Raf kinase activity requires more than Ras-induced translocation to the plasma membrane. Proposed events leading to full activation of Raf-1 include Raf-1 phosphorylation by tyrosine kinases (such as Src) and/or serine/threonine kinases (such as PKC), as well as Raf-1 interaction with other cofactors (such as the β and ζ members of the 14-3-3 protein family).[147] In fibroblasts, PKC is capable of activating fully Raf-1 and its downstream MAP kinase pathway, completely independent of Ras.[148] The βγ complex of G$_i$ (particularly β$_1$γ$_2$) has also been shown to activate Ras, possibly through a cytoplasmic tyrosine kinase.[149] Direct interactions between βγ complexes and Sos or Ras-GAP have also been proposed, in light of the independent observations that both Sos and Ras-GAP contain pleckstrin homology (PH) domains and that free βγ dimers interact with the β-adrenergic receptor kinase (βARK) through a PH-encompassing region.[145]

Thus, emerging evidence suggests that the Ras—Raf-1 connection is a critical focal point in several cellular signaling mechanisms mediating both proliferative and antiproliferative responses (Fig. 2-3). Regarding the latter, cAMP and its analogs are capable of inhibiting growth factor-induced mitogenic actions in many cell types, including fibroblasts, adipocytes, and human arterial smooth muscle cells.[145] This antiproliferative effect is paralleled by the ability of cAMP-dependent protein kinase (PKA) to antagonize RTK activation of MAP kinase. PKA can directly phosphorylate c-Raf-1, predominantly at Ser$_{43}$, and the phosphorylated c-Raf-1 demonstrates a decreased affinity for binding to Ras-GTP.[150]

FIGURE 2-3 Schematic of identified signal transduction pathways for receptor tyrosine kinases (RTKs). Compounds are as designated in the text. Solid lines depict positive interactions, and dashed lines depict inhibitory pathways. In the Ras activation cycle, Grb2-Sos potentiates the exchange of GTP for GDP, and the Ras GTPase activating protein GAP stimulates the conversion of Ras-bound GTP back to GDP. The diagram also notes that other, as yet identified, factor(s) appear to be involved in activating the serine/threonine kinase, Raf-1.

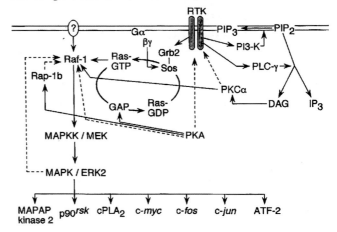

In addition, cAMP has been shown to inhibit activation of the Raf-1—MAP kinase cascade induced by 12-O-tetra-decanoylphorbol-13-acetate (an activator of PKC) or purified PKC-α, which is felt to induce MAP kinase activity independent of Ras activation.[151,152] Lastly, it recently has been shown that a Ras-like GTPase termed *Rap1a* is phosphorylated in vivo in response to cAMP-inducing agents.[145] Rap1a has the same Raf-1 binding region as Ras, and so may compete with Ras for Raf-1 binding or may inactivate Raf-1 by regulating the relocation of Raf-1 from the plasma membrane to the cytosol.[145] Thus, PKA may inhibit activation of Raf-1 at three different levels:

1. By attenuating the binding affinity for Ras-GTP through phosphorylation of Ser$_{43}$
2. By decreasing the catalytic activity of Raf-1 through phosphorylation of other residues
3. By promoting the Rap1a—Raf-1 interaction through phosphorylation of Rap1a

Activated Raf-1 phosphorylates and activates the dual-specificity kinase MAP kinase kinase (MAPKK, alternately termed *MEK* or *ERK kinase*), which subsequently phosphorylates and activates the mitogen-activated protein kinases p44^{MAPK} and p42^{MAPK}, also known as extracellular-signal-regulated kinases 1 and 2 (ERK1 and ERK2), respectively. How a single MAPKK is able to phosphorylate both a threonine and tyrosine residue in a Thr-Glu-Tyr sequence to activate MAPK remains unknown. Nevertheless, among the identified substrates for activated MAP kinases are certain serine/threonine kinases, such as ribosomal S6 kinase (p90^{rsk})[153] and MAPK-activated protein kinase-2,[154] cytoplasmic phospholipase A$_2$,[155] and several transcription factors, including c-myc, c-fos, c-jun, and ATF-2.[146] In addition, the downstream MAP kinases ERK1 and ERK2 have been shown to also phosphorylate c-Raf-1, although the latter phosphorylation does not appear to alter the activity of the kinase. It has been proposed that ERK-phosphorylation may result in dissociation of activated Raf-1 from the plasma membrane, thereby providing a negative feedback loop causing Raf-1 inactivation.[146]

REGULATION OF RECEPTOR TYROSINE KINASE SIGNALING

It is increasingly apparent that RTKs can interact with several critical cell signaling pathways to elicit their effects (Fig. 2-3). In part, the interaction with specific substrates depends upon the RTK's pattern of autophosphorylation, but how this pattern may vary with growth factor binding is unknown. For example, the PDGF receptor can be autophosphorylated on 8 tyrosine residues in the cytoplasmic domain of the RTK. Phosphorylated tyrosine residues 579 and 581[156] and 857[157] have been implicated in the interaction between the PDGFβR and the Src family of cytoplasmic tyrosine kinases. In contrast, phosphorylation of tyrosines 740 and 771 is essential for the binding and activation of PI3-K.[158,159] Ras-GAP binds to phosphotyrosine 771,[133] the tyrosine phosphatase SH-PTP2/Syp/PTP1D binds to phosphotyrosine

1009,[133] and PLC-γ binds to phosphotyrosines 1009 and 1021.[133,160] It remains unclear whether all these signaling pathways are activated with PDGF-receptor binding, or whether specific pathways can be preferentially recruited under certain conditions. To that end, PDGF-BB has been shown to stimulate to formation of Ins(1,4,5)P$_3$ and DAG and to induce changes in intracellular pH and Ca^{2+} in vascular smooth muscle cells. In contrast, PDGF-AA stimulated only DAG formation, and did so with a different time course than that observed in PDGF-AB or -BB responses.[161,162] Thus, some response selectivity may be tissue specific, related to relative proportions of the substrates within the tissue, the types of PDGF receptor dimers that are formed (i.e., $\alpha\alpha$, $\alpha\beta$, and/or $\beta\beta$) and, perhaps, colocalization of certain effectors or cofactors in the plasma membrane region around the growth receptor.

Moreover, although common downstream signaling pathways are shared between subclasses of RTK, in some circumstances, activation of two or more RTK subclasses results in additive effects,[163] whereas in others, activation of one receptor (e.g., the PDGFR) elicits downregulation of another receptor (e.g., the EGFR).[13] Also largely uncertain are the relationships between RTKs and G proteins. As discussed, the $\beta\gamma$ complex of G$_i$ can potentially induce Ras activation and, thereby, augment a RTK mitogenic response. It has also been shown, however, that several RTK-mediated effects are inhibited by pertussis toxin, which inactivates α_i proteins. Pertussis toxin ablates EGF-induced phosphatidylinositol metabolism in hepatocytes,[164] several of the effects of insulin in cultured BC3H-1 murine myocytes,[165] and MCSF-1-induced phosphorylation in human neutrophils.[166] How G$_i$ proteins may be involved in these pertussis toxin-sensitive responses is unknown. At least some of the metabolic actions of insulin may be mediated through a novel, 66-kDa GTP-binding protein, designated G$_{ir}$, that is phosphorylated by the IR tyrosine kinase and ADP-ribosylated by pertussis toxin.[167] Finally, the mechanisms whereby the MAP-kinase cascade and other RTK-activated pathways are turned off and/or downregulated largely remain obscure. Antagonistic and inhibitory processes likely will involve novel signaling pathways, including certain phosphatases and serine/threonine kinases, as discussed below.

Receptor Serine/Threonine Kinases

Analogous to the receptor tyrosine kinases, there also exists a class of transmembrane molecules with extracellular receptor domains linked to cytoplasmic serine/threonine kinase activity. These receptor serine/threonine kinases (RSTKs) transduce the biologic effects of a superfamily of biologic factors comprising the activins/inhibins, bone morphogenetic proteins (BMPs) and other decapentaplegic (dpp)/Vg-related factors, Müllerian inhibiting substance (MIS), and the well-characterized cytokine, transforming growth factor β (TGF-β). TGF-β exists in three mammalian isoforms (TGF-β1, TGF-β2, and TGF-β3) encoded by separate genes.[168] Similar factors (TGF-β4 and TGF-β5) have also been cloned from chick and frog embryos, respectively. Each TGF-β isoform is structurally similar to TGF-β1, which is a 25-kDa homodimer of two disulfide-linked subunits.[169] TGF-βs are expressed ubiquitously and exert a variety of biologic actions, including:

1. Stimulating the proliferation of several mesenchymal cell types, including fibroblasts
2. Inhibiting the proliferation of other cell types, including epithelial and lymphoid cells
3. Modulating mesenchymal tissue differentiation
4. Increasing cellular integrin expression
5. Inducing the synthesis of extracellular-matrix proteins
6. Signaling the chemotaxis of monocytes and fibroblasts

The cellular actions of TGF-β are mediated through two main types of RSTK, which have been termed *TβR-I* and *TβR-II*. Types I and II TGF-β receptor are 53-kDa and 70- to 85-kDa proteins, respectively, that consist of a short extracellular domain, a transmembrane domain, and a long cytoplasmic domain containing the serine/threonine kinase catalytic moiety and a short carboxy-terminal segment.[170] Various cell lines also express a larger, third type of non-RSTK TGF-β receptor (also called *betaglycan*) that is a 200- to 400-kDa glycoprotein with heparan sulfate glycosaminoglycan chains and other proteoglycan residues attached to a core protein.[171,172] Unlike the type I and II receptors, type III TGF-β receptors exists do not directly participate in cellular signaling.[172] Instead, existing evidence suggests that type III receptors are involved in ligand presentation to type II receptors. Accordingly, TβR-II binding affinity for TGF-βs (particularly TGF-β2, which otherwise has minimal affinity) is substantially increased in cells coexpressing TβR-III with the types I and II TGF-β RSTKs.[173,174]

TYPE I AND TYPE II RECEPTOR SERINE/THREONINE KINASES

All TGF-β signal transduction is mediated through TβR-I and TβR-II receptors (Fig. 2-4). These two receptors, like all RSTKs, share certain characteristic features, including (1) a short extracellular domain containing several conserved cysteine residues and a cluster of three cysteins just upstream from the transmembrane region; (2) a single, short membrane-spanning domain; and (3) a long cytoplasmic portion that primarily consists of the kinase domain. The kinase activity may be of dual specificity, since both type I and II RSTKs are autophosphorylated on tyrosine in addition to serine/threonine residues.[175]

Type II RSTKs were the first to be cloned and sequenced. They include the TGF-β receptor, TβR-II, as well as a receptor for BMPs (termed *DAF-4*) and three distinct activin receptors (ActR-II, ActR-IIB, and Atr-II).[169] TβR-II binds TGFβ-1 and TGFβ-3 with high affinity but only binds TGFβ-2 in the presence of the type III receptor. Recent evidence has implicated a second type II RSTK with selective high affinity for TGFβ-2, but this receptor remains to be fully characterized.[176] TβR-II has a structure similar to all type II RSTKs which, in addition to the above common features, includes a juxtamembrane spacer region prior to the kinase domain and a short carboxy-terminal tail.[175]

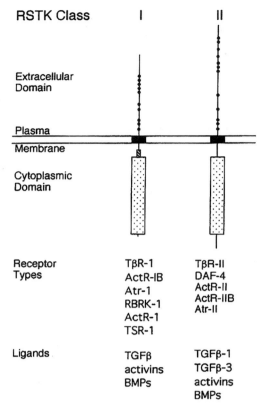

FIGURE 2-4 Classes of receptor serine/threonine kinases (RSTKs). Representative receptors and specific ligands for each RSTK class are listed below the schematized receptors. Stippled boxes symbolize the *serine/threonine kinase domain(s)*, preceded by a *GS domain* (slashed box) in the Type I receptors; dots represent conserved *cysteine residues*. Abbreviations: transforming growth factor-β (TGFβ) and its receptors (TβR-I and TβR-II); bone morphogenetic proteins (BMPs).

Type I RSTKs are more diverse and heterogeneous. The TGF-β receptor TβR-I (also called *ALK5, R4,* or *RPK2*) belongs to the type I RSTK family, as do the activin receptors ActR-IB (also called *ALK4* or *R2*) and Atr-1, and the BMP receptor RBRK-1 (also called *ALK3*). In addition, however, there exist at least two receptors with high affinity for both activins and TGF-βs; that is, ActR-1 (also termed *Tsk7L, SKR1, ALK2,* or *R1*) and TSR-1 (also termed *ALK1* or *R3*).[169] In comparison to type II RSTKs, all type I family receptors have shorter extracellular domains and carboxy-tails, and their cytoplasmic juxtamembrane spacer regions include a highly conserved SGSGSGLP motif (the *GS domain*) just adjacent to the kinase domain that is absent in type II receptors.[175]

Studies with cell mutants lacking TGF-β responsiveness have revealed that both receptors are required for TGF-β signal transduction[177,178] and that the cytoplasmic regions of the receptors are not interchangeable.[179] In addition, whereas TβR-II receptors can bind TGF-β, type I receptors require the type II receptor for ligand binding.[177] The above findings, coupled with studies of receptor autophosphorylation, have led to the following model of RSTK activation.

Type II receptors have been shown to form stable homodimeric complexes with constitutively active kinase in the presence or absence of ligand.[180,181] It has been proposed that TGF-β first binds to the TβR-II homodimer and that this interaction promotes the formation of a heterotetrameric receptor complex with two type I receptor molecules. Each type II RSTK can interact with divers type I receptors, and some type I receptors can interact with more than one type II receptor.[169] Within this multiplicity of interaction, ligand specificity (i.e., TGF-β vs activin versus BMP) is determined by the type II receptor. Whereas the type I receptor may enhance ligand binding affinity,[182] its primary role may be to modulate recruitment of specific signal transduction pathways.

SIGNAL TRANSDUCTION IN RECEPTOR SERINE/THREONINE KINASES

The heteromeric interaction of type I and type II RSTKs likely results in transphosphorylation of each other's cytoplasmic domains.[175] Similar autophosphorylation of dimerized receptors allows tyrosine kinase receptors to interact with their downstream substrates, but it is unclear whether an analogous mechanism plays a role in RSTK signaling. In many systems, the activities of both type I and type II kinases in the receptor complex are necessary for signaling, in that receptor complexes containing TβR-I or TβR-II molecules with point mutations in the ATP-binding site that abolish kinase activity fail to transmit TGF-β-mediated growth inhibition.[178,183] The antiproliferative effect of TGF-β appears to be distinct from effects on extracellular matrix production, however, in that the latter typically requires only a functional type I receptor, along with the extracellular domain of a type II receptor to provide ligand interaction with the type I RSTK.[170,175,184] Thus, transfection of a truncated type II receptor into a lung epithelial cell line (Mv1Lu cells) was found to inhibit the antiproliferative effects of TGF-β in a dominant-negative fashion but had no effect on other TGF-β-induced responses.[185]

As observed above, TGF-β is a potent modulator of cell proliferation, but its effects are quite variable. Indeed, TGF-β may either stimulate or inhibit cell growth, depending upon the cell type, the presence of other growth factors, and the preexisting state of activation of the cells.[186] Moreover, the actions of TGF-β on cell growth may be directly mediated or may be induced via the modulation of other growth factor responses. In this regard, it has been shown that TGF-β upregulates the number of PDGF-β receptor subunits but downregulates the number of α subunits in murine NIH/3T3 fibroblasts and in human smooth muscle cells.[187,188] Accordingly, in these cell types, the mitogenic response to PDGF-BB is minimally affected, but the response to PDGF-AA is markedly attenuated by exposure to TGF-β. Furthermore, TGF-β is capable of inducing the synthesis and release of PDGF, and so can indirectly stimulate proliferation of NRK949F cells[189] and smooth muscle cells[188,190] that are capable of responding to PDGF in an autocrine fashion. Since slightly lower concentrations of TGF-β are needed to stimulate PDGF release than to induce downregulation of

the PDGF-α receptor, TGF-β typically demonstrates a biphasic dose-response relationship affecting cell proliferation.[188]

Emerging evidence also suggests that at least some of the direct proliferative effects of TGF-β-related RSTKs are mediated through the G-protein system. For example, the mitogenic effects of TGF-β1 in AKR-2B fibroblasts appear to be mediated by G_i proteins, since pertussis toxin inhibits TGF-β-induced proliferation and *c-sis* and *c-myc* proto-oncogene expression in this cell line.[191] Conversely, TGF-β is growth inhibitory in lung epithelial cells, and this action is also lost in a mutant cell type possessing the three TGF-β receptor types but having impaired receptor-G-protein coupling.[192] Downstream events that are induced in cells that are growth-arrested by TGF-β include activation of Ras,[193] induction of protein phosphatase 1 activity,[194] and phosphorylation of the cAMP response element binding protein/transcription factor CREBP.[195] How these signaling events are activated following receptor activation remains unclear, as do the potential mechanistic roles of these pathways in the antiproliferative effects of TGF-β.

The antiproliferative effect of TGF-β appears to be cell cycle-dependent, in that the cytokine arrests the growth of epithelial cells when administered during early G1 but is less efficient in late G1. Moreover, the growth inhibitory effect is lost once cells progress through the G1 → S transition.[196,197] In light of our present understanding of cell cycle regulation, the consideration has been raised that these cycle-dependent effects may be mediated through inhibition of cell cyclins and associated cyclin-dependent kinases (CDKs). Derynck[175] has proposed a model, as illustrated in Fig. 2-5, wherein TGF-β acts by inhibiting the induction of the cyclin-D associated kinase CDK4, as has been demonstrated in human keratinocytes[197] and mink lung epithelial cells.[198] TGF-β may also, at least in some cell types, inhibit the subsequent induction of cyclin E and its partner CDK2. Both CDK4 and CDK2 are major phosphorylators of a critical cell cycle regulator, RB (retinoblastoma protein, named from the tissue in which it was first identified). In quiescent cells, RB

FIGURE 2-5 Schematic of potential sites of action of transforming growth factor-β (TGF-β) inhibition of cell mitogenesis. Solid lines depict positive interactions, and dashed lines depict inhibitory pathways. Abbreviations: cyclin-dependent kinase (CDK); retinoblastoma protein (RB).

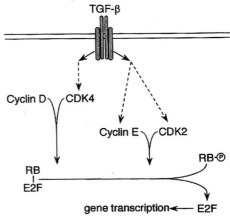

exists in an underphosphorylated state in complex to the transcription factor E2F. Following RB phosphorylation, E2F is released and activates a specific set of genes required for G1 → S transition.[199] Accordingly, it has been shown that in cells responding to TGR-β by late G1 growth arrest, RB is maintained in its underphosphorylated form.[196]

Even less is known about the non-growth-cycle effects of TGF-β and its receptors. In contrast to some of its mitogenic actions, TGF-β-stimulated extracellular matrix gene expression does not appear to be mediated through the G-protein system, in that the effect is not inhibited by pertussis toxin. Instead, induction of matrix gene expression by TGF-β appears to involve direct action on a nuclear 1 binding site within the promoter region of the procollagene I gene.[191,200] The specific signaling pathway involved in this action has yet to be elucidated. Nevertheless, it has been shown that TGF-β modulates extracellular matrix deposition at several points, including:

1. Increased transcription, translation, and processing of such matrix components as chondroitin/dermatan sulfate proteoglycans,[201,202] fibronectin,[203,204] and hyaluronan[205]
2. Decreased synthesis of matrix-degrading enzymes, including procollagenases[206] and type-1 plasminogen activator inhibitor[207]
3. Regulation of molecules involved in cell-cell and cell-matrix interactions, such as integrins,[208] the fibronectin receptor,[209] and the vitronectin receptor.[210]

In accordance with its presumed role in lung injury repair and fibrosis, induction of TGF-β gene expression has been shown to precede other aspects of tissue remodeling (e.g., collagen or proteoglycan gene expression) in animals exposed to bleomycin.[211–213] Pulmonary sources of TGF-β in response to injury include fibroblasts[212] as well as pulmonary endothelial cells.[214]

Thus, considerably less is known about RSTK than RTK signal transduction pathways. Analogous to the tyrosine kinase activity of RTKs, the serine/threonine kinase activity is essential for receptor function. It is likely, therefore, that the pattern of RSTK autophosphorylation will mediate the interactions with specific intracellular substrates, analogous to the SH2 domain-containing mediators of RTK signaling. Given the complexity of cellular responses modulated by RSTK receptors, however, considerably more information is required before we can understand how TGF-β and related factors exert their multiple activities.

Receptor Protein Tyrosine Phosphatases

Still less is known about the third class of enzyme-linked receptors, the receptor protein tyrosine kinases (RPTPs). Seven distinct RPTPs have been isolated from human, mouse, and *Drosophila* cDNA libraries,[215,216] and these receptors appear to be widely expressed, except for the hematopoietic receptor CD45. Unlike RTKs such as the EGF and PDGF receptors, purified RPTPs demonstrate considerable activity against artificial substrates in the absence of ligand, suggesting that these enzymes may be constitutively active in vivo.[217,218] This high intrinsic activity has con-

founded the search for potential ligands and has lead to the speculation that ligand binding may inhibit rather than activate the enzyme or may modulate the enzyme's function by redistributing it within the membrane.[219] Originally thought to function as "off" switches for RTK activity, there is emerging evidence that the role of RPTPs in cellular homeostasis and responses is far more complex. Because the function of this newly characterized group of receptors in pulmonary development, physiology, and response to injury is unknown, the present discussion of this class of enzyme-coupled receptor must be limited to a description of the enzyme classes and to our general understanding of their function.

RECEPTOR PROTEIN TYROSINE PHOSPHATASE STRUCTURE

Like the tyrosine kinase and serine/threonine kinase receptors, RPTPs are single transmembrane molecules that have been classified into at least five types based on the structures of their extracellular domains. The intracellular region of each RPTP contains a protein tyrosine phosphatase domain located 78 to 95 amino acid residues from the transmembrane segment and exhibiting 30 to 40 percent sequence homology with the cytoplasmic protein tyrosine phosphatase, PTP1B.[220] Like the smaller cytoplasmic protein tyrosine phosphatases (PTPs), enzymatic activity of RPTPs is dependent upon a conserved residue in their catalytic domains. Of interest, the catalytic domain exists in tandem duplication in most RPTPs. The reasons for and effects of this duplication have not been determined. In type I and type II RPTPs, only the first catalytic site (i.e., closest to the plasma membrane) appears to have intrinsic enzymatic activity.[221] The second catalytic site may require additional regulatory molecules to display its activity, or it may be involved in substrate regulation.[220] In contrast, the second catalytic domain of type IV RPTPs has intrinsic enzymatic activity which is reduced in comparison to the first domain but which is increased by the presence of the first catalytic domain.[222] Finally, class III RPTPs lack the second catalytic site completely.

Since the intracellular portion is similar between these receptors, it is the structure of the extracellular domain that determines the classification of the RPTPs (Fig. 2-6). The type I family is represented by CD45 (also known as *leukocyte common antigen, LCA*), a 180- to 220-kDa glycoprotein of multiple isoforms arising from differential splicing of sequences at the amino terminus.[223] CD45 proteins are densely expressed on all hematopoietic cells except erythrocytes and erythroblasts. The extracellular region of CD45 shows no structural similarity to other known proteins, but the portion does contain cysteine-rich segments that may be involved in ligand binding. It has been demonstrated that CD45 participates in lymphocyte signaling by inducing tyrosine$_{505}$ dephosphorylation in and the consequent activation of a src-family cytoplasmic tyrosine kinase, p56^{lck} [224,225] which in turn phosphorylates tyrosines on the ζ-chain of the TCR-CD3 complex.[226]

Type II RPTPs include the leukocyte common antigen-related receptor (LAR), the human receptors HPTPδ,

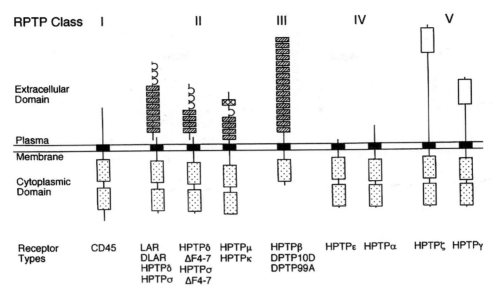

FIGURE 2-6 Classes of receptor protein tyrosine phosphatases (RPTPs). Representative receptors for each RPTP class are listed below the schematized receptors (specific ligands are unknown). Stippled boxes symbolize the *protein tyrosine phosphatase* *domain(s)*; semicircles symbolize *immunoglobulin-like domains*; striped boxes symbolize *fibronectin type III homology domains*; crossed box symbolizes a *meprin homology domain*; open boxes symbolize regions of sequence homolgy to *carbonic anhydrase.*

HPTPσ, HPTPμ, and HPTPκ, and two *Drosophila* RPTPs (DLAR and DPTP).[227] Recent in situ hybridization studies have demonstrated LAR to be uniformly expressed in all epithelial cells of day-14 and day-18 fetal rat lungs.[228] Like CD45, type II receptors have a double cytoplasmic kinase domain, but their extracellular portions differ in the incorporation of several immunoglobulin-like (IG) and fibronectin (FN) type III homology domains. The LAR and HPTPδ receptors have three amino-terminal IG-like domains and eight downstream FN III homology domains.[229] DLAR is similar, with three IG followed by nine FN III domains. In contrast, the DPTP receptor contains only two IG-like motifs and two FN III homology sequences,[215] and the HPTPμ and HPTPκ receptors contain one IG-like domain and four FN III repeats,[230] along with an MAM (meprin) homology domain amino-terminal to the IG-like motif. Type II RPTPs appear to be expressed on the cell surface as two noncovalently associated subunits derived from intracellular processing of a proprotein.[229] This class of receptors is complicated further by the recent finding that HPTPσ and HPTPδ each exist in a "long" form and a "short" form lacking fibronectin repeats 4 to 7, and that both long and short isoforms exist that lack short sequences within the second IG-domain, IG2-IG3 spanning region, and the fifth fibronectin repeat.[229]

No endogenous ligands for type II RPTPs have been identified to date. Indeed, given the presence of FN III domains in neural cell adhesion molecules (NCAMs) and the MAM motif in other transmembrane adhesion proteins (e.g., meprin and A5), it has been proposed that type II RPTPs could have adhesive functions in the cell. In this regard, HPTPμ has recently been identified as its own ligand, with the interaction of HPTPμ proteins facilitating homophilic cell-cell adhesion in insect Sf9 cells following baclovirus-mediated expression.[231,232] Moreover, naturally occurring HPTPμ has been shown to mediate cell-cell aggregation in a

lung cell line.[231] The homophilic adhesion mediated by type II RPTPs appears to be independent of the receptors' tyrosine phosphatase activities, however.[231] Whether such RPTPs merely have adhesive function, or whether their interaction induces a signal response coupled through their cytoplasmic phosphatase domains (e.g., cell-contact inhibition of cell growth) remains to be elucidated.

The type III RPTPs (HPTPβ, DPTP10D, and DPTP99A) may also play a role in cell-cell interaction, in that their extracellular sequences contain multiple FN III repeats (e.g., 16 FN III domains in HPTPβ). Unlike type II RPRPs, however, HPTPβ contains no IG-like motifs, and its intracellular portion is shortened by the absence of the second kinase region.[215,233]

Type IV RPTPs consist of two proteins termed HPTPα and HPTPε.[233] These proteins have very short extracellular regions (e.g., 123 amino acids for HPTPα) with no sequence homology to other proteins and no obvious ligand binding structure. Coupled with the absence of known ligands for these "receptors," it may be more appropriate to consider HPTPα and HPTPε as membrane-fixed enzymes rather than as receptor molecules. By analogy to the CD3 complex of T cells, type IV RPTPs may interact with other receptor proteins on the cell membrane and transmit a signal through the protein-RPTP complex, independent of any type IV-specific ligand. Independent evidence suggests that HPTPα may activate the cytoplasmic tyrosine kinase c-Src in rat embryonic fibroblasts[234] and in embryonal carcinoma cells[235] through dephosphorylation of the inhibitory phosphotyrosine 527 on c-Src. In turn, c-Src may mediate the constitutive phosphorylation of Tyr$_{789}$ on HPTPα, which then forms part of a consensus binding site for the SH3-SH2-SH3 adaptor protein Grb2.[236] RPTPα has been coimmunoprecipitated with Grb2 from NIH 3T3 cells but, of interest, such immunoprecipitates lacked the Ras guanine nucleotide releasing factor Sos, which is typically complexed with Grb2.[236] The absence of Sos implies that Grb2 associated with HPTPα cannot activate Ras and that HPTPα may exert inhibitory effects on Ras-mediated signaling.

The fifth group of RPTPs is comprised of four related proteins, the neural-specific human HPTPζ, mouse RPTPβ, rat PTP18, and HPTPγ, which is expressed in kidney, brain, and lung.[237] The unique property of type V RPTPs is that their extracellular domains contain a region bearing strong similarity to the enzyme carbonic anhydrase.[238] Two of the three essential histidyl residues in carbonic anhydrase required for its enzymatic activity are missing in these receptor regions, however, giving rise to the supposition that this domain may have ligand-recognition rather than enzymatic function in the RPTPs.[238]

Conclusions

Over the past decade, the cellular repertoire of receptors has grown increasingly complex. As signal transduction mechanisms for G-protein-coupled receptors were being elucidated, an entire new class or receptor was being characterized—that which contained its effector enzyme within the receptor molecule. Several of these receptors were found to transduce the signals of an emerging class of cytokines known colloquially as growth factors. As a group, the enzyme-linked receptors may be thought of as mediating longer-term responses to stimuli, involving cell proliferation or differentiation rather than the more immediate responses transduced by the G-protein-coupled receptors. It is clear, however, that the true cellular picture is far more complicated than this simple aphorism. The receptor tyrosine kinases are capable of mediating more immediate responses via such substrates as phosphatidylinositol 3′-kinase and phospholipase C. Conversely, several of the G-protein-coupled receptors and their ligands have been found to have potent mitogenic effects in a myriad of tissues, including those from the lung. Through shared substrates and pathways, enzyme-linked and G-protein-coupled receptors can influence each other's activities. Moreover, within the class of enzyme-linked receptors, there is considerable potential interaction between the tyrosine and serine/threonine kinases as well as the protein tyrosine phosphatases. Substantially more work needs to be done for us to understand how these diverse receptors work in concert to orchestrate the symphony of cellular responses.

References

RECEPTOR TYROSINE KINASES

1. van der Geer P, Hunter T, Lindberg RA: Receptor protein-tyrosine kinases and their signal transduction pathways. *Annu Rev Biol* 1994; 10:251–337.
2. White MF: Structure and function of tyrosine kinase receptors. *J Bioenerg Biomembr* 1991; 23:63–82.
3. Ullrich A, Schlessinger J: Signal transduction by receptors with tyrosine kinase activity. *Cell* 1990; 61:203–212.
4. Lemmon MA, Schlessinger J: Regulation of signal transduction and signal diversity by receptor oligomerization. *Trends Biol Sci* 1994; 19:459–463.
5. Yarden Y, Ullrich A: Molecular analysis of signal transduction by growth factors. *Biochemistry* 1988; 27:3113–3119.
6. Fantl WJ, Johnson DE, Williams LT: Signalling by receptor tyrosine kinases. *Annu Rev Biochem* 1993; 62:453–481.
7. Schultz S, Chinkers M, Garbers DL: The guanylate cyclase/receptor family of proteins. *FASEB J* 1989; 3:2026–2035.
8. Adamson ED, Meek J: The ontogeny of epidermal growth factor receptors during mouse development. *Dev Biol* 1984; 103:62–70.
9. Warburton D, Seth R, Shum L, et al.: Epigenic role of epidermal growth factor expression and signalling in embryonic mouse lung morphogenesis. *Dev Biol* 1992; 149:123–133.
10. Johnson MD, Gray ME, Carpenter G, et al.: Ontogeny of epidermal growth factor receptor/kinase and of lipocortin-1 in the ovine lung. *Pediatr Res* 1989; 25:535–541.
11. Johnson MD, Gray ME, Carpenter G, et al.: Ontogeny of epidermal growth factor receptor and lipocortin-1 in fetal and neonatal human lungs. *Hum Pathol* 1990; 21:182–191.
12. Carpenter G: Receptors for epidermal growth factor and other polypeptide mitogens. *Annu Rev Biochem* 1987; 56:881–914.
13. Schlessinger J: The epidermal growth factor as a multifunctional allosteric protein. *Biochemistry* 1988; 27:3119–3123.
14. Carpenter G, Cohen S: Epidermal growth factor. *J Biol Chem* 1990; 265:7709–7712.
15. Wen D, Peles E, Cupples R, et al.: Neu differentiation factor: A transmembrane glycoprotein containing an EGF domain and an immunoglobulin homology unit. *Cell* 1992; 69:559–572.
16. Huang SS, Huang JS: Purification and characterization of the neu/erb B2 ligand-growth factor from bovine kidney. *J Biol Chem* 1992; 267:11508–11512.
17. Lax I, Burgess WH, Bellot F, et al.: Localization of a major receptor-binding domain for epidermal growth factor by affinity labeling. *Mol Cell Biol* 1988; 8:1831–1834.
18. Soderquist AM, Carpenter G: Glycosylation of the epidermal growth factor receptor in A-431 cells. *J Biol Chem* 1984; 259:12586–12594.
19. Wada T, Qian X, Greene MI: Intermolecular association of the p185[neu] protein and EGF receptor modulates EGF receptor function. *Cell* 1990; 61:1339–1347.
20. Walton GM, Chen WS, Rosenfeld MG, Gill GN: Analysis of deletions of the carboxy terminus of the epidermal growth factor receptor reveals self-phosphorylation at tyrosine 992 and enhanced in vivo tyrosine phosphorylation of cell substrates. *J Biol Chem* 1990; 265:1750–1754.
21. Hsu C-Y, Hurwitz DR, Mervic M, Zilberstein A: Autophosphorylation of the intracellular domain of the epidermal growth factor receptor results on different effects on its tyrosine kinase activity with various peptide substrates. *J Biol Chem* 1991; 266:603–608.
22. King AC, Cuatrecasas P: Resolution of high and low affinity epidermal growth factor receptors. *J Biol Chem* 1982; 257:3053–3060.
23. Defize LHK, Boonstra J, Meisenhelder J, et al.: Signal transduction by epidermal growth factor occurs through the subclass of high affinity receptors. *J Cell Biol* 1989; 109:2495–2507.
24. Strandjord TP, Clark JG, Madtes DK: Expression of TGF-α, EGF, and EGF receptor in fetal rat lung. *Am J Physiol* 1994; 267 (*Lung Cell Mol Physiol* 11):L384–L389.
25. Catterton WZ, Escobedo MB, Sexson WR, et al.: Effect of epidermal growth factor on lung maturation in fetal rabbits. *Pediatr Res* 1979; 13:104–108.
26. Sundell HW, Gray ME, Serenius FS, et al.: Effects of epidermal growth factor on lung maturation in fetal lambs. *Am J Pathol* 1980; 100:707–726.

27. Plopper CG, St George JA, Read LC, et al.: Acceleration of alveolar type II cell differentiation in fetal rhesus monkey lung by administration of EGF. *Am J Physiol* 1992; 262 (*Lung Cell Mol Physiol* 6): L313–L321.

28. Seth R, Shum L, Wu F, et al.: Role of epidermal growth factor expression in early mouse embryo lung branching morphogenesis in culture: Antisense oligonucleotide inhibitory strategy. *Dev Biol* 1993; 158:555–559.

29. Stahlman MT, Orth DN, Gray ME: Immunocytochemical localization of epidermal growth factor in the developing human respiratory system and in acute and chronic lung disease in the neonate. *Lab Invest* 1989; 60:539–547.

30. Oliver AM: Epidermal growth factor receptor expression in human foetal tissues is age-dependent. *Br J Cancer* 1988; 58:461–463.

31. Madtes DK, Busby HK, Strandjord TP, Clark JG: Expression of transforming growth factor-α and epidermal growth factor receptor is increased following bleomycin-induced lung injury in rats. *Am J Respir Cell Mol Biol* 1994; 11:540–551.

32. Kheradmand F, Folkesson HG, Nitenberg G, Matthay MA: The role of transforming growth factor-α (TGF-α) in alveolar epithelial cell repair: clinical and experimental evidence. *Am J Respir Crit Care Med* 1994; 149:A61.

33. Liu C, Woo A, Tsao M-S: Expression of transforming growth factor-alpha in primary human colon and lung carcinomas. *Br J Cancer* 1990; 62:425–429.

34. Tateishi M, Ishida T, Mitsudomi T, et al.: Immunohistochemical evidence of autocrine growth factors in adenocarcinoma of the human lung. *Cancer Res* 1990; 50:7077–7080.

35. Hwang DL, Tay Y-C, Lin SS, Lev-Ran A: Expression of epidermal growth factor receptors in human lung tumors. *Cancer* 1986; 58:2260–2263.

36. Veale D, Kerr N, Gibson GJ, Harris AL: Characterization of epidermal growth factor receptor in primary human non-smal cell lung cancer. *Cancer Res* 1989; 49:1313–1317.

37. Retsch-Bogart GZ, Stiles AD, Moats-Staats BM, et al.: Canine trachial epithelial cells express the type 1 insulin-like growth factor receptor and proliferate in response to insulin-like growth factor 1. *Am J Respir Cell Mol Biol* 1990; 3:227–234.

38. Noveral JP, Bhala A, Hintz RL, Grunstein MM, Cohen P. Insulin-like growth factor axis in airway smooth muscle cells. *Am J Physiol* 1994; 267 (*Lung Cell Mol Physiol* 11):L761–L765.

39. Kahn CR, White MF, Shoelson SE, Backer JM, Araki E, Cheatham B, Csermely P, Folli F, Goldstein BJ, Huertas P, Rothenberg PL, Saad MJA, Siddle K, Sun X-J, Wilden PA, Yamada K, Kahn SA: The insulin receptor and its substrate: molecular determinants of early events in insulin action. *Rec Progress Hormone Res* 1993; 48:291–339.

40. Lee J, Pilch PF: The insulin receptor: structure, function, and signaling. *Am J Physiol* 1994; 266 (*Cell Physiol* 35): C319–C334.

41. Shoelson SE, Boni-Schnetzler M, Pilch PF, Kahn CR: Autophosphorylation within insulin receptor β-subunits can occur as an intramolecular process. *Biochemistry* 1991; 30:7740–7746.

42. Frattali AL, Treadway JL, Pessin JE: Transmembrane signaling by the human insulin receptor kinase. Relationship between intramolecular β subunit trans- and cis-autophosphorylation and substrate kinase activation. *J Biol Chem* 1992; 267:19521–19528.

43. Sun XJ, Rotherberg P, Kahn CR, Backer JM, Araki E, Wilden PA, Cahill DA, Goldstein BJ, White MF: Structure of the insulin receptor substrate IRS-1 defines a unique signal transduction protein. *Nature* (London) 1991; 352:73–77.

44. Myers MG Jr, Sun XJ, Cheatham B, Jachna BR, Glasheen EM, Backer JM, White MF: IRS-1 is a common element in insulin and IGF-1 signaling to the phosphatidylinositol 3'-kinase. *Endocrinology* 1993; 132:1421–1430.

45. Goldring MB, Goldring SR: Cytokines and cell growth control. *Crit Rev Eukar Gene Express* 1991; 1:301–326.

46. Wallen LD, Han VKM: Spatial and temporal distribution of insulin-like growth factors I and II during development of rat lung. *Am J Physiol* 1994; 267 (*Lung Cell Mol Physiol* 11):L531–L542.

47. Moxham CD, Duronio V, Jacobs S. Insulin-like growth factor I receptor β subunit heterogeneity: Evidence for hybrid tetramers composed of insulin-like growth factor I and insulin receptor heterodimers. *J Biol Chem* 1989; 264:13238–13244.

48. Yang CM, Chou S-P: Primary culture of canine tracheal smooth muscle cells in serum-free medium: effects of insulin-like growth factor 1 and insulin. *J Receptor Res* 1993; 13:943–960.

49. Lund PK, Moats-Staats BM, Hynes MA, Simmons JG, Jansen M, D'Ercole AJ, Van Wyk JJ: Somatomedin-C/insulin-like growth factor-I and insulin-like growth factor-II mRNAs in rat fetal and adult tissues. *J Biol Chem* 1986; 261:14539–14544.

50. Nakanishi Y, Mulshine JL, Kasprzyk PG, Natale RB, Maneckjee R, Avis I, Treston AM, Gazdar AF, Minna JD, Cuttitta F: Insulin-like growth factor-I can mediate autocrine proliferation of human small cell lung cancer cell lines in vitro. *J Clin Invest* 1988; 82:354–359.

51. Yarden Y, Escobedo JA, Kuang W-J, Yang-Feng TL, Daniel TO, Tremble TM, Chen EY, Ando ME, Harkins RN, Francke U, Fried VA, Ullrich A, Williams LT: Structure of the receptor for platelet-derived growth factor helps define a family of closely related growth factor receptors. *Nature* (*London*) 1986; 323:226–252.

52. Nicola NA: Hematopoietic cell growth factors and their receptors. *Annu Rev Biochem* 1989; 58:45–77.

53. Hart CE, Seifert RA, Ross R, Bowen-Pope DF: Synthesis, phosphorylation, and degradation of multiple forms of the platelet-derived growth factor receptor studied using a monoclonal antibody. *J Biol Chem* 1987; 262:10780–10785.

54. Zerwez H-G, Risau W: Polarized secretion of platelet-derived growth factor-like chemotactic factor by endothelial cells in vitro. *J Cell Biol* 1987; 105:2037–2041.

55. Sjölund M, Hedin U, Sejerson T, Heldin C-H, Thyberg J: Arterial smooth muscle cells express platelet-derived growth factor (PDGF) A chain mRNA, secrete a PDGF-like mitogen, and bind exogenous PDGF in a phenotype- and growth state-dependent manner. *J Cell Biol* 1988; 106:403–413.

56. Raines EW, Bowen-Pope DF, Ross R: Platelet derived growth factor. In *Peptide Growth Factors and Their Receptors*. Part I. MB Sporn and AB Roberts, editors. New York: Springer-Verlag, 1991; pp 173–262.

57. Han RN, Mawdsley C, Souza P, Tanswell AK, Post M: Platelet-derived growth factors and growth-related genes in rat lung. III. Immunolocalization during fetal development. *Pediatr Res* 1992; 31:323–329.

58. Caniggia I, Liu J, Han R, Buch S, Funa K, Tanswell K, Post M: Fetal lung epithelial cells express receptors for platelet-derived growth factor. *Am J Respir Cell Mol Biol* 1993; 9:54–63.

59. Jassal D, Han RN, Caniggia I, Post M, Tanswell AK: Growth of distal fetal rat lung epithelial cells in a defined serum free medium. *In Vitro Cell Dev Biol* 1991; 27:625–632.

60. Buch S, Jassal D, Cannigia I, Edelson J, Han R, Liu J, Tanswell K, Post M: Ontogeny and regulation of platelet-derived growth factor gene expression in distal fetal rat lung epithelial cells. *Am J Respir Cell Mol Biol* 1994; 11:251–261.

61. Souza P, Sedlackova L, Kuliszewski M, Wang J, Liu J, Tseu I, Tanswell AK, Post M: PDGF-A antisense oligonucleotide inhibits embryonic lung growth and branching morphogenesis. *Am Rev Respir Dis* 1994; 149:A254.

62. Fabisiak JP, Kelley J: Platelet-derived growth factor. In *Cytokines of the Lung*, J Kelley (ed). New York, NY: Marcel Dekker, Inc., 1993; pp 3–39.

63. Shaw RJ, Benedict SH, Clark RA, King TE: Pathogenesis of pulmonary fibrosis in interstitial lung disease. Alveolar macrophage PDGF(B) gene activation and up-regulation by interferon gamma. *Am Rev Respir Dis* 1991; 143:167–173.

64. Martinet Y, Rom WN, Grotendorst GR, Martin GR, Crystal RG: Exaggerated spontaneous release of platelet-derived growth factor by alveolar macrophages from patients with idiopathic pulmonary fibrosis. *N Engl J Med* 1987; 317:202–209.

65. Witkop CJ, Townsend D, Bittermann PB, Harmon K: The role of ceroid in lung and gastrointestinal disease in Hermansky-Pudlak syndrome. *Adv Exp Med Biol* 1989; 266:283–296.

66. Antoniades HN, Bravo MA, Avila RE, Galanopoulos T, Neville-Golden J, Maxwell M, Selman M: Platelet-derived growth factor in idiopathic pulmonary fibrosis. *J Clin Invest* 1990; 86:1055–1064.

67. Connolly DT: Vascular permeability factor: a unique regulator of blood vessel formation. *J Cell Biochem* 1991; 47:219–223.

68. Dionne CA, Crumley G, Bellot F, Kaplow JM, Searfoss G, Ruta M, Burgess WH, Jaye M, Schlessinger J: Cloning and expression of two distinct high-affinity receptors cross-reacting with acidic and basic fibroblast growth factors. *Embo J* 1990; 9:2685–2692.

69. Champion-Arnaud P, Ronsin C, Gilbert E, Gesnel MC, Houssaint E, Breathnach R: Multiple mRNAs code for proteins related to the BEK fibroblast growth factor receptor. *Oncogene* 1991; 6:979–987.

70. Miki T, Fleming TP, Bottaro DP, Rubin JS, Ron D, Aaronson SA: Expression of cDNA cloning of the KGF receptor by creation of a transforming autocrine loop. *Science (Wash DC)* 1991; 251:72–75.

71. Bellot F, Crumley G, Kaplow JM, Schlessinger J, Jaye M, Dionne CA: Ligand-induced transphosphorylation between different FGF receptors. *Embo J* 1991; 10:2849–2854.

72. Ueno H, Gunn M, Dell K, Tseng A Jr, Williams LT: A truncated form of fibroblast growth factor receptor 1 inhibits signal transduction by multiple types of fibroblast growth factor receptor. *J Biol Chem* 1992; 267:1470–1476.

73. Jones R, Wang CC, Powell PP: Developmental expression of mRNAs encoding acidic and basic fibroblast growth factors & fibroblast growth factor receptors 1, 2, and 3 in rat lung. *Am J Respir Dis* 1993; 147:A942.

74. Herbert JM, Basilico C, Goldfarb M, Haub O, Martin GR: Isolation of cDNAs encoding four mouse FGF family members and characterization of their expression patterns during embryogenesis. *Dev Biol* 1990; 138:454–463.

75. Gonzales A-M, Buscaglia M, Ong M, Baird A: Distribution of basic fibroblast growth factor in the 18-day rat fetus: Localization in the basement membranes of diverse tissues. *J Cell Biol* 1990; 110:753–765.

76. Mason RJ, Leslie CC, McCormick-Shannon K, Deterding RR, Nakamura T, Rubin JS, Shannon JM: Hepatocyte growth factor is a growth factor for rat alveolar type II cells. *Am J Respir Cell Mol Biol* 1994; 11:561–567.

77. Chinkers M, Garbers DL, Chang M-S, Lowe DG, Chin H, Goeddel DV, Schultz S: A membrane form of guanylate cyclase is an atrial natriuretic peptide receptor. *Nature (London)* 1989; 338:78–83.

78. Debant A, Clauser E, Panzio G, Filloux C, Auzan C, Contreres J, Rossi B: Replacement of insulin receptor tyrosine residues 1162 and 1163 does not alter the mitogenic effect of the hormone. *Proc Natl Acad Sci USA* 1988; 85:8032–8036.

79. Kazlauskas A, Cooper JA: Phosphorylation of the PDGF β subunit creates a tight binding site for phosphatidylinositol 3 kinase. *Embo J* 1990; 9:3279–3286.

80. Hall A: *ras* and GAP—Who's controlling whom? *Cell* 1990; 61:921–923.

81. Honegger A, Dull TJ, Szapary D, Komoriya A, Kris R, Ullrich A, Schlessinger J: Kinetic parameters of the protein tyrosine kinase activity of EGF-receptor mutants with individually altered autophosphroylation sites. *Embo J* 1988; 7:3053–3060.

82. Khazaie K, Dull TJ, Graf T, Schlessinger J, Ullrich A, Beug H, Vennström B: Truncation of the human EGF receptor leads to differential transforming potentials in primary avian fibroblasts and erythroblasts. *Embo J* 1988; 7:3061–3071.

83. Davis RJ: Independent mechanisms account for the regulation by protein kinase C of the epidermal growth factor receptor affinity and tyrosine-protein kinase activity. *J Biol Chem* 1988; 263:9462–9469.

84. Downward J, Waterfield MD, Parker PJ: Autophosphorylation and protein kinase C phosphorylation of the epidermal growth factor receptor. Effect on tyrosine kinase activity and ligand binding affinity. *J Biol Chem* 1985; 260:14538–14546.

85. Stadtmauer L, Rosen OM: Increasing the cAMP content of IM-9 cells alters the phosphorylation state and protein kinase activity of the insulin receptor. *J Biol Chem* 1986; 261:3402–3407.

86. Jacobs S, Cuatrecasas P: Phosphorylation of receptors for insulin and insulin-like growth factor I. Effects of hormones and phorbol esters. *J Biol Chem* 1986; 261:934–939.

87. Lewis RE, Cao L, Perregaux D, Czech MP: Threonine 1336 of the human insulin receptor is a major target for phosphorylation by protein kinase C. *Biochemistry* 1990; 29:1807–1813.

88. Glenney JR Jr, Chen WS, Lazar CS, Walton GM, Zokas MR, Rosenfeld MG, Gill GN: Ligand-induced endocytosis of the EGF receptor is blocked by mutational inactivation and by microinjection of anti-phosphotyrosine antibodies. *Cell* 1988; 52:675–684.

89. Honegger AM, Schmidt A, Ullrich A, Schlessinger J: Separate endocytotic pathways of kinase-defective and -active EGF receptor mutants expressed in the same cells. *J Cell Biol* 1990; 110:1541–1548.

90. Goldfine I:The insulin receptor: molecular biology and transmembrane signalling. *Endocr Rev* 1987; 8:235–255.

91. Russell DS, Gherzi R, Johnson EL, Chou C-K, Rosen OM: The protein-tyrosine kinase activity of the insulin receptor is necessary for insulin-mediated receptor down-regulation. *J Biol Chem* 1987; 262:11833–11840.

92. Carpenter G: Receptor tyrosine kinase substrates: *src* homology domains and signal transduction. *FASEB J* 1992; 6:3283–3289.

93. Schlessinger J: SH2/SH3 signaling proteins. *Curr Opin Genet Dev* 1994; 4:25–30.

94. Cohen GB, Ren R, Baltimore D: Modular binding domains in signal transduction proteins. *Cell* 1995; 80:237–248.

95. Koch CA, Anderson D, Moran MF, Ellis C, Pawson T: SH2 and SH3 domains: elements that control interactions of cytoplasmic signaling proteins. *Science (Wash DC)* 1991; 252:668–674.

96. Songyang Z, Shoelson SE, Chaudhuri M, Gish G, Pawson T, Haser WG, King F, Roberrts T, Ratnofsky S, Lechleider RJ, Neel BG, Birge RB, Fajardo JE, Chou MM, Hanafusa H, Schaffhausen B, Cantley LC: SH2 domains recognize specific phosphopeptide sequences. *Cell* 1993; 72:767–778.

97. Kazlauskas A: Receptor tyrosine kinases and their targets. *Curr Opin Genet Dev* 1994; 4:5–14.

98. Taylor SJ, Chase HZ, Rhee SG, Exton JH: Activation of the β1 isoenzyme of phospholipase C by α subunits of the Gq class of G proteins. *Nature (London)* 1991; 350:516–518.

99. Margolis B, Rhee SG, Felder S, Mervic M, Lyall R, Levitzki A, Ullrich A, Zilberstein A, Schlessinger J: EGF induces tyrosine phosphorylation of phospholipase C-II: a potential mechanism of EGF receptor signaling. *Cell* 1989; 57:1101–1107.

100. Meisenhelder J, Suh P-G, Rhee SG, Hunter T: Phospholipase

C-γ is a substrate for the PDGF and EGF receptor protein-tyrosine kinases in vivo and in vitro. *Cell* 1989; 57:1109–1122.

101. Wahl MI, Nishibe S, Suh P-G, Rhee SG, Carpenter G: Epidermal growth factor stimulates tyrosine phosphorylation of phospholipase C-II independently of receptor internatlization and extracellular calcium. *Proc Natl Acad Sci USA* 1989; 86:1568–1572.

102. Vega QC, Cochet C, Filhol O, Chang C-P, Rhee SG, Gill GN: A site of tyrosine phosphorylation in the C terminus of the epidermal growth factor receptor is required to activate phospholipase C. *Moll Cell Biol* 1992; 12:128–135.

103. Kumjian DA, Wahl MI, Rhee SG, Daniel TO: Platelet-derived growth factor (PDGF) binding promotes physical association of PDGF receptor with phospholipase C. *Proc Natl Acad Sci USA* 1989; 86:8232–8236.

104. Wahl MI, Olashaw NE, Nishibe S, Rhee SG, Pledger WJ, Carpenter G: Platelet-derived growth factor induces rapid and sustained tyrosine phosphorylation of phospholipase C-γ in quiescent BALB/c 3T3 cells. *Mol Cell Biol* 1989; 9:2934–2943.

105. Valius M, Kazlauskas A: Phospholipase C-γ1 and phosphatidylinositol 3 kinase are the downstream mediators of the PDGF receptor's mitogenic signal. *Cell* 1993; 73:321–324.

106. Guo D, Jia Q, Song H-Y, Warren RS, Donner DB: Vascular endothelial cel growth factor promotes tyrosine phosphorylation of mediators of signal transduction that contain SH2 domains. Association with endothelial cell proliferation. *J Biol Chem* 1995; 270:6729–6733.

107. Morrison DK, Kaplan DR, Rapp U, Roberts TM: Signal transduction from membrane to cytoplasm: growth factors and membrane-bound oncogene products increase Raf-1 phosphorylation and associated protein kinase activity. *Proc Natl Acad Sci USA* 1988; 85:8855–8859.

108. Burgess WH, Dionne CA, Kaplow J, Mudd R, Friesel R, Zilberstein A, Schlessinger J, Jayne M: Characterization and cDNA cloning of phospholipase C-γ, a major substrate for heparin-binding growth factor 1 (acidic fibroblast growth factor)-activated tyrosine kinase. *Mol Cell Biol* 1990; 10:4770–4777.

109. Bardelli A, Maina F, Gout I, Fry MJ, Waterfield MD, Comoglio PM, Ponzetto C: Autophosphorylation promotes complex formation of recombinant hepatocyte growth factor receptor with cytoplasmic effectors containing SH2 domains. *Oncogene* 1992; 7:1973–1978.

110. Nishibe S, Wahl MI, Wedegaertner PB, Kim JJ, Rhee SG, Carpenter G: Selectivity of phospholipase C phosphorylation by the epidermal growth factor receptor, the insulin receptor, and their cytoplasmic domains. *Proc Natl Acad Sci USA* 1990; 87:424–428.

111. Downing JR, Margolis BL, Zilberstein A, Ashmun RA, Ullrich A, Sherr CJ, Schlessinger J: Phospholipase C-γ, a substrate for PDGF receptor kinase, is not phosphorylated on tyrosine during the mitogenic response to CSF-1. *EMBO J* 1989; 8:3345–3350.

112. Kolch W, Heidecker G, Kochs G, Hummel R, Vahidi H, Mischak H, Finkenzeller G, Marmé D, Rapp U: Protein kinase Cα activates Raf-1 by direct phosphorylation. *Nature (London)* 1993; 364:249–252.

113. Parker PJ, Waterfield MD: Phosphatidylinositol 3-kinase: a novel effector. *Cell Growth Diff* 1992; 3:747–752.

114. Hu P, Mondino A, Skolnik EY, Schlessinger J: Cloning of a novel, ubiquitously espressed human phosphatidylinositol 3-kinase and identificaiton of its binding site on p85. *Mol Cell Biol* 1993; 13:7677–7688.

115. Carter AN, Downes CP: Phosphatidylinositol 3-kinase is activated by nerve growth factor and epidermal growth factor in PC12 cells [published erratum appears in *J Biol Chem* 1992; 267:23434] *J Biol Chem* 1992; 267:14563–14567.

116. Joly M, Kazlauskas A, Fay F, Corvera S: Disruption of PDGF

117. receptor trafficking by mutation of its PI-3 kinase binding sites. *Science* (Wash DC) 1994; 263:684–687.

117. Shearman MS, Herbst R, Schlessinger J, Ullrich A: Phosphatidylinositol 3′-kinase associates with p145^{c-kit} as part of a cell type characteristic multimeric signalling complex. *EMBO J* 1993; 12:3817–3826.

118. Liu X, Marengere LE, Koch CA, Pawson T: The v-Src SH3 domain binds to phosphatidylinositol 3′-kinase. *Mol Cell Biol* 1993; 13:5225–5232.

119. Pleiman CM, Clark MR, Timson-Gauen LK, Winitz S, Coggeshall KM, Johnson GL, Shaw AS, Cambier JC: Mapping of sites on the Src family protein tyrosine kinases, p55^{blkT}, p59^{fyn}, p56^{lyn}, which interact with the effector molecules, phospholipase C-γ2, microtubule-associated protein kinase, GTPase-activiting protein, and phosphatidylinositol 3-kinase. *Mol Cell Biol* 1993; 13:5877–5887.

120. Backer JM, Myers MG Jr, Sun X-J, Chin DJ, Shoelson SE, Miralpeix M, White MF: Association of IRS-1 with insulin receptor and the phosphatidylinositol 3′-kinase. Formation of binary and ternary signaling complexes in intact cells. *J Biol Chem* 1993; 268:8204–8212.

121. Shoelson SE, Chatterjee S, Chaudhuri M, White MF: YMXM motifs of IRS-1 define substrate specificity of the insulin receptor kinase. *Proc Natl Acad Sci USA* 1992; 89:2027–2031.

122. Myers MG Jr, Backer JM, Sun XJ, Shoelson S, Hu P, Schlessinger J, Yoakim M, Schaffhausen B, White MF: IRS-1 activates phosphatidylinositol 3′-kinase by associating with *src* homology 2 domains of p85. *Proc Natl Acad Sci USA* 1992; 89:10350–10354.

123. Kelly KL, Ruderman NB: Insulin-stimulated phosphatidylinositol 3-kinase. Association with a 185-kDa tyrosine-phosphorylated protein (IRS-1) and localization in a low density membrane vesicle. *J Biol Chem* 1993; 268:4391–4398.

124. Ruderman NB, Kapeller R, White MF, Cantley LC: Activation of phosphatidylinositol 3-kinase by insulin. *Proc Natl Acad Sci USA* 1990; 87:1411–1415.

125. Auger KR, Serunian LA, Soltoff SP, Libby P, Cantley LC: PDGF-dependent tyrosine phosphorylation simulates production of novel polyphosphoinositides in intact cells. *Cell* 1989; 57:167–175.

126. Nakanishi H, Brewer KA, Exton JH: Activation of the ζ isoenzyme of protein kinase C by phosphatidylinositol 3,4,5-triphosphate. *J Biol Chem* 1993; 268:13–16.

127. Berra E, Diaz-Meco MT, Dominguez I, Municio MM, Sanz I, Lozano J, Chapkin RS, Moscat J: Protein kinase Cζ isoform is critical for mitogenic signal transduction. *Cell* 1993; 74:555–563.

128. Chung J, Grammer TC, Lemon KP, Kazlauskas A, Blenis J: PDGF-dependent regulation of pp70-S6 kinase is coupled to receptor-dependent binding and activation of phosphoinositide 3-kinase. *Nature (London)* 1994; 370:71–75.

129. Wennstrom S, Siegbahn A, Yokote K, Avridsson A-K, Heldin CH, Mori S, Claesson-Welsh L: Membrane ruffling and chemotaxis transduced by the PDGF-β receptor require the binding site for phosphotidylinositol 3′ kinase. *Oncogene* 1994; 9:651–660.

130. Ridley AJ, Paterson HF, Johnston CL, Diekmann D, Hall A: The small GTP-binding protein rac regulates growth factor-induced membrane ruffling. *Cell* 1992; 70:401–410.

131. Vogel W, Lammers R, Huang J, Ullrich A: Activation of a phosphotyrosine phosphatase by tyrosine phosphorylation. *Science* 1993; 259:1611–1614.

132. Yi T, Ihle JN: Association of hematopoietic cell phosphatase with c-Kit after stimulation with the c-Kit ligand. *Mol Cell Biol* 1993; 13:3350–3358.

133. Kazlauskas A, Feng G-S, Pawson T, Valius M: The 64kDa protein that associates with the PDGF receptor subunit via tyrosine 1009 is the SH2 containing phosphotyrosine phosphatase

Syp/SH-PTP2/PTP1D/SH-PTP3. *Proc Natl Acad Sci USA* 1993; 90:6969–6943.

134. Feng GS, Hui CC, Pawson T: SH2-containing phosphotyrosine phosphatase as a target of protein-tyrosine kinases. *Science (Wash DC)* 1993; 259:1607–1611.

135. Lechleider RJ, Freeman RMJ, Neel BG: Tyrosyl phosphorylation and growth factor receptor association of the human *corkscrew* homologue, SH-PTP2. *J Biol Chem* 1993; 268:13434–13438.

136. Li W, Nishimura R, Kashishian A, Batzer AG, Kim WJ, Cooper JA, Schlessinger J: A new function for a phosphotyrosine phosphatase: linking GRB2-Sos to a receptor tyrosine kinase. *Mol Cell Biol* 1994; 14:509–517.

137. Buday I, Downward J: Epidermal growth factor regulates p21^ras through the formation of a complex of receptor, Grb2 adaptor protein, and Sos nucleotide exchange factor. *Cell* 1993; 73:611–620.

138. Skolnik EY, Lee C-H, Batzer A, Vicentini LM, Zhou M, Daly R, Myers MJ Jr, Backer JM, Ullrich A, White MF, Schlessinger J: The SH2/SH3 domain-containing protein GRB2 interacts with tyrosine-phosphorylated IRS-1 and Shc: implications for insulin control of Ras signalling. *Embo J* 1993; 12:1929–1936.

139. Zhang X-F, Settleman J, Kyriakis JM, Takeuchi-Suzuki E, Elledge SJ, Marshall MS, Bruder JT, Rapp UR, Avruch J: Normal and oncogenic p21^ras proteins bind to the amino-terminal regulatory domain of c-Raf-1. *Nature (London)* 1993; 364:308–313.

140. Molloy CJ, Bottaro DP, Fleming TP, Marshall MS, Gibbs JB, Aaronson SA: PDGF induction of tyrosine phosphorylation of GTPase activating protein. *Nature (London)* 1989; 342:711–714.

141. Kaplan DR, Morrison DK, Wong G, McCormick F, Williams LT: PDGF β-receptor stimulates tyrosine phosphorylation of GAP and association of GAP with a signaling complex. *Cell* 1990; 61:125–133.

142. Macdonald SG, Crews CM, Wu L, Driller J, Clark R, Erikson RL, McCormick F: Reconstruction of the Raf-1-MEK-ERK signal transduction pathway in vitro [published erratum appears in *Mol Cell Biol* 1994; 14:2223–2224]. *Mol Cell Biol* 1993; 13:6615–6620.

143. Leevers SJ, Paterson HF, Marshall CJ: Requirement for Ras in Raf activation is overcome by targeting Raf to the plasma membrane. *Nature (London)* 1994; 369:411–414.

144. Stokoe D, Macdonald SG, Cadwallader K, Symons M, Hancock JF: Activation of Raf as a result of recruitment to the plasma membrane. *Science (Wash DC)* 1994; 264:1463–1467.

145. Burgering BMT, Bos JL: Regulation of Ras-mediated signalling: more than one way to skin a cat. *Trends Biochem Sci* 1995; 20:18–22.

146. Daum G, Eisenmann-Tappe I, Fries H-W, Troppmair J, Rapp UR: The ins and outs of Raf kinases. *Trends Biochem Sci* 1994; 19:474–479.

147. Freed E, Symons M, Macdonald SG, McCormick F, Ruggieri R: Binding of 14-3-3 proteins to the protein kinase Raf and effects on its activation. *Science (Wash DC)* 1994; 265:1713–1716.

148. de Vries-Smits AMM, Burgering BMT, Leevers SJ, Marshall CJ, Bos JL: Involvement of p21^ras in activation of extracellular signal-regulated kinase 2. *Nature (London)* 1992; 357:602–604.

149. Hordijk PL, Verlaan I, van Corven EJ, Moolenaar WH: Protein tyrosine phosphorylation induced by lysophosphatidic acid in Rat-1 fibroblasts. Evidence that phosphorylation of map kinase is mediated by the G_i-p21ras pathway. *J Biol Chem* 1994; 269:645–651.

150. Wu J, Dent P, Jelinek T, Wolfman A, Weber MJ, Sturgill TW: Inhibition of the EGF-activated MAP kinase signaling pathway by adenosine 3′,5′-monophosphate. *Science (Wash DC)* 1993; 262:1065–1069.

151. Burgering BM, Pronk GJ, van Weeren PC, Chardin P, Bos JL: cAMP antagonizes p21^ras-directed activation of extracellular signal-regulated kinase 2 and phosphorylation of mSos nucleotide exchange factor. *Embo J* 1993; 12:4211–4220.

152. Hafner S, Adler HS, Mischak H, Janosch P, Heidecker G, Wolfman A, Pippig S, Lohse M, Ueffing M, Kolch W: Mechanism of inhibition of Raf-1 by protein kinase A. *Mol Cell Biol* 1994; 14:6696–6703.

153. Erikson RL: Structure, expression, and regulation of protein kinases involved in the phosphorylation and ribosomal protein S6. *J Biol Chem* 1991; 266:6007–6010.

154. Stokoe D, Campbell DG, Nakielny S, Hidaka H, Leevers SJ, Marshall CJ, Cohen P: MAPKAP kinase-2: a novel protein kinase activated by mitogen-activated protein kinase. *Embo J* 1992; 11:3985–3994.

155. Lin LL, Wartmann M, Lin AY, Knopf J, Seth A, Davis R: cPLA2 is phosphorylated and activated by MAP kinase. *Cell* 1993; 72:269–278.

156. Mori SM, Rönnstrand L, Yokote K, Engstrom A, Courtneidge SA, Claesson-Welsh L, Heldin CH: Identification of two juxtamembrane autophosphorylation sites in the PDGFβ-receptor: involvement in the interaction with Src family tyrosine kinases. *Embo J* 1993; 12:2257–2264.

157. Courtneidge SA, Kypta RM, Cooper JA, Kazlauskas A: Platelet-derived growth factor sequences important for binding of src family tyrosine kinases. *Cell Growth and Differ* 1991; 2:483–486.

158. Escobedo JA, Kaplan DR, Kavanaugh WM, Turek CW, Williams LT: A phosphatidylinositol 3-kinase binds to platelet-derived growth factor receptors through a specific receptor sequence containing phosphotyrosine. *Mol Cell Biol* 1991; 11:1125–1132.

159. Kazlauskas A, Kashishian A, Cooper JA, Valius N: GTPase activating proteins and phosphatidylinositol-3 kinase bind to distinct regions of the platelet-derived growth factor β subunit. *Mol Cell Biol* 1992; 12:2534–2455.

160. Rönnstrand L, Mori S, Arridsson A-K, Eriksson A, Wernstedt C, Hellman U, Claeson-Welsh L, Heldin C-H: Identification of two C-terminal autophosphorylation sites in the PDGFβ-receptor: involvement in the interaction with phospholipase C-γ. *Embo J* 1992; 11:3911–3919.

161. Block LH, Emmons LR, Vogt E, Sachinidis A, Vetter W, Hoppe J: Ca^{2+}-channel blockers inhibit the action of recombinant platelet-derived growth factor in vascular smooth muscle cells. *Proc Natl Acad Sci USA* 1989; 85:2388–2392.

162. Sachinidis A, Locher R, Vetter W, Tatje D, Hoppe J: Different effects of platelet-derived growth factor isoforms on rat vascular smooth muscle cells. *J Biol Chem* 1990; 265:10238–10243.

163. van Zoelen EJ, Oostwaard TM, de Laat SW: PDGF-like growth factor induces EGF-potentiated phenotypic transformation of nromal rat kidney cells in the absence of TGF β. *Biochem Biophys Res Commu* 1987; 141:1229–1235.

164. Johnson RM, Garrison JC: Epidermal growth factor and angiotensin II stimulate formation of inositol 1,4,5- and inositol 1,3,4-triphosphate in hepatocytes. Differential inhibition by pertussis toxin and phosbol 12-myrisate 13-acetate. *J Biol Chem* 1987; 262:17285–17293.

165. Luttrell LM, Hewlett EL, Romero G, Rogol AD: Pertussis toxin treatment attenuates some effects of insulinin BC3H-1 murine myocytes. *J Biol Chem* 1988; 263:6134–6141.

166. Gomez-Cambronero J, Yamazaki M, Metwally F, Molski TF, Bonak VA, Huang CK, Becker EL, Sha'afi RI: Granulocyte-macrophage colony-stimulating factor and human neutrophils: role of guanine nucleotide regulatory proteins. *Proc Natl Acad Sci USA* 1989; 86:3569–3573.

167. Srivastava SK, Varma TK, Sinha AC, Singh US: Guanosine 5′-(γ-thio) triphosphate (GTPγS) inhibits phosphorylation of insulin receptor and a novel GTP-binding protein, G_ir, from human placenta [published erratum appears in *Febs Lett* 1994; 348:220] *Febs Lett* 1994; 340:124–128.

RECEPTOR SERINE/THREONINE KINASES

168. Derynck R, Lindquist PB, Lee A, Wen D, Tamm J, Graycar JL, Rhee L, Mason AJ, Miller DA, Coffey RJ, Moses HL, Chen EY: A new type of transforming growth factor-β, TGF-β3. *Embo J* 1988; 7:3737–3743.

169. Massagué J, Attisano L, Wrana JL: The TGF-β family and its composite receptors. *Trends Cell Biol* 1994; 4:172–178.

170. Massagué J: Receptors for the TGF-β family. *Cell* 1992; 69:1067–1070.

171. Andres JL, Stanley K, Cheifetz S, Massagué J: Membrane-anchored and soluble forms of betaglycan, a polymorphic proteoglycan than binds transforming growth factor-β. *J Cell Biol* 1989; 109:3137–3145.

172. Segarini PR, Rosen DM, Seyedin SM: Binding of transforming growth factor-β to cell surface proteins varies with cell type. *Mol Endocrinol* 1989; 3:261–272.

173. Lopez-Casillas F, Wrana JL, Massagué J: Betaglucan presents ligand to the TGFβ signaling receptor. *Cell* 1993; 73:1435–1444.

174. Moustakas A, Yin HY, Henis YI, Plamondon J, O'Connor-McCourt MD, Lodish HF: The transforming growth factor β receptors types I, II, and III form hetero-oligomeric complexes in the presence of ligand. *J Biol Chem* 1993; 268:22215–22218.

175. Derynck R: TGF-β-receptor-mediated signaling. *Trends Biol Sci* 1994; 19:548–553.

176. Lawler S, Candia AF, Ebner R, Shum L, Lopez AR, Moses HL, Wright CVE, Derynck R: The murine type II TGF-β receptor has a coincident embryonic expression and binding preference for TGF-β1. *Development* 1994; 120:165–175.

177. Laiho M, Weis FMB, Boyd FT, Ignotz RA, and Massagué J: Responsiveness to transforming growth factor-β (TGF-β) restored by genetic complementation between cells defective in TGF-α receptors I and II. *J Biol Chem* 1991; 266:9108–9112.

178. Wrana JL, Attisano J, Zentella A, Doody J, Laiho M, Wang X-F, Massagué J: TGFβ signals through a heteromeric protein kinase receptor complex. *Cell* 1992; 71:1003–1014.

179. Okadome T, Yamashita H, Franzen P, Moren A, Heldin CH, Miyazono K: Distinct roles of the intracellular domains of transforming growth factor-β type I and type II receptors in signal transduction. *J Biol Chem* 1994; 269:30753–30756.

180. Chen R-H, Derynck R: Homomeric interactions between type II transforming growth factor-β receptors. *J Biol Chem* 1994; 269:22868–22874.

181. Henis YI, Moustakas A, Lin HY, Lodish HF: The types II and III transforming growth factor-β receptors form homo-oligomers. *J Cell Biol* 1994; 126:139–154.

182. Attisano L, Cárcamo J, Ventura F, Weis FMB, Massagué J, Wrana J: Identification of human activan and TGF β type 1 receptors that form heteromeric complexes with type II receptors. *Cell* 1993; 75:671–680.

183. Bassing CH, Yingling JM, Howe DJ, Wang T, He WW, Gustafson ML, Shah P, Donahoe PK, Wang XF: A transforming growth factor beta type I receptor that signals to activate gene expression. *Science* 1994; 263:87–89.

184. Cate RL, Mattaliano RJ, Hession C, Tizard R, Farber NM, Cheung A, Ninfa EG, Frey AZ, Chow DJ, Fisher RA, Bertonis JM, Torres G, Wallner BP, Ramachandran KL, Ragin RC, Manganaro TF, LacLaughlin DT, Donahoe PK: Isolation of the bovine and human genes for Müllerian inhibiting substance and expression of the human gene in animal cells. *Cell* 1986; 45:685–698.

185. Chen R-H, Ebner R, Derynck R: Inactivation of the type II receptor reveals two receptor pathways for the diverse TGF-β activities. *Science* 1993; 260:1335–1338.

186. Lyons RM, Moses HL: Transforming growth factors and regulation of cell proliferation. *Eur J Biochem* 1990; 187:467–473.

187. Gronwald RGK, Seifert RA, Bowen-Pope DF: Differential regulation of expression of two platelet-derived growth factor receptor subunits by transforming growth factor-β. *J Biol Chem* 1989; 264:8120–8125.

188. Battegay EJ, Raines EW, Seifert RA, Bowen-Pope DF, Ross R: TGF-β induces bimodal proliferation of connective tissue cells via complex control of an autocrine PDGF loop. *Cell* 1990; 63:515–524.

189. Leof AB, Proper JA, Goustin AS, Shipley GD, Dicorleto PE, Moses HL: Induction of c-*sis* mRNA and activity similar to platelet-derived growth factor by transforming growth factor β: A proposed model for indirect mitogenesis involving autocrine activity. *Proc Natl Acad Sci USA* 1986; 83:2453–2457.

190. Majack RA, Majesky MW, Goodman LV: Role of PDGF-A expression in the control of vascular smooth muscle cell growth by transforming growth factor-β. *J Cell Biol* 1990; 111:239–247.

191. Howe PH, Cunningham MR, Leof EB: Distinct pathways regulate transforming growth factor β1-stimulated proto-oncogene and extracellular matrix gene expression. *J Cell Physiol* 1990; 142:39–44.

192. Howe PH, Cunningham MR, Leof EB: Inhibition of mink lung epithelial cell proliferation by transforming growth factor-β is coupled through a pertussis toxin-sensitive substrate. *Biochem J* 1990; 266:537–543.

193. Mulder KM, Morris SL: Activation of p21^{ras} by transforming growth factor β in epithelial cells. *J Biol Chem* 1992; 267:5029–5031.

194. Gruppuso PA, Mikumo R, Brautigan DL, Braun L: Growth arrest induced by transforming growth factor beta 1 is accompanied by protein phosphatase activation in human keratinocytes. *J Biol Chem* 1991; 266:3444–3448.

195. Kramer IM, Koornneef I, de Laat SW, ven der Eijnden-van Raaij AJM: TGF-β$_1$ induces phosphorylation of the cyclic AMP responsive element binding protein in ML-CC164 cells. *Embo J* 1991; 10:1083–1089.

196. Laiho M, DeCaprio JA, Ludlow JW, Livingston DM, Massagué J: Growth inhibition by TGF-β linked to expression of retinoblastoma protein phosphorylation. *Cell* 1990; 62:175–185.

197. Geng Y, Weinberg RA: Transforming growth factor beta effects on expression of G1 cyclins and cyclin-dependent kinases. *Proc Natl Acad Sci USA* 1993; 90:10315–10319.

198. Ewen ME, Sluss HK, Whitehouse LL, Livingston DM: TGF beta inhibition of Cdk4 synthesis is linked to cell cycle arrest. *Cell* 1993; 74:1009–1020.

199. Sherr CJ: The ins and outs of *RB*: coupling gene expression to the cell cycle clock. *Trends Cell Biol* 1994; 4:15–18.

200. Rossi R, Karsenty G, Roberts AB, Roche NS, Sporn MB, de Crombrugghe B: A nuclear 1 binding site mediates the transcriptional activation of a type 1 collagen promoter by transforming growth factor-β. *Cell* 1988; 52:405–414.

201. Bassols A, Massagué J: Transforming growth factor beta regulates the expression and structure of extracellular matrix chondroitin/dermatan sulfate proteoglycans. *J Biol Chem* 1988; 263:3039–3045.

202. Westergren-Thorsson G, Schmidtchen A, Särnstrand B, Franson L-À, Malmström A: Transforming growth factor α induces selective increase of proteoglycan production and changes in the copolymeric structure of dermatan sulfate in skin fibroblasts. *Eur J Biochem* 1991; 205:277–286.

203. Ignotz RA, Endo T, Massagué J: Regulation of fibronectin and type I collagen mRNA levels by transforming growth factor-beta. *J Biol Chem* 1987; 262:6443–6446.

204. Varga J, Rosenbloom J, Jimenez SA: Transforming growth factor β (TGF-β) causes a persistent increase in steady-state amounts of type I and type II collagen and fibronectin mRNAs in normal human dermal fibroblasts. *Biochem J* 1987; 247:597–604.

205. Westergren-Thorsson G, Särnstrand B, Frannson L-Å, Malmström A: TGF-β enhances the production of hyaluronan in human lung but not in skin fibroblasts. *Exp Cell Res* 1990; 186:192–195.

206. Overall CM, Wrana JL, Sodek J: Independent regulation of collagenase, 72-kDa progelatinase, and metalloendoproteinase inhibitor expression in human fibroblasts by transforming growth factor-β. *J Biol Chem* 1989; 264:1860–1869.

207. Keski-Oja J, Raghow R, Sawdey M, Loskutoff DJ, Postlethwaite AE, Kang AH, Moses HL: Regulations of mRNAs for type-1 plasminogen activator inhibitor, fibronectin, and type I procollagen by transforming growth factor-β. Divergent responses in lung fibroblasts and carcinoma cells. *J Biol Chem* 1988; 263:3111–3115.

208. Heino J, Ignotz RA, Hemler ME, Crouse C, Massagué J: Regulation of cell adhesion receptors by transforming growth factor-beta. Concomitant regulation of integrins that share a common beta 1 subunit. *J Biol Chem* 1989; 264:380–388.

209. Roberts CJ, Birkenmeier TM, McQuillian JJ, Akiyama SK, Yamada SS, Chen WT, Yamada KM, McDonald JA: Transforming growth factor beta stimulates the expression of fibronectin and of both subunits of the human fibronectin receptor by cultured human lung fibroblasts. *J Biol Chem* 1988; 263:4586–4592.

210. Ignotz RA, Heino J, Massagué J: Regulation of cell adhesion receptors by transforming growth factor-β. Regulation of vitronectin receptor and LFA-1. *J Biol Chem* 1989; 264:389–392.

211. Hoyt DG, Lazo JS: Alterations in pulmonary mRNA encoding procollagens, fibronectin, and transforming growth factor-β precede bleomycin-induced pulmonary fibrosis in mice. *J Pharmacol Exp Ther* 1988; 246:765–771.

212. Breen E, Absher M, Kelley J, Phan S, Cutroneo KR: Bleomycin regulation of TGF-β mRNA in rat lung fibroblasts. *Am J Respir Cell Mol Biol* 1992; 6:146–152.

213. Westergren-Thorsson G, Hernnäs J, Särnstrand B, Oldberg Å, Heinegård D, Malmström A: Altered expression of small proteoglycans, collagen, and transforming growth factor-β_1 in developing bleomycin-induced pulmonary fibrosis in rats. *J Clin Invest* 1993; 92:632–637.

214. Phan SH, Gharaee-Kermani M, Wolber F, Ryan US: Stimulation of rat endothelial cell transforming growth factor-β production by bleomycin. *J Clin Invest* 1991; 87:148–154.

RECEPTOR PROTEIN TYROSINE PHOSPHATASES

215. Fischer EH, Charbonneau H, Tonks NK: Protein tyrosine phosphatases: A diverse family of intracellular and transmembrane enzymes. *Science (Wash DC)* 1991; 253:401–406.

216. Saito H, Streuli M: Molecular characterization of protein tyrosine phosphatases. *Cell Growth and Differ* 1991; 2:59–65.

217. Tonks NK, Diltz CD, Fischer EH: CD45, an integral membrane protein tyrosine phosphatase. *J Biol Chem* 1990; 265:10674–10680.

218. Daum G, Zander NF, Morse B, Hurwitz D, Schlessinger J, et al: Characterization of a human recombinant receptor-linked protein tyrosine phosphatase. *J Biol Chem* 1991; 266:12211–12215.

219. Charbonneau H, Tonks NK: 1002 protein phosphatases. *Annu Rev Cell Biol* 1992; 8:463–493.

220. Cool DE: Protein tyrosine phosphatases: A multigene family of diverse structure and function. In Kelley J (ed.), *Cytokines of the Lung* (New York: Marcel Dekker, 1993), pp 181–198.

221. Streuli M, Krueger NX, Thai T, Tang M, Saito H: Distinct functional roles of the two intracellular phosphatase like domains of the receptor-linked protein tyrosine phosphatases LCA and LAR. *Embo J* 1990; 9:2399–2407.

222. Wang Y, Pallen CJ: The receptor-like protein tyrosine phosphatase HPTPα has two active catalytic domains with distinct substrate specificities. *Embo J* 1991; 10:3231–3237.

223. Charbonneau H, Tonks NK, Walsh KA, Fischer EH: the leukocyte comman antigen (CD45): a putative receptor-linked protein tyrosine phosphatase. *Proc Natl Acad Sci USA* 1988; 85:7182–7186.

224. Mustelin T, Altman A: Dephosphorylation and activation of the T-cell tyrosine kinase pp56^{lck} by the leukocyte common antigen (CD45). *Oncogene* 1990; 5:809–814.

225. Ostergaard HL, Towbridge IS: Coclustering CD45 and CD4 or CD8 alters the phosphorylation and kinase activity of p56^{lck}. *J Exp Med* 1990; 172:347–350.

226. Klausner RD, Samelson LE: T-cell antigen receptor activation pathways: the tyrosine kinase connection. *Cell* 1991; 64:875–878.

227. Streuli M, Kreuger NX, Tsai AYM, Saito H: A family of receptor-linked protein tyrosine phosphatases in humans and *Drosophila*. *Proc Natl Acad Sci USA* 1989; 86:8698–8702.

228. Katsura H, Williams MC, Brody JS, Yu Q: Receptor protein tyrosine phosphatase in lung development. *Am Rev Respir Dis* 1993; 147:A940.

229. Pulido R, Krueger NX, Serra-Pagès C, Saito H, Streuli M: Molecular characterization of the human transmembrane protein-tyrosine phosphatase δ. Evidence for tissue-specific expression of alternative human transmembrane protein-tyrosine phosphatase δ isoforms. *J Biol Chem* 1995; 270:6722–6728.

230. Jiang Y-P, Wang H, D'Eustachio P, Musacchio JM, Schlessinger J, Sap J: Cloning and characterization of R-RTP-κ, a new member of the receptor protein tyrosine phosphatase family with a proteolytically cleaved cellular adhesion molecule-like extracellular region. *Mol Cell Biol* 1993; 13:2942–2951.

231. Brady-Kalnay SM, Flint AJ, Tonks NK: Homophilic binding of PTPμ, a receptor-type protein tyrosine phosphatase, can mediate cell-cell aggregation. *J Cell Biol* 1993; 122:961–972.

232. Gebbink MFBG, Zondag GCM, Wubbolts RW, Beijersbergen RL, van Etten I, Moolenaar WH: Cell-cell adhesion mediated by a receptor-like protein tyrosine phosphatase. *J Biol Chem* 1993; 268:16101–16104.

233. Kreuger NK, Streuli M, Saito H: Structural diversity and evolution of human receptor-like protein tyrosine phosphatases. *Embo J* 1990; 9:3241–3252.

234. Zheng XM, Wang Y, Pallen CJ: Cell transformation and activation of pp60^{c-src} by overexpression of a protein tyrosine phosphatase. *Nature (London)* 1992; 359:336–339.

235. den Hertog J, Pals CEGM, Peppelenbosch MP, Tertoolen LGJ, de Laat SW, Kruijer W: Receptor protein tyrosine phosphatase α activates pp60^{c-src} and is involved in neuronal differentiation. *Embo J* 1993; 12:3789–3798.

236. den Hertog, Tracy S, Hunter T: Phosphorylation of receptor protein-tyrosine phosphatase α on Tyr789, a binding site for the SH3-SH2-SH3 adaptor prtein GRB-2 in vivo. *Embo J* 1994; 13:3020–3032.

237. Mourey RJ, Dixon JE: Protein tyrosine phosphatases: characterization of extracellular and intracellular domains. *Curr Opin Genet Dev* 1994; 4:31–39.

238. Walton KM, Dixon JE: Protein tyrosine phosphatases. *Annu Rev Biochem* 1993; 62:101–120.

Chapter 3

RECEPTORS 3: NUCLEAR HORMONE RECEPTORS

CRAIG M. SCHRAMM AND MICHAEL M. GRUNSTEIN

This chapter discusses the large superfamily of intracellular, regulatory receptors that includes receptors for the three groups of steroids [adrenal corticosteroids (glucocorticoid and mineralocorticoid), sex steroids (estrogen, progesterone, and androgen), and vitamin D_3], thyroid hormone (T_3), retinoic acid (RA), and certain oncogenes such as v-*erbA* (the avian erythroblastosis virus, which has captured a gene encoding for thyroid receptor and uses the mutated molecule for its own oncogenesis). All the major members of this superfamily have been cloned, and their complementary DNAs (cDNA) have been sequenced. The exploration of cDNA libraries for related sequences has led to the characterization of more than 40 orphan receptors whose cloned cDNAs clearly belong to this receptor superfamily but whose ligands have not been identified. All these receptors are present in minute quantities, typically only 1000 to 10,000 receptor molecules per cell.[1] Such cellular levels appear to vary with development,[2] aging,[3] and the cell cycle.[4] Despite their low abundance, these receptors are capable of transducing widespread cellular responses.

Like the enzyme-linked receptors and, to a lesser extent, the G-protein coupled receptors, these receptor molecules modulate the complex network of gene expression that mediates cellular differentiation, development, and longer-term adaptive responses to stimuli. Because the effects elicited by stimulation of these receptors generally involve gene transcription, the members of this receptor superfamily have been referred to as hormone- or ligand-responsive transcription factors (LTFs). For simplicity, they are specified here as *nuclear hormone receptors* (NHRs). Unlike the previously considered families of receptors, however, NHRs are entirely intracytoplasmic or intranuclear, with no portion of the receptor molecule extending beyond the cell membrane to effect ligand binding. Accordingly, their activation requires entry of a hormone into the cell. This entry is generally by passive diffusion but, under certain circumstances, active transport may also occur.[5] Alternatively, some of these orphan receptors may respond to intracellular ligands, such as products of metabolic pathways, thereby establishing what has been termed *intracrine* gene regulatory pathways.[6] Following ligand binding, the myriad effects of these NHRs and their hormones in the lung are beyond the scope of this chapter. Rather, the ensuing discussion focuses on the structure-function relationship of these receptors and current understanding of the molecular basis of their regulation of gene activity.

General Structure of Nuclear Hormone Receptors

A schematic of selected members of the human NHR superfamily, based on amino acid sequence homology to the glucocorticoid receptor (GR), is shown in Fig. 3-1. Protease degradation and molecular cloning studies have identified

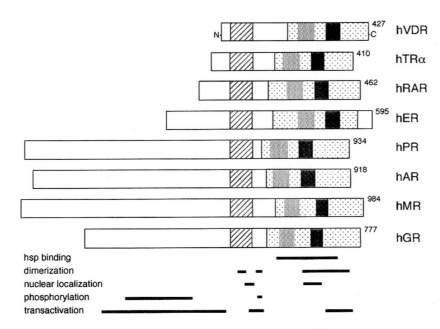

FIGURE 3-1 Schema of selected nuclear hormone receptors, aligned with the DNA-binding domain (*striped area*) of the glucocorticoid receptor. Numbers to right designate the amino acid length of the receptor proteins. Bars on the bottom of the figure indicate areas of the glucocorticoid receptor believed to be involved with various steps in receptor regulation and activation. Abbreviations designate human receptor proteins for vitamin D₃ (hVDR), thyroid hormone (hTRα), retinoic acid (hRAR), estrogen (hER), progesterone (hPR), androgen (hAR), mineralocorticoid (hMR), and glucocorticoid (hGR).

three distinct functional domains of conserved amino acids within these receptors. The most highly conserved region is a centrally located sequence of 66 to 68 amino acids that constitutes the receptor's DNA-binding domain (DBD, also referred to as region I, Fig. 3-1, striped segment). The sequence homology is so striking for this region that many receptor-encoding genes were cloned by screening cDNA libraries with probes against it. The DBD is a true domain, at least for the GR, in that it folds into a stable form and retains its function in isolation from the remainder of the receptor.[7] The structure of the DBD distinguishes the NHR/LTF superfamily from other transcription factors by the presence of two peptide projections known as *zinc fingers*, that is, loops that are stabilized by tetrahedral coordination of four cysteines around a zinc ion. The zinc finger domain is principally responsible for the recognition of specific genomic sequences known as *response elements*. The latter are enhancer elements in the regulatory (usually 5' flanking) region of specific steroid-inducible genes.

The two other relatively invariant regions lie within the carboxy-terminal, ligand-binding domain (LBD, Fig. 3-1, stippled segment). The LBD is a large (≈250 amino acid), functionally complex area that contains sequences important for the following essential NHR functions: (1) association with accompanying proteins, (2) dimerization, (3) nuclear translocation, (4) gene transactivation, and (5) intermolecular silencing for thyroid and retinoic acid receptors.[8] The entire LBD has substantial homology between receptors for glucocorticoids, mineralocorticoids, androgen, and progesterone (a trait that accounts for the modest cross-sensitivity of these receptors toward each steroid ligand), but is more variable for the thyroid hormone, retinoic acid, and vitamin D₃ receptors. Nevertheless, this region contains two highly conserved subdomains throughout the NHR superfamily. The more central subdomain (region II; Fig. 3-1, darker stippled segment) is a 42 amino acid sequence potentially

involved in the inactivation of transcription in the absence of ligand binding.[9] Deletions within this domain of the GR result in proteins with constitutive transactivating capacity.[10] The more carboxy-terminal conserved sequence (region III; Fig. 3-1, darkest stippled segment) lies within the putative dimerization domain and likely regulates ligand-dependent NHR dimerization, a step necessary to gene transcription. The ligand- and DNA-binding domains are separated by a hinge region (Fig. 3-1, central open segment) containing a short sequence of basic amino acids[11] that may participate in regulating the nuclear localization of the receptor.[12,13]

Proteins of $M_r \geq 40,000$ require a nuclear localization signal (NLS) to mediate passage through nuclear pores. The GR contains two such NLSs. One signal (NL1) is located just to the carboxy side of the DNA binding domain, in the receptor's hinge region. NL1 of the GR contains the sequence Thr-Lys-Lys-Lys-Ile-Lys-Gly, which resembles the well characterized NLS of the SV40 large T antigen (Pro-Lys-Lys-Lys-Arg-Lys-Val).[14] When fused to β-galactosidase, NL1 acts constitutively to transport the fusion protein to the nucleus. Similar constitutively active NLS present in receptors for progesterone (PR),[15] estrogen (ER),[16] and androgen (AR)[17] account for the nuclear localization in the unliganded sex steroid receptors. In contrast, NL1 of the native GR requires hormone binding for its activation. A second localization signal (NL2) is present within the hormone binding domain of the GR and it, too, is hormone-dependent.[14] Thus, in the absence of hormone, the GR is localized to the cytoplasm, whereas sex steroid receptors (i.e., PR, ER, AR) are predominantly intranuclear in location.

In contrast to the carboxy end, the amino-terminal halves of NHRs are extremely variable both in size (25 amino acids in the vitamin D₃ receptor versus 603 in the mineralocorticoid receptor, Fig. 3-1) and in sequence. This region houses the transcriptional regulatory motifs of the receptor molecule[18]; its variability imparts specificity to gene activation following ligand binding to the LTF. Activating sequences have been identified as being rich in acidic amino acids (as in an 82-residue sequence in the GR), glutamines, or prolines.[19] Deletion of the entire region reduces the ability of GRs and PRs to induce gene activation by 50 to 85 percent.[18,20]

Alternative splicing of the amino end of NHRs results in isoforms that contribute to the functional diversity of these receptor responses. The human glucocorticoid receptor (hGR) exists in two major isoforms of 777 and 742 amino acids in length (GRα and GRβ, respectively) formed by alternative splicing of an mRNA encoded from a single gene on chromosome 5.[21] (See also Chapter 55) Similarly, differential splicing of PR mRNA results in isoforms of 934 and 806 amino acids, with the shorter form lacking a highly acidic region within the amino-terminal domain.[22] The later alternative splicing is due to the differential activity of alternate promoters, which induce transcription of different first exons and subsequent amino-terminal sequences.[9]

Additional diversity is achieved for human T_3 and retinoic acid receptors (hTR and hRAR, respectively) by gene duplication as well as alternative splicing. Two linked hTR and hRAR loci have been identified on chromosomes 17 and 3 (hTRα and hRARα, and hTRβ and hRARβ, respectively).[23–25] A third hRAR locus (hRARγ) is present on chromosome 12,[26] and a fourth unrelated retinoic acid-binding receptor (RXR) has also been identified.[27] Furthermore, at least 7 different isoforms of RARγ have been characterized, which are formed by alternative splicing or in response to different promoters.[28,29] These RARs are expressed in a tissue-specific manner and likely play key roles in tissue morphogenesis and differentiation. TRα also exists in 3 alternative splicing-derived isoforms, but only TRα1 can bind T_3. The other isoforms, Trα2 and TRα3, are nonetheless capable of binding DNA and, thus, may act as intranuclear molecular antagonists of thyroid hormone action.[9] Indeed, it has been shown that the ratio of TRα2 to TRα1 determines tissue responsiveness to thyroid hormone.[30] TRα2 may itself be regulated at the transcriptional level by Rev-TRα, a third gene product that is encoded by the DNA strand opposite to that which encodes TRα1/α2.[31]

Cellular Localization and Complexing Proteins

With the exception of the adrenal steroid receptors (GR and MR), NHRs are predominantly intranuclear. Receptors for thyroid hormone, retinoic acid, and vitamin D have been shown to be transported directly from their cytoplasmic areas of synthesis to intranuclear sites in hormone-free cells.[32,33] It is believed that, even in their unliganded state, these receptors are transferred to their appropriate response elements in the genome. In some circumstances, such unliganded receptors may serve as inhibitors of transcription.[14] Similarly, receptors for the sex steroids (PR, ER, and AR) are also relocated to the nucleus following their cytoplasmic synthesis. In contrast to TRs and RARs, however, the sex steroid receptors are believed to exist in a loosely bound, inactive state within the nucleus until they are bound by hormone, whereupon they move to high-affinity binding sites in association with their transcriptional response elements.[14] Recent studies with PR deletional mutants have indicated that the nuclear localization of PR results from a dynamic equilibrium between diffusion into the cytoplasm and active transport back into the nucleus.[34] Conversely, GRs basally exist in the cytoplasm of hormone-free cells and are translocated to the nucleus only upon ligand binding.[35,36]

Under nonactivated conditions, the GR is present in the cytoplasm as a multimolecular, heterooligomeric 9S complex of M_r approximately 330,000. Both sex steroid- and glucocorticoid-binding receptors have been shown to exist as parts of large heterooligomeric complexes with several other proteins, including the heat shock proteins hsp90 and hsp 70, the immunophilin hsp56, and proteins p50 and p23. The latter proteins are members of a group of *chaperone proteins*, whose function is to oversee the fundamental molecular processes ensuring the proper folding of newly synthesized proteins and the correct assembly of multiprotein complexes. It is believed that the glucocorticoid and sex hormone receptors have appropriated a usually transient interaction and form more long-lasting complexes with these chaperone proteins to maintain an otherwise unstable conformation that promotes hormone binding to the NHR. A brief review of each component protein is given below.

HEAT SHOCK PROTEIN 90

hsp90 is a ubiquitous and highly expressed protein, accounting for approximately 1 percent of all cytoplasmic proteins in unstressed cells and increasing in synthesis after heat shock. It consists of two isoforms of slightly different M_r (e.g., hsp84 and hsp86 in the mouse; hsp90α and hsp90β in human tissues) that are products of separate genes.[37] hsp90 is an essential component of unstimulated GR, MR, ER, PR, and AR complexes. It is present within the cytoplasm in great stoichiometric excess to the NHRs, and hsp90 has been found complexed with 2 additional heat shock proteins, hsp70 and hsp56, independent of an NHR.[38] hsp90 exists as a homodimer in its purified form[39] and in complex with NHRs. The NHR protein is believed to interact asymmetrically with the hsp90 dimer, more directly with one hsp90 molecule than the other.[40] In this regard, although both hsp90 isoforms are recovered in the GR heterocomplex,[39,41,42] it has yet to be determined whether the NHR interacts preferentially with a particular isoform.

A highly conserved 20-amino-acid sequence within the LBD of NHRs (residues 583 to 602 in the mouse GR) has been proposed to be an essential site for interaction with hsp90[43]; however, this region is conserved in TR and RAR, neither of which displays stable binding to hsp90.[44,45] Moreover, a mutant GR lacking this region (Δ574 to 632) is bound to hsp90 within the cell.[46] Additional observations with the GR[46] and the PR[47] suggest that either there are multiple hsp contact sites within the LBD, or that hsp90 binding depends on a general property of the unfolded receptor protein that involves a diffuse region of the LBD.[37] Functions attributed to hsp90 in complex with steroid receptors include the following:

1. Protecting the receptor from denaturation[46]
2. Stabilizing hormone binding by promoting a high-affinity binding state for the GR[48,49]
3. Interacting with the carboxy-terminal portion of the DBD to inhibit DNA binding and transcriptional activity[50]
3. Regulating the distribution of GR within the cytosol through interactions of hsp90 with actin[51] and microtubules[52]

Despite the above functions ascribed to hsp90, not all NHRs require hsp90 for ligand binding. As noted above, hsp90 confers a high-affinity binding configuration to the GR, but glucocorticoid binding can subsequently be maintained in the absence of the heat shock protein. In fact, hsp90 appears normally to dissociate from the receptor in the presence of hormone, possibly through an ATP-dependent process.[53] In contrast, the persistence of hsp90 within an NHR heterocomplex is essential to preserving a ligand-binding configuration for the sex steroid receptors. Lastly, receptors for T_3, RA, and vitamin D_3 never seem to be associated with hsp90. Indeed, based on their binding affinity for hsp90 and cellular localization, Pratt and coworkers have proposed a classification system for NHRs,[54] as shown in Table 3-1.

HEAT SHOCK PROTEIN 70

hsp70 exists as a family of closely related ATP-binding proteins of 70 to 76 kDa M_r. Some of these proteins are expressed constitutively (hsc70), whereas others are highly inducible by heat shock (hsp70). hsp70 has been identified in complexes of chick oviduct and human PRs[55,56] and in association with hsp90 and mouse GR overexpressed in Chinese hamster ovary cells.[54] In contrast, hsp70 has not been found as a component of native GR heterocomplexes in L cells,[42,54] WEHI mouse lymphoma cells,[57] and cultured human HeLa cells,[58] except for trace amounts in immunoadsorbed GR complexes from L-cell cytosol.[37] Like hsp90, hsp70 interacts with the NHR's LBD, probably also by a general structural quality of the entire hormone-binding region.[47]

The co-location of the hsp70 and hsp90 binding sites within the LBD of steroid receptors suggests that hsp70 may have a fundamental role in receptor-hsp90 complex formation. It is thought that members of the hsp70 protein family bind to hydrophobic regions of other proteins in an ATP-dependent manner and induce an "unfolded" state of the associated protein. Accordingly, it has been postulated that hsp70 may participate in the catalysis of NHR heterocomplex assembly.[59] Several independent observations, including that hsp70 exists in tissues as a complex with hsp60 and hsp90 and that the addition of the anti-hsp70 monoclonal antibody N27 to in vitro reconstitution systems inhibits hsp90 binding,[60] have led to the speculation that hsp70 may interact transiently with the NHR to promote the stabilization of the early SR-hsp90 complex through the unfoldase activity of hsp70.[61]

Alternatively, hsp70 may mediate the translocation of SHs across the nuclear membrane. Large proteins often must be transformed into unfolded states to cross organellar membranes.[59] The unfoldase activity of hsp70 has been implicated in the passage of proteins across mitochondrial and endoplasmic reticular membranes.[37] In this regard, the differential recovery of receptors complexed to hsp70 may be a function of their cellular location. Thus, the cytoplasmic GR in hormone-free cells is not complexed to hsp70, whereas the predominantly nuclear GR in overexpressing CHO cells[54] and the largely nuclear PR[62] are found in association with hsp70 because these receptors have entered the nucleus by an hsp70-dependent mechanism.

HEAT SHOCK PROTEIN 56

A third member of the NHR heterocomplex is the immunophilin, hsp56 (also called p59). *Immunophilins* are proteins with intrinsic rotamase (peptidyl-prolyl *cis-trans*-isomerase) activity[37,63] and specific, high-affinity binding for immunosuppressive agents such as cyclosporin (cyclophilins), rapamycin, and FK506. hsp56 is a FK506-binding type of immunophilin with homology to carboxy-terminal sequences of other FK506-binding proteins.[64] There exists some species difference in regard to the size of this protein as well, with M_r ranging from 55 to 59 kDa.[37] Nevertheless, the

TABLE 3-1   Classification of Nuclear Hormone Receptors

	Class I	Class II	Class III
Hormone ligands	Retinoic acid Thyroid hormone Vitamin D_3	Glucocorticoid Mineralocorticoid	Progesterone Estrogen Androgen
hsp90			
Stable complex	No	Yes	Yes
Required for steroid- binding configuration	No	No	Yes
Cellular location of unliganded receptors	Nuclear, tightly bound to response elements	Cytoplasmic	Nuclear, loosely bound in docking complex with hsp90

protein has been found in multiple steroid receptor complexes prepared from rabbit (GR, PR, ER, AR[65]), calf uterus (GR, PR, ER, AR[66]), and human MCF7 cells (GR, PR[67]). From various cross-linking experiments, it has been shown that hsp56 interacts with both hsp90 and the NHR's LBD at undetermined sites.[57,58] The function of hsp56 within the NHR heterocomplex remains to be identified but does not appear to involve its rotamase activity since FK506, which inhibits the rotamase activity of immunophilins[63] has no effect of GR function in vitro or on glucocorticoid-mediated transcriptional activation in intact cells.[37]

ADDITIONAL HEAT SHOCK PROTEINS

Four additional proteins have been found in association with various NHRs. A 54- and a 50-kDa protein (p54 and p50, respectively, have been identified as components of the avian PR complex. To date, no specific functions have been ascribed to these proteins. Certain binding characteristics suggest an interaction between p50 and hsp90,[68] and both of these proteins rapidly dissociate from the receptor heterocomplex upon in vivo hormone treatment. A 50-kDa protein is also co-immunoadsorbed from rat hepatic cytosol with monoclonal antibodies against hsp90,[38] but it is unclear whether this protein is similar to the chick PR complex.[37] A slightly larger protein, p60, has been associated with hsp90 and hsp70 in intermediate complexes with GR, ER, and PR.[60] Like hsp70, p60 is believed to possess chaperone properties involved in protein folding and assembly.

The chick PR complex also contains a 23-kDa protein,[67] which has been found in the L-cell GR complex as well.[37] A protein of similar size and pI can also be immunoadsorbed from human IM-9 cells as part of the hsp56-hsp90-hsp70 complex.[68] p23 is an acidic phosphoprotein with an ATP binding site. It has no sequence homology to any known

protein, and so no clues can be derived as to its function.[67] Nevertheless, when reconstitution systems are depleted of p23, they no longer support the formation of PR complexes, suggesting that p23 is an essential intermediary component in the assembly of at least some NHR heterocomplexes.[69]

Formation of the heterocomplex between NHRs and heat shock proteins is an enzymatic process believed to be at least partially mediated by hsp70.[37] Receptors that are dissociated from hsp90 have undergone a conformational change that prevents the receptor protein from directly interacting with hsp90. This process is conceptualized by an inward folding of the LBD into the molecule (Fig. 3-2). It is speculated that hsp70 recognizes the folded state of the NHR and catalyzes an ATP-dependent unfolding of the receptor protein. The unfolded state of the receptor is thermodynamically unstable, but it is stabilized through interaction of the exposed LBD with the hsp90 component of the complex.[70] In the case of the GR, interaction of the unfolded receptor with hsp90 may trigger the dissociation of hsp70 from the receptor-protein heterocomplex. The remaining hsp90 inactivates the transactivating portion of the receptor protein, either by inducing a conformational change in the NHR's gene transcription site[71] or by "docking" to the receptor and stearically preventing its active site from interacting with its response elements.[37] Nevertheless, it is this inactive form of NHR in complex with hsp90 that provides an open LBD accessible to hormone binding (Fig. 3-2). Hormone binding to the receptor induces a different refolding of the LBD and the dissociation of the NHR from hsp90. This dissociation, in turn, removes the inhibitory influence on the receptor's active site and allows for steroid-induced responses to occur.

The roles of each of these proteins within the NHR heterocomplex are unknown. It has been shown, however, that the heterocomplex is associated with both cytoplasmic and nuclear NHRs. Accordingly, Pratt and Scherrer[14] have

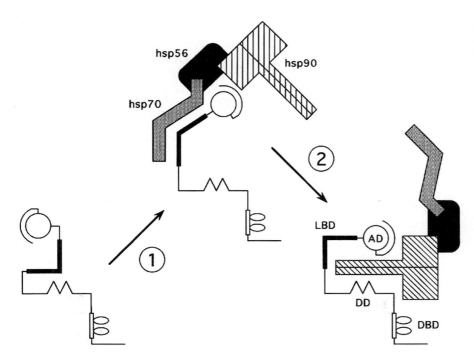

FIGURE 3-2 Conceptualization of heat-shock protein participation in nuclear hormone receptor (NHR) ligand binding. The uncomplexed NHR exists in a folded configuration wherein the ligand binding domain (LBD, *heavy bar*) is "folded" within the receptor and unavailable for ligand binding. Association of the NHR with hsp70 (here shown as part of a preexisting cytoplasmic complex with hsp56 and dimerized hsp90) results in an unfolding of the NHR. This unfolding allows the hsp90 to form a complex with the NHR, stabilizing an NHR configuration that exposes the LBD for ligand binding. Note that in some circumstances, hsp70 and hsp56 may dissociate from the NHR-hsp90 heterocomplex. AD = activation domain; DD = dimerization domain; DBD = DNA-binding domain.

hypothesized that an additional function of the chaperone protein complex is to act as a "transportosome," a structure that transports steroid receptors and other proteins from site to site within the cell. These investigators have proposed that the associated proteins hsp56 and p50 function as direction-determining proteins, with hsp56 directing inward movement to the nucleus and p50 directing outward movement to the cell periphery.[14]

The DNA Binding Domain

Proteolysis experiments initially suggested that an independent domain mediated DNA binding in the rat GR.[72] The subsequent cloning of the human GR demonstrated a region rich in cysteine, arginine, and lysine residues[21] that was homologous to the cysteine-rich domain of the *Xenopus* transcription factor TFIIIA.[73] This DNA-binding domain was found to lie within a 66- to 68-residue region that is conserved throughout the NHRs (Fig. 3-1). Eighteen of the 68 residues within this region are invariant for all NHRs across all species, including nine cysteines. The first eight of these cysteine residues are tetrahedrally coordinated around two zinc ions, forming the two zinc fingers that characterize the NHR-type of transcription factors (Fig. 3-3). The NHR zinc fingers differ from those found in other eukaryotic transcription factors in that the zinc ions in the latter either are coordinated by two histidines and two cysteines (e.g., in TFIIIA, ADR1, and Xfin)[74] or share cysteine ions (e.g., GAL4[75]).

The DBD can be subdivided into two portions, each containing a zinc finger. The amino-terminal portion begins with a short segment of antiparallel β sheet that helps to orient the residues for making contact with the phosphate backbone to the DNA.[8] The amino acids are arranged in an R

configuration about the first zinc ion. This portion ends with an α-helical structure (residues 457 to 469) that contains a region referred to as the *P-box* (Fig. 3-3). The amino acids within the *P box* are critical for receptor recognition of specific DNA sequences, termed the receptor's *response elements*. The carboxy-portion of the DBD contains the second zinc finger in an S configuration. The five amino acids interspersed between the two amino-terminal cysteines make up a so-called *D box*, which regulates receptor dimerization (Fig. 3-3). The C-terminal region contains another α helix extending from proline 493 to glycine 504, which appears to have secondary effects on DNA binding. The two α helices are aligned perpendicular to each other and form a compact core of several conserved hydrophobic and aromatic residues that appears to be a common element to the NHR DBDs.[76,77]

Steroid Hormone Response Elements

The investigation of glucocorticoid-responsive DNA sequences (glucocorticoid response elements, or GREs) in various genes identified a conserved, 15-base-pair sequence of two 6-nucleotide imperfectly inverted repeats, or palindromes, separated by a three-base pair spacer. The consensus sequence for such GREs is given by the following: 5'-GGTACAnnnTGTTCT-3', where n is any nucleotide.[78,79] The bases to the left of the spacer are conventially identified with negative numerals (e.g., A-1, C-2, A-3, T-4, G-5, G-6), while the right-sided bases are positive (e.g., T1, G2, T3, T4, C5, T6). Considerable variation is found in the left half-site of GREs, and only the C-2 nucleotide is highly conserved. By contrast, most of the right half-site of GREs is conserved, except for occasional substitutions of cysteine for the T4. Deviations from the consensus sequence may be important for grading of affinity and/or activity of the GREs. A similar, inverted palindromic estrogen response ele-

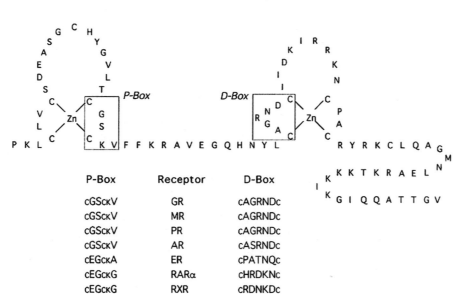

P-Box	Receptor	D-Box
cGSckV	GR	cAGRNDc
cGSckV	MR	cAGRNDc
cGSckV	PR	cAGRNDc
cGSckV	AR	cASRNDc
cEGckA	ER	cPATNQc
cEGckG	RARα	cHRDKNc
cEGckG	RXR	cRDNKDc
cEGckG	TRβ	cKYEGKc
cEGckG	VDR	cPFNGDc

FIGURE 3-3 Schema of the DNA-binding domain (DBD) of the glucocorticoid receptor. The two zinc fingers are invariant between all NHRs. Interreceptor variation in P-box and D-box residues is listed for receptors for glucocorticoids (GR), mineralocorticoids (MR), progesterone (PR), androgen (AR), estrogen (ER), retinoic acid (RARα and RXR), thyroid hormone (TRβ), and vitamin D$_3$ (VDR).

ment (ERE) has been identified in genes responding to estrogen, with the sequence: 5'-AGGTCAnnnTGACCT-3'.[80] EREs are more highly conserved than GREs, and no substitutions are found in positions T1, G2, A3, C5, C−2, T−3, and A−6.[81] Receptors for androgen and progesterone recognize the same response elements as GRs, that is, DNA sequences containing TGTCCT or TGTTCT half-sites.[81] Although the three nucleotides imposed between the palindromic hexamers may be any base pairs, the presence of these three nucleotides is critical, since increasing or decreasing the spacing completely abolishes transactivation of a responsive gene.[82,83] The three nucleotides serve to position properly the NHR molecules for them to dimerize, and NHR dimerization is essential to gene transactivation, as discussed below.

The intranuclear receptors TR, RAR, and VDR activate transcription from response elements composed of ERE half-sites (i.e., TGACCT hexamers), but for these receptor response elements the EREs usually are arranged as direct repeats, not as palindromes, and are separated by a spacer region of variable length. Umesono et al.[84] have proposed a "3,4,5 rule" for predicting the binding specificity of these receptors: VDR activates transcription from a response element with three base pairs separating the direct-repeat (DR) ERE half-sites (a structure termed DR3); TR recognizes EREs with four-base pair spacers (DR4); and RAR interacts with five-base pair-spaced EREs (DR5). DR2 response elements have also been shown to mediate transactivation by RXR-RAR heterodimers.[85] The direct-repeat orientation of these response elements, in contrast to the palindromic orientation of GREs and EREs, suggests that TR, VDR, and RAR bind to DNA as asymmetric dimers in a head-to-tail configuration, unlike the symmetric head-to-head binding of the adrenal and sex steroid receptors.

Two additional fundamental differences between TR, RAR, and VDR and the other NHRs are that (1) TR, RAR, and VDR bind to their respective response elements as heterodimers with RXR (i.e., as TR-RXR, RAR-RXR, and VDR-RXR),[86-88] although certain RXR-specific ligands (e.g., 9-*cis*-retinoic acid) can induce formation of RXR-RXR homodimers that activate separate RXR homodimeric-specific genes[89] and RXR independent TR[90] and VDR[91] signaling have been reported; and (2) TR-RXR, RAR-RXR, and VDR-RXR binding to their respective response elements is independent of ligand. Based on the latter property, these heterodimers may have dual functions, serving as transcriptional activators in the presence of ligand but as gene repressors in the absence of ligand.[92] Accordingly, certain retinoids that promote RXR homodimer formation have been found to inhibit T_3-mediated effects. Treatment with such retinoids sequesters RXR molecules into homodimers, thereby limiting their availability for TR-RXR dimerization, which is necessary to transduce the T_3-stimulated response.[93]

The NHR components discriminating between GRE and ERE binding have been mapped to the N terminal of the steroid receptor DBD, in the region of the P box. The three amino acids with the P box confer specific positive and negative influences on DNA binding. The first site contains a glycine in GR (Gly[439]) and a glutamine in ER. The glutamine residue is capable of forming hydrogen bonds with the C4 cysteine in EREs,[94] but its carbonyl group exerts a negative stearic interaction with the methyl group of the T4 thymine in GREs.[81] Similarly, the valine at position 443 of the GR (versus alanine in the ER) forms a hydrophobic attraction with the methyl group of T3 in the GRE,[95] whereas its interaction is negative with A3 in the ERE.[81] Thus, Glu[439] and Val[443] exert both positive and negative interactions with the correct and incorrect response elements, respectively. In contrast, Ser[440] seems to confer GRE specificity to GRs by forming a hydrogen bond with an arginine at site 470 in the GR DBD.[95] The resultant GR DBD structure favors the overall interaction with GREs and restricts binding to EREs.[81] The importance of these P-box amino acids is illustrated in receptor mutation studies, wherein the substitution of the three P-box ER residues (i.e., Glu, Gly, and Ala) with the corresponding GR residues (Gly, Ser, and Val) results in a mutant ER receptor that transactivates GRE—but not ERE—reporter genes.[96]

The net effect of such amino acid–nucleotide interactions is the establishment of considerable DNA binding-site specificity to the DBD. The P-box sequence cGSckV (major determinants in capitals) has been shown to recognize the TGTTCT half-site of GREs whereas the sequences cEGckG, cEGckS, cEAckA, cESckG, cDGckG, and cEGckA recognize the AGGTCA half-site of EREs.[8] Since dimerization of the NHR is required to induce gene transcription, the repetition of the recognition site within the response element in either a direct or inverted orientation determines the receptor binding specificity and alignment. Accordingly, the steroid receptors (i.e., GR, ER, PR, AR, and MR) interact with palindromic response elements as symmetric homodimers,[97,98] whereas the other nuclear receptors (i.e., TR, RAR, and VDR) bind to direct repeat response elements as asymmetric heterodimers with RXR.[86-88]

NHR Dimerization

Receptor dimerization is believed to be regulated by an area in the C-terminal half of the ligand binding domain that contains leucine-rich sequences which may form coil-coil interactions as the receptor dimerizes,[99,100] similar to the leucine-zipper motifs that mediate heterodimerization of the proto-oncogene products c-Fos and c-Jun to form the transcription factor AP-1. NHR dimerization is also modulated by the D-box region within the DNA-binding domain. The role of the receptor ligand in DNA binding is not entirely clear but, at least for the adrenal and sex steroid receptors, which bind to DNA only as homodimers, it has been proposed that hormone binding induces a conformational change in the NHR that exposes the major dimerization sites in the LBD region and brings the two D boxes into approximation. Two D-box residues, Arg[479] and Asp[481], are then able to form symmetric interreceptor salt bridges, and the carbonyl oxygen of Ala[477] can form a hydrogen bond with the NH of Ile[483].[101] The subsequently dimerized receptor is capable of binding to its DNA response element with high affinity. That GR, PA, and AR bind to identical DNA response elements is at variance with the distinct effects elicited by their corresponding hormones. The specific cellular responses induced by these hormones must, therefore, be regulated by other mechanisms, including:

1. Differential expression of the receptors within the tissue
2. Varied expression or activity of metabolizing enzymes, such as 11-β-hydroxysteroid dehydrogenase, which catalyzes the conversion of active cortisol to inactive cortisone and thereby regulates the access of cortisol to both MRs and GRs
3. Positive and negative genomic interactions with other transcription factors
4. Gene-specific differences in chromatin structure around the DNA response elements

The activation of NHRs by ligand binding is termed *transformation*. As noted earlier, the adrenal and sex steroidal receptors exist in the absence of hormone as 8S to 10S heterocomplexes with various heat-shock proteins. Following hormone binding, the receptor dissociates from the heat-shock proteins and dimerizes. This dimerization confers on the receptor to ability to bind to its DNA response elements with high enough affinity ($K_d \approx 1$ nM) to transactivate target genes. Although unliganded receptors also can bind to DNA, they do so with much lower affinity and are incapable of initiating gene transcription. Once bound to a response element, the NHR dimer can couple with a second dimer or another transcription factor at an adjacent response element to create a more stable complex ($K_d \approx 0.01$ pM) capable of greater transcriptional regulation.[102] Hormone antagonists also elicit NHR dimerization and the establishment of high-affinity DNA binding. Nevertheless, the bound antagonist-associated dimer is unable to induce transcription.

Hormonal Activation of Gene Transcription

These observations, coupled with several conformational and mutagenesis studies, have led to a general model wherein the NHR exists in the absence of hormone in a conformation that masks or somehow otherwise represses one or more intrinsic activation domains (Fig. 3-4A). The association with heat-shock proteins may help maintain this otherwise unstable structure, although it should be noted that removing heat-shock proteins is not sufficient to convert a receptor from a hormone-dependent to a constitutively active molecule.[8] Agonist binding alters the conformation of the receptor, resulting in two essential changes: (1) exposure of the dimerization domains, which allows receptor dimerization and high-affinity binding to DNA to occur; and (2) removal of the inhibition of the activation domains, which enables them to activate gene transcription (Fig. 3-4B).

Antagonists have been shown to bind to different sites than agonists in GRs and PRs[103] as well as ERs.[104] It has been proposed that antagonist binding results in a different conformational change in the receptor, such that the dimerization site is exposed but the activation domains remain inhibited (Fig. 3-4C). Accordingly, antagonist-bound receptors can dimerize and bind to DNA, but they are not able to activate gene transcription.[8] In support of this model, deletion of a C-terminal inhibitory region in hPR has been shown to result in a receptor mutant that allows transactivation by the antagonist RU486[105] (Fig. 3-4D).

A variation of the above model must account for the observation that TR, RAR, RXR, VDR, and most orphan receptors are found bound to specific DNA recognition sites in the absence of ligand. These receptors do not associate with heat-shock proteins and are able to form homodimers or het-

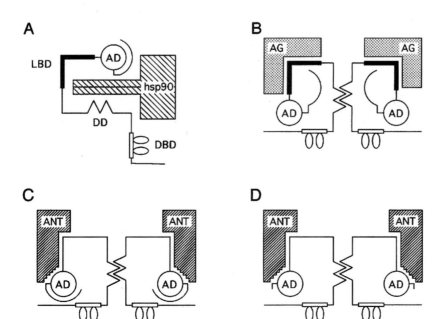

FIGURE 3-4 Conceptualization of steroid hormone receptor transformation. *A.* The unactivated NHR protein is present in a heterocomplex with hsp90 (as in Fig. 3-1). *B.* Agonist binding to the ligand-binding domain (LBD; *heavy bar*) induces a conformational change that (1) exposes the dimerization domain (DD) for NHR dimerization; (2) exposes the DNA-binding domain (DBD) for interaction with the NHR's specific DNA response elements; (3) removes an inhibitory C-terminal region from an activation domain (AD), allowing the latter to initiate gene transcription. *C.* Antagonists bind to a different region than the agonist LBD and induce a different conformational change, such that the dimerization and DNA-binding domains are exposed, but the inhibitory region is not removed from the activation domain. *D.* In a mutant receptor molecule lacking the C-terminal inhibitory region, antagonist binding results in dimerization, DNA-binding, and transactivation.

erodimers with RXR in the absence of hormone. Most likely, these unstimulated receptors exist in a conformation that constitutively exposes the dimerization domain, thereby allowing them to bind to DNA. They cannot transactivate genes without hormone, however, and so it is proposed that agonist binding induces a conformational change on the DNA-bound receptor that frees its activation domain and initiates transcription (analogous to Fig. 3-4*B*).

Regulation of Nuclear Hormone Receptors

PHOSPHORYLATION

All NHR molecules are phosphoproteins, such that when cultured cells or tissues are incubated with ^{32}P orthophosphate, NHRs are phosphorylated in the absence of ligand.[106] The addition of hormone results in receptor hyperphosphorylation, which occurs rapidly (<30 min) and is associated with receptor transformation. Antagonists do not elicit this NHR hyperphosphorylation, an observation which suggests that hormone-dependent phosphorylation contributes to the transformation of NHRs. In in vitro systems, NHRs can be phosphorylated by several kinases, including protein kinase A, protein kinase C, casein kinase II, a DNA-dependent protein kinase, serine-proline-directed kinases, and several tyrosine kinases.[106,107] Whether these enzymes also regulate NHR phosphorylation and function in vivo and, if so, how these kinases are activated following hormone binding and receptor transformation are questions that remain unanswered. Four of the seven hormone-dependent phosphorylation sites in the amino-terminal domain of GRs are in consensus sequences for the cell-cycle regulatory kinases, p34 CDC2 kinases.[108] The latter may account for some of the cell cycle–dependent changes in sensitivity to glucocorticoids reported in many systems.

The principal hormone-dependent phosphorylation sites lie within the amino-terminal portion of the GR, ER, PR, and AR; an additional site is within the hinge region of the PR. All but one of these sites in the GR are in the amino-terminal transactivation domain,[109] supporting the notion that receptor hyperphosphorylation is important to ligand-induced NHR transformation. The VDR is also phosphorylated in its hinge region, but additional sites in its LBD and DBD have been identified.[106,107] For the ER, the hormone-dependent phosphorylation sites all appear to be serine residues,[110] but a tyrosine residue within the LBD (i.e., Tyr^{537}) must be phosphorylated to allow estradiol binding. Receptors for glucocorticoids, progesterone, androgen, and vitamin D_3 are also phosphorylated on serines, and some phosphorylation of threonine residues has also been reported.[107]

Based largely on analogies to other transcription factors, the following functions have been associated with phosphorylation of NHRs:

1. Modulation of receptor association with heat-shock proteins (GR[108])
2. Activation of hormone-binding (ER[111])
3. Regulation of nuclear translocation and transporting (GR[112])
4. Subnuclear localization
5. Receptor dimerization
6. Modulation of binding to hormone response elements (ER[113] and VDR)[114]
7. Potentiation of gene transcription (ER[110])
8. Regulation of receptor turnover and recycling (GR[115])

The role of phosphorylation in NHR function remains unclear, however, since hyperphosphorylation of NHRs has not been directly linked to increased transcriptional activity. Indeed, antagonists induce similar increases in ER and PR phosphorylation but do not increase gene transactivation,[116,117] and a constitutively active PR mutant is not hyperphosphorylated.[116]

By contrast, other studies have demonstrated that agents that stimulate intracellular phosphorylation pathways can activate NHRs in the absence of ligand.[8,106,107] For example, the stable cAMP analog, 8-bromoadenosine 3',5'-cyclic monophosphate (8-bromo-cAMP), and cAMP inducers have been shown to activate the chicken PR and rat PR in a hormone-independent manner.[117-119] Similarly, dopamine, acting through D_1 receptors, can activate chicken PR and human ER in the absence of their steroid ligands.[120] Moreover, certain RTK-associated cytokines (e.g., EGF, TGFα, and IGF-1) can stimulate transcription of estrogen-responsive genes by directly activating hER.[8,117,119,121] Thus, under certain circumstances, NHRs may serve as more pleiotropic transcription factors, recruited by other cell pathways to transduce specific effects.

NHRs also are capable of interacting with other transcription factors to up- or downregulate gene transcription. The best characterized of these interactions is with the transcription factor, activator protein-1 (AP-1), which is a heterodimer of the protooncogene proteins c-Fos and c-Jun.[121] AP-1 mediates the proliferative signal induced by various protein kinase C-activating, G-protein-coupled and enzyme-linked receptors by binding to specific DNA sites (AP-1 response elements) and inducing gene transactivation. Ligand-bound TRs and RARs have been shown to interfere with activity of AP-1, while the latter is capable of inhibiting TR and RAR function. This mutual antagonism is believed to result from direct protein-protein interactions between TR/RAR and AP-1.[123] Similarly, the glucocorticoid dexamethasone has been shown to inhibit AP-1 DNA binding in human lung tissue,[124] likely through analogous GR-AP-1 protein-protein interactions.[125] In addition, longer-term dexamethasone treatment downregulated the expression of both c-fos and c-jun mRNA and the subsequent nuclear levels of c-Fos and c-Jun proteins.[124]

DEACTIVATION AND DOWNREGULATION

After it has exerted its gene-regulating effects, the activated nuclear GR appears to be recycled back to the cytoplasm, where it is deactivated.[126] The latter process may involve dephosphorylation, since a nuclear phosphatase has been shown to inactivate hormone binding to the calf uterus ER by dephosphorylating phosphotyrosine 537.[127] The dephosphorylated ER is reconverted to an estradiol-binding form by a specific calcium-calmodulin-dependent tyrosine kinase termed estrogen receptor kinase.[111] Conversely, treatment of rat fibroblasts with the phosphatase inhibitor, okadaic acid, resulted in inefficient nuclear retention of agonist-bound GRs, redistribution of the GRs into the cytoplasm, and an inability of the GRs to recycle and reenter the nucleus with persistent agonist exposure.[115]

Prolonged treatment with corticosteroids results in downregulation of GRs in most animal tissues and cell lines. Such ligand-dependent downregulation has been attributed to increased receptor protein turnover[128] as well as decreased receptor mRNA levels. In some systems, prolonged glucocorticoid exposure promotes the degradation of GR mRNA.[129] More commonly, however, the decreased mRNA levels result from hormone-dependent decreased transcription of the GR gene.[128,130] Similar effects have been observed with the rabbit PR and human ER and AR cDNAs.[131–133] The transcriptional inhibition does not seem to be mediated by a separate glucocorticoid-inducible gene product, since neither actinomycin D nor cycloheximide attenuate the downregulatory response.[129] Instead, agonist-dependent downregulation of NHR gene transcription appears to be due to specific intragenic sequences identified with the PR, hER, hAR, and hGR genes that are involved in homologous hormone-induced downregulation.[131–134] These regions do not contain sequences resembling response elements associated with genes that are positively regulated by the steroids, but it should be noted that negative GRE or ERE consensus sequences have not yet been established. The glucocorticoid receptor antagonist RU486 is equally effective as the agonist dexamethasone in inhibiting GR cDNA transcription. Although RU486 also is as effective as dexamethasone in inducing nuclear translocation of the ligand-bound GR,[129] RU486 neither stimulates transcription of positive glucocorticoid-regulated genes nor inhibits expression of the POMC gene, which is under negative GR regulation.[135] On the basis of these and related studies, it is likely that glucocorticoid-induced GR downregulation is mediated by a fundamentally different mechanism than other GR effects on gene transcription.

Conclusions

Cells utilize a number of diverse signaling pathways to respond to extracellular stimuli. Several pathways transduce short-term, reactive responses through the generation of second messengers and modulation of intracellularion concentrations. Other responses are more intermediate to long-term in nature, and involve cellular proliferation, differentiation, and/or protein synthesis. The nuclear hormone receptors are unique signaling molecules in that they are capable of relaying directly extracelluar stimuli to intranuclear response sites. Nevertheless, there are large gaps in the understanding of how this process is accomplished. Somehow, fairly ubiquitous receptors sharing common signal transduction systems must mediate the specific tissue- and development-dependent responses to these hormones.

Moreover, interactions between NHR-mediated and other cell-signaling pathways are just beginning to be discerned. It has been noted how several kinases, some of which are activated by G-protein-coupled and enzyme-linked receptor signaling systems, can phosphorylate steroid receptor proteins, leading to altered function or even ligand-independent activation of the NHRs. On the other hand, glucocorticoids, in addition to promoting fetal lung maturation, are capable of modulating the expression and subsequent related responses of many important regulatory proteins in the lung, including receptors (e.g., β-adrenergic,[136] neurokinin 1,[137] and vasopressin receptors[138]), ion channels (e.g., amiloride-sensitive Na^+ channel[139]) ion pumps (e.g., Na^+,K^+-ATPase[140]), growth factors (e.g., epidermal growth factor,[141] tumor necrosis factor-α,[142] and transforming growth factor-β1[143]), and key regulatory enzymes (e.g., neutral endopeptidase[144] and fatty acid synthetase[145]). Accordingly, activation of nuclear hormone receptors can influence markedly many other receptor signaling pathways in the lung. Further understanding of the interplay between these systems and their cross-regulatory mechanisms will provide new fundamental insights into lung development and the pathophysiology and therapy of lung disease.

References

1. Evans RM: The steroid and thyroid hormone superfamily. *Science (Wash DC)* 1988; 240:889.
2. Giannopoulos G: Variations in the levels of cytoplasmic glucocorticoid receptors in lungs of various species at different developmental stages. *Endocrinology* 1973; 94:450.
3. Chang WC, Roth GO: Changes in the mechanisms of steroid action during aging. *J Steroid Biochem* 1979; 11:889.
4. Cidlowski JA, Michaels GA: Alteration in glucocorticoid receptor binding site number during the cell cycle in HeLa cells. *Nature (Lond)* 1977; 266:643.
5. Rao GO: Mode of entry of steroid and thyroid hormones into cells. *Mol Cell Endocrin* 1981; 21:97.
6. O'Malley BW: Editorial: Did eukaryotic steroid receptors evolve from intracrine gene regulators? *Endocrinology* 1989; 125:1119.
7. Freedman LP, Luisi BF, Korszun ZR, et al.: The function and structure of the metal coordination sites within the glucocorticoid receptor DNA binding domain. *Nature (Lond)* 1988; 334:543.
8. Tsai M-J, O'Malley BW: Molecular mechanisms of action of steroid/thyroid receptor superfamily members. *Ann Rev Biochem* 1994; 63:451.
9. Fuller PJ: The steroid receptor superfamily: Mechanisms of diversity. *FASEB J* 1991; 5:3092.
10. Godowski PJ, Rusconi S, Miesfeld S, Yamamoto KR: Glucocorticoid receptor mutants are constitutive activators of transcriptional enhancement. *Nature (Lond)* 1987; 325:365.
11. Rusconi S, Yamamoto KR: Functional dissection of the hormone and DNA binding activities of the glucocorticoid receptor. *EMBO J* 1987; 6:1309–1315.
12. Picard D, Yamamoto KR: Two signals mediate hormone-dependent nuclear localization of the glucocorticoid receptor. *EMBO J* 1987; 6:3333.
13. Akner G, Wilkstrom AC, Mossberg K, et al.: Morphometric studies of the localization of the glucocorticoid receptor in mammalian cells and of glucocorticoid hormone-induced effects. *J Histochem Cytochem* 1994; 42:645.

14. Pratt WB, Scherrer LC: Heat shock proteins and the cytoplasmic-nuclear trafficking of steroid receptors, in Moudgil (ed): *Steroid Hormone Receptors.* Boston, Birkhäuser, 1993: 215–246.

15. Guiochon-Mantel A, Loosfelt H, Lescop P, et al.: Mechanisms of nuclear localization of the progesterone receptor: Evidence for interaction between monomers. *Cell* 1989; 57:1147.

16. Picard D, Kumar V, Chambon P, Yamamoto KR: Signal transduction by steroid hormones: Nuclear localization is differentially regulated in estrogen and glucocorticoid receptors. *Cell Regul* 1990; 1:291.

17. Simental JA, Sar M, Lane MV, et al.: Transcriptional activation and nuclear targeting signals of the human androgen receptor. *J Biol Chem* 1991; 266:510.

18. Tora L, Gronemeyer H, Turcotte B, Gaub M-P, Chambon P: The *N*-terminal region of the chicken progesterone receptor specifies target gene activation. *Nature (Lond)* 1988; 333:185–188.

19. Mitchell PJ, Tijan R: Transcriptional regulation in mammalian cells by sequence-specific DNA binding proteins. *Science (Wash DC)* 1989; 348:458.

20. Allan GF, Leng X, Tsai SY, et al.: Hormone and antihormone induce distinct conformational changes which are central to steroid receptor activation. *J Biol Chem* 1991; 267:19513.

21. Hollenberg SM, Weinberger C, Ong ES, et al.: Primary structure and expression of a functional human glucocorticoid receptor cDNA. *Nature (Lond)* 1985; 318:635.

22. Kastner P, Krust A, Turcotte B, et al.: Two distinct estrogen-regulated promoters generate transcripts encoding the two functionally different human progesterone forms A and B. *EMBO J* 1990; 9:1603.

23. de The H, Marchio A, Tiollais P, Dejean A: Differential expression and ligand regulation of the retinoic acid receptor α and β genes. *EMBO J* 1989; 8:429.

24. Sakurai A, Taheda K, Ain K, et al.: Generalized resistance to thyroid hormone associated with a mutation in the ligand-binding domain of the human thyroid receptor β. *Proc Natl Acad Sci USA* 1989; 86:8977.

25. Usala SJ, Tennyson GE, Bale AE, Lash RW, Gesundheit N, Wondisford FE, Accili D, Hauser P, Weintraub BD: A base mutation of the c-erbA β thyroid hormone receptor in a kindred with generalized thyroid hormone resistance. *J Clin Invest* 1990; 85:93.

26. Giguére V, Shago M, Zirngibl R, Tate P, Rossant J, Varmuza S: Identification of a novel isoform of the retinoic acid receptor γ expressed in the mouse embryo. *Mol Cell Biol* 1990; 10:2335.

27. Mangelsdorf DJ, Ong ES, Dyck JA, Evans RM: Nuclear receptor that identifies a novel retinoic acid response pathway. *Nature (Lond)* 1990; 345:224.

28. Kastner PL, Krust A, Mendelsohn C, et al.: Murine isoforms of retinoic acid receptor γ with specific patterns of expressions. *Proc Natl Acad Sci USA* 1990; 87:2700.

29. Wahli W, Martinez E: Superfamily of steroid nuclear receptors: Positive and negative regulators of gene expression. *FASEB J* 1991; 5:2243.

30. Koenig RJ, Lazar MA, Hodin RA, et al.: Inhibition of thyroid hormone action by a non-hormone binding c-erbA protein generated by alternative mRNA splicing. *Nature (Lond)* 1989; 337:659–661.

31. Lazar MA, Hodin RA, Cardona G, Chin WW: Gene expression from the c-erbAα/Rev-erbAα genomic locus. *J Biol Chem* 1990; 265:12859.

32. Spindler SR, MacLeod KM, Ring J, Baxter JD: Thyroid hormone receptors: Binding characteristics and lack of hormonal dependency for nuclear localization. *J Biol Chem* 1975; 250:4113.

33. Nervi C, Grippo JF, Sherman MI, et al.: Identification and characterization of nuclear retinoic acid binding activity in human myeloblastic leukemia HL-60 cells. *Proc Natl Acad Sci USA* 1989; 86:5854.

34. Guiochon-Mantel A, Lescop P, Christin-Maitre S, et al.: Nucleocytoplasmatic shuttling of the progesterone receptor. *EMBO J* 1991; 10:3851.

35. Papamichail M, Tsokos G, Tsawdaroglou N, Sekeris CE: Immunochemical demonstration of glucocorticoid receptors in different cell types and their translocation from the cytoplasm to the cell nucleus in the presence of dexamethasone. *Exp Cell Res* 1980; 125:490.

36. Wikstrom AC, Bakke O, Okret S, et al.: Intracellular localization of the glucocorticoid receptor: Evidence for cytoplasmic and nuclear localization. *Endocrinology* 1987; 120:1232.

37. Pratt WB: Role of heat-shock proteins in steroid receptor function, in Parker MG (ed): *Steroid Hormone Action.* Oxford, IRL Press, 1993:64–93.

38. Perdew GH, Whitelaw ML: Evidence that the 90-kDa heat shock protein (hsp90) exists in cytosol in heteromeric complexes containing hsp70 and three other proteins with M_r 63,000, 56,000, and 50,000. *J Biol Chem* 1991; 266:6708.

39. Minami Y, Kawasake H, Miyata Y, et al.: Analysis of native forms and isoform compositions of the mouse 90-kDa heat shock protein, hsp90. *J Biol Chem* 1991; 266:10099.

40. Lefebvre P, Sablonniere B, Tbarka N, et al.: Study of the heteromeric structure of the untransformed glucocorticoid receptor using chemical cross-linking and monoclonal antibodies against the 90K heat-shock protein. *Biochem Biophy Res Commun* 1989; 159:667.

41. Mendel DB, Orti E: Isoform composition and stoichiometry of the ~90-kDa heat shock protein associated with glucocorticoid receptors. *J Biol Chem* 1988; 263:6695.

42. Bresnick EH, Dalman FC, Pratt WB: Direct stoichiometric evidence that the untransformed M_r 300,000, 9S, glucocorticoid receptor is a core unit derived from a larger heteromeric complex. *Biochemistry* 1990; 29:520.

43. Danielsen M, Northrop JP, Ringold GM: The mouse glucocorticoid receptor: Mapping of functional domains by cloning, sequencing and expression of wilt-type and mutant receptor proteins. *EMBO J* 1986; 5:2513.

44. Dalman FC, Koenig RJ, Perdew GH, et al.: In contrast to the glucocorticoid receptor, the thyroid receptor is translated in the DNA-binding state and is not associated with hsp90. *J Biol Chem* 1990; 265:3615.

45. Dalman FC, Sturzenbecker LJ, Levin AA, et al.: The retinoic acid receptor belongs to a subclass of nuclear receptors that do not form 'docking' complexes with hsp90. *Biochemistry* 1991; 30:5605.

46. Housley PR, Sanchez ER, Danielsen M, et al.: Evidence that the conserved region in the steroid binding domain of the glucocorticoid receptor is required for both optimal binding of hsp90 and protection from proteolytic cleavage. A two-site model for hsp90 binding to the steroid binding domain. *J Biol Chem* 1990; 265:12778.

47. Schowalter DB, Sullivan WP, Maihle NJ, et al.: Characterization of progesterone receptor binding to the 90- and 70-kDa heat shock proteins. *J Biol Chem* 1991; 266:21165.

48. Bresnick EH, Dalman FC, Sanchez ER, Pratt WB: Evidence that the 90-kDa heat shock protein is necessary for the steroid binding conformation of the L cell glucocorticoid receptor. *J Biol Chem* 1989; 265:4992.

49. Denis M, Gustafsson J-A: The Mr = 90,000 heat shock protein, an important modulator of ligand and DNA-binding properties of the glucocorticoid receptor. *Cancer Res* 1989; *Suppl* 49:2275s.

50. Lebeau M-C, Binart N, Cadepond F, et al.: Steroid receptor associated proteins: Heat shock protein 90 and p59 immunophilin,

in Moudgil VK (ed): *Steroid Hormone Receptors.* Boston, Birkhäuser, 1993:261.

51. Koyasu S, Nishida E, Kadowaki T, et al.: Two mammalian heat shock proteins, hsp90 and hsp100, are actin-binding proteins. *Proc Natl Acad Sci USA* 1986; 83:8054.

52. Redmond T, Sanchez ER, Bresnick EH, et al.: Immunofluorescence colocalization of the 90-kDa heat shock protein and microtubules in interphase and mitotic mammalian cells. *Eur J Cell Biol* 1989; 50:66.

53. Smith DF, Stensgard BA, Welch WJ, Toft DO: Assembly of progesterone receptor with heat shock proteins and receptor activation are ATP mediated events. *J Biol Chem* 1992; 267:1350.

54. Sanchez ER, Hirst M, Scherrer LC, et al.: Hormone-free mouse glucocorticoid receptors overexpressed in Chinese hamster ovary cells are localized to the nucleus and are associated with both hsp70 and hsp90. *J Biol Chem* 1990; 265:20123.

55. Kost SL, Smith DF, Sullivan WP, et al.: Binding of heat shock proteins to the avian progesterone receptor. *Mol Cell Biol* 1989; 9:3829.

56. Onate SA, Estes PA, Welch WJ, et al.: Evidence that heatshock protein-70 associated with progesterone receptors is not involved in receptor-DNA binding. *Mol Endocrinol* 1991; 5:1993.

57. Rexin M, Busch W, Gehring U: Protein components of the non-activated glucocorticoid receptor. *J Biol Chem* 1991; 266:24601.

58. Alexis MN, Mavridou I, Mitsiou DJ: Subunit composition of the untransformed glucocorticoid receptor in the cytosol and in the cell. *Eur J Biochem* 1992; 204:75.

59. Rothman JE: Popypeptide chain binding proteins: Catalysts of protein folding and related processes in cells. *Cell* 1989; 59:591.

60. Smith DF, Toft DO: Steroid receptors and their associated proteins. *Mol Endocrinol* 1993; 7:4.

61. Hutchinson KA, Czar MJ, Scherrer LC, Pratt WB: Monovalent cation selectivity for ATP-dependent association of the glucocorticoid receptor with hsp70 and hsp90. *J Biol Chem* 1992; 267:14047.

62. Perrot-Applanat M, Logeat F, Groyer-Picard MT, Milgrom E: Immunocytochemical study of mammalian progesterone receptor using monoclonal antibodies. *Endocrinology* 1985; 116:1473.

63. Schreiber SL: Chemistry and biology of the immunophilins and their immunosuppressive ligands. *Science (Wash DC)* 1991; 251:283.

64. Yem AW, Tomasselli AG, Heinrikson RL, et al.: The hsp56 component of steroid receptor complexes binds to immobilized FK506 and shows homology to FKBP-12 and FKBP-13. *J Biol Chem* 1992; 267:2868.

65. Tai PK, Maeda Y, Nakao K, et al.: A 59-kilodalton protein associated with progestin, estrogen, androgen, and glucocorticoid receptors. *Biochemistry* 1986; 25:5269.

66. Renoir JM, Radanyi C, Faber LE, Baulieu EE: The non-DNA-binding heterooligomeric form of mammalian steroid hormone receptors contains a hsp90-bound 59-kilodalton protein. *J Biol Chem* 1990; 265:10740.

67. Smith DF, Faber LE, Toft DO: Purification of unactivated progesterone receptor and identification of novel receptor-associated proteins. *J Biol Chem* 1990; 265:3996.

68. Sanchez ER, Faber LE, Henzel WJ, Pratt WB: The 56-59 kilodalton protein identified in untransformed steroid receptor complexes is a unique protein that exists in cytosol in a complex with both the 70- and 90-kilodalton heat shock proteins. *Biochemistry* 1990; 29:5145.

69. Johnson JL, Toft DO: A novel chaperone complex for steroid receptors involving heat shock protein, immunophilins and p23. *J Biol Chem* 1994; 269:24989.

70. Pratt WB, Hutchinson KL, Scherrer LC: Steroid receptor folding by heat shock proteins and composition of the receptor heterocomplex. *Trends Endocrinol Metab* 1992; 3:326.

71. Picard D, Salser SJ, Yamamoto KR: A movable and regulable inactivation function within the steroid binding domain of the glucocorticoid receptor. *Cell* 1988; 54:1073,

72. Wrange O, Gustafsson J-Å: Separation of the hormone- and DNA-binding sites of the hepatic glucocorticoid receptor by means of proteolysis. *J Biol Chem* 1978; 253:856.

73. Miller J, McLachlan AD, Klug A: Repetitive zinc-binding domains in the protein transcription factor IIIA from Xenopus oocytes. *EMBO J* 1985; 4:1609.

74. Berg J: Zinc fingers and other metal-binding domains. *J Biol Chem* 1990; 265:6513.

75. Marmomstein R, Carey M, Ptashne M, Harrison SC: DNA recognition by GAL4: Structure of a protein-DNA complex. *Nature (Lond)* 1992; 356:408.

76. Hard T, Kellenbach E, Boelens R, et al.: ^{1}H-NMR studies of the glucocorticoid receptor DNA-binding domain: Sequential assignments and identification of secondary structure elements. *Biochemistry* 1990; 29:9015.

77. Schwabe JWR, Neuhaus D, Rhodes D: Solution structure of the DNA binding domain of the oestrogen receptor. *Nature (Lond)* 1990; 348:458.

78. Strähle U, Klock G, Schütz G: A DnA sequence of 15 base pairs is sufficient to mediate both glucocorticoid and progesterone induction of gene expression. *Proc Natl Acad Sci USA* 1987; 84:7871.

79. Beato M, Chalepakis G, Schauer M, Slater EP: DNA regulatory elements for steroid hormones. *J Steroid Biochem* 1989; 32:737.

80. Walker P, Germond JE, Brown-Luedi M, et al.: Sequence homologies in the region preceding the transcription initiation site of the liver estrogen-responsive vitellogenin and apo- VLDLII genes. *Nucleic Acids Res* 1984; 12:8611.

81. Zilliacus J, Wright APH, Carlstedt-Duke J, Gustafsson J-Å. Structural determinants of DNA-binding specificity by steroid receptors. *Mol Endocrinol* 1995; 9:389.

82. Dahlman-Wright K, Siltata-Roos H, Carlstedt-Duke J, Gustafsson J-Å: Protein-protein interactions facilitate DNA binding by the glucocorticoid receptor DNA binding domain. *J Biol Chem* 1990; 265:14030.

83. Nordeen SK, Suh BJ, Kuhnel B, Hutchinson CA: Structural determinants of a glucocorticoid receptor recognition element. *Mol Endocrinol* 1990; 4:1866.

84. Umesono K, Murakami KK, Thompson CC, Evans RM: Direct repeats as selective response elements for the thyroid hormone, retinoic acid, and vitamin D_3 receptors. *Cell* 1991; 65:1255.

85. Giguére V: Retinoic acid receptors and cellular retinoid binding proteins: Complex interplay in retinoid signaling. *Endocr Rev* 1994; 15:61.

86. Yu VC, Delsert C, Andersen B, et al.: RXRβ: A coregulator that enhances binding of retinoic acid, thyroid hormone, and vitamin D receptors to their cognate response elements. *Cell* 1991; 67:1251.

87. Kliewer SA, Umesono K, Mangelsdorf DJ, Evans RM: Retinoid X receptor interacts with nuclear receptors in retinoic acid, thyroid hormone and vitamin D_3 signalling. *Nature* 1992; 355:446.

88. Hermann T, Hoffmann B, Zhang X-K, et al.: Heterodimeric receptor complexes determine 3,5,3'-triiodothyronine and retinoid signaling specificities. *Mol Endocrinol* 1992; 6:1153.

89. Lehmann JM, Jong L, Fanjul A, et al.: Retinoids selective for retinoid X receptor response pathways. *Science (Wash DC)* 1992; 258:1944.

90. Hallenbeck PL, Marks MS, Lippoldt RE, et al.: Heterodimerization of thyroid hormone (TH) receptor with H-2RIIBP (RXRβ) enhances DNA binding and TH-dependent transcriptional activation. *Proc Natl Acad Sci USA* 1992; 89:5572.

91. Carlberg C, Bendik I, Wyss A, et al.: Two nuclear signaling pathways for vitamin D. *Nature (Lond)* 1993; 361:657.

92. Graupner G, Willis KN, Tzukerman M, et al.: Dual regulatory role for thyroid-hormone receptors allows control of retinoic-acid receptor activity. *Nature (Lond)* 1989; 340:653.

93. Lehmann JM, Zhang X-K, Graupner G, Hermann T, Hoffmann B, Pfahl M: Formation of RXR homodimers leads to repression of T₃ response: Hormonal cross-talk by ligand induced squelching. *Mol Cell Biol* 1993; 13:7698.

94. Schwabe JW, Chapman L, Finch JT, Rhodes D: The crystal structure of the estrogen receptor DNA-binding domain bound to DNA: How receptors discriminate between their response elements. *Cell* 1993; 75:567.

95. Luisi BF, Xu WX, Otwinowski Z, et al.: Crystallographic analysis of the interaction of the glucocorticoid receptor with DNA. *Nature (Lond)* 1991; 352:497.

96. Mader S, Kumar V, de Verneuil H, Chambon P: Three amino acids of the oestrogen receptor are essential to its ability to distinguish an oestrogen from a glucocorticoid-responsive element. *Nature (Lond)* 1989; 338:271.

97. Tsai SY, Carlstedt-Duke J, Weigel NL, et al.: Molecular interactions of steroid hormone receptor with its enhancer element: Evidence for receptor dimer formation. *Cell* 1988; 55: 361.

98. Chalepakis G, Schauer M, Cao XA, Beato M: Efficient binding of glucocorticoid receptor to its responsive element requires a dimer and DNA flanking sequences. *DNA Cell Biol* 1990; 9:355.

99. Fawell SE, Lees JA, White R, Parker MG: Characterization and colocalization of steroid binding and dimerization activities in the mouse estrogen receptor. *Cell* 1990; 60:953.

100. Forman BM, Samuels HH: Interaction among a subfamily of nuclear hormone receptors: The regulatory zipper model. *Mol Endocrinol* 1990; 4:1293.

101. Freedman LP: Structure and function of the steroid receptor zinc finger region, in Parker MG (ed): *Steroid Hormone Action*, Oxford, IRL Press, 1993:141–165.

102. Tsai SY, Tsai M-J, O'Malley BW: Cooperative binding of steroid hormone receptors contributes to transcriptional synergism at target enhancer elements. *Cell* 1989; 57:443.

103. Benhamou B, Garcia T, Lerouge T, et al.: A single amino acid that determines the sensitivity of progesterone receptors to RU486. *Science (Wash DC)* 1992; 255:206.

104. Pakdel F, Katzenellenbogen BS: Human estrogen receptor mutants with altered estrogen and antiestrogen ligand discrimination. *J Biol Chem* 1992; 267:3429.

105. Vegeto E, Allan GF, Schrader WT, et al.: RU486 antagonism is dependent on the conformation of the carboxy-terminal tail of the human progesterone receptor. *Cell* 1992; 69:703.

106. Orti E, Bodwell JE, Munck A: Phosphorylation of steroid hormone receptors. *Endo Rev* 1992; 13:105.

107. Kuiper GGJM, Brinkman AO: Steroid hormone receptor phosphorylation: Is there a physiological role? *Mol Cell Endocrinol* 1994; 100:103.

108. Bodwell JE, Hu LM, Hu JM, et al.: Glucocorticoid receptors: ATP-dependent cycling and hormone-dependent hyperphosphorylation. *J Steroid Biochem Mol Biol* 1993; 43:31.

109. Bodwell JE, Orti E, Coull JM, et al.: Identification of phosphorylated sites in the mouse glucocorticoid receptor. *J Biol Chem* 1991; 266:7549.

110. Ali S, Metzger D, Bornert JM, Chambon P: Modulation of transcriptional activation by ligand-dependent phosphorylation of the human oestrogen receptor A/B region. *EMBO J* 1993; 12:1153.

111. Castoria G, Migliaccio A, Green S, et al.: Properties of a purified estradiol-dependent calf uterus tyrosine kinase. *Biochemistry* 1993; 32:1740.

112. Orti E, Hu L-M, Munck A: Kinetics of glucocorticoid receptor phosphorylation in intact cells. Evidence for hormone-induced hyperphosphorylation after activation and recycling of hyper-phosphorylated receptors. *J Biol Chem* 1993; 268:7779.

113. Denton RR, Koszewski NJ, Notides AC: Estrogen receptor phosphorylation. Hormonal dependence and consequence on specific DNA binding. *J Biol Chem* 1992; 267:7263.

114. Hsieh JC, Jurutka PW, Nakajima S, et al.: Phosphorylation of the human vitamin D receptor by protein kinase C. *J Biol Chem* 1993; 268:15118.

115. DeFranco DB, Qi M, Borror KC, et al.: Protein phosphatase types 1 and/or 2A regulate nucleocytoplasmic shuttling of glucocorticoid receptors. *Mol Endocrinol* 1991; 5:1215.

116. Chauchereau A, Loosfelt H, Milgrom E: Phosphorylation of transfected wild type and mutated progesterone receptors. *J Biol Chem* 1991; 226:18280.

117. Aronica SM, Katzenellenbogen BS: Stimulation of estrogen receptor-mediated transcription and alteration in the phosphorylation state of the rat uterine estrogen receptor by estrogen, cyclic adenosine monophosphate, and insulin-like growth factor-I. *Mol Endocrinol* 1993; 7:743.

118. Denner LA, Weigel NL, Maxwell BL, et al.: Regulation of progesterone receptor-mediated transcription by phosphorylation. *Science (Wash DC)* 1990; 250:1740.

119. Zhang Y, Bai W, Allgood VE, Weigel NL: Multiple signaling pathways activate the chicken progesterone receptor. *Mol Endocrinol* 1994; 8:577.

120. Power RF, Mani SK, Codina J, et al.: Dopaminergic and ligand-independent activation of steroid hormone receptors. *Science (Wash DC)* 1991; 254:1636.

121. Ignar-Trowbridge DM, Teng CT, Ross KA, et al.: Peptide growth factors elicit estrogen receptor-dependent transcriptional activation of an estrogen-responsive element. *Mol Endocrinol* 1993; 7:992.

122. Ransome LJ, Verma IM: Nuclear proto-oncogenes Fos and Jun. *Ann Rev Cell Biol* 1991; 6:539.

123. Pfahl M: Molecular mechanisms of thyroid hormone and retinoid acid action, in Moudgil VK (ed): *Steroid Hormone Receptors*, Boston, Birhäuser, 1993:197–211.

124. Adcock IM, Brown CR, Shirasake H, Barnes PJ: Effects of dexamethasone on cytokine and phorbol ester stimulated c-Fos and c-Jun DNA binding and gene expression in human lung. *Eur Respir J* 1994; 7:2117.

125. Yang-Yen H-F, Chambard J-C, Sun Y-L, Smeal T, Schmidt TJ, Drouin J, Karin M: Transcriptional interference between c-Jun and the glucocorticoid receptor: Mutual inhibition of DNA binding due to direct protein-protein interaction. *Cell* 1990; 62:1205.

126. Ichii S, Yoshida A: Effect of colchicine on the depletion and replenishment of cytoplasmic glucocorticoid receptor in rat liver after administration of glucocorticoid. *Endocrinol Japon* 1985; 32:225.

127. Auricchio F: Phosphorylation of steroid receptors. *J Steroid Biochem* 1989; 32:613.

128. Dong Y, Poellinger L, Gustafsson J-Å, Okret S: Regulation of glucocorticoid receptor expression: Evidence for transcriptional and post-transcriptional mechanism. *Mol Endocrinol* 1988; 2:1256.

129. Burnstein KL, Jewell CM, Sar M, Cidlowski JA: Intragenic sequences of the human glucocorticoid receptor complementary DNA mediate hormone-inducible receptor messenger RNA down-regulation through multiple mechanisms. *Mol Endo* 1994; 8:1764.

130. Rosewicz S, McDonald AR, Maddux BA, et al.: Mechanism of glucocorticoid receptor down regulation by glucocorticoids. *J Biol Chem* 1988; 263:2581.

131. Savouret JF, Bailey A, Misrahi M, et al.: Characterization of the

hormone response element involved in the regulation of the progesterone receptor. *EMBO J* 1991; 10:1875.

132. Kaneko KJ, Furlow JD, Gorski J: Involvement of the coding sequence for the estrogen receptor gene in autologous ligand-dependent down-regulation. *Mol Endocrinol* 1993; 7:879.

133. Burnstein KL, Maiorino CA, Cameron DJ: Sequences present within the human androgen receptor cDNA confer ligand-inducible receptor mRNA down regulation. *J Cell Biochem* 1994; 18B(suppl):K206 (abstract).

134. Alksnis M, Barkhem T, Stromstedt P-E, et al.: High level expression of functional full length and truncated glucocorticoid receptor in Chinese hamster ovary cells. *J Biol Chem* 1991; 264:14601.

135. Drouin J, Trifiro MA, Plante RK, et al.: Glucocorticoid receptor binding to a specific DNA sequence is required for hormone dependent repression of proopiomelanocortin gene transcription. *Mol Cell Biol* 1989; 9:5314.

136. Verbeeck MA, Sutanto W, Burbach JP: Regulation of vasopressin messenger RNA levels in the small cell lung carcinoma cell line GLC-8: Interactions between glucocorticoids and second messengers. *Mol Endocrin* 1991; 5:795.

137. Adcock IM, Peters M, Gelder C, et al.: Increased tachykinin receptor gene expression in asthmatic lung and its modulation by steroids. *J Mol Endocrinol* 1993; 11:1.

138. Mak JC, Nishikawa M, Barnes PF: Glucocorticosteroids increase beta 2-adrenergic receptor transcription in human lung. *Am J Physiol* 1995; 268:L41.

139. Champigny G, Voilley N, Lingueglia E, et al.: Regulation of expression of the lung amiloride-sensitive Na^+ channel by steroid hormones. *EMBO J* 1994; 13:2177.

140. Celsi G, Wang ZM, Akusjarvi G, Aperia A: Sensitive periods for glucocorticoids' regulation of $Na^+,K^{(+)}$-ATPase mRNA in the developing lung and kidney. *Pediatr Res* 1993; 33:5.

141. Oberg KC, Carpenter G: Dexamethasone and retinoic acid regulate the expression of epidermal growth factor receptor mRNA by distinct mechanisms. *J Cell Physiol* 1991; 149:244.

142. Jaskoll T, Boyer PD, Melnick M: Tumor necrosis factor-α and embryonic mouse lung morphogenesis. *Develop Dynamics* 1994; 201:137.

143. Shull S, Meisler N, Absher M, Phan S, Cutroneo K: Glucocorticoid-induced down regulation of transforming growth factor-β1 in adult rat lung fibroblasts. *Lung* 1995; 173:71.

144. Borson DB, Gruenert DC: Glucocorticoids induce neutral endopeptidase in transformed human tracheal epithelial cells. *Am J Physiol* 1991; 260:L83.

145. Gonzales LW, Ballard PL, Gonzales J: Glucocortocoid and cAMP increase fatty acid synthetase mRNA in human fetal lung explants. *Biochim Biophys Acta* 1994; 1215:49.

Chapter 4

CELL-TO-CELL INTERACTION: AN OVERVIEW

MARC B. HERSHENSON

Ephedrine in a crude state has been used in Chinese medicine for thousands of years.[1] Nevertheless, it may be asserted that pulmonary pharmacology as currently conceived originated at the turn of the century, with the elucidation of the chemical structure of the suprarenal extract epinephrine.[2] First recognized as a vasopressor, epinephrine was soon demonstrated to have bronchodilator effects both in vivo and in vitro.[3] Interestingly, the use of adrenal extracts for the treatment of asthma was first advocated in 1898, before the bronchodilator properties of the drug were characterized.[4] By the 1920s, epinephrine had become the most commonly used and efficacious medication for the treatment of asthma.[4]

At about that time, Dale and Laidlaw[5] investigated the physiologic effects of the ergot extract β-iminazolylethylamine. On administering this drug to animals, the investigators recorded an intense vasodepressor action, as well as "the acute obstruction of air entry," which they attributed to "bronchial spasm." Furthermore, Dale and Laidlaw noted the similarity between the effects of β-iminazolylethylamine

and those of various tissue extracts, which previously had been demonstrated by Popielski to produce profound hypotension when injected intravenously.[5] However, it was not until 1927 that this substance, later renamed *histamine* for its apparent presence in a variety of tissue extracts, was demonstrated exclusively to occur naturally in the lung.[6] Histamine soon was implicated in the pathogenesis of anaphylaxis[7]; 10 years later, the first "anti-histamines" were developed.[8]

Thus, the science and practice of pulmonary pharmacology and therapeutics evolved by means of strong interactions between pharmacologists, physiologists, and physicians. In a more recent example, Clements[9] demonstrated the presence of a surface-tension–lowering substance in lung extracts. Almost concurrently, it was argued by Mead and Collier[10] that surface forces operating at the gas-liquid interface in the lungs might be responsible for the major part of the volume-pressure hysteresis. Avery and Mead[11] further asserted that the loss of "surfactant" might be responsible for the respiratory distress syndrome of premature infants.

Shortly thereafter, dipalmitoylphosphatidylcholine was identified as the most active principle in surfactant.[12] Today, surfactant preparations are used widely in the treatment of premature infants with respiratory distress syndrome.

In recent years, neurotransmitters, neuropeptides, eicosanoids, cytokines, growth factors, and other novel substances have been isolated from the lung tissue of animals and humans. With each discovery, there arises the hope that the new agents or their antagonists will be useful in the treatment of pulmonary diseases. This chapter surveys the cellular sources of these substances and the interactions between these cell types.

Target Cells

The clear characterization of cell-to-cell interactions requires the identification of the target cells, that is, the cell types whose function is influenced by signals (neurotransmitters, hormones, cytokines, eicosinoids, growth factors, etc.) originating from other cells. It may be argued, for example, that the airway myocyte is the principal target cell in the tracheobronchial tree. Airway myocytes are targets of intercellular signals from neurons, epithelial cells, eosinophils, and other cell types. Transduction of these intercellular signals leads to smooth muscle contraction or relaxation, depending on the stimulus. Some intercellular signals also may promote the growth of airway smooth muscle. This elementary portrayal of airway cell-to-cell interactions underestimates the intricacy of such interactions, however. There are instances in which multiple, contradictory signals originate from the same source; in which transmission from one cell type to the target cell requires the presence of a third cell type; and in which a given cell type serves as both the recipient and the initiator of intercellular signals. Examples of these phenomena follow. Of course, more complete discussions of specific pulmonary cell types and their interactions are to be found in later chapters of this book.

A Survey of Cell-to-Cell Interactions in the Airways

INTERACTIONS BETWEEN NEURONS AND MYOCYTES: NEUROTRANSMITTERS

Airway caliber depends in large part on the contractile state of airway myocytes. Airway myocytes are directly innervated by (1) efferent parasympathetic postganglionic fibers (cholinergic fibers), and (2) afferent capsaicin-sensitive sensory nerves (C fibers). In addition, sympathetic nerves influence airway tone by altering cholinergic neurotransmission via prejunctional β receptors on postganglionic neurons.[13] Parasympathetic innervation is mediated by the neurotransmitter acetylcholine and is excitatory in nature (i.e., it induces smooth muscle contraction). Stimulation of prejunctional β₂-adrenergic receptors by epinephrine inhibits cholinergic neurotransmission. Sensory nerve stimulation,

which follows chemical or physical irritation of the airways, results in the antidromic release of tachykinins (primarily substance P and neurokinin A), leading to bronchoconstriction.[14]

In recent years, it has been demonstrated that electrical stimulation of airway nerves may result in responses that are not blocked by either anticholinergic agents or β-adrenergic receptor antagonists; these nonadrenergic, noncholinergic (NANC) responses are mediated in part by sensory C fibers (see above). Other, inhibitory NANC responses may be mediated by parasympathetic postganglionic fibers.[15] The neurotransmitters involved remain unclear; vasoactive intestinal peptide[16] and nitric oxide[17] are likely candidates (Fig. 4-1). Interestingly, there is some evidence that these NANC neurotransmitters, which inhibit smooth muscle contraction, may be cotransmitted with acetylcholine from the same postganglionic nerve fiber.[15,18] Cotransmission of excitatory and inhibitory substances might fine-tune or brake excessive airway constrictor responses.

Although increased cholinergic tone has been hypothesized to play a pathogenetic role in asthma, evidence for this proposition is lacking. However, sensory nerve stimulation, with consequent release of tachykinins, is thought to contribute to hyperpnea and irritant-induced asthma.[14]

INTERACTIONS BETWEEN ADRENAL MEDULLARY CHROMAFFIN CELLS AND MYOCYTES: EPINEPHRINE

Circulating epinephrine released by the adrenal medulla may inhibit airway smooth muscle contraction by modulation of parasympathetic postganglionic nerves (see above). Plasma epinephrine levels are not increased in patients with asthma, however, suggesting that epinephrine release is unlikely to be an important defense against bronchoconstriction.

FIGURE 4-1 Nitric oxide is responsible for nonadrenergic, noncholinergic (i-NANC) relaxation in human airway smooth muscle. Electrical field stimulation of human lower tracheal segments pretreated with atropine and propranolol induced relaxation which was inhibited by L-N^G-nitroarginine methyl ester (L-NAME), an inhibitor of nitric oxide synthase. This inhibition was specifically reversed by L-arginine. (*From Belvisi et al.,*[17] *with permission.*)

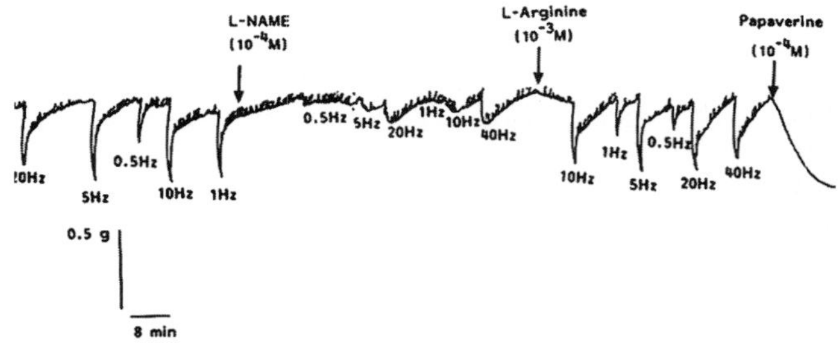

INTERACTIONS BETWEEN EPITHELIAL CELLS AND MYOCYTES: EICOSINOIDS, NITRIC OXIDE, AND OTHER MEDIATORS

Experiments demonstrating alterations in airway responsiveness after damage to or removal of epithelium are consistent with the notion that the airway epithelium elaborates substances that modulate airway smooth muscle contraction. Epithelial removal has often been noted to increase airway responsiveness, implying the presence of epithelium-associated factors that induce airway relaxation. These include prostaglandin E$_2$, which induces airway relaxation[19] and is the major cyclo-oxygenase product of human tracheal smooth muscle cells in primary culture,[20] nitric oxide[21] and "epithelium-derived relaxant factor" (EpDRF). The latter substance is distinct from nitric oxide and is nonprostanoid in nature.[22] It is conceivable that the loss of such relaxant factors contributes to airways hyperresponsiveness in asthma, a disease in which airway epithelial damage is a feature[23] (Fig. 4-2).

It also is possible that epithelium-derived constrictor substances play a role in the pathogenesis of airways hyperresponsiveness. Prostaglandins F$_{2\alpha}$ and D$_2$ are elaborated by human epithelial cells in culture,[20] and have been demonstrated to induce smooth muscle contraction in human airways.[24,25] The possible importance of epithelium-derived prostanoids is suggested by experiments using one model of airway hyperresponsiveness, hyperoxic exposure. Either removal of epithelium or inhibition of cyclo-oxygenase abolishes the stimulatory effects of both in vivo O$_2$ exposure and in vitro hydrogen peroxide exposure on tracheal cylinder stress generation[26,27] (Fig. 4-3). An intact epithelium also is required for the bronchoconstrictor effect induced by major basic protein (MBP), an eosinophil-derived cationic protein.[28] In the latter study, removal of epithelium did not increase tracheal responsiveness to alternative bronchoconstrictor substances, suggesting that MBP does not act by inhibiting EpDRF release; instead, MBP likely augments airway responses by inducing the elaboration of bronchoconstrictor prostanoids from the airway epithelium, such as prostaglandin F$_{2\alpha}$.[29]

INTERACTIONS BETWEEN NEUROENDOCRINE CELLS AND MYOCYTES: SEROTONIN AND NEUROPEPTIDES

A subgroup of epithelial cells, termed *pulmonary neuroendocrine cells*, populate the conducting airways and rarely are found in the alveolar ducts and alveoli. These granule-containing secretory cells exist primarily in the form of innervated clusters (neuroepithelial bodies) lying on the epithelial basement membrane. Serotonin, gastrin-releasing peptide, calcitonin, calcitonin-gene–related peptide, and endothelin have each been identified in the granules of pulmonary neu-

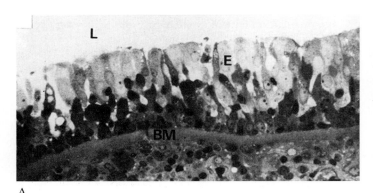

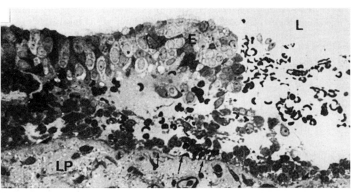

FIGURE 4-2 Airway epithelial damage in patients with asthma. Light micrographs (×300) of the airway epithelia from (*A*) a control subject and (*B*) a patient with asthma. The intralobar airway from the asthmatic patient demonstrates shedding of the pseudostratified columnar epithelium. *Arrows* point to epithelial basement membrane; L, lumen; E, epithelium; LP, laminan propria. (*From Laitinen et al.,*[23] *with permission*).

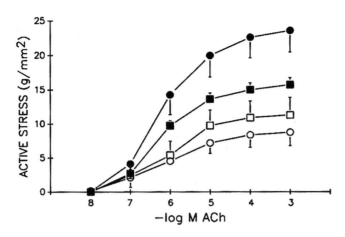

FIGURE 4-3 Hyperoxic exposure of immature rats increases tracheal smooth muscle stress generation in vitro. Untreated tracheal cylinders from O_2-exposed rats generated significantly greater active stress in response to methacholine than cylinders from control animals (*open bars*). Epithelial removal (*solid bars*) or indomethacin pretreatment (*hatched bars*) reversed the observed hyperresponsiveness, which suggests that the response involves the elaboration of an epithelium-derived prostanoid. Treatment with Zileuton, a 5-lipoxygenase inhibitor, had no effect on cholinergic responsiveness. (*From Hershenson et al.,*[26] *with permission.*)

roendocrine cells. Release of these granules appears to be directed away from the airway lumen, toward underlying airway capillaries, sensory nerves, or smooth muscle cells.[30] On the basis of the mitogenic actions of the mediators involved,[31–33] as well as the greater rate of cellular DNA synthesis in airway regions contiguous to neuroepithelial bodies[34] (Fig. 4-4), it is likely that pulmonary neuroendocrine cells promote the growth of the developing airway. In addition, the bronchomotor and vasomotor actions of these neuropeptides, combined with the release of granules and the proliferation of neuroendocrine cells observed in response to alterations in alveolar gas composition,[35] suggests that neuroendocrine cells function as airway "receptors," controlling bronchomotor and vasomotor tone in response to alterations in airway gas or chemical composition.

An increase in the number of pulmonary neuroendocrine cells has been observed in the airways of patients with bronchopulmonary dysplasia and cystic fibrosis, as well as following prolonged mechanical ventilation.[35] Neuroendocrine cell hyperplasia in these instances may be the result of abnormal gas exchange, or it may represent attempts at airway regeneration following epithelial injury. It also is conceivable that, in infants with bronchopulmonary dysplasia,

abnormal neuroendocrine cell proliferation or granule release could play a primary pathogenetic role in the airway smooth muscle hyperplasia observed in this disease.[36]

INTERACTIONS BETWEEN EOSINOPHILS AND MYOCYTES: EICOSANOIDS, PLATELET-ACTIVATING FACTOR, CATIONIC PROTEINS, AND REACTIVE OXYGEN INTERMEDIATES

Eosinophils elaborate a variety of lipid bronchoconstrictor substances, including leukotriene C_4 and platelet-activating factor[37,38] (Fig. 4-5). Further, eosinophil activation may result in the release of major basic protein and reactive oxygen intermediates,[37] both of which induce epithelium-dependent bronchoconstriction.[26,27] As noted above, it appears that MBP acts by increasing epithelial production of bronchoconstrictor substances such as prostaglandin $F_{2\alpha}$.[29] Finally, release of such compounds may indirectly augment bronchoconstriction by promoting the release of tachykinin from sensory nerves.[39]

It is conceivable that reactive oxygen intermediates produced by eosinophils enhance the growth as well as the contraction of airway smooth muscle. Hydrogen peroxide

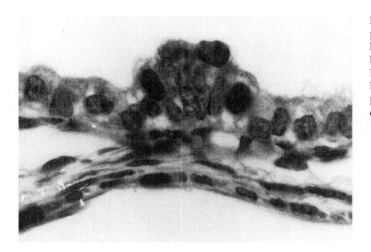

FIGURE 4-4 Neuroepithelial bodies elaborate substances that promote epithelial cell proliferation. Immunostaining of fetal hamster airway epithelium after injection of the mother with bromodeoxyuridine (BrdU), a thymidine analog, demonstrates BrdU uptake (large, dark-staining nuclei), indicative of new DNA synthesis, in epithelial cells located adjacent to a neuropithelial body (clustered vertical nuclei, center). (*From Hoyt et al.,*[34] *with permission.*)

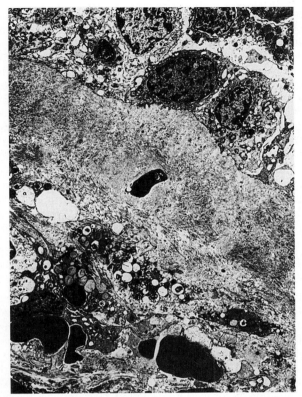

FIGURE 4-5 Electron micrograph demonstrating eosinophils in the lamina propria of an airway from a patient with asthma (×5000). Note the heterogeneity of the eosinophil granules, consistent with the variety of substances elaborated by these cells. (*From Beasley R, Roche WR, Roberts JA, Holgate ST: Cellular events in the bronchi in mild asthma and after bronchial provocation.* Am Rev Respir Dis *1989; 139:806.*)

gen-induced airways disease. Finally, airway tissues from asthmatic patients demonstrate epithelial and subepithelial eosinophil infiltration as well as epithelial damage,[23] likely resulting from the elaboration of eosinophil MBP, the presence of which has been demonstrated in the bronchial wall of asthmatic lung tissue.[45]

INTERACTIONS BETWEEN MAST CELLS AND MYOCYTES: HISTAMINE, LIPID MEDIATORS, PROTEASES, AND PROTEOGLYCANS

A number of mediators have been identified in the granules of airway mast cells, including histamine, leukotrienes C_4, D_4, and E_4, prostaglandin D_2, and platelet-activating factor. The effects of histamine on airway smooth muscle are well known, and the influences of lipid mediators on airway muscle already have been mentioned. Recently, however, attention has been focused on the role of mast cell proteases (including tryptase and β-hexosaminidase) and proteoglycans (including heparin) on airway function. Mast cell tryptase has been shown to substantially increase the tension generated by canine airways in response to histamine.[46] Both tryptase and β-hexosaminidase have been demonstrated to have mitogenic activity for airway smooth muscle cells.[47,48] Heparin, on the other hand, may have anti-inflammatory[49] and antiproliferative effects[50,51] A highly anionic protein, heparin may also neutralize cationic proteins such as eosinophil MBP.

Mast cell degranulation plays a pivotal role in the acute, immediate bronchospastic reaction to inhaled antigen. However, it has been suggested that the recent paradoxical increase in the asthma morbidity and mortality relates to the failure to control the *late* asthmatic response to inhaled antigen, a response involving the participation of additional leukocytes, including neutrophils, lymphocytes, eosinophils, monocytes, and basophils.

increases the activation of mitogen-activated protein (MAP) kinase in cultured bovine tracheal myocytes[40] (Fig. 4-6). MAP kinase, which consists of a family of 40- to 46-kDa cytosolic serine/threonine kinases, participates in the transduction of mitogenic signals to the cell nucleus. The activation of MAP kinase by the reactive oxygen intermediate H_2O_2 therefore may be significant for the pathogenesis of chronic, severe asthma, which is characterized by excessive smooth muscle mass.[41]

In recent years the important role of eosinophils and their secretory products in airways hyperresponsiveness has been elucidated. Blockade of eosinophil adhesion or production (by treatment with antibodies against intercellular adhesion molecule-1 or anti-interleukin-5, respectively) has been demonstrated to blunt allergen-induced hyperresponsiveness in animals.[42,43] Eosinophils and eosinophil products are increased in the bronchoalveolar lavage fluid of allergen-sensitized animals and asthmatic subjects.[38] Oxygen-radical scavengers prevent airways hyperresponsiveness following ovalbumin challenge in sensitized guinea pigs,[44] suggesting that reactive oxygen intermediates produced by eosinophils and other cell types are involved in the pathogenesis of aller-

FIGURE 4-6 Mitogen-activated protein (MAP) kinase, a family of 40- to 46-kDa cytosolic serine/threonin kinases involved in the transduction of mitogenic signals to the cell nucleus, is activated by hydrogen peroxide. In the kinase renaturation assay shown here, cell lysates from bovine tracheal myocytes treated with hydrogen peroxide demonstrated activation of both the 42-kDa and the 44-kD MAP kinases. (*From Abe et al.,*[40] *with permission.*)

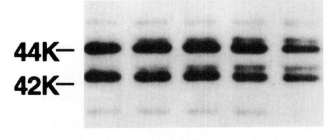

AIRWAY NEUTROPHILS, LYMPHOCYTES, AND MACROPHAGES

Neutrophils, lymphocytes, and macrophages have been noted in the bronchoalveolar lavage fluid of subjects 4 to 6 h after antigen challenge. Although the precise roles of these cells in the late asthmatic response have not yet been determined, these leukocytes are capable of elaborating a large variety of reactive substances into the airways, including proteases, oxygen intermediates, lipid mediators, tumor necrosis factors, interleukins, and platelet-derived growth factor (PDGF). The effects of many of these substances have been outlined above.

Cell-to-Cell Interactions in the Alveoli

In the lung parenchyma, unlike the airways, it is difficult to select a single cell type that is the target for most of the intercellular signals. One may argue, however, that alveolar epithelial type II cells and lung fibroblasts are important recipients of such signals. The main signaling outcomes following stimulation of type II cells and fibroblasts are cell proliferation and the biosynthesis of phospholipids and proteins. In the case of type II cells, surfactant is the main biosynthetic product, whereas for lung fibroblasts, collagen and other extracellular matrix proteins are synthesized. The remainder of this chapter presents a few examples of cell-to-cell interactions in the lung parenchyma. More complete discussions of specific pulmonary cell types and their interactions are found in later chapters.

INTERACTIONS AMONG ALVEOLAR MACROPHAGES, LUNG FIBROBLASTS, AND ALVEOLAR TYPE II EPITHELIAL CELLS CULMINATING IN CELL GROWTH

Inflammatory insults to the lung (as occur in experimental oxygen toxicity, experimental oleic acid injury, and the adult respiratory distress syndrome) generally result in the proliferation of both alveolar epithelial type II cells and lung fibroblasts.[52,53] One of the first studies to examine the role of growth factors in excess lung cell proliferation was performed by Davis and colleagues,[54] who in 1983 demonstrated increased alveolar macrophage-derived PDGF bioactivity in the bronchoalveolar lavage fluid of 14 adult volunteers exposed to greater than 95 percent O_2. Since that time, lung fibroblasts have been demonstrated to be an additional source of PDGF,[55] a potent mitogen for mesenchymal cells. Recently, hyperoxic exposure has been found to induce transforming growth factor-α synthesis in lung fibroblasts[56] (Fig. 4-7), the elaboration of which may promote both lung fibroblast and type II cell proliferation.[56,57] Finally, a variety of other fibroblast-derived polypeptide growth factors are capable of promoting their own growth (*autocrine* growth factors) as well as that of alveolar epithelial type II cells. These include insulin-like growth factor-1,[58] keratinocyte growth factor, and hepatocyte growth factor/scatter factor.[59]

CELL-TO-CELL INTERACTIONS IN THE FETAL LUNG CULMINATING IN SURFACTANT BIOSYNTHESIS

The cell-to-cell interactions leading to surfactant production are somewhat unique in the respiratory system. Although surfactant synthesis depends on local communication (from fibroblasts to alveolar type II epithelial cells), it also is largely influenced by signals from distant organs (i.e., hormones).

A principal regulator of surfactant biosynthesis in the developing lung is fibroblast pneumonocyte factor (FPF). On stimulation by corticosteroids, FPF factor stimulates the synthesis of phosphatidylcholine, phosphatidylglycerol, and surfactant proteins from fetal type II cells[60,61]; thus, corticosteroids are administered during premature labor to speed the synthesis of lung surfactant. The FPF pathway is influenced by an abundance of additional hormones, including androgens, thyroid hormones, and insulin. Androgens and insulin inhibit corticosteroid-induced FPF synthesis by lung fibroblasts,[62,63] thereby retarding surfactant synthesis in male fetuses and infants of diabetic mothers. Androgens also decrease the responsiveness of type II cells to FGF.[62] Thyroid hormones, on the other hand, increase the responsiveness of type II cells to FPF,[64] thereby increasing lung maturation. Unfortunately, the precise chemical and molecular nature of FPF is still unknown.

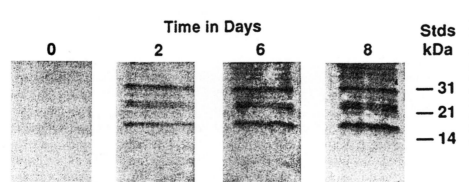

Time in Days

0   2   6   8

Stds kDa

— 31
— 21
— 14

FIGURE 4-7 Exposure of guinea pigs to 100 percent oxygen induces cultured lung fibroblasts to synthesize transforming growth factor-α (TGF-α), a growth factor for lung fibroblasts and alveolar type II epithelial cells. In the immunoblot shown here, fibroblast lysates from guinea pigs exposed to increasing periods of in vivo hyperoxic exposure demonstrate synthesis of three TGF-α isoforms. (*From Vivekananda J, et al.,*[56] *with permission.*)

Conclusion

The development and implementation of effective therapy for pulmonary disease requires an understanding of the cell-to-cell interactions among airway and lung cells. In the remainder of this book, the individual contributions of specific pulmonary cell types to respiratory disease processes will be considered.

References

1. Chen KK, Schmidt CF: Ephedrine and related substances. *Medicine* 1930; 9:1.
2. Barger G, Dale HH: Chemical structure and sympathomimetic action of amines. *J Physiol (Lond)* 1910; 41:19.
3. Trendelenburg P: Physiologische und pharmakologische untersuchungen an der isolierten bronchialmusckulatur. *N S Arch Exp Pathol Pharmakol* 1912; 69:79.
4. Walzer M: The treatment of asthma, in Coca AF, Walzer M, Thommon AA (eds): *Asthma and Hay Fever in Theory and Practice*. Springfield, IL, CC Thomas, 1931.
5. Dale HH, Laidlaw PP: The physiological action of β-iminazolylethylamine. *J Physiol (Lond)* 1910; 21:318.
6. Best CH, Dale HH, Dudley HW, Thorpe WV: The nature of the vasodilator constituents of certain tissue extracts. *J Physiol (Lond)* 1927; 62:397.
7. Lewis T: *The Blood Vessels of the Human Skin and Their Responses*. London, Shaw & Sons, Ltd., 1927.
8. Staub AM, Bovet D: Action de la thymoxyéthyldiéthylamine (929F) et des ethers phénoliques sur le choc anaphylactique du coyabe. *C R Soc Biol (Paris)* 1937; 125:818.
9. Clements JA: Surface tension of lung extracts. *Proc Soc Exp Biol Med* 1957; 95:170.
10. Mead J, Collier C: Relation of volume history of lungs to respiratory mechanics in anesthetized dogs. *J Appl Physiol* 1959; 14:669.
11. Avery ME, Mead J: Surface properties in relation to atelectasis and hyaline membrane disease. *Am J Dis Child* 1959; 97:517.
12. Brown ES: Isolation and assay of dipalmitoyl lecithin in lung extracts. *Am J Physiol* 1964; 207:402.
13. Barnes PJ: Neural control of human airways in health and disease. *Am Rev Respir Dis* 1986; 134:1289.
14. Solway J, Leff AR: Sensory neuropeptides and airway function. *J Appl Physiol* 1991; 71:2077.
15. Watson N, Maclagan J, Barnes PJ: Vagal control of guinea pig tracheal smooth muscle: lack of involvement of VIP or nitric oxide. *J Appl Physiol* 1993; 74:1964.
16. Palmer JBD, Cuss FMC, Barnes PJ: VIP and PHM and their role in non-adrenergic inhibitory responses in isolated human airways. *J Appl Physiol* 1986; 61:1322.
17. Belvisi MG, Stretton CD, Miura M, et al.: Inhibitory NANC nerves in human tracheal smooth muscle: a quest for the neurotransmitter. *J Appl Physiol* 1992; 73:2505.
18. Dev RD, Altemus B, Michalkiewicz M: Distribution of vasoactive intestinal peptide- and substance P-containing nerves originating from the neurons of airway ganglia from cat bronchi. *J Comp Neurol* 1991; 304:330.
19. Melillo E, Woolley KL, Manning PJ, et al.: Effect of inhaled PGE_2 on exercise-induced bronchoconstriction in asthmatic subjects. *Am J Respir Crit Care Med* 1994; 14:1138.
20. Churchill L, Chilton FH, Resau JH, et al.: Cyclooxygenase metabolism of endogenous arachidonic acid by cultured human tracheal epithelial cells. *Am Rev Respir Dis* 1989; 140:449.
21. Nijkamp FP, Van der Linde HJ, Folkerts G: Nitric oxide synthesis inhibitors induce airway hyperresponsiveness in the guinea pig in vivo and in vitro: role of the epithelium. *Am Rev Respir Dis* 1993; 149:727.
22. Morrison KJ, Gao Y, Vanhoutte PM: Epithelial modulation of airway smooth muscle. *Am J Physiol* 1990; 258:L254.
23. Laitinen LA, Heino M, Laitinen A, et al.: Damage of the airway epithelium and bronchial reactivity in patients with asthma. *Am Rev Respir Dis* 1985; 131:599.
24. Jongejan R, De Jongste J, Raatgeep R, et al.: Effect of epithelial denudation, inflammatory mediators and mast cell activation on the sensitivity of isolated human airways to methacholine. *Eur J Pharmacol* 1991; 203:187.
25. Al Jarad N, Hui KP, Barnes N: Effects of a thromboxane receptor antagonist on prostaglandin D_2 and histamine-induced bronchoconstriction in man. *Br J Clin Pharmacol* 1994; 37:97.
26. Hershenson MB, Wylam ME, Punjabi N, et al.: Exposure of immature rats to hyperoxia increases tracheal smooth muscle stress generation in vitro. *J Appl Physiol* 1994; 76:743.
27. Gao Y, Vanhoutte PM: Products of cyclooxygenase mediate the responses of the guinea pig trachea to hydrogen peroxide. *J Appl Physiol* 1993; 74:2105.
28. Brofman JD, White SR, Blake JS, et al.: Epithelial augmentation of trachealis constriction caused by major basic protein of eosinophils. *J Appl Physiol* 1989; 66:1867.
29. White SR, Sigrist KS, Spaethe S: Prostaglandin secretion by guinea pig tracheal epithelial cells caused by eosinophil major basic protein. *Am J Physiol* 1993; 265:L234.
30. Hoyt RF, Sorokin SP, Feldman H: Small granule (neuro)endocrine cells in the infracardiac lobe of a hamster lung: number, subtypes and distribution. *Exp Lung Res* 1982; 3:273.
31. Lee S-L, Wang WW, Lanzillo JJ, Fanburg BL: Serotonin produces both hyperplasia and hypertrophy of bovine pulmonary artery smooth muscle cells in culture. *Am J Physiol* 1994; 266:L46.
32. White SR, Hershenson M, Sigrist KS, et al.: Proliferation of guinea pig tracheal epithelial cells elicited by calcitonin gene-related peptide. *Am J Respir Cell Mol Biol* 1993; 8:592.
33. Noveral JP, Rosenberg SM, Anbar RA, et al.: Role of endothelin-1 in regulating proliferation of cultured airway smooth muscle cells. *Am J Physiol* 1992; 263:L317.
34. Hoyt RF, McNelly NA, McDowell EM, Sorokin SP: Neuroepithelial bodies stimulate proliferation of airway epithelium in fetal hamster lung. *Am J Physiol (Lung Cell Mol Physiol)* 1991; 260:L234.
35. Johnson DA, Georgieff MK: Pulmonary neuroendocrine cells. *Am Rev Respir Dis* 1989; 140:1807.
36. Margraf LR, Tomashefski JF, Bruce MC, Dahms BB: Morphometric analysis of the lung in BPD. *Am Rev Respir Dis* 1991; 143:391.
37. Henderson WR: Eicosanoids and platelet activating factor in allergic respiratory diseases. *Am Rev Respir Dis* 1991; 143:S86.
38. Piacentini GL, Kaliner MA: The potential roles of leukotrienes in bronchial asthma. *Am Rev Respir Dis* 1991; 143:S100.
39. Martins MA, Shore SA, Drazen JM: Release of tachykinins by histamine, methacholine, PAF, LTD_4 and substance P from guinea pig lungs. *Am J Physiol* 1991; 261:L449.
40. Abe MK, Chao OT-S, Solway J, et al.: Hydrogen peroxide stimulates mitogen-activated protein kinase activation in bovine tracheal myocytes: implications for human airway disease. *Am J Respir Cell Mol Biol*, in press.
41. James A, Pare P, Hogg J: The mechanics of airway narrowing in asthma. *Am Rev Respir Dis* 1989; 139:242.
42. Wegner CD, Gundel RH, Reilley P, et al.: Intercellular adhesion molecule-1 (ICAM-1) in the pathogenesis of asthma. *Science* 1990; 247:456.
43. Mauser PJ, Pitman A, Witt A, et al.: Inhibitory effect of the TRFK-

S anti-IL-5 antibody in a guinea pig model of asthma. *Am Rev Respir Dis* 1993; 148:1623.

44. Ikuta N, Sugiyama S, Takagi K, et al.: Implication of oxygen radicals on airway hyperresponsiveness after ovalbumin challenge in guinea pigs. *Am Rev Respir Dis* 1992; 145:561.

45. Filley WV, Holley KE, Kephart GM, Gleich GJ: Identification by immunofluorescence of eosinophil major basic protein in lung tissues of patients with bronchial asthma. *Lancet* 1982; 2:11.

46. Sekizawa K, Caughey GH, Lazarus SC, et al.: Mast cell tryptase causes airway smooth muscle hyperresponsiveness in dogs. *J Clin Invest* 1989; 83:179.

47. Jones CA, Caughey GH, Brown JK: Tryptase-induced mitogenesis in airway smooth muscle cells: synergistic interactions with other mast cell mediators. (Abstract) *Am J Respir Crit Care Med* 1994; 149:A300.

48. Lew DB, Nebigil C, Malik KU: Dual regulation by cAMP of β-hexosaminidase-induced mitogenesis in bovine tracheal myocytes. *Am J Respir Cell Mol Biol* 1992; 7:614.

49. Bowler SD, Smith SM, Lavercombe PS: Heparin inhibits the immediate response to antigen in the skin and lungs of allergic subjects. *Am Rev Respir Dis* 1993; 147:160.

50. Johnson PRA, Armour CL, Carey D, Black JL: The effect of heparin on human airway smooth muscle growth in culture. (Abstract) *Am J Respir Crit Care Med* 1994; 149:A300.

51. Halayko AJ, Delacruz R, Stephens NL: Heparin sulfate inhibits proliferation of cultured airway smooth muscle cells but does not prevent phenotypic modulation. (Abstract) *Am J Respir Crit Care Med* 1994; 149:A300.

52. Crapo JD, Barry BE, Foscue HA, Shelburn T: Structural and biochemical changes in rat lungs occurring during exposures to lethal and adaptive doses of oxygen. *Am Rev Respir Dis* 1980; 122:123.

53. Coalson JJ, King RJ, Winter VT, et al.: O₂ and pneumonia-induced lung injury: I. Pathological and morphometric studies. *J Appl Physiol* 1989; 67:346.

54. Davis WB, Rennard SI, Bitterman PB, Crystal RG: Pulmonary oxygen toxicity. Early reversible changes in human alveolar structures induced by hyperoxia. *N Engl J Med* 1983; 309:878.

55. Fabisiak JP, Absher M, Evans JN, Kelley J: Spontaneous production of PDGF A-chain homodimer by rat lung fibroblasts in vitro. *Am J Physiol* 1992; 263:L185.

56. Vivekananda J, Lin A, Coalson JJ, King RJ: Acute inflammatory injury in the lung precipitated by oxidant stress induces fibroblasts to synthesize and release transforming growth factor-α. *J Biol Chem* 1994; 269:25057.

57. Ryan RM, Mineo-Kuhn MM, Kramer CM, Finkelstein JN: Growth factors alter neonatal type II alveolar cell proliferation. *J Appl Physiol* 1994; 266:L17.

58. Stiles AD, D'Ercole J: The insulin-like growth factors and the lung. *Am J Respir Cell Mol Biol* 1990; 3:93.

59. Panos RJ, Rubin JS, Csaky KG, et al.: Keratinocyte growth factor and hepatocyte growth factor/scatter factor are heparin-binding growth factors for alveolar type II cells in fibroblast-conditioned medium. *J Clin Invest* 1993; 92:969.

60. Post M, Smith BT: Effect of fibroblast pneumocyte factor on the synthesis of surfactant phospholipids in type II cells from the fetal rat lung. *Biochim Biophys Acta* 1984; 793:297.

61. Liley HG, White R, Benson BJ, Ballard PL: Glucocorticoids both stimulate and inhibit production of pulmonary surfactant protein A in fetal human lung. *Proc Natl Acad Sci USA* 1988; 85:9096.

62. Torday JS: Dihydrotestosterone inhibits fibroblast pneumocyte factor-mediated synthesis of saturated phosphatidylcholine by fetal rat lung cells. *Biochim Biophys Acta* 1985; 835:23.

63. Carlson KS, Smith BT, Post M: Insulin acts on the fibroblast to inhibit glucocorticoids stimulation of lung maturation. *J Appl Physiol* 1984; 57:1577.

64. Smith BT, Sabry K: Glucocorticoid-thyroid synergism in lung maturation: a mechanism involving epithelial-mesenchymal interaction. *Proc Natl Acad Sci USA* 1983; 80:1951.

AUTONOMIC INNERVATION

Chapter 5

SYMPATHETIC INNERVATION
RALPH J. ALTIERE AND GREG LINDSAY

Regulation of lung function by autonomic nerves is well established.[1–3] Autonomic neural control of lung function is provided by efferent motor nerves, which directly provoke responses in target tissues,[4] and by afferent sensory nerves, which detect chemical and mechanical stimuli[5] and can evoke airway responses either by a local axon reflex, by the release of substances from nerve endings directly at the site of activation, or by a central nervous system reflex involving activation of efferent motor nerves (parasympathetic cholinergic nerves, sympathetic adrenergic nerves, or nonadrenergic, noncholinergic inhibitory nerves[3,6,7]). This chapter focuses on one of the efferent motor pathways, sympathetic adrenergic nerves. Other components of autonomic efferent and afferent neural pathways are described in Chaps. 6 through 9.

As with other organ systems, adrenergic control of lung function involves the two components of the sympathetic nervous system: direct innervation of tissues by postganglionic sympathetic nerve fibers, which release norepinephrine, and indirect sympathetic input through the circulating catecholamines epinephrine and norepinephrine, which are released from the adrenal medulla. Because the neural component of the sympathetic system ramifies extensively and serves many effector tissues throughout the body, and because the system also includes the circulating catecholamines, sympathetic activation elicits a widespread response involving many organ systems.[6,8,9] The heart is stimulated, blood pressure increases, there is greater mental awareness, metabolism is accelerated, and airways dilate. These actions of catecholamines are mediated by α- and β-adrenoceptors located on cell surfaces. Norepinephrine acts principally on α-adrenoceptors of all subtypes and on β$_1$-drenoceptors, but it has weak activity on β$_2$-adrenoceptors. Epinephrine has potent effects on all α- and β-adrenoceptors. As described later, both α- and β-adrenoceptors are found on many lung cells, and both norepinephrine and epinephrine, therefore, can evoke significant physiologic responses in various lung tissues. The cellular mechanisms that mediate these responses are described in Chap. 1. In general, α-adrenoceptor activation provokes excitatory responses, such as smooth muscle contraction, whereas β-adrenoceptor activation often leads to inhibitory effects, such as smooth muscle relaxation. More specific actions of sympathetic nervous system mediators will be described below. On the basis of the known physiologic effects of endogenous catecholamines, as well as the use for nearly a century of epinephrine to treat asthma and the now widespread use of β$_2$-adrenoceptor agonists as bronchodilators, it has been assumed that the sympathetic nervous system plays an important part in the regulation of lung function, especially of airway smooth muscle tone. Only recently, however, has research provided a clearer picture of this role.

In airway diseases such as asthma and COPD, numerous factors contribute to the disease and its exacerbations. These factors include airway smooth muscle hyperresponsiveness, airway wall edema, increased mucus secretion, impaired mucociliary transport, and excessive mediator release—all of which may be manifestations of underlying inflammation. Neural inputs to the lungs can affect all of these events. Accordingly, this chapter is organized to address the physiologic role of the sympathetic nervous system acting through α- or β-adrenoceptor activation on several major target functions: airway smooth muscle tone, mucus secretion and epithelial fluid transport, blood flow and vascular permeability, regulation of neurotransmission, and release of mediators from inflammatory cells. It is important to note that there are many species differences in autonomic innervation and function, so that extrapolation of findings from one species to another is difficult. The traditional view of the role of sympathetic adrenergic innervation in human lungs, especially in the control of airway smooth muscle tone, has been redefined in light of research conducted over the past 15 years.

Sympathetic Innervation of the Lungs

Direct innervation of the lungs has been studied for more than 300 years.[1,3] The general pattern of human lung innervation was described earlier in this century.[1,3,10–12] Parasympathetic nerves send long preganglionic fibers to the lungs, where they form synapses with short postganglionic nerves in intrinsic ganglia embedded in the tissues. By contrast, preganglionic sympathetic nerves synapse in paravertebral and other peripheral ganglia, from which long postganglionic nerves are sent to target tissues. Postganglionic sympathetic nerve fibers from the middle and inferior cervical ganglia and the upper four to five thoracic ganglia (arising from the upper six thoracic segments of the spinal cord) form anterior and posterior plexuses at the lung hilus and intermingle with parasympathetic nerves to form nerve plexuses around airways and blood vessels. The hilar plexus splits into two principal nerve networks, the peribronchial and periarterial nerve plexuses. The peribronchial plexus subdivides into extrabronchial nerves, which lie external to the cartilage of the airways, and subchondrial nerves, which lie between cartilage and epithelium. Ganglion cells belonging to parasympathetic nerves can be seen throughout the peribronchial plexus down to small bronchi and are localized primarily in the extrabronchial nerves. Autonomic nerves also innervate regions down to the respiratory bronchioles and innervate submucosal glands. Periarterial nerves innervate bronchial vessels down to arterioles.

Since these early studies, more extensive investigations have yielded a more detailed picture of lung sympathetic innervation. Recent advances in histochemical and ultrastructural techniques for nerve identification, pharmacologic methods for examining autonomic receptors, and physiologic methods for measuring the functional effects of autonomic nerve activity have provided important new information on adrenergic innervation and function, especially in human lungs.[3] Comparative studies have shown considerable species variation in the sympathetic innervation of the airways.[1,13,14] For example, cat airways have a dense sympathetic innervation,[15] whereas primate airways receive sparse adrenergic innervation.[16] Human lung tissue contains very little norepinephrine in comparison with other organs such as the heart and systemic blood vessels, suggesting sparse sympathetic innervation.[17] More recent studies, which directly assessed adrenergic innervation patterns, confirm that human airways, like those of other primates, are sparsely innervated by sympathetic nerves. Fluorescence histochemical studies show a relatively high density of adrenergic nerve fibers around submucosal glands[18,19] and bronchial arteries[13,18] but few adrenergic fibers in bronchial smooth muscle.[13,18,20] A similar distribution of adrenergic nerve fibers was found using a different technique more specific for adrenergic nerves.[21] Electron microscopic studies have confirmed these findings. Small, dense-cored granules characteristic of adrenergic neurons are found in glands[19,22] and airway ganglia,[23] but relatively few of them are associated with human airway smooth muscle.[19,22–24] Thus, histochemical and ultrastructural evidence demonstrates that human airway smooth muscle receives little or no adrenergic innervation, whereas glands and blood vessels are more densely innervated by sympathetic nerves.

These findings suggest that sympathetic nerves exert little control over smooth muscle tone in human airways. However, ultrastructural studies show that human airway smooth muscle has numerous gap junctions between adjacent cells,[23,25] suggesting that the smooth muscle cells are electrically coupled and may act as a unit. Therefore, it has been suggested[24,26] that the innervation of only a few smooth muscle cells or the overflow of norepinephrine from sympathetic nerves innervating bronchial or pulmonary blood vessels or submucosal glands could have physiologically significant regulatory effects on human bronchial smooth muscle, either directly or through the inhibition of cholinergic neurotransmission.[2] This notion, however, is not supported by functional studies in airway smooth muscle, which confirm a close correlation between patterns of sympathetic innervation and effects of sympathetic nerve activation in various species. In species that have a relatively dense sympathetic innervation, nerve activation causes bronchodilation, whereas in species that, like humans, have little or no sympathetic innervation to airway smooth muscle, activation of sympathetic nerves produces little or no effect.

Airway Smooth Muscle

Many studies have been conducted in various mammalian species, including humans, to determine the physiologic role of the sympathetic nervous system in regulating airway smooth muscle tone. Both norepinephrine and epinephrine act on cell-surface α- and β-adrenoceptors in airways,[27,28] and much work has focused on responses evoked by activation of these receptors.

β-ADRENOCEPTORS

FUNCTIONAL STUDIES

Studies conducted in vitro on isolated tissues and in vivo have demonstrated functional sympathetic innervation causing β-adrenoceptor–mediated relaxation of airway smooth muscle in various mammalian species. Electrical stimulation of sympathetic nerves to the lungs of cats provokes a bronchodilator response that is abolished by treatment with the β-adrenoceptor antagonist propranolol.[29] Similarly, electrical field stimulation of isolated segments of cat trachea or intrapulmonary bronchi also provokes a relaxant response that can be attenuated by treatment with propranolol and guanethidine, which blocks release of norepinephrine.[30] The relaxant response that remains after elimination of adrenergic nerve influences represents the nonadrenergic, noncholinergic inhibitory nervous system, which is carried in the vagus nerve bundle and not in sympathetic nerve tracts. This inhibitory nervous system is described in Chap 8. Several experimental approaches have been used in other species to demonstrate various degrees of sympathetic adrenergic innervation to airway smooth muscle.[7,13] Electrical field stimulation experiments show functional sympathetic innervation to guinea pig trachea but not to intrapulmonary bronchi,[13,31,32] which is consistent with the distribution of sympathetic adrenergic nerves in this species.[33] In addition, cocaine, which blocks neuronal uptake of norepinephrine, potentiates the relaxant response to norepinephrine in guinea pig trachea but not lung strips, indicating the presence of adrenergic nerves in trachea but not in intrapulmonary bronchi.[34] Electrical field stimulation studies also demonstrate functional sympathetic innervation to dog[35-37] and sheep airways,[38] ferret trachea,[39] and airways of several other species.[13]

Similar studies consistently demonstrate the absence of functional sympathetic adrenergic nerves to airway smooth muscle in primates. Adrenergic blockade by propranolol or guanethidine treatment has no effect on electrical field stimulation–evoked relaxant responses in baboon airways,

although the nerve toxin tetrodotoxin abolishes the response indicating it is of neural origin.[40] In contrast to dog airways, where tyramine, which acts by releasing norepinephrine from adrenergic nerve terminals, causes a propranolol-sensitive reversal of histamine-induced tone,[37] tyramine does not cause relaxation of baboon airways.[40] Similarly, monkey airways do not exhibit a functional sympathetic adrenergic nerve system.[13,41] These findings are consistent with morphologic studies demonstrating that there are adrenergic nerves in dog airways but a preponderance of nonadrenergic, noncholinergic nerve profiles and sparse adrenergic innervation in the airway smooth muscle of monkey and baboon.[42]

Similar studies in human isolated airway segments also consistently have shown the absence of functional sympathetic adrenergic innervation, as in nonhuman primates. Electrical field stimulation of human airways evokes cholinergic contraction, which is inhibited by atropine, followed by relaxation. The relaxant response is unaffected by β-adrenoceptor blockade with propranolol but is abolished by tetrodotoxin, indicating a nerve-mediated response.[13,20,43-45] Similarly, cocaine does not enhance norepinephrine-induced responses in human airways[34]; this also indicates a lack of adrenergic innervation to human airways. Furthermore, bronchoconstriction per se, unless accompanied by hypoxemia or hypotension, does not elicit a reflex sympathetic bronchodilator response in human airways.[6] Other evidence suggesting the presence of adrenergic nerves in human bronchi has been reported.[25] Imipramine causes a small leftward shift in the norepinephrine concentration-response curve, presumably by inhibiting norepinephrine uptake into adrenergic nerve terminals, and a combination of tyramine and electrical field stimulation provokes the release of norepinephrine. Given the evidence described above for adrenergic innervation of glands and blood vessels but the absence of direct adrenergic innervation of human airway smooth muscle, it is likely that these results reflect the uptake and release of norepinephrine from the nerve supply of blood vessels. This conclusion is supported by the finding that tyramine does not evoke bronchodilation in human subjects with mild asthma, despite the fact that these individuals bronchodilate in response to infused β-adrenoceptor agonist.[46] This suggests further that sympathetic nerves do not regulate resting bronchomotor tone in humans.

Morphologic and physiologic evidence indicates that human airway smooth muscle, like that of other primates, does not have a direct functional sympathetic adrenergic innervation. These findings do not preclude the possibility that activity of sympathetic nerves innervating submucosal glands, blood vessels, or ganglia may affect human airway smooth muscle indirectly by overflow of released norepinephrine or by alteration of secretions, vascular leakage, or cholinergic nerve activity (see below).

The lack of direct sympathetic innervation might suggest that β-adrenoceptor mechanisms are of relatively minor importance in the regulation of human airway smooth muscle. Two important facts refute this idea. First, β-adrenoceptor agonists are potent bronchodilators that are used widely to treat bronchospasm associated with asthma and other obstructive airway diseases. More detailed information on the pharmacology and therapeutic use of these bronchodilators is given in Chaps. 41 through 48. Second, β-adrenoceptor antagonists cause bronchoconstriction in asthmatic subjects but not in normal subjects. These observations suggest that sympathetic drive may not influence resting airway smooth muscle tone—that is, that there is no basal sympathetic bronchodilator tone[47–49]—but that there may be enhanced adrenergic drive to the airways of asthmatics and COPD patients.[49–53] Moreover, β-adrenoceptor antagonists may increase bronchial hyperresponsiveness in asthmatic subjects.[54] Subsequent studies have revealed that β-adrenoceptor antagonist-induced bronchoconstriction appears to be related, at least in part, to enhanced release of acetylcholine[55–58] (see "β-Adrenoceptor Function in Asthma," below). Thus, activation or blockade of airway β-adrenoceptors has important influences on regulating airway smooth muscle tone in disease states.

β-ADRENOCEPTOR DISTRIBUTION

The knowledge that β-adrenoceptors mediate potent airway smooth muscle relaxant effects stimulated a considerable amount of research aimed at characterizing these receptors on airway smooth muscle.[8,28,58–61] Radioligand binding studies using whole-lung homogenates have shown a high density of β-adrenoceptors in the lungs of many species,[28,62–64] including humans.[65,66] However, the distribution of receptors within the lung could not be determined from such studies. Localization studies using autoradiographic techniques have found β-adrenoceptors on many different cell types, including smooth muscle, glands, epithelium, and blood vessels, in the lungs of numerous species[67–72] and in human airway smooth muscle.[73,74] The density of β-adrenoceptors was shown to be inversely related to airway diameter —that is, density increases as airway caliber decreases.[68,75,76] The demonstration of β-adrenoceptors in airways from the trachea to the terminal bronchioles correlates with the efficacy of β-adrenoceptor agonists as relaxants in these tissues.[34,43,77–79]

Additional insight into β-adrenoceptor function in the airways is gained from determination of β-adrenoceptor subtype distribution. Beta adrenoceptors have been classified into β$_1$- and β$_2$-subtypes,[80] and each type of tissue was believed to possess a single receptor subtype. Beta$_3$-adrenoceptors have since been identified but have no known function in the airways.[81] Initially, airways were believed to contain only β$_2$-adrenoceptors. Subsequent investigations showed that there could be more than one β-adrenoceptor subtype in a single tissue and led to the concept of "neuronal" and "hormonal" receptors. It has been proposed that β$_1$-adrenoceptors are the sites of action for norepinephrine released from sympathetic adrenergic nerves ("neuronal" β-adrenoceptors) and that β$_2$-adrenoceptors are targets for circulating epinephrine ("hormonal" β-adrenoceptors),[82,83] and that both subtypes could be present in the same tissue. This hypothesis implies that there should be a direct relationship between the density of adrenergic nerves and the density of "neuronal" β$_1$-adrenoceptors in a given tissue. Experimental data from airway smooth muscle demonstrate such a relationship. Relaxation of guinea pig tracheal smooth muscle is mediated by both β$_1$- and β$_2$-

adrenoceptors,[84,85] with β$_2$-adrenoceptors predominating. Radioligand binding studies also show a mixture of β$_1$- and β$_2$-adrenoceptors in this tissue in a ratio of approximately 15:85.[86] More recent studies indicate that the abundance of β$_1$-adrenoceptors decreases from cervical to thoracic trachea in the guinea pig[59] and that relaxations are mediated solely by β$_2$-adrenoceptors in guinea pig peripheral lung strips.[34] These findings are consistent with the distribution of sympathetic adrenergic nerves in guinea pig airways—that is, sympathetic innervation that decreases in density from the upper to the lower trachea and is absent in the peripheral airways. Neuronal β$_1$-adrenoceptors have an identical pattern. Similar receptor heterogeneity is found in dog trachea, where β$_1$-adrenoceptors make up about 20 percent of the total β-adrenoceptor population.[63] Functional studies in this tissue demonstrate that the relaxations elicited by activation of sympathetic nerves are mediated by β$_1$-adrenoceptors but that responses to exogenous β-adrenoceptor agonists are mediated by β$_2$-adrenoceptors. These observations, also, are consistent with the hypothesis that β$_1$-adrenoceptors represent neuronal receptors that respond primarily to norepinephrine released from adrenergic nerves, whereas β$_2$-adrenoceptors represent hormonal receptors that respond to endogenous agonists such as circulating epinephrine. Other studies have shown that β$_1$-adrenoceptors predominate in cat trachea,[87] as would be expected from the relatively dense adrenergic innervation in the airways of this species. Similarly, β$_1$-adrenoceptors predominate in the airways of other species.[88–90]

As described previously, airway smooth muscle in humans has no functional sympathetic adrenergic innervation. Receptor characterization studies have found, as would be expected, that this tissue also lacks β$_1$-adrenoceptors. Functional studies in vitro have shown that relaxation in central and peripheral human airways in response to β-adrenoceptor agonists is mediated solely by β$_2$-adrenoceptors.[34,91] In vivo studies in humans yield similar results. Intravenous administration of the β$_1$-adrenoceptor agonist, prenalterol, increases the pulse rate in asthmatics but fails to evoke bronchodilation, whereas the β$_2$-adrenoceptor agonist, terbutaline, induces a pronounced bronchodilation.[92] Further, isoproterenol, which acts at both β$_1$- and β$_2$-adrenoceptors, produces no greater maximal bronchodilation than a β$_2$-adrenoceptor agonist alone.[93] Autoradiographic analysis of β-adrenoceptor subtypes in human airways confirms the evidence from functional studies and demonstrates the presence of only β$_2$-adrenoceptors in bronchial smooth muscle.[76] More recent molecular studies demonstrate expression of the β$_2$-adrenoceptor gene both in airway smooth muscle in situ and in cultured human airway smooth muscle.[94] Beta$_1$-adrenoceptors have also been found in human lungs by radioligand binding and autoradiographic studies; they appear to be located predominantly in alveolar walls in the peripheral lung.[59,76]

Human airway smooth muscle appears, therefore, to possess only β$_2$-adrenoceptors. Similarly, other cell types in human lung, including submucosal gland cells, epithelial cells, neurons, and mast cells, all appear to have predominantly or solely β$_2$-adrenoceptors.[60] It is reasonable to conclude from the distribution of β-adrenoceptor subtypes in human lungs and the absence of sympathetic innervation to human airway smooth muscle that adrenergic regulation of human airways most likely is provided by circulating catecholamines acting on "hormonal" β_2-adrenoceptors.

CIRCULATING CATECHOLAMINES

Both norepinephrine and epinephrine are secreted from the adrenal medulla glands. Advances in measurement techniques have made it possible to determine plasma catecholamine content more accurately and to determine the role of circulating catecholamines in regulating airway smooth muscle tone.[95,96] The norepinephrine in plasma originates as overflow from sympathetic nervous system activity.[97] At physiologic concentrations, norepinephrine has no significant effects on airway function,[98,99] suggesting that it does not function as a circulating hormone in humans. This concept is supported by the receptor selectivity profile of norepinephrine, which acts primarily on α-adrenoceptors and β_1-adrenoceptors but has relatively low activity on β_2-adrenoceptors. Norepinephrine-induced relaxation of airway smooth muscle occurs principally in airways containing β_1-adrenoceptors[8] (see preceding section). Given that human airway smooth muscle contains almost exclusively β_2-adrenoceptors, it is unlikely that circulating norepinephrine would act as a bronchodilator in humans. Epinephrine, on the other hand, has substantial β_2-adrenoceptor activity as well as α- and β_1-adrenoceptor activity. Within its expected physiologic range of plasma concentrations in humans, epinephrine produces metabolic effects[100,101] and elicits bronchodilation in normal subjects[102] and in asthmatics.[103] Epinephrine also protects against histamine- and methacholine-induced bronchoconstriction, although bronchoconstriction per se does not enhance catecholamine secretion.[104,105] Thus, epinephrine acts as the principal circulating sympathoadrenal hormone.

As noted previously, β-adrenoceptor antagonists cause bronchoconstriction in asthmatic but not in normal subjects. This observation suggests that asthmatic airways may be under greater sympathetic drive to protect against bronchoconstrictor influences, which, in view of the absence of functional airway smooth muscle sympathetic innervation, might be provided by circulating epinephrine. However, studies have shown that circulating plasma epinephrine concentrations are no greater in asthmatics than in normal subjects and that bronchoconstriction alone does not increase plasma epinephrine concentrations,[105,106] including bronchoconstriction induced by propranolol.[107] These observations do not support the concept of greater sympathetic drive in asthmatics, even during active bronchoconstriction, but they do suggest that normal circulating plasma concentrations of epinephrine may protect against bronchoconstriction. Circulating epinephrine concentrations also cycle in parallel with diurnal variations in airway function—that is, the lowest plasma concentrations occur in the early morning hours, when nocturnal asthma tends to occur.[108,109] Thus, it is questionable whether epinephrine at its usual plasma concentrations can cause airway smooth muscle relaxation, but it may exert other beneficial actions, such as reducing the release of mediators from mast cells or other inflammatory cells. However, this also is uncertain[58,60] (see below). Alternatively, as noted already, epinephrine may act to reduce cholinergic neurotransmission (see below). This possibility is supported by the findings that atropine inhibits propranolol-induced bronchoconstriction,[55–57] an effect that would be significant if cholinergic autoreceptors, which inhibit acetylcholine release, are dysfunctional[57,58] (see below). The exact mechanism notwithstanding, current evidence suggests that at normal physiologic plasma concentrations, epinephrine helps to protect airways against bronchoconstriction.

Secretion of epinephrine also may be abnormal in asthmatics, an effect that would weaken the responses that counteract bronchoconstrictor stimuli such as enhanced cholinergic nerve activity or inflammatory mediator action. In normal subjects, exercise causes an increase in plasma catecholamine concentrations. In asthmatics, however, exercise sufficient to induce bronchoconstriction does not cause an increase in plasma epinephrine concentrations,[110–111] and the increase in plasma cAMP (an indirect measure of β-adrenoceptor stimulation by epinephrine) is blunted relative to that of normal subjects.[110,112] More vigorous exercise, however, increases plasma catecholamine concentrations in asthmatics.[113] Conversely, bronchoconstriction caused by hyperventilation,[110] antigen,[114] methacholine[105] or propranolol,[107] or even acute severe asthma requiring hospitalization[115] does not cause an increase in plasma epinephrine concentrations. These findings suggest that a defect in the initiation of epinephrine release from the adrenal medulla may exist in asthmatics and that a strong systemic stimulus other than bronchoconstriction may be required to activate the sympathoadrenal system and overcome this dysfunction. Thus, normal plasma concentrations of epinephrine appear to provide some degree of defense against potential bronchoconstrictor stimuli, but failure to increase epinephrine secretion during bronchoconstriction may contribute to the bronchospasm. These events, however, are not likely to be a primary defect in asthma, as chronic β-adrenoceptor blockade fails to induce bronchoconstriction or airways hyperreactivity in normal subjects.[60]

β-ADRENOCEPTOR FUNCTION IN ASTHMA

Given the apparent importance of β-adrenoceptors in the regulation of airway tone by endogenous circulating epinephrine and, more importantly, by exogenously administered β-adrenoceptor agonists, it has been hypothesized that asthma and bronchial hyperresponsiveness are associated with dysfunction of the β-adrenoceptor system.[116] This hypothesis has stimulated much research. Some of the results suggest that β-adrenoceptor mechanisms are dysfunctional in asthma, whereas other results suggest that they are normal.[28,60,117,118] One complicating factor is that altered β-adrenoceptor function is found in experiments on isolated tissue samples, but little evidence obtained in vivo from asthmatic subjects supports this finding.[119] Nevertheless, recent data suggest that reduced β-adrenoceptor function occurs in asthmatic human airways independent of β-adrenoceptor agonist therapy[120–123] which, paradoxically, is associated with either no change or an increase in the density of both β-adrenoceptors[124–126] and their mRNA.[127] Similar findings of impaired β-adrenoceptor function associated with increased β-adrenoceptor density have been reported in a dog model of airways hyperreactivity.[128] Moreover, the frequency of β-adrenoceptor polymorphisms appears to be the same in normal and asthmatic subjects.[129] Together, these findings suggest that impaired β-adrenoceptor coupling to G proteins, rather than a defect in the β-adrenoceptor itself, may explain the apparent β-adrenoceptor dysfunction in asthma. The question of the mechanisms responsible for impaired β-adrenoceptor function is a major focus of current research. Possible dysfunction of β-adrenoceptors notwithstanding, β-adrenoceptor agonists generally prove to be effective bronchodilators in asthma, indicating that β-adrenoceptor dysfunction may contribute to but probably is not a primary factor underlying asthma or airways hyperreactivity. Nevertheless, the chronic use of β-adrenoceptor agonists in the treatment of asthma remains controversial, mainly because of the effects of β-adrenoceptor agonists on airway functions other than smooth muscle tone.[130–132]

α-ADRENOCEPTORS

Norepinephrine and epinephrine act on α- as well as β-adrenoceptors. This fact has prompted a considerable amount of investigation into potential α-adrenoceptor–mediated effects in airway smooth muscle. Studies have demonstrated the presence of α-adrenoceptors in airway smooth muscle and, as for sympathetic innervation and β-adrenoceptors, have shown considerable species variation in the airway effects of α-adrenoceptor activation or blockade. The role of α-adrenoceptors in regulating human airway smooth muscle tone is not completely resolved, but α-adrenoceptor mechanisms appear to have minor significance relative to other events controlling human airway function.[3,8,28,59,60]

α-ADRENOCEPTOR DISTRIBUTION

Alpha-adrenoceptors have been identified and localized in airway smooth muscle. Alpha-adrenoceptor–mediated contractions are observed in diseased human airways and in human airways exposed to endotoxin.[133,134] Studies using radioligand binding methods have identified α-adrenoceptors in the lungs of numerous mammalian species, including humans, and an increase in α-adrenoceptor density in disease states has been postulated.[65,135–139] Autoradiographic studies have localized α-adrenoceptors to airway smooth muscle, as well as to other lung tissues such as glands and blood vessels. In several species, there is a higher density of α-adrenoceptors in bronchioles than in larger airways, but, in general, airway smooth muscle has many fewer α-adrenoceptors than β-adrenoceptors.[75,140,141] In human lung, α-adrenoceptors are also found in relatively low density compared to β-adrenoceptors throughout the lung, but there is no apparent differential distribution between large and small airways.[142,143] These findings correlate with functional studies (see below) demonstrating weak effects of α-adrenoceptor agonists on airway smooth muscle.

Just as β-adrenoceptors exist in different molecular forms or subtypes, α-adrenoceptors exist as two major subtypes, α₁ and α₂. Additional subtypes of both α₁- and α₂-adrenoceptors also have been characterized. Numerous studies have identified α₁-adrenoceptors in airways of several species, including humans.[136,138,140–143] Postsynaptic α₁- and α₂-adrenoceptors are found in canine airway smooth muscle; in this species, unlike others, α₂-adrenoceptors appear to predominate in this location.[144,145] Nonasthmatic human airways appear to lack postjunctional α₂-adrenoceptors[146] and, similarly, there is no evidence for α₂-adrenoceptor–mediated actions in asthmatic human airways.[147] These studies provide a partial characterization of postjunctional α-adrenoceptors in human airways. Additional studies are needed to fully characterize α-adrenoceptors on airway smooth muscle and other structures in normal and diseased human airways.

FUNCTIONAL STUDIES

Functional studies conducted in vivo and in isolated airways in vitro have investigated the potential physiologic or pathophysiologic role of α-adrenoceptors in regulating airway smooth muscle function. In guinea pig, cat, rabbit, and rat trachea, norepinephrine evokes contraction, but only in the presence of β-adrenoceptor blockade, demonstrating the predominance of β-adrenoceptor–mediated relaxation over α-adrenoceptor–mediated contraction.[148] Many other studies have been performed with dog airways. Alpha-adrenoceptor–induced contraction is observed in isolated dog trachea only in the presence of β-adrenoceptor blockade and precontraction induced by histamine, KCl, or methacholine,[134,149,150] an effect that appears to involve a postreceptor mechanism, possibly through calcium channels.[151] When studied in situ in the intact animal in the presence of β-adrenoceptor blockade, canine tracheal smooth muscle contracts in response to α-adrenoceptor agonists without precontraction induced by another agonist,[144,152–154] but precontraction with histamine or serotonin potentiates the α-adrenoceptor–mediated contractile response.[151,154] Moreover, prostaglandins appear to regulate α-adrenoceptor function.[155] In dogs, in which α-adrenoceptors are more abundant in smaller than in larger airways, norepinephrine correspondingly elicits stronger contractions in small airways than in central airways under conditions of β-adrenoceptor blockade.[156,157] As noted previously, α₂-adrenoceptors predominate in canine airway smooth muscle, and these receptors respond not only to exogenously administered α-adrenoceptor agonists but also to norepinephrine released from sympathetic nerves.[145] In summary, α-adrenoceptors present on airway smooth muscle mediate contractile responses most readily under conditions in which β-adrenoceptors are blocked and tissues are precontracted. At least in dogs, norepinephrine released by stimulation of sympathetic nerves can activate airway α-adrenoceptors to produce contractile effects.

In human airways, α-adrenoceptor agonists have variable effects. Generally, α-adrenoceptor agonists such as norepinephrine and phenylephrine cause relatively weak contractile responses in nondiseased human isolated bronchi, but only after β-adrenoceptor blockade.[133,134,158] As in the case of dog airways, α-adrenoceptor–mediated contractions are potentiated by precontraction with histamine or KCl. Moreover, bronchi from diseased lungs (pneumonia, COPD, pulmonary fibrosis) have enhanced α-adrenergic contraction, suggesting that α-adrenoceptor function is increased in diseased airways. This finding is not observed consistently, however.[143,147]

Similarly, α-adrenoceptor agonists cause varied effects in human subjects. Several investigators found that asthmatic subjects bronchoconstrict in response to α-adrenoceptor agonists, while normal subjects do not respond.[133,159–161] Inhibition of the bronchoconstrictor effect of methoxamine by the α₁-adrenoceptor antagonist, prazosin, suggests that α₁-adrenoceptors mediate the response.[162] However, ipratropium bromide also blocks this response, suggesting that methoxamine may stimulate irritant receptors and trigger a vagal reflex response.[163] Still, other investigators did not observe bronchoconstriction induced by phenylephrine.[164]

The effects of α-adrenoceptor antagonists also are equivocal. Early studies with nonselective α-adrenoceptor antagonists are difficult to interpret because these agents have antihistaminic and cardiovascular effects. Studies with inhaled prazosin show no effect on resting airway tone in asthmatic subjects,[165,166] indicating that α₁-adrenoceptors do not influence the degree of airways obstruction in asthmatics[167] and that α-adrenoceptor antagonists are ineffective in treating asthma.[168] There is, however, some indication that the α-adrenoceptor antagonists phentolamine and prazosin may attenuate exercise-induced asthma.[165,166,169,170] This finding is difficult to understand, because it is unlikely that airway smooth muscle α-adrenoceptors are activated by endogenous catecholamines, given the lack of sympathetic innervation to airway smooth muscle in humans and the observations that circulating catecholamines appear to protect against and not cause bronchoconstriction (see above). One explanation may be that airway blood flow is reduced by increased sympathetic activity (see below), thereby reducing airway warming and facilitating airway cooling, which may lead to bronchoconstriction in asthmatics. Treatment with an α-adrenoceptor antagonist could then prevent vasoconstriction, increase blood flow, and enhance airway warming.[60] Conversely, the α₁-adrenoceptor agonist methoxamine also has been reported to reduce exercise-induced asthma.[171] It is difficult to reconcile the observations that both antagonists and agonists of α-adrenoceptors may attenuate exercise-induced asthma. The latter result suggests that airway wall edema contributes to exercise-induced asthma and that, by producing vasoconstriction in bronchial blood vessels, α-adrenoceptor agonists reduce airway lumen restriction by wall edema and thus increase airflow. If this mechanism is important in asthma, it is reasonable to assume that α-adrenoceptor agonists would be beneficial in the treatment of this disease. In general, however, α-adrenoceptor agonists have not proven useful in the treatment of asthma, and, in fact, they may cause bronchospasm (see above). These conflicting results may reflect differences in α-adrenoceptor subtypes in different airway wall tissues. More complete characterization of the α-adrenoceptor subtypes on blood vessels in the bronchial circulation and those on airway smooth muscle may provide avenues for development of more selective agents that can induce vasoconstriction without the potential for activating airway smooth muscle receptors to induce bronchospasm. Results obtained to date

with α-adrenoceptor agonists and antagonists suggest that α-adrenoceptor regulation of airway smooth muscle tone is complex and, more important, does not appear to be a major factor in airway diseases such as asthma.

Sympathetic nerves have been shown to innervate tissues other than airway smooth muscle in the human lung, including submucosal glands, blood vessels, and neuronal ganglia. The distribution of sympathetic nerves to these other tissues suggests potentially important physiologic roles. The functional significance of sympathetic innervation to these tissues is explored in the sections that follow.

Mucus Secretion

Mucus secretion and mucociliary transport not only are important in maintaining normal airway function but also are critical factors contributing to airway diseases such as asthma, COPD, and cystic fibrosis. Submucosal glands are innervated by autonomic nerves, which can modulate secretory processes.[172] Epithelial cells, while devoid of efferent autonomic innervation, have autonomic receptors, which, when activated, can modulate their function.

SYMPATHETIC INNERVATION AND ADRENOCEPTOR DISTRIBUTION

Innervation of bronchial submucosal glands by sympathetic adrenergic nerves differs among species. Glands in cat trachea contain adrenergic nerves,[173] as do glands in the sheep, but goat, calf, and pig airways have no adrenergic innervation to submucosal glands.[174] As determined by histochemical and electron microscopic studies, human bronchial submucosal glands are innervated by sympathetic adrenergic and other autonomic nerves.[18,19,22,24] Physiologic studies involving electrical stimulation of airway segments containing submucosal glands also demonstrate the presence of functional adrenergic nerves in the glands. Electrical stimulation of sympathetic nerves evokes an increase in secretion of bronchial glands in the trachea of cats[175,176] and ferrets.[177,178] By contrast, electrical field stimulation of human bronchus evokes a cholinergically mediated increase in glandular secretion but no adrenergically mediated changes.[179] This finding is unusual given the presence of adrenergic nerves in submucosal glands, as well as the localization of adrenoceptors on these glands (see below), and the demonstrated stimulatory effects of α- and β-adrenoceptor agonists on mucus secretion in human bronchi.[180] It was suggested that adrenergic innervation may act to modulate cholinergic nerve activity,[179] or, alternatively, that the lack of effects of sympathetic stimulation may be related to the large variability observed in human airway responses.[60] In addition to the demonstration of sympathetic innervation, both α- and β-adrenoceptors have been localized to tracheal submucosal glands.[181] Serous cells have a higher density of α- than β-adrenoceptors, whereas mucous cells have a higher density of β- than α-adrenoceptors. Human submucosal glands have few β₁-adrenoceptors compared to β₂-adrenoceptors.[76] In humans, epithelial cells lining the airway lumen are not innervated by sympathetic nerves and, as expected, possess only β_2-adrenoceptors.[76,182] Similarly, rabbit epithelial cells have predominantly β_2-adrenoceptors.[183]

ADRENOCEPTOR-MEDIATED EFFECTS

Consistent with the presence of both sympathetic innervation and adrenoceptors in submucosal glands, α- and β-adrenoceptor agonists stimulate secretions from these glands.[184] Several investigators have shown that these agonists evoke preferential secretion either of fluid or of mucus glycoprotein. In cat trachea, α-adrenoceptor agonists stimulate the secretion of fluid with a low concentration of protein and sulfur but a high concentration of lysozyme, a component of serous cells. By contrast, β-adrenoceptor agonists stimulate secretion of a relatively small amount of fluid containing high concentrations of protein and sulfur, indicative of mucous cell secretion.[185] In addition, α-adrenoceptor agonists preferentially deplete serous cells rather than mucous cells,[186] and β-adrenoceptor agonists cause marked degranulation of mucous cells.[187] Similarly, α-adrenoceptor agonists evoke secretions low in viscosity and elasticity and high in volume, whereas β-adrenoceptor agonists evoke secretions high in viscosity and low in volume.[188] In human bronchial submucosal glands, both α- and β-adrenoceptor agonists, including norepinephrine, induce secretion of fluid and mucins.[183,189] Extrapolating from animal and human studies, it is reasonable to suggest that norepinephrine released from sympathetic nerves in submucosal glands acts principally on α-adrenoceptors to produce copious amounts of watery fluid and represents a sympathetic reflex effect to dilute inhaled irritants. Conversely, circulating epinephrine acts on β-adrenoceptors to cause a more viscous secretion.[190] However, activation of β-adrenoceptors on epithelial cells also stimulates chloride ion transport and the secretion of water into the airway lumen, resulting in a less viscous fluid.[61,191,192] Moreover, β-adrenoceptor agonists also increase mucociliary transport.[193–197] Activation of α_1-adrenoceptors on human tracheal epithelial cells stimulates NaCl(K) cotransport, the mechanism that supplies epithelial cells with the chloride used for chloride secretion.[198]

Thus, α- and β-adrenoceptor agonists, including endogenous norepinephrine and epinephrine as well as exogenously administered agents, potentially can increase the secretion of fluid and mucin from submucosal glands, enhance the secretion of fluid from epithelial cells, and increase mucociliary clearance, all of which serve to remove inhaled particles trapped in the airway mucus. These modulatory influences are complex and are not yet fully resolved in human airways. Moreover, defects in these modulatory influences are observed in disease states. Recent studies in cystic fibrosis epithelial cells suggest a defect in the adenylyl cyclase-cAMP system, the intracellular mechanism that is activated by β-adrenoceptor agonists.[199] Activation of adenylyl cyclase by isoproterenol and/or forskolin and inhibition of cAMP degradation by isobutylmethylxanthine fails to stimulate chloride secretion in cystic fibrosis cells. By contrast, the α_1-adrenoceptor mechanisms linked to NaCl(K) cotransport apparently operate normally in cystic fibrosis epithelial cells.[198]

Neuromodulation

The release of neurotransmitters from airway neurons is regulated in a complex manner through the interaction of numerous substances released from a variety of cell types. Peripheral autonomic nerve impulses are modulated both in ganglia, where ganglionic synaptic transmission is regulated, and at neuroeffector junctions, where local modulatory control of autonomic transmission may occur on both sides of the junction. At the neuronal terminals, the amount of transmitter substance released can be increased or decreased, and at the effector cells, the responses can be enhanced or attenuated.[200] Both types of neuroregulation can be important in the physiologic control of airway function and may be particularly relevant in airway diseases, such as asthma and COPD.[201]

Modulation of norepinephrine release from sympathetic nerve terminals is less important in the control of airway caliber in humans than in other species because of the lack of direct functional sympathetic adrenergic innervation to airway smooth muscle in humans. However, activation of sympathetic nerves may influence profoundly the release of transmitters from other neural pathways.

TYPES OF MODULATION

In 1977, Westfall classified the various types of local modulation of transmitter release at neuroeffector junctions into four general types: automodulation, transneuronal modulation, transjunctional modulation, and hormonal modulation.[202,203] *Automodulation* is the process by which a released transmitter modulates subsequent release of transmitter by activating receptors on the axon terminals of the neuron, thereby establishing a feedback control loop. The receptors involved in this loop are called *autoreceptors*. *Transneuronal modulation* refers to modulation of the release of transmitter from one type of neuron by a transmitter released from terminals of another type of neuron. This type of modulation requires that the terminals of the two kinds of neurons be reasonably close together. In the airways, transneuronal modulation between adrenergic and cholinergic terminals may be important in regulating airway caliber by affecting the release of acetylcholine. More recently, transneuronal modulation arising from the juxtaposition of nerve terminals containing nonadrenergic, noncholinergic transmitters to adrenergic and cholinergic terminals also has been characterized.[200] *Transjunctional modulation* occurs when substances released from effector cells feed back on nerve terminals to affect subsequent transmitter release. For example, effector cells in the airways are capable of releasing various inflammatory mediators, such as prostaglandins and leukotrienes, that can influence neurotransmission. *Hormonal modulation* is the alteration by hormones of transmitter release through activation of specific receptors located on nerve terminals. By acting on prejunctional β-adrenoceptors, circulating epinephrine may play an important role in modulating the release of acetylcholine from cholinergic nerve terminals in the airways. It is important to note that any of the substances involved in neuromodulation may, and often do, engage in more than one type of local modulatory control.[200]

AUTOMODULATION

Autoregulation at postganglionic parasympathetic nerve terminals in the airways is well documented.[204] However, the role of prejunctional autoreceptors on adrenergic nerves in human airways has not been explored, most likely because the effects mediated by adrenergic nerves, such as bronchial blood flow and mucus secretion, are difficult to measure.[201] In nasal blood vessels, the release of both norepinephrine and neuropeptide (NPY) from sympathetic nerves is modulated by prejunctional α_2-receptors. The release of these transmitters in response to sympathetic nerve stimulation is decreased by α_2-adrenoceptor agonists but increased by α_2-adrenoceptor antagonists. NPY also may act at Y2 autoreceptors on sympathetic nerves, inhibiting the release of NPY and norepinephrine, but this possibility has not been specifically addressed in the airways. Presynaptic β_2-adrenoceptors are present on sympathetic nerve fibers in human pulmonary arteries; however, it is not certain whether similar receptors are present on sympathetic nerves that supply bronchial vessels or submucosal glands.[201]

TRANSNEURONAL MODULATION

Neurally mediated cholinergic responses in airways of several species, including humans, are inhibited presynaptically by agonists of α_2-,[205,206] β_1-,[207] or β_2-adrenoceptors.[208] In addition, there are close associations between adrenergic and cholinergic nerve profiles in human airways.[209] These observations suggest that sympathetic nerves may modulate the release of acetylcholine from postganglionic parasympathetic nerves. However, tyramine, which releases norepinephrine from sympathetic nerves, has no effect on cholinergic neurotransmission in human airways.[3] This result likely is due to the sparse innervation of human airway smooth muscle by adrenergic nerves. Airway nonadrenergic, noncholinergic excitatory nerves, which are sensory in origin, also possess prejunctional α_2-adrenoceptors, which function to inhibit neurotransmitter release.[210,211] Activity of these nerves may be of particular importance, as the pulmonary axon reflex is considered to contribute to the pathophysiology of bronchial asthma.[3] Thus, catecholamines may have antiasthmatic actions through inhibition of an axon-reflex mechanism in peripheral airways. It is not entirely clear whether these prejunctional receptors are activated by norepinephrine released from sympathetic nerves or by circulating epinephrine. The possibility that nonadrenergic, noncholinergic inhibitory nerve-mediated relaxation is modulated by adrenoceptor agonists also has been studied in guinea pig tracheal muscle,[206,212] but no significant effect of α- or β-adrenoceptor agonists on nonadrenergic, noncholinergic relaxation was found.

The sparseness of the adrenergic innervation of airway smooth muscle does not preclude a role for sympathetic nerves in modulating cholinergic transmission. Sympathetic postganglionic fibers innervate parasympathetic ganglia in the airways, suggesting that sympathetic input influences ganglionic processing.[213] It has been known for a long time that catecholamines modulate ganglionic transmission.[214] Both depression and, less consistently, facilitation of ganglionic transmission, mediated, respectively, by α- and β-adrenoceptors, have been observed.[215-217] Exogenous norepinephrine inhibits transmission in airway ganglia of the ferret.[218] This effect is inhibited by phentolamine, indicating that it is mediated by α-adrenoceptors.

TRANSJUNCTIONAL MODULATION

Sympathetic nerve activation may lead to inhibition of transjunctional neuromodulation in the airways by reducing the release of mediators from effector cells. Catecholamines are known to inhibit mediator release from several inflammatory cell types[58] (see below), which may be important to ganglionic neurotransmission, since mast cells are often found surrounding parasympathetic ganglia in the airways.[219] As noted above, sympathetic nerves terminate in parasympathetic genglia, where they can affect ganglionic transmission directly and by modulating mast cell secretion. In addition to their direct effects, several inflammatory mediators may cause bronchoconstriction by enhancing release of excitatory transmitters. For example, histamine can directly activate afferent nerves in the airways and also can increase the release of acetylcholine from postganglionic nerves.[220,221] Other substances that are released from inflammatory cells in the airways and may affect neurotransmission include serotonin, prostaglandins, thromboxanes, bradykinin, platelet activating factor, and nitric oxide.

HORMONAL MODULATION

In the absence of a functional sympathetic nerve supply to human airway smooth muscle, sympathetic control of airway caliber is provided by circulating epinephrine, which can activate pre- and postsynaptic β_2-adrenoceptors in human airways. Presynaptic β_2-adrenoceptors on cholinergic nerve terminals appear to attenuate acetylcholine release.[208] The clinical relevance of presynaptic β_2-adrenoceptors relates to bronchoconstriction induced by β-adrenoceptor antagonists, as noted previously. Beta-adrenoceptor antagonists may inhibit the action of circulating epinephrine to reduce acetylcholine release, resulting in enhanced transmitter release, leading to bronchoconstriction. This idea is supported by the demonstration of an inhibitory effect of anticholinergic drugs on bronchoconstriction induced by β-adrenoceptor antagonists in asthmatic subjects.[56] This effect may be amplified in asthmatics because of defective presynaptic M_2-autoreceptors, which normally would prevent an increase in acetylcholine release.[58,222] Epinephrine also may be responsible for inhibiting the release of tachykinin from sensory nerves in the airways through activation of β_2-adrenoceptors.[210,211]

Studies exploring the process of neurotransmitter release have led to a better understanding of the actions of existing drugs and provided information useful in the development of new drugs. However, knowledge of the processes whereby neurotransmission is modulated in the airways remains incomplete. Further studies are needed to provide a better understanding of the complex mechanisms underlying neuroregulation of the airways in health and disease.

Lung Vasculature

The lung vasculature differs from that of other organs in that it is divided into two distinct circulations, pulmonary and bronchial, which differ in size, origin, and function.[223,224] The blood vessels of these two circulations are specialized to serve specific needs. These specializations include the architecture of the regional beds, the density of innervation, the neurotransmitters released from the nerves, and the specific types of receptors located on vascular smooth muscle cells and endothelial cells.[225] The pulmonary circulation, which receives the entire venous return of the body, functions principally in gas exchange and in selected metabolic functions. By contrast, the bronchial circulation normally receives only about 1 percent of the cardiac output[226] and serves primarily to supply nutrients and remove metabolic wastes from lung tissue. The bronchial circulation supplies blood to the airways from the large central bronchi to the terminal bronchioles.[223]

INNERVATION

The innervation of both lung circulations is similar to the pattern observed in other systemic vascular beds, with sympathetic nerves providing the principal nervous control of vascular tone. Catecholamine-containing nerve terminals are present in the adventitia of pulmonary arteries and veins of humans and extend to the microcirculation.[227,228] Stimulation of sympathetic nerves causes contraction of isolated vessels and decreased compliance and increased pulmonary vascular resistance in vivo.[228] In the intact, perfused pulmonary vascular bed, stimulation of these nerves induces a frequency-dependent increase in perfusion pressure and pulmonary vascular resistance.[229,230] The pulmonary vasculature is somewhat unusual in that it receives parasympathetic cholinergic innervation as well as sympathetic innervation.[231,232] The bronchial circulation appears to have principally sympathetic adrenergic innervation throughout its length from large arteries to arterioles.[13,18]

The two circulations also differ in the primary mechanisms that influence blood flow. Pulmonary vascular tone is under powerful control by local mechanisms that cause vasoconstriction in response to acute hypoxia, a response that does not appear to involve adrenergic nerves.[233,234] However, sympathetic nerves are believed to participate in the reflex increase in pulmonary vascular resistance or the decrease in compliance associated with stimulation of carotid and aortic chemoreceptors.[234–236] Sympathetic nerves also are likely to be involved in the pulmonary vasoconstriction observed in cold exposure,[234] reperfusion,[237] pulmonary embolism,[238,239] and neurogenic pulmonary edema.[240,241] The neurogenic component of pulmonary vascular contraction is mediated principally by sympathetic nerves innervating α-adrenoceptors.[242,243] Relaxation responses in the pulmonary vasculature can be achieved through activation of several types of neurohumoral receptors. Beta-adrenoceptors on pulmonary vessels mediate relaxation and are activated primarily by circulating epinephrine. Cholinergic receptors also can mediate relaxation responses in the pulmonary vasculature. Neurogenic relaxation is mediated, at least in part, by release of a nonadrenergic, noncholinergic transmitter, perhaps nitric oxide.[242,244]

BRONCHIAL CIRCULATION

α-ADRENOCEPTORS

In contrast to the pulmonary circulation, the primary control mechanism regulating tone in the bronchial circulation is the sympathetic nervous system.[245] Stimulation of sympathetic nerves to the bronchial vasculature of dogs produces a powerful vasoconstriction.[246–248] As in the pulmonary circulation, this response appears to be mediated by α-adrenoceptors.[249–251] The use of α$_1$-adrenoceptor agonists for treatment of airway inflammation has been advocated.[252] Diseases such as asthma are accompanied by significant microvascular leakage, which results in plasma exudation into the airway lumen and leads to airway wall edema and thickening of the bronchial mucosa. These changes may contribute to airway hyperresponsiveness. Alpha$_1$-adrenoceptor agonists diminish microvascular leakage by producing bronchial vasoconstriction, thus reducing blood flow to areas of increased permeability. Whether activation of the sympathetic nervous system occurs under these conditions, and whether it is effective in attenuating the consequences of inflammation and vascular leakage, are questions that require further study.

β-ADRENOCEPTORS

β-adrenoceptors also are present on bronchial arteries in large numbers.[73] These receptors may respond to either neurally released or circulating catecholamines and mediate vasodilation in bronchial vessels. Exogenously applied β-adrenoceptor agonists cause a large increase in bronchial blood flow, an effect blocked by propranolol.[249,250,253,254] It appears that β$_2$-adrenoceptors predominate, although both β$_1$- and β$_2$-adrenoceptors are present in isolated bronchial arteries.[255] In sheep and dog bronchial circulations, injection of the β$_2$-adrenoceptor–specific agonist salbutamol elicits a reduction in perfusion pressure, indicating vasodilation.[251,256]

Recently, research has focused on the effects of sensory neuropeptides on the bronchial vasculature, particularly in relation to the extravasation of protein into the interstitial space—that is, neurogenic inflammation and edema.[245] Plasma extravasation is a key feature of several inflammatory diseases, including asthma.[257] Experimental evidence indicates that inflammation causes plasma leakage by producing gaps between endothelial cells, mainly in the postcapillary venules.[258] In addition to the widely accepted idea that sympathomimetic drugs exert anti-inflammatory actions through α-adrenoceptor–mediated vasoconstriction and, hence, decreased blood flow to inflamed tissues, it is now apparent that these drugs also act to decrease vascular permeability through β-adrenoceptor–mediated mechanisms.[259] In experiments in which large doses of inflammatory mediators are given, the vascular leakage effect may be significantly attenuated by endogenous circulating epinephrine or by addition of exogenous β$_2$-adrenoceptor agonists.[260] Beta$_2$-adrenoceptor agonists inhibit plasma leakage produced by a variety of inflammatory mediators, including histamine,[261–264] bradykinin,[261,265,266] substance P,[265,266] platelet-activating factor,[265–267] and allergen.[268,269]

Evidence also suggests that activation of the sympathetic nervous system can attenuate plasma exudation and edema through the actions of inflammatory mediators. To induce plasma exudation, inflammatory mediators such as bradykinin and histamine must be given locally.[270,271] If administered systemically, these substances reduce blood pressure, causing a reflex sympathetic activation and release of epinephrine from the adrenal medulla, which activates β_2-adrenoceptors to inhibit plasma exudation. Beta$_2$-adrenoceptor agonists reduce capsaicin-, bradykinin-, and histamine-induced exudation of plasma into the lumen of guinea pig trachea.[261,270] These agonists are effective even though they also increase mucosal blood flow, an effect that would be expected to enhance plasma exudation. Several mechanisms have been proposed to account for the anti-edema effects of β_2-adrenoceptor agonists, including inhibition of mast cell degranulation,[260] a direct effect on the vascular endothelium,[270] and the inhibition of inflammatory-mediator release from sensory nerves.[261,272] Considering the evidence that conditions such as bronchoconstriction in asthma are not sufficient to activate the sympathetic nervous system (see above), it is unlikely that this system is activated by inflammatory conditions in the airways, although direct evidence has yet to be found. However, conditions that activate the sympathetic nervous system, including release of epinephrine from adrenal glands, as described above, can result in attenuation of neurogenic or other inflammation-induced plasma exudation and thereby reduce pulmonary wall edema. From this brief review, it is apparent that the bronchial circulation plays an important role in the pathophysiology of airway disease. Further research into the nervous and other mechanisms that regulate bronchial vascular control are needed to elucidate completely the role this system plays in airway function in health and disease.

Mediator Release

Several prominent inflammatory cells appear to play an integral part in airway diseases such as asthma. These cells include mast cells, eosinophils, neutrophils, macrophages, and lymphocytes. The role of sympathetic adrenergic nerves and catecholamines in regulating the secretory and other properties of these inflammatory cells has been investigated for more than two decades.[58] Evidence suggests that adrenergic receptors mediate inhibitory and excitatory effects in some of these cells.

MAST CELLS

Activation of β_2-adrenoceptors inhibits immune-degranulation of mast cells in human lung fragments[273–275] and in isolated human lung mast cells.[276,277] Sympathetic nervous system activation inhibits secretion from mast cells in dog airways but not from systemic mast cells.[273] Once immune-degranulation of mast cells has been initiated, sympathetic stimulation can cause sufficient release of epinephrine from

adrenal glands to partially reverse the bronchoconstriction and hypotension of anaphylactic shock, but it is no longer sufficient to inhibit mast cell degranulation. It is estimated that 10 times more epinephrine is required to inhibit degranulation than to promote bronchodilation. The inhibition of bronchoconstriction and mast cell degranulation induced by sympathetic stimulation is blocked by β-adrenoceptor antagonists,[278] a finding consistent with the action of β-adrenoceptor agonists on mast cell secretion.

In humans, inhaled salbutamol inhibits the increase in plasma histamine caused by allergen exposure in asthmatic subjects[279] but has a relatively small effect on urinary excretion of leukotriene E$_4$.[280] Evidence that inhaled β-adrenoceptor agonists inhibit mast cell secretion in vivo in humans is provided by the findings that nebulized salbutamol (a β-adrenoceptor agonist) is more potent against cAMP-induced bronchoconstriction, which is mediated by release of histamine from mast cells,[281] than against histamine- or methacholine-induced bronchoconstriction.[282] Unlike the bronchodilator effect on airway smooth muscle, the inhibition of mast cell secretion in human airways by β-adrenoceptor agonists readily exhibits tachyphylaxis.[283,284] These findings demonstrate that β-adrenoceptor agonists inhibit mast cell secretion, which can be beneficial in asthma because it reduces the quantity of bronchoconstrictor and inflammatory mediators released from mast cells in the airways. Whether the sympathetic nervous system acts to inhibit mast cell secretion in human airways during allergen-induced bronchospasm is not known. However, considering the magnitude of the stimulus required to enhance the release of epinephrine from the adrenal glands (see above), and given that bronchoconstriction alone is insufficient to increase epinephrine release, it is unlikely that the sympathetic system plays a major role in regulating mast cell secretion under the usual conditions associated with asthma. However, these findings may have important implications for the treatment of asthma with β-adrenoceptor agonists.

Alpha-adrenoceptor activation does not affect mast cell secretion in dog airways,[278] which is consistent with the demonstrated absence of α-adrenoceptors on canine mastocytoma cells.[285] The role of α-adrenoceptors in regulating human airway mast cell secretion is not yet resolved, although activation of α-adrenoceptors augments IgE-induced secretion of mediators from peripheral human lung fragments.[286] As noted in the previous section, sympathetic nerves terminate in airway ganglia, where numerous mast cells are found in addition to postganglionic parasympathetic nerve cell bodies.[3] The effects of sympathetic stimulation on these mast cells are unclear.

OTHER INFLAMMATORY CELLS

Human blood eosinophils and guinea pig peritoneal eosinophils possess β_2-adrenoceptors.[287] Activation of β_2-adrenoceptors inhibits the leukotriene B$_4$–induced production of hydrogen peroxide and release of thromboxane A$_2$ from guinea pig peritoneal eosinophils.[58,288] Formoterol, a β_2-adrenoceptor agonist, also inhibits superoxide anion generation in antigen-challenged bronchoalveolar lavage eosinophils from the guinea pig.[289] However, tachyphylaxis to the inhibitory effects of β-adrenoceptor agonists develops rapidly.[287] These findings suggest that β2-adrenoceptor agonists may be beneficial in asthma by inhibiting some eosinophil functions, but it is not known whether sympathetic activation can elicit the same effects in vivo.

Similarly, neutrophils have β2-adrenoceptors that mediate inhibition of neutrophil responsiveness, for example, leukotriene B4 production,[290,291] aggregation,[292] superoxide anion generation, and lysosomal enzyme release.[293] As with eosinophils, tachyphylaxis to the inhibitory effects of β-adrenoceptor agonists develops readily in neutrophils.[294] Human alveolar macrophages also possess β2-adrenoceptors,[295] which do not appear to have an inhibitory effect on mediator secretion[61] but may inhibit cytoplasmic motility.[296] Peripheral blood lymphocytes also express β2-adrenoceptors that exhibit rapid tachyphylaxis.[58,61] Their function in vivo in relation to lung disease is not clear.

To summarize, inflammatory cells express β2-adrenoceptors, and activation of these receptors can inhibit various cell functions, including mediator release. However, in nearly all cases, these receptors show rapid tachyphylaxis, suggesting that they may have little physiologic role in regulating cellular function in health or disease.[58] It is not known whether activation of the sympathetic nervous system, specifically, sympathoadrenal stimulation causing release of epinephrine, results in activation of these cellular β2-adrenoceptors.

Future Research

Current research efforts are focused less on physiologic effects of sympathetic adrenergic activation and more on cellular mechanisms involving regulation of adrenoceptors and control of cell growth and proliferation in both airway smooth muscle and epithelial cells. As far as these cell types are concerned, regulation by the sympathetic system would involve circulating epinephrine, because, as already described, neither human airway smooth muscle nor epithelial cells are innervated by sympathetic nerves, and both cell types in humans express almost exclusively β2-adrenoceptors.

Airway wall remodeling in asthma has become a major focus of investigation.[297] Recent evidence suggests that adrenergic agonists can regulate growth and proliferation of airway wall cells. In rabbit tracheal smooth muscle cells in culture, activation of α1- and α2-adrenoceptors, which are negatively coupled to the adenylyl cyclase-cAMP signal transduction pathway, stimulates cell growth. By contrast, activation of β-adrenoceptors, which are positively coupled to the adenylyl cyclase-cAMP system, inhibits growth.[298] Whether sympathoadrenal activation and circulating epinephrine also can affect growth and proliferation of airway smooth muscle in vivo is not known. In rabbit tracheal epithelial cells, a high density of β2-adrenoceptors is expressed in both columnar and basal epithelial cells.[299] Columnar cells exhibit highly differentiated functions that are under catecholamine control, such as salt and water secretion and mucociliary clearance as described previously. The function of β2-adrenoceptors on basal cells is not known, but it has been suggested that these receptors may mediate catecholamine regulation of basal cell proliferation. In human tracheal submucosal glands in organ culture, epinephrine promotes growth and differentiation,[300] although the adrenoceptor mediating these effects has not been characterized. The question of the involvement of the sympathoadrenal system in these processes in vivo awaits further investigation.

Another area of research receiving considerable attention is the regulation of adrenoceptor expression and function in airway cells. Numerous conditions contribute to the regulation of β-adrenoceptor expression or function, including homologous desensitization, cytokine concentrations, and hypoxia. The desensitization of β-adrenoceptors has been studied for many years and continues to be an important and active area of interest. Exposure to β-adrenoceptor agonists has been shown to decrease variably the expression of mRNA for β-adrenoceptors in guinea pig lung,[301] to desensitize the β-adrenoceptor-adenylyl cyclase system in rabbit airway epithlium[302] and human airway epithelium,[303] or not to desensitize β2-adrenoceptors in guinea pig tracheal smooth muscle.[304] Airways from asthmatic subjects or asthma models exhibit impaired function but no change or an increase in β-adrenoceptor density (see above). Other regulatory mechanisms also are being investigated. Cytokines impair β-adrenoceptor function in guinea pig tracheal[305] and human tracheal smooth muscle.[306] Chronic hypoxia upregulates β-adrenoceptors in rat lungs.[307] The influence of muscarinic receptor activation, especially of the M2-subtype receptor, on β-adrenoceptor function continues to be an area of active research. M2-Muscarinic receptor activation inhibits β-adrenoceptor–mediated relaxation in dog airway smooth muscle.[308] Conversely, muscarinic receptor activation does not alter β-adrenoceptor function in guinea pig tracheal epithelial cells.[309] The interaction of these receptor mechanisms may prove to be important in human airway smooth muscle, where acetylcholine released from cholinergic nerves can act on smooth muscle muscarinic receptors to reduce β-adrenoceptor function and reduce airway smooth muscle relaxation elicited by endogenous sympathoadrenal catecholamines or exogenously administered β-adrenoceptor agonists. The significance of these autonomic receptor interactions in regulating human airway smooth muscle function in vivo awaits further investigation.

Summary

The sympathetic nervous system plays a vital role in regulating numerous physiologic functions in multiple organ systems. In human lung, the sympathetic nervous system innervates many structures, including submucosal glands, blood vessels, and other nerves, but, most notably, does not innervate airway smooth muscle or epithelial cells. Circulating catecholamines, particularly epinephrine, can act at adrenergic receptors on many cell types, including airway smooth muscle, to elicit important physiologic effects, such as airway smooth muscle relaxation, enhanced mucus secretion and mucociliary transport, vasoconstriction, and regulation of neural activity. Evidence suggests that in humans the sympathoadrenal system can beneficially influence airway function in health and disease but that most likely it is not the major determinant for regulating airway function.

References

1. Richardson JB: Nerve supply to the lungs. *Am Rev Respir Dis* 1979; 119:785.
2. Nadel JA, Barnes PJ: Autonomic regulation of the airways. *Ann Rev Med* 1984; 35:451.
3. Barnes PJ: Neural control of human airways in health and disease. *Am Ref Respir Dis* 1986; 134:1289.
4. Andersson RGG, Grundström N: Innervation of airway smooth muscle: Efferent mechanisms. *Pharmacol Ther* 1987; 32:107.
5. Coleridge HM, Coleridge JCG: Pulmonary reflexes: Neural mechanisms of pulmonary defense. *Ann Rev Physiol* 1994; 56:69.
6. Leff, AR: Endogenous regulation of bronchomotor tone. *Am Rev Respir Dis* 1988; 137:1198.
7. Diamond L, Altiere RJ: Airway nonadrenergic noncholinergic inhibitory nervous system, in Lenfant C (ed): *Lung Biology in Health and Disease*, vol. 33: *The Airways. Neural Control in Health and Disease*. New York, Marcel Dekker, 1988:343.
8. Leff AR: Role of the adrenergic nervous system in asthma, in Lenfant C (ed): *Lung Biology in Health and Disease*, vol 49: *Asthma. Its Pathology and Treatment*. New York, Marcel Dekker, 1991:357.
9. Lefkowitz RJ, Hoffman BB, Taylor P: Neurohumoral transmission: The autonomic and somatic motor nervous systems, in Gilman AG, Rall TW, Nies AS, Taylor P (eds): *Goodman and Gilman's the Pharmacological Basis of Therapeutics*, 8th ed. New York, Pergamon, 1990:84.
10. Larsell G, Dow RS: The innervation of the human lung. *Am J Anat* 1933; 52:125.
11. Gaylor JB: The intrinsic nervous mechanism of the human lung. *Brain* 1934; 57:143.
12. Spencer H, Leof D: The innervation of the human lung. *J Anat* 1954; 98:599.
13. Doidge JM, Satchell DG: Adrenergic and non-adrenergic inhibitory nerves in mammalian airways. *J Auton Nerv Syst* 1982; 5:83.
14. Gabella G: Innervation of airway smooth muscle: Fine structure. *Ann Rev Physiol* 1987; 49:583.
15. Silva DG, Ross G: Ultrastructural and fluorescence histochemical studies on the innervation of the tracheo-bronchial muscle of normal cats treated with 6-hydroxydopamine. *J Ultrastruct Res* 1974; 47:310.
16. El-Bermani, AI: Pulmonary noradrenergic innervation of rat and monkey: A comparative study. *Thorax* 1978; 33:167.
17. Anton AH, Sayre DF: A study of the factors affecting the aluminium oxide-trihydroxyindole procedure for the analysis of catecholamines. *J Pharmacol Exp Ther* 1962; 138:360.
18. Partanen M, Laitinen A, Hervonen A, et al.: Catecholamine- and acetylcholinesterase-containing nerves in human lower respiratory tract. *Histochemistry* 1982; 76:175.
19. Pack RJ, Richardson PS: The aminergic innervation of the human bronchus: A light and electron microscopic study. *J Anat* 1984; 138:493.
20. Richardson J, Béland J: Nonadrenergic inhibitory nervous system in human airways. *J Appl Physiol* 1976; 41:764.
21. Sheppard MN, Kurian SS, Henzen-Longmans SC, et al.: Neurone-specific enolase and S-100: New markers for delineating the innervation of the respiratory tract in man and other mammals. *Thorax* 1983; 38:333.
22. Laitinen A, Partanen M, Hervonen A, Laitinen LA: Electron microscopic study on the innervation of the human lower respiratory tract: Evidence of adrenergic nerves. *Eur J Respir Dis* 1985; 67:209.
23. Richardson JB, Ferguson CC: Neuromuscular structure and function in the airways. *Fed Proc* 1979; 38:202.
24. Laitinen LA: Detailed analysis of neural elements in human airways, in Lenfant C (ed): *Lung Biology in Health and Disease*, vol. 33: *The Airways. Neural Control in Health and Disease*. New York, Marcel Dekker, 1988:35.
25. Daniel EE, Davis C, Jones T, Kannan MS: Control of airway smooth muscle, in Hargreave FE (ed): *Airway Reactivity. Mechanisms and Clinical Relevance*. Mississagua, Ontario, Canada, Astra, 1980:80.
26. Laitinen LA, Laitinen A: Innervation of airway smooth muscle. *Am Rev Respir Dis* 1987; 136:S38.
27. Barnes PJ: Adrenergic receptors of normal and asthmatic airways. *Eur J Respir Dis* 1984; 65(suppl 135):72.
28. Goldie RG, Paterson JW, Lulich KM: Adrenoceptors in airway smooth muscle. *Pharmacol Ther* 1990; 48:295.
29. Diamond L, O'Donnell M: A nonadrenergic vagal inhibitory pathway to feline airways. *Science* 1980; 208:185.
30. Altiere RJ, Szarek JL, Diamond L: Neural control of relaxation in cat airways smooth muscle. *J Appl Physiol* 1984; 57:1536.
31. Kalenberg S, Satchell DG: The inhibitory innervation of the guinea-pig trachea: A study of its adrenergic and non-adrenergic components. *Clin Exp Pharmacol Physiol* 1979; 6:549.
32. Grundström N, Andersson RGG, Wikberg JES: Pharmacological characterization of the autonomous innervation of guinea pig tracheobronchial smooth muscle. *Acta Pharmacol Toxicol* 1981; 49:150.
33. O'Donnell SR, Saar N, Wood LJ: The density of adrenergic nerves at various levels in the guinea-pig lung. *Clin Exp Pharmacol Physiol* 1978; 5:325.
34. Zaagsma J, van der Heijden PJCM, van der Schaar MWG, Bank CMC: Comparison of functional β-adrenoceptor heterogeneity in central and peripheral airway smooth muscle of guinea pig and man. *J Receptor Res* 1983; 3:89.
35. Suzuki H, Morita K, Kuriyama H: Innervation and properties of the smooth muscle of the dog trachea. *Jpn J Physiol* 1976; 26:303.
36. Kannan MS, Daniel EE: Structural and functional study of control canine tracheal smooth muscle. *Am J Physiol* 1980; 238:C27.
37. Russell J: Noradrenergic inhibitory innervation of canine airways. *J Appl Physiol* 1980; 48:16.
38. Sheller JR, Brigham KL: Bronchomotor responses of isolated sheep airways to electrical field stimulation. *J Appl Physiol* 1982; 53:1088.
39. McWilliam PN, Gray SJ: The innervation of tracheal smooth muscle in the ferret. *J Auton Nerv Syst* 1990; 30:233.
40. Middendorf WF, Russell JA: Innervation of airway smooth muscle in the baboon: Evidence for a nonadrenergic inhibitory system. *J Appl Physiol* 1980; 48:947.
41. Altiere RJ, Szarek JL, Diamond L: Neural regulation of bronchomotor tone in the intact monkey. *Physiologist* 1984; 27:244.
42. Knight DS, Hyman AL, Kadowitz PJ: Innervation of intrapulmonary airway smooth muscle of the dog, monkey and baboon. *J Auton Nerv Syst* 1981; 3:31.
43. Davis C, Kannan MS, Jones TR, Daniel EE: Control of human airway smooth muscle: In vitro studies. *J Appl Physiol* 1982; 53:1080.
44. Taylor SM, Paré PD, Schnellenberg RR: Cholinergic and nonadrenergic mechanisms in human and guinea pig airways. *J Appl Physiol* 1984; 56:958.
45. Palmer JB, Cuss FM, Barnes PJ: VIP and PHM and their role in nonadrenergic inhibitory responses in isolated human airways. *J Appl Physiol* 1986; 61:1322.

46. Ind PW, Scriven AJI, Dollery CT: Use of tyramine to probe pulmonary noradrenaline release in asthma. *Clin Sci* 1983; 64:9.

47. Zaid G, Beall GN: Bronchial response to beta-adrenergic blockage. *N Engl J Med* 1966; 275:580.

48. Tattersfield AE, Leaver DG, Pride NB: Effect of beta-adrenergic blockage and stimulation on normal human airways. *J Appl Physiol* 1973; 35:613.

49. Richardson PS, Sterling GM: Effects of beta-adrenergic receptor blockade on airway conductance and lung volume in normal and asthmatic subjects. *Br Med J* 1969; 3:143.

50. Benson MK, Berrill WT, Sterling GM, et al.: Cardioselective and non-cardioselective beta-blockers in reversible obstructive airways disease. *Postgrad Med J* 1977; 53(Suppl 3):143.

51. McNeill RS: Effect of a beta-adrenergic blocking agent, propranolol, on asthmatics. *Lancet* 1964; 2:1101.

52. McNeill RS, Ingram CG: Effect of propranolol on ventilatory function. *Am J Cardiol* 1966; 18:473.

53. van Herwaarden CLA: β-Adrenoceptor blockade and pulmonary function in patients suffering from chronic obstructive pulmonary disease. *J Cardiovasc Pharmacol* 1983; 5:46.

54. Townley RG, McGeady S, Bewtra A: The effect of beta-adrenergic blockade on bronchial sensitivity to acetyl-beta-methacholine in normal and allergic rhinitis subjects. *J Allergy Clin Immunol* 1976; 57:358.

55. Grieco MH, Pierson RN: Mechanism of bronchoconstriction due to beta-adrenergic blockade. *J Allergy Clin Immunol* 1971; 48:143.

56. Ind PW, Dixon CMS, Fuller RW, Barnes PJ: Anticholinergic blockade of beta-blocker induced bronchoconstriction. *Am Rev Respir Dis* 1989; 139:1390.

57. Okayama M, Shen T, Midorikawa J, et al.: Effect of pilocarpine on propranolol-induced bronchoconstriction in asthma. *Am J Respir Crit Care Med* 1994; 149:76.

58. Barnes PJ: β-Adrenoceptors on smooth muscle, nerves and inflammatory cells. *Life Sci* 1993; 52:2101.

59. Zaagsma J, van Amsterdan RGM, Brouwer F, et al.: Adrenergic control of airway function. *Am Rev Resir Dis* 1987; 136:S45.

60. Barnes PJ: Adrenergic regulation of airway function, in Lenfant C (ed): *Lung Biology in Health and Disease*, vol. 33: *The Airways. Neural Control in Health and Disease*. New York, Marcel Dekker, 1988:57.

61. Nijkamp FP, Engels F, Hendricks PAJ, van Oosterhout AJM: Mechanisms of β-adrenergic receptor regulation in lungs and its implications for physiological responses. *Physiol Rev* 1992; 72:323.

62. Rugg EL, Barnett DB, Nahorski SR: Coexistence of beta$_1$ and beta$_2$-adrenoceptors in mammalian lung: Evidence from direct binding studies. *Mol Pharmacol* 1978; 14:996.

63. Barnes PJ, Nadel JA, Skoogh BE, Roberts JM: Characterization of β-adrenoceptor subtypes in canine airway smooth muscle by radioligand binding and physiological responses. *J Pharmacol Exp Ther* 1983; 225:456.

64. Engel G, Hoyer D, Berthold R, Wagner H: (±[^{125} Iodo]-cyanopindolol, a new ligand for β-adrenoceptors: Identification and quantitation of subclass of β-adrenoceptors in guinea-pig. *Naunyn-Schmiedebergs Arch Pharmacol* 1981; 317:277.

65. Barnes PJ, Karliner JS, Dollery CT: Human lung adrenoceptors studied by radioligand binding. *Clin Sci* 1980; 58:457.

66. Engel G: Subclasses of beta-adrenoceptors: A quantitative estimation of beta$_1$ and beta$_2$-adrenoceptors in guinea pig and human lung. *Postgrad Med J* 1981; 57(Suppl 1):77.

67. Barnes PJ, Basbaum CB, Nadel JA, Roberts JM: Localization of β-adrenoceptors in mammalian lung by light microscopic autoradiography. *Nature* 1982; 299:444.

68. Barnes PJ, Basbaum CB: Mapping of adrenergic receptors in the trachea by autoradiography. *Exp Lung Res* 1983; 5:183.

69. Barnes PJ, Jacobs M, Roberts JM: Glucocorticoids preferentially increase fetal alveolar beta-adrenoceptors: Autoradiographic evidence. *Pediatr Res* 1984; 18:1191.

70. Finkel MS, Quirion R, Pert C, Petterson RE: Characterization and autoradiographic distribution of the β-adrenergic receptor in rat lung. *Pharmacology* 1984; 29:247.

71. Goldie RG, Papadimitriou JM, Paterson JW, et al.: Autoradiographic localization of β-adrenoceptors in pig lung using [^{125}I]iodocyanopindolol. *Br J Pharmacol* 1986; 88:621.

72. Henry PJ, Rigby PJ, Goldie RG: Distribution of β$_1$- and β$_2$-adrenoceptors in mouse trachea and lung: A quantitative autoradiographic study. *Br J Pharmacol* 1990; 99:136.

73. Carstairs JR, Nimmo AJ, Barnes PJ: Autoradiographic localization of beta-adrenoceptors in human lung. *Eur J Pharmacol* 1984; 103:189.

74. Spina D, Rigby PJ, Paterson JW, Goldie RG: Autoradiographic localisation of β-adrenoceptors in asthmatic human lung. *Br J Pharmacol* 1989; 97:701.

75. Barnes PJ, Basbaum CB, Nadel JA: Autoradiographic localization of autonomic receptors in airway smooth muscle: Marked differences between large and small airways. *Am Rev Respir Dis* 1983; 127:758.

76. Carstairs JR, Nimmo AJ, Barnes PJ: Autoradiographic visualization of beta-adrenoceptor subtypes in human lung. *Am Rev Respir Dis* 1985; 132:541.

77. Goldie RG, Paterson JW, Wale JL: Pharmacological responses of human and porcine lung parenchyma, bronchus and pulmonary artery. *Br J Pharmacol* 1982; 76:515.

78. Guillot C, Fornaris M, Badier M, Orehek J: Spontaneous and provoked resistance to isoproterenol in isolated human bronchi. *J Allergy Clin Immunol* 1984; 74:713.

79. Finney MJB, Karlsson J-A, Persson CGA: Effects of bronchoconstrictors and bronchodilators on a novel human airway preparation. *Br J Pharmacol* 1985; 85:29.

80. Lands AM, Arnolds A, McAuliff JP, et al.: Differentiation of receptor systems activated by sympathomimetic amines. *Nature* 1967; 214:597.

81. Emorine L, Blin N, Strosberg AD: The human β$_3$-adrenoceptor: The search for a physiological function. *Trends Pharmacol Sci* 1994; 15:3.

82. Ariëns EJ, Simonis AM: Receptors and receptor mechanisms, in Saxena RR, Forsythe RP (eds): *β-Adrenoceptor Blocking Agents*. Amsterdam, Elsevier, 1976:1.

83. Ariëns EJ, Simonis AM: Physiological and pharmacological aspects of adrenergic receptor classification. *Biochem Pharmacol* 1983; 32:1539.

84. Levy GP, Apperly GH: Recent advances in the pharmacological subclassification of β-adrenoceptors, in Szabadi E, Bradshaw CM, Devan P (eds): *Recent Advances in the Pharmacology of Adrenoceptors*. Amsterdam, Elsevier, 1978:201.

85. Zaagsma J, Oudhof R, van der Heijden PJCM, Plantje JF: Subheterogeneity of β-adrenoceptors in the pulmonary and the cardiac system of the guinea pig, in Usdin E, Kopin I, Barchas J (eds): *Catecholamines: Basic and Clinical Frontiers*. New York, Pergamon, 1979:435.

86. Carswell H, Nahorski SR: β-Adrenoceptor heterogeneity in guinea-pig airways: Comparison of functional and receptor labelling studies. *Br J Pharmacol* 1983; 79:965.

87. O'Donnell SR, Wanstall JC: Relaxation of cat trachea by

β-adrenoceptor agonists can be mediated by both β$_1$ and β$_2$-adrenoceptors and potentiated by inhibitors of extraneuronal uptake. *Br J Pharmacol* 1983; 78:417.

88. Toda N, Hayashi S, Hatano Y, et al.: Selectivity and steric effects of metoprolol isomers on isolated rabbit atria, arteries and tracheal muscles. *J Pharmacol Exp Ther* 1978; 207:311.

89. Goldie RG, Paterson JW, Wale JL: Classification of β-adrenoceptors in isolated bronchus of the pig. *Br J Pharmacol* 1983; 79:177.

90. Henry PJ, Goldie RG: β$_1$-Adrenoceptors mediate smooth muscle relaxation in mouse isolated trachea. *Br J Pharmacol* 1990; 99:131.

91. Goldie RG, Paterson JW, Spina D, Wale JL: Classification of beta-adrenoceptors in human isolated bronchus. *Br J Pharmacol* 1984; 81:611.

92. Löfdahl C-G, Svedmyr N: Effects of prenalterol in asthmatic patients. *Eur J Clin Pharmacol* 1982; 23:297.

93. Barnes PJ, Pride NB: Dose-response curves to inhaled beta-adrenoceptor agonists in normal and asthmatic subjects. *Br J Clin Pharmacol* 1983; 15:677.

94. Hamid QA, Mak JC, Sheppard MN, et al.: Localization of β$_2$-adrenoceptor messenger RNA in human and rat lung using in situ hybridization: Correlation with receptor auroradiography. *Eur J Pharmacol (Mol Pharmacol)* 1991; 206:133.

95. Barnes PJ: Endogenous plasma adrenaline in asthma. *Eur J Respir Dis* 1984; 64:559.

96. Barnes PJ: Endogenous catecholamines and asthma. *J Allergy Clin Immunol* 1986; 77:791.

97. Brown MJ, Jenner DA, Allison DJ, Dollery CT: Variations in individual organ release of noradrenaline measured by an improved radioenzymatic technique; limitations of peripheral venous measurements in the assessment of sympathetic nervous activity. *Clin Sci* 1981; 61:585.

98. Berkin KE, Inglis GC, Ball SG, Thomson NC: Airway responses to low concentrations of adrenaline and noradrenaline in normal subjects. *Q J Exp Physiol* 1985; 70:203.

99. Larsson K, Martinsson A, Hjemdahl P: Influence of circulating α-adrenoceptor agonists on pulmonary function and cardiovascular variables in patients with exercise induced asthma and healthy subjects. *Thorax* 1986; 41:552.

100. Cryer PE: Physiology and pathophysiology of the human sympathoadrenal neuroendocrine system. *N Engl J Med* 1980; 303:436.

101. FitzGerald GA, Barnes P, Hamilton CA, Dollery CT: Circulating adrenaline and blood pressure: The metabolic effects and kinetics of infused adrenaline in man. *Eur J Clin Invest* 1980; 10:401.

102. Warren JB, Dalton N: A comparison of the bronchodilator and vasopressor effects of exercise levels of adrenaline in man. *Clin Sci* 1983; 64:475.

103. Barnes PJ, FitzGerald GA, Dollary CT: Circadian variation in adrenergic responses in asthmatic subjects. *Clin Sci* 1982; 62:349.

104. Warren JB, Dalton N, Turner C, Clark TJH: Protective effects of circulating epinephrine within the physiological range on the airway response to inhaled histamine in non-asthmatic subjects. *J Allergy Clin Immunol* 1984; 74:683.

105. Sands MF, Douglas FL, Green J, et al.: Homeostatic regulation of bronchomotor tone by sympathetic activation during bronchoconstriction in normal and asthmatic humans. *Am Rev Respir Dis* 1985; 132:993.

106. Barnes PJ, Ind PW, Brown MJ: Plasma histamine and catecholamines in stable asthmatic subjects. *Clin Sci* 1982; 62:661.

107. Ind PW, Barnes PJ, Durham SR, Kay AB: Propranolol-induced bronchoconstriction in asthma: Beta-receptor blockade and mediator release. *Am Rev Respir Dis* 1984; 129:A10.

108. Barnes PJ, FitzGerald G, Brown M, Dollery C: Nocturnal asthma and changes in circulating epinephrine, histamine and cortisol. *N Engl J Med* 1980; 303:263.

109. Bates ME, Clayton M, Calhoun W, et al.: Relationship of plasma epinephrine and circulating eosinophils to nocturnal asthma. *Am J Respir Crit Care Med* 1994; 149:667.

110. Barnes PJ, Brown MJ, Silverman M, Dollery CT: Circulating catecholamines in exercise and hyperventilation-induced asthma. *Thorax* 1981; 36:435.

111. Warren JB, Keynes RJ, Brown MJ, et al.: Blunted sympathoadrenal response to exercise in asthmatic subjects. *Br J Dis Chest* 1982; 76:147.

112. Hartley JPR, Davies CJ, Money RDH, et al.: Plasma cyclic nucleotide levels in exercise-induced asthma. *Thorax* 1981; 36:823.

113. Larsson K, Hjemdahl P, Martinsson A: Sympathoadrenal reactivity in exercise-induced asthma. *Chest* 1982; 82:561.

114. Larsson K, Grunneberg R, Hjemdahl P: Bronchodilation and inhibition of allergen-induced bronchoconstriction by circulatory epinephrine in asthmatic subjects. *J Allergy Clin Immunol* 1985; 75:586.

115. Ind PW, Causon RC, Brown MJ, Barnes PJ: Circulating catecholamines in acute asthma. *Br Med J* 1985; 290:267.

116. Szentivanyi A: The beta adrenergic theory of the atopic abnormality in bronchial asthma. *J Allergy* 1968; 42:203.

117. DeJongste JC, Mons H, Bonta IL, Kerrebijn KF: In vitro responses of airways from an asthmatic patient. *Eur J Respir Dis* 1987; 71:23.

118. DeJongste JC, Jongejan RC, Kerrebijn KF: Control of airway caliber by autonomic nerves in asthma and in chronic obstructive pulmonary disease. *Am Rev Respir Dis* 1991; 143:1421.

119. Beach JR, Young CL, Harkawat R, et al.: Effects on airway responsiveness of six weeks treatment with salmeterol. *Pulm Pharmacol* 1993; 6:155.

120. Cerrina J, Ladurie MLR, Labat C, et al.: Comparison of human bronchial muscle responses to histamine in vivo with histamine and isoproterenol agonists in vitro. *Am Rev Respir Dis* 1986; 134:57.

121. Goldie RG, Spina D, Hanry PJ, et al.: In vitro responsiveness of human asthmatic bronchus to carbachol, histamine, β-adrenoceptor agonists and theophylline. *Br J Clin Pharmacol* 1986; 22:669.

122. Bai TR: Abnormalities in airway smooth muscle in fatal asthma. *Am Rev Respir Dis* 1990; 141:552.

123. Bai TR: Abnormalities in airway smooth muscle in fatal asthma: A comparison between trachea and bronchus. *Am Rev Respir Dis* 1991; 143:441.

124. van Koppen CJ, Rodrigues de Miranda JF, Beld AJ, et al.: Beta-adrenoceptor binding and induced relaxation in airway smooth muscle from patients with chronic airflow obstruction. *Thorax* 1989; 44:28.

125. Sharma RK, Jeffry PK: Airway β-adrenoceptor number in cystic fibrosis and asthma. *Clin Sci* 1990; 78:409.

126. Bai TR, Mak JCW, Barnes PJ: A comparison of β-adrenergic receptors and in vitro relaxant responses to isoproterenol in asthmatic airway smooth muscle. *Am J Respir Cell Mol Biol* 1992; 6:647.

127. Bai TR, Zhou D, Aubert J-D, et al. Expression of β-adrenergic receptor mRNA in peripheral lung in asthma and chronic

obstructive pulmonary disease. *Am J Respir Cell Mol Biol* 1993; 8:325.

128. Emala C, Black C, Curry C, et al.: Impaired β-adrenergic receptor activation of adenylyl cyclase in airway smooth muscle in the Basenji-Greyhound dog model of airway hyperresponsiveness. *Am J Respir Cell Mol Biol* 1993; 8:668.

129. Reihsaus E, Innis M, MacIntyre N, Liggett SB: Mutations in the gene encoding for the β₂-adrenergic receptor in normal and asthmatic subjects. *Am J Respir Cell Mol Biol* 1993; 8:334.

130. Barrett TE, Strom BL: Inhaled beta-adrenergic receptor agonists in asthma: More harm than good? *Am J Respir Crit Care Med* 1995; 151:574.

131. Wanner A: Is the routine use of inhaled β-adrenergic agonists appropriate in asthma treatment? Yes. *Am J Respir Crit Care Med* 1995; 151:597.

132. Sears MR: Is the routine use of inhaled β-adrenergic agonists appropriate in asthma treatment? No. *Am J Respir Crit Care Med* 1995; 151:600.

133. Simonsson BG, Svedmyr N, Skoogh B-E, et al.: In vivo and in vitro studies on alpha-receptors in human airways: Potentiation with bacterial endotoxin. *Scand J Respir Dis* 1972; 53:227.

134. Kneussl MP, Richardson JB: Alpha-adrenergic receptors in human and canine tracheal and bronchial smooth muscle. *J Appl Physiol* 1978; 45:307.

135. Szentivanyi A: The conformational flexibility of adrenoceptors and the constitutional basis of atopy. *Triangle* 1979; 18:109.

136. Barnes PJ, Karliner J, Hamilton C, Dollery C: Demonstration of alpha₁-adrenoceptors in guinea pig lung using [³H]prazosin. *Life Sci* 1979; 25:1207.

137. Barnes PJ, Dollery CT, MacDermot J: Increased pulmonary α-adrenergic and reduced β-adrenergic receptors in experimental asthma. *Nature* 1980; 285:569.

138. Latifpour J, Bylund DB: Characterization of alpha-adrenergic receptors in rat lung membranes: Presence of alpha₁- but not alpha₂-receptors. *Biochem Pharmacol* 1981; 30:2623.

139. Raaijmakers JAM, Wassink GA, Kreukniet J, Terpstra GK: Adrenoceptors in lung tissue: Characterization, modulation and relations with pulmonary function. *Eur J Respir Dis* 1984; 65(Suppl 135):215.

140. Barnes PJ, Basbaum CB, Nadel JA, Roberts JM: Pulmonary α-adrenoceptors: Autoradiographic localization using [³H]prazosin. *Eur J Pharmacol* 1983; 88:57.

141. Xue QF, Maurere R, Engel G: Selective distribution of beta- and alpha₁-adrenoceptors in rat lung visualized by autoradiography. *Arch Int Pharmacodyn Ther* 1983: 266:308.

142. Goldie RG, Spina D, Lulich KM, Paterson JW: Role of α-adrenoceptors in the lung, in Hollinger MA (ed): *Focus on Pulmonary Pharmacology and Toxicology*, vol 1. Boca Raton, FL, CRC Press, 1988:91.

143. Spina D, Rigby PJ, Paterson JW, Goldie RG: α₁-Adrenoceptor function and autoradiographic distribution in human asthmatic lung. *Br J Pharmacol* 1989; 97:701.

144. Leff AR, Munoz NM: Evidence for two subtypes of alpha adrenergic receptors in canine airway smooth muscle. *J Pharmacol Exp Ther* 1981; 217:530.

145. Barnes PJ, Skoogh B-E, Nadel JA, Roberts JM: Postsynaptic alpha₂-adrenoceptors predominate over alpha₁-adrenoceptors in canine tracheal smooth muscle and mediate neuronal and hormonal alpha-adrenergic contraction. *Mol Pharmacol* 1983; 23:570.

146. Grundström N, Andersson RGG: Inhibition of the cholinergic neurotransmission in human airways via prejunctional alpha-2-adrenoceptors. *Acta Physiol Scand* 1985; 125:513.

147. Goldie RG, Lulich KM, Paterson JW: Bronchial alpha-adrenoceptor function in asthma. *Trends Pharmacol Sci* 1985; 6:469.

148. Fleisch JH, Maling HM, Brodie BB: Evidence for existence of alpha-adrenergic receptors in the mammalian trachea. *Am J Physiol* 1970; 218:596.

149. Ohno Y, Watanabe M, Kasuya Y: Manifestation of latent alpha-excitatory response in the canine tracheal smooth muscle preparation—relation to basal tone. *Arch Int Pharmacodyn Ther* 1981; 230:601.

150. Leff AR, Tallet J, Munoz NM, Shoulberg N: Physiological antagonism caused by adrenergic stimulation of canine tracheal muscle. *J Appl Physiol* 1986; 60:216.

151. Barnes PJ, Skoogh B-E, Brown JK, Nadel JA: Activation of alpha-adrenergic responses in tracheal smooth muscle: A postreceptor mechanism. *J Appl Physiol* 1983; 54:1469.

152. Beinfield WH, Seifter J: Contraction of dog trachealis muscle in vivo: Role of α-adrenergic receptors. *J Appl Physiol* 1980; 48:329.

153. Leff AR, Munoz NM: Interrelationship between alpha- and beta-adrenergic agonists and histamine in canine airways. *J Allergy Clin Immunol* 1981; 68:300.

154. Brown JK, Shields R, Jones C, Gold WM: Augmentation of α-adrenergic contractions in the trachealis of living dogs. *J Appl Physiol* 1983; 54:1558.

155. Tallet J, Munoz NM, Fried R, Leff AR: Endogenous modulation of α-adrenergic contraction in canine tracheal muscle. *J Appl Physiol* 1986; 61:464.

156. Leff AR, Munoz NM, Hendrix SG: Comparative distribution of smooth muscle postsynaptic contractile responses in canine trachea and bronchus in vivo. *J Pharmacol Exp Ther* 1983; 224:259.

157. Leff AR, Munoz NM, Hendrix SG: Parasympathetic and adrenergic contractile responses in canine trachea and bronchus. *J Appl Physiol* 1983; 55:113.

158. Mathe AA, Astrom A, Persson N-A: Some bronchoconstricting and bronchodilating responses of human isolated bronchi: Evidence for the existence of alpha-adrenoceptors. *J Pharm Pharmacol* 1971; 23:905.

159. Patel KR, Kerr JW: The airways response to phenylephrine after blockade of alpha and beta receptors in extrinsic bronchial asthma. *Clin Allergy* 1973; 3:439.

160. Snashall PD, Boother FA, Sterling GM: The effect of alpha-adrenoceptor stimulation on the airways of normal and asthmatic man. *Clin Sci Mol Med* 1978; 54:283.

161. Black JL, Salome CM, Yan K, Shaw J: Comparison between airways response to an alpha-adrenoceptor agonist and histamine in asthmatic and non-asthmatic subjects. *Br J Clin Pharmacol* 1982; 14:464.

162. Black JL, Salome C, Yan K, Shaw J: The action of prazosin and propylene glycol on methoxamine-induced bronchoconstriction in asthmatic subjects. *Br J Clin Pharmacol* 1984; 18:349.

163. Black JL, Vicenc K, Salome CM: Inhibition of methoxamine-induced bronchoconstriction by ipratropium bromide and disodium cromoglycate in asthmatic subjects. *Br J Clin Pharmacol* 1985; 20:41.

164. Thomson NC, Daniel EE, Hargreave FE: Role of smooth muscle alpha₁-receptors in nonspecific bronchial responsiveness in asthma. *Am Rev Respir Dis* 1982; 126:521.

165. Barnes PJ, Ind PW, Dollery CT: Inhaled prazosin in asthma. *Thorax* 1981; 36:378.

166. Barnes PJ, Wison NM, Vickers H: Prazosin, an alpha₁-adrenoceptor antagonist, partially inhibits exercise-induced asthma. *J Allergy Clin Immunol* 1981; 68:411.

167. Jenkins C, Breslin ABX, Marlin GE: The role of alpha and beta-adrenoceptors in airway hyperresponsiveness to histamine. *J Allergy Clin Immunol* 1985; 75:364.

168. Ind PW, Dollery CT: Pulmonary adrenoceptors and asthma. *Agents Actions* 1983; 13:213.

169. Bleecker ER, Chahal KS, Permutt S: The effect of alpha adrener-

gic blockade on non-specific airways reactivity and exercise induced asthma. *Eur J Respir Dis* 1983; 64(Suppl 128): 258.

170. Walden SM, Bleecker ER, Chahal K, et al.: Effect of alpha-adrenergic blockade on exercise-induced asthma and conditioned air. *Am Rev Respir Dis* 1984; 130:357.

171. Dinh Xuan AT, Chaussain M, Regnard J, Lockhart A: Pretreatment with an inhaled α_1-adrenoceptor agonist, methoxamine, reduces exericse-induced asthma. *Eur Respir J* 1989; 2:409.

172. Rogers DF, Dewar A: Neural control of airway mucus secretion. *Biomed Pharmacother* 1990; 44:447.

173. Murlas C, Nadel JA, Basbaum CB: Anatomic characteristics of adrenergic efferent nerves to the tracheal glands of cats. *J Auton Nerv Syst* 1980; 2:23.

174. Mann SP: The innervation of mammalian bronchial smooth muscle: The localisation of catecholamines and cholinesterases. *Histochem J* 1971; 3:319.

175. Gallagher IT, Kent PW, Passatore M, et al.: The composition of tracheal mucus and the nervous control of its secretion in the cat. *Proc R Soc Lond (Biol)* 1975; 192:49.

176. Peatfield AC, Richardson PS: The control of mucus secretion into the lumen of the cat by α- and β-adrenoceptors, and their relative inducement during sympathetic nerve stimulation. *Eur J Pharmacol* 1982; 81:617.

177. Borson DB, Chinn RA, Davis B, Nadel JA: Adrenergic and cholinergic nerves mediate fluid secretion from tracheal glands of ferrets. *J Appl Physiol* 1980; 49:1027.

178. Borson DB, Charlin M, Gold BD, Nadel JA: Neural regulation of $^{35}SO_4$ macromolecule secretion from tracheal glands of ferrets. *J Appl Physiol* 1984; 57:457.

179. Baker B, Peatfield AC, Richardson PS: Nervous control of mucin secretion into human bronchi. *J Physiol (Lond)* 1985; 365:297.

180. Phipps RJ, Williams IP, Richardson PS, et al.: Sympathetic drugs stimulate the output of glycoprotein from human bronchi in vitro. *Clin Sci* 1982; 63:23.

181. Barnes PJ, Basbaum CB: Mapping of adrenergic receptors in the trachea by autoradiography. *Exp Lung Res* 1983; 5:183.

182. Davis PB, Silski CL, Kercsmar CM, Infeld M: Beta-adrenergic receptors on human tracheal epithelial cells in primary culture. *Am J Physiol* 1990; 258:C71.

183. Mardini IA, Higgins NC, Zhou S, et al.: Functional behavior of the β_2-adrenergic receptor-adenylyl cyclase system in rabbit airway epithelium. *Am J Respir Cell Mol Biol* 1994; 11:287.

184. Wagner U, von Wichert P: Control of mucus secretion in airways. *Respiration* 1991; 58:1.

185. Phipps RJ, Nadel JA, Davis B: Effect of alpha-adrenergic stimulation on mucus secretion and on ion transport in cat trachea in vitro. *Am Rev Respir Dis* 1980; 121:359.

186. Basbaum CB, Ueki I, Brezina L, Nadel JA: Tracheal submucosal gland serous cells stimulated in vitro with adrenergic and cholinergic agonists: A morphometric study. *Cell Tissue Res* 1981; 220:481.

187. Basbaum CB, Finkbeiner WE: Mucus-producing cells of the airways, in Lenfant C (ed): *Lung Biology in Health and Disease*, vol. 41: *Lung Cell Biology*. New York, Marcel Dekker, 1989:37.

188. Likauf GD, Ueki IF, Nadel JA: Autonomic regulation of viscoelasticity of cat tracheal gland secretions. *J Appl Physiol* 1984; 56:426.

189. Pack RJ, Richardson PS, Smith ICH, Webb SR: The functional significance of the sympathetic innervation of mucous glands in the bronchi of man. *J Physiol (Lond)* 1988; 403:211.

190. Kaliner MA, Borson DB, Nadel JA, et al.: Respiratory mucus in Lenfant C (ed): Lung Biology in Health and Disease, vol. 33: *The Airways. Neural Control in Health and Disease*. New York, Marcel Dekker, 1988:575.

191. Smith PL, Welsh MJ, Stoff SJ, Frizzell RA: Chloride secretion by canine tracheal epithelium: I. Role of intracellular cAMP levels. *J Membr Biol* 1982; 70:215.

192. Knowles M, Murray G, Shallal J, et al.: Bioelectric properties and ion flow across excised human bronchi. *J Appl Physiol* 1984; 56:868.

193. Verdugo P, Johnson NT, Tam PY: β-Adrenergic stimulation in respiratory ciliary activity. *J Appl Physiol* 1980; 48:868.

194. Wong LB, Miller IF, Yeats DB: Regulation of ciliary beat frequency by autonomic mechanisms: In vitro. *J Appl Physiol* 1988; 65:1895.

195. Wanner A: Autonomic control of mucociliary function, in Lenfant C (ed): *Lung Biology in Health and Disease*, vol. 33: *The Airways. Neural Control in Health and Disease*. New York, Marcel Dekker, 1988:551.

196. Sanderson MJ, Dirksen ER: Mechanosensitive and β-adrenergic control of the ciliary beat frequency of mammalian respiratory tract cells in culture. *Am Rev Respir Dis* 1989; 139:432.

197. Satir P, Sleigh MA: The physiology of cilia and mucociliary interactions. *Annu Rev Physiol* 1990; 52:137.

198. Liedtke CM: The role of protein kinase C in α-adrenergic regulation of NaCl(K) cotransport in human airway epithelial cells. *Am J Physiol* 268 (Lung Cell Mol Physiol 12) 1995:L414.

199. Grubb B, Lazarowski E, Knowles M, Boucher R: Isobutylmethylxanthine fails to stimulate chloride secretion in cystic fibrosis airway epithelia. *Am J Respir Cell Mol Biol* 1993; 8:454.

200. Rand MJ, Majewski H, Story DF: Modulation of neuroeffector transmission, in Antonaccio, MJ (ed): *Cardiovascular Pharmacology*, 3rd ed. New York, Raven Press, 1990:229.

201. Barnes PJ: Modulation of neurotransmission in airways. *Pharmacol Rev* 1992; 72:699.

202. Westfall TC: Local regulation of adrenergic neurotransmission. *Physiol Rev* 1977; 57:659.

203. Rand MJ, Majewski H, Wong-Dusting H, et al.: Modulation of neuroeffector transmission. *J Cardiovasc Pharmacol* 1987; 10(Suppl 2):S33.

204. Maclagan J: Presynaptic control of airway smooth muscle. *Am Rev Respir Dis* 1987; 136:S54.

205. Grundström N, Andersson RGG, Wikberg JES: Prejunctional alpha-2 adrenoceptors inhibit contraction of tracheal smooth muscle by inhibiting cholinergic neurotransmission. *Life Sci* 1981; 28:2981.

206. Thompson DC, Diamond L, Altiere RJ: Presynaptic alpha adrenoceptor modulation of neurally mediated cholinergic excitatory and nonadrenergic noncholinergic inhibitory responses in guinea pig trachea. *J Pharmacol Exp Ther* 1990; 254:306.

207. Danser AHJ, Van Den Ende R, Lorenz RR, et al.: Prejunctional β1-adrenoceptors inhibit cholinergic neurotransmission in canine bronchi. *J Appl Physiol* 1987; 62:785.

208. Rhoden KJ, Meldrum LA, Barnes PJ: Inhibition of cholinergic neurotransmission in human airways by β_2-adrenoceptors. *J Appl Physiol* 1988; 65:700.

209. Daniel EE, Kannan M, Davis C, Posey-Daniel V: Ultrastructural studies on the neuromuscular control of human tracheal and bronchial muscle. *Respir Physiol* 1986; 63:109.

210. Grundström N, Andersson RGG: In vivo demonstration of α_2-adrenoceptor mediated inhibition of the excitatory nonadrenergic neurotransmission in guinea pig airways. *Naunyn Schmiedeberg's Arch Pharmacol* 1985; 328:236.

211. Grundström N, Andersson RGG, Wikberg JES: Inhibition of the excitatory non-adrenergic non-cholinergic neurotransmission in the guinea pig tracheo-bronchial tree mediated by α_2-adrenoceptors. *Acta Pharmacol Toxicol* 1984; 54:8.

212. Kamikawa Y: Autonomic regulation of airway smooth muscle. *Respir Res* 1987; 6:1384.

213. Jacobowitz D, Kent KM, Fleisch JH, Cooper T: Histofluorescent study of catecholamine-containing elements in cholinergic ganglion from the calf and dog lung. *Proc Soc Exp Biol Med* 1973; 144:464.

214. Marrazzi AS: Electrical studies on the pharmacology of autonomic synapses: II. The action of a sympathomimetic drug (epinephrine) on sympathetic ganglia. *J Pharmacol Exp Ther* 1939; 65:395.

215. Haefely WE: Effects of catecholamines in the cat superior cervical ganglion and their postulated role as physiological modulators of ganglionic transmission, in Akert K, Waser PG (eds): *Progress in Brain Research: Mechanisms of Synaptic Transmission*. Amsterdam, Elsevier, 1969:61.

216. Volle RL: Ganglionic actions of anticholinesterase agents, catecholamines, neuromuscular blocking agents, and local anaesthetics, in Kharkevich DA (ed): *Pharmacology of Ganglionic Transmission*. New York, Springer-Verlag, 1980:385.

217. Brown DA, Caulfield MP: Adrenoceptors in ganglia, in Kunos G (ed): *Adrenoceptors and Catecholamine Action*. New York, Wiley, 1981: 99.

218. Baker DG, Basbaum CB, Herbert DA, Mitchell RA: Transmission of airway ganglia of ferrets: Inhibition by norepinephrine. *Neurosci Lett* 1983; 41:139.

219. Grillo MA, Nadel JA: Vital staining of tracheal ganglia. *Physiologist* 1980; 23:77.

220. Sampson SR, Vidruk EH: The nature of the receptor mediating stimulant effects of histamine on rapidly adapting vagal effects in the lung. *J Physiol (Lond)* 1979; 287:509.

221. Shore S, Irvin CG, Shenaker T, Martin JG: Mechanisms of histamine-induced contraction of canine airway smooth muscle. *J Appl Physiol* 1983; 55:22.

222. Barnes PJ: Muscarinic receptor subtypes: Implications for lung disease. *Thorax* 1989; 44:161.

223. Deffebach ME, Charan NB, Lakshminarayan S, Butler J: The bronchial circulation: Small, but a vital attribute of the lung. *Am Rev Resir Dis* 1987; 135:463.

224. Lenfant C (ed): *Lung Biology in Health and Disease*, vol. 38: *Pulmonary Vascular Physiology and Pathophysiology*. New York, Marcel Dekker, 1989.

225. Bevan RD: Influence of adrenergic innervation on vascular growth and mature characteristics. *Am Rev Respir Dis* 1989; 140:1478.

226. Staub NC: The respiratory system, in Berne RM, Levy MN (eds): *Physiology*, 3rd ed. St. Louis, Mosby Year Book, 1993.

227. Hebb C: Motor innervation of the pulmonary blood vessels of mammals, in Fishman AP, Hecht HH (eds): *The Pulmonary Circulation and Interstitial Space*. Chicago, University of Chicago Press, 1969:195.

228. Downing SE, Lee JC: Nervous control of the pulmonary circulation. *Annu Rev Physiol* 1980; 42:199.

229. Kadowitz PJ, Hyman AL: Effect of sympathetic nerve stimulation on pulmonary vascular resistance in the dog. *Circ Res* 1973; 32:221.

230. Kadowitz PJ, Knight DS, Hibbs RG, et al.: Influence of 5- and 6-hydroxydopamine on adrenergic neurotransmission and nerve terminal morphology in the canine pulmonary vascular bed. *Cir Res* 1976; 39:191.

231. Fillenz M: Innervation of pulmonary and bronchial vessels of the dog. *J Anat* 1970; 106:449.

232. Amenta F, Cavallotti C, Ferrante F, Tonelli F: Cholinergic innervation of the human pulmonary circulation. *Acta Anat* 1983; 117:58.

233. Fishman AP: Hypoxia on the pulmonary circulation: How and where it acts. *Circ Res* 1976; 38:221.

234. McLean JR: Pulmonary vascular innervation, in Bergofsky EH (ed): *Abnormal Pulmonary Circulation*. London, Churchill Livingstone, 1986:27.

235. Daly IDB, Hebb C: Innervation of the lungs, in Daly IDB, Hebb C (eds): *Pulmonary and Vascular Systems*. Baltimore, William & Wilkins, 1966:89.

236. Szidon JP, Flint JF: Significance of sympathetic innervation of pulmonary vessels in response to acute hypoxia. *J Appl Physiol* 1977; 43:65.

237. Clougherty PW, Nyhan DP, Chen BB, et al.: Autonomic nervous system pulmonary vasoregulation after hypoperfusion in conscious dogs. *Am J Physiol* 1988; 254:H976.

238. Price KC: Pulmonary vasomotion resulting from miliary embolism of the lungs. *Am J Physiol* 1955; 182:183.

239. Kabins SA, Fridman J, Kandelman M, Weisberg H: Effects of sympathectomy on pulmonary embolism-induced lung edema. *Am J Physiol* 1962; 202:687.

240. Colice GL, Matthay MA, Bass E, Matthay RA: Neurogenic pulmonary edema. *Am Rev Respir Dis* 1984; 130:941.

241. Malik AB: Mechanisms of neurogenic pulmonary edema. *Circ Res* 1985; 57:1.

242. Barnes PJ, Liu SF: Regulation of pulmonary vascular tone. *Pharm Rev* 1995; 47:87.

243. Kobayashi Y, Amenta F: Neurotransmitter receptors in the pulmonary circulation with particular emphasis on pulmonary endothelium. *J Auton Pharmacol* 1994; 14:137.

244. Kubota E, Hamasaki Y, Sata T, et al.: Autonomic innervation of pulmonary artery: Evidence for a nonadrenergic noncholinergic inhibitory system. *Exp Lung Res* 1988; 14:349.

245. Widdicombe JG, Webber SE: Neuroregulation and pharmacology of the tracheobronchial circulation, in Lenfant C (ed): *Lung Biology in Health and Disease*, vol 57: *The Bronchial Circulation*. New York, Marcel Dekker, 1992:249.

246. De Letona JML, De La Mata RC, Aviado DM: Local and reflex effects of bronchial artery injection of drugs. *J Pharmacol Exp Ther* 1961; 133:295.

247. Aviado DM: Pharmacology of the bronchial circulation, in Uvnas B (ed): *First International Pharmacology Meeting*. London, Pergamon Press, 1963:125.

248. Murao H: Nervous regulation of the bronchial vascular system. *Jpn Circ J* 1965; 29:855.

249. Himori N, Tiara N: A method for recording smooth muscle and vascular responses of the blood-perfused dog trachea in situ. *Br J Pharmacol* 1976; 56:293.

250. Barker JA, Chediak AD, Baier HJ, Wanner A: Bronchial circulation in asthma. *Respiration* 1988; 48:199.

251. Laitinen LA, Laitinen MA, Widdicombe JG: Dose-related effects of pharmacological mediators on tracheal vascular resistance in dogs. *Br J Pharmacol* 1987; 92:703.

252. Barnes PJ, Boschetto P, Rogers DF, et al.: Effects of treatment on airway microvascular leakage. *Eur Respir J [Suppl]* 1990; 12:663s.

253. Lung MA, Wang JCC, Cheng KK: Bronchial circulation: An autoperfusion method for assessing its vasomotor activity and the study of alpha adrenoceptors in the bronchial artery. *Life Sci* 1976; 19:577.

254. Parsons GH, Kramer GC, Link DP, et al.: Studies of reactivity and distribution of bronchial blood flow in sheep. *Chest* 1985; 87:180S.

255. Arwolo RPA, Eyre P: Preliminary pharmacological characterization of the bovine isolated artery strip: A new preparation. *Br J Pharmacol* 1980; 68:283.

256. Webber SE, Salonen RO, Widdicombe JG: Effects of antigen on

tracheal circulation and smooth muscle in sheep of different ages. *J Appl Physiol* 1989; 67:1256.

257. Persson CGA: Plasma exudation and asthma. *Lung* 1988; 166:1.

258. Persson CGA, Erjefalt IA-L: Inflammatory leakage of macromolecules from the vascular compartment into the tracheal lumen. *Acta Physiol Scand* 1986; 126:615.

259. Persson CGA, Erjefalt IA-L: Nonneural regulation of plasma exudation in airways, in Lenfant C (ed): *Lung Biology in Health and Disease*, vol 57: *The Bronchial Circulation*. New York, Marcel Dekker, 1992:523.

260. Tomioka K, Yamada T, Ida H: Anti-allergic activities of the β-adrenoceptor stimulant formoterol (BD 40A). *Arch Int Pharmacodyn* 1981; 250:279.

261. Advenier C, Qian Y, Koune JD, et al.: Formoterol and salbutamol inhibit bradykinin- and histamine-induced airway microvascular leakage in guinea-pig. *Br J Pharmacol* 1992; 105:792.

262. O'Donnell SR, Persson CGA: Beta-adrenoceptor mediated inhibition by terbutaline of histamine effects on vascular permeability. *Br J Pharmacol* 1978; 62:321.

263. Tokuyama K, Lotvall JO, Lofdahl CG, et al.: Inhaled formoterol inhibits histamine-induced airflow obstruction and airway microvascular leakage. *Eur J Pharmacol* 1991; 193:35.

264. Whelan CJ, Johnson M, Vardey CJ: Comparison of the anti-inflammatory properties of formoterol, salbutamol and salmeterol in guinea-pig skin and lung. *Br J Pharmacol* 1993; 110:613.

265. Bowden JJ, Sulakvelidze I, McDonald DM: Inhibition of neutrophil and eosinophil adhesion to venules of the rat trachea by the β2-adrenergic agonist formoterol. *J Appl Physiol* 1994; 77:397.

266. Sulakvelidze I, McDonald DM: The anti-edema action of formoterol in the rat trachea does not depend on capsaicin sensitive sensory nerves. *Am J Respir Crit Care Med* 1994; 149:232.

267. Underwood SL, Lewis SA, Raeburn D: RP-58802B, a long-acting β2-adrenoceptor agonist: Assessment of antiasthma activity in the guinea-pig in vivo. *Pulm Pharmacol* 1992; 5:203.

268. Erjefalt I, Persson CGA: Long duration and high potency of antiexudative effects of formoterol in guinea-pig tracheo-bronchial airways. *Am Rev Respir Dis* 1991; 144:788.

269. Inagaki N, Miura T, Daikoku M, et al.: Inhibitory effects of β-adrenergic stimulants on increased vascular permeability caused by passive cutaneous anaphylaxis, allergic mediators, and mediator releasers in rats. *Pharmacology (Basel)* 1989; 39:19.

270. Erjefalt I, Perrson CGA: Pharmacological control of plasma exudation into tracheobronchial airways. *Am Rev Respir Dis* 1991; 143:1008.

271. Grega GJ, Maciejco JJ, Raymond RM, Sak PD: The interrelationship among histamine, various vasoactive substances, and macromolecular permeability in the canine forelimb. *Circ Res* 1980; 46:264.

272. Hui KP, Ventresca P, Brown AC, et al.: Modulation of neurally mediated microvascular leakage in guinea-pig airways by β2-adrenoceptor agonists. *Agents Actions* 1992; 36:29.

273. Garrity ER, Stimler NP, Munoz NM, et al.: Sympathetic modulation of the biochemical and physiological response to immune degranulation in canine bronchial airways in vitro. *J Clin Invest* 1985; 75:2038.

274. Orange RP, Austen WG, Austen KF: Immunological release of histamine and slow-reacting substance of anaphylaxis from human lung: I. Modulation by agents influencing cellular levels of 3',5'-adenosine monophosphate. *J Exp Med* 1971; 134:136.

275. Butchers PR, Skidmore IF, Vardey CJ, Wheeldon AM: Characterization of the receptor mediating the anti-anaphylactic effects of beta-adrenoceptor agonists in human lung tissue in vitro. *Br J Pharmacol* 1980; 71:663.

276. Peters JE, Schulman ES, Schleimer RP, et al.: Dispersed human lung mast cells: Pharmacologic aspects and comparison with human lung tissue fragments. *Am Rev Respir Dis* 1982; 126:1034.

277. Church MK, Hiroi J: Inhibition of IgE-dependent histamine release from human dispersed lung mast cells by anti-allergic drugs and salbutamol. *Br J Pharmacol* 1987; 90:421.

278. White SR, Stimler-Gerard NP, Munoz NM, et al.: Effect of beta-adrenergic blockade and sympathetic stimulation on the canine bronchial mast cell response to immune degranulation in vivo. *Am Rev Respir Dis* 1989; 139:73.

279. Howarth PH, Durham SR, Lee TH, et al.: Influence of albuterol, cromolyn sodium and ipratropium bromide on the airway and circulating mediator responses to allergen bronchial provocation in asthma. *Am Rev Respir Dis* 1985; 132:986.

280. Taylor IK, O'Shaughnessy KM, Choudry NB, et al.: A comparative study in atopic subjects with asthma of the effects of salmeterol and salbutamol on allergen-induced bronchoconstriction, increase in airway reactivity and increase in urinary leukotriene E4 excretion. *J Allergy Clin Immunol* 1992; 89:575.

281. Cushley MJ, Holgate ST: Adenosine induced bronchoconstriction in asthma: Role of mast cell mediator release. *J Allergy Clin Immunol* 1985; 75:272.

282. Phillips GD, Finnerty JT, Holgate ST: Comparative protective effect of the inhaled β-agonist salbutamol (albuterol) on bronchoconstriction provoked by histamine, methacholine, and adenosine 5'-monophosphate in asthma. *J Allergy Clin Immunol* 1990; 85:755.

283. van der Heijden PJCM, van Amsterdam JGC, Zaagsma J: Desensitization of smooth muscle and mast cell adrenoceptors in the airways of guinea pig. *Eur J Respir Dis* 1984; 65(Suppl 135):128.

284. O'Connor BJ, Aikman SL, Barnes PJ: Tolerance to the non-bronchodilator effects of inhaled β2-agonists. *New Engl J Med* 1992; 327:1204.

285. Phillips MJ, Barnes PJ, Gold WM: Characterization of purified dog mastocytoma cells: Autonomic membrane receptors in pharmacological modulation of histamine release. *Am Rev Respir Dis* 1985; 132:1019.

286. Kaliner MA, Orange RP, Austen KF: Immunological release of histamine and slow reacting substance of anaphylaxis from human lung: IV. Enhancement by cholinergic and alpha-adrenergic stimulation. *J Exp Med* 1972; 136:556.

287. Yukawa T, Ukena D, Kroegel C, et al.: Beta2-adrenergic receptors on eosinophils: Binding and functional studies. *Am Rev Respir Dis* 1990; 141:1446.

288. Rabe KF, Giembycz M, Dent G, et al.: Salmeterol is a competitive antagonist at β-adrenoceptors mediating inhibition of respiratory burst in guinea pig eosinophils. *Eur J Pharmacol* 1993; 231:305.

289. Okada C, Sugiyama H, Eda R, et al.: Effect of formoterol on superoxide anion generation from bronchoalveolar cells after antigen challenge in guinea pigs. *Am J Respir Cell Mol Biol* 1993; 8:509.

290. Galant SP, Durisetti L, Underwood S, Insel PA: Decreased beta-adrenergic receptors on polymorphonuclear leukocytes after adrenergic therapy. *N Engl J Med* 1978; 299:933.

291. Szefler SJ, Edwards CK, Haslett C, et al.: Effects of cell isolation procedures and radioligand selection on the characterization of human leukocyte beta-adrenergic receptors. *Biochem Pharmacol* 1987; 36:1589.

292. Weisdorf DJ, Jacobs HS: Beta-adrenergic blockade: Augmentation of neutrophil-mediated inflammation. *J Lab Clin Med* 1987; 109:120.

293. Nielson CP: β-Adrenergic modulation of the polymorphonu-

clear leukocyte respiratory burst is dependent upon the mechanism of cell activation. *J Immunol* 1987; 139:2392.

294. Busse WW, Sosman JM: Isoproterenol inhibition of isolated neutrophil function. *J Allergy Clin Immunol* 1984; 73:404.

295. Liggett SB: Identification and characterization of a homogeneous population of β_2-adrenergic receptors on human alveolar macrophages. *Am Rev Respir Dis* 1989; 139:552.

296. Fukushima T, Sekizawa K, Jin Y, et al.: Effects of β-adrenergic receptor activation on alveolar macrophage cytoplasmic motility. *Am J Physiol* 265 (Lung Cell Mol Physiol 9) 1993:L67.

297. Stewart AG, Tomlinson PR, Wilson J: Airway wall remodelling in asthma: A novel target for the development of anti-asthma drugs. *Trends Pharmacol Sci* 1993; 14:275.

298. Noveral JP, Grunstein MM: Adrenergic receptor-mediated regulation of cultured rabbit airway smooth muscle cell proliferation. *Am J Physiol* 267 (Lung Cell Mol Physiol 11) 1994:L291.

299. Kelsen SG, Zhou S, Anakwe O, et al.: Expression of the β-adrenergic receptor-adenylyl cyclase system in basal and columnar airway epithelial cells. *Am J Physiol* 267 (Lung Cell Mol Physiol 11) 1994:L4546.

300. Merten MD, Tournier J-M, Mecklar Y, Figarella C: Epinephrine promotes growth and differentiation of human tracheal gland cells in culture. *Am J Respir Cell Mol Biol* 1993; 9:172.

301. Nishikawa M, Mak JCW, Shirasaki H, et al.: Long-term exposure to norepinephrine results in down-regulation and reduced mRNA expression of pulmonary β-adrenergic receptors in guinea pigs. *Am J Respir Cell Mol Biol* 1994: 10:91.

302. Mardini IA, Higgins NC, Zhou S, et al.: Functional behavior of the β-adrenergic receptor-adenylyl cyclase system in rabbit airway epithelium. *Am J Respir Cell Mol Biol* 1994; 11:287.

303. Penn RB, Kelson SG, Benovic JL: Regulation of β-agonist- and prostaglandin E_2-mediated adenylyl cyclase activity in human airway epithelial cells. *Am J Respir Cell Mol Biol* 1994; 11:496.

304. Wang Z-L, Bramley AM, McNamara A, et al.: Chronic fenoterol exposure increases in vivo and in vitro airway responses in guinea pigs. *Am J Respir Crit Care Med* 1994; 149:960.

305. Wills-Karp M, Uchida Y, Lee JY, et al.: Organ culture with proinflammatory cytokines reproduces impairment of the β-adrenoceptor-mediated relaxation in tracheas of a guinea pig antigen model. *Am J Respir Cell Mol Biol* 1993; 8:153.

306. Nogami M, Romberger DJ, Rennard SI, Toews ML: TGF-β1 modulates β-adrenergic receptor number and function in cultured human tracheal smooth muscle cells. *Am J Physiol* 266 (Lung Cell Mol Physiol 10) 1994:L187.

307. Brinkrant DJ, Davis PB, Ernsberger P: Visualization of high- and low-affinity β-adrenergic receptors in rat lung: Upregulation by chronic hypoxia. *Am J Physiol* 265 (Lung Cell Mol Physiol 9) 1993:L389.

308. Fernandes LB, Fryer AD, Hirshman CA: M2 muscarinic receptors inhibit isoproterenol-induced relaxation of canine airway smooth muscle. *J Pharmacol Exp Ther* 1992; 262:119.

309. Yang J, Emala CW, Hirshman CA, et al.: Characterization of GTP-binding proteins coupled to inhibition of adenylyl cyclase in guinea pig tracheal epithelial cells. *Am J Respir Cell Mol Biol* 1994; 10:665.

Chapter 6

PARASYMPATHETIC INNERVATION OF THE AIRWAYS

DAVID B. JACOBY AND ALLISON D. FRYER

Introduction

The parasympathetic, cholinergic nerves in the vagi provide the dominant autonomic control of the airways. Stimulating the vagus nerves electrically releases acetylcholine onto muscarinic receptors, contracting airway smooth muscle and causing bronchoconstriction. Defective control of the parasympathetic nerves supplying the lungs may lead to increased release of acetylcholine in airways diseases, such as asthma and chronic obstructive pulmonary disease.

Certain peptides, prostaglandins, and leukotrienes potentiate acetylcholine release from parasympathetic nerves in the lungs. Conversely, acetylcholine release can be inhibited significantly by norepinephrine from sympathetic nerves and by an assortment of prostaglandins, opioids, and peptides. Furthermore, acetylcholine can inhibit its own release through prejunctional autoreceptors on the parasympathetic nerves. In this chapter, the parasympathetic control of airway smooth muscle and the evidence for the local control of acetylcholine release from the pulmonary parasympathetic nerves are described.

Cholinergic Innervation of the Airways

Electrical stimulation of the vagus nerves constricts the airways.[1–10] Dixon and Brody demonstrated that anticholinergic agents like atropine blocked the bronchoconstriction resulting from both muscarine and vagal stimulation.[1] It later was demonstrated that electrical stimulation of the vagus nerves releases acetylcholine in the lung.[11] When the addition of anticholinesterases potentiated vagally induced bronchoconstriction[2,3] and the inhibitory effect of atropine on vagally induced bronchoconstriction was confirmed,[2] it

was concluded that the vagus nerves supplying the lung are cholinergic (i.e., that the neurotransmitter released from the vagus nerve is acetylcholine) and that vagally induced bronchoconstriction is mediated by muscarinic acetylcholine receptors. Cholinergic nerves also supply the airway submucosal glands and stimulate secretion through muscarinic receptors.[12]

The recurrent laryngeal nerve (a branch of the thoracic vagus) supplies the parasympathetic innervation of the trachea.[13,14] The parasympathetic ganglia are most dense near the trachealis muscle and lie in chains along each side of it (see Fig. 6-1).[15] The intrapulmonary airways are supplied by branches of the vagus that enter the lung at the hilum, where they synapse in the bronchi with parasympathetic ganglionic cells located in both extrachondrial and subchondrial plexuses. In both trachea and lung, the postganglionic nerves are nonmyelinated and supply airway smooth muscle and glands.[16]

The cholinergic innervation of the lungs is most dense in the area of the hilum of the lung.[13] It decreases in the smaller bronchi, and while human infant bronchi with diameters as small as 1 mm contain parasympathetic ganglia,[16] cholinergic nerves are nonexistent in cat and dog airways < 0.8 mm in diameter and in the parenchyma.[13]

The density of muscarinic receptors also decreases in the more distal airways, and the terminal bronchioles are almost devoid of muscarinic receptors.[17,18] Therefore, electrical stimulation of the vagus nerves causes a greater degree of contraction in the intermediate bronchi, those bronchi with diameters of 1 to 5 mm in dogs and 0.8 to 2.0 mm in cats, than in either the main bronchi or the trachea.[8,9,19,20] It is significant that cholinergic nerves have their greatest effects in intermediate airways since there is evidence that these airways are the sites of maximal resistance to airflow.[21]

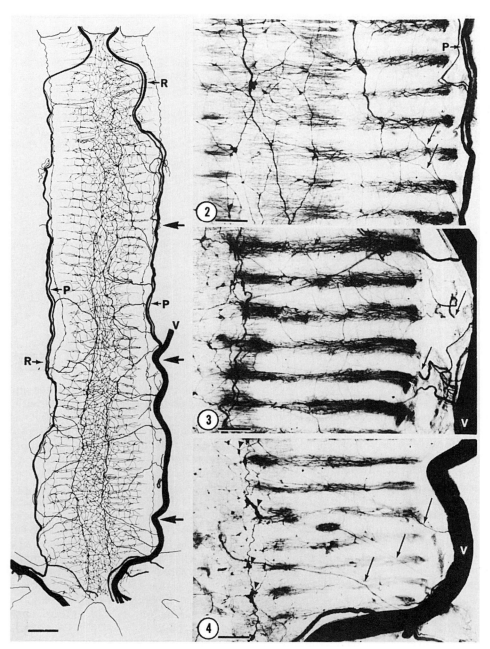

FIGURE 6-1 Staining a ferret trachea for acetylcholinesterase reveals a network of parasympathetic nerve fibers. A tracing of these stained nerves is shown on the left from larynx (*top*) to the carina (*bottom*) of a newborn ferret. The vagus nerves (V), the recurrent laryngeal nerves (R), and the pararecurrent laryngeal nerves (P) are shown. Panels 2 to 4 on the right are photomicro-graphs of the trachea taken in the region of the corresponding arrows. Axons in the deep muscle plexus run horizontally and tend to give the muscle a striated appearance in these three photographs. Branches of the pararecurrent laryngeal nerve (arrows, photo 2) and vagus (arrows, photos 3,4) are shown. (*From Baker et al.,*[15] *with permission.*)

CHOLINERGIC CONTROL OF AIRWAY SMOOTH MUSCLE

In all species studied, the airways are constricted tonically. It is the parasympathetic nerves that maintain this tone since atropine or sectioning of the vagi leads to bronchodilation.[2–5,8,22,23] Vagal nerve stimulation can increase resistance by 500 to 1000 percent in cats.[3,24]

By contrast, in many species including humans, the sympathetic nerves probably have no direct effects on airway smooth muscle. Rather, they modulate cholinergic neurotransmission. Concurrent stimulation of the sympathetic nerves with the cholinergic nerves reduces vagally induced bronchoconstriction but does not reverse it,[3,8,25] and when the vagus nerves are cut, electrical stimulation of the sympathetic nerves has no effect on airway smooth muscle.[4,8,26] Thus, the cholinergic nerves, not the sympathetic nerves, are responsible for the maintenance of tone in the airways and for bronchoconstriction tone.

MUSCARINIC RECEPTORS ON AIRWAY SMOOTH MUSCLE

The receptors responsible for vagally mediated bronchoconstriction are muscarinic since the effects of vagal nerve stimulation are blocked by the muscarinic receptor antagonist atropine. The use of radioligand binding on slide-mounted tissue sections has allowed quantification of muscarinic receptors in the lung. Within the trachea and bronchi, muscarinic receptors have been localized to the smooth muscle, epithelium, submucosal glands, and parasympathetic ganglia. Bronchial smooth muscle contains significantly fewer receptors than tracheal muscle, and muscarinic receptor density decreases with bronchial size. In most species, the alveoli contain very few muscarinic receptors, while in some species (ferret and guinea pig), the alveoli have no apparent muscarinic receptors.[18,27–29] Muscarinic receptors have been described in rat alveoli type II pneumocytes, which respond to agonists with increased intracellular Ca^{2+}.[29] There are also muscarinic receptors in human lung parenchyma[28,30]; however, they probably are not innervated by cholinergic nerves, and their function is not known.

Genes for five subtypes of muscarinic receptor, designated M_1 to M_5, have been identified,[31–33] although only three subtypes (M_1 to M_3) can be distinguished pharmacologically (for classification of receptor subtypes see Chap. 7). Ligand-binding studies reveal M_2- and M_3-muscarinic receptors on airway smooth muscle.[34,35] This has been confirmed using Northern blot analysis to detect mRNA for M_2- and M_3-receptors.[30,36] Receptor ligand-binding assays demonstrate that the number of M_3 receptors is $\leq$ the number of M_2 receptors; 15 to 26 percent are M_3 in the cow trachea,[35,37–39] 30 percent are M_3 in rat airway smooth muscle,[40] while in dog and guinea pig trachea, the proportion of M_2 to M_3 receptors is almost equal.[41,42]

Functional studies indicate that M_3-muscarinic receptors mediate airway smooth muscle contraction.[41,43–50] M_3 receptors in the ileal, uterine, and bladder smooth muscle also mediate contraction.[51] Stimulation of M_3-muscarinic receptors in airway smooth muscle stimulates the turnover of membrane phosphoinositides.[45,52] This occurs because the receptors are coupled through G proteins to phospholipase C, which catalyzes the breakdown of the membrane phospholipid phosphatidylinositol 4,5-bisphosphate to inositol trisphosphate (which releases Ca^{2+} from the sarcoplasmic reticulum), and diacylglycerol, which activates protein kinase C and may increase the sensitivity of the smooth muscle contractile proteins to activation by Ca^{2+}.[52–59]

Although it is known that M_3-receptors mediate both turnover of membrane phosphoinositides and smooth muscle contraction, there are differences between occupancy of the receptors, turnover of phosphoinositide, and contraction. Contraction of airway smooth muscle is several orders of magnitude more sensitive to acetylcholine than is turnover of phosphoinositide.[54] Maximum contraction occurs when 20 percent of receptors are occupied, while the maximum increase in phosphoinositide turnover does not occur until all receptors are occupied. Some of these discrepancies can be explained by the presence of spare receptors in airway smooth muscle. However, muscarinic receptors can be linked to many intracellular processes including inhibition of adenylate cyclase (see below), activation of phospholipases A and D and nitric oxide synthase, stimulation of cyclic guanosine monophosphate (cGMP) production, and regulation of several ion channels.[60] It may be a combination of various pathways that ultimately results in contraction of airway smooth muscle.

Stimulating the remaining 50 to 80 percent of muscarinic receptors on airway smooth muscle, the M_2-receptors, inhibits β-adrenoreceptor-induced relaxation of airway smooth muscle.[61,62] It is known that stimulation of M_2-muscarinic receptors in airway smooth muscle leads to inhibition of adenylyl cyclase through an inhibitory, pertussis-sensitive G protein (G_i).[52,63–66] Thus, the cholinergic nerves can directly inhibit catecholamine-mediated relaxation of airway smooth muscle.

ACETYLCHOLINESTERASE

The effects of acetylcholine on airway smooth muscle are limited as it is broken down by acetylcholinesterase. Decreasing cholinesterase activity would, therefore, increase vagally mediated bronchoconstriction. This may be relevant to certain disease states, as it has been shown that acetylcholinesterase activity is decreased after allergen sensitization[67] or inhalation of ozone.[68–70]

Control of Acetylcholine Release

The release of acetylcholine from pulmonary cholinergic nerves is controlled by a variety of substances, including neurotransmitters, amines, prostaglandins, and peptides. Whether these substances are important physiologically, as well as pharmacologically, still is debated, but many of them are endogenous in the lung and exert their effects at concentrations that could occur in the area of the cholinergic nerves. Local control of acetylcholine release from the cholinergic nerves supplying the airways may be important in regulating basal airway tone and for determining the degree of bronchoconstriction during vagally mediated reflexes.

Traditionally, the effect of a mediator on acetylcholine release has been tested by determining the effect of the mediator on the smooth muscle response to electrical stimulation of the vagus nerve. This then is compared to the effect of the mediator on the smooth muscle response to exogenous acetylcholine. If the mediator inhibits or enhances vagally induced contraction of the airway smooth muscle but has little or no effect on acetylcholine-induced contractions, it is concluded that it either inhibited or enhanced acetylcholine release (respectively) from the vagus nerves. Direct measurement of acetylcholine release from airway vagal fibers has been used recently to confirm the prejunctional control of acetylcholine release.

EFFECTS OF INFLAMMATORY MEDIATORS

Inflammation of the airways is a characteristic of many conditions associated with increased vagally mediated bronchoconstriction. A variety of inflammatory mediators may affect acetylcholine release from airway parasympathetic nerves.

HISTAMINE

Histamine contracts airway smooth muscle directly and also stimulates airway irritant receptors to initiate a vagally mediated reflex bronchoconstriction.[71] Histamine potentiates acetylcholine release and vagally induced bronchoconstriction in dogs[72-74] and may also cause acetylcholine release itself in the absence of nerve depolarization.[75] In humans and guinea pigs, histamine may also inhibit acetylcholine release, an effect that is mediated by H_3-receptors.[76,77] (See also Chap. 11)

PLATELET-ACTIVATING FACTOR

Bronchoconstriction caused by platelet-activating factor (PAF) is attenuated by atropine.[78] Acetylcholine-induced bronchoconstriction is unaffected by PAF.[79] It has therefore been assumed that PAF increases acetylcholine release. However, PAF probably has no direct effect on the nerves, because when it is injected only into the tracheal arteries, it has no effect on vagally induced bronchoconstriction.[80] This raises the possibility that inflammatory cells, when stimulated by PAF, release mediators that affect acetylcholine release. It has been demonstrated that many of the effects of PAF are mediated via the generation of lipoxygenase products.[81]

BRADYKININ

Atropine inhibits bradykinin-induced bronchoconstriction.[82,83] However, it is the tachykinins and cyclooxygenase products released by bradykinin, rather than bradykinin itself, that affect cholinergic neurotransmission.[83,84] Inhalation of bradykinin also may stimulate afferent nerves,[85] causing reflex bronchoconstriction (Chap. 15).

PROSTAGLANDINS AND LEUKOTRIENES

Inhibiting prostaglandin (PG) synthesis in dogs induces wheezing,[86] while aspirin can induce bronchoconstriction in some asthmatics.[87] While many mechanisms may play a role in these responses, the inhibitory effects of prostaglandins on cholinergic neurotransmission have been demonstrated in most species studied,[88-91] including humans.[92]

Repeated electrical stimulation of airway vagal fibers causes a gradual decrease in the evoked smooth muscle contraction. When tissues are treated with the cyclooxygenase inhibitor indomethacin, this attenuation is blocked.[91,93] Indomethacin[94,95] or blockade of prostaglandin receptors[96] also potentiates vagally induced bronchoconstriction in vivo. Thus, airway prostaglandins[91,97] inhibit acetylcholine release from the cholinergic nerves.

These inhibitory prostaglandins in the airways include PGE_2,[88,89,92,96] PGE_1,[90,93] $PGF_{2\alpha}$,[96] PGA_1, PGA_2, and PGB_2. Both PGE_2 and PGE_1 inhibit acetylcholine release completely in the nM range. Leukotriene E_4 also has been shown to inhibit cholinergic neurotransmission,[81,98] while thromboxane A_2,[99-101] PGD_2,[102] and leukotrienes B_4, C_4, and D_4[81,98] potentiate the release of acetylcholine in the airways.

Inhibition of acetylcholine release by PGE_2 also can be demonstrated by direct measurement of acetylcholine. The inhibition of acetylcholine release by endogenous prostaglandins also is evident from studies in which these measurements show increased acetylcholine release after treatment with indomethacin.[103,104]

Ganglionic neurotransmission can be potentiated by PGD_2, an effect that likely results from the resting membrane potential of the ganglion cells becoming less negative. This effect may be particularly relevant to the response to antigen challenge, which causes release of PGD_2 and potentiates ganglionic transmission.[105]

EOSINOPHIL PROTEINS

The eosinophil is ubiquitous in the airways of patients with asthma. Eosinophil influx also occurs in the airway parasympathetic nerves in antigen-challenged guinea pigs (unpublished observation). The eosinophil contains several proteins that may interact with M_2-muscarinic receptors on the parasympathetic nerves to increase acetylcholine release (see below).

ENDOTHELIN

Endothelin (ET) is a peptide produced in the airways by the airway epithelium. It is a potent bronchoconstrictor itself but also potentiates the release of acetylcholine from vagal fibers.[106] This effect appears to be mediated by ET_B receptors on the nerves.[107,108]

EFFECTS OF NEUROTRANSMITTERS

A complex interplay exists between the cholinergic, adrenergic, and nonadrenergic, noncholinergic nerves. Peptide neurotransmitters such as vasoactive intestinal peptide (VIP) and the tachykinins may have important effects both on the nerves and the airway smooth muscle. Catecholamines may inhibit acetylcholine release by interaction with multiple receptors. Gamma amino butyric acid (through the $GABA_B$ receptor),[109] β-endorphin,[110] and μ- and δ-opioid receptor agonists[111] also inhibit cholinergic neurotransmission. Gamma amino butyric acid through the $GABA_A$ receptor,[112] somatostatin,[113] corticotropin-releasing factor,[114] 5-hydroxytryptamine,[115] and adenosine[116,117] all potentiate cholinergic neurotransmission.

VASOACTIVE INTESTINAL PEPTIDE

Vasoactive intestinal peptide is present in the airway nerves.[118] VIP antagonists enhance cholinergic neurotransmission in the cat,[119,120] suggesting that endogenous VIP is released simultaneously with acetylcholine and that it inhibits acetylcholine release.[119,121,122]

TACHYKININS

Substance P increases unstimulated acetylcholine release from the cholinergic nerves supplying the lungs.[123-125] This effect is not affected by ganglionic blockade or by tetrodotoxin. Thus the acetylcholine release occurs independently of action potentials and is not the result of a reflex. Similar results were obtained in vivo, where atropine, but not vagotomy, inhibited substance P–induced bronchoconstriction.[126]

Substance P also potentiates stimulus-evoked acetylcholine release. The degree of potentiation appears to be species-dependent. In rabbits 10^{-7} M substance P causes a 275 percent increase in the bronchoconstriction response to electrical stimulation of the vagus, while in guinea pigs the potentiation is approximately 40 percent.[127,128] In human bronchus, the tachykinin neurokinin A (NK A) causes a small potentiation of cholinergic contractions but only in the presence of K^+ channel antagonists.[129] This potentiation of cholinergic contractions by tachykinins is separate from the increased leak of acetylcholine described above since it is blocked by tetrodotoxin.[128] Furthermore, endogenous tachykinins potentiate cholinergic contractions induced by nicotine or vagal nerve stimulation, as these can be inhibited by depletion of substance P or by treatment with a substance P an-tagonist.[125,130] Conversely, cholinergic contractions are potentiated by inhibitors of the enzyme neutral endopeptidase, which breaks down substance P, and by capsaicin-stimulated release of substance P.[123,131] In vivo, electrical stimulation of the capsaicin-sensitive nerves, which contain tachykinins, enhances cholinergic contractions of airway smooth muscle by 50 percent.[105] Thus, tachykinins have a significant excitatory effect on cholinergic neurotransmission. Using selective neurokinin receptor antagonists, the receptors on the parasympathetic nerves have been classified as NK_1 receptors.[132] (See Chap. 17)

Cholinergic neurotransmission is enhanced during infection with respiratory viruses (e.g., influenza and parainfluenza). These infections decrease the activity of neutral endopeptidase, the enzyme that normally breaks down the tachykinins.[133] Thus, increased levels of endogenous tachykinins could enhance vagally induced bronchoconstriction, contributing to the airway hyperreactivity seen with some viral infections.

CATECHOLAMINES

While stimulation of the parasympathetic nerves leads to contraction of airway smooth muscle, stimulation of the sympathetic nerves (in most species) opposes this bronchoconstriction. These nervous systems may oppose each other at the level of airway nerves. Norepinephrine can inhibit acetylcholine release from parasympathetic nerves, while acetylcholine can inhibit norepinephrine release from sympathetic nerves.[134]

Airway smooth muscle contraction induced by electrical field stimulation, but not that induced by exogenous acetylcholine, can be inhibited dramatically by either norepinephrine or isoproterenol. Thus, adrenergic agonists inhibit acetylcholine release from postganglionic parasympathetic nerves.[135–143] Both norepinephrine and isoproterenol inhibit the excitatory junction potentials (EJPs) elicited by electrical field stimulation of canine trachea,[137] providing electrophysiologic evidence that catecholamines inhibit cholinergic neurotransmission by acting prejunctionally to inhibit acetylcholine release.

There are catecholamine-containing nerve fibers in the pulmonary parasympathetic ganglia.[144,145] Electrical stimulation of the sympathetic nerves inhibits vagally mediated tracheal tone completely in anesthetized cats but reduces tone induced by exogenous acetylcholine by only 50 percent.[138] Thus, it is possible that local concentrations of endogenous norepinephrine are sufficient to affect cholinergic neurotransmission. Norepinephrine in concentrations between 10^{-5} M and 10^{-4} M, depending on the species, can inhibit vagally induced bronchoconstriction almost completely. While circulating concentrations of catecholamines never reach these concentrations endogeneously, it is likely that local release of catecholamines plays a role in regulation of acetylcholine release.

Different types of adrenoreceptor are responsible for catecholamine-induced inhibition of cholinergic neurotransmission in different species. In dogs, the effect is mediated by β-adrenergic receptors,[135,137] specifically β_1 receptors,[136] while in guinea pigs, α_2-adrenergic receptors inhibit cholinergic neurotransmission.[139–141] In humans, the effect of catecholamines on parasympathetic nerves has been reported to be mediated through β_2-adrenergic receptors.[143] However, when β-adrenoreceptors are blocked with propranolol, inhibition of acetylcholine release by α-adrenergic receptors can be demonstrated.[142] Nonetheless, given the high potency of isoproterenol for this effect, it seems most likely that inhibition of acetylcholine release by catecholamines is mediated predominantly through β-adrenergic receptors in the human lung.

Catecholamines also inhibit transmission at the parasympathetic ganglion, blocking release of acetylcholine from the preganglionic nerve. This effect can be reversed by phentolamine, indicating that it is mediated by α-adrenergic receptors.[146]

INHIBITORY M$_2$-MUSCARINIC RECEPTORS ON PARASYMPATHETIC NERVES

Perhaps the most important mechanism for the inhibition of acetylcholine release from the parasympathetic nerves is provided by acetylcholine itself, which stimulates prejunctional autoreceptors to inhibit acetylcholine release. In the airways, acetylcholine release from the cholinergic nerves is controlled by inhibitory M_2-muscarinic autoreceptors (see Fig. 6-2).[147] These autoreceptors on the postganglionic vagal fibers provide a negative feedback mechanism whereby acetylcholine released from the vagus nerve inhibits further release of acetylcholine.

OVERVIEW OF M$_2$-RECEPTOR FUNCTION

Autoradiographic binding to tissue sections of bovine, guinea pig, and human lung as well as cultures of postganglionic, parasympathetic nerves from the trachea demonstrate dense labeling of muscarinic receptors in airway ganglia and nerve axons.[28,148–150] Direct measurement of acetylcholine release confirms that blocking these autoreceptors increases acetylcholine release.[151,152] Furthermore, M_2-receptors can be demonstrated on cultured airway parasympathetic neurons immunohistologically, and mRNA encoding the M_2-receptor can be demonstrated in these cells

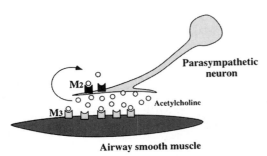

FIGURE 6-2 Release of acetylcholine from parasympathetic nerve fibers contracts airway smooth muscle by acting on M_3 receptors. At the same time, acetylcholine feeds back onto inhibitory M_2 receptors on the nerve ending, decreasing the further release of acetylcholine.

using the polymerase chain reaction (Fryer and Jacoby, unpublished observations).

Pharmacologic experiments demonstrate that vagally induced bronchoconstriction is altered by selective muscarinic agonists and antagonists at doses that do not affect acetylcholine-induced bronchoconstriction. Inhibitory M_2-muscarinic autoreceptors are present on the airway nerves of every species studied thus far, including guinea

pigs,[52,147,153–155] cats,[156,157] rats,[158] dogs,[46,159] and humans.[160] They may be dysfunctional in humans with asthma.[161,162]

Blocking the M_2-receptors increases acetylcholine release and potentiates vagally induced bronchoconstriction 10-fold.[147,151,152] Conversely, stimulating the M_2 receptors with muscarinic agonists inhibits vagally induced bronchoconstriction in the guinea pig as much as 80 percent (Fig. 6-3).[147] In human bronchi, the muscarinic agonist, pilocarpine, inhibits electrical field stimulation–induced contraction by 96 percent, demonstrating that the M_2-muscarinic receptors also exert a marked degree of inhibition in human lung.[160]

M_2-RECEPTOR DYSFUNCTION IN DISEASE

Loss of function of the M_2-receptor has the same effect as blocking it pharmacologically. Acetylcholine release is increased, and vagally mediated bronchoconstriction is potentiated. Such a situation may exist in the airways of patients with asthma.[161,162]

In guinea pigs, M_2-receptor function is lost after acute infection with parainfluenza virus,[163] sensitization and challenge with ovalbumin,[164] and acute exposure to ozone[70] (Fig. 6-4). Different mechanisms may lead to M_2-receptor dysfunction in each of these models, but vagally mediated bronchoconstriction is increased in all.

FIGURE 6-3 Pilocarpine inhibits vagally mediated bronchoconstriction. Pulmonary inflation pressure (Ppi), blood pressure, and heart rate were measured in anesthetized, ventilated guinea pigs. Electrical stimulation of both vagus nerves (V.S. and at the black diamonds) causes a decrease in heart rate and bronchoconstriction (measured as a rise in pulmonary inflation pressure; top trace represents the increase in inflation pressure at a higher gain). The muscarinic agonist, pilocarpine (1 to 100 µg/kg i.v.), stimulates the M_2-muscarinic receptors in the parasympathetic nerves and inhibits the release of acetylcholine, thus also inhibiting vagally mediated bronchoconstriction.

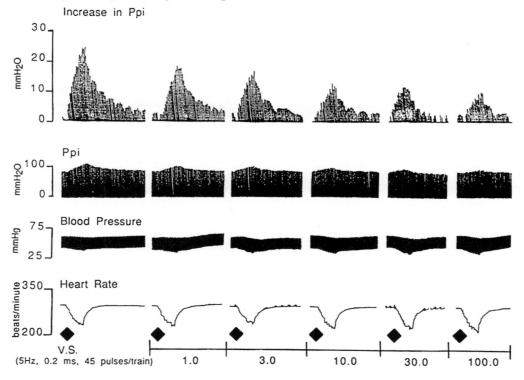

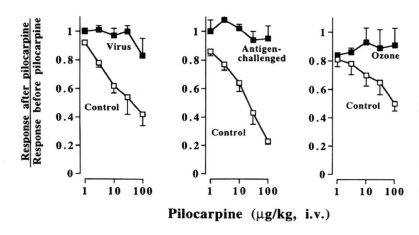

FIGURE 6-4 M$_2$-muscarinic receptor function is lost after viral infection (*left*), antigen challenge (*middle*), and ozone exposure (*right*). Results are expressed as the ratio of the response to vagal stimulation after pilocarpine to the response before pilocarpine. In control animals (open squares), pilocarpine inhibited vagally induced bronchoconstriction; however, in each model of hyperresponsiveness, pilocarpine is no longer able to suppress the response to vagal stimulation (closed squares).

Ozone Inhalation and the Role of Inflammation

Although it has been recognized for some time that inhalation of ozone causes airway inflammation,[165,166] the role of inflammation in causing airway hyperresponsiveness has been debated.[167,168] For ozone-induced M$_2$-receptor dysfunction in guinea pigs, the time course of M$_2$-receptor damage and recovery parallels closely the development and resolution of airway inflammation.[70] M$_2$-receptor dysfunction develops immediately upon ozone exposure and resolves (along with inflammation) by 14 weeks after exposure. Furthermore, in guinea pigs treated with cyclophosphamide to deplete inflammatory cells, M$_2$-receptor function is preserved after exposure to ozone.[169] This suggests that inflammatory cells or mediators are important in the pathogenesis of the loss of M$_2$-receptor function.

Antigen-Induced M$_2$-Receptor Dysfunction and Eosinophil Proteins

Exposure to antigen increases the magnitude of the excitatory postjunctional potentials in the airway smooth muscle[170] as well as acetylcholine release from the parasympathetic nerves in the lungs.[171] After inhalation of antigen, the function of the neuronal M$_2$-receptors largely is lost in guinea pigs.[164] Because antigen inhalation causes airway inflammation that is composed largely of eosinophils, it appears possible that a product of eosinophils might be responsible for M$_2$-receptor dysfunction. Such a hypothesis is also attractive because of the presence of eosinophilic inflammation in the airways of asthmatics.[172] Furthermore, blocking the influx of eosinophils into the airways using an antibody to interleukin-5 prevents antigen-induced loss of M$_2$-receptor function.[173]

Some positively charged proteins are antagonists for M$_2$- but not for M$_3$-muscarinic receptors.[174] Eosinophils recruited into the lungs during an inflammatory response release positively charged proteins such as eosinophil major basic protein and eosinophil peroxidase,[175–177] both of which are allosteric antagonists for M$_2$- but not for M$_3$-muscarinic receptors.[178] In guinea pigs made hyperresponsive by sensitization and challenge with an antigen, administration of either heparin or poly-1-glutamate, both of which bind to and neutralize major basic protein in vitro, reverses the

hyperresponsiveness (Fig. 6-5) and completely restores the function of the M$_2$-muscarinic receptor.[179] Thus, it is possible that positively charged proteins released from inflammatory cells bind to the neuronal M$_2$ receptor, blocking the negative feedback control of acetylcholine release that it provides. Further support for the involvement of eosinophils in antigen-induced M$_2$-receptor dysfunction is provided by the observation that the parasympathetic nerves are infiltrated with eosinophils in antigen-challenged guinea pigs (Fig. 6-6).

Viral Infections and the Role of Neuraminidase

Viral infections of the airways exacerbate both asthma and chronic obstructive pulmonary disease. Furthermore, in previously normal individuals, viral infections cause temporary airway hyperresponsiveness.[180–182] The temporary hyperresponsiveness to histamine in virus-infected airways can be blocked by atropine in humans[180] and by vagotomy in guinea pigs.[183] Thus, virus-induced hyperresponsiveness is reflex mediated through the vagus nerves. The efferent, parasympathetic limb of the reflex arc is affected since airway smooth muscle contraction in response to electrical stimulation of the vagus is potentiated during viral infections.[183] Infection of guinea pigs with parainfluenza virus causes loss of M$_2$-receptor function.[163]

Multiple mechanisms may be involved in virus-induced M$_2$-receptor dysfunction. M$_2$-muscarinic receptors contain negatively charged sialic acid residues that are crucial to agonist binding.[184] Removal of the sialic acid by the enzyme neuraminidase reduces agonist affinity for the M$_2$-receptor. Neuraminidase is present in influenza and parainfluenza viruses.[185,186] Exposure of M$_2$-receptors to parainfluenza virus in vitro causes a 10-fold decrease in agonist affinity, an effect that can be blocked by a neuraminidase inhibitor and mimicked by an equivalent concentration of purified *Clostridium perfringens* neuraminidase.[187]

Viral infections also cause airway inflammation. Because of the importance of airway inflammation in the attenuation of M$_2$-receptor function that follows exposure to ozone or antigen, the role of inflammation in virus-induced M$_2$-receptor dysfunction has been determined. Depleting leukocytes by pretreating guinea pigs with cyclophosphamide before

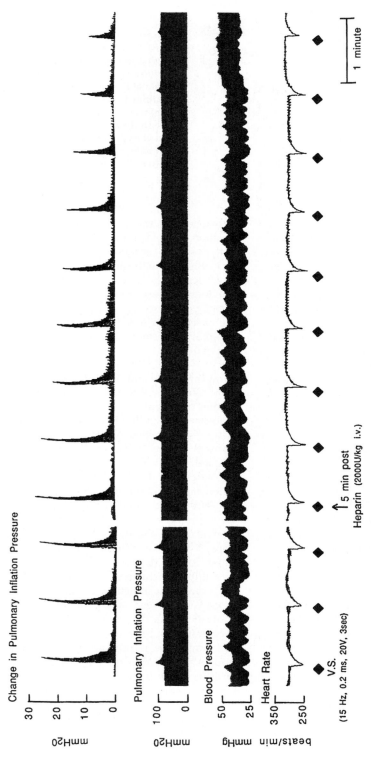

FIGURE 6-5 In antigen-challenged guinea pigs, heparin (2000 units/kg, i.v.) acutely restores M_2-receptor function, causing a 50 percent decrease in the response to vagal stimulation. Pulmonary inflation pressure, blood pressure, and heart rate were measured in anesthetized, ventilated guinea pigs. Electrical stimulation of both vagus nerves (V.S. and at the black diamonds) causes bronchoconstriction (measured as a rise in pulmonary inflation pressure; top trace represents the change in inflation pressure at a higher gain) and bradycardia. The first three responses to vagal nerve stimulation on the left of the figure are in the absence of heparin. The remaining responses are post-heparin. The response to pilocarpine is lost in antigen-challenged guinea pigs (see Fig. 6-4); however, heparin restores the ability of pilocarpine to suppress vagally mediated bronchoconstriction (not shown), thus demonstrating that heparin can restore the function of the inhibitory M_2-muscarinic receptor. Heparin has no effect on vagally mediated bronchoconstriction in animals that have not been challenged with antigen. (*From Fryer and Jacoby,*[179] *with permission.*)

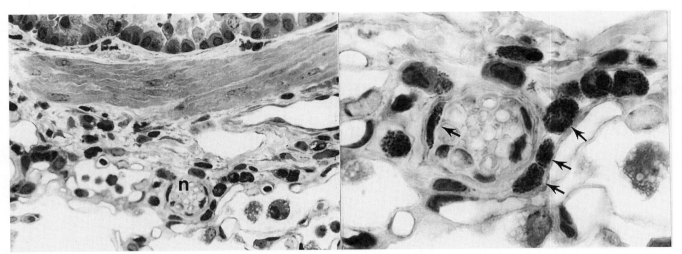

FIGURE 6-6 Antigen challenge of sensitized guinea pigs causes infiltration of the airway parasympathetic nerves with eosinophils. A representative section from one guinea pig lung is shown under low (*left*) and high (*right*) magnification. A nerve bundle (labeled n) is clearly seen lying directly under the airway smooth muscle. In this antigen-challenged guinea pig, eosinophils not only surround the nerves but have also infiltrated the nerve bundle (arrows). In control guinea pigs, this influx of eosinophils is not present (not shown). Magnification bars represent 42 μm (*left*) and 20 μm (*right*). (*From Elbon et al.,*[173] *with permission.*)

infecting them with virus prevented M_2-receptor dysfunction in about half of the animals.[188] It is likely to be significant that the viral content of those animals that lost M_2-receptor function despite depletion of leukocytes was approximately 10-fold greater than in those animals in which M_2-receptor function was preserved. Thus, both leukocyte-dependent mechanisms (in animals with mild viral infections) and leukocyte-independent mechanisms (in animals with severe viral infections) may contribute to virus-induced M_2-receptor dysfunction.

Long-Term Alterations in M_2-Receptor Function

Airway inflammation and viral infections may cause both acute and long-term alterations in M_2-receptor function. After either viral infection or ozone exposure, M_2-receptor function appears to return to normal within 2 to 4 weeks.[189,190] However, subtle, but potentially important, changes in M_2-receptor function persist, as revealed by the effects of both cycloxygenase inhibitors and nitric oxide synthase inhibitors.

In pathogen-free guinea pigs, the function of M_2-receptors is completely independent of prostaglandin production and is unaffected by indomethacin.[95] However, in nonpathogen-free guinea pigs, indomethacin potentiates vagally induced bronchoconstriction and markedly inhibits M_2-receptor function.[191] Thus, the function of M_2-receptors in the lung is dependent on cyclooxygenase and, presumably, on prostaglandins. This change in receptor function can be demonstrated 1 to 2 months after either viral infection[190] or ozone exposure (Fryer, unpublished observation). Similarly, inhibiting nitric oxide synthase does not affect M_2-receptor function in pathogen-free guinea pigs but does inhibit M_2-receptor function markedly after recovery from either ozone exposure or viral infection[192] (Fryer, unpublished observation).

THERAPEUTIC IMPLICATIONS OF INHIBITORY M_2 RECEPTORS

Because blocking inhibitory M_2 receptors on the parasympathetic nerves increases the release of acetylcholine, currently available anticholinergic bronchodilators (atropine, ipratropium, and glycopyrrholate) are suboptimal. These medications decrease the effects of released acetylcholine on the excitatory M_3-receptors on the airway smooth muscle, causing bronchodilation, but at the same time they decrease the effect of released acetylcholine on the inhibitory M_2-receptors on the nerves. Thus, while decreasing the bronchoconstrictor response to acetylcholine, these drugs markedly increase the release of acetylcholine from the airway nerves.[152,193]

Several studies have demonstrated the physiologic relevance of this increase in acetylcholine release. In guinea pigs, the response to vagal stimulation is increased by ipratropium bromide given intravenously (see Fig. 6-7). Greater doses are required to decrease the response to vagal stimulation.[194]

More recently, it has been shown that ipratropium bromide, when administered to anesthetized dogs, constricted the airways at doses of 2 to 4 puffs and dilated the airways only at much greater doses (16 puffs) (Dr. Robert Brown, personal communication). When dogs were pretreated with the M_2-receptor antagonist gallamine, the M_2 blockade caused a similar degree of bronchoconstriction as did the ipratropium, but subsequent administration of ipratropium did not cause any further bronchoconstriction. Hence, it may be concluded preliminarily that ipratropium-induced bronchoconstriction results from its effect on neuronal M_2 receptors.

This effect of both atropine and ipratropium has been confirmed using direct measurement of acetylcholine release. Atropine (3×10^{-7} M) nearly doubles the amount of acetyl-

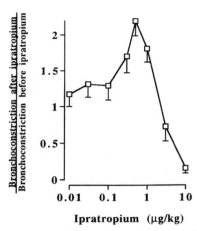

FIGURE 6-7 Ipratropium (0.01 to 1.0 μg/kg i.v.) blocks M_2 receptors and potentiates vagally mediated bronchoconstriction (open squares; solid line). Results are expressed as the ratio of the response to vagal stimulation after ipratropium to the response before ipratropium. Doses higher than 1.0 μg/kg i.v. ipratropium also block M_3 receptors on airway smooth muscle, thus inhibiting bronchoconstriction induced by both i.v. acetylcholine (not shown) and vagal nerve stimulation. (*From Fryer and Maclagan,*[194] *with permission.*)

choline released from rabbit trachea, while ipratropium (3×10^{-8} M) increases acetylcholine release by 50 percent.[193]

To avoid this deleterious effect of nonselective anticholinergics, some effort has been invested in developing selective M_3-receptor antagonists. Unfortunately, the high degree of homology among the different subtypes of muscarinic receptors has hampered the development of highly selective antagonists. The most widely used M_3-selective drugs currently available are hexahydro-sila-difenidol and *p*-fluoro-hexahydro-sila-difenidol. Direct measurement of acetylcholine release reveals that these compounds can block acetylcholine-induced airway smooth muscle contraction without increasing acetylcholine release.[193]

More recently, another anticholinergic agent, Ba 679 BR (tiotropium bromide), has been used experimentally. Receptor ligand-binding studies show that Ba 679 BR has similar affinities for M_2- and M_3-receptors. However, Ba 679 BR dissociates rapidly from M_2-receptors and very slowly from M_3-receptors. The result of this is that immediately after treatment, Ba 679 BR increases acetylcholine release, but after several hours, there is no longer any effect on M_2-receptors, and acetylcholine release returns to baseline. At this point, however, the binding of Ba 679 BR to M_3-receptors still is maximal, and the response of the smooth muscle to acetylcholine still is inhibited. Thus, Ba 679 BR is a selective M_3-antagonist.[195]

Conclusions

The cholinergic nerves provide the dominant control of smooth muscle tone in the lungs. Release of acetylcholine from the cholinergic nerves is affected by a variety of mediators and neurotransmitters including acetylcholine itself, which contribute to maintenance of normal autonomic tone in the lungs. Abnormalities in the control of acetylcholine release by any of these mechanisms, as well as changes in the function of inhibitory M_2-receptors on the parasympathetic nerves, may play an important role in vagally mediated bronchoconstriction in airways diseases.

References

1. Dixon WE, Brody TG: Contributions to the physiology of the lungs. Part 1, The bronchial muscles and their innervation and the action of drugs upon them. *J Physiol* 1903; 29:97.
2. Colebatch H, Halmagyi F: Effect of vagotomy and vagal stimulation on lung mechanics and circulation. *J Appl Physiol* 1963; 18:881.
3. Olsen CR, Colbatch HJH, Mebel PE, et al.: Motor control of pulmonary airways studied by nerve stimulation. *J Appl Physiol* 1965; 20:202.
4. Green M, Widdicombe JG: The effects of ventilation of dogs with different gas mixtures on airway caliber and lung mechanics. *J Physiol* 1966; 186:363.
5. Karczewski W, Widdicombe JG: The effect of vagotomy, vagal cooling and efferent vagal stimulation on breathing and lung mechanics of the rabbit. *J Physiol* 1969; 201:259.
6. Woolcock AJ, Macklem PT, Hogg JC, Wilson NJ: Influence of autonomic nervous system on airway resistance and elastic recoil. *J Appl Physiol* 1969; 26:814.
7. Woolcock AJ, Macklem PT, Hogg JC, et al.: Effect of vagal stimulation on central and peripheral airways in dogs. *J Appl Physiol* 1969; 26:806.
8. Cabezas GA, Graf PD, Nadel JA: Sympathetic versus parasympathetic nervous regulation of airways in dogs. *J Appl Physiol* 1971; 31:651.
9. Nadel JA, Cabezas GA, Austin JHM: In vivo roentgenographic examination of parasympathetic innervation of small airways: Use of tantalum and fine focal spot X-ray tube. *Invest Radiol* 1971; 6:9.
10. Suzuki H, Morita K, Kuriyama H: Innervation and properties of the smooth muscle of the dog trachea. *Jpn J Pharmacol* 1976; 26:303.
11. Carlyle RF: The responses of the guinea-pig isolated intact trachea to transmural stimulation and the release of an acetylcholine-like substance under conditions of rest and stimulation. *Br J Pharmacol* 1964; 22:126.
12. Borson DB, Chinn RA, Davis B, Nadel JA: Adrenergic and cholinergic nerves mediate fluid secretion from tracheal glands of ferrets. *J Appl Physiol* 1980; 49:1027.
13. Richardson JB: Nerve supply to the lungs. *Am Rev Respir Dis* 1979; 119:785.
14. Richardson JB: Recent progress in pulmonary innervation. *Am Rev Respir Dis* 1983; 128:S65.
15. Baker DG, McDonald DM, Basbaum CB, Mitchell RA: The architecture of nerves and ganglia of the ferret trachea as revealed by acetylcholinesterase histochemistry. *J Comp Neurol* 1986; 246:513.
16. Larsell O, Dow RS: The innervation of the human lung. *Am J Anat* 1933; 52:125.
17. Murlas C, Nadel JA, Roberts JM: The muscarinic receptors of airway smooth muscle: Their characteristics in vitro. *J Appl Physiol* 1982; 52:1084.
18. Barnes PJ, Nadel JA, Roberts JM, Basbaum CB: Muscarinic receptors in lung and trachea: Autoradiographic localization

using [3H] quinuclidinyl benzylate. *Eur J Pharmacol* 1983; 86:103.

19. Russell JA: Responses of isolated canine airways to electric stimulation and acetylcholine. *J Appl Physiol* 1978; 45:690.

20. Inoue H, Ishii M, Fuyuki T, et al.: Sympathetic and parasympathetic nervous control of airway resistance in dog lungs. *J Appl Physiol* 1983; 54:1496.

21. Nadel JA: Autonomic regulation of the airways, in Nadel JA (ed): *Physiology and Pharmacology of the Airways.* New York, Marcel Dekker, 1980; 217.

22. Widdicombe JG: Action potentials in parasympathetic and sympathetic efferent fibers to the trachea and lungs of dogs and cats. *J Physiol* 1966; 186:56.

23. Severinghaus JW, Stupfel M: Respiratory dead space increase following atropine in man, and atropine, vagal or ganglionic blockade and hypothermia in dogs. *J Appl Physiol* 1955; 8:81.

24. Blaber LC, Fryer AD: The response of the cat airways to histamine in vivo and in vitro. *Br J Pharmacol* 1985; 84:309.

25. Mitchell RA, Herbert DA, Baker DG: Inspiratory rhythm in airway smooth muscle tone. *J Appl Physiol* 1985; 58:911.

26. Daly MD, Mount LE: The origin, course and nature of bronchomotor fibers in the cervical sympathetic nerves of the cat. *J Physiol* 1951; 113:43.

27. Cheng JB, Townley RG: Comparison of muscarinic and beta adrenergic receptors between bovine peripheral lung and tracheal smooth muscles: A striking difference. *Life Sci* 1982; 30:2079.

28. Mak JCW, Barnes PJ: Autoradiographic visualization of muscarinic receptor subtypes in human and guinea-pig lung. *Am Rev Respir Dis* 1990; 141:1559.

29. Keeney SE, Oelberg DG: Alpha 1-adrenergic and muscarinic receptors in adult and neonatal rat type II pneumocytes. *Lung* 1993; 171:355.

30. Mak JCW, Baraniuk JN, Barnes PJ: Localization of muscarinic receptor subtype mRNAs in human lung. *Am J Respir Cell Mol Biol* 1992; 7:344.

31. Bonner TI, Buckley NJ, Young AC, Brann MR: Identification of a family of muscarinic receptor genes. *Science* 1987; 237:527.

32. Peralta EG, Ashkenazi A, Winslow JW, et al.: Distinct primary structures, ligand-binding properties and tissue-specific expression of four human muscarinic acetylcholine receptors. *EMBO J* 1987; 6:3923.

33. Buckley NJ, Bonner TI, Brann MR: Localization of a family of muscarinic receptor mRNAs in rat brain. *J Neurosci* 1988; 12:4646.

34. van Koppen CJ, Rodrigues de Miranda JF, Beld AJ, et al.: Characterization of the muscarinic receptor in human tracheal smooth muscle. *Naunyn Schmiedebergs Arch Pharmacol* 1985; 331:247.

35. Madison JM, Jones CA, Tom-Moy M, Brown JK: Affinities of pirenzepine for muscarinic cholinergic receptors in membranes isolated from bovine tracheal mucosa and smooth muscle. *Am Rev Respir Dis* 1987; 135:719.

36. Maeda A, Kubo T, Mishina M, Numa S: Tissue distribution of mRNAs encoding muscarinic acetylcholine receptor subtypes. *FEBS Lett* 1988; 239:339.

37. Roffel AF, in't Hout WG, de Zeeuw RA, Zaagsma J: The M2 selective antagonist AF-DX 116 shows high affinity for muscarine receptors in bovine tracheal membranes. *Naunyn Schmiedebergs Arch Pharmacol* 1987; 335:593.

38. Roffel AF, Elzinga CR, Meurs H, Zaagsma J: Allosteric interactions of three muscarine antagonists at bovine tracheal smooth muscle and cardiac M2 receptors. *Eur J Pharmacol* 1989; 172:61.

39. Lucchesi A, Scheid CR, Romano FD, et al.: Ligand binding and G protein coupling of muscarinic receptors in airway smooth muscle. *Am J Physiol* 1990; 258:C730.

40. Fryer AD, El-Fakahany EE: Identification of three muscarinic receptor subtypes in rat lung using binding studies with selective antagonists. *Life Sci* 1990; 47:611.

41. Haddad E-B, Landry Y, Gies J-P: Muscarinic receptor subtypes in guinea-pig airways. *Am J Physiol* 1991; 261:L327.

42. Yang CM: Characterization of muscarinic receptors in dog tracheal smooth muscle cells. *J Auton Pharmacol* 1991; 11:51.

43. Roffel AF, Elzinga CR, Van Amsterdam RG, et al.: Muscarinic M2 receptors in bovine tracheal smooth muscle: Discrepancies between binding and function. *Eur J Pharmacol* 1988; 153:73.

44. Gies JP, Bertrand C, Vanderheyden P, et al.: Characterization of muscarinic receptors in human, guinea-pig and rat lung. *J Pharmacol Exp Ther* 1989; 250:309.

45. Roffel AF, Meurs H, Elzinga CRS, Zaagsma J: Characterization of the muscarinic receptor subtype involved in phosphoinositide metabolism in bovine tracheal smooth muscle. *Br J Pharmacol* 1990; 99:293.

46. Brichant JF, Warner DO, Gunst SJ, Rehder K: Muscarinic receptor subtypes in canine trachea. *Am J Physiol* 1990; 258:L349.

47. Janssen LJ, Daniel EE: Pre- and postjunctional muscarinic receptors in canine bronchi. *Am J Physiol* 1990; 259:L304.

48. Howell RE, Laemont K, Gaudette R, et al.: Characterization of the airway smooth muscle muscarinic receptor in vivo. *Eur J Pharmacol* 1991; 197:109.

49. Itabashi S, Aikawa T, Sekisawa K, et al.: Pre- and postjunctional muscarinic receptor subtypes in dog airways. *Eur J Pharmacol* 1991; 204:235.

50. Mahesh VK, Nunan LM, Halonen M, et al.: A minority of muscarinic receptors mediate rabbit tracheal smooth muscle contraction. *Am J Respir Cell Mol Biol* 1992; 6:279.

51. Mitchelson F: Muscarinic receptor differentiation. *Pharmacol Ther* 1988; 37:357.

52. Yang CM, Chou SP, Sung TC: Muscarinic receptor subtypes coupled to generation of different second messengers in isolated tracheal smooth muscle cells. *Br J Pharmacol* 1991; 104:613.

53. Hashimoto T, Mirata M, Ito Y: A role for inositol 1,4,5-triphosphate in the initiation of agonist-induced contractions of dog tracheal smooth muscle. *Br J Pharmacol* 1985; 86:191.

54. Grandordy BM, Cuss FM, Sampson AS, et al.: Phosphatidylinositol response to cholinergic agonists in airway smooth muscle: Relationship to contractile and muscarinic receptor occupancy. *J Pharmacol Exp Ther* 1986; 238:273.

55. Meurs H, Roffel AF, Postema JB, et al.: Evidence for a direct relationship between phosphoinositide metabolism and airway smooth muscle contraction induced by muscarinic agonists. *Eur J Pharmacol* 1988; 156:271.

56. Baron CB, Pring M, Coburn RF: Inositol lipid turnover and compartmentation in canine trachealis smooth muscle. *Am J Physiol* 1989; 256:C-375.

57. Chilvers ER, Barnes PJ, Nahorski SR: Characterization of agonist-stimulated incorporation of myo-[3H]inositol into inositol phospholipids and [3H]inositol phosphate formation in tracheal smooth muscle. *Biochem J* 1989; 262:739.

58. Meurs H, Timmermans A, Van Amsterdam GM, et al.: Muscarinic receptors in human airway smooth muscle are coupled to phosphoinositide metabolism. *Eur J Pharmacol* 1989: 156:271.

59. Al-Hassani MH, Garcia JGN, Gunst SJ: Differences in Ca^{2+} mobilization by muscarinic agonists in tracheal smooth muscle. *Am J Physiol* 1993; 264:L53.

60. Hosey MM: Diversity of structure, signaling and regulation within the family of muscarinic cholinergic receptors. *FASEB J* 1992; 6:845.

61. Fernandes LB, Fryer AD, Hirshman CA: M2 muscarinic receptors inhibit isoproterenol-induced relaxation of canine airway smooth muscle. *J Pharmacol Exp Ther* 1992; 262:119.

62. Watson N, Eglen RM: Effects of muscarinic M_2- and M_3-receptor stimulation and antagonism on responses to isoprenaline of guinea-pig trachea in vitro. *Br J Pharmacol* 1994; 112:179.

63. Torphy TJ, Zheng C, Peterson SM, et al.: Inhibitory effect of methacholine on drug-induced relaxation, cyclic-AMP accumulation and cyclic-AMP-dependent protein kinase activation in canine tracheal smooth muscle. *J Pharmacol Exp Ther* 1985; 233:409.

64. Jones CA, Madison JM, Tom-Moy M, Brown JK: Muscarinic cholinergic inhibition of adenylate cyclase in airway smooth muscle. *Am J Physiol* 1987; 253:C97.

65. Sankary RM, Jones CA, Madison JM, Brown JK: Muscarinic cholinergic inhibition of cyclic AMP accumulation in airway smooth muscle. *Am Rev Respir Dis* 1988; 57:801.

66. Pyne NJ, Grady MW, Shehnaz D, et al.: Muscarinic blockade of β-adrenoceptor-stimulated adenylyl cyclase, the role of stimulatory and inhibitory guanine-nucleotide binding regulatory proteins (Gs and Gi). *Br J Pharmacol* 1992; 107:881.

67. Mitchell RW, Kelly E, Leff AR: Reduced activity of acetylcholinesterase in canine tracheal smooth muscle homogenates after active immune-sensitization. *Am J Respir Cell Mol Biol* 1991; 5:56.

68. Buckley RD, Hackney JD, Clark K, Posin C: Ozone and human blood. *Arch Environ Health* 1975; 30:40.

69. Gordon T, Taylor BF, Amdur MO: Ozone inhibition of tissue cholinesterase in guinea-pigs. *Arch Environ Health* 1981; 36:284.

70. Schultheis A, Bassett D, Fryer A: Ozone-induced airway hyperresponsiveness and loss of neuronal M2 muscarinic receptor function. *J Appl Physiol* 1994; 76:1088.

71. Loring SH, Drazen JM, Ingram RH: Canine pulmonary response to aerosol histamine: Direct versus vagal effects. *J Appl Physiol* 1977; 42:946.

72. Benson MK, Graf PD: Bronchial reactivity: Interaction between vagal stimulation and inhaled histamine. *J Appl Physiol* 1977; 43:643.

73. Kikuchi Y, Okayama H, Okayama M, et al.: Interaction between histamine and vagal stimulation on tracheal smooth muscle in dogs. *J Appl Physiol* 1984; 56:590.

74. Loring SH, Drazen JM, Snapper JR, Ingram RH: Vagal and aerosol histamine interactions on airway responses in dogs. *J Appl Physiol* 1978; 45:40.

75. Shore S, Irvin CG, Shenkier T, Martin JG: Mechanisms of histamine-induced contraction of canine airway smooth muscle. *J Appl Physiol* 1983; 55:22.

76. Ichinose M, Barnes PJ: Inhibitory histamine H3-receptors on cholinergic nerves in human airways. *Eur J Pharmacol* 1989; 163:383.

77. Ichinose M, Stretton CD, Schwartz JC, Barnes PJ: Histamine H3-receptors inhibit cholinergic neurotransmission in guinea-pig airways. *Br J Pharmacol* 1989; 97:13.

78. Leff AR, White SR, Munoz NM, et al.: Parasympathetic involvement in PAF-induced contraction in canine trachealis in vivo. *J Appl Physiol* 1987; 62:599.

79. Robertson DN, Coyle AJ, Rhoden KJ, et al.: The effect of platelet-activating factor on histamine and muscarinic receptor function in guinea-pig airways. *Am Rev Respir Dis* 1988; 137:1317.

80. Bethel RA, Curtis SP, Lien DC, et al.: Effect of PAF on parasympathetic contraction of canine airways. *J Appl Physiol* 1989; 66:2629.

81. Tashiro K, Xie Z, Ito Y: Effects of PAF on excitatory neuro-effector transmission in dog airways. *Br J Pharmacol* 1992; 107:956.

82. Fuller RW, Dixon CMS, Cuss FMC, Barnes PJ: Bradykinin-induced bronchoconstriction in humans. *Am Rev Respir Dis* 1987; 135:176.

83. Ichinose M, Belvisi MG, Barnes PJ: Bradykinin-induced bronchoconstriction in guinea-pig in vivo: role of neural mechanisms. *J Pharmacol Expt Thera* 1990; 253:594.

84. Saria A, Martling CR, Yan Z, et al.: Release of multiple tachykinins from capsaicin-sensitive sensory nerves in the lung by bradykinin, histamine, dimethylphenyl piperazinium, and vagal nerve stimulation. *Am Rev Respir Dis* 1988; 137:1330.

85. Kaufman MP, Coleridge HM, Coleridge JCG, Baker DG: Bradykinin stimulates afferent vagal C-fibers in intrapulmonary airways of dogs. *J Appl Physiol* 1980; 48:511.

86. Ito Y, Tajima K: Spontaneous activity in the trachea of dogs treated with indomethacin: An experimental model for aspirin-related asthma. *Br J Pharmacol* 1981; 73:563.

87. Lee TH: Mechanism of aspirin sensitivity. *Am Rev Respir Dis* 1992; 145:S34.

88. Black JL, Johnson PRA, Alfredson M, Armour CL: Inhibition by prostaglandin E2 of neurotransmission in rabbit but not human bronchus—a calcium-related mechanism? *Prostaglandins* 1989; 37:317.

89. Daniel E, Davis C, Sharma V: Effects of endogenous and exogenous prostaglandin in neurotransmission in canine trachea. *Can J Physiol Pharmacol* 1987; 65:1433.

90. Nakanishi H, Yoshida H, Suzuki T: Inhibitory effects of prostaglandin E1 and E2 on cholinergic transmission in isolated canine tracheal muscle. *Jpn J Pharmacol* 1976; 26:669.

91. Walters EH, O'Byrne PM, Fabbri LM, et al.: Control of neurotransmission by prostaglandins in canine trachealis smooth muscle. *J Appl Physiol* 1984; 57:129.

92. Ito Y, Suzuki H, Aizawa H, et al.: Pre-junctional inhibitory action of prostaglandin E2 on excitatory neuro-effector transmission in the human bronchus. *Prostaglandins* 1990; 39:639.

93. Ito Y, Tajima K: Actions of indomethacin and prostaglandins on neuro-effector transmission in the dog trachea. *J Physiol* 1981; 319:379.

94. Bethel RA, McClure CL: Cyclooxygenase inhibitors increase canine tracheal muscle response to parasympathetic stimuli in situ. *J Appl Physiol* 1990; 68:2597.

95. Fryer AD, Okanlami OA: Neuronal M_2 muscarinic receptor function in guinea-pig lungs is inhibited by indomethacin. *Am Rev Respir Dis* 1993; 147:559.

96. Inoue T, Ito Y, Takeda K: Prostaglandin-induced inhibition of acetylcholine release from neuronal elements of dog tracheal tissue. *J Physiol* 1984; 349:553.

97. Orehek J, Douglas JS, Bouhuys A: Contractile responses to the guinea-pig trachea in vitro: Modification by prostaglandin synthesis-inhibiting drugs. *J Pharmacol Exp Ther* 1975; 194:554.

98. Xie Z, Hakoda H, Ito Y: Airway epithelial cells regulate membrane potential neurotransmission and muscle tone of the dog airway smooth muscle. *J Physiol* 1992; 449:619.

99. Chung KF, Evans TW, Graf PD, Nadel JA: Modulation of cholinergic neurotransmission in canine airways by thromboxane mimetic U46619. *Eur J Pharmacol* 1985; 117:373.

100. Munoz NL, Shioya T, Murphy TM, et al.: Potentiation of vagal contractile response by thromboxane mimetic U-46619. *J Appl Physiol* 1986; 61:1173.

101. Tamaoki J, Sekizawa K, Osborne ML, et al.: Platelet aggregation increases cholinergic neurotransmission in canine airway. *J Appl Physiol* 1987; 62:2246.

102. Tamaoki J, Sekizawa K, Graf PD, Nadel JA: Cholinergic neuromodulation by prostaglandin D_2 in canine airway smooth muscle. *J Appl Physiol* 1987; 63:1396.

103. Deckers IA, Rampart M, Bult H, Herman AG: Evidence for the involvement of prostaglandins in modulation of acetylcholine release from canine bronchial tissue. *Eur J Pharmacol* 1989; 167:415.

104. Shore S, Collier B, Martin JG: Effect of endogenous

prostaglandins on acetylcholine release from dog trachealis muscle. *J Appl Physiol* 1987; 62:1837.

105. Myers AC, Undem BJ, Weinreich D: Influence of antigen on membrane properties of guinea pig bronchial ganglion neurons. *J Appl Physiol* 1991; 71:970.

106. McKay KO, Armour CL, Black JL: Endothelin-3 increases transmission in the rabbit pulmonary parasympathetic system. *J Cardiovasc Pharmacol* 1993; 22 (suppl 8):S181.

107. Takimoto M, Inui T, Okada T, Urade Y: Contraction of smooth muscle by activation of endothelin receptors on autonomic neurons. *FEBS Lett* 1993; 324:277.

108. Henry PJ, Goldie RG: Potentiation by endothelin-1 of cholinergic nerve-mediated contractions in mouse trachea via activation of ET_B receptors. *Br J Pharmacol* 1995; 114:563.

109. Tamaoki J, Graf PD, Nadel JA: Effect of gamma-aminobutyric acid on neurally mediated contraction of guinea-pig trachealis smooth muscle. *J Pharmacol Exp Ther* 1987; 243:86.

110. Horii S, Tamaoki J, Kanemura T, et al.: Effects of β-endorphin and dynorphin A on cholinergic neurotransmission in canine airway smooth muscle. *Eur J Pharmacol* 1990; 182:497.

111. Belvisi MG, Stretton CD, Barnes PJ: Modulation of cholinergic neurotransmission in guinea-pig airway by opioids. *Br J Pharmacol* 1990; 100:131.

112. Shirakawa J, Taniyama K, Tanaka C: Gamma-aminobutyric acid-induced modulation of acetylcholine release from the guinea-pig lung. *J Pharmacol Exp Ther* 1987; 243:364.

113. Sekizawa K, Graf PD, Nadel JA: Somatostatin potentiates cholinergic neurotransmission in ferret trachea. *J Appl Physiol* 1989; 67:2397.

114. Tamaoki J, Sakai N, Kobayashi K, et al.: Corticotropin-releasing factor potentiates the contractile response of rabbit airway smooth muscle to electrical field stimulation but not to acetylcholine. *Am Rev Respir Dis* 1989; 140:1331.

115. Hahn HL, Wilson AG, Graf PD, et al.: Interaction between serotonin and efferent vagus nerves in dog lungs. *J Appl Physiol* 1978; 44:144.

116. Grundstrom N, Andersson RGG, Wikberg JES: Investigations on possible presynaptic effect of adenosine and noradrenaline on cholinergic neurotransmission in guinea-pig trachea. *Acta Pharmacol Toxicol* 1981; 49:158.

117. Gustafsson LE, Wiklund NP, Cederqvist B: Apparent enhancement of cholinergic transmission in rabbit bronchi via adenosine A2 receptors. *Eur J Pharmacol* 1986; 120:179.

118. Matsuzaki Y, Hamasaki Y, Said SI: Vasoactive intestinal peptide: A possible transmitter of nonadrenergic relaxation of guinea pig airways. *Science* 1980; 210:1252.

119. Hakoda H, Ito Y: Modulation of cholinergic neurotransmission by the peptide VIP, VIP antiserum and VIP antagonists in dog and cat trachea. *J Physiol* 1990; 428:133.

120. Xie Z, Hirose T, Hakoda H, Ito Y: Effects of vasoactive intestinal polypeptide antagonists on cholinergic neurotransmission in dog and cat trachea. *Br J Pharmacol* 1991; 104:938.

121. Aikawa T, Sekizawa K, Itabashi S, et al.: Nonadrenergic inhibitory nerves attenuate neurally mediated contraction in cat bronchi. *J Appl Physiol* 1990; 69:1594.

122. Ellis JL, Farmer SG: Modulation of cholinergic neurotransmission by vasoactive intestinal peptide and peptide histidine isolucine in guinea-pig tracheal smooth muscle. *Pulm Pharmacol* 1989; 2:107.

123. Sekizawa K, Tamaoki J, Graf PD, et al.: Enkephalinase inhibitor potentiates mammalian tachykinin-induced contraction in ferret trachea. *J Pharmacol Exp Ther* 1987; 243:1211.

124. Tanaka DT, Grunstein MM: Mechanisms of substance P-induced contraction of rabbit airway smooth muscle. *J Appl Physiol* 1984; 57:1551.

125. Kizawa Y, Takayanagi I: Substance P-containing nerves mediate

126. nicotine-induced contractions of rabbit bronchial smooth muscle. *Gen Pharmacol* 1988; 19:265.

126. Joos GF, Pauwels RA, van der Straeten ME: The mechanism of tachykinin-induced bronchoconstriction in the rat. *Am Rev Respir Dis* 1988; 137:1038.

127. Hall AK, Barnes PJ, Meldrum LA, Maclagan J: Facilitation by tachykinins of neurotransmission in guinea-pig pulmonary parasympathetic nerves. *Br J Pharmacol* 1989; 97:274.

128. Tanaka DP, Grunstein MM: Effect of substance P on neurally mediated contraction of rabbit airway smooth muscle. *J Appl Physiol* 1986; 60:458.

129. Black JL, Johnson PRA, Alouan L, Armour CL: Neurokinin A with K^+ channel blockade potentiates contraction to electrical stimulation in human bronchus. *Eur J Pharmacol* 1990; 180:311.

130. Stretton D, Belvisi M, Barnes PJ: The effect of sensory nerve depletion on cholinergic neurotransmission in guinea-pig airways. *J Pharmacol Exp Ther* 1992; 260:1073.

131. Aizawa H, Miyazaki N, Inoue H, et al.: Effect of endogenous tachykinins on neuro-effector transmission of vagal nerve in guinea-pig tracheal tissue. *Respiration* 1990; 57:338.

132. Watson N, Maclagan J, Barnes PJ: Demonstration of a facilitatory role of endogenous tachykinins in cholinergic neurotransmission in guinea-pig trachea. *Br J Pharmacol* 1992; 105:78P.

133. Jacoby DB, Tamaoki J, Borson DB, Nadel JA: Influenza infection causes airway hyperresponsiveness by decreasing enkephalinase. *J Appl Physiol* 1988; 64:2653.

134. Pendry Y, Maclagan J: Evidence for inhibition of sympathetic neurotransmission by endogenously released acetylcholine in the guinea-pig trachea. *Br J Pharmacol* 1991; 104:817.

135. Vermeir PA, Vanhoutte PM: Inhibitory effects of catecholamines in isolated canine bronchial smooth muscle. *J Appl Physiol* 1979; 46:787.

136. Danser AHJ, van den Ende R, Lorenze RR, et al.: Prejunctional β_1-adrenoceptors inhibit cholinergic transmission in canine bronchi. *J Appl Physiol* 1987; 62:785.

137. Ito Y, Tajima K: Dual effects of catecholamines on pre- and postjunctional membranes in the dog trachea. *Br J Pharmacol* 1982; 75:433.

138. Baker DG, Don H: Catecholamines abolish vagal but not acetylcholine tone in the intact cat trachea. *J Appl Physiol* 1987; 63:2490.

139. Grundstrom N, Andersson RGG, Wikberg JES: Prejunctional alpha2-adrenoceptors inhibit contraction of tracheal smooth muscle by inhibiting cholinergic neurotransmission. *Life Sci* 1981; 28:2981.

140. Thompson DC, Diamond L, Altiere RJ: Presynaptic alpha modulation of neurally mediated cholinergic excitatory and non-adrenergic noncholinergic inhibitory responses in guinea pig trachea. *J Pharmacol Exp Ther* 1990; 254:306.

141. Womer D, Diamond L, Thompson DC, Altiere RJ: Airway cholinergic neural responses modulated by atypical presynaptic alpha2-adrenoceptors. *Am Rev Respir Dis* 1991; 143:A358.

142. Grundstrom N, Andersson RGG: Inhibition of the cholinergic neurotransmission in human airways via prejunctional alpha-2-adrenoceptors. *Acta Physiol Scand* 1985; 125:513.

143. Rhoden KJ, Meldrum LA, Barnes PJ: Inhibition of cholinergic neurotransmission in human airways by β2-adrenoceptors. *J Appl Physiol* 1988; 65:700.

144. Jacobowitz D, Kent KM, Fleisch JH, Cooper T: Histofluorescent study of catecholamine-containing elements in cholinergic ganglia from calf and dog lung. *Proc Soc Exp Bio Med* 1973; 144:464.

145. Knight DS: A light and electron microscopic study of feline intrapulmonary ganglia. *J Anat* 1980; 131:413.

146. Baker DG, Bausbaum CB, Herbert DA, Mitchell RA: Transmission in airway ganglia of ferrets, inhibition by noradrenaline *Neurosci Lett* 1983; 4:139.

147. Fryer AD, Maclagan J: Muscarinic inhibitory receptors in pulmonary parasympathetic nerves in the guinea-pig. *Br J Pharmacol* 1984; 83:973.

148. van Koppen CJ, Blanksteijn M, Klaassen BM, et al.: Autoradiographic visualization of muscarinic receptors in pulmonary nerves and ganglia. *Neurosci Lett* 1987; 83:237.

149. van Koppen CJ, Blanksteijn M, Klaassen BM, et al.: Autoradiographic visualization of muscarinic receptors in human bronchi. *J Pharmacol Exp Ther* 1988; 244:760.

150. James S, Bailey D, Burnstock G: Autoradiographic visualization of muscarinic receptors on rat paratracheal neurones in dissociated cell culture. *Brain Res* 1990; 513:74.

151. Kilbinger H, Schneider R, Siefken H, et al.: Characterization of prejunctional muscarinic autoreceptors in guinea-pig trachea. *Br J Pharmacol* 1991; 103:1757.

152. Baker D, Don H, Brown J: Direct measurement of acetylcholine release in guinea-pig trachea. *Am J Physiol* 1992; 263:L142.

153. Doelman CJA, Sprong RC, Nagtegaal JE, et al.: Prejunctional muscarinic receptors on cholinergic nerves in the guinea-pig airway are of the M2 subtype. *Eur J Pharmacol* 1991; 193:117.

154. Faulkner D, Fryer AD, Maclagan J: Post-ganglionic muscarinic receptors in pulmonary parasympathetic nerves in the guinea-pig. *Br J Pharmacol* 1986; 88:181.

155. Fryer AD, Maclagan J: Pancuronium and gallamine are antagonists for pre- and post-junctional muscarinic receptors in the guinea-pig lung. *Naunyn Schmiedebergs Arch Pharmacol* 1987; 335:367.

156. Blaber LC, Fryer AD, Maclagan J: Neuronal muscarinic receptors attenuate vagally induced contraction of feline bronchial smooth muscle. *Br J Pharmacol* 1985; 86:723.

157. Killingsworth CR, Mingfu Y, Robinson NE: Evidence for the absence of a functional role for muscarinic M2 inhibitory receptors in cat trachea in vivo: Contrast with in vitro results. *Br J Pharmacol* 1992; 105:263.

158. Aas P, Maclagan J: Evidence for prejunctional M2 muscarinic receptors in pulmonary cholinergic nerves of the rat. *Br J Pharmacol* 1990; 101:73.

159. Ito Y, Yoshitomi T: Autoregulation of acetylcholine release from vagus nerves terminals through activation of muscarinic receptors in the dog trachea. *Br J Pharmacol* 1988; 93:636.

160. Minette P, Barnes PJ: Prejunctional inhibitory muscarinic receptors on cholinergic nerves in human and guinea-pig airways. *J Appl Physiol* 1988; 64:2532.

161. Ayala LE, Ahmed T: Is there loss of a protective muscarinic receptor in asthma? *Chest* 1989; 96:1285.

162. Minette PJ, Lammers JWJ, Dixon CMS, et al.: A muscarinic agonist inhibits reflex bronchoconstriction in normal but not asthmatic subjects. *J Appl Physiol* 1989; 67:2461.

163. Fryer AD, Jacoby DB: Parainfluenza virus infection damages inhibitory M2 muscarinic receptors on pulmonary parasympathetic nerves in the guinea-pig. *Br J Pharmacol* 1991; 102:267.

164. Fryer AD, Wills-Karp M: Dysfunction of M2 muscarinic receptors in pulmonary parasympathetic nerves after antigen challenge in guinea-pigs. *J Appl Physiol* 1991; 71:2255.

165. Holtzman MJ, Fabbri LM, O'Byrne PM, et al.: Importance of airway inflammation for hyperresponsiveness induced by ozone in dogs. *Am Rev Respir Dis* 1983; 127:686.

166. Bassett DJP, Bowen-Kelly E, Brewster EL, et al.: A reversible model of acute lung injury based on ozone exposure. *Lung* 1988; 166:355.

167. Murlas CG, Roum JH: Sequence of pathologic changes in the airway mucosa of guinea-pigs during ozone-induced bronchial hyperreactivity. *Am Rev Respir Dis* 1985; 131:314.

168. Murlas C, Roum JH: Bronchial hyperreactivity occurs in steroid treated guinea-pigs depleted of leucocytes by cyclophosphamide. *J Appl Physiol* 1985; 58:1630.

169. Gambone LM, Elbon CL, Fryer AD: Ozone-induced loss of neuronal M2 muscarinic receptor function is prevented by cyclophosphamide. *J Appl Physiol* 1994; 77:1492.

170. McCaig DJ: Comparison of autonomic responses in the trachea isolated from normal and albumin-sensitive guinea-pigs. *Br J Pharmacol* 1987; 92:809.

171. Larsen GL, Fame TM, Renz H, et al.: Increased acetylcholine release in tracheas from allergen-exposed IgE-immune mice. *Am J Physiol* 1994; 266:L263.

172. Holgate ST, Wilson JR, Howarth PH: New insights into airway inflammation by endobronchial biopsy. *Am Rev Respir Dis* 1992; 145:S2.

173. Elbon CL, Jacoby DB, Fryer AD: The function of pulmonary M2 receptors in antigen challenged guinea-pigs is protected by pretreatment with an antibody to IL-5. *Am J Respir Cell Mol Biol* 1995; 12:320.

174. Hu J, Wang S-Z, Forray C, El-Fakahany EE: Complex allosteric modulation of cardiac muscarinic receptors by protamine: A potential model for putative endogenous ligands. *Mol Pharmacol* 1992; 42:311.

175. Barker RL, Loegering DA, Ten RM, et al.: Eosinophil cationic protein cDNA: Comparison with other toxic cationic proteins and ribonucleases. *J Immunol* 1989; 143:952.

176. Frigas E, Loegering DA, Solley GO, et al.: Elevated levels of the eosinophil granule MBP in the sputum of patients with bronchial asthma. *Mayo Clin Proc* 1981; 56:345.

177. Wasmoen TL, Bell MP, Loegering DA, et al.: Biochemical and amino acid sequence analysis of human eosinophil granule major basic protein. *J Biol Chem* 1988; 263:12559.

178. Jacoby DB, Gleich GJ, Fryer AD: Human eosinophil major basic protein is an endogenous allosteric antagonist at the inhibitory muscarinic M2 receptor. *J Clin Invest* 1993; 91:1314.

179. Fryer AD, Jacoby DB: Function of pulmonary M2 muscarinic receptors in antigen challenged guinea-pigs is restored by heparin and poly-1-glutamate. *J Clin Invest* 1992; 90:2292.

180. Empey DW, Laitinen LA, Jacobs L, et al.: Mechanisms of bronchial hyperreactivity in normal subjects following upper respiratory tract infection. *Am Rev Respir Dis* 1976; 113:523.

181. Little JW, Hall WJ, Douglas RG, et al.: Airway hyperreactivity and peripheral airway dysfunction in influenza A infection. *Am Rev Respir Dis* 1978; 118:295.

182. Aquilina AT, Hall WJ, Douglas RG, Utell MJ: Airway reactivity in subjects with viral upper respiratory tract infections: The effects of exercise and cold air. *Am Rev Respir Dis* 1980; 122:3.

183. Buckner CK, Songsiridej V, Dick EC, Busse WW: In vivo and in vitro studies of the use of the guinea pig as a model for virus-provoked airway hyperreactivity. *Am Rev Respir Dis* 1985; 132:305.

184. Gies J-P, Landry Y: Sialic acid is selectively involved in the interaction of agonists with M2 muscarinic acetylcholine receptors. *Biochem Biophys Res Commun* 1988; 150:673.

185. Laver WG: The structure of influenza viruses: III. Disruption of the virus particle and separation of neuraminidase activity. *Virology* 1963; 20:251.

186. Scheid A, Caliguiri LA, Compans RW, Choppin PW: Isolation of paramyxovirus glycoproteins: Association of both hemagglutinating and neuraminidase activities with the larger SV5 glycoprotein. *Virology* 1972; 50:640.

187. Fryer AD, El-Fakahany EE, Jacoby DB: Parainfluenza virus type 1 reduces the affinity of agonists for muscarinic receptors in guinea-pig heart and lung. *Eur J Pharmacol* 1990; 181:51.

188. Fryer AD, Yarkony KA, Jacoby DB: The effect of leukocyte depletion on M2 muscarinic receptor function in parainfluenza virus-infected guinea-pigs. *Br J Pharmacol* 1994; 112:588.

189. Sorkness R, Clough J, Castleman W, Lemanske RF: Persistent abnormalities in lung physiology and airway parasympathetic

conduction after parainfluenza type 1 infection in adult rats. *Am Rev Respir Dis* 1992; 145:A462.

190. Kahn R, Fryer A, Jacoby DB: Effect of indomethacin on inhibitory M2 muscarinic receptor function in guinea-pig airways: Influence of previous viral infections. *Am Rev Respir Dis* 1994; 149:A899.

191. Okanlami OA, Hirshman CA, Fryer AD: Pulmonary M2 receptor function depends on cyclooxygenase products in normal but not in specific pathogen free guinea-pigs. *Am Rev Respir Dis* 1992; 145:A615.

192. Yarkony KA, Fryer AD: The effects of nitric oxide synthase inhibitors on neuronal M2 muscarinic receptors in the lung. *Am J Respir Crit Care Med* 1994; 149:A860.

193. Loenders B, Rampart M, Herman AG: Selective M3 muscarinic receptor antagonists inhibit smooth muscle contraction in rabbit trachea without increasing the release of acetylcholine. *J Pharmacol Exp Ther* 1992; 263:773.

194. Fryer AD, Maclagan J: Ipratropium bromide potentiates bronchoconstriction induced by vagal nerve stimulation in the guinea-pig. *Eur J Pharmacol* 1987; 139:187.

195. Takahashi T, Belvisi MG, Patel H, et al.: Effect of BA679 BR, a novel long-lasting anti-cholinergic agent, on cholinergic neurotransmission in guinea pig and human airways. *Am J Respir Crit Care Med* 1994; 150:1640.

MUSCARINIC RECEPTORS

JAMES N. BARANIUK

Parasympathetic, cholinergic reflexes are the most potent tonically active regulators of bronchoconstriction and submucosal gland exocytosis and secretion in the airways. The actions of acetylcholine (ACh) on end-organs and the release of ACh from postganglionic neurons are regulated by specific muscarinic receptor subtypes. Four receptors have been defined by pharmacologic ligand binding studies (M$_1$ to M$_4$), whereas five (and possibly seven) muscarinic receptor genes (m$_1$ to m$_5$) have been cloned.[1–3] Acetylcholine is synthesized in peripheral nerves by choline acetyltransferase and stored in secretory vesicles. The actions of ACh are limited by degradation by acetylcholinesterase, an enzyme that is widely expressed in airway cells.

Cholinergic Ganglia and Efferent Nerves

Preganglionic vagal efferent fibers originate in the dorsal motor nucleus of the brainstem and innervate laryngeal and tracheobronchial parasympathetic ganglia. Nasal cavity, ethmoid sinus, and anterior nasopharyngeal parasympathetic innervation is derived from preganglionic seventh nerve motor fibers that originate in the superior salivatory nucleus and synapse in the sphenopalatine ganglion and then pass with sympathetic neurons through the Vidian canal. Brainstem parasympathetic nuclei are capable of inducing independent nasal, laryngeal, and tracheobronchial efferent responses. This contrasts with the generalized, all-or-nothing response of the sympathetic nervous system. Additional glossopharyngeal, vagal, and spinal accessory motor neurons innervate pharyngeal, laryngeal, and upper esophageal striated muscle and participate in the gag reflex.

Tracheobronchial ganglia contain between 6 and 20 individual neuron cell bodies. Preganglionic neurons release ACh that stimulates nicotinic receptor ion channels to induce postganglionic neural depolarization. These ganglia are also innervated by nociceptive sensory neurons that contain substance P, neurokinin A, calcitonin gene related peptide and possibly other neurotransmitters that may act on "excitatory" autoreceptors to stimulate postganglionic cell depolarization.[1,2] Prostaglandins and leukotrienes may promote the actions of excitatory autoreceptors by reducing the threshold for depolarization. Sympathetic neurons that innervate parasympathetic ganglia release norepinephrine, and probably neuropeptide Y, that may act on "inhibitory" α_2-adrenergic or NPY autoreceptors to decrease the frequency of postganglion cell depolarization.[1] Circulating epinephrine may act on β_2-adrenergic autoreceptors. Other inhibitory autoreceptors include muscarinic M$_2$, GABA$_B$, histamine H$_3$, and μ-opioid receptors.[1,2] These inhibitory autoreceptors may open a potassium channel that hyperpolarizes the ganglion making it more difficult to induce depolarization. In this fashion, the ganglion cell can be thought of as an electrical "filter" that integrates incoming inhibitory

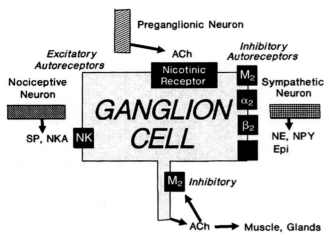

FIGURE 7-1 Ganglion cell regulation. Preganglionic neurons release ACh that activates nicotinic receptors to depolarize the ganglion cell. Neuropeptides released from nociceptive sensory neurons may also activate the ganglion via excitatory autoreceptors. Inhibitory autoreceptors activated by sympathetic neurotransmitters and other mediators may suppress ganglion depolarization. M₂ autoreceptors on postganglionic nerves may reduce ACh release.

and excitatory signals to "decide" its own rate of depolarization, subsequent ACh release, and tonic cholinergic bronchoconstrictor and glandular secretion tone (Fig. 7-1).

Postganglionic fibers innervate glands and some vessels in the nasal, pharyngeal, laryngeal, and tracheobronchial mucosa.[4–7] In bronchi, these neurons are most dense in the proximal airways, with decreasing densities in the smaller, more distal bronchi and bronchioles and are essentially nonexistent in the alveoli. Submucosal smooth muscle and glands are densely innervated, whereas bronchial epithelium and vessels have very little cholinergic innervation. In addition to ACh, these neurons may contain vasoactive intestinal peptide (VIP), VIP-related peptides (PHM), and constitutively active nitric oxide synthetase.[8,9]

Autoradiographic radioligand binding studies indicate that muscarinic receptors are located on airway smooth muscle, submucosal glands, parasympathetic ganglia, and nerve bundles.[10–15] There is little binding to epithelium and vessels. In human lung, muscarinic receptors are distributed over both proximal and distal airways and are present in alveoli.

Muscarinic receptors are expressed in the developing respiratory tract, but only weak bronchoconstrictor responses are generated. This may be the result of delayed G-protein expression or other intracellular events.[16]

Pharmacology of Muscarinic Receptors

Although five muscarinic receptor genes (M₁ to M₅) have been cloned, only four of these (M₁ to M₄) have been defined by pharmacologic means.[2,3,17,18] Currently available agonists and antagonists do not have sufficient selectivity to absolutely discriminate between receptor subtypes (Table 7-1). Pirenzepine (M₁), gallamine and AF DX-116 (M₂), 4-DAMP (M₃), and himbascine (M₂ and M₄) have been used to define particular functions, but this task is complex since multiple subtypes may be present on endorgans. For example, in guinea pig ileal smooth muscle, M₂ receptors account for approximately 80 percent of the total binding capacity, yet M₃ receptor stimulation (20 percent of tissue muscarinic receptors) accounts for essentially all the cholinergically induced contraction.[3]

Muscarinic Receptor Structure

The five cloned muscarinic receptors belong to the rhodopsin family of G-protein related receptors that bind sensory molecules (light, odorants), biogenic amines (muscarinic, dopamine, epinephrine, norepinephrine, histamine, serotonin), glycoprotein hormones including thyrotropin-releasing hormone (TRH) and (FSH) follicle-stimulating hormone, neuropeptides and peptide hormones (substance P, bradykinin, gastrin-releasing peptide, cholecystokinin,

TABLE 7-1 Pharmacology of Muscarinic Receptors

Receptor	Ligands	G Protein	G-Protein Effect
M₁	Pirenzepine Telenzepine	G$_q$	Stimulate PLC, release IP₃ and DAG
M₂	AF DX-116 Gallamine Methoctramine Himbascine AQRA741 (Pilocarpine is an agonist)	G$_i$	Inhibit adenylyl cyclase
M₃	4-DAMP p-F-HHSiD Zamifenacin	G$_q$	Stimulate PKC, release IP₃ and DAG
M₄	Himbascine	G$_i$	Inhibit adenyly/cyclase
M₅	Not defined	G$_q$	Stimulate PLC

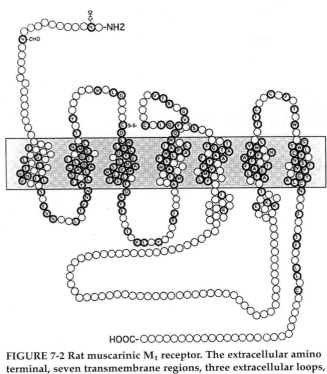

FIGURE 7-2 Rat muscarinic M₁ receptor. The extracellular amino terminal, seven transmembrane regions, three extracellular loops, three intracellular loops, and an intracellular carboxy terminal. Amino acids conserved in all five muscarinic receptors are shown in dark circles. (From Fraser and Lee,[19] with premission.)

many others), IL-8, and other mediators.[19] These proteins have a characteristic structure with glycosylated extracellular NH₂ terminal, seven transmembrane regions (Tm1 to Tm7), three extracellular loops (E1 to E3), three intracellular or cytoplasmic loops (C1 to C3), and an intracellular COOH tail (Fig. 7-2).

The seven transmembrane regions are amphipathic helical cylinders that are stacked parallel to each other as they span the membrane. The intra- and extracellular loops are like tethers that group the cylinders together. Two cysteines in E1 and E2 form a disulfide bond that constrains the side-by-side orientation of Tm2, Tm3, Tm4, and Tm5.[20] Amino acid interactions between adjacent cylinders determine the spacing of the cylinders. Amino acids that project from the cylinders into the oblong space between the seven cylinders form the ACh binding pocket and may promote intercylinder interactions. These interacting amino acids generate a "charged pit" within the otherwise hydrophobic helices and membrane lipid environment, and determine the specificity and avidity of ligand binding.

The helices are not completely cylindrical. Prolines in Tm5, Tm6, and Tm7 are highly conserved among these receptors. Proline disrupts, or "breaks" alpha helices, and may warp Tm5, Tm6, and Tm7, perhaps allowing them to stack next to each other within the membrane like stackable chairs. Point mutations of each of these prolines reduces the membrane expression of these receptors, suggesting that these bends are essential for receptor packaging or transport into the membrane. Substitution of proline[540] to alanine

reduces the ability of carbachol to induce signal transduction but does not alter ligand binding, suggesting that the transmembrane regions have two functions: ligand binding in the portions of the helices near the extracellular surface and transduction of ligand-binding-induced conformation changes to the intracellular portions of the receptor.[19]

Other highly conserved amino acids include the cluster glycine-aspartate-x-x-valine in Tm1; an aspartate in Tm2; aspartate-arginine-tyrosine near the intracellular end of Tm3; tryptophans in Tm4, Tm6, and Tm7; and, in muscarinic and adrenergic receptors, a conserved cluster of tryptophan-x-x-x-aspartate in Tm3 that plays a role in amine ligand binding.[19]

Based on the adrenergic receptor model and affinity labeling experiments,[20–22] the carboxyl group of the highly conserved aspartate[105] in Tm3 of the rat M₁-receptor (Fig. 7-2) appears essential for binding the cationic onium (amine) of ACh and muscarinic agonists and antagonists. Point mutation to asparagine reduced ligand binding capacity.[19] Tryptophans at positions 191 in Tm4 and 503 in Tm6 may provide hydrogen bonds that stabilize the acetyl moiety in the ligand binding site since their point mutation to phenylalanine reduces ligand binding affinities.[23,24] Asn[382] may also contribute to this task.

In contrast, Hibert et al.,[25] working with computer-generated molecular models, has proposed that Asp[308] of rat M₂-receptors interacts by electrostatic interactions with the charged amine group of ACh, while hydrogen bonds from Asn[627] stabilize the ester in the acetyl group. Trp[413] and Leu[621] are proposed to cluster around this ester-Asn[617] interaction by forming a hydrophobic pocket. Trp[304], Ala[504], Ala[507], Phe[508], Trp[613], Pro[615], and Tyr[616] would form the "sides" of the ligand binding site. Binding of ACh is proposed to alter the configuration of these aromatic amino acids by shifting the positions of Tyr[715], Asp[209], and Asp[308] and the spatial orientation of Tm1, Tm2, and Tm7. In turn, ratcheting of hydrophobic and charged groups within the Tm regions would shift Asn[721] and Pro[722] in Tm7 and induce a realignment of C3 and C-terminal tail that may promote G-protein binding.

Each C3 has a unique sequence. The M₃-receptor has an amphipathic alpha helix that is essential for G-protein interaction. Mutations that alter the C3 helical structure prevent G-protein activation.[26] The precise G proteins that associate with each muscarinic receptor are still being defined, but it appears that M₁, M₃, and M₅ receptors bind with Gq proteins that activate phospholipase C, while M₂ and M₄ receptors bind Gi proteins that inhibit adenylyl cyclase (Table 7-1).[2,3,27] The COOH tails contain phosphorylation sites that may regulate the binding of G proteins or lead to receptor desensitization or "tachyphylaxis."[19]

These data suggest that the ligand binding site consists of a pocket formed by adjacent surfaces of the transmembrane helices, that ligand binding induces conformational rotations or shifts in position of these helices relative to each other, and that these conformational changes are translated to the third intracellular (C3) G-protein binding region, or C-terminal tail to promote G-protein binding. While the ligand binding regions of the five muscarinic receptors are relatively highly conserved, the intracytoplasmic C3 loop and C terminal are very divergent, suggesting that differences in G-protein binding specificities are the principal differences between the receptor subtypes.

M_1-Receptors

M_1 receptors and m_1 mRNA have been demonstrated by radioligand binding studies, Northern blotting, and in situ hybridization in human alveoli and by autoradiography in human nasal mucosa (see Table 7-2).[11,12,15,28,29] The significance of the alveolar receptors is unclear, since this tissue is not innervated by cholinergic nerves. M_1-receptors predominate in neuronal tissues and are present in parasympathetic[12,14] and sympathetic peripheral neurons.[1] These receptors may be functionally important, since pirenzepine, an M_1-antagonist, blocks the bronchoconstriction induced by electrical vagus nerve stimulation in vitro[30,31] and by inhalation of SO_2,[32] an agent thought to activate nociceptive sensory nerves that recruit parasympathetic bronchoconstrictor reflexes. Pirenzepine does not block the effects of inhaled methacholine. Although M_1-binding sites have been noted on submucosal glands in the bronchial and nasal mucosae[12,15,33,34] pirenzepine has no effect on cholinergic glandular secretion. The identity of these glandular receptors has not been confirmed at the mRNA level, as m_1 mRNA has not been localized to these sites.[12]

M_1 receptors can activate both G_{qa} and G_{11a} to initiate phosphoinositol metabolism.[2]

M_2-Receptors

M_2-receptors regulate cholinergic ganglion and bronchial smooth-muscle function. M_2-receptors are coupled to a pertussis-toxin-sensitive G_i protein, which inhibits adenylyl cyclase and decreases intracellular cAMP levels.[1–3] Alterations in M_2-receptor functions may lead to cholinergic hyperresponsiveness.

SMOOTH MUSCLE

M_2-binding sites and m_2 mRNA have been demonstrated in cultured human tracheal smooth-muscle cells and airway smooth muscle.[28,35] M_2-receptor binding with inhibition of adenylyl cylase does not alter smooth-muscle contraction. However, M_2-receptor activation antagonizes the effects of β_2-adrenergic receptor stimulation and leads to bronchoconstriction, since the β_2-adrenoceptor effects are mediated by stimulation of adenylyl cyclase and increased cAMP production (Fig. 7-3). Thus, in the presence of high sympathetic tone, parasympathetic cholinergic reflexes would lead to relative bronchoconstriction by activating M_3-receptors (smooth-muscle contraction) and M_2-receptors (antagonism of β_2-receptor-induced bronchodilation). Increased parasympathetic tone would limit the bronchodilator efficacy of β_2-adrenergic agonists.

M_2-receptor stimulation does not appear to affect PGE_1- or PGE_2-induced cAMP formation suggesting that these are coupled to different adenylyl cyclase isoforms.[36] In some systems, M_2-receptors may be linked to a pertussin-toxin-sensitive G protein that may activate an ion channel to induce smooth-muscle contraction.[2,3]

GANGLIONIC AUTORECEPTORS

"Inhibitory" M_2-autoreceptors decrease the release of ACh from parasympathetic ganglia in guinea pig trachea.[37-39] Pilocarpine, an M_2-agonist, inhibits SO_2-induced bronchoconstriction in humans in vivo.[40] M_2-receptors may also inhibit norepinephrine release from sympathetic nerves.[41]

Inhibitory M_2-autoreceptors on ganglion cells may be modified in disease states. Influenza infection of guinea pigs can increase bronchial responses to methacholine. The neuraminidase of the influenza virus is capable of cleaving sialic acid residues from M_2-receptors, thereby inactivating the receptors.[42,43] This mechanism could contribute to some cases of postviral bronchospasm.

TABLE 7-2 Autoradiographic Localization of Muscarinic Receptors in Human Nasal and Trachaeobronchial Airways

Subtype	Localization	Function
M_1	Parasympathetic ganglia	Facilitate neurotransmission
	Nasal submucosal glands	Exocytosis?
	Alveolar walls	?
M_2	Postganglionic cholinergic nerves	Inhibit ACh release
	Airway smooth muscle	Inhibit adenylyl cyclase and antagonize adrenergic bronchodilation
	Sympathetic nerves	Inhibit norepinephrine release
M_3	Airway smooth muscle	Contraction
	Submucosal glands	Exocytosis
	Goblet cells?	Exocytosis
	Epithelial cells	Increased ciliary beat frequency?
	Endothelial cells	Release of ntric oxide and vasodilation
M_4	Alveolar Walls[a]	?
	Airway smooth muscle[a]	?
	Postganglionic cholineric nerves	Inhibit ACh release

[a] Rabbit only

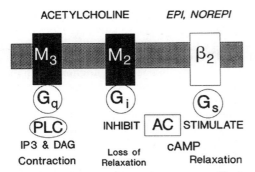

FIGURE 7-3 Acetylcholine released from postganglionic neurons can stimulate M_3-receptors that induce smooth muscle contractions or M_2-receptors that inhibit adenylyl cyclase (AC). This action of M_2-receptors on cAMP formation may antagonize the effects of β_2-adrenergic agonists and promotes bronchoconstriction.

Allergic reactions are characterized by eosinophilia and release of eosinophil cationic proteins. Eosinophil major basic protein (MBP) and peroxidase (EPO), but not eosinophil cationic protein (ECP) or eosinophil-derived neurotoxin (EDN), can bind selectively and inactivate M_2-receptors and lead to ganglionic dysfunction.[44] Heparin can antagonize ECP-M_2 binding. Eosinophil protein-M_2-receptor interactions could play a role in allergic asthma.

Ozone may also alter M_2-receptor function.[45] Inhalation of O_3 for 8 weeks by pathogen-free guinea pigs induces (1) cholinergic hyperresponsiveness, (2) loss of M_2-receptor mediated attenuation of cholinergic-reflex-induced bronchoconstriction, and (3) the development of a requirement for prostaglandins for proper functioning of M_2-receptors.[46] The mechanism of the prostaglandin dependency is unclear.

Dependence on prostaglandins for autoreceptor function is of interest, since some asthmatic and rhinitis-sinusitis patients have aspirin sensitivity. Blockade of cyclooxygenase leads to decreased prostaglandin synthesis and shunting of arachidonic acid to leukotriene formation, which leads to severe, acute bronchospasm or rhinitis.[47]

The combination of M_2-autoreceptor dysfunction plus β_2-adrenergic antagonists could be a very dangerous situation since both the inhibitory influences of epinephrine or norepinephrine and M_2-autoreceptors on ganglion cell transmission would be missing. β_2-adrenoceptors on smooth-muscle cells would also be blocked, again promoting bronchoconstriction. M_2-receptors are absent from human alveoli and nasal mucosa.[15,28]

M_3-Receptors

M_3-receptors mediate cholinergic bronchoconstriction and glandular secretion in the human respiratory tract.[1,3]

M_3-receptor stimulation activates a pertussis-toxin-insensitive G_q protein that activates phospholipase C (PLC) to release inositol 1,4,5-trisphosphate (IP_3) and diacylglycerol.[3,48,49] IP_3 releases calcium from intracellular stores, whereas diacylglycerol (DAG) activates protein kinase C (PKC). The two actions lead to smooth-muscle contrac-

tion[3] in airway, gastrointestinal, urinary bladder, vascular, and other tissues. Other functions include release of endothelium-dependent relaxing factor, tracheal epithelium-derived relaxing factor, stimulation of guinea pig ileal electrolyte secretion, and rapid induction of E-cadherin by a small cell lung carcinoma cell line.[3,50]

M_3-binding sites and m_3 mRNA are distributed throughout the large and small airways and are localized in high concentration to smooth-muscle and submucosal gland cells where their function is to induce smooth-muscle contraction and exocytosis, respectively,[11,12,15,28,34] M_3-selective antagonists inhibit cholinergically induced smooth-muscle contraction and exocytosis from human tracheobronchial and nasal glands.[3,33,34]

M_3-receptors are expressed in lower densities on nasal and bronchial epithelium and endothelium where they are thought to contribute to goblet cell secretion, ion and water transport, and vasodilation.[51,52]

The development of more selective M_3-antagonists will help to better define the actions of these receptors and will have therapeutic benefit as bronchodilators by selectively inhibiting the bronchoconstriction induced by parasympathetic tone (M_3-receptor-mediated) without blocking regulatory ganglionic M_2-autoreceptors.

M_4-Receptors

M_4-receptors and m_4 mRNA have been identified in rabbit lung. In situ hybridization localizes it to alveolar walls and bronchial smooth muscle.[28,53] The function of these receptors is not known. M_4-receptors also have been postulated to modulate postganglionic cholinergic nerves in guinea pig trachea.[54] In human bronchial mucosa, m_4 mRNA has not been identified.[28]

M_5-Receptors

Selective ligands for M_5-receptors have not been developed; m_5 mRNA does not appear to be present in human respiratory tissues.[28]

Physiology of Nasal Cholinergic Reflexes

Parasympathetically released acetylcholine is paramount in stimulating submucosal gland secretion in human nasal mucosa.[55,56] About 55 percent of the muscarinic receptors are of the M_3 type, whereas the remainder are M_1.[15] M_1 binding sites are present on epithelium and submucosal glands. M_3-receptors and m_3 mRNA have been identified by autoradiography[15] and in situ hybridization,[57] respectively, on the epithelium, submucosal glands, and endothelium. M_2 binding sites are apparently not present in human nasal mucosa. M_4 sites were not examined.

Methacholine stimulates both serous and mucous cell exocytosis, an effect that is inhibited by M_3-antagonists, and weakly inhibited by M_1-antagonists.[34] In vivo, cholinergic reflexes act on resistance vessels to increase superficial blood flow, but there is little effect on capacitance vessels (sinusoids) that control mucosal thickness, or postcapillary venules that are the site of vascular permeability.

Stimulation of nasal nociceptive sensory nerves by cold, dry air, capsaicin, histamine, bradykinin, or allergic reactions recruits parasympathetic reflexes.[55,58–60] These reflexes are the most important mechanism regulating glandular serous and mucous cell exocytosis, a finding clearly demonstrated in unilateral provocation models. For example, unilateral histamine provocation leads to the direct activation of H_1-receptors on vessels to stimulate arterial dilation, sinusoidal filling with obstruction to nasal airflow, and vascular permeability with the secretion of a fluid enriched by albumin, IgG and other plasma proteins.[55,60] Nociceptive sensory nerves are stimulated to transmit sensations of itch and trigger protective reflexes, including sneezing. Bilateral, cholinergic reflexes stimulate glandular secretion of mucous cell mucoglycoproteins and serous cell lysozyme, lactoferrin, secretory IgA, and other enzymes. The noncholinergic component of the reflex-mediated nasal obstruction has not been well quantitated.

The muscarinic antagonists atropine and ipratropium bromide effectively reduce glandular secretion and "dry" the mucosa, but have no effect on sneezing or vascular congestion.[61] Selective M_3-receptor antagonists may have clinical utility in rhinitis where parasympathetic glandular secretion is a significant cause of patient discomfort. However, reduction in glandular secretion volume could reduce the amounts of serous-cell-derived antimicrobial and lubricating proteins on the mucosal surface, and lead to drying of the surface, irritation, and sensory nerve stimulation. Use of cholinergic antagonists in asthma is discussed elsewhere in this text.

Other Colocalized Neurotransmitters

In addition to acetylcholine, the postganglionic neurons contain other colocalized neurotransmitters including vasoactive intestinal peptide (VIP), PHI/PHM (PHI–peptide with Histidine at the N-terminal and Isolencine at the C-terminal: PHM–peptide with histidine at the N-terminal and methionine at the C-terminal) that are closely related to VIP, and possibly nitric oxide.[8,9] These ganglia appear to have some "plasticity," since they can be induced to alter their neurotransmitter phenotype. After heart-lung transplant, for example, NPY can be induced by these cells.[62] It remains undetermined if there are analogous changes during airway inflammatory diseases such as asthma.

VIP nerve fibers innervate smooth muscle, glands, and some vessels.[7,55,60] VIP binding sites are present on epithelium, glands, and vessels, suggesting roles in secretion and vasodilation. In vitro, VIP stimulates glandular secretion in many models, but in human bronchial explants inhibits mucous secretion.[63,64] Anti-VIP antibodies may play a pathologic role in some cases of chronic bronchitis.[64] An absence of VIP nerve fibers has been described in status asthmaticus[65] and cystic fibrosis.[66] Increased VIP nerve fiber density has been demonstrated in vasomotor rhinitis (chronic choliner-

gic rhinitis).[67] In vivo, VIP may be more active as a vasodilator than as a secretogogue since atropine blocks essentially all gland secretion but only partially blocks neurogenically induced blood flow.[59,68]

VIP and PHM also influence postganglionic ACh release.[69] ACh is released at low nerve impulse frequency rates, whereas at high rates, acetylcholine and VIP are released. VIP may augment the postsynaptic acetylcholine-induced secretory response in glands (eg., cat salivary glands[68]), but may also have presynaptic inhibitory effects to limit neuropeptide release.

Hyperresponsiveness

Hyperresponsiveness to methacholine is a characteristic finding in asthma (bronchoconstriction) and rhinitis (glandular secretion), but the molecular mechanisms remain elusive.[1,70–72] Compared with normal subjects, asthmatics are more sensitive to SO_2, which stimulates nociceptive sensory nerves and parasympathetic reflexes and propranolol, which blocks β_2-adrenergic receptors. However, asthmatics are less responsive to pilocarpine, which stimulates M_2-receptors and reduces parasympathetic bronchoconstrictor tone. These findings suggest decreases in inhibitory M_2-autoreceptor function with consequent increases in cholinergic reflex bronchoconstriction.[39,40,73] However, there is no evidence to indicate that alterations in muscarinic receptor density, affinity, expression, signal coupling and transduction, or phosphoinositol turnover exist in asthmatic or rhinitis tissues.[74–78] Mast cell degranulation does not alter muscarinic receptor expression in human lung fragments in vitro.[79] These studies would not detect small changes in receptor subtype expression on ganglia in airways.

Summary

M_3- and M_2-receptors appear to predominate in the human respiratory tract; m_1 mRNA is present in unidentified alveolar cells, but not bronchi. The mRNA for m_3 is found in bronchial epithelium, endothelium, glands, and smooth muscle; m_2 mRNA is found in smooth muscle and ganglion cells, while m_4 and m_5 mRNA are not detectable. M_3-receptor activation is the major tonically active stimulus for smooth-muscle contraction and glandular exocytosis. M_3-receptor antagonists are potentially therapeutically beneficial. They are selective inhibitors of glandular secretion and vasodilation in human nasal mucosa and bronchoconstriction in human bronchi, which may be free of side effects caused by actions on M_2- and other subtype receptors. M_2-receptors appear to be critical for the regulation of parasympathetic ganglion function since M_2-autoreceptor stimulation may reduce acetylcholine release. On smooth muscle, M_2-agonists may enhance cholinergically induced contraction by antagonizing cAMP formation and the relaxant effects of β_2-adrenergic agonists. These M_2-autoreceptor events may be therapeutically diverse, since ganglionic effects promote bronchodilation and reduce cholinergically induced glandular secretion, whereas smooth muscle effects promote bronchoconstriction. These issues will be resolved by clinical studies as new selective muscarinic receptor agonists and antagonists are developed.

References

1. Barnes PJ: Modulation of neurotransmission in airways. *Physiol Rev* 1993; 72:699.
2. Caulfield MP: Muscarinic receptors—characterization, coupling and function. *Pharmacol Ther* 1993; 58:319.
3. Eglen RM, Reddy H, Watson N, Challiss RAJ: Muscarinic acetylcholine receptor subtypes in smooth muscle. *TiPS* 1994; 15:114.
4. Laitinen LA, Laitinen A: Innervation or airway smooth muscle. *Am Rev Respir Dis* 1987; 136:S38.
5. Richardson JB: Nerve supply to the lungs. *Am Rev Respir Dis* 1979; 119:785.
6. Partanen M, Laitinen A, Hervonen A, Toivanen M, Laitinen LA: Catecholine- and acetylcholinesterase-containing nerves in human lower respiratory tract. *Histochem* 1992; 76:175.
7. Uddman R, Sundler F: Innervation of the upper airways. *Clin Chest Med* 1986; 7:201.
8. Said SI, Mutt V: Vasoactive intestinal peptide and related peptides. *Ann NY Acad Sci* 1988; 527:1.
9. Kummer W, Fischer A, Lang RE, et al.: Nitric oxide and guanylyl cyclases: Correlation with neuropeptides, in Kaliner MA, Barnes PJ, Kunkel GHH, Baraniuk JN (eds): *Neuropeptides in Respiratory Medicine*. New York, Marcel-Dekker, 1994: 641–652.
10. Barner PJ, Nadel JA, Roberts JM, Basbaum CB: Muscarinic receptors in lung and trachea: Autoradiographic localization using [^{3}H]quinuclidinyl benzilate. *Eur J Pharmacol* 1983; 86:103,
11. Mak JCW, Barnes PJ: Muscarinic receptor subtypes in human and guinea pig lung. *Eur J Pharmacol* 1989; 164:223.
12. Mak JCW, Barnes PJ: Autoradiographic visualization of muscarinic receptor subtypes in human and guinea pig lung. *Am Rev Respir Dis* 1990; 141:1559.
13. van Koppen CJ, Rodrigues de Miranda JF, Beld AJ, et al.: Characterization of the muscarinic receptor in human tracheal smooth muscle. *Arch Pharmacol* 1985; 331:247.
14. van Koppen CJ, Blankesteijn WM, Klassen ABM, et al.: Autoradiographic visualization of muscarinic receptors in human bronchi. *J Pharmacol Exp Ther* 1988; 244:760.
15. Okayama M, Baraniuk NJ, Merida M, Kaliner MA: Autoradiographic localization of muscarinic receptor subtypes in human nasal mucosa. *J Allergy Clin Immunol* 1992: 89:1144.
16. Haxhiu-Poskurica B, Ernsberger P, Haxhiu MA, et al: Development of cholinergic innervation and muscarinic receptor subtypes in piglet trachea. *Am J Physiol* 1993; 264:L606.
17. Buckley NJ, Bonner TI, Buckley CM, Brann MR: Antagonist binding properties of five cloned muscarinic receptors expressed in CHO-K1 cells. *Mol Pharmacol* 1989; 35:469.
18. Dorje F, Wess J, Lambrecht G, et al.: Antagonist binding profiles of five cloned human muscarinic receptor subtypes. *J Pharmacol Exp Ther* 1991; 256:727.
19. Fraser CM, Lee NH: Molecular characterization of autonomic and neuropeptide receptors, in Kaliner MA, Barnes PJ, Kunkel GHH, Baraniuk JN: *Neuropeptides in Respiratory Medicine*. New York, Marcel-Dekker 1994: 225–250.
20. Kurtenbach E, Curtis CAM, Pedder EK: Muscarinic acetylcholine receptors. Peptide sequencing identifies residues involved in antagonist binding and disulfide bond formation. *J Biol Chem* 1990; 265:13702.
21. Curtis CAM, Wheatlry M, Bansal S: Propyl benzilycholine mustard labels an acidic residue in transmembrane helix 3 of the muscarinic receptor. *J Biol Chem* 1989; 264:489.
22. Fraser CM, Wang C-D, Robinson DA: Site-directed mutagenesis of m$_1$ muscarinic receptors: Conserved aspartic acids play important roles in receptor function. *Mol Pharmacol* 1989; 36:840.
23. Wess J, Nanavati S, Vogel Z: Functional role of proline and tryptophan residues highly conserved among G protein-coupled receptors studied by mutational analysis of the m$_3$ muscarinic receptor. *EMBO J* 1992; 12:331.
24. Norvald G, Hacksell U: Binding site modelling of the muscarinic m$_1$ receptor: A combination of homology-based and indirect approaches. *J Med Chem* 1993; 36:967.
25. Hibert MF, Trumpp-Kallmeyer S, Bruinvels A, Hoflack J: Three-dimensional models of neurotransmitter G-binding protein-coupled receptors. *Mol Pharm* 1991; 40:8.
26. Duerson K, Carroll R, Clapham D: Alpha-helical distorting substitution disrupt coupling between m$_3$ muscarinic receptor and G proteins. *FEBS Lett* 1993; 324:103.
27. Yang CM, Chow S-P, Sung T-C: Muscarinic receptor subtypes coupled to generation of different second messengers in isolated tracheal smooth muscle cells. *Be J Pharmacol* 1991; 104:613.
28. Bloom JW, Halonen M, Yamamura HI: Characterization of muscarinic cholinergic receptor subtypes in human peripheral lung. *J Pharmacol Exp Ther* 1988; 244:625.
29. Mak JCW, Baranuik JN, Barnes PJ: Localization of muscarinic receptor subtype messenger RNA's in human lung. *Am J Respir Cell Mol Biol* 1992; 7:344.
30. Beck KC, Vettermann J, Flavahan NA, Rehder K: Muscarinic M$_1$ receptors mediate the increase in pulmonary resistance during vagus nerve stimulation in dogs. *Am Rev Respir Dis* 1987; 137:1135.
31. Bloom JW, Yamamura HI, Baumgartner C, Halonen M: A muscarinic receptor with high affinity for pirenzepine mediates vagally induced bronchoconstriction. *Eur J Pharmacol* 1987; 133:21.
32. Lammers J-WJ, Minette P, MuCusker M, Barnes PJ: The role of pirenzepine-sensitive (M$_1$) muscarinic receptors in vagally mediated bronchoconstriction in humans. *Am Rev Respir Dis* 1989: 139:446.
33. Johnson CW, Rieves RO, Logun C, Shelhamer JH: Cholinergic stimulation of mucin type glycoprotein release from human airways in vitro is inhibited by an antagonist of the M$_3$ muscarinic receptor subtype. *Am J Respir Cell Mol Biol* 1994, in press.
34. Mullol J, Baraniuk JN, Logun C, et al.: M$_1$ and M$_3$ muscarinic antagonists inhibit human nasal glandular secretion in vitro. *J Appl Physiol* 1992; 73:2069.
35. Maeda A, Kubo T, Mishina M, Numa S: Tissue distribution in mRNAa encoding mescarinic acetylcholine receptor subtypes. *FEBS Lett* 1988; 239:339.
36. Griffin MT, Ehlert FJ: Specific inhibition of isoproterenol cyclic AMP accumulation by M$_2$ muscarinic receptors in rat intestinal smooth muscle. *J Pharm Exp Ther* 1992; 263:221.
37. Kilbinger H, Schoreider R, Siefken H, et al.: Characterization of prejunctional muscarinic autoreceptors in the guinea-pig trachea. *Br J Pharmacol* 1991; 103:1757.
38. Fryer AD, Maclagan J: Muscarinic inhibitory receptors in pulmonary parasympathetic nerves in the guinea pig. *Br J Pharmacol* 1984; 83:973.
39. Minette PA, Barnes PJ: Prejunctional inhibitory muscarinic receptors on cholinergic nerves in human and guinea pig airways. *J Appl Physiol* 1988; 64:2532.
40. Minette PAH, Lanners J, Dixon CMS, et al.: A muscarinic agonist inhibits reflex bronchoconstriction in normal but not in asthmatic subjects. *J Appl Physiol* 1989; 67:2461.

41. Racke K, Hey C, Wessler I: Endogenous noradrenaline release from guinea pig isolated trachea is inhibited by activation of M_2 receptors. *Br J Pharmacol* 1992; 107:3.

42. Fryer AD, Jacoby DB: Parainfluenza virus infection damages inhibitory M_2 muscarinic receptors on pulmonary parasympathetic nerves in the guinea-pig. *Br J Pharmacol* 1991; 102:267.

43. Haddad E-B, Gies JP: Neuraminidase reduces the super-high-affinity [^{3}H]oxotremorine-M binding sites in guinea pig. *Eur J Pharmacol* 1992; 211:L327.

44. Jacoby DB, Gleich GJ, Fryer AD: Human eosinophil major basic protein is an endogenous, allosteric antagonist at the inhibitory muscarinic M_2 receptor. *Am Rev Respir Dis* 1992; 145:A436 (abstract).

45. Schultheis A, Bassett DJP, Fryer AD: Ozone induced airway hyperresponsiveness is due to temporary loss of neuronal M_2 muscarinic receptor function. *Am Rev Respir Dis* 1992; 145:A615.

46. Fryer A, Okanlami O, Neuronal M_2 muscarinic receptor function in guinea pig lungs in inhibited by indomethacin. *Am Rev Respir Dis* 1993; 147:500.

47. Stechschulte DJ: Leukotrienes in asthma and allergic rhinitis. *N Engl J Med* 1990; 323:1769.

48. Grandordy BM, Cuss FM, Sampson AS, et al.: Phosphatidylinositol response to cholinergic agonists in airway smooth muscle: Relationship to contaction and muscarinic receptor occupancy. *J Pharmacol Exp Ther* 1986; 238:273.

49. Chilvers ER, Batty IH, Barnes PJ, Nahorski SR: Formation of inositol polyphosphates in airway smooth muscle after muscarinic receptor stimulation. *J Pharmacol Exp Ther* 1990; 252:786.

50. Williams CL, Hayes VY, Hummmel AM, et al.: Regulation of E-cadherin-mediated adhesion by muscarinic acetylcholine receptors in small cell carcinoma. *J Cell Biol* 1993; 121:643.

51. McCormack DG, Mak JC, Minette P, Barnes PJ: Muscarinic receptor subtypes mediating vasodialation in the pulmonary artery. *Eur J Pharmacol* 1993; 158:293.

52. Tokuyama K, Kuo H-P, Rohode JAL, et al.: Neural control of goblet cell secretion in guinea pig airways. *Am J Physiol (Lung Cell Mol Physiol)* 1990; 259:L108.

53. Mak JCW, Haddad EB, Buckley NJ, Barnes PJ: Visualization of muscarinic m_4 mRNA and M_4 receptor subtype in rabbit lung. *Life Sci* 1993; 53:1501.

54. Kilbinger H, von Barbeleben RS, Siefken H: Is the presynaptic muscarinic autoreceptor in the guinea-pig trachea an M_2 receptor: *Life Sci* 1993; 52:577, (abstract).

55. Raphael GR, Baraniuk JN, Kaliner MA: How and why the nose runs. *J Allergy Clin Immunol* 1991; 87:457.

56. van Megen YJB, Klaassen ABM, Rodrigues de Miranda JF, et al.: Alterations of muscarinic acetylcholine receptors in the nasal mucosa of allergic patients in comparison with nonallergic individuals. *J Allergy Clin Immunol* 1991; 87:521.

57. Baraniuk JN, Kaliner MA, Barnes PJ: Muscarinic m_3 receptor mRNA in situ hybridization in human nasal mucosa. *Am J Rhinol* 1992; 6:145.

58. Naclerio RM: Allergic rhinitis. *New England J Med* 1991; 325:860.

59. Stjarne P, Lacroix JS, Anggard A, Lundberg JM: Compartment analysis of vascular effects of neuropeptides and capsaicin in the pig nasal mucosa. *Acta Physiol Scand* 1991; 141:335.

60. Baraniuk JN: Neural control of human nasal secretion. *Pulm Pharmacol* 1991; 4:20.

61. Mygind N, Borum P: Anticholinergic treatment of watery rhinorrhea. *Am J Rhinol* 1990; 4:1.

62. Springall DR, Polak JM, Howard T: Persistence of intrinsic neurones and possible phenotypic changes after extrinsic denervation of human respiratory tract by heart-lung transplantation. *Am Rev Respir Dis* 1990; 141:1538.

63. Coles SJ, Said SI, Reid LM: Inhibition by vasoactive intestinal peptides of glycoconjugate and lysozyme secretion by human airways in vitro. *Am Rev Respir Dis* 1981; 124:531.

64. Marom Z, Goswami SK: Respiratory mucus hypersecretion (bronchorrea): A case discussion—possible mechanism(s) and treatment. *J Allergy Clin Immunol* 1991; 87:1050.

65. Ollerenshaw S, Jarvis D, Woolcock A., et al.: Absence of immunoreactive vasoactive intestinal peptide in tissue from the lungs of patients with asthma. *N Engl J Med* 1989; 320:1244.

66. Heinz-Erian P, Dey RD, Said SI: Deficient vasoactive intestinal peptide innervation in sweat glands of cystic fibrosis patients. *Science* 1985; 229:1407.

67. Kurian SS, Blank MA, Sheppard MN: Vasoactive intestinal polypeptide (VIP) in vasomotor rhinitis. *Clin Biochem* 1983; 11:425.

68. Lundberg JM, Angaard A, Fahrenkrug J: Complementary role of vasoactive intestinal peptide (VIP) and acetylcholine for cat submandibular gland blood flow and secretion. *Acta Physiol Scand* 1981; 113:329.

69. Hokfelt T, Fuxe K, Pernow B: Coexistence of neuronal messengers: A new principle in chemical transmission. *Prog Brain Res* 1987; 68:1.

70. Druce HM, Wright RH, Kossoff D, Kaliner MA: Cholinergic nasal hyperreactivity in atopic subjects. *J Allergy Clin Immunol* 1985; 76:445.

71. Devillier P, Dessanges JF, Rakatosihanaka J, et al.: Nasal response to substance P and methacholine in subjects with and without allergic rhinitis. *Eur Respir J* 1988; 1:356.

72. Stjarne P, Lundblad L, Lundberg JM, Anggard A: Capsaicin and nicotine sensitive afferent neurones and nasal secretion in healthy human volunteers and in patients with vasomotor rhinitis. *Br J Pharmacol* 1989; 96:693.

73. Ahmed T: Is there loss of protective muscarinic receptor mechanism in asthma? *Chest* 1989; 96:1285.

74. Robertson DN, Rhoden KJ, Grandordy B, et al.: The effect of platelet activating factor on histamine and muscarinic receptor function in guinea pig airways. *Am Rev Respir Dis* 1988; 137:1317.

75. Roberts JA, Raeburn D, Rodger IW, Thomson NC: Comparison of in vivo airway responsiveness and in vitro smooth muscle sensitivity to methacholine. *Thorax* 1984; 39:837.

76. van Koppen CJ, Rodrigues de Miranda JF, Beld AJ, et al.: Muscarinic receptor sensitivity in airway smooth muscle of patients with obstructive airway disease. *Arch Int Pharmacodyn Ther* 1988; 295:238.

77. van Koppen CJ, Lammers J-WJ, Rodrigues de Miranda JF, et al.: Muscarinic receptor binding in central airway musculature in chronic airflow limitation. *Pulm Pharmacol* 1988; 2:131.

78. Whicker SD, Armour CL, Black JL: Responsiveness of bronchial smooth muscle from asthmatic patients to relaxant and contractile agonists. *Pulm Pharmacol* 1988; 1:25.

79. Casale TB: Acute effects of in vitro mast cell degranulation on human lung muscarinic receptors. *Am Rev Respir Dis* 1993; 147:940.

Chapter 8

THE NONADRENERGIC, NONCHOLINERGIC EXCITATORY NERVOUS SYSTEM

JULIAN SOLWAY, DANIEL W. RAY, AND
SHANNON S. CARSON

Functional Identification of Nonadrenergic, Noncholinergic Excitatory Innervation in Lungs

Structural Identification of Nonadrenergic, Noncholinergic Excitatory Innervation

Summary

Functional Identification of Nonadrenergic, Noncholinergic Excitatory Innervation in Lungs

The existence of a nonadrenergic, noncholinergic (NANC) excitatory innervation of the lungs was first suggested by observations of Hawkins and Paton[1] in the late 1950s. They reported that exposure of guinea pig bronchus to nicotine elicited a two-phase bronchoconstriction. The first phase was rapid in onset and was blocked by treatment with atropine, implying that muscarinic neurotransmission accounted for this initial contraction. After a brief intervening relaxation (probably NANC inhibition; see Chap. 9, there ensued a second prolonged contraction of slow onset that was unaffected by atropine, physostigmine, or mepyramine but was blocked by hexamethonium or cocaine. Because of the influence of hexamethonium on this response, Hawkins and Paton attributed this phenomenon to an unknown ganglionic activity. However, it now seems likely, in retrospect, that what they observed was the consequence of nicotine-induced release of contractile neuropeptides from sensory C-fiber nerve endings within the bronchial preparation.

Through the next two decades, cholinergic control of the contractile apparatus within airways was the subject of thorough investigation (see Chap. 9). Yet, it was not until 1981 that Grundström and colleagues[2] rediscovered the NANC excitatory phenomenon with their sentinel demonstration that electrical field stimulation (EFS) of isolated guinea pig hilar bronchus results in a contraction that contains both atropine-sensitive and atropine-insensitive components. The entire contraction could be prevented by preteatment with tetrodotoxin, a sodium channel antagonist that inhibits neural conduction. This finding implicated neural activity and

neurotransmitter release in the response to EFS. Thus, Grundström's findings implicated both cholinergic and noncholinergic neural mechanisms in EFS-induced bronchial contraction.

These diverse mechanisms of bronchoconstriction are illustrated clearly in data from Myers and Undem,[3] in which contraction of an isolated guinea pig bronchial preparation with intact vagal innervation was examined during and after electrical stimulation of the vagus nerve (Fig. 8-1). During the application of stimulating current, the guinea pig bronchus (whose intrinsic tone was reduced by cyclooxygenase blockade with indomethacin) developed an initial spike of tension that persisted for the duration of vagal stimulation, then waned into a second more modest but sustained phase of force generation that persisted for several minutes following cessation of electrical vagal stimulation. The initial tension spike could be blocked by administration of hexamethonium or atropine prior to electrical stimulation of the vagus nerve, but neither muscarinic nor nicotinic blockade inhibited the subsequent prolonged phase of force generation, indicating that the latter does not stem primarily from cholinergic activity and that it does not involve ganglionic neurotransmission. Studies in living animals from other investigators also have demonstrated that electrical stimulation of the cut vagus nerves elicits bronchoconstriction that is resistant to atropine or ganglionic blocking agents.[4-8] Together, these reports clearly demonstrated that there must be another NANC excitatory innervation of the lungs that functions in vivo.

The identity of this NANC excitatory innervation of sensory C-fiber afferent nerves was established over the next 2 years by Szolcsanyi and coworkers[10,11] and by Lundberg and associates in Sweden.[4,6-9] It had been shown that the airways are innervated with C-fiber nerves that contain substance P, one of a family of neuropeptides (called

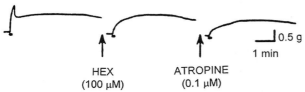

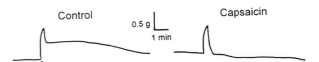

FIGURE 8-1 Contractile responses in guinea pig bronchus elicited by vagus nerve stimulation (bar, 24 V, 0.8 ms, 16 Hz, 10 s) at 30-min intervals. Left tracing: no pretreatment; note that a two-phase contraction is present. Middle tracing: addition of hexamethonium reduces the initial phase of contraction. Right tracing: addition of hexamethonium plus atropine abolishes the initial phase of contraction but has no influence upon the second, long-lasting phase. (*Adapted from Myers and Undem,[3] with permission.*)

FIGURE 8-2 Effect of capsaicin pretreatment on right vagus nerve stimulation of bronchial smooth muscle contraction. In the control preparation, right vagus nerve stimulation elicits a two-phase contraction. Capsaicin pretreatment, which disrupts sensory C-fiber function, ablates the second phase of vagus nerve stimulation-induced contraction, demonstrating that C-fiber neuropeptide release accounts for this component of the bronchoconstriction observed in the control preparation. (*Adapted from Undem et al.[21] with permission.*)

"tachykinins"; see Chap. 10) synthesized by sensory C fibers and stored—along with the nontachykinin calcitonin gene-related peptide (CGRP)—in vesicles located in varicosities within the sensitive nerve terminals.[12–14] A distinguishing characteristic of sensory C fibers is their sensitivity to capsaicin, the pungent agent of chili peppers.[14] By activating what is now known as the vanilloid receptor[15–18] located on C-fiber nerve membranes, capsaicin stimulates calcium (and other di- and monovalent cations) influx, which acutely initiates conduction of an action potential along the C-fiber axon and simultaneously effects the external release of preformed sensory neuropeptides from storage granules.[14] Besides its acute effect on C-fiber conduction and neuropeptide release, capsaicin also can disrupt C-fiber function through a phenomenon known as "desensitization" when applied locally to C-fiber axons.[18–20] When given locally or systemically in large doses, capsaicin exhibits neurotoxicity for C fibers, resulting in long-term (weeks) or even permanent C-fiber dysfunction and tachykinin depletion. By contrast, capsaicin has no direct influence on other nerves comprising the autonomic innervation of the lung.

Both Szolcsanyi et al. and Lundberg et al. exploited these selective properties of capsaicin to evaluate the possibility that C fibers within the guinea pig bronchus constitute the NANC innervation. They desensitized C fibers by local application of capsaicin to the isolated vagi (which contains the afferent innervation of the central airways, see below) or disrupted sensorineural function by systemic capsaicin pretreatment and found that these interventions blocked the atropine-resistant bronchial contractions induced by electrical vagal nerve stimulation in vivo or electrical field stimulation in vitro (see Fig. 8-2).[21] Thus, the NANC excitatory pathway described by Grundström[2] could be explained by the function of capsaicin-sensitive afferent nerves. Pharmacologic proof of this notion came when these and other investigators showed that substance P and neurokinin A—tachykinins released from stimulated sensory C-fiber endings[22]—were potent constrictors of guinea pig bronchus,[23,24] and that NANC contractions of guinea pig airway smooth muscle could be blocked by administration of tachykinin (or "neurokinin") receptor antagonists.[6] The finding that afferent nerves locally release bronchoactive substances with quite "motor" effects has altogether changed

our view of these C-fiber nerves from "sensory" to "sensorimotor."[25] Human bronchial smooth muscle also contracts when exposed to neurokinin A or substance P,[26–30] but the physiologic importance of NANC excitatory innervation is more uncertain, given the much more modest tachykininergic innervation of human airways compared with rodent species (see below).

The synthesis, release, and mechanisms of action of sensory neuropeptides are discussed in greater detail in Chaps. 10 and 17. Briefly, the tachykinins are a family of small peptide mediators that, when released locally from sensory C-fiber endings, stimulate diverse neurokinin receptor subtypes on target cell membranes to cause their local end-organ effects.[31] A wide range of physical and chemical stimuli provoke endogenous sensory neuropeptide release,[22] and both endogenously released and exogenously administered tachykinins elicit a wide range of effector responses within the airways, including broncho-constriction,[23] bronchovascular hyperpermeability and vasodilation,[32,33] mucous gland secretion and enhanced mucociliary function,[34–37] facilitation of cholinergic neurotransmission through pre- and postganglionic mechanisms,[3,38,39] and local recruitment and activation of inflammatory cells from the systemic circulation.[40–42] Given these diverse actions, which may all promote airway hyperresponsiveness, it has been proposed that the NANC excitatory C-fiber system may play some role in asthma.[43]

Structural Identification of Nonadrenergic, Noncholinergic Excitatory Innervation

The neural pathways that supply the sensorimotor innervation of the lung have been revealed in elegant studies that incorporate immunohistochemical detection of sensory neuropeptides, neural ligation/neurotransmitter depletion, and retrograde tracer techniques. Carefully performed immunohistochemical studies have demonstrated that, in general, substance P, neurokinin A, and CGRP are all colocalized within storage granules of C-fiber nerve endings.[44–46] Thus, for the most part (because each can exist outside of C fibers),

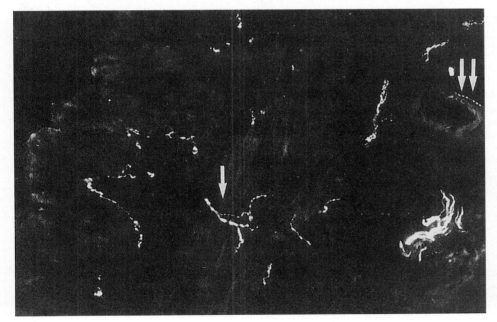

FIGURE 8-3 Immunohistochemical stains of rat lung for substance P (*A*) or CGRP (*B*). *A*. Numerous fibers are evident here, some of which penetrate the airway epithelium (*arrow*). *B*. Immunoreactive nerve fibers are seen in bronchial smooth muscle (*single arrow*) or at the perimeter of a blood vessel (*double arrow*). Original magnifications, ×400. (*Adapted from Springall and Polak,*[47] *with permission.*)

the distribution of any of these substances reflects the distribution of C fibers. In rodent airways, immunohistochemically detected C fibers are abundant, with nerve endings found surrounding airway smooth muscle, bronchial blood vessels, and submucosal glands and within airway epithelium (see Fig. 8-3).[47–49] The innervation of human airways with C fibers is decidedly less prominent,[49–51] reflecting the 10-fold lesser SP content compared to guinea pig airways.[5] Substance P-immunoreactive fibers have been observed around local ganglion cells, within the bronchial smooth muscle layer, under and within bronchial epithelium, and in surrounding blood vessels,[49] though some investigators have reported only sparse tachykinin immunoreactivity

within human airways.[47,51] There is controversy as to whether airway tachykinin content is increased or decreased in asthma. In one study, the length and thickness of SP-containing nerves was increased in the airways of asthmatic subjects.[52] However, in another study, central airway SP content was reduced in asthmatic humans compared with normal control subjects.[53]

Surgical interruption/neural ligation studies and retrograde tracer studies in animals have revealed that the trachea and main bronchi receive afferent C-fiber innervation through the vagus nerves, from cell bodies within the jugular and nodose ganglia[54]; the jugular ganglion may be the more important source of tachykininergic airway innervation, for injection of Fast Blue dye into the airway mucosa labels jugular—but not nodose—ganglion substance P-containing cells.[55] Most C fibers innervating these most central airways travel within the right vagus nerve.[4,21] The lower airways and lung receive afferent nerve supply in animals both from the vagal sensory ganglia and from neurons within the thoracic spinal dorsal root ganglia,[4,7,54,55] whose axons are distributed through the stellate ganglion along with sympathetic pulmonary nerves. In guinea pigs, stellatectomy reduces lower airway substance P content by about 35 percent,[7] and tachykinin depletion from vagal afferent nerves by local capsaicin application reduces lung SP content by about 60 percent,[4] reflecting the relative contributions of spinal and vagal afferents in this species.

Summary

Functional studies have established the existence of an excitatory nervous system whose activation results in bronchoconstriction that occurs independent of cholinergic neurotransmission. This NANC excitatory system has been identified as the tachykinin-containing C-fiber afferent innervation of the lung through pharmacologic and denervation studies. A variety of natural stimuli of C fibers initiate conduction into the central nervous system; these impulses represent the afferent limb of long central reflexes that can result in cough, cholinergic bronchoconstriction, and other respiratory responses.[56] However, these stimuli also cause C fibers to release their preformed neuropeptides within the airways, where they act upon a host of target cells to mediate acute and longer-term airway responses. The precise role of the NANC excitatory system in normal and pathologic human airway function remains to be established, but the constellation of effects seen in animal models raises some possibility that sensory neuropeptides contribute to that pathophysiology of airways disease.

References

1. Hawkins DF, Paton WDM: Responses of isolated bronchial muscle to ganglionically active drugs. *J Physiol* 1958; 144:193.
2. Grundström N, Andersson RGG, Wikberg JES: Pharmacological characterization of the autonomic innervation of guinea pig tracheobronchial smooth muscle. *Acta Pharmacol Toxicol* 1981; 49:150.
3. Myers AC, Undem BJ: Functional interactions between capsaicin-sensitive and cholinergic nerves in the guinea pig bronchus. *J Pharm Exp Ther* 1991; 259:104.
4. Lundberg JM, Brodin E, Saria A: Effects and distribution of vagal capsaicin-sensitive substance P neurons with special reference to the trachea and lungs. *Acta Physiol Scand* 1983; 119:243.
5. Martling CR: Sensory nerves containing tachykinins and CGRP in the lower airways: Functional implications for bronchoconstriction, vasodilatation and protein extravasation. *Acta Physiol Scand Suppl* 1987; 563:1.
6. Lundberg JM, Saria A, Brodin E, et al.: A substance P antagonist inhibits vagally induced increase in vascular permeability and bronchial smooth muscle contraction in the guinea pig. *Proc Nat Acad Sci USA* 1983; 80:1120.
7. Saria A, Martling CR, Dalsgaard CJ, Lundberg JM: Evidence for substance P-immunoreactive spinal afferents that mediate bronchoconstriction. *Acta Physiol Scand* 1985; 125:407.
8. Lundberg JM, Brodin E, Hua X, Saria A: Vascular permeability changes and smooth muscle contraction in relation to capsaicin-sensitive substance P afferents in the guinea pig. *Acta Physiol Scand* 1984; 120:217.
9. Saria A, Martling CR, Yan A, et al.: Release of multiple tachykinins from capsaicin-sensitive sensory nerves in the lung by bradykinin, histamine, dimethylphenyl piperazinium, and vagal nerve stimulation. *Am Rev Respir Dis* 1988; 137:1330.
10. Szolcsanyi J, Bartho L: Capsaicin-sensitive non-cholinergic excitatory innervation of the guinea pig tracheobronchial smooth muscle. *Neurosci Lett* 1982; 34:247.
11. Szolcsanyi J: Tetrodotoxin-resistant non-cholinergic contraction evoked by capsaicinoids and piperine on the guinea pig trachea. *Neurosci Lett* 1983; 42:83.
12. Helke CJ, Drause JE, Mantyh PW, et al.: Diversity in mammalian tachykinin peptidergic neurons: multiple peptides, receptors and regulatory mechanisms. *FASEB J* 1990; 4:1606.
13. Steenbergh PH, Hoppener JW, Zandberg J, et al.: Structure and expression of the human calcitonin/CGRP genes. *FEBS Lett* 1986; 209:97.
14. Theriault E, Otsuka M, Jessell T: Capsaicin-evoked release of substance P from primary sensory neurons. *Brain Res* 1979; 170:209.
15. Fitzgerald M: Capsaicin and sensory neurones—A review. *Pain* 1983; 15:109.
16. Szallasi A, Blumberg PM: Resiniferatoxin and its analogs provide novel insights into the pharmacology of the vanilloid (capsaicin) receptor. *Life Sci* 1990; 47:1399.
17. Bevan S, Szolcsanyi J: Sensory neuron-specific actions of capsaicin: Mechanisms and applications. *Trends Pharmacol Sci* 1990; 11:330.
18. Bevan S, James IF, Rang HP, et al.: The mechanism of action of capsaicin—A sensory neurotoxin, in Jenner P (ed): *Neurotoxins and Their Pharmacological Applications.* New York: Raven Press, 1987:261.
19. Taylor DCM, Pierau FK, Szolcsanyi J: Long lasting inhibition of horseradish peroxidase (HRP) transport in sensory nerves induced by capsaicin treatment of the receptive field. *Brain Res* 1984; 298:45.
20. Jessel TM, Iversen L, Cuello AC: Capsaicin-induced depletion of substance P from primary sensory neurones. *Brain Res* 1978; 152:183.
21. Undem BJ, Myers AC, Barthlow H, Weinreich D: Vagal innervation of guinea pig bronchial smooth muscle. *J Appl Physiol* 1990; 69:1336.
22. Solway J, Leff AR: Sensory neuropeptides and airway function. *J Appl Physiol* 1991; 71:2077.
23. Manzini S, Conti S, Maggi CA, et al.: Regional differences in the motor and inflammatory responses to capsaicin in guinea pig airways: Correlation with content and release of substance P-like immunoreactivity. *Am Rev Respir Dis* 1989; 140:936.
24. Shore SA, Drazen JM: Enhanced airway responses to substance P after repeated challenge in guinea pigs. *J Appl Physiol* 1989; 62:955.
25. Maggi CA, Meli A: The sensory-efferent function of capsaicin-sensitive sensory neurons. *Gen Pharmacol* 1988; 19:1.
26. Naline EP, Devillier P, Drapeau G, et al.: Characterization of neurokinin effects and receptor selectivity in human isolated bronchi. *Am Rev Respir Dis* 1989; 140:679.
27. Frossard N, Barnes PJ: Effects of tachykinins on small human airways. *Neuropeptides* 1991; 19:157.
28. Joos GF, Pauwels RA, van der Straeten ME: Effect of inhaled substance P and neurokinin A in the airways of normal and asthmatic subjects. *Thorax* 1987; 42:779.

29. Martling CR, Theodorsson-Norheim E, Lundberg JM: Occurrence and effects of multiple tachykinins: Substance P, neurokinin A, and neuropeptide K in human lower airways. *Life Sci* 1987; 40:1633.

30. Cheung D, Timmers MC, Zwinderman AH, et al.: Neutral endopeptidase activity and airway hyperresponsiveness to neurokinin A in asthmatic subjects in vivo. *Am Rev Respir Dis* 1993; 148(6, pt 1):1467.

31. Holzer P: Local effector functions of capsaicin-sensitive sensory nerve endings: Involvement of tachykinins, calcitonin gene-related peptide, and other neuropeptides. *Neuroscience* 1988; 24:739.

32. McDonald DM, Mitchell RA, Gabella G, Haskell A: Neurogenic inflammation in the rat trachea: II. Identity and distribution of nerves mediating the increase in vascular permeability. *J Neurocytol* 1988; 17:605.

33. Salonen RO, Webber SE, Widdicombe JG: Effects of neuropeptides and capsaicin on the canine tracheal vasculature in vivo. *Br J Pharmacol* 1988; 95:1262.

34. Coles, SJ, Neill KH, Reid LM: Potent stimulation of glycoprotein secretion in canine trachea by substance P. *J Appl Physiol* 1984; 57:1323.

35. Nagaki M, Ishihara H, Shimura S, et al.: Tachykinins induce a $[Ca^{2+}]i$ rise in the acinar cells of feline tracheal submucosal gland. *Respir Physiol* 1994; 98:111.

36. Tamaoki J, Ueki IF, Widdicombe JH, Nadel JA: Stimulation of Cl secretion by neurokinin A and neurokinin B in canine tracheal epithelium. *Am Rev Respir Dis* 1988; 137:899.

37. Lindberg S, Dolata J: NK1 receptors mediate the increase in mucociliary activity produced by tachykinins. *Eur J Pharmacol* 1993; 231:375.

38. Belvisi MG, Patacchini R, Barnes PJ, Maggi CA: Facilitatory effects of selective agonists for tachykinin receptors on cholinergic neurotransmission: Evidence for species differences. *Br J Pharmacol* 1994; 111:103.

39. Tanaka DT, Grunstein MM: Maturation of neuromodulatory effect of substance P in rabbit airways. *J Clin Invest* 1990; 85:345.

40. DeRose V, Robbins RA, Snider RM, et al.: Substance P increases neutrophil adhesion to bronchial epithelial cells. *J Immunol* 1994; 152:1339.

41. Davies D, Medeiros MS, Keen J, et al.: Eosinophil chemotactic peptide sequences in rat alpha-CGRP: Activation of a novel trophic action by neutral endopeptidase 24.11. *Ann NY Acad Sci* 1992; 657:405.

42. Kroegel C, Geinbycz MA, Barnes PJ: Characterization of eosinophil activation by peptides: Differential effects of substance P, mellitin, and f-Met-Leu-Phe. *J Immunol* 1990; 145:2581.

43. Barnes PJ: Asthma as an axon reflex. *Lancet* 1986; 1:242.

44. Martling CR, Saria A, Fischer JA, et al.: Calcitonin gene-related peptide and the lung: Neuronal coexistence with substance P, release by capsaicin and vasodilatory effect. *Regul Pept* 1988; 20:125.

45. Dey RD, Altemus JB, Zervos I, Hoffpauir J: Origin and colocalization of CGRP- and SP-reactive nerves in cat airway epithelium. *J Appl Physiol* 1990; 68:770.

46. Lundberg JM, Saria A, Theodorsson-Norheim E, et al.: Multiple tachykinins in capsaicin-sensitive afferents: Occurrence, release and biological effects with special reference to irritation of the airways, in Håkanson R, Sundler F, (ed): *Tachykinin Antagonists*. Amsterdam, Elsevier, 1985: 159–169.

47. Springall DR, Polak JM: Neuropeptides in the lower airways investigated by modern microscopy, in Kaliner MA, Barnes PJ, Kunkel GHH, Baraniuk JN (eds): *Neuropeptides in Respiratory Medicine*. New York: Marcel Dekker, 1994:693.

48. Holzer P, Bucsics A, Lembeck F: Distribution of capsaicin-sensitive nerve fibres containing immunoreactive substance P in cutaneous and visceral tissues of the rat. *Neurosci Lett* 1982; 31:253.

49. Lundberg JM, Hökfelt T, Martling CR, et al.: Substance P-immunoreactive sensory nerves in the lower respiratory tract of various mammals including man. *Cell Tissue Res* 1984; 235:251.

50. Baraniuk JN, Lundgren JD, Mullol J, et al.: Substance P and neurokinin A in human nasal mucosa. *Am J Respir Cell Mol Biol* 1991; 4:228.

51. Howarth PH, Djukanovic R, Wilson JW, et al.: Mucosal nerves in endobronchial biopsies in asthma and non-asthma. *Int Arch Allergy Appl Immunol* 1991; 94:330.

52. Ollerenshaw SL, Jarvis DL, Sullivan CE, Woolcock AJ: Substance P immunoreactive nerves in airways from asthmatics and non-asthmatics. *Eur Respir J* 1991; 4:673.

53. Lilly CM, Bai TR, Shore SA, et al.: Neuropeptide content of lungs from asthmatic and non-asthmatic patients. *Am J Respir Crit Care Med* 1995; 151:548.

54. Springall DR, Cadieux A, Oliveira H, et al.: Retrograde tracing shows that CGRP-immunoreactive nerves of rat trachea and lung originate from vagal and dorsal root ganglia. *J Auton Nerv Syst* 1987; 20:155.

55. Kummer W, Fischer A, Kurkowski R, Heym C: The sensory and sympathetic innervation of guinea-pig lung and trachea as studied by retrograde neuronal tracing and double-labelling immunohistochemistry. *Neuroscience* 1992; 49:715.

56. Sant' Ambrogio G: Afferent pathways for the cough reflex. *Bull Eur Physiopathol Respir* 1987; 23(Suppl. 10):19S.

Chapter 9 _____

THE AIRWAY NONADRENERGIC, NONCHOLINERGIC INHIBITORY NERVOUS SYSTEM

LOUIS DIAMOND AND RALPH J. ALTIERE

Evidence for Airway NANC Inhibitory Nerves

Species Distribution

Anatomic Organization

Pharmacologic Characteristics

Putative NANC Inhibitory Neurotransmitters

Functional Significance

In mammalian species, the circumferential layers of smooth muscle located in the submucosal region of the tracheobronchial tree are regulated by autonomic nerves that originate in the central nervous system. When activated, these nerves release either excitatory or inhibitory neurotransmitters from postganglionic nerve terminals closely associated with airway smooth muscle tissue. The resulting muscular contraction or relaxation leads to a change in the caliber of the airways and a corresponding change in airways resistance, lung distensibility, or both, depending on the level of the tracheobronchial tree at which the release of neurotransmitter occurs.

Until relatively recently, the autonomic postganglionic nerves responsible for airway smooth muscle relaxation were thought to be composed exclusively of sympathetic neurons using noradrenaline as their neurotransmitter. This view persisted for many years despite numerous early reports of airway smooth muscle relaxation following parasympathetic vagal nerve stimulation. However, in the absence of pharmacologic tools able to show that these responses were not noradrenergically mediated, these reports largely were ignored. Shortly after the introduction of specific β-adrenoceptor blocking agents in the 1970s, reports began to appear of neurally induced relaxations of isolated airway smooth muscle preparations that occurred in the presence of atropine and were insensitive to the blocking actions of β-adrenoceptor antagonists. Although many candidate transmitters have been studied, the chemical compound responsible for these relaxation responses still is not known with certainty, and the nerves that release the compound are still called *nonadrenergic, noncholinergic* (NANC) inhibitory nerves.

This chapter describes briefly the evidence for the existence of NANC inhibitory nerves in the airways, their occurrence in various species, their anatomic organization, some of their distinguishing pharmacologic characteristics, what is known regarding the chemical nature of their neurotransmitter, and their possible physiologic and/or pathophysiologic significance. For a more critical appraisal of the literature on airway NANC inhibitory nerves and a broader historical perspective, the interested reader is referred to a more comprehensive treatise on this topic.[1]

Evidence for Airway NANC Inhibitory Nerves

The existence of NANC inhibitory nerves has been confirmed in the airways of at least 12 mammalian species, including humans, using a variety of in vitro, in situ, and in vivo techniques. In vitro studies have been performed on airway tissues isolated from the trachea and bronchi as well as from more distal regions of the tracheobronchial tree. Typically, fresh preparations are mounted between metal-plate electrodes in constant-temperature tissue baths, where they are bubbled with oxygen and bathed with other essential nutrients. A voltage is applied to the electrodes, and current is allowed to flow through the tissue. By carefully regulating the electrical stimulation parameters, neural elements in the airway tissue can be depolarized selectively and caused to release their neurotransmitters. The neurotransmitters in turn stimulate receptors on airway smooth muscle cell membranes, causing changes in muscle tension that can be recorded using appropriate physiologic instruments. This technique, known as *electrical field stimulation* (EFS), has been used extensively to demonstrate and characterize NANC inhibitory nerves in the airways. It is important to note that EFS can discriminate between nerves and muscle but not between different types of intrinsic autonomic nerves. Thus, EFS elicits the release of transmitter substances simultaneously from all autonomic nerves in the tissue being stimulated.

To demonstrate the presence of functional NANC inhibitory nerves in an airway tissue using EFS, a tonic background is created first by adding a contractile agonist to the bath. Electrical stimulation then results in a biphasic response consisting of a contraction followed by a relaxation. The contraction phase can be eliminated by pretreatment with a cholinergic antagonist such as atropine. In the guinea pig, which has both an inhibitory and an excitatory NANC system (see Chap. 8), it is necessary also to desensitize the tissue with capsaicin to eliminate the contraction phase completely. Depending on the species and specific airway tissue being studied, the relaxation phase may be unaffected or may be abolished partially or totally by subsequent pretreatment with a β-adrenoceptor blocking agent. Relaxation responses that persist in the presence of β-adrenergic blockade are assumed to have been caused by release of a NANC inhibitory mediator. It is easy to confirm that these responses are neurally derived by showing that they disappear following treatment with tetrodotoxin, an agent that selectively prevents depolarization of neuronal cell membranes.

In situ and in vivo methods also have been used to demonstrate NANC inhibitory nerves in airways.[1] Unlike in vitro methods, which directly measure changes in airway smooth muscle tone, these methods rely on indirect indices of tone, such as tracheal intraluminal pressure or airflow resistance, to assess changes in the contractile state of airway smooth muscle. In a typical experiment, anesthetized animals are pretreated with atropine and propranolol, and airway smooth muscle tone is enhanced with a contractile agonist such as histamine or serotonin. Under these conditions, a decrease in tracheal intraluminal pressure or airflow resistance upon electrical stimulation of the extrinsic neural pathways is taken as evidence for the existence of an NANC inhibitory system. In general, the results obtained with in situ and in vivo techniques have been consistent with those of in vitro techniques. There are a few notable exceptions, however. In most of those cases, in vitro results indicate the presence of NANC inhibitory nerves, but in situ or in vivo results fail to provide corroboration. The most plausible explanation for this type of discordance is that extrinsic NANC inhibitory nerves may travel to airways by a pathway different from the one being stimulated.

Species Distribution

NANC inhibitory nerves first were demonstrated in the isolated trachea of the guinea pig.[2-5] Many other mammalian species have been examined since, and most have been found to have NANC inhibitory nerves.[6] Currently, there are both in vitro and in situ or in vivo data supporting the existence of NANC inhibitory nerves in cat, guinea pig, monkey, and human airways. There also are in vitro data showing that NANC inhibitory nerves are present in the airways of the baboon, cow, chicken, ferret, horse, pig, sheep, and rabbit. The only species studied to date in which NANC inhibitory nerves have not been found are the dog, rat, and swine. In the dog, the inhibitory innervation of the airways is entirely sympathetic; in the rat, the airways seem to have no functional inhibitory innervation. With the exception of humans and nonhuman primates, species that have an airway NANC inhibitory system also appear to have a redundant sympathetic inhibitory system. Human and nonhuman primate airways have only a NANC inhibitory system.

Anatomic Organization

The NANC inhibitory nerves that supply airway smooth muscle resemble other autonomic nerves in that they have both preganglionic and postganglionic components[7-10] and can be activated reflexively through the stimulation of specific afferent pathways.[11-14] However, the central integrating mechanisms that control NANC inhibitory outflow to the airways are not known. Also unknown are the precise locations of the ganglia where NANC preganglionic fibers communicate with NANC postganglionic fibers. In contrast with cholinergic ganglia, which lie in the airway wall, NANC ganglia may reside outside the airways. For example, it has been shown recently that preganglionic fibers responsible for NANC relaxations of guinea pig trachealis muscle synapse on ganglion neurons extrinsic to the trachea and likely in or near the esophagus.[15] Other nerve fibers projecting to the guinea pig trachea and thought to be NANC in nature have been shown to arise directly from the sympathetic stellate ganglia.[16]

Because NANC inhibitory nerves are activated upon stimulation of the vagi or branches thereof, they are considered part of the parasympathetic nervous system. Hence, questions such as the following have arisen: (1) is the NANC inhibitory transmitter colocalized with acetylcholine in cholinergic nerve terminals? (2) can release of the NANC transmitter occur independently of release of the cholinergic transmitter—that is, are parasympathetic NANC and parasympathetic cholinergic neurons distinct functional entities? and (3) does acetylcholine in some way modulate the release of or physiologic response to the NANC transmitter? Although some evidence has been presented to show that at least one putative NANC neurotransmitter is colocalized with acetylcholine in airway cholinergic nerves,[17,18] a definitive answer to the first question awaits final identification of the airway NANC neurotransmitter.

As regards the second question, electrophysiologic data indicate that NANC inhibitory and cholinergic excitatory neurons involved in the regulation of airway smooth muscle do indeed have distinguishing properties, such as different stimulus thresholds and conduction velocities, that allow them to function independently of one another.[15,19] It has not been possible to examine the effects of acetylcholine on the quantity of transmitter released from NANC inhibitory nerves in the airways, but the question of whether acetylcholine modulates physiologic responses to the NANC inhibitory transmitter has been addressed using an acetylcholinesterase inhibitor to enhance the effects of acetylcholine and hemicholinium to deplete airway nerves of acetylcholine.[20] These treatments neither enhance nor diminish NANC relaxations, and, thus, it may be concluded that acetylcholine does not modulate NANC responses in the airways.

The pattern of distribution of NANC inhibitory nerves in the tracheobronchial tree has been studied in vitro by comparing NANC relaxation responses to electrical field stimulation in airways obtained from different regions of the tracheobronchial tree and in vivo by monitoring changes in selected indices of airway mechanical function following stimulation of extrinsic NANC nerves. Additional evidence on the pattern of distribution of NANC nerves has been obtained by anatomic means, primarily by immunohistochemical localization of putative neurotransmitters. Collectively, these approaches have revealed a general pattern of abundance in large, central airways and a gradual or abrupt disappearance toward the peripheral bronchi and bronchioles. The most studied species with respect to the longitudinal distribution of airway NANC inhibitory nerves is the guinea pig. Several laboratories have reported that NANC innervation is more prominent in the cervical trachea than in the thoracic trachea[2,21] and is absent in the bronchi.[1,22] However, the putative NANC inhibitory neurotransmitter NO has been detected in peripheral bronchi of the guinea pig,[23] and it is possible that NANC excitatory responses, which are strong in the lower airways of this species, may mask NANC inhibitory responses.[24] Functional and anatomic studies on human isolated airways have demonstrated the presence of NANC inhibitory innervation from the trachea to the bronchioles.[25–28]

Pharmacologic Characteristics

Numerous pharmacologic agents have been evaluated for their ability to modulate responses to NANC inhibitory nerve stimulation. Many of these compounds were selected for study because they had been shown previously to act either prejunctionally or postjunctionally to modulate cholinergically or noradrenergically mediated responses. For the most part, studies of this type have yielded negative results. For example, studies that have investigated presynaptic modulation of NANC inhibitory neurotransmission by prostaglandins,[4,28-30] adenosine,[31] γ-aminobutyric acid,[32] substance P,[33] enkephalins,[34] α-adrenoceptor agonists,[35] or nedocromil sodium[36] have failed to demonstrate any suppressive or facilitative actions. Similarly, endogenously released acetylcholine has been shown not to alter NANC inhibitory responses in the airways.[20] In contrast, many substances, including prostanoids, α-adrenoceptor agonists, neuropeptide Y, and muscarinic cholinergic agonists have been found to have inhibitory effects on both cholinergic and NANC excitatory neurotransmission in the airways.[6,37]

These findings lend support to two hypotheses: (1) NANC inhibitory neurotransmission occurs independently of cholinergic neurotransmission (because modulation of one fails to influence the other), and (2) when cholinergic or NANC excitatory neurotransmission is suppressed, NANC inhibitory neurotransmission is unaffected, a condition that favors the maintenance of patent airways with low resistance to airflow.

Two pharmacologic interventions are able to modulate NANC inhibitory neurotransmission in the airways through presynaptic mechanisms. The N-type voltage-sensitive calcium channel blocker ω-conotoxin has been shown to attenuate NANC inhibitory responses in guinea pig trachea without altering the postsynaptic relaxant mechanisms evoked by sodium nitroprusside.[38] These results suggest that, like other types of autonomic nerves, NANC inhibitory nerves are regulated by presynaptic N-type voltage-sensitive calcium channels. NANC inhibitory responses in guinea pig trachea are also inhibited by the loop diuretics furosemide and bumetanide. These agents do not affect postsynaptic relaxation responses to vasoactive intestinal peptide (VIP) or nitroprusside, again suggesting a presynaptic site of action on NANC inhibitory nerves.[36] The mechanism by which furosemide and bumetanide produce their effects on NANC inhibitory nerves remains undefined.

Postsynaptic mechanisms also may modulate NANC inhibitory responses in the airways. For example, antigen challenge in sensitized cats has been shown to inhibit NANC relaxation responses, an effect that is reversed by the peptidase inhibitor leupeptin.[39] These results suggest that antigen challenge promotes peptidase activity, which in turn inhibits NANC relaxation responses. Support for this concept has come from studies demonstrating that peptidase inhibition potentiates relaxation responses to VIP in human bronchi.[40,41] In contrast, peptidase inhibition has not been found to alter NANC relaxation responses in guinea pig trachea, despite evidence confirming that peptidase inhibition enhances VIP-induced relaxations.[42] These results suggest that the NANC inhibitory transmitter in guinea pig trachea may not be susceptible to the same peptidases as exogenous VIP.

Other postsynaptic mechanisms have been shown to alter NANC inhibitory responses in the airways. Activation of the NANC excitatory system, with subsequent release of tachykinins, has been found to blunt NANC relaxation responses in guinea pig trachea, suggesting a functional interaction between mediators of the two nervous systems.[42] Inhibition of smooth muscle cyclic nucleotide phosphodiesterases has been demonstrated to potentiate NANC relaxation responses in guinea pig and human airways. In guinea pig trachea, inhibition of phosphodiesterase III (which metabolizes cAMP) potentiates NANC relaxation responses.[43] In human airways, NANC relaxation responses are potentiated primarily by inhibition of phosphodiesterase IV (which also metabolizes cAMP) and, to a limited extent, also by inhibitors of phosphodiesterase V (which metabolizes cGMP).[44] From these results, it appears that different phosphodiesterase isozymes may predominate in the airways of different species.[6]

Putative NANC Inhibitory Neurotransmitters

To date, no laboratory has been able to document the release of a transferrable, pharmacologically active relaxant substance from airway NANC inhibitory nerves following their stimulation. Although the very existence of a NANC inhibitory transmitter in the airways remains hypothetical, that has not deterred speculation and experimentation directed at identifying its chemical nature. Initially, much attention was focused on purines and peptides, because large granular vesicles seen by electron microscopy in axon varicosities associated with airway smooth muscle were believed to be sites of synthesis and storage for these types of compounds. In addition, the purines had gained widespread acceptance as inhibitory neurotransmitters in the gastrointestinal tract, and the gut and tracheobronchial tree have a similar embryonic origin. Although data substantiating a transmitter role for purines in guinea pig airways have been presented,[4,45] more conclusive evidence has been advanced to indicate that purines do not function as inhibitory transmitters in the airways of the guinea pig or of several other species that have a NANC inhibitory system.[22,28,31,46–51]

Of the several peptides that have been identified in airway tissue and circumstantially linked with the airway NANC inhibitory system, the most extensively studied is vasoactive intestinal peptide. As part of its broad spectrum of biologic activity, VIP has the ability to relax mammalian airway smooth muscle and hence to mimic the effects of airway NANC inhibitory nerve stimulation. In addition, it has been shown that when the guinea pig trachealis muscle is either desensitized to VIP by means of prolonged incubation with the peptide or preincubated with VIP antiserum, it loses part of its ability to relax in response to NANC inhibitory nerve stimulation.[31,46,52,53] Further, when the guinea pig trachealis muscle is pretreated with the proteolytic agent α-chymotrypsin, which breaks down VIP and abolishes relaxation responses to the peptide, relaxation responses to NANC inhibitory nerve stimulation are diminished concurrently.[54–56] These apparently confirmatory findings in the guinea pig trachealis muscle have not, however, been successfully and consistently reproduced in airway tissues from other species known to possess an airway NANC inhibitory system, including humans.[27,51,57–59] Moreover, there is evidence that the guinea pig trachea retains some ability to relax in response to NANC inhibitory nerve stimulation after it has been maximally relaxed by exposure to a high concentration of VIP or, vice versa, to VIP after it has been maximally relaxed by NANC inhibitory nerve stimulation.[49,60] The weight of current evidence suggests that VIP may have a transmitter role in guinea pig airways and possibly in the airways of other species, but that it probably is not the sole inhibitory NANC neurotransmitter in any species so far studied.

With the advent of the general concept of gaseous neurotransmission and the coincident identification of NO as the endothelium-derived vascular smooth muscle relaxant factor in the late 1980s, numerous investigators undertook studies to evaluate NO as a possible transmitter of airway NANC inhibitory responses. These studies have yielded results that, while still inconclusive, strongly suggest that NO does play a role in mediating airway NANC inhibitory responses in some species. Humans and guinea pigs have been studied the most,[27,51,55,56,59] but significant data also have been obtained in cats, pigs, and horses.[58,61,62]

Nitric oxide meets two of the principal criteria necessary to establish a substance as a neurotransmitter. First, the enzyme responsible for its biosynthesis from L-arginine, nitric oxide synthase (NOS), has been localized to nerve terminals associated with airway smooth muscle. Second, administration of NO has been shown to produce effects on airway smooth muscle that mimic those produced by NANC inhibitory nerve stimulation. Through the use of histochemical and immunocytochemical techniques, the presence of NOS-containing nerve fibers associated with smooth muscle cells has been confirmed in guinea pig trachea[23] and in large, cartilaginous human airways.[63] Both tissues are known to have a functional NANC inhibitory system. Further, application of authentic NO to isolated airways has been shown to mimic the relaxant response observed when intrinsic NANC nerves are stimulated, and inhalation of authentic NO has been found to cause bronchodilation similar to that which occurs when extrinsic NANC nerves are stimulated.[64] However, the potency of NO as an airway smooth muscle relaxant varies between species and between airway segments within a given species.[65]

Perhaps the most compelling evidence that NO participates in the airway NANC inhibitory system comes from experiments in which NOS inhibitors have been used to prevent the biosynthesis of NO. Several L-arginine analogs have been shown to be competitive inhibitors of NOS. When airway tissues known to have a NANC inhibitory system are treated with these compounds, relaxant responses to NANC nerve stimulation typically are either diminished or abolished. In those instances where NANC responses are blunted but not eliminated by NOS inhibition, it is presumed the NANC system loses two or more inhibitory transmitters. That appears to be the case in the cat, pig, and guinea pig. In the airways of the horse, NOS inhibitors completely abolish NANC relaxations,[62] suggesting that in this species NO is the sole NANC inhibitory neurotransmitter. The situation in human airways is unclear. Virtually total abolition of NANC responses by NOS inhibition has been reported by two groups of investigators,[27,51,66] whereas another group using the same NOS inhibitor has reported a much smaller degree of inhibition.[59]

Not all of the experimental data gathered to date support NO as the airways NANC inhibitory transmitter. For example, NOS-containing nerves have been found in rat intrapulmonary airways[63] and in ferret trachea,[67] but functional NANC inhibitory nerves are absent from both these sites.[45,68,69] Relaxations induced by NANC nerve stimulation in cat bronchi, unlike those in cat trachea, have been shown to be resistant to the effects of NOS inhibitors.[70] In guinea pig trachea, hydroquinone, which inhibits NO by acting as a free-radical scavenger or as a generator of superoxide anions, has been found to nearly abolish relaxations induced by exogenous NO without having discernible effects on relaxations induced by NANC nerve stimulation.[71] Given these conflicting reports, it seems prudent to continue to question the transmitter role of NO in the airways NANC inhibitory system until more conclusive data become available. It also would be wise to pursue experiments to determine if NO functions as a neuromodulator in the airways, either by altering the release of autonomic neurotransmitters or by communicating or modifying responses to them. Interestingly, a neuromodulatory role for NO has been suggested by one study that showed attenuation of VIP-induced relaxations in guinea pig lungs pretreated with a NOS inhibitor[72] and by another study that showed VIP- and NOS-containing neurons innervating parasympathetic cholinergic ganglia but not smooth muscle in ferret trachea.[73]

Functional Significance

The discovery of NANC inhibitory nerves in the airways aroused interest in their possible physiologic and/or pathophysiologic significance. While it is conceivable these nerves are mere evolutionary vestiges that have persisted in various species because of their innocuousness, that seems unlikely in view of the fact that they are the only inhibitory nerves present in primate airways and that they possess afferent connections which allow them to be activated reflexively. Efforts have been made to account for several perplexing airway phenomena by attributing functional significance to NANC inhibitory nerves. For example, the observation that healthy airway smooth muscle contracts to a much greater extent in vitro than in vivo in response to the same spasmogenic stimulus[74–77] may be due, in part, to the loss of tonic or reflex NANC inhibitory control when airway tissues are removed from the intact organism. Similarly, the failure of asthmatic subjects to reach a response plateau, like normal subjects, when challenged with increasing concentrations of a bronchoconstrictive stimulus could, in theory, be explained partly by a deficiency in NANC inhibitory nerve function.[78]

Collectively, the evidence supporting the notion that a defect in the NANC inhibitory system is responsible for hyperreactive airway disease is less than compelling. An effort to induce airway hyperreactivity in nonasthmatic subjects by pharmacologically removing the NANC inhibitory pathway by means of ganglionic blockade with hexamethonium did not result in increased airway responsiveness to inhaled methacholine.[79] Some workers have been able to demonstrate that the NANC inhibitory system has the capacity to counteract induced bronchoconstriction,[80,81] but whether or not the system actually functions in that way under physiologic conditions is unknown. One study found diminished NANC relaxation responses in airway tissues obtained from an asthmatic subject,[82] but a subsequent investigation failed to confirm this finding.[83] Another study, using immunohistochemical techniques, found that VIP was absent from airway neurons of asthmatic subjects.[84] A more recent investigation that measured the actual VIP content of

human trachea and lung parenchyma, however, found no disease-related differences in VIP tissue levels.[85]

While an inherent defect in the NANC inhibitory nervous system may not account for the airway hyperreactivity that characterizes asthma, the possibility remains that NANC function may become compromised during acute exacerbations of the disease. This concept is supported by recent findings showing impairments of NANC inhibitory function following antigen inhalation in actively sensitized cats[39] and rabbits.[86] In theory, these functional impairments could result from the accelerated destruction of NANC neurotransmitters by peptidases and free radicals released from inflammatory cells on antigen stimulation.

The availability of NOS inhibitors has made it possible to explore the question of whether or not airway reactivity increases when NO biosynthesis is suppressed. In the guinea pig, aerosol administration of a NOS inhibitor markedly increased airway responses to histamine, carbachol, and methacholine.[87] Thus, insofar as these increases in airway responses reflect downregulation of the NANC inhibitory system, NANC inhibitory nerves may indeed play an important role in maintaining normal airway reactivity. Further, it has been suggested that the joint operation of NANC inhibitory nerves and NANC excitatory nerves plays an essential role in stabilizing the airways and preventing excessive changes in the contractile state of airway smooth muscle.[88]

References

1. Diamond L, Altiere RJ: Airway nonadrenergic noncholinergic inhibitory nervous system, in Lenfant C (ed): *Lung Biology in Health and Disease*, vol. 33: *The Airways. Neural Control in Health and Disease*. Marcel Dekker, New York, 1988:343.
2. Coburn RF, Tomita T: Evidence for nonadrenergic inhibitory nerves in guinea pig trachealis muscle. *Am J Physiol* 1973; 224:1072.
3. Coleman RA: Evidence for non-adrenergic inhibitory nervous pathway in guinea-pig trachea. *Br J Pharmacol* 1973; 48:360.
4. Coleman RA, Levy GP: A non-adrenergic inhibitory pathway in guinea-pig trachea. *Br J Pharmacol* 1974; 52:167.
5. Richardson JB, Bouchard T: Demonstration of a nonadrenergic inhibitory nervous system in the trachea of the guinea pig. *J Allergy Clin Immunol* 1975; 56:473.
6. Ellis JL, Undem BJ: Pharmacology of non-adrenergic, non-cholinergic nerves in airway smooth muscle. *Pulm Pharmacol* 1994; 7:205.
7. Chesrown SE, Venugopalan CS, Gold WM, Drazen JM: In vivo demonstration of nonadrenergic inhibitory innervation of the guinea pig trachea. *J Clin Invest* 1980; 65:314.
8. Yip P, Palombini B, Coburn RF: Inhibitory innervation to the guinea pig trachealis muscle. *J Appl Physiol* 1981; 50:374.
9. Irvin CG, Boileau R, Tremblay J, et al.: Bronchodilation: Noncholinergic nonadreneregic mediation demonstrated in vivo in the cat. *Science* 1980; 207:791.
10. Diamond L, O'Donnell M: A nonadrenergic vagal inhibitory pathway to feline airways. *Science* 1980; 208:185.
11. Szarek JL, Gillespie MN, Altiere R, Diamond L: Reflex activation of the nonadrenergic noncholinergic inhibitory nervous system in feline airways. *Am Rev Respir Dis* 1986; 133:1159.

12. Michoud M-C, Amyot R, Jeanneret-Grosjean A, Couture J: Reflex decrease of histamine-induced bronchoconstriction after laryngeal stimulation in humans. *Am Rev Respir Dis* 1987; 136:618.

13. Inoue H, Ichinose M, Miura M, et al.: Sensory receptors and reflex pathways of nonadrenergic inhibitory nervous system in feline airways. *Am Rev Respir Dis* 1989; 139:1175.

14. Lammers J-W, Minette B, McCusker MT, et al.: Capsaicin-induced bronchodilation in mild asthmatic patients: Possible role of nonadrenergic inhibitory system. *J Appl Physiol* 1989; 67:856.

15. Canning BJ, Undem BJ: Evidence that distinct neural pathways mediate parasympathetic contractions and relaxations of guinea-pig trachealis. *J Physiol* 1993; 471:25.

16. Bowden JJ, Gibbins IL: Vasoactive intestinal peptide and neuropeptide Y coexist in non-noradrenergic sympathetic neurons to guinea pig trachea. *J Auton Nerv Syst* 1992; 38:1.

17. Laitinen A, Partanen M, Hervonnee A, et al.: VIP-like immunoreactive nerves in human respiratory tract: Light and electron microscopic study. *Histochemistry* 1985; 82:313.

18. Lundberg JM, Lundblad L, Martling C-R, et al.: Coexistence of multiple peptides and classical transmitters in airway neurons: Functional and pathophysiological aspects. *Am Rev Respir Dis* 1987; 136:S16.

19. Lama A, Delpierre S, Jammes Y: The effects of electrical stimulation of myelinated and non-myelinated vagal motor fibres on airway tone in the rabbit and the cat. *Respir Physiol* 1988; 74:265.

20. Altiere RJ, Szarek JL, Diamond L: Neurally mediated nonadrenergic relaxation in cat airways occurs independent of cholinergic mechanisms. *J Pharmacol Exp Ther* 1985; 234:590.

21. Ellis JL, Undem BJ: Non-adrenergic, non-cholinergic contractions in the electrically field stimulated guinea-pig trachea. *Br J Pharmacol* 1990; 101:875.

22. Grundström N, Andersson RGG, Wikberg JES: Pharmacological characterization of the autonomic innervation of the guinea pig tracheobronchial smooth muscle. *Acta Pharmacol Toxicol* 1981; 49:150.

23. Fischer A, Mundel P, Mayer B, et al.: Nitric oxide synthase in guinea pig lower airway innervation. *Neurosci Lett* 1993; 149:157.

24. Undem BJ, Myers AC, Barthlow H, Weinreich D: Vagal innervation of guinea pig bronchial smooth muscle. *J Appl Physiol* 1990; 69:1336.

25. Richardson J, Beland J: Nonadrenergic inhibitory nervous system in human airways. *J Appl Physiol* 1976; 41:764.

26. Taylor SM, Pare PD, Schellenberg RR: Cholinergic and nonadrenergic mechanisms in human and guinea pig airways. *J Appl Physiol* 1984; 56:958.

27. Ellis JL, Undem BJ: Inhibition by L-N^G-nitro-L-arginine of non-adrenergic-noncholinergic-mediated relaxations of human isolated central and peripheral airways. *Am Rev Respir Dis* 1992; 146:1543.

28. Davis C, Kannan MS, Jones TR, Daniel EE: Control of human airway smooth muscle: In vitro studies. *J Appl Physiol* 1982; 53:1080.

29. Kamikawa Y, Shimo Y: Pharmacological differences of nonadrenergic inhibitory response and of ATP-induced relaxation in guinea-pig tracheal strip-chain. *J Pharm Pharmacol* 1976; 28:854.

30. Altiere RJ, Szarek JL, Diamond L: Neural control of relaxation in cat airways smooth muscle. *J Appl Physiol* 1984; 57:1536.

31. Ellis JL, Farmer SG: The effects of vasoactive intestinal peptide (VIP) antagonists, and VIP and peptide histidine isoleucine antisera on non-adrenergic, non-cholinergic relaxations of tracheal smooth muscle. *Br J Pharmacol* 1989; 96:513.

32. Tamaoki J, Graf PD, Nadel JA: Effect of gamma-aminobutyric acid on neurally mediated contraction of guinea pig trachealis smooth muscle. *J Pharmacol Exp Ther* 1987; 243:86.

33. Thompson DC, Diamond L, Altiere RJ: Functional interactions between VIP, nonadrenergic noncholinergic inhibitory nervous responses and substance P in guinea pig airways. *Am Rev Respir Dis* 1989; 139:A236.

34. Altiere RJ, Thompson DC, Diamond L: Selectivity of opioid inhibition of neurotransmission in airway smooth muscle. *Am Rev Respir Dis* 1990; 141:A181.

35. Thompson DC, Diamond L, Altiere RJ: Presynaptic alpha adrenoceptor modulation of neurally mediated cholinergic excitatory and nonadrenergic noncholinergic inhibitory responses in guinea pig trachea. *J Pharmacol Exp Ther* 1990; 254:306.

36. Verleden GM, Pype JL, Demedts MG: Furosemide and bumetanide, but not nedocromil sodium, modulate nonadrenergic relaxation in guinea pig trachea in vitro. *Am J Respir Crit Care Med* 1994; 149:138.

37. Barnes PJ: Modulation of neurotransmission in airways. *Physiol Rev* 1992; 72:699.

38. Altiere RJ, Diamond L, Thompson DC: Omega-conotoxin-sensitive calcium channels modulate autonomic neurotransmission in guinea pig airways. *J Pharmacol Exp Ther* 1992; 260:98.

39. Miura M, Ichinose M, Kimura K, et al.: Dysfunction of nonadrenergic noncholinergic inhibitory system after antigen inhalation in actively sensitized cat airways. *Am Rev Respir Dis* 1992; 145:70.

40. Tam EK, Franconi GM, Nadel JA, Caughey GH: Protease inhibitors potentiate smooth muscle relaxation induced by vasoactive intestinal peptide in isolated human bronchi. *Am J Respir Cell Mol Biol* 1990; 2:449.

41. Hulsmann AR, Jongjan RC, Raatgeep HR, et al.: Epithelium removal and peptidase inhibition enhance relaxation of human airways to vasoactive intestinal peptide. *Am Rev Respir Dis* 1993; 147:1483.

42. Thompson DC, Diamond L, Altiere RJ: Enzymatic modulation of vasoactive intestinal peptide and nonadrenergic noncholinergic inhibitory responses in guinea pig trachea. *Am Rev Respir Dis* 1990; 142:1119.

43. Rhoden KJ, Barnes PJ: Potentiation of nonadrenergic neural relaxation in guinea pig airways by a cyclic AMP phosphodiesterase inhibitor. *J Pharmacol Exp Ther* 1990; 252:396.

44. Fernandes LB, Ellis JL, Undem BJ: Potentiation of nonadrenergic noncholinergic relaxation of human isolated bronchus by selective inhibitors of phosphodiesterase isozymes. *Am J Respir Crit Care Med* 1994; 150:1384.

45. Satchell DG: Adenosine deaminase antagonizes inhibitory responses to adenosine and non-adrenergic, non-cholinergic inhibitory nerve stimulation in isolated preparations of guinea-pig trachea. *Br J Pharmacol* 1984; 83:323.

46. Ito Y, Takeda K: Non-adrenergic inhibitory nerves and putative transmitters in the smooth muscle of cat trachea. *J Physiol (Lond)* 1982; 330:497.

47. Cameron AR, Johnson CF, Kirkpatrick CT, Kirkpatrick MCA: The quest for the inhibitory neurotransmitter in bovine tracheal smooth muscle. *Q J Exp Physiol* 1983; 68:413.

48. Coleman RA: Purine antagonists in the identification of adenosine-receptors in guinea-pig trachea and the role of purines in non-adrenergic inhibitory neurotransmission. *Br J Pharmacol* 1980; 69:359.

49. Karlsson JA, Persson CGA: Neither vasoactive intestinal peptide (VIP) nor purine derivatives may mediate non-adrenergic tracheal inhibition. *Acta Physiol Scand* 1984; 122:589.

50. Irvin CG, Martin RR, Macklem PT: Nonpurinergic nature and efficacy of nonadrenergic bronchodilation. *J Appl Physiol* 1982; 52:562.

51. Belvisi MG, Stretton CD, Miura M, et al.: Inhibitory NANC nerves in human tracheal smooth muscle: A quest for the neurotransmitter. *J Appl Physiol* 1992; 73:2505.

52. Venugopalan CS, Said SI, Drazen JM: Effect of vasoactive intesti-

nal peptide on vagally mediate tracheal pouch relaxation. *Respir Physiol* 1984; 56:205.

53. Matsuzaki Y, Hamasaki Y, Said SI: Vasoactive intestinal peptide: A possible transmitter of nonadrenergic relaxation of guinea pig airways. *Science* 1980; 210:1252.

54. Ellis JL, Farmer SG: Effects of peptidases on non-adrenergic, noncholinergic inhibitory responses of tracheal smooth muscle: A comparison with effects on VIP- and PHI-induced relaxation. *Br J Pharmacol* 1989; 96:521.

55. Tucker JF, Brave SR, Charalambous L, et al.: L-N^G-nitro-L-arginine inhibits non-adrenergic, non-cholinergic relaxations of guinea-pig isolated tracheal smooth muscle. *Br J Pharmacol* 1990; 100:663.

56. Li CG, Rand MJ: Evidence that part of the NANC relaxant response of guinea-pig trachea to electrical field stimulation is mediated by nitric oxide. *Br J Pharmacol* 1991; 102:91.

57. Altiere RJ, Diamond L: Effect of α-chymotrypsin on the nonadrenergic noncholinergic inhibitory system in cat airways. *Eur J Pharmacol* 1985; 114:75.

58. Fisher JT, Anderson JW, Waldron MA: Nonadrenergic noncholinergic neurotransmitter of feline trachealis: VIP or nitric oxide? *J Appl Physiol* 1993; 74:31.

59. Bai TR, Bramley AM: Effect of inhibitor of nitric oxide synthase on neural relaxation of human bronchi. *Am J Physiol* 1993; 264:L425.

60. Karlsson JA, Persson CGA: Evidence against vasoactive intestinal peptide (VIP) as a dilator and in favour of substance P as a constrictor in airway neurogenic responses. *Br J Pharmacol* 1983; 79:634.

61. Kannan MS, Johnson DE: Nitric oxide mediates the neural nonadrenergic noncholinergic relaxation of pig tracheal smooth muscle. *Am J Physiol* 1992; 262:L511.

62. Yu M, Wang Z, Robison NE, LeBlanc PH: Inhibitory nerve distribution and mediation of NANC relaxation by nitric oxide in horse airways. *J Appl Physiol* 1994; 76:339.

63. Kobzik L, Bredt DS, Lowenstein CJ, et al.: Nitric oxide synthase in human and rat lung: Immunocytochemical and histochemical localization. *Am J Respir Cell Mol Biol* 1993; 9:371.

64. Dupuy PM, Shore SA, Drazen JM, et al.: Bronchodilator action of inhaled nitric oxide in guinea pigs. *J Clin Invest* 1992; 90:421.

65. Altiere RJ, Diamond L, Thompson DC: Species variation in airway sensitivity to nitric oxide and nonadrenergic noncholinergic inhibitory nerve activation. *Am J Respir Crit Care Med* 1994; 149:A594.

66. Belvisi MG, Stretton CD, Yacoub M, Barnes PJ: Nitric oxide is the endogenous neurotransmitter of bronchodilator nerves in humans. *Eur J Pharmacol* 1992; 210:221.

67. Dey RD, Mayer B, Said SI: Colocalization of vasoactive intestinal peptide and nitric oxide synthase in neurons of the ferret trachea. *Neuroscience* 1993; 54:839.

68. McWilliam PN, Gray SJ: The innervation of tracheal smooth muscle in the ferret. *J Auton Nerv Syst* 1990; 30:233.

69. Mahey R, Lindsay GW, Thompson DC, Altiere RJ: Cyclic nucleotide second messengers in the non-adrenergic non-cholinergic inhibitory system in airways smooth muscle. *FASEB J* 1995; 9:A677.

70. Diamond L, Lantta J, Thompson DC, Altiere RJ: Nitric oxide synthase inhibitors fail to affect cat airway nonadrenergic non-cholinergic inhibitory (NANCI) responses. *Am Rev Respir Dis* 1992; 145:A382.

71. Hobbs AJ, Tucker JF, Gibson A: Differentiation by hydroquinone of relaxations induced by exogenous and endogenous nitrates in non-vascular smooth muscle: Role of superoxide anions. *Br J Pharmacol* 1991; 104:645.

72. Lilly CM, Stamler JS, Gaston B, et al.: Modulation of vasoactive intestinal peptide pulmonary relaxation by NO in tracheally superfused guinea pig lungs. *Am J Physiol* 1993; 265:L410.

73. Zhu W, Dey R: Fluoro-Ruby as an anterograde and retrograde axonal marker for the study of ferret paratracheal parasympathetic ganglia. *FASEB J* 1995; 9:A698.

74. Roberts JA, Raeburn D, Rogers IW, Thomson NC: Relationship between in vivo airway responsiveness and in vitro smooth muscle sensitivity to methacholine in man. *Thorax* 1983; 38:705.

75. Vincenc KS, Black JL, Yan K, et al.: Comparison of in vivo and in vitro responses to histamine in human airways. *Am Rev Respir Dis* 1983; 128:875.

76. Armour CL, Black JL, Berend N, Woolcock AJ: The relationship between bronchial hyperresponsiveness to methacholine and airway smooth muscle structure and reactivity. *Respir Physiol* 1984; 58:223.

77. Armour CL, Lazar NM, Schellenberg RR, et al.: A comparison of in vivo and in vitro human airway reactivity to histamine. *Am Rev Respir Dis* 1984; 129:907.

78. Boonsawat W, Salome CM, Woolcock AJ: Effect of allergen inhalation on the maximal response plateau of the dose-response curve to methacholine. *Am Rev Respir Dis* 1992; 146:565.

79. Sterk PJ, Daniel EE, Zamel N, Hargreave FE: Limited maximal airway narrowing in nonasthmatic subjects: Role of neural control and prostaglandin release. *Am Rev Respir Dis* 1985; 132:865.

80. Miura M, Inoue H, Ichinose M, et al.: Effect of nonadrenergic noncholinergic inhibitory stimulation on the allergic reaction in cat airways. *Am Rev Respir Dis* 1990; 141:29.

81. Inoue H, Aizawa H, Miyazaki N, et al.: Possible roles of the peripheral vagal nerve in histamine-induced bronchoconstriction in guinea-pigs. *Eur Respir J* 1991; 4:860.

82. de Jongste JC, Mons H, Bonta IL, Kerrebijn KF: In vitro responses of airways from an asthmatic patient. *Eur J Respir Dis* 1987; 71:23.

83. Adcock IM, Belvisi MG, Stretton CD, et al.: Inhibitory NANC responses and VIP mRNA levels in asthmatic and denervated human lung. *Am Rev Respir Dis* 1991; 143:A355.

84. Ollerenshaw S, Jarvis D, Woolcock A, et al.: Absence of immunoreactive vasoactive intestinal polypeptide in tissue from the lungs of patients with asthma. *N Engl J Med* 1989; 320:1244.

85. Lilly CM, Bai TR, Shore SA, et al.: Neuropeptide content of lungs from asthmatic and nonasthmatic patients. *Am J Respir Crit Care Med* 1995; 151:548.

86. Fame TM, Colasurdo GN, Loader JE, et al.: Decrease in the airways' nonadrenergic noncholinergic inhibitory system in allergen sensitized rabbits. *Pediatr Pulmonol* 1994; 17:296.

87. Nijkamp FP, van der Linde HJ, Folkerts G: Nitric oxide synthesis inhibitors induce airway hyperresponsiveness in the guinea pig in vivo and in vitro: Role of epithelium. *Am Rev Respir Dis* 1993; 148:727.

88. Lindén A, Skoogh B-E: NANC responses-role in control of airway tone. *Respir Med* 1994; 88:249.

MEDIATORS OF INFLAMMATION

Chapter 10

INTRODUCTION TO MEDIATORS OF INFLAMMATION

JEFFERY M. DRAZEN

IgE Structure and Function

The High-Affinity IgE Receptor

Mast Cell and Basophil Activation

Histamine

Proteolytic Enzymes

Substance P

Cytokines

Mediators Synthesized on Cellular Activation

Platelet Activating Factor

Secondary Microenvironmental Changes

The evolution of adoptive immunity allowed the immune system to recognize specific foreign antigens and to clonally proliferate molecules (i.e., immunoglobulins, T-cell receptors) that can physically bind to these antigens. In infections, adoptive immunity is manifested by the binding of antibody to the infectious agent, an event that aids in the neutralization and destruction of that agent. For reasons that are not entirely clear, an alternative process has evolved in which the recognition of specific foreign antigen results in the production of IgE antibody that sensitizes certain cells (i.e., mast cells and basophils); presentation of the antigen activates the effector systems in these sensitized cells, so that mediators of immediate hypersensitivity are synthesized and released. This process, which is known as type I, or immediate, hypersensitivity, is thought to be the basis for the reactions that lead to asthma and allergic airway diseases. (Recent reviews on this subject can be found in Refs. 1 to 3.)

The two major phases of the immune hypersensitivity response are outlined in Table 10-1. In the first phase the introduction of antigen into an appropriate microenviron-ment results in cellular sensitization with IgE, whereas in the second phase, the reintroduction of antigen results in an immediate hypersensitivity response.[4]

Immediate hypersensitivity responses can occur in many organ systems and can produce different physiologic syndromes. The syndromes of greatest importance to the respiratory system include allergic rhinitis, which affects the upper airways, and asthma, which affects the pulmonary airways. In their most severe form, immediate hypersensitivity reactions are expressed as anaphylaxis, which results in circulatory compromise and respiratory insufficiency. Although the locus of response differs, the same sequence of biologic events accounts for anaphylaxis and allergic rhinitis. This sequence is reviewed in detail below.

IgE Structure and Function

IgE is synthesized when specific antigens—those to which allergic reactions are commonly elicited—are presented by

TABLE 10-1   Phases of the Allergic Process

Phase I

Host is exposed to antigen.
Antigen-presenting cells process antigen and present it to T cells.
T cells bearing the T_{H2} phenotype recognize antigen and proliferate.
B cells emerge with capacity to differentiate into plasma cells producing IgE directed against the antigen.
The IgE produced binds to specific IgE receptors on target cells.

Phase II

Host is reexposed to antigen.
Antigen binds to IgE on target cells resulting in aggregation of IgE receptors.
Aggregation of IgE receptors triggers release of mediators of hypersensitivity
IgE-receptor complexes reappear on surface of target cells to initiate a further cycle of response.

macrophages to T cells in an environment that supports the emergence of T_{H2} cells.[5,6] These T-helper cells, by virtue of their restricted cytokine profile (i.e., the production of IL-4, and IL-5 and IL-10), render conditions favorable to the emergence of B cells with the capacity to differentiate into IgE-forming plasma cells.

The molecular structure of IgE is similar to that of other immunoglobulins (Fig. 10-1). There are two light chains, either kappa (κ) or lambda (λ) that are the same as in other immunoglobulins; in addition, there are two heavy chains of the epsilon (ε) class that are found only in IgE. As in other immunoglobulin molecules, the light chains in IgE confer antigenic specificity, while the heavy chains confer class specificity. The interchain structures—that is, the bonds

among the chains resulting in antibody formation—are covalent disulfide bonds; in this regard, IgE again resembles other immunoglobulins.

IgE is found in low concentrations in the plasma of normal human blood. A concentration of 100 IU/m is considered the upper limit in normal plasma samples; individuals with allergies may have higher concentrations of IgE in their plasma.[7] Assays for antigen-specific forms of IgE have been developed, and the amount of antibody to a particular allergen can be quantitated accurately.[8] The latter ability is attributable in part to the somewhat limited number of distinct antigens in response to which IgE molecules are commonly formed. Hence, the assays can be used to determine the level of IgE antibody to specific allergens in the plasma of potentially allergic individuals.

The High-Affinity IgE Receptor

IgE binds to the surface of mast cells and basophils through the high-affinity IgE receptor (Fig. 10-1).[9] In this designation Fc_ϵ indicates that the receptor binds the Fc_ϵ portion of IgE, R stands for the receptor, and I stands for the high-affinity receptor. $Fc_\epsilon RII$, a lower-affinity IgE receptor, is found on B cells, eosinophils, and macrophages. Its specific role in atopic diseases is not known. $Fc_\epsilon RI$ is a heterotetrameric structure composed of two identical γ chains, one α chain and one β chain. Each of the chains has a membrane-spanning unit. The α chain is largely extracellular and is the unit that actually binds IgE, whereas the β and γ chains are largely intracellular and are thought to be responsible for signal transduction via this unit.

IgE binds with high affinity to $Fc_\epsilon RI$ on the surface of mast cells and basophils. There are approximately 100,000 high-affinity IgE receptors on the surface of each cell. The concen-

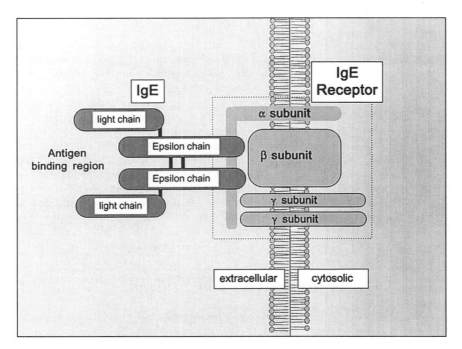

FIGURE 10-1 Schematic diagram showing a representative IgE molecule and $F_{C\epsilon}RI$, the high-affinity IgE receptor.

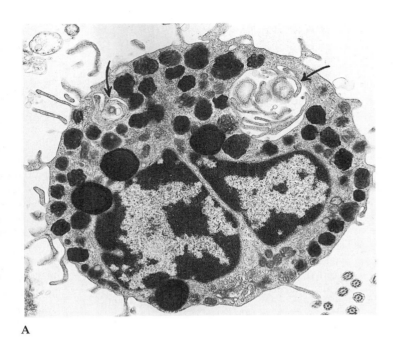

A

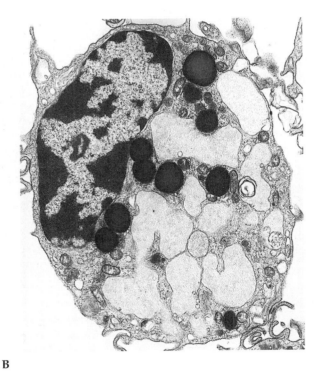

B

FIGURE 10-2 Electron micrographs of nonactivated (*A*) and activated (*B*) human mast cells. The latter cells were activated by the addition of anti-IgE to mast cells isolated from human lung. (*From Dvorak,*[11,12] *with permission.*)

Mast Cell and Basophil Activation

The major biologic result of the coupling of antigen to IgE and the subsequent intracellular events is the release and synthesis of mediators from mast cells and basophils (See recent review by Galli.[10]) Electron micrographs of "resting" and "activated" human lung mast cells are shown in Fig. 10-2.[11,12] Mediators are biomolecules whose field of action is the local microenvironment; thus they are distinguished from hormones, which, by definition, act both locally and at a distance. A number of mediators released or synthesized as a result of mast cell activation exert diverse biologic effects.[10] Many of the subsequent chapters in this section deal with biologic effects arising from specific mast-cell- or basophil-derived mediators. In this section some of the mediators known to be contained in, released by, or synthesized by Fc$_\epsilon$RI-bearing cells on activation will be reviewed briefly.

Histamine

Histamine, β-imidazolylethylamine, is a potent bronchoconstrictor agonist. In addition, it dilates and increases the permeability of the microvasculature and promotes the secretion of mucus. Histamine, most likely complexed with heparin, resides within mast-cell granules that are actively extruded within minutes of the interaction between antigen and IgE.

Proteolytic Enzymes

Mast cells contain proteases commonly known as tryptase and chymase.[13,14] An individual mast cell may contain

tration of IgE is low in the plasma; however, of the total number of IgE molecules available to bind antigen in the body, the majority are bound to Fc$_\epsilon$ receptors. When antigen interacts with IgE molecules such that Fc$_\epsilon$RI molecules are aggregated, the host cell, that is, mast cell or basophil, is activated.

mostly tryptase, mostly chymase, or similar amounts of the two molecules. The proteolytic profiles or tryptase and chymase are distinct, yet the specific endogenous substrates against which they are directed are not known. Moreover, the importance of these proteolytic enzymes in furthering the immediate hypersensitivity response has not been established. It has been speculated that they may cleave bioactive peptides from circulating plasma precursors and inactivate molecules with a predominant homeostatic role.

Substance P

Substance P, an 11-amino-acid peptide, is released from mast cells after activation.[15] In the microenvironment of the airway, substance P can transduce—through action at NK_1 or NK_2 receptors—the constriction of airway smooth muscle as well as vascular leak. The expression of proinflammatory actions by this peptide is limited by its proteolytic cleavage and inactivation by a neutral-pH active protease (E.C.3.4.24.11).

Cytokines

During the activation of mast cells and basophils, various cytokines (the most important being IL-4), are released into the microenvironment. This event promotes further synthesis of IgE and perpetuation of the allergic reaction.[16]

Mediators Synthesized on Cellular Activation

One of the consequences of the interaction of specific antigen and IgE is the elevation of intracellular calcium concentrations. This change results in the activation of a number of enzyme systems, which in turn results in the synthesis of active biomolecules. Among such molecules are eicosanoids,[17] which are biologically active molecules derived from arachidonic acid. Two major classes of bioactive eicosanoids are produced by activated mast cells and basophils. The first class consists of prostaglandins (including the prophologistic prostaglandins PGD_2 and $PGF_{2\alpha}$) as well as thromboxane A_2. In addition, mast cells and baso-phils produce the homeostatic prostaglandin PGE_2. The second class consists of the leukotrienes, which are the products of the lipoxygenation of arachidonic acid, at the 5 position. The cysteinyl leukotrienes include the sulfur-containing amino acid cysteine and compose the molecular entities that make up the material formerly known as slow-reacting substance of anaphylaxis (SRS-A). In addition, the dihydroxy leukotriene B_4 (LTB_4), a chemotactic agent likely of importance in creating the microenvironment recognized in immediate hypersensitivity reactions, is formed. Other eicosanoids that are produced, including hydroxyeicosatetraenoic acids (HETEs), may have a chemotactic role in promoting the cellular microenvironment of the immediate hypersensitivity response.

Platelet Activating Factor

Platelet activating factor (PAF) is a derivative of phosphocholine with an ether link in the *sn*-1 position and an acetyl group in the *sn*-2 position. PAF has multiple biologic effects, mediated through action at specific receptors including increasing microvascular permeability, causing platelet aggregation, and promoting eosinophil chemotaxis.[18,19]

Secondary Microenvironmental Changes

The release of both preformed and newly synthesized mediators has two effects on the microenvironment of the mast cell or basophil. First, the released mediators may change the biology of the microenvironment in which they become available. In the airways, for example, their presence may result in muscular bronchoconstriction, edema of the airway wall, and mucus secretion, all of which will be recognized physiologically as airway obstruction. Furthermore, the mediators, either directly or through their physiological actions, can promote the release of secondary mediators such as tachykinins. The release of tachykinins can result in the spread of inflammation beyond the site of local release through an axon reflex.

A secondary effect of the mediators released, many of which have chemotactic properties, is to change the cellular makeup of the microevironment in which the immediate hypersensitivity has occurred. The release of LTB_4 and PAF as well as the cleavage of chemotactic factors from plasma substrates by mast-cell proteases results in the migration into the lesion of eosinophils, neutrophils, and a variety of mononuclear cells. Eosinophils contain a variety of toxic proteins that can be released into the microenvironment, with the consequent promotion of tissue damage due to the immediate hypersensitivity response. Prominent among these proteins are eosinophilic major basic protein, eosinophilic cationic protein, and eosinophil-derived neurotoxin.

Thus, the mediators produced either directly or indirectly as a result of the IgE antibody response not only are responsible for the physiological changes associated with immediate hypersensitivity responses but also provide the stimuli producing the altered cellular milieu that characterizes this condition.

References

1. Borish L, Joseph BZ: Inflammation and the allergic response. *Med Clin North Am* 1992; 76:765.
2. Church MK, Okayama Y, Bradding P: The role of the mast cell in acute and chronic allergic inflammation. *Ann NY Acad Sci* 1994; 725:13.
3. Plaut M: Cytokines and modulation of diseases of immediate hypersensitivity. *Ann NY Acad Sci* 1993; 685:512.
4. Maggi E, Romagnani S, Ricci M: Regulation mechanisms of IgE synthesis and their deregulation in atopy. *Allergol Immunopathol (Madr)* 1992; 20:165.

5. Geha RS: Regulation of IgE synthesis in humans. *J Allergy Clin Immunol* 1992; 90:143.

6. Sutton BJ, Gould HJ: The human IgE network. *Nature* 1993; 366:421.

7. VanArsdel PP Jr, Larson EB: Diagnostic tests for patients with suspected allergic disease. Utility and limitations. *Ann Intern Med* 1989; 110:304.

8. Aas K: The radioallergosorbent test (RAST): diagnostic and clinical significance. *Ann Allergy* 1974; 33:251.

9. Ravetch JV, Kinet JP: Fc receptors. *Annu Rev Immunol* 1991; 9:457.

10. Galli SJ: New concepts about the mast cell. *N Engl J Med* 1993; 328:257.

11. Dvorak A: Human mast cells, in Beck F, Hild W, Kriz W, et al. (eds): *Advances in Anatomy, Embryology and Cell Biology.* Berlin, Springer-Verlag, 1989:50–119.

12. Dvorak A: Morphologic expressions of maturation and function can affect the ability to identify mast cells and basophils in man, guinea pig and mouse, in Befus AD, Bienenstock J, Denburg JA (eds): *Mast Cell Differentiation and Heterogeniety.* New York, Raven, 1986:95–126.

13. Barrett KE, Metcalfe DD: Heterogeneity of mast cells in the tissues of the respiratory tract and other organ systems. *Am Rev Respir Dis* 1987; 135:1190.

14. Schwartz LB, Metcalfe DD, Miller JS, et al.: Tryptase levels as an indicator of mast-cell activation in systemic anaphylaxis and mastocytosis. *N Engl J Med* 1987; 316:1622.

15. Lilly CM, Drazen JM, Shore SA: Peptidase modulation of airway effects of neuropeptides. *Proc Soc Exp Biol Med* 1993; 203:388.

16. Holgate S: Mediator and cytokine mechanisms in asthma. *Thorax* 1993; 48:103.

17. Samuelsson B: Leukotrienes: Mediators of immediate hypersensitivity reactions and inflammation. *Science* 1983; 220:568.

18. Shukla SD: Platelet-activating factor receptor and signal transduction mechanisms. *FASEB J* 1992; 6:2296.

19. Shimizu T, Honda Z, Nakamura M, et al.: Platelet-activating factor receptor and signal transduction. *Biochem Pharmacol* 1992; 44:1001.

Chapter 11

HISTAMINE

REBECCA BLUMENTHAL AND JONATHAN MOSS

Histamine is an endogenous vasoactive amine formed from the chemical or enzymatic decarboxylation of L-histidine.[1] More than 80 percent of histamine is stored in mast cells or basophils. Mast cells are present in many tissues, especially those that come into frequent contact with the external environment, such as the skin, upper and lower airways, lungs, and the gastrointestinal tract. Together with basophils, mast cells represent the initial cellular elements of allergic and chemically mediated reactions. Although mast cells are a single class of cells, they exhibit functional and structural heterogeneity between tissues and species.[2,3] Histochemical, ultrastructural, and functional differences in mast cell content and release mechanisms have been identified that correspond to the wide spectrum of symptoms in reactions. Upon release from mast cells by chemical or immunologic mechanisms, histamine can exert significant effects on a wide variety of tissues in the respiratory, cardiovascular, central nervous, gastrointestinal, and genitourinary systems.

Pharmacology of Histamine

HISTAMINE SYNTHESIS

ENDOGENOUS/CELLULAR CONTRIBUTION
Although the pharmacology of histamine synthesis has been well understood for many years, the cellular location of its synthesis has been difficult to study with conventional fluorescence techniques. The development of a specific antibody to the histidine decarboxylase enzyme (HDC, L-histidine decarboxylase, EC 4.1.22) a decade ago and the more recent development of cDNA probes have allowed localization of histamine biosynthesis at a cellular level.[4,5] Most histamine, perhaps >80 percent, is located in mast cells, but there is evidence for storage, if not synthesis, in basophils, neurons, and endothelial cells.

EXOGENOUS/DIETARY CONTRIBUTION
Although histamine is enzymatically synthesized from L-histidine, a growing body of evidence suggests dietary sources of histamine or its precursor are relevant to human pathophysiology.[6] For example, when hemoglobin is released into the stomach, as in upper gastrointestinal bleeding, a significant portion of the hemoglobin is converted to histidine (about 7 percent of the amino acids in hemoglobin) and then decarboxylated to histamine. The resultant histamine can be measured by increase in plasma concentrations or is manifested as a decrease in systemic vascular resistance, which may be attenuated by prophylaxis with H_1 and H_2 antagonists. Thus, gastric lavage can lead to significant improvement in systemic vascular resistance. As a result, there is a resurgence of interest in histamine-free foods, particularly in Europe.[7–10]

HISTAMINE STORAGE IN MAST CELLS

As is the case for many biogenic amines, histamine is stored within granules, most often in mast cells. Although histamine is distributed widely throughout the body, its greatest concentration is in the skin, respiratory tract, and gastrointestinal mucosa.[1] Some of the confusion involving the biologic functions of histamine derives from the fact that histamine does not exist in isolation within the storage granules. Depending upon the location of the mast cells, there may be an ionic complex with either heparin or chondroitin sulfate in the granule. In addition to heparin and chondroitin sulfate, eosinophilic and neutrophilic chemotactic factors, prostaglandin D_2 (PGD_2), and leukotrienes B_4, C_4, and D_4 are also released. Thus, many studies of immunologic reactions overstate the importance of histamine when many other potent biologic compounds may also be released.[11]

HISTAMINE RELEASE FROM MAST CELLS

IMMUNOLOGIC/ANAPHYLACTIC MECHANISMS
Although pharmacologists have used a variety of cytolytic agents to examine mast cell release, most clinicians are familiar with release by immunologic, complement, or chemical mechanisms (Fig. 11-1). The sequence by which immunologic release occurs is well understood: Mast cells or basophils are degranulated by cross-linking adjacent IgE molecules located on the cell membrane. After initial sensitization and subsequent reexposure, IgE binds to and causes degranulation of mast cells. With IgE-mediated stimulation of human mast cells, the mast cell granules swell, form a scroll pattern, and appear, in electron micrographs, as electron-dense clumps with little stainable matrix. Granules then become ropelike and soluble and release their contents. Extruded granules never are observed intact outside the mast cells.[12] Studies with human mast cells have demonstrated that such release requires ATP and is contingent upon an elevation in free calcium. Perhaps less well appreciated is the extraordinary geographic variation when a 10-fold difference in specific IgE has been documented.[13]

NONIMMUNOLOGIC MECHANISMS
The mechanism of histamine release by nonimmunologic means is less well understood. Under some circumstances, mast cell release involves activation of phospholipase via G proteins (leading ultimately to the production of both 1,4,5-triphosphate and diacylglycerol) and granular fusion. Less well understood are the mechanisms by which common drugs, including opioids and neuromuscular blockers, also cause histamine release. There is some evidence based on chemical structure that simple cationic exchange may be important in this mechanism. Unlike immunologic release, in which the mast cell is degranulated, chemically mediated release is selective for preformed mediators.[14]

HISTAMINE CATABOLISM

As with most biogenic amines, the half-life of histamine in plasma is very short. Normal plasma concentrations are <1 ng; recent radioimmunoassay (RIA) and high performance liquid chromatography (HPLC) methods of measurement suggest concentrations of 200 pg/ml.[15] Studies of release by drugs suggest a half-life in plasma of 1 min. Upon its release, there are two pathways for catabolism of histamine. The primary route of catabolism is through histamine N-methyltransferase (HNMT). This enzyme methylates the telenitrogen in the imidazole ring, resulting in the formation of biologically inactive N-methylhistamine, which subsequently can be degraded. The secondary pathway is through diamine oxidase (DAO), which is a relatively nonspecific enzyme. Except in certain ovarian carcinomas and during the third trimester of pregnancy, DAO is the secondary route of catabolism. Because under normal conditions there is a surplus of inactivating enzymes, very little histamine, perhaps <1 percent, is recovered in the urine.[1,16] For these reasons, tryptase, an enzyme contained in granules of many mast cells but not blood elements and coreleased with histamine, has been used as a marker for histamine release. Plasma tryptase has a half-life of approximately 3 h and thus confers a significant advantage in evaluating clinically important histamine release.[17–19]

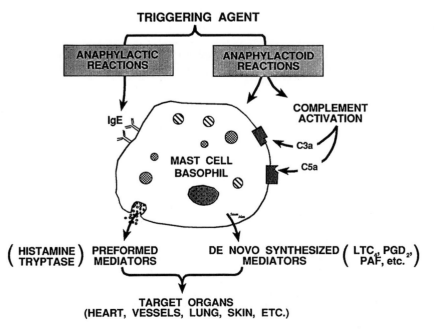

FIGURE 11-1 Mast Cell. LTC_4 = leukotriene C_4; PGD_2 = prostaglandin D_2; PAF = platelet-activating factor; IgE = immunoglobulin E. (*From Marone et al.: Mechanisms of activation of human mast cells and basophils.* Ann F Anesth Reanim 1993; 12:116, with permission.)

It is increasingly appreciated that many common intravenous drugs, including neuromuscular antagonists and antibiotics, can inhibit either DAO or HNMT enzymes. While there are few clinical data to substantiate important interaction, a growing body of evidence from mammalian investigations suggests that such inhibition of catabolism increases lethality of histamine-releasing agents or states. In the case of steroidal muscle relaxants, HNMT inhibition may be irreversible.[20,21]

Histamine Receptors

RECEPTORS

Like other biologic transmitters, histamine acts according to the nature and distribution of its receptors. The actions of histamine are determined by three, and possibly four, distinct receptors. Both the H_1- and H_2-receptors have been cloned within the past 5 years. Analysis of their sequences suggest that they are widely separated in phylogeny and function. The development of relatively specific H_1- and H_2-antagonists has permitted extensive identification of their roles in human physiology.

MECHANISMS OF SIGNAL TRANSDUCTION

While cloning data have provided unequivocal structural evidence for discrete H_1- and H_2-receptors, there are significant differences in the way in which the H_1- and H_2-receptors transduce their signals.[22] The H_1-receptors initiate smooth-muscle action from breakdown of inositol phosphates. They also act on endothelial cells to promote the release of nitric oxide and other relaxant factors. In contrast, the H_2-receptors activate adenylyl cyclase as the second messenger, resulting in gastric acid secretion, vasodilation, inotropic and chronotropic responses, and neuronal activation.[16,23]

In recent years, there has been enthusiasm for a role of the H_3-receptor. With the development of potent and specific agonists and antagonists and some refinement of imaging techniques, a growing body of evidence suggests an important role for histamine in consciousness and awareness.[24] In animal models, the H_3-receptor inhibits the release of catecholamines presynaptically and influences release in the parasympathetic nervous system. More recently, an intracellular histamine receptor (H_{IC}) has been described. The H_{IC}-receptor plays a role in modulating mitosis and may be influenced by a variety of antidepressants and antihistamines.[25–27]

Physiologic Roles of Histamine

The physiologic effects of histamine are complex. Unlike many biogenic amines, histamine acts differently in humans than in experimental animals. There is considerable species-to-species and tissue-to-tissue variation in the structure and content of mast cells, as well as considerable variation between mast cell histamine content and release.[3,28,29] Thus, it is often difficult to extrapolate from studies of animals or isolated tissue to human pathophysiologic states. This difficulty has led to confusion in understanding the biologic roles of histamine. Changes in heart rate, blood pressure, and gastric acid secretion, however, correlate with histamine liberation.

CARDIOVASCULAR EFFECTS

Both H_1- and H_2-receptors exert profound cardiovascular effects, including chronotropic, inotropic, and antidromic effects, and can significantly alter fibrillation threshold. The action of histamine on the heart mirrors the action of catecholamines, with the H_1-receptor acting like the α-adrenergic receptor, and the H_2-receptor acting like the β-adrenergic receptor.[30] In addition, both H_1- and H_2-receptors participate, although independently, in the decrease in systemic vascular resistance caused by histamine-releasing drugs.[2,31–35] The role of histamine in the cardiovascular system is underscored by epidemiologic studies of life-threatening anaphylactic and anaphylactoid reactions, in which cardiovascular collapse is the most frequent and serious feature (Table 11-1).

RESPIRATORY EFFECTS

H_1-receptors also have been identified in bronchiolar smooth muscle, but they appear to be of less consequence there than in the cardiovascular system. Although bronchoconstriction may be mediated by H_1-receptors, the tendency in recent years has been to focus on other transmitters for the dominant role in clinical asthma. The relative ineffectiveness of H_1-antihistamines in attenuating asthma, the lack of bronchospasm in many serious hypersensitivity reactions,[36–38] and the weakness of histamine as a pharmacologic agent for bronchoconstriction suggest that histamine plays a modest role in human asthma. Histamine does, however, play an important role in the overall inflammatory response. Cuta-

TABLE 11-1   Features of Life-Threatening Anaphylaxis during Anesthesia[a]

Clinical Features	n	Sole Feature	Worst Feature
Cardiovascular collapse	389	44	351
Bronchospasm	161	13	75
Transient	72		
Asthmatics	72		
Cutaneous			
Rash	55		
Erythema	201		
Urticaria	37		
More than one	29		
Angioedema	107	5	13
Generalized edema	30		
Pulmonary edema	13	1	5
Gastrointestinal	35		

NOTE: Total number of patients $n = 422$.
[a] Subjective symptoms (metallic taste, itch, feeling of doom) cannot be tabulated.

neous manifestations are mediated by both H_1- and H_2-receptors,[39,40] and gastric acid secretion is mediated primarily by the H_2 receptor.

As a bronchoconstrictor, histamine is only 1/4000 as potent as other endogenous compounds such as leukotrienes. Recent initiatives in the development of medications for asthma have focused on lipoxygenase inhibition.[41] The role of histamine on the bronchi is confounded by the well-described release of catecholamines from the adrenal medulla and sympathetic neurons.[42] Although the administration of exogenous histamine through injection or inhalation or release from endogenous stores can activate H_1-receptors to produce bronchial smooth-muscle constriction, histamine challenge tests often fail to replicate the extent or symptoms of endogenous release and are of little import in healthy individuals. However, in animal models of asthma, such as basenji-greyhound dogs,[43] and in some patients with asthma, bronchoconstriction caused by histamine is more severe.[44–46] The H_1-receptor also can increase airway secretion. Although an H_1-receptor has been demonstrated in the bronchi, evidence is sparse for the existence of functional H_2-receptors there.[47] The large number of patients with airway disease who tolerate H_2-antagonists for concomitant ulcer disease suggests that antagonism of any putative H_2-pulmonary receptors is not a significant clinical problem.

TISSUE AND SPECIES MAST CELL HETEROGENEITY

There are few studies of histamine in isolated human pulmonary mast cells.[3,28,29] Those that have been performed support the clinical observations that both release and content of mast cells vary considerably between tissues. Recent studies have characterized the biochemical and functional differences between human sinus, skin, and lung mast cells[2] (Fig. 11-2). Among the tissue-specific mast cell properties found were (1) decreased tryptase content in sinus versus skin and lung mast cells (histamine was constant); (2) no response by sinus mast cells to compound 48/80, a nonspecific mast cell degranulating agent, or substance P–released

arachidonic acid; and (3) release of histamine by sinus mast cells after adenosine exposure.[48] For example, the administration of the muscle relaxant atracurium results in a high incidence of cutaneous manifestations,[40] whereas propofol (perhaps because of its solvent) is more highly associated with bronchospasm.[49,50] Some drugs commonly used to treat asthma exploit the functional and structural differences of mast cells. Thus, cromolyn may be active in preventing release of histamine from human lung and intestinal mast cells but inactive in basophils and skin mast cells.[2]

GASTROINTESTINAL AND NEUROLOGIC EFFECTS

Despite the problems in extrapolation from in vitro studies, unequivocal evidence supports the role of histamine as one of the prime mediators in inflammation, gastric acid secretion, and anaphylactic shock. A growing body of evidence also suggests that histamine is an important central neurotransmitter influencing consciousness, and that it acts as an autonomic neuromodulator, perhaps by the recently discovered H_3-receptors.

HISTAMINE'S ROLE IN THE NASAL MUCOSA

Although the physiologic significance of histamine in the lungs is minimal, it plays a key role in the pathophysiology of upper airway disease and is especially important in the nasal mucosa. In part because of its accessibility, considerable knowledge exists regarding the nasal mucosa. The nasal mucosa consists of epithelial and subepithelial layers and is lined with pseudostratified columnar epithelium resting on a basement membrane that separates it from the deeper submucosal structures. The pseudostratified epithelium contains goblet cells, nonciliated columnar cells with microvilli, basal cells, ciliated columnar cells, and occasional intraepithelial mast cells.[51] On the epithelial surface, the outer layer of bilayered fluid traps foreign particles, and the inner layer provides antimicrobial secretions. Below the epithelial base-

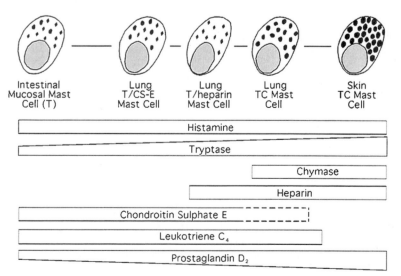

Intestinal
Mucosal Mast
Cell (T)

Lung
T/CS-E
Mast Cell

Lung
T/heparin
Mast Cell

Lung
TC Mast
Cell

Skin
TC Mast
Cell

Histamine

Tryptase

Chymase

Heparin

Chondroitin Sulphate E

Leukotriene C$_4$

Prostaglandin D$_2$

FIGURE 11-2 Mast cell populations in humans form a continuum based on cytochemical properties. *Horizontal bars* indicate the existence and amount of various mediators synthesized by the mast cell subtypes. CS-E: chondroitin sulphate E. (*From Barrett and Pearce,*[2] *with permission.*)

ment membrane is a submucosa rich in glands (mucous, seromucous, and serous) and abundantly populated by mast cells.[12]

LOCATION AND DISTRIBUTION OF THE MAST CELL

There are about 10 mast cells/mm³ in nasal basement membrane. These mast cells, rich in tryptase and chymase, are located in close proximity to nerves and blood vessels and are occasionally seen between epithelial cells. Neurovascular function is affected by mast cells in the nose. Most nasal mast cells are found in the superficial 200 μm of mucosa, clustered between the basement membrane and in the epithelium. The number of mast cells in normal individuals is 7000/mm³ in the tissue and 50/mm³ in the epithelium.[12] The total number of mucosal mast cells counted in tissue sections does not change significantly with the onset of pollen season, because mucosal mast cells migrate about 4 to 5 days after pollen exposure and are redistributed from the submucosa into the epithelium.[52]

MECHANISMS AND SEQUELAE OF NASAL HISTAMINE RELEASE

In contrast to the lungs, the upper respiratory tract is very sensitive to the effects of histamine, whether exogenous or immunologically released. Within minutes of antigen exposure, mast cells release histamine and a plethora of other biologically active compounds including leukotriene C_4 and PGD_2, which induce vasodilation, cause leakage of intravascular proteins into submucosa, smooth-muscle contraction, goblet and glandular secretion, stimulation of irritant (itch and sneeze) nerve receptors, and reflex stimulation of cholinergic glands.[53] Over a few minutes, about 1000 secretory granule contents are discharged from each mast cell. Some of these released substances activate secondary pathways such as kinin and complement, while others act as chemotactic factors for neutrophils and eosinophils.[12] In contrast, in nonimmunologic anaphylactoid reactions, only preformed mediators, such as histamine, are released. Of the preformed and rapidly synthesized mast cell mediators, histamine, adenosine, neutrophil chemotactic factor, mast cell tryptase and chymase, PGD_2, and leukotrienes have been identified in nasal secretions.[12] As in the skin and lungs, tryptase levels in the nasal mucosa serve as excellent markers of mast cell release.[54] As the concentration of allergen increases in the nasal mucosa, so does the measured level of histamine.[55] The immediate phase response is caused in large part by histamine; the late phase response is characterized by an increase in other mediators.[56]

NEUROVASCULAR CONSEQUENCES OF NASAL HISTAMINE RELEASE

Nasal blood flow and secretion are regulated through a complex interaction of glandular and neurovascular elements. The nose is one of the most vascular organs in the body, with total blood flow per cubic centimeter of tissue exceeding that in muscle, brain, and liver. Although the veins and venules in the nasal mucosa are predominantly innervated by sympathetic nerves, the glands in the nose and their arterial supply are also innervated by cholinergic fibers. Cholinergic stimulation causes arteriolar dilation, enhancing passive dif-

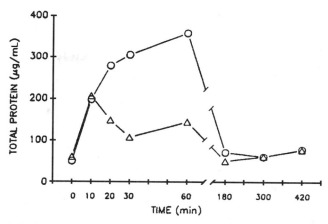

FIGURE 11-3 Total protein in nasal lavages after unilateral nasal allergen challenge (*n* = 8 subjects). Allergen was applied to the ipsilateral side of the nose at time zero, and nasal lavages were collected serially from both sides of the nose for 7 h. Symbols represent geometric mean values (*n* = 8). Ipsilateral protein secretion (○) was significantly greater than contralateral secretion (△) across the entire time course (*p* < 0.001 for side-to-side comparison by analysis of variance). (*From Raphael et al.,*[57] *with permission.*)

fusion of plasma protein, and induces active secretion from serous and mucous glands. Histamine stimulation produces a profound ipsilateral protein secretion, enriched in the serum proteins albumin and IgA, and a smaller contralateral protein secretion in the glands. The ipsilateral response may reflect release of mast cell mediators, as evidenced by increases in these mediators in secretions obtained from allergen-challenged sites.[57] In contrast, the contralateral response may not depend on local mediator release but on reflex stimulation of cholinergic efferent nerves (the nasonasal reflex)[58] (Figs. 11-3 and 11-4). The contralateral secretory response can be significantly inhibited by surgical transection of the vidian nerve, the major cholinergic nerve

FIGURE 11-4 Albumin secretion in nasal lavages after allergen challenge. Ipsilateral (○) and contralateral (△) symbols represent geometric mean values (*n* = 8); the asterisks (*) represent *p* values (*p* ≤ 0.02) for side-to-side comparisons at specific points. (*From Raphael et al.,*[57] *with permission.*)

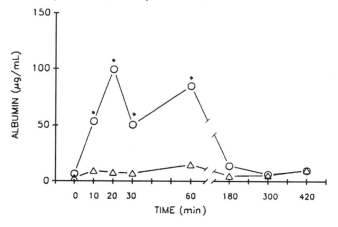

supplying the nose.[59] Recent studies have demonstrated that histamine concentrations, mast cell density, and clinical symptoms decrease after vidian neurectomy.[59]

MEDIATORS THAT MIMIC HISTAMINE'S ACTIONS IN THE NASAL MUCOSA

As in the lung, mediators other than histamine may play an important role in nasal pathophysiology and mimic its action. In addition to containing the classic neurotransmitters, the three types of nerve fibers innervating the nose (sensory, cholinergic, and sympathetic) also contain neuropeptides. Two such mediators, vasoactive intestinal peptide (VIP) and substance P, have been described.[12] VIP coexists with acetylcholine in separate granules in postganglionic parasympathetic nerve terminals.[60] Acetylcholine is released preferentially by low-frequency stimulation, and VIP by high-frequency stimulation. VIP also has a positive modulatory effect on cholinergic receptors. It augments the effects of cholinergic stimulation by enriching selectively serous cell products in nasal secretions and eliciting cutaneous plasma extravasation and vasodilation. VIP-binding sites have been found on submucosal glands, on epithelium, and in the walls of arterioles and veins in human nasal mucosa, as well as in pulmonary vascular and bronchial smooth muscle.[61] Increased immunohistochemical staining of VIP in the nasal mucosa has been reported in patients with allergic diathesis and nasal obstruction. Thus, VIP derived from parasympathetic nerve fibers may function in serous cell secretion in human nasal mucosa and in regulation of vasomotor tone.[62]

In addition to VIP, several tachykinins in airway sensory nerves, including substance P, are released upon irritation and mimic the effects of histamine. Substance P is a neurotransmitter released from sensory nerve endings (C-fibers) by prostaglandins and bradykinin. After nerve stimulation by bradykinin and antidromic conduction of impulses down the nerve collaterals, neuropeptide (substance P) is released. Substance P induces vasodilation, protein extravasation, edema, mucous hypersecretion, and inflammatory cell infiltration.[63] In addition, substance P acts directly on the vasculature (nasal sinusoids); causing blockage of the nasal mucosa. Capsaicin, which ablates sensory C-fibers that secrete substance P, has been found to reduce the frequency of sneezing in animals but not in humans.[64]

The Role of Histamine in Clinical Pathology

RHINITIS

CLASSIFICATION

An issue that confounds both the clinical and experimental literature on nasal histamine is the classification of rhinitis. Allergic rhinitis is common, affecting at least 10 percent of the population to some degree. It can be seasonal or perennial. Seasonal allergic rhinitis may be recognized as hay fever and is associated with inflamed conjunctival and nasal membranes and bronchial symptoms. It is caused by an IgE-mediated reaction to inhalant pollen allergens, leading to mediator release, mucosal edema, and direct reflex vasodilation. Treatment typically involves antihistamines. Perennial allergic rhinitis is also common, but patients suffering from it have year-round nasal stuffiness, especially at night.[65] Vasomotor rhinitis seems identical to nasal allergy, but is ten times less common. In pure vasomotor rhinitis, skin tests and serum IgE concentration are negative. Treatment with antihistamine and vasoconstrictor combinations is far less successful in this syndrome. Possible therapeutic interventions are cryosurgery, electrocautery, or parasympathetic neurectomy.

CLINICAL SYMPTOMS

Over the past 15 years, considerable progress has been made in defining how individual components of the allergic reaction cause clinical symptoms. The cardinal symptoms of allergic rhinitis include pruritus, sneezing, rhinorrhea, and nasal congestion. Pruritus and sneezing are induced by sensory nerve stimulation, whereas congestion results from vasodilation with engorgement of cavernous sinusoids. Histamine is capable of inducing all features of acute allergic rhinitis except the late phase reaction[12] (Table 11-2).

TREATMENT MODALITIES AND LIMITATIONS

Most symptoms of allergic rhinitis can be attenuated by treatment with H_1-antagonists and topical corticosteroids.[12] However, even with the newer and more potent generations of H_1-antagonists, uniform therapeutic success has not been achieved. The lack of efficacy of antihistamines is attributed to low receptor affinity, as well as significant cross-reactivity with other receptors. Antihistamines may have effects on other receptors (serotonin) and exhibit local anesthetic activity. Many of the most commonly used antihistamines (terfenadine, chlorpheniramine, and ceftizine) block H_1-receptors with low affinity (about 30 percent.[66] In addition, the utility of many traditional histamines is limited by their central activity and by cardiac and other side effects.

Topical corticosteroids often are used in conjunction with antihistamines for treatment of allergic rhinitis. Topical corticosteroids decrease symptom score, inflammatory cell number, tryptase concentration, and reactivity of the nasal mucosa to histamine[67] in both the immediate and late phase reactions. By contrast, systemically administered corticosteroids have no effect on the appearance of immediate symptoms or mediator concentrations, except for a reduction in kinins. However, systemic corticosteroids reduce symptom score, concentration of histamine, kinins, and albumin in the late phase of the allergic reaction after antigen challenge.[68] Clinically, both topical and systemic corticosteroids are effective in treating allergic rhinitis, but because the side effects of systemic corticosteroids outweigh their benefits, topical corticosteroids are utilized as first-line agents for allergic rhinitis.[67,68]

PHENOMENON OF PRIMING

One phenomenon, which appears unique to the nasal mucosa, is known as *priming*; that is, on repeated nasal provocations less allergen is required to produce clinical symptoms. Priming correlates with persistence of rhinitis symptoms after the pollen season and synergistic effects of

TABLE 11-2   Allergic Rhinitis

Symptom	Pathologic Feature	Proposed Mediator
Pruritus	Sensory nerve stimulation	Histamine (H_1)
		Prostaglandins
Nasal obstruction	Mucosal edema due to vascular permeability and vasodilation	Histamine (H_1)
		Kinins
		Leukotrienes C_4, D_4, E_4
		TNF-α
		CGRP
		Substance P
Sneezing	Sensory nerve stimulation	Histamine (H_1)
		Leukotrienes C_4, D_4, E_4
Rhinorrhea	Increased secretion of mucus	Histamine (via muscarinic reflex)
		Leukotrienes C_4, D_4, E_4
		Substance P
		VIP
Hyperirritability and prolonged congestion	Late phase reaction	Inflammatory factors
		Eicosanoids
		Chemotactic factors
		Interleukins 1, 5, 6, 8 and TNF-α
		PAF

NOTE: TNF-α = tumor necrosis factor d; CGRP = calcitonin gene–related peptide; VIP = vasoactive intestinal peptide; PAF = platelet-activating factor.
SOURCE: From Raphael G, et al.,[57] with permission.

multiple pollen exposures. On a cellular basis, it can be explained by proliferation of mast cells, increase in their capability for release, and nonspecific effects of nasal inflammation.[68]

ANAPHYLACTIC AND ANAPHYLACTOID REACTIONS

DRUG-INDUCED ANAPHYLAXIS

There are few subjects as poorly understood as the complex issue of anaphylactic and anaphylactoid reactions to anesthetics and drugs used in the intensive care unit (ICU).[37,69–71] Large epidemiologic studies from France, Australia, and elsewhere have demonstrated that over half of life-threatening reactions in the perioperative period are immune in nature, the other half being chemically mediated.[36,38] A major biologic difference is that in chemically mediated reactions, only the preformed mediators are released, whereas in immune reactions, mast cells degranulate. Such studies in the perioperative period are particularly instructive because patients are monitored during the reactions.[42,71,72]

With regard to immune reactions in this setting, muscle relaxants, particularly succinylcholine, represent the most common allergens. Muscle relaxants account for 70 percent of life-threatening immune reactions in the perioperative period. Antibiotics, local anesthetics, and opioids rarely precipitate such reactions (Fig. 11-5). On the other hand, many anesthetic and ICU drugs (including the curariform relaxants, morphine, meperidine, and many plasma substitutes) can cause a dose-dependent release of histamine from mast cells.[73,74] These chemical reactions may mimic acute type I hypersensitivity reactions, but they are much more likely to be manifest by hypotension. Prospective studies reveal that

although histamine is released in both species of reactions, the cardiovascular changes occurring with chemically mediated histamine release may be completely prevented by chemoprophylaxis with H_1- and H_2-antagonists.[32,75,76] There is considerable debate as to whether such pretreatment alters immunologically mediated reactions, although the large-scale chympopapain trials, in which adverse reactions were IgE-mediated, suggest a reduction in the severity but not the incidence of reactions when patients were pretreated with H_1- and H_2-antagonists.[77] This finding is consistent with the increased appreciation that, although many mediators are released during immune reactions, histamine plays an important, and perhaps primary, role.

CLINICAL SYMPTOMS

The experience in monitored life-threatening perioperative anaphylactic reactions reveals that cardiovascular collapse is the most frequent and severe symptom (see Table 11-1). While cutaneous manifestations and bronchospasm occur in fully half of these cases, the cardiovascular manifestations predominate. This is consistent with the relative contribution of histamine in the cardiovascular and respiratory systems.

OTHER CASES OF ANAPHYLAXIS

While these monitored reactions to medications provide useful information on the pathophysiology of drug-induced anaphylaxis, other causes for such reactions (including food, exercise, and Hymenoptera) occur more frequently in the general patient population. These reactions elicit similar responses to the drug-induced reactions described above, except that the psychological prodrome (a sense of impending doom) and subjective symptoms (itch, metallic taste) can be appreciated before cardiovascular collapse.

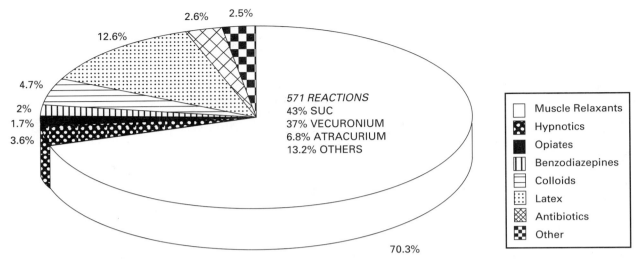

FIGURE 11-5 Incidence of drugs responsible for life-threatening perioperative anaphylaxis. SUC: succinylcholine (*From Laxenaire et al.*: Ann Fr Anesth Reanim *1993; 31:232, with permission.*)

Reactions to radiocontrast media are often attributed to histamine release but may have several etiologies.[78–80] It is typically believed that 5 percent of patients may experience some reactions to conventional contrast agents,[81–83] with approximately 0.5 percent to 1 percent experiencing a reaction in which a therapeutic intervention is necessary. Adverse reactions to radiocontrast media are diverse and are likely to be associated with multiple different pathogenic mechanisms. Nonidiosyncratic reactions (nausea, vomiting, burning, warmth, and mental status changes) are believed to be due to the inherent toxicity of radiocontrast media, including the high osmolality (up to 2000 mosmol/kg).[84] Idiosyncratic reactions (urticaria, angioedema, bronchospasm, dyspnea, hypotension, and shock) are not dose-related and can occur with 1 mL or less of agent. Multiple mechanisms have been proposed, although a unifying hypothesis has not been established; complement[78,85] and bradykinin activation,[86] histamine liberation,[85] and central nervous system toxicity[87] have all been postulated. Antibody-mediated mechanisms also may be involved,[79] although this too is controversial.[80,88,89]

Summary

The biogenic amine histamine is dispersed in many human and animal tissues and has been the subject of intensive research. Because of the considerable species and tissue heterogeneity in structure and function, extrapolation of animal in vitro investigations to human pathophysiology has been difficult. The actions of histamine are mediated by three, or possibly four, distinct histamine receptors that differ in phylogeny and function. Through these receptors, histamine exerts profound cardiovascular effects and causes alterations in the nasal mucosa and skin. In contrast, the physiologic significance of histamine in the lungs is minimal. Clinically, the actions of histamine are best exemplified by acute allergic rhinitis and anaphylactic reactions.

References

1. Beaven M: Histamine: Its role in physiological and pathological processes. *Monogr Allergy* 1978; 13:1.
2. Barrett K, Pearce F: Heterogeneity of mast cells, in Uvnäs B (ed): *Handbook of Experimental Pharmacology.* New York, Springer, 1991; 93.
3. Stellato C, dePaulis A, Cirillo R, et al.: Heterogeneity of human mast cells and basophils in response to muscle relaxants. *Anesthesiology* 1991; 74:1078.
4. Watanabe T, Taguchi Y, Maeyama K, Wada H: Formation of histamine: Histamine decarboxylase, in Uvnäs B (ed): *Handbook of Experimental Pharmacology.* New York, Springer, 1991; 145.
5. Yamatodani A, Inagaki N, Panula P, et al.: Structure and functions of the histaminergic neurone system, in Uvnäs B (ed): *Handbook of Experimental Pharmacology.* New York, Springer, 1991; 243.
6. Slorach S: Histamine in food, in Uvnäs B (ed): *Handbook of Experimental Pharmacology.* New York, Springer, 1991; 511.
7. Sattler J, Lindlar R, Lorenz W, et al.: Elevated plasma histamine concentration in upper GI bleeding: Which mechanisms are involved? *Hepatogastroenterology* 1990; 37:267.
8. Sattler J, Hesterberg R, Klotter H-J, Lorenz W: A new complex shock model in pigs for upper gastrointestinal (GI) bleeding: Hemorrhage, instillation of blood and drug-induced diamine oxidase (DAO) inhibition. *Circ Shock* 1988; 24:283.
9. Sattler J, Häfner D, Klotter H-J, et al.: Food-induced histaminosis as an epidemiological problem: Plasma histamine elevation of haemodynamic alterations after oral histamine administration and blockade of diamine oxidase (DAO). *Agents Actions* Apr 1989; 27 (1–2):212–214.
10. Sattler J, Lorenz W, Kubo K, et al.: Food-induced histaminosis under diamine oxidase (DAO) blockade in pigs: Further evidence of the key role of elevated plasma histamine levels as

demonstrated by successful prophylaxis with antihistamines. *Agents Actions* 1989; 27:212.

11. Bochner BS, Lichtenstein L: Anaphylaxis. *N Engl J Med* 1991; 324:1785.

12. White M, Kaliner M: Mediators of allergic rhinitis. *J Allergy Clin Immunol* 1992; 90:699.

13. Agre K, Wilson R, Brim M, McDermott D: Chymodiactin post-marketing surveillance. Demographic and adverse experience data in 29,075 patients. *Spine* 1984; 9:479.

14. Gomperts B: Control of the exocytotic mechanism in rat mast cells, in Uvnäs B (ed): *Handbook of Experimental Pharmacology.* New York, Springer, 1991; 119.

15. Lorenz W, Neugebauer E, Unväs B, et al.: Munich consensus development conference on histamine determination, in Unväs B (ed): *Handbook of Experimental Pharmacology.* New York, Springer, 1991; 81.

16. Moss J: The impact of histamine research on clinical anesthesia and surgery. *Agents Actions* Special Conference Issue 1992; C135.

17. Laroche D, Vergnaud M, Sillard B, et al.: Biochemical markers of anaphylactoid reactions to drugs. *Anesthesiology* 1991; 75:945.

18. Laroche D, Lefrancois C, Gerard J, et al.: Early diagnosis of anaphylactic reactions to neuromuscular blocking drugs. *Br J Anaesth* 1992; 69:611.

19. Schwartz L, Metcalve D, Miller J, et al.: Tryptase levels as an indicator of mast-cell activation in systemic anaphylaxis and mastocytosis. *N Engl J Med* 1987; 316:1622.

20. Futo J, Kupferberg J, Moss J, et al.: Vecuronium inhibits histamine N-methyltransferase. *Anesthesiology* 1988; 69:92.

21. Futo J, Kupferberg J, Moss J: Neuromuscular relaxants inhibit HNMT in vitro. *Biochem Pharmacol* 1990; 39:415.

22. Gantz I, Schaffer M, DelValle J, et al.: Molecular cloning of a gene encoding the histamine H_2 receptor. *Proc Natl Acad Sci USA* 1991; 88:429.

23. Garrison J: Histamine, bradykinin, 5-hydroxytryptamine, and their antagonists, in Gillman A, Rall T, Nies A, Taylor P (eds): *The Pharmacological Basis of Therapeutics,* 8th ed. New York, Pergamon, 1990; 575.

24. Schwartz J-C, Arrang J-M, Bouthenet M-L, et al.: Histamine receptors in brain, in Uvnäs B (ed): *Handbook of Experimental Pharmacology.* New York, Springer, 1991; 191.

25. Brandes L, LaBella F, Glavin G, et al.: Histamine as an intracellular messenger (review). *Biochem Pharmacol* 1990; 40:1677.

26. Brandes L, Arron R, Bogdanovic R, et al.: Stimulation of malignant growth in rodents by antidepressant drugs at clinically relevant doses. *Cancer Res* 1992; 52:3796.

27. Brandes L, Somons K, Bracken S, Warrington R: Results of a clinical trial in humans with refractory cancer of the intracellular histamine antagonist, N, N-diethyl-2-[4-(phenylmethyl) phenoxy] ethanamine-HCl, in combination with various single antineoplastic agents. *J Clin Oncol* 1994; 12:1281.

28. Stellato C, Casolaro V, Ciccarelli A, et al.: General anaesthetics induce only histamine release selectively from human mast cells. *Br J Anaesth* 1991; 67:751.

29. Stellato C, Cirillo R, dePaulis A, et al.: Human basophil/mast cell releasability: IX. Heterogeneity of the effects of opioids on mediator release. *Anesthesiology* 1992; 77:932.

30. Bristow M, Ginsberg R, Harrison D: Histamine and the human heart: The other receptor system. *Am J Cardiol* 1982; 49:249.

31. Levi R, Owen D, Trzeciakowski J: Actions of histamine on the heart and vasculature, in Ganellin R, Parsons M (eds) *Pharmacology of Histamine Receptors.* London, 1982; 236.

32. Owen D: Physiology and pharmacology of histamine: Cardiovascular studies in man, in Moss J (ed): *Clinics in Anesthesiology, Vasoactive Amines.* Philadelphia, Saunders, 1984; 384.

33. Rosow C, Moss J, Philbin D, Savarese J: Histamine release during morphine and fentanyl anesthesia. *Anesthesiology* 1982; 56:93.

34. Savarese J, Ali H, Basta S, et al.: The cardiovascular effects of mivacurium chloride (BW B1090U) in patients receiving nitrous oxide-opiate-barbiturate anesthesia. *Anesthesiology* 1989; 70:386.

35. Levi R, Rubin L, Gross S: Histamine in cardiovascular function and dysfunction: Recent developments, in Uvnäs B (ed): *Handbook of Experimental Pharmacology.* New York, Springer, 1991; 347.

36. Fisher M, Baldo B: The incidence and clinical features of anaphylactic reactions during anaesthesia in Australia. *An Fr Anesth Reanim* 1993; 12:97.

37. Laxenaire M, Moneret-Vautrin D: Allergy and anesthesia. *Curr Opin Anaesth* 1992; 5:436.

38. Laxenaire M, Moneret-Vautrin D, Boileau S, Moeller R: Adverse reactions to intravenous agents in anaesthesia in France. *Klin Wochenschr* 1982; 60:1006.

39. Levy L, Brister N, Shearin A, et al.: Wheal and flare responses to opioids in humans. *Anesthesiology* 1989; 70:756.

40. Doenicke A, Moss J, Lorenz W, et al.: Are hypotension and rash after atracurium really due to histamine release? *Anesth Analg* 1994; 78:976.

41. Stechschulte D: Leukotrienes in asthma and allergic rhinitis. *N Engl J Med* 1990; 323:1769.

42. Moss J, Fahmy N, Sunder N, Beaven M: Hormonal and hemodynamic profile of an anaphylactic reaction in man. *Circulation* 1981; 63:210.

43. Mehr E, Hirshman C, Lindeman K: Mechanism of action of atracurium on airways. *Anesthesiology* 1992; 76:448.

44. Findlay S, Lichtenstein L: Basophil "releasability" in patients with asthma. *Am Rev Respir Dis* 1980; 122:53.

45. Akagi K, Townley R: Spontaneous histamine release and histimine content in normal subjects and subjects with asthma. *J Allergy Clin Immunol* 1989; 83:742.

46. Laxenaire M, Matta E, Gueant J, et al.: Basophil histamine release in atopic patients after *in vivo* provocation with thiopental, Diprivan, and chlormethiazole. *Acta Anaesthesiol Scand* 1991; 35:706.

47. Foreman J: Histamine H_2 receptors and lung function, in Uvnäs B (ed): *Handbook of Experimental Pharmacology.* New York, Springer, 1991; 285.

48. Mita H, Ishii T, Yamada T, et al.: Further characterization of dispersed human sinus mast cell. *Life Sci* 1993; 53:775.

49. Laxenaire M, Mata-Bermejo E, Moneret-Vautrin D, Gueant J: Life-threatening anaphylactoid reactions to propofol (Diprivan). *Anesthesiology* 1992; 77:275.

50. De Leon-Cassasola O, Weis A, Lema M: Anaphylaxis due to propofol. *Anesthesiology* 1992; 77:384.

51. Naclerio R, Proctor D: Allergy: Principles and practice, in Middleton E (ed): *The Anatomy and Physiology of the Upper Airway.* St. Louis, Mosby, 1988; 579.

52. Enerbäck L, Pipkorn U, Granerus G: Intraepithelial migration of nasal mucosal mast cells in hay fever. *Int Arch Allergy Appl Immunol* 1986; 80:44.

53. Borish L, Joseph B: Inflammation and the allergic response. *Med Clin North Am* 1992; 76:765.

54. Juliusson S, Holmberg K, Baumgarten C, et al.: Tryptase in nasal lavage fluid after local allergen challenge. *Allergy* 1990; 46:459.

55. Enterbäck L, Karlsson: Nasal mast cell response to natural allergan exposure. *Int Arch Allergy Appl Immunol* 1989; 88:209.

56. Georgitis J, Stone B, Gottschlich G: Inflammatory cells and mediator release during ragweed challenge: Correlation between histamine content in nasal secretions and appearance of inflammatory cells. *Ann Allergy* 1992; 68:413.

57. Raphael G, Igarashi Y, White M, Kaliner M: The pathophysiology of rhinitis. *J Allergy Clin Immunol* 1991; 88:33.

58. Raphael G, Meredith S: The pathophysiology of rhinitis. *Am Rev Respir Dis* 1989; 139:791.

59. Rucci L, Riccaradi R: Vidian nerve resection, histamine turnover and mucosal mast cell function in patients with chronic hypertopic non-allergic rhinitis. *Agents Actions* 1989; 28:224.

60. Mosimann B, White M: Substance P, calcitonin gene-related peptide, and vasoactive intestinal peptide increase in nasal secretions after allergen challenge in atopic patients. *J Allergy Clin Immunol* 1993: 92:95.

61. Uddman R, Malm L: VIP increases in nasal blood during stimulation of the vidian nerve. *Acta Otolaryngol* 1981; 91:135.

62. Baraniuk J, Lundgren J, Okayama M, et al.: Vasoactive intestinal peptide in human nasal mucosa. *J Clin Invest* 1990; 86:825.

63. Nieber K, Baungarten C: The possible role of substance P in the allergic reaction, based on two different provocation models. *Int Arch Allergy Appl Immunol* 1991; 94:334.

64. Kokumai S, Imamura T, Masayama K, et al.: Effect of capsaicin as a neuropeptide-releasing substance on sneezing reflex in type I allergic animal model. *Int Arch Allergy Appl Immunol* 1992; 98:256.

65. Badhwar A, Druce H: Allergic rhinitis. *Med Clin North Am* 1992; 76:789.

66. Naclerio R, Proud D: The effect of ceftirizine on early allergic response. *Laryngoscope* 1989; 99:596.

67. Sim T, Hilsmeier K, Alam R, et al.: Effect of topical corticosteroids on the recovery of histamine releasing factors in nasal washings of patients with allergic rhinitis. *Am Rev Respir Dis* 1992; 145:1316.

68. Baroody F, Naclerio R: Smell and taste in human disease, in Getchell T (ed): *Allergic Rhinitis*. New York, Raven, 1991; 529.

69. Moss J: Adverse drug reactions caused by histamine, in Barash P (ed): *ASA Refresher Courses in Anesthesiology*. Philadelphia, Lippincott, 1992; 155.

70. Weiss M, Hirshman C: Anaphylactic reactions and anesthesia, in Rogers M, Covino B, Tinker J, Longnecker D (eds): *Principles and Practice of Anesthesiology*. St. Louis, Mosby, 1992; 2457.

71. Alessi R, Moss J: A clinician's guide to allergy and anesthesia. *Semin Anesth* 1993; 12:211.

72. Beaupré P, Roizen M, Cahalan M, et al.: Hemodynamic and two-dimensional transesophageal echocardiographic analysis of an anaphylactic reaction in a human. *Anesthesiology* 1984; 60:482.

73. Moss J, Rosow C: Histamine release by narcotics and muscle relaxants in humans. *Anesthesiology* 1983; 59:330.

74. Moss J, Rosow C, Savarese J, et al.: Role of histamine in the hypotensive action of d-tubocurarine in man. *Anesthesiology* 1981; 55:19.

75. Philbin D, Moss J, Akins C, et al.: The use of H_1 and H_2 histamine antagonists with morphine anesthesia: A double-blind study. *Anesthesiology* 1981; 55:292.

76. Lorenz W, Ennis M, Doenicke A, Dick W: Perioperative uses of histamine antagonists. *J Clin Anesth* 1990; 2:345.

77. Moss J, Roizen M, Nordby E, et al.: Decreased incidence and mortality of anaphylaxis to chymopapain. *Anesth Analg* 1985; 64:1197.

78. Arroyave C, Bhat K, Crown R: Activation of the alternative pathway of the complement system by radiographic contrast media. *J Immunol* 1976; 117:1866.

79. Brasch R: Evidence supporting an antibody mediation of contrast media reactions. *Invest Radiol* 1980; 15:S29.

80. Carr D, Walker A: Contrast media reactions: Experimental evidence against the allergy theory. *Br J Radiol* 1984; 57:469.

81. Ansell G, Tweedie M, West C, et al.: The current status of reactions to intravascular contrast media. *Invest Radiol* 1980; 15(S):532.

82. Shehadi W: Adverse reactions to intravascularly administered contrast media. *Am J Roentgenol* 1975; 124:145.

83. Witten D, Hirsch F, Hartman G: Acute reactions to urographic contrast medium. *Am J Roentgenol* 1973; 119:832.

84. Eggleston P, Kagey-Sobotka A, Lichtenstein L: A comparison of the osmotic activation of basophils and human lung mast cells. *An Rev Respir Dis* 1987; 135:1043.

85. Cogen F, Norman M, Dunsky E, et al.: Histamine release and complement changes following injection of contrast media in humans. *J Allergy Clin Immunol* 1979; 64:299.

86. Lasser E: A coherent biochemical basis for increased reactivity to contrast material in allergic patients: A novel concept. *Am J Roentgenol* 1987; 149:1281.

87. Lalli A: Contrast media reactions: Data, analysis and hypothesis. *Radiology* 1980; 134:1.

88. Lieberman P, Siegel R, Taylor W: Anaphylactoid reactions to iodinated contrast media. *J Allergy Clin Immunol* 1978; 62:174.

89. Siegel R, Lieberman P: Measurement of histamine, complement components and immune complexes during patient reactions to iodinated contrast material. *Invest Radiol* 1976; 11:98.

Chapter 12
PROSTAGLANDINS/ THROMBOXANE
(THE PROSTANOIDS)

NILDA MARIA MUÑOZ

Introduction

Prostaglandins (PGs) and thromboxane are families of oxygenated fatty acids that are produced in pathologic processes and have a variety of physiologic and cellular activities, such as effects on airway smooth muscle[1–3] and inflammatory cells.[4–5] Some studies have suggested that the production of PGs during anaphylaxis in conducting airways could play a vital regulatory role in the control of airway narrowing.[1–3] Others have regarded PGs and thromboxane as mediators of airway hyperresponsiveness[1–3] and airway inflammation.[6–7] Unfortunately, it seems that the modulatory role of PGs and thromboxane in humans is as variable as that seen in experimental animals.[3] The purpose of this chapter is to review briefly the important investigations concerning relevant aspects of the bioactivity of these compounds.

Nomenclature and Classifications

Eicosanoids is a collective name for unsaturated lipids derived from 20-carbon essential fatty acids ($C_{20:4\ n=6}$) or similar polyunsaturated fatty acids, through the cyclooxygenase or lipoxygenase metabolic pathways. The biosynthetic pathway of PGs, thromboxanes, leukotrienes, lipoxins, and related hydroperoxy-fatty acid compounds is generally referred to as the *arachidonic acid cascade*. Lipid compounds termed *prostanoids* are the products of cyclooxygenase that contain the oxygenated polyunsaturated 20-carbon aliphatic monocarboxylic acids with a cyclopentane ring (PG) and an oxane ring (thromboxane).

Prostaglandins are designated by the following: (1) letters A to J, which represent the position of the cyclopentane ring; (2) numerical subscripts 1 to 3, which indicate the number of the double bonds in the alkyl side chain; and (3) α or β subscripts, which denote the orientation of the hydroxyl group at the C9-keto group. Thromboxane, so named after its first isolation from thrombocytes, contains a bicyclic oxane-oxetane ring structure. The unstable thromboxane, designated A$_2$, undergoes a rapid, nonenzymatic degradation to an inactive and stable compound, thromboxane B$_2$.

Consequently, there are two classifications of PGs: the E series and the F series. These types of compound derive from the metabolism of PGG and PGH series have three members: E$_1$, E$_2$, E$_3$ for the E series and F$_{1\alpha}$, F$_{2\alpha}$, F$_{3\alpha}$ for the F series.[8] In general, PGEs exert a bronchodilator action, while PGFs contract airway smooth muscle from different species, including humans.[9–11] The chemical structures of the naturally occurring prostaglandins are summarized in Fig. 12-1.

Transformation of Prostaglandin H$_2$ into Bioactive Prostanoids

The enzymatic conversion of arachidonic acid to biologically active prostaglandins and related prostanoids is outlined in Fig. 12-2. Phospholipase A$_2$ (PLA$_2$) is a phosphatidyl-glycerol-2-acylhydrolase responsible for the liberation of arachidonic acid, a biosynthetic precursor of putative inflammatory mediators. Production of prostanoids and related compounds results from release of arachidonate, which is catalyzed by PLA$_2$. Arachidonate is catalyzed by cyclooxygenase to PGG$_2$ and then by endoperoxidase (PGH synthase) to PGH$_2$.[12–14]

There are two major types of PLA$_2$ enzymes, the extracellular or low molecular mass (14 to 18 kDa) forms, termed as secretory PLA$_2$ (i.e., pancreatic and non-pancreatic) and the intracellular or high molecular (85-110 kDa) forms, termed as cPLA$_2$ for their cytosolic origin.[14–15] Under alkaline pH and high Ca^{2+} concentration, PLA$_2$ has been shown to be optimally active in arachidonic acid generation.[14] There are two

I: Primary Prostaglandins

A. Prostaglandin E series

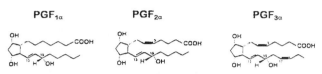

B. Prostaglandin F series

II: Secondary Prostaglandins (Pentane ring structure)

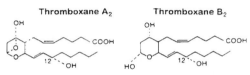

III: Thromboxanes

FIGURE 12-1 Chemical structures of the naturally occuring prostanoids. *I.* Primary prostaglandins. *II.* Secondary prostaglandins. *III.* Thromboxanes.

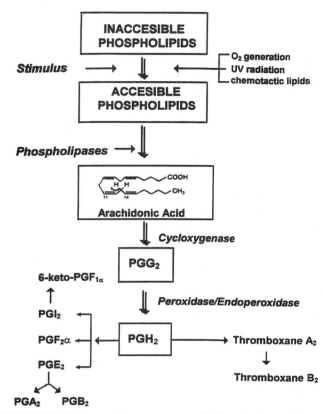

FIGURE 12-2 Major cyclooxygenase metabolites in the arachidonic acid cascade. Generation of prostaglandin synthase (PGH$_2$) from arachidonic acid and subsequent enzymatic conversions to prostaglandins and thromboxanes.

other phospholipases, PLC and PLD, that have been implicated in the release of arachidonic acid.[12,14] The pathways of these phospholipases involved in arachidonate generation for prostanoid formation are outlined in Fig. 12-3. In general, PLA$_2$ acts mainly on phosphatidylcholine (PC) and phosphatidylethanolamine (PE), while PLC acts principally through phosphatidylinositol (PI) and initial conversion by PLD of PE or PC to phosphatidic acid.

Theoretically, any source of arachidonic acid can function as an essential source for prostanoid formation. Given the expanding physiologic and pathologic roles of PG and thromboxane, interest in their oxidative metabolism by PGH synthase continues to increase. Mainly located on microsomal, nuclear, and plasma membranes, PGH synthase activity has two catalytic functions: (1) cyclooxygenase activity that catalyzes the production of PGG$_2$, and (2) peroxidase activity catalyzing a two-electron reduction of PGG$_2$ to PGH$_2$.[12–14] Although the half-life of PGH$_2$ is 4 to 5 min, this endoperoxide has the ability to aggregate platelets and contract airway smooth muscle.[1,14] Most importantly, the biologically active PGs and thromboxane are formed enzymatically and nonenzymatically from PGH$_2$ synthase.[12–14] For example, the conversion of PGH$_2$ to PGF$_{2\alpha}$ and PGI$_2$ to 6-keto PGF$_{1\alpha}$ appears to be a nonenzymatic process,[12,13] while conversion of PGE$_2$ to PGF$_{2\alpha}$ and to PGD$_2$ is formed through enzymes, prostaglandin 9-keto reductase

and endoperoxide isomerase, respectively. PGH$_2$ synthase also serves as an intermediate in the production of thromboxane A$_2$ and B$_2$, while PGA and PGB are products of simple dehydration and isomerization of PGE series.[14]

Two newly recognized PGH$_1$ and PGH$_2$ synthase isoenzymes (often referred to as COX-1 and COX-2) have been characterized.[16,17] In addition, PGH synthase has now been sequenced completely. The deduced amino acid sequence is highly conserved (90 percent homology) in a variety of cell types (i.e., macrophages, fibroblast, endothelial cells).[18–20] Recent studies have shown evidence that increased PGs and thromboxane syntheses occur as a result of increased transcription of PGH synthase protein, suggesting an indirect effect of PGH synthase expression.[18,19] Other investigations have shown that an anti-inflammatory inhibitor, a glucocorticoid, that selectively inhibits the induction and activity of PGH$_2$ synthase may, in turn, decrease prostaglandin synthesis.[20–22]

Generation and Biologic Actions of Prostanoids

AIRWAY SMOOTH MUSCLE

In the airways, PGD$_2$, PGF$_{2\alpha}$, PGE$_2$, and PGI$_2$ are released in the greatest amount.[1,23] The mode of action of PGs on airway

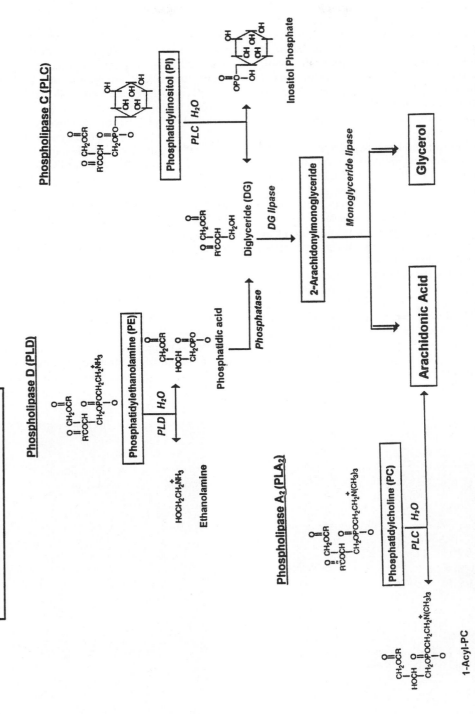

FIGURE 12-3 The phospholipase pathways: formation of arachidonic acid. The principal source of arachidonate for prostanoid synthesis is through phospholipase A_2 phospholipase C, and phospholipase D.

smooth muscle remains complex, depending not only upon the route of administration but also upon the dose of agonists and upon the size of the airway.[23–27] $PGF_{1\alpha}$ and $PGF_{2\alpha}$ caused tissue injury and contraction of isolated tracheal airway smooth muscle from canines, guinea pigs, and cats.[28–30] When studied in vivo in humans, $PGF_{2\alpha}$ evoked a biphasic response: relaxation was induced by aerosol inhalation at lower doses and was converted to bronchoconstriction with higher doses.[31] These data are consistent with the findings of Shioya et al.,[26] in which higher concentrations of intravenous $PGF_{2\alpha}$ resulted in constriction during progressive dilation in more central airways (Fig. 12-4). Others have found that repeated administration of $PGF_{2\alpha}$, like histamine, induced tachyphylaxis in human bronchial strips,[32,33] while in dogs, histamine at concentrations below 1 nM enhanced the bronchoconstrictor effect of $PGF_{2\alpha}$.[28] During this period of high metabolic activity, there is an increase in Ca^{2+} concentration, suggesting that perhaps both $PGF_{2\alpha}$ and histamine affect the equilibrium of smooth-muscle membrane excitability. Such findings may be biologically important in immunologic reactions since both mediators of inflammation are release primarily in lung tissue.

The predominant effect of thromboxane A_2 is transient airway smooth-muscle contraction when given by aerosol in guinea pigs[1,6] or selectively into the isolated canine tracheal circulation.[6,24] In addition to its direct effect, this compound has a potentiating effect on muscarinic stimulation by either increasing postganglionic contraction or by enhancing its cholinergic neurotransmission.[6,24] In vitro, bronchial smooth muscle from asthmatic patients is contracted by thromboxane A_2 more than that from normal individuals, with a potency and efficacy that are greater than those of $PGF_{2\alpha}$ and histamine.[6,34]

Like $PGF_{2\alpha}$, the relaxant PGs produce a paradoxical effect on airway smooth muscle.[1,6,34–37] In most instances, E series PGs exert a bronchodilatory effect,[35–37] although contraction was observed occasionally when their effect was studied in isolated human airways.[37] On the other hand, very little has been studied concerning the effect of $PGF_{2\beta}$ on airway smooth muscle. Studies suggest that $PGF_{2\beta}$ is a less potent relaxing agent than PGE_2, but the magnitude of response seems identical.[38] Baum and coworkers[38] have reported that $PGF_{2\beta}$ relaxes both the naturally occurring spontaneous tone of isolated guinea pig trachea and tissue strips previously exposed to either histamine or $PGF_{2\alpha}$. Other PGs, PGE_1 and PGA_1, and the PG analog, 9-oxo-15-ϵ-hydroxyprostanoic acid, also antagonized contraction caused by muscarinic stimulation of isolated airways from experimental animals and humans.[6,37,39–40] In contrast, PGI_2 is without effect or induces minimal bronchodilation,[41,42] while PGD_2, released from activated mast cells, contracts airway smooth muscle.[23,43]

RESIDENT AND INFLAMMATORY CELLS

The characteristic features of airway inflammation are caused by either activated resident cells (i.e., mast cells, alveolar macrophages, airway epithelium) or inflammatory cells (i.e., eosinophils, neutrophils, mononuclear cells) present in the airways and pulmonary vasculature and by the media-

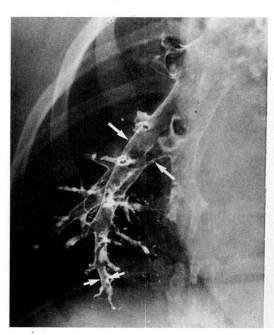 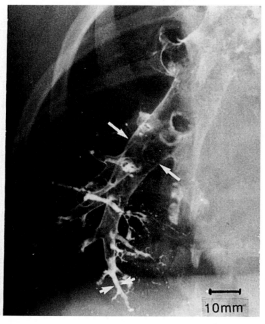

**FIGURE 12-4 Tantalum bronchography of canine lung after intravenous infusion of $PGF_{2\alpha}$. *Left panel:* Control airway. *Right panel:* Greatest airway response after $PGF_{2\alpha}$. Arrows indicate the dilation of generation 2 airway and coexisting constriction in generation 5 airways. (*From Shioya et al.,[26] with permission.*)

tors they release. These cells have the capacity to synthesize one or more prostanoids, which are believed to play an important role in the pathogenesis of a variety of airway diseases, particularly in the clinical features of asthma. However, the regulatory role of prostanoids in the inflammatory process is difficult to evaluate, and the importance of PGs in acute cellular inflammation of asthma has been questioned. Nonsteroidal anti-inflammatory drugs do not cause improvement in the disease, and such drugs may cause bronchoconstriction in sensitive subjects, perhaps as a result of shunting the cylooxygenase pathways and redirecting the arachidonic acid metabolism to lipoxygenase pathways.

MAST CELLS

Human mast cells challenged with anti-IgE release a variety of mediators, including cyclooxygenase metabolites (i.e., PGE_2, $PGF_{2\alpha}$, PGD_2, and PGI_1), but PGs alone do not stimulate mast cells to induce the release of histamine or platelet-activating factor (PAF). Bioactive PGs released during anaphylactic reaction cause marked bronchoconstriction[1,5,6]; however, it is difficult to evaluate the magnitude of this contribution to the anaphylactic reaction because of simultaneous release of other biologically active substances such as histamine, bradykinin, and leukotrienes.[44–46] Under normal conditions, as well as during anaphylactic reactions, experiments with purified human mast cells and lung fragments demonstrated that increase vasodilatation, vasopermeability, and airway smooth-muscle contraction are, at least in part attributed to anti-IgE-induced synthesis of PGs.[44,47,48] Studies in vivo in humans have suggested that anti-IgE-induced release and function of histamine are antagonized by antihistamine and that the action of antihistamine is mimicked by PGE_2.[49] Conversely, the bioactivity of endogenous histamine is not apparent in the presence of $PGF_{2\alpha}$ or PGD_2.[49] In some instances, treatment with indomethacin enhances both the inhibitory effect of PGE_2 and the stimulatory effect of $PGF_{2\alpha}$. These experimental data suggest that PGs have a dual action on mast cells, such that the PGE series antagonizes the antigen-induced histamine release, while the PGF series counteracts these effects. Although PG synthesis may play a role in the regulation of anaphylactic reactions, other concepts derived from early findings suggested that mast cells are unlikely to play a critical role in bronchial hyperresponsiveness and chronic asthma since other inflammatory cells may play a more significant role in the chronic inflammatory state in human asthma.

NEUTROPHILS

Neutrophils are particularly active producers of PGs; however, the role of neutrophils in the pathogenesis of asthma remains uncertain. Neutrophils are mostly found in patients with chronic obstructive pulmonary disease and bronchiectasis and apparently do not contribute significantly to bronchial airway hyperresponsiveness. Active products that are derived from molecular oxygen and that normally contribute to the microbicidal system of phagocytic vacuoles are released by activation of neutrophils. This, in turn, causes release of thromboxane A_2.[50] As a potent chemotactic agent,[2,3,6] thromboxane A_2 may participate in the bronchoobstructive reaction of patients with allergic asthma. This is suggested because both eosinophils and neutrophils are recruited into the airway after bronchial challenge, although eosinophils remain longer in the airway (>24 h) than neutrophils (<4 h).[6,51]

EOSINOPHILS

Studies of the bioactivity of PGs in eosinophils have been limited to a few investigations. It has been documented that activation of eosinophils caused the release of active eosinophilic granular proteins,[52–54] 5-lipoxygenase metabolites,[52,53,55] free oxygen radicals,[52,56] and PAF[57] but not prostanoids. However, recent studies have demonstrated that PGD_2 is the most effective of the PGs at inhibiting luminol-enhanced chemiluminescence caused by formyl-met-leu-phe-stimulated eosinophils.[58] When studied in vitro, PGD_2 acts as a chemokinetic agent in that it enhances the activated opsonized zymosan-induced human eosinophil migration.[58] Similarly, in dogs in vivo, PGD_2 promotes accumulation of eosinophils in airway lumen, which is inhibited by SK&F 88046, a nonspecific PG receptor antagonist.[58] In addition, others have reported that human eosinophils generate leukotriene C_4 in response to PAF,[52,59] while in guinea pig eosinophils, PAF stimulates thromboxane A_2 production.[60] Theoretically, PGs secreted by eosinophils could play a significant role in allergic asthma, but this remains undefined.

EPITHELIAL CELLS

Epithelial cells are important in the uptake or degradation of inflammatory mediators, and the epithelium itself may release an epithelial-derived relaxing factor, possibly PGE_2. Epithelial denudation increases the sensitivity of guinea pig, canine, bovine, and porcine airways to histamine and muscarinic stimulation.[61–64] In human airways, however, the role of PGE_2 seems doubtful. Activated, cultured epithelial cells release 15-lipoxygenase products but not PGE_2.[65] Furthermore, indomethacin does not alter the intrinsic tone of human airways[52] but completely abolishes the spontaneous tone of guinea pig tracheal airways.[56] Finally, pretreatment with nordihydroguaiaretic acid inhibits the endothelial-derived relaxing factor but has no effect on the airway contracted response after disrupting the epithelium.[3,5,6] Altogether, the present data support the concept that the epithelium-derived relaxing factor is as yet unidentified, particularly in humans.

ADHESION MOLECULES

It is of considerable interest that while PGs and thromboxane do not upregulate the expression of adhesion molecules, there is convincing evidence that prostanoids might play a significant modulatory role in cell-cell interactions. Recently, Andrews et al.[66] have reported that lymphocyte function-associated antigen 1 (LFA-1) and intercellular adhesion molecule 1 (ICAM-1) adhesion molecules in gastric mucosa were significantly increased after treatment with nonsteroidal anti-inflammatory drug and indomethacin, suggesting that this increase in the expression of adhesion molecules may be associated with the inhibition of prostanoids synthesis. This result raises some questions regarding the involvement of prostanoids in the upregulation of adhesion molecule in airways that may warrant further investigations.

Conclusions

The specific mode of action of PGs and their relationship to autonomic control mechanisms in the lungs still are undefined. Relaxant PGs have not been developed as bronchodilating agents for a number of reasons. These compounds have a short half-life and it is also known that several of the PGs are chemically unstable. When given to asthmatic patients, PGs induce cough by irritating the upper airway. In vitro, PG inhibitors do not relax human bronchial spontaneous tone, while in the guinea pig, indomethacin abolishes the tracheal airway tone and PGI_2 relaxes tracheal contraction induced by muscarinic stimulation. In clinical trials, PGI_2 failed to demonstrate a protective effect on asthmatic patients before antigen challenge, and ingestion of aspirin, nonsteroidal anti-inflammatory drugs, or other cyclooxygenase inhibitors can cause severe asthmatic bronchoconstriction. The mechanisms of aspirin sensitivity of some asthmatic patients are yet to be defined. Several drugs are now available to inhibit the production and action of mediators of inflammation. However, these drugs have not been successful in suppressing asthmatic bronchoconstriction.

References

1. Gardiner PJ: Eicosanoids and airway smooth muscle. *Pharmacol Ther* 1989; 44:1.
2. Kumlin M: Studies on the metabolism of eicosanoids with respect to their roles in human lung. *Acta Physiol Scand* 1991; 141 (suppl 596):1.
3. Robinson C, Holgate ST: Regulation by prostanoids, in Crystal RG, West JB, Barnes PJ, et al. (eds): *The Lung: Scientific Foundation*. New York, Raven Press, 1991; 941.
4. Raible DG, Schulman ES, DiMuzio J, et al.: Mast cell mediators: Prostaglandin D_2 and histamine activate human eosinophils. *J Immunol* 1992; 148:3536.
5. Smith HR, Larsen GL, Cherniak RM: Inflammatory cells and eicosanoid mediators in subjects with late asthmatic responses and increases in airway responsiveness. *J Allergy Clin Immunol* 1992; 89:1076.
6. Shore SA, Austen KF, Drazen JM: Eicosanoids and the lung; in Massaro D (ed): *Lung Cell Biology*. New York, Marcel Dekker, 1989; 1011.
7. Zurier RB: Role of prostaglandin E in inflammation and immune responses. *Adv Prostaglaudin Thromboxane Leukot Res* 1990; 21:947.
8. Gardiner PJ: Classification of prostanoids receptors. *Adv Prostaglandin Thromboxane Leukot Res* 1990; 20:110.
9. Melillo E, Wooley KL, Manning PJ, et al.: Effect of PGE_2 on exercise-induced bronchoconstriction in asthmatic subjects. *Am J Respir Crit Care Med* 1994; 149(5):1138.
10. Leff AR, Muñoz NM, Tallet J, et al.: Augmentation of parasympathetic contraction in tracheal and bronchial airways by prostaglandin $F_{2\alpha}$ in situ. *J Appl Physiol* 1985; 58:1558.
11. Beasley R, Varley J, Robinson C, Holgate ST: Cholinergic-mediated bronchoconstriction induced by prostaglandin D_2, its initial metabolite 9α, 11β-PGF_2 and $PGF_{2\alpha}$ in asthma. *Am Rev Respir Dis* 1987; 136:1140.
12. DeWitt DL: Prostaglandin endoperoxide synthase: Regulation of enzyme expression. *Biochim Biophys Acta* 1991; 1083:121.
13. Smith WL, Marnett LJ: Prostaglandin endoperoxide synthase: Structure and catalysis. *Biochem Biophys Acta* 1991; 1083:1.
14. Smith WL: Prostanoid biosynthesis and mechanisms of action. *Am J Physiol* 1992; 263:F181.
15. Davidson FF, Dennis EA: Evolutionary relationships and implication for the regulation of phospholipase A_2 from snake venom to human secretory forms. *J Mol Evol* 1990; 31:228.
16. Xie W, Chipman JG, Robertson DL, et al.: Expression of a mitogen-response gene encoding prostaglandin synthase I regulated by mRNA splicing. *Proc Natl Acad Sci USA* 1991; 88:2692.
17. Hla T, Neilson K: Human cycloxygenase-2 cDNA. *Proc Natl Acad Sci USA* 1992; 89:7384.
18. O'Sullivan MG, Chilton FH, Huggins EM, McCall CE: Lipopolysaccharide priming of alveolar macrophages for enhanced synthesis of prostanoids involves induction of a novel prostaglandin H synthase. *J Biol Chem* 1992; 267:14547.
19. Lin AH, Bienkowski MJ, Gorman RR: Regulation of prostaglandin H synthase on RNA levels and prostaglandin biosynthesis by platelet-derived growth factor. *J Biol Chem* 1989; 264:17370.
20. Masferrer JL, Seibert K, Zweifel B, Needleman P: Endogenous glucocorticoids regulate an inducible cycloxygenase enzyme. *Proc Natl Acad Sci USA* 1992; 89:3917.
21. O'Banion MK, Winn VD, Young DA: cDNA cloning and functional acitivity of a glucocorticoid-regulated inflammatory cyclooxygenase. *Proc Natl Acad Sci USA* 1992; 89:4888.
22. O'Banion MK, Sadowski HB, Winn V, Young DA: A serum- and glucocorticoid-regulated 4-kilobase mRNA encodes a cyclooxygenase-related protein. *J Biol Chem* 1991; 266:23261.
23. Steel J, Platshon L, Kaliner M: Prostaglandin generation by human and guinea pig lung tissue: Comparison of parenchymal and airway responses. *J Allergy Clin Immunol* 1979; 64:287.
24. Muñoz NM, Shioya T, Murphy TM, et al.: Potentiation of vagal efferent contractile response on canine tracheal smooth muscle by the thromboxane mimetic-U46619. *J Appl Physiol* 1986; 61:1173.
25. Black JI, Armour CL, Vincenc KS, Johnson PRA: A comparison of the contractile activity of PGD_2 on isolated bronchus. *Prostaglandins* 1986; 32:25.
26. Shioya T, Solway J, Muñoz NM, et al.: Distribution of airway contractile responses within the major diameter bronchi during exogenous bronchoconstriction. *Am Rev Respir Dis* 1987; 135:1105.
27. Schulman ES, Adkinson NF, Newball HH: Cyclooxygenase metabolites in human lung anaphylaxis: Airway vs parenchyma. *J Appl Physiol* 1982; 53:585.
28. Wasserman MA: Bronchopulmonary responses to prostaglandin $F_{2\alpha}$, histamine and acetylcholine in the dog. *Eur J Pharmacol* 1975; 32:146.
29. Banovcin P, Visnovsky P: Effect of prostaglandin $F_{2\alpha}$ on the contractile tissues of the respiratory system of the cat in experimental airway inflammation. *Physiol Res* 1991; 40:75.
30. Granstrom E: Metabolism of prostaglandin $F_{2\alpha}$ in guinea pig lung. *Eur J Biochem* 1971; 20:451.
31. Fish JE, Newball HH, Norman PS, Peterman VI: Novel effects of $PGF_{2\alpha}$ in airway function in asthmatic subjects. *J Appl Physiol* 1983; 54:105.
32. Walters EH: Prostaglandins and the control of airways responses to histamine in normal and asthmatic subjects. *Thorax* 1983; 38:188.

33. Haye-Legrand I, Cerrina J, Raffstein B: Histamine contraction of isolated human airway muscle preparations: Role of prostaglandins. *J Pharmacol Exp Ther* 1986; 239:536.

34. Richards IM, Oostreen SA, Griffin RL, Bunting S: Pulmonary pharmacology of synthetic thromboxane A_2. *Adv Prostaglandin Thromboxane Leukot Res* 1987; 17:1067.

35. Pavord ID, Wisniewski A, Mather R, et al.: Effect of inhaled prostaglandin E_2 on bronchial reactivity to sodium metabisulfite and metacholine in patients with asthma. *Thorax* 1991; 46:633.

36. Choudry NB, Fuller RW, Pride NB: Sensitivity of the human cough reflex: Effect of inflammatory mediators prostaglandin E_2, bradykinin, and histamine. *Am Rev Respir Dis* 1989; 140:137.

37. Walters EH, Davies BH: Dual effects of prostaglandin E_2 on normal airways smooth muscle in vivo. *Thorax* 1982; 37:918.

38. Baum T, Wendt RL, Peters JR, et al.: Comparison of activities of two prostaglandin stereoisomers: $PGF_{2\alpha}$ and $PGF_{2\beta}$. *Eur J Pharmacol* 1974; 25:92.

39. Kawakami Y, Uchiyama K, Irie T, Murao M: Evaluation of aerosols of prostaglandin E_1 and E_2 as bronchodilators. *Eur J Clin Pharmacol* 1973; 6:127.

40. Smith AP, Cuthbert MF, Dunlop LS: Effects of inhaled prostaglandin E_1, E_2, and $F_{2\alpha}$ on the airway resistance of healthy and asthmatic man. *Clin Sci Mol Med* 1975; 48:421.

41. Hardy CC, Bradding P, Robinson C, Holgate ST: Bronchoconstrictor and antibronchoconstrictor properties of inhaled prostacyclin in asthma. *J Appl Physiol* 1988; 64:1567.

42. Wasserman MA, DuCharme DW, Wendling MG, et al.: Bronchodilator effects of prostacyclin (PGI_2) in dogs and guinea pigs. *Eur J Pharmacol* 1980; 66:53.

43. Hardy CC, Robinson C, Tattersfield AE, Holgate ST: The bronchoconstrictor effect of the inhaled prostaglandin D_2 in normal asthmatic men. *N Engl J Med* 1984; 311:209.

44. Holgate ST, Burns GB, Robinson C, Church MK: Anaphylactic- and calcium-dependent generation of prostaglandin D_2, thromboxane B_2, and other cyclooxygenase products of arachidonic acid by dispersed human lung cells and relationship to histamine release. *J Immunol* 1984; 133:2138.

45. Naclero RM, Meier HL, Kagey-Sabotka A, et al.: Mediator release after nasal airway challenge with allergen. *Am Rev Respir Dis* 1983; 128:597.

46. Madonna A, Tedeski A, Brasia C, et al.: Mediator releases after endobronchial antigen challenge in patients with respiratory allergy. *J Allergy Clin Immunol* 1990; 85:906.

47. Armstrong RA, Matthews JS, Jones RL, Wilson NH: Characterization of PGE_2 receptors mediating increased vascular permeability in inflammation. *Adv Prostaglandin Thromboxane Leukot Res* 1990; 21:375.

48. Spannhake EW, Kadowitz PJ, Kleeberger SR: Influence of mediators of anaphylaxis on collateral ventilation and the lung periphery of the dog. *J Pharmacol Exp Ther* 1985; 234:491.

49. Braunstein G, Labat C, Brunelleschi S, et al.: Evidence that histamine sensitivity and responsiveness of guinea pig isolated trachea are modulated by epithelial PGE_2 production. *Br J Pharmacol* 1988; 95:300.

50. Muñoz NM, Leff AR: Blockade of eosinophil migration by 5-lipoxygenase and cyclooxygenase inhibition in explanted guinea pig trachealis. *Am J Physiol:* Lung Cell Mol Biol 1995; 268:L446.

51. Stewart AG: Biological properties of platelet activating factor, in Cunningham FM (ed): *Lipid Mediators.* San Diego, Academic, 1994; 223.

52. Rabe KF, Muñoz NM, Vita AJ, et al.: Contraction of human bronchial smooth muscle caused by activated human eosinophils. *Am J Physiol* 1994; 267:L326.

53. Muñoz NM, Vita AJ, Neeley SP, et al.: Beta adrenergic modulation of formyl-methionine-leucine-phenylalanine-stimulated secretion of eosinophil peroxidase and leukotriene C_4. *J Pharm Exp Ther* 1994; 268:139.

54. Muñoz NM, Rabe KF, Vita AJ, et al.: Paradoxical blockade of beta-adrenergically mediated inhibition of stimulated eosinophil secretion by salmeterol. *J Pharm Exp Ther* 1995; 273:850.

55. Weller PF, Lee CW, Foster DW, et al.: Generation and metabolism of 5-lipoxygenase pathway leukotrienes by human eosinophils: Predominant production of leukotriene C4. *Proc Natl Acad Sci USA* 1983; 80:7626.

56. Galens S, Muñoz NM, Rabe KF, et al.: Assessment of agonist- and cell-mediated responsiveness in microsection explants of airways by computerized video micrometry. *Am J Physiol* 1995; 12:L519.

57. Lee T, Lenihan DJ, Malone B, et al.: Increased biosynthesis of platelet activating factor in activated eosinophils. *J Biol Chem* 1984; 139:801.

58. Emery DL, Djokic TD, Graf PO, Nadel JA: Prostaglandin D_2 causes accumulation of eosinophils in the lumen of the dog trachea. *J Appl Physiol* 1989; 67:959.

59. Bruijnzeel PI, Koenderman L, Kok PT, et al.: Platelet activating factor (PAF-acether) induced leukotriene C_4 formation and luminol-dependent chemiluminescence by human eosinophils. *Pharmacol Res Commun* 1986; 18:61.

60. Hirata K, Pele JP, Robidoux C, Sirois P: Guinea pig lung eosinophils: Purification and prostaglandin production. *J Leukoc Biol* 1989; 45:523.

61. Strek ME, White SR, Ndukwu IM, et al.: Physiological significance of epithelial removal on guinea pig tracheal smooth muscle response to acetylcholine and serotonin. *Am Rev Respir Dis* 1993; 147:1477.

62. Brofman JD, White SR, Blake J, et al.: Epithelial augmentation of trachealis contraction caused by major basic protein of eosinophils. *J Appl Physiol* 1989; 66:1867.

63. Barnes PJ, Cuss FM, Palmer JB: The effect of airway epithelium on smooth muscle contractility in bovine trachea. *Br J Pharmacol* 1985; 65:685.

64. Stuarts-Smith K, Vanhoute PM: Airway epithelium modulates the responsiveness of porcine bronchial smooth muscle. *J Appl Physiol* 1988; 65:721.

65. Hunter JA, Finkbeiner WE, Nadel JA, et al.: Predominate generation of 15-lipoxygenase metabolites of arachidonic acid by epithelial cells from human trachea. *Proc Natl Acad Sci USA* 1985; 82:4633.

66. Andrews FJ, Malcontenti-Wilson C, O'Brien PE: Effect of nonsteroidal anti-inflammatory drugs on LFA-1 and ICAM-1 expression in gastric mucosa. *Am J Physiol* 1994; 266:G656.

LEUKOTRIENES

JEFFREY M. DRAZEN

Leukotrienes are synthesized in the course of immediate hypersensitivity reactions when mast cells or basophils are appropriately activated.[1–3] Leukotrienes can also be produced outside the context of immediate-type hypersensitivity by other cells, such as eosinophils or alveolar macrophages, when these cells are suitably activated. To appreciate the pulmonary pharmacology of the leukotrienes, it is important to examine the biochemistry of their formation, their pharmacologic characteristics in the airways, their recovery in asthmatic conditions, and the effects of inhibiting their action or synthesis in induced or spontaneous asthma.

Biochemistry of Leukotriene Synthesis

Leukotrienes are derivatives of arachidonic acid (Fig. 13-1), an abundant naturally occurring polyunsaturated 20-carbon fatty acid (5,8,11,14-*cis*-eicosatetraenoic acid) commonly found esterified in the *sn*-2 position of cell-membrane phospholipids.[1] Recent data suggest that the arachidonic acid that is eventually transformed into the leukotrienes is derived from perinuclear membranes.[4] The increase in the intracellular calcium concentration that occurs on cellular activation initiates a series of events leading to the translocation of phospholipase A_2.[5–10] The catalytic action of phospholipase A_2 results in the cleavage of arachidonic acid from the *sn*-2 position of phospholipids, and the acid so liberated then serves as the substrate for 5-lipoxygenase. However, for 5-lipoxygenase to be active catalytically, it must be translocated from the cytosol to the perinuclear membrane.[11–13] This translocation results from the action of 5-lipoxygenase activating protein (FLAP) in the presence of increased intracellular calcium.[11,14] FLAP is an integral membrane protein that exhibits a high affinity for the activated form of 5-lipoxygenase and can also serve as an arachidonic acid–

binding protein.[12,15] It has been speculated that, when arachidonic acid is liberated from membrane phospholipids, it is sequestered by FLAP and presented to 5-lipoxygenase. This enzyme operates on arachidonic acid twice in succession, first to form 5-hydroperoxyeicosatetraenoic acid (5-HPETE) and then to convert 5-HPETE to the unstable epoxide known as leukotriene A_4 (LTA$_4$). Unless sequestered in a lipid environment, LTA$_4$ is rapidly degraded nonenzymatically to 5,12-dihydroxy fatty acids having little or no known biologic activity.[1]

In the presence of appropriate enzymes, LTA$_4$ is converted to the biologically active leukotrienes. In neutrophils, the main enzyme operating on LTA$_4$ is LTA$_4$ epoxide hydrolase.[16] In the intracellular microenvironment, this enzyme converts LTA$_4$ into leukotriene B_4 (LTB$_4$; 5S-12R-dihydroxy-6,14,-*cis*-8,10-*trans*-eicosatetraenoic acid). It is interesting that, in the extracellular microenvironment, LTA$_4$ epoxide hydrolase functions as an aminopeptidase with unknown substrate specificity; its action may contribute to the perpetuation of inflammation in immediate hypersensitivity responses.

In eosinophils and mast cells, LTA$_4$ is a substrate for leukotriene C_4 (LTC$_4$) synthase,[17] which adds the tripeptide glutathione at the C6 position to form LTC$_4$ (5S-hydroxy-6R-glutathionyl-7,9-*trans*-11,14-*cis*-eicosatetraenoic acid). It now is recognized that LTC$_4$ synthase also is a highly hydrophobic integral membrane protein, which probably resides in the perinuclear membrane. Thus, when LTA$_4$ is produced by 5-lipoxygenase, it can remain in the perinuclear environment as it is enzymatically processed into the bioactive molecule LTC$_4$. Both LTB$_4$ and LTC$_4$ are intracellular products. The mechanism by which LTB$_4$ leaves the cell is not known. In contrast, it is well established that LTC$_4$ leaves the cell through the action of a specific transmembrane transporter.[18] Outside the cell, LTB$_4$ acts at specific receptors, known as *BLT receptors*, to initiate chemotactic and other

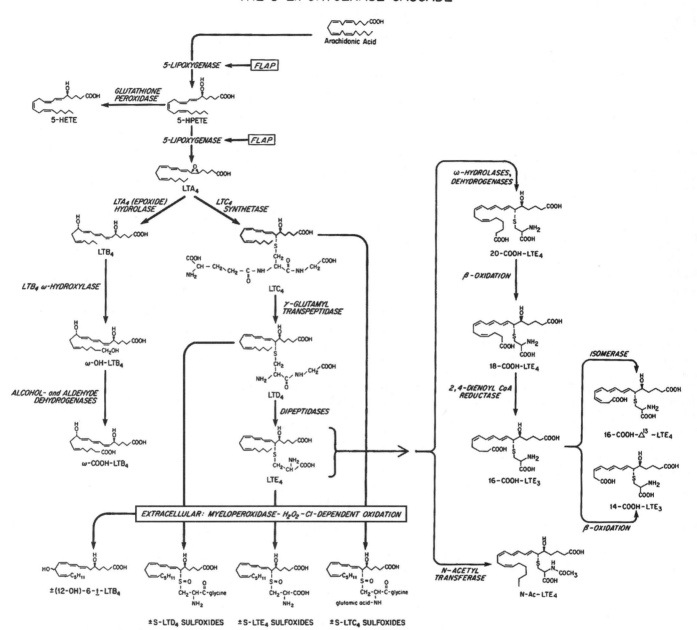

FIGURE 13-1 Biochemical pathways leading to the formation and inactivation of the leukotrienes.

responses; LTC$_4$ becomes a substrate for γ-glutamyl-transpeptidase,[19,20] which cleaves the glutamic acid moiety to form leukotriene D$_4$ (LTD$_4$; 5S-hydroxy-6R-cysteinylgly-cyl-7,9-$trans$-11,14-cis-eicosatetraenoic acid). LTD$_4$ serves as a substrate for a variety of dipeptidases that cleave the glycine moiety to form the 6-cysteinyl analog of LTC$_4$ known as leukotriene E$_4$ (LTE$_4$). The three naturally occurring human leukotrienes containing cysteine, known as the cysteinyl leukotrienes (LTC$_4$, LTD$_4$, and LTE$_4$) together constitute

what was previously called $slow-reacting\ substance\ of\ anaphy-laxis$ (SRS-A).[2]

In the extracellular microenvironment, LTC$_4$ can be N-acetylated; alternatively, it is subject to ω-hydroxylation and subsequent β-elimination, the result being the formation of a series of biologically inactive molecules.[21] Approximately 15 percent of bioavailable LTC$_4$ appears in the urine as LTE$_4$. The cysteinyl leukotrienes are also inactivated by a myelo-peroxidase-dependent pathway, which yields LTB$_4$ and the respective leukotriene sulfoxide—for example, 2 moles of LTC_4 are broken down to yield a mole LTB_4 and a mole of LTC_4-sulfoxide.[22]

Biologic Effects of the Cysteinyl Leukotrienes

Cysteinyl leukotrienes effect obstruction, glandular secretion, and microvascular leakage in airways. The similarity between these activities and the profile of physiologic abnormalities in asthma suggests that cysteinyl leukotrienes may be important asthmatic mediators.[23,24] In isolated human bronchi, LTC_4 and LTD_4 are potent contractile agonists. Airways 2 to 4 mm in diameter from normal subjects respond to these agonists, with IC_{50} values of 1 to 50 nM.[25] Thus, these agents are approximately 1000 to 10,000 times more potent than histamine at eliciting airway contraction. However, bronchi from asthmatic subjects respond to the same concentrations of cysteinyl leukotrienes as bronchi from nonasthmatic subjects. This observation suggests that alteration in the sensitivity of airway smooth muscle to the leukotrienes is not part of the basic disorder of asthma.

When leukotrienes are administered by aerosol to nonasthmatic subjects, airways obstruction ensues.[24] After aerosol exposure to LTC_4, this effect appears in approximately 10 to 15 min and peaks in 15 to 25 min. By contrast, exposure to aerosols of LTD_4 or LTE_4 results in immediate airway obstruction. The nebulized concentrations of the cysteinyl leukotrienes required to effect a given degree of airway narrowing are 3000 to 10,000 times lower than the concentrations of histamine or methacholine required. For example, in nonasthmatic subjects, the average nebulized concentration required for a 30 percent decrease in the maximal expiratory flow rate, measured from a partial flow volume curve, is 10 to 100 nM for histamine or methacholine, 12.7 µM for LTC_4, 11.3 µM for LTD_4, and 300 µM for LTE_4. LTE_4 thus is about 30 times less potent as a bronchoconstrictor agonist than LTC_4 or LTD_4.[26,27] Subjects with asthma are hyperresponsive to the cysteinyl leukotrienes, as they are to other bronchoconstrictor agonists. However, their hyperresponsiveness to the cysteinyl leukotrienes is less pronounced than that to histamine or methacholine. For example, in a group of asthmatic subjects who were 100 times more responsive to histamine than a group of nonasthmatic subjects, the difference for leukotrienes was approximately 10-fold. These findings suggest that specific airways may respond to each of these agonists in a characteristic way.[28]

Evidence for selective airways responses to the leukotrienes has been derived from studies in which subjects breathe either air or helium/oxygen mixtures, and the main site of physiological airways responses is identified. In such studies, nonasthmatic subjects respond to inhaled LTC_4 primarily with a peripheral airways response, while asthmatic subjects show both a central and a peripheral airways response.[29] Thus, one can postulate that part of the asthmatic lesion is a specific central-airways hyperresponsiveness to LTC_4.

A variety of antagonists to the $CysLT_1$ receptor for cysteinyl leukotrienes have been developed. In isolated tissue strips, these antagonists have pA_2 values of 7 to 10.[30] In human subjects in vivo, $CysLT_1$ receptor antagonists have been developed that shift the response to inhaled LTD_4 by a factor ranging from 4 to over 200 (Fig. 13-2).[31,32] Indeed, because of their potent ability to antagonize the action of LTD_4 at its receptor, these agents have been used in pharmacologic studies of asthma.

Recovery of Leukotrienes

Approximately 5 to 15 percent of biologically available LTC_4 appears in the urine unchanged as LTE_4.[21,33,34] Thus, the level of urinary LTE_4 is an index of cysteinyl leukotriene production. When individuals with allergic asthma are exposed to aerosols of specific allergens to which they are known to be sensitive, the "early-phase" bronchoconstrictor response is accompanied by an increase in urinary excretion of LTE_4.[35–41] A number of investigators have found a relation between the amount of LTE_4 recovered in the urine and the magnitude of the decrease in flow rate resulting from the allergen exposure. During the "late-phase" asthmatic response, however, elevated amounts of LTE_4 have not been recovered from the urine.[37]

During spontaneous episodes of acute asthma, approximately two-thirds of patients presenting for treatment have elevated levels of LTE_4 in their urine.[42] It is important to note that among patients with such elevated levels, all those with reversible airway narrowing (most likely caused by muscular airway constriction) were included. These variations in urinary LTE_4 are consistent with the hypothesis that leukotrienes are physiologically important in some but not all asthma patients.

Effects of Leukotriene Receptor Antagonists and Synthesis Inhibitors on Airways Obstruction

The most compelling evidence that leukotrienes play a role in the biology of asthma comes from studies with three kinds of pharmacologic agents: (1) agents that inhibit the action of LTD_4 and LTE_4 on the $CysLT_1$ receptor, (2) agents that inhibit the synthesis of leukotrienes by inhibiting the action of 5-lipoxygenase, and (3) agents that prevent the translocation of 5-lipoxygenase to the perinuclear membrane by binding to FLAP. More than a half dozen agents that can interrupt the 5-lipoxygenase pathway have been studied (Fig. 13-3). The agents that inhibit the action of LTD_4 or LTE_4 at its receptor vary in potency by approximately 25-fold.[31,32] In contrast, the agents that inhibit the *synthesis* of the cysteinyl leukotrienes have similar potencies. All three classes of agents have been used in chronic stable asthma and in clinical trials of induced asthma as well as of the reduction of the bronchoconstriction that develops when asthmatic patients are not treated with bronchodilators.

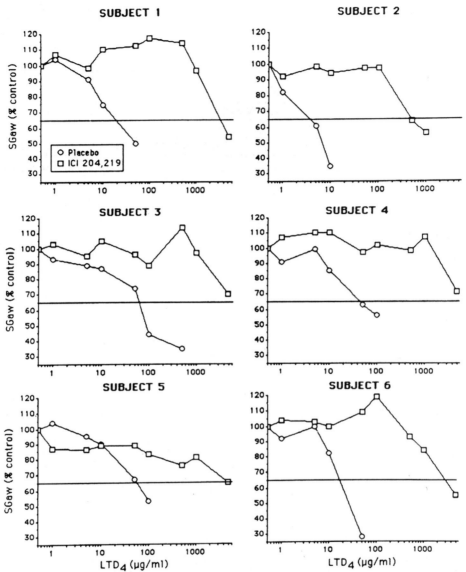

FIGURE 13-2 Effects of a potent CysLT$_1$ receptor antagonist on LTD$_4$-induced airway obstruction. In each panel, the squares represent the airways obstructive response to inhaled aerosols generated from solutions of LTD$_4$ with no pretreatment, while the circles represent the response after pretreatment with 40 mg of ICI 204219, a CysLT$_1$ receptor antagonist. Concentrations of LTD$_4$ approximately 100 times greater are required in the nebulizer after pretreatment to achieve the same degree of airways narrowing. (From Smith et al.,[32] with permission.)

Inhibition of Induced Asthma

Agents that inhibit the 5-lipoxygenase pathway have been studied in cold air- or exercise-induced asthma, antigen-induced asthma, or aspirin-induced asthma. In cold air- or exercise-induced asthma, all of the agents studied, despite their varied inhibitory potencies, resulted in a decrease of approximately 50 percent in the bronchoconstrictor response to cold air exposure or standard exercise challenge. When subjects with asthma induced by exposure to a specific allergen are pretreated with such an agent, the magnitude of the inhibitory response is closely related to the capacity of that agent to inhibit either the action or the synthesis of leukotrienes. However, none of the agents studied to date has resulted in a *total* attenuation of the bronchoconstrictor response elicited by antigen stimulation. In contrast, in patients with aspirin-induced asthma, blockade of the 5-lipoxygenase pathway is associated with total inhibition of physiologic responses.[43] For example, when patients with known aspirin sensitivity are given an oral aspirin challenge in the presence of an inhaled leukotriene receptor antagonist, the airways physiologic response is inhibited, while the

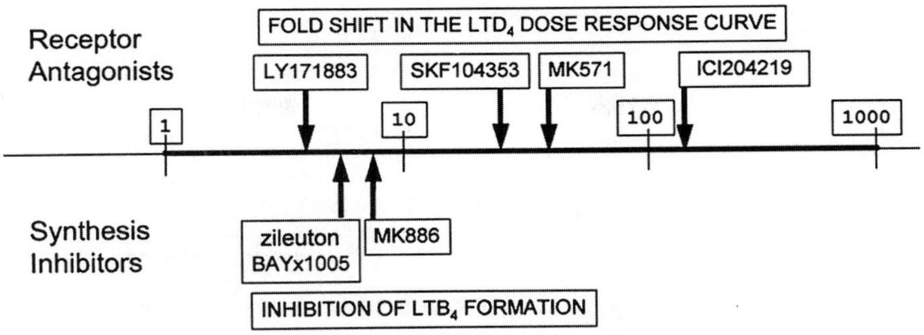

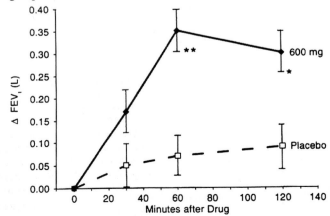

FIGURE 13-3 Agents shown in clinical trials to act on the 5-lipoxygenase pathway. $CysLT_1$ receptor antagonists are shown above the line, and agents that inhibit the synthesis of 5-lipoxygenase products are shown below the line. The potency of $CysLT_1$ receptor antagonists is measured by comparing the shift in LTD_4 dose-response curves before and after treatment with the agent in question. The potency of agents that inhibit the formation of leukotrienes is measured by examining the decrease in the production of LTB_4 in whole blood on challenge ex vivo with calcium ionophore.

nonairways physiologic responses are not. When subjects with aspirin-sensitive asthma are given an inhaled challenge with lysine aspirin after the administration of a systemic leukotriene receptor antagonist, the physiologic responses in the lung are blocked. Most important, oral aspirin challenge after pretreatment with a 5-lipoxygenase inhibitor results in a total abrogation of physiologic responses, including a loss of the bronchoconstrictor response as well as the naso-ocular, gastrointestinal, and dermal responses observed in this setting.

The variety of the responses to agents that inhibit the 5-lipoxygenase pathway under conditions of various physiologic challenges suggests a unique form of asthmatic heterogeneity—that is, a heterogeneity in the asthmatic responses, with different stimuli eliciting different panels of bronchoactive agents, which in some cases include leukotrienes and in others do not. Allergen-induced asthma appears to be predominantly a leukotriene-mediated response, while aspirin-induced asthma appears to be almost exclusively a leukotriene-mediated response.

Inhibition of Asthmatic Airways Obstruction

Individuals with moderate asthma develop airways obstruction when their asthma medications are withheld. The reversal of airways obstruction induced in this fashion has been examined by various investigators. Administration of agents that inhibit the action of LTD_4 at its receptor or the synthesis of the leukotrienes is associated with a 10 to 20 percent increase in the forced expiratory volume in the first second (FEV_1)[44-46] (Fig. 13-4). The onset of this effect coincides with the known onset of the effect of the specific agents administered. Furthermore, neither normal subjects nor patients with mild asthma exhibit improved airway function when such agents are administered. These data indicate that patients with moderate to severe asthma are continuously producing leukotrienes, which are in part responsible for their baseline airways obstruction.

Studies of Chronic Asthma

A number of trials with LTD_4 receptor antagonists or leukotriene synthesis inhibitors in moderate asthma have been conducted. In these trials patients are given a placebo, in a single-blind manner, for a "run-in" period that lasts from 7 to 14 days. There is then an active-treatment period of 4 to 6 weeks, which is followed, in some cases, by a "withdrawal" period. The results of trials conducted to date have been remarkably similar. During the first month of treatment, the FEV_1 improves by 10 to 15 percent, and this improvement is associated with a 30 percent decrease in asthma symptoms, a decrease in nighttime awakenings, improvement in morning and evening peak flow rates, and a decrease in β-agonist use. The similarity of the data for a variety of pharmacologically distinct agents constitutes strong evidence that the leukotrienes are important media-

FIGURE 13-4 Bronchodilator response observed within 2 h after systemic administration of Zileuton, an inhibitor of 5-lipoxygenase, to patients with mild asthma. The response effect in the treatment group is significantly greater than that in the control group. (*From Israel et al.,*[42] *with permission.*)

tors of the biologic events that give rise to asthmatic airways obstruction and symptoms. Longer trials have shown that these effects persist.[46,47] An additional benefit is that patients require fewer courses of oral prednisone for "rescue" from severe episodes of asthma.

Summary

The cysteinyl leukotrienes are potent airway contractile agonists and can be recovered from bodily fluids of patients with asthma. The inhibition of their synthesis or action is beneficial in this disease. Taken together, these data strongly support the importance of the leukotrienes in asthma.

References

1. Samuelsson B: Leukotrienes: mediators of immediate hypersensitivity reactions and inflammation. *Science* 1983; 220:568.
2. Samuelsson B, Dahlen SE, Lindgren JA, et al.: Leukotrienes and lipoxins: structures, biosynthesis, and biological effects. *Science* 1987; 237:1171.
3. Lewis RA, Austen KF, Soberman RJ: Leukotrienes and other products of the 5-lipoxygenase pathway. Biochemistry and relation to pathobiology in human diseases. *N Engl J Med* 1990; 323:645.
4. Woods JW, Evans JF, Ethier D, et al.: Lipoxygenase and 5-lipoxygenase activating protein are localized in the nuclear envelope of activated human leukocytes. *J Exp Med* 1993; 178:1935.
5. Waite M: Phospholipases, enzymes that share a substrate class. *Adv Exp Med Biol* 1990; 279:1.
6. Weiss J, Wright G: Mobilization and function of extracellular phospholipase A_2 in inflammation. *Adv Exp Med Biol* 1990; 275:103.
7. van den Bosch H, Aarsman AJ, van Schaik RH, et al.: Structural and enzymological properties of cellular phospholipases A2. *Biochem Soc Trans* 1990; 18:781.
8. Kaiser E, Chiba P, Zaky K: Phospholipases in biology and medicine. *Clin Biochem* 1990; 23:349.
9. Dennis EA, Rhee SG, Billah MM, Hannum YA: Role of phospholipase in generating lipid second messengers in signal transduction. *FASEB J* 1991; 5:2068.
10. Ferguson JE, Hanley MR: The role of phospholipases and phospholipid-derived signals in cell activation. *Curr Opin Cell Biol* 1991; 3:206.
11. Miller DK, Gillard JW, Vickers PJ, et al.: Identification and isolation of a membrane protein necessary for leukotriene production. *Nature* 1990; 343:278.
12. Dixon RA, Diehl RE, Opas E, et al.: Requirement of a 5-lipoxygenase-activating protein for leukotriene synthesis. *Nature* 1990; 343:282.
13. Abramovitz M, Wong E, Cox ME, et al.: 5-Lipoxygenase-activating protein stimulates the utilization of arachidonic acid by 5-lipoxygenase. *Eur J Biochem* 1993; 215:105.
14. Reid GK, Kargman S, Vickers PJ, et al: Correlation between expression of 5-lipoxygenase-activating protein, 5-lipoxygenase, and cellular leukotriene synthesis. *J Biol Chem* 1990; 265:19818.
15. Mancini JA, Abramovitz M, Cox ME, et al.: 5-Lipoxygenase-activating protein is an arachidonate binding protein. *FEBS Lett* 1993; 318:277.
16. Orning L, Gierse JK, Fitzpatrick FA: The bifunctional enzyme leukotriene-A(4) hydrolase is an arginine aminopeptidase of high efficiency and specificity. *J Biol Chem* 1994; 269:11269.
17. Lam BK, Penrose JF, Freeman GJ, Austen KF: Expression cloning of a cDNA for human leukotriene C_4 synthase, an integral membrane protein conjugating reduced glutathione to leukotriene A_4. *Proc Natl Acad Sci USA* 1994; 91:7663.
18. Lam BK, Owen WF Jr, Austen KF, Soberman RJ: The identification of a distinct export step following the biosynthesis of leukotriene C4 by human eosinophils. *J Biol Chem* 1989; 264:12885.
19. Wetmore LA, Gerard NP, Herron DK, et al.: Leukotriene receptor on U-937 cells: discriminatory responses to leukotrienes C4 and D4. *Am J Physiol* 1991; 261:L164.
20. Wetmore LA, Gerard C, Drazen JM: Human lung expresses unique gamma-glutamyl transpeptidase transcripts. *Proc Natl Acad Sci USA* 1993; 90:7461.
21. Sala A, Voelkel N, Maclouf J, Murphy RC: Leukotriene E4 elimination and metabolism in normal human subjects. *J Biol Chem* 1990; 265:21771.
22. Lee CW, Lewis RA, Tauber AI, et al.: The myeloperoxidase-dependent metabolism of leukotrienes C4, D4, and E4 to 6-trans-leukotriene B4 diastereoisomers and the subclass-specific S-diastereoisomeric sulfoxides. *J Biol Chem* 1983; 258:15004.
23. Piper PJ: Leukotrienes and the airways. *Eur J Anaesthesiol* 1989; 6:241.
24. Drazen JM: Inhalation challenge with sulfidopeptide leukotrienes in human subjects. *Chest* 1986; 89:414.
25. Snyder DW, Krell RD: Pharmacological evidence for a distinct leukotriene D4 receptor in guinea-pig trachea. *J Pharmacol Exp Ther* 1984; 231:616.
26. Davidson AB, Lee TH, Scanlon PD, et al.: Bronchoconstrictor effects of leukotriene E4 in normal and asthmatic subjects. *Am Rev Respir Dis* 1987; 135:333.
27. O'Hickey SP, Arm JP, Rees PJ, et al.: The relative responsiveness to inhaled leukotriene E4, methacholine and histamine in normal and asthmatic subjects. *Eur Respir J* 1988; 1:913.
28. Adelroth E, Morris MM, Hargreave FE, O'Byrne PM: Airway responsiveness to leukotrienes C4 and D4 and to methacholine in patients with asthma and normal control. *N Engl J Med* 1986; 315:480.
29. Pichurko BM, Ingram RH Jr, Sperling RI, et al.: Localization of the site of the bronchoconstrictor effects of leukotriene C4 compared with that of histamine in asthmatic subjects. *Am Rev Respir Dis* 1989; 140:334.
30. Drazen JM, Austen KF: Leukotrienes and airway responses. *Am Rev Respir Dis* 1987; 136:985.
31. Phillips GD, Rafferty P, Robinson C, Holgate ST: Dose-related antagonism of leukotriene D4-induced bronchoconstriction by p.o. administration of LY-171883 in nonasthmatic subjects. *J Pharmacol Exp Ther* 1988; 246:732.
32. Smith LJ, Geller S, Ebright L, et al.: Inhibition of leukotriene D4-induced bronchoconstriction in normal subjects by the oral LTD4 receptor antagonist ICI 204,219. *Am Rev Respir Dis* 1990; 141:988.
33. Orning L, Kaijser L, Hammarstrom S: In vivo metabolism of leukotriene C4 in man: urinary excretion of leukotriene E4. *Biochem Biophys Res Commun* 1985; 130:214.
34. Wescott JY, Voelkel NF, Jones K, Wenzel SE: Inactivation of leukotriene C4 in the airways and subsequent urinary leukotriene E4 excretion in normal and asthmatic subjects. *Am Rev Respir Dis* 1993; 148:1244.
35. Taylor GW, Taylor I, Black P, et al.: Urinary leukotriene E4 after antigen challenge and in acute asthma and allergic rhinitis. *Lancet* 1989; 1:584.
36. Sladek K, Dworski R, Fitzgerald GA, et al.: Allergen-stimulated release of thromboxane A2 and leukotriene E4 in humans. Effect of indomethacin. *Am Rev Respir Dis* 1990; 141:1441.
37. Manning PJ, Rokach J, Malo JL, et al: Urinary leukotriene E4 levels during early and late asthmatic responses. *J Allergy Clin Immunol* 1990; 86:211.

38. Tagari P, Rasmussen JB, Delorme D, et al.: Comparison of urinary leukotriene E4 and 16-carboxytetranordihydro leukotriene E4 excretion in allergic asthmatics after inhaled antigen. *Eicosanoids* 1990; 3:75.

39. Kumlin M, Dahlen B, Bjork T, et al.: Urinary excretion of leukotriene-E4 and 11-dehydro-thromboxane-B2 in response to bronchial provocations with allergen, aspirin, leukotriene-D4, and histamine in asthmatics. *Am Rev Respir Dis* 1992; 146:96.

40. Westcott JY, Smith HR, Wenzel SE, et al.: Urinary leukotriene-E4 in patients with asthma—effect of airways reactivity and sodium cromoglycate. *Am Rev Respir Dis* 1991; 143:1322.

41. Smith CM, Christie PE, Hawksworth RJ, et al.: Urinary leukotriene-E4 levels after allergen and exercise challenge in bronchial asthma. *Am Rev Respir Dis* 1991; 144:1411.

42. Drazen JM, Obrien J, Sparrow D, et al.: Recovery of leukotriene-E4 from the urine of patients with airway obstruction. *Am Rev Respir Dis* 1992; 146:104.

43. Israel E, Fischer AR, Rosenberg MA, et al.: The pivotal role of 5-lipoxygenase products in the reaction of aspirin-sensitive asthmatics to aspirin. *Am Rev Respir Dis* 1993; 148:1447.

44. Hui KP, Barnes NC: Lung function improvement in asthma with a cysteinyl-leukotriene receptor antagonist. *Lancet* 1991; 337:1062.

45. Impens N, Reiss TF, Teahan JA, et al.: Acute bronchodilation with an intravenously administered leukotriene-D(4) antagonist, MK-679. *Am Rev Respir Dis* 1993; 147:1442.

46. Israel E, Rubin P, Kemp JP, et al.: The effect of inhibition of 5-lipoxygenase by zileuton in mild to moderate asthma. *Ann Intern Med* 1993; 119:1059.

47. Spector SL, Smith LJ, Glass M, et al.: Effects of 6 weeks of therapy with oral doses of ICI 204,219, a leukotriene D_4 receptor antagonist, in subjects with bronchial asthma. *Am J Respir Crit Care Med* 1994; 150:618.

PLATELET-ACTIVATING FACTOR

JONATHAN D. PLITMAN
JAMES R. SNAPPER

Platelet-activating factor (PAF) was originally identified as a product of stimulated rabbit basophils that induced histamine release from platelets.[1] It has since been recognized as an extraordinarily potent lipid mediator whose protean actions may participate in many inflammatory phenomena. Platelet-activating factor comprises a group of related glycerophospholipids, which typically bear an alkyl group at the *sn*-1 position, a short acyl group at the *sn*-2 position, and a phosphocholine polar head group. The molecular structure of the "classic" principal PAF species (1-*O*-alkyl-2-acetyl-*sn*-glycero-3-phosphocholine, with an alkyl chain of 16 or 18 carbons in length) was elucidated in the late 1970s.[2,3] This structure (Fig. 14-1) has been referenced by a number of names, including Paf-acether, acetylglycerylether phosphorylcholine (AGEPC), and alkyl-PAF.

It is important to note that many closely related PAF analogs are produced as well.[4] These include PAFs with acyl or alkenyl *sn*-1 moieties, analogs with longer chains esterified at the *sn*-2 position, varieties with polar heads other than choline, and biosynthetic intermediates, such as alkyl-acetylglycerols, which might themselves act as mediators. The analog bearing an *sn*-1 acyl linkage (1-acyl-2-alkyl-*sn*-glycero-3-phosphocholine, or acyl-PAF) is of particular interest, in that in some cell types (e.g., endothelial cells, basophils, mast cells), acyl-PAF production may equal or exceed that of alkyl-PAF under certain circumstances.[5–7] Acyl-PAFs have proinflammatory actions, although their potency appears low compared with the highly potent alkyl-PAF.[8–10] Acyl-PAF compounds may thus serve in and of themselves as endogenous competitive PAF antagonists or, if present in sufficiently high local concentrations, as inflammatory agonists. Knowledge of the (patho)physiologic significance of acyl-PAF (as well as that of the other PAF analogs) remains limited, but the existence of these compounds is a useful reminder that PAF biology is complex and incompletely understood. Future pharmacologic research will define the significance of PAF molecular heterogeneity; investigations to date have focused primarily on alkyl-PAF. The term PAF in this chapter will hereinafter refer to alkyl-PAF except where otherwise specified.

PAF Biosynthesis and Catabolism

This area has been the subject of considerable investigation and extensive review.[11,12] Platelet-activating factor is the product of two distinct biosynthetic pathways. In the "remodeling" pathway the starting material is a membrane-associated lipid glycero-3-phosphocholine, while in the "de novo" pathway a non-choline-containing alkylglycero-3-phosphate precursor is utilized. It appears that the remodeling pathway is principally responsible for the accelerated production of PAF in response to inflammatory stimuli, while the de novo pathway produces the physiologic "background" levels of PAF present in the absence of inflammation.

The remodeling pathway is a two-step process (Fig. 14-2). The first step is the hydrolytic removal of the 2-acyl moieties [typically, arachidonic acid (AA)] of membrane-bound 1-alkyl-2-acyl-*sn*-glycero-3-phosphocholines, resulting in

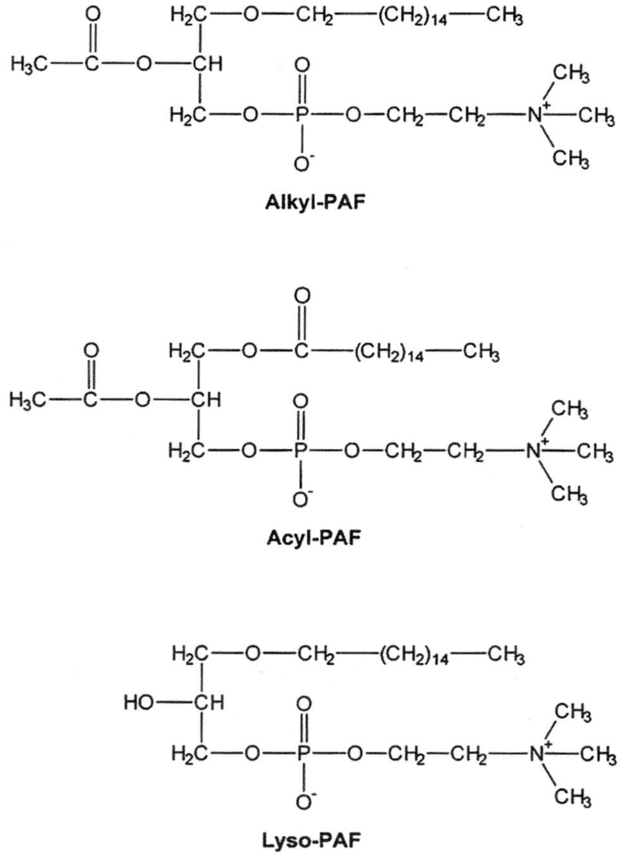

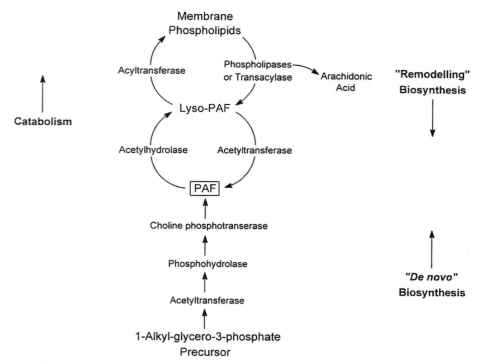

Alkyl-PAF

Acyl-PAF

Lyso-PAF

FIGURE 14-1 Molecular structures of representative PAF species.

FIGURE 14-2 Biosynthesis and catabolism of PAF.

1-alkyl-2-lyso-*sn*-glycero-3-phosphocholine, or lyso-PAF (see structure in Fig. 14-1). This reaction is catalyzed by a phospholipase A$_2$– (PLA$_2$) like enzyme that is selective for 2-arachidonoyl or 2-polyenoic precursors; inflammatory cells depleted of AA lose the ability to synthesize PAF by the remodeling process. The resultant lyso-PAF is then acetylated at the *sn*-2 position by an acetyl CoA–requiring lyso-PAF acetyltransferase. The acetyltransferase reaction appears to be an important regulatory step and is activated by calcium ions and protein kinase–mediated phosphorylation of the enzyme.

In that the initial *sn*-2 hydrolysis liberates a fatty acid, PAF synthesis can be accompanied by the release of free AA, which, as the substrate for the production of eicosanoids, could amplify the inflammatory effects of PAF. Platelet-activating factor production by neutrophils appears closely temporally linked to that of leukotriene B$_4$ (LTB$_4$),[13] and both PAF and LTB$_4$ production can be attenuated by single drugs, albeit ones with rather diverse anti-inflammatory actions, such as dexamethasone.[14] Eicosanoids do appear to be significant secondary mediators in many PAF-induced phenomena (see below), but the relationship between PAF and eicosanoid synthesis is probably quite complex. Exogenous PAF stimulates eicosanoid production,[15] and PAF may thus activate AA metabolism by paracrine or autocrine effects unrelated to the coliberation of AA and lyso-PAF by PLA$_2$. Furthermore, production of the lyso-PAF intermediate also can occur through the actions of a transacylase[16,17]; here, the *sn*-2 arachidonoyl moiety is not liberated as free AA, but rather is transferred to another lyso-phospholipid molecule. Inflammatory cells also can take up extracellular lyso-PAF. Transcellular traffic in preformed lyso-PAF could thus be an important "short-cut" to PAF synthesis at inflammatory sites in which, for example, activated platelets (that release considerable lyso-PAF) interact with granulocytes.[18]

De novo PAF synthesis (Fig. 14-2) begins with the 2-acetylation of a non-choline-containing PAF precursor, 1-alkyl-2-lyso-*sn*-glycero-3-phosphate. The acetyltransferase that catalyzes this step is dissimilar to the analogous enzyme of the remodeling pathway. The product of this reaction is dephosphorylated to 1-alkyl-2-acetyl-*sn*-glycerol, to which a phosphocholine polar head group is then transferred from CDP-choline via a choline phosphotransferase. The rate-limiting steps appear to be acetylation and the production of CDP-choline by cytidylyltransferase. In what may represent a counterregulatory mechanism, calcium ions, which stimulate remodeling synthesis of PAF, inhibit the enzymes of the de novo pathway.

Platelet-activating factor is rapidly catabolized to lyso-PAF in various tissues. In the isolated-perfused lung, type II pneumocytes and Clara cells seem to be the primary sites of action[19]; alveolar macrophages also take up and degrade PAF.[20] The primary catabolic enzyme is a ubiquitous, specific, highly active PAF acetylhydrolase, which catalyzes the hydrolytic removal of the *sn*-2 acetyl group. The enzyme exists in intracellular and extracellular forms, which differ in molecular weight and certain chemical properties, but have similar catalytic actions. Plasma concentrations of PAF hydrolytic activity can change in disease states; of note, PAF acetylhydrolase seems to be decreased in asthma.[21] The lyso-

PAF produced by PAF hydrolysis may be recycled into the membrane as alkylarachidonoylglycerophosphocholine (the starting material for remodeling biosynthesis of PAF) or be further degraded.

Cellular Sources of PAF

Platelet-activating factor is synthesized by a variety of inflammatory and noninflammatory cells.[11,12] Neutrophils synthesize large amounts of PAF in response to a number of stimuli, including calcium ionophore, opsonized zymosan, the chemotactic peptide *N*-formyl-L-methionyl-L-leucyl-L-phenylalanine (FMLP), and cytokines. While bacterial lipopolysaccaharide (LPS) does not cause neutrophils to produce PAF per se, it has a priming effect, heightening PAF production in response to subsequent stimulation with FMLP.[23] Activated eosinophils produce considerable amounts of PAF.[24] Alveolar macrophages release PAF in response to calcium ionophore or phagocytic stimuli,[25] including LPS.[26] In each of these cell types, alkyl-PAF production predominates. Anti-IgE–stimulated human lung mast cells synthesize considerable amounts of acyl-PAF.[5,6,27] The same may be true of basophils,[6] although the ability of human basophils to release PAF has not been universally observed. Airways epithelial cells have been observed to produce PAF.[28] Human endothelial cells exposed to calcium ionophore, thrombin, leukotrienes, and cytokines produce PAF, and acyl-PAF seems to predominate. While acyl-PAF is quantitatively the principal product, smaller amounts of the extremely potent alkyl-PAF may be more biologically significant. Platelets and lymphocytes seem to synthesize, at most, modest amounts of PAF.

PAF Receptors

Platelet-activating factor binds to specific, high-affinity sites, which are present in lung[29] as well as in many individual cell and tissue types, including inflammatory cells and smooth muscle.[30] The biologic actions of PAF appear related to the degree of receptor binding.[31] The receptors are membrane-bound proteins,[30] and the cDNA of lung, heart, and neutrophil receptors has been cloned.[32–34] The receptor may have multiple conformational states with varying affinity for PAF,[35] and receptor subclasses may mediate different aspects of the cellular response to PAF.[36] From a pharmacological point of view, however, there appears to be functionally only one type of high-affinity PAF receptor, which is subject to blockade by a variety of structurally diverse antagonists.

Rapid tachyphylaxis to the effects of PAF can occur,[1,37] but its mechanism is unclear. Various studies of effects of PAF on its receptors have reported a decrease in number of sites,[38] a decrease in binding avidity,[39] and a possible inhibition of receptor-response coupling.[40]

It is important to note that much PAF remains associated with its cells of origin[41–44] and that cells also can take up ambient PAF.[19,45] Intracellular PAF receptors exist,[46,47] and PAF may serve as an intracellular messenger modulating metabolic functions of inflammatory cells.[48–51] Anti-PAF

TABLE 14-1   PAF Receptor Antagonists

Type	Examples
Naturally Occurring	
Gingkgolides	BN 52020, BN 52021, BN 52022, BN 52063
Lignans	Kadsurenone, fargesin, veraguensin
Semisynthetic or synthetic	
Phospholipid analogs	CV-3988, CV-6209, E5880, SDZ 63-675, SRI 63-441
Lignan analogs	L-652,731, L-659,989
Benzodiazepine derivatives	Alprazolam, WEB 2086, WEB 2170, BN 50739
Calcium channel blockers	Verapamil, diltiazem
Imidazolyl derivatives	PCA-4248, UK-74,505, SDZ 64-412, BB-882
Pyridyl derivatives	RP 59227, RP 66681, SM-10661, ABT-299

drugs, which can traverse the plasma membrane, may thus have enhanced efficacy.

PAF Antagonists

Platelet-activating factor receptor antagonists have been the subject of extensive development and investigation, and copious review material on their structures and properties is available.[52,53] The principal classes of these compounds and representative members thereof are listed in Table 14-1. Typically, the drugs are competitive antagonists at the PAF receptor, although irreversible inhibitors exist.

Many of the naturally occurring drugs were isolated from Chinese traditional medicines. The gingkolides are terpenoids found in the tree *Gingko biloba* and are used in a chinese herbal medicine called *ba-guo* for the treatment of hypertension. Of them, gingkolide B (BN 52021) is the most potent. Kadsurenone was found in the herbal anti-asthma medicine *haifenteng*, a product of the plant *Piper futokadsurae*. Herbal products of the tree *Magnolia biondii* contain fargesin and related compounds. Modification of the structures of these natural compounds has led to the synthesis of many novel, potent PAF antagonists such as L-652,731 and L-659,989.

Many synthetic PAF receptor blockers exist. Some phospholipid analogs have mixed PAF agonist/antagonist properties; those considered of the greatest potential utility have minimal or no agonist properties. The discovery that certain hypnotic benzodiazepines are PAF antagonists has led to the development of a series of analogs whose relative hydrophilicity and limited affinity for the benzodiazepine receptor allows them to act as PAF antagonists with minimal or no sedating properties. The archetype of these compounds is WEB 2086. The calcium channel blockers verapamil and diltiazem also have PAF-blocking activity. While the class 1 imidazolyl calcium channel drugs (for example, nifedipine) lack significant action at the PAF receptor, imidazolyl PAF antagonists have been created. Pyridyl PAF antagonists are also the subjects of active research.

In light of the ability of PAF to stimulate the production of many other inflammatory mediators, mixed-function drugs may prove of use. Such drugs include the PAF antagonist/antihistamine SCH 37370, the PAF antagonist/5-lipoxygenase inhibitor L-653,150, and the PAF antagonist/antioxidant BN 50739. Compounds that interfere with the production of PAF through acetyltransferase inhibition are in development.

Biologic Effects of PAF

INDIVIDUAL CELL TYPES

The effects of PAF on various cell types are summarized in Table 14-2.[54] Species differences in these effects exist. Guinea pig and rabbit platelets respond to PAF more readily than human platelets, while rat platelets, which lack specific PAF surface receptors, are insensitive to PAF.[55,56]

The most significant action of PAF on the neutrophil may be its ability to enhance responsiveness to subsequent stim-

TABLE 14-2   Responses of Inflammatory Cells to PAF

Response	Neutrophil	Eosinophil	Macrophage	Platelet
Aggregation	+	?	~+	+
Adhesion	+	+	?	+
Arachidonate mobilization	+	+	+	+
↑ intracellular Ca^{2+}	+	+	+	+
Chemotaxis	+	+	+	—
Degranulation	±	+	—	+
Priming	+	+	+	—
Superoxide generation	±	+	+	?

SOURCE: Adapted with permission from Stewart.[54]

uli. Neutrophils primed by PAF at very low concentrations (as low as 10^{-12} molar) show significantly enhanced oxidant production,[57] production of eicosanoids,[58] and ability to damage cultured endothelium[59] in response to stimulation with FMLP and other agonists. Platelet-activating factor is a particularly effective stimulator of eosinophil chemotaxis,[60] degranulation,[61] and oxidant generation.[62] With specific regard to intrapulmonary cells, PAF enhances alveolar macrophage production of the proinflammatory cytokine tumor necrosis factor.[63]

Platelet-activating factor induces structural abnormalities in endothelial cells[64] and can increase endothelial permeability to macromolecules.[65] As noted above, stimulated endothelial cells produce PAF, and most of this PAF remains associated with the cells. The local presence of PAF at endothelial surfaces may promote adherence and activation of effector cells such as neutrophils[66] with possible subsequent endothelial damage.

There is evidence that PAF also may attract lymphocytes to the respiratory tract.[67] The effects of PAF on lymphocyte proliferation, however, are complex and probably indirect; both stimulation and suppression can be observed in different models.[68]

EFFECTS ON SPECIFIC TISSUES AND ORGANS

SYSTEMIC VASCULATURE

The ability to decrease systemic blood pressure is a hallmark of PAF.[3] While receptor-mediated, this effect is probably dependent in significant part on secondary mediators such as eicosanoids[69–71] or nitric oxide.[72,73] Platelet-activating factor-induced hypotension is complex. Decreased cardiac output in response to PAF is typical and results from myocardial depression[74–76] as well as reduced left ventricular filling pressure caused by peripheral vasodilation[69,72] or pulmonary vasoconstriction.[71,77] Platelet-activating factor is an arterial vasodilator in various in vitro and in situ preparations,[72,73,79] and systemic administration of PAF in vivo reduces systemic vascular resistance in rats and cats.[72,78,79] On the other hand, PAF-induced hypotension occurs despite increased systemic vascular resistance in dogs, pigs, and sheep.[69,70,75,77]

Platelet-activating factor can also cause vascular hyperpermeability at many sites.[80,81] This action has particularly significant potential pathogenetic significance in the pulmonary and bronchial vascular systems (see below).

PULMONARY VASCULATURE

Platelet-activating factor has profound effects on the pulmonary circulation, causing vasoconstriction and increased vascular permeability. In the isolated-perfused lung, PAF causes pulmonary hypertension, increased vascular resistance and lung edema which are both receptor-mediated[82,83] and dependent on production of thromboxane A_2[84] and leukotrienes C_4 and D_4.[85,86] Acute intravenous administration of PAF to rabbits causes inflammatory cell aggregation in the pulmonary microvasculature, vasoconstriction, and endothelial damage.[87] Chronic PAF administration to rabbits causes pulmonary hypertension and vascular narrowing[88,89]

as well as increased pulmonary vascular responsiveness to the vasoconstrictor agonists.[90]

In the intact sheep, PAF administration causes pulmonary hypertension and increased fluid and protein transit across the lung with a concomitant increase in production of thromboxane.[91–94] Cyclooxygenase or thromboxane synthase inhibition attenuates these effects. The source of the thromboxane in this model is unclear, as platelet depletion only modestly attenuates the hypertension, and granulocyte depletion has no effect.[91,92]

In porcine tissues in vitro, pulmonary venous smooth muscle appears more responsive than pulmonary arterial smooth muscle to the constrictive effects of PAF.[95] The increased hydrostatic driving pressure created by venoconstriction has been shown to be of considerable importance in the PAF-induced efflux of fluid and solute from the pulmonary vasculature.[96]

The effects of PAF on pulmonary vascular tone may be biphasic. At low concentrations, PAF dilates pulmonary vessels,[97] and PAF antagonists can increase pulmonary vascular resistance in the isolated perfused rat lung.[98] Low basal concentrations of PAF may thus serve to reduce pulmonary vascular pressures. As is typical of PAF, secondary mediators (e.g., endothelium-derived factors) are likely involved.[99]

AIRWAYS

Bronchial Vasculature

Platelet-activating factor potently enhances the leakage of plasma tracers from the microvasculature of the airways,[100,101] probably by a combination of increased permeability and constriction of postcapillary venules. Plasma leakage and airway edema induced by PAF could have significant effects on airways function (see below). While the effect of exogenous PAF is blocked by PAF-receptor antagonists,[100–102] the PAF-antagonist WEB 2086 failed to attenuate the increased dye leakage seen after administration of ovalbumin to sensitized guinea pigs.[103] Eicosanoids such as thromboxane A_2 may be involved in the vascular leak.[102,104]

Airways Epithelium

Exogenous PAF can induce inflammation and structural abnormalities of the epithelial lining of the airspace. Introduction of PAF into the airspace causes the accumulation of inflammatory cells[105,106] associated with damage to the airways mucosa.[105,107,108] Such phenomena can be attenuated by PAF-receptor antagonists[107,108] as well as various anti-asthma drugs.[109]

Platelet-activating factor has several actions that could increase the amount of fluid within the airway lumen, thus potentially increasing airways responsiveness and airway narrowing (see below). Platelet-activating factor can increase airway mucin secretions[110] and can diminish mucociliary transport.[111] Platelet-activating factor also increases transepithelial secretion of chloride ions (and hence water) in canine large airways.[112]

Airways Smooth Muscle

Exogenous PAF causes receptor-dependent activation of airways smooth muscle in vitro possibly through activation of platelets or other leukocytes[113,114] and is an in vivo bronchoconstrictor in various species[91,115] including humans. Release of secondary mediators such as serotonin and eicosanoids probably is involved.[116–120] Bronchoconstriction in humans caused by inhaled PAF is blunted by nedocromil, which inhibits mediator release[121] and also by PAF-receptor antagonists.[122,123]

Although PAF causes bronchoconstriction, PAF-induced airway narrowing is probably multifactorial in mechanism, involving activation of inflammatory cells, microvascular changes, and airway edema as well as smooth muscle activation per se. Human airway responses to inhaled PAF and to inhaled methacholine do not correlate strongly,[124,125] and PAF may, in fact, be a more effective bronchial provocative agent than methacholine in selected human subjects when responsiveness is measured by particularly sensitive means.[126] Inhaled salbutamol (which abolishes bronchoconstriction induced by methacholine) has only a limited ability to reduce PAF-induced airway narrowing in normal humans.[127]

Airways Responsiveness

Hyperresponsiveness of the airways to nonantigenic agonists such as histamine or methacholine (i.e., "nonspecific" airways hyperresponsiveness, or NAHR), is a phenomenon frequently associated with asthma.[128] In addition to its ability to cause bronchoconstriction per se, PAF can induce NAHR in various nonhuman species[129–131]; this effect is blocked by PAF antagonists.[131,132] The increased responsiveness is attenuated by broadly acting anti-inflammatory drugs such as nedocromil[133] and corticosteroids.[134] Inflammatory cell activation by PAF[135,136] with the release of secondary mediators is apparently important.[129,137]

Post-PAF NAHR might occur by at least three mechanisms, all of which are speculative. First, PAF could enhance the responsiveness of the smooth muscle itself. Platelet-activating factor acutely increases the contractile response of airway smooth muscle in vitro or in situ to other stimuli,[138,139] but in vivo studies of PAF administration with subsequent isolation of airways tissues for in vitro analysis have shown no differences in responsiveness to contractile agonists between tissues from PAF-treated animals and controls.[140,141] Prior exposure to PAF does not alter the affinity or density of lung muscarinic receptors, histamine H_1-receptors, or β-adrenergic receptors in vitro,[140,142,143] although contradictory data for the β-adrenergic receptor exist.[144]

Second, by damaging the airways epithelium, PAF may increase the access of inhaled agonists to their sites of action, although, in various studies, airways permeability has not been observed to correlate well with responsiveness to inhaled agonists.[145,146] Epithelial damage also might deprive the airways of substances such as certain eicosanoids (such as prostaglandin E_2), nitric oxide, or the tachykinin-degrading enzyme neutral endopeptidase, which might attenuate bronchoconstriction.

Third, PAF may cause edema of the airway lining within the perimeter of the smooth muscle. This could occur as a result of altered bronchial vascular tone (i.e., engorgement of small vessels as a result of postcapillary venular constric-

tion) and of vascular hyperpermeability with resultant intraluminal, mucosal, and submucosal edema. The thickened airway lining, consisting principally of water, would be essentially incompressible, and thus would tend to amplify the degree of luminal narrowing caused by any given degree of smooth muscle tone.[128,147,148]

Studies of the ability of inhaled PAF to induce or increase NAHR in humans have produced mixed results. The original observation that inhaled PAF could induce significant subsequent NAHR in normal humans[124] has been reproduced[114,126,127,149,150] and contradicted[151–155] with roughly equal frequency. In studies in which induced NAHR occurs, it appears to be blocked well by nedocromil,[150] only weakly by salbutamol,[127] and not at all by theophylline.[149] Several studies concur that inhaled PAF does not increase the degree of NAHR in asthmatics.[125,126,153] Platelet-activating factor antagonists also have failed to modify consistently the NAHR of asthmatics, as is discussed below.

It is important to note that the variable results with regard to PAF and NAHR in humans do not, specifically exclude a potential role for PAF in asthma. Studies on the effects of isolated exposures to inhaled PAF on airway responsiveness do not replicate NAHR in real life, which involves prolonged action by responsiveness-enhancing (probably inflammatory) stimuli at specific loci in the bronchial microenvironment.[128] While NAHR typically accompanies asthma,[156,157] it also occurs in a significant portion of the "normal" asymptomatic population,[158,159] and some studies have failed to show a tightly coupled relationship between the degree of NAHR and symptoms in asthmatics.[160–163] Nonspecific airway hyperresponsiveness may be better viewed as a frequent laboratory marker of asthma, but one that is a result, rather than the cause, of the disease.

The Role of PAF in Specific Diseases

ASTHMA

Platelet-activating factor has proinflammatory properties that potentially could induce asthma. These include recruitment of inflammatory cells to the airspace, stimulation of production of various mediators and oxidants, activation of airways smooth muscle, injury to the bronchial epithelium, stimulation of airways secretions, impairment of mucociliary clearance, and induction of bronchial plasma leakage and edema. Intravenous administration of PAF to guinea pigs induces morphologic changes in the lungs, such as increased infiltration by eosinophils and mast cells, submucosal airways edema, muscular hypertrophy, and contraction of bronchi and bronchioli,[135,164] which are similar to those observed in human asthma.[165]

There is considerable circumstantial evidence that human asthma is accompanied by heightened PAF activity. While assaying PAF in biologic fluids is a task fraught with difficulty, PAF has been detected in bronchoalveolar lavage fluid obtained from asthmatics, while the lavages of control patients and patients with emphysema do not appear to contain PAF.[67] Furthermore, blood concentrations of PAF in asthmatics increase during symptomatic episodes[166,167] or after inhaled antigen challenge,[168] and decrease after successful asthma immunotherapy.[166] As noted above, symptomatic asthmatics also seem to have reduced blood concentrations of the catabolic enzyme PAF acetylhydrolase.[21] Lung tissue from asthmatics contains increased amounts of PAF-receptor mRNA,[169] which could reflect amplification of the actions of PAF. Neutrophils and alveolar macrophages from asthmatics also appear to have a heightened ability to release PAF.[166,170] Eosinophils from these individuals also have an increased chemotactic response to PAF.[171] Inhalation of PAF by asthmatics causes bronchospasm, hypoxemia, and ventilation-perfusion abnormalities.[172]

Animal studies of acute antigen-induced bronchospasm and the subsequent development of NAHR are a frequently employed model of human asthma. Such antigenic stimulation results in the production of PAF (and other mediators) in the lung,[173] and induction of tachyphylaxis by serial administration of PAF reduces the bronchospastic response of sensitized guinea pigs to antigen challenge.[174] Gingkolide PAF antagonists such as BN 52021 and BN 52063 reduce bronchoconstriction and airways hyperresponsiveness caused by antigen challenge in sensitized guinea pigs and rabbits.[175–178] Both the heterocyclic antagonists SDZ 64-412 and SM-10661 and the phospholipid analog CV-6209 block antigen-induced NAHR in guinea pigs.[179,180] The benzodiazepine derivative WEB 2086 exerts similar effects in sheep, reducing antigen-induced late (but not early) bronchoconstriction and subsequent NAHR.[181,182] Efficacy may be less against non-antigen-induced phenomena, as the lignan derivative L-659,989 failed to reduce airways hyperresponsiveness induced by ozone exposure in guinea pigs.[183]

An early pilot study in human asthmatics showed that three days of therapy with BN 52063 reduced early bronchoconstriction after antigen challenge, and there was a tendency toward some reduction of subsequent airways hyperresponsiveness.[184] BN 52021 also appeared to blunt allergen-induced bronchospasm, but in only three of seven patients tested; the response to methacholine was unaffected.[185] Other studies to date have been less encouraging. BN 52063 did not reduce bronchospasm induced by isocapnic hyperventilation of cold, dry air or by exercise.[186] UK-74,505 did not alter antigen-induced spirometric responses or hyperresponsiveness to inhaled histamine in eight asthmatics.[187] A crossover study of one week's therapy with WEB 2086 in eight atopic asthmatics showed no benefit from the drug in terms of attenuation of bronchospasm or increased histamine responsiveness after antigen inhalation.[188] In a group of atopic asthmatics on stable doses of inhaled corticosteroids, the addition of WEB 2086 to the regimen for six weeks did not enhance the ability of patients to tolerate reduced corticosteroid doses.[189]

Thus, despite a compelling theoretical role for PAF drugs in asthma, human studies remain unconvincing. All of these trials, however, are preliminary. As is the case with inhaled corticosteroids, therapy for weeks or months might be required to achieve maximum benefit. Longer trials or trials using drugs that are more potent, penetrate the intracellular milieu more effectively, or have mixed anti-inflammatory actions, may be more revealing.

ACUTE RESPIRATORY DISTRESS SYNDROME AND SEPSIS

The acute respiratory distress syndrome (ARDS)* is associated with high-permeability pulmonary edema, pulmonary hypertension, reduced lung compliance, and increased airways resistance.[191–194] Animal models of the syndrome are associated with increased airways responsiveness,[195] and such hyperresponsiveness has been documented in human ARDS survivors.[196] A role for PAF in all of these phenomena can be envisioned. Acute respiratory distress syndrome is the pulmonary manifestation of a systemic inflammatory state, which can be induced by a variety of insults.[197] The most common and most lethal cause of ARDS is sepsis,[198,199] and lung dysfunction is detectable by sensitive measures in most septic patients.[200] In this section, ARDS and gram-negative sepsis generally are treated interchangeably.

Administration of exogenous PAF produces physiologic abnormalities that resemble ARDS in isolated-perfused lungs[84] and in intact animals.[91–93] Administration of LPS to animals results in increased PAF production,[26,201] and increased concentrations of PAF have been noted in bronchoalveolar lavage specimens from ARDS patients.[202] Platelet-activating factor thus has been frequently incriminated in the genesis of septic lung injury and ARDS. The injurious effects of LPS and PAF on the lung appear, in fact, to be synergistic.[203,204] Platelet-activating factor activates secondary mechanisms of injury, which have been of particular interest in the study of septic injury, such as eicosanoid production (see above), production of proinflammatory cytokines,[204–206] and the induction of nitric oxide synthase.[207] Platelet-activating factor seems to be released early in the complex cascade of mediators initiated by LPS exposure.[208] It thus may be a key mediator in ARDS and sepsis, but the therapeutic "window of opportunity" for the use of anti-PAF drugs after the initial insult may be brief.

Numerous studies have demonstrated the ability of an assortment of PAF antagonists to attenuate various aspects of LPS-induced lung injury in rats,[201,204,209] guinea pigs and hamsters,[210,211] sheep,[212,213] and swine.[214–217] Such drugs have also had beneficial effects in studies of cytokine-induced lung dysfunction, another prevalent model of septic injury.[218–220] In a large prospective trial in human sepsis, the gingolide anti-PAF drug BN 52021 appeared protective only in the subset of subjects with documented gram-negative infection.[221] A follow-up trial is currently in progress. Trials involving more potent and selective PAF antagonists such as ABT-299 and BB-882[222–224] may yield a clear insight into the utility of PAF-receptor antagonists in sepsis and ARDS.

Conclusion

Platelet-activating factor has a wide variety of potent proinflammatory effects in the lung, and a convincing theoretical case can be made for its involvement in various diseases,

* The older term "adult respiratory distress syndrome" is a misnomer, in that the syndrome clearly can occur in children. A recent international consensus conference concluded that the designation "acute" is preferable.[190]

including asthma and ARDS. None of the currently available PAF antagonists has, to date, proved categorically useful in humans. Such proof may await larger and more prolonged trials, particularly those involving very potent PAF antagonists and novel drugs such as PAF acetyltransferase inhibitors.

References

1. Benveniste J, Henson PM, Cochrane CG: Leukocyte-dependent histamine release from rabbit platelets. The role of IgE, basophils, and a platelet-activating factor. *J Exp Med* 1972; 136:1356.
2. Demopoulos CA, Pinckard RN, Hanahan DJ: Platelet-activating factor. Evidence for 1-*O*-alkyl-2-acetyl-*sn*-glyceryl-3-phosphorylcholine as the active component (a new class of lipid chemical mediators). *J Biol Chem* 1979; 254:9355.
3. Blank ML, Snyder F, Byers LW, et al.: Antihypertensive activity of an alkyl ether analog of phosphatidylcholine. *Biochem Biophys Res Commun* 1979; 90:1194.
4. McManus LM, Woodard DS, Deavers SI, Pinckard RN: PAF molecular heterogeneity: pathobiological implications. *Lab Invest* 1993; 69:639.
5. Triggiani M, Hubbard WC, Chilton FH: Synthesis of 1-acyl-2-acetyl-*sn*-glycero-3-phosphocholine by an enriched preparation of the human lung mast cell. *J Immunol* 1990; 144:4773.
6. Triggiani M, Schleimer RP, Warner JA, Chilton FH: Differential synthesis of 1-acyl-2-acetyl-*sn*-glycero-3-phosphocholine and platelet-activating factor by human inflammatory cells. *J Immunol* 1991; 147:660.
7. Clay KL, Johnson C, Worthen GS: Biosynthesis of platelet activating factor and 1-*O*-acyl analogues by endothelial cells. *Biochim Biophys Acta* 1991; 1094:43.
8. Triggiani M, Goldman DW, Chilton FH: Biological effects of 1-acyl-2-acetyl-*sn*-glycero-3-phosphocholine in the human neutrophil. *Biochim Biophys Acta* 1991; 1084:41.
9. Pinckard RN, Showell HJ, Castillo R, et al.: Differential responsiveness of human neutrophils to the autocrine actions of 1-*O*-alkyl-homologs and 1-acyl analogs of platelet-activating factor. *J Immunol* 1992; 148:3528.
10. Columbo M, Horowitz EM, Patella V, et al.: A comparative study of the effects of 1-acyl-2-*sn*-glycero-3-phosphocholine and platelet activating factor on histamine and leukotriene C_4 release from human leukocytes. *J Allergy Clin Immunol* 1993; 92:325.
11. Snyder F: Platelet-activating factor and related acetylated lipids as potent biologically active cellular mediators. *Am J Physiol* 1990; 259:C697.
12. Snyder F: Biosynthesis and catabolism of platelet-activating factor, in Cunningham FM (ed): *Lipid Mediators*. London, Academic Press, 1994:181–192.
13. Sisson JH, Prescott SM, McIntyre TM, Zimmerman GA: Production of platelet-activating factor by stimulated human polymorphonuclear leukocytes. Correlation of synthesis with release, functional events, and leukotriene B_4 metabolism. *J Immunol* 1987; 138:3918.
14. Fradin A, Rothhut B, Poincelot-Canton B, et al.: Inhibition of eicosanoid and PAF formation by dexamethasone in rat inflammatory polymorphonuclear neutrophils may implicate lipocortin 's'. *Biochim Biophys Acta* 1988; 963:248.
15. Lin AH, Morton DR, Gorman RR: Acetyl glyceryl ether phosphorylcholine stimulates leukotriene B_4 synthesis in human polymorphonuclear leukocytes. *J Clin Invest* 1982; 70:1058.
16. Uemura Y, Lee TC, Snyder F: A coenzyme A–independent transacylase is linked to the formation of platelet-activating factor (PAF) by generating the lyso-PAF intermediate in the remodeling pathway. *J Biol Chem* 1991; 266:8268.
17. Venable ME, Nieto ML, Schmitt JD, Wykle RL: Conversion of 1-*O*-[^{3}H]alkyl-2-arachidonoyl-*sn*-glycero-3-phosphorylcholine to lyso platelet-activating factor by the CoA-independent transacylase in membrane fractions of human neutrophils. *J Biol Chem* 1991; 266:18691.
18. Coeffier E, Delautier D, Le Couedic JP, et al.: Cooperation between platelets and neutrophils for paf-acether (platelet-activating factor) formation. *J Leukoc Biol* 1990; 47:234.
19. Haroldsen PE, Voelkel NF, Henson JE, et al.: Metabolism of platelet-activating factor in isolated perfused rat lung. *J Clin Invest* 1987; 79:1860.
20. Robinson M, Snyder F: Metabolism of platelet-activating factor by rat alveolar macrophages: lyso-PAF as an obligatory intermediate in the formation of alkylarachidonoyl glycerophosphocholine species. *Biochim Biophys Acta* 1985; 837:52.
21. Miwa M, Miyake T, Yamanaka T, et al.: Characterization of serum platelet-activating factor (PAF) acetylhydrolase. Correlation between deficiency of serum PAF acetylhydrolase and respiratory symptoms in asthmatic children. *J Clin Invest* 1988; 82:1983.
22. Bratton DL, Clay KL, Henson PM: Cellular sources of platelet-activating factor and related lipids, in Cunningham FM (ed): *Lipid Mediators*. London, Academic Press, 1994:193–219.
23. Worthen GS, Seccombe JF, Clay KL, et al.: The priming of neutrophils by lipopolysaccharide for production of intracellular platelet-activating factor. Potential role in mediation of enhanced superoxide secretion. *J Immunol* 1988; 140:3553.
24. Lee T, Lenihan DJ, Malone B, et al.: Increased biosynthesis of platelet-activating factor in activated human eosinophils. *J Biol Chem* 1984; 259:5526.
25. Arnoux B, Duval D, Benveniste J: Release of platelet-activating factor (PAF-acether) from alveolar macrophages by the calcium ionophore A23187 and phagocytosis. *Eur J Clin Invest* 1980; 10:437.
26. Rylander R, Beijer L: Inhalation of endotoxin stimulates alveolar macrophage production of platelet-activating factor. *Am Rev Respir Dis* 1987; 135:83.
27. Schleimer RP, MacGlashan DW, Jr., Peters SP, et al.: Characterization of inflammatory mediator release from purified human lung mast cells. *Am Rev Respir Dis* 1986; 133:614.
28. Holtzman MJ, Ferdman B, Bohrer A, Turk J: Synthesis of the 1-*O*-hexadecyl molecular species of platelet-activating factor by airway epithelial and vascular endothelial cells. *Biochem Biophys Res Commun* 1991; 177:357.
29. Hwang SB, Lam MH, Shen TY: Specific binding sites for platelet-activating factor in human lung tissues. *Biochem Biophys Res Commun* 1985; 128:972.
30. Hwang SB, Lee CS, Cheah MJ, Shen TY: Specific receptor sites for 1-*O*-alkyl-2-*O*-acetyl-*sn*-glycero-3-phosphocholine (platelet activating factor) on rabbit platelet and guinea pig smooth muscle membranes. *Biochemistry* 1983; 22:4756.
31. Hwang SB, Li CL, Lam MH, Shen TY: Characterization of cutaneous vascular permeability induced by platelet-activating factor in guinea pigs and rats and its inhibition by a platelet-activating factor receptor antagonist. *Lab Invest* 1985; 52:617.
32. Honda Z, Nakamura M, Miki I, et al.: Cloning by functional expression of platelet-activating factor receptor from guinea-pig lung. *Nature* 1991; 349:342.
33. Nakamura M, Honda Z, Izumi T, et al.: Molecular cloning and expression of platelet-activating factor receptor from human leukocytes. *J Biol Chem* 1991; 266:20400.

34. Sugimoto T, Tsuchimochi H, McGregor CG, et al.: Molecular cloning and characterization of the platelet-activating factor receptor gene expressed in the human heart. *Biochem Biophys Res Commun* 1992; 189:617.

35. Hwang SB, Lam MH: L-659,989: a useful probe in the detection of multiple conformational states of PAF receptors. *Lipids* 1991; 26:1148.

36. Kroegel C, Yukawa T, Westwick J, Barnes PJ: Evidence for two platelet activating factor receptors on eosinophils: dissociation between PAF-induced intracellular calcium mobilization degranulation and superoxides anion generation in eosinophils. *Biochem Biophys Res Commun* 1989; 162:511.

37. O'Flaherty JT, Lees CJ, Miller CH, et al.: Selective desensitization of neutrophils: further studies with 1-O-alkyl-sn-glycero-3-phosphocholine analogues. *J Immunol* 1981; 127:731.

38. Kloprogge E, Akkerman JW: Binding kinetics of PAF-acether (1-O-alkyl-2-acetyl-sn-glycero-3-phosphocholine) to intact human platelets. *Biochem J* 1984; 223:901.

39. Chesney CM, Pifer DD, Huch KM: Desensitization of human platelets by platelet activating factor. *Biochem Biophys Res Commun* 1985; 127:24.

40. Homma H, Hanahan DJ: Attenuation of platelet activating factor (PAF)-induced stimulation of rabbit platelet GTPase by phorbol ester, dibutyryl cAMP, and desensitization: concomitant effects on PAF receptor binding characteristics. *Arch Biochem Biophys* 1988; 262:32.

41. Prescott SM, Zimmerman GA, McIntyre TM: Human endothelial cells in culture produce platelet-activating factor (1-alkyl-2-acetyl-sn-glycero-3-phosphocholine) when stimulated with thrombin. *Proc Natl Acad Sci USA* 1984; 81:3534.

42. Lynch JM, Henson PM: The intracellular retention of newly synthesized platelet-activating factor. *J Immunol* 1986; 137:2653.

43. Cluzel M, Undem BJ, Chilton FH: Release of platelet-activating factor and the metabolism of leukotriene B_4 by the human neutrophil when studied in a cell superfusion model. *J Immunol* 1989; 143:3659.

44. Burke LA, Crea AE, Wilkinson JR, et al.: Comparison of the generation of platelet-activating factor and leukotriene C_4 in human eosinophils stimulated by unopsonized zymosan and by the calcium ionophore A23187: the effects of nedocromil sodium. *J Allergy Clin Immunol* 1990; 85:26.

45. Bratton DL, Dreyer E, Kailey JM, et al.: The mechanism of internalization of platelet-activating factor in activated human neutrophils. Enhanced transbilayer movement across the plasma membrane. *J Immunol* 1992; 148:514.

46. Marcheselli VL, Rossowska MJ, Domingo MT, et al.: Distinct platelet-activating factor binding sites in synaptic endings and in intracellular membranes of rat cerebral cortex. *J Biol Chem* 1990; 265:9140.

47. Hwang SB: Function and regulation of extracellular and intracellular receptors of platelet activating factor. *Ann N Y Acad Sci* 1991; 629:217.

48. Stewart AG, Phillips WA: Intracellular platelet-activating factor regulates eicosanoid generation in guinea-pig resident peritoneal macrophages. *Br J Pharmacol* 1989; 98:141.

49. Stewart AG, Dubbin PN, Harris T, Dusting GJ: Evidence for an intracellular action of platelet-activating factor in bovine cultured aortic endothelial cells. *Br J Pharmacol* 1989; 96:503.

50. Tool AT, Verhoeven AJ, Roos D, Koenderman L: Platelet-activating factor (PAF) acts as an intercellular messenger in the changes of cytosolic free Ca^{2+} in human neutrophils induced by opsonized particles. *FEBS Lett* 1989; 259:209.

51. Stewart AG, Dubbin PN, Harris T, Dusting GJ: Platelet-activating factor may act as a second messenger in the release of icosanoids and superoxide anions from leukocytes and endothelial cells. *Proc Natl Acad Sci USA* 1990; 87:3215.

52. Hwang SB: Platelet-activating factor: Receptors and receptor antagonists, in Cunningham FM (ed): *Lipid Mediators*. London, Academic Press, 1994:297–360.

53. Koltai M, Guinot P, Hosford D, Braquet PG: Platelet-activating factor antagonists: scientific background and possible clinical applications. *Adv Pharmacol* 1994; 28:81.

54. Stewart AG: Biological properties of platelet-activating factor, in Cunningham FM (ed): *Lipid Mediators*. London, Academic Press, 1994:221–295.

55. Cargill DI, Cohen DS, Van Valen RG, et al.: Aggregation, release and desensitization induced in platelets from five species by platelet activating factor (PAF). *Thromb Haemost* 1983; 49:204.

56. Inarrea P, Gomez-Cambronero J, Nieto M, Crespo MS: Characteristics of the binding of platelet-activating factor to platelets of different animal species. *Eur J Pharmacol* 1984; 105:309.

57. Dewald B, Baggiolini M: Activation of NADPH oxidase in human neutrophils. Synergism between fMLP and the neutrophil products PAF and LTB_4. *Biochem Biophys Res Commun* 1985; 128:297.

58. Tanizawa H, Tai HH: Synergism between chemotactic peptide and platelet-activating factor in stimulating thromboxane B_2 and leukotriene B_4 biosynthesis in human neutrophils. *Biochem Pharmacol* 1989; 38:2559.

59. Vercellotti GM, Yin HQ, Gustafson KS, et al.: Platelet-activating factor primes neutrophil responses to agonists: role in promoting neutrophil-mediated endothelial damage. *Blood* 1988; 71:1100.

60. Wardlaw AJ, Moqbel R, Cromwell O, Kay AB: Platelet-activating factor. A potent chemotactic and chemokinetic factor for human eosinophils. *J Clin Invest* 1986; 78:1701.

61. Kroegel C, Yukawa T, Dent G, et al.: Stimulation of degranulation from human eosinophils by platelet-activating factor. *J Immunol* 1989; 142:3518.

62. Zoratti EM, Sedgwick JB, Vrtis RR, Busse WW: The effect of platelet-activating factor on the generation of superoxide anion in human eosinophils and neutrophils. *J Allergy Clin Immunol* 1991; 88:749.

63. Dubois C, Bissonnette E, Rola-Pleszczynski M: Platelet-activating factor (PAF) enhances tumor necrosis factor production by alveolar macrophages. Prevention by PAF receptor antagonists and lipoxygenase inhibitors. *J Immunol* 1989; 143:964.

64. Grigorian GY, Ryan US: Platelet-activating factor effects on bovine pulmonary artery endothelial cells. *Circ Res* 1987; 61:389.

65. Handley DA, Arbeeny CM, Lee ML, et al.: Effect of platelet activating factor on endothelial permeability to plasma macromolecules. *Immunopharmacology* 1984; 8:137.

66. Lewis MS, Whatley RE, Cain P, et al.: Hydrogen peroxide stimulates the synthesis of platelet-activating factor by endothelium and induces endothelial cell-dependent neutrophil adhesion. *J Clin Invest* 1988; 82:2045.

67. Stenton SC, Court EN, Kingston WP, et al.: Platelet-activating factor in bronchoalveolar lavage fluid from asthmatic subjects. *Eur Respir J* 1990; 3:408.

68. Denizot Y, Dupuis F, Praloran V: Effects of platelet-activating factor on human T and B cells—an overview. *Res Immunol* 1994; 145:109.

69. Yamanaka S, Miura K, Yukimura T, et al.: Putative mechanism of hypotensive action of platelet-activating factor in dogs. *Circ Res* 1992; 70:893.

70. Olson NC, Kruse-Elliott KT, Johnson LW: Effect of 5-lipoxygenase and cyclooxygenase blockade on porcine hemodynamics during continuous infusion of platelet-activating factor. *Prostaglandins Leukot Essent Fatty Acids* 1993; 49:549.

71. Laurindo FR, Goldstein RE, Davenport NJ, et al.: Mechanisms of hypotension produced by platelet-activating factor. *J Appl Physiol* 1989; 66:2681.

72. Bellan JA, Minkes RK, Hood JS, et al.: Analysis of pulmonary and systemic vascular responses to platelet-activating factor in the cat. *Am J Physiol* 1992; 263:H234.

73. Moritoki H, Hisayama T, Takeuchi S, et al.: Involvement of nitric oxide pathway in the PAF-induced relaxation of rat thoracic aorta. *Br J Pharmacol* 1992; 107:196.

74. Levi R, Burke JA, Guo ZG, et al.: Acetyl glyceryl ether phosphorylcholine (AGEPC). A putative mediator of cardiac anaphylaxis in the guinea pig. *Circ Res* 1984; 54:117.

75. Kenzora JL, Perez JE, Bergmann SR, Lange LG: Effects of acetyl glyceryl ether of phosphorylcholine (platelet activating factor) on ventricular preload, afterload, and contractility in dogs. *J Clin Invest* 1984; 74:1193.

76. Sybertz EJ, Watkins RW, Baum T, et al.: Cardiac, coronary and peripheral vascular effects of acetyl glyceryl ether phosphoryl choline in the anesthetized dog. *J Pharmacol Exp Ther* 1985; 232:156.

77. Toyofuku T, Kobayashi T, Koyama S, Kusama S: Pulmonary vascular response to platelet-activating factor in conscious sheep. *Am J Physiol* 1988; 255:H434.

78. Sanchez Crespo M, Alonso F, Inarrea P, Egido J: Non-platelet-mediated vascular actions of 1-O-alkyl-2-acetyl-sn-3-glyceryl phosphorycholine (a synthetic PAF). *Agents Actions* 1981; 11:565.

79. Siren AL, Feuerstein G: Effects of PAF and BN 52021 on cardiac function and regional blood flow in conscious rats. *Am J Physiol* 1989; 257:H25.

80. Morley J, Page CP, Paul W: Inflammatory actions of platelet-activating factor (Pafacether) in guinea-pig skin. *Br J Pharmacol* 1983; 80:503.

81. Sirois MG, Jancar S, Braquet P, et al.: PAF increases vascular permeability in selected tissues: effect of BN-52021 and L-655,240. *Prostaglandins* 1988; 36:631.

82. Casals-Stenzel J, Franke J, Friedrich T, Lichey J: Bronchial and vascular effects of Paf in the rat isolated lung are completely blocked by WEB 2086, a novel specific Paf antagonist. *Br J Pharmacol* 1987; 91:799.

83. Imai T, Vercellotti GM, Moldow CF, et al.: Pulmonary hypertension and edema induced by platelet-activating factor in isolated, perfused rat lungs are blocked by BN52021. *J Lab Clin Med* 1988; 111:211.

84. Heffner JE, Shoemaker SA, Canham EM, et al.: Acetyl glyceryl ether phosphorylcholine-stimulated human platelets cause pulmonary hypertension and edema in isolated rabbit lungs. Role of thromboxane A$_2$. *J Clin Invest* 1983; 71:351.

85. Voelkel NF, Worthen S, Reeves JT, et al.: Nonimmunological production of leukotrienes induced by platelet-activating factor. *Science* 1982; 218:286.

86. Davidson D, Drafta D: Prolonged pulmonary hypertension caused by platelet-activating factor and leukotriene C$_4$ in the rat lung. *J Appl Physiol* 1992; 73:955.

87. McManus LM, Pinckard RN: Kinetics of acetyl glyceryl ether phosphorylcholine (AGEPC)-induced acute lung alterations in the rabbit. *Am J Pathol* 1985; 121:55.

88. Ohar JA, Pyle JA, Waller KS, et al.: A rabbit model of pulmonary hypertension induced by the synthetic platelet-activating factor acetylglyceryl ether phosphorylcholine. *Am Rev Respir Dis* 1990; 141:104.

89. Ohar JA, Waller KS, DeMello D, Lagunoff D: Administration of chronic intravenous platelet-activating factor induces pulmonary arterial atrophy and hypertension in rabbits. *Lab Invest* 1991; 65:451.

90. Ohar JA, Waller KS, Dahms TE: Platelet-activating factor induces selective pulmonary arterial hyperreactivity in isolated perfused rabbit lungs. *Am Rev Respir Dis* 1993; 148:158.

91. Christman BW, Lefferts PL, King GA, Snapper JR: Role of circulating platelets and granulocytes in PAF-induced pulmonary dysfunction in awake sheep. *J Appl Physiol* 1988; 64:2033.

92. Burhop KE, Garcia JG, Selig WM, et al.: Platelet-activating factor increases lung vascular permeability to protein. *J Appl Physiol* 1986; 61:2210.

93. Burhop KE, van der Zee H, Bizios R, et al.: Pulmonary vascular response to platelet-activating factor in awake sheep and the role of cyclooxygenase metabolites. *Am Rev Respir Dis* 1986; 134:548.

94. Trochtenberg DS, Lefferts PL, King GA, et al.: Effects of thromboxane synthase and cyclooxygenase inhibition on PAF-induced changes in lung function and arachidonic acid metabolism. *Prostaglandins* 1992; 44:555.

95. Pritze S, Simmet T, Peskar BA: Effect of platelet-activating factor on porcine pulmonary blood vessels in vitro. *Naunyn Schmiedebergs Arch Pharmacol* 1991; 344:495.

96. Sakai A, Chang SW, Voelkel NF: Importance of vasoconstriction in lipid mediator–induced pulmonary edema. *J Appl Physiol* 1989; 66:2667.

97. Voelkel NF, Chang SW, Pfeffer KD, et al.: PAF antagonists: different effects on platelets, neutrophils, guinea pig ileum and PAF-induced vasodilation in isolated rat lung. *Prostaglandins* 1986; 32:359.

98. Haynes J, Chang SW, Morris KG, Voelkel NF: Platelet-activating factor antagonists increase vascular reactivity in perfused rat lungs. *J Appl Physiol* 1988; 65:1921.

99. McMurtry IF, Morris KG: Platelet-activating factor causes pulmonary vasodilation in the rat. *Am Rev Respir Dis* 1986; 134:757.

100. Evans TW, Chung KF, Rogers DF, Barnes PJ: Effect of platelet-activating factor on airway vascular permeability: possible mechanisms. *J Appl Physiol* 1987; 63:479.

101. O'Donnell SR, Erjefalt I, Persson CG: Early and late tracheobronchial plasma exudation by platelet-activating factor administered to the airway mucosal surface in guinea pigs: effects of WEB 2086 and enprofylline. *J Pharmacol Exp Ther* 1990; 254:65.

102. Sirois MG, Plante GE, Braquet P, Sirois P: Role of eicosanoids in PAF-induced increases of the vascular permeability in rat airways. *Br J Pharmacol* 1990; 101:896.

103. Evans TW, Dent G, Rogers DF, et al.: Effect of a Paf antagonist, WEB 2086, on airway microvascular leakage in the guinea-pig and platelet aggregation in man. *Br J Pharmacol* 1988; 94:164.

104. Tokuyama K, Lotvall JO, Morikawa A, et al.: Role of thromboxane A$_2$ in airway microvascular leakage induced by inhaled platelet-activating factor. *J Appl Physiol* 1991; 71:1729.

105. Camussi G, Pawlowski I, Tetta C, et al.: Acute lung inflammation induced in the rabbit by local instillation of 1-O-octadecyl-2-acetyl-sn-glyceryl-3-phosphorylcholine or of native platelet-activating factor. *Am J Pathol* 1983; 112:78.

106. Wardlaw AJ, Chung KF, Moqbel R, et al.: Effects of inhaled PAF in humans on circulating and bronchoalveolar lavage fluid neutrophils. Relationship to bronchoconstriction and changes in airway responsiveness. *Am Rev Respir Dis* 1990; 141:386.

107. Lellouch-Tubiana A, Lefort J, Simon MT, et al.: Eosinophil recruitment into guinea pig lungs after PAF-acether and allergen administration. Modulation by prostacyclin, platelet depletion, and selective antagonists. *Am Rev Respir Dis* 1988; 137:948.

108. Takizawa H, Ishii A, Suzuki S, et al.: Bronchoconstriction induced by platelet-activating factor in the guinea pig and its inhibition by CV-3988, a PAF antagonist: serial changes in findings of lung histology and bronchoalveolar lavage cell population. *Int Arch Allergy Appl Immunol* 1988; 86:375.

109. Sanjar S, Aoki S, Boubekeur K, et al.: Eosinophil accumulation in pulmonary airways of guinea-pigs induced by exposure to an aerosol of platelet-activating factor: effect of anti-asthma drugs. *Br J Pharmacol* 1990; 99:267.

110. Goswami SK, Ohashi M, Stathas P, Marom ZM: Platelet-activating factor stimulates secretion of respiratory glycoconjugate from human airways in culture. *J Allergy Clin Immunol* 1989; 84:726.

111. Nieminen MM, Moilanen EK, Nyholm JE, et al.: Platelet-activating factor impairs mucociliary transport and increases plasma leukotriene B_4 in man. *Eur Respir J* 1991; 4:551.

112. Tamaoki J, Sakai N, Isono K, et al.: Effects of platelet-activating factor on bioelectric properties of cultured tracheal and bronchial epithelia. *J Allergy Clin Immunol* 1991; 87:1042.

113. Popovich KJ, Sheldon G, Mack M, et al.: Role of platelets in contraction of canine tracheal muscle elicited by PAF in vitro. *J Appl Physiol* 1988; 65:914.

114. Kaye MG, Smith LJ: Effects of inhaled leukotriene D_4 and platelet-activating factor on airway reactivity in normal subjects. *Am Rev Respir Dis* 1990; 141:993.

115. Vargaftig BB, Lefort J, Wal F, et al.: Non-steroidal anti-inflammatory drugs if combined with anti-histamine and anti-serotonin agents interfere with the bronchial and platelet effects of "platelet-activating factor" (PAF-acether). *Eur J Pharmacol* 1982; 82:121.

116. Murphy TM, Munoz NM, Moss J, et al.: PAF-induced contraction of canine trachea mediated by 5-hydroxytryptamine in vivo. *J Appl Physiol* 1989; 66:638.

117. Underwood DC, Kadowitz PJ: Analysis of bronchoconstrictor responses to platelet-activating factor in the cat. *J Appl Physiol* 1989; 67:377.

118. Spencer DA, Evans JM, Green SE, et al.: Participation of the cysteinyl leukotrienes in the acute bronchoconstrictor response to inhaled platelet activating factor in man. *Thorax* 1991; 46:441.

119. Taylor IK, Ward PS, Taylor GW, et al.: Inhaled PAF stimulates leukotriene and thromboxane A_2 production in humans. *J Appl Physiol* 1991; 71:1396.

120. Kidney JC, Ridge SM, Chung KF, Barnes PJ: Inhibition of platelet-activating factor–induced bronchoconstriction by the leukotriene D_4 receptor antagonist ICI 204,219. *Am Rev Respir Dis* 1993; 147:215.

121. Hayes JP, Chung KF, Barnes PJ: Attenuation of platelet-activating factor induced bronchoconstriction by nedocromil sodium. *Eur Respir J* 1992; 5:1193.

122. Roberts NM, McCusker M, Chung KF, Barnes PJ: Effect of a PAF antagonist, BN52063, on PAF-induced bronchoconstriction in normal subjects. *Br J Clin Pharmacol* 1988; 26:65.

123. Adamus WS, Heuer HO, Meade CJ, Schilling JC: Inhibitory effects of the new PAF acether antagonist WEB-2086 on pharmacologic changes induced by PAF inhalation in human beings. *Clin Pharmacol Ther* 1990; 47:456.

124. Cuss FM, Dixon CM, Barnes PJ: Effects of inhaled platelet-activating factor on pulmonary function and bronchial responsiveness in man. *Lancet* 1986; 2:189.

125. Chung KF, Barnes PJ: Effects of platelet activating factor on airway calibre, airway responsiveness, and circulating cells in asthmatic subjects. *Thorax* 1989; 44:108.

126. Rubin AH, Smith LJ, Patterson R: The bronchoconstrictor properties of platelet-activating factor in humans. *Am Rev Respir Dis* 1987; 136:1145.

127. Chung KF, Dent G, Barnes PJ: Effects of salbutamol on bronchoconstriction, bronchial hyperresponsiveness, and leucocyte responses induced by platelet activating factor in man. *Thorax* 1989; 44:102.

128. Plitman JD, Snapper JR: Nonspecific airway hyperresponsiveness: mechanisms and meaning, in Simmons DH, Tierney DF (eds): *Current Pulmonology*, vol 13. Chicago, Mosby-Year Book, 1992:143–192.

129. Chung KF, Aizawa H, Leikauf GD, et al.: Airway hyperresponsiveness induced by platelet-activating factor: role of thromboxane generation. *J Pharmacol Exp Ther* 1986; 236:580.

130. Christman BW, Lefferts PL, Snapper JR: Effect of platelet-activating factor on aerosol histamine responsiveness in awake sheep. *AM Rev Respir Dis* 1987; 135:1267.

131. Dixon EJ, Wilsoncroft P, Robertson DN, Page CP: The effect of Paf antagonists on bronchial hyperresponsiveness induced by Paf, propranolol or indomethacin. *Br J Pharmacol* 1989; 97:717.

132. Coyle AJ, Urwin SC, Page CP, et al.: The effect of the selective PAF antagonist BN 52021 on PAF- and antigen-induced bronchial hyper-reactivity and eosinophil accumulation. *Eur J Pharmacol* 1988; 148:51.

133. Soler M, Mansour E, Fernandez A, et al.: PAF-induced airway responses in sheep: effects of a PAF antagonist and nedocromil sodium. *J Allergy Clin Immunol* 1990; 85:661.

134. Mansour E, Abraham WM, Ahmed T: Attenuation of platelet-activating factor–induced airway responses with methylprednisolone succinate in sheep. *J Appl Physiol* 1992; 72:1529.

135. Mencia-Huerta JM, Touvay C, Pfister A, Braquet P: Effect of long-term administration of platelet-activating factor on pulmonary responsiveness and morphology in the guinea pig. *Int Arch Allergy Appl Immunol* 1989; 88:154.

136. Bethel RA, Worthen GS, Henson PM, Lien DC: Effects of neutrophil depletion and repletion on PAF-induced hyperresponsiveness of canine trachea. *J Appl Physiol* 1992; 73:2413.

137. Anderson GP, Fennessy MR: Lipoxygenase metabolites mediate increased airways responsiveness to histamine after acute platelet activating factor exposure in the guinea-pig. *Agents Actions* 1988; 24:8.

138. Sasaki M, Herd CM, Page CP: Effect of heparin and a low-molecular weight heparinoid on PAF-induced airway responses in neonatally immunized rabbits. *Br J Pharmacol* 1993; 110:107.

139. Johnson PR, Armour CL, Black JL: The action of platelet activating factor and its antagonism by WEB 2086 on human isolated airways. *Eur Respir J* 1990; 3:55.

140. Robertson DN, Coyle AJ, Rhoden KJ, et al.: The effect of platelet-activating factor on histamine and muscarinic receptor function in guinea pig airways. *Am Rev Respir Dis* 1988; 137:1317.

141. Coyle AJ, Spina D, Page CP: PAF-induced bronchial hyperresponsiveness in the rabbit: contribution of platelets and airway smooth muscle. *Br J Pharmacol* 1990; 101:31.

142. Barnes PJ, Grandordy BM, Page CP, et al.: The effect of platelet activating factor on pulmonary β-adrenoceptors. *Br J Pharmacol* 1987; 90:709.

143. Agrawal DK, Bergren DR, Byorth PJ, Townley RG: Platelet-activating factor induces nonspecific desensitization to bronchodilators in guinea pigs. *J Pharmacol Exp Ther* 1991; 259:1.

144. Agrawal DK, Townley RG: Effect of platelet-activating factor on β-adrenoceptors in human lung. *Biochem Biophys Res Commun* 1987; 143:1.

145. Elwood RK, Kennedy S, Belzberg A, et al.: Respiratory mucosal permeability in asthma. *Am Rev Respir Dis* 1983; 128:523.

146. Kennedy SM, Elwood RK, Wiggs BJ, et al.: Increased airway mucosal permeability of smokers. Relationship to airway reactivity. *Am Rev Respir Dis* 1984; 129:143.

147. Moreno RH, Hogg JC, Paré PD: Mechanics of airway narrowing. *Am Rev Respir Dis* 1986; 133:1171.

148. Wiggs BR, Bosken C, Paré PD, et al.: A model of airway narrowing in asthma and in chronic obstructive pulmonary disease. *Am Rev Respir Dis* 1992; 145:1251.

149. Chung KF, Lammers JW, McCusker M, et al.: Effect of theophylline on airway responses to inhaled platelet-activating factor in man. *Eur Respir J* 1989; 2:763.

150. Di Maria GU, Bellofiore S, Ciancio N, et al.: Nedocromil sodium inhibits the increase in airway reactivity induced by platelet activating factor in humans. *Chest* 1992; 102:123.

151. Hopp RJ, Bewtra AK, Agrawal DK, Townley RG: Effect of platelet-activating factor inhalation on nonspecific bronchial reactivity in man. *Chest* 1989; 96:1070.

152. Spencer DA, Green SE, Evans JM, et al.: Platelet activating factor does not cause a reproducible increase in bronchial responsiveness in normal man. *Clin Exp Allergy* 1990; 20:525.

153. Hopp RJ, Bewtra AK, Nabe M, et al.: Effect of PAF-acether inhalation on nonspecific bronchial reactivity and adrenergic response in normal and asthmatic subjects. *Chest* 1990; 98:936.

154. Lai CK, Jenkins JR, Polosa R, Holgate ST: Inhaled PAF fails to induce airway hyperresponsiveness to methacholine in normal human subjects. *J Appl Physiol* 1990; 68:919.

155. Gebremichael I, Leuenberger P: Platelet-activating factor does not induce bronchial hyperreactivity in nonasthmatic subjects. *Respiration* 1992; 59:193.

156. Cockcroft DW, Killian DN, Mellon JJ, Hargreave FE: Bronchial reactivity to inhaled histamine: a method and clinical survey. *Clin Allergy* 1977; 7:235.

157. Hopp RJ, Bewtra AK, Nair NM, Townley RG: Specificity and sensitivity of methacholine inhalation challenge in normal and asthmatic children. *J Allergy Clin Immunol* 1984; 74:154.

158. Weiss ST, Tager IB, Weiss JW, et al.: Airways responsiveness in a population sample of adults and children. *Am Rev Respir Dis* 1984; 129:898.

159. Woolcock AJ, Peat JK, Salome CM, et al.: Prevalence of bronchial hyperresponsiveness and asthma in a rural adult population. *Thorax* 1987; 42:361.

160. Josephs LK, Gregg I, Mullee MA, Holgate ST: Nonspecific bronchial reactivity and its relationship to the clinical expression of asthma. A longitudinal study. *Am Rev Respir Dis* 1989; 140:350.

161. Pattemore PK, Asher MI, Harrison AC, et al.: The interrelationship among bronchial hyperresponsiveness, the diagnosis of asthma, and asthma symptoms. *Am Rev Respir Dis* 1990; 142:549.

162. Djukanović R, Roche WR, Wilson JW, et al.: Mucosal inflammation in asthma. *Am Rev Respir Dis* 1990; 142:434.

163. Expert Panel on the Management of Asthma: *Guidelines for the Diagnosis and Management of Asthma.* National Institutes of Health, Bethesda, MD, 1991.

164. Lellouch-Tubiana A, Lefort J, Pirotzky E, et al.: Ultrastructural evidence for extravascular platelet recruitment in the lung upon intravenous injection of platelet-activating factor (PAF-acether) to guinea-pigs. *Br J Exp Pathol* 1985; 66:345.

165. Dunnill MS: The pathology of asthma, with special reference to changes in the bronchial mucosa. *J Clin Pathol* 1960; 13:27.

166. Hsieh KH, Ng CK: Increased plasma platelet-activating factor in children with acute asthmatic attacks and decreased in vivo and in vitro production of platelet-activating factor after immunotherapy. *J Allergy Clin Immunol* 1993; 91:650.

167. Kurosawa M, Yamashita T, Kurimoto F: Increased levels of blood platelet-activating factor in bronchial asthmatic patients with active symptoms. *Allergy* 1994; 49:60.

168. Chan-Yeung M, Lam S, Chan H, et al.: The release of platelet-activating factor into plasma during allergen-induced bronchoconstriction. *J Allergy Clin Immunol* 1991; 87:667.

169. Shirasaki H, Nishikawa M, Adcock IM, et al.: Expression of platelet-activating factor receptor mRNA in human and guinea pig lung. *Am J Respir Cell Mol Biol* 1994; 10:533.

170. Arnoux B, Joseph M, Simoes MH, et al.: Antigenic release of paf-acether and beta-glucuronidase from alveolar macrophages of asthmatics. *Bull Eur Physiopathol Respir* 1987; 23:119.

171. Warringa RA, Mengelers HJ, Kuijper PH, et al.: In vivo priming of platelet-activating factor–induced eosinophil chemotaxis in allergic asthmatic individuals. *Blood* 1992; 79:1836.

172. Felez MA, Roca J, Barbera JA, et al.: Inhaled platelet-activating factor worsens gas exchange in mild asthma. *Am J Respir Crit Care Med* 1994; 150:369.

173. Parente L, Fitzgerald MF, Moncada S: Anaphylactic release of platelet activating factor acether and eicosanoids from lungs of guinea pigs sensitized to ovalbumin aerosol. *Adv Prostaglandin Thromboxane Leukot Res* 1987; 17A:171.

174. Cirino M, Lagente V, Lefort J, Vargaftig BB: A study of BN 52021 demonstrates the involvement of PAF-acether in IgE-dependent anaphylactic bronchoconstriction. *Prostaglandins* 1986; 32:121.

175. Lagente V, Touvay C, Randon J, et al.: Interference of the PAF-acether antagonist BN 52021 with passive anaphylaxis in the guinea-pig. *Prostaglandins* 1987; 33:265.

176. Touvay C, Etienne A, Braquet P: Inhibition of antigen-induced lung anaphylaxis in the guinea-pig by BN 52021 a new specific paf-acether receptor antagonist isolated from *Gingko biloba. Agents Actions* 1986; 17:371.

177. Braquet P, Touqui L, Shen TY, Vargaftig BB: Perspectives in platelet-activating factor research. *Pharmacol Rev* 1987; 39:97.

178. Coyle AJ, Page CP, Atkinson L, et al.: Modification of allergen-induced airway obstruction and airway hyperresponsiveness in an allergic rabbit model by the selective platelet-activating factor antagonist, BN 52021. *J Allergy Clin Immunol* 1989; 84:960.

179. Ishida K, Thomson RJ, Beattie LL, et al.: Inhibition of antigen-induced airway hyperresponsiveness, but not acute hypoxia nor airway eosinophilia, by an antagonist of platelet-activating factor. *J Immunol* 1990; 144:3907.

180. Morooka S, Uchida M, Imanishi N: Platelet-activating factor (PAF) plays an important role in the immediate asthmatic response in guinea-pig by augmenting the response to histamine. *Br J Pharmacol* 1992; 105:756.

181. Abraham WM, Stevenson JS, Garrido R: A possible role for PAF in allergen-induced late responses: modification by a selective antagonist. *J Appl Physiol* 1989; 66:2351.

182. Soler M, Sielczak MW, Abraham WM: A PAF antagonist blocks antigen-induced airway hyperresponsiveness and inflammation in sheep. *J Appl Physiol* 1989; 67:406.

183. Tan WC, Bethel RA: The effect of platelet activating factor antagonist on ozone-induced airway inflammation and bronchial hyperresponsiveness in guinea pigs. *Am Rev Respir Dis* 1992; 146:916.

184. Guinot P, Brambilla C, Duchier J, et al.: Effect of BN 52063, a specific PAF-acether antagonist, on bronchial provocation test to allergens in asthmatic patients. A preliminary study. *Prostaglandins* 1987; 34:723.

185. Hsieh KH: Effects of PAF antagonist, BN 52021, on the PAF-, methacholine-, and allergen-induced bronchoconstriction in asthmatic children. *Chest* 1991; 99:877.

186. Wilkens JH, Wilkens H, Uffmann J, et al.: Effects of a PAF-antagonist (BN 52063) on bronchoconstriction and platelet activation during exercise induced asthma. *Br J Clin Pharmacol* 1990; 29:85.

187. Kuitert LM, Hui KP, Uthayarkumar S, et al.: Effect of the platelet-activating factor antagonist UK-74,505 on the early and late response to allergen. *Am Rev Respir Dis* 1993; 147:82.

188. Freitag A, Watson RM, Matsos G, et al.: Effect of a platelet activating factor antagonist, WEB 2086, on allergen induced asthmatic responses. *Thorax* 1993; 48:594.

189. Spence DP, Johnston SL, Calverley PM, et al.: The effect of the orally active platelet-activating factor antagonist WEB 2086 in the treatment of asthma. *Am J Respir Crit Care Med* 1994; 149:1142.

190. Bernard GR, Artigas A, Brigham KL, et al.: The American-European Consensus Conference on ARDS. Definitions, mechanisms, relevant outcomes, and clinical trial coordination. *Am J Respir Crit Care Med* 1994; 149:818.

191. Ashbaugh DG, Bigelow DB, Petty TL, Levine BE: Acute respiratory distress in adults. *Lancet* 1967; 2:319.

192. Murray JF, Matthay MA, Luce JM, Flick MR: An expanded definition of the adult respiratory distress syndrome. *Am Rev Respir Dis* 1988; 138:720.

193. Snapper JR: Lung mechanics in pulmonary edema. *Clin Chest Med* 1985; 6:393.

194. Wright PE, Bernard GR: The role of airflow resistance in patients with the adult respiratory distress syndrome. *Am Rev Respir Dis* 1989; 139:1169.

195. Hutchison AA, Hinson JM, Jr., Brigham KL, Snapper JR: Effect of endotoxin on airway responsiveness to aerosol histamine in sheep. *J Appl Physiol* 1983; 54:1463.

196. Simpson DL, Goodman M, Spector SL, Petty TL: Long-term follow-up and bronchial reactivity testing in survivors of the adult respiratory distress syndrome. *Am Rev Respir Dis* 1978; 117:449.

197. Rinaldo JE: The adult respiratory distress syndrome, in Tierney DF (ed): *Current Pulmonology*, vol 15. St. Louis, Mosby-Year Book, 1994:137–156.

198. Pepe PE, Potkin RT, Reus DH, et al.: Clinical predictors of the adult respiratory distress syndrome. *Am J Surg* 1982; 144:124.

199. Fowler AA, Hamman RF, Good JT, et al.: Adult respiratory distress syndrome: risk with common predispositions. *Ann Intern Med* 1983; 98:593.

200. Wheeler AP, Swindell B, Carroll F, et al.: The lung in sepsis: data from the ibuprofen human sepsis multicenter trial. (abstract) *Chest* 1993; 104:56S.

201. Chang SW, Feddersen CO, Henson PM, Voelkel NF: Platelet-activating factor mediates hemodynamic changes and lung injury in endotoxin-treated rats. *J Clin Invest* 1987; 79:1498.

202. Matsumoto K, Taki F, Kondoh Y, et al.: Platelet-activating factor in bronchoalveolar lavage fluid of patients with adult respiratory distress syndrome. *Clin Exp Pharmacol Physiol* 1992; 19:509.

203. Salzer WL, McCall CE: Primed stimulation of isolated perfused rabbit lung by endotoxin and platelet activating factor induces enhanced production of thromboxane and lung injury. *J Clin Invest* 1990; 85:1135.

204. Rabinovici R, Esser KM, Lysko PG, et al.: Priming by platelet-activating factor of endotoxin-induced lung injury and cardiovascular shock. *Circ Res* 1991; 69:12.

205. Rabinovici R, Bugelski PJ, Esser KM, et al.: Tumor necrosis factor-α mediates endotoxin-induced lung injury in platelet activating factor-primed rats. *J Pharmacol Exp Ther* 1993; 267:1550.

206. Thivierge M, Rola-Pleszczynski M: Platelet-activating factor enhances interleukin-6 production by alveolar macrophages. *J Allergy Clin Immunol* 1992; 90:796.

207. Szabo C, Wu CC, Mitchell JA, et al.: Platelet-activating factor contributes to the induction of nitric oxide synthase by bacterial lipopolysaccharide. *Circ Res* 1993; 73:991.

208. Klosterhalfen B, Horstmann-Jungemann K, Vogel P, et al.: Time course of various inflammatory mediators during recurrent endotoxemia. *Biochem Pharmacol* 1992; 43:2103.

209. Chang SW, Fernyak S, Voelkel NF: Beneficial effect of a platelet-activating factor antagonist, WEB 2086, on endotoxin-induced lung injury. *Am J Physiol* 1990; 258:H153.

210. Rylander R, Beijer L, Lantz RC, et al.: Modulation of pulmonary inflammation after endotoxin inhalation with a platelet-activating factor antagonist (48740 RP). *Int Arch Allergy Appl Immunol* 1988; 86:303.

211. Lantz RC, Keller GE, Burrell R: The role of platelet-activating factor in the pulmonary response to inhaled bacterial endotoxin. *Am Rev Respir Dis* 1991; 144:167.

212. Christman BW, Lefferts PL, Blair IA, Snapper JR: Effect of platelet-activating factor receptor antagonism on endotoxin-induced lung dysfunction in awake sheep. *Am Rev Respir Dis* 1990; 142:1272.

213. Sessler CN, Glauser FL, Davis D, Fowler AA: Effects of platelet-activating factor antagonist SRI 63-441 on endotoxemia in sheep. *J Appl Physiol* 1988; 65:2624.

214. Olson NC, Joyce PB, Fleisher LN: Role of platelet-activating factor and eicosanoids during endotoxin-induced lung injury in pigs. *Am J Physiol* 1990; 258:H1674.

215. Siebeck M, Weipert J, Keser C, et al.: A triazolodiazepine platelet activating factor receptor antagonist (WEB 2086) reduces pulmonary dysfunction during endotoxin shock in swine. *J Trauma* 1991; 31:942.

216. Dobrowsky RT, Voyksner RD, Olson NC: Effect of SRI 63-675 on hemodynamics and blood PAF levels during porcine endotoxemia. *Am J Physiol* 1991; 260:H1455.

217. Byrne K, Sessler CN, Carey PD, et al.: Platelet-activating factor in porcine Pseudomonas acute lung injury. *J Surg Res* 1991; 50:111.

218. Hocking DC, Phillips PG, Ferro TJ, Johnson A: Mechanisms of pulmonary edema induced by tumor necrosis factor-α. *Circ Res* 1990; 67:68.

219. Horvath CJ, Kaplan JE, Malik AB: Role of platelet-activating factor in mediating tumor necrosis factor α-induced pulmonary vasoconstriction and plasma-lymph protein transport. *Am Rev Respir Dis* 1991; 144:1337.

220. Rabinovici R, Sofronski MD, Renz JF, et al.: Platelet activating factor mediates interleukin-2-induced lung injury in the rat. *J Clin Invest* 1992; 89:1669.

221. Dhainaut JF, Tenaillon A, Letulzo Y, et al.: Efficacy of PAF antagonist (BN 52021) in reducing mortality of patients with severe gram-negative sepsis. (abstract) *Circ Shock* 39 Suppl 1993; 1:42.

222. Davidsen SK, Summers JB, Albert DH, et al.: N-(acyloxyalkyl) pyridinium salts as soluble prodrugs of a potent platelet activating factor antagonist. *J Med Chem* 1994; 37:4423.

223. Formela LJ, Wood LM, Whittaker M, Kingsnorth AN: Amelioration of experimental acute pancreatitis with a potent platelet-activating factor antagonist. *Br J Surg* 1994; 81:1783.

224. Galloway SW, Formela L, Kingsnorth AN, et al.: A double-blind placebo controlled study of lexipafant (a potent PAF antagonist) in acute pancreatitis. (abstract) *European Pancreatic Club Proceedings* 1994; 10.

Chapter 15 _____
BRADYKININ
PAULA L. WATSON

JAMES R. SNAPPER

Bradykinin, a peptide composed of nine amino acids, is widely distributed in mammalian tissues and body fluids. It produces inflammatory effects including vasodilation, increased microvascular permeability, bronchoconstriction, and pain. These properties have led to much investigation into its role in various inflammatory diseases as well as the potential use of bradykinin antagonists in the treatment of these disorders. The following discussion will include information regarding the production, mechanism of action, and metabolism of bradykinin, as well as its possible role in lung diseases including asthma, sepsis, small-cell lung cancer, and angiotensin-converting enzyme (ACE) inhibitor-induced cough.

Formation and Metabolism

Bradykinin (Arg–Pro–Pro–Gly–Phe–Ser–Pro–Phe–Arg) is formed along with kallidin (Lys–Arg–Pro–Pro–Gly–Phe–Ser–Pro–Phe–Arg) from two precursor proteins known as *kininogens*. Bradykinin and kallidin produce similar physiologic effects and are often discussed collectively. The kininogens are present in high-molecular-weight (MW 110,000) and low-molecular-weight (MW 50,000) forms. They circulate in plasma at concentrations of approximately 270 μg/ml. These kininogens are activated by either plasma or tissue kallikrein which, like the kininogens, are derived from inactive proenzymes. High-molecular-weight kininogen contains a binding site for prekallikrein, the inactive form of plasma kallikrein, and circulates bound to this enzyme. This close association makes high-molecular-weight kininogen the preferred substrate for plasma kallikrein, and their interaction results in the formation of bradykinin. The initiation of this activation pathway occurs when Hageman factor is activated by substances such as collagen, immune complexes, or by contact with the negatively charged surfaces of heparin and mucous glycoproteins.

Tissue kallikrein is present in most tissues and in glandular secretions. It has no specificity for either low-molecular-weight or high-molecular-weight kininogen and leads to the production of kallidin when activated. Kallidin, which is active at both β_1 and β_2 receptors, also may be metabolized by aminopeptidase M to form bradykinin.[1,2] Bradykinin is relatively inactive on β_1 receptors. Thus, the conversion of kallidin to bradykinin potentially could lead to a significant change in kinin-produced effects. Tryptase from mast cells[3] and neutrophil-derived proteinases have been shown to cleave kininogens to active kinins, but the activity of these enzymes is felt to be insignificant when compared with the activity of kallikreins.

Once formed, bradykinin and kallidin act locally and are rapidly inactivated. The half-life of bradykinin and kallidin are both <30 s,[4] and a single pass through the lung results in 80 percent to 90 percent inactivation. Several different peptidases have been found to metabolize bradykinin. Angiotensin-converting enzyme is membrane-bound and found primarily in endothelial cells and renal tubular epithelium. It cleaves the C-terminal dipeptide, Phe-Arg, to form an inactive peptide. Neutral endopeptidase is found on bronchial epithelium, fibroblasts, and alveolar cells. Inhibition of this enzyme has been shown to enhance bradykinin-induced bronchoconstriction in the guinea pig both in vitro[5] and in vivo.[6] Carboxypeptidase N is a metallopeptide that cleaves the carboxyl-terminal Arg to form des Arg[9] bradykinin, which is active at β_1 receptors but not β_2 receptors. It is membrane-bound and found in abundance in plasma.

Other enzymes are responsible for the inactivation of bradykinin. The membrane-bound carboxypeptidase M, found on pulmonary endothelial cells and alveolar cells, removes the C-terminal Arg; deamidase also removes the C-terminal Arg; membrane-bound aminopeptidase P cleaves the Arg-Pro bond[7,8]; and prolyl endopeptidase cleaves the Pro-Gly bond. Dipeptidylamino-peptidase IV, which cleaves the Pro–Gly bond of des-Arg-bradykinin, also has been isolated from human tissues.[9]

Receptors and Antagonists

The kinins mediate many of their effects through activation of specific receptors. There are two major classes of bradykinin receptors: β_1 and β_2. Their classification is based on the relative potencies of agonists and antagonists. β_1 agonist potencies are: des-Arg[10]-kallidin > des-Arg[9]-bradykinin = kallidin ≫ bradykinin; and β_2 agonist potencies are: bradykinin = kallidin ≫ des-Arg[10]-kallidin > des-Arg[9] bradykinin. The study of tissue response to synthetic antagonists over the past few years has suggested the existence of β_2 subtypes and the possibility of a β_3 receptor.

Beta$_1$ receptors are predominately found in vascular smooth muscle. They are most responsive to the des-Arg-kinins formed during the metabolism of bradykinin and kallidin by the carboxypeptidase enzymes. The physiologic role of β_1 receptors has not been fully established. They are synthesized de novo following tissue injury and following exposure to lipopolysaccharide. They have been shown to mediate hyperalgesia in animal models of inflammation[10] and also to mediate the contraction of rabbit aorta.[11] Beta$_1$ receptors appear to play little role in airway disease.

The majority of physiologic effects produced by bradykinin occur through activation of β_2 receptors. These effects include bronchoconstriction, arterial vasodilation, increased microvascular permeability, the activation of sensory nerves, and the stimulation of prostaglandin and nitric oxide production. Beta$_2$ receptors appear to be widely distributed as evidenced by autoradiography of human and guinea pig lung. Bronchial and pulmonary vessels of all sizes are labeled densely, with the greatest density occurring over the endothelial cells, and there is also labeling over epithelial cells and airway smooth muscle, which is greatest in the small airways. There is also autoradiographic labeling of β_2 receptors around submucosal glands and nerve fibers surrounding bronchial vessels.[12]

Early β_2 antagonists were developed by substituting the D-phenylalanine for L-proline in position 7.[13] The use of these antagonists in the study of physiologic functions is limited because of their low potency, actions as partial agonists, susceptibility to enzyme degradation (and the subsequent production of β_1 agonists[14]), and the ability to induce histamine release from mast cells.[15]

The next generation of antagonists synthesized contained unnatural amino acids, which made them less susceptible to enzymatic degradation.[16,17] The prototype of this group is Hoe 140, (D-Arg-[Hyp[3],Thi[5],D-Tic[7],D-Phe[8]]BK), which is two to three times more potent than any previously described antagonist[17] and has no agonist activity; however, it is noncompetitive in some systems, and it also causes the release of histamine.

Evaluation of tissues with the early antagonists, such as [Thi[5,8],D-Phe[7]]bradykinin, revealed differences in affinities depending on the tissue tested. This led to the subdivision of β_2 receptors into two subtypes, a "neuronal form" and a "smooth muscle form."[18] Continued evaluation has failed to

show different subtypes within a species. However, interspecies differences in β_2 receptor affinities has been consistently found. Regoli and colleagues evaluated vascular and peripheral tissues in four species and demonstrated no significant differences between tissues. There was interspecies variability, which could be divided into two groups based on affinities for β_2 antagonists. Human and rabbit tissues had similar pharmacologic properties, and rat and guinea pig tissues were alike. Regoli proposed that β_2 subtypes should be named β_{2A} and β_{2B}, respectively.[19]

Recently a new class of antagonists has been developed. The prototype of this class, WIN 64338, represents the first synthetic nonpeptide bradykinin antagonist.[20] It is β_2 selective, highly potent, and demonstrates competitive inhibition, which will make it a good tool for the study of receptor physiology. Other non-peptide antagonists have been found in nature. The rhizome from *Mandevilla velutina*, a native plant in Brazil, has been used in the treatment of snake bites for years. Steroid glycoids, purified from its extract, inhibit bradykinin-induced contraction in the rat uterus and in the guinea pig ileum.[21]

Farmer and coworkers proposed the existence of a β_3 receptor based on the inability of β_1- and β_2-receptor antagonists to prevent bradykinin-induced smooth muscle contraction in the guinea pig trachea. These antagonists also failed to displace [³H]-bradykinin binding in this tissue.[22] Pyne and Pyne provided further evidence of a β_3 receptor, as β_2 antagonists inhibited bradykinin-induced phospholipase C activity but not phospholipase D activity.[23] The nonpeptide antagonist WIN 64338 also had no effect in preventing bradykinin-induced contraction of the guinea pig trachea.[24] However, HOE 140 was found to inhibit this contraction and displace [³H]-BK binding.[25] The existence of β_3 receptors continues to be controversial.

The β_1 receptor[26] and β_2 receptor from several tissues, including the human lung fibroblast[27] and rat uterus,[18] have been cloned. Their sequences indicated that the receptor contains seven transmembrane regions and is a member of the superfamily of G protein–coupled receptors. Binding of bradykinin to its receptor has been shown to induce activation of phospholipases A_2, C, and D. Through activation of these second messengers, bradykinin causes the production of eicosanoids, nitric oxide,[28] and initiates mitogenesis.[29]

Bradykinin is a potent stimulator of type C sensory nerve fibers,[30] which, when activated, will lead to cholinergic axon reflexes and local release of sensory neuropeptides.[31] This effect is inhibited by β_2 antagonists. These sensory neuropeptides, such as substance P and neurokinin A, also cause microvascular leakage and bronchoconstriction. It is often difficult to distinguish between the direct effects of bradykinin and the effects mediated by sensory neuropeptides and prostaglandins.

Bradykinin in Asthma

Asthma is characterized by reversible airway constriction, hyperresponsiveness to various stimuli, and inflammation. Bradykinin, because of its ability to cause bronchoconstriction and inflammation, has long been considered to be a possible mediator of asthma. Over the years, experimental evidence has accumulated to support its role in this complex disease.

Bradykinin has been shown to cause bronchoconstriction in asthmatics but not in normal subjects.[32] Asthmatics also have been demonstrated to have increased concentrations of kinins in plasma[33] and in bronchoalveolar lavage (BAL) fluid.[33,34] Furthermore, these BAL kinin concentrations are greater in symptomatic than in asymptomatic asthmatics,[34] and asymptomatic subjects increase their concentrations following allergen challenge.[34]

Allergen-induced airway disease is characterized by an early and a late phase. In a sheep model, Abraham and colleagues demonstrated that a β_2-receptor antagonist had no effect on bronchoconstriction or mediator release during the early phase. There was a significant decrease in the late phase bronchoconstriction, which was accompanied by a decrease in inflammatory mediators as well as a decrease in BAL neutrophils.[35] This would suggest that bradykinin may play an important role in initiation of the late-phase response. However, human subjects have failed to demonstrate a late-phase response following bradykinin inhalation.[36] The role of bradykinin, if any, in late-phase bronchoconstriction and mediator release in humans is yet to be determined.

Bradykinin also has been implicated in the sodium metabisulfite (MBS) reaction. Sodium metabisulfite is a food and wine preservative that causes bronchoconstriction in some asthmatics, the mechanism of which remains undefined. Using an allergic sheep model, Mansour and coworkers demonstrated that MBS increased BAL kinin concentrations by nine times baseline; β_2 antagonism prevented this increase as well as the bronchoconstriction.[37]

Bradykinin-induced bronchoconstriction is maximal at 3 to 10 min and resolves within 60 min. The bronchoconstriction is not produced at β_1 agonists[38] but is inhibited by β_2 antagonists,[39,40] indicating that the response is mediated by the β_2 receptor. Unlike histamine, repeated challenges with bradykinin result in significant tachyphylaxis.[32]

The mechanism through which bradykinin produces bronchoconstriction in asthmatics is not fully understood. Bradykinin causes airway microvascular leakage[39,41] leading to airway edema, which may contribute to bronchoconstriction. More importantly, bradykinin causes secondary effects such as a stimulation of eicosanoid production, the release of mast cell mediators,[42] and the stimulation of sensory afferent nerves with the subsequent release of tachykinins and activation of the cholinergic reflex.

In humans, the bronchoconstrictor effect appears to be mediated through indirect mechanisms, as bradykinin is only a weak constrictor of isolated human bronchi.[32] Ipratropium bromide, pretreatment with capsaicin (which depletes sensory nerves of tachykinins), and cromolyn sodium all significantly reduce the bronchoconstriction of inhaled bradykinin, implicating activation of sensory neurons and release of mast cell mediators as possible mechanisms.[32] The tachykinin-receptor antagonist FK-224 has been shown to attenuate bradykinin-induced bronchoconstriction, further implicating sensory nerve activation as a mediating event.[43] Aspirin, a cyclooxygenase inhibitor that prevents prostaglandin and thromboxane production, does not reduce bradykinin-induced bronchoconstriction.[32]

In guinea pigs, bronchoconstriction secondary to intravenous and instilled bradykinin[44] is reduced by pretreatment with indomethacin and atropine. Pretreatment with OKY-046, a selective thromboxane synthetase inhibitor, also attenuated this effect, implicating involvement of thromboxane in this process.[44]

Besides its bronchoconstrictive effects, bradykinin also may contribute to the cough seen in asthmatics. Upon inhalation, it produces a cough in both asthmatics and normal subjects.[32] It may increase sputum production, as it has been shown to stimulate mucous secretion[45] and also increase chloride secretion by airway epithelial cells,[46] leading to increased water content in airway fluids.

Bradykinin in Upper Airway Disease

The characteristics that make bradykinin important in the pathogenesis of lower airway disease also implicate a possible role for the mediator in inflammatory disease of the upper airways. Supporting evidence has been found for kinin involvement in allergic rhinitis and in rhinovirus infections.

Increased kinin concentrations are found in nasal lavage fluids during both the early- and late-phase reactions to allergens.[47,48] Bradykinin also has been implicated in the production of cold-air–induced nasal congestion. Patients who previously reported cold-induced symptoms were found to have increased kinin concentrations in nasal lavage fluids following challenge with cold, dry air.[49] In both instances, the increased concentrations correlated with release of other inflammatory mediators and with the onset of clinical symptoms. With the release of other mediators in the studies, it is difficult to determine which, if any, symptoms are caused directly by bradykinin. A human in vivo study failed to demonstrate any contribution by histamine or the cholinergic pathway to bradykinin-induced nasal symptoms.[50] It does appear that allergen-induced nasal obstruction is caused by activation of the β_2 receptor, as Hoe 140 attenuates this effect.[51]

Nasal challenge with bradykinin has been shown to produce symptoms resembling those of a rhinovirus infection.[52] These symptoms include unilateral nasal obstruction (on the side of bradykinin administration), rhinorrhea, and a sore throat that persists up to 4 h. No increase in histamine release was found during this challenge, suggesting that bradykinin did not produce its symptoms by activating mast cells or basophils. Rhinovirus infection is associated with increased kinin concentrations in nasal lavage fluids of humans[53,54] and in ferrets.[55] The similarity between humans and ferrets in their response to rhinovirus allows for the study of experimental bradykinin-receptor antagonists in an animal model.

Kinins have been shown to increase vascular permeability and increase mucous secretion in human nasal mucosa,[45] which may contribute to rhinitis symptoms. The increased mucous secretion is blocked by the β_1-receptor antagonist des-Arg-Leu-BK and by inhibition of arachidonic product formation by indomethacin.[45] This suggests that the increase is likely caused by β_1-receptor activation leading to the stimulation of cyclooxygenase metabolism of arachidonic acid. Failure of the β_2-receptor antagonist D-Arg[0][Hyp[3],D-Phe[7]]-BK to block the increased vascular permeability suggests that this action of the kinins is mediated selectively by activation of the β_1 receptor.[56]

Autoradiography of human nasal mucosa revealed binding in small arteries and venous sinusoids and on submucosal fibers.[45] While the identity of these fibers is unknown, the authors speculate that they may represent sensory nerve fibers. No binding was found on submucosal glands or goblet cells, further suggesting an indirect mechanism for the etiology of increased mucous secretion.

Further study of rhinitis with bradykinin receptor antagonists will be needed to define the role of kinins in upper airway disease.

Bradykinin and the ACE-Inhibitor Cough

Angiotensin-converting enzyme inhibitors are frequently used in the treatment of hypertension and heart failure. It was not until several years after their clinical introduction that the development of a nonproductive cough was recognized as a side effect of these agents. Early studies reported the incidence to be only 1 percent to 4 percent, but subsequent trials have indicated an incidence as high as 31 percent.[57]

The ACE-inhibitor cough develops anywhere from a few hours to 1 year following drug initiation, with the usual time being from 3 to 4 weeks. This highly variable induction time often obscures the true etiology of the cough. It is often worse at night and occurs more commonly in women than in men. It also is more frequently reported in nonsmokers than in smokers. The cough generally resolves within 4 days after discontinuation of the drug. However, it may continue for as long as 1 month.

The etiology of the ACE-inhibitor cough remains unknown. One hypothesis is that ACE inhibition slows bradykinin degradation and leads to an accumulation of the peptide in lung tissue. Therapeutic doses of ACE inhibitors have not been shown to cause a significant increase in plasma bradykinin concentrations. However, the lung contains a large amount of ACE, and serum concentrations may not adequately reflect tissue levels. Indeed, ACE inhibitors augment the wheal and flare response to intradermally administered bradykinin.[58] This reaction also was associated with the development of a dry cough.

Bradykinin produces several effects that may contribute to the ACE-inhibitor cough. The cough could be a result of increased microvascular permeability leading to edema. More likely, it is secondary in indirect effects such as stimulation of J receptors and sensory afferent C fibers,[30] or the induction of arachidonic acid product formation.

Evidence of J receptor involvement has been demonstrated. Inhalation of bradykinin and capsaicin, a C-fiber stimulus, cause a dry cough similar to the ACE-inhibitor cough.[32,59] ACE inhibition causes increased sensitivity in inhaled capsaicin.[59] There also is evidence suggesting eico-

sanoid involvement, as cyclooxygenase inhibitors have been shown to decrease the cough response.[60,61]

There is little evidence that ACE inhibition leads to bronchoconstriction. Several patients with preexisting asthma have reported exacerbations after beginning an ACE inhibitor.[62] However, the majority of patients who develop this cough have no evidence of asthma, and several studies have reported no significant change in pulmonary function tests after use of the ACE inhibitor.[57,63,64]

While the kinins appear to be involved in the pathophysiology of ACE-inhibitor cough, they are unlikely to be the sole etiology. Substance P, a neuropeptide released from sensory nerves upon stimulation, also is metabolized by ACE. It is known to cause bronchoconstriction and stimulate eicosanoid production, making it a possible contributor to the pathophysiology. Continued investigation is needed to determine the exact role of bradykinin in this disorder.

Bradykinin in Lung Cancer

Lung cancer is the most common lethal malignancy in the United States. Small-cell lung cancer (SCLC) comprises approximately 25 percent of all cases. Small-cell lung cancer is characterized by the presence of neurosecretory granules and the production of multiple neuropeptides, including vasopressin, gastrin-releasing peptide, neurotensin, and cholecystokinin. It is speculated that these peptides, as well as bradykinin (which is produced extracellulary in the damaged tissue surrounding tumors), function as autocrine and paracrine growth factors for lung cancer.

Kinins have been demonstrated to promote DNA synthesis and function as mitogens in human lung fibroblasts.[65,66] They have been found in malignant effusions[67] and in increased concentrations in the plasma of patients with advanced cancer.[68] These observations have led to further evaluation of bradykinin and the neuropeptides in the regulation of tumor growth in an effort to develop novel treatment methods. The majority of the work has been performed in SLCL cell lines, although some evaluation of non-small-cell lung cancer (NSCLC) and breast tumors also has been performed.

As previously discussed, bradykinin is one of many peptides known to act through specific receptors coupled to G proteins. Activation of these receptors ultimately results in a release of intracellular Ca^{2+}. The increase in intracellular Ca^{2+} is associated with increased mitogenesis[69,70] and initiation of transcription of *fos* and *myc* oncogenes.[71,72]

Bradykinin and several neuropeptides, when applied to SCLC cell lines, cause a dose-dependent increase in Ca^{2+} concentrations and also increase the colony growth of these cell lines.[29] The response of various SCLC cell lines to the different peptides is highly variable and has been found to correlate with the presence or absence of specific receptors.[73] Bunn and colleagues demonstrated that only 83 percent of the cells from a single SCLC cell line responded to any single peptide. This maximal response occurred with bradykinin. However, in most cell lines tested, bradykinin produced effects in <50 percent of cells.[74] Non-small-cell lung cancer was found to respond less often, and only minimal response was seen in breast cancer cell lines. The heterogeneous response of SCLC and NSCLC cell lines to peptides indicates that the inhibition of any single peptide is unlikely to be effective in the treatment of this disease. Since these peptides all appear to work through release of intracellular Ca^{2+}, the inhibition of this step is being investigated as a method to prevent their mitogenic effects.

Ligand binding studies suggest that the mitogenic response of lung cancer is most likely mediated by β_2 receptors. β_2 receptors were found in both healthy lung tissue and in non-small-cell lung cancer. There was no evidence of β_1 receptors in these tissues.[75]

Bradykinin and Sepsis

Sepsis syndrome, characterized by hypotension, increased vascular permeability, tachycardia, and respiratory distress, occurs in greater than 400,000 individuals in the United States per year. Forty percent of those affected will progress to septic shock and 60 percent to 80 percent of these patients will die. The pathogenesis of this disease involves the activation and interaction of multiple mediators, including Hageman factor, the kinins, arachidonic acid metabolites, and multiple cytokines, including tumor necrosis factor-α (TNF-α), interleukin-1 (IL-1), and interleukin-6 (IL-6).

Endotoxin, by damaging endothelial cells, leads to activation of the kallikrein/kinin system. Decreased kinin precursors, as well as increased bradykinin levels in plasma, have been documented in humans and in animal models. Several studies indicate that endotoxin also causes a decrease in angiotensin-converting enzyme in animal models and in human endothelial cell cultures.[76–78] Human clinical trials also have shown decreased ACE levels in patients with acute respiratory distress syndrome (ARDS) and sepsis.[79–81] A decrease of this enzyme may lead to decreased bradykinin degradation, exacerbating any effect of bradykinin on hypotension and inflammation.

In a guinea pig model of septic shock, Khan and co-workers showed that lethal shock was associated with a 46 percent consumption of Hageman factor, 100 percent consumption of prekallikrein, and 85 percent consumption of high-molecular-weight kininogen. Furthermore, if any of these components were depleted, the guinea pigs became resistant to the same lethal dose of pseudomonal elastase. Pretreatment with a β_2-receptor antagonist prevented shock in these animals.[82]

Bradykinin stimulates the production of prostacyclin and nitric oxide through activation of the β_2 receptor. Both of these mediators are potent vasodilators that have been implicated in the pathophysiology of sepsis. The induction of these mediators may explain the mechanism of bradykinin-induced hypotension.

Animal studies of endotoxin-induced sepsis have shown an attenuation of hypotension and a decrease in mortality when the animals were pretreated with β_2-receptor antagonists.[83] Unfortunately, when the antagonist was given either concomitantly or following endotoxin, these benefits were not seen. Human studies evaluating the effects of bradykinin antagonists in sepsis are under way.[84]

Conclusion

Considerable evidence suggests that bradykinin and related kinins may be important mediators in the pathogenesis of lung diseases. Pharmacologic tools currently becoming available will allow for the critical assessment of the importance of kinins in a variety of disease processes. It is abundantly clear that there are important interactions between the kinins and other mediator systems. It is perhaps naïve to imply that bradykinin will prove important only in a pathologic cascade. It is equally likely that the kinins are responsible for homeostasis and that only under very aberrant conditions do they contribute to disease.

Acknowledgment

This work was supported by grants HL 46971 and HL 07123 from the National Heart, Lung, and Blood Institute, National Institutes of Health.

References

1. Guijmaraes JA, Borges DR, Prado ES, Prado JL: Kinin-converting aminopeptidase from human serum. *Biochem Pharmacol* 1973; 22:3157.
2. Palmieri FE, Petrelli JJ, Ward PE: Vascular, plasma membrane aminopeptidase M. *Biochem Pharmacol* 1985; 34:2309.
3. Proud D, Siekierski ES, Bailey GS: Identification of human lung mast cell kininogenase as tryptase and relevance of tryptase kininogenase activity. *Biochem Pharmacol* 1988; 37:1473.
4. Ferreirra SH, Vane JR: Half-lives of peptides and amines in the circulation. *Nature* 1967; 215:1237.
5. Frossard N, Stretton CD, Barnes PJ: Modulation of bradykinin responses in airway smooth muscle by epithelial enzymes. *Agents Actions* 1990; 31:204.
6. Ichinose M, Barnes PJ: The effect of peptidase inhibitors on bradykinin-induced bronchoconstriction in guinea-pigs in vivo. *Brit J Pharmacol* 1990; 101:77.
7. Simmons WH, Orawski AT: Membrane-bound aminopeptidase P from bovine lung; its purification, properties, and degradation of bradykinin. *J Biol Chem* 1992; 267:4897.
8. Ryan JW, Berryer P, Chung AY, Sheffy DH: Characterization of rat pulmonary vascular aminopeptidase P in vivo: role in the inactivation of bradykinin. *J Pharmacol Exp Therapeut* 1994; 269:941.
9. Behal FJ, Sidorowicz W, Heins J, Barth A: Human lung kinin catabolism. *Fed Proc* 1983; 42:1021.
10. Dray A, Perkins M: Bradykinin and inflammatory pain. *Trends Neurosci* 1993; 16:99.
11. Schachter M: Kallikreins (kininogenases)—a group of serine proteases with bioregulatory actions. *Pharm Rev* 1980; 31:1.
12. Mak JC, Barnes PJ: Autoradiographic visualization of bradykinin receptors in human and guinea pig lung. *Eur J Pharmacol* 1991; 194:37.
13. Vavrek R, Stewart JM: Competitive antagonists of bradykinin. *Peptides* 1985; 6:161.
14. Regoli D, Drapeau G, Rovero P, et al.: Conversions of kinins and their antagonists into B_1 receptor activators and blockers in isolated vessels. *Eur J Pharmacol* 1986; 127:219.
15. Devillier P, Renoux M, Drapeau G, Regoli D: Histamine release from rat peritoneal mast cells by kinin antagonists. *Eur J Pharmacol* 1988; 149:137.

16. Lembeck F, Griesbacher T, Eckgardt M, et al.: New, long-acting, potent bradykinin antagonist. *Brit J Pharmacol* 1991; 102:297.

17. Hock FJ, Wirth K, Albus J, et al.: Hoe 140 a new potent and long acting bradykinin-antagonist: in vitro studies. *Brit J Pharmacol* 1991; 102:769.

18. McEachern AE, Shelton ER, Bhakta S, et al.: Expression cloning of a rat B$_2$ bradykinin receptor. *Proc Natl Acad Sci U S A* 1991; 88:7724.

19. Regoli D, Gobeil F, Nguyen QT, et al.: Bradykinin receptor types and B$_2$ subtypes. *Life Sci* 1994; 55:735.

20. Sawutz DG, Salvino JM, Dolle RE, et al.: The nonpeptide WIN 64338 is a bradykinin B$_2$ receptor antagonist. *Proc Natl Acad Sci U S A* 1994; 91:4693.

21. Calixto JB, Pizzolatti MG, Yunes RA: The competitive antagonistic effect of compounds from *Mandevilla velutina* on kinin-induced contractions of rat uterus and guinea-pig ileum in vitro. *Brit J Pharmacol* 1988; 94:1133.

22. Farmer SC, Burch RM, Meeker SA, Wilkins DE: Evidence for a pulmonary B$_3$ receptor. *Mol Pharm* 1989; 36:1.

23. Pyne S, Pyne NJ: Differential effects of B$_2$ receptor antagonists upon bradykinin-stimulated phospholipase C and D in guinea-pig cultured tracheal smooth muscle. *Brit J Pharmacol* 1993; 110:477.

24. Farmer SG, DeSiato MA: Effects of novel nonpeptide bradykinin B$_2$ receptor antagonist on intestinal and airway smooth muscle: further evidence for the tracheal B$_3$ receptor. *Brit J Pharmacol* 1994; 112:461.

25. Field JL, Hall JM, Mortan IKM: Putative novel bradykinin B$_3$ receptors in the smooth muscle of the guinea-pig taenia caeci and trachea. *Agents Actions* 1992; 38(suppl):540.

26. Menke JG, Borkowski JA, Bierilo KK, et al.: Expression cloning of a human B$_1$ bradykinin receptor. *J Biol Chem* 1994; 269: 21583.

27. Hess JF, Borkowski JA, Young GS, et al.: Cloning and pharmacological characterization of a human bradykinin (BK-2) receptor. *Biochem Biophys Res Commun* 1992; 184:260.

28. Liao JK, Homcy CJ: The G proteins of the G alpha$_i$ and G alpha$_q$ family couple the bradykinin receptor to the release of endotheluim-derived relaxing factor. *J Clin Invest* 1993; 92:2168.

29. Sethi T, Rozengurt E: Multiple neuropeptides stimulate clonal growth of small cell lung cancer: effects of bradykinin, vasopressin, cholecystokinin, galanin, and neurotensin. *Cancer Res* 1991; 51:3621.

30. Kaufman MP, Coleridge JCG, Baker DG: Bradykinin stimulates afferent vagal c-fibers in intrapulmonary airways of dogs. *J Appl Physiol* 1980; 48(3):511.

31. Saria A, Martling C, Yan Z, et al.: Release of multiple tachykinins from capsaicin-sensitive sensory nerves in the lung by bradykinin, histamine, dimethylphenyl piperazinium, and vagal nerve stimulation. *Am Rev Respir Dis* 1988; 137:1330.

32. Fuller RW, Dixon CM, Cuss FM, Barnes PJ: Bradykinin-induced bronchoconstriction in humans. *Am Rev Respir Dis* 1987; 135:176.

33. Abe K, Watanabe N, Kumagnai N, et al.: Circulating plasma kinin in patients with branchial asthma. *Experientia* 1967; 23:626.

34. Baumgarten CR, Lehmkuhl B, Brunnee T, et al.: Bradykinin and other inflammatory mediators in BAL-fluid from patients with active pulmonary inflammation. *Agents Actions* 1992; 38(suppl):475.

35. Abraham WM, Burch RM, Farmer SG, et al.: A bradykinin antagonist modifies allergen-induced mediator release and late bronchial responses in sheep. *Am Rev Respir Dis* 1991; 143:787.

36. Polosa R, Rajakulasingam K, Prosperini G, et al.: Effect of inhaled bradykinin on indices of airway responsiveness in asthmatic subjects. *Eur Respir J* 1994; 7:1490.

37. Mansour E, Ahmed A, Cortes A, et al.: Mechanisms of metabisulfite-induced bronchoconstriction: evidence for bradykinin B$_2$-receptor stimulation. *J Appl Physiol* 1992; 72:1831.

38. Polosa R, Holgate ST: Comparative airway response to inhaled bradykinin, kallidin, and [des-Arg^9]bradykinin in normal and asthmatic subjects. *Am Rev Respir Dis* 1990; 142:1367.

39. Ichinose M, Barnes PJ: Bradykinin-induced airway microvascular leakage and bronchoconstriction are mediated via a bradykinin B$_2$ receptor. *Am Rev Respir Dis* 1990; 142:1104.

40. Wirth KJ, Gehring D, Scholkens BA: Effect of Hoe 140 on bradykinin-induced bronchoconstriction in anesthetized guinea pigs. *Am Rev Respir Dis* 1993; 148:702.

41. Nakajima N, Ichinose M, Takahashi T, et al.: Bradykinin-induced airway inflammation. *Am J Respir Crit Care Med* 1994; 149:694.

42. Ishizaka T, Iwata M, Ishizaka K: Release of histamine and arachidonate from mouse mast cells induced by glycosylation-enhancing factor and bradykinin. *J Immunol* 1985; 134:1880.

43. Ichinose M, Nakajima N, Takahashi T, et al.: Protection against bradykinin-induced bronchoconstriction in asthmatic patients by neurokinin receptor antagonist. *Lancet* 1992; 340:1248.

44. Arakawa H, Kawikova I, Lofdahl CG, Lotvall J: Bradykinin-induced airway responses in guinea pig: effects of inhibition of cyclooxygenase and thromboxane synthetase. *Eur J Pharmacol* 1992; 229:131.

45. Baraniuk JN, Lundgren JD, Mizoguchi H, et al.: Bradykinin and respiratory mucous membranes. *Am Rev Respir Dis* 1990; 141:706.

46. Leikauf GD, Ueki IF, Nadel JA, Widdicombe JH: Bradykinin stimulates Cl secretion and prostaglandin E$_2$ release by canine tracheal epithelium. *Am J Physiol* 1985; 248:F48.

47. Naclerio RM, Proud D, Togias AG, et al.: Inflammatory mediators in late antigen-induced rhinitis. *N Engl J Med* 1985; 313:65.

48. Proud D, Togias A, Naclerio RM, et al.: Kinins are generated in vivo following nasal airway challenge of allergic individuals with allergen. *J Clin Invest* 1983; 72:1678.

49. Togias, AG, Naclerio RM, Proud D, et al.: Nasal challenge with cold, dry air results in release of inflammatory mediators: Possible mast cell involvement. *J Clin Invest* 1985; 76:1374.

50. Rajakulasingam K, Polosa R, Lau LCK, et al.: The influence of terfenadine and ipratropium bromide alone and in combination on bradykinin-induced nasal symptoms and plasma protein leakage. *Clin Exp Allergy* 1992; 22:717.

51. Austin CE, Foreman JC, Scadding GK: Reduction by Hoe 140, the B$_2$ kinin receptor antagonist, of antigen-induced nasal blockage. *Brit J Pharmacol* 1995.

52. Proud D, Reynolds CJ, Lacapra S, et al.: Nasal provocation with bradykinin induces symptoms of rhinitis and a sore throat. *Am Rev Respir Dis* 1988; 137:613.

53. Naclerio RM, Gwaltney JM, Hendley JO, et al.: Kinins are generated during rhinovirus colds. *Clin Res* 1985; 33:613.

54. Naclerio RM, Proud D, Lichtenstein LM, et al.: Kinins are generated during experimental rhinovirus colds. *J Infect Dis* 1988; 157:133.

55. Barnett JKC, Cruse LW, Proud D: Kinins are generated in nasal secretions during influenza A infections in ferrets. *Am Rev Respir Dis* 1990; 142:162.

56. Pongracic JA, Naclerio RM, Reynolds CJ, Proud D: A competitive kinin receptor antagonist, [D-Arg^0,Hyp^3,D-Phe^7]-bradykinin, does not affect the response to nasal provocation with bradykinin. *Br J Clin Pharmacol* 1991; 31:287.

57. Town GI, Hallwright GP, Maling TJB, O'Donnell TV: Angiotensin converting enzyme inhibitors and cough. *N Z Med J* 1987; 100:161.

58. Ferner RE, Simpson JM, Rawlins MD: Effects of intradermal bradykinin after inhibition of angiotensin converting enzyme. *Br Med J* 1987; 294:1119.

59. Barber ND, Gibbs JSR, Barrett P, Fox KM: Increased cough reflex associated with angiotensin converting enzyme inhibitor cough. *Br Med J* 1987; 295:1025.

60. Nicholls MG, Gilchrist NL: Sulindac and cough induced by converting enzyme inhibitors. *Lancet* 1987; i:872.

61. Fogari R, Zoppi A, Tettamanti F, et al.: Effects of nifedipine and indomethacin on cough induced by angiotensin-converting enzyme inhibitors: a double-blind, randomized, cross-over study. *J Cardiovasc Pharmacol* 1992; 19:670.

62. Popa V: Captopril-related (and -induced?) asthma. *Am Rev Respir Dis* 1987; 136:999.

63. Peacock AJ, Waller D, Oliver RM: Effects of captopril on pulmonary and renal function in patients with chronic airflow obstruction. *Thorax* 1988; 43:832P.

64. Boulet LP, Milot J, Lampron N, Lacourciere Y: Pulmonary function and airway responsiveness during long-term therapy with captopril. *JAMA* 1989; 261:413.

65. Owen NE, Villereal ML: Lys-bradykinin stimulates Na^+ influx and DNA synthesis in cultured human fibroblasts. *Cell* 1983; 32:979.

66. Goldstein RH, Wall M: Activation of protein formation and cell division by bradykinin and des-Arg^9-bradykinin. *J Biol Chem* 1984; 259:9263.

67. Wunderer G, Walter I, Eschenbacher B, et al.: Ile–Ser–Bradykinin is an aberrant permeability factor in various human malignant effusions. *Biol Chem Hoppe-Seyler* 1990; 371:977.

68. Matsumura Y, Marou K, Kimura M, et al.: Kinin-generating cascade in advanced cancer patients and in vitro study. *Jpn J Cancer Res* 1991; 82:732.

69. Rozengurt E: Early signals in the mitogenic response. *Science* 1986; 234:161.

70. Rozengurt E: Neuropeptides as cellular growth factors: role of multiple signalling pathways. *Eur J Clin Invest* 1991; 21:123.

71. McCaffrey P, Ran W, Campisi J, Rosner MR: Two independent growth factor–generated signals regulate c-*fos* and c-*myc* mRNA levels in Swiss 3T3 cells. *J Biol Chem* 1987; 262:1442.

72. Letterio JJ, Coughlin SR, Williams LT: Pertussis toxin–sensitive pathway in the stimulation of c-*myc* expression and DNA synthesis by bombesin. *Science* 1986; 234:1117.

73. Sethi T, Herget T, Wu SV, et al.: CCKA and CCKB receptors are expressed in small cell lung cancer lines and mediate Ca^{2+} mobilization and clonal growth. *Cancer Res* 1993; 53:5208.

74. Bunn PA Jr, Chan D, Dienhart DG, et al.: Neuropeptide signal transduction in lung cancer: clinical implications of bradykinin sensitivity and overall heterogeneity. *Cancer Res* 1992; 52:24.

75. Trifilieff A, Lach E, Dumont P, Gies JP: Bradykinin binding sites in healthy and carcinomatous human lung. *Brit J Pharmacol* 1994; 111:1228.

76. Cookson WOCM, Wiseman MS, Shale DJ: Angiotensin converting enzyme and endotoxin induced lung damage in the mouse. *Thorax* 1985; 40:774.

77. Hollinger MA: Effect of endotoxin on mouse serum angiotensin-converting enzyme. *Am Rev Respir Dis* 1983; 127:756.

78. Watanabe K, Lam G, Keresztes RS, Jaffe EA: Lipopolysaccharides decrease angiotension converting enzyme activity expressed by cultured human endothelial cells. *J Cell Physiol* 1992; 150:433.

79. Fourrier F, Chopin C, Wallaert B, et al.: Angiotensin-converting enzyme in human adult respiratory distress syndrome. *Chest* 1983; 83:593.

80. Fourrier F, Chopin C, Wallaert B, et al.: Compared evolution of plasma fibronectin and angiotensin-converting enzyme levels in septic ARDS. *Chest* 1985; 87:191.

81. Bedrossian CWM, Woo J, Miller WC, Cannon DC: Decreased angiotensin-converting enzyme in the adult respiratory distress syndrome. *Am J Clin Pathol* 1978; 70:244.

82. Khan MMH, Yamamoto T, Araki H, et al.: Role of Hageman factor/kallikrein-kinin system in pseudomonal elastase-induced shock model. *Biochim Biophys Acta* 1993; 1157:119.

83. Wilson DD, de Garavilla L, Kuhn W, et al.: D-Arg-(Hyp^3-D-Phe^7)-bradykinin, a bradykinin antagonist, reduces mortality in a rat model of endotoxic shock. *Circ Shock* 1989; 27:93.

84. Stone R: Search for sepsis drugs goes on despite past failures. *Science* 1994; 264:365.

Chapter 16

ADENOSINE

GORDON DENT AND KLAUS F. RABE

Adenosine (9-β-D-ribofuranosyl-6-aminopurine) is a ribonucleoside formed by the hydrolytic dephosphorylation of the ribonucleotide adenosine 5'-monophosphate (adenylic acid; AMP) through the action of the ubiquitous ectoenzyme 5'-nucleotidase (5'-ribonucleotide phosphohydrolase; EC 3.1.3.5; CD73; see Fig. 16-1). Production of adenosine occurs throughout the body and is increased in tissues undergoing oxygen deprivation or when adenosine triphosphate (ATP) utilization is increased (e.g., during contraction of muscle or secretion by glandular or immune cells).[1] Similarly, the cell surface receptors that mediate the biologic actions of adenosine occur on almost all cells.[2] Early studies revealed the extensive physiologic actions of adenosine in regulation of local blood flow and activity of neurons and cardiac conducting cells (generally supporting a role for this mediator in balancing tissue oxygen consumption with availability), and the ability of drugs such as caffeine and other methylxanthines to block the effects of adenosine suggested the existence of specific receptors for the nucleoside.[3] The fact that methylxanthines had been effectively used for several decades in the treatment of reversible and chronic airway obstruction had led to an interest in the role of adenosine in the etiology of diseases such as asthma, and a result of this interest has been the identification of multiple subtypes of adenosine receptors and the development of drugs that antagonize specific receptor subtypes with differing degrees of selectivity.[3] The actions of adenosine in the airways and on the inflammatory cells involved in asthma pathology, and the role of adenosine receptors and their antagonists in the study of these actions, form the material of this chapter.

Adenosine Metabolism

Adenosine is produced during the breakdown of the purine ribonucleotides AMP and inosine 5'-monophosphate (IMP) (see Fig. 16-1). Free AMP arises from the enzymatic degradation of nucleic acids and the phosphodiesteric cleavage of the intracellular "second messenger" adenosine 3',5'-cyclic monophosphate (cyclic AMP), as well as from the metabolism of ATP in energy-dependent processes such as muscle contraction. AMP released from cells undergoes hydrolysis of the 5'-ribose phosphate bond to produce adenosine that may be either salvaged by nucleoside kinase-dependent phosphorylation to produce AMP or degraded further by the action of adenosine deaminase to produce another purine nucleoside, inosine. Inosine, as well as its corresponding nucleotide IMP, can be converted to hypoxanthine, which is oxidized by xanthine oxidase to generate xanthine and, finally, the excretory product uric acid.

During periods of high metabolic activity, such as the contraction of muscles, there is a large increase in the transfer of phosphate from ATP to phosphocreatine, leading to stimulation of oxygen consumption and respiration of fuel molecules. Some of the adenosine diphosphate (ADP) formed as a result of ATP breakdown undergoes conversion by adenylate kinase to produce AMP and ATP; during hypoxia, the regeneration of ATP from ADP by the action of creatine kinase is decreased as a result of depletion of phosphocreatine stores, so that more ADP undergoes conversion to AMP. Thus, concentrations of AMP are greatly increased at sites of physiologic stress, and the adenosine derived from the ectonucleotidase-catalyzed breakdown of AMP may be involved in resolving the local stress condition through mechanisms such as inhibiting contraction of vascular smooth muscle or discharge of pacemaker cells in the hypoxic working heart.[1] Conditions of physiologic stress also may occur at sites of inflammation, such as the asthmatic lung, as reflected in the increased levels of adenosine measurable in the plasma of asthmatic subjects after allergen inhalation.[4] Interestingly, the basal concentration of adenosine in the bronchoalveolar lavage (BAL) fluid of asthmatics is significantly higher than in normal subjects; such an eleva-

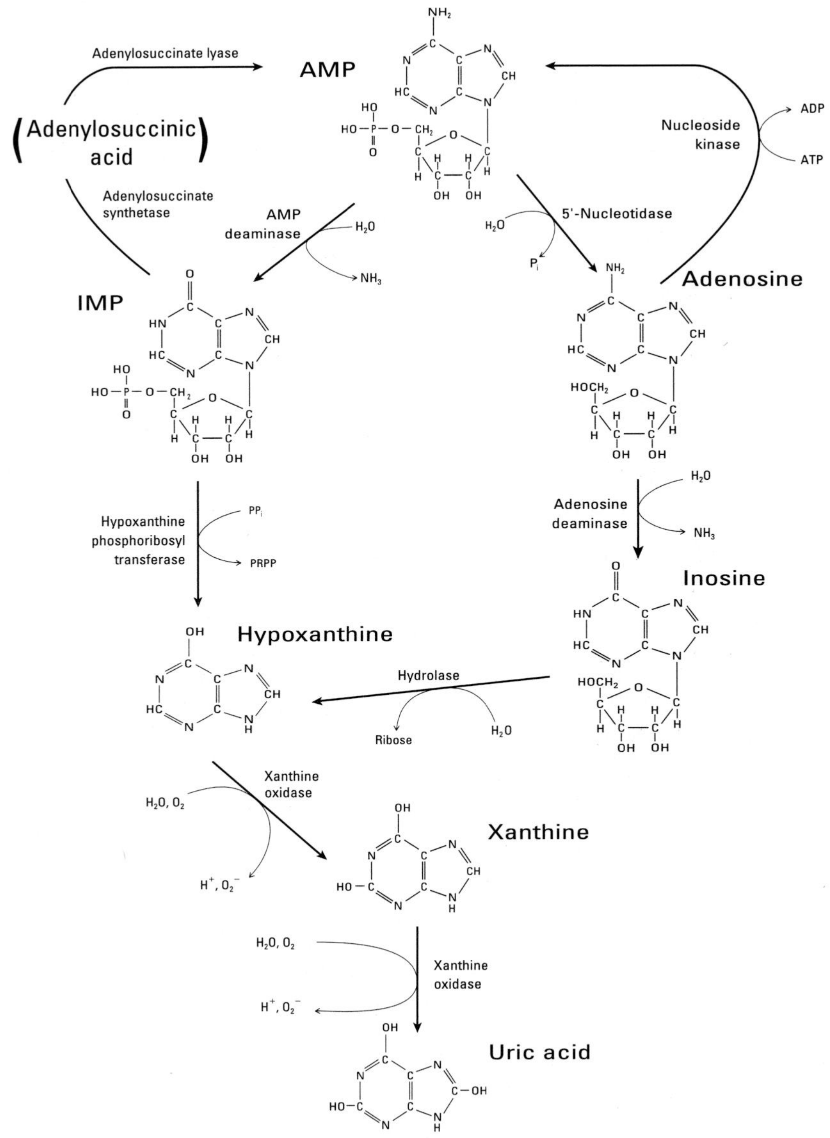

FIGURE 16-1 Adenosine metabolism. Abbreviations: ADP, adenosine 5′-diphosphate; AMP, adenosine 5′-monophosphate; ATP, adenosine 5′-triphosphate; IMP, inosine 5′-monophosphate; P_i, phosphate; PP_i, pyrophosphate; PRPP, 5-phosphoribose-1-pyrophosphate.

tion is also exhibited in nonasthmatic smokers and appears to correlate with local inflammation.[5]

Adenosine Receptors (P_1 Purinoceptors)

Purine nucleosides and nucleotides in extracellular spaces act on cells through the activation of specific cell-surface receptors. These receptors—known collectively as *purinoceptors*—are divided into two classes on the basis of their affinity for purine agonists: P_1-purinoceptors are activated preferentially by adenosine and have low affinity for AMP, ADP, and ATP; P_2-receptors respond preferentially to ATP, and

have lower affinity for ADP and no response to AMP and adenosine.[3]

P_1-purinoceptors are subclassified further on biochemical and pharmacologic grounds, as shown in Table 16-1. Early studies of the cellular actions of adenosine identified opposing actions on the generation of intracellular cyclic AMP: activation of A_1-receptors leads to inhibition of the cyclic AMP-synthesizing enzyme adenylyl cyclase, while A_2-receptor activation activates the enzyme.[6] The development of a range of adenosine analogs and xanthine derivatives with differing affinities for the receptor classes as agonists and antagonists, respectively, has revealed a further subdivision of A_2-receptors into A_{2a}- and A_{2b}-subtypes, as well as disclosing the existence of a third class of receptors (A_3) that

TABLE 16-1   P$_1$-Purinoceptor Classes

	A$_1$	A$_{2a}$	A$_{2b}$	A$_3$
Effectors	↓ cyclic AMP ↑ IP$_3$ ↑ K$^+$ ↓ Ca^{2+}	↑ cyclic AMP	↑ cyclic AMP	↓ cyclic AMP
Agonists: high affinity	CPA, CHA	CGS 21,680 R-PIA	NECA NECA, Ado	APNEA
intermediate affinity	NECA, Ado 2-Cl-Ado	2-Cl-Ado R-PIA	2-Cl-Ado Ado, R-PIA	NECA R-PIA
low affinity	CGS 21,680	CPA, CHA	CGS 21,680	CGS 21,680 Ado
Antagonists: high affinity	DPCPX XAC	XAC, CSC CGS 15,943 KF 17,837	XAC, 8-PT DPCPX CGS 15,943	BW-A 522
intermediate affinity	CPT, 8-PT CGS 15,943	CPT, 8-PT DPCPX	8-pSPT	
low affinity	Theophylline IBMX, 8-pSPT KF 17,387 Caffeine	Theophylline IBMX, 8-pSPT Caffeine	Theophylline IBMX KF 17,387 Caffeine	8-PT, XAC IBMX

Adenosine receptor (P$_1$-purinoceptor) classes. Adapted from Fredholm *et al.*[3] **Abbreviations:** 8-pSPT, 8-*p*-sulfophenyltheophylline; 8-PT, 8-phenyltheophylline; Ado, adenosine; APNEA, N^6-2-(4-aminophenyl)ethyladenosine; BW-A 522, 3-(3-iodo-4-aminobenzyl)-8-(4-oxyacetyl)-1-propylxanthine; CGS 15,943, 9-chloro-2-(2-furanyl)-5,6-dihydro-[1,2,4]-triazolo[1,5]quinazolin-5-imine monomethanesulfonate; CGS 21,680, 2-[*p*-(2-carbonylethyl)phenylethylamino]-5'-N-ethylcarboxamidoadenosine; CHA, N^6-cyclohexyladenosine; CPA, N^6-cyclopentyladenosine; CPT, 8-cyclopentyltheophylline; DPCPX, 1,3-dipropyl-8-cyclopentylxanthine; IBMX, 3-isobutyl-1-methylxanthine; KF 17,387; 1,3-dipropyl-8-(3,4-dimethoxystyryl)-7-methylxanthine; NECA, 5'-N-ethylcarboxyamidoadenosine; R-PIA, N^6-(R-phenylisopropyl)adenosine; XAC, xanthine amine congener (8-4-[(2-aminoethylaminocarbonylmethyloxy)phenyl]-1,3-dipropylxanthine).

is present in large quantities in the lung.[7] The A$_3$-receptor has a low affinity for adenosine but appears to mediate some important functions of the mediator in allergic and inflammatory reactions (see below).

In addition to these cell-surface receptors, adenosine and certain adenine derivatives, such as 2',5'-dideoxyadenosine, also bind to an intracellular site (named the *P-site*) on the catalytic subunit of adenylyl cyclase and thus inhibit the enzyme.[3]

Physiologic Actions of Adenosine

BRONCHOCONSTRICTION

The predominant effect of adenosine, when studied in isolated guinea pig trachea, is prolonged smooth muscle relaxation,[8,9] although a transient contraction also can be observed.[8] Relaxation is induced by concentrations of adenosine < 1 μM in the presence of dipyridamole, a drug that blocks cellular reuptake of adenosine, although in the absence of this agent concentrations greater than 100 μM are required.[10]

When studied in vivo in humans, adenosine has little or no effect on the airway caliber of normal individuals. However, inhalation of aerosolized adenosine leads to a concentration-related bronchoconstriction in patients with either allergic (extrinsic) or nonallergic (intrinsic) asthma when concentrations greater than 67 μg/ml (approximately 200 to 250 μM) are inhaled during normal tidal breathing at 16 breaths/min for 1 min (Fig. 16-2). Similarly, adenosine inhalation has no effect on airway caliber in normal rabbits

and causes bronchodilation in normal guinea pigs. However, adenosine causes marked bronchoconstriction in rabbits actively sensitized to IgE-dependent (ragweed) allergens or guinea pigs sensitized to IgG-dependent (ovalbumin) allergens.[12,13] This phenomenon does not reflect nonspecific hyperresponsiveness: sensitized guinea pigs exhibit normal bronchoconstriction in response to inhalation of the muscarinic agonist carbachol, while guinea pigs rendered hyperresponsive by inhalation of platelet activating factor or ozone display increased responses to both carbachol and adenosine.[13]

In vitro studies of airways reinforce these in vivo findings. Adenosine contracts bronchial rings from ragweed-sensitized rabbits and tracheal spirals from ovalbumin-sensitized guinea pigs but has no effect on normal rabbit bronchi and relaxes normal guinea pig trachea.[9,12] Bronchial smooth muscle from asthmatic humans also is contracted in vitro by adenosine more effectively than that from nonasthmatic patients, while no difference in responsiveness to histamine or leukotriene C$_4$ (LTC$_4$) is observed (Fig. 16-3).[14] The response of asthmatic airways to adenosine is abolished by a combination of histamine and cysteinyl leukotriene receptor antagonists, suggesting that adenosine exerts its bronchoconstrictor action indirectly through the release of histamine and leukotrienes from a cellular source that is either absent or unresponsive to adenosine in nonasthmatic airways.[14]

Bronchoconstrictor responses to adenosine in asthmatic humans are enhanced by dipyridamole, indicating that the effect is mediated by a cell-surface receptor.[15] The receptor subtype mediating adenosine-induced bronchoconstriction in vivo has not been studied in humans, but the rank order

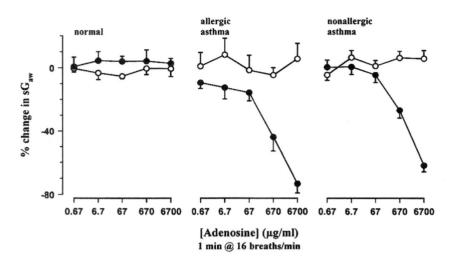

FIGURE 16-2 Adenosine causes bronchoconstriction in asthmatic subjects but not in normals. Effects of increasing doses of nebulized adenosine (●) or time-matched saline inhalations (○) on specific airway conductance (sG_{aw}) in normals, allergic asthmatics, and nonallergic asthmatics. Data are taken from Cushley et al.[11]

of potency of adenosine analogs causing bronchoconstriction has been evaluated in sensitized rabbits.[12] This order (CPA > NECA > CGS 21,680 > adenosine; see Table 16-1 for abbreviations) suggests the participation of A_1-receptors, although the low potency of adenosine, as compared with CGS 21,680, may point to some involvement of A_3-receptors. In guinea pig airways, relaxant responses to adenosine are blocked by 8-phenyltheophylline (8-PT), a methylxanthine P_1-purinoceptor antagonist with moderate to high affinity at A_2- and A_1-receptors (Table 16-1), but this drug, which has very low affinity at A_3-receptors,[3] is ineffective against the contraction induced by adenosine in airways of sensitized guinea pigs.[9] This suggests that the contraction may be mediated by A_3-receptors in this system, although no direct confirming evidence is yet available.

Bronchoconstriction also can be induced in asthmatic subjects by inhalation of AMP,[4] which undergoes rapid metabolism by 5'-ectonucleotidase to produce adenosine.[16] AMP is often used for studies of the actions of adenosine in humans, owing to its greater aqueous solubility, but even at the highest concentrations achievable bronchoconstriction is very rarely observed in nonasthmatic subjects.[17] It is interesting to note that responsiveness to AMP increases following aller-

gen challenge,[18] and that AMP responsiveness is elevated in patients exhibiting more than 15 percent circadian variation in peak expiratory flow rate (PEFR).[19] Bronchial responsiveness to AMP itself also exhibits greater diurnal variation than does methacholine responsiveness.[19] These observations, along with the evidence for an indirect action of adenosine in vitro (see above), point to a bronchoconstrictor mechanism for adenosine that is related to immunologic responses and is independent of smooth muscle. This indirect mechanism appears to be common to adenosine and bradykinin, since prior inhalation of bradykinin leads to cross-tachyphylaxis (desensitization) to AMP but not to histamine.[20]

ACTIONS ON INFLAMMATORY CELLS

MAST CELLS
Bronchoconstriction induced in asthmatic patients by inhalation of AMP is inhibited by histamine H_1-receptor antagonists, similarly to in vitro contraction of asthmatic airways caused by adenosine (see above). The H_1-antagonist terfenadine blocks more than 80 percent of the response to a con-

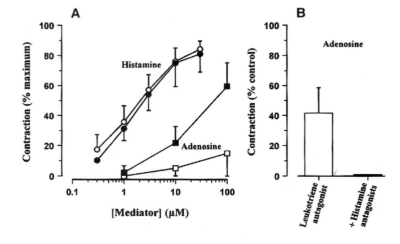

FIGURE 16-3 Adenosine contracts asthmatic human airways in vitro. (*A*) Contraction of normal (open symbols) and asthmatic (closed symbols) human bronchi in vitro by histamine (circles) and adenosine (squares), expressed as percentage of maximal contraction induced by histamine + acetylcholine. (*B*) Contraction of asthmatic human bronchi in vitro by adenosine after treatment of tissues with the sulfidopeptide leukotriene receptor antagonist ICI 198,615 alone (open bar) or with the histamine H_1- and H_2-receptor antagonists mepyramine and metiamide (solid bar), expressed as percentage of contraction induced by adenosine in the absence of drugs. Data are taken from Björck et al.[14]

centration of AMP that causes a 30 percent decrease in FEV_1 (PC_{30}) in placebo-treated patients, at a dose that abolishes the response to PC_{30} histamine and causes a twofold reduction in the response to allergen.[21] The difference in sensitivity of the AMP and allergen responses to inhibition by terfenadine, as well as their different time courses, suggests that allergen and AMP exert bronchoconstrictor actions through different mechanisms. Rapid tachyphylaxis develops to adenosine both in sensitized guinea pig airways in vitro and in human airways in vivo. Sensitized guinea pig tracheal spirals, which contract in response to an initial application of adenosine, exhibit reduced contractions or even relaxations upon subsequent adenosine application.[9] Similarly, repeated inhalations of AMP by atopic, nonasthmatic humans lead to a diminution and eventual loss of bronchoconstriction responses, which is not associated with loss of sensitivity to histamine.[22] Thus, either downregulation of adenosine receptors occurs upon repeated challenge or responses to adenosine rely on release of a preformed mediator, so that replenishment of stores is required before further responses can be evoked. In the light of these data, it has been proposed that release of histamine from lung mast cells accounts for the bronchoconstrictor action of adenosine.

Adenosine alone does not stimulate the release of histamine from human lung mast cells in vitro but does enhance histamine release induced by anti-IgE (Fig. 16-4*A*) or calcium ionophore, as well as anti-IgE-induced synthesis of LTC_4.[23] Since this action of adenosine was mimicked (with greater potency) by the adenosine analogs NECA and R-PIA (see Table 16-1 for abbreviations), it was assumed that the mechanism was mediated by A_2-receptors, at which NECA is more potent than it is at A_1-receptors.[23,24] In experiments with lung fragments, adenosine had no effect on histamine release induced by calcium ionophore or the plant lectin concanavalin A under normal conditions. In the presence of xanthine amine congener (XAC; an A_1- and A_2-receptor antagonist), however, enhancement of histamine release by adenosine did become apparent.[25] These data suggest that adenosine has a dual action on mast cells: an inhibition of mediator release mediated by an XAC-sensitive receptor and an enhancement of release mediated by an XAC-insensitive receptor. Since cyclic AMP has been demonstrated to sup-press mast cell activation,[26] it appears likely that the inhibitory action of adenosine is mediated by A_2-receptors, which increase intracellular cyclic AMP by activating adenylyl cyclase (Table 16-1). The receptor mediating augmentation of responses may be of the A_3-type, since A_3-receptors are insensitive to XAC, but no definite evidence for this is yet available.

The nucleoside transport inhibitor N-(p-nitrobenzyl)-6-thioinosine (NBTI), which blocks reuptake of adenosine into the cell, causes enhancement of stimulated histamine release from both human lung fragments and rat peritoneal mast cells,[25,27] and suggests that there is release of adenosine from the mast cells, which causes enhancement of cell activation when removal of the extracellular adenosine is blocked. Under these conditions, addition of exogenous adenosine inhibits calcium ionophore- or concanavalin A-induced histamine release. The high extracellular adenosine concentrations thus achieved preferentially stimulate A_2-receptors, thereby leading to increased cyclic AMP and inhibition of cell function.[25] This concentration dependence is confirmed by findings that adenosine and its analogs NECA and R-PIA enhance anti-IgE-induced release of histamine and LTC_4 at low concentrations,[24,28] while higher concentrations inhibit the response.[24] Although the rank order of agonist potencies (NECA > R-PIA > adenosine) for both phases of the adenosine response is characteristic of A_2-receptor-mediated actions, the inhibitory action appears to predominate when the intracellular cyclic AMP concentration rises above a certain level, suggesting that the stimulatory action of adenosine may be independent of cyclic AMP modulation and, therefore, independent of A_2-receptors.[16]

More detailed research has been conducted into the actions of adenosine on rat, mouse, and hamster mast cells, and the results of these experiments point toward an important role for the A_3-receptor in mediating the response-enhancing action of adenosine.[29] For example, the enhancement of rat peritoneal mast cell mediator release by adenosine is not inhibited by 8-PT, although the A_2-receptor-mediated increase in cyclic AMP is reduced.[17] It remains to be determined whether this action also is mediated by A_3-receptors in human mast cells, although the abundance of A_3-receptors in human lung (which contains very small

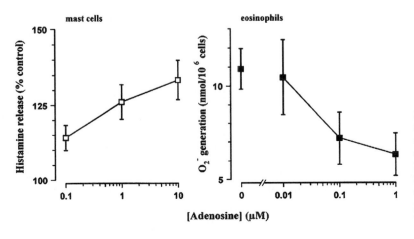

FIGURE 16-4 Adenosine enhances mediator release from human lung mast cells and inhibits oxygen radical generation by human eosinophils. (*A*) Enhancement of anti-IgE-induced histamine release from human lung mast cells by adenosine. Data are taken from Peachell *et al.*[23] (*B*) Inhibition of opsonized zymosan-induced superoxide anion radical release form human peripheral blood eosinophils by adenosine. Data are taken from Yukawa *et al.*[32]

numbers of A_1-receptors)[30] suggests some role for this purinoceptor subtype in pulmonary physiopathology.

EOSINOPHILS

Eosinophils have been implicated in the pathogenesis of bronchial asthma by their presence in the airways during late asthmatic reactions and by the ability of their granule proteins and reactive oxygen metabolites to induce hyperresponsiveness of airway smooth muscle.[31] Very little is known about the actions of adenosine on eosinophil function. In one study, fairly low concentrations of adenosine have been shown to suppress the stimulated generation of superoxide anion radical ($\cdot O_2^-$) by eosinophils obtained from either human peripheral blood (Fig. 16-4B) or guinea pig peritoneal cavity. This action is mimicked by NECA with a greater potency than by R-PIA, suggesting the participation of an A_2-receptor. A modulatory role for adenosine in the eosinophil response is indicated by the ability of 8-PT to enhance the opsonized zymosan-induced $\cdot O_2^-$ generation in the absence of exogenous adenosine. It appears, therefore, that activated eosinophils release adenosine that acts on cell-surface A_2-receptors in a "negative-feedback" loop to suppress further cell activation.[32]

NEUTROPHILS

The actions of adenosine on neutrophils—which are the major cell type mediating acute inflammation and which participate in the airway inflammatory reactions of diseases, such as pneumonia, chronic bronchitis, and emphysema, have been studied extensively. Neutrophils themselves release adenosine during the process of secretion of granule proteins[2] and, as described above for mast cells, this endogenous adenosine appears to exert a biphasic modulation of neutrophil activation.

Low concentrations of adenosine promote both the migration of neutrophils in response to chemotactic peptides [N-formylmethionylphenylalanine (fMLP) and the complement fragment C5a] and the adherence of the cells to endothelial layers in vitro. These low concentrations also cause an enhancement of phagocytosis of opsonized particles by neutrophils. At higher concentrations, however, adenosine inhibits neutrophil adherence and release of oxygen radical, although the ability of adenosine to inhibit neutrophil degranulation remains controversial. Adenosine also inhibits the "priming" (i.e., the induction of increased responsiveness to chemotactic factors) of neutrophils by agents such as platelet activating factor and tumor necrosis factor.[2]

Biochemical and pharmacologic studies of neutrophil responses to adenosine have indicated the presence of two receptor classes. Pertussis toxin, which inactivates the guanine nucleotide-binding regulatory protein (G protein) coupling receptors to inhibition of adenylyl cyclase (G_i), reverses the enhancement of fMLP-induced neutrophil chemotaxis by adenosine.[33] This finding indicates the presence on neutrophils of a G_i-coupled adenosine receptor of the A_1- or A_3-subtype. The presence of A_2-receptors on neutrophils also has been demonstrated by the ability of A_2-receptor agonists to increase neutrophil cyclic AMP content.[34] Since cyclic AMP inhibits neutrophil $\cdot O_2^-$ genera-

tion through a mechanism involving cyclic AMP-dependent protein kinase (protein kinase A), it is likely that the suppression of oxygen-radical release by adenosine is mediated by A_2-receptors. However, the attenuation of neutrophil $\cdot O_2^-$ release by adenosine is unaffected by inhibition of protein kinase A. Furthermore, the suppression of oxygen radical generation by adenosine is not enhanced by a cyclic AMP phosphodiesterase (PDE) inhibitor even though this combination of drugs produces a much greater increase in intracellular cyclic AMP.[34] The role of A_2-receptors in the modulation of neutrophil function remains, therefore, uncertain.[2]

ACTIONS ON NERVE FUNCTIONS

Along with enhancing and inhibiting inflammatory cell mediator release, adenosine also displays biphasic actions on nerve-mediated responses in the airways of experimental animals. In vitro, adenosine potentiates the contraction of rabbit bronchi in response to transmural electrical stimulation[35]; in vivo, the bronchoconstriction induced in guinea pigs by capsaicin (which provokes the release of peptide neurotransmitters such as substance P from the terminals of unmyelinated sensory nerve fibers) is suppressed by adenosine.[36] The latter, inhibitory action of adenosine is mimicked by A_{2a}-receptor agonists (NECA and CGS 21,680) but not by a selective A_1-agonist (CHA; see Table 16-1). While NECA and CGS 21,680 (but not CHA) can be shown to block capsaicin-induced release of substance P from guinea pig lung, the adenosine analogs have no effect on the bronchoconstriction induced by exogenous substance P, implying that the action of adenosine is on transmitter release from the nerves and not on the response of airway smooth muscle to the transmitter.

Pharmacologic Modulation of Adenosine Responses

The bronchoconstriction induced by aerosolized AMP is inhibited by treatment of patients with inhaled budesonide for 14 days. This corticosteroid is substantially more effective against AMP responses than against those to inhaled methacholine or sodium metabisulfite, another indirect bronchoconstrictor agent.[37] Clearly, therefore, corticosteroids have specific inhibitory actions in the pathways through which adenosine exerts its bronchoconstrictor action in addition to its general modification of bronchial hyperreactivity in asthma. Responses to adenosine in asthmatic subjects are also inhibited by the loop diuretics furosemide and bumetanide—drugs that also protect against bronchoconstriction induced by other indirect stimuli such as bradykinin, metabisulfite, and allergen.[38]

The bronchoconstrictor response to inhaled AMP is reduced by treatment of asthmatic patients with disodium cromoglycate or nedocromil sodium—drugs that suppress mast cell release of mediator and inhibit neural reflexes in the peptidergic sensory nerves.[16] There is very little evidence of a direct action of cromoglycate or nedocromil at adenosine receptors, and it appears likely that these drugs act more generally against indirect bronchoconstrictor stimuli.

The ability of methylxanthines to antagonize the actions of adenosine has long been recognized, and this property of the methylxanthines has been proposed to underlie their effectiveness in the treatment of obstructive lung diseases.[17] Interpretation of studies of the inhibition of bronchoconstriction by methylxanthines such as theophylline is complicated by the well-characterized inhibition of PDE by such drugs, a property that also causes bronchodilation (see Chap. 50). Theophylline inhibits bronchoconstriction induced by inhaled adenosine more effectively than that induced by histamine or methacholine,[39,40] but this could reflect the indirect nature of the adenosine response. Methylxanthines suppress the stimulated release of mediators from mast cells and other inflammatory cells and, consequently, may exert a double inhibitory action—inhibition of mediator release and inhibition of smooth muscle contraction—on adenosine-induced bronchoconstriction. The ability of methylxanthines to relax airways is unrelated to their potency in antagonizing adenosine[41]; this may be due to a combination of proinflammatory and anti-inflammatory actions of adenosine. Enprofylline (3-propylxanthine), which is far less potent than theophylline as an adenosine antagonist, is more potent than theophylline as a bronchodilator and inhibitor of allergen-induced bronchoconstriction in asthmatic patients (see Chap. 51), suggesting that adenosine antagonism is not the most important mechanism of action by methylxanthine in the treatment of asthma.[16,17,41]

Summary

Adenosine is of interest in the field of pulmonary pharmacology because of its capacity to induce bronchoconstriction in asthmatic patients but not in normal subjects. Some possible mechanisms through which this effect may be mediated have been proposed, but the precise pathways involved have not been identified. Similarly, no definite role for adenosine in the pathology of asthma is recognized; bronchoconstriction can be provoked in severe asthmatic patients by intravenous administration of dipyridamole, but it remains questionable whether the extracellular adenosine concentrations achieved by this procedure can be realized under physiologic conditions.[16] Research into the role of adenosine has been hampered by the lack of specificity of the available methylxanthine adenosine antagonists, which all exhibit some degree of PDE inhibition. The development of new adenosine receptor-blocking xanthines with very low potency as PDE inhibitors may allow better characterization of the participation of adenosine in pulmonary disease processes.[42]

References

1. Rall TW: Drugs used in the treatment of asthma: the methylxanthines, cromolyn sodium, and other agents, in Gilman AG, Rall TW, Nies AS, Taylor P (eds): Goodman & Gilman's *The Pharmacological Basis of Therapeutics*, 8th ed. New York, Pergamon, Chap 25, pp 618–637, 1990.
2. Cronstein BN: Adenosine, an endogenous anti-inflammatory agent. *J Appl Physiol* 76:5, 1994.
3. Fredholm BB, Abbracchio MP, Burnstock G, et al.: Nomenclature and classification of purinoceptors. *Pharmacol Rev* 46:143, 1994.
4. Mann JS, Holgate ST, Renwick AG, Cushley MJ: Airway effects of purine nucleosides and nucleotides and release with bronchial provocation in asthma. *J Appl Physiol* 61:1667, 1986.
5. Driver AG, Kukoly CA, Ali S, Mustafa SJ: Adenosine in bronchoalveolar lavage fluid in asthma. *Am Rev Respir Dis* 148:91, 1993.
6. Wolff J, Londos C, Cooper DMF: Adenosine receptors and the regulation of adenylate cyclase. *Adv Cyclic Nucleotide Res* 14:199, 1994.
7. Salvatore CA, Jacobson MA, Taylor HE, et al.: Molecular cloning and characterization of the human A_3 adenosine receptor. *Proc Natl Acad Sci USA* 90:10365, 1993.
8. Coleman RA: Effects of some purine derivatives on the guinea pig trachea and their interaction with drugs that block adenosine uptake. *Br J Pharmacol* 57:51, 1976.
9. Thorne JR, Broadley KJ: Adenosine-induced bronchoconstriction of isolated lung and trachea from sensitized guinea-pigs. *Br J Pharmacol* 106:978, 1992.
10. Kenakin T: Concentrations of drugs, in *Pharmacological Analysis of Drug-Receptor Interaction*, 2d ed. New York, Raven Press, Chap. 5, pp 137–175, 1993.
11. Cushley MJ, Tattersfield AE, Holgate ST: Inhaled adenosine and guanosine on airway resistance in normal and asthmatic subjects. *Br J Clin Pharmacol* 15:161, 1983.
12. Ali S, Mustafa SJ, Metzger WJ: Adenosine-induced bronchoconstriction and contraction of airway smooth muscle from allergic rabbits with late-phase airway obstruction: evidence for an inducible adenosine A_1 receptor. *J Pharmacol Exp Ther* 268:1328, 1994.
13. Thorne JR, Broadley KJ: Adenosine-induced bronchoconstriction in conscious hyperresponsive and sensitized guinea pigs. *Am J Respir Crit Care Med* 149:392, 1994.
14. Björck T, Gustafsson LE, Dahlén SE: Isolated bronchi from asthmatics are hyperresponsive to adenosine, which apparently acts indirectly by liberation of leukotrienes and histamine. *Am Rev Respir Dis* 145:1087, 1992.
15. Crimi N, Palermo F, Oliveri R, et al.: Enhancing effect of dipyridamole inhalation on adenosine-induced bronchospasm in asthmatic patients. *Allergy* 43:179, 1988.
16. Polosa R, Ng WH, Church MK: Adenosine, a positive modulator of the asthmatic response, in Barnes PJ, Rodger IW, Thomson NC (eds): *Asthma: Basic Mechanisms and Clinical Management*, 2d ed. London, Academic Press, Chap 18, pp 288–296, 1992.
17. Church MK, Featherstone RL, Cushley MJ, et al.: Relationships between adenosine, cyclic nucleotides, and xanthines in asthma. *J Allergy Clin Immunol* 78:670, 1986.
18. Aalbers R, Kaufman HF, Groen H, et al.: Allergen-induced changes in adenosine 5'-monophosphate bronchial responsiveness: effect of nedocromil sodium. *Ann Allergy* 69:339, 1992.
19. Oosterhoff Y, Koeter GH, de Monchy JG, Postma DS: Circadian variation in airway responsiveness to methacholine, propranolol, and AMP in atopic asthmatic subjects. *Am Rev Respir Dis* 147:512, 1993.
20. Polosa R, Rajakulasingam K, Church MK, Holgate ST: Repeated inhalation of bradykinin attenuates adenosine 5'-monophosphate (AMP) induced bronchoconstriction in asthmatic airways. *Eur Respir J* 5:700, 1992.
21. Rafferty P, Beasley R, Southgate P, Holgate S: The role of histamine in allergen and adenosine-induced bronchoconstriction. *Int Arch Allergy Appl Immunol* 82:292, 1987.
22. Daxum Z, Rafferty P, Richards R, et al.: Airway refractoriness to adenosine 5' monophosphate after repeated inhalation by atopic non-asthmatic subjects. *J Allergy Clin Immunol* 83:152, 1989.

23. Peachell PT, Columbo M, Kagey-Sobotka A, et al.: Adenosine potentiates mediator release from human lung mast cells. *Am Rev Respir Dis* 138:1143, 1988.

24. Peachell PT, Lichtenstein LM, Schleimer RP: Differential regulation of human basophil and lung mast cell function by adenosine. *J Pharmacol Exp Ther* 256:717, 1991.

25. Ott I, Lohse MJ, Klotz KN, et al.: Effects of adenosine on histamine release from human lung fragments. *Int Arch Allergy Appl Immunol* 98:50, 1992.

26. Peachell PT, MacGlashan DW Jr, Lichtenstein LM, Schleimer RP: Regulation of human basophil and lung mast cell function by cyclic adenosine monophosphate. *J Immunol* 140:571, 1988.

27. Lohse MJ, Maurer K, Klotz KN, Schwabe U: Synergistic effects of calcium-mobilizing agents and adenosine on histamine release from rat peritoneal mast cells. *Br J Pharmacol* 98:1392, 1989.

28. Marone G, Cirillo R, Genovese A, et al.: Human basophil/mast cell releasability: VII. Heterogeneity of the effect of adenosine on mediator secretion. *Life Sci* 45:1745, 1989.

29. Linden J: Cloned adenosine A₃ receptors: pharmacological properties, species differences and receptor functions. *Trends Pharmacol Sci* 15:298, 1994.

30. Joad JP, Kott KS: Effect of adenosine receptor ligands on cAMP content in human airways and peripheral lung. *Am J Respir Cell Mol Biol* 9:134, 1993.

31. Gleich GJ, Adolphson CR: The eosinophilic leukocyte: structure and function. *Adv Immunol* 39:177, 1986.

32. Yukawa T, Kroegel C, Chanez P, et al.: Effect of theophylline and adenosine on eosinophil function. *Am Rev Respir Dis* 140:327, 1989.

33. Rose FR, Hirschhorn R, Weissmann G, Cronstein BN: Adenosine promotes neutrophil chemotaxis. *J Exp Med* 167:1186, 1988.

34. Cronstein BN, Kramer SB, Rosenstein ED, et al.: Occupancy of adenosine receptors raises cyclic AMP alone and in synergy with occupancy of chemoattractant receptors and inhibits membrane depolarization. *Biochem J* 252:709, 1988.

35. Gustafsson LE, Wiklund NP, Cederqvist B: Apparent enhancement of cholinergic transmission in rabbit bronchi via adenosine A₂ receptors. *Eur J Pharmacol* 120:179, 1986.

36. Morimoto H, Yamashita M, Imazumi K, et al.: Effects of adenosine A₂ receptor agonists on the excitation of capsaicin-sensitive afferent sensory nerves in airway tissues. *Eur J Pharmacol* 240:121, 1993.

37. O'Connor BJ, Ridge SM, Barnes PJ, Fuller RW: Greater effect of inhaled budesonide on adenosine 5'-monophosphate-induced than on sodium-metabisulfite-induced bronchoconstriction in asthma. *Am Rev Respir Dis* 146:560, 1992.

38. Rajakulasingam K, Polosa R, Church MK, et al.: Effect of inhaled furosemide on responses of airways to bradykinin and adenosine 5'-monophosphate in asthma. *Thorax* 49:485, 1994.

39. Cushley MJ, Tattersfield AE, Holgate ST: Adenosine-induced bronchoconstriction in asthma: antagonism by inhaled theophylline. *Am Rev Respir Dis* 129:380, 1984.

40. Mann JS, Holgate ST: Specific antagonism of adenosine-induced bronchoconstriction in asthma by oral theophylline. *Br J Clin Pharmacol* 19:685, 1985.

41. Persson CGA, Karlsson J-A: In vitro responses to bronchodilator drugs, in Jenne JW, Murphy S (eds): *Drug Therapy for Asthma: Research and Clinical Practice (Lung Biology in Health and Disease, vol. 31)*, New York, Marcel Dekker, Chap 4, pp 129–176, 1987.

42. Ukena D, Schudt C, Sybrecht GW: Adenosine receptor-blocking xanthines as inhibitors of phosphodiesterase isozymes. *Biochem Pharmacol* 45:847, 1993.

Chapter 17 _____

THE SENSORY NEUROPEPTIDES

SHANNON S. CARSON, M.D. AND JULIAN SOLWAY

Sensory Neuropeptide Synthesis

Tachykinin Receptors

Airway Responses to Tachykinins

Stimulation of Sensory Neuropeptide Release

Enzymatic Modulation of Tachykinins

Neurokinin Receptor Antagonists

Clinical Pharmacology in Humans

The sensory neuropeptides include the tachykinins [e.g., substance P (SP), neurokinin A (NKA), neuropeptide K (NPK), and neuropeptide-γ (NPγ)] as well as calcitonin-gene-related peptide (CGRP). These peptide mediators are synthesized by sensory C-fiber nerves and are packaged together in synaptic vesicles stored within the varicosities at nerve terminals. They are released locally, within the innervated tissue, as a result of various types of noxious physical or chemical nerve stimulation. When released from C-fibers within the airway wall, the sensory neuropeptides act at cell surface receptors to provoke bronchoconstriction (in most species other than the mouse), bronchovascular vasodilation and hyperpermeability, enhanced respiratory secretion, and inflammatory cell recruitment and activation. The role that these agents play in human airways disease is yet to be clearly identified, but this remains a subject of intense investigation. This chapter reviews the structure and function of the sensory neuropeptides, factors that control their release and subsequent inactivation, and contributions to airway inflammation.

Sensory Neuropeptide Synthesis

The tachykinins are a family of short peptides (10 to 36 amino acid residues) that share a common carboxy-terminal sequence including an amidated C-terminal methionine (Table 17-1)[1,2] SP and NKA are synthesized as products of the preprotachykinin (PPT)-I gene. Alternative splicing of the seven exons in the PPT-I gene results in three different mRNA species: α-PPT-I, β-PPT-I and γ-PPT-I.[1] A fourth variant, δ-PPT-I, has also been described in rat intestine.[3] Synthesis of the individual peptides results from posttrans-

lational processing of the distinct mRNA encoded products as outlined in Table 17-1. α-PPT-I excludes exon 6 and encodes SP alone; β-PPT-I includes all seven exons and encodes SP, NKA, and NPK; γ-PPT-I excludes exon 4 and encodes SP, NKA, and NPγ. NPK and NPγ are N-terminal elongations of NKA. δ-PPT-I excludes exons 6 and 7, and, like α-PPT-I mRNA, encodes SP alone; however, its expression in nerves innervating the lung has not been studied. NPK undergoes intraneuronal proteolytic conversion to NKA; therefore, it does not appear in synaptic vesicles and is probably not released endogenously. Neurokinin B is synthesized from a separate PPT gene, PPT-II, but this gene is not expressed in airway C-fibers, which therefore do not contain NKB. The regulation of neurokinin gene expression has not yet been established fully.[1] PPT-I expression in the basal ganglia is influenced by dopamine or methamphetamine, and in the rat anterior pituitary, thyroid hormone downregulates PPT-I expression. In primary sensory neuron cultures, nerve growth factor is necessary for the synthesis of SP, and it increases PPT mRNA transcription in a dose-dependent manner.[4] Interleukin-1β (IL-1β) increases SP and PPT mRNA in superior cervical ganglia cultured as explants,[5] and this action is blocked both by depolarization of the ganglia and by glucocorticoids.[6] This effect of IL-1β is apparently mediated through its actions on supporting cells within the ganglia, as IL-1β has no effect on cultured neurons that have been dissociated from these supporting cells.[6] Interestingly, a recent report documents increased PPT-I expression in the nodose ganglia after pulmonary allergen challenge in sensitized guinea pigs.[7]

Two genes encode the 37-amino acid human CGRP,[8] CALC-I and CALC-II. Their mRNA products (α-CGRP and β-CGRP, respectively) are both transcribed in neurons.

TABLE 17-1 Mammalian Sensory Neuropeptides

Peptide	Gene	mRNA	Structure (1-letter code)
SP	PPT-I	$\alpha, \beta, \gamma, \delta$ PPT-I	RPKPQQFFGLM-NH$_2$
NKA (1–10)		β, γ PPT-I	HKTDSFVGLM-NH$_2$
NPK		β PPT-I	DADSSIEKQVALLKALYGHGQISHKRHKTDSFVGLM-NH$_2$
NP γ		γ PPT-I	DAGHGQISHKRHKTDSFVGLM-NH$_2$
NKB	PPT-II	PPT-II	DMHDFFVGLM-NH$_2$
CGRP-I	CALC-I	α-CGRP	ACDTATCVTHRLAGLLSRSGGVVKNNFVPTNVGSKAF-NH$_2$
CGRP-II	CALC-II	β-CGRP	ACNTATCVTHRLAGLLSRSGGMVKSNFVPTNVGSKAF-NH$_2$

Reprinted with permission from References 1 and 2.

Alternative processing of mRNA from the CALC-I gene results in transcription of calcitonin from its exon 4 or CGRP from its exon 5. In contrast to SP, neural CGRP content does not increase in response to nerve growth factor in primary nerve culture, indicating differential regulation of tachykinin and CGRP expression.[9] CGRP does not have the carboxy-terminal amino acid sequence characteristic of the tachykinins, but it is often colocalized with tachykinins in airway sensory nerves.[10–12] Each of the neurokinins is synthesized in the cell body and transported along the axon to the nerve terminals.

Terminal varicosities of airway sensory C-fiber nerves are located beneath and within the epithelium, airway smooth muscle, submucosal bronchial glands, and bronchial blood vessels, and SP-immunoreactivity has been detected within intramural tracheobronchial ganglion cells.[13,14] Although C-fiber axons originating within the trachea travel in the vagus nerves (mostly the right vagus) to cell bodies within the jugular and nodose ganglia (mostly the jugular ganglion in the guinea pig[15]), bronchial C-fibers have cell bodies both in these vagal ganglia and in the thoracic spinal dorsal root ganglia. Fibers from dorsal root ganglion cells are distributed with sympathetic fibers to the lung bilaterally. In general, C-fiber axons exhibit immunoreactivity for all the PPT-I tachykinins, as well as for CGRP, which appear colocalized within secretory granules. However, CGRP also exists independently in some nerve fibers as well as in mucosal neuroendocrine cells and neuroepithelial bodies in the intrapulmonary airways.[16] There are substantial differences in airway SP content among species, which may suggest differences in the roles that tachykinins play in controlling airway function. While normal humans appear to have 10-fold less SP content that normal guinea pigs,[14] there is controversy about whether the airways of asthmatic patients contain increased[17] or reduced[18] amounts of substance P compared with airways from normal human lungs. In all species, the central airways appear to contain greater concentrations of neurokinins than does the peripheral lung.

Tachykinin Receptors

Tachykinin (or neurokinin, NK) receptors are complex membrane bound molecules that interact with guanine nucleotide regulatory proteins. They are similar in structure and function to β-adrenergic receptors and muscarinic receptors, but differences in the extracellular ligand binding domains confer affinity for neurokinins as opposed to small amine agonists.[19] Phosphoinositide generation is the main second-messenger system linked to their activation.

There are three classes of neurokinin receptors—NK-1, NK-2, and NK. These differ in their order of affinity for natural tachykinins as outlined in Table 17-2.[21] All three tachykinin receptors probably recognize the common C terminus of the tachykinins; receptor subtype specificity may reside in differing affinities for the more N-terminal amino acid residues.[22] Until the development of subtype-specific receptor antagonists (see below), the order of potency of natural or selective synthetic agonists was used as an indicator of the predominant receptor subtype mediating a tachykinin response within a given tissue.

Tachykinin receptors also differ in their abilities to mediate the various end actions of the tachykinins. In general, NK-1 receptors mediate systemic arterial vasodilation and promote exocrine secretions; NK-2 stimulation causes smooth muscle constriction; and NK-3 activation modulates the release of acetylcholine in peripheral organs.[20,23] Differences in responses to receptor-specific agonists or antagonists indicate receptor population differences among species for a given tissue.[24] In particular, two types of NK-2 receptors (designated NK-2A and NK-2B) have been identified in rabbit pulmonary artery (NK-2A) or hamster trachea (NK-2B). Furthermore, recent evidence points to the existence of two types of NK-1 receptors that occur in different species; guinea pig and human NK-1 receptors are similar, but differ in affinity for various NK-1 antagonists from rat and mouse NK-1 receptors, which are also similar in antagonist affinities.[25] Even within guinea pig trachea, there may be NK-1 receptor heterogeneity.[26] Tachykinin receptors are found in both large and small airways in animals and humans and are concentrated beneath the epithelium, in airway smooth muscle, in small vessels within the lamina propria, and, in humans, in deep submucosal glands.[27,28] Similarly, SP binding sites are also found within the epithelium, submucosal glands, and small vessels in human nasal mucosa.[29] A recent study reported increased lung mRNA level for NK-1 but not NK-2 receptors in the lungs of asthmatic patients.[30] Interestingly, incubation of these asthmatic tissues with dexamethasone attenuates the increase in NK-1 receptor gene expression. The number of NK-1 receptors, and their affinity for certain agonists, have been shown to decrease in guinea pigs 7 days after infection with parain-

TABLE 17-2   Pharmacology of NK-1, NK-2, and NK-3 Tachykinin Receptors

	NK-1	NK-2	NK-3
Agonists' order of potency	SP > NKA = NKB	NKA > NKB ≫ SP	NKB > NKA ≫ SP
Selective agonists	SP methylester [Sar^9] SP sulfone [Pro^9] SP sulfone [Pro^9] SP Septide GR 73,632	[Nle^{10}] NKA (4-10) [βAla^8] NKA (4-10) [Lys^5, MeLeu^9, Nle^{10}] NKA (4-10) GR64,349	Senktide [MePhe^7] NKB
Monoreceptorial bioassays for tachykinin receptors	Dog carotid artery Guinea pig vas deferens Rabbit jubular vein Rabbit vena cava Mouse bronchus Guinea pig urethra	Rabbit pulmonary artery Rat vas deferens Hamster trachea Human bronchus Human colon Human urinary bladder	Rat portal vein

Reprinted with permission from Reference 21.

fluenza type 3 virus, despite an increase in substance P-mediated physiologic effects (see "Enzymatic Modulation of Tachykinins," below).[31]

There are two receptors for CGRP. Like tachykinin receptors,[125] I-CGRP binding sites are found throughout the lung, but are most dense within bronchial and pulmonary blood vessels of all sizes and in alveolar walls.[20] These distributions of tachykinin and CGRP receptors closely parallel the tachykinin and CGRP-mediated actions among airway tissue components (see below).

Airway Responses to Tachykinins

Sensory neuropeptides influence airway function on both acute and more chronic time scales. Immediate effects include bronchoconstriction, vascular changes, glandular and epithelial secretory stimulation, and modulation of cholinergic neurotransmission. Longer-term consequences of airway exposure to sensory neuropeptides are granulocyte recruitment, development of airway constrictor hyperresponsiveness, and probable enhancement of epithelial repair. These responses are considered further below.

Whether endogenously released or exogenously administered, tachykinins cause acute airflow obstruction in most animal airways.[12,13,32–34] NKA is 20 to several hundred times more potent than substance P in provoking bronchoconstriction. NKA primarily stimulates NK-2 receptor-mediated phosphoinositide hydrolysis that increases the formation of inositol-1,4,5-triphosphate, which in turn releases calcium ions from intracellular stores in airway smooth muscle.[35] NK-1 receptors may also contribute to this response in guinea pigs.[20] Human airways obtained from surgical specimens also constrict when exposed in vitro to capsaicin (which releases endogenous tachykinins) or to synthetic tachykinins.[23] Interestingly, the contractile response to NKA is significantly greater in smaller human bronchi than in more proximal airways.[36] Both SP and NKA aerosols cause

dose-dependent bronchoconstriction in asthmatic patients, but these agents have little or no effect in normal human subjects.[37] As in isolated human bronchi, NKA is more potent than SP when inhaled. The bronchoconstrictor effect of nebulized NKA in asthmatic patients is inhibited by pretreatment with nedocromil sodium or sodium cromoglycate, possibly by inhibiting secondary release of mast-cell products or by some other mechanism.[38,39]

Endogenous tachykinin release or exogenous administration in the airways also causes rapid development of mucosal microvascular hyperpermeability and plasma extravasation.[40,41] SP is more potent than NKA or NKB in mediating this effect, and NK-1 receptors have been localized to postcapillary venules in the airway submucosa. The axial distribution of plasma extravasation along rat airways is primarily central with relative sparing of the peripheral airways; this parallels the density of SP receptors topographically along the rat airways.[27] It has not yet been proven that tachykinins can cause microvascular leak in human airways, although SP injected into human skin can cause a wheal, indicating the capacity to cause microvascular leak in human postcapillary venules.[42]

Sensory neuropeptides also have significant effects on airway blood flow. SP is the most powerful vasodilator of these species,[43] and its action appears to be endothelium-dependent.[44] CGRP generally causes endothelium-independent vasodilation by a direct effect on vascular smooth muscle,[45] though it may also stimulate a parallel dilator mechanism through stimulation of endothelial prostacyclin synthesis.[46] Its effect follows a prolonged time course, and CGRP may play the dominant physiologic role in regulating airway blood flow.[47] The vasodilation and vascular hyperpermeability caused by sensory neuropeptides are known collectively as "neurogenic inflammation."[48]

Substance P administration stimulates submucosal gland secretion mediated by NK-1 receptors. Rather than causing increased mucus production, SP instead appears to constrict submucosal gland secretory tubules, causing them to expel mucus stored within.[49] SP also influences bronchial epithelial chloride secretion[50] and mucociliary activity,[51] though these actions may be indirect. NKA also causes mucous glycoprotein secretion through a mechanism involving increases in calcium ion concentration within acinar cells.[52]

Tachykinins can potentiate release of acetycholine from efferent fibers in rabbits and ferrets by a prejunctional effect on postganglionic parasympathetic nerves,[53,54] mediated by action at NK-1 and/or NK-2 receptors. A similar effect is noted in guinea-pig bronchus.[55] Thus, tachykinins may enhance sensitivity to cholinergically mediated airway responses.

Endogenous tachykinin release caused by intravenous or aerosol capsaicin administration or electrical vagal nerve stimulation results in the recruitment of circulating granulocytes into the airway wall.[56] Initially, neutrophils and eosinophils adhere to postcapillary venules—the site of endothelial cell retraction and microvascular hyperpermeability. Some of the adherent cells then traverse the endothelium and migrate into the airway wall.[57] SP is a chemoattractant for human polymorphonuclear leukocytes. Unlike most other tachykinin effects, which depend on the carboxy-terminal amino acid residues, chemotaxis is a property that resides in the amino-terminal end of SP and does not involve tachykinin receptors. The contribution of adherent granulocytes to the pathogenesis of neurogenic inflammation is uncertain. There is also evidence that SP induces the release of neutrophil chemotactic factors from bronchial epithelial cells in culture[58] and causes increased adherence of neutrophils to bronchial epithelial cells.[59]

CGRP or its degradation products also may cause recruitment of eosinophils to the airways. Rat CGRP-1 is chemotactic for guinea pig eosinophils, and this activity is substantially increased by tryptic digestion. The structure of residues 32 to 35 of rat CGRP-1 is identical to the tetrapeptide identified as the eosinophil chemotactic factor of anaphylaxis (ECF-A), Val-Gly-Ser-Glu.[60] In high concentrations, SP can cause degranulation of eosinophils.[61] As mentioned earlier, there is indirect evidence that tachykinins may cause release of histamine or other mediators from mast cells in the airway, based upon the blunted bronchoconstrictor effects of nebulized SP or NKA by pretreatment with nedocromil sodium or cromolyn sodium. However, SP does not stimulate histamine release from mast cells isolated from the lung or other sites except for the skin.[62]

Inhalation of substance P or endogenous release of sensory neuropeptides caused by capsaicin exposure have each been shown to induce non-specific bronchoconstrictor hyperresponsiveness that lasts ≥24 h in guinea pigs,[63,64] and inhalation of neurokinin A evokes a similar response in monkeys.[65] The mechanism by which this occurs is unknown, but could conceivably relate to airway wall changes attributable to neuropeptide-induced granulocyte influx and/or neurogenic plasma extravasation. Evidence from animal studies also implicates sensory neuropeptides in the generation of allergen-induced hyperresponsiveness.[66] A recent preliminary report suggests that products released from activated eosinophils can stimulate tachykinin release from C-fiber nerves in primary culture.[67]

While many of these effects of sensory neuropeptide release appear detrimental to airway function, there are important potential beneficial effect of these peptides as well. For example, CGRP induces tracheal epithelial cell migration[68] and proliferation[69] in vitro, factors that might promote repair of the epithelial denudation characteristic of asthmatic airways. Recent experiments in which tracheal epithelial cells were cocultured with sensory neurons suggests that tachykinins also promote epithelial proliferation.[70] Thus, although speculative, it may be that C-fiber endings exposed when epithelial cells are shed become stimulated, release their neuropeptides, and promote epithelial migration and proliferation to repair mucosal integrity in asthmatic airways. Intact sensorineural function also apparently moderates the inflammation induced by instillation of endotoxin into rat trachea.[71]

Stimulation of Sensory Neuropeptide Release

Sensory neuropeptides are released locally upon stimulation of the sensitive terminals of C-fibers.[2] A wide range of chemical and physical stimuli can elicit this response, and as with the release of other neurotransmitters, sensory neuropeptide release can be inhibited pharmacologically. Electrical stimulation of nerve bundles carrying sensory C-fibers can result in release of tachykinins or CGRP from their nerve terminals in vivo; electrical field stimulation (EFS) in organ bath or tissue preparations similarly provokes neuropeptide release in vitro. In the former circumstance, electrical impulses pass from the site of stimulation along the axons to the nerve terminals, in a direction away from the cell body ("antidromic conduction"). An impulse generated within a nerve terminal can proceed in the usual ("orthodromic") direction toward the cell body, then spread down an arborized branch to another nerve terminal without passing through a cell body in what is referred to as an "axon reflex." In either case, or during direct depolarization of nerve terminals by EFS, storage granules containing sensory neuropeptides are released locally when intracellular free calcium concentration increases as a consequence of nerve terminal depolarization.[12,53]

A wide range of chemical agents also can stimulate conduction within and neuropeptide release from C-fibers. One chemical commonly used experimentally is capsaicin,[72] the chemical irritant in chili peppers. In everyday experience, accidental exposure of the eye to pepper causes two responses. First, the eye hurts, reflecting the generation of electrical impulses within scleral C-fibers that are transmitted centrally and perceived as pain. Second, the eye turns red, reflecting the vasodilation and hyperemia caused by local sensory neuropeptide release. Addition of capsaicin to fluid perfusing the pulmonary circulation[73] of isolated guinea pig lungs increases SP, NKA, and/or CGRP release in the effluents. Administration of intravenous or aerosolized capsaicin acutely induces bronchoconstriction and airway plasma extravasation in animals in vivo,[40] and tracheal or bronchial tissue strips exposed to capsaicin demonstrate noncholinergic contraction in vitro.[14] Capsaicin elicits these responses by binding to the vanilloid receptor found on C-fiber membranes,[74] thus opening a cation conductance channel permeable to both monovalent and divalent cations.[75] The resulting cationic influx depolarizes the nerve, and initiates the release of storage granules that contain tachykinins and CGRP.[72] Stimulation by capsaicin leads to a refractory state that may be reversible, but this desensitization can be irreversible upon overwhelming exposure to capsaicin. This causes increased calcium and sodium concentrations within the cell[76] and subsequent neurotoxicity. Systemic administration of capsaicin to animals in large doses releases neuropeptides acutely and causes massive bronchoconstriction in guinea pigs; this also depletes the airway sensory C-fibers of their neuropeptides. In adult animals, the resulting dysfunction of sensory C-fibers may last for a few weeks, but in neonates capsaicin "pretreatment" can induce lifelong tachykinin depletion.[77] Prior to the development of specific neurokinin receptor antagonists, chronic capsaicin pretreatment served as a useful tool for discerning the contribution of sensory neuropeptides to physiologic or pathophysiologic airway responses in animals.

Using competitive inhibitors of the vanilloid receptor, it has been shown that several agents including bradykinin and lipoxin A_4 stimulate C-fibers without involving the vanilloid receptor.[78] Nicotine in cigarette smoke increases firing rate in vagal C-fiber afferent nerves[79] and stimulates increases in the release of SP from isolated guinea pig bronchi. Histamine can stimulate tachykinin release,[73,80] and leukotriene D_4 can potentiate C-fiber mediated bronchoconstriction[81] or possibly elicit tachykinin release itself.[82,83] Other evidence that sensory neuropeptides may mediate acute bronchial responses to allergen challenge in sensitized airways is equivocal, and there is evidence both for[84,85] and against important participation[86] in various preparations. However, guinea pigs sensitized and repeatedly challenged with antigen show an increase in bronchial reactivity to cholinergic stimulation. Since this effect is ablated in animals depleted of sensory neuropeptides,[66] it seems likely that allergen challenge does stimulate sensory C-fibers.[66,87] Indeed, recent reports document increased recovery of SP in bronchoalveolar lavage fluid from atopic human subjects after acute allergen challenge.[88–90]

There are also physical stimuli that can activate C-fibers. Among the most common is mechanical stimulation, which in the airways, provokes C-fiber-initiated cough.[91] Isocapnic hyperpnea of dry gas elicits bronchoconstriction[92] and bronchovascular hyperpermeability[93] in a number of animal species.[92–97] In guinea pigs, hyperpnea-induced bronchoconstriction depends critically on tachykinin release from airway sensory nerves.[98] The mechanism by which dry gas hyperpnea elicits tachykinin release may be related to water loss from the airway as hypertonic aerosol inhalation has been shown to cause neuropeptide-dependent airway plasma extravasation,[99] and sensory nerves in primary culture release tachykinins in response to a hypertonic environment, but not in response to a decrease in temperature.[100] At present, it remains unknown whether dry gas hyperpnea (a well-described precipitant of bronchoconstriction in humans with exercise-induced asthma) also stimulates C-fiber neuropeptide release in human asthmatic subjects.

There are several compounds that inhibit C-fiber neuropeptide release by stimulating receptor sites on nerve terminals. Perhaps most notably, morphine and other opioids inhibit C-fiber afferent-initiated cough and bronchoconstrictor reflexes[101] and inhibit release of tachykinins in response to various stimuli that otherwise cause noncholinergic bronchoconstriction and neurogenic plasma extravasation.[102] Morphine acts by "prejunctional" stimulation of μ- and δ-receptors, which inhibit sensory neuropeptide release; it does not antagonize neurokinin receptors and has no influence on the effects of exogenously administered tachykinins. Other C-fiber membrane receptors capable of inhibiting neuropeptide release include histamine H_3 receptors, GABA-B receptors, P_1 purinoceptors, α_2-adrenoreceptors, and neuropeptide Y_2 receptors.[103] In addition, cromolyn sodium appears to inhibit capsaicin-induced C-fiber activation.[104]

Enzymatic Modulation of Tachykinins

Enzymatic cleavage and inactivation represents an important mechanism controlling the physiologic activity of sensory neuropeptides within the airways. Several enzymes in the lung can act upon tachykinins as substrates; these include mast cell-derived chymases and tryptases, serine proteases, aminopeptidases, carboxypeptidases, neutral endopeptidase (NEP), and angiotensin-converting enzyme (ACE). However, evidence to date indicates that only two have likely important physiological roles in vivo—NEP and ACE.[105–114] NEP and ACE are zinc metalloendopeptidases that are bound to cell membranes by single hydrophobic domains.[106,107] NEP immunoreactivity can be demonstrated in airway epithelium, smooth muscle and submucosal glands, as well as alveolar epithelium and vascular endothelium.[108–110] Within the lung, ACE is expressed primarily by vascular endothelium. ACE inactivates only SP, which explains the longer half-life of NKA in plasma. NEP, on the other hand, cleaves both SP and NKA. The C-terminal dipeptide is removed from both peptides, which eliminates their bronchoactive properties.[111] NEP and ACE are both located in various other tissues besides the lung, and both are known to cleave a variety of other peptide substrates besides tachykinins. Degradation of CGRP in the lung has not been evaluated thoroughly, though CGRP can be a substrate for NEP.[112]

NEP can be inhibited by the chemical agents thiorphan or phosphoramidon. NEP inhibition enhances bronchial responses to SP or NKA administered intravenously or intraluminally, including bronchoconstriction,[105,111] neurogenic plasma extravasation,[56] mucus secretion,[113] and neutrophil and eosinophil adhesion to endothelium[114] in animals. Recent reports show that NEP inhibition also potentiates the bronchoconstrictor responses to NKA in normal and asthmatic human subjects.[115,116] As NEP is concentrated within airway epithelium, removal of airway epithelium enhances airway reactivity to tachykinins by removing functional NEP and therefore slowing tachykinin degradation.[117] Neutral endopeptidase activity is decreased by respiratory viral infections.[118] *Mycoplasma pulmonis* infection,[119] cigarette smoke,[120] and toluene diisocyanate.[121] The fact that each of these agents are known to increase airway hyperresponsiveness provides further evidence that NEP is an important modulator of tachykinin activity in the airway, and that tachykinins may participate substantially in the regulation of airway function. Interestingly, NEP expression appears to be increased by corticosteroid treatment in vitro.[122]

Neurokinin Receptor Antagonists

Tachykinin receptor antagonists have been available since the early 1980s, but only in the last few years have improvements in their selectivities and potencies made them truly useful tools for dissecting the roles of individual receptor subtypes in various airway responses in animal experiments. Experience with neurokinin receptor antagonists in humans is extremely limited.

The first tachykinin receptor antagonists contained D-amino acid substitions in substance P.[123] These agents, such as Spantide I, competitively blocked NK-1 and NK-2 receptors (along with bombesin receptors, endothelin receptors, and growth-hormone-releasing receptors), but also exhibited partial agonist activity, local anesthetic properties, and ability to degranulate mast cells. Their poor specificity and substantial side effects limited their usefulness.

Improvements in receptor selectivity and activity of peptide antagonists were achieved through several approaches. Cyclization of SP analogs, multiple substitutions within truncated linear tachykinin sequences, incorporation of large side groups, or introduction of non-amino acids into the peptide chain all achieved receptor subtype selectivity and improved potency in second-generation peptide antagonists.[124] Interestingly, short 2- or 3-amino acid antagonists have also been developed; the dipeptide FK888 is a potent and rather selective NK-1 blocker.[125]

The latest series of neurokinin receptor antagonists is based on multicyclic nonpeptide structures, most of which are selective inhibitors of NK-1 receptors. Although the first such compound, CP-96,345, exhibited an important non-NK-1 receptor activity—blockage of L-type calcium channels[126]—subsequent compounds have been developed that lack this adverse effect. These have proved extremely useful in dissecting the roles of NK-1 receptors in tachykinin-mediated airway responses. For example, whereas initial studies using (+/−) CP-96,345 suggested that NK-1 receptors of guinea pigs, might participate in hyperpnea-induced bronchoconstriction of guinea pigs,[127] subsequent investigations revealed that CP-99,994 (an NK-1 antagonist which lacks calcium channel activity in the doses used) had no effect.[128] Instead, only SR-48,968 (a nonpeptide NK-2 antagonist) blocked this response.[128] Thus, NK-2 but not NK-1 receptors mediate hyperpnea-induced bronchoconstriction in guinea pigs. Figure 17-1[21] shows the chemical structures of recently developed nonpeptide neurokinin receptor antagonists.

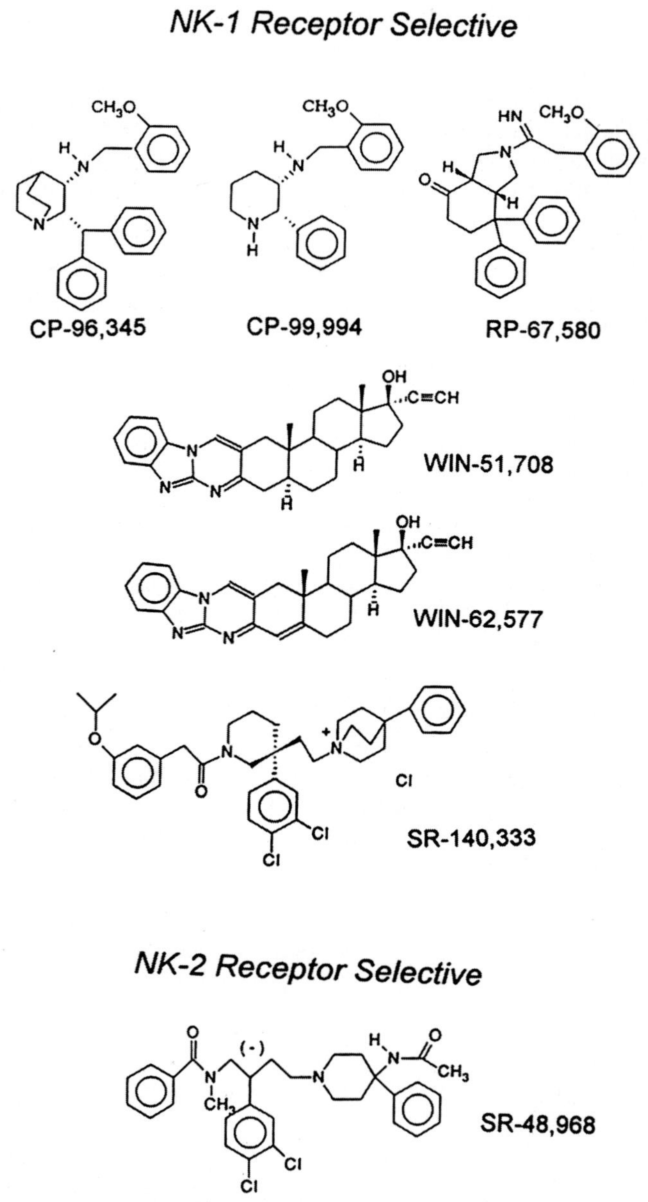

FIGURE 17-1 The chemical structures of recently developed nonpeptide neurokinin receptor antagonists. (*Adapted from Meini and Maggi,*[21] *with permission.*)

Clinical Pharmacology in Humans

Clinical application of neurokinin receptor antagonists has been extremely limited. The first published report demonstrated that FK224—a cyclic peptide that associates with both NK-1 and NK-2 receptors—slightly but significantly blunted bradykinin aerosol-induced bronchoconstriction in asthmatic human subjects.[129] It previously had been shown that bradykinin stimulates tachykinin release from airway sensory nerves,[130] and this finding for the first time appeared to confirm the physiologic importance of endogenous tachykinin release in a human airway response.

Subsequent studies with FK224 demonstrated that this agent does not block NKA-induced bronchoconstriction in asthmatic subjects,[131] suggesting that its effect against bradykinin-induced bronchoconstriction may have been through blockade of NK-1 receptors.

In the only other available report of studies in human asthmatic subjects, the selective NK-1 antagonist CP-99,994 was shown to be ineffective in preventing the bronchoconstriction or cough induced by hypertonic saline aerosol inhalation.[132] While the reason for this lack of efficacy is unknown, it may relate in part to the predominance of NK-2 receptors on human airway smooth muscle.[133]

References

1. Helke CJ, Drause JE, Mantyh PW, Couture R, and Bannon MJ: Diversity in mammalian tachykinin peptidergic neurons: multiple peptides, receptors and regulatory mechanisms. *FASEB J.* 1990; 4:1606–1615.
2. Solway J and Leff AR: Sensory neuropeptides and airway function. *J Appl Physiol* 1991; 71(6):2077–2087.
3. Khan I and Collins SM: Fourth isoform of preprotachykinin messenger RNA encoding for substance P in the rat intestine. *Biochem Biophys Res Comm* 1994; 202(2):796–802.
4. Lindsay RM, Harmar AJ: Nerve growth factor regulates expression of neuropeptide genes in sensory neurons. *Nature* 1989; 337:362–4.
5. Hart RP, Shadiack AM, and Jonakait GM: Substance P expression is regulated by interleukin-1 in cultured sympathetic ganglia. *J Neurosci Res* 1991; 29:282–291.
6. Shadiack AM, Hart RP, Carlson CD, and Jonakait GM: Interleukin-1 induces substance P in sympathetic ganglia through the induction of leukemia inhibitory factor (LIF). *J Neurosci* 1991; 13(6):2601–2609.
7. Fischer A, Philippin B, Saria A, McGregor G, Kummer W: Neuronal plasticity in sensitized and challenged guinea pigs: neuropeptides and neuropeptide gene expression. *Am J Resp and Crit Care Med* 1994; 149:A890.
8. Steenbergh PH, Hoppener JW, Zandberg J, Visser A, Lips DJ, and Jansz HS: Structure and expression of the human calcitonin/CGRP genes. *FEBS Letters* 1986; 209:97–103.
9. MacLean DB, Bennett B, Morris M, and Wheeler FB: Differential regulation of calcitonin gene-related peptide and substance P in cultured neonatal rat vagal sensory neurons. *Brain Research* 1989; 478:349–355.
10. Martling CR, Saria A, Fischer JA, Hökfelt T, and Lundberg JM: Calcitonin gene-related peptide and the lung: neuronal coexistence with substance P, release by capsaicin and vasodilatory effect. *Regul Pept* 1988; 20:125–139.
11. Dey RD, Altemus JB, Zervos I, and Hoffpauir J: Origin and colocalization of CGRP- and SP-reactive nerves in cat airway epithelium. *J Appl Physiol* 1990; 68:770–778.
12. Lundberg JM, Saria A, Theodorsson-Norheim E, Brodin E, Hua X, Margling CR, Games R, and Hökfelt T: Multiple tachykinins in capsaicin-sensitive afferents; occurence, release and biological effects with special reference to irritation of the airways. In: *Tachykinin Antagonists*, Håkanson R and Sundler F, eds.). Elsevier, Amsterdam, pp. 159–169.
13. Lundberg JM, Brodin E, and Saria A: Effects and distribution of vagal capsaicin-sensitive substance P neurons with special reference to the trachea and lungs. *Acta Physiol Scand* 1983; 119:243–252.
14. Martling CR: Sensory nerves containing tachykinins and CGRP in the lower airways. Functional implications for bronchoconstriction, vasodilatation and protein extravasation. *Acta Physiol Scand Suppl* 1987; 563:1–57.
15. Kummer W, Fischer A, Kurkowski R, and Heym C: The sensory and sympathetic innervation of guinea-pig lung and trachea as studied by retrograde neuronal tracing and double-labelling immunohistochemistry. *Neuroscience* 1992; 49(3):715–737.
16. Cadieux A, Springall DR, Mulderry PK, et al.: Occurrence, distribution, and ontogeny of CGRP immunoreactivity in the rat lower respiratory tract: effect of capsaicin treatment and surgical denervation. *Neuroscience* 1986; 19:605–627.
17. Ollerenshaw SL, Jarvis DL, Sullivan CE, Woolcock AJ: Substance P Immunoreactive nerves in airways from asthmatics and non-asthmatics. *Eur Resp J* 1991; 4:673–82.
18. Lilly CM, Bai TR, Shore SA, Hall AE, and Drazen JM: Neuropeptide content of lungs from asthmatic and non-asthmatic patients. *Am J Respir Crit Care Med* 1995; 151:548–553.
19. Fraser CM and Lee NH: Molecular characterization of autononic and neuropeptide receptors. In: *Neuropeptides in Respiratory Medicine*. Eds. Kaliner MA, Barnes PJ, Kunkel GH, and Baraniuk JN. Marcel Dekker, Inc. 1994; pp. 225–250.
20. Regoli D, Drapeau G, Dion S, and D'Orleans-Juste P: Pharmacological receptors for substance P and neurokinins. *Life Sci* 1987; 40:109–117.
21. Meini S and Maggi CA: Tachykinin receptor antagonists. Chapter 12 in: *Neuropeptides in Respiratory Medicine*, ed. Kaliner MA, Barnes PJ, Kunkel GHH, and Baraniuk JN. Marcel-Dekker, New York, 1994, 693 pp.
22. Schwyzer R: Membrane-assisted molecular mechanism of neurokinin receptor subtype selection. *EMBO J* 1987; 6:2255.
23. Naline EP, Devillier P, Drapeau G, Toty L, Bakdach H, Regoli H, and Advenier C: Characterization of neurokinin effects and receptor selectivity in human isolated bronchi. *Am Rev Respir Dis* 1989; 140:679–686.
24. Maggi CA, Patacchinin R, Guiliani S, et al.: Competitive antagonists discriminate between NK2 tachykinin receptor subtypes. *Br J Pharmacol* 1990; 100:588–92.
25. Gitter BD, Waters DC, Bruns RF, Mason NR, Nixon JA, Howbert JJ: Species differences in affinities of non-peptide antagonists for substance P receptors. *Eur J of Pharmacol* 1991; 197(2-3):237–238.
26. Zeng XP, Burcher E: Use of selective antagonists for further characterization of tachykinin NK-2, NK-1 and possible "septide-selective" receptors in guinea pig bronchus. *J Pharm Exp Ther* 1994; 270(3):1295–1300.
27. Sertl K, Wiedermann CJ, Kowalski ML, Hurtado S, Plutchok J, Linnoila I, Pert CB, and Kaliner MA: Substance P: the relationship between receptor distribution in rat lung and the capacity of substance P to stimulate vascular permeability. *Am Rev Respir Dis* 1988; 138:151–158.
28. Springall DR and Polak JM: Neuropeptides in the lower airways investigated by modern microscopy. Chapter 3 in: *Neuropeptides in Respiratory Medicine*, ed. Kaliner MA, Barnes PJ, Kunkel GHH, and Baraniuk JN. Marcel-Dekker, New York, 1994, 693 pp.
29. Baraniuk JN, Lundgren JD, Mullol J, Okayama M, Merida M, Kaliner M: Substance P and neurokinin A in human nasal mucosa. *Am J Respir Cell Mol Biol* 1991; 4:228–236.
30. Adcock IM, Peters M, Gelder C, Shirasaki H, Brown CR, and Barnes PJ: Increased tachykinin receptor gene expression in asthmatic lung and its modulation by steroids. *J Mol Endocrin* 1993; 11(1):1–7.
31. Kudlacz EM, Shatzer SA, Farrell AM, and Baugh LE: Parainfluenza virus type 3 induced alterations in tachykinin NK1 receptors, substance P levels and respiratory functions in guinea pig airways. *Eur J of Pharmacol* 1994; 270(4):291–300.

32. Manzini S, Conti S, Maggi CA, Abelli L, Somma V, Del-Bianco E, and Geppetti P: Regional differences in the motor and inflammatory responses to capsaicin in guinea pig airways. Correlation with content and release of substance P-like immunoreactivity. *Am Rev Respir Dis* 1989; 140:936–941.

33. Shore SA, and Drazen J: Enhanced airway responses to substance P after repeated challenge in guinea pigs. *J Appl Physiol* 1989; 62:955–961.

34. Manzini S: Bronchodilatation by tachykinins and capsaicin in the mouse main bronchus. *Br J of Pharmacol* 1992; 105(4):968–72.

35. Grandordy BM, Frossard N, Rhoden KJ, Barnes PJ: Tachykinin-induced phosphoinositide breakdown in airway smooth muscle and epithelium: relationship to contraction. *Mol Pharmacol* 1988; 33:515–519.

36. Frossard N, Barnes PJ: Effects of tachykinins on small human airways. *Neuropeptides* 1991; 19:157–162.

37. Joos GF, Pauwels RA, and van der Straeten ME: Effect of inhaled substance P and neurokinin A in the airways of normal and asthmatic subjects. *Thorax* 1987; 42:779–83.

38. Joos GF, Pauwels RA, and van der Straeten ME: The effect of nedocromil sodium on the bronchoconstrictor effect of neurokinin A in subjects with asthma. *J Allergy Clin Immunol* 1989; 83:663–668.

39. Crimi N, Palermo F, Oliveri R, Palermo B, Polosa R, and Mistretta A: Protection of nedocromil sodium on bronchoconstriction induced by inhaled neurokinin A (NKA) in asthmatic patients. *Clin Exp Allergy* 1992; 22(1):75–81.

40. Lundberg JM, Brodin E, Hua X, and Saria A: Vascular permeability changes and smooth muscle contraction in relation to capsaicin-sensitive substance P afferents in the guinea-pig. *Acta Physiol Scanda* 1984; 120:217–227.

41. McDonald DM, Mitchell RA, Gabella G, and Haskell A: Neurogenic inflammation in the rat trachea. II. Identity and distribution of nerves mediating the increase in vascular permeability. *J Neurocytol* 1988; 17:605–628.

42. Crossman DC, Dashwood MR, Taylor GW, Wellings R, and Fuller RW: Sodium cromoglycate: evidence of tachykinin antagonist activity in the human skin. *J Appl Physiol* 1993; 75(1):167–72.

43. Matran R, Alving K, Martling CR, Lacroix JS, and Lundberg JM: Effects of neuropeptides and capsaicin on tracheobronchial blood flow of the pig. *Acta Physiol Scand* 1989; 135:335–342.

44. Bolton TB and Clapp LH: Endothelial-dependent relaxant actions of carbachol and substance P in arterial smooth muscle. *Br J Pharmacol* 1986; 87:713–723.

45. McCormack DG, Mak JC, Coupe MD, and Barnes PJ: Calcitonin gene-related peptide vasodilation of human pulmonary vessels. *J Appl Physiol* 1989; 67(3):1265–1270.

46. Crossman D, McEwan J, MacDermott J, MacIntyre I, and Dollery CT: Human calcitonin gene-related peptide activates adenylate cyclase and releases prostacyclin from human umbilical vein endothelial cells. *Br J Pharmacol* 1987; 92(4):695–701.

47. Salonen RO, Webber SE, and Widdiconbe JG: Effects of neuropeptides and capsaicin on the canine tracheal vasculature in vivo. *Br J Pharmacol* 1988; 95:1262–1270.

48. Janscó N: Role of the nerve terminals in the mechanism of inflammatory reactions. *Bull Millard Filmore Hosp. (Buffalo, NY)* 1960; 7:53–77.

49. Coles SJ, Neill KH, and Reid LM: Potent stimulation of glycoprotein secretion in canine trachea by substance P. *J Appl Physiol* 1984; 57:1323–1327.

50. Tamaoki J, Ueki IF, Widdicombe JH, and Nadel JA: Stimulation of Cl secretion by neurokinin A and neurokinin B in canine tracheal epithelium. *Am Rev Respir Dis* 1988; 137:899–902.

51. Lindberg S, Dolata J: NK1 receptors mediate the increase in

52. Nagaki M, Ishihara H, Shimura S, Sasaki T, Takishima T, and Shirato K: Tachykinins induce a $[Ca^{2+}]i$ rise in the acinar cells of feline tracheal submucosal gland. *Respir Physiol* 1994; 98(1):111–120.

53. Tanaka DT, and Grunstein MM: Maturation of neuromodulatory effect of substance P in rabbit airways. *J Clin Invest* 1990; 85:345–350.

54. Belvisi MG, Patacchini R, Barnes PJ, Maggi CA: Facilitatory effects of selective agonists for tachykinin receptors on cholinergic neurotransmission: evidence for species differences. British Journal of Pharmacology. 1994; 111(1):103–10.

55. Myers AC and Undem BJ: Functional interactions between capsaicin-sensitive and cholinergic nerves in the guinea pig bronchus. *J Pharm Exp Therap* 1991; 259(1):104–109.

56. Umeno E, Nadel JA, Huang H, and McDonald DM: Inhibition of neutral endopeptidase potentiates neurogenic inflammation in the rat trachea. *J Appl Physiol* 1989; 66(6):2647–2652.

57. Umeno E, Nadel JA, and McDonald DM: Neurogenic inflammation of the rat trachea: fate of neutrophils that adhere to venules. *J Appl Physiol* 1990; 69(6):2131–6.

58. Von Essen SG, Rennard SI, O'Neill D, Ertl RF, Robbins RA, Koyama S, and Rubinstein I: Bronchial epithelial cells release neutrophil chemotactic activity in response to tachykinins. *Am J Physiol* 263(*Lung Cell Mol Physiol* 2 Pt 1): 1992; L226–31.

59. DeRose V, Robbins RA, Snider RM, Spurzem JR, Thiele GM, Rennard SI, and Rubinstein I: Substance P increases neutrophil adhesion to bronchial epithelial cells. *J Immunol* 1994; 152(3):1339–46.

60. Davies D, Medeiros MS, Keen J, Turner AJ, Haynes LW: Eosinophil chemotactic peptide sequences in rat alpha-CGRP. Activation of a novel trophic action by neutral endopeptidase 24.11. *Ann N.Y. Acad Sci* 1992; 657:405–11.

61. Kroegel C, Geinbycz MA, Barnes PJ: Characterization of eosinophil activation by peptides. Differential effects of substance P, melittin, and f-Met-Leu-Phe. *J Immunol* 1990; 145: 2581–2587.

62. Lawrence ID, Warner JA, Cohan VL, Hubbard WC, Kagey-Sobotka A, and Lichtenstein LM: Purification and characterization of human skin mast cells. Evidence for human mast cell heterogeneity. *J Immunol* 1987; 139:3062–3069.

63. Hsiue TR, Garland A, Ray DW, Hershenson MB, Leff AR, and Solway J: Endogenous sensory neuropeptide release enhances nonspecific airway responsiveness in guinea pigs. *Am Rev Respir Dis* 1992; 146(1):148–153.

64. Umeno E, Hirose T, Nichima S: Pretreatment with aerosolized capsaicin potentiates histamine-induced bronchoconstriction in guinea pigs. *Am Rev Respir Dis* 1992; 146(1):159–62.

65. Tamura G, Sakai K, Taniguchi Y, et al. Neurokinin A-induced bronchial hyperresponsiveness to methacholine in Japanese monkeys. *Tohuko J Exp Med* 1989; 159:69–73.

66. Matsuse T, Thompson RJ, Chen XR, Salari H, and Schellenberg RR: Capsaicin inhibits airway hyperresponsiveness but not lipoxygenase activity or eosinophilia after repeated aersolized antigen in guinea pigs. *Am Rev Respir Dis* 1991; 144:368–372.

67. Garland A, Jordan JE, Neeley S, White SR, Necheles J, Alger LE, Leff AR, and Solway J: Effects of eosinophil products upon sensory c-fiber neurons in cell culture. *Am Rev Respir Dis* 1993; 147(4, Part 2):A816.

68. Sanghavi JN, Rabe KF, Kim JS, Magnussen H, Leff AR, White SR: Migration of human and guinea pig airway epithelial cells in response to calcitonin gene-related peptide. *Am J Respir Cell Mol Biol* 1994; 11(2):181–187.

69. White SR, Hershenson M, Sigrist K, Zimmerman A, and Solway

J: Proliferation of guinea pig tracheal epithelial cells induced by calcitonin gene related peptide. *Am J Respir Cell Mol Biol* 1993; 8:592–596.

70. White SR, Garland A, Gitter B, Rodger I, Alger LE, Necheles J, Raila A, and Solway J: Proliferation of guinea pig tracheal epithelial cells in co-culture with rat dorsal root ganglion neural cells. *Am J Physiol: Lung Cell Mol Physiol* (in press, 1995)

71. Long NC, Frevert CW, Shore SA: Capsaicin pretreatment increases inflammatory response to intratracheal instilation of endotoxin in rats. *Regulatory Peptides* 1993; 46:208–10.

72. Theriault E, Otsuka M, and Jessell T: Capsaicin-evoked release of substance P from primary sensory neurons. *Brain Research* 1979; 170:209–213.

73. Saria A, Martling CR, Yan A, Theodorsson-Norgeim E, Gamse R, and Lundberg JM: Release of multiple tachykinins from capsaicin-sensitive sensory nerves in the lung by bradykinin, histamine, dimethylphenyl piperazinium, and vagal nerve stimulation. *Am Rev Respir Dis* 1988; 137:1330–1335.

74. Szallasi A, and Blumberg PM: Resiniferatoxin and its amalogs provide novel insights into the pharmacology of the vanilloid (capsaicin) receptor. *Life Sci* 1990; 47:1399.

75. Bevan S, and Szolcsanyi J: Sensory neuron-specific actions of capsaicin: mechanisms and applications. *Trends Pharmacol Sci* 1990; 11:330.

76. Bevan S, James IF, Rang HP, Winter J, and Wood JN: The mechanism of action of capsaicin—a sensory neurotoxin. In: *Neurotoxins and Their Pharmacological Applications.* Ed. Jenner P. Raven Press, New York. 1987.

77. Holzer P, Bucsics, and Lembeck F: Distrolution of capsaicin-sensitive nerve fibres containing immunoreactive substance P in cutaneous and visceral tissues of the rat. *Neurosci Lett* 1982; 31:253–257.

78. Meini S, Evangelista S, Geppetti P, Szallasi A, Blumberg PM, and Manzini S: Pharmacological and neurochemical evidence for the activation of capsaicin-sensitive nerves by lipoxin A4 in guinea pig bronchus. *Am Rev Respir Dis* 1992; 146:930–934.

79. Lee LY, Kou YR, Frazier DT, Beck ER, Pisarri TE, Coleridge HM, and Coleridge JC: Stimulation of vagal pulmonary C-fibers by a single breath of cigarette smoke in dog. *J Appl Physiol* 1989; 66:2032–2038.

80. Martins MA, Shore SA, Drazen JM: Release of tachykinins by histamine, methacholine, PAF, LTD4, and substance P from guinea pig lungs. *Am J Physiol* 1991: 261(*Lung Cell Mol Physiol* 6 Pt 1):L449–55.

81. Ellis JL and Undem BJ: Role of peptidoleukotrienes in capsaicin-sensitive sensory fibre-mediated responses in guinea-pig airways. *J Physiol* 1991; 436:469–84.

82. Bloomquist EI and Kream RM: Leukotriene D4 acts in part to contract guinea pig ileum smooth muscle by releasing substance P. *J Pharm Exp Ther* 1987; 523–528.

83. Bloomquist EI and Kream RM: Release of substance P from guinea pig trachea by leukotriene D4. *Exp Lung Res* 1990; 16(6):645–59.

84. Alving K, Matran R, Lacroix JS, and Lundberg JM: Capsaicin and histamine antagonist-sensitive mechanisms in the immediate allergic reaction of pig airways. *Acta Physiol Scand* 1990; 138(1): 49–60.

85. Sestini P, Dolovich M, Vancheri C, Stead RH, Marshall JS, Perdue M, Gauldie J, and Bienenstock J: Antigen-induced lung solute clearance in rats is dependent on capsaicin-sensitive nerves. *Am Rev Respir Dis* 1989; 139(2):401–406.

86. Ingenito EP, Pliss LB, Martins MA, and Ingram RH Jr.: Effects of capsaicin on mechanical, cellular, and mediator responses to antigen in sensitized guinea pigs. *Am Rev Respir Dis* 1991; 143(3):572–7.

87. Hsiue TR, Leff AR, Garland A, Hershenson MB, Ray DW, and Solway J: Impaired sensorineural function after allergen-induced mediator release. *Am Rev Respir Dis* 1993; 148: 447–454.

88. Nieber K, Baumgarten C, Witzel A, Rathsack R, Oehme P, Brunnee T, Kleine-Tebbe J, and Kunkel G: The possible role of substance P in the allergic reaction, based on two different provocation models. *Int Arch Allergy Appl Immunol* 1991; 94(1-4):334–8.

89. Nieber K, Baumgarten CR, Rathsack R, Furkert J, Oehme P, and Kunkel G: Substance P and beta-endorphin-like immunoreactivity in lavage fluids of subjects with and without allergic asthma. *J Allergy Clin Immunol* 1992; 90(4 Pt 1):646–52.

90. Nieber K, Baumgarten C, Rathsack R, Furkert J, Laake E, Muller S, and Kunkel G: Effect of azelastine on substance P content in bronchoalveolar and nasal lavage fluids of patients with allergic asthma. *Clin Exp Allergy* 1993; 23(1):69–71.

91. Sant'Ambrogio G: Afferent pathways for the cough reflex. *Bull Eur Physiopathol Respir* 23, *Suppl.* 1987; 10:19S–23S.

92. Ray DW, Hernandez C, Munoz N, Leff AR, and Solway J: Bronchoconstriction elicited by isocapnic hyperpnea in guinea pigs. *J Appl Physiol* 1988; 65:934–939.

93. Garland A, Ray DW, Doerschuk CM, Alger L, Eappen S, Hernandez C, Jackson M, and Solway J: The role of tachykinins in hyperpnea-induced bronchovascular hyperpermeability in guinea pigs. *J Appl Physiol* 1991; 70:27–35.

94. Freed AN, Bromberger-Barnea B, and Menkes HA: Dry air-induced constriction in lung periphery: a canine model of exercise-induced asthma. *J Appl Physiol* 1985; 59:1986–1990.

95. Koyama S, Ohtsuka A, and Horie T: Eucapnic hyperventilation-induced bronchoconstriction in rabbits. *Tohuko J Exp Med* 1992; 168:611–619.

96. Jammes Y, Barthelemy P, and Delpierre S: Respiratory effects of cold air breathing in anesthetized cats. *Respir Physiol* 1983; 54:41–54.

97. Biagini RE, Clark JC, Moorman WJ, and Knecht EA: Evaluation of the onset and duration of response to cold air inhalation challange in cynomolgus monkeys (Macaca fascicalaris). *J Appl Toxicol* 1991; 44(1):1–6.

98. Ray DW, Hernandez A, Leff AR, Drazen JM, and Solway J: Tachykinins mediate bronchoconstriction elicited by isocapnic hyperpnea in guinea pigs. *J Appl Physiol* 1989; 63:1108–1112.

99. Umeno E, McDonald DM, and Nadel JA: Hypertonic saline increases vascular permeability in the rat trachea by producing neurogenic inflammation. *J Clin Invest* 1990; 85:1905–1908.

100. Garland A, Jordan JE, Necheles J, Alger LE, Scully MM, Miller RJ, Ray DW, White SR, and Solway J: Hypertonicity, but not hypothermia, elicits substance P release from rat C-fiber neurons in primary culture. *J Clin Invest*, (in press, 1995).

101. Fuller RW, Karlsson JA, Choudry NB, and Pride NB: Effect of inhaled and systemic opiates on responses to inhaled capsaicin in humans. *J Appl Physiol* 1988; 65:1125–1130.

102. Belvisi MG, Rogers DF, and Barnes PJ: Neurogenic plasma extravasation: inhibition by morphine in guinea pig airways in vivo. *J Appl Physiol* 1989; 66:268–272.

103. Barnes PJ, Baraniuk JN, and Belvisi MG: Neuropeptides in the respiratory tract. Part II. *Am Rev Respir Dis* 1991; 144:1391–1399.

104. Dixon M, Jackson DM, and Richards IM: The action of sodium cromoglycate on "C" fibre endings in the dog lung. *Br J Pharmacol* 1980; 70:11–13.

105. Martins MA, Shore SA, Gerard NP, Gerard C, and Drazen JM: Peptidase modulation of the pulmonary effects of tachykinins in tracheal superfused guinea pig lungs. *J Clin Invest* 1990; 85:170–176.

106. Erdos EG, and Skidgel RA: Neutral endopeptidase 24.11

(enkephalinase) and related regulators of peptide hormones. *FASEB J* 1989; 3:145–151.

107. Skidgel RA and Erdos EG: Biochemistry of angiotensin converting enzyme. In: *The Renin Angiotensin System*. Vol. 1. Eds. Robertson JIS, and Nicholls MG. Gower Medical Publ., London, pp10.1–10.10, 1993.

108. Nadel JA: Regulation of neurogenic inflammaton by neutral endopeptidase. *Am Rev Respir Dis* 1992; 145:S48.

109. Johnson AR, Ashton J, Schulz WW, and Erdos EG: Neutral metalloendopeptidase in human lung tissue and cultured cells. *Am Rev Respir Dis* 1985; 132:564.

110. Llorens-Cortes C, Huang H, Vicart P, Gasc GM, Paulin D, and Corvol P: Identification and characterization of neutral endopeptidase in endothelial cells fromvenous and arterial orign. *J Biol Chem* 1992; 267:14012–14018.

111. Shore SA and Drazen JM: Degradative enzymes modulate airway responses to intravenous neurokinins A and B. *J Appl Physiol* 1989: 67:2504–2511.

112. Katayama M, Nadel JA, Bunnett NW, DiMarin GU, Haxhin M, Borson DB: Catabolism of calcitonin gene-related peptide and substance P by neutral endopeptidase. *Peptides* 1991; 12:563–7.

113. Borson DB, Corrales R, Varsano S, Gold M, Viro N, Caughey G, Ramachandran J, and Nadel JA: Enkephalinase inhibitors potentiate substance P-induced secretion of $^{35}SO_4$-macromolecules from ferret trachea. *Exp Lung Res* 1987; 12:21–36.

114. Baluk P, Bertrand C, Geppetti P, McDonald DM, Nadel JA: The NK-1 receptor antagonist, CP-96,345 inhibits the adhesion of neutrophils and eosiniphils in rat trachea. *Am Rev Respir Dis* 1993; 147:A475.

115. Crimi N, Palermo F, Oliveri R, Polosa R, Magri S, Mistretta A: Inhibition of neutral endopeptidase potentiates bronchoconstriction induced by neurokinin A in asthmatic patients. *Clin Exp Allergy* 1994; 24(2):115–20.

116. Cheung D, Timmers MC, Zwinderman AH, den Hartigh J, Dijkman JH, and Sterk PJ: Neutral endopeptidase activity and airway hyperresponsiveness to neurokinin A in asthmatic subjects in vivo. *Am Rev Respir Dis* 1993; 148(6 Pt 1):1467–73.

117. Frossard N, Rhoden KJ, Barnes PJ: Influence of epithelium on guinea pig airway responses to tachykinins: role of endopeptidase and cyclooxygenase. *J Pharmacol Exp Ther* 1989; 248: 292–298.

118. McDonald DM: Infections intensify neurogenic plasma extravasation in the airway mucosa. *Am Rev Respir Dis* 1992; 146(5 Pt 2):S40–4.

119. McDonald DM: Respiratory tract infections increase susceptibility to neurogenic inflammation in the rat trachea. *Am Rev Respir Dis* 1988; 137:1432–1440.

120. Dusser DJ, Djokic TD, Borson DB, and Nadel JA: Cigarette smoke induces bronchoconstrictor hyperresponsiveness to substance P and inactivates airway neutral endopeptidase in the guinea pig. Possible role of free radicals. *J Clin Invest* 1989; 84:900–906.

121. Sheppard D and Scypinski L: A tachykinin receptor antagonist inhibits and an inhibitor of tachykinin metabolism potentiates toluene diisocyanate-induced airway hyperresponsiveness in guinea pigs. *Am Rev Respir Dis* 1988; 138(3):547–551.

122. Lang Z, Murlas CG: Dexamethasone increases airway epithelial cell neutral endopeptidase by enhancing transcription and new protein synthesis. *Lung* 1993; 171:161–72.

123. Folkers K, Hakanson R, Horig H, Xu JC, and Leander S: Biological evaluation of SP antagonists. *Br J Pharmacol* 1984; 83:449–456.

124. Maggi CA, Patacchini R, Rovero P, and Giachetti A: Tachykinin receptors and receptor antagonists. *J Autonom Pharmacol* 1993; 13:23–93.

125. Fujii T, Murai M, Morimoto H, Hagiwara D, Miyake H, and Matsuo A: Effect of novel SP antagonist, FK888, on airway constriction and airway edema in guinea pigs. *Neuropeptides* 1992; 22:24.

126. Schmidt AW, McLean S, and Heym J: The substance P receptor antagonist CP-96,345 interacts with Ca^{2+} channels. *Eur J Pharmacol* 1992; 219:491–492.

127. Solway J, Kao BM, Jordan JE, Gitter B, Rodger IW, Howbert JJ, Alger LE, Necheles J, Leff AR, and Garland A: Tachykinin receptor antagonists inhibit hyperpnea-induced bronchoconstriction in guinea pigs. *J Clin Invest* 1993; 92(1):315–323.

128. Solway J, Ray DW, Gitter BD, Rodger IW, Alger LE, and Garland A: NK-2, but not NK-1, receptor blockage inhibits hyperpnea-induced bronchoconstriction (HIB) in guinea pigs. *Am Rev Respir Dis* 1994; 149(4, Part 2):A892.

129. Ichinose M, Nakajima N, Takahashi T, Yamauchi H, Inoue H, and Takishima T: Protection against bradykinin-induced bronchoconstriction in asthmatic patients by a neurokinin receptor antagonist. *Lancet* 1992; 340(8830):1248–1251.

130. Perney TM: Substance P release, calcium homeostasis, and phospholipid metabolism in dorsal root ganglion neurons *in vitro*. *Ph D Thesis, University of Chicago*, 1989.

131. Joos GF, van Schoor J, Kips JC, and Pauwels RA: The effect of inhaled FK224, an NK-1 and NK-2 receptor antagonist, on neurokinin A-induced bronchoconstriction in asthmatics. *Am J Respir Crit Care Med* 1994; 149(4, Pt. 2):A890.

132. Fahy JV, Wong HH, Geppetti P, Nadel JA, and Boushey HA: Effect of an NK-1 receptor antagonist (CP-99,994) on hypertonic saline-induced bronchoconstriction and cough in asthmatic subjects. *Am J Respir Crit Care Med* 1994; 149(4, Pt. 2):A1057.

133. Joos GF, Germonpre PR, Kips JC, Peleman RA, and Pauwels RA: Sensory neuropeptides and the human lower airways: present state and future directions. *Eur Resp J* 1994; 7(6):

AIRWAY SMOOTH MUSCLE

Chapter 18 _____
REGULATION OF SMOOTH MUSCLE CONTRACTION

RICHARD W. MITCHELL

Airway and Vascular Smooth Muscle

Multiunit, Single-Unit, and Intermediate Smooth Muscle

Smooth Muscle versus Skeletal Muscle Contraction

Contractile Proteins

Regulation of Contraction in Smooth Muscle

Airway and Vascular Smooth Muscle

In the lung, smooth muscle is found in the airways, vasculature, and lymphatics. Smooth muscle contracts and relaxes; the level of tone determines the caliber of the bronchi and vessels (Fig. 18-1). The *tone* (degree of contraction) is determined by the intracellular concentration of calcium ($[Ca^{2+}]_i$), where $[Ca^{2+}]_i$ is a dynamic product of intrinsic neural, hormonal, and inflammatory cell influences and extrinsic chemical insults or therapies. The importance of bronchiolar smooth muscle is demonstrated by the quantity of pharmacologic therapies directed toward alleviating or preventing the symptoms associated with asthma and chronic obstructive pulmonary disease (COPD). Prophylactic therapies include the use of corticosteroids for the reduction of airway inflammation, cromolyn sodium to stabilize mast cell membranes, and methylxanthines to inhibit phosphodiesterases and thus augment smooth-muscle myocyte cyclic adenosine monophosphate (cyclic AMP) concentration. During early and late phases of asthmatic attacks, aerosolized β-adrenergic receptor agonists, which stimulate the production of cyclic AMP, are the mainstay of asthma therapies.

Airway, pulmonary vascular, and, to some extent, lymphatic smooth muscle, are controlled intrinsically by neural mechanisms. These smooth muscle beds contract directly to cholinergic (acetylcholine) and catecholamine (α-adrenergic) neurotransmitters and relax to β-adrenergic receptor agonists. However, the vasculature and lymphatics relax in response to acetylcholine in the presence of an intact endothelium (see Chap. 20).

The endothelium is intimately involved in vascular and lymphatic (Chap. 20) smooth muscle intrinsic tone through the production of nitric oxide (NO), which is a potent vasorelaxant. Nitric oxide induces relaxation through a cyclic guanosine monophosphate (cyclic GMP) mediated mechanism in these tissues. It also has been shown for lymphatic vessels that endothelial cells have nodal projections (myoendothelial junctions) that make contact with the underlying smooth muscle and probably regulate tone by a direct cell-cell mechanism. Similarly, it has been demonstrated that the epithelium can release relaxant[1] and contractile[2] arachidonate metabolites that can modulate the tone of the airway smooth muscle (see Chap. 12).

Other intrinsic mechanisms for the control of smooth muscle tone in the lungs involve the release of inflammatory mediators from mast cells, neutrophils, and eosinophils. In addition to the effects of histamine, prostaglandin, and leukotriene release from these cells on smooth muscle tone, the eosinophils may release inflammatory peptides, such as major basic protein, which may affect the degree of smooth muscle tone through presynaptic neural mechanisms, direct smooth muscle effects, or through the epithelium.[3]

Multiunit, Single-Unit, and Intermediate Smooth Muscle

Smooth muscle has been categorized into multiunit, single unit, and intermediate types, based on the density of innervation and the ability of the tissue to propagate membrane

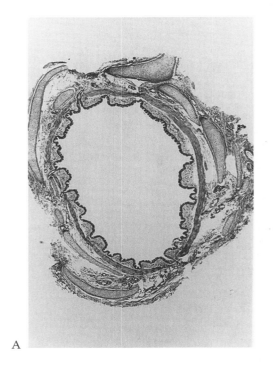

A

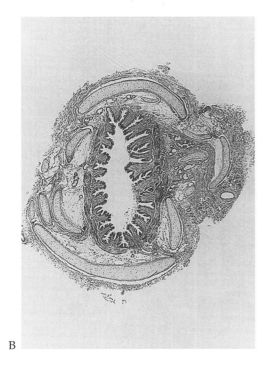

B

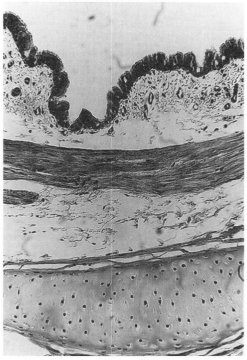

C

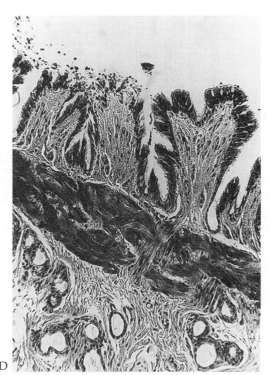

D

FIGURE 18-1 Regulation of airway caliber by the smooth muscle. Panels *A* and *B* are 5-μm sections (30×) of contiguous bronchial rings (4-mm diameter) taken from the same canine airway. The airway in panel *A* was relaxed using a β-adrenergic receptor agonist, and the airway in panel *B* was contracted maximally with a muscarinic receptor agonist. Contraction of the smooth muscle, which lies just under the epithelium and mucosa, significantly reduced the lumenal area of the bronchus, increasing the depth of the infolding of the epithelial and mucosal layers and dis-placing the surrounding lunate cartilage plaques. Panel *C* is a 200× magnification of the same airway section in panel *A*, showing epithelium, smooth muscle, secretory glands, and cartilage plaque. The smooth muscle cells, which lie in parallel with each other, are fusiform in shape with cigar-shaped nuclei. Panel *D* is a 200× magnification of the same airway section in panel *B*. The smooth muscle cells do not appear as uniform as in panel *C*, have lost their fusiform shape, and appear as a wavy band of tissue. *(Photographs courtesy of Andrew Halayko.)*

depolarizing pulses and, thus, waves of contraction from cell to cell.[4] Multiunit smooth muscle has a rich neural network with individual myocytes being innervated. There is little cell-to-cell communication based on the observations that (1) there are few, if any, gap junctions or nexuses (low impedance areas of the sarcolemma that allow the propagation of electrical pulses from one smooth muscle cell to the next); (2) the tissue has a high membrane resistance; and (3) no action potentials can be observed.[5] When artificially stretched, multiunit smooth muscles do not demonstrate a rebound myogenic contractile response. The larger blood vessels contain multiunit smooth muscle.

Single-unit smooth muscles demonstrate a sparse neural network, many gap junctions, and low electrical resistance, allowing the tissue to contract as a syncytium. Depolarizing electrical pulses (including action potentials) are easily transmitted throughout the tissue and the membrane potential displays oscillations.[6] Single-unit smooth muscles demonstrate spontaneous contractile activity and myogenic responses, and can be found in the intestines, ureters, the term-pregnant uterus, and in smaller blood vessels.

Originally, the smooth muscle of the airways was characterized as the intermediate type.[4] The smooth muscle of the *upper* airways is characteristically more multiunit; tracheal smooth muscle has relatively few gap junctions, displays no action potentials or myogenic responses, but has a relatively sparse innervation.[7] For these reasons, airway smooth muscle has been categorized as the intermediate type. However, in the presence of K^+-channel blocking agents such as tetraethylammonium, canine tracheal smooth muscle has been shown to demonstrate (1) membrane depolarization with the decreased permeability to K^+, resulting in a decreased electrical resistance and increased electrical conduction velocity through the tissue; (2) spontaneous electrical activity; and (3) myogenic contractile activity—characteristics of single-unit smooth muscle.[8]

Like the smaller blood vessels, it has been speculated that the smaller bronchioles may demonstrate single-unit–type electrical and contractile responses. It is known that the innervation of airway smooth muscle decreases distally from the trachea, and sixth- to seventh-generation bronchi dissected from lung resections demonstrate spontaneous active tone and some myogenic response to quick stretch.[9] It has been suggested, on the basis of in vivo human studies and in vitro studies using K^+-channel blockers, that, in airway hyperresponsive diseases such as asthma, the smooth muscle may change from a more multiunit to a more single-unit type by a quantitative change in the excitability of the tissue.[10]

Smooth Muscle versus Skeletal Muscle Contraction

Contraction of smooth muscle, like skeletal muscle, results from the interaction of the two contractile proteins, α-actin and myosin. Calcium is required for contraction in both smooth and skeletal muscle. However, unlike skeletal (striated) muscle, regulation of contraction is myosin-linked (rather than actin-linked), and there is no apparent, organized sarcomere structure in smooth muscle. The deficiency of sarcomeres accounts for the lack of striations observed under light microscopy. Smooth muscle also lacks troponin, a regulatory protein in skeletal muscle associated with the thin actin filament, which, in the presence of calcium, allows the myosin heads to bind with actin and form cross bridges (actin-linked regulation). In smooth muscle, calcium for contraction binds with calmodulin, which begins a cascade of regulatory steps necessary before the interaction of actin and myosin.

Unlike skeletal muscle, actomyosin adenosine triphosphatase (ATPase) is calcium-activated in smooth muscle. In skeletal muscle, calcium (Ca^{2+}) inhibits actomyosin ATPase activity. In the presence of minimal cytosolic Ca^{2+}, magnesium is the major constituent divalent cation that inhibits actomyosin ATPase. Generally, in skeletal muscle magnesium inhibits the enzyme activity more than Ca^{2+}; but, with activation and high cytosolic Ca^{2+} concentrations, the inhibition of actomyosin ATPase activity is reduced and contraction-coupling occurs. In smooth muscle, purified actomyosin demonstrates almost no ATPase activity, unless in the presence of calcium. Thus, calcium in smooth muscle is a direct activator of the enzyme. This fact indicates a role for alterations in calcium metabolism in smooth muscle disease states such as vascular hypertension, asthma, chronic obstructive pulmonary disease, and the associated vessel dysfunction observed in sepsis.

Contractile Proteins

In skeletal muscle, globular actin monomers are linked together to form the *thin filament*: a double-stranded, α-helical protein with a half-pitch rotation every seven monomers (Fig. 18-2). One tropomyosin molecule is associated with every seven actin monomers and, in association with one Ca^{2+}-sensitive troponin complex per seven actin monomers, regulates the binding of myosin molecule heads to the actin filament (cross bridges). In skeletal muscle actin filaments are anchored to Z-discs, which delineate each sarcomere and maintain the crystalline-like structure of the actin and myosin filaments in this tissue. In smooth muscle, actin is found in α-helices with associated tropomyosin-like skeletal muscle, but troponin is absent (Fig. 18-2). Actin filaments are found passing through dense bodies in smooth muscle myocytes and anchoring to dense bands on the sarcolemmal membrane. The dense bodies are linked by intermediate filaments, which give some degree of organization to the interdigitation of the actin and myosin contractile filaments. This less-structured organization with dense bodies and dense bands probably is what allows smooth muscle to be able to shorten down to 25 percent of the normal resting body length compared with skeletal muscle, which can shorten maximally to 75 percent of original length.[6] Although the gross structures of skeletal and smooth muscle differ, the similar interaction between actin and myosin is responsible for the qualitative similarities the two types of muscle display in both their biophysical (mechanical) properties and relationships between length, stress, and velocity.[11]

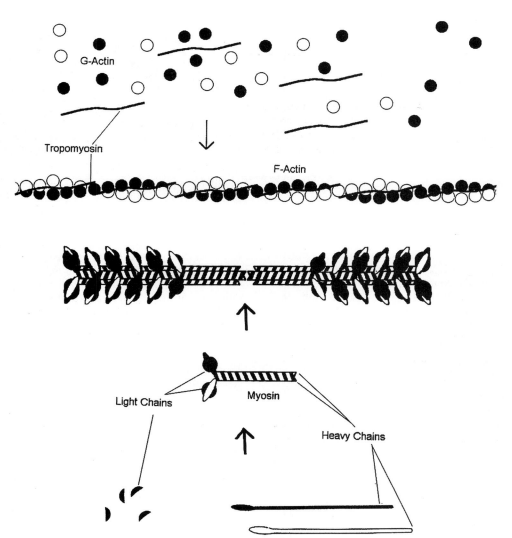

FIGURE 18-2 Structure of actin and myosin filaments. Globular actin (G-actin) monomers are linked together to form the thin filament (F-actin): a double-stranded, α-helical protein with a half-pitch rotation every seven monomers. One tropomyosin molecule is associated with every seven actin monomers. Myosin monomers contain six protein chains. Two heavy chains form the cross-bridge heads at one end of the molecule, and the other ends of the heavy chains are twisted into a helix that shapes the tail of the monomer. Four light chains are associated with the two heads of the heavy chains. The thick myosin filament is formed from monomers with the tails of the heavy chains entwined such that there is a central bare region with the myosin heads projecting out distally from the center. The myosin heads can bind to actin filaments, and the resulting actomyosin can hydrolyze ATP (actomyosin ATPase) in the presence of increased cytosolic calcium. The energy derived from the splitting of ATP to ADP and inorganic phosphate is used to cause an angular rotation of the myosin head while attached to actin, and thus slide the two filaments past each other.

Myosin monomers contain six protein chains (Fig. 18-2). Two heavy chains form the cross-bridge heads at one end of the molecule, and the other ends of the heavy chains are twisted into a helix that shapes the tail of the monomer. Four light chains are associated with the two heads of the heavy chains. The thick myosin filament is formed from monomers with the tails of the heavy chains entwined such that there is a central bare region with the myosin heads projecting out distally from the center. The myosin heads can bind to actin filaments and the resulting actomyosin can hydrolyze adenosine triphosphate (ATP). The energy derived from the splitting of ATP to adenosine diphosphate (ADP) and inorganic phosphate (P_i) is used to cause an angular rotation of the myosin head while attached to actin, and thus slide the two filaments past each other.

Regulation of Contraction in Smooth Muscle

In all smooth muscles after activation, Ca^{2+} for contraction enters the cytosol either from intracellular stores in the sarcoplasmic reticulum or from extracellular sites through receptor-operated and voltage-dependent calcium channel mechanisms at the sarcolemma. The surface area of the sarcolemma is increased greatly by *caveoli*, which are surface pits that appear like pinocytotic vesicles. Isolated caveoli have been shown to demonstrate structural, biochemical, and physiological similarities with the sarcolemma.[12] Electron microscopy has shown that caveoli communicate with the extracellular space.[13] This greatly augmented cell surface area probably facilitates the exchange of materials, including Na^+, K^+, Ca^{2+}, and water, between the intracellular and extracellular space.

In the cytosol, Ca^{2+} binds to calmodulin, a ubiquitous protein similar in molecular structure to the troponin-C found in skeletal muscle (Fig. 18-3). Four Ca^{2+} ions bind to each calmodulin molecule, which increases the calmodulin affinity for the enzyme myosin light-chain kinase (MLCK). The Ca^{2+}–calmodulin complex binds to MLCK; the Ca^{2+}–calmodulin–MLCK can now phosphorylate the light chains on the myosin heads.

Phosphorylation of the light chains is necessary for the initiation of contraction of smooth muscle[14] but not for the maintenance of contraction in the presence of increased $[Ca^{2+}]_i$.[15] Myosin light-chain phosphatases dephosphorylate the light chains and greatly reduce the activity of the actomyosin ATPase, slowing down the making and breaking of the cross bridges.[16,17] These slowly cycling cross bridges (or

FIGURE 18-3 Regulation of contraction in smooth muscle. The increase in intracellular cytosolic calcium concentration ($[Ca^{2+}]_i$), either through release from intracellular stores or from extracellular sources through receptor-operated channel (ROC) and/or voltage-dependent channel (VDC) mechanisms (excitation), begins a cascade of regulatory steps that initiates cross-bridge cycling. The Ca^{2+} that enters the cytosol has two modes of action. First, four Ca^{2+} ions bind to calmodulin; the $4Ca^{2+}$–calmodulin moiety then activates myosin light-chain kinase (MLCK). Active MLCK, at the expense of ATP molecules, phosphorylates the 20-kDa myosin light chains on the myosin head. Phosphorylation of the light chains activates the myosin head to bind with the actin filament and form actomyosin, which has the capacity to hydrolyze ATP to ADP (ATPase activity). Second, Ca^{2+} is needed to activate actomyosin ATPase directly. (In smooth muscle, actomyosin has almost no ATPase activity in the absence of Ca^{2+}.) Myosin light-chain phosphatase (MLCP) dephosphorylates the myosin light chains, but, in the continued presence of high $[Ca^{2+}]_i$, cross-bridge cycling continues, albeit at a much slower rate (see Fig. 18-4). Not until $[Ca^{2+}]_i$ is reduced, by resequestration into the sarcoplasmic reticulum or extrusion to the extracellular space, (see Figs. 19-1 and 19-3), does relaxation occur.

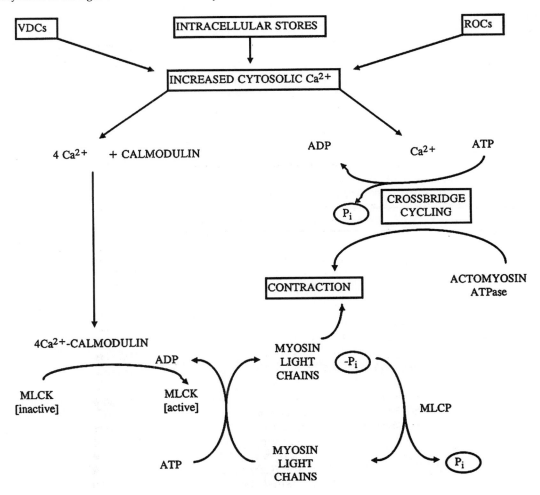

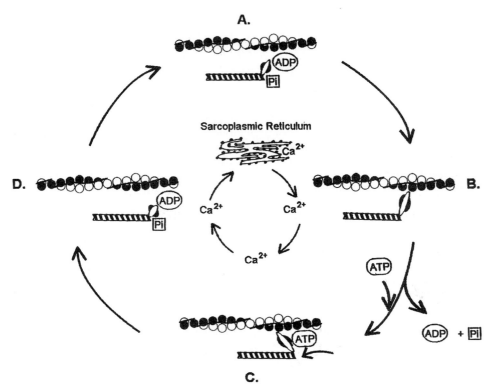

FIGURE 18-4 The cross-bridge cycle. (*A*) In the relaxed state (minimal cytosolic Ca^{2+}), the myosin head of the heavy chain has associated with it a molecule each of ADP and inorganic phosphate (P_i). This conformation of the myosin head has a high affinity for actin. (*B*) In the presence of increased $[Ca^{2+}]_i$ and subsequent phosphorylation of the myosin light chains, the myosin head binds to the actin filament. The binding of the myosin head to actin causes the release of products ADP and P_i. (In the absence of ATP, the cross-bridge cycle would stop here and the muscle would remain in rigor.) (*C*) The binding of another ATP molecule to the myosin head causes a conformational change in the hinge region of myosin, resulting in the rotation of the head and the movement of the thin actin filament in relation to the thick filament. (*D*) The affinity of myosin for actin is reduced with this conformational change and, with the splitting of the ATP to ADP and P_i, the cross bridge is broken and the cycle completed. In the continued presence of elevated Ca^{2+}, the cross-bridge cycle continues with the myosin head binding to the next actin monomer, causing the thick and thin contractile filaments to slide further past each other.

latch bridges) require little energy to maintain contraction.[18] This is an efficient mechanism by which a reduced airway or vessel caliber can be maintained with little energy expenditure in the presence of increased $[Ca^{2+}]_i$. Relaxation occurs with reduction in cytosolic $[Ca^{2+}]_i$ and deactivation of the actomyosin ATPase.

During the cross-bridge cycle and in the relaxed state (reduced $[Ca^{2+}]_i$), the myosin head of the heavy chain has associated with it a molecule each of ADP and P_i (Fig. 18-4). This conformation of the myosin head has a high affinity for actin. In the presence of increased $[Ca^{2+}]_i$ and subsequent phosphorylation of the myosin light chains, the myosin head binds to the actin filament. The binding of the myosin head to actin causes the release of products ADP and P_i. (In the absence of ATP, the cross-bridge cycle would stop here and the muscle would remain in rigor.) The binding of another ATP molecule to the myosin head causes a conformational change in the hinge region of myosin, resulting in the rotation of the head and the movement of the thin actin filament in relation to the thick filament. The affinity of myosin for actin is reduced with this conformational change and, with the splitting of the ATP to ADP and P_i, the cross bridge is

broken and the cycle completed. With sustained, increased $[Ca^{2+}]_i$, the cross-bridge cycle continues with the myosin head binding to the next actin monomer, causing the thick and thin contractile filaments to slide further along past each other. Thus, contraction and relaxation, shortening and elongation of smooth muscle, are dependent on the regulation of $[Ca^{2+}]_i$.

References

1. Hay DWP, Farmer SG, Raeburn D, et al.: Airway epithelium modulates the reactivity of guinea-pig respiratory muscle. *Eur J Pharmacol* 1986; 129, 11.
2. Ndukwu IM, Solway J, Arbetter K, et al.: Immune sensitization augments epithelium-dependent spontaneous tone in guinea pig trachealis. *Am J Physiol* 1994; 266 (*Lung Cell Mol Physiol* 1994; 10):L485.
3. White SR, Ohno S, Munoz NM, et al.: Epithelium-dependent contraction of airway smooth muscle caused by eosinophil MBP. *Am J Physiol* 1990; 259 (*Lung Cell Mol Physiol* 1990; 3):L294.
4. Burnstock G: Purinergic nerves. *Pharmacol Rev* 1972; 24:509.

5. Kirkpatrick CT: Excitation and contraction in bovine tracheal smooth muscle. *J Physiol (Lond)* 1975; 244:263.

6. Abe Y, Tomita T: Cable properties of smooth muscle. *J Physiol (Lond)* 1968; 196:87.

7. Stephens NL: State of the art: Airway smooth muscle. *Am Rev Resp Dis* 1987; 135:960.

8. Kroeger EA, Stephens NL: Effect of tetraethylammonium on tonic airway smooth muscle: Initiation of phase electrical activity. *Am J Physiol* 1975; 228:633.

9. Ito Y, Suzuki H, Aizawa H, et al.: The spontaneous electrical and mechanical activity of human bronchial smooth muscle; its modulation by drugs. *Br J Pharmacol* 1989; 98:1249.

10. Akasaka K, Konno K, Ono Y: Electromyographic study of bronchial smooth muscle in bronchial asthma. *Tohoku J Exp Med* 1975; 117:55.

11. Stephens NL: Physical properties of contractile systems, in Daniel EE, Paton DM (eds): *Methods in Pharmacology*, vol 3. New York, Plenum Press, 1975:555–591.

12. Daniel EE, Davis C, Jones T: Control of airway smooth muscle, in Hargreave FE (ed): *Airway Reactivity: Mechanisms and Clinical Relevance.* Hamilton, Canada, McMaster University Press, 1979: 80–107.

13. Gabella G: Smooth muscle membrane allied structures, in Stephens NL (ed). *Smooth Muscle Contraction.* New York, Marcel Dekker, 1984: 21–45.

14. Kamm KE, Stull JT: Activation of smooth muscle contraction: relation between myosin phosphorylation and stiffness. *Science* 1986; 232:80.

15. Dillon PF, Aksoy MO, Driska SP, Murphy RA: Myosin phosphorylation and the cross bridge cycle in arterial smooth muscle. *Science* 1981; 211:495.

16. Cohen P: The structure and regulation of protein phosphatases. *Ann Rev Biochem* 1989; 58:453.

17. Pato MD, Kerc E: Regulation of smooth muscle phosphatase-II by divalent cations. *Mol Cell Biochem* 1991; 101:31.

18. Wendt IR, Gibbs CL: Energy expenditure of longitudinal smooth muscle of rabbit urinary bladder. *Am J Physiol* 1987; 252 (*Cell Physiol* 1987; 21):C88.

Chapter 19

REGULATION OF INTRACELLULAR CALCIUM CONCENTRATION IN AIRWAY SMOOTH MUSCLE

RICHARD W. MITCHELL

Dynamic Calcium Flux in Airway Smooth Muscle

As noted in Chap. 18, the regulation of the cytosolic intracellular calcium concentration ($[Ca^{2+}]_i$) is a dynamic process. Calcium can enter the cell *passively* down a very powerful concentration gradient; extracellular Ca^{2+} concentration approximates 2×10^{-3} M, whereas the resting $[Ca^{2+}]_i$ is normally 10^{-7} M (Fig. 19-1). Also driven by this concentration gradient, Ca^{2+} can enter the cytosol either from the cell exterior through receptor-operated channel (ROC) or voltage-dependent channel (VDC) mechanisms, or from the sarcoplasmic reticulum.[1] The release of Ca^{2+} stores from the sarcoplasmic reticulum comes about through the second messenger inositol triphosphate (IP$_3$) after activation of ROCs by contractile agonists.[2]

An increase in $[Ca^{2+}]_i$, in addition to initiating contraction through calmodulin and myosin light-chain kinase (MLCK) and activating actomyosin adenosine triphosphatase (ATPase) (see Chap. 18), immediately activates the processes that cause a reduction in $[Ca^{2+}]_i$, and thus, relaxation. Calcium pumps on the sarcoplasmic reticulum begin to drive Ca^{2+} back into storage using energy-dependent [adenosine triphosphate (ATP)–requiring] mechanisms.[3]

Calcium-activated K^+ channels (K_{Ca}) open, allowing relatively more K^+ to exit the myocytes down a concentration gradient, and thus, hyperpolarizing the cell membrane and decreasing the ability of Ca^{2+} to enter the cell (Fig. 19-1).[4] This process also favors the entrance of Na^+ ions down this concentration gradient and, in association with membrane ATP–dependent Na^+–K^+ pumps (which pump the Na^+ back across the sarcolemma to the extracellular space against the concentration gradient for Na^+), promotes the extrusion of Ca^{2+} by an Na^+–Ca^{2+} cotransporter exchange mechanism (Fig. 19-1).[5]

Therefore, the maintenance of a given level of active tone in airway smooth muscle is dependent on a balance of Ca^{2+} entry and extrusion. Interference or enhancement of any of these processes will either cause greater tone or relax the myocytes. For example, cardiac glycosides, such as ouabain, can inhibit the Na^+–K^+ pump causing (en passant) membrane depolarization. With depolarization, the entry of Ca^{2+} down the concentration gradient through VDCs is facilitated, $[Ca^{2+}]_i$ increases, and contraction occurs. However, the entry of Ca^{2+} across the sarcolemma through VDCs and the resultant increase in smooth muscle tone can be retarded by VDC blockers, such as nifedipine. Under normal conditions, and notwithstanding the importance of these ion exchange mechanisms and the vast number of Na^+–K^+

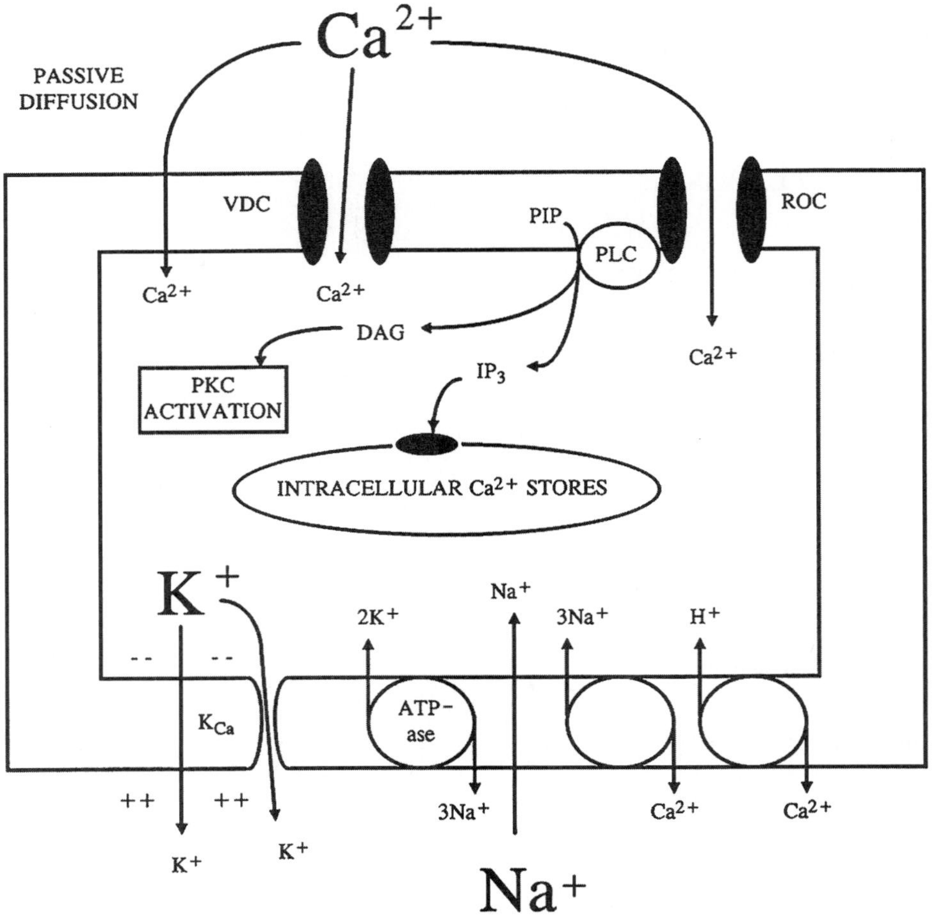

FIGURE 19-1 Dynamic Ca^{2+} flux in airway smooth muscle. The level of airway smooth muscle tone is determined by the concentration of cytosolic free calcium ($[Ca^{2+}]_i$). In turn, the dynamic $[Ca^{2+}]_i$ is a result of the amount of calcium entering the cytosol, either from the extracellular space or from intracellular stores, and the amount of calcium exiting the cytosol either by resequestration into the sarcoplasmic reticulum or extrusion back out of the myocyte. Calcium enters smooth muscle cells from the extracellular space (1) passively down a concentration gradient, (2) through voltage-dependent channel (VDC) mechanisms with depolarization of the sarcolemma, and (3) through receptor-operated channel (ROC) mechanisms in the presence of receptor-specific contractile agonists. Agonist occupation of receptors that mediate contraction also releases intracellular stores of Ca^{2+} through activation of phospholipase C (PLC), which metabolizes membrane phosphoinositides (PIP) to form inositol triphosphate (IP_3) and diacyl glycerol (DAG). The second messenger IP_3 causes the release of sarcoplasmic reticular Ca^{2+}, and DAG acti-vates the enzyme protein kinase C (PKC), which may be responsible for the prolonged tonic contractions observed in airway smooth muscle. Increased $[Ca^{2+}]_i$ immediately sets in motion the mechanisms to lower this concentration; ATP-dependent Ca^{2+} pumps are activated to reuptake Ca^{2+} into the sarcoplasmic reticulum or to extrude Ca^{2+} across the sarcolemma to the extracellular space against concentration gradients. The Ca^{2+} is exchanged for 2 H^+ ions. An Na^+–Ca^{2+} exchange mechanism also pumps Ca^{2+} to the extracellular space, utilizing the concentration gradient for Na^+ as a power source. In turn, the concentration gradient for Na^+ is maintained by the Na^+–K^+ pump, an ATPase that translocates these ions at the expense of energy from ATP. Calcium in the cytosol also activates Ca^{2+}-activated K^+ channels (K_{Ca}), causing an increase in the diffusion of K^+ down its concentration gradient, hyperpolarization of the sarcolemma, and decreasing the ability of Ca^{2+} to enter the myocyte either passively or through VDC mechanisms.

ATPases and Na^+–Ca^{2+} cotransporters that exist on airway myocytes to reduce $[Ca^{2+}]_i$, the amount of Ca^{2+} entering the cell eventually overwhelms extrusion mechanisms and causes contraction.

There are several new lines of drug therapy that are being developed with the goal to reduce $[Ca^{2+}]_i$ in airway smooth muscle cells. These include K^+-channel activators. Specific K^+-channel activators (as opposed to K^+-channel blockers that augment airway smooth muscle responsiveness) may stabilize (by hyperpolarization) smooth muscle cell membranes to reduce active tone or stabilize mast cells, eosinophils, and neutrophils to reduce the release of inflammatory mediators. There also are sarcoplasmic reticular IP_3-receptor antagonists being developed that may offer another route by which reduction in airway smooth muscle tone may be induced in disease states such as asthma.

Neural Pathways Affecting Airway Caliber

The dominant neural input to the airways is the parasympathetic nervous system,[6] which, when stimulated, causes contraction of the airway smooth muscle through the release of acetylcholine from the postganglionic en passage neural net observed in electron micrographs. (There are no true neuromuscular junctions in airway smooth muscle. Neural nodes are found as neuronal outpouchings that contain neurotransmitter in vesicles.) Acetylcholine activates muscarinic M_3-receptors on the smooth muscle membrane, which leads to increased $[Ca^{2+}]_i$. The release of acetylcholine is, in part, regulated by "presynaptic" muscarinic M_2-receptors, which, when activated by acetylcholine, inhibit further release. There is also mounting evidence that postsynaptic muscarinic M_1-receptors may be present; however, their exact role is unknown. Ganglionic transmission of nerve impulses from the central nervous system to the postganglionic innervation of the airways is mediated by postganglionic muscarinic M_1-receptors.

Sympathetic nerves are found in close association with parasympathetic fibers. In fact, electron micrographs demonstrate both clear (acetylcholine) and dense-cored (norepinephrine) "synaptic" vesicles within the same neural nodes. The interaction of these two neural networks in airway smooth muscle still is understood poorly, but the effect of norepinephrine release and subsequent activation of relaxant β-adrenergic receptors probably plays a minor role in the control of tone because of the dominance of the parasympathetic input.[6] There also is evidence for α-adrenergic receptors on airway smooth muscle; these receptors are activated in the presence of increased basal active tone to cause further contraction. A definitive role for α-adrenergic receptors in the airways has yet to be determined.

Nonadrenergic, noncholinergic inhibitory ($NANC_i$) nerves are present in the airways, but vary considerably in their significance from species to species. Electrical field stimulation of guinea pig trachealis strips in vitro demonstrates significant relaxation of spontaneous tone or agonist-elicited contraction that is sensitive to tetrodotoxin, an Na^+-channel blocker that inhibits neuronal transmission, but the electrically induced relaxations are not sensitive to β-adrenergic or muscarinic receptor blockage.[7] Human bronchial ring preparations do not demonstrate significant relaxation to electrical stimulation, indicating a sparse $NANC_i$ neural input. Recent studies of porcine trachealis muscle suggest that the neurotransmitter may be nitric oxide (NO).

Contraction also can be elicited through the release of substance P (SP) and neurokinin A (NKA) from sensory C fibers found in the airways—a nonadrenergic, noncholinergic contractile ($NANC_c$) system found in many species.[8] Release of these tachykinins causes a neurogenic inflammatory response in the airway, which includes increased vascular permeability, direct and indirect (neutrophil-mediated) inflammation and sloughing of the epithelium, and contraction of the airway smooth muscle. Tachykinins have been shown to be released by capsaicin, an extract that gives red peppers their characteristic hot flavor.[9]

Substance P and NKA contract airway smooth muscle directly and cause the release of other neurotransmitters, including acetylcholine, from cholinergic nerves to add indirectly to airway smooth muscle tone. Inhibition of neutral endopeptidase (NEP), an epithelium-associated enzyme that metabolizes the tachykinins, causes augmentation of contractile responses of airway to SP, NKA, and capsaicin. In the presence of NEP inhibitors or in the absence of epithelium (due to some inflammatory process), released tachykinins would be unopposed in causing constriction of the bronchioles.

Increased $[Ca^{2+}]_i$ through Receptor-Operated Channel Mechanisms

Not only is there a substantial variety of receptors on airway smooth muscle that respond to neurally mediated activation, but there also are other receptors that can modulate smooth muscle tone by affecting $[Ca^{2+}]_i$. Inflammatory cells, such as mast cells, may contain serotonin, histamine, leukotrienes, and prostanoids that can be released upon antigen challenge and cause contraction. Receptor-linked activation of airway myocytes involves G protein–mediated sarcolemmal membrane events (Fig. 19-2). With contractile receptor occupation, G proteins are activated on the myocyte membranes to inhibit (G_i) adenylyl cyclase or stimulate (G_s) phospholipase C (PLC); PLC metabolizes phosphoinositide to form inositol triphosphate (IP_3). The IP_3 formed mobilizes Ca^{2+} from intracellular stores by binding to IP_3 receptors on the sarcoplasmic reticulum,[10] thus leading to increased $[Ca^{2+}]_i$ and contraction.[2]

Diacylglycerol (DAG), the other by-product of PLC activation, activates protein kinase C (PKC), which, in turn, is responsible for phosphorylating several membrane-bound intracellular enzymes.[11] It has been suggested that PKC is responsible for (1) the prolonged tonic contraction of airway smooth muscle observed with muscarinic activation, in contrast to IP_3-mediated release of sarcoplasmic reticular Ca^{2+} for the initiation of contraction; and/or (2) increasing the sensitivity of contractile proteins, such that Ca^{2+} and PKC may act synergistically to increase the responsiveness of airway smooth muscle. Also, PKC may phosphorylate β-adrenergic receptors and G_s, impairing the coupling of the receptor to adenylyl cyclase.[12] It has been demonstrated in guinea pig lung strips that PKC activation, either through muscarinic receptor activation or directly by using tumor-promoting phorbol esters, results in reduced relaxation responses to β-adrenergic receptor agonists.

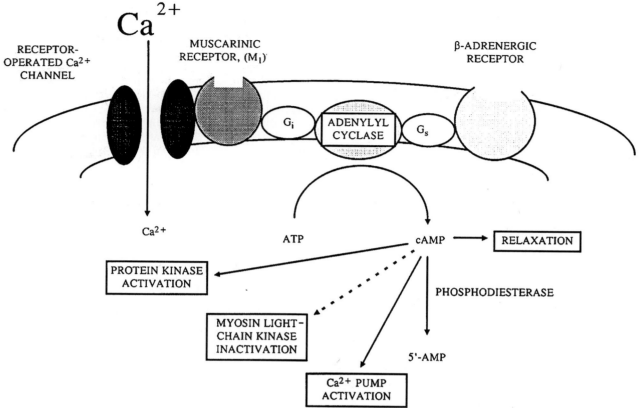

FIGURE 19-2 Factors affecting cAMP-mediated relaxation in airway smooth muscle. Cyclic AMP induces relaxation of airway smooth muscle through inactivation of myosin light-chain kinase (see Fig. 18-2), initiation of Ca^{2+} extrusion mechanisms, and activation of protein kinase (see Fig. 18-2). β-adrenergic receptor activation increases cytosolic cyclic AMP concentrations through adenylyl cyclase; however, the sensitivity to β-adrenergic receptor agonists and the efficacy of the relaxation process is dependent on the agonist (and its receptor) that elicited contraction. Relaxation through cyclic AMP mechanisms is relatively resistant to contraction of the airways caused by muscarinic agonists, as compared with contractions caused by histamine or serotonin. The functional antagonism to relaxation is not only a result of the greater coupling of muscarinic receptors to phospholipase C (and the production of IP_3), but also the muscarinic receptor–mediated inhibition of adenylyl cyclase. Adenylyl cyclase is activated with β-adrenergic receptor activation through a stimulatory guanine nucleotide regulatory protein (G_s). Adenylyl cyclase is inhibited through an inhibitory G protein (G_i) that is linked to muscarinic receptors, which may be of the M_1 subtype. The rate of cyclic AMP production, therefore, is dependent on the relative degrees of occupation of receptors mediating contraction and relaxation. Other than through β-adrenergic receptor agonists, intracellular cyclic AMP concentrations can be elevated by inhibition of phosphodiesterase. Methylxanthines, such as theophylline, cause relaxation by reducing the ability of airway smooth muscle myocytes to metabolize cyclic AMP to 5′-adenosine monophosphate.

Increased $[Ca^{2+}]_i$ through Voltage-Dependent Channel Mechanisms

Calcium can enter smooth muscle myocytes from the extracellular space through VDCs; the amount of Ca^{2+} entering is related to the degree of depolarization. Substituting K^+ for Na^+ in the physiological perfusate that bathes airway smooth muscle preparations in vitro will cause contraction that is blocked by VDC blockers such as nifedipine or verapamil.[13] Concentration-response curves to K^+ are sigmoidal in shape; that is, qualitatively similar to agonist-receptor relationships.

Histamine causes contraction of airway myocytes through H_1-receptors with the subsequent depolarization of the sarcolemma and secondary increases in $[Ca^{2+}]_i$. The bimodal contractile response to histamine (an initial phasic contraction followed by a sustained contraction) can be completely blocked by histamine H_1-receptor antagonists, such as pyrilamine maleate. In the presence of VDC blockers or in the absence of extracellular Ca^{2+}, only the initial phasic contractile response to histamine is observed; this phasic response is significantly blunted, indicating poor coupling of the H_1-receptor to G_s and PLC. With reintroduction of Ca^{2+} into the extracellular bathing medium, the secondary, sustained phase of contraction is observed.

That the maintenance of $[Ca^{2+}]_i$ is a dynamic process is demonstrated by the phenomenon known as *pharmacomechanical coupling of contraction.* It has been demonstrated in canine tracheal smooth muscle that 127 mM K^+ substitution for Na^+ will depolarize completely the tissue and cause a contraction (electromechanical coupling). However, at this maintained plateau of contraction and independent of extracellular Ca^{2+}, introduction of other agonists (e.g., acetylcholine) to the organ bath causes a further contraction (pharmacomechanical coupling) through G_s, PLC, and the liberation of IP_3.[14] Therefore, active tone in airway smooth muscle is a summation of the contractile (and relaxant) influences on $[Ca^{2+}]_i$.

Relaxation of Airway Smooth Muscle: Mechanisms Reducing $[Ca^{2+}]_i$

The most prevalent and potent method of relaxing the airway smooth muscle is through activation of β-adrenergic receptors and adenylyl cyclase. In asthmatics, β-adrenergic receptor agonists are the most common drugs used to reverse airway constriction and alleviate the increased work of breathing. These receptors are coupled to adenylyl cyclase through G_s.[12] Adenylyl cyclase converts ATP to cyclic adenosine monophosphate (cyclic AMP); cyclic AMP causes relaxation of airway myocytes by binding to the Ca^{2+}–calmodulin–myosin light-chain kinase (MLCK) complex (see Chap. 18). The binding of cyclic AMP to this complex greatly reduces the affinity of Ca^{2+} and MLCK for calmodulin, causing Ca^{2+}–calmodulin to separate from MLCK and Ca^{2+} to be lost from calmodulin. The cyclic AMP also activates protein kinase (Fig. 19-3). Protein kinase, in turn, may phosphorylate several regulatory proteins to bring about relaxation by (1) inhibiting Ca^{2+} entry, (2) inhibiting phosphoinositol metabolism and PKC, (3) augmenting Ca^{2+} extrusion mechanisms, and (4) phosphorylating MLCK. The sarcolemmal and sarcoplasmic reticular Ca^{2+}-pump mechanisms then are able to reduce $[Ca^{2+}]_i$ and begin the relaxation process.

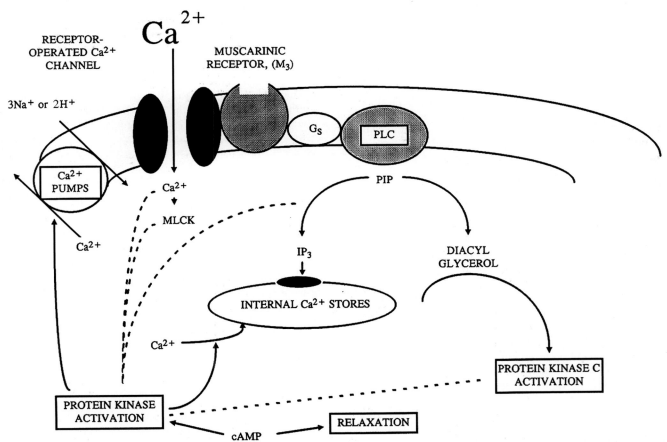

FIGURE 19-3 Mechanisms reducing tone in airway smooth muscle. In addition to the pump mechanisms that reduce cytosolic free Ca^{2+} and lead to relaxation (see Fig. 19-1), an increased concentration of cyclic adenosine monophosphate (cyclic AMP) induces relaxation through inactivation of myosin light-chain kinase (MLCK) directly or through activation of protein kinase (--- = inhibition). Protein kinase phosphorylates several regulatory proteins to bring about relaxation. Protein kinase may phosphorylate receptor-operated Ca^{2+} channels, reducing the ability of this ion to enter from the extracellular space. Protein kinase phosphorylation of phospholipase C (PLC) and protein kinase C inhibit inositol triphosphate (IP_3) formation and the tonic contractile effects of protein kinase C, respectively; phosphorylation of MLCK also reduces the ability of this enzyme to increase cross-bridge cycling. Protein kinase also augments Ca^{2+} extrusion mechanisms, both across the sarcolemma and back into the sarcoplasmic reticulum.

Relaxation of smooth muscle by β-adrenergic receptor activation is relatively resistant to contraction of the airways caused by muscarinic agonists, as compared with contraction caused by histamine or serotonin (see Fig. 19-2). The functional antagonism to relaxation is a result of (1) the greater coupling of muscarinic receptors to PLC and the production of IP$_3$, and (2) the muscarinic receptor–mediated inhibition through G$_i$ of adenylyl cyclase.[15,16]

Other than β-adrenergic receptor agonists, agents that increase intracellular cyclic AMP concentrations augment relaxation. Forskolin is a compound that bypasses the β-adrenergic receptor and stimulates adenylyl cyclase directly to increase cyclic AMP. Methylxanthines, such as theophylline, cause relaxation by reducing the ability of airway smooth muscle myocytes to metabolize cyclic AMP by inhibiting phosphodiesterase (Fig. 19-2). There are at least five different phosphodiesterases in airway smooth muscle cells.

In skeletal muscle, studies have estimated that one-third of the ATP consumed during contraction is metabolized in pumping Ca^{2+} back into the sarcoplasmic reticulum. In smooth muscle, ATP-dependent Ca^{2+} pumps may be activated by cAMP or by increased [Ca^{2+}]$_i$ to reuptake Ca^{2+} into the sarcoplasmic reticulum or across the sarcolemma to the extracellular space against concentration gradients. The Ca^{2+} is exchanged for 2 H$^+$ ions.[17] There also exists an Na$^+$–Ca^{2+} exchange mechanism at the sarcolemma that is not directly ATP-dependent, but relies on the ATP-dependent Na$^+$–K$^+$ pump, which maintains gradients across the sarcolemma for these ions by pumping 2 K$^+$ into the cell for every 3 Na$^+$ pumped out.[5] For every 3 Na$^+$ that now enter the airway myocyte down the concentration gradient created by the Na$^+$–K$^+$ pump, 1 Ca^{2+} is extruded. In the presence of ouabain, which inhibits the Na$^+$–K$^+$ pump, the gradients are not maintained, Ca^{2+} extrusion is decreased, and the sarcolemma slowly depolarizes, allowing more Ca^{2+} to enter the myocytes through VDCs, thus causing contraction.

Increased [Ca^{2+}]$_i$ also causes calcium-activated K$^+$ (K$_{Ca}$) channels to open and allow K$^+$ to exit the myocyte, thus inducing a relative hyperpolarization of the sarcolemma. Activation of K$_{Ca}$ channels also may come about through increase in intracellular cAMP concentrations, PKA activation, and the phosphorylation of the channels. Hyperpolarization of the sarcolemma reduces the ability of Ca^{2+} to enter the myocyte, thus causing relaxation. Quaternary ammonium bases, such as tetraethylammonium, block K$^+$ channels, leading to membrane depolarization, which is associated with spike potentials and spontaneous contractions.[18] Drugs such as 4-aminopyridine have a similar mode of action on these channels, increasing the excitability of airway smooth muscle myocytes.

Cromakalim (BRL 34915) is a recently developed pharmacologic agent that opens K$^+$ channels, allowing the ion to exit the cell, increasing the outward K$^+$ current, thus hyperpolarizing airway myocytes and causing relaxation (or preventing contraction).[19] Glibenclamid is a K$^+$-channel blocker that competitively inhibits the action of cromakalim, suggesting that cromakalim activates ATP-sensitive K$^+$ channels

(K$^+_{ATP}$).[20] Cromakalim also inhibits contraction caused by receptor activation (IP$_3$-mediated release of intracellular Ca^{2+} stores) by acetylcholine, histamine, and NKA, suggesting that this agent may have other actions on the airway myocyte, including activation of sarcoplasmic reticular Ca^{2+}-pumps to reduce [Ca^{2+}]$_i$. The efficacy of cromakalim to relax airway smooth muscle is similar to β-adrenergic receptor agonists. This has generated the development of new K$^+$-channel activators as bronchodilators for use in asthma.

Influence of the Epithelium on Airway Smooth Muscle

The epithelium is not only an effective barrier that has been demonstrated to block airway smooth muscle contraction of intralumenally administered contractile agents,[21] but also is a local source for relaxing factors.[22] It has been demonstrated in vitro for several species that removal of the epithelium (or inhibition by indomethacin of cylooxygenase, the enzyme that metabolizes arachidonic acid to prostanoids) augments smooth muscle contraction independent of a barrier effect. There is evidence to suggest that the epithelium-derived relaxing factor is prostaglandin E$_2$ (PGE$_2$), and that PGE$_2$ production by the epithelium is augmented in the presence of products of inflammation, such as bradykinin. However, despite the significant amount of PGE$_2$ produced by the epithelium and the fact that airway smooth muscle responsiveness to other agonists is augmented with epithelium removal or cyclooxygenase blockade in vitro, the shifts in efficacy and sensitivity may not be physiologically significant in vivo.

Recent evidence also points to the fact that epithelium-derived contractile factors (again, arachidonate metabolites) may be increased in inflammatory states caused by immune sensitization.[7] Tracheal smooth muscle strips with an intact epithelium demonstrate augmented spontaneous tone, increased responsiveness to acetylcholine, and diminished relaxation with β-adrenergic receptor activation after in vivo immune-sensitization of guinea pigs. All these changes were reversed with removal of the epithelium or inhibition of cyclooxygenase.

References

1. Bolton TB: The mechanism of action of transmitters and other substances in smooth muscle. *Physiol Rev* 1979; 59:606.
2. Berridge MJ: Inositol triphosphate and diacyl glycerol: Two interacting second messengers. *Annu Rev Biochem* 1987; 56:159.
3. Sands H, Mascali J: Effects of cyclic AMP and of protein kinase on the calcium uptake by various tracheal smooth muscle organelles. *Arch Int Pharmacodyn Ther* 1978; 236:180.
4. McCann JD, Welsh MJ: Calcium-activated potassium channels in canine airway smooth muscle. *J Physiol (Long)* 1986; 372:113.
5. Bullock CG, Fettes JJF, Kirkpatrick CT: Tracheal smooth muscle—second thoughts on sodium calcium exchange. *J Physiol* 1981; 318:46.
6. Barnes PJ: Cholinergic control of airway smooth muscle. *Am Rev Respir Dis* 1987; 136:S42.
7. Ndukwu IM, Solway J, Arbetter K, et al.: Immune sensitization

augments epithelium-dependent spontaneous tone in guinea pig trachealis. *Am J Physiol* 1994; 266 (*Lung Cell Mol Physiol* 1994, 10):L485.

8. Martling CR: Sensory nerves containing tachykinins and CGRP in the lower airway: Functional implications for bronchoconstriction, vasodilation, and protein extravasation. *Acta Physiol Scand Suppl* 1987; 563:1.

9. Holzer P, Bucsics A, Lembeck F: Distribution of capsaicin-sensitive nerve fibres containing immunoreactive substance P in cutaneous and visceral tissues of the rat. *Neurosci Lett* 1982; 31:253.

10. Twort CHC, van Breeman C: Human airway smooth muscle in cell culture: Control of the intracellular calcium store. *Pulm Pharmacol* 1989; 2:45.

11. Nishizuka Y: The role of protein kinase C in the cell surface signal transduction and tumour promotion. *Nature* 1984; 308:693.

12. Grandordy BM, Mak JC, Barnes PJ: Modulation of airway smooth muscle beta-adrenergic function by a muscarinic agonist. *Life Sciences* 1994; 54:185.

13. Weiss GB, Pang IH, Goodman FR: Relationship between ^{45}Ca transients, different calcium components and responses to acetylcholine and potassium in airway smooth muscle. *J Pharmacol Exp Ther* 1985; 233:389.

14. Baron CB, Coburn RF: Phorbol ester modulates inositol phospholipid turnover during contraction of canine trachealis muscle. *Ann N Y Acad Sci* 1987; 494:80.

15. Jones CA, Madison JM, Tom-Moy M, Brown JK: Muscarinic cholinergic inhibition of adenylate cyclase in airway smooth muscle. *Am J Physiol* 1987; 253:C97.

16. Mitchell RW, Koenig SM, Popovich KJ, et al.: Pertussis toxin augments β-adrenergic relaxation of muscarinic contraction in canine trachealis. *Am Rev Respir Dis* 1993; 147:327.

17. Hogaboom GK, Fedan JS: Calmodulin stimulation of calcium uptake and (Ca^{2+}–Mg^{2+}) ATPase activities in microsomes from canine tracheal smooth muscle. *Biochem Biophys Res Commun* 1981; 125:905.

18. Kroeger EA, Stephens NL: Effect on tetraethylammonium on tonic airway smooth muscle: Initiation of phasic electrical activity. *Am J Physiol* 1975; 228:633.

19. Kume H, Taai A, Tokuno H, Tomita T: Regulation of Ca^{2+}–dependent K^+ channel activity in tracheal myocytes by phosphorylation. *Nature* 1989; 341:152.

20. Black JL, Barnes PJ: Potassium channels and airway function: New therapeutic prospects. *Thorax* 1990; 45:213.

21. Mitchell HW, Fisher JT, Sparrow MP: The integrity of the epithelium is a major determinant of the responsiveness of the dog bronchial segment to mucosal provocation. *Pulm Pharmacol* 1993; 6:263.

22. Hay DWP, Farmer SG, Raeburn D, et al.: Airway epithelium modulates the reactivity of guinea-pig respiratory smooth muscle. *Eur J Pharmacol* 1986; 129:11.

Chapter 20

LUNG LYMPHATIC SMOOTH MUSCLE

RICHARD W. MITCHELL

Lymphatic Vessels in the Lung

There is an extensive network of lymphatic vessels associated with the pleural lining and occurring within the peribronchial and perivascular sheaths (peribronchovascular lymphatics) in the lung.[1] These vessels are responsible for collecting and draining fluid and particulates from the interstitial spaces so as to maximize gas diffusion across the alveoli.[2] The peribronchovascular lymphatics lie in the sheath of connective tissue that surrounds the interlobular veins, and, as the veins branch and narrow in diameter toward the periphery of the lung, so do these lymph vessels. Lymph flows in these vessels from the periphery toward the hilus of the lung, starting at or near the level of the alveolar duct and emptying into the thoracic duct.[3]

Pulmonary collecting lymphatics receive fluid and particulates from the lymphatic capillaries. The collecting lymphatics have numerous valves along their length to maintain a unidirectional flow to the lymph. These vessels have three layers or tunicae: intima, media, and adventitia. The tunica intima lines the inside of the collecting lymphatics and is composed of endothelial cells. The outer tunica adventitia is mainly composed of fibroblasts and collagen fibers that surround the smooth muscle layer(s) of the tunica media.

Smooth muscle layers are often found to be spiral in shape; this is particularly true at or near junctions of collecting vessels and lymphatic capillaries. Larger collecting vessels may have several layers of smooth muscle, some discontinuous. Smooth muscle of the lymphatics is of the single-unit type, where there are many gap junctions, a sparse innervation, and the tissues demonstrate spontaneous active tone. Associated with the spontaneous tone are cyclical depolarizations of the sarcolemma.

Smooth muscle myocytes in the lymphatics also have intimate contact with endothelial cells, the areas of contact known as myoendothelial junctions.[4] As in the vasculature, the endothelium can modulate the tone of the smooth muscle; acetylcholine applied intraluminally results in relaxation of the lymphatic smooth muscle by a mechanism that may involve both nitric oxide production and the myoendothelial junction.[5]

Lymphatic Valves

Valves are found at regular intervals along the pulmonary collecting lymphatics, usually at the sites where smaller vessels drain into larger collecting lymphatics, and are responsible for giving lymph its unidirectional flow.[6] Lymphatic valves consist of specialized endothelial cells. These cells are a duplication of the endothelium that surrounds the wall of the vessel, and appear as a bicuspid valve. The two leaflets produced are lined with flattened endothelial cells. Those endothelial cells composing the leaflets have actin filaments as one of their cellular constituents.[7] These actin filaments are contractile in nature, allowing dilation and contraction of the valve as the amount of lymph flowing through the system changes, and, as the fluid volume changes, so does the vessel diameter. Actin filaments, in association with microtubules and intermediate filaments found in the endothelial leaflet cells, give structural support to the valve.

Control of Lymphatic Smooth Muscle

Because the lymphatics of the lung are important in reducing lung interstitial fluid, it is useful to understand how lung fluid clearance by these tissues is affected by drug therapies and mediators of inflammation. However, little is known about the control of pulmonary collecting lymphatics in humans. Most studies on the control of lymphatic vessels and the smooth muscle found in the tunica media have been conducted on bovine and porcine lymphatics, including vessels from the mesentery and the thoracic duct.[8–12]

Most collecting lymphatics display spontaneous and phasic electrical activity, with action potentials preceding spontaneous contractile responses.[9] These phasic responses travel as a wave through the tissue. Electrical and contractile activity have been demonstrated to be propagated either orthograde or retrograde in vitro for bovine mesenteric vessels. The frequency of the spontaneous electrical activity can be significantly increased by contractile agonists and reduced by β-adrenergic receptor-specific agents[10] or by atrial natriuretic peptide (bovine mesenteric lymphatics).[11] Both these mechanisms for relaxation have been shown to be independent of the endothelium, and both β_1- and β_2-adrenergic receptor agonists have been demonstrated to attenuate spontaneous contractions or relax vessels precontracted by 5-hydroxytryptamine (serotonin).[10] The mechanism of relaxation to atrial natriuretic peptide may involve synthesis of guanosine 3′,5′-cyclic monophosphate in lymphatic myocytes.

Bovine mesenteric lymphatics have nerves in their walls.[12] Electrical field stimulation causes an increase in frequency of the spontaneous contractions inherent in this tissue. The increase in frequency can be blocked by α-adrenergic receptor antagonists. In addition to noradrenaline and serotonin, lymphatic vessels have been shown to contract in response to the inflammatory mediators histamine, prostaglandin $F_{2\alpha}$, and the thromboxane A_2 mimetic U-44069.[13] However, several studies have demonstrated regional differences (among lymphatic beds and species) in the sensitivity to, and efficacy of, these inflammatory contractile agonists.

In a fashion similar to the modulation of vascular smooth muscle tone by the endothelium, the endothelium of lymphatic vessels mediates responses to acetylcholine and bradykinin.[5,14] Porcine tracheobronchial lymphatic vessels with an intact endothelium and precontracted to histamine relax to acetylcholine and bradykinin in a concentration-dependent fashion. These relaxant responses could be inhibited by mechanical denudation of the endothelium.

Thus, while little is known about pulmonary lymphatic vessels and the smooth muscle contained within them in humans, in vitro studies utilizing other species and tissue beds have demonstrated the potential importance of this tissue as a pharmacologic target for the administration of drug therapies to augment lung fluid clearance.

References

1. Leak LV: Structure of the blood and lymphatic vascular system in the lungs, in Witschi H, Nettlesheim P, (eds.): *Mechanisms in Respiratory Toxicology*. Boca Raton, FL: CRC Press, 1982:77–159.
2. Guyton AC, Taylor AE, Brace RA: A synthesis of interstitial fluid regulation and lymph formation. *Fed Proc Am Soc Exp Biol* 1976; 35:1881.
3. Lauweryns JM: The lymphatic vessels of the neonatal rabbit lung. *Acta Anat* 1966; 63:427.
4. Leak LV: Pulmonary lymphatics and their role in the removal of interstitial fluid and particulate matter, in Brian JD, Procter DF, Reid LM (eds): *Respiratory Defense Mechanisms, Part II*. New York, Marcel Dekker, 1977: 631–685.
5. Ferguson MK: Modulation of lymphatic smooth muscle contractile responses by the endothelium. *J Surg Res* 1992; 52:359.
6. Leak LV: Lymphatic removal of fluids and particles in mammalian lung. *Proceedings of the Symposium on Experimental Models for Pulmonary Research*. EPA Bulletin, 1979: 89–114.
7. Lauweryns JM, Baert JH, DeLoecker W: Fine filaments in lymphatic endothelial cells. *J Cell Biol* 1976; 68:163.
8. Ferguson, MK, Williams U, Leff AR, Mitchell, RW: Length-tension characteristics of bovine tracheobronchial lymphatic smooth muscle. *Lymphology* 1993; 26:19.
9. McHale NG, Meharg MK: Co-ordination of pumping in isolated bovine lymphatic vessels. *J Physiol* 1992; 450:503.
10. Ikomi F, Kawai Y, Ohhashi T: Beta-1 and beta-2 adrenoceptors mediate smooth muscle relaxation in bovine isolated mesenteric lymphatics. *J Pharmacol Exp Ther* 1991; 259:365.
11. Ohhashi T, Watanabe N, Kawai Y: Effects of atrial natriuretic peptide on isolated bovine mesenteric lymph vessels. *Am J Physiol* 1990; 2599:H42.
12. McHale NG: Lymphatic innervation (review). *Blood Vessels* 1990; 27:127.
13. Sjoberg T, Steen S: Contractile properties of lymphatics from the human lower leg. *Lymphology* 1991; 16.
14. Bohlen HG, Lash JM: Intestinal lymphatic vessels release endothelial-dependent vasodilators. *Am J Physiol* 1992; 262:H813.

Chapter 21

PULMONARY VASCULAR PHARMACOLOGY

MARK E. WYLAM

Introduction

In the past few years, there has been a renewed interest in the systems that regulate the pulmonary vasculature and an increased awareness of the clinical potential of pharmacologic manipulation of the pulmonary circulation. Much has been learned about the physiologic role of the endothelium, vasoactive substances, and neural modulation of the pulmonary vasculature. However, the mechanisms by which these influences interact to control the matching of ventilation to perfusion remain to be elucidated. Consequently, even less is known about the way that lung injury influences these regulatory processes.

Alteration in pulmonary vascular tone may be mediated either directly, by changes in membrane ion channels and intracellular pH, or secondarily by peptide and lipid mediators. Hemodynamic stresses can interact with the vascular wall cells, particularly the endothelium, and cause changes in pulmonary tone (if the stress is acute) and structure (under chronic conditions). These same signals may promote vessel wall hypertrophy. Similarly, alterations in local oxygen tension (hypoxia or hyperoxia) and inflammatory mediators may alter the pulmonary vascular tone or vascular structure. As pulmonary vascular tone modulating signals may alter the vascular cell phenotype and lead to chronic functional and structural alterations, an ultimate understanding will require an integrated molecular approach.

Structure of the Pulmonary Circulation

There are 17 branching orders in the human pulmonary arterial system. The pulmonary arteries run with the airways but give off many more branches than an airway. Two main types of arterial branching can be distinguished.[1] *Conventional* describes the pulmonary branch that runs with an airway, dividing as the airway, and distributing to the capillary bed beyond the terminal bronchiolus. *Supernumerary* describes the additional branches that arise from the pulmonary artery between the conventional branches and supply the capillary bed of alveoli immediately around the pulmonary artery. The ratio of conventional to supernumerary branches is 1:2 in the prelobular region and becomes 1:3 along the pre- and intra-acinar region of the intralobular artery. The venous branching pattern resembles the arteries in that there are many more venous tributaries than airway branches.

The walls of the large pulmonary arteries, which are thinner than those of the systemic arteries, consist of smooth muscle inserting into short elastic fibers; this enables the vessel to distend rather than actively constrict or dilate. The terminal branches of the pulmonary arteries also have a larger internal diameter and a thinner wall than corresponding systemic arteries. Between the large arteries and the terminal branches are small muscular pulmonary arteries, which are the predominant site of changes in pulmonary vascular tone.

Hakim and Kelly[2] determined that only a small pressure gradient exists between arteries and veins 30 to 50 μm in diameter, whereas the largest pressure decrease across the pulmonary circulation occurs in vessels larger than 0.9 mm. Medial thickening, which occurs in the small arteries, develops in patients with pulmonary hypertension and potentiates the increase in resistance produced by active vasoconstriction. This decreases the ability of the vessels to distend passively and increases the contribution that the small arteries make to the vascular resistance.

Infusion of vasodilator agents does little to decrease the already low pulmonary vascular tone in the normal state. As the pulmonary circulation receives the entire cardiac output into a low-impedance circuit, it is likely that the low degree of vascular tone is maintained both by the absence of active vasoconstrictor influence and by the presence of active vasodilator influences.

Mechanical Influences on the Pulmonary Circulation

The pulmonary vascular bed operates at a minimal energy cost, thus minimizing oxygen consumption by the heart to move blood through the pulmonary vascular bed. Accordingly, the pressure decrease across the pulmonary bed is 20 percent of that of the systemic vasculature. It is likely that mechanical factors and circulating vasoactive factors contribute to the maintenance of a relatively low vascular tone. Moreover, as a result of the low pressures within the system, the pulmonary vasculature is more susceptible to mechanical factors that modify the pressure–blood flow relationship in the lungs, in turn affecting gas exchange. Mechanical influences include the relationship between transpulmonary and vascular pressures and the changing alignment of blood vessels within lung parenchyma.

The hemodynamic effects of these transient cyclic changes in transpulmonary pressure and their dependence on the volumetric conditions of the pulmonary circulation are well described by the regional distribution of pulmonary blood flow.[3] The transmural pressure in the pulmonary vasculature is influenced by the alveolar pressure. This is especially true in the pulmonary capillaries; thus, changes in pulmonary vascular resistance (PVR) are not necessarily an accurate reflection of active changes in vascular myocyte tone. Most clinical studies of pulmonary hemodynamics have simplified the definition of the resistance as the pressure decrease across a segment of the pulmonary vasculature divided by the flow through it. Measurement of the pressure decrease may be difficult in patients where the downstream left atrial pressure may be misrepresented by the pulmonary artery occlusion pressure, especially in patients with chronic obstructive pulmonary disease (COPD).[4] This has led to the use of pulmonary arterial pressure/flow curves and pulmonary vascular resistance/flow curves to detect *active* changes in pulmonary vascular myocyte tone, so that the effects of the changes in both flow and pressure on resistance can be assessed.[5]

In summary, it is important to realize that mechanical influences produced by positive pressure ventilation can exceed and overwhelm the important local regulatory mechanisms mediated by the neural, humoral, and pharmacologic regulation.

Intracellular Regulation of Pulmonary Vascular Tone

CALCIUM ACTIVATION OF VASCULAR SMOOTH MUSCLE

The cellular mechanisms for the regulation of pulmonary myocyte activation are not defined fully. Cytoplasmic calcium plays a role in activating a host of cellular functions in smooth muscle, including smooth-muscle contraction[6] and growth factor release. Two major classes of calcium channels are expressed in vascular smooth muscle (VSM): voltage-dependent (VD) channels on the plasmalemma and intracellular calcium (Ca_i) release channels on the endoplasmic reticulum. The VD channel is activated by depolarization of the plasmalemma, allowing extracellular calcium (Ca_e) entry. This channel belongs to the supergene family that includes the voltage-operated potassium and sodium channels. These three cation channels share a common transmembrane topography. The major Ca_i release channel is the inositol 1,4,5-trisphosphate receptor (IP_3R) on the endoplasmic reticulum. The IP_3R is activated by inositol 1,4,5-trisphosphate (IP_3), a second messenger generated at the plasmalemma. Also present is the ryanodine receptor (RYR) calcium release channel of the sarcoplasmic reticulum. The RYR channel is found to a lesser degree in VSM than in skeletal muscle, and its role in the pulmonary circulation is not known.

The following is a model of smooth-muscle cell Ca^{2+} activation proposed to describe the mechanisms by which Ca_i is regulated when the cell is stimulated by agonist or depolarization. The Ca_i store comprises two Ca^{2+} pools: A-store, which is sensitive to IP_3, and C-store, insensitive to IP_3 but sensitive to Ca_i. The A-store is refilled by Ca^{2+} from the C-store and reuptake of Ca_i. The uptake rate is dependent on the degree of filling in the A-store. The C-store, activated by Ca_i, is replenished by Ca_e. IP_3 generated by an agonist changes the A-store permeability, discharging its Ca^{2+} into the cytosol. Depolarization activates Ca_e entry through the L-type channels.[7]

MECHANISMS OF RELAXATION

Changes in cytoplasmic concentrations of free-ionized Ca^{2+} regulate the relaxation of VSM. Aside from changing the intrinsic rate of energy use within the cell, interventions that reduce the strength of contraction of VSM must in general alter either the Ca_i concentration, change the calcium requirements of the contractile apparatus, or exert both effects. Relaxation of VSM is influenced by myocyte membrane potential (regulating Ca_e entry) and Ca_i handling modulated by at least three important second messengers: cyclic adenosine 3′,5′-monophosphate (cAMP), cyclic guanine 3′,5′-monophosphate (cGMP), and IP_3. These substances modulate Ca_i at multiple steps in excitation-contraction coupling. Whereas in pulmonary VSM, diacylglycerol (DAG) appears to play an important role in the regulation of myofilament calcium requirements during contraction, two distant mechanisms exist to produce pulmonary VSM relaxation: cyclic nucleotide– and myocyte membrane potential–mediated relaxation. Overall, Ca^{2+} homeostasis is maintained through the action of sarcolemmal mechanisms that extrude Ca^{2+} into the extracellular space; these mechanisms include a sodium-calcium exchange mechanism and an energy-dependent Ca^{2+} pump. Alterations in electrophysiologic properties, sarcoplasmic reticulum function, energy use and supply, and contractile element interactions are potential pathophysiologic mechanisms in the regulation of PVR in the disease state. These abnormalities may be affected differentially by therapeutic agents that act on the pulmonary vasculature; therefore, it is important to understand the underlying cellular abnormalities and subcellular actions of inotropic, vasoconstrictor, and vasodilatory drugs to apply rational therapeutics in the clinical setting.

CYCLIC NUCLEOTIDE–MEDIATED RELAXATION

Both cAMP and cGMP elicit vasodilation of preconstricted pulmonary vascular tissue.[8] Cyclic AMP is activated by β-adrenoreceptors and prostacyclin (PGI_2). Cyclic GMP is activated by nitric oxide (NO) (see below) and hence by vasoactive drugs that release NO. Though the mechanism of activation of each of these systems is reasonably well understood, the relative physiologic importance of these two cyclic nucleotides in VSM is not understood fully. However, in isolated rings of rat pulmonary artery, agents that elicit relaxation through cGMP (sodium nitroprusside and nitroglycerin) or β-adrenergically stimulated cAMP (isoproterenol) are significantly more sensitive than agents that elicit relaxation through the prostaglandin receptor activation (PGE_1) of cAMP or phosphodiesterase inhibition (amrinone). Certain kinases are activated following increased intracellular cAMP concentration. Following increased concentration of protein kinase A (PKA), isolated perfused rat pulmonary vasculature relaxes, an effect that includes the indirect gating of a non-ATP-sensitive K^+ channel.[9]

Cyclic GMP–dependent kinases follow increased concentrations of cGMP and are proposed to induce arterial smooth-muscle relaxation by either (1) decreasing myoplasmic Ca^{2+}, (2) decreasing the Ca^{2+} sensitivity of phosphorylation, or (3) uncoupling smooth-muscle force generation from myosin phosphorylation.[10]

MEMBRANE POTENTIAL–MEDIATED RELAXATION

Hyperpolarization of myocyte membranes leads to pulmonary smooth-muscle relaxation in vitro. The in vivo regulation of membrane potential (MP) is largely unknown. However, in vitro K^+ channels are associated with repolarization of excitable cells after depolarization. As outward K^+ conductance determines resulting MP, opening of K^+ channels results in membrane hyperpolarization. At least four or five major classes of K^+ channels exist.

Voltage-gated K^+ channels open and close in response to membrane potential change; depolarizing or hyperpolarizing signals can increase channel opening to generate outward or inward rectification, respectively. Ligand-gated K^+ channels are modulated by neurotransmitters, ions (Ca^{2+}), or by nucleotides (ATP)-acting either at intra- or extracellular sites. G protein–coupled K^+ channels are ligand sensitive and are coupled to neurotransmitter and hormone receptors by pertussis toxin–sensitive G proteins.

During the past decade, a group of chemically heterogeneous compounds, known as K^+ channel openers, has emerged. These compounds open the ligand-gated K^+ channels (ATP-sensitive K^+ channels) in the sarcolemma of VSM cells, which leads to hyperpolarization of the cell membrane and relaxation of the tissue. Experimental evidence suggests that the mechanisms by which hyperpolarization affects pulmonary VSM contraction include (1) the prevention of Ca^{2+} entry through voltage-operated calcium channels, (2) the reduction of agonist-induced accumulation of IP_3 and, consequently, reduction of Ca^{2+} mobilization from intracellular stores, and (3) a decrease in the calcium sensitivity of the contractile apparatus. Hyperpolarization also may cause vasorelaxation by mechanisms that are not linked to the opening of the plasmalemmal K^+ channels, such as the modulation of local neurotransmitter release.[11] The patch-clamp technique has shown that ATP-sensitive K^+ channels regulate resting potential. It is possible that intracellular ATP concentrations directly modulate the resting potential by inhibition of K^+ channels.[12] ATP-sensitive K^+ channels are activated by substances such as pinacidil, cromakalim, nicorandil, and calcitonin gene–related peptide and have a greater relaxant effect on pulmonary vascular as compared to airway smooth muscle.[13] These K^+ channels are inhibited by glibenclamide, 4-aminopyridine, and tetraethylammonium (TEA), which block the delayed rectifier K^+ channel, and are modulated by changes in Ca_i and magnesium that may alter membrane potential and hence the contractile state of smooth muscle.[14]

Activation of the large conductance Ca^{2+}-activated K^+ channels may mediate the pulmonary smooth-muscle contraction elicited by four distinct types of stimuli (agonist-induced cytosolic Ca^{2+}, membrane potential, membrane stretch, and fatty acids).[15] The ratio of the reduced form of nicotinamide adenine dinucleotide (NADH) to NAD determines the intracellular redox potential; these potentials contribute to the activity of Ca^{2+}-activated K^+ channels, with NADH inhibiting and NAD activating the channel.[16]

VASODILATION ELICITED BY CALCIUM-CHANNEL ANTAGONISTS

In pulmonary VSM, contractions elicited by K^+ are abolished in Ca^{2+}-free medium and by Ca^{2+}-channel antagonists. However, contractions caused by norepinephrine, histamine, or serotonin are inhibited only partially by Ca^{2+}-channel antagonists. As such, the effect of Ca^{2+}-channel antagonists on pulmonary smooth-muscle tone depends upon Ca_e entry. Mechanical stretching increases Ca^{2+} influx and efflux in cultured pulmonary arterial smooth-muscle cells. This stretch-stimulated Ca^{2+} influx does not require sodium influx and is mediated in part by a pathway sensitive to verapamil.[17]

Neural Influence on the Pulmonary Circulation

The pulmonary vasculature is innervated by the autonomic nervous system. The exact role of the nervous system in regulation of pulmonary blood flow is unclear, but under physiologic conditions, there is substantial evidence that the nervous system modifies pulmonary blood flow. Afferents from both the sympathetic nervous system (SNS) and parasympathetic (PSNS) nervous system are sparse in the human but more numerous in the cat and guinea pig.[18] Anatomically, nerve trunks are found only with the larger arteries and veins and run in the adventitia of the vessels. Nerve fibers are not seen in the alveolar wall vessels. Developmental changes occur; at birth, only two-thirds of the pulmonary arteries are innervated to the level of the alveolar duct. This increases to near full innervation by age 2.5 years, and the pulmonary arteries are innervated fully in adulthood. The pulmonary veins are innervated to a much lesser degree throughout life. Since almost all of the intrapulmonary nerves are sympathetic, the paucity of nerves with vasoconstrictor potential at parturition might facilitate the rapid maintenance and remodeling of the pulmonary bed after birth.

Sympathetic input activates both α- and β-adrenergic receptors. Electrical stimulation of the sympathetic nerves causes vasoconstriction with increases in PVR as great as 70 percent. The segmental distribution of this vascular resistance increase is not entirely established. Although the pulmonary venous constriction is less intense than the arterial constriction, pulmonary veins of 2.5 to 3.0 mm participate and may account for ≥50 percent of the increase in PVR. At resting tone, the vasoconstrictor effect of sympathetic nerve stimulation is mediated primarily by α_1-adrenoreceptors. As basal tone is increased, subsequent SNS stimulation leads to modulated tone through α_2- and β_2-adrenergic responses.

Given the overall paucity of direct innervation of the pulmonary vasculature, nonneural adrenergic receptors likely have a significant effect on tone. Norepinephrine (NE) constricts both large and small pulmonary arteries and veins.[19] However, when pulmonary vascular tone is increased and α-adrenoreceptors are blocked, administration of NE or sympathetic nerve stimulation causes dose- and frequency-dependent *decreases* in PVR mediated by β-adrenoreceptor activation. These decreases in PVR are blocked with propranolol. Epinephrine and isoproterenol likewise have marked vasodilator activity in the pulmonary vascular bed when pulmonary vascular tone is increased.[20]

To describe the influence of the SNS during normoxia and hypoxia, Tucker eliminated SNS influence by treating dogs with the sympatholytic agent 6-hydroxydopamine.[21] Pulmonary vascular hemodynamics during normoxia and responses to hypoxia were unchanged, indicating that canine PVR is under little basal sympathetic influence. Moreover, a nonadrenergic sympathetic tone is likely to be modulated by dopamine in the pulmonary circulation. This is evident by studies[22] indicating nerve fibers in the guinea pig lung exhibiting immunoreactivity for both tyrosine hydroxylase and dopamine decarboxylase, which is consistent with innervation of pulmonary resistance vessels by dopaminergic sympathetic axons. Finally, the SNS contributes a significant trophic effect on the development of the structure of the pulmonary vasculature during growth.[23]

The role of the PSNS is more complex. Moreover, in some species, the vagus nerve contains both sympathetic and parasympathetic fibers. Stimulation of the vagus nerve in the cat leads to pulmonary vasodilation when the PVR is increased.[24] This vasodilation is mediated by muscarinic receptor activation following acetylcholine release, which causes an increase in cGMP concentration in vascular myocytes. As this effect is blocked by both methylene blue and NO synthase inhibitors, parasympathetic vasodilation may be mediated by endothelial release of NO. The PSNS does not appear to contribute to hypoxic pulmonary vasoconstriction (HPV), as bilateral cervical vagotomy and atropine administration do not impair human or feline pulmonary vascular responses to hypoxia.[25]

The significance of pulmonary vascular innervation has been elucidated by the advent of human lung transplantation. Lung transplantation has established that innervation of the lung is not essential for maintenance of gas exchange, ventilatory responses to hypoxia, or breathing patterns during sleep and wakefulness.[26,27] However, the ventilatory responses to hypercarbia are blunted following transplantation. The long-term effects of the neural disruption following lung transplantation, including the neural-trophic role of the SNS innervation on vascular homeostasis, are not known.

NONADRENERGIC, NONCHOLINERGIC INNERVATION

For many years, norepinephrine and acetylcholine were thought to be the only autonomic neurotransmitters, but many airway and pulmonary vascular responses could not be associated unambiguously with one or the other. Now, neuropeptides are known to exist as cotransmitters within autonomic nerve fibers as well as in separate nerves that arise within airway ganglia.[28] This system has become known as the *nonadrenergic, noncholinergic* (NANC) *neural regulation system* (see Chaps. 8 and 9). Allen and colleagues investigated a series of peptides: vasoactive intestinal peptide (VIP), the neurokinins/tachykinins, substance P, and calcitonin gene–related peptide (CGRP). These neuropeptides coexist with other neuropeptides and classic neuropeptides in NANC sensory neurons.[29] In addition, the neuropeptide tyrosine is found in all sympathetic nerves. NANC innervation influences the vascular permeability of pulmonary vessels in addition to modulating pulmonary vascular tone.

VASOACTIVE INTESTINAL PEPTIDE

VIP is a 28-amino acid peptide that was extracted originally from porcine duodenum as a vasodilator peptide.[30] It is localized to several types of nerves in the respiratory tract, particularly to nerves and ganglia in airways and pulmonary vessels. Most commonly, it is found associated with the small muscular arteries immediately proximal to the respiratory unit. The cells that give rise to intrinsic VIP-ergic motor nerves are largely cholinergic.[31] Binding of VIP to its receptor activates adenylyl cyclase and thus cAMP formation. Its actions are, therefore, similar to those of β-adrenoreceptor agonists.[32] VIP is a potent dilator of systemic and pulmonary vessels. In vitro, VIP relaxes pulmonary vessels in many species, including humans.[33] This action is independent of endothelial cells, indicating that VIP acts directly on vascular myocytes rather than indirectly through an endothelial relaxant factor.[34] Relative to airway smooth muscle, the density of VIP receptors is significantly greater on human pulmonary vessels, which may explain why VIP is about 10-fold more potent as a vasodilator than a bronchodilator in vitro. As VIP has significant action on bronchial blood vessels, it may provide a mechanism for increasing blood flow to contracted smooth muscle. VIP is also a potent vasodilator of nasal vessels.[35] As it is one of the mediators of NANC vasodilation, it may contribute to nasal congestion and enhanced airway blood flow during parasympathetic reflex stimulation.[36]

TACHYKININS

Tachykinins are a family of peptides with a common C-terminal sequence (See Ch. 17). They include neurokinin A (NKA) and neurokinin B (NKB), substance P, and CGRP.[37] Tachykinin effects are mediated through specific receptors referred to as NK-1 through NK-3.[38] The signal transduction of tachykinins on VSM is not well studied. However, their action in airway smooth muscle is stimulation of phosphoinositide hydrolysis, thus increasing the formation of IP_3 and release of Ca^{2+}.[39] In canine and porcine trachea, both substance P and NKA markedly increase blood flow.[40] They also dilate canine bronchial vessels in vitro by an endothelium-dependent mechanism.[41] Both CGRP and VIP act as arterial dilators and have synergistic effects.[42] Finally, as tachykinins may interact with inflammatory and immune cells, their pulmonary vascular effects likely are involved with products of inflammation.[43]

In addition to the effects of neuropeptides on vascular resistance, they likely have two additional effects on the pulmonary circulation—increased vascular permeability and chemotaxis. Increased vascular permeability is the hallmark of neurogenic inflammation. Among the tachykinins, substance P is most potent at causing leakage in guinea pig airway by stimulating NK-1 receptors localized to postcapillary venules in airway submucosa.[44] Whether tachykinins cause microvascular leakage in human airways is not certain; however, they cause a wheal when injected intradermally. In addition to an increase in vascular permeability, adherence of neutrophils to venular walls and subsequent migration of polymorphonuclear cells into the interstitium occur following stimulation of NANC neurons. This effect is most pronounced with the release of substance P and NKA from sensory neurons following vagal stimulation.[45] Indeed, a recent study suggests that the leak of plasma proteins through airway capillaries may be partly under cholinergic control.[46] As vascular leak and neutrophil recruitment are components of lung inflammation, neuropeptides released from sensory NANC neurons may mediate, at least in part, the inflammatory process.[47]

CALCITONIN GENE–RELATED PEPTIDE

The 37-amino acid peptide has two forms, A-CGRP and B-CGRP, that differ by three amino acids; both are potent vasodilators.[48] CGRP is an effective dilator of human pulmonary vessels in vitro and acts directly on receptors on VSM.[49] It also dilates canine bronchial vessels potently in vitro and produces a marked and long-lasting increase in airway blood flow in anesthetized dogs. It is possible that CGRP may be the predominant mediator of arterial vasodilation in response to sensory nerve stimulation in the nose and bronchi.[50]

NEUROPEPTIDE Y

Neuropeptide Y (NPY) is a 36-amino acid peptide that is a cotransmitter with NE in adrenergic nerves and usually amplifies its effects.[51] NPY binding sites are present on arterial smooth muscle and arteriosinusoidal anastamoses in human nasal mucosa.[52] NPY is a potent vasoconstrictor in most vascular beds, leading to prolonged reduction in tracheal blood flow in anesthetized dogs.[41] It has no direct effect on canine bronchial vessels in vitro. NPY vasoconstriction may lessen microvascular leak by the reduction in perfusion of permeable postcapillary venules.

NEUROGENIC PULMONARY EDEMA

The intracisternal administration of veratrine to chloralose-anesthetized dogs produces neurogenic pulmonary edema (NPE). The double-occlusion pulmonary catheter technique indicates that 74 percent of this increase in PVR is caused by an increase in pulmonary venous tone.[53] This pattern of venoconstriction is similar to that observed during the infusion of exogenous catecholamines and suggests that catecholamines, or centrally mediated sympathetic nervous system output, mediate venoconstriction and are responsible for NPE. It also is plausible that increases in endothelial permeability may contribute to the development of NPE.

Physiologic Regulation of Pulmonary Vascular Smooth Muscle

ENDOGENOUS REGULATORS

ANGIOTENSIN II

Angiotensin II (ANG II) is an octopeptide formed by the enzymatic activity of angiotensin-converting enzyme (ACE; located in the pulmonary capillary endothelium) on circulating ANG I and causes pulmonary vasoconstriction. The vasoconstriction is mediated by activation of G proteins and protein kinase C with release of DAG and both Ca_i and Ca_e mobilization. ANG I and ANG III also possess pulmonary pressor activity that is mediated by ANG II receptors. In humans, the pulmonary circulation exhibits a greater sensitivity to ANG II in comparison to the systemic circulation.[54]

Pressor responses to angiotensin I are reduced by captopril (ACE inhibitor), while pressor responses to ANG II and III increase.[55] In a rat model of chronic hypoxia, ANG II infusion prevents chronic hypoxic pulmonary hypertension, associated right ventricular hypertrophy, and vascular changes that may be related to release of vasodilator prostaglandins.[56] Moreover, chronic hypoxia is associated with a significant inhibition of transpulmonary conversion of ANG I and ANG II, which may diminish the role of ANG in producing pulmonary vasoconstriction.[57] ANG II does not seem to be involved directly in acute hypoxic vasoconstriction.[58]

PLATELET-ACTIVATING FACTOR

Platelet-activating factor (PAF) is a highly potent lipid mediator that has been implicated in inflammation and allergy. It is released from a variety of cells in vitro, including leukocytes and endothelial cells.[59] The precise mechanism of action of PAF is not known; however, eicosanoids, especially lipooxygenase products, play a major role in mediating PAF effects in the lung.[60] PAF causes vasoconstriction in high doses when basal tone is low and vasodilation when the dose is low and basal tone is increased.[60] PAF antagonists inhibit the development of monocrotaline- and hypoxia-induced pulmonary hypertension.[61,62] Moreover, the chronic administration of PAF induces a state of pulmonary arterial hyperreactivity to selected vasoconstricting agents.[63]

ENDOTHELIN

Endothelins (ETs) are a family of novel regulatory peptides. ETs are 21-amino acid peptides produced within the pulmonary endothelium; they also are released from macrophages and epithelial cells.[64] The ETs are formed from a precursor, "big endothelin," which is stimulated by epinephrine, ANG II, arginine vasopressin, transforming growth factor beta, thrombin, interleukin 1, and hypoxia. ETs bind to a specific receptor, which activates phospholipase C and causes the formation of IP_3 and DAG. In certain vessels, they also are linked to a VD calcium channel through a G protein. This explains why Ca^{2+} antagonists inhibit ET-induced contractions in some vessels.[65] The release from pulmonary endothelium is modulated by a variety of chemical and physical stimuli and regulated at the level of transcription or translation. At low concentrations (10 to 100 pmol), ET is a transient pulmonary vasodilator; at greater concentrations, a vasoconstrictor response predominates. ET concentration is increased in a number of inflammatory lung conditions[66,67] and, hence, may serve to modulate the pulmonary circulation during lung injury. Moreover, ETs can enhance vascular permeability, and plasma ET-1 concentrations are increased in patients with pulmonary hypertension, an event that has yet to be defined as causal.[68]

ENDOTHELIUM-DERIVED HYPERPOLARIZING FACTOR

In vascular tissue, including the lung, many agonists that elicit endothelium-dependent relaxation hyperpolarize the smooth-muscle membrane. This hyperpolarization is resistant to inhibitors of the action of NO, thereby suggesting that it is elicited by an unidentified substance called *endothelium-derived hyperpolarizing factor* (EDHF). EDHF-induced hyperpolarization is produced by an increase in K^+ permeability of the smooth-muscle membrane, which in turn, leads to closure of VOCs.[69] Release of EDHF requires an increase in endothelial Ca^{2+} either through intracellular release or from influx from the external milieu. The influence of EDHF in the isolated rat pulmonary circulation was reported by Hasunuma et al.[70] They noted that K^+-channel blockers (TEA and glibenclamide) prolonged the recovery of hypoxia-elicited vasoconstriction. Moreover, TEA, but not glibenclamide, increased basal pulmonary perfusion pressure and the peak response to hypoxia.[70] As these effects were noted to be endothelial dependent, they suggested a role for EDHF in the control of rat pulmonary vascular reactivity.

PROSTAGLANDINS

The profile of prostaglandins (PGs) from the pulmonary circulation is evaluated by examining the effluent from isolated perfused lungs. As in many other vascular beds, prostacyclin is the major metabolite of arachidonic acid released into the effluent. Other cyclooxygenase derivatives released are thromboxane A_2 (TXA_2), $PGF_{2\alpha}$, and PGE_2. Hypoxia, increased left atrial pressure, hyperinflation, and sympathetic stimulation all result in increased PGI_2 release. Because PGI_2 is released in relatively large amounts, it likely is responsible for the relatively low vascular tone in the pulmonary circulation. Inhibitors of prostaglandin synthesis are likely to produce their net effect relative to the balance between TXA_2 and PGI_2 on influencing pulmonary vascular tone.[71] In as much as oxygen is involved in the synthesis of prostaglandins from arachidonic acid, alterations of in vivo oxygen tension may alter the prostaglandin profile. Madden et al. noted that both PGI_2 and TXA_2 production are decreased during pulmonary endothelial cell culture during hypoxia.[72]

ATRIAL NATRIURETIC FACTOR

Originally discovered in cardiac atria, atrial natriuretic factor (ANF) synthesis has been detected recently in the lung. The biologically active 28-amino acid peptide is released into the bloodstream from granules within cardiac atria.[73] The ANF receptor is an integral part of the guanylate cyclase molecule, which mediates the physiologic actions of ANF. The whole ANF system is present in the lungs. ANF is synthesized and released by lung tissue, and ANF R_1 transducing receptors, which mediate its several biologic effects, and R_2 receptors, which eliminate ANF from the plasma (but are not coupled to secondary messengers), are present as well.[74] Lung ANF concentrations are coupled to salt and water intake. Water deprivation decreases, and salt intake increases lung ANF concentrations in rats.[75] In the pulmonary vasculature, ANF has been localized to the pulmonary veins. This is not surprising since in many mammals, cardiac muscle cells extend to the pulmonary vein adventitia—more so in extrapulmonary than in intrapulmonary veins. ANF synthesis is stimulated by several factors including glucocorticoid and thyroid hormones, hemodynamic overload (possibly mediated by vascular stretch), as well as hydration status.[76,77]

ANF induces vascular relaxation mediated by increased myocyte cGMP. The peptide exerts a greater dilator effect on pulmonary than on systemic arteries.

As opposed to endogenous NO and exogenous nitrovasodilators, ANF induces vasodilation, which is endothelium-independent, slow in onset, sustained, and not inhibited by methylene blue.[78] ANF activates the particulate form of cGMP, whereas endogenous NO activates primarily the soluble form of this enzyme. The potent vasodilator effect is enhanced in pulmonary arteries when vascular resistance is increased by vasoconstriction or hypoxia.[78,80] The elevation of cGMP decreases the concentration of Ca_i and is responsible for vascular relaxation.

Patients with primary or secondary pulmonary hypertension present with an increased plasma concentrations of ANF. These concentrations correlate with right atrial pressure, pulmonary artery occlusion pressure, and with the degree of hypoxemia.[81,82] It remains uncertain which parameter is directly responsible for the increase in ANF release. Chronic ANF infusion appears to attenuate the development of chronic pulmonary hypertension and vascular remodeling in hypoxia-adapted rats.[83] Thus, endogenous ANF may play a protective role by attenuating HPV through its dilator effect and reducing vascular remodeling through its antimitogenic actions.

ADENOSINE

Adenosine is a purine nucleoside with vasodilator activity in the pulmonary circulation. When it was infused into the pulmonary artery of seven patients with primary pulmonary hypertension, there was a dose-dependent reduction in PVR. The decrease in systemic vascular resistance was only about 10.5 percent of the decrease in PVR. This indicates that, in humans, adenosine has a preferential vasodilator effect on the pulmonary circulation.[84] In patients who respond to calcium-channel antagonists with a decrease in PVR, adenosine augments this effect.[85] In the intact cat lung, adenosine leads to pulmonary vasoconstriction following activation of P_1-purinergic receptors coupled to a pertussis toxin–sensitive G protein.[86] The selective effect of adenosine on the pulmonary circulation likely is due to its substantial extraction during passage through the pulmonary vascular bed.[87]

BRADYKININ

Bradykinin (BK) is a potent vasodilating and natriuretic peptide that is potentiated by ACE inhibitors. The main degradation pathway of BK in the lungs is through the action of kinases (hence enhanced action by captopril) at the carboxy terminus, and sequential cleavage by aminopeptidase P followed by dipeptidylaminopeptidase IV at the amino terminus.[88] BK exerts a dual action on the pulmonary circulation. In the isolated rat lung, BK causes a transient decrease in HPV. However, pretreatment with endothelial NO synthase inhibitors produces vasoconstriction, uncovering a direct action of BK on pulmonary VSM.[89] The duration of the response to BK is enhanced by zaprinast (cGMP phophodiesterase inhibitor), suggesting that response to BK involves increases in cGMP concentration.[85] Moreover, the action of endothelial NO release may lead to feedback inhibition of the endothelium-dependent relaxation caused by an increase

in cGMP concentrations.[33]

Hypoxic Regulation of the Pulmonary Circulation

In 1946, von Euler and Liljestrand were the first to show that acute hypoxia induces pulmonary vasoconstriction.[90] Although a local decrease in tissue P_{O_2} produces systemic vasodilation, alveolar hypoxia is a potent arteriolar constrictor in the pulmonary circulation, which reduces perfusion with respect to ventilation. It is likely that the response to hypoxia may involve a system with many pathways and much redundancy such that blockade of the production of a single agent has only a minor effect on HPV. Until the cardinal regulator of HPV is identified, it remains speculative that the concerted action of multiple regulators of the pulmonary circulation will modify pulmonary vascular tone during both normoxic and hypoxic conditions. These regulators include the products of arachidonic acid metabolism, PAF, adenosine, and endothelium-derived relaxing factor (EDRF), along with the influence of neural pathways and K^+ channel–determined membrane potential, all acting together in a "microenvironment" bounded by the alveolus and endothelium.

EFFECTS OF HYPOXIA ON ISOLATED PULMONARY ARTERY RINGS IN VITRO

The response of arteries to hypoxia *in vitro* can be contraction, relaxation, or a biphasic response. These studies have been performed in tissue baths where the P_{O_2} is decreased rapidly by gassing the buffer with N_2.[91–94] There is no consensus on whether hypoxia affects pulmonary artery smooth-muscle cells solely or whether, in addition, some other cell type senses hypoxia and produces a mediator that causes pulmonary vasoconstriction. In most of these experiments, the contractile response to hypoxia requires the pulmonary artery rings to be preconstricted with an agonist or is enhanced if they are.[93,94] This might be expected if the contractile response to hypoxia were mediated solely by the withdrawal of active vasodilator influence rather than activation of a contractile mechanism. Moreover, these in vitro studies do not show a graded contractile response over the physiologically relevant range of oxygen tensions that produce HPV in vivo.[93,94] In vivo, the physiologic threshold of HPV is an alveolar oxygen tension of approximately 80 mmHg. However, values less than 40 mmHg are required to initiate HPV in vitro, and often HPV does not occur until an oxygen tension in the experimental condition reaches near zero mmHg.[93,94] It is possible that this relationship is observed because most researchers have used vascular rings from conduit-sized, nonflow controlling vessels of the proximal pulmonary circulation. However, one study performed in vitro using cat pulmonary artery rings (<300 μM I.D.) has reported sensitivity to oxygen tesions comparable to that found in vivo.[95] These vessels required no exogenous preconstrictor agent, and VSM contraction was seen in a bath

P_{O_2} of 200 to 250 mmHg. Recently, isolated pulmonary artery smooth-muscle cells have shown to respond to hypoxia.[96]

ROLE OF ENDOTHELIUM IN HYPOXIC CONTRACTION

Holden and McCall[97] reported that the hypoxic contraction in porcine pulmonary artery depended completely upon the endothelium. DeMey and Vanhoutte found hypoxic contraction in canine pulmonary artery was only partially endothelium-dependent.[98] These differences may be explained, in large part, by a careful notation of blood vessel caliber. In larger vessels, removal of endothelium has been reported to result in a 48 to 80 percent reduction in the pulmonary artery hypoxic response.[93] The significance of this finding is unclear, as these vessels produce a biphasic contractile response to hypoxia; the in vivo significance of this response is questionable. Only the transient initial phase of contraction appears to be endothelium-dependent, whereas the sustained contraction phase that follows an initial relaxation is endothelium independent.[94] By contrast, hypoxic contraction has been reported neither abolished[99] nor enhanced[100] by removal of the endothelium.

RELEASE OF PROSTANOIDS

In cultured cells, hypoxia reduces prostacyclin production by smooth muscle.[101] By contrast, hypoxia can either increase or decrease prostacyclin release from the endothelium.[102] This might explain why there are variable effects of cyclooxygenase inhibitors on hypoxic constriction in pulmonary artery rings. Indomethacin abolishes pulmonary venoconstriction to hypoxia in sheep but results in enhancement of arterial constriction.[103] In animal models of hypoxic respiratory failure, indomethacin decreases intrapulmonary shunt, possibly by enhancing HPV. This effect is synergistic with the influence of positive end-expiratory pressure (PEEP).[104] Unfortunately, the use of indomethacin in human lung injury has not produced this significant potential benefit. These effects may be related to maturation, as a marked enhancement of hypoxic reactivity by indomethacin occurs in younger lambs, suggesting that cyclooxygenase products exert a vasodilatory modulation of hypoxic vasoconstriction that decreases with age.[105] Recently, studies have reported that 5-lipoxygenase products, cyclooxygenase products, and free radicals are not involved in mediating hypoxic contractions in isolated rat pulmonary arterial rings.[94]

RELEASE OF NITRIC OXIDE

Hypoxia decreases basal and stimulated NO release from the endothelium of bovine pulmonary artery and cultured endothelial cells.[106] This may account for the small transient contraction observed in relatively large isolated pulmonary artery rings in vitro in response to modest hypoxia. By contrast, several other studies have shown that release of NO from the endothelium serves to limit the magnitude of hypoxia-induced contraction.[107] Though the exact modulators of EDRF in the intact pulmonary circulation are not known, there is likely an increased basal NO tone caused by shear stress–stimulated release. Therefore, modulation of endothelial-derived NO would be expected to be more important in the vasoconstrictor response to hypoxia in vivo than in isolated rings in an organ bath. Recent investigations also have demonstrated that HPV is augmented significantly by drugs that inhibit NO-synthase (NOS).[108] The complexity of hypoxic modulation of NO production recently was demonstrated by Shaul and Wells, who noted that a decrease in oxygen tension (680 to 150 mmHg attenuates NO production in fetal pulmonary endothelial cells but not in fetal systemic endothelium.[109] This decrease was not caused by oxygen or L-arginine substrate limitation and may involve oxygen modulation of cytosolic calcium mobilization.

PRODUCTION OF ENDOTHELIN

Prolonged hypoxia can stimulate endothelin formation. In rats, plasma endothelin concentrations increase 60 min after exposure to alveolar hypoxia.[110] In systemic beds such as the rat mesentery, a 30-min perfusion with an hypoxic gas causes a 71 percent increase in plasma endothelin concentration compared to control tissues.[111] It also is possible that other vasoconstrictors are released from vascular ring preparations during hypoxia as a diffusable mediator that is not endothelin.[112]

ROLE OF MYOCYTE MEMBRANE POTENTIAL

Changes in myocyte membrane potential correspond to hypoxia-induced changes in pulmonary vascular tone. In the cat, hypoxia causes small pulmonary artery rings to contract in parallel with membrane depolarization from -51 to -37 mV.[92] Conversely, in the systemic dog carotid artery, a decrease in P_{O_2} to 20 mmHg produced depolarization and contraction, while a P_{O_2} between 30 and 80 mmHg induced membrane hyperpolarization and relaxation.[113]

ROLE OF INTRA- AND EXTRACELLULAR CALCIUM

Both intracellular and extracellular stores of Ca^{2+} appear to mediate hypoxic contraction of pulmonary artery rings. Recent data[95] suggest that a change in Ca^{2+} concentration, rather than a change in the Ca^{2+} sensitivity of the contractile apparatus, is involved in the response to hypoxia. In sheep and human vessels, the Ca^{2+}-channel antagonist, verapamil, does not reduce hypoxic contraction.[114] Diltiazem, however, abolishes hypoxic contraction of dog cerebral artery rings.[115] Moreover, other studies indicate that the omission of calcium from extracellular buffers attenuates hypoxic contraction. As membrane fluidity is altered by omission of Ca_e, one must be cautious in differentiating membrane effects caused by reduced Ca_e from the effects caused by reduced transcellular Ca^{2+} entry based on concentration gradients.[116] BAY K 8644 (a Ca^{2+}-channel agonist) potentiates HPV but increases resting tone. Likewise, inhibition of the sodium-calcium exchange mechanism[117] or inhibition of calcium ATPases[118] enhance pulmonary smooth muscle tone during normoxia, and each may be impaired somewhat during hypoxia to augment myocyte contraction. Therefore, the effect of Ca^{2+}-channel agents on basal smooth-muscle activation (i.e., resting tone) has not been dissociated from the effect on hypoxic contraction. Finally, in the isolated rat lung, the role of Ca^{2+} as influenced by cGMP and cAMP recently has been studied through the use of specific phospodiesterase (PDE) inhibitors.[119] During normoxia, none of the currently available PDE inhibitors significantly influences baseline pulmonary perfusion pressure. However, during hypoxia, inhibition of the cGMP-inhibitable cAMP PDE (indolidan) seems to play a larger role than inhibition of the cGMP PDE (zaprinast) or inhibition of the cGMP-insensitive cAMP PDE (rolipram) [see also Chaps. 49 and 62].

MODULATION THROUGH K^+ CHANNELS

Reduction of oxygen tension from normoxic levels to hypoxic levels directly inhibits K^+ currents in isolated canine pulmonary myocytes. This K^+-channel inhibition leads to membrane depolarization, leading to smooth muscle contraction. Nisoldipine or buffering of intracellular calcium prevents this hypoxic inhibition of K^+ currents, suggesting that a Ca^{2+}-sensitive K^+ channel may be responsible for the hypoxic response.[120] It is unlikely that intracellular ATP concentration mediates these effects because the experiments were performed with ATP present in the dialysis solution of the patch-clamp electrodes.

THE EFFECTS OF CHRONIC HYPOXIA ON ENDOTHELIAL AND SMOOTH-MUSCLE CELLS

Apart from the acute effects of hypoxia on endothelial and smooth-muscle tone, chronic hypoxia may influence the same cells to remodel the pulmonary circulation. In vitro data indicate that hypoxic pulmonary and nonpulmonary endothelial cells secrete decreased amounts of NO because of decreased expression of the endothelial NO synthase (eNOS) gene.[121] As NO is known to downregulate smooth-muscle proliferation, it is possible that decreased NO release in hypoxia removes the negative NO influence on smooth-muscle proliferation and leads to enhanced smooth-muscle proliferation in the pulmonary circulation. Likewise, increased production of vasoconstrictors accompanies the hypoxic state.[122] In addition to the effects of ET-1[123] and platelet-derived growth factor[124] as powerful vasoconstrictor agents, both are known to be potent smooth-muscle mitogens. Thus, the endothelial cell is a source of potent agents that can affect smooth-muscle tone and proliferation. Using the erythropoietin gene[125] as a model for the oxygen-sensing mechanism, it has been suggested that a heme-binding protein may be involved as the smooth-muscle oxygen sensor.

Changes in the configuration of this putative heme-protein complex, capable of binding oxygen, may transduce oxygen tension into a cascade of intracellular signals that eventually transduce a nuclear DNA-protein interaction and affect gene transcription.

Intra- and Extracellular pH

It is well known that intracellular pH has a role in modulating pulmonary artery contractile responses. The relative importance of pH and P_{CO_2} in the modulation of such tone, however, still is debated.

Local effects of pH on VSM contractility indicate that the basic effect of acidosis is the inhibition of K^+ channels and L-type Ca^{2+} channels.[126,127] Inhibition of K^+ channels results in membrane depolarization, opening of L-type Ca^{2+} channels, increase in Ca^{2+} influx, and muscle contraction. Direct inhibition of Ca^{2+} channels results in an opposite effect. Thus, the effect of acidosis is determined by the relative potency of these two contradictory events. This may be the reason why acidosis induces contraction in polarized muscle, whereas it inhibits contraction in depolarized muscle.[128] Such an explanation may describe differences between the behavior of systemic vessels and those of the pulmonary and cerebral circulation. As such, extracellular acidosis or alkalosis may influence pulmonary vascular tone depending on the balance of other factors modulating pulmonary vascular tone, i.e., the degree of active tone affected by hypoxia. In addition, measurements of cytosolic Ca^{2+} concentrations simultaneously with muscle tension suggest that acidosis increases Ca^{2+} sensitivity of contractile elements. To some degree, it is likely that intracellular pH alters intracellular ionized Ca^{2+} concentration without changing total cytosolic Ca^{2+} content.

Alteration in intracellular pH of smooth muscle may have other effects. For example, an increase in Ca_i caused by acidification may be explained by cell buffering such that, as cytosolic H^+ increases, it displaces Ca_i from internal buffers with similar affinities for Ca^{2+} and H^+. Moreover, a reduction in extracellular pH may reduce specific agonist-receptor binding.[129] Finally, alkalosis leads to enhanced synthesis of vasodilator prostaglandins, although inhibition of cyclooxygenase fails to block the alkalosis-induced attenuation of PVR.

A similar understanding of the influence of pH on pulmonary vascular tone follows from studies in the isolated, perfused rat lung, where the addition/removal of NH_4Cl (producing alternately corresponding intracellular alkalosis and acidosis) decreases/increases pulmonary arterial perfusion pressure.[130] In intact animals, most studies suggest that both systemic metabolic alkalosis and respiratory alkalosis inhibit HPV, whereas systemic respiratory acidosis has no effect, and metabolic acidosis enhances HPV.[131–133] This would indicate that CO_2 has a pH-independent vasodilating effect.

In adult humans, Bindslev et al.[134] determined that hyperventilation caused a 3.5-fold attenuation of HPV. Conversely, increasing P_{CO_2} from 30 to 50 mmHg by adding CO_2 to a breathing circuit during general anesthesia increased the PVR index by 44 percent. Infusion of 0.2 N HCl caused a parallel change in the PVR index as pulmonary H^+ concentration increased while the P_{CO_2} was held constant. In newborn infants with persistent pulmonary hypertension and in infants with pulmonary hypertension following surgery to correct congenital heart disease, hypocarbic alkalosis produces significant reductions in the PVR index. As hypocapnia without alkalosis does not reduce the PVR index in experimental settings, the likely stimulus is extracellular pH relative to intracellular pH.[135] As such, the use of hyperventilation may provide only transient relief of pulmonary hypertension as intracellular pH decreases.[136]

Effect of Inflammation on the Pulmonary Circulation

The mechanism of hypoxemia in pneumonia was recently reinvestigated by Gea et al.[137] They studied 23 patients with mild to severe arterial hypoxemia and/or increased alveolar-arterial O_2 difference. In subjects who were breathing spontaneously, only small amounts of intrapulmonary shunt (7 ± 2%) and moderate ventilation/perfusion (V_A/Q) mismatching were present. In contrast, in patients who required mechanical ventilation, shunt was larger (22 ± 5%), and a greater proportion of perfusion went to low V_A/Q units (11 ± 5%). These same investigators also examined the gas-exchange abnormalities in patients with hepatic cirrhosis. In this condition, marked by a low systemic vascular resistance and elevated cardiac output, a widened V_A/Q distribution was noted, with an excess perfusion going to low V_A/Q units.[138] In both pneumonia and cirrhosis, the data suggest that an attenuation of physiologic HPV accounts for the gas-exchange abnormalities.

Local and circulating inflammatory mediators are increased in both pneumonia and cirrhosis. These conditions often are associated with lipopolysaccharide (LPS) and inflammatory cytokines capable of producing lung injury in situ with attenuation of HPV[139] and with alteration in cellular integrity.[140] As NO is capable of altering vascular reactivity and causing cytotoxicity,[141] it may contribute to disease processes of the lung characterized by immune activation or inflammation. Both LPS and a combination of cytokines produce an increase in nitrite from cultured rat pulmonary artery smooth-muscle cells. Northern blot analysis reveals that inducible NO synthase (iNOS) activity is responsible for the increase in nitrite accumulation.[142] Future studies likely will explore the role of iNOS in producing increased permeability and a loss of HPV in clinical lung injury.

It is equally possible that attenuated *endothelial*-derived NO may alter the pulmonary circulation in these same conditions. Recently, it has been reported that tumor necrosis factor enhances HPV in the isolated rat lung circulation by inducing endothelial dysfunction.[143] Thus, NO may elicit a dual vascular dysfunction in lung injury. First, through iNOS induction, NO may cause areas of inappropriate pulmonary vasodilation. This vasodilation may worsen gas exchange. However, a local reduction of NO, controlled by the constitutive endothelial NOS, may cause other areas of inappropriate pulmonary vasoconstriction by removal of a tonic vasodilator influence. Such a removal of vasodilator influence actually may accentuate HPV and improve gas exchange. In a heterogeneous group of human lung diseases (primary pulmonary hypertension, COPD, idiopathic pulmonary fibrosis, or liver cirrhosis–related hypoxemia), diminished pulmonary vascular tone (via exogenous vasodilators) or increased pulmonary vascular tone (via almitrine) leads to a parallel deterioration or enhancement of ventilation-perfusion matching, respectively.[144]

Nitric Oxide

Interaction between the vascular endothelium and the tone of underlying smooth muscle was demonstrated first by Furchgott and Zawadzki in 1980.[145] They observed that a vasodilator, such as acetylcholine, has either no effect or causes vasoconstriction when applied to vessels without endothelium. They demonstrated that endothelial cells elaborate an extremely labile nonprostanoid vasodilator, which they termed *endothelium-derived relaxing factor*. These studies quickly were followed by observations of others that vascular relaxation caused by a number of agents, including organic nitrates, nitroprusside, acidified nitrite, and nitric oxide, was mediated by the accumulation of cGMP. The effect of all of these agents could be inhibited by methylene blue, methemoglobin, or hemoglobin. Following the suggestion by Furchgott and the demonstration by Ignarro et al.[146] that EDRF might, in fact, be NO, Palmer and coworkers reported a series of cascade bioassay experiments demonstrating that an NO-like compound was released from cultured endothelial cells.[147] Ignarro's team, studying native endothelium from pulmonary artery and vein, arrived at the same conclusion.[148] The endothelial mediator (or mediators) that elicits this behavior thus was identified as NO or a very similar nitrosocompound synthesized from L-arginine.[149]

NO is a well-suited local transcellular effector molecule because of its small size, lipophilic nature, and short duration of action. In vascular endothelial cells, NO is synthesized from the terminal quanidino nitrogen of L-arginine by eNOS and diffuses rapidly into subjacent vascular myocytes. Within the myocyte, it binds to the heme-iron complex within soluble guanylate cyclase. The resulting nitrosylheme activates, by conformational change, the guanylate cyclase, stimulating the production of cGMP leading to relaxation of the VSM. As NO, which diffuses readily into the vasculature, binds avidly to hemoglobin leading to the formation of methemoglobin, its biologic activity is limited to local sites of production.

Normal endothelium maintains a continuous release of NO, which can be stimulated by a variety of endothelial agonists including acetylcholine (ACh), bradykinin, histamine, and thrombin. In addition, its production can be promoted by certain mechanical forces such as shear stress exerted along the endothelial surface of the blood vessel. NO also is the active form of commonly used nitrovasodilators such as nitroglycerin and sodium nitroprusside. Through inhibitor studies in both animals and humans, L-arginine analogs such as L-*N*-mono-methyl-arginine, competitively inhibit NOS, resulting in a rapid, dramatic increase in blood pressure, which can be reversed by administering L-arginine.[150] When endothelial production of both NO and prostacyclin is blocked in vessels with an intact endothelium, a limited residual response to vasodilating agents exists, which is endothelium-dependent. This observation indicates the presence of an additional relaxing factor (EDHF) (see above).[151]

Multiple NO synthases have been characterized and their genes identified, and rapid progress has been made to identify alterations in NO synthesis and effect.[152] The constitutive isoform isolated from the cerebellum weighs 150 kDa, is regulated by calcium and calmodulin, and is present in the cytosolic fraction of the cell. The constitutive isoform isolated from vascular endothelium is 135 kDa; it also is regulated by Ca^{2+} but is membrane bound. The inducible isoform isolated from LPS-interferon–γ treated murine macrophages is a 130-kDa protein and is found in the cytosol. This isoform has not shown a dependence on Ca^{2+}; however, there is some evidence suggesting that this NOS contains tightly bound calmodulin and is activated by very low levels of Ca^{2+}.

The exact role of NO and EDHF in the regulation of the pulmonary circulation is not known. The complexity of the overall role of NO in the lung is underscored by the numerous distinct anatomic compartments within human lungs that contain NOS. Uniform labeling of human epithelium in large, cartilaginous airways occurs with anti-iNOS, in nerve elements and large-vessel endothelium with anti-eNOS, and in human alveolar macrophages with anti-iNOS.[153] The complexity of understanding the physiologic role in vivo is demonstrated by the dual vasodilatory/vasoconstrictor nature that many known endogenous vasoactive drugs may play. For example, in intact human pulmonary arterial rings, histamine relaxes tissues preconstricted with serotonin—a response that is obliterated in endothelium-denuded tissues.[154] In fact, endothelial denudation uncovers a direct effect of histamine on myocyte activation with resulting smooth-muscle contraction. NANC neurons mediate vasodilation in guinea pig pulmonary artery by both endothelium-dependent and endothelium-independent mechanisms. The endothelium-independent mechanism is mediated by NO.[155]

In addition, NO may function as a negative feedback modulator of endothelial cell function by inhibiting NOS in vascular endothelial cells. As this has been demonstrated in isolated bovine endothelial cells,[156] it might be expected that when exogenous NO is administered in vivo, either as a precursor NO donor compound (such as nitroglycerin) or as authentic NO by inhalation, there may be a downregulation of endogenous NO activity that may cause a rebound vasoconstrictor influence when NO administration is withdrawn.[157] This downregulated activity of NO may be related to downregulation of NO synthesis or an effect of a sustained increase in myocyte concentrations of cGMP.[158] Moreover, the site of NO production in vivo in disease states may not arise solely from the endothelium. For example, in rat pulmonary artery smooth muscle, LPS and cytokines

cause induced expression of the inducible NO synthase gene, which may contribute to lung injury and gas-exchange abnormalities in sepsis.[159] Nakayama et al. recently showed that the inducible NOS in rat pulmonary artery smooth muscle is regulated by de novo synthesis of tetrahydrobiopterin.[160] As NO may be induced by cytokine stimulation in pneumonia, it may contribute to the diminished hypoxic pulmonary vasoconstriction. However, if so, it appears that, in established pneumonia, the late administration of L-arginine analogs may not improve the attenuated hypoxic pressure response.[161]

The role of NO in modulating pulmonary vascular tone first was suggested by Rodman et al. in 1990.[91] Previously, having found that hypoxic contraction of the rat pulmonary artery was dependent (in large part) on the presence of a functioning endothelium, they noted that cGMP decreased in endothelium-intact rings during normoxia by greater than 50 percent. As cAMP concentrations decreased only slightly during hypoxia, they concluded that, in isolated rat pulmonary arteries, hypoxia is caused largely by decreased EDRF activity. Indeed, infusion of NOS inhibitors [*N*-omega-nitro-L-arginine (L-NNA), *N*-omega-nitro-L-arginine methyl ester (L-NAME)] into the intact feline pulmonary circulation increases perfusion pressure during constant-flow conditions and inhibits vasodilator responses to endothelial-dependent vasodilators (ACh, BK, substance P).[162] However, many other studies have noted that NO is not the sole regulator of hypoxic pulmonary vasoconstriction but, rather, an endogenous *modulator* of the hypoxic pressor response.[163] In fact, there is evidence to suggest that NO activity is increased during acute alveolar hypoxia, attenuating pulmonary vasopressor response. In chronic hypoxic pulmonary hypertension, experimental data and studies performed in humans demonstrate impairment of NO synthesis and/or release. These events promote excessive pulmonary vasoconstriction and also might permit mitogenesis and proliferation of various cell types within the vascular wall.[164]

Following studies indicating that NO modulates pulmonary vascular tone, animal and human studies indicated that NO could be administered by inhalation to alter pulmonary hemodynamics and gas exchange. Under normal conditions, NO inhalation does not alter pulmonary hemodynamics. However, within minutes of adding 10 to 80 ppm NO to inspired gas of awake, spontaneously breathing lambs, pulmonary hypertension caused either by the thromboxane analog U46619 or by hypoxemia is reversed.[165] In a study of healthy adults, HPV (induced by breathing 12% oxygen) increased mean pulmonary artery pressure (PAP) (from 14.7 ± 0.8 to 19.8 ± 0.9 mmHg) and was reversed after adding 40 ppm NO to the inspired gas. These effects are not accompanied by any alteration in systemic vascular resistance, as NO is readily inactivated by hemoglobin. As breathing 40 ppm in 21% O_2 caused no significant change in PAP, cardiac output, or Pa_{O_2}; again, it is likely that the normal pulmonary circulation is near fully vasodilated.[166]

After identifying NO as a regulator of PVR, it was logical to determine whether its deficiency would produce chronic pulmonary hypertension. However, rats administered *N*-nitro-L-arginine (NOS substrate inhibitor) for 3 weeks under both normoxic or hypoxic conditions do not develop the vascular and hemodynamic changes or the increased medial thickening of hypoxic pulmonary hypertension.[167]

The role of NO in lung injury is likely to be complex. LPS and tumor necrosis factor are known to attenuate endothelial-derived NO.[168,169] Moreover, these same agents induce NOS in vascular myocytes. The net effects are complex to predict in the intact circulation because attenuated endothelial-derived NO may decrease perfusion locally, while iNOS expression in myocytes may increase local blood flow. As drugs to effect eNOS or iNOS specifically are not available, the relative contribution of these enzymes to effects on ventilation-perfusion ratios in acute lung injury are unclear.

THERAPUTIC USE OF INHALED NO

INFANTS

Persistent pulmonary hypertension (PPHN) is a syndrome that may be idiopathic or may be associated with fetal asphyxia, meconium aspiration, neonatal pneumonia/sepsis, or congenital diaphragmatic hernia. The main feature is sufficient pulmonary hypertension leading to right-to-left shunting through a patent foramen ovale and ductus arteriosus. As such, the hypoxemia in these patients is refractory to oxygen therapy. Conventional therapy includes mechanical hyperventilation, hyperoxia, metabolic alkalemia, extracorporeal membrane oxygenation (ECMO), and vasodilator pharmacotherapy. Vasodilator therapy is associated with systemic hypotension because of vasodilation of the systemic circulation.

Several studies have examined the effect of inhaled NO on infants with PPHN. In each, inhalation of 10 to 80 ppm NO showed rapid improvement in oxygenation with reduction in systemic blood pressure, and this likely averted the need for ECMO in selected patients.[166,170] Infants and children with congenital heart disease complicated by chronic pulmonary hypertension also have been studied.[171] As hyperoxia and alkalosis can produce pulmonary vasodilation independent of the effects of NO, the ultimate theraputic strategy in the treatment of PPHN may include some combination of each of these therapies.[172]

ADULTS

As in infants, inhaled NO is a selective pulmonary vasodilator in adults with either COPD or cardiac disease. It is likely that the extent of NO-induced reduction in pulmonary hypertension may be related to the level of baseline pulmonary hypertension. Moreover, NO inhalation has only a slight influence on gas exchange in COPD as measured by the multiple inert gas technique.[173] This suggests that the vasodilatory effect occurs only in well-ventilated areas. In many adults with mild-to-moderate pulmonary hypertension, acute lung disease or acute thromboembolic disease may produce right heart cardiac output–limited states. The major treatment must be aimed at the condition causing the acute exacerbation of chronic hypertension. Treatment with vasodilator drugs may result in systemic hypotension, which may impair coronary blood flow to the right ventricle and precipitate circulatory collapse. Inhalation of NO is an

interesting new approach to the treatment of this syndrome, but its value has not been evaluated in randomized controlled trials to date.

Theoretically, in an injured lung with pulmonary hypertension, inhaled NO produces local vasodilation of well-ventilated lung units and may "steal" blood flow away from underventilated units. In the adult respiratory distress syndrome, inhaled NO reduces pulmonary hypertension and improves arterial oxygenation,[174] but whether these modest differences in pulmonary artery pressure and gas exchange contribute to improved outcome is unclear.

SIDE EFFECTS OF NO

In an oxygen environment, NO forms other more oxidized compounds such as NO_2.[175] Though NO is endogenous and concentrations of NO_2 <1 ppm likely are safe, there are no long-term studies on the safety of NO in humans. Thus, in the experimental use of NO, the following are recommended: (1) commercially purchased stock tanks of NO in nitrogen should be used; (2) systems used to blend and deliver NO must monitor proximal airway concentrations of NO and NO_2, (3) exhaust gases should be scavenged, (4) blood concentrations of methemoglobin should be measured frequently, and (5) the lowest concentration of NO to produce the desired clinical effect should be used, in conjunction with frequent attempts to wean slowly.[176]

Exogenous Mediators on the Pulmonary Circulation

VASODILATORS

Vasodilators have been used primarily to treat patients with pulmonary hypertension (PH). Many studies are difficult to evaluate because of the focus of many investigators on measuring PVR as an end point. Indeed, PVR may decline in patients treated with exogenous vasodilators, but often this is caused by an increase in cardiac output related to augmented venous return and the recruitment of previously poorly perfused lung units. Often, a decrease in PVR is associated with impaired HPV, causing worsening oxygenation.[177] Unexpected, sudden decreases in cardiac output may cause syncope and sudden death, as inadvertent systemic venodilation and attendant diminished venous return follow systemic vasodilator treatment. As the specific activity of exogenous vasodilators on the pulmonary circulation may not be apparent without invasive monitoring, drugs used for this condition often are administered initially in the catheterization laboratory. Often, a test of acute pulmonary vasodilator response potential is assessed by administering 100% oxygen or potent, titratable, short-acting intravenous agents such as PGE_1 or PGI_2.[178,179] The role of inhaled NO (10 ppm) to assess this potential appears to be as effective as PGI_2 and offers several advantages.[180]

ANESTHETICS

The effects of anesthetics on the pulmonary circulation were reviewed recently.[181] Many inhalational anesthetic agents, such as diethyl ether and halothane, attenuate HPV.[182] The nature of these agents limits their clinical usefulness outside of the surgical arena. More recently, intravenous geneal anesthetics have more frequent use in the operating room and critical care units. One such agent, propofol neither affects canine pulmonary vascular tone nor attenuates HPV.[183]

CALCIUM-CHANNEL AGONISTS

Rich and Brundage[184] used calcium-channel antagonists to show that substantial reductions in pulmonary arterial pressure and PVR are associated with regression of right ventricular hypertrophy in patients with primary PH. They were able to achieve a 50 percent decrease in PVR and 33 percent decrease in PAP in 8 out of 13 patients following the administration of oral calcium-channel antagonist. These patients initially were given a test dose of 60 mg diltiazem or 20 mg nifedipine, followed by consecutive hourly doses of the same until the goal was achieved or hypotension developed. They were subsequently maintained on high-dose therapy of up to 720 mg/day diltiazem or 240 mg/day nifedipine to produce regression of right ventricular hypertrophy. In a follow-up study, Rich et al. noted that in the 26 percent of patients who responded as above to high doses of calcium-channel antagonists, an improved survival over a 5-year period was noted.[185]

ZAPRINAST

Zaprinast is a cGMP-specific phosphodiesterase inhibitor (see Chaps. 49 and 62). Under baseline conditions, intravenous infusions into isolated, constant-perfused cat lung produce small decreases in pressure. However, when tone is elevated by agonist infusion, zaprinast leads to a dose-dependent decrease in perfusion pressure. This effect is reduced by pretreatment with eNOS inhibitors and prolongs markedly the vasodilation caused by NO. Vasodilator responses to adenosine, albuterol, and pinacidil are not affected by zaprinast.[186] These data suggest that zaprinast prolongs cGMP production in the lung. Future studies in humans likely will evaluate the role of zaprinast in pulmonary hypertension as a sole agent or in combination with "low-dose" or intermittent inhaled NO.

PROSTACYCLIN

Intravenous PGI_2 is a potent pulmonary vasodilator in PH. However, dose-dependent systemic vasodilation, an increase in intrapulmonary shunt, and hypoxemia limit its clinical application. Continuous infusion of PGI_2 into the isolated pulmonary circulation causes sustained cardiovascular depression via a vagal reflex mechanism that is probably mediated by pulmonary C-fibers.[187] Another clinical limitation is its relative ineffectiveness as a pulmonary vasodilator during coexisting hypercapnia.[188] The complex influence of PGI_2 infusion (12.5 to 35.0 ng/kg/min) on gas exchange during the adult respiratory distress syndrome (ARDS) was recently analyzed using the multiple inert gas elimination technique in nine patients.[189] PGI_2 reduced the pulmonary artery pressure from 35.6 to 28.8 mmHg and the pulmonary capillary occlusion pressure from 22.9 to 19.7 mmHg. However, despite a marked deterioration of V_A/Q matching

with an increase in true intrapulmonary shunt from 28.6 to 38.6 percent, the Pa_{O_2} was unchanged because of increased mixed venous oxygen content (venous P_{O_2} increased from 37.0 to 41.9 mmHg). This caused a 35 percent increase in the systemic oxygen delivery rate. Thus, infusions of PGI_2 in patients with ARDS may reduce pulmonary perfusion pressures (though not commonly necessary in current management strategies of ARDS) without deleterious effects on arterial pressures, but *only* in patients who have limited systemic oxygen delivery.

NITROVASODILATORS

Organic nitrates and compounds that liberate NO intracellularly (nitroglycerin, nitroprusside, isosorbide dinitrate) are non-specific smooth muscle relaxants; they activate cGMP-mediated smooth muscle relaxation through NO.[190] These agents have been used in adults with primary and secondary PH, and infants with idiopathic PH and PH secondary to sepsis. However, the lack of selective action in the pulmonary circulation makes their use problematic. Indeed, it is possible that the decrease in pulmonary vascular pressures observed after the administration of nitroglycerin results from a shift in the pulmonary vascular pressure-volume relationship caused by systemic venodilation, resulting in a reduction in the unstressed (distending) pulmonary blood volume.[191] In the adult respiratory distress syndrome, nitrovasodilators may worsen gas exchange by inhibiting vasoconstriction in edematous lung units.[192]

ANGIOTENSIN-CONVERTING ENZYME INHIBITORS

The lack of specific pulmonary vasodilation following administration of ACE inhibitors in patients with primary PH first was noted by Rich et al. in 1982.[193] Likewise, in patients with COPD, captopril combined with oxygen produced no significant clinical benefit at rest or during exercise following an 8-week trial.[194,195] More recently, in a select group of patients with connective tissue disease–associated PH, a significant and sustained reduction in pulmonary vascular resistance and mean pulmonary artery pressure was observed.[196]

VASOCONSTRICTORS

ALMITRINE

Almitrine bimesylate, a peripheral chemoreceptor agonist, has been reported in some studies to enhance HPV. In addition to its well-known ventilatory effect, a small rise in pulmonary arterial pressure or PVR occasionally is observed with chronic administration. Although the mechanism of action is unknown, it may improve ventilation/perfusion relationships, by redistribution of pulmonary perfusion. In isolated rat lungs, almitrine potentiates HPV.[197] In a recent, controlled double-blind study in patients with stable COPD, almitrine increased Pa_{O_2} by 20 percent and PVR by 48 percent. This effect was reversed following sublingual administration of nifedipine.[198] Following a 6-month administration at a low daily dose of 75 mg, tests showed that the agent may be safe with regard to previously noted toxicity to peripheral nerve function.[199] This dose also produced a 15 mmHg increase in arterial oxygen tension and amelioration of hypercapnia, with only a slight increase in mean PAP.

CYCLOOXYGENASE INHIBITORS

In acute lung injury, cyclooxygenase inhibitors have been reported to accentuate pulmonary hypertension and to improve gas exchange in an oleic acid model of lung injury.[200] In canine models of pneumonia[201] or ARDS,[200,202] arterial hypoxemia is improved in association with a decrease in pulmonary shunt through consolidated lung units following administration of acetylsalicylic acid or indomethacin. Moreover, the HPV response remains intact.[202] Though clinical information on the use of indomethacin to reduce shunt in human lung disease is limited, its use to cause closure of the ductus arteriosus in preterm infants does *not* cause significant alterations in newborn gas exchange. Indeed, pretreatment of fetal lambs with indomethacin does not alter the increase in pulmonary blood flow caused at birth by an increase in alveolar oxygen tension.[203]

In a study of 10 adults with chronic lung disease and resting room air hypoxemia, a 50 mg infusion of indomethacin caused pronounced effects on the pulmonary circulation, which were observed 3 h after administration.[204] Mean systemic arterial pressure increased from 76 ± 4 to 86 ± 4 mmHg (P < 0.01), whereas mean PAP was unchanged. However, systemic and PVR indexes increased from 22 ± 2 to $27.5 \pm 2\,U/m^2$ and from 11.9 ± 2 to $13.4 \pm 2\,U/m^2$, respectively. The Pa_{O_2} also increased from 49.5 ± 4 to 57.5 ± 4 mmHg. Moreover, in combination with hydralazine, indomethacin diminished the systemic vasodilating effect of hydralazine but preserved its pulmonary vasodilatory effect. Clearly, the role of cyclooxygenase inhibitors on pulmonary hemodynamics and gas exchange deserves a cautious interpretation. For example, in an experimental model of pulmonary embolism,[205] several different coclooxygenase inhibitors appear to aggravate pulmonary hypertension and worsen gas exchange by altering the distribution of V_A/Q to lung units with a greater than normal V_A/Q. Recently, inhaled PGI_2 was noted to reverse the hypoxic vasoconstriction in dogs, and clinically relevant systemic vasodilation was prevented.[206]

ADRENERGIC AGONISTS AND ANTAGONISTS

The pulmonary circulation contains postjunctional α_1- and α_2-adrenoreceptors, which mediate vasoconstriction, and β_2-adrenoreceptors, which cause vasodilation.[207] Intravenous infusion of β-adrenergic agonists has long been known to cause pulmonary vasodilation. In patients with cardiopulmonary/respiratory failure, this may cause a decrease in systemic blood pressure and cardiac output. Recently, β-adrenergic mechanisms were shown to attenuate HPV in cats.[208] As "intense" therapy with inhalation β-adrenergic agonists has evolved in the treatment of obstructive airways diseases, a pulmonary vascular effect is often noted as an increase in V_A/Q mismatching. Rodriguez-Roisen et al. noted a high level of hypoxic pulmonary vascular response in mechanically ventilated patients with asthma; it is possible that worsening hypoxemia thus may

result from β-adrenergic attenuation of HPV.[209] Though clinical experience with α-adrenergic antagonists is limited, α-adrenergic blockade is tried occasionally in the management of pulmonary hypertension in neonates. Tolazoline, which is structurally related to phentolamine, has some α-adrenergic blockade and is occasionally useful.

DOPAMINE

In intact lambs, dopamine alone increases the proportion of pulmonary blood flow to low V_A/Q regions during alveolar hypoxia without increasing PVR index.[210] However, in combination with PEEP in adult humans with acute respiratory failure, dopamine maintains the beneficial effects of PEEP on gas exchange and favorably increases the distribution of pulmonary blood flow toward high V_A/Q regions.[211] Apart from species differences, the discrepancy between these two studies suggests that dopamine causes pulmonary vasodilation directly. Indeed, singularly, dopamine may increase shunt by increasing cardiac output. However, errors in determining the variables used to determine the PVR calculation may erroneously identify a drug as a vasodilator when in fact it is not. This complex relationship, involving direct effects of dopamine on pulmonary vessels versus calculated changes in PVR caused by systemic effects on cardiac output, was recently examined by Ducas et al.[212] They examined directly the pulmonary pressure-flow characteristics in dogs following acute reductions in cardiac output produced by the injection of an autologous blood clot. They concluded that though dopamine decreases calculated PVR, it improves cardiac output without affecting pulmonary perfusion-flow characteristics.

Summary

The pulmonary circulation provides intimate control of the matching of alveolar ventilation to alveolar perfusion, contributing to efficient gas exchange. Though the pulmonary vasculature contains basic components common to other organ circulatory systems (endothelial cells, vascular smooth-muscle cells), the pulmonary vasculature is governed by a unique neural-humoral-local regulation. This regulatory control allows the pulmonary circulation to provide controlled alveolar perfusion in a low-pressure, low-resistance circuit. A more complete understanding of this regulation awaits the identification of the oxygen-sensing mechanisms that provide for the finely tuned regulation of hypoxic pulmonary vasoconstriction in health. Moreover, a fuller understanding of inflammatory mediator influence on dysregulated pulmonary blood flow and abnormal vascular remodeling will aid in the management of acute and chronic lung disease.

References

1. Elliot FM, Reid L: Some new facts about the pulmonary artery and its branching pattern. *Clin Radiol* 1965; 16:193.
2. Hakim TS, Kelly S: Occlusion pressures vs. micropipette pressures in the pulmonary circulation. *J Appl Physiol* 1989; 67(3):1277.

3. West JB, Bollery CT, Naimark A: Distribution of blood flow in isolated lung: Relation to vascular and alveolar pressures. *J Appl Physiol* 1964; 19:713.

4. Lockhart A, Tzareva M, Nader F, et al.: Elevated pulmonary artery wedge pressure at rest and during exercise in chronic bronchitis—fact or fancy? *Clin Sci* 1969; 37:503.

5. Fishman AP: Respiratory gases in the regulation of pulmonary circulation. *Physiol Rev* 1961; 41:214.

6. Morgan JP, Perreault CL, Morgan KG: The cellular basis of contraction and relaxation in cardiac and vascular smooth muscle. *Am Heart J* 1991; 121(3 pt 1):961.

7. Wong AY, Klassen GA: A model of calcium regulation in smooth muscle cell. *Cell Calcium* 1993; 14(3):227.

8. Fullerton DA, Hahn AR, Banerjee A, Harken AH: Pulmonary vascular smooth muscle relaxation by cGMP- versus cAMP-mediated mechanisms. *J Surg Res* 1994; 57(2):259.

9. Hayes J, Robinson J, Saunders L, et al.: Role of cAMP-dependent protein kinase in cAMP-mediated vasodilation. *Am J Physiol* 1992; 262(2 pt 2):H511.

10. McDaniel NL, Chen XL, Singer HA, et al.: Nitrovasodilators relax arterial smooth muscle by decreasing $[Ca^{2+}]i$ and uncoupling stress from myosin phosphorylation. *Am J Physiol* 1992; 263(2 pt 1):C461.

11. Quast U: Do the K^+ channel openers relax smooth muscle by opening K^+ channels? *Trends Pharmacol Sci* 1993; 14(9):332.

12. Clapp LH, Gurney AM: ATP-sensitive K^+ channels regulate resting potential of pulmonary arterial smooth muscle cells. *Am J Physiol* 1992; 262(3 pt 2):H916.

13. Dumas M, Dumas JP, Advenier C, Giudicelli: Effects of three K^+ channel openers on airways and pulmonary circulation in the isolated guinea-pig lung. *Eur J Pharmacol* 1993; 239(1–3):141.

14. Gelband CH, Ishikawa T, Post JM, et al.: Intracellular divalent cations block smooth muscle K^+ channels. *Circ Res* 1993; 73(1):24.

15. Kirber MT, Ordway RW, Clapp LH, et al.: Both membrane stretch and fatty acids directly activate large conductance Ca^{2+}-activated K^+ channels in vascular smooth muscle cells. *FEBS Lett* 1992; 297(1–2):24.

16. NADH and NAD modulate Ca^{2+}-activated K^+ channels in small pulmonary arterial smooth muscle cells of the rabbit. *Eur J Physiol* 1994; 427(3–4):378.

17. Bialecki RA, Kulik TJ, Colcucci WE: Stretching increases calcium influx and efflux in cultured pulmonary arterial smooth muscle cells. *Am J Physiol* 1992; 263(5 pt 1):L602.

18. Partanen M, Laitinen A, Hervonen A, et al.: Catecholamine and acetylcholinesterase-containing nerves in human lower respiratory tract. *Histochem* 1982; 76(2):175.

19. Dawson CA, Linehan JH, Rickaby DA, Krenz GS: Effect of vasoconstriction on longitudinal distribution of pulmonary vascular pressure and volume. *J Appl Physiol* 1991; 70(4):1607.

20. Hyman AL, Nandiwada P, Knight DS, Kadowitz PJ: Pulmonary vasodilator responses to catecholamines and sympathetic nerve stimulation in the cat. Evidence that vascular beta-2 adrenoreceptors are innervated. *Circ Res* 1987;48(3):407.

21. Tucker A: Pulmonary and systemic vascular responses to hypoxia after chemical sympathectomy. *Cardiovasc Res* 1979; 13(8):469.

22. Bakhle YS, Mann R, Bell C: Evidence that blood vessels in guinea-pig lung are supplied by both noradrenergic and dopaminergic axons. *J Auto Nerv Sys* 1988; 26(2):169.

23. Bevan RD: Influence of adrenergic innervation on vascular growth and mature characteristics. *Am Rev Respir Dis* 1989; 140(5):1478.

24. McMahon TJ, Kadowitz PJ: Methylene blue inhibits neurogenic cholinergic vasodilator responses in the pulmonary vascular bed of the cat. *Am J Physiol* 1992; 263(5 pt 1):L575.

25. Lejeune P, Vachiery JL, Leeman M, et al.: Absence of parasympathetic control of pulmonary vascular pressure-flow plots in hyperoxic and hypoxic dogs. *Respir Physiol* 1989; 78(2):123.

26. Sanders MH, Owens GR, Sciurba FC, et al.: Ventilation and breathing pattern during progressive hypercapnia and hypoxia after human heart-lung transplantation. *Am Rev Respir Dis* 1989; 140(1):38.

27. Sanders MH, Constantino JP, Owens GR, et al.: Breathing during wakefulness and sleep after human heart-lung transplantation. *Am Rev Respir Dis* 1989; 140(1):45.

28. Uddman R, Sundler F: Neuropeptides in the airways. A review. *Am Rev Respir Dis* 1987; 136:53.

29. Allen KM, Wharton J, Pollak JM, Haworth S: A study of nerves containing peptides in the pulmonary vasculature of healthy infants and children and of those with pulmonary hypertension. *Br Heart J* 1989; 62:353.

30. Said SI: Vasoactive peptides in the lung, with special reference to vasoactive intestinal peptide. *Exp Lung Res* 1982; 3:343.

31. Coburn RF: Neural coordination of excitation of ferret trachealis muscle. *Am J Physiol* 1984; 246:C459.

32. Frandsen EK, Krishina GA, Said SI: Vasoactive intestinal polypeptide promotes cyclic adenosine 3′,5′-monophosphate accumulation in guinea pig trachea. *Br J Pharmacol* 1987; 62:367.

33. Said SL, Mutt V: Long acting vasodilator peptide from lung tissue. *Nature* 1969; 224:699.

34. Greenberg B, Rhoden K, Barnes PJ: Effect of vasoactive intestinal peptide and peptide histidine isoleucine in human and bovine pulmonary arteries. *Blood Ves* 1987; 24:45.

35. Lung MA, Widdicombe JG: Lung reflexes and nasal vascular resistance in the anaesthetized dog. *J Physiol* 1987; 386:465.

36. Lundberg JM, Anggard A, Emson P, et al.: Vasoactive intestinal polypeptide and cholinergic mechanisms in cat nasal mucosa. Studies on choline acetyltransferase and release of VIP. *Proc Natl Acad Sci USA* 1981; 78:5255.

37. Nakanishi S: Substance P precursor and kininogen: Their structures, gene organizations, and regulation. *Physiol Rev* 1987; 67:1117.

38. Regoli D, Drapeau G, Dion S, D'Orleaans-Juste P: Receptors for substance P and related neurokininis. *Pharmacology* 1989; 38(1):1.

39. Grandordy BM, Frossard N, Rhoden KJ, Barnes PJ: Tachykinin-induced phosphoinositide breakdown in airway smooth muscle and epithelium: Relationship to contraction. *Mol Pharmacol* 1988; 33:515.

40. Salonen RO, Webber SE, Widdicombe JG: Effects of neuropeptides and capsaicin on the canine tracheal vasculature in vivo. *Br J Pharmacol* 1988; 95:1262.

41. McCormack DG, Salonen RO, Barnes PJ: Effect of sensory neuropeptides on canine bronchial and pulmonary vessels in vitro. *Life Sci* 1989; 45:2405.

42. Gamse R, Saria A: Potentiation of tachykinin-induced plasma extravasation by calcitonin gene-related peptide. *Eur J Pharmacol* 1985; 114:61.

43. McGillis JP, Organist ML, Payan DG: Substance P and immunoregulation. *Fed Proc* 1987; 14:120.

44. Sertl K, Wiedermann CJ, Kowalski ML, et al.: Substance P: The relationship between receptor distribution in rat lung and the capacity of substance P to stimulate vascular permeability. *Am Rev Respir Dis* 1988; 138(1):151.

45. McDonald DM: Neurogenic inflammation in the rat trachea. I. Changes in venules, leukocytes and epithelial cells. *J Neurocytol* 1988; 17:583.

46. Kowalski ML, Didler A, Kaliner MA: Neurogenic inflammation in the airways. 1. Neurogenic stimulation induced plasma protein extravasation into the rat airway lumen. *Am Rev Respir Dis* 1989; 140(1):101.

47. Nadel JA: Mechanisms of inflammation and potential role in the pathogenesis. *Allergy Proc* 1991; 12(2):85.

48. Steenberg PH, Hoppener JW, Zandberg J, et al.: Structure and expression of the human calcitonin/CGRP genes. *FEBS Lett* 1986; 209(1):97.

49. McCormack DG, Mak JC, Coupe MO, Barnes PJ: Calcitonin gene-related peptide vasodilation of human pulmonary vessels: Receptor mapping and functional studies. *J Appl Physiol* 1989; 67:1265.

50. Matran R, Alving K, Martling CR, et al.: Effects of neuropeptides and capsaicin on tracheobronchial blood flow in the pig. *Acta Physiol Scand* 1989; 135:335.

51. Potter EK: Neuropeptide Y as an autonomic neurotransmitter. *Pharmacol Ther* 1988; 37:251.

52. Baraniuk JN, Castellino S, Lundgren JD, et al.: Neuropeptide Y (NPY) in human nasal mucosa. *Am J Respir Cell Mol Biol* 1990; 3(2):165.

53. Maron MB: Pulmonary vasoconstriction in a canine model of neurogenic pulmonary edema. *J Appl Physiol* 1990; 68(3):912.

54. Lipworth BJ, Dagg KD: Vasoconstrictor effects of angiotensin II on the pulmonary vascular bed. *Chest* 1994; 105(5):1360.

55. Cheng DY, DeWitt BJ, McMahon TJ, Kadowitz PJ: Comparison of pressor responses to angiotensin I, II, III in pulmonary vascular bed of cats. *Am J Physiol* 1994; 266(6 pt 2):J2247.

56. Rabinovitch M, Mullen M, Rosenberg HC, et al.: Angiotensin II prevents hypoxic pulmonary hypertension and vascular changes in rat. *Am J Physiol* 1988; 254(3 pt 2):H500.

57. Jackson RM, Narkates AJ, Oparil S: Impaired pulmonary conversion of angiotensin I to angiotensin II in rats exposed to chronic hypoxia. *J Appl Physiol* 1986; 60(4):1121.

58. Shepard JM, Joyner WL, Gilmore JP: Hypoxia does not alter angiotensin converting enzyme activity in hamster pulmonary microvessels. *Circ Res* 1987; 61(2):228.

59. Chao W, Olson MS: Platelet-activating factor: Receptors and signal transduction. *Biochem J* 1993; 292 (pt 3):617.

60. Toga H, Hibler S, Ibe BO, Raj JU: Vascular effects of platelet-activating factor in lambs: Role of cyclo- and lipoxygenase. *J Appl Physiol* 1992; 73(6):2559.

61. Ono S, Westcott JY, Voelkel NF: PAF antagonists inhibit pulmonary vascular remodeling induced by hypobaric hypoxia in rats. *J Appl Physiol* 1992; 73:1084.

62. Ono S, Voelkel NF: PAF antagonists inhibit moncrotaline-induced lung injury and pulmonary hypertension. *J Appl Physiol* 1991; 71:2483.

63. Ohar JA, Waller KS, Dahms TE: Platelet-activating factor induces selective pulmonary arterial hyperreactivity in isolated perfused rabbit lungs. *Am Rev Respir Dis* 1993; 148:158.

64. Filep JG: Endothelin peptides: Biological actions and pathophysiological significance in the lung. *Life Sci* 1993; 52(2):119.

65. Luscher TF: Endothelin: Systemic arterial and pulmonary effects of a new peptide with potent biological properties. *Am Rev Respir Dis* 1992; 146(5 pt 2):S56.

66. Langleben D, DeMarchie M, Laporta D, et al.: Endothelin-1 in acute lung injury and the adult respiratory distress syndrome. *Am Rev Respir Dis* 1993; 148(6 pt 1):1646.

67. Druml W, Steltzer H, Waldhausl W, et al.: Endothelin-1 in adult respiratory distress syndrome. *Am Rev Respir Dis* 1993; 148(5):1169.

68. Deleuze PH, Adnot S, Shiiya N, et al.: Endothelin dilates bovine pulmonary circulation and reverses hypoxic pulmonary vasoconstriction. *J Cardiovasc Pharmacol* 1992; 19(3):354.

69. Nagao T, Vanhoutte PM: Endothelium-derived hyperpolarizing factor and endothelium-dependent relaxations. *Am J Respir Cell Mol Biol* 1993; 8:1.

70. Hasunuma K, Yamaguchi T, Rodman DM, et al.: Effects of inhibitors of EDRF and EDHF on vasoreactivity of perfused rat lungs. *Am J Physiol* 1991; 260(2 pt):L97.

71. Tod ML, Rubin LJ: Pulmonary vascular responses to thromboxane and prostacyclin. *J Appl Physiol* 1992; 73(6):2717.

72. Madden MC, Vender RL, Friedman M: Effect of hypoxia on prostacyclin production in cultured pulmonary artery endothelium. *Prostaglandins* 1986; 31(6):1049.

73. DeBold AJ, Borenstein HB, Veress AT, Sonnenberg H: A rapid and potent natriuretic response to intravenous injection of atrial myocardial extract in rats. *Life Sci* 1981; 28:89.

74. Chinkers M, Garbers DL, Chang MS, et al.: A membrane form of guanylate cyclase is an atrial natriuretic peptide receptor. *Nature* 1989; 338:78.

75. Widimsky J Jr, Kuchel O, Debinski W, Thibault G: Dissociation between right atrial pressure and plasma atrial natriuretic factor following prolonged high salt intake. *Can J Physiol Pharmacol* 1990; 68:408.

76. Matsubara H, Niru Y, Umeda Y, et al.: Atrial natriuretic peptide gene expression and its secretion by pneumocytes derived from neonatal rat lungs. *Biochem Biophys Res Commun* 1988; 156:619.

77. Currie MG, Oehlenschlager WF, Kurtz DT: Profound elevation of ventricular and pulmonary atriopeptin in a model of heart failure. *Biochem Biophys Res Commun* 1987; 148:1158.

78. Ignaro LJ, Wood KS, Harbison RG, Kadowitz PJ: Atriopeptin II relaxes and elevates cGMP in bovine pulmonary artery but not vein. *J Appl Physiol* 1986; 60:1128.

79. Cigarini I, Adnot S, Chabrier PE, et al.: Pulmonary vasodilator responses to atrial natriuretic factor and sodium nitroprusside. *J Appl Physiol* 1989; 67:2269.

80. Jin H, Yang RH, Thornton RM, et al.: Atrial natriuretic peptide lowers pulmonary arterial pressure in hypoxia-adapted rats. *J Appl Physiol* 1988; 65:1729.

81. Adnot S, Chabrier PE, Andrivet P, et al.: Atrial natriuretic peptide concentrations and pulmonary hemodynamics in patients with pulmonary artery hypertension. *Am Rev Respir Dis* 1987; 136:951.

82. Winter RF, Davidson AC, Treacher D, et al.: Atrial natriuretic peptide concentrations in hypoxic pulmonary hypertension: Relation to haemodynamic and blood gas variables and response to supplemental oxygen. *Thorax* 1989; 44(1):58.

83. Jin H, Yan RH, Chen YF, et al.: Atrial natriuretic peptide attenuates the development of pulmonary hypertension in rats adapted to chronic hypoxia. *J Clin Invest* 1990; 85:115.

84. DeWitt BJ, Cheng DY, McMahon TJ, et al.: Analysis of responses to bradykinin in the pulmonary vascular bed of the cat. *Am J Physiol* 1994; 266(6 pt 2):H2256.

85. Lippton HL, Hao Q, Hauth T, Hyman A: Mechanisms of signal transduction for adenosine and ATP in pulmonary vascular bed. *Am J Physiol* 1992; 262(3 pt 2):H926.

86. Inbar S, Schrader BJ, Kaufmann E, et al.: Effects of adenosine in combination with calcium channel blockers in patients with primary pulmonary hypertension. *J Am Coll Cardiol* 1993; 21(2):414.

87. Utterback DB, Staples ED, White SE, et al.: Basis for the selective reduction of pulmonary vascular resistance in humans during infusion of adenosine. *J Appl Physiol* 1994; 76(2):724.

88. Pesquero JB, Jubilut GN, Lindsey CJ, Paiva AC: Bradykinin metabolism pathway in the rat pulmonary circulation. *J Hypertens* 1992; 10(12):1471.

89. McMahon TJ, Hood JS, Bellan JA, Kadowitz PJ: N-omega-nitro-L-arginine methyl ester selectively inhibits pulmonary

vasodilator responses to acetylcholine and bradykinin. *J Appl Physiol* 1991; 71(5):2026.

90. von Euler US, Liljestrand G: Observations on the pulmonary arterial blood pressure in the cat. *Acta Physiol Scand* 1946; 12:301.

91. Rodman DM, Yamaguchi T, Hasunuma K, et al.: Effects of hypoxia on endothelium-dependent relaxation of rat pulmonary artery. *Am J Physiol* 1990; 259(4 pt 1):L207.

92. Madden JA, Dawson CA, Harder DR: Hypoxia-induced activation in small isolated pulmonary arteries from the cat. *J Appl Physiol* 1985; 59:1389.

93. Rodman M, Yamaguchi T, O'Brien RF, McMurtry IF: Hypoxic contraction of isolated rat pulmonary artery. *J Pharmacol Exp Ther* 1988; 248:952.

94. Bennie RE, Packer CS, Powell DR, et al.: Biphasic contractile response of pulmonary artery to hypoxia. *Am J Physiol* 1991; 261(pt 5):L156.

95. Vadula MS, Kleinman JG, Madden JA: Effect of hypoxia and norepinephrine on cytoplasmic free Ca^{2+} in pulmonary and cerebral arterial myocytes. *Am J Physiol* 1993; 265(6 pt 1):L591.

96. Madden JA, Vadula MS, Kurup VP: Effects of hypoxia and other vasoactive agents on pulmonary and cerebral artery smooth cells. *Am J Physiol* 1992; 263(3 pt 1):L384.

97. Holden WE, McCall E: Hypoxia-induced contraction of porcine pulmonary artery strips depend on intact endothelium. *Exp Lung Res* 1984; 7:101.

98. DeMey JG, Vanhoutte PM: Heterogeneous behavior of the canine arterial and venous wall. Importance of the endothelium. *Circ Res* 1982; 51:439.

99. Mathew R, Burke-Wolin T, Gewitz MH, Wolin MS: O_2 and rat pulmonary artery tone: Effects of endothelium, Ca^{2+}, cyanide, and monocrotaline. *J Appl Physiol* 1991; 71(1):30.

100. Yuan XJ, Tod ML, Rubin LJ, Blaustein MP: Contrasting effects of hypoxia on tension in rat pulmonary and mesenteric arteries. *Am J Physiol* 1990; 259:H281.

101. Makary A, Pataki M, Toth E, Lusztig G: The effect of hypoxia and hypokinesia on prostacyclin (PGI_2) production of vessel wall. *Exp Pathol* 1987; 32(4):251.

102. Madden MC, Vender RL, Friedman M: Effect of hypoxia on prostacyclin production in cultured pulmonary artery endothelium. *Prostaglandins* 1986; 31(6):1049.

103. Raj JU, Chen P: Role of eicosanoids in hypoxic vasoconstriction in isolated lamb lungs. *Am J Physiol* 1987; 253 (3 pt 2):H626.

104. Ali J, Duke K: Does indomethacin affect shunt and its response to PEEP in oleic acid pulmonary edema. *J Appl Physiol* 1987; 62(6):2187.

105. Gordon JB, Tod ML, Wetzel RC, et al.: Age-dependent effects of indomethacin on hypoxic vasoconstriction in neonatal lamb lungs. *Pediatr Res* 1988; 23(6):580.

106. Warren JB, Maltby, MacCormack D, Barnes PJ: Pulmonary endothelium-derived relaxing factor is impaired in hypoxia. *Clin Sci* 1989; 77(6):671.

107. Johns RA, Linden JM, Peach MJ: Endothelium-dependent relaxation and cyclic GMP accumulation in rabbit pulmonary artery are selectively impaired by moderate hypoxia. *Circ Res* 1989; 65(6):1508.

108. Robertson BE, Warren JB, Nye PC: Inhibition of nitric oxide synthesis potentiates hypoxic vasoconstriction in isolated rat lungs. *Exp Physiol* 1990; 75(2):255.

109. Shaul PW, Wells LB: Oxygen modulates nitric oxide production selectively in fetal pulmonary endothelial cells. *Am J Respir Cell Mol Biol* 1994; 11:432.

110. Shirakami G, Nakao K, Saito Y, et al.: Acute pulmonary alveolar hypoxia increases lung and plasma endothelin-1 levels in conscious rats. *Life Sci* 1991; 48(10):969.

111. Rakugi H, Tabuchi Y, Nakamaru M, et al.: Evidence for endothelin-1 release from resistance vessels of rats in response to hypoxia. *Biochem Biophys Res Commun* 1990; 169:793.

112. Vanhoutte PM, Luscher TM, Graser T: Endothelium-dependent contractions. *Blood Ves* 1991; 28(1-3):74.

113. Siegel G, Grote I: in Acker II (ed): *Oxygen Sensing in Tissues.* Berlin, Springer, 1988; 131.

114. Demirvurek AT, Wadsworth RM, Kane KA, Peacock AJ: The role of endothelium in hypoxic constriction of human pulmonary artery rings. *Am Rev Respir Dis* 1993; 147(2):283.

115. Daut J, Maier-Rudolph W, von Beckerath N, et al.: Hypoxic dilation of coronary arteries is mediated by ATP-sensitive potassium channels. *Science* 1990; 247(4984):1341.

116. Bohr DF, Webb RC: Vascular smooth muscle membrane on hypertension. *Ann Rev Pharmacol Toxicol* 1988; 28:389.

117. Salvaterra CG, Rubin LJ, Schaeffer J, Blaustein: The influence of the transmembrane sodium gradient on the responses of pulmonary arteries to decreases in oxygen tension. *Am Rev Respir Dis* 1989; 139:933.

118. Farrukh IS, Michael JR: Cellular mechanisms that control pulmonary vascular tone during hypoxia and normoxia. *Am Rev Respir Dis* 1992; 145:1389.

119. Haynes J Jr, Kithas PA, Taylor AE, Strada SJ: Selective inhibition of cGMP-inhibitable cAMP phosphodiesterase decreases pulmonary vasoreactivity. *Am J Physiol* 1991; 261(2 pt 2):H487.

120. Post JM, Hume JR, Archer SL, Weir EK: Direct role for potassium channel inhibition in hypoxic pulmonary vasoconstriction. *Am J Physiol* 1992; 262(Cell Physiol 31):C882.

121. McQuillan LP, Leung GK, Marsden PA, et al.: Hypoxia inhibits expression of endothelial constitutive NOS via transcriptional and post-transcriptional mechanisms. *Am J Physiol* 1994; 267(5 pt 2):H1921.

122. Kourembanas S, McQuillan LP, Leung GK, Faller DV: Nitric oxide regulates the expression of vasoconstrictors and growth factors by vascular endothelium under both normoxia and hypoxia. *J Clin Invest* 1993; 92:99.

123. Kourembanas S, Marsden PA, McQuillan LP, Faller DV: Hypoxia induces endothelin gene expression and secretion in cultured human endothelium. *J Clin Invest* 1991; 8:1054.

124. Kourembanas S, Hannan RL, Faller DV: Oxygen tension regulates the expression of the platelet-derived growth factor-β chain gene in human endothelial cells. *J Clin Invest* 1990; 86:670.

125. Goldberg MA, Dunning SP, Bunn HF: Regulation of the erythropoietin gene: Evidence that the oxygen sensor is a heme protein. *Science* 1988; 242:1412.

126. Siegel G, Emden J, Wenzel K, et al.: Potassium channel activation in vascular smooth muscle. *Adv Exp Med Biol* 1992; 311:53.

127. Sperelakis N: Properties of calcium channels in cardiac muscle and vascular smooth muscle. *Mol Cell Biochem* 1990; 99(2):97.

128. Karaki H, Kitajima S, Ozaki H: Effects of pH on vascular smooth muscle contraction. *Jpn J Clin Med* 1992; 50(9):2106.

129. Bronstein EH, Procelli RJ: Effects of hydrogen ion concentration on *in vitro* pulmonary vascular reactivity. *Exp Lung Res* 1988; 14(6):837.

130. Krampetz IK, Rhoades RA: Intracellular pH: Effect on pulmonary arterial smooth muscle. *Am J Physiol* 1991; 260(6 pt 1):L516.

131. Brimioulle S, Lejeune P, Vachiery JL, et al.: Effects of acidosis and alkalosis on hypoxic pulmonary vasoconstriction in dogs. *Am J Physiol* 1990; 258(2 pt 2):H347.

132. Lejeune P, Brimioulle S, Leeman M, et al.: Enhancement of

hypoxic pulmonary vasoconstriction by metabolic acidosis in dogs. *Anesthesiology* 1990; 73(2):256.

133. Loeppky JA, Scotto P, Riedel CE, et al.: *J Appl Physiol* 1992; 72(5):1787.

134. Bindslev L, Jolin-Carlsson A, Santesson J, Gottlieb I: Hypoxic pulmonary vasoconstriction in man: Effects of hyperventilation. *Acta Anaesthesiol Scand* 1985; 29(5):547.

135. Schreiber MD, Heymann MA, Soifer SJ: Increased arterial pH, not decreased PaCO2, attenuates hypoxia-induced pulmonary vasoconstriction in newborn lambs. *Pediatr Res* 1986; 20(2):113.

136. Gorden JB, Martinez FR, Keller PA, et al.: Differing effects of acute and prolonged alkalosis on hypoxic pulmonary vasoconstriction. *Am Rev Respir Dis* 1993; 148:1651.

137. Gea J, Roca J, Torres A, et al.: Mechanisms of abnormal gas exchange in patients with pneumonia. *Anesthesiology* 1991; 75(5):782.

138. Augusti AG, Roca J, Bosch J, et al.: Effects of propranolol on arterial oxygenation and oxygen transport to tissues. *Am Rev Respir Dis* 1990; 142(2):306.

139. Hutchinson AA, Ogletree ML, Snapper JR, Brigham KL: Effect of endotoxemia on hypoxic pulmonary vasoconstriction in unanesthetized sheep. *J Appl Physiol* 1985; 58:1463.

140. Meyrick B, Christman B, Jesmok G: Effects of recombinant tumor necrosis factor-alpha on cultured pulmonary artery and lung microvascular endothelial monolayers. *Am J Pathol* 1991; 138:93.

141. Hibbs JB Jr, Taintor RR, Vavrin Z, Rachlin EM: Nitric oxide: A cytotoxic activated macrophage effector molecule. *Biochem Biophys Res Commun* 1988; 157:87.

142. Johnson BA, Lowenstein CJ, Schwarz MA, et al.: Culture of pulmonary microvascular smooth muscle cells from intraacinar arteries of the rat: Characterization and inducible production of nitric oxide. *Am J Respir Cell Mol Biol* 1994; 10:604.

143. Fang S, Dewar A, Crawley DE, et al.: Effect of tumor necrosis factor on hypoxic pulmonary vasoconstriction. *J Appl Physiol* 1992; 72(3):1044.

144. Agusti AGN, Rodriguez-Roisin R: Effect of pulmonary hypertension on gas exchange. *Eur Respir J* 1993; 6:1371.

145. Furchgott RF, Zawadzki JV: The obligatory role of endothelial cells in the relaxation of arterial smooth muscle by acetylcholine. *Nature* 1980; 288(5789):373.

146. Ignarro LJ, Buga GM, Wood KS, et al.: Endothelium-derived relaxing factor produced and released from artery and vein is nitric oxide. *Proc Natl Acad Sci USA* 1987; 84(24):9265.

147. Palmer RMJ, Ferrige AG, Moncada S: Nitric oxide release accounts for the biological activity of endothelium-derived relaxing factor. *Nature* 1987; 327:524.

148. Ignarro LJ, Byrns BE, Buga GM, Wood KS: Endothelium-derived relaxing factor from pulmonary artery and vein possesses pharmacologic and chemical properties identical to those of nitric oxide radical. *Circ Res* 1987; 61(6):866.

149. Palmer RMJ, Ashton DS, Moncada S: Vascular endothelial cells synthesize nitric oxide from L-arginine. *Nature* 1988; 333(6174):664.

150. Kilbourn RG, Jubran A, Gross SS, et al.: Reversal of endotoxin-mediated shock by NG-methyl-L-arginine, an inhibitor of nitric oxide synthesis. *Biochem Biophys Res Commun* 1990; 172:1132.

151. Komori K, Vanhoutte PM: Endothelium-derived hyperpolarization factor. *Blood Ves* 1990; 27(2-5):238.

152. Morgan JM, McCormack DG, Griffiths MJ, et al.: Adenosine as a vasodilator in primary pulmonary hypertension. *Circulation* 1991; 84(3):1145.

153. Kobzik L, Bredt DS, Lowenstein CJ, et al.: Nitric oxide synthase in human and rat lung: Immunocytochemical and histochemical localization. *Am J Respir Cell Mol Biol* 1993; 9:371.

154. Ortiz JL, Labat C, Norel X, et al.: Histamine receptors on human isolated pulmonary arterial muscle preparations: Effects of endothelial cell removal and nitric oxide inhibitors. *J Pharmacol Exp Ther* 1992; 260(2):762.

155. Liu SF, Crawley DE, Rohde JA, et al.: Role of nitric oxide and guanosine 3',5'-cyclic monophosphate in mediating nonadrenergic, noncholinergic relaxation in guinea-pig pulmonary arteries. *Br J Pharmacol* 1992; 107(3):861.

156. Assreuy J, Cunha FQ, Liew FY, Moncada S: Feedback inhibition of nitric oxide synthase activity by nitric oxide. *Br J Pharmacol* 1993; 108:833.

157. Buga GM, Griscavage JM, Rogers NE, Ignarro LJ: Negative feedback regulation of endothelial cell function by nitric oxide. *Circ Res* 1993; 73(5):808.

158. Archer SL, Rist K, Nelson DP, et al.: Comparison of the hemodynamic effects of nitric oxide and endothelium-dependent vasodilators in intact lungs. *J Appl Physiol* 1990; 68(2):735.

159. Thomae KR, Geller DA, Billiar TR, et al.: Antisense oligodeoxynucleotide to inducible nitric oxide synthase inhibits nitric oxide synthesis in rat pulmonary artery smooth muscle cells in culture. *Surgery* 1993; 114(2):272.

160. Nakayama DK, Geller DA, Di Silvio M, et al.: Tetrahydrobiopterin synthesis and inducible nitric oxide production in pulmonary artery smooth muscle. *Am J Physiol* 1994; 266(4 pt 1):L455.

161. McCormack DG, Paterson NA: Loss of hypoxic pulmonary vasoconstriction in chronic pneumonia is not mediated by nitric oxide. *Am J Physiol* 1993; 265(5 pt 2):H1523.

162. Cheng DY, DeWitt BJ, McMahon TJ, Kadowitz PJ: Comparative effects of L-NNA and alkyl esters of L-NNA on pulmonary vasodilator responses to ACh, BK, and SP. *Am J Physiol* 1994; 266(6 pt 2):H2416.

163. Persson MG, Gustafsson LE, Wiklund NP, et al.: Endogenous nitric oxide as a probable modulator of pulmonary circulation and hypoxic pressor response in vivo. *Acta Physiol Scand* 1990; 140(4):449.

164. Dinh-Xuan AAT: Endothelial modulation of pulmonary vascular tone. *Eur Respir J* 1992; 5(6):757.

165. Frostell C, Fratacci MD, Wain JC, et al.: Inhaled nitric oxide: A selective pulmonary vasodilator reversing hypoxic pulmonary vasoconstriction. *Circulation* 1991; 83(6):2038.

166. Frostell CG, Blomqvist J, Hedenstierna G, et al.: Inhaled nitric oxide selectively reverses human hypoxic pulmonary vasoconstriction without causing systemic vasodilation. *Anesthesiology* 1993; 78(3):427.

167. Hampl V, Archer SL, Nelson DP, Weir EK: Chronic EDRF inhibition and hypoxia: Effects on pulmonary circulation and systemic blood pressure. *J Appl Physiol* 1993; 75(4):1748.

168. Umans JG, Wylam ME, Samsel RW, et al.: Effects of endotoxin in vivo on endothelial and smooth-muscle function in rabbit and rat aorta. *Am Rev Respir Dis* 1993; 148(6 pt 1):1638.

169. Johnson A, Ferro TJ: TNF-alpha augments pulmonary vasoconstriction via the inhibition of nitrovasodilator activity. *J Appl Physiol* 1992; 73(6):2483.

170. Kinsella JP, Neish SR, Shaffer E, Abman SH: Low-dose inhalational nitric oxide in persistent pulmonary hypertension of the newborn. *Lancet* 1992; 340:819.

171. Roberts JD Jr, Lang P, Bigatello LM, et al.: Inhaled nitric oxide in congenital heart disease. *Circulation* 1993; 87:447.

172. Fineman JR, Wong J, Soifer SJ: Hyperoxia and alkalosis produce pulmonary vasodilation independent of endothelium-derived nitric oxide in newborn lambs. *Pediatr Res* 1993; 33(4 pt 1):341.

173. Moinard J, Manier G, Pillet O, Castaing Y: Effect of inhaled nitric oxide on hemodynamics and V_A/Q inequalities in patients with chronic obstructive pulmonary disease. *Am J Respir Crit Care Med* 1994; 149:1482.

174. Rossaint R, Falke KJ, Lopez F, et al.: Inhaled nitric oxide for the

adult respiratory distress syndrome. *N Engl J Med* 1993; 328:399.

175. Stamler JS: Redox signalling: Nitrosylation and related target interactions of nitric oxide. *Cell* 1994; 78:931.

176. Zapol WM, Rimar S, Gillis N, et al.: Nitric oxide and the lung. *Am J Respir Crit Care Med* 1994; 149:1375.

177. Rich S, Martinez, Lam W, et al.: Reassessment of the effects of vasodilator drugs in primary pulmonary hypertension: Guidelines for determining a pulmonary vasodilator response. *Am Heart J* 1985; 105:119.

178. Rubin LJ, Groves BM, Reeves JT, et al.: Prostacyclin-induced pulmonary vasodilation in primary pulmonary hypertension. *Circulation* 1982; 66(2):334.

179. Long W, Rubin LJ: Prostacyclin and prostaglandin E$_1$ treatment of pulmonary hypertension. *Am Rev Respir Dis* 1987; 136:773.

180. Sitbon O, Brenot F, Denjean A, et al.: Inhaled nitric oxide as a screening vasodilator agent in primary pulmonary hypertension. *Am J Respir Crit Care Med* 1995; 151:384.

181. Eisenkraft JB: Effects of anaesthetics on the pulmonary circulation. *Br J Anaesthesiol* 1990; 65(1):63.

182. Bjertnaes LJ: Hypoxia-induced pulmonary vasoconstriction in man: Inhibition due to diethyl ether and halothane anesthesia. *Acta Anaesthesiol Scand* 1978; 2:570.

183. Naeije R, Lejeune P, Leeman M, et al.: Effects of propofol on pulmonary and systemic arterial pressure-flow relationships in hyperoxic and hypoxic dogs. *Br J Anaesthesiol* 1989; 62(5):532.

184. Rich S, Brundage BH: High-dose calcium channel-blocking therapy for primary pulmonary hypertension: Evidence for long-term reduction in pulmonary arterial pressure and regression of right ventricular hypertrophy. *Circulation* 1987; 76(1):135.

185. Rich S, Kaufmann E, Levy PS: The effect of high doses of calcium-channel blockers on survival in primary pulmonary hypertension. *N Engl J Med* 1992; 327(2):76.

186. McMahon TJ, Ignarro LJ, Kadowitz PJ: Influence of zaprinast on vascular tone and vasodilator responses in cat pulmonary vascular bed. *J Appl Physiol* 1993; 74(4):1704.

187. Allen DA, Schertel ER, Bailey JE: Reflex cardiovascular effects of continuous prostacyclin administration into an isolated *in situ* lung in the dog. *J Appl Physiol* 1993; 74(6):2928.

188. Bush A, Busst CM, Knight WB, Shinebourne EA: Interactions between alveolar hypercapnia and epoprostenol on the pulmonary circulation: Clinical and pharmacological implications. *Pulm Pharmacol* 1990; 3(4):167.

189. Radermacher P, Santak B, Wust HJ, et al.: Prostacyclin for the treatment of pulmonary hypertension in the adult respiratory distress syndrome: Effects on pulmonary capillary pressure and ventilation-perfusion distributions. *Anesthesiology* 1990; 72(2):238.

190. Ignarro LJ, Kadowitz PJ: The pharmacological and physiological role of cyclic GMP in vascular smooth muscle relaxation. *Annu Rev Pharmacol Toxicol* 1985; 25:171.

191. Smiseth OA, Manyari DE, Scott-Douglas NW, et al.: The effect of nitroglycerin on pulmonary vascular capacitance in dogs. *Am Heart J* 1991; 121(5):1454.

192. Glauser FL, Polatty RC, Sessler CN: Worsening oxygenation in the mechanically ventilated patient: Causes, mechanisms, and early detection. *Am Rev Respir Dis* 1988; 138:458.

193. Rich S, Martinez J, Lam K, Rosen K: Captopril as treatment for patients with pulmonary hypertension: Problem of variability in assessing chronic drug treatment. *Br Heart J* 1982; 48:272.

194. Pison CM, Wolf JE, Levy PA, et al.: Effects of captopril combined with oxygen therapy at rest and on exercise in patients with chronic bronchitis and pulmonary hypertension. *Respiration* 1991; 58(1):9.

195. Zielinski J, Hawrylkiewicz I, Gorecka D, et al.: Captopril effects on pulmonary and systemic hemodynamics in chronic cor pulmonale. *Chest* 1986; 90(4):562.

196. Alpert MA, Pressly TA, Mukerji V, et al.: Short- and long-term hemodynamic effects of captopril in patients with pulmonary hypertension and selected connective tissue disease. *Chest* 1992; 102(5):1407.

197. Gottschall EB, Fernyak S, Wuertemberger G, Voelkel NF: Almitrine mimics hypoxic vasoconstriction in isolated rat lungs. *Am J Physiol* 1992; 63(2 pt 2):H383.

198. Saadjian A, Philip-Joet F, Barret A, et al.: Nifedipine inhibits the effects of almitrine in patients suffering from pulmonary artery hypertension secondary to chronic obstructive pulmonary disease. *J Cardiovasc Pharmacol* 1993; 21(5):797.

199. Bohning W, Winkelmann B, Worth H, et al.: Long-term therapy with almitrine dimesilate has no effect on pulmonary hemodynamics at rest and during stress. *Pneumologie* (suppl) 1990; 1:444.

200. Leeman M, Lejeune P, Hallemans R, et al.: Effects of increased pulmonary vascular tone on gas exchange in canine oleic acid pulmonary edema. *J Appl Physiol* 1988; 65(2):662.

201. Light RB: Indomethacin and acetylsalicylic acid reduce intrapulmonary shunt in experimental pneumococcal pneumonia. *Am Rev Respir Dis* 1986; 134(3):520.

202. Leeman M, Delcroix M, Vachiery JL, et al.: Blunted hypoxic vasoconstriction in oleic acid lung injury: Effect of cyclooxygenase inhibitors. *J Appl Physiol* 1992; 72(1):251.

203. Morin FC, Egan EA, Norfleet WT: Indomethacin does not diminish the pulmonary vascular response of the fetus to increased oxygen tension. *Pediatr Res* 1988; 24(6):696.

204. Adnot S, Defouilloy C, Brun-Buisson C, et al.: Effects of indomethacin on pulmonary hemodynamics and gas exchange in patients with pulmonary artery hypertension; interference with hydralazine. *Am Rev Respir Dis* 1987; 136(6):1343.

205. Delcroix M, Melot C, Lejeune P, et al.: Cyclooxygenase inhibition aggravates pulmonary hypertension and deteriorates gas exchange in canine pulmonary embolism. *Am Rev Respir Dis* 1992; 145(4 pt 1):806.

206. Welte M, Zwissler B, Habazettl H, Messmer K: PGI$_2$ aerosol versus nitric oxide for selective pulmonary vasodilation in hypoxic pulmonary vasoconstriction. *Eur Surg Res* 1993; 25(5):329.

207. Hyman Al, Kadowitz PJ: Enhancement of alpha- and beta-adrenoceptor responses by elevations in vascular tone in pulmonary circulation. *Am J Physiol* 1986; 250(6 pt 2):H1109.

208. Shirai M, Shindo T, Ninomiya I: Beta-adrenergic mechanisms attenuated hypoxic pulmonary vasoconstriction during systemic hypoxia in cats. *Am J Physiol* 1994; 266(5 pt 2):H1777.

209. Rodriguez-Roisin R, Ballester E, Roca J, et al.: Mechanisms of hypoxemia in patients with status asthmaticus requiring mechanical ventilation. *Am Rev Respir Dis* 1989; 139:732.

210. Truog WE, Standaert TA: Effect of dopamine infusion on pulmonary gas exchange in lambs. *Biol Neonate* 1984; 46(5):220.

211. Matamis D, Lemaire F, Harf A, et al.: Redistribution of pulmonary blood flow induced by positive end-expiratory pressure and dopamine infusion in acute respiratory failure. *Am Rev Respir Dis* 1984; 129(1):39.

212. Ducas J, Stitz M, Gu S, et al.: Pulmonary vascular pressure-flow characteristics. Effects of dopamine before and after pulmonary embolism. *Am Rev Respir Dis* 1992; 146(2):307.

The role and importance of the bronchial circulation are incompletely defined.[1] Its blood flow consists of <1 percent of the cardiac output, and in most species no obvious derangement is noted when the bronchial circulation is completely obliterated. The bronchial circulation also is a source of hemoptysis and may contribute to the increased airway blood flow and microvascular hyperpermeability found in many diseases of the airways.[2] The bronchial circulation may be important in regulation of air-space fluid, nourishment of the ciliated columnar epithelium, and conditioning of the inspired air. Its presence may prevent pulmonary infarction, aid in lung repair following injuries or infection, and modulate airway smooth muscle tone by minimizing airway dehydration that would otherwise accompany respiratory water loss. In addition, there is increasing evidence that the bronchial circulation may be important in various disease states such as asthma. During bronchoconstriction, bronchial blood flow increases, and an increase in bronchial blood flow precedes the late asthmatic reaction in sheep.[3] Transport of mediators to and from the airway wall and the development of mucosal edema may also involve the bronchial circulation.

Anatomy

Although in the adult lung the bronchial circulation consists of only 1 to 2 percent of the cardiac output,[4] the bronchial blood flow is important to development of the lungs in the fetus and contributes to gas exchange in many types of congenital cardiac abnormalities. The existence of a systemic arterial supply to the lung was first noted by Galen.[2] Leonardo de Vinci described the function of the bronchial circulation as nutrient vessels of the lung.[5] In the early 1900s, detailed anatomic studies of the human bronchial circulation were performed utilizing injection and casting techniques,[6,7] and more recently angiography has been employed.[8]

The arterial origin of the bronchial arteries is variable both within and among species. Human bronchial arteries normally arise directly from the aorta or intercostobronchial trunk[9] and usually number from two to four.[6] Typically, one bronchial artery originates on the right from the third intercostal artery (directly from the aorta), and two bronchial arteries originate on the left (from the ventral aspect of the aorta at the level of the fifth and sixth vertebrae)[10] (Fig. 22-1). A common arterial pattern is for each lung to be supplied by two posterior bronchial arteries arising directly or indirectly from the aorta. This pattern occurs in 20 to 30 percent of the population.[9] The proximal extrapulmonary branches form an intercommunicating circular arc near the hilum surrounding the main stem bronchi from which the true intrapulmonary bronchial arteries radiate.

The intrapulmonary bronchial arteries extend along the bronchial tree within the peribronchial connective tissue. At least two divisions are present along each bronchus, one on either side of the bronchial wall. The divisions communicate extensively with the bronchial adventitia, sending branches through the bronchial wall and forming two vascular plexuses, one submucosal and the other peribronchial (Fig. 22-2). In some species (sheep[10] and dogs[11]), the submucosal plexus comprises a significant volume of the subepithelial tissue within the airways. The peribronchial plexus follows bronchial vessels, which penetrate the bronchial wall and terminate in an intercommunicating capillary network in the submucosa. The bronchial arteries extend peripherally as far as the terminal bronchioles and can be seen extending to the alveolar ducts and occasionally into the lung parenchyma around alveolar sacs. More proximally, the bronchial arteries may send branches to the tracheal wall; the middle third of the esophagus; the visceral pleura over mediastinal and

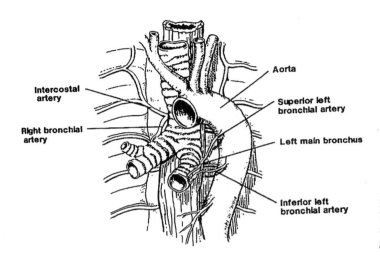

Aorta

Intercostal artery

Superior left bronchial artery

Right bronchial artery

Left main bronchus

Inferior left bronchial artery

FIGURE 22-1 Origins of the bronchial circulation. Usually one bronchial artery arises on the right and two on the left, each supplying their respective main bronchus. (*From Butler,*[1] *with permission.*)

diaphragmatic surfaces; the paratracheal, carinal, hilar, and intrapulmonary lymph nodes; and occasionally the parietal layer of the pericardium and thymus.[12,13] Moreover, the vasa vasorum of the aortic arch, pulmonary arteries, and pulmonary veins is supplied by branches of bronchial arteries.

The venous return of the bronchial circulation is less well characterized but is unique in that a dual venous drainage pattern exists. Bronchial arterial inflow is returned to the central circulation primarily through the pulmonary circulation. This arises from extensive anastomoses of the bronchial arterial circulation with pulmonary circulation at precapillary, capillary, and postcapillary sites and thus drains into the left atrium through the pulmonary veins. This circulation is referred to as the bronchopulmonary anastomotic flow[14] (Fig. 22-3). A lesser portion of bronchial flow drains through bronchial veins to the right heart through the azygos and hemiazygos systems. This flow contains predominately the

extrapulmonary intrathoracic venous drainage. Approximately 25 to 33 percent of the bronchial arterial supply returns to the right atrium by the bronchial veins, and 67 to 75 percent flows into the left atrium through pulmonary veins.[15]

Recently, large vascular sinuses have been identified in large airways.[16] These 50- to 400-μM, thin-walled, interconnecting vessels have an uncertain significance. They could serve as a vascular reservoir of fluid within the airways, and may be important in absorption of drugs from the airways. Controversy still exists concerning the presence and significance of bronchopulmonary arterial anastomoses, which are direct vascular connections between pulmonary and bronchial arteries.[17] Evidence indicates they occur sporadically and infrequently in normal lungs; however, they are more easily identified in the lungs of infants and may increase considerably in a number of pathologic conditions.

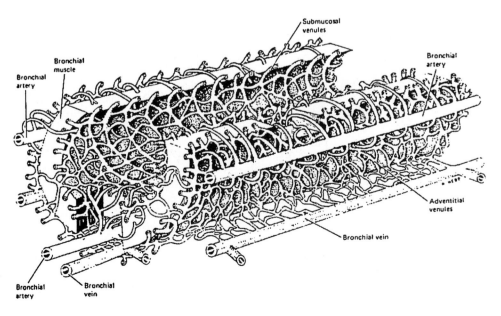

Submucosal venules

Bronchial muscle

Bronchial artery

Bronchial artery

Bronchial artery

Adventitial venules

Bronchial vein

Bronchial artery   **Bronchial vein**

FIGURE 22-2 The bronchial vascular plexus arises from the branches of the bronchial arteries that penetrate the bronchial wall. A dense capillary network intercommunicates within the submucosa. (*From Fishman,*[105] *with permission.*)

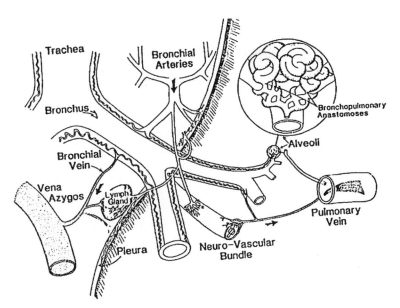

FIGURE 22-3 The dual venous return of the bronchial circulation. Bronchial venous return, the lesser system, returns blood to the right heart via the azygos and hemi-azygos systems. The greater system is the extensive bronchopulmonary anastomotic flow, which returns blood via the pulmonary veins. The bronchopulmonary anastomotic flow is thus influenced by the relative pulmonary venous, alveolar, and bronchial arterial pressures. (*From Deffebach et al.,*[99] *with permission.*)

Regulation of Bronchial Vascular Tone

MECHANICAL ASPECTS OF PHYSIOLOGIC REGULATION OF BRONCHIAL VASCULAR TONE

The bronchial blood flow is directly influenced by mechanical stresses produced by lung volume changes and indirectly through changes in the downstream pulmonary vascular pressures. Thus bronchial blood flow is dependent on the alveolar pressure, azygos vein pressure, and pulmonary vascular pressure. Substantial changes in bronchial vascular resistance can be imposed by the application of positive end-expiratory pressure (PEEP). Likewise, increased pulmonary capillary pressure can cause a significant decrease in bronchial perfusion and hence affect airway reactivity to exogenous substances (Fig. 22-4).

Several investigations have shown that increases in lung volume and airway pressure with the application of PEEP cause significant increases in bronchial vascular resistance. Lung inflation decreases bronchial blood flow in dogs,[18] sheep,[19] and humans.[20] At greater lung volumes, the relative proportion of bronchial arterial flow that is drained by systemic veins is increased.[21] Baile et al.[21] demonstrated that these increases in bronchial vascular resistance were most apparent in lung parenchyma and bronchi and less significant in larger airways outside the lung. Cassidy and Haynes[19] showed that the decrease in bronchial blood flow with the application of PEEP was much greater than what might be expected if the pressure gradient for flow were simply decreased by the increase in alveolar pressure. They suggested some neural reflex or mediator-induced response to explain the large increase in bronchial vascular resistance with PEEP. To test whether active vascular constriction were involved during PEEP, Wagner and Mitzner[22] measured bronchial perfusion pressure at constant controlled flow before and after the smooth muscle relaxant papaverine was infused. They concluded that elevation of left atrial pressure with PEEP causes an increase in active bronchial smooth muscle tone and that increase in airway pressure caused by PEEP produces increased bronchial vascular resistance. Thus, substantial changes in bronchial vascular resistance can be imposed by the application of PEEP. Likewise, pathologic increases in pulmonary capillary perfusion pressure may cause decreases in bronchial vascular perfusion.

NEURAL REGULATION OF BRONCHIAL VASCULAR TONE

PARASYMPATHETIC NERVE STIMULATION

The role of the parasympathetic nervous system in the control of the bronchial circulation is unclear. The bronchial circulatory system of many species is innervated by cholinergic neurons.[23,24] Cholinergic nerves are seen in close association with the blood vessel walls.[25] Vagal nerve transection may cause decreased[23] bronchial blood flow.[26] One difficulty in this interpretation is changes in systemic blood pressure that follow transection of cervical vagi[27] (resulting in increased tracheal vascular resistance) or the superior laryngeal nerves[28] (resulting in decreased tracheal vascular resistance). In addition, these nerves may contain sympathetic motor fibers.

In other experiments, stimulation of the distal end of transected vagi increased bronchial blood flow in dogs.[29] In this species, vasodilation of the tracheal vascular system following superior laryngeal nerve stimulation was decreased by atropine,[30] suggesting, at least in part, a cholinergic vasodilatory influence. Thus, nerve transection and stimulation suggest that parasympathetic motor nerves elicit airway vasodilation by cholinergic mechanisms. As this vasodilation following parasympathetic nerve stimulation is only halved by atropine and incompletely attenuated by the ganglionic blocker hexamethonium, the residual vasodilator response may be due to antidromic stimulation of sensory nerves[28] (see below).

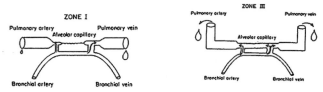

FIGURE 22-4 *A.* In zone 1 lung conditions, bronchopulmonary anastomoses favor bronchial flow (approximately 80 percent) to the pulmonary venous side. *B.* In zone 3 lung conditions, alveolar capillaries are patent; retrograde flow of bronchial arterial inflow into the upstream arm (pulmonary arterial side) of the alveolar capillary bed exists, and anastomotic blood flow both flow into the pulmonary vein. (*From Butler et al.,*[106] *with permission.*)

CHOLINERGIC AGONISTS

In isolated bovine bronchial arteries, cholinergic agonists cause contractions that are inhibited by atropine.[31,32] Moreover, nicotine causes contractions that are inhibited by both atropine and hexamethonium, suggesting that the contractile effect is caused by endogenous acetylcholine released from postganglionic nerves in the blood vessel wall.[32] The subtype of muscarinic receptor mediating contraction of bovine bronchial artery is not known.[33] In contrast to bovine bronchial arteries, isolated canine bronchial arteries do not contract in response to acetylcholine. Muscarinic contraction of bronchial arterial smooth muscle is species-specific. As vagal stimulation causes arterial dilation in the intact canine bronchial circulation (see above), isolated canine bronchial arteries do not contract in response to acetylcholine. However, in isolated rings of canine bronchial artery, acetylcholine causes concentration-dependent relaxation in preconstricted rings only in those preparations that have an intact endothelium. These results (combined with prejunctional inhibition of norepinephrine release) could partially explain the increase in bronchial arterial flow caused by intraarterial infusion of acetylcholine.[34] In the canine bronchial artery, atropine is a potent, competitive inhibitor of endothelium-dependent relaxation, indicating that the response is coupled to activation of muscarinic receptors.[28] As pirenzepine (M_1-muscarinic subtype antagonist) does not alter the concentration-response curve to acetylcholine in canine bronchial arteries, it can be concluded that acetylcholine does not act on M_1-muscarinic receptors.[33] However, the selective, M_3-muscarinic antagonist 4-DAMP is a potent inhibitor of acetylcholine-elicited endothelial-dependent relaxation. These results suggest that the bronchial circulation is similar to the canine coronary circulation[35] in which M_3-muscarinic receptors on endothelial cells mediate vascular relaxation. The subtype of muscarinic receptor mediating this vasodilation in the bovine bronchial artery has not been reported.

NONADRENERGIC, NONCHOLINERGIC NERVE STIMULATION

Sensory neuropeptides may be important in the noncholinergic component of parasympathetic vasodilation of the bronchial circulation.[36] In isolated canine bronchial artery, calcitonin gene-related peptide is a potent relaxant. Substance P has a bimodal effect; at low concentrations, it causes vasodilation of preconstricted arteries, and in high concentrations, it contracts vessels above resting tone.[37] This bimodal effect is probably due to release of an endothelial-derived vasodilator at low concentrations, which competes with a less sensitive direct effect, causing constriction of the bronchial artery smooth muscle at higher concentrations. Neurokinins A and B cause only relaxation. The importance of parasympathetic modulation of the bronchial circulation may differ depending on the location of the bronchial circulation. In contrast to the upper trachea, where the parasympathetic vasodilatory components of both the cholinergic and noncholinergic mechanisms predominate, the vagal blood flow regulation in the peripheral airways is determined entirely by the local release of the aforementioned neuropeptides from capsaicin-sensitive nerves.[38] As such, inhalation of sensory nerve irritants, such as cigarette smoke, may cause a marked increase in bronchial blood flow through the release of these local mediators. Until specific antagonist are developed, however, any specific role of particular peptide mediators in health and disease remains speculative.

SYMPATHETIC NERVE STIMULATION

The tracheobronchial circulation has a predominately greater input from the sympathetic nervous system relative to the parasympathetic system, which produces a significant vasoconstriction.[34] This is in distinct contrast to the bronchial airway smooth muscle, where sympathetic innervation is relatively sparse.[39] Vasoconstriction has been shown to occur in the dog following stimulation of sympathetic nerves, which results in an increase in perfusion pressure during constant flow.[40] The predominant mechanism for this vasoconstriction is stimulation of α-adrenergic receptors. In isolated rings of canine bronchial artery, transmural nerve stimulation causes contraction, which is abolished by tetrodotoxin, phenoxybenzamine, or phentolamine, suggesting that the contraction is mediated by the release of norepinephrine from adrenergic nerve endings in the vessel wall.[33]

EXOGENOUS ADRENERGIC AGONISTS

Infusion of epinephrine, norepinephrine, or phenylephrine in dogs[41,42] or sheep[43,44] significantly decreases bronchial blood flow. In the dog, this effect is blocked by phentolamine, suggesting mediation by α receptors.[45] In isolated rings of canine bronchial artery, norepinephrine produces concentration-dependent increases in tension, which are inhibited by the selective α_1-adrenergic antagonist prazosin.[46] β-adrenergic receptors also are found on bronchial arteries.[44,45] As in the pulmonary circulation, exogenously applied β-adrenergic agonist causes a significant vasodilation, which is blocked by propranolol. This effect is probably mediated by β_2-subtype adrenoreceptors.[47,48] In the horse, during and immediately following exercise, the bronchial artery flow is increased. Similarly, exogenously administered do-butamine causes β_2-adrenergically mediated bronchial arterial dilation response.

NONNEURAL FACTORS REGULATING BRONCHIAL VASCULAR TONE

HISTAMINE
Histamine increases bronchial artery blood flow in dogs[41] and sheep[49] and may contribute to the pathogenesis of antigen-induced bronchial obstruction by promoting mucosal edema or the clearance of inflammatory mediators. Aerosolized administration of histamine causes a vasodilation in the bronchial vascular bed of sheep that is mediated by H_2 receptors.[49] In the isolated human bronchial artery, histamine evokes a concentration-dependent effect, causing relaxation at lower concentrations and contraction at higher concentrations. In both cases H_1 receptors are the subtype involved.[50] This H_1-receptor-mediated relaxation is abolished by removal of the endothelium of the bronchial artery and is probably caused by endothelial release of nitric oxide. The vasodilator effect of histamine at lesser concentrations may contribute to the inflammatory response in the airway wall in asthma by increasing blood flow to hyperpermeable postcapillary venules.

SEROTONIN
Serotonin (5-hydroxytryptamine, 5HT) is formed by the decarboxylation of tryptophan, which is stored in neurosecretory granules. Exogenously applied 5HT has a potent bronchoconstricting effect and causes vasoconstriction of the pulmonary circulation.[51] These effects are mediated by $5HT_1$ receptors (inhibitory),[52] $5HT_2$ receptors (excitatory),[53] and $5HT_3$ receptors[54] present on neurons, leading to neurotransmitter release. Isolated perfused canine[23] or sheep[52] bronchial arteries respond variably to injections of 5HT, with increased bronchial blood flow in some cases and vasodilation in others. This vasoconstriction is blocked by ketanserin ($5HT_2$-receptor antagonist) and by methysergide (combined $5HT_1$- and $5HT_2$-receptor antagonist), indicating a $5HT_1$-mediated vasodilation.[52]

BRADYKININ
Bradykinin, generated by the action of kininogenase from kininogens, is a potent vasodilator of the dog tracheal circulation when perfused at constant flow[47] and of the pig[55] when measured by a transonic flow probe. In the sheep, both bradykinin and lys-bradykinin cause long-lasting increases in tracheal blood flow.[56] This effect is not blocked by indomethacin but is prevented by prior perfusion with hemoglobin-containing solutions, suggesting that the effect is caused by the endothelial release of nitric oxide.

CYCLOOXYGENASE AND LIPOXYGENASE PRODUCTS
Arachidonic acid (AA) is the precursor for prostaglandins, thromboxanes, leukotrienes, and several hydroxyacids. The synthesis of arachidonic acid from membrane phospholipids by the action of phospholipase A_2 is the rate-limiting step. Arachidonic acid then is oxidized to form prostaglandins, thromboxane A_2, and prostacyclin. Lipoxygenation of AA initiates the formation of leukotrienes and hydroeicosatetraenoic acids (HPETE). 5-Lipoxygenase then converts HPETE to various leukotrienes. PGE_1, PGF_{2a}, and PGD_2 are all po-tent vasodilators of the canine tracheal circulation.[47] (See Chap. 13.) PGI_2 increases bronchial blood flow in dogs when given as an infusion.[57] Leukotrienes C_4 and D_4 decrease bronchial blood flow in the sheep,[55] while vasodilator prostanoids contribute to the increase in bronchial blood flow that accompanies allergen-mediated bronchoconstriction.[3] Leukotrienes cause microvascular hyperpermeability.[59]

THE INFLUENCE OF HYPOXIA ON THE BRONCHIAL CIRCULATION
The bronchial vasculature vasodilates in response to a systemic hypoxic challenge. The direct effect of decreased PO_2 on the bronchial vascular smooth muscle, a release of a dilator substance, or neural activation due to hypoxic exposure are all probable causes of this vasodilation.[60] Cyclooxygenase blockade prevents the dilation of bronchopulmonary anastomoses during hypoxia,[61] and selective carotid body stimulation with hypoxic blood can cause increases in bronchial blood flow.[62] Wagner and Mitzner.[60] found that although brief episodes of hypoxia in the sheep lead to bronchial vasodilation during severe, prolonged hypoxia (Pa_{O_2} = 45 mmHg for 30 min), bronchovascular resistance returns to baseline and exceeds control levels. They also found that the major site of resistance of the bronchial circulation during prolonged hypoxia is in the small arteries and arterioles and in vessels connecting the peribronchial plexus with the submucosal plexus and that this resistance was not due to prostaglandins. However, Charan et al.[61] found that systemic hypoxemia (and systemic hypercarbia) increase bronchopulmonary anastomotic blood flow. They also concluded that cyclooxygenase products mediate this response. However, cyclooxygenase inhibitors also significantly decreased bronchopulmonary anastomotic flow during normoxia. Thus AA metabolites may modulate the normoxic bronchial circulation and influence subsequent responses to hypoxemia and hypercarbia. The significance of the hypoxia-mediated increase in bronchopulmonary anastomotic flow is suggested by its potential to minimize ischemic lung damage during obliteration of the pulmonary circulation caused by pulmonary emboli. Experimental studies indicate that bronchial flow increases markedly over the few days after pulmonary arterial obstruction[63] due to a subsequent hypertrophy of the bronchial vascular bed.[64]

BRONCHIAL CIRCULATION IN DISEASE

ASTHMA
In models of airway inflammation, three major vascular manifestations occur: hyperemia, endothelial hyperpermeability, and tissue edema.[65] These mechanisms include the actions of leukocytes and inflammatory mediators on vas-

cular endothelial cells and vascular myoctyes. The major functional consequences are increased blood flow and microvascular hyperpermeability. The increased blood flow is thought to result from vasodilation of small bronchial arteries. Bradykinin can increase vascular permeability.[66] Likewise, histamine, sensory autonomic nerve stimulation, and neuropeptides can cause intercellular gaps in postcapillary venules.[67]

In an allergic model of asthma in sheep, inhalation challenge with specific antigen caused an increase in total bronchial arterial flow, which corresponded to an immediate increase in airway resistance.[65] Pharmacologic studies have shown that this increase in blood flow is independent of the increase in airway resistance.[65] Similarly, intravenous administration of ovalbumin has been shown to increase the extravasation of Evans blue dye in the conducting airways of sensitized guinea pigs.[68] Histamine, through both H_1 and H_2 receptors,[69] bradykinin,[70] sulfidopeptide leukotrienes,[71] prostaglandins E_1 and F_{2a},[72] PAF,[47] and oxygen radicals[73] all have been implicated in the bronchial vasodilation and hyperpermeability. The direct role of the cholinergic and adrenergic nervous system is less clear than the role of sensory neuropeptides in mediating the bronchial vascular response in models of asthma.[74]

In 1983, McFadden[75] reported blanching of the tracheobronchial mucosa when normal subjects hyperventilated frigid air, suggesting that human bronchial vessels may constrict when subjected to tissue cooling. This may serve further to decrease airway temperature while improving water conservation. Decreasing bronchial blood flow promotes bronchoconstriction in sheep[76] during cold/dry-gas hyperpnea and prolongs the recovery from histamine-induced peripheral bronchoconstriction in dog lungs.[77] In human asthmatic subjects intraairway temperature increases more rapidly following cessation of exercise than in subjects without asthma.[78] This suggests that restoration of bronchial blood flow (and consequent tissue rewarming) occurs more quickly in asthmatic subjects and may be responsible for bronchoconstriction. The mechanism by which airway cooling or drying leads to bronchovascular vasodilation remains unknown. Bilateral vagotomy has no effect on this response, nor do adrenergic neural inputs.[79] Topical lidocaine anesthesia applied to the tracheal mucosa attenuates local increases in blood flow—an effect that probably is caused by suppression of a sensory neuronal axon reflex that leads to neuropeptide release.[80] Neuropeptides induce bronchial vascular dilation, and lidocaine inhibits neuropeptide release. Ray and associates have demonstrated that tachykinin release from airway sensory nerves mediates this response. Thus, it is plausible that mucosal heat and/or water loss causes neuropeptide release, which then modulates mucosal blood flow. Mucosal water loss also may lead to inflammatory mediator secretion from mast cells.[82] Finally, Ingenito and coworkers.[83] found increase in eicosanoid mediator in bronchoalveolar lavage fluid at the peak of hyperpnea-induced bronchoconstriction in guinea pigs.

CHRONIC OBSTRUCTIVE AND INFECTIOUS LUNG DISEASE

Morphologic data have been reported on the bronchial circulation in chronic airway diseases, including bronchiectasis[84] and chronic lung abscess,[85] which affect blood flow to a greater degree than chronic bronchitis[86] and emphysema.[87] Sufficient data are available to suggest that the bronchial vasculature proliferates and hypertrophies in such diseases as bronchiectasis, cystic fibrosis, lung abscess, tuberculosis, and empyema. In most of these cases except lung abscess, the bronchial blood flow also increases. In chronic bronchitis and emphysema, autopsy studies indicate hypertrophy of the bronchial arterial system and prominent anastomoses with the pulmonary circulation.[88] However, in regions where destruction and dilation of lung acini occur, narrowed and obliterated branches of intrapulmonary bronchial arteries are observed.[89] It is possible that the vascular lesions in emphysema precede the pathologic changes in the air-conducting tissues; injection of sclerosing substances in the bronchial arteries causes emphysematous changes in the horse.[90] However, similar studies in sheep do not produce this effect.[91]

The mediators involved in morphologic change of the bronchial circulation in chronic obstructive lung disease are not known. It is possible that the edema, hyperperfusion, and release of mediators from the vascular endothelium may all contribute to the physiologic reduction in airway lumenal diameter. For example, increased blood flow and edema formation could obstruct peripheral bronchi by increasing the thickness of the airway wall. Despite a role in contributing to airflow obstruction, it is possible that the bronchial circulation is important for host defense mechanisms in certain lung infections, especially in poorly ventilated areas of the lung where the native pulmonary circulation is reduced. For therapy of obstructive lung diseases, the increased bronchial blood flow could be of advantage by enhancing the delivery of systemic drugs to the diseased airways or of disadvantage by promoting the clearance of inhaled drugs from the airways.

PHARMACOLOGIC MANAGEMENT OF BRONCHIAL BLEEDING

Before the advent of angiography, it was believed that the pulmonary arteries were the principal source of pulmonary hemorrhage except in alveolar hemorrhage syndromes. It now is known that the pulmonary, bronchial, and non-bronchial systemic arteries communicating through trans-pleural collaterals each may be involved in complex arrangements in congenital, inflammatory, and neoplastic lung processes.[92] However, the source of bleeding is the bronchial arteries in 90 percent of these cases.[93] Cessation of bleeding with bronchial artery embolization does not necessarily prove that the bronchial vessel was the culprit, as the bleeding may have derived from a pulmonary artery with which the bronchial vessel had anastomosed. Tuberculosis, bronchiectasis, fungal cavities, and cystic fibrosis are the clinical conditions most often associated with bronchial bleeding. In tuberculosis, the majority of bleeding occurs in cavitary disease.[94] The source of bleeding may be bronchial hypervascularization, erosion of vessels by cavities or lymph nodes, or related to bronchiectasis. In classical cylindrical bronchiectasis, the bronchial hypervascularization is characterized by large, sinuous arteries with spindle-shaped and saccular microaneurysms.[95] The bronchopulmonary anastomoses are numerous, sometimes affecting distal pulmonary arteries. Aneurysms in the proximal bronchial arteries may rupture into a bronchus or other intrathoracic structures. Intracavitary aspergilloma is a relatively frequent cause of bronchial bleeding.[96] Definitive treatment is surgery; however, the morbidity is high. The related occurrence of cavitation, bleeding, and recovery of granulocytes in patients with chemotherapy-related fungal cavitary pneumonia suggests that a proteolytic enzyme from the leukocytes may contribute to bronchial vessel wall destruction. In lung abscess cavities, the mechanism of bleeding is either erosion through the wall of a large bronchial artery in the abscess cavity or capillaries in the granulation tissue of the wall, which is supplied by highly developed bronchial arteries.[85]

The indication for vasoocclusion or embolization is severe bronchial bleeding that resists medical treatment in a patient who cannot be managed surgically.[97] The location of the bronchial arterial ostia first is identified by dye injection in the aorta above the takeoff of the bronchial arteries. The choice of embolic material includes Gelfoam, which is easy to use, low in cost, and biodegradable.[98] However, the frequency of recanalization after Gelfoam has led to the use of nonresorbable material such as isobutyl-2-cyanoacrylate. Polyvinyl alcohol and lyophilized dura mater are also used in bronchial arteries. Systemic administration of indomethacin, which may inhibit the production of relevant vasodilating prostaglandins, has been tried, but its effect on platelet aggregation and prolongation of bleeding time discourage its use.[99] As Adamkiewicz's artery, which supplies the anterior spinal artery, arises from intercostal arteries, a risk of vascular spinal cord injury may occur during bronchial arteriography.[100]

LUNG TRANSPLANTATION

In the 20 years following Hardy's[101] initial attempt, it has become clear that airway ischemia was one of the major problems associated with clinical lung transplantation. The lung is the only solid organ transplanted without the routine reestablishment of its systemic arterial circulation. However, early on, Derom[102] noted a 61 percent complication rate of bronchial necrosis and stenosis in 82 canine left lung autotransplantations. To improve blood supply to the anastomotic airway, Cooper[103] perfected the technique of bronchial omentopexy during lung reimplantation. Injection studies documented the revascularization of the bronchial mucosa within 5 days. Additional studies, in totally ischemic bronchial allografts, confirmed the ability of the omentum to revascularize an ischemic bronchus.[104] The consequence of bronchial wall ischemia, including stenosis to the anasto-

mosis and dehiscence, was subsequently reduced to approximately 14 percent. More recently the bronchial anastomosis is made using a telescoping technique, which permits healing without the need for omentopexy.[105]

References

1. Butler J: *The Bronchial Circulation.* New York, Marcel Dekker, 1992.
2. Fick RB Jr, Metzger WJ, Richerson HB, et al.: Increased bronchovascular permeability after allergen exposure in sensitive asthmatics. *J Appl Physiol* 1987; 63:1147.
3. Long WM, Yerger LD, Martinez H, et al.: Modification of bronchial blood flow during allergic airway responses. *J Appl Physiol* 1988; 65:272.
4. Wu CH, Lindsey DC, Traber DL, et al.: Measurement of bronchial blood flow with radioactive microspheres in awake sheep. *J Appl Physiol* 1989; 65:1131.
5. Cudkowicz L: Leonardo da Vinci and the bronchial circulation. *Br J Tuberc* 1953; 47:23.
6. Cauldwell EW, Siekert RG, Linenger RE, et al.: The bronchial arteries: An anatomic study of 150 cadavers. *Surg Gynecol Obstet* 1948; 86:395.
7. Tobin CE: The bronchial arteries and their connection with other vessels in the human lung. *Surg Gynecol Obstet* 1952; 95:741.
8. Newton TH, Preger L: Selective bronchial arteriography. *Radiology* 1965; 84:1043.
9. Liebow AA: Patterns of origin and distribution of the major bronchial arteries in man. *Am J Anat* 1965; 117:19.
10. Marchand P, Gilroy JC, Wilson VH: An anatomical study of the bronchial vascular system and its variations in disease. *Thorax* 1950; 5:207.
11. Laitinen A, Laitinen LA, Moss R, Widdicombe JG: Organization and structure of the tracheal and bronchial blood vessels in the dog. *J Anat* 1989; 166:133.
12. Charan NB, Turk GM, Czartolomny J, Andreazuk T: Systemic arterial blood supply to the trachea and lung in sheep. *J Appl Physiol* 1987; 62:2283.
13. Viamonte M Jr, Viamonte M, Camacho M, Liebow AA: Corrosion cast studies of the bronchial arteries. *Surg Radiol Anat* 1989; 11:215.
14. Murata K, Itoh H, Todo G, et al.: Bronchial venous plexus and its communication with the pulmonary circulation. *Invest Radiol* 1986; 21:25.
15. Malik AB: Pulmonary microembolism. *Physiol Rev* 1983; 63:1114.
16. Hill P, Goulding D, Webber SE, Widdicombe JG: Blood sinuses in the submucosa of the large airways of the sheep. *J Anat* 1989; 162:235.
17. Wagenoort CA, Wagenwoort N: Arterial anastomoses, bronchopulmonary arteries and pulmobronchial arteries in perinatal lungs. *Lab Invest* 1967; 16:13.
18. Auld PAM, Rudolph AM, Golinko RJ: Factors affecting bronchial collateral flow in the dog. *Am J Physiol* 1960; 198:1166.
19. Cassidy SS, Haynes MS: The effects of ventilation with positive end-expiratory pressure on the bronchial circulation. *Respir Physiol* 1986; 66:269.
20. Agostoni P, Arena V, Biglioli P, et al.: Increase in alveolar pressure reduces systemic-to-pulmonary bronchial blood flow in humans. *Chest* 1989; 69:1081.
21. Baile EM, Albert RK, Kirk W, et al.: Positive end-expiratory

pressure decreases bronchial blood flow in the dog. *J Appl Physiol* 1984; 56:1289.

22. Wagner EM, Mitzner WA: Effect of left atrial pressure on bronchial vascular hemodynamics. *J Appl Physiol* 190; 69:837.

23. Horisberger G, Rodbard S: Direct measurement of bronchial artery flow. *Circ Res* 1960; 8:1149.

24. Partanen M, Laitinen A, Hervonen A, et al.: Catecholamine- and acetylcholinesterase-containing nerves in human lower respiratory tract. *Histochemistry* 1982; 76:175.

25. Barnes PJ: Muscarinic receptors in the lung. *Postgrad Med J* 1987; 63:13.

26. Jindal SK, Kakshminarayanan S, Kirk W, Butler J: Effect of cervical vagotomy on anatomotic bronchial blood flow after pulmonary artery obstruction in dogs. *Indian J Med Res* 1985; 91:83.

27. Salonen RO, Webber SE, Widdicombe JG: Effects of neuropeptides and capsaicin on the canine tracheal vasculature in vivo. *Br J Pharmacol* 1988; 95:1262.

28. Laitinen LA, Laitinen MVA, Widdicombe JG: Parasympathetic nervous control of tracheal vascular resistance in the dog. *J Physiol* 1987; 385:135.

29. Murano H: Nervous regulation of the bronchial vascular system. *Jpn Circ J* 1965; 29:855.

30. Martran R, Alving K, Martling CR, et al.: Vagally mediated vasodilation by motor and sensory nerves in the tracheal and bronchial circulation of the pig. *Acta Physiol Scand* 1989; 135:29–35.

31. Arowolo ROA, Eyre P: Preliminary pharmacological characterization of the bovine isolated bronchial artery strip: A new preparation. *Br J Pharmacol* 1980; 68:283.

32. Tracy WR, Alexander DI, Eyre P, Singh A: Cholinergic properties of the bronchial artery and contribution of the endothelium. *Artery* 1983; 12:244.

33. O'Rourke ST, Vanhoutte PM: Adrenergic and cholinergic regulation of bronchial vascular tone. *Am Rev Respir Dis* 1992; 146:S11.

34. De Letona JML, De La Mata RC, Aviado DM: Local and reflex effects of bronchial artery injection of drugs. *J Pharmacol Exp Ther* 1961; 133:295.

35. O'Rourke ST: Cholinergic stimulus-response coupling in coronary artery endothelium. *Circulation* 1989; 80:278.

36. Matran R: Neural control of lower airway vasculature: Involvement of classical transmitters and neuropeptides. *Acta Physiol Scand* 1991; 601:1.

37. McCormack DG, Salonen RO, Barnes PJ: Effect of sensory neuropeptides on canine bronchial and pulmonary vessels in vitro. *Life Sci* 1990; 45:2405.

38. Persson CGA, Erjefalt I: Non-neural and neural regulation of plasma exudation in airways, in Kaliner MA, Barnes PJ (eds): *The Airways: Neural Control in Health and Disease*. New York: Marcel Dekker, 1988:523–550.

39. Pack RJ, Richardson PS: The aminergic innervation of the human bronchus: A light and electron microscope study. *J Anat* 1984; 138:493.

40. Sahin G, Webber SE, Widdicombe JG: Nervous control of tracheal vascular resistance. *Clin Respir Physiol* 1987; 23:384S.

41. Bruner HD, Schmidt CF: Blood flow in the bronchial artery of the anesthetized dog. *Am J Physiol* 1947; 148:647.

42. Lung MA, Wang JC, Cheng KK: Bronchial circulation: An autoperfusion method for assessing its vasomotor activity and the study of alpha adrenoceptors in the bronchial artery. *Life Sci* 1976; 19:577.

43. Charan NB, Turk GM, Ripley R: Measurement of bronchial blood flow and bronchovascular resistance in sheep. *J Appl Physiol* 1985; 59:305.

44. Parsons GH, Kramer GC, Link DP, et al.: Studies of reactivity and distribution of bronchial blood flow in sheep. *Chest* 1985; 87:180s.

45. Himori N, Taira N: A method for recording smooth muscle and vascular responses of the blood-perfused dog trachea in situ. *Br J Pharmacol* 1976; 56:293.

46. O'Rourke ST, Vanhoutte PM: Adrenergic and cholinergic responsiveness of isolated canine bronchial arteries. *Am J Physiol* 1990; 259:H156.

47. Laitinen LA, Laitinen MA, Widdicombe JG: Dose-related effects of pharmacological mediators on tracheal vascular resistance in dogs. *Br J Pharmacol* 1987; 92:703.

48. Webber SE, Salonen RO, Widdicombe JG: Effects of antigen on tracheal circulation and smooth muscle in sheep of different ages. *J Appl Physiol* 1989; 67:1256.

49. Long WM, Sprung CL, Fawal HE, et al.: Effects of histamine on bronchial artery blood flow and bronchomotor tone. *J Appl Physiol* 1985; 59:254.

50. Liu S, Yacoub M, Barnes PJ: Effect of histamine on human bronchial arteries in vitro. *Arch Pharmacol* 1990; 342:90.

51. Raffestin B, Cerina J, Boullet C, et al.: Response and sensitivity of isolated human pulmonary muscle preparations to pharmacological agents. *J Pharmacol Exp Ther* 1985; 264:186.

52. Weber SE, Salonen RO, Widicombe JG: Receptors mediating the effects of 5-hydroxytryptamine on the tracheal vasculature and smooth muscle of sheep. *Br J Pharmacol* 1990; 99:21.

53. Selig WM, Bloomquist MA, Cohen ML, Fleish JH: Serotonin-induced pulmonary responses—the perfused guinea-pig lung: Evidence for 5HT receptor-mediated pulmonary vascular and airway smooth muscle constriction. *Pulm Pharmacol* 1988; 1:93.

54. Richardson BP, Engle G: The pharmacology and function of $5HT_3$-receptors. *Trends Neurol Sci* 1986; 2:424.

55. Matran R, Alving K, Martling CR, et al.: Effects of neuropeptides and capsaicin on tracheobronchial blood flow in the pig. *Acta Physiol Scand* 1989; 135:335.

56. Corfield DR, Webber SE, Hanafi Z, Widdicombe JG: The actions of bradykinin and lys-bradykinin on tracheal blood flow and smooth muscle in anaesthetised sheep. *Pulm Pharmacol* 1991; 4:85.

57. Deffebach M, Agostoni P, Lakshminarayan S, Butler J: Prostacyclin increases bronchial blood flow in the dog. *Am Rev Respir Dis* 1986; 133:162.

58. Long WM, Yerger LD, Sprung CL, et al.: Differential effects of lipoxygenase and cyclooxygenase products on antigen-induced late phase increases on bronchomotor tone and bronchial artery blood flow. *Am Rev Respir Dis* 1986; 133:175.

59. Woodward DF, Weichman BM, Gill CA, Wasserman MA: The effect of synthetic leukotrienes on tracheal microvascular permeability. *Prostaglandins* 1983; 25:131.

60. Wagner EM, Mitzner WA: Effect of hypoxia on bronchial circulation. *J Appl Physiol* 1988; 65:1627.

61. Charan NB, Lakshminarayan S, Ibert RK, et al.: Hypoxia and hypercarbia increase bronchial blood flow through bronchopulmonary anastomoses in anesthetized dogs. *Am Rev Respir Dis* 1986; 134:89.

62. Alsberge M, Magno M, Lipschutz M: Carotid body control of bronchial circulation in sheep. *J Appl Physiol* 1988; 65:1152.

63. Mathes ME, Holman E, Reichert FL: A study of the bronchial, pulmonary and lymphatic circulations of the lung under various pathological conditions experimentally produced. *J Thorac Surg* 1932; 1:339.

64. Weibel ER: Early stages in the development of collateral circulation to the lung in the rat. *Circ Res* 1960; 8:353.

65. Dukanovic R, Roche W, Wilson J, et al.: Mucosal inflammation in asthma. *Am Rev Respir Dis* 1990; 142:434.

66. Weiner R, d'Altura BM: Serotonin-braykinin synergism in the mammalian capillary bed. *Proc Soc Exp Biol Med* 1967; 124:494.

67. Majno G, Shea SM, Levelthal M: Endothelial contraction induced by histamine-type mediators. *J Cell Biol* 1969; 42:647.

68. Evans TW, Rogers DF, Aursudkij B, et al.: Inflammatory mediators involved in antigen-induced airway microvascular leakage in guinea pigs. *Am Rev Respir Dis* 1988; 138:395.

69. Chediak AD, Waner A: Effects of histamine on tracheal mucosal perfusion, water content and airway smooth muscle in sheep. *Respir Physiol* 1991; 84:231.

70. Gabbiani G, Babonnel MC, Majno G: Intra-arterial injections of histamine, serotonin, or bradykinin: A topographic study of vascular leakage. *Proc Soc Exp Biol Med* 1970; 135:447.

71. Lee TH, Austen KF, Lieitch AG, et al.: The effects of fish-oil-enriched diet on pulmonary mechanics during anaphylaxis. *Am Rev Respir Dis* 1985; 132:1204.

72. Svensjo E: Bradykinin and prostaglandin E_1, E_2 and F_2-induced macromolecular leakage in the hamster cheek pouch. *Prostagland Med* 1987; 1:397.

73. Lewis RE, Granger HJ: Neutrophil-dependent mediation of microvascular permeability. *Fed Proc* 1986; 45:109.

74. Barker JA, Chediak AD, Baier HJ, Wanner A: Tracheal mucosal blood flow responses to autonomic agonist. *J Appl Physiol* 1988; 65:829.

75. McFadden ER: Respiratory heat and water exchange: Physiological and clinical implications. *J Appl Physiol* 1983; 54:331.

76. Wagner EM, Mitzner WA, Bleecker ER: Role of the bronchial circulation in cold air induced bronchospasm (abstr). *Am Rev Respir Dis* 1986; 133:A174.

77. Kelly L, Kolbe J, Mitzner W, Spannahake EW, et al.: Bronchial blood flow affects recovery from constriction in dog lung periphery. *J Appl Physiol* 1986; 60:1954.

78. Gilbert IA, Fouke JM, McFadden ER: Heat and water flux in the intratoracic airways and exercise-induced asthma. *J Appl Physiol* 1987; 63:1681.

79. Baile EM, Osborne S, Pare PD: Effect of autonomic blockade on tracheobronchial blood flow. *J Appl Physiol* 1986; 62:520.

80. Baile EM, Godden DJ, Pare DP: Mechanism for increase in tracheobronchial blood flow induced by hyperventilation of dry air in dogs. *J Appl Physiol* 1990; 68:105.

81. Ray DW, Hernandez C, Leff AR, et al.: Tachykinins mediated bronchoconstriction elicited by isocapnic hyperpnea in guinea pigs. *J Appl Physiol* 1989; 66:1108.

82. Eggleston PA, Kagey-Sobotka A, Lichtenstein LM: A comparison of the osmotic activation of basophils and human lung mast cells. *Am Rev Respir Dis* 1987; 135:1043.

83. Igenito EP, Bliss LB, Ingram RH, Pichurko BM: Bronchoalveolar lavage cell and mediator responses to hyperpnea-induced bronchoconstriction in the guinea pig. *Am Rev Respir Dis* 1990; 141:1162.

84. Liebow AA, Hales MR, Lindskog GE: Enlargement of the bronchial arteries and their anastomoses with the pulmonary arteries in bronchiectasis. *Am J Pathol* 1949; 25:211.

85. Charan NB, Turk GM, Dhand R: The role of bronchial circulation in lung abscess. *Am Rev Respir Dis* 1985; 131:121.

86. Nakamura T, Katori R, Miyasawa K, et al.: Bronchial blood flow in patients with chronic pulmonary disease and its influences upon respiration and circulation. *Dis Chest* 1961; 39:193.

87. Cudkowicz L, Armstrong JB: The bronchial arteries in pulmonary emphysema. *Thorax* 1953; 8:46.

88. Woods DA, Miller M: The role of the dual pulmonary circulation in various pathologic conditions of the lung. *J Thorac Surg* 1938; 7:649.

89. Cudkowicz L: Bronchial arterial circulation in men: Normal anatomy and responses to disease, in Moser K (ed): *Pulmonary Vascular Diseases*: vol 14. New York: Marcel Dekker, 1980:112–232.

90. McLaughlin RF, Edwards DW: Naturally occurring emphysema, the fine gross and histopathological counterpart of human emphysema. *Am Rev Respir Dis* 1966; 93:22.

91. Ricketts HJ, Carrington CB: Experimental bronchial artery occlusions in sheep, in Proceedings of the 11th Aspen Emphysema Conference. *Bethesda, U.S. DHEW*, 1968:187–189.

92. Conlan AA, Hurwitz SS, Kriege L, et al.: Massive hemoptysis: Review of 123 cases. *J Thorac Cardiovas Surg* 1983; 85:120.

93. Remy J, Remy-Jardin M, Voisin C: Endovascular management of bronchial bleeding, in Butler J (ed): *The Bronchial Circulation*. New York: Marcel Dekker, 1992:667–723.

94. Telku B, Felleke: Massive hemoptysis in tuberculosis. *Tubercle* 1982; 63:213.

95. Crockett FB, Vass CN: A comparison of the role of the bronchial arteries in bronchiectasis and in experimental ligation of the pulmonary artery. *Thorax* 1951; 6:268–275.

96. Albelda SM, Talbot GH, Gerson SL, et al.: Pulmonary cavitation and massive hemoptysis in invasive pulmonary aspergillosis. *Am Rev Respir Dis* 1985; 131:115.

97. Crocco JA, Rooney JJ, Fankushen DS, et al.: Massive hemoptysis. *Arch Intern Med* 1988; 121:495.

98. Stoll JF, Bettmann MA: Bronchial artery embolization to control hemoptysis: A review. *Cardiovasc Intervent Radiology* 1988; 11:263.

99. Deffebach ME, Charan NB, Lakshminarayan S, Butler J: The bronchial circulation: Small, but a vital attribute of the lung. *Am Rev Respir Dis* 1987; 135:463–481.

100. Miller FJ, Mineau DE: Transcatheter arterial embolization: Major complications and their prevention. *Cardiovas Intervent Radiol* 1983; 6:141–149.

101. Hardy JD, Webb WR, Dalton ML, Walker GR: Lung homotransplantation in man: Report of the initial case. *JAMA* 1963; 188:1065–1074.

102. Derom F, Barbier F, Ringoir S, et al.: Ten-month survival after lung homotransplantation in man. *J Thorac Cardiovasc Surg* 1971; 61:835.

103. Cooper JD and the Toronto Lung Transplant Group: Unilateral lung transplantation for pulmonary fibrosis. *N Eng J Med* 1986; 314:1140–1145.

104. Patterson GA, Todd TJ, Cooper JD, et al.: Airway complications following double lung transplantation. *J Thorac Cardiovasc Surg* 1990; 99:14–20.

105. Miller JD, DeHoyos.: An evaluation of the role otomentopexy and early perioperative corticosteroid administration in clinical lung transplantation. *J Thorac Cardiovasc Surg* 1993; 105:247–252.

Chapter 23 _____

DOPAMINE, DOBUTAMINE, AND DOPEXAMINE

PATRICK MURRAY

MARK E. WYLAM

Dopamine
    Development
    Receptor types
    Sites of action
    Clinical pharmacology

Dobutamine
    Cardiovascular and pulmonary vascular effects of DB
    Renal vascular effects of DB
    Metabolism and side effects of DB

Dopexamine

The primary role of the circulation is to provide energy sources to all systemic organs, and to remove waste products of metabolism. Diseases of the circulation may involve the central pump or influence the distribution of cardiac output producing intra- or interorgan maldistribution of blood flow. As complex interrelationships exist and control the cardiovascular system in health, the management of disease states requires a detailed understanding of pharmacologic compounds that have significant action on this system. This chapter reviews the pharmacology of two widely used catecholamines, dopamine and dobutamine, and introduces dopexamine, an agent that may combine the useful pharmacologic properties of this newly synthesized catecholamine (Fig. 23-1).

Dopamine

Dopamine (3,4-dihydroxyphenethylamine; DA) is an endogenous catecholamine synthesized from dihydroxyphenylalanine by the enzyme dopa decarboxylase. Noradrenergic nerves in the central and peripheral sympathetic nervous systems contain dopamine β-hydroxylase, which catalyzes the conversion of DA to norepinephrine (NE). In these neurons, DA is stored in neuronal vesicles, and may be co-released with NE. Dopamine also may be released singularly by dopaminergic neurons, which lack dopamine β-hydroxylase. In addition to functioning as a central and peripheral neurotransmitter, DA has direct effects on endocrine function and on renal tubular reabsorp-

tive processes. Dopamine, in a dose-dependent manner, may activate specific peripheral DA receptors (vascular and renal tubular), myocardial β_1-adrenergic receptors, and vascular α_1- and α_2-adrenergic receptors; thus, it has developed widespread use as therapy for systemic hypoperfusion states. A putative renoprotective effect underlies the commonly practiced routine use of DA for therapy of patients developing (or at risk of developing) acute renal failure.

DEVELOPMENT

Dopamine was synthesized in 1910 independently by Mannich and Jacobsohn[1] and Barger and Ewins.[2] Cardiovascular research over the next 30 years noted that DA was a less potent vasopressor than other adrenergic amines. In 1942, Holtz and Credner reported that DA decreased blood pressure at low doses in the guinea pig and rabbit; however, blood pressure increased at relatively higher doses.[3] This dose-dependent shift in the action of DA was subsequently demonstrated in the cat, dog, and unanesthetized human being. The vasodepressor effect was not effected by β-adrenergic antagonist, atropine, or antihistamines.[4] However, the pressor effect was consistently prevented by α-adrenergic antagonist. Goldberg and colleagues subsequently used other selective dopaminergic agonists and antagonists to demonstrate the existence of a specific peripheral vascular dopamine receptor. Vasodilation was seen with the administration of low-dose dopamine, which was masked by a vasoconstrictor effect caused by adrenergic receptor activation at greater doses.[5–7]

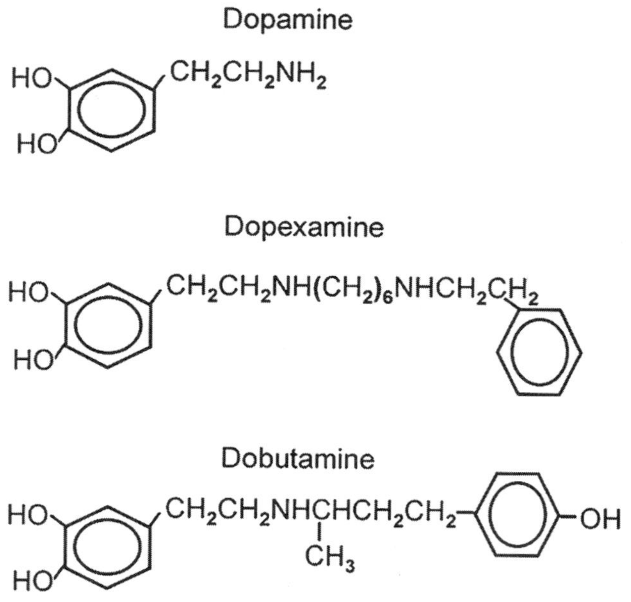

Dopamine

Dopexamine

Dobutamine

FIGURE 23-1 Chemical structures of endogenous and synthetic vasoactive catecholamines.

RECEPTOR TYPES

In 1979, Kebabian and Calne proposed a classification of dopamine receptor subtypes (D_1 and D_2) based on biochemical and pharmacologic criteria.[8] D_1-receptors, of which the bovine parathyroid DA receptor is the prototype, stimulate adenylyl cyclase (AC) and are located postsynaptically. D_2-receptors, typified by DA receptors on anterior pituitary mammotroph cells, do not stimulate AC, and are located pre- and postsynaptically. The classification of dopamine receptors in the CNS has since been expanded, through DA receptor homogenization and gene cloning with expression in cell lines, to include three D_1-type (D_{1A}, D_{1B}, D_5) and four D_2-type (D_{2short}, D_{2long}, D_3, D_4) dopamine receptors.[9]

Dopamine receptor structure and signal transduction processes have been partially elucidated. Dopamine receptors belong to a large family of cell-surface receptor proteins, which includes adrenergic and muscarinic acetylcholine receptors and a variety of peptide hormones. They contain seven transmembrane domains, and are coupled to G proteins.[9,10] The D_{1A}, D_{1B}, and D_5-receptors interact with a G protein (G_s) and stimulate AC. Adenylyl cyclase converts ATP into the second messenger cyclic AMP, which binds to and activates protein kinase A (PKA). D_2 receptor activation conversely inhibits adenylyl cyclase, through interaction with a (pertussis toxin–sensitive) G protein (G_i). The simplest model of signal transduction of DA effects at D_1- and D_2-receptors is through G protein–mediated regulation of cellular cyclic AMP concentrations, and the net effects of resultant phosphorylation by cyclic AMP–dependent protein kinase (PKA) and dephosphorylation by phosphoprotein phosphatases.[11,12] Based on this schema, a 32,000 dalton phosphoprotein called DARPP-32 has been proposed as an intracellular "third messenger" for dopamine.[13] Phosphory-

lation by PKA of DARPP-32 is stimulated in vitro by DA and cyclic AMP and can be blocked by DA antagonists. The phosphorylated form of DARPP-32 is a potent inhibitor of protein phosphatase-1, thus inhibiting dephosphorylation of other phosphoproteins and amplifying their physiological effects. Biochemical and immunohistochemical techniques show colocalization of DARPP-32 and D_1-receptor binding in brain regions. DARPP-32 also has been detected in ocular and adipose tissues, adrenal and parathyroid glands, and in the kidney of several species (mRNA in medullary thick ascending limb more than renal cortex, with none in renal vessels, glomeruli, or inner medulla). A recent study found that protein phosphatase activity in the renal proximal tubule was not inhibited by the D_1-agonist, fenoldopam, unlike previous findings in the medullary thick ascending limb and the brain striatum.[14]

Many alternative/complementary signal tranduction mechanisms have been demonstrated for both D_1-type and D_2-type receptors. D_1-receptors have been found to stimulate phospholipase C (PLC), thus increasing phosphatidyl inositol hydrolysis, diacylglycerol and inositol triphosphate generation, and, ultimately, protein kinase C (PKC) activation and intracellular calcium mobilization. These D_1-receptors may activate AC.[15] D_2-type receptors are universally coupled to pertussis toxin–insensitive G proteins and have been variously shown to activate K^+ channels, phospholipase A_2, and PLC, rather than inhibiting adenylyl cyclase.[9] In fact, though pharmacologically similar to the D_2-receptor, the recently cloned D_3- and D_4-receptors have undefined signal transduction pathways, which do not seem linked to AC.

In 1979, Goldberg and colleagues divided the peripheral (outside the CNS) dopamine receptors into two groups, DA_1- and DA_2-based on synaptic localization (corresponding to D_1- and D_2-classes) and physiological studies of the peripheral effects of dopamine and related agonists/antagonists.[16–18] DA_1-receptors are postsynaptic and have pharmacologic properties (AC linkage, greater affinity for D_1-agonists and antagonists) approximating D_{1A}, D_{1B}, and D_5-receptors. DA_2-receptors are presynaptic or postsynaptic in location and inhibit AC activity or phosphoinositide turnover; their overall pharmacologic properties approximating D_2-receptors.

Peripheral dopamine receptors are found in the cardiovascular system, adrenergic nerve endings, renal tubules, and certain endocrine organs. Radioligand binding and functional studies demonstrate that DA_1-receptors are found in greatest numbers in the renal and mesenteric vascular beds,[9,19,20] as well as in cerebral,[21,22] coronary, pulmonary,[23,24] skeletal muscle, and cutaneous vessels.[25] In vascular tissue, DA_1 stimulation activates AC, increasing cyclic AMP and (presumably via protein kinase A–mediated protein phosphorylation) causes vascular smooth muscle relaxation.[26] Protein kinase C activation recently was shown to augment DA_1-stimulated cyclic AMP generation in cultured vascular smooth muscle cells.[27] Alternatively, PLC stimulation mediates DA_1 effects,[28] which may be G protein–linked without AC or PLC involvement.[29]

Nonvascular DA_1-receptors along the nephron (see below) modulate tubular function and stimulate renin release, with segmental variation in linkages to AC–PKA, PLA_2, PLC, and

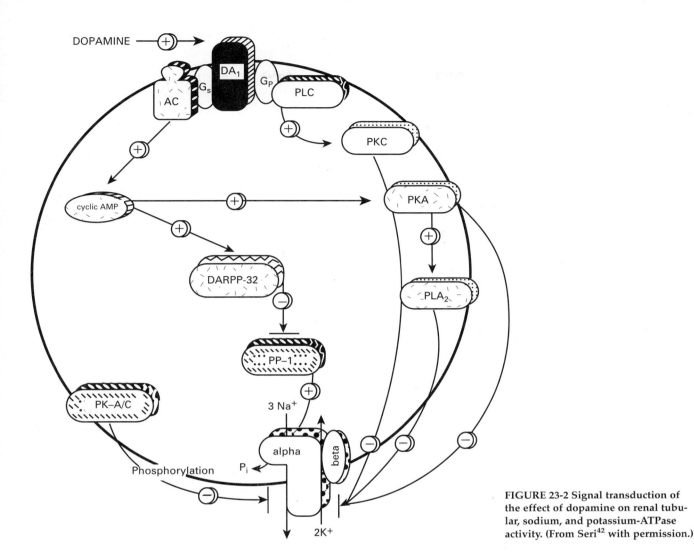

FIGURE 23-2 Signal transduction of the effect of dopamine on renal tubular, sodium, and potassium-ATPase activity. (From Seri[42] with permission.)

PKC (Fig. 23-2).[30,31] DA_2-receptor stimulation inhibits AC or phosphoinositide turnover. Presynaptic DA_2-receptors are particularly abundant in the renal and mesenteric vascular beds[32,33] where decreased AC activity inhibits NE release, causing vasodilation. Stimulation of vascular postsynaptic DA_2-receptors in the intimal layer of the renal, mesenteric, and cerebral vasculature also causes vasodilation.[22] D_2-like receptors recently localized in the rabbit pulmonary vascular tree are of undetermined functional significance.[34] In the kidney, nonvascular postsynaptic DA_2 receptors are found along the nephron and in the juxtaglomerular apparatus. DA_{2k} is a unique D_2-like receptor found in the inner medulla, where it increases prostaglandin E_2 production through phospholipase A_2 stimulation, without AC linkage.[35]

SITES OF ACTION

The effects of DA administration vary according to species, dose, and the basal hemodynamic and volume status of the experimental subjects.

SYSTEMIC HEMODYNAMIC EFFECTS

In anesthetized dogs,[4,36–38] intravenous DA administration at low doses (2 to 4 μg/kg per min) has little or no inotropic effect but produces a slight vasodepressor (hypotensive) effect. At intermediate doses (8 to 16 μg/kg per min), myocardial contractility, heart rate, and blood pressure increase. Further increase in the dose (32 to 64 μg/kg per min), leads to a marked increase in myocardial contractility, heart rate, and arterial pressure. Intravenous DA infusions administered to normal adult human subjects (from 2.6 to 11.6 μg/kg per min) produce increased cardiac output, decreased systemic vascular resistance, and little or no change in heart rate or mean arterial blood pressure.[36,39,40] Dopamine appears to act exclusively at DA-receptors at a dose of ≤ 1 μg/kg per min, with a predominant effect on DA-receptors in a dose range of 0.5 to 2.0 μg/kg per min, causing a reduction in systemic vascular resistance, a decrease in blood pressure, an increase in heart rate, and diuresis/natriuresis.[41] Increased renal, mesenteric, and coronary blood flow are accompanied by lesser cerebral and pulmonary arterial vasodilation.[36,42] With further increases (beginning at 2 to 4 μg/kg per min) β_1-adrenergic receptor stimulation increases cardiac output through both inotropic and chronotropic effects. Up to 50 percent of the positive inotropic effect of DA has been attributed to release (through a predominantly β_2-adrenergically mediated indirect effect) of stored NE from cardiac adrenergic nerve endings.[36,43] Beginning at 5μg/kg per min, α-adrenergic receptor activation causes vasoconstriction, so that at 10 μg/kg per min arterial blood pressure is increased. Venoconstriction caused by stimulation of serotonin and α-adrenoceptors reduces venous capacitance in animal and human subjects at DA infusion rates of only 2 to 6 μg/kg per min in human subjects.[36,42] Dopamine-elicited contraction in isolated gastroepiploic vein from human omentum was converted to a typical D_1-mediated relaxation by treatment with phentolamine.[44] By contrast, gastroepiploic arteries from the same subjects relaxed with dopamine, and monkey veins (mesenteric, renal, portal, vena cava) demonstrated a contraction, which phentolamine converted to relaxation only in the former two vessels. As noted above, the dose ranges within which these effects occur vary among individuals and according to the patient's age, hemodynamic status, and associated level of neurohumoral regulatory system activation.

RENAL EFFECTS

Physiologic Renal Actions of Dopamine

Renal proximal tubular cells contain aromatic L-amino acid decarboxylase (L-AAAD), which forms dopamine from circulating L-dopa.[45] Volume expansion increases local dopamine production by L-AAAD, and dopamine receptor antagonism impairs the natriuretic response to some forms of volume expansion.[46,47] These data suggest a physiologic role for dopamine as a natriuretic hormone.[48] Direct renal tubular effects of dopamine in vitro (see below) support this suggestion.

Localization of Renal Dopamine Receptors

Dopamine receptor subtypes have been localized to specific segments of the nephron and renal vasculature through the use of autoradiography, radioligand binding, and studies of adenylyl cyclase linkage.[9] Both DA_1- and DA_2-receptors are present throughout the renal arterial vasculature (predominantly DA_1), as well as in the brush-border and basolateral membranes of the proximal tubule. DA_1-receptors are scant in the glomeruli (where predominantly DA_2-receptors have been found), but are otherwise found in a nonhomogeneous pattern along the rest of the nephron, including the proximal tubule, juxtaglomerular cells, thick ascending limb, distal tubule, and cortical collecting duct.[49,50] As noted above, the DA_{2k}-receptor is found only in inner medullary collecting duct cells.

Renal Hemodynamic Effects

Administration of dopamine or selective DA_1- or DA_2-agonists causes renal vasodilation and increased renal blood flow (RBF; 20 percent to 40 percent) in dogs (1 to 10 μg/kg per min) and in normal human subjects (0 to 3 μg/kg per min), accompanied by a lesser (5 percent to 20 percent) increment in glomerular filtration rate (GFR).[36–40,42,43,45,51–53] Estimates of the relative magnitude of vasodilatory effects on the main renal, arcuate, and interlobular arteries, and on the afferent and efferent arterioles, vary among different experimental preparations.[54,55] In isolated glomerular preparations, dopamine vasodilates the afferent and efferent arterioles equally, so that glomerular hydrostatic pressure does not increase in proportion to increased blood flow, and the potential increment in GFR is dissipated accordingly. In experimental subjects, dopamine also directly stimulates renin production. The preferential efferent arteriolar vasoconstrictor effect of subsequently augmented angioten-sin II production tends to preserve increased glomerular hydrostatic pressure, thus increasing GFR. High-dose dopa-mine stimulates α adrenoceptors and decreases both RBF and GFR.

Renal Tubular Effects

Low doses of dopamine produce natriuresis and diuresis in animal and human subjects, even in the absence of increased GFR. Some of this effect is attributable to diminished urinary concentrating capacity following "urea washout" and dissipation of medullary hypertonicity due to increased medullary blood flow.l[42,56] Most is attributed to blockade of renal tubular sodium reabsorption, which is caused by the inhibitory effects of dopamine on the luminal Na/H exchanger in the proximal convoluted tubule (PCT) and on the basolateral Na-K-ATPase in the PCT, thick ascending loop of Henle, (Fig. 23-3) (TALH), distal tubule, and cortical collecting tubule.[12,57–59] Stimulation of the DA_{2k}-receptor increases prostaglandin E_2 production in the inner medullary collecting duct, thus inhibiting the effect of antidiuretic hormone (ADH) and Na-K-ATPase activity, which causes diuresis and natriuresis.[9,42] Dopamine also inhibits adrenocortical secretion of aldosterone and pituitary prolactin release; the former is a natriuretic effect, and the latter a natriuretic and diuretic effect (since prolactin modulates both aldosterone and ADH effects).[42,60] Conversely, high-dose dopamine stimulates tubular α-adrenergic receptors,[61] thus increasing tubular sodium and water reabsorption.

PULMONARY HEMODYNAMIC EFFECTS

The pulmonary vascular effects of DA administration vary according to species, age, and the presence or absence of preexisting pulmonary hypertension. The former two factors influence the relative activation of DA_1-versus α-adrenergic receptors at any given DA dose (as noted above, the functional significance of pulmonary vascular DA_2-receptors is unknown at this point). Dopamine has been variously noted to increase pulmonary vascular resistance[17,62] or pulmonary vascular pressure (without affecting resistance) in dogs, where only pulmonary vasorelaxation was elicited by the selective DA_1-agonist fenoldopam. Rabbit studies in vitro and in vivo indicate that DA, DA_1-agonist, and (to a lesser extent) DA_2-agonist are both endothelium-dependent and -independent pulmonary arterial vasodilators.[63,64] Normal human studies have not specifically studied the pulmonary vasculature, but it appears that DA increases pulmonary blood flow with little change in pressure in subjects without

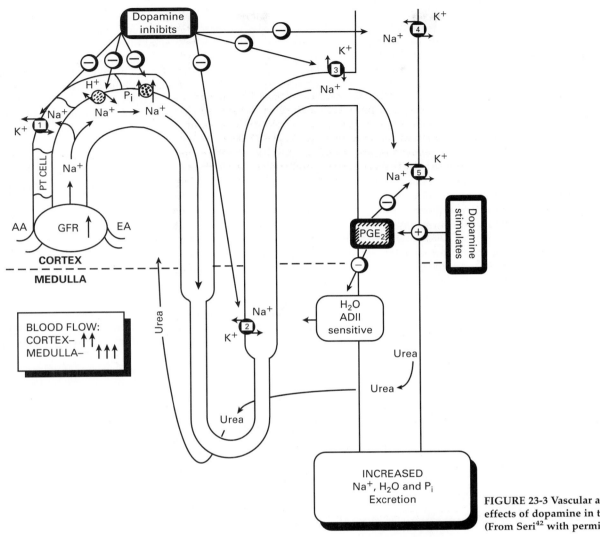

FIGURE 23-3 Vascular and tubular effects of dopamine in the kidney. (From Seri[42] with permission.)

preexisting pulmonary hypertension, suggesting a vasodilatory effect (even in neonates).[65,66] In adults with acute respiratory distress syndrome (ARDS), DA decreases pulmonary vascular resistance,[67] whereas pulmonary artery pressures further increase in infants and adults with preexisting pulmonary hypertension (in whom DA also has been noted to enhance hypoxic vasoconstriction).[68–72]

ENDOCRINE AND OTHER EFFECTS

Dopamine stimulates renin release from the juxtaglomerular apparatus, but this is not translated into augmented aldosterone secretion due to the inhibitory effect of DA on zona glomerulosa aldosterone secretion.[42,60] Inhibition of prolactin secretion by DA may have clinical relevance with respect to sodium and water homeostasis (as noted above) and neonatal pulmonary alveolar surfactant concentrations.[42] Dopamine inhibits pituitary secretion of growth hormone, gonadotropins, and thyrotropin (TSH); the latter effect is complicated by the difficulty of differentiating DA-induced hypothyroidism from euthyroid-sick syndrome or even neonatal hypothyroidism.[42,73] Nausea and emesis are common side effects of DA administration. These effects are thought to result from stimulation of specific DA receptors in the chemoreceptor trigger zone of the medulla.[16] Dopamine directly inhibits gastrointestinal motility and causes ileus through stimulation of specific D_{1A}- and D_{1B}-receptors.[16,74] Stimulation of DA_2-receptors in the carotid bodies causes hypoventilation,[75] specifically reducing hypoxic ventilatory drive.[76,77] Dopamine decreases superoxide anion production by (neonatal) polymorphonuclear leukocytes, without altering their mobility or bactericidal function.[42,78] The clinical relevance of this phenomenon is unknown.

CLINICAL PHARMACOLOGY

Dopamine is administered by intravenous infusion and has a terminal elimination half-life of 6 to 9 min. Elimination kinetics are variably estimated as first order (linear) or saturable.[79,80] Dopamine is metabolized by monoamine oxidase in neurons, and by catechol-*O*-methyltransferase in the liver, kidney, and pulmonary endothelium, with some unmetabolized renal excretion.

THERAPEUTIC INDICATIONS

Dopamine is widely used in the therapy of systemic hypoperfusion (shock) states. The utility of DA as an inotropic and/or vasopressor agent must be considered in the context of shock etiology and pathophysiology. Patients with *cardiogenic shock* caused by left or right ventricular systolic dysfunction may benefit from the systemic or pulmonary arterial vasodilatory effects of low-dose DA, which reduces afterload. Larger doses may add additional inotropic effect through release of myocardial NE stores and stimulation of myocardial β_1-adrenergic receptors. Patients with depleted myocardial NE stores (chronic congestive heart failure[80]) are more likely to benefit from dobutamine administration, as are those with myocardial ischemia, in whom DA appears to increase myocardial oxygen utilization without a proportional augmentation of coronary blood flow (achieved with dobutamine[81]). Of additional concern in patients with systolic or diastolic (i.e., ventricular noncompliance) ventricular dysfunction, the venoconstrictor effect elicited by moderate DA doses may aggravate cardiogenic pulmonary edema by reducing venous capacitance. Finally, the development of pulmonary or systemic arterial α-adrenergic receptor stimulation and vasoconstriction increases ventricular afterload and may occur at a relatively low and unpredictable DA dose. At such doses, DA may be chosen for hemodynamic support in cardiogenic shock when hypotension is aggravated by the vasodilator effect of dobutamine.[82] *Hypovolemic shock* is always best-treated with volume resuscitation alone, but the systemic arterial vasoconstrictor effect and, in particular, the venoconstrictor effect of DA are sometimes useful as temporizing measures pending adequate volume administration and/or hemostasis. *Septic shock* is characterized by a generalized vasodilation that is relatively vasopressor-resistant, large requirements for volume resuscitation (due to vasodilation and diffuse capillary leak), and high cardiac output with a frequent component of relative myocardial depression (caused by circulating inflammatory mediators[83]); all of these defects occur in a hypermetabolic setting where tissue oxygen requirements are increased. Dopamine may have salutary effects in treatment of this syndrome by reducing venous capacitance, maintaining an adequate mean arterial blood pressure, augmenting depressed myocardial function, and, possibly, improving renal and splanchnic perfusion. Unfortunately, attainment of an acceptable mean arterial blood pressure with vasoconstrictor therapy without providing adequate circulating volume may mask inadequate tissue oxygen delivery and ongoing multiorgan injury. Of additional concern, DA therapy in a porcine model of hypovolemic shock aggravates ischemic gut injury, presumably through α-adrenergic receptor–mediated vasoconstriction[84]; these data challenge the assumption that low-dose DA predictably improves splanchnic and renal perfusion in hypoperfusion states.

Dopamine is used most commonly at low dose to prevent or treat acute renal failure, but there is little direct evidence to support this therapy.[85,86] In animal models, DA affords no additional protection over saline in preventing nephrotoxic insult,[87] and, although DA was shown to ameliorate renal hypoperfusion in a dog model of (NE-induced) renal isch-

emia, GFR was not measured in this study.[88] Furthermore, clinical studies of prophylactic DA administration prior to or during ischemic renal insults have yielded negative[89–91] or conflicting[92–93] results. Studies purporting to demonstrate improvement in renal function or prognosis with DA treatment of established ARF have lacked adequate size or randomization to be definitive,[94,95] and the commonly achieved endpoint of improved urine output does not necessarily accompany improvements in GFR or even renal blood flow.[96]

Several renal effects of DA suggest potential benefit in the setting of renal hypoperfusion-increased renal blood flow, blunted tubuloglomerular feedback (renal vasoconstriction in response to natriuresis[97]), diversion of renal blood flow to the medullary region (which is borderline hypoxic at baseline), and blockade of tubular sodium reabsorption (which is responsible for the majority of renal oxygen consumption[98]). Unfortunately, experimental evidence has not confirmed the expected benefit. In light of the above effects and negative experimental data, it should be noted that the net effect of DA therapy on renal oxygen consumption depends on the balance of oxygen delivery (blood flow and hemoglobin saturation) and oxygen consumption (renal tubular reabsorptive work, a function of filtered sodium load and ultimately of GFR). It is therefore conceivable that DA-induced blockade of proximal tubular sodium reabsorption might even precipitate ischemia in the corresponding ascending loop of Henle, through increased distal sodium delivery, unless medullary blood flow increased proportionately or DA equally inhibited loop sodium reabsorption.

Dopamine is also used commonly in conjunction with intravascular volume loading to induce hypertensive hypervolemia to overcome cerebral vasospasm and provide cerebral perfusion following subarachnoid hemorrhage and aneurysm clipping.[99] Obviously, the potential for DA-induced cerebral vasospasm is somewhat less predictable than is desirable in this setting.

ADVERSE EFFECTS

Extravasation of drug with tissue injury due to vasoconstriction may be treated successfully with local injection of phentolamine. Tachycardia, arrhythmia, and myocardial ischemia may all be precipitated by DA, and improve with dose reduction. Digital/extremity gangrene due to vasoconstriction is more common in the pediatric population. For reasons described above, other side effects include hypothyroidism, gastrointestinal dysfunction, hypoventilation, and volume depletion.[100]

Dobutamine

Dobutamine   (±-4-[2-[[3-(*p*-hydroxyphenyl)-1-methylpropyl]amino]ethyl]pyrocatechol; DB) was developed by systematic modification of the catecholamine molecule in search of an agent that would have selective inotropic activity with little peripheral vascular effect.[101] Dobutamine has a larger substitution on the amino terminus of the catecholamine molecule, and, like isoproterenol, is administered as a racemic mixture of the positive and negative enantiomer. This is because DB possesses an asymmetric carbon atom. The negative enatiomer is a potent, selective α_1-adrenergic agonist, and the positive enatiomer potently stimulates β_1- and β_2-adrenoceptors.[102] The net hemodynamic effect of DB is determined by its direct action at these receptors, combined with a reflexive decrease in sympathetic nervous tone when an associated DB-elicited increase in cardiac output occurs.[103]

The inotropic effect of DB generally is attributed to stimulation of myocardial β_1-adrenoceptors.[104,105] However, it has been proposed that the α_1-adrenoceptor–mediated effects may contribute to the inotropic selectivity of this compound.[106,107] Evidence to support this includes (1) the α_1-adrenoceptor–mediated effects are more potent than the β_1-adrenoceptor–mediated effects[107]; (2) myocardial α_1-adrenoceptors exist and mediate a positive inotropic response with little increase in heart rate[109]; (3) the negative enatiomer of DB is the more selective steroisomer as an inotropic agent[107,110]; and finally (4) the inotropic effect of DB is attenuated, in part, by α-adrenoceptor antagonist,[110] and α-adrenoceptor antagonist also decreases left ventricular dp/dt_{max}.[111] The location of the α_1-adrenoceptor involved in increasing cardiac output is not known. Myocardial adrenoceptors have been proposed,[108,110] but it also is possible that the site of action of α-adrenoceptor activation is on systemic veins leading to a venoconstriction with increasing systemic venous return. Supplementation of myocardial perfusion may partly explain the ability of DB to produce sustained improvement of cardiac function in patients with congestive heart failure following short-term infusion.[131] The low chronotropic/inotropic ratio of cardiac responses to DB has been attributed in part to preferential action of DB on ventricular inotropic receptors relative to atrial chronotropic receptors.[120] However, this is not the case in anesthetized vagotomized dogs, suggesting that, at least in part, the low chronotropic effect of the drug in normal dogs is probably caused by the activation of the baroreceptor reflex in response to the increased pulse pressure.[121]

The possibility that the action of DB may arise from the contribution of a metabolite is not discounted. The major metabolite of DB is 3-O-methyldobutamine, which is formed enzymatically by catechol-O-methyltransferase.[112] The positive enantiomer of this metabolite is a relatively potent and highly selective α_1-adrenoceptor antagonist.[113] High concentrations of 3-O-methyldobutamine circulate in the blood as the conjugate. The possibility that lower levels of 3-O-methyldobutamine may exist and exert a α_1-adrenoceptor inhibitory effect must be considered.[113]

CARDIOVASCULAR AND PULMONARY VASCULAR EFFECTS OF DB

At clinically used infusion rates (5 to 20 μg/kg per min), the predominant effect of DB is cardiac, with an increase in contractility and a relatively smaller increase in heart rate. Dobutamine typically decreases, or has little effect on, systemic and pulmonary vascular resistance and decreases left ventricular end-diastolic pressure.[114,115] In contrast to DA,

which can increase pulmonary capillary wedge pressure by postsynaptic pulmonary vascular α adrenoceptors, DB elicits little pulmonary vasoconstriction because of the activation of β-adrenoceptors mediating pulmonary vasodilation. In fact, the effect of DB in the pulmonary circulation is a balance between the α_1- and β-adrenoceptor activities. In the isolated autoperfused canine pulmonary circulation, DB (100 μg/kg per min) increased pulmonary pressure 15 percent above baseline, while DA elicited increases in perfusion pressure 10-fold greater than baseline.[117] This relatively small pulmonary vasoconstrictor response is more prominent after β-adrenoceptor blockade, which indicates that DB stimulates both postjunctional vascular α- and β-adrenoceptors, such that a small net effect occurs.[118]

Dobutamine, like other inotropes, can increase intrapulmonary shunt.[116] This results from an indirect effect of augmenting cardiac output, which increases perfusion of poorly ventilated lung units.[116] Moreover, a deterioration in arterial oxygenation is needed in anesthetized dogs that are breathing a hypoxic gas mixture (F_IO_2, 0.1 percent). The main mechanisms that have been invoked to explain this are an increase in venous admixture caused by an increased pulmonary blood flow and an inhibition of hypoxic pulmonary vasoconstriction.[123] In clinical use, the net effect on gas exchange will be determined by this effect and on the influence of changes in cardiac output, and left ventricular end diastolic pressure on the hydraulic gradients influencing lung water and on mixed venous oxygen saturation. An example of the complexity of this relationship is illustrated by the investigation of the effect of DB on oxygenation in adults with acute pulmonary embolism. Administration of DB improved oxygen transport and tissue oxygenation, but the PaO_2 remained constant, or even decreased in some cases because of an increase $\dot{V}A/Q$ mismatch.[124] In general, in mixed populations of critically ill postoperative surgical patients, DB causes a greater increase in oxygen delivery with less adverse effect on intrapulmonary shunt than that produced by DA.[126,127]

Since the inotropic action of DB does not depend on myocardial stores of norepinephrine, it is a more suited inotrope in the cardiac transplant recipient than DA.[126] Dobutamine often will increase cardiac output, and oxygen delivery in volume-resuscitated patients with septic shock; however, the certainty of improved oxygen delivery does not necessarily translate into improved splanchnic organ perfusion.[128] Schumacker and colleagues[129] have shown that DB does not interfere with the ability of the isolated canine jejunum to extract oxygen during limited oxygen supply.

RENAL VASCULAR EFFECTS OF DB

In addition to enhanced myocardial blood flow, DB infusion increases blood flow to the stomach and skeletal muscle in dogs.[122] Concomitantly, vascular resistance in these organs also decreases. Although DB lacks a selective renal vascular effect, it often enhances urine output by improving cardiac output, and thus renal perfusion.[119] Dobutamine has no significant effects on total body oxygen consumption and arterial concentrations of glucose, lactate, pyruvate, and fatty acids. Thus, unlike other catecholamines, DB in clinically used doses does not activate the β-adrenergic receptors that mediate the glycogenolytic, lipolytic, and calorigenic effects.[122]

METABOLISM AND SIDE EFFECTS OF DB

Dobutamine is cleared rapidly by catechol-O-methyltransferase and rapidly redistributed from the plasma compartment.[125] In stable adults with congestive heart failure, there is a good correlation between the DA dose, plasma concentration, and hemodynamic effects.[129] Dysrhythmias are the most frequent side effect, although less frequent than with DA or isoproterenol.[130] Other side effects include excessive tachycardia, headaches, anxiety, tremors, and excessive increases or decreases in blood pressure.[115]

Dopexamine

Dopexamine hydrochloride (DX) is a relatively new synthetic catecholamine that has been used clinically in Europe in recent years and which bears structural resemblance to both DA and albuterol.[132,133] Dopexamine has a systemic and pulmonary vasodilator effect caused by β₂-adrenergic receptor stimulation and a lesser agonist activity at peripheral DA receptors (predominantly DA₁, with approximately one-third the potency of DA).[134] Dopexamine also has a positive inotropic effect, mainly attributable to two mechanisms: (1) blocking reuptake of NE by sympathetic nerves, and (2) a baroreceptor-mediated release of NE due to hypotension (provoked by the above vasodilatory effects); stimulation of myocardial β₂-adrenergic receptors does not appear to contribute importantly to this inotropic effect.[135] Dopexamine has insignificant β₁-adrenergic receptor activity and no α-adrenergic receptor activity.

Dopexamine increases cerebral, coronary, splanchnic (including mesenteric and hepatic beds), renal, and skeletal muscle blood flows.[136–139] Increased cardiac output is achieved without a significant increase in myocardial oxygen consumption.[140,141] No specific information is available regarding the effects of DX on GFR or renal tubular sodium reabsorption, though a specific (DA₁-mediated) renal vasodilator effect is well-documented.[45,142,143]

Clinically, DX has been used successfully to augment cardiac output in patients with chronic left ventricular dysfunction,[142,143] following coronary artery bypass surgery,[144] in experimental myocardial infarction,[145] and in acute myocardial infarction with left ventricular dysfunction.[146,147] Recent studies have found that DX reduces mortality when used to increase oxygen delivery perioperatively in high-risk surgical patients,[148,149] and selectively augments splanchnic perfusion in patients with sepsis syndrome.[150] Since no α-adrenergic receptor effect is elicited, venoconstriction and mesenteric/renal arterial vasoconstriction do not occur at any dose, and tissue injury does not follow extravasation (so that DX may be safely administered by peripheral vein). Dopexamine therefore combines useful pharmacologic effects of both DA and DB, and offers specific benefits over either agent.

References

1. Mannich C, Jacobsohn W: Uber oxyphenyl-alkylamine und dioxylalkylamine. *Ber Deut Chem Ges* 1910; 43:189–197.
2. Barger G, Ewins AJ: Some phenolic derivatives of β-phenylethylamine. *J Chem Soc (London)* 1910; 97:2253–2261.
3. Holtz P, Credner K: Die enzymatische entstehung von oxytyramin im organismus und die physiologische bedeutung der dopadecarboxylase. *Naunyn Schmiedebergs Arch Pharmacol* 1942; 200:356–388.
4. McDonald RH, Goldberg LI: Analysis of the cardiovascular effects of dopamine in the dog. *J Pharmacol Exp Ther* 1963; 140:60–66.
5. Yeh BK, McNay JL, Goldberg LI: Attenuation of dopamine renal and mesenteric vasodilation by haloperidol: evidence for a specific dopamine receptor. *J Pharmacol Exp Ther* 1969; 168(2):303–309.
6. Goldberg LI, Toda N: Dopamine induced relaxation of isolated canine renal, mesenteric, and femoral arteries contracted with prostaglandin F₂ₐ. *Circ Res* 1975; 36–37 (suppl I):I-97-102.
7. Brodde OE: Vascular dopamine receptors: demonstration and characterization by in vitro studies. *Life Sci* 1982; 31:289–306.
8. Kebabian JW, Calne DB: Multiple receptors for dopamine. *Nature* 1979; 277:93–96.
9. Jose PA, Raymond JR, Bates MD, et al.: The renal dopamine receptors. *J Am Soc Nephrol* 1992; 2:1265–1278.
10. Felder RA, Felder CC, Eisner GM, Jose PA: The dopamine receptor in adult and maturing kidney. *Am J Physiol* 1989; 257:F315–327.
11. Bertorello A, Aperia A: Regulation of Na⁺–K⁺-ATPase activity in kidney proximal tubules: involvement of GTP binding proteins. *Am J Physiol* 1989; 256:F57–62.
12. Felder CC, Campbell T, Albrecht F, Jose PA: Dopamine inhibits Na⁺–H⁺ exchanger activity in renal BBMV by stimulation of adenylate cyclase. *Am J Physiol* 1990; 259:F297–303.
13. Meister B, Aperia A: Molecular mechanisms involved in catecholamine regulation of sodium transport. *Semin Nephrol* 1993; 13(1), 41–49.
14. Slobodyansky E, Aoki Y, Gaznabi AKM, et al.: Dopamine and protein phosphatase activity in renal proximal tubules. *Am J Physiol* 1995; 268:F279–284.
15. Felder CC, Jose PA, Axelrod J: The dopamine agonist, SKF 82526, stimulates phospholipase-C activity independent of adenylate cyclase activity. *J Pharmacol Exp Ther* 1989; 248(1):171–175.
16. Goldberg LI, Volkman PH, Kohli JD: A comparison of the vascular dopamine receptor with other dopamine receptors. *Annu Rev Pharmacol Toxicol* 1978; 18:57–79.
17. Goldberg LI: Dopamine: receptors and clinical applications. *Clin Physiol Biochem* 1985; 3:120–126.
18. Goldberg LI, Kohli JD, Glock D: Conclusive evidence for two subtypes of peripheral dopamine receptors, in Woodruff GN, Poat JA, Roberts PJ (eds): *Dopaminergic Systems and Their Regulation*. London, Eng, Macmillan, 1986; 195–212.
19. Missale C, Castelletti L, Memo M, et al.: Identification and characterization of postsynaptic D₁- and D₂-dopamine receptors in the cardiovascular system. *J Cardiovasc Pharmacol* 1988; 11:643–650.
20. Hall AS, Bryson SE, Vaughan PF, et al.: Pharmacological characterization of the dopamine receptor coupled to cyclic AMP

formation expressed by rat mesenteric artery vascular smooth muscle cells in culture. *Br J Pharmacol* 1993; 110(2):681–6.

21. Amenta F, Cavalloti C, DeRossi M, Mione MF: Dopamine-sensitive cAMP generating system in rat extracerebral arteries. *Eur J Pharmacol* 1984; 97:105–9.

22. Amenta F, Collier WL, Ricci A: Autoradiographic localization of vascular dopamine receptors. *Am J Hypertension* 1990; 3(6 pt 2):34S–36S.

23. Ricci A, Collier WL, Amenta F: Endothelial dopamine DA-1 receptor sites in the rabbit pulmonary artery: autoradiographic demonstration. *J Pharmacol Exp Ther* 1992; 261(2):830–4.

24. Kobayashi Y, Ricci A, Amenta F: Autoradiographic localization of dopamine D1-like receptors in the rabbit pulmonary circulation. *Eur J Pharmacol* 1994; 253(3):201–6.

25. Murphy MB, Elliot WJ: Dopamine and dopamine receptor agonists in cardiovascular therapy. *Crit Care Med* 1990; 18(1):S14–18.

26. Somlyo AP, Somlyo AV: Signal transduction and regulation in smooth muscle. *Nature* 1994; 372:231–236.

27. Yasunari K, Kohno M, Murakawa KI, et al.: Interaction between a phorbol and dopamine DA_1 receptors on vascular smooth muscle. *Am J Physiol* 1993; 264:F24–30.

28. Felder CC, Albrecht F, Eisner GA, Jose PA: The signal transducer for the dopamine-1 regulated sodium transport in renal cortical brush border membrane vesicles. *Am J Hypertension* 1990; 3:47S–50S.

29. Felder CC, Albrecht FE, Campbell T, et al.: cAMP-independent, G protein–linked inhibition of Na^+/H^+ exchange in renal brush border by D_1 dopamine agonists. *Am J Physiol* 1993; 264:F1032–1037.

30. Satoh T, Cohen HT, Katz AI: Intracellular signalling in the regulation of renal Na-K-ATPase (I. Role of cyclic AMP and phospholipase A_2). *J Clin Invest* 1992; 89:1496–1500.

31. Satoh T, Cohen HT, Katz AI: Different mechanisms of renal Na-K-ATPase regulation by protein kinases in proximal and distal nephron. *Am J Physiol* 1993; 265:F399–405.

32. Ricci A, Amenta F: Autoradiographic localization of dopamine DA-2 receptor sites in rat mesenteric vascular tree. *J Pharmacol Exp Ther* 1990; 254(2):750–5.

33. Dupont AG, Vanderniepen P, LeFebvre RA, Bogaert MG: Pharmacological characterization of neuronal dopamine receptors in the rat hindquarters, renal and superior mesenteric vascular beds. *J Auton Pharmacol* 1986; 5:305–9.

34. Kobayashi Y, Ricci A, Rossodivita I, Amenta F: Autoradiographic localization of dopamine D2-like receptors in the rabbit pulmonary vascular tree. *Naunyn Schmiedebergs Arch Pharmacol* 1994; 349(6):559–64.

35. Huo TL, Ye MQ, Healy DP: Characterization of a dopamine receptor (DA_{2k}) in the kidney inner medulla. *Proc Natl Acad Sci U S A* 1991; 88:3170–74.

36. Goldberg LI: Cardiovascular and renal actions of dopamine: potential clinical applications. *Pharmacol Rev* 1972; 24(1):1–29.

37. Meyer MB, McNay JL, Goldberg LI: Effects of dopamine on renal function and hemodynamics in the dog. *J Pharmacol Exp Ther* 1967; 156(1):186–192.

38. Robie NW, Goldberg LI: Comparative systemic and renal hemodynamic effects of dopamine and dobutamine. *Am Heart J* 1975; 90(3):340–345.

39. Horwitz D, Fox SM, Goldberg LI: Effects of dopamine in man. *Circ Res* 1962; X:237–243.

40. McDonald RH, Goldberg LI, McNay JL, Tuttle EP: Effects of dopamine in man: augmentation of sodium excretion, glomerular filtration rate, and renal plasma flow. *J Clin Invest* 1964; 43(6):1116–1124.

41. D'Orio V, El Allaf D, Juchmes J, Marcelle R: The use of low doses of dopamine in intensive care medicine. *Arch Int Physiol Biochem* 1984; 92:S11.

42. Seri I: Cardiovascular, renal, and endocrine actions of dopamine in neonates and children. *J Pediatr* 1995; 126(3):333–344.

43. Lass NA, Glock D, Goldberg LI: Cardiovascular and renal hemodynamic effects of intravenous infusions of the selective DA_1 agonist, fenoldopam, used alone or in combination with dopamine and dobutamine. *Circulation* 1988; 78:1310–5.

44. Okamura T, Yamazaki M, Toda N: Responses to dopamine of isolated human and monkey veins compared with those of arteries. *J Pharmacol Exp Ther* 1991; 258(1):275–9.

45. Lee MR: Dopamine and the kidney: ten years on. *Clin Sci* 1993; 84:357–375.

46. Bass AS, Murphy MB: Role of endogenous dopamine in the natriuresis accompanying various sodium challenges. *Am J Hypertension* 1990; 3:90S–92S.

47. Hansell P, Fasching A: The effect of dopamine receptor blockade on natriuresis is dependent on the degree of hypervolemia. *Kidney Int* 1991; 39:253–258.

48. Vyas SJ, Jadhav AL, Eichberg J, Lokhandwala MF: Dopamine receptor-mediated activation of phospholipase C is associated with natriuresis during high salt intake. *Am J Physiol* 1992; 262:F494–498.

49. Takemoto F, Satoh T, Cohen HT, Katz AI: Localization of dopamine-1 receptors along the microdissected rat nephron. *Pflugers Arch* 1991; 419:243–248.

50. Felder RA, Blecher M, Eisner GM, Jose PA: Cortical tubular and glomerular dopamine receptors in the rat kidney. *Am J Physiol* 1984; 246:F557–568.

51. Olsen NV, Hansen JM, Ladafoged SD, et al.: Renal tubular reabsorption of sodium and water during infusion of low-dose dopamine in normal man. *Clin Sci* 1990; 78:503–507.

52. Siragy HM, Felder RA, Howell NL, et al.: Evidence that dopamine-2 mechanisms control renal function. *Am J Physiol* 1990; 259:F793–800.

53. Schwartz LB, Gewertz BL: The renal response to low dose dopamine. *J Surg Res* 1988; 45:574–588.

54. Edwards RM: Response of isolated renal arterioles to acetylcholine, dopamine, and bradykinin. *Am J Physiol* 1985; 248:F183–189.

55. Steinhausen M, Weis S, Fleming J, et al.: Responses of in vivo microvessels to dopamine. *Kidney Int* 1986; 30:361–370.

56. Hardaker WT, Wechsler AS: Redistribution of renal intracortical blood flow during dopamine infusion in dogs. *Circ Res* 1973; XXXIII:437–444.

57. Aperia A, Bertorello A, Seri I: Dopamine causes inhibition of Na^+-K^+-ATPase activity in rat proximal convoluted tubule segments. *Am J Physiol* 1987; 252:F39–F45.

58. Seri I, Kone BC, Gullans SR, et al.: Influence of Na^+ intake on dopamine-induced inhibition of renal cortical Na^+-K^+-ATPase. *Am J Physiol* 1990; 258:F52–F60.

59. Takemoto F, Cohen HT, Satoh T, Katz AI: Dopamine inhibits Na/K-ATPase in single tubules and cultured cells from distal nephron. *Pflugers Arch* 1992; 421:302–306.

60. Missale C, Lombardi C, Sigala S, Spano P: Dopaminergic regulation of aldosterone secretion. *Am J Hypertension* 1990; 3:93S–95S.

61. Bello-Reuss E: Effect of catecholamines on fluid reabsorption by the isolated proximal convoluted tubule. *Am J Physiol* 1980; 238:F347–352.

62. Shebuski RJ, Smith JM, Ruffolo RR: Comparison of the renal and pulmonary hemodynamic effects of fenoldopam, dobutamine, dopamine, and norepinephrine in the anesthetized dog. *Pharmacology* 1988; 36(1):35–43.

63. Polak MJ, Taylor DA: Functional ontogeny of pulmonary vascular DA1 dopamine receptors in the isolated perfused rabbit lung. *Pediat Res* 1994; 35(2):228–232.

64. Yamauchi M, Kobayashi Y, Shimoura K, et al.: Endothelium-

dependent and -independent relaxation by dopamine in the rabbit pulmonary artery. *Clin Exp Pharmacol Physiol* 1992; 19(6):401–410.

65. Goldberg LI, Hsieh Y-Y, Resnekov L: Newer catecholamines for treatment of heart failure and shock: an update on dopamine and a first look at dobutamine. *Prog Cardiovasc Dis* 1977; 19:327–340.

66. Keeley SR, Bohn DJ. The use of inotropic and afterload-reducing agents in neonates. *Clin Perinatol* 1988; 15:469–89.

67. Malloy WD, Dobson K, Girling L, et al.: Effects of dopamine on cardiopulmonary function and left ventricular volume in patients with acute respiratory failure. *Am Rev Respir Dis* 1984; 130:396–9.

68. Holloway EL, Palumbo RA, Harrison DC: Acute circulatory effects of dopamine in patients with pulmonary hypertension. *Br Heart J* 1975; 37:482–485.

69. Zaritsky A, Chernow B: The use of catecholamines in pediatrics. *J Pediatr* 1984; 105:341–50.

70. Lang P, Williams RG, Norwood WI, Castaneda AR: The hemodynamic effects of dopamine in infants after corrective cardiac surgery. *J Pediatr* 1980; 96:630–4.

71. Furman WR, Summer WR, Kennedy TP, Sylvester JT: Comparison of the effects of dobutamine, dopamine, and isoproterenol on hypoxic pulmonary vasoconstriction in the pig. *Crit Care Med* 1982; 10:371–374.

72. Mentzer RM Jr, Alegre CA, Nolan SP: The effects of dopamine and isoproterenol on the pulmonary circulation. *J Thorac Cardiovasc Surg* 1976; 71:807–14.

73. Leebaw W, Lee L, Woolf P: Dopamine affects basal and augmented pituitary hormone secretion. *J Clin Endocrinol Metab* 1978; 47:480–486.

74. Marmon LM, Albrecht F, Canessa LM, et al.: Identification of dopamine 1A receptors in the rat small intestine. *J Surg Res* 1993; 54(6):616–20.

75. Welsh MJ, Heistad DD, Abboud FM: Depression of ventilation by dopamine in man: evidence for an effect on the chemoreceptor reflex. *J Clin Invest* 1978; 61:708–713.

76. Olson LG, Hensley MJ, Saunders NA: Ventilatory responses to hypercapnic hypoxia during dopamine infusion in humans. *Am Rev Respir Dis* 1982; 126:783–787.

77. Ward DS, Bellville JW: Reduction of hypoxic ventilatory drive by dopamine. *Anesth Analg* 1982; 61:333–337.

78. Matsuoka T: A sedative effect of dopamine on the respiratory burst in neonatal polymorphonuclear leukocytes. *Pediatr Res* 1990; 28:24–7.

79. Jamberg PO, Bengtsson L, Ekstrand J, Hamberger B: Dopamine infusion in man. Plasma catecholamine levels and pharmacokinetics. *Acta Anaesth Scand* 1981; 25:328–331.

80. Zaritsky AL: Catecholamines, inotropic medications, and vasopressor agents, in Chernow B (ed): *Essentials of Critical Care Pharmacology*. Baltimore: Williams & Wilkins, 1994: 255–272.

81. Fowler MB, Alderman EL, Oester SN, et al.: Dobutamine and dopamine after cardiac surgery: greater augmentation of myocardial blood flow with dobutamine. *Circulation* 1984; 70 (suppl I):I103–I111.

82. Califf RM, Bengston JR: Cardiogenic shock. *N Eng J Med* 1994; 330:1724–30.

83. Parrillo JE: Pathogenetic mechanisms of septic shock. *N Engl J Med* 1993; 328:1471–77.

84. Segal JM, Phang T, Walley KR: Low-dose dopamine hastens onset of gut ischemia in a porcine model of hemorrhagic shock. *J Appl Physiol* 1992; 73:1159–1164.

85. Szerlip HM: Renal-dose dopamine: fact and fiction. *Ann Intern Med* 1991; 115:153–154.

86. Vendegna TR, Anderson RJ: Are dopamine and/or dobutamine renoprotective in intensive care unit patients? *Crit Care Med* 1994; 22:1893–1894.

87. Conger JD, Falk SA, Yuan BH, Schrier RW: Atrial natriuretic peptide and dopamine in a rat model of ischemic acute renal failure. *Kidney Int* 1989; 35:1126–1132.

88. Schaer GL, Fink MP, Parrillo JE: Norepinephrine alone versus norepinephrine plus low-dose dopamine: enhanced renal blood flow with combination pressor therapy. *Crit Care Med* 1985; 13:492–496.

89. Baldwin L, Henderson A, Hickman P: Effect of postoperative low-dose dopamine on renal function after elective major vascular surgery. *Ann Intern Med* 1994; 120:744–747.

90. Grundmann R, Kindler J, Meider G, et al.: Dopamine treatment of human cadaver kidney graft recipients: a prospectively randomized trial. *Lancet* 1980; ii:827–828.

91. Wenstone R, Campbell JM, Booker PD, et al.: Renal function after cardiopulmonary bypass in children: comparison of dopamine with dobutamine. *Br J Anaesth* 1991; 67:591–594.

92. Polson RJ, Park GR, Lindop MJ, et al.: The prevention of renal impairment in patients undergoing orthotopic liver grafting by infusion of low dose dopamine. *Anaesthesia* 1987; 42:15–19.

93. Swygert TH, Roberts LC, Valek TR, et al.: Effect of intraoperative low-dose dopamine on renal function in liver transplant recipients. *Anesthesiology* 1991; 75:571–576.

94. Lumlertgul D, Keoplung M, Sitprija V, et al.: Furosemide and dopamine in malarial acute renal failure. *Nephron* 1989; 52:40–44.

95. Graziani G, Cantaluppi A, Casati S, et al.: Dopamine and furosemide in oliguric acute renal failure. *Nephron* 1984; 37:39–42.

96. Duke GJ, Briedis JH, Weaver RA: Renal support in critically ill patients: low-dose dopamine or low-dose dobutamine? *Crit Care Med* 1994; 22:1919–1925.

97. Schnermann J, Todd KM, Briggs JP: Effect of dopamine on the tubuloglomerular feedback mechanism. *Am J Physiol* 1990; 258:790–798.

98. Brezis M, Rosen S: Hypoxia of the renal medulla—its implications for disease. *N Engl J Med* 1995; 332:647–655.

99. Darby JM, Yonas H, Marks EC, et al.: Acute cerebral blood flow response to dopamine-induced hypertension after subarachnoid hemorrhage. *J Neurosurg* 1994; 80:857–64.

100. Polansky D, Eberhard N, McGrath R: Dopamine and polyuria (letter). *Ann Intern Med* 1987; 107:941.

101. Tuttle RR, Mills J: Dobutamine: development of a new catecholamine to selectively increase cardiac contractility. *Circ Res* 1975; 36:185–196.

102. Ruffolo RR Jr, Yaden EL: Vascular effects of the steroisomers of dobutamine. *J Pharmacol Exp Ther* 1983; 224:46–50.

103. Liang CS, Hood WB: Dobutamine infusion in conscious dogs with and without autonomic nervous system inhibition: effects of systemic hemodynamics, regional blood flows and cardiac metabolism. *J Pharmacol Exp Ther* 1979; 211:698–705.

104. Robie NW, Nutter DO, Moody C, McNay JL: In vivo analysis of adrenergic receptor activity of dobutamine. *Circ Res* 1974; 34:663–671.

105. Kenakin TP: An in vitro quantitative analysis of the α-adrenoceptor partial agonist activity of dobutamine and its relevance to inotropic selectivity. *J Pharmacol Exp Ther* 1981; 216:210–219.

106. Ruffolo RR Jr, Spradlin TA, Pollock GD, et al.: α- and β-adrenergic effects of the steroisomers of dobutamine. *J Pharmacol Exp Ther* 1981; 219:447–452.

107. Ruffolo RR Jr, Yaden EL: Vascular effects of the steroisomers of dobutamine. *J Pharmacol Exp Ther* 1983; 224:46–50.

108. Ruffolo RR Jr, Messick K: Systemic hemodynamic effects of dopamine, (+)-dobutamine and the (+)- and (−)-enantiomers

of dobutamine in anesthetized normotensive rats. *Eur J Pharmacol* 1985; 109:173–181.

109. Ruffolo RR Jr, Messick K: Inotropic selectivity of dobutamine enantiomers in pithed rat. *J Pharmacol Exp Ther* 1985; 235:344–348.

110. Maccarrone C, Malta E, Raper C: β-adrenoceptor selectivity of dobutamine: In vivo and in vitro studies. *J Cardiovasc Pharmacol* 1984; 6:132–141.

111. Murphy PJ, Williams TL, Kau DLK: Disposition of dobutamine in the dog. *J Pharmacol Exp Ther* 1976; 119:423–431.

112. Ruffolo RR Jr, Messick K, Horng JS: Interactions of the enantiomers of 3-O-methyldobutamine with α- and β-adrenoceptors in vitro. *Naunyn Schmeidebergs Arch Pharmacol* 1985; 329: 244–252.

113. Loeb HS, Bredakis J, Gunnar RM: Superiority of dobutamine over dopamine for augmentation of cardiac output in patients with chronic low output cardiac failure. *Circulation* 1977; 55:375–381.

114. Leier CV, Unverferth DV: *Dobutamine Ann Intern Med* 1983; 99:490–496.

115. Ruffolo RR Jr, Goldberg MR, Morgan EL: Interaction of epinephrine, norepinephrine, dopamine and their corresponding α-methyl-substituted derivatives with alpha- and beta-adrenoceptors in pithed rat. *J Pharmacol Exp Ther* 1984; 230:595–600.

116. Jardin F, Sportiche M, Bazin M, et al.: Dobutamine: a hemodynamic evaluation in human septic shock. *Crit Care Med* 1981; 9:329–332.

117. Shebuski RJ, Smith JM, Ruffolo RR, Jr: Comparison of the renal and pulmonary hemodynamic effects of fenoldopam, dobutamine, dopamine and norepinephrine in the anesthetized dog. *Pharmacology* 1988; 36:35–43.

118. Shebuski RJ, Fujita T, Ruffolo RR Jr: Evaluation of alpha-1 and alpha-2 adrenoceptor-mediated vasoconstriction in the in situ autoperfused pulmonary circulation of the anesthetized dog. *J Pharmacol Exp Ther* 1986; 238:217–222.

119. Leier CV, Hebran PT, Huss P, et al.: Comparative systemic and regional hemodynamic effects of dopamine and dobutamine in patients with cardiomyopathic heart failure. *Circulation* 1978; 58:466–475.

120. Tuttle RR, Hillman CC, Toomery RE: Differential β-adrenergic sensitivity of atrial and ventricular tissue assessed by chronotropic, inotropic, and cyclic AMP responses to isoprenaline and dobutamine. *Cardiovasc Res* 1976; 10:452–458.

121. Gero J, Gerova M: Significance of the individual parameters of pulsating pressure in stimulation of vasoreceptors, in *Baroreceptor and Hypertension*. Kezdi P (ed): Oxford, Eng, Pergamon Press, 1967; 17–30.

122. Liang C-S, Hood WB Jr: Dobutamine infusions in conscious dogs with and without autonomic nervous system inhibition: effects on systemic hemodynamics, regional blood flows and cardiac metabolism. *J Pharmacol Exp Ther* 1979; 211:698–705.

123. Lemaire F: Effect of catecholamines on pulmonary right-to-left shunt. *Int Anesthesiol Clin* 1983; 21:43–58.

124. Manier G, Castaing Y: Influence of cardiac output on oxygen exchange in acute pulmonary embolism. *Am Rev Respir Dis* 1992; 145:130–136.

125. Murphy PJ, Williams GL, Kau DLK: Disposition of dobutamine in the dog. *J Pharmacol Exp Ther* 1976; 199:423–431.

126. Edwaards H, Olafsson O, Yman AI, et al.: Dobutamine in the rejecting heart transplant patient. *Crit Care Med* 1981; 9:498–499.

127. Shoemaker WC, Appel PL, Kram HB: Oxygen transport measurements to evaluated tissue perfusion and titrate therapy: dobutamine and dopamine effects. *Crit Care Med* 1991; 19:672–688.

128. Vincent JL, Roman A, Kahn RJ: Dobutamine administration in septic shock: addition to a standard protocol. *Crit Care Med* 1990; 18:689–693.

129. Leier CV, Unverferth DV, Kates RE: The relationship between plasma dobutamine concentrations and cardiovascular responses in cardiac failure. *Am J Med* 1979; 66:238–242.

130. Sonnenblick EH, Frishman WH, LeJental TH: Dobutamine. A new synthetic cardioactive sympathetic amine. *N Engl J Med* 1979; 300:17–22.

131. Liang CS, Sherman LG, Doherty JU, et al.: Sustained improvement in patients with congestive heart failure after short-term infusion of dobutamine. *Circulation* 1984; 69:113–119.

132. Smith GW, O'Connor SE: An introduction to the pharmacologic properties of Dopacard (dopexamine hydrochloride) *Am J Cardiol* 1988; 62:9C–17C.

133. Perrin G, Papazian L, Martin C: Dopexamine: a new dopaminergic agonist. *Annales Francaises d'Anesthesie et de Reanimation* 1993; 12(3):308–320.

134. Brown RA, Dixon J, Farmer JB, et al.: Dopexamine: a novel agonist at peripheral dopamine receptors and β-adrenoceptors. *Br J Pharmacol* 1985; 85:599–608.

135. Goldberg LI, Bass AS: Relative significance of dopamine receptors, beta adrenoceptors and norepinephrine uptake inhibition in the cardiovascular actions of dopexamine hydrochloride. *Am J Cardiol* 1988; 62:37C–40C.

136. Brown RA, Farmer JB, Hall JC, et al.: The effects of dopexamine on the cardiovascular system of the dog. *Br J Pharmacol* 1985; 85:609–619.

137. Biro GP, Douglas JR, Keon WJ, Taichman GC: Changes in regional blood flow distribution induced by infusions of dopexamine hydrochloride or dobutamine in anesthetized dogs. *Am J Cardiol* 1988; 62:30C–36C.

138. Amenta F, Ricci A, Napoleone P, et al.: Anatomical localization of the binding and functional characterization of responses to dopexamine hydrochloride in the rat mesenteric vasculature. *Pharmacology* 1991; 42:211–222.

139. Van Kesteren RG, Heethaar RM, Charbon GA, et al.: Comparison of effects of dopamine hydrochloride and dopexamine hydrochloride on abdominal and femoral hemodynamics in anesthetized dogs. *Circ Shock* 1993; 40:227–233.

140. Dawson JR, Thompson DS, Signy M, et al.: Acute haemodynamic and metabolic effects of dopexamine, a new dopaminergic agonist, in patients with chronic heart failure. *Br Heart J* 1985; 54:313–320.

141. De Marco T, Kwasman M, Lau D, Chatterjee K: Dopexamine hydrochloride in chronic congestive heart failure with improved cardiac performance without increased metabolic cost. *Am J Cardiol* 1988; 62:57C–62C.

142. Magrini F, Foulds R, Roberts N, et al.: Renal hemodynamic effects of dopexamine hydrochloride. *Am J Cardiol* 1988; 62:53C–56C.

143. Mousdale S, Clyburn PA, Mackie AM, et al.: Comparison of the effects of dopamine, dobutamine, and dopexamine upon renal blood flow: a study in normal healthy volunteers. *Br J Clin Pharmacol* 1988; 25:555–560.

144. Van Der Starre PJA, Rosseel PMJ: Dopexamine hydrochloride after coronary artery bypass grafting. *Am J Cardiol* 1988; 62:78C–82C.

145. Parratt JR, Wainwright CL, Fagbemi O: Effect of dopexamine hydrochloride in the early stages of experimental myocardial infarction and comparison with dopamine and dobutamine. *Am J Cardiol* 1988; 62:18C–23C.

146. Svenson G, Strandberg LE, Lindvall B, et al.: Haemodynamic response to dopexamine hydrochloride in postinfarction heart failure: lack of tolerance after continuous infusion. *Br Heart J* 1988; 60:489–496.

147. Tan LB, Littler WA, Murray RG: Beneficial haemodynamic effects of intravenous dopexamine in patients with low-output heart failure. *J Cardiovasc Pharmacol* 1987; 10:280–286.

148. Boyd O, Grounds RM, Bennett ED: The use of dopexamine hydrochloride to increase oxygen delivery postoperatively. *Anesth Analg* 1993; 76:372–376.

149. Boyd O, Grounds RM, Bennett ED: A randomized clinical trial of the effect of deliberate perioperative increase in oxygen delivery on mortality in high-risk surgical patients. *JAMA* 1993; 270:2699–2707.

150. Smithies M, Yee TH, Jackson L, et al.: Protecting the gut and liver in the critically ill: effects of dopexamine. *Crit Care Med* 1994; 22:789–795.

CYTOKINES IN THE LUNG

Chapter 24
CYTOKINES IN AIRWAYS
KIMM J. HAMANN

Cytokines initially were discovered in the mid-1960s as biologically active proteins released from sensitized lymphocytes and originally were termed *lymphokines* to denote their source.[1] The term *monokines* also was used when factors were isolated from monocytes or unfractionated mononuclear cell populations. After several years, it became clear that several cell types can produce and release these factors, and the term *cytokine* was proposed to reflect this fact.[2] At the Second International Lymphokine Workshop held in 1979, a more functionally derived term, *interleukin*, was proposed for certain of these proteins to indicate their ability to act as signals between different populations of leukocytes.[3] Nevertheless, the term *cytokine* has come to be the most widely used as well as the least restrictive term. Cytokines now include protein regulators produced by a variety of cells and found in the extracellular medium, which have important roles in normal physiologic as well as pathophysiologic responses and also have therapeutic potential.[4] This chapter presents an overview of the cytokine network of the lung and reviews the major changes in cytokine expression and activity during the pathogenesis of asthma. The discussion will focus mainly on the interleukins that regulate the interaction of cells relevant to the inflammatory processes characteristic of human asthma. While many of the properties of interleukins are shared by other groups of protein mediators, such as growth factors, the discussion of the latter will be limited primarily to those of the relationships that may shed light on the functions of cytokines in the asthmatic lung.

The Cytokine Network of the Lung

Underlying the stable composition of the mature lung is a high metabolic turnover at both the cellular and the molecular levels, even in the absence of injury or disease.[5] Presumably, these changes were regulated, at least in part, by cytokines and growth factors. These proteins may stimulate or suppress cellular activities, such as growth and differentiation, and they may regulate cell-cell and cell-matrix interactions through relatively simple or very complex pathways involving cytokine cascades. Furthermore, cytokines may interact in such a way that their effects in combination may differ from the effects they would have individually. The complexity of these interactions, compounded by the pleiotropy of most cytokines, makes an exhaustive review of their activities impractical. Therefore, this chapter focuses on the interactions that have major consequences for lung biology, particularly during the inflammatory processes of asthma.

INTERLEUKIN-1

Interleukins 1 and 2 (IL-1 and IL-2) were the first cytokines to be classified as interleukins—that is, as proteins acting as biochemical messengers between leukocytes.[3] IL-1 is produced by several cell types, but primarily by monocytes and macrophages.[6] It has a broad range of biologic activities on many different target cells, including lymphocytes, monocytes, and endothelial cells (Table 24-1). IL-1 exists as two distinct forms, IL-1α and IL-1β, which are products of two different genes. Although IL-1α and IL-1β have only 26 percent sequence identity,[7] they share the same receptor,[8] and their biologic activities appear to overlap extensively. IL-1

TABLE 24-1   Interleukins, Colony-Stimulating Factors, and Growth Factors[a]

Cytokine	Biochemistry[b]	Cellular Sources	Targets/Effects
Interleukins			
IL-1α	159 aa; 17.5 kDa	Monocytes, macrophages, fibroblasts,	Activates T and B lymphocytes,
IL-1β	153 aa; 17.3 kDa glycoproteins	vascular endothelium, eosinophils, and others	endothelial cells, epithelial cells; induces fibroblast secretion of PDGF, prostaglandin, collagenase
IL-2	133 aa; 15.5 kDa glycoprotein	T lymphocytes	Stimulates growth & differentiation of T cells, B cells, monocytes, macrophages, natural killer cells
IL-3	133 aa; 20–32 kDa glycoforms	T cells, mast cells, eosinophils	Hematopoietic growth factor for erythroid & myeloid lineages; activates some of these cells
IL-4	129 aa; 18–20 kDa glycoprotein	T cells, mast cells, B-cell lines	Multiple biologic effects on T cells, B cells, monocytes, endothelial cells, fibroblasts
IL-5	115 aa; 40–45 kDa glycoprotein	T cells, mast cells, eosinophils	Hematopoietic and activator of eosinophils, urine B cells
IL-6	184 aa; 21–26 kDa glycoprotein	T cells, B cells, macrophages, fibroblasts, endothelial cells, eosinophils	Multiple effects on T cells, B cells, & hematopoiesis
IL-7	152 aa; 25 kDa glycoprotein	Thymic and bone marrow stromal cells	Stimulates immature and mature lymphocytes
IL-8	72–77 aa; ~8 kDa non-glycosylated isoforms	Monocytes, macrophages, T cells, fibroblasts, endothelial cells, eosinophils, neutrophils	Neutrophil activator & chemoattractant; less potent chemoattractant for T cells, basophils
IL-9	126 aa; 32–39 kDa glycoprotein	T lymphocytes	T-cell and mast cell growth factor; enhances B-cell IgE production
IL-10	160 aa; nonglycosylated noncovalent homodimer	T (T$_H$2) cells, B cells, monocytes, macrophages	Inhibits T$_H$1 cytokine production; costimulates growth of T cells, B cells, mast cells, & progenitor cells
IL-11	178 aa; nonglycosylated(?); no disulfide bonds	Fibroblasts, bone marrow, & lung fibroblast cell lines	Acts synergistically with IL-3, IL-4, stem cell factor in hematopoiesis
IL-12	35 & 40 kDa subunits; heterodimeric glycoprotein	B cells, macrophages, monocytes	Induces IFN-γ and TNF production by T cells & natural killer cells and stimulates their growth
IL-13	112 aa; 14–40 kDa glycoforms	Activated T cells	Multiple effects on monocytes/macrophages, B cells
IL-14	483 aa; 50–60 kDa glycoprotein	T cells, B-cell lines	Induces proliferation of activated B cells; inhibits Ig synthesis

generally is considered to be a proinflammatory cytokine, and in vivo it can produce fever, neutrophilia, muscle proteolysis, and increased concentrations of acute-phase proteins.[6] IL-1 can have several effects on lymphocytes: it stimulates T-cell proliferation, IL-2 release, and IL-2 receptor expression, and it regulates B-cell growth and antibody production.[6]

IL-1 concentrations are increased in the bronchoalveolar lavage (BAL) fluids of nonallergic asthmatics,[9] and this mediator may perpetuate the hyperresponsiveness of asthmatic airways. In a rat model, inhalation of IL-1 resulted in neutrophil infiltration of the airways and increased hyperresponsiveness to bradykinin.[10] Human bronchial epithelial cells responded to in vitro exposure to the asthmogenic substance toluene diisocyanate by increasing the secretion of IL-1β (and IL-6),[11] and hamster tracheal epithelial cells increased production of an intracellular form of IL-1α after

stimulation with pertussis toxin.[12] IL-1, in turn, is able to stimulate airway epithelial cells to produce IL-8 and granulocyte/macrophage colony-stimulating factor (GM-CSF),[13,14] both of which, as outlined below, can amplify the inflammatory processes during asthma. Human alveolar macrophages secrete IL-1β,[15] and human lung fibroblasts can be stimulated synergistically by IL-1 (α and β) and tumor necrosis factor to synthesize both forms of IL-1.[16,17] IL-1 can upregulate adhesion molecules, such as ICAM-1 or VCAM-1, on endothelial cells and enhance adhesion and migration of eosinophils[18] and other inflammatory cells into the pulmonary tissues, or it can act in an autocrine fashion to amplify the reaction. Recently, in another rat model, IL-1β has been shown to induce eosinophil accumulation through the local generation (in skin) of secondary inflammatory mediators such as IL-8 and platelet-activating factor (PAF).[19] Whether these interactions can contribute to airway

TABLE 24-1   Continued

Cytokine	Biochemistry[b]	Cellular Sources	Targets/Effects
Interleukins			
IL-15	114 aa; 14–15 kDa glycoprotein	Blood mononuclear cells, epithelial cells, kidney, lung, and other tissues	Stimulates proliferation of activated T cells; costimulates secretion of IgM, IgG, IgA
GM-CSF	144 aa; 20–30 kDa glycoprotein	T cells, endothelial cells, macrophages, fibroblasts	Promotes proliferation, differentiation, activation, and survival of granulocytes, macrophages
Chemokines			
α subfamily	The "C-X-C" chemokines with an amino acid separating the first two cysteines; includes IL-8 (above)	Monocytes/macrophages fibroblasts, T cells, neutrophils, endothelial cells	As a group, induce differential migration of various cell types; IL-8 is primarily a neutrophil attractant/activator
β subfamily	The "C-C" chemokines; no amino acid separating the first two cysteines		
RANTES	68 aa; 8kDa	T lymphocytes, macrophages	Chemotactic (& activator?) for eosinophils, T cells, monocytes
MIP-1α	70 aa; 8–200 kDa aggregates	T cells, B cells, macrophages, neutrophils	Chemoattractant for B cells, some T cells, and eosinophils
MCP-1	76 aa; 8–18 kDa glycoprotein	Monocytes, endothelial cells, smooth muscle cells, T cells, fibroblasts	Chemoattracts & activates monocytes; activates basophils
Growth factors			
TGF-β	112 aa; 25 kDa	Platelets, most nucleated cells	Regulates cell proliferation and differentiation
PDGF	Homo- or heterodimer: AA, AB, or BB chains; ~ 30 kDa	Platelets, macrophages, endothelial cells	Stimulates growth & chemotaxis of fibroblasts, smooth muscle cells
EFG	53 aa; 6 kDa	Macrophages/monocytes	Stimulates growth of many nonhematopoietic cells
FGF	Family of 15–32 kD polypeptides	Many sources; monocytes, endothelial cells	Variety of roles in cell growth, differentiation, tissue repair, & angiogenesis
IGF-I	Insulin-like A and B domains: 70 aa	Most tissues	Involved in normal growth; physiologic & pathologic states

[a] This table lists cytokines that are potentially important to the immunologic maintenance or inflammatory cell interactions of the lung. Not all of these cytokines have yet been localized to the lung.
[b] Molecular weights usually vary according to degree of glycosylation and/or cellular source. Natural IL-3, for example, consists of a heterogeneous mixture of different molecular species or "glycoforms."

eosinophilia in asthma remains to be determined. To add further to the potential complexity of IL-1 interactions in asthma, eosinophils themselves may be capable of synthesizing and releasing IL-1.[20]

The relevance of IL-1 to asthma has been underscored by the recent discovery of an IL-1 receptor antagonist (IL-1ra).[21–23] This molecule inhibits the proinflammatory effects of IL-1 and can be produced by alveolar macrophages.[24] Recombinant IL-1ra has inhibitory effects on experimental allergic inflammation of the airways in guinea pigs,[25,26] and it holds some promise as a potential therapeutic agent in asthma.[27]

INTERLEUKIN-2

IL-2 is secreted primarily by helper (CD4+) T lymphocytes following antigen- or mitogen-induced activation. In turn, IL-2 binds to its receptor (IL-2R = CD25) in an autocrine or paracrine fashion and stimulates the proliferation of antigen-specific T cells.[28] While levels of IL-2 expression in BAL cells from allergic asthmatics do not appear to be elevated above those from some nonasthmatic, nonallergic subjects,[29] a recent comparison of allergic and nonallergic asthmatics revealed significantly elevated amounts of IL-2 in BAL fluids form nonallergic asthmatics.[30] IL-2 and other cytokines upregulate the release of endothelin-1, a potent broncho-constrictor, from guinea pig airway epithelial cells.[31] Administration of IL-2 to sensitized rats caused an inflammatory infiltrate, which included eosinophils, mast cells, and lymphocytes, to appear around the airways and increased the lung resistance during both the early and late response.[32] IL-2 can also stimulate increased production of GM-CSF (see below) and contribute to increased eosinophil survival and accumulation in the pulmonary tissues.[33]

Recent evidence suggests that IL-2 can stimulate eosinophils directly through IL-2R on their surface and is a potent chemoattractant (about 100- to 1000-fold more potent than PAF or C5a).[34] The concentrations of soluble IL-2R, which correlate with the expression of IL-2R on T cells, are greater in symptomatic than in asymptomatic asthmatics.[35] These findings, coupled with studies that indicate increased numbers of CD25+ (IL-2R+) T cells in asthmatics,[30,36] suggest that IL-2 plays a role in the inflammatory processes, specifically those directly involving T cells, in intrinsic asthma and perhaps in allergic asthma as well.

INTERLEUKIN-3, INTERLEUKIN-5, AND GRANULOCYTE/MACROPHAGE COLONY-STIMULATING FACTOR

IL-3, IL-5, and GM-CSF are important cytokines affecting eosinophil development and activation; because a great deal of recent evidence suggests eosinophils play a central role in asthma,[18,37–40] the participation of these cytokines in asthma has been the subject of numerous recent studies. IL-3 stimulates the colony formation and development of a number of hematopoietic lineages, including those of neutrophils, eosinophils, mast cells, and monocytes, and was originally termed *multicolony stimulating factor* (multi-CSF).[41] IL-3 is produced by activated T cells and mast cells, but also by stimulated eosinophils.[42,43] Beyond early hematopoietic regulation of inflammatory cell types involved in asthma, the direct participation of IL-3 in this disease is unclear. Nevertheless, several studies have demonstrated upregulation of mRNA and protein expression for IL-3 (and IL-5 and GM-CSF) in infiltrating cells of asthmatic airways[18,30] and allergic inflammations.[44,45] Furthermore, IL-3 may be involved in the migration of eosinophils and neutrophils in pulmonary tissues. Adhesion of eosinophils to endothelial cells can be enhanced by treatment with IL-3,[46] and eosinophils preincubated ("primed") with IL-3 show prolonged survival and increased chemotactic responsiveness to other activators.[47,48] During later interactions in pulmonary inflammation, IL-3 potentially can act as a secretagogue for both eosinophils and neutrophils.[49]

Much more evidence exists for active roles of IL-5 and GM-CSF in the eosinophilic inflammation in asthma, although many of the effects of IL-3 on eosinophils are also seen with GM-CSF and IL-5.[47–49] Like IL-3, GM-CSF is a multipotent cytokine involved in normal hematopoiesis, but it can also regulate the activities of mature granulocytes and macrophages, as well as those of endothelial cells and fibroblasts, which express the high-affinity GM-CSF receptor.[50] GM-CSF can be synthesized and released by several cell types in the lung, including T cells, macrophages, mast cells, and eosinophils. Activation of CD4+ T cells in the airways of asthma patients results in a T_H2-like profile of cytokine expression (Fig. 24-1), which includes increases in cells expressing GM-CSF.[44,51] Epithelial cells in the airways of asthmatics also express GM-CSF mRNA.[52,53] Interestingly, corticosteroids used in the treatment of asthma decrease GM-CSF expression in human lung tissue.[53,54] Peripheral blood mononuclear cells from asthmatics secrete increased

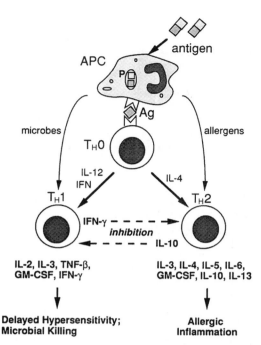

FIGURE 24-1 Diagram of the development of CD4+ T-cell subsets T_H1 and T_H2. Following antigen/microbe uptake and intracellular processing (P) by antigen-presenting cells (APC), antigen (Ag) presentation associated with class II MHC leads to the production of CD4+ T cells, sometimes initially into a T_H0 population. Restimulation with antigen (*thin arrows*) leads to differentiation into T_H1 and T_H2 subsets. Early release of IL-12 and IFN-γ from macrophages may promote the development of T_H1 cells, while release of IL-4 from, for example, mast cells may promote T_H2 differentiation. Furthermore, release of these cytokines from the respective subsets may be a self-amplifying mechanism. In addition, IL-10 can suppress T_H1 cells, while IFN-γ can block the development of T_H2 cells. T_H1 cells are involved primarily in cell-mediated immunity against intracellular microbes and in delayed hypersensitivity reactions. T_H2 cells are upregulated in helminthic infections and allergic reactions. Imbalances in the proportions and/or activities of T_H1 and T_H2 may be important in the development of diseases, such as asthma, in which the T_H2 profile predominates (see refs 30, 44, 51).

amounts of GM-CSF,[55] and GM-CSF mRNA and protein can be detected in activated human eosinophils.[56,57] In addition, mRNA for GM-CSF has been detected in the sputum of asthmatic patients by the polymerase chain reaction (PCR).[58] In addition to its hematopoietic activities, GM-CSF can regulate surface molecule expression and mediator functions of human neutrophils and eosinophils.[59,60] Alveolar macrophages can release GM-CSF to prime eosinophils for increased leukotriene C_4 release[61]; GM-CSF can enhance calcium ionophore-induced release of proteins from human eosinophil granules.[62] While normal eosinophils respond to GM-CSF with augmented superoxide anion generation, eosinophils from asthmatics are refractory to this enhancement, suggesting in vivo priming of the cells by this factor.[63]

IL-5 has a unique role in the production of eosinophils and appears to be the principal cytokine mediator associated with the eosinophilic inflammation in asthma.[64,65] IL-5 is a product of the T_H2 type of T cells and can be produced by airway mast cells[66] and by eosinophils themselves as well.[57,67] Airways challenge in allergic asthmatics increases the expression of IL-5 mRNA[29,57] and leads to increased levels of IL-5 protein.[68,69] IL-5 specifically upregulates the integrin Mac-1 and downregulates L-selectin on the surface of eosinophils,[69a] potentially enhancing eosinophil migration into inflamed tissues. Anti-IL-5 neutralizing antibodies completely block the characteristic eosinophilia associated with parasitic infections[70,71]; therefore, this approach has attracted attention with respect to the eosinophilic inflammation in asthma. In guinea pig models, administration of anti-IL-5 prevented lung and BAL-fluid eosinophilia in eosinophilic inflammation induced by allergen[72] or Sephadex[73] and had no effect on the accumulation of neutrophils and mononuclear cells.[73] Furthermore, in similar models, blockade of IL-5 can inhibit antigen-induced[74] or virus-induced[75] airway hyperresponsiveness and prevent the loss of M_2-muscarinic receptor function.[76]

Known effects of IL-5 on cells other than eosinophils are limited to mouse B cells, in which IL-5 can act as a priming stimulus for resting B cells,[77] perhaps by upregulating IL-2 receptors on these cells.[78] Human basophils also may possess IL-5 receptors,[79] and IL-5 may prime them for increased histamine and leukotriene production,[80] but any role in human asthma for IL-5-mediated regulation of cells other than eosinophils remains to be determined.

INTERLEUKIN-4

IL-4 is another cytokine that is considered a typical product of the T_H2-type lymphocytes.[45,51] In addition to T cells, mast cells and basophils also can synthesize and release IL-4.[81] IL-4 is uniquely important in the induction of the T_H2 subpopulation of T cells[82] through the upregulation of the IL-1 receptor; this activity may amplify the immune response.[83] As outlined in discussion of other cytokines above and shown in Fig. 24-1, the IL-4-mediated regulation of the T_H2 helper cells has important implications for humoral immunity as well as mast cell and eosinophil development. One of the most important activities of IL-4 is its regulation of immunoglobulin production by B cells. IL-4 specifically directs isotope switching to IgE and augments IgG_1 production,[84] and this property may be critical in responses to allergen challenge. Anti-IL-4 antibodies block the development of IgE in a number of immune responses in vivo[85] and mutation of the IL-4 gene in mice results in the lack of IgE and impaired IgG_1 production in these animals.[86] In addition to the central role of IL-4 in the production of IgE, IL-4 may also be an important factor in promoting the migration of eosinophils, lymphocytes, and other cells into pulmonary tissues by upregulating endothelial-cell VCAM-1,[87] to which VLA-4 on the former cell types specifically binds.[88] IL-4 mRNA expression is associated with the late-phase reaction in atopic patients,[45] and IL-4 is increased in the BAL fluid of allergic asthmatics.[30] The number of airway mast cells stain-

ing for IL-4 is increased in asthmatic subjects,[66] and allergen challenge of mast-cell-deficient mice produced fewer lung and BAL-fluid eosinophils than in normal littermates.[89] IL-4 also may have anti-inflammatory activity in that it can inhibit the production of IL-1, TNF,[90] and IL-8,[91] although this regulation probably is more complex than previously realized and may depend on kinetic and costimulatory factors.[92]

INTERLEUKIN-6

Along with IL-1 and TNF (see below), IL-6 often is considered a member of the "inflammatory triad,"[93] is produced by a variety of activated cells, and acts on a number of different targets (Table 24-1). IL-6 originally was recognized as a B-cell differentiation factor that induces the final maturation of these cells into antibody-producing cells. It also was called *interferon-β_2,*[94] as well as *hepatocyte-stimulatory factor* for its induction of acute-phase proteins in liver cells.[95] Recently, IL-6 has gained attention as a proinflammatory cytokine that may be involved in pathogenic processes in the lung. Both IL-1 and TNF are potent inducers of lung fibroblast IL-6 production,[96] and IL-6 itself may act synergistically to amplify some of the tissue effects of IL-1.[97] Release of IL-6 from alveolar macrophages from asthmatic subjects is increased during the late-phase reaction following allergen challenge.[98] Both alveolar macrophages and peripheral blood mononuclear cells from asthmatic patients secrete IL-6 after IgE-dependent stimulation.[99] Cultures of human (and guinea pig) respiratory epithelial cells also release increased amounts of IL-6 after exposure to inflammatory stimuli, including the cyokines IL-1 and TNF.[100] Glucocorticoids used in asthma treatments downregulate the expression of IL-6 (and some other cytokines) in lung fibroblasts.[101]

INTERLEUKIN-8 AND RANTES

IL-8 previously was known as neutrophil activation protein-1 (NAP-1), and it is a potent chemoattractant for neutrophils.[102] RANTES, a chemoattractant for eosinophils,[103] is a related cytokine; it, IL-8, and several other structurally related proteins constitute the family of cytokines known as *intercrines* or *chemokines* (Table 24-1). The chemokine family currently consists of at least 14 rather small (8 to 10 kDa) cytokines, and it has been divided into two subfamilies, α and β, on the basis of protein structure.[104] The proteins of both families have four conserved cysteine residues. In the α subfamily, the first two of these cysteines are separated by one other amino acid (Cys-X-Cys), and the subfamily therefore sometimes is called the *C-X-C subfamily*. In the β subfamily, the first two cysteines are directly adjacent (Cys-Cys), and the subfamily sometimes is termed the *C-C subfamily*.[104] While the C-X-C subfamily contains several members, including melanoma growth-stimulatory activator (MGSA/GROα), neutrophil-activating protein 2 (NAP-2), and platelet factor 4 (PF4),[105] IL-8 is the α chemokine that has thus far attracted the most attention as an important factor in pulmonary inflammation during asthma.[106] Production of IL-8 by alveolar macrophages from asthmatics has been shown to be increased fourfold following stimulation (and 20-fold greater than other cytokines tested).[107] IL-8 can be synthesized by several other types of airway cells, including fibroblasts,[108] bronchial epithelial cells,[109] and eosinophils themselves.[110] TNF and IL-1 released by lipopolysaccharide-stimulated alveolar macrophages can induce production of IL-8 by lung fibroblasts,[108] while direct stimulation of these fibroblasts by lipopolysaccharide had no effect on IL-8 transcription or release.[108,111] Because of its chemotactic activity for neutrophils, as well as perhaps for primed eosinophils,[27,112] the role of IL-8 in vivo has been examined recently in animal models of pulmonary inflammation. Intranasal administration of IL-8 to guinea pigs induced a significant increase in BAL-fluid neutrophils (but not eosinophils) and enhanced the bronchial responsiveness to histamine in a dose-dependent manner.[113] Furthermore, treatment with a thromboxane receptor antagonist significantly inhibited this hyperresponsiveness, a finding that supports a role for thromboxane A_2 in neutrophil-induced bronchial hyperreactivity.[113] In rats, administration of anti-IL-8 blocked glycogen-induced neutrophil accumulation in the lungs and prevented inflammatory lung injury.[114]

RANTES and members of the β chemokine subfamily are chemotactic for eosinophils,[103,115] monocytes,[116,117] and memory T cells,[117] but not for neutrophils. RANTES is produced by macrophages, T lymphocytes, platelets, and by stimulated endothelial cells. Interferon-γ (IFN-γ) and TNF-α were shown to act synergistically to induce the in vitro production of RANTES by human umbilical vein endothelial cells.[118] This synergy apparently was caused by "sensitization" or priming of the endothelial cells by IFN-γ to respond to TNF-α, and it was present at the mRNA level. Interestingly, the T_H2-type cytokines IL-4 and IL-13 significantly inhibited the production of RANTES, but IL-10 had no effect.[118] These observations underscore the potential complexity of cytokine networks, which probably exist in many pathophysiologic processes in the lung and elsewhere. Because RANTES is a chemoattractant for eosinophils and memory T cells, it may be an important cytokine in human allergic reactions, including atopic asthma, in which these cells are characteristically involved.[103,119] RANTES also can activate human eosinophils, inducing the release of granular cationic proteins and stimulating the respiratory burst in these cells.[120] RANTES also may upregulate surface adhesion molecules like β2-integrins on eosinophils[119] and basophils[120] and thereby enhance their adhesion to endothelial cells during the beginning of their migration into inflammatory sites. Other β chemokines have been examined for their effects on the activation and migration of eosinophils. Like RANTES, macrophage inflammatory protein-1α (MIP-1α) induces migration and degranulation, but it does not cause a respiratory burst in eosinophils.[121] The monocyte chemoattractant protein-1 (MCP-1) is expressed by alveolar macrophages during chronic lung injury[122] and probably is an important mediator of mononuclear cell accumulation during inflammatory processes in the lung.[123] However, MCP-1 does not appear to be active on human eosinophils.[121] The chemokines likely will remain the subject of intense study over the next few years, and additional roles for these important cytokines in the lung, particularly

during inflammatory processes such as asthma, will be recognized (see also Chap. 27).

OTHER INTERLEUKINS

To date, a total of 15 cytokines are designated as interleukins (Table 24-1). Except in the cases discussed above, little is known regarding the relationship of these interleukins to the normal function of the lung or to the immunologic or pathophysiologic aspects of asthma. Several of these interleukins directly affect lymphocyte development or differentiation and, therefore, may affect indirectly humoral or cellular immune responses in the lung. IL-7 was identified initially as a B-cell growth factor in bone marrow, but it also is found in the spleen and thymus and acts as a growth factor for immature thymocytes[124] and mature peripheral T cells.[125] Recently, a human lung cancer cell line was shown to produce IL-7,[126] and the administration of IL-7 to melanoma-bearing mice increased natural killer cell activity and reduced lung metastases.[127] Finally, IL-7 gene expression was detected in BAL-fluid cells from lung transplant patients.[128] Thus, it seems clear that IL-7 can be produced by cells in the lung, but any role for IL-7 in the pathophysiology of asthma is speculative at present. IL-9 originally was identified as a murine growth factor (then termed P40) for some T-cell clones,[129] but recently it has been shown to enhance IL-4-induced IgE and IgG production by human B cells.[130] In addition, IL-9 can induce mast cell differentiation by stimulating IL-6 production, and it can upregulate the expression of the high-affinity IgE receptor.[131] Consequently, IL-9 may be involved in the regulation of allergic inflammation, including asthma, but it has not yet been examined in this regard. The regulation of IL-9 synthesis again illustrates the complexity of the cytokine network; a hierarchical model for IL-9 production was proposed recently which involves IL-2, TGF-β, IL-4, IFN-γ, and combinations of these cytokines.[132]

IL-10 is an important regulatory cytokine in T-cell interactions (Fig. 24-1) and probably plays a role in T-cell subset interactions during pulmonary disease. IL-10 was discovered as a mediator produced by murine T_H2 cells, which suppressed cytokine production of T_H1 cells.[133] It is now clear that IL-10 also can be produced by B cells,[134] monocytes, and macrophages[135] and can affect cell types other than T cells.[136] Because the T_H2 cytokine profile typically is associated with allergic asthma,[30] IL-10 probably is among the interleukins released in this disease, but its precise role in asthma is not known. However, there is evidence that IL-10 production in the lungs may participate in mechanisms that protect the lung from some types of inflammatory injury.[137] Like the related interleukin IL-6, IL-11 is a pleiotropic cytokine that acts on several targets in the hematopoietic system and elsewhere.[138–140] The IL-6 type cytokines also can stimulate neurons to increase the production of tachykinins,[141] which may be important in the pathophysiology of asthma.[142] Thus, IL-11 recently has attracted attention as a pulmonary cytokine that may be an important regulator of epithelial and periepithelial inflammation and physiology.[143,144] Mast cells are prevalent at epithelial surfaces in the respiratory tract and are involved in the pathogenesis of allergic reactions. Histamine is a major mediator released by mast cells and has been shown to regulate IL-11 production by human lung fibroblasts; further, histamine interacts with TGF-β and IL-1 to augment the production of fibroblast IL-11.[144]

Interleukin-12 is a heterodimeric cytokine which has costimulatory activity for T-cell proliferation and enhances both IFN-γ production in the lung[145] and the cytolytic activity of natural killer cells and activated T cells.[131,146] While IL-12 can stimulate the development of T_H1 T cells[147] and can suppress IgE production stimulated by the T_H2-type cytokine IL-4,[148] any roles for IL-12 in modulating the immune responses in allergic pulmonary inflammation remain to be demonstrated.

Interleukin-13 is produced specifically by activated T cells[149] and shares some sequence homology (~25 percent)[150] and certain biologic activities with IL-4. IL-13 has been shown to costimulate B cells to proliferate[149] and to cause immunoglobulin switching leading to an increase in IgE synthesis.[151] IL-13 also can regulate cell surface molecules, including integrins, on monocytes and can inhibit the production of proinflammatory cytokines such as IL-1, IL-6, and TNF-α by activated human monocytes.[152] The production of IL-1ra (see discussion above) by alveolar macrophages is significantly augmented by IL-13, and IL-13 also suppressed the production of TNF-α, IL-1, and IL-6 by stimulated alveolar macrophages.[153] While IL-13 does not stimulate T cells, as does IL-4,[131] the activities that IL-13 shares with IL-4 may be due to signaling by a receptor subunit shared by the two cytokines.[154]

Interleukin-14 is a recently discovered cytokine that is produced by both CD4+ T cells (T_H1 and T_H2) and CD8+ T cells upon stimulation. IL-14 induces the proliferation of a subpopulation of B cells and may have a role in the development and maintenance of B-cell memory. To date, the receptor for IL-14 has been found only on B cells,[155] and no studies of IL-14 activity in specific pulmonary diseases have been reported.

Interleukin-15 is the latest addition to the interleukin class and, like IL-14, is produced by both CD4+ and CD8+ T cells after activation.[156] IL-15 mRNA has been found in a wide variety of tissues, including lung; fibroblast and epithelial cells lines as well as monocytes synthesize significant quantities of it in vitro.[157] In a relationship similar to that between IL-13 and IL-4, studies suggest that IL-15 uses two of the subunits (β and γ) of the IL-2 receptor[156,158] and shares many activities with IL-2. Both interleukins stimulate the proliferation of T cells andlymphokine-activated killer (LAK) cells; however, recent evidence indicates that IL-2 and IL-15 use the β receptor subunit by different mechanisms.[156] While administration of IL-2 to rats causes an inflammatory infiltrate and airway hyperresponsiveness, there are no reports to date of similar studies using IL-15.

TUMOR NECROSIS FACTOR-α

TNF-α is an important proinflammatory cytokine; it is produced by macrophages primarily, but also by mast cells, epithelial cells, and many other cell types.[159] TNF was named for its capacity to cause hemorrhagic necrosis of cer-tain tumors in vivo[93]; it has also been called *cachectin* and *macrophage cytoxic factor*, among other names.[50] More recently, however, TNF-α has attracted attention for a variety of other biologic activities, including modulation of adhesion molecule expression on endothelial cells and activation of granulocytes. TNF-α also stimulates the proliferation of fibroblasts and induces the production of other cytokines, such as IL-2 and IL-6.[93] TNF-α mRNA expression is increased in allergic inflammation in asthmatics,[160] and mucosa from mildly atopic asthmatic subjects contains significantly larger numbers of mast cells staining for TNF-α than tissue from normal subjects.[66] Bronchoalveolar leukocytes from asthmatic patients release increased amounts of TNF-α after stimulation with lipopolysaccharide (LPS) or phytohemagglutinin/phorbol 12-myristate 13-acetate (PHA/PMA) in vitro,[107,161] as do monocytes and macrophages from subjects with occupational and allergic asthma after bronchoprovocation.[98,162] IgE triggering leads to increased expression of TNF-α mRNA in macrophages in vitro[99] and in epithelial cells in vivo.[163,164] Human tissue eosinophils from nasal polyps[165,166] and peripheral blood eosinophils from patients with hypereosinophilic syndrome[165] produce TNF-α; TNF-α, in turn, may stimulate eosinophils to increase oxidant production and cytotoxicity.[167] TNF induces bronchial epithelial cells to produce cytokines such as GM-CSF, IL-6, and IL-8,[13] as well as the enzyme nitric oxide synthase, which is expressed in asthmatic airways.[168] Upregulation of the expression of the adhesion molecules ICAM-1, VCAM-1, and E-selectin on the surface of epithelial and endothelial cells following stimulation with TNF[169-172] has important implications for inflammatory cell migration into pulmonary tissues and epithelial damage during asthma. Culturing of guinea pig tracheas with TNF-α (or IL-1β) in vitro reproduces the impairment of β-adrenoceptor-mediated relaxation seen in the intact animal model of asthma.[173] In rats, infusion of TNF causes bronchial hyperreactivity,[174] and, in normal human volunteers, administration of TNF-α caused an inflammatory cell influx and augmented airway reactivity.[175] Recently, studies of the effects of corticosteroids on monocytes from asthmatics demonstrated that TNF production by cells from corticosteroid-sensitive patients was inhibited but that cells from corticosteroid-resistant subjects released the same amount of TNF-α as they had before treatment.[176] Treatment of blood monocytes and alveolar macrophages with theophylline inhibits both gene expression and release of TNF-α.[177] These findings suggest at least a correlative relationship in vitro and in vivo between TNT levels and the symptomatology or therapy of asthma.

INTERFERON-γ

While IFN-γ has been studied for 30 years for its antiviral activity, recently this cytokine attracted attention for its involvement in inflammatory diseases such as asthma. IFN-γ is synthesized and released by T_H1 cells and has been scrutinized for its inhibitory effects on T_H2 cells (Fig. 24-1). Indeed, because evidence suggests that a T_H2-type profile exists in asthma,[30,44,51,178] the therapeutic value of IFN-γ has been investigated recently in a number of model systems. In vitro, IFN-γ can inhibit both cell priming for IL-4 production[179] and B-cell production of IgE.[180] Moreover, the in vitro development of T_H2 lymphocyte clones is blocked by IFN-γ.[181] Administration of aerosolized IFN-γ to sensitized mice prevents antigen-induced eosinophil and CD4+ T-cell infiltration in the trachea.[182] In a perfused rabbit lung preparation, PAF-induced lung responses, including increased pulmonary arterial and peak airway pressures and total pulmonary vascular resistance, were attenuated by IFN-γ pretreatment.[183] Steroid-sensitive asthmatics respond well to prednisone, and this response is associated with an increase in IFN-γ mRNA; after treatment of steroid-resistant asthmatics, there was a decrease in cells positive for IFN-γ mRNA.[184] On the other hand, IFN-γ now is recognized to possess a variety of activities that could be considered proinflammatory. For example, treatment of human tracheal epithelial cells with IFN-γ results in increased ICAM-1 expression and ICAM-1-dependent neutrophil adherence to the cells.[185] IFN-γ can activate alveolar macrophages to release proinflammatory cytokines both in vitro and in vivo,[99,185–187] and it can act synergistically with IL-1 to increase IL-8 generation by human lung microvascular endothelial cells.[188] Furthermore, recent patient studies have not demonstrated therapeutic benefits from IFN administration,[189] and inhalation of IFN has even impaired lung ventilation in some asthmatics.[190] Thus, studies of the therapeutic usefulness of IFN-γ as an anti-inflammatory cytokine yield equivocal results, probably because of the complexity of the cytokine network in the lung. Further studies will be necessary to fully evaluate such a therapeutic approach to subduing the inflammatory processes in human asthma.

GROWTH FACTORS IN THE LUNG: TGF-β, PDGF, EFG, FGF, AND IGF-I

Although growth factors often are grouped with the cytokines, and, in fact, often are considered cytokines, production of "classic" growth factors tends to be constitutive, and the major activities of these factors are targeted at nonimmune or nonhematopoietic cells.[191] Nevertheless, the expression and activities of these protein mediators are important in the lung and in the pathophysiologic responses in the pulmonary tissue in asthma; therefore, some of these factors will be considered briefly here. Transforming growth factor-β (TGF-β) is a cytokine found in the lung and other organs, where it is secreted as an inactive protein complex.[5] Following proteolytic activation[192] and dimer formation, mature TGF-β plays a wide variety of roles in biologic processes. Most cells are capable of producing TGF-β, including lung fibroblasts[193] and eosinophils.[194] TGF-β can induce or inhibit cell growth, depending on the degree of differentiation, the cell type, and the presence of other cytokines.[5,131] It is a potent mitogen for fibroblasts in the presence of platelet-derived growth factor (PDGF) or in autoimmune diseases with lung involvement[195]; however, in the presence of epidermal growth factor (EGF), TGF-β inhibits fibroblast growth.[196] TGF-β also induces extracellular matrix formation[197] and, recently, TGF-β was shown to increase the production of fibronectin by bronchial epithelial

cells.[198] Given the complexity of TGF-β interactions, it is not surprising that clarification of its role(s) in asthma await additional studies.

Platelet-derived growth factor (PDGF) is a 30-kDa cationic protein originally isolated from the alpha granules of platelets; it can exist as a homo- or heterodimer of A and/or B chains, each dimer isoform inducing and binding to homo- or heterodimeric complexes of the PDGF α and β receptors.[199] Responses of cells to PDGF depend on the stimulating isoform and the receptor types expressed.[131] PDGF is expressed in alveolar macrophages,[200] and its production can be upregulated by IFN-γ[201] and dexamethasone.[202] While PDGF is found in the lung and can stimulate fibroblast and smooth muscle proliferation[203] as well as eosinophil degranulation and the respiratory burst,[204] a recent study found no correlation between PDGF and structural changes in airways of patients with asthma or chronic obstructive pulmonary disease (COPD)[205]; thus, its importance in asthma is not clear.

Epidermal growth factor is a small (~6kDa) polypeptide which stimulates the proliferation of several epithelial tissues[131] and may affect the growth of other cell types as well. Secretion of EGF by macrophages may be stimulated by IFN-γ,[206] and EGF has been hypothesized to play a role in smooth muscle hyperplasia in asthma.[207] Interestingly, salbutamol reduces the mitogenic responses of cultured airway smooth muscle cells to EGF through activation of the $β_2$-adrenoceptor.[208] The fibroblast growth factor (FGF) family consists of a number of proteins ranging in size from 15 to 32 kDa and sharing 30 to 70 percent amino acid sequence identity.[131] As their name indicates, FGFs stimulate the proliferation of fibroblasts and may be involved in fibrogenesis in the airways.[27] FGFs also have a role in tumor vascularization,[209] and they may stimulate angiogenesis in the lung during chronic asthma.[27] Expression of insulin-like growth factor-I (IGF-I) is seen in most tissues; it is involved primarily in normal growth of the lung, but it may be involved in tissue repair and pulmonary fibrosis as well.[5] IGF-I is released by human airway epithelial cells[210] and by alveolar macrophages[211,212] in culture and is active in stimulating fibroblast proliferation. Like TGF-β and some other factors, IGF-I can modulate the production of extracellular matrix molecules such as collagen[213] and play a role in airway remodeling.

Conclusion

The study of interleukins and other cytokines in the normal human lung and during the inflammatory processes of bronchial asthma and remodeling processes still is in its infancy. Clearly, several cytokines are involved in the pathophysiology of asthma, and the lung contains a diversity of cells that produce these cytokines under various, incompletely defined conditions. New cytokines are discovered each year, and novel activities of known cytokines are frequently revealed by in vitro and in vivo experimentation. Assessment and clarification of the roles of cytokines in lung disease and their potential as therapeutic agents or targets of therapy are laudable and challenging goals. The complexity of the cytokine network and the intricate and sometimes paradoxical cellular responses to combinations or sequences of cytokines will complicate this pursuit. Nevertheless, an organized, multipronged approach, using techniques ranging from classic cell culture to in vivo testing and the latest molecular manipulations, should provide many answers in the coming years.

References

1. Dumonde DC, Wolstencroft RA, Panayi GS, et al.: 'Lymphokines': non-antibody mediators of cellular immunity generated by lymphocyte activation. *Nature* 169; 224:38.
2. Cohen S, Bigazzi PE, Yoshida T: Similarities of T cell function in cell mediated immunity and antibody production. *Cell Immunol* 1974; 12:150.
3. Aarden LA, Brunner TK, Cerottini JC, et al.: Revised nomenclature for antigen-nonspecific T cell proliferation and helper factors. *J Immunol* 1979; 123:2928.
4. Balkwell FR, Burke F: The cytokine network. *Immunol Today* 1989; 10:299.
5. Kelley J: Cytokines of the lung. *Am Rev Respir Dis* 1990; 141:765.
6. Dinarello CA: Interleukin-1 and biologically related cytokines. *Adv Immunol* 1989; 44:153.
7. March CJ, Mosley B, Larsen A, et al.: Cloning, sequence and expression of two distinct human interleukin complementary DNAs. *Nature* 1985; 315:641.
8. Dower SK, Kronheim SR, Hopp TK, et al.: The cell surface receptors for interleukin-1 alpha and interleukin-1 beta are identical. *Nature* 1986; 324:266.
9. Mattoli S, Mattoso VL, Soloperto M, et al.: Cellular and biochemical characteristics of bronchoalveolar lavage fluid in symptomatic nonallergic asthma. *J Allergy Clin Immunol* 1991; 84:794.
10. Tsukagochi H, Sakamoto T, Xu W, et al.: Interleukin-1β-induced airway hyperresponsiveness and inflammation in Brown Norway rats: role of active sensitization. *Am Rev Respir Dis* 1993; 147:A1013.
11. Mattoli S, Colotta F, Fincato G, et al.: Time course of Il-1 and IL-6 synthesis and release in human bronchial epithelial cell cultures exposed to toluene diisocyanate. *J Cell Physiol* 1991; 149:260.
12. Heiss LN, Moser SA, Unanue ER, Goldman WE: Interleukin-1 is linked to the respiratory epithelial cytopathology of pertussis. *Infect Immun* 1993; 61:3123.
13. Cromwell O, Hamid Q, Corrigan CJ, et al.: Expression and generation of interleukin-8, IL-5, and granulocyte colony stimulating factor by bronchial epithelial cells and enhancement by IL-1β and tumor necrosis factor-α. *Immunology* 1992; 77:330.
14. Kwon OJ, Collins PD, Au B, et al.: Glucocorticoid inhibition of TNF-α-induced IL-8 gene expression in human primary cultured epithelial cells. *Immunology* 1994; 81:379.
15. Borish L, Mascali JJ, Dishuck J, et al.: Detection of alveolar macrophage-derived IL-1β in asthma. *J Immunol* 1992; 149:3078.
16. Elias JA, Reynolds MM, Kotloff RM, Kern JA: Fibroblast interleukin 1β: Synergistic stimulation by recombinant interleukin and tumor necrosis factor and posttranscriptional regulation. *Proc Natl Acad Sci USA* 1989; 86:6171.
17. Elias JA, Reynolds MM: Interleukin-1 and tumor necrosis factor synergistically stimulate lung fibroblast interleukin-1α production. *Am J Respir Cell Mol Biol* 1990; 3:13.
18. Bochner BS, Undem BJ, Lichtenstein LM: Immunological aspects of allergic asthma. *Annu Rev Immunol* 1994; 12:295.
19. Sanz M-J, Weg VB, Bolanowski MA, Nourshargh S: IL-1 is a potent inducer of eosinophil accumulation in rat skin: Inhibition of response by a platelet activating factor antagonist and an anti-IL-8 antibody. *J Immunol* 1995; 154:1364.
20. del Pozo V, de Andres B, Martin E, et al.: Murine eosinophils and IL-1 mRNA detection by in situ hybridization: production and release of IL-1 from peritoneal eosinophils. *J Immunol* 1990; 144:3117.
21. Hannum CH, Wilcox CJ, Arend WP, et al.: Interleukin-1 receptor antagonist activity of a human interleukin-1 inhibitor. *Nature* 1990; 343:336.
22. Eisenberg SP, Evans RJ, Arend WP, et al.: Primary structure and functional expression from complementary DNA of a human interleukin-1 receptor antagonist. *Nature* 1990; 343:341.
23. Arend WP: Interleukin-1 receptor antagonist: a new member of the interleukin 1 family. *J Clin Invest* 1991; 88:1445.
24. Gosset P, Lassalle P, Tonnel AB, et al.: Production of an interleukin-1 inhibitory factor by human alveolar macrophages from mammals and allergic asthmatic patients. *Am Rev Respir Dis* 1988; 138:40.
25. Selig W, Tocker J: Effect of interleukin-1 receptor antagonist on antigen-induced pulmonary responses in guinea-pigs. *Eur J Pharmacol* 1992; 213:331.
26. Watson ML, Smith D, Bourne AD, et al.: Cytokines contribute to airway dysfunction in antigen-challenged guinea pigs: inhibition of airway hyperreactivity, pulmonary eosinophil accumulation and tumor necrosis factor generation by pretreatment with an interleukin-1 receptor antagonist. *Am J Respir Cell Mol Biol* 1993; 8:365.
27. Barnes PJ: Cytokines as mediators of chronic asthma. *Am J Respir Crit Care Med* 1994; 150:S42.
28. Smith KA: T-cell growth factor. *Immunol Rev* 1980; 51:337.
29. Krishnaswamy G, Liu MC, Su S-N, et al.: Analysis of cytokine transcripts in the bronchoalveolar lavage cells of patients with asthma. *Am J Respir Cell Mol Biol* 1993; 9:279.
30. Walker C, Bauer W, Braun RK, et al.: Activated T cells and cytokines in bronchoalveolar lavages from patients with various lung diseases associated with eosinophilia. *Am J Respir Crit Care Med* 1994; 150:1038.
31. Calderon E, Gomez-Sanchez CE, Cozza EN, et al.: Modulation of endothelin-1 production by a pulmonary epithelial cell line: I. Regulation by glucocorticoids. *Biochem Pharmacol* 1994; 48:2065.
32. Renzi PM, Sapienza S, Wasterman S, et al.: Effect of interleukin-2 on the airway response to antigen in the rat. *Am Rev Respir Dis* 1992; 146:163.
33. Nakamura Y, Ozaki T, Kamei T, et al.: Increased granulocyte/macrophage colony-stimulating factor by mononuclear cells from peripheral blood of patients with bronchial asthma. *Am Rev Respir Dis* 1993; 147:87.
34. Rand TH, Silberstein DS, Kornfeld H, Weller PF: Human eosinophils express functional interleukin-2 receptors. *J Clin Invest* 1991; 88:825.
35. Park CS, Lee SM, Uh ST, et al.: Soluble interleukin-2 receptor and cellular profiles in bronchoalveolar lavage fluid from patients with bronchial asthma. *J Allergy Clin Immunol* 1993; 91:623.
36. Corrigan CJ, Kay AB: CD4+ lymphocyte activation in acute severe asthma: relationship to disease severity. *Am Rev Respir Dis* 1990; 140:970.
37. Gleich, GJ: The eosinophil and bronchial asthma: current understanding. *J Allergy Clin Immunol* 1990; 85:422.
38. Bousquet J, Chanez P, Lacoste JY, et al.: Eosinophilic inflammation in asthma. *N Engl J Med* 1990; 323:1033.
39. Calhoun WJ, Sedgwick J, Busse WW: The role of eosinophils in the pathophysiology of asthma. *Ann NY Acad Sci* 1991; 629:62.

40. Hamann KJ, White SR, Gundel RH, Gleich GJ: Interactions between respiratory epithelium and eosinophil granule proteins in asthma: the eosinophil hypothesis, in Farmer SG, Hay DWP (eds): *The Airway Epithelium: Structure and Function in Health and Disease.* New York, Marcel Dekker, 1991:255.

41. Arai K, Lee F, Miyajima A, et al.: Cytokines: coordinators of immune and inflammatory responses. *Annu Rev Biochem* 1990; 59:783.

42. Kita H, Ohnish T, Okubo Y, et al.: Granulocyte/macrophage colony-stimulating factor and interleukin 3 release from human peripheral blood eosinophils and neutrophils. *J Exp Med* 1991; 174:745.

43. Fujisawa T, Atsuta J, Ichimi R, et al.: Interferon-γ induces interleukin-3 release from peripheral blood eosinophils. *J Allergy Clin Immunol* 1993; 91:175.

44. Robinson DR, Hamid Q, Ying S, et al.: Predominant T$_H$2-like bronchoalveolar lavage T-lymphocyte population in atopic asthma. *N Engl J Med* 1992; 326:298.

45. Kay AB, Ying S, Varney V, et al.: Messenger RNA expression of the cytokine gene cluster, interleukin 3 (IL-3), IL-4, IL-5, and granulocyte/macrophage colony-stimulating factor in allergen-induced late-phase cutaneous reactions in atopic subjects. *J Exp Med* 1991; 173:775.

46. Wardlaw AJ: Eosinophil adhesion receptors. *Behr Inst Mitt* 1993; 92:178.

47. Rothenberg ME, Owen WF Jr, Silberstein DS, et al.: Human eosinophils have prolonged survival, enhanced functional properties and become hypodense when exposed to human interleukin 3. *J Clin Invest* 1988; 81:1986.

48. Warringa RA, Koenderman L, Kok PTM, et al.: Modulation and induction of eosinophil chemotaxis by granulocyte-macrophage colony-stimulating factor and IL-3. *Blood* 1991; 77:2694.

49. Carlson M, Peterson C, Venge P: The influence of IL-3, IL-5, and GM-CSF on normal human eosinophil and neutrophil C3b-induced degranulation. *Allergy* 1993; 48:437.

50. Callard R, Gearing A: *The Cytokine Facts Book.* New York, Academic Press, 1994.

51. Robinson D, Hamid Q, Bentley A, et al.: Activation of CD4+ T cells, increased T$_H$2-type cytokine mRNA expression, and eosinophil recruitment in bronchoalveolar lavage after allergen inhalation challenge in patients with atopic asthma. *J Allergy Clin Immunol* 1993; 92:313.

52. Churchill L, Friedman B, Schleimer RP, Proud D: Production of granulocyte-macrophage colony-stimulating factor by cultured human tracheal epithelial cells. *Immunology* 1992; 75:189.

53. Sousa AR, Poston RN, Lane SJ, et al.: Detection of GM-CSF in asthmatic bronchial epithelium and decrease by inhaled corticosteroids. *Am Rev Respir Dis* 1993; 147:1557.

54. Kato M, Schleimer RP: Antiinflammatory steroids inhibit granulocyte/macrophage colony-stimulating factor production by human lung tissue. *Lung* 1994; 172:113.

55. Nakamura Y, Ozaki T, Kamgi T, et al.: Increased granulocyte-macrophage colony-stimulating factor production by mononuclear cells from peripheral blood of patients with bronchial asthma. *Am Rev Respir Dis* 1993; 147:87.

56. Moqbel R, Hamid Q, Ying S, et al.: Expression of messenger RNA and immunoreactivity for the granulocyte/macrophage colony-stimulating factor in activated human eosinophils. *J Exp Med* 1991; 174:749.

57. Broide DH, Paine MM, Firestein GF: Eosinophils express interleukin 5 and granulocyte/macrophage colony-stimulating factor mRNA at sites of allergic inflammation in asthmatics. *J Clin Invest* 1992; 90:1414.

58. Gelder CM, Morrison JFJ, Southcott AM, et al.: Polymerase chain reaction cytokine profiles of induced sputum from asthmatic subjects. *Am Rev Respir Dis* 1993; 147:A786.

59. Lopez AF, Williamson DJ, Gamble JR, et al.: Recombinant human granulocyte-macrophage colony-stimulating factor stimulates in vitro mature human neutrophil and eosinophil function, surface receptor expression, and survival. *J Clin Invest* 1988; 78:1220.

60. Naccache PH, Faucher N, Borgeat P, et al.: Granulocyte-macrophage colony-stimulating factor modulates the excitation-response coupling sequence in human neutrophils. *J Immunol* 1988; 140:3541.

61. Howell CJ, Pujol J-L, Crea AEG, et al.: Identification of an alveolar macrophage-derived activity in bronchial asthma that enhances leukotriene C$_4$ generarion by human eosinophils stimulated by ionophore A23187 as a granulocyte-macrophage colony-stimulating factor. *Am Rev Respir Dis* 1989; 140:1340.

62. Fabian I, Kletter Y, Mor S, et al.: Activation of human eosinophil and neutrophil functions by haematopoietic growth factors: comparisons of IL-1, IL-3, IL-5 and GM-CSF. *Br J Haematol* 1992; 80:137.

63. Schauer U, Leinhaas C, Jager R, Rieger CHL: Enhanced superoxide generation by eosinophils from asthmatic children. *Int Arch Allergy Appl Immunol* 1991; 96:317.

64. Sanderson CJ: Interleukin-5, eosinophils and disease. *Blood* 1992; 79:3101.

65. Weller PF. Cytokine regulation of eosinophil function. *Clin Immunol Immunopathol* 1992; 62:S55.

66. Bradding P, Roberts KJA, Britten KM, et al.: Interleukin-4, -5 and -6 and tumor necrosis factor-α in normal and asthmatic airways: evidence for the human mast cell as a source of these cytokines. *Am J Respir Cell Mol Biol* 1994; 10:471.

67. Desreumaux P, Janin A, Colombel JF, et al.: Interleukin 5 messenger RNA expression by eosinophils in the intestinal mucosa of patients with coeliac disease. *J Exp Med* 1992; 175:293.

68. Sedgwick JB, Calhoun WJ, Gleich GJ, et al.: Immediate and late airway response of allergic rhinitis patients to segmental antigen challenge: characterization of eosinophil and mast cell mediators. *Am Rev Respir Dis* 1991; 144:1274.

69. Ohnishi T, Kita H, Weiler D, et al.: IL-5 is the predominant eosinophil-active cytokine in the antigen-induced pulmonary late-phase reaction. *Am Rev Respir Dis* 1993; 147:901.

69a. Neeley SP, Hamann KJ, White SR, et al.: Selective upregulation of expression of surface adhesion molecules Mac-1, L-selectin, and VLA-4 on human eosinophils and neutrophils. *Am J Respir Cell Mol Biol* 1993; 8:633.

70. Coffman RL, Seymour BW, Hudak S, et al.: Antibody to interleukin-5 inhibits helminth-induced eosinophilia in mice. *Science* 1989; 245:308.

71. Okudaira H, Nogami M, Matsuzaki G, et al.: T-cell-dependent accumulation of eosinophils in the lung and its inhibition by monoclonal anti-interleukin-5. *Int Arch Allergy Appl Immunol* 1991; 94:171.

72. Gulbenkian AR, Egan RW, Fernandez X, et al.: Interleukin-5 modulates eosinophil accumulation in allergic guinea pig lung. *Am Rev Respir Dis* 1992; 148:263.

73. Das AM, Williams TJ, Lobb R, Nourshargh S: Lung eosinophilia is dependent on IL-5 and the adhesion molecules CD18 and VLA-4 in a guinea-pig model. *Immunology* 1995; 84:41.

74. Mauser PJ, Pitman A, Fernandez X, et al.: The effects of anti-IL-5 on antigen-induced airway hyperreactivity and pulmonary eosinophilia in guinea pigs. *Am Rev Respir Dis* 1992; 145:A859.

75. van Oosterhoot AJM, van Ark I, Folkerts G, et al.: Antibody to interleukin-5 inhibits virus-induced airway hyperresponsive-

ness to histamine in guinea pigs. *Am J Respir Crit Care Med* 1995; 151:177.

76. Elbon CL, Jacoby DB, Fryer AD: Pretreatment with an antibody to interleukin-5 prevents loss of pulmonary M_2 muscarinic receptor function in antigen-challenged guinea pigs. *Am J Respir Cell Mol Biol* 1995; 12:320.

77. O'Garra A, Warren DJ, Holman M, et al.: Interleukin 4 (B-cell growth factor II eosinophil differentiation factor) is a mitogen and differentiation factor for preactivated murine B lymphocytes. *Proc Natl Acad Sci USA* 1986; 83:5228.

78. Loughnan MS, Nossal GJ: Interleukins 4 and 5 control expression of IL-2 receptor on murine B cells through independent induction of its two chains. *Nature* 1989; 340:76.

79. Lopez AF, Eglinton JM, Lyons AB, et al.: Human interleukin 3 inhibits the binding of granulocyte-macrophage colony-stimulating factor and interleukin 5 to basophils and strongly enhances their functional activity. *J Cell Physiol* 1990; 145:69.

80. Bischoff SC, Brunner T, DeWeck AL, Dahinden CA: Interleukin 5 modifies histamine release and leukotriene generation by human basophils in response to diverse agonists. *J Exp Med* 1990; 172:1577.

81. Plaut M, Pierce JH, Watson CJ, et al.: Mast cell line produce lymphokines in response to cross-linkage of $Fc_\epsilon RI$ or to calcium ionophores. *Nature* 1989; 339:64.

82. Ricci M: IL-4: a key cytokine in atopy. *Clin Exp Allergy* 1994; 24:801.

83. Koch K, Ye K, Clark BD, Dinarello CA: Interleukin 4 (IL-4) upregulates gene and surface IL-1 receptor type I in murine T helper type II cells. *Eur J Immunol* 1992; 22:153.

84. Gauchat J-F, Lebman DA, Coffman RL, et al.: Structure and expression of germline ϵ transcripts in human B cells induced by interleukin-4 to switch to IgE production. *J Exp Med* 1990; 172:463.

85. Finkelman FD, Holmes J, Katona IM, et al.: Lymphokine control of in vivo immunoglobulin isotype selection. *Annu Rev Immunol* 1990; 8:303.

86. Kuhn R, Rajewsky K, Muller W: Generation and analysis of interleukin-4 deficient mice. *Science* 1991; 254:707.

87. Schleimer RP, Sterbinsky SA, Kaiser J, et al.: Interleukin-4 induces adherence of human eosinophils and basophils but not neutrophils to endothelium: association with expression of VCAM-1. *J Immunol* 1992; 148:1086.

88. Hemler ME: VLA proteins in the integrin family: structures, functions, and their role on leukocytes. *Annu Rev Immunol* 1990; 8:365.

89. Kung TT, Stelts D, Zurcher JA, et al.: Mast cells modulate allergic pulmonary eosinophilia in mice. *Am J Respir Cell Mol Biol* 1995; 12:404.

90. Essner R, Rhoades K, McBride WH, et al.: IL-4 down-regulates IL-1 and TNF gene expression in human monocytes. *J Immunol* 1989; 142:3857.

91. Standiford TJ, Strieter RM, Chensue SW, et al.: IL-4 inhibits expression of IL-8 from stimulated human monocytes. *J Immunol* 1990; 145:1435.

92. D'Andrea A, Ma X, Aste-Amezaga, et al.: Stimulatory and inhibitory effects of interleukin (IL)-4 and IL-13 on the production of cytokines by human peripheral blood mononuclear cells: priming for IL-12 and tumor necrosis factor α production. *J Exp Med* 1995; 181:537.

93. Hamblin AS: *Cytokines and Cytokine Receptors*, 2d ed. Oxford, Oxford University Press, 1993.

94. Tosato G, Seaman KB, Goldman ND, et al.: Monocyte-derived human B-cell growth factor identified as interferon-β_2 (BSF-2, IL-6). *Science* 1988; 239:502.

95. Gauldie J, Richard C, Harnish D, et al.: Interferon-β_2/BSF-2 shares identity with monocyte derived hepatocyte stimulating factor and regulates the major acute phase response in liver cells. *Proc Natl Acad Sci USA* 1987; 84:7251.

96. Elias JA, Lentz V: IL-1 and tumor necrosis factor synergistically stimulate fibroblast IL-6 production and stabilize IL-6 messenger RNA. *J Immunol* 1990; 145:161.

97. Elias JA, Trinchieri G, Beck JM, et al.: A synergistic interaction of IL-6 and IL-1 mediates the thymocyte-stimulating activity produced by recombinant IL-1-stimulated fibroblasts. *J Immunol* 1989; 142:509.

98. Gosset P, Tsicopoulos A, Wallaert B, et al.: Increased secretion of tumor necrosis factor α and interleukin-6 by alveolar macrophages consecutive to the development of the late asthmatic reaction. *J Allergy Clin Immunol* 1991; 88:561.

99. Gosset P, Tsicopoulos A, Wallaert B, et al.: Tumor necrosis factor α and interleukin-6 production by human mononuclear phagocytes from allergic asthmatics after IgE-dependent stimulation. *Am Rev Respir Dis* 1992; 146:768.

100. Adler KB, Fischer BM, Wright DT, et al.: Interactions between respiratory epithelial cells and cytokines: relationships to lung inflammation. *Ann NY Acad Sci* 1994; 725:128.

101. Tobler A, Meier R, Seitz M, et al.: Glucocorticoids downregulate gene expression of GM-CSF, NAP-1/IL-8, and IL-6, but not of M-CSF in human fibroblasts. *Blood* 1992; 79:45.

102. Yoshimura T, Matsushima K, Tanaka S, et al.: Purification of a human monocyte-derived neutrophil chemotactic factor that has peptide sequence similarity to other host defense cytokines. *Proc Natl Acad Sci USA* 1987; 84:9233.

103. Kameyoshi Y, Dörschner A, Mallet AI, et al.: Cytokine RANTES released by thrombin-stimulated platelets is a potent attractant for human eosinophils. *J Exp Med* 1992; 176:587.

104. Taub DD, Oppenheim JJ: Review of the chemokine meeting. The Third International Symposium of Chemotactic Cytokines. *Cytokine* 1993; 5:175.

105. Walz A, Dewald B, von Tscharner V, Baggiolini M: Effects of the neutrophil-activating peptide NAP-2, platelet basic protein, connective tissue-activating peptide III, and platelet factor 4 on human neutrophils. *J Exp Med* 1989; 170:1745.

106. Kunkel SL, Standiford T, Kasahara K, Strieter RM: Interleukin-8 (IL-8): the major neutrophil chemotactic factor in the lung. *Exp Lung Res* 1991; 17:17.

107. Hallsworth MP, Soh CP, Lane SJ, et al.: Selective enhancement of GM-CSF, TNF-α, IL-1β and IL-8 production by monocytes and macrophages of asthmatic subjects. *Eur Respir J* 1994; 7:1096.

108. Rolfe MW, Kunkel SL, Standiford TJ, et al.: Pulmonary fibroblast expression of interleukin-8: a model for alveolar macrophage-derived cytokine networking. *Am J Respir Cell Mol Biol* 1991; 5:493.

109. Nakamura H, Yoshimura K, Jaffe HA, Crystal RG: Interleukin-8 gene expression in human bronchial epithelial cells. *J Biol Chem* 1991; 266:19611.

110. Braun RK, Franchini M, Erard F, et al.: Human peripheral blood eosinophils produce and release interleukin-8 on stimulation with calcium ionophore. *Eur J Immunol* 1993; 23:956.

111. Xing Z, Hordana M, Braciak T, et al.: Lipopolysaccharide induces expression of granulocyte/macrophage colony-stimulating factor, interleukin-8, and interleukin-6 in human nasal, but not lung, fibroblasts: evidence for heterogeneity within the respiratory tract. *Am J Respir Cell Mol Biol* 1993; 9:255.

112. Shute J: Interleukin-8 is a potent eosinophil chemoattractant. *Clin Exp Allergy* 1994; 24:203.

113. Xiu Q, Fujimara M, Nomura M, et al.: Bronchial hyperresponsiveness and airway neutrophil accumulation induced by inter-

leukin-8 and the effect of the thromboxane A$_2$ antagonists S-1452 in guinea pigs. *Clin Exp Allergy* 1995; 25:51.

114. Mulligan MS, Jones ML, Bolanowski MA, et al.: Inhibition of lung inflammatory reactions in rats by an anti-human IL-8 antibody. *J Immunol* 1993; 150:5585.

115. Alam R, Stafford S, Forsythe P, et al.: RANTES is a chemotactic and activating factor for human eosinophils. *J Immunol* 1993; 150:3442.

116. Yoshimura T, Yuhki N, Moore SK, et al.: Human monocyte chemoattractant protein-1 (MCP-1): full-length cDNA cloning, expression in mitogen-stimulated blood mononuclear leukocytes, and sequence similarity to mouse competence gene JE. *FEBS Lett* 1989; 244:487.

117. Schall TJ, Bacon K, Toy KJ, Goeddel DV: Selective attraction of monocytes and T lymphocytes of the memory phenotype by cytokine RANTES. *Nature* 1990; 347:669.

118. Marfaing-Koka A, Devergne O, Gorgone G, et al.: Regulation of the production of the RANTES chemokine by endothelial cells: Synergistic induction of IFN-γ plus TNF-α and inhibition by IL-4 and IL-13. *J Immunol* 1995; 154:1870.

119. Zhang L, Redington AE, Holgate ST: RANTES: a novel mediator of allergic inflammation? *Clin Exp Allergy* 1994; 24:899.

120. Bacon KB, Flores-Romo L, Aubry J-P, et al.: Interleukin-8 and RANTES induce the adhesion of the human basophilic cell line KU-812 to human endothelial cell monolayers. *Immunology* 1994; 82:473.

121. Rot A, Krieger M, Brunner T, et al.: RANTES and macrophage inflammatory protein 1α induce the migration and activation of normal human eosinophil granulocytes. *J Exp Med* 1992; 176:1489.

122. Brieland JK, Jones ML, Flory CM, et al.: Expression of monocyte chemoattractant protein-1 (MCR-1) by rat alveolar macrophages during chronic lung injury. *Am J Respir Cell Mol Biol* 1993; 9:300.

123. Kunkel SL, Chensue SW, Strieter RM, et al.: Cellular and molecular aspects of granulomatous inflammation. *Am J Respir Cell Mol Biol* 1989; 1:439.

124. Henney CS: Interleukin 7: effects on early events in lymphopoiesis. *Immunol Today* 1989; 10:170.

125. Londei M, Verhoef A, Hawrylowicz C, et al.: Interleukin 7 is a growth factor for mature human T cells. *Eur J Immunol* 1990; 20:425.

126. Kuriya S, Ogata K, Hamaguchi H, et al.: A novel megakaryocyte potentiator produced by MC-1 human lung cancer cell line. *Pathobiology* 1993; 61:256.

127. Wu B, Shen RN, Wang WX, et al.: Antitumor effect of interleukin 7 in combination with local hyperthermia in mice bearing b16a melanoma cells. *Stem Cells* 1993; 11:412.

128. Whitehead BF, Stoehr C, Wu CJ, et al.: Cytokine gene expression in human lung transplant recipients. *Transplant* 1993; 56:956.

129. Uyttenhove C, Simpson RJ, Van Snick J: Functional and structural characterization of P40, a mouse glycoprotein with T-cell growth factor activity. *Proc Natl Acad Sci USA* 1988; 85:6934.

130. Dugas B, Renauld J-C, Pène J, et al.: Interleukin-9 potentiates the interleukin-4-induced immunoglobulin (IgG, IgM and IgE) production by normal human B lymphocytes. *Eur J Immunol* 1993; 23:1687.

131. Nicola NA: *Guidebook to Cytokines and Their Receptors*. Oxford, Oxford University Press, 1994.

132. Schmitt E, Germann T, Goedert S, et al.: IL-9 production of naive CD4+ T cells depends on IL-2, is synergistically enhanced by a combination of TGF-β and IL-4, and is inhibited by IFN-γ. *J Immunol* 1993; 153:3989.

133. Fiorentino DF, Bond MW, Mosmann TR: Two types of mouse helper T cell: IV. T$_H$2 clones secrete a factor that inhibits cytokine production by T$_H$1 clones. *J Exp Med* 1989; 170:2081.

134. O'Garra A, Stapleton G, Dhar V, et al.: production of cytokines by mouse B cells: B lymphomas and normal B cells produce interleukin 10. *Int Immunol* 1990; 2:821.

135. de Waal Malefyt R, Abrams J, Bennett B, et al.: IL-10 inhibits cytokine synthesis by human monocytes: an autoregulatory role of IL-10 produced by monocytes. *J Exp Med* 1991; 174:1209.

136. Howard M, O'Garra A, Ishida H, et al.: Biological properties of interleukin 10. *J Clin Immunol* 1992; 12:239.

137. Mulligan MS, Jones ML, Vaporciyan AA, et al.: Protective effects of IL-4 and IL-10 against immune complex-induced lung injury. *J Immunol* 1993; 151:5666.

138. Paul SR, Bennett F, Calvetti JA, et al.: Molecular cloning of a cDNA encoding interleukin 11, a stromal cell-derived lymphopoietic and hematopoietic cytokine. *Proc Natl Acad Sci USA* 1990; 87:7512.

139. Musashi M, Yang Y-C, Paul SR, et al.: Direct and synergistic effects of interleukin 11 on murine hemopoiesis in culture. *Proc Natl Acad Sci USA* 1991; 88:765.

140. Baumann H, Schendel P: Interleukin-11 regulates the hepatic expression of the same protein genes as interleukin-6. *J Biol Chem* 1991; 266:20424.

141. Bazan JF: Neuropoietic cytokines in the hematopoietic fold. *Neuron* 1991; 7:197.

142. Barnes PJ: Airway neuropeptides, in Busse WW, Holgate ST (eds): *Asthma and Rhinitis*. Cambridge, Blackwell Scientific, 1995:667.

143. Elias JA, Zheng T, Einarsson O, et al.: Epithelial interleukin-11: Regulation by cytokines, respiratory syncytial virus and retinoic acid. *J Biol Chem* 1994; 269:22761.

144. Zheng T, Nathanson MH, Elias JA: Histamine augments cytokine-stimulated IL-11 production by human lung fibroblasts. *J Immunol* 1994; 153:4742.

145. Gladue RP, Laquerre AM, Magna HA, et al.: In vivo augmentation of IFN-γ with a rIL-12 human/mouse chimera: pleiotropic effects against infectious agents in mice and rats. *Cytokine* 1994; 6:318.

146. Mehrotra PT, Wu D, Crim JA, et al.: Effects of IL-12 on the generation of cytotoxic activity in human CD8+ T lymphocytes. *J Immunol* 1993; 151:2444.

147. Hsieh CS, Macatonia SE, Tripp CS, et al.: Development of T$_H$1 CD4+ T cells through IL-12 produced by *Listeria*-induced macrophages. *Science* 1993; 260:547.

148. Kiniwa M Gately M, Gubler U, et al.: Recombinant interleukin-12 suppresses the synthesis of immunoglobulin E by interleukin-4 stimulated human lymphocytes. *J Clin Invest* 1992; 90:262.

149. McKenzie AN, Culpepper JA, de Waal Malefyt R, et al.: Interleukin 13, a T-cell-derived cytokine that regulates human monocyte and B-cell function. *Proc Natl Acad Sci USA* 1993; 90:3735.

150. Minty A, Chalon P, Derocq J-M, et al.: Interleukin-13 is a new human lymphokine regulating inflammatory and immune responses. *Nature* 1993; 362:248.

151. Punnonen J, Aversa G, Cocks BG, et al.: Interleukin 13 induces interleukin 4-independent IgG4 and IgE synthesis and CD23 expression by human B cells. *Proc Natl Acad Sci USA* 1993; 90:3730.

152. de Waal Malefyt R, Figdor C, Huijbens R, et al.: Effects of IL-13 on phenotype, cytokine production and cytotoxic function of human monocytes. *J Immunol* 1993; 151:6370.

153. Yanagawa H, Sone S, Haku T, et al.: Contrasting effects of interleukin-13 on interleukin-1 receptor antagonist and proinflammatory cytokine production by human alveolar macrophages. *Am J Respir Cell Mol Biol* 1995; 12:71.

154. Zurawski SM, Vega F Jr, Huyghe B, Zurawski G: Receptors for interleukin-13 and interleukin-4 are complex and share a novel

component that functions in signal transduction. *EMBO J* 1993; 12:3899.

155. Ambrus JL Jr, Jurgensen CH, Brown EJ, et al.: Identification of a receptor for high molecular weight human B cell growth factor. *J Immunol* 1988; 141:861.

156. Grabstein KH, Eisenman J, Shanebeck K, et al.: Cloning of a T cell growth factor that interacts with the β chain of the interleukin-2 receptor. *Science* 1994; 264:965.

157. Armitage RJ, Macduff BM, Eisenman J, et al.: IL-15 has stimulatory activity for the induction of B cell proliferation and differentiation. *J Immunol* 1995; 154:483.

158. Giri JG, Ahdieh M, Eisenman J, et al.: Utilization of the β and γ chains of the IL-2 receptor by the novel cytokine IL-15. *EMBO J* 1994; 13:2822.

159. Aggarwal BB: Tumor necrosis factor, in Gutterman JU, Aggarwal BB (eds): *Human Cytokines: Handbook for Basic and Clinical Researchers.* New York, Blackwell, 1992:270.

160. Ying S, Robinson DS, Varnet V, et al.: TNF alpha mRNA expression in allergic inflammation. *Clin Exp Allergy* 1991; 21:745.

161. Cembrzynska-Nowak M, Szlarz E, Inglot AD, Teodorczyk-Injeyan JA: Elevated release of tumor necrosis factor-α and interferon-γ by bronchoalveolar leukocytes from patients with bronchial asthma. *Am Rev Respir Dis* 1993; 147:291.

162. Siracusa A, Vecchiarelli A, Brugnami G, et al.: Changes in interleukin-1 and tumor necrosis factor production by peripheral blood monocytes after specific bronchoprovocation test in occupational asthma. *Am Rev Respir Dis* 1992; 146:408.

163. Ohno I, Ohkawara Y, Yamauchi K, et al.: Production of tumor necrosis factor with IgE receptor triggering from sensitized lung tissue. *Am J Respir Cell Mol Biol* 1990; 3:285.

164. Ohkawara Y, Yamauchi K, Tanno Y, et al.: Identification of TNF-producing cells in sensitized human lung after IgE receptor triggering. *Am Rev Respir Dis* 1991; 143:A201.

165. Costa JJ, Matossian K, Resnick MB, et al.: Human eosinophils can express the cytokines tumor necrosis factor-α and macrophage inflammatory protein-1α. *J Clin Invest* 1993; 91:2673.

166. Finotto S, Ohno I, Marshall JS, et al.: TNF-α production by eosinophils in upper airways inflammation (nasal polyposis). *J Immunol* 1994; 153:2278.

167. Slungaard A, Vercellotti GM, Walker G, et al.: Tumor necrosis factor α/cachetin stimulates eosinophil oxidant production and toxicity towards human endothelium. *J Exp Med* 1990; 171:2025.

168. Hamid Q, Springall DR, Riveros-Moreno V, et al.: Induction of nitric oxide synthase in asthma. *Lancet* 1993; 342:1510.

169. Pober JS, Cotran RS: Cytokines and endothelial cell biology. *Physiol Rev* 1990; 70:427.

170. Thornhill MH, Wellicome SM, Mahiouz DL, et al.: Tumor necrosis factor combines with IL-4 of IFN-γ to selectively enhance endothelial cell adhesiveness for T cells: the contribution of vascular adhesion molecule-1-dependent and -independent binding mechanisms. *J Immunol* 1991; 146:592.

171. Tosi MF, Stark JM, Smith CW, et al.: Induction of ICAM-1 expression on human airway epithelial cells by inflammatory cytokines: effects of neutrophil-epithelial cell adhesion. *Am J Respir Cell Mol Biol* 1992; 7:214.

172. Lassalle P, Gosset P, Delneste Y, et al.: Modulation of adhesion molecule expression on endothelial cells during the late asthmatic reaction: role of macrophage-derived tumour necrosis factor-α. *Clin Exp Immunol* 1993; 94:105.

173. Wills-Karp M, Uchida Y, Lee JY, et al.: Organ culture with proinflammatory cytokines reproduces impairment of the β-adrenoceptor-mediated relaxation in tracheas of a guinea pig antigen model. *Am J Respir Cell Mol Biol* 1993; 8:153.

174. Kips JC, Tavernier J, Pauwels RA: Tumor necrosis factor causes bronchial hyperresponsiveness in rats. *Am Rev Respir Dis* 1992; 145:332.

175. Yates DH, Barnes PJ, Thomas PS: Tumor necrosis factor α alters human bronchial reactivity and induces inflammatory cell influx. *Am Rev Respir Dis* 1993; 147:A1011.

176. Vecchiarelli A, Siracusa A, Cenci E, et al.: Effect of corticosteroid treatment on interleukin-1 and tumour necrosis factor secretion by monocytes from subjects with asthma. *Clin Exp Allergy* 1992; 22:365.

177. Spatafora M, Chiappara G, Merendino AM, et al.: Theophylline suppresses the release of tumour necrosis factor-α by blood monocytes and alveolar macrophages. *Eur Respir J* 1994; 7:223.

178. Del Prete G: Human T_H1 and T_H2 lymphocytes: their role in the pathophysiology of atopy. *Allergy* 1992; 47:450.

179. Goldstein RA, Paul WE, Metcalfe DD, et al.: NIH conference: asthma. *Ann Intern Med* 1994; 121:698.

180. Romagniani S: Regulation and deregulation of human IgE synthesis. *Immunol Today* 1990; 11:316.

181. Maggi E, Parronchi P, Manetti R, et al.: Reciprocal effects of IFN-γ and IL-4 on the in vitro development of human T_H1 and Th2 clones. *J Immunol* 1992; 148:2142.

182. Nakajima H, Iwamoto I, Yoshida S: Aerosolized interferon-γ prevents antigen-induced eosinophil recruitment in mouse trachea. *Am Rev Respir Dis* 1993; 148:1102.

183. Huang YC, Kennedy TP, Su YF, et al.: Protection against platelet-activating factor-induced injury by interferon inducer in perfused rabbit lung. *J Appl Physiol* 1993; 74:251.

184. Leung DY, Martin RJ, Szefler SJ, et al.: Disregulation of interleukin 4, interleukin 5 and interferon gamma gene expression in steroid-resistant asthma. *J Exp Med* 1995; 181:33.

185. Look DC, Rapp SR, Keller BT, Holzman MJ: Selective induction of intracellular adhesion molecule-1 by interferon-γ in human airway epithelial cells. *Am J Physiol* 1992; 263:L79.

186. Gifford GE, Lohmann-Matthess M-L: Gamma interferon priming of mouse and human macrophages for induction of tumor necrosis factor production by bacterial lipopolysaccharide. *J Natl Cancer Inst* 1987; 78:121.

187. Jaffe HA, Buhl R, Mastrangeli A, et al.: Organ-specific cytokine therapy: local activation of mononuclear phagocytes by delivery of an aerosol of recombinant interferon-γ to the human lung. *J Clin Invest* 1991; 88:297.

188. Brown Z, Gerritsen ME, Carley WW, et al.: Chemokine gene expression and secretion by cytokine-activated human microvascular endothelial cells: Differential regulation of monocyte chemoattractant protein-1 and interleukin-8 in response to interferon-γ. *Am J Pathol* 1994; 145:913.

189. Boguniewicz M, Schneider LC, Milgrom H, et al.: Treatment of steroid-dependent asthma with recombinant interferon-γ. *J Allergy Clin Immunol* 1992; 89:288.

190. Krasnowski M, Malolepszy J, Liebhart E, Inglot AD: Inhaled natural human interferon-α induces bronchospastic reactions in asthmatics. *Arch Immunol Ther Exp* 1992; 40:75.

191. Vilcek J, Le J: Immunology of cytokines: an introduction, in Thompson A (ed): *The Cytokine Handbook.* New York, Academic Press, 1988:1.

192. Lyons RM, Keski-Oja J, Moses HL: Proteolytic activation of latent transforming growth factor-β from fibroblast-conditioned medium. *J Cell Biol* 1988; 106:1659.

193. Kelley J, Fabisiak JP, Hawes K, Abscher M: Cytokine signalling in the lung: transforming growth factor-β secretion by lung fibroblasts. *Am J Physiol* 1991; 260:L123.

194. Ohno I, Lea RG, Flanders KC, et al.: Eosinophils in chronically inflamed human upper airway tissues express tranforming growth factor $β_1$ (TGF-$β_1$). *J Clin Invest* 1992; 89:662.

195. Deguchi Y: Spontaneous increase of transforming growth fac-

tor-β production by bronchoalveolar mononuclear cells of patients with systemic autoimmune diseases affecting the lung. *Ann Rheum Dis* 1992; 51:362.

196. Roberts AB, Anzano MA, Wakefield LM, et al.: Type-β transforming growth factor: a bifunctional regulator of cellular growth. *Proc Natl Acad Sci USA* 1985; 82:119.

197. Massagué J: The tranforming growth factor-beta family. *Annu Rev Cell Biol* 1990; 6:597.

198. Romberger DJ, Beckmann JD, Claassen L, et al.: Modulation of fibronectin production of bovine bronchial epithelial cells by transforming growth factor-β. *Am J Respir Cell Mol Biol* 1992; 7:149.

199. Seifert RA, Hart CE, Philips PE, et al.: Two different subunits associate to create isoform-specific platelet-derived growth factor receptors. *J Biol Chem* 1989; 264:8771.

200. Mornex JF, Martinet Y, Yamauchi K, et al.: Spontaneous expression of the c-*sis* gene and release of a platelet-derived growth factor-like molecule by human alveolar macrophages. *J Clin Invest* 1986; 78:61.

201. Wangoo A, Taylor IK, Haynes AR, Shaw RJ: Up-regulation of alveolar macrophage platelet-derived growth factor-B (PDGF-B) mRNA by interferon-gamma from *Mycobacterium tuberculosis* antigen (PPD)-stimulated lymphocytes. *Clin Exp Immunol* 1993; 94:43.

202. Haynes AR, Shaw RJ: Dexamethasone-induced increase in platelet-derived growth factor (B) mRNA in human alveolar macrophages and myelomonocytic HL60 macrophage-like cells. *Am J Respir Cell Mol Biol* 1992; 7:198.

203. Hirst SJ, Barnes PJ, Twort CHC: Quantifying proliferation of cultured human and rabbit airway smooth muscle cells in response to serum and platelet-derived growth factor. *Am J Respir Cell Mol Biol* 1992; 7:574.

204. Bach MK, Brashler JR, Stout BK, et al.: Activation of human eosinophils by platelet-derived growth factor. *Int Arch Allergy Immunol* 1992; 97:121.

205. Aubert J-D, Hayashi S, Hards J, et al.: Platelet-derived growth factor and its receptor in lungs from patients with asthma and chronic airflow obstruction. *Am J Physiol* 1994; 266:L655.

206. Kumar RK, O'Grady R, Li W, Rajkovic I: Secretion of epidermal growth factor-like molecular species by lung parenchymal macrophages: induction by interferon-gamma. *Growth Factors* 1993; 9:223.

207. Stewart AG, Grigoriadis G, Harris T: Mitogenic actions of endothelin-1 and epidermal growth factor in cultured airway smooth muscle. *Clin Exp Pharmacol Physiol* 1994; 21:277.

208. Tomlinson PR, Wilson JW, Stewart AG: Inhibition by salbutamol of the proliferation of human smooth muscle cells grown in culture. *Br J Pharmacol* 1994; 111:641.

209. Kandel J, Bossy-Wetzel E, Radvanyi F, et al.: Neovascularization is associated with a switch to the export of bFGF in the multistep development of fibrosarcoma. *Cell* 1991; 66:1095.

210. Cambrey AD, Kwon OJ, McAnulty RJ, et al.: Release of fibroblast proliferative activity from cultured human airway epithelial cells: a role for insulin-like growth factor 1 (IGF-1). *Am Rev Respir Dis* 1993; 147:A272.

211. Bitterman, PB, Adelburg S, Crystal RG: Mechanisms of pulmonary fibrosis: Spontaneous release of the alveolar macrophage-derived growth factor in the interstitial lung disorders. *J Clin Invest* 1983; 72:1801.

212. Rom WN, Basset P, Fells GA, et al.: Alveolar macrophages release an insulin-like growth factor I-type molecule. *J Clin Invest* 1988; 82:1685.

213. Sara VR, Hall K: Insulin-like growth factors and their binding proteins. *Physiol Rev* 1990; 70:591.

Chapter 25

PHARMACOLOGIC MODULATION OF CYTOKINES AND THEIR ROLE IN THE PATHOGENESIS OF SEPSIS

LARRY C. CASEY

Sepsis is the thirteenth leading cause of death in the United States, and the rate of mortality from it has not decreased despite the use of supportive therapy and modern antibiotics.[1] The cascade of events leading from bacterial infection to the development of organ failure and death are poorly understood. Previous work suggested that the lipopolysaccharide (LPS) portion of the cell wall of gram-negative bacteria was the agent by which gram-negative bacteria started the cascade causing organ failure and death. However, in the past 8 years, evidence has accumulated to indicate that LPS is not in itself responsible for the adverse effects of sepsis. Instead, LPS stimulates the production and release of endogenous mediators, the actions of which are responsible for the pathophysiologic changes and mortality associated with sepsis. Cytokines, which are polypeptides produced by many different cell types, have been implicated as important mediators in the pathogenesis of sepsis. This chapter provides an overview of the major cytokines implicated in sepsis.

Tumor Necrosis Factor

OVERVIEW

Tumor necrosis factor-α (TNF-α) was the first cytokine implicated in the pathogenesis of septic shock.[2] TNF-α and TNF-β are two closely related proteins sharing similar biologic activities. TNF-α is produced by monocytes and macrophages, whereas TNF-β is produced by activated T cells. TNF-α is the main form produced in sepsis, and this discussion will be limited to it. TNF-α is a 17-kDa polypeptide that exists in multimers of two or three identical subunits and contains several potential glycosylation sites.[3] TNF-α also exists as an integral membrane protein. Membrane-bound TNF-α is a 26-kDa polypeptide translation product, which includes an uncleaved 76-amino-acid residual signal sequence that is normally cleaved off to yield the 17-kDa secreted form.[4]

TNF RECEPTORS

There are two types of TNF receptors, a 55 kDa form and a 75 kDa form. The 75 kDa receptor has a greater affinity for TNF than does the 55 kDa receptor. Aggregation of the receptors mediated by the binding of dimeric or trimeric TNF is thought to initiate the transmembrane signaling process. While the transmembrane signaling process may be different for the two receptors, a critical step is the induction of the transcription factor NF-kB.[5] TNF receptors can be shed from the cell surface by proteolytic cleavage. The soluble forms of the TNF receptors can be detected in serum and urine.[6] The release of soluble forms of the receptors results in the loss of cell-surface receptors as well as in the generation of competitors for ligand binding, resulting in the "neutralization" of circulating TNF activity.[7] The ability of soluble TNF receptors to inhibit TNF activity has led to clinical trials using soluble TNF receptors in patients with sepsis.

ROLE OF TNF IN SEPSIS

TNF was the first cytokine implicated in the pathogenesis of sepsis. Cerami and Beutler made this discovery in a search for the factor responsible for the severe weight loss (cachexia) observed in patients with chronic infections.[2] They determined that a monocyte-derived factor was responsible and subsequently cloned and sequenced this protein, which was identical to the sequence of tumor necrosis factor. To investigate the role of cachectin/TNF in the pathogenesis of sepsis, Beutler and colleagues demonstrated that a strain of mice known to be resistant to the effects of LPS were deficient in synthesizing TNF in response to LPS and that the infusion of TNF into the LPS-resistant mice reproduced the pathophysiology of sepsis similarly to the infusion of LPS into "normal" mice.[8] In other studies, it was shown that antibodies to TNF prevented LPS-induced mortality in mice and that if the genetically resistant mice (C3H/HeJ) were given a bone marrow transplant from a sensitive mouse (C3H/FeJ), the resistant mouse became sensitive to LPS.[9,10] Additional studies confirmed the ability of antibodies to TNF to prevent LPS-induced mortality in animals infused with LPS or nonhuman primates infused with live *E. coli*.[11] Thus, the evidence implicating TNF in the pathogenesis of sepsis was very strong: (1) TNF was detectable in animals infused with LPS; (2) animals deficient in TNF were tolerant to the effects of LPS; (3) the infusion of TNF into animals produced the same pathophysiology as

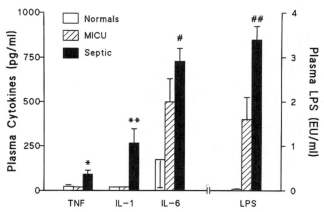

FIGURE 25-1 Comparison of plasma LPS, TNF-α, IL-1β, and IL-6 concentrations in patients with the sepsis syndrome ($n = 97$), patients in the medical intensive care unit (MICU) who did not have sepsis ($n = 20$), and normal healthy controls ($n = 20$). Plasma samples were obtained immediately after the identification of patients with the sepsis syndrome and critically ill patients without sepsis who were in the MICU. The three groups differed in plasma concentrations of TNF-α, IL-1β, IL-6, and LPS ($p < 0.001$ for all comparisons). Plasma TNF-α, IL-1β, IL-6, and LPS concentrations were increased in patients with sepsis as compared with both critically ill patients without sepsis ($p <$ for all comparisons) and normal controls ($p < 0.001$ for all comparisons). (*From Casey et al.,*[13] *with permission.*)

the infusion of LPS; and (4) antibodies to TNF prevented the adverse effects of LPS infusion. The inverse correlation between plasma levels of TNF and survival in patients with meningococcal bacteremia also gave strong support to a primary role of TNF in the pathogenesis of sepsis.[12]

Plasma or serum concentrations of TNF are elevated in patients with sepsis. The magnitude of the elevation may in part depend on the severity and acuity of the sepsis. For instance, in fulminant bacterial meningitis, serum TNF concentrations are increased and correlate with mortality.[12] Bacterial meningitis closely resembles animal models of sepsis using infusions of LPS or large amounts of bacteria. In contrast, patients with less fulminant forms of sepsis, such as the sepsis syndrome, do not have a dramatic increase in circulating concentrations of TNF (Fig. 25-1).[13] Furthermore, in patients with the sepsis syndrome, there is not a correlation between plasma concentrations of TNF and survival (Fig. 25-2). There are a number of potential explanations for these differences. The time course of the appearance of TNF in plasma is the same for either a bolus injection of LPS or a continuous LPS infusion: there is a rapid increase reaching a peak in 1 to 2 h followed by a return to undetectable levels by 4 to 6 h.[14] Since fever develops in response to the secretion of cytokines, in clinical sepsis, there may be a delay between the onset of sepsis, the development of fever, and the notification of the physician. Thus, by the time a physician becomes aware that the patient is septic, plasma levels of TNF may have already peaked and returned toward normal. Thus, the failure to detect circulating TNF in septic patients does not mean that TNF was not present, nor does

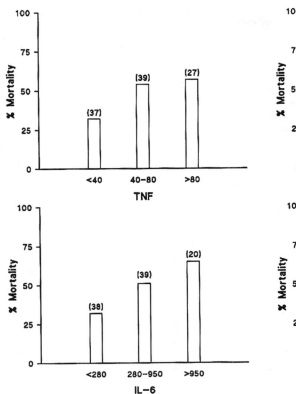

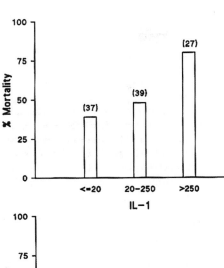

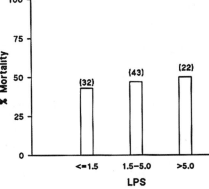

FIGURE 25-2 Relations between categorized levels of TNF-α, IL-1β, and LPS and mortality from the sepsis syndrome. Mortality increased with increasing categorized plasma levels of TNF-α ($p = 0.047$), IL-1β ($p < 0.01$), and IL-6 ($p < 0.01$), but not LPS ($p < 0.2$). The number of patients in each category is indicated at the top of each bar. (*From Casey et al.,*[13] *with permission.*)

it mean that TNF does not play a role in sepsis. Other problems related to the detection of TNF include the presence of circulating soluble receptors. Depending on the type of assay being used, soluble receptors may interfere with TNF detection. This problem will be discussed later.

The overwhelming data implicating TNF as a mediator of the pathophysiologic consequences of sepsis led to clinical trials using either monoclonal antibodies (mAbs) to TNF-α or soluble TNF receptors. Unfortunately, these trials have been disappointing, in that these agents did not improve survival. In fact, a dose-dependent increase in mortality was associated with the use of anti-TNF mAbs.[15] Although there are numerous explanations for the discrepancy between animal models and clinical trials, some of the animal data were seemingly ignored. For instance, using a murine model in which peritonitis was produced by cecal ligation and puncture, anti-TNF IgG *increased* mortality, whereas the infusion of TNF into the mice treated with anti-TNF mAb *decreased* mortality.[16] At autopsy, it was found that the mice in which TNF was inhibited using TNF antibodies had diffuse peritonitis, whereas, in the mice that also received an infusion of TNF, the abscess was contained. These data illustrate that the simple concept of a single toxic mediator that is released during sepsis and accounts for multiorgan failure and death is not correct. Cytokine release is a normal and beneficial response to infection, and, while excessive and unregulated production may result in organ injury and death, the release of cytokines is an essential component of the inflammatory response, and efforts to totally block this response are likely to cause more harm than good.

Interleukin-1

OVERVIEW

Interleukin-1 (IL-1) originally was called by a variety of names, the two most common being *lymphocyte activating factor* and *endogenous pyrogen*. There are two forms of interleukin-1, IL-1α and IL-1β, both with molecular weights of about 17 kDa. These two polypeptides can be separated on the basis of their isoelectric points (p*I*); the p*I* of IL-1α is 5.0, whereas that of IL-1β is 7.0. IL-1β has been studied the most in sepsis and thus will be the focus of this discussion. IL-1β is synthesized initially as a 32-kDa propeptide of 269 amino acids, which undergoes C-terminal cleavage to produce the mature form of 153 amino acids. The IL-1 precursor lacks a hydrophobic signal peptide, and the mechanism of IL-1 secretion is still under investigation.[17]

IL-1 RECEPTORS

There are two distinct IL-1 receptors, type I and type II. The type I receptor is an 80-kDa protein belonging to the Ig superfamily of receptors. It has three extracellular Ig-like domains, a short transmembrane domain, and a large cytoplasmic domain. The type II receptor is also a member of the Ig superfamily; it has an extracellular ligand-binding domain composed of three Ig-like domains, a single transmembrane domain, and a short cytoplasmic domain. Type I and type II receptors bind IL-1α and IL-1β with different affinities.[18] Binding of IL-1 to its receptors induces signal transduction through a phosphorylation pathway that results in the activation of the nuclear transcription factors AP-1 and NF-kB.[19]

There is a circulating soluble inhibitor of IL-1 activity, the interleukin-1 receptor antagonist (IL-1ra or IRAP). IL-1ra binds to the IL-1 receptor with an affinity similar to that of IL-1, but even at high concentrations, IL-1ra has no IL-1-like activity. IL-1ra is produced by the same cells as IL-1.[20] Circulating plasma levels of IL-1ra rise later than those of IL-1; thus, as with the role of soluble TNF receptors in neutralizing TNF activity, IL-1ra may function to block further IL-1 activity by blocking the IL-1 receptor.[21] The ability of IL-1ra to inhibit the effects of IL-1 have led to clinical trials using IL-1ra in sepsis.

ROLE OF IL-1 IN SEPSIS

The animal data suggesting a role for IL-1 in mediating sepsis are similar to the findings with TNF. The infusion of IL-1 causes hypotension in rabbits and a leukocytic infiltration in the lungs.[22] IL-1 can be detected after the infusion of LPS, but inconsistently and at low concentrations.[23] Nevertheless, the infusion of IL-1ra significantly improved survival in animal models of sepsis.[24] These results provided the strongest evidence that IL-1 played a major role in the pathogenesis of sepsis and led to clinical trials using IL-1ra in septic patients.

In patients with the sepsis syndrome, IL-1 rarely is detected (Fig. 25-1), but, when it is, there is a significant correlation with mortality (Fig. 25-2).[13] The failure of IL-1ra to improve survival in patients with sepsis does not necessarily mean that IL-1 is not important in sepsis.[25] It is just as likely that the studies were not designed to test the hypothesis adequately. The problem of experimental design in sepsis trials is addressed later.

Interleukin-6

OVERVIEW

Interleukin-6 (IL-6) is a 22 to 29 kDa protein that has previously been called *B cell growth factor*, *plasmacytoma growth factor*, and *hepatocyte stimulating factor*. IL-6 is produced by activated monocytes and macrophages, endothelial cells, astrocytes, fibroblasts, and activated B and T lymphocytes.[26] The variation in molecular weight is the result of post-translational modification. Variable glycosylation and/or serine phosphorylation may affect the biological activity of IL-6.[27,28] IL-6 drives the acute-phase response.

IL-6 RECEPTORS

The IL-6 receptor consists of two chains, a ligand-binding 80-kDa protein and a non-ligand–binding signal-transducing protein, gp 130. The low-affinity subunit includes a signal

peptide as well as an Ig-superfamily domain.[29] There is also a secreted form of the IL-6 receptor. Unlike the soluble TNF receptors and IL-ra, which neutralize or block circulating TNF and IL-1 activities, respectively, the soluble IL-6 receptor enhances IL-6 activity by transporting IL-6 to the gp 130 signal transducer unit of the IL-6 receptor.[30]

ROLE OF IL-6 IN SEPSIS

Most studies investigating the relationship between plasma levels of IL-6 and mortality in septic patients have found a direct correlation between IL-6 and mortality[13,31] However, while the intravenous infusion of IL-6 causes fever, it produces no adverse hemodynamic changes or other changes suggestive of sepsis or multisystem organ failure.[32] Thus, it appears that IL-6 may not be a direct mediator, but may be a marker of systemic inflammation and reflect the net effects of previously produced TNF and IL-1. This hypothesis is supported by the observation that inhibition of either TNF or IL-1 production attenuate IL-6 formation. An alternative explanation is that IL-6 is toxic only when present with other cytokines. This issue of cytokine synergy has not been addressed adequately.

Interleukin-8

OVERVIEW

Interleukin-8 (IL-8) is a 10-kDa peptide described as a neutrophil chemotactic factor produced by monocytes stimulated with LPS. IL-8 has gone by several names, including *leukocyte adhesion inhibitor*, *neutrophil activation protein*, and *neutrophil chemotactic factor*. IL-8 has been grouped into a superfamily of 10 or more proinflammatory cytokines, designated the *chemokine family*. The chemokines have been divided into the CC and CXC subfamilies according to the spacing of conserved cysteine residues in the primary amino acid sequences. Members of the CXC family include macrophage inflammatory proteins (MIP-1α and MIP-1β), monocyte chemotactic and activating factor (MCAF), and RANTES (regulated upon activation, normal T-cell–expressed and presumably secreted). The members of the CXC subfamily include IL-8, MGSA/Gro, platelet factor 4, and β-thromboglobulin. Four distinct N-terminal variants of IL-8 are generated from a common precursor peptide of 99 amino acids by specific proteolytic cleavage at different sites. IL-8 is produced by a variety of different cells, including endothelial cells, mitogen-granulocytopenia followed by granulocytosis.[33]

IL-8 RECEPTORS

There are two high-affinity IL-8 receptors. The type I receptor binds only IL-8, whereas the type II receptor binds IL-8, MGSA/Gro, and NAP-2. These receptors belong to a superfamily whose members contain seven transmembrane domains and are coupled to the guanine nucleotide-binding proteins (G proteins). Signal transduction involves a receptor-coupled G protein, mobilization of intracellular calcium stores, activation of protein kinase C, and receptor internalization.[34,35]

ROLE OF IL-8 IN SEPSIS

The precise role of IL-8 in the pathogenesis of sepsis still is being investigated. IL-8 is detectable in patients with sepsis, and in one study, the concentrations correlated with mortality.[36,37] IL-8 is detected in bronchoalveolar fluid in patients with acute lung injury.[38]

Other Cytokines Possibly Involved in Sepsis

A number of other cytokines may be involved in the pathogenesis of sepsis, but the data are too limited at this time to discuss their role. Some additional cytokines that may be involved in sepsis are IL-10, IL-12, MIP-1α, MIP-1β, GM-CSF, G-CSF, and leukemia inhibitory factor (LIF). Another factor that is not a cytokine but which may play a major role in the pathogenesis of sepsis is the calcitonin gene related protein (CGRP), which may be responsible for hypotension during sepsis.[39]

Synergistic Interactions between Cytokines during Sepsis

A number of recent studies support the concept of synergistic interactions between cytokines in the causation of tissue injury. TNF-α and IL-1β given in small doses individually produce no hemodynamic changes, but, when given together, they cause severe lung injury and hypotension.[22] Similarly, when LPS is combined with TNF-α in doses that are tolerated individually, they cause lethal shock in mice.[40] Other examples of synergistic interactions between LPS, TNF-α, and IL-1β include protection from fatal hyperoxia and stimulation of fibroblast prostaglandin E$_2$.[41,42] In a clinical study of the role of cytokines in the pathogenesis of sepsis, the correlation between plasma levels of LPS, TNF-α, IL-1β, or IL-6 and mortality were not as strong as the correlation between an LPS-cytokine score and mortality (Fig. 25-3).[13] These data suggest that combinations of LPS and cytokines, even at low concentrations, are as much of a risk as a large increase in the concentrations of any one cytokine. These data also indicate that there may be a need to monitor a profile of cytokines rather than just one cytokine in sepsis.

Strategies for Interrupting the Cytokine Cascade during Sepsis

There are a number of different approaches for blocking LPS stimulation of cytokine production, including neutralizing cytokines that already have been produced and modulating the end-organ effects of cytokines (Fig. 25-4).

LPS binds to a plasma protein called LPS-binding protein (LBP), and this complex then binds to CD14 receptors on

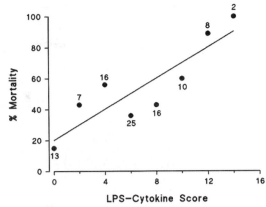

FIGURE 25-3 Relationship between lipopolysaccharide-cytokine score and mortality from the sepsis syndrome. A unit increase in the lipopolysaccharide-cytokine score was associated with a 5 percent increase in mortality (*p* < 0.001). The numbers under the points represent the number of patients with that score. (*From Casey et al.,[13] Reprinted from the Ann Intern Med 119:771–778, 1993, with permission.*)

monocytes. The binding of the LPS-LBP complex to CD14 causes signal transduction by mechanisms that are still under investigation but include tyrosine phosphorylation, protein kinase C, and the nuclear transcription factor NF-kB.[43]

One way to prevent LPS stimulation of cytokine generation is to block the binding of LPS to LBP. LBP is an acute-phase reactant, and plasma concentrations become very high during sepsis. Antibody to LBP blocks LPS-LBP binding and prevents CD14 stimulation. As an alternative approach, there is a naturally occurring protein produced by neutrophils called *bactericidal permeability-increasing protein* (BPI).[44] BPI binds to LPS and prevents LPS-LBP interaction, thus blocking CD14 stimulation. Another approach is to block CD14 with monoclonal antibodies. In vitro, antibodies to CD14 prevent LPS stimulation of cytokine generation. Monocyte expression of CD14 also can be regulated. CD14 is linked to the membrane by a phosphatidylinositol linkage, and, thus, can be cleaved from the membrane by phospholipase C.[45] Soluble CD14 is present in plasma, but its molecular weight is less than that of CD14 cleaved from the membrane by phospholipase C, suggesting that it has been cleaved by a protease. Soluble CD14 is capable of binding to LPS-LBP complexes and stimulating endothelial cells (which do not express CD14), but not monocytes or macrophages. Thus, even though monocyte CD14 may be downregulated by shedding, LPS can still activate endothelial cells via the binding of soluble CD14 to LPS-LBP to produce the CD14-LPS-LBP complex, which binds to and stimulates endothelial cells.[46]

When the LPS-LBP complex binds to CD14, a transmembrane signaling event takes place that involves tyrosine kinase and protein kinase C. Inhibitors of tyrosine kinase prevent LPS-induced mortality.[47] Similar beneficial effects have been seen with inhibitors of protein kinase C and inhibitors of phosphodiesterase.[48,49] Corticoteroids may be beneficial, but only if given as pretreatment. Corticosteroid-

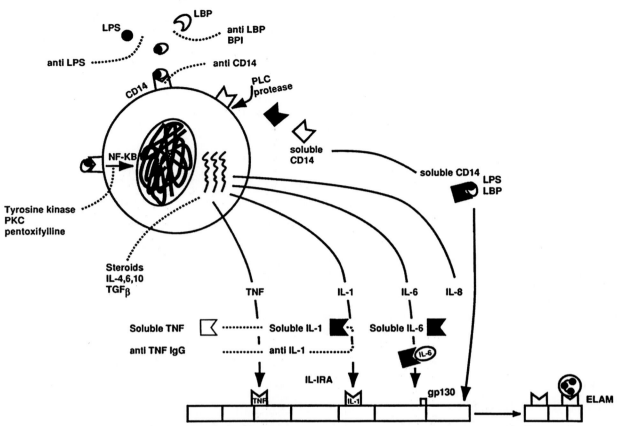

FIGURE 25-4 Diagram of the mechanism by which LPS interacts with monocytes to stimulate cytokine production and the ways in which cytokine production can be inhibited or neutralized. LPS binds to a plasma protein, LBP, and this complex then binds to CD14 on monocytes. BPI also prevents LPS from binding to CD14. The mechanism(s) of signal transduction are unclear but involve tyrosine phosphorylation, protein kinase C, and the induction of nuclear transcription factors, including NF-kB. Inhibitors of tyrosine kinase and protein kinase C can block LPS stimulation of cytokine synthesis, as can activators of cAMP. Cytokine synthesis can be inhibited by corticosteroids if they are given prior to induction of TNF mRNA. IL-4, IL-6, IL-10, and TGF-β also can inhibit TNF and IL-1 synthesis. Once TNF and IL-1 are secreted from the cell (possibly by proteases), their activity can be "neutralized" by circulating soluble receptors. In addition, there is a naturally occurring IL-1 receptor antagonist that blocks IL-1 activity. Once cytokines bind to cell receptors, they induce cell activation, as indicated by the expression of leukocyte adhesion molecules and the conversion of the surface of endothelial cells into a prothrombotic state.

pretreatment prevents the induction of TNF mRNA and subsequent transcription of TNF protein. However, if TNF mRNA is already present, corticosteroids will not prevent the stimulation of TNF protein synthesis by LPS.[8] This observation may explain why corticosteroids have failed in clinical trials, because by the time a patient is recognized as being septic, the induction of TNF mRNA already has occurred. Pentoxifylline is a potent inhibitor of phosphodiesterase and is effective in inhibiting cytokine generation and preventing organ injury and death in animal models of sepsis.[50] Some cytokines also act as inhibitors of TNF and IL-1 synthesis. IL-4, IL-6, IL-10, and TGF-β all inhibit TNF and IL-1 synthesis, and, thus, may play a role in downregulating TNF-α and IL-1β synthesis during sepsis. TNF and IL-1 may be cleaved from the cell membrane by proteolytic activity, and, thus, antiproteases might prevent the release of TNF and IL-1 from the cell membrane, resulting in greater amounts of cell-

associated TNF and IL-1 but lesser plasma concentrations. Once cytokines are released, a variety of mechanisms are available for inhibiting their activity.

There are endogenous inhibitors of cytokine activity, such as soluble cytokine receptors.[51] TNF receptors are shed from the membrane and neutralize TNF bioactivity. Since there are two types of TNF receptors, there are two soluble receptors, type I and type II. These receptors bind and neutralize circulating TNF bioactivity.[7] Clinical trials have been conducted using soluble TNF receptors or modified versions of the receptors but have failed thus far to demonstrate efficacy. Possible reasons why clinical trials have failed are discussed later.

Another naturally occurring inhibitor of cytokine activity is IL-1ra. IL-1ra is secreted by monocytes in response to LPS. IL is a 52 to 66-kDa protein which blocks the ability of IL-1 to stimulate cellular responses to IL-1. In vivo, IL-1ra is effective in blocking the activity of IL-1 in various animal models of disease. In several studies on circulating IL-1β during sepsis in humans, concentrations rarely exceed 500 pg/mL, whereas concentrations of IL-1ra exceed the concentrations of IL-1β by 100 fold, but IL-1ra does not appear until after the release of IL-1β.[13,23] Sepsis seems to stimulate a small increase in IL-1β, followed by a large increase in IL-1ra. Thus, it is thought that endogenously produced IL-1ra helps to limit the severity of the inflammatory response. Since only about 10 percent of the IL-1 receptors need to be occupied to elicit an IL-1 response, it is thought that the IL-1ra response still may be inadequate under conditions of severe infection. For this reason, a multicenter trial using IL-1ra in sepsis was undertaken; this trial did not show efficacy.[25] Potential reasons for the failure of IL-1ra as well as TNF antibodies and soluble TNF receptors are discussed later.

It is likely that by the time a patient is recognized as being septic, cytokines have already been produced and induced their biologic responses. Thus, devising strategies for blocking cytokine synthesis or neutralizing cytokines may not be as useful as developing an ability to assess their end-organ effects and to modulate the activation of cells already stimulated by the cytokines.

Problems with Cytokine Measurement

Numerous potential problems are associated with measuring cytokines and interpreting the results.[52] Blood concentrations of cytokines depend on a balance between net production, clearance, and/or inactivation and metabolism. For example, a cytokine released into the blood may be bound immediately to a cell receptor and thus no longer be measurable in plasma. Substantial data suggest that cytokine production is compartmentalized, so blood concentrations do not necessarily reflect cytokine production in the lung or spinal fluid. Even in the lung, cytokine production is likely to be different at different sites—the airway, the alveolus, the interstitium, and the intravascular space.

There are also factors in blood that interfere with cytokine measurements. The presence of soluble receptors or receptor antagonists may interfere with the assay results. Biologic assays measure biologic activity. Thus, even if a large amount of a cytokine is present, if there is an equal or greater amount of a soluble receptor or receptor antagonist, no activity will be detected. Some ELISA assays use neutralizing antibodies. These assays also are influenced by the presence of soluble receptors, as the soluble receptors compete for the same site as the antibody, and the net results depend on the relative avidities of the antibody and the soluble receptor. To compound this problem, serial dilution of the plasma before the assay may cause the measured concentration to be greater in the more dilute solutions, because the affinity of the soluble receptor may be such that in very dilute solutions, it no longer binds to the cytokine, and the cytokine thus becomes available for binding to the antibody. Other ELISA assays use nonneutralizing antibodies; these assays are not influenced by the presence of soluble receptors, and serial dilution of plasma should result in serial reduction in

cytokine concentration. However, which is it more important to measure—the total amount of circulating cytokine, or the amount of circulating "free" cytokine? The answer is not known, but it makes sense that the more important information would be the amount of biologically active cytokine, which is not being neutralized by natural host defenses.

Sample preparation is also very important.[52] The original description of TNF activity used serum. However, allowing blood to clot to form serum can introduce new artifacts, and using EDTA plasma is better. It is also important to keep the blood on ice and to separate the plasma from the cellular component as quickly as possible. Allowing blood to remain at room temperature for several hours can result in the loss of measurable cytokines. For instance, the addition of LPS to heparinized whole blood in a test tube at room temperature causes an increase in plasma TNF-α to about 10,000 pg/ml. However, after 16 h, the same blood contains an undetectable amount of TNF-α (unpublished observation). Thus, care in sample collection and processing is important.

Why Clinical Sepsis Trials Have Failed

In the past 10 years, many millions of dollars have been spent in multicenter clinical trials attempting to improve survival in sepsis, but all these trials have failed. The agents that have been tested and have failed include corticosteroids, anti-LPS antibody, anti-TNF antibody, soluble TNF receptors, and IL-ra. Another clinical trial is about to begin, testing the use of an inhibitor of nitric oxide production. Why have all these trials failed? Is it because the basic hypothesis that these mediators are important in the pathogenesis of sepsis is wrong, or are the trials themselves designed so that they could never show a beneficial effect? It may be that the trials themselves are fundamentally flawed.

Consider the use of a similar approach for testing hypertension treatments. One wants to see if an antihypertensive drug improves survival. Patients with demonstrated increased blood pressures are not enrolled. Instead, a group of patients is selected that might have hypertension, for instance, obese patients. These patients are started on either the antihypertensive drug or placebo and then followed long-term to assess their outcome. Since blood pressure was never measured, it is likely that many of the patients in both groups were not hypertensive, and thus there is no reason to expect them to do better with or without the antihypertensive drug. Furthermore, some of the patients treated with the antihypertensive drug who did not have hypertension will probably develop hypotension and suffer associated morbidity or mortality. How could an antihypertensive drug ever show efficacy if blood pressure is never measured and the drug not titrated to properly control the hypertension? How could a neutralizing antibody to LPS be effective if only one-third of the patients enrolled (the criterion for enrollment being the presence of septic syndrome) actually have gram-negative sepsis—meaning that two-thirds of the patients should not have received the drug? [Even worse, the anti-LPS antibodies used in clinical trials do not even prevent gram-negative bacterial stimulation of cytokine production.] Why use an inhibitor to TNF if excess TNF activity is not present? Why use an IL-1 receptor antagonist if IL-1 concentrations in the blood not only are low but are 100 times less than the concentration of naturally produced IL-1ra already present in the blood? Is it safe to block TNF-α when animal studies show increased mortality in mice with peritonitis when an antibody to TNF is given? Is it safe to block nitric oxide production when animal models of sepsis show that doing so causes seizures and worsening myocardial function?

Cytokines are clearly important mediators that are released during sepsis and contribute to the pathophysiology of sepsis and multisystem organ failure. However, there is great concern that pharmaceutical companies may abandon sepsis research because of the "high financial risk," when, in fact, the multicenter trials have used inappropriate patient populations and poor experimental designs.

References

1. Center for Disease Control: Increase in national hospital discharge survey rates for septicemia—United States, 1979–1987. *MMWR* 1990; 39:31.

2. Beutler B, Cerami A: Cachectin: more than a tumor necrosis factor. *N Engl J Med* 1987; 316:379.

3. Beutler B, Cerami A: The biology of cachectin/TNF—a primary mediator of the host response. *Annu Rev Immunol* 1989; 7:625.

4. Kriegler M, Perez C, DeFay K, et al.: A novel form of TNF/cachectin is a cell surface cytotoxic transmembrane protein: ramifications for the complex physiology of TNF. *Cell* 1988; 53:45.

5. Tartaglia LA, Goedeel DV: Two TNF receptors. *Immunol Today* 1992; 13:151.

6. Heller RA, Song K, Onasch MA, et al.: Complementary DNA cloning of a receptor for tumor necrosis factor and demonstration of a shed form of the receptor. *Proc Natl Acad Sci USA* 1990; 87:6151.

7. van Zee KJ, Kohno T, Fischer E, et al.: Tumor necrosis factor soluble receptors circulate during experimental and clinical inflammation and can protect against excessive tumor necrosis factor α in vitro and in vivo. *Proc Natl Acad Sci USA* 1992; 89:4845.

8. Beutler B, Krochin N, Milsark IW, et al.: Control of cachectin (tumor necrosis factor) synthesis: mechanisms of endotoxin resistance. *Science* 1976; 232:977.

9. Beutler B, Milsark IW, Cerami AC: Passive immunization against cachectin/tumor necrosis factor protects mice from the lethal effect of endotoxin. *Science* 1985; 229:869.

10. Mannel DN, Rosenstreich DL, Mergenhagen SE: Mechanism for lipopolysaccharide-induced tumor necrosis: requirement for lipopolysaccharide-sensitive lymphoreticular cells. *Infect Immun* 1979; 24:573.

11. Tracey KJ, Fong Y, Hesse DG, et al.: Anti-cachectin/TNF monoclonal antibodies prevent septic shock during lethal bacteremia. *Nature* 1987; 330:662.

12. Waage A, Halstensen A, Espevik T: Association between tumor necrosis factor in serum and fatal outcome in patients with meningococcal disease. *Lancet* 1987; 1:355.

13. Casey LC, Balk RA, Bone RC: Plasma cytokine and endotoxin levels correlate with survival in patients with sepsis syndrome. *Ann Intern Med* 1993; 119:771.

14. Waage A: Production and clearance of TNF in rats exposed to endotoxin and dexamethasone. *Clin Immunol Immunopathol* 1987; 45:348.

15. Wherry J, Wenzel R, Abraham E, et al.: A controlled randomized double blind clinical trial of monoclonal antibody to human tumor necrosis factor (TNF Mab) in patients with sepsis syndrome. *Chest* 1993; 104:48S.

16. Echtenacher B, Falk W, Mannel DN, Krammer PH: Requirement of endogenous tumor necrosis factor/cachectin for recovery from experimental peritonitis. *J Immunol* 1990; 145:3762.

17. Dinarello C: Biology of interleukin-1. *Chem Immunol* 1992; 51:1.

18. Sims JE, Acres RB, Grubin CE, et al.: Cloning the interleukin 1 receptor from human T cells. *Proc Natl Acad Sci USA* 1989; 86:8946.

19. Iwasaki T, Uehara Y, Graves L, et al.: Herbimycin A blocks IL-1-induced NF-kappa B DNA-binding activity in lymphoid cells lines. *FEBS Lett* 1992; 298:240.

20. Hannum CH, Wilcox CJ, Arend WP, et al.: Interleukin-1 receptor antagonist activity of a human interleukin-1 inhibitor. *Nature* 1990; 343:336.

21. Rogy MA, Coyle SM, Oldenburg HS, et al.: Persistently elevated soluble tumor necrosis factor receptor and interleukin-1 receptor antagonist levels in critically ill patients. *J Am Coll Surg* 1994; 178:132.

22. Okusaw S, Gelfand JA, Ikejima T, et al.: Interleukin-1 induces a shock-like state in rabbits. Synergism with tumor necrosis factor and the effect of cyclooxygenase inhibitors. *J Clin Invest* 1988; 81:1162.

23. Cannon JG, Tompkins RG, Gelfand JA, et al.: Circulating interleukin-1 and tumor necrosis factor in septic shock and experimental endotoxin fever. *J Infect Dis* 1990; 161:79.

24. Wakabayaski G, Gelfand JA, Burke JF, et al.: A specific receptor antagonist for interleukin-1 prevents Escherichia coli-induced shock in rabbits. *FASEB J* 1991; 5:338.

25. Fisher CJ, Stolman GJ, Opal SM, et al.: Inital evaluation of human recombinant interleukin-1 receptor antagonist in the treatment of sepsis syndrome: a randomized, open-labeled, placebo-controlled multicenter trial. The IL-1RA Sepsis Syndrome Study Group. *Crit Care Med* 1994; 22:12.

26. Van Snick J: Interleukin-6: an overview. *Annu Rev Immunol* 8:253–278, 1990.

27. Wong GG, Clark SC: Multiple actions of interleukin 6 within a cytokine network. *Immunol Today* 1988; 9:137.

28. May LT, Santhanam U, Tatter SB, et al.: Phosphorylation of secreted forms of human beta 2-interferon/hepatocyte stimulating factor/interleukin-6. *Biochem Biophys Res Commun* 1988; 152:1144.

29. Hirano T: Interleukin-6 and its relation to inflammation and disease. *Clin Immunol Immunopathol* 1992; 62:S60.

30. Honda M, Yamamoto S, Cheng M, et al.: Human soluble IL-6 receptor: its detection and enhanced release by HIV infection. *J Immunol* 1992; 148:2175.

31. Hack CE, De Groat ER, Felt-Bersma RJ, et al.: Increased plasma levels of interleukin-6 in sepsis. *Blood* 1989; 74:1704.

32. Preiser JC, Schmartz D, Van der Linden P, et al.: Interleukin-6 administration has no acute hemodynamic or hematologic effect in the dog. *Cytokine* 1991; 3:1.

33. Oppheim JJ, Zachariae CO, Mukaida N, Matsushima K: Properties of the novel proinflammatory supergene "intercrine" cytokine family. *Annu Rev Immunol* 1993; 9:617.

34. Holmes WE, Lee J, Kunag WJ, et al.: Structure and functional expression of a human interleukin-8 receptor. *Science* 1991; 253:1278.

35. Murphy PM, Tiffany HL: Cloning of complementary DNA encoding a functional human interleukin-8 receptor. *Science* 1991; 1280.

36. Zee KJ, De Foege LE, Fischer E, et al.: IL-8 in septic shock, endotoxemia, and after IL-1 administration. *J Immunol* 1991; 146:3478.

37. Marty C, Missett B, Tamion F, et al.: Circulating interleukin-8

concentrations in patients with multiple organ failure of septic and non-septic origin. *Crit Care Med* 1994; 22:673.

38. Chollet-Martin S, Montravers P, Gilbert C, et al.: High levels of interleukin-8 in the blood and alveolar spaces of patients with pneumonia and adult respiratory distress syndrome. *Infect Immun* 1993; 61:4553.

39. Arden WA, Fiscus RR, Wang X, et al.: Elevations in circulating calcitonin gene-related peptide correlate with hemodynamic deterioration during endotoxin shock in pigs. *Circ Shock* 1994; 42:147.

40. Rothstein JL, Schreiber H: Synergy between tumor necrosis factor and bacterial products causes hemodynamic necrosis and lethal shock in normal mice. *Proc Natl Acad Sci USA* 1988; 85:607.

41. White CW, Ghezzi P, Dinarello CA: Recombinant tumor necrosis factor/cachectin and interleukin-1 pretreatment decreases lung oxidized glutathione accumulation, lung injury, and mortality in rats exposed to hyperoxia. *J Clin Invest* 1987; 79:868.

42. Elias JA, Gustilo K, Baeder W, Freundlich B: Synergistic stimulation of fibroblast prostaglandin by recombinant interleukin-1 and tumor necrosis factor. *J Immunol* 1987; 138:3812.

43. Tobias PS, Mathison J, Mintz D, et al.: Participation of lipopolysaccharide-binding protein in lipopolysaccharide-dependent macrophage activation. *Am J Respir Cell Mol Biol* 1992; 7:239.

44. Appelmelk BJ, An YQ, Thijs BG, et al.: Recombinant human bactericidal/permeability-increasing protein (rBPI23) is a universal lipopolysaccharide-binding ligand. *Infect Immun* 1993; 62:3564.

45. Haziot A, Chen S, Ferrero E, et al.: The monocyte differentiation antigen, CD14, is anchored to the cell membrane by a phosphatidylinositol linkage. *J Immunol* 1988; 141:547.

46. Read MA, Cordle SR, Veach RA, et al.: Cell-free pool of CD14 mediates activation of transcription factor NF-kappa B by lipopolysaccharide in human endothelial cells. *Proc Natl Acad Sci USA* 1993; 90:9887.

47. Novogrodasky A, Vanichkin A, Patya M, et al.: Prevention of lipopolysaccharide-induced lethal toxicity by tyrosine kinase inhibitors. *Science* 1994; 264:1319.

48. Inaba H, Filkins JP: Antagonism of endotoxic glucose dyshomeostasis by protein kinase C inhibitors. *Am J Physiol* 1991; 261:R26.

49. Shapira L, Takashiba S, Champagne C, et al.: Involvement of protein kinase C and protein tyrosine kinase in lipopolysaccharide-induced TNF-alpha and IL-1 beta production by human monocytes. *J Immunol* 1994; 153:1818.

50. Schade UF: Pentoxifylline increases survival in murine endotoxin shock and decreases formation of tumor necrosis factor. *Circ Shock* 1990; 31:11.

51. Fernandez-Botran R: Soluble cytokine receptors: their role in immunoregulation. *FASEB J* 1991; 5:2567.

52. Dinarelo CA, Cannon JG: Cytokine measurement in septic shock. *Ann Intern Med* 1993; 119:853.

Chapter 26

CYTOKINES AND INTERSTITIAL LUNG DISEASE

LYNN T. TANOUE AND JACK A. ELIAS

Cellular Events in the Interstitial Disorders
  Lung injury
  Vascular permeability alterations, thrombosis, and thrombolysis
  Leukocyte margination and entry into the interstitium
  Activation and proliferation of leukocytes
  The repair response

Associations Between Cytokines and Interstitial Lung Disorders

Systemic Sarcoidosis

Bleomycin-Induced Pulmonary Fibrosis

Idiopathic Pulmonary Fibrosis

Hypersensitivity Pneumonitis

Therapeutic Implications

The interstitial diseases of the lung are a heterogeneous group of > 100 diseases and disorders. In many cases, the cause has been nicely defined. For the majority of patients, however, no cause has been identified and as a result, at least 35 different idiopathic disease syndromes have been elucidated (reviewed in Refs. 1 and 2). The natural histories of these disorders also are quite variable, with some resolving spontaneously, some chronically remitting and relapsing, and others progressing rapidly to respiratory failure and death. There are, however, a number of features that are common to all. Every interstitial disorder is characterized, in varying degree, by (1) lower respiratory tract inflammation, which can be granulocytic and/or mononuclear and granulomatous and/or nongranulomatous; (2) increased numbers of mesenchymal cells, such as fibroblasts and myofibroblasts; and (3) excessive and/or abnormal connective tissue accumulation.[1,2]

The inflammatory and fibrotic responses characteristic of the interstitial disorders are responsible for the morbidity and mortality of these diseases. The inflammatory response is thought to be at least partially amenable to treatment with immunosuppressives such as corticosteroids. In contrast, the fibrotic changes are presumed to be irreversible and are, as a result, a cause of grave concern. The close approximation of inflammatory cells, fibroblasts, and fibrosis in the biopsies from these patients led many years ago to the hypothesis that the inflammation seen in these lungs is responsible for the generation of the fibrotic response. Evidence supporting this hypothesis has been accumulating since the 1920s, when

it was demonstrated that mononuclear cells play an important role in wound healing. However, only recently have the complexity of the inflammatory and fibrotic responses and the role that cytokines play in these responses begun to be appreciated. The understanding of cytokine biology has increased greatly during the last two decades. As a result, it is impossible in this limited format to review all the information that is pertinent to this large number of disorders. In this chapter, the basic principles of pulmonary injury and repair that are relevant to the interstitial disorders are highlighted, and selected cytokine–interstitial lung disorder associations pertinent to these principles are featured.

Cellular Events in the Interstitial Disorders

The impressive heterogeneity of the interstitial disorders is indicative of the variety of different mechanisms involved in their initiation and perpetuation. Studies of these diseases and animal models of these disorders have, however, provided evidence for a clear series of cellular events that appears to be involved in their pathogenesis. They include lung injury; alterations in vascular permeability, with exposure of the interstitial and alveolar spaces to blood components; the influx of inflammatory cells into the pulmonary interstitium; leukocyte activation and proliferation; and fibroproliferative repair and fibrosis. Cytokines appear to play important roles in each of these steps, as outlined below.

LUNG INJURY

A wide variety of agents—including oxidants, hyperoxia, immune complexes, dusts, toxins, and antimetabolites—can produce interstitial lung damage. The responses elicited can be acute or chronic. The acute injury is characterized by diffuse alveolar damage, varying degrees of epithelial and endothelial injury, inflammation, and fibrin-rich alveolar exudates (hyaline membranes). The subsequent organizing (chronic) phase is characterized by type II pneumocyte proliferation, inflammation, and varying degrees of intraalveolar and interstitial fibrosis. Because immune mechanisms are believed to be important in the pathogenesis of many interstitial disorders, immune insults such as repeated antigen challenge[3,4] and immune complexes[5,6] have been used to attempt to model these diseases. These agents successfully induce lung injury in appropriately sensitized animals but have not resulted in progressive interstitial or fibrotic responses. In contrast, models of progressive interstitial pneumonitis and fibrosis have been successfully established with a variety of agents including bleomycin, ozone, silica, and cadmium.[1,7] Although the explanation for these different outcomes is not totally clear, it is believed that epithelial and endothelial damage are prominent features of the injuries that cause progressive lung disease.[7] Cytokines clearly play an important role in these processes, as evidenced by studies in which acute lung injury has been generated by the intrapulmonary administration of inflammatory cytokines such as interleukin-1 (IL-1) and tumor necrosis factor (TNF)[8–10] and studies demonstrating that lung injury can be ameliorated by a cytokine blockade such as that caused by the IL-1-receptor antagonist[11] and anti-TNF antibodies.[12] Cytokine-cytokine interactions also appear to be important in lung injury, since low concentrations of IL-1 and TNF, which by themselves do not cause lung injury, interact when combined to damage respiratory structures.[8]

VASCULAR PERMEABILITY ALTERATIONS, THROMBOSIS, AND THROMBOLYSIS

As a result of pulmonary injury, platelets are activated, releasing platelet-derived cytokines such as platelet-derived growth factor (PDGF), transforming growth factor-β (TGF-β). Serum components, platelets, and platelet-derived cytokines are then deposited in the interstitium and alveolar space. If clearance of the alveolar space is delayed, thrombosis, reorganization, and alveolar fibrosis can ensue.[7] Plasmin is a major mediator of the clearance of the alveolus. Its levels depend on the levels of local plasminogen activator, antiplasmins, and plasminogen activator inhibitors.[13] Alveolar macrophages and epithelial cells play an important role in this process, since alveolar macrophages produce urokinase-type plasminogen activator and plasminogen activator inhibitor-2, while epithelial cells produce urokinase-type plasminogen activator and plasminogen activator inhibitor-1.[13,14] TNF and TGF-β appear to play an important

role in this regulation, since both increase epithelial cell expression of plasminogen activator inhibitor-1.[13,15]

LEUKOCYTE MARGINATION AND ENTRY INTO THE INTERSTITIUM

The tissue inflammation that appears after pulmonary injury is, at least in part, the result of leukocyte migration from the intravascular compartment to the interstitial space of the lung. To accomplish this, leukocytes marginate to the endothelium and eventually pass into the interstitium. Leukocyte margination is now known to require the intricate interplay of adhesion molecules on both leukocytes and endothelial cells. It is also known that cytokines, such IL-1, TNF, and IL-4, when produced at sites of local inflammation, play an important role in this process by regulating adhesion molecule expression. The ability of IL-1 to regulate intercellular adhesion molecule-1 (ICAM-1), endothelial leukocyte adhesion molecule-1 (ELAM-1), and gp140 is well documented,[16] as is the ability of IL-4 to regulate the expression of vascular cell adhesion molecule-1 (VCAM-1) on endothelial cells.[17] As a result of interactions between these molecules—for example, ICAM-1 binding to lymphocyte function associated antigen-1 (LFA-1, CD11a/CD18 complex) and endothelial VCAM-1 binding to leukocyte very late activation antigen-4 (VLA-4)—white blood cells adhere to the vessel wall. This process is, however, not permanent. Its reversibility allows inflammatory cells to pass through the endothelium along chemotactic gradients. A number of cytokines have been implicated in the generation of these chemotactic gradients. Prominent in this regard have been the chemokine family of chemotactic agents, including IL-8, macrophage inflammatory protein-1α (MIP-1α), and monocyte chemotactic protein-1 (MCP-1), which attract granulocytes and/or monocytes to sites of inflammation.[18,19] The orderly progression of granulocytic to monocytic inflammatory responses that is frequently seen may result from the sequential production of chemotactic agents that selectively attract granulocytes and monocytes (for example, complement fragment C5a and MCP-1).[20]

ACTIVATION AND PROLIFERATION OF LEUKOCYTES

The lung is exposed constantly to inhaled antigens and particulates, the majority of which are cleared without inducing an inflammatory response. The mechanisms that suppress and/or prevent pulmonary inflammation in response to these particulate and antigen loads are not fully understood. However, studies of the cytokine profile of normal human macrophages have provided some relevant insights, since they have demonstrated that, on a per-cell basis, normal alveolar macrophages elaborate less soluble IL-1-β[21] and significantly greater quantities of the potentially suppressive cytokines IL-6 and the IL-1-receptor antagonist.[22–25] By contrast, injuries of appropriate intensity do cause severe inflammation in the lung. The alterations required to allow an inflammatory response also are poorly understood. The inflammatory response, however, appears to be associated with the influx of monocytes into the lung.[26] This results in the enhanced local production of IL-1 which, through its ability to directly affect target cells and interact in a synergistic fashion with IL-2, IL-6, TGF-β, and TNF, then may initiate and augment local inflammatory reactions.

The majority of the alveolar macrophages in the lung are derived from circulating blood monocytes. They enter the lung along chemotactic gradients and have a limited, but definite, capacity to proliferate locally. When appropriately stimulated (e.g., noxious stimuli, infectious agents, etc.), they produce TNF, IL-6, IL-8, TGF-β, insulinlike growth factor-1 (IGF-1), PDGF, modest amounts of IL-1-β, MCP-1, and IL-12. The chemokines (for example, IL-8) in conjunction with IL-1, TNF, and other chemotactic agents recruit neutrophils and eventually monocytes to the pulmonary tissues. These cytokines also interact with antigen-presenting cells (such as alveolar macrophages and dendritic cells) to activate T lymphocytes in the presence of appropriate antigen. The cytokines that are produced have many autocrine effects. The IL-2 stimulates lymphocyte proliferation and the generation of cytotoxic T (CT) lymphocytes and NK (natural killer) cells. The IL-3 stimulates hematopoiesis, the interferon-γ (IFN-γ) activates local macrophages and CT and NK cells, and the IL-4 stimulates immunoglobulin switching, augmenting IgE production. In addition, IL-4, IL-5, and IL-6, in combination, induce the proliferation and terminal differentiation of B lymphocytes into antibody-producing plasma cells; IL-5 stimulates eosinophil growth and differentiation; and IL-1, TNF, IL-6, and IL-11 stimulate the elaboration of acute-phase proteins and act as endogenous pyrogens. Stromal cells also appear to play an active role in these inflammatory responses, since they respond to a variety of cytokines, including IL-1, TNF, and TGF-β and produce a wide array of biologically active molecules including IL-6, IL-11, IL-1-α, pro-IL-1-β, colony-stimulating factors, stem-cell factor, insulinlike growth factors, and hepatocyte growth factor/scatter factor.[27] Interestingly, in most circumstances, stromal cells do not produce inflammatory cytokines in response to specific stimuli but instead respond to any agent that induces local macrophages and T cells to produce IL-1, TNF, and TGF-β. For this reason, it is believed that stromal cells play a different role in the inflammatory response than antigen-responsive cells such as monocytes, macrophages, and T cells, with the latter serving to initiate antigen/stimulus-specific inflammatory responses and the former serving to nonspecifically amplify inflammatory responses through their ability to generate proinflammatory signals.

Recent advances in T-lymphocyte biology have demonstrated that mouse and probably human T lymphocytes can be divided into two major classes, based on the profile of the cytokines they secrete. T_H1 clones produce IL-2, IFN-γ, and lymphotoxin, while T_H2 clones induce IL-4, IL-5, IL-6, IL-10, and IL-13.[28] Inflammatory responses that are T_H2 cell–predominant appear to be largely B-cell and antibody-based, whereas responses that are T_H1-predominant appear to be manifestations of delayed-type hypersensitivity. Cross-talk between T_H1 and T_H2 lymphocytes appears to determine which response predominates with IFN-γ, a T_H1 cell product inhibiting T_H2 cells and IL-10, a T_H2 factor inhibiting T_H1-cell production.[28]

THE REPAIR RESPONSE

The restoration of normal lung architecture after pulmonary injury requires the resolution of tissue inflammation, fibroblast proliferation, and matrix molecule deposition; the clearance of intraalveolar clot; and the reepithelization of the basement membrane. Cytokines have been implicated in each of these processes.

RESOLUTION OF TISSUE INFLAMMATION

In spite of their obvious importance, the processes that turn off an inflammatory response once appropriate healing has occurred are poorly understood. The data that are available, however, have implicated $TGF-\beta_1$, IL-4, and IL-6 in this process. TGF-β is well recognized as an inhibitor of a variety of macrophage, T-lymphocyte, and B-lymphocyte functions[29,30] while stimulating granulation tissue accumulation and tissue fibrosis.[31] IL-4 inhibits macrophage production of a variety of cytokines, including IL-1, IL-6, IL-8, TNF, and GM-CSF and endothelial-cell production of IL-8,[32,33] thus diminishing B-lymphocyte-, T-lymphocyte- and granulocyte-mediated inflammatory responses. Interestingly, IL-13, a newly discovered cytokine with many IL-4-like properties, has also been shown to inhibit macrophage cytokine production.[34] IL-6 long has been known to be a stimulator of the acute-phase response which is presumed to be a host response designed to limit tissue injury. More recently, IL-6 has been shown to inhibit tissue inflammation and fibrosis in a murine model of hypersensitivity pneumonitis[25] and to inhibit macrophage TNF and IFN-γ production.[24]

FIBROBLAST PROLIFERATION AND MATRIX MOLECULE DEPOSITION

It is well known clinically that many inflammatory responses heal without residual scarring or loss of organ function. In contrast, many of the interstitial lung disorders progress relentlessly through a fibrotic phase, which causes significant morbidity and mortality. A variety of cytokines have been implicated in the pathogenesis of this fibrotic phase. Platelet aggregation at sites of injury results in TGF-β, PDGF, and epidermal growth factor (EGF) release, and vascular permeability alterations allow serum growth factors and coagulation factors to enter the alveolar and interstitial spaces of the lung. This activates fibroblasts and provides a thrombin meshwork upon which fibrosis may be structured. In addition, macrophage activation results in IL-1, TNF, $TGF-\beta_1$, IFN-γ, PDGF, TGF-α, IGF-1, and basic fibroblast growth factor (bFGF) release; T-cell activation results in TGF-β, IFN-γ, IL-4, and lymphotoxin elaboration. Under appropriate circumstances, PDGF, bFGF, IL-1, TNF, TGF-β, IFN-γ, EGF, TGF-α, and IGF-1 can stimulate fibroblast proliferation and/or collagen production. PDGF, TGF-β, and IL-4 also stimulate fibroblast chemotaxis,[35] and IL-1, TNF, IFN-γ, and TGF-β augment fibroblast production of hyaluronic acid.[1,36] Interestingly, IFN-γ, TNF, and IL-1, under appropriate circumstances, can also inhibit fibroblast proliferation and/or collagen production.[37-39] In addition, cytokine-cytokine interactions appear to play a role in inhibiting the fibrotic response, since TNF interacts with IL-1 or IFN-γ to synergistically inhibit fibroblast proliferation and collagen production.[37,39] IL-1 also negates the stimulatory effects of TGF-β on fibroblasts matrix molecule production.[40]

CLEARANCE OF INTRAALVEOLAR CLOT

As noted above, the clearance of intraalveolar clot depends on the balance of plasminogen, plasminogen activator, and plasminogen-activator inhibitors and is under the influence of cytokines such as TNF and TGF-β$_1$.[13–15]

REPAIR AND REEPITHELIZATION OF THE ALVEOLAR BASEMENT MEMBRANE

Many of the injuries that lead to interstitial pulmonary disorders cause alveolar epithelial damage and alter basement membrane integrity. Thus, restoration of the integrity and reepithelization of the basement membrane are key components of the recovery from these insults. When successfully accomplished, healing occurs with restoration of normal or near-normal architecture. When the damage is so extensive as to preclude and/or delay these reparative processes, tissue fibrosis frequently ensues.[1,7] The reepithelization process involves alveolar-type II pneumocyte proliferation and differentiation into type I alveolar lining cells. A variety of cytokines, including TGF-α, EGF, and IGF-1,

are involved in this process. Fibroblasts and alveolar macrophages also produce factors involved in the growth and chemotaxis of alveolar epithelial cells. Recent studies have demonstrated that hepatocyte growth factor/scatter factor and keratinocyte growth factor are important mediators of these latter processes.[41]

Associations Between Cytokines and Interstitial Lung Disorders

Any attempt to understand the contributions that cytokines make in complex diseases like the interstitial disorders must take into account the fact that cytokine production at a site of injury may represent (1) a normal healing and repair response; (2) an abnormal response that contributes to injury and disease pathogenesis; or (3) dysregulation that is of only minor biologic significance (see Table 26-1). To differentiate amongst these options, one must determine whether (1) the cytokine is present at an appropriate site at an appropriate time in the evolution of the pathologic response; (2) the cytokine mediates relevant biologic processes; (3) treatment with antibodies or antagonists that specifically negate the biologic effects of the cytokine, alter the pathologic response;

TABLE 26-1 Cytokine-Disease Associations

Disease	Cytokine Association	Reference Number
Sarcoidosis	↑ IL-1	44,57
	↑ IL-1-receptor antagonist	51
	↑ TNF	45,58
	↑ GM-CSF	47,61
	↑ IFN-γ	48
	↑ IGF-1	50
	↑ MCP-1	53
	↑ IL-8	53
	↑ MIP-1α	52
	↑ IL-6	46,54,60
	↑ PDGF	49
	↑ IL-2	59
Bleomycin-induced lung injury	↑ TGF-β	64–66
	↑ IL-1	11,67
	↑ TNF	12,67
Idiopathic pulmonary fibrosis	↑ IL-2	71
	↑ IFN-γ	72
	↑ IL-8	74
	↑ TGF-β	75,79
	↑ IL-1	51
	↑ PDGF	76
	↑ IGF	77
	↑ MIP-1α	52,73
	↑ MCP-1	53,80
	↑ TNF	78
Hypersensitivity pneumonitis	↑ IL-1	85,87
	↑ IL-6	85
	↑ TNF	85,87
	↑ IL-3	82
	↑ GM-CSF	82
	↑ TGF-β	84
	↑ PDGF	88

and (4) the cytokine can reproduce a component of the pathologic event that is being studied. The answer to all four of these questions must be yes, to allow one to conclude that dysregulated production of the cytokine in question is a major component of the pathogenesis of the noted pathologic process. A large number of examples of dysregulated cytokine production have been documented in interstitial lung disorders. Unfortunately, for most, the role that the cytokine plays in disease pathogenesis has not been adequately defined. As a result, it is best to think of these findings as cytokine-disease associations that still warrant further investigation.

Systemic Sarcoidosis

Sarcoidosis is a multisystem granulomatous disorder which, despite decades of effort, has remained etiologically elusive (see also Chaps. 29 and 112). It is characterized pathologically by noncaseating granulomas composed of histiocytes, multinucleated giant cells, lymphocytes, and plasma cells. This granulomatous response is associated with mononuclear interstitial pneumonitis and varying degrees of pulmonary fibrosis. In-trathoracic structures are involved most frequently, with parenchymal lung involvement and/or lymph node (hilar, mediastinal) involvement in 90 to 100 percent of cases. In many patients, the disease appears to resolve spontaneously. In others, it can stabilize, remit, and relapse or proceed inexorably to severe scarring and pulmonary destruction. Approximately 20 percent of patients with sarcoidosis suffer a permanent loss of lung function, and a ≤ 5 percent mortality rate, most frequently due to respiratory failure and cor pulmonale, has been reported (reviewed in Ref. 42).

In an attempt to clarify the pathogenesis of sarcoidosis, bronchoalveolar lavage (BAL) has been applied extensively to this disorder. These studies have demonstrated an increased inflammatory response at sites of sarcoidosis tissue inflammation. This response is characterized by T-helper lymphocyte proliferation and activation, macrophage activation, and prominent cytokine dysregulation. The studies also have demonstrated a striking dichotomy between the activation seen in tissues and the depressed cell-mediated immune response and anergy frequently seen in the peripheral circulation of these patients, making sarcoidosis a prototypical example of immune compartmentalization.

The insults that cause systemic sarcoidosis lead to macrophage and lymphocyte accumulation in the lung. Macrophage accumulation results, at least in part, from the influx of small monocytelike cells[26] and an enhanced ability of alveolar macrophages to proliferate locally.[43] Once in the lung, the alveolar macrophages are activated, acquiring enhanced antigen-presenting capacities and ICAM-1 and LFA-1 expression, which likely promote endothelial adhesion and the maintenance of interstitial pulmonary inflammation. This activation also increases the ability of these cells to produce IL-1, TNF, GM-CSF, IFN-γ, IGF-1, PDGF, and IL-6[44–50] and may augment their production of the IL-1-receptor antagonist.[51] Studies of the BAL fluid from patients with sarcoidosis have also demonstrated increased levels of

MIP-1α,[52] IL-8,[53] and MCP-1[53]; immunohistochemical studies have demonstrated TGF-β, TNF, IFN-β, IL-1, and the IL-1-receptor antagonist in sarcoid granuloma[54–56]; and in situ hybridization has demonstrated increased levels of IL-1 and TNF mRNA in granulomatous tissue.[57,58] As a result of these studies, it is reasonable to believe that the pleotropic molecules IL-1 and TNF are cornerstones of this inflammatory response. Particularly important in this regard are the abilities of IL-1 and TNF to contribute to the lymphocyte proliferation and activation that are characteristic of this disorder. IGF-1 and PDGF likely serve as fibroblast mitogens; GM-CSF may contribute to the heightened macrophage proliferation seen in the lungs of these patients; IFN-γ may contribute to macrophage activation in this disorder; and MCP-1, MIP-1α, and IL-8 likely attract leukocytes to sites of inflammation. IL-1, TNF, and IL-6 induce fever and stimulate the acute-phase response seen in these patients. IL-6 also augments the terminal differentiation of B cells and thus may contribute to the elevated immunoglobulin levels seen in this disorder. The role that IL-6 plays is somewhat more quizzical, since it may contribute to the inflammatory response or actually serve to suppress macrophage cytokine production and tissue inflammation.[24,25]

T-cell activation and infiltration is a cardinal feature of sarcoidosis. The lymphocytes in the lungs of patients with sarcoidosis are largely T4+, Leu8-, 5/9+, and T17-. They spontaneously produce IL-2[59] and express increased amounts of IFN-γ[48] and monocyte chemotactic factors. The dysregulated production of IL-2 is felt to play a key role in this disorder, since IL-2 acts in an autocrine and/or paracrine fashion to stimulate T-lymphocyte proliferation and macrophage activation.

A major issue in the management of patients with sarcoidosis is the differentiation of symptoms and physiologic defects that are the result of active inflammation from those that are the result of fibrosis. The importance of this issue stems from the belief that anti-inflammatory agents can reverse inflammation-based but not fibrosis-based abnormalities and can prevent the development of tissue fibrosis. As a result, a number of investigators have attempted to determine whether BAL cytokine concentrations provide a means of prognostication. Although BAL samples a dynamic process at only a single point in time, a number of studies suggest that it can provide useful information. Specifically, the concentrations of IL-6, TNF-α, and IL-1 in BAL fluid may parallel disease activity in sarcoidosis.[54,60] Similarly, mRNA concentrations of GM-CSF in BAL cells have been reported to correlate with disease status during the year prior to study.[61] In the latter report, GM-CSF mRNA levels also correlated with the degree of BAL lymphocytic alveolitis and serum angiotensin converting enzyme levels. Although it is still unclear whether measurement of cytokine levels in a single BAL can truly predict disease progression,[62] further investigation appears to be warranted.

Bleomycin-Induced Pulmonary Fibrosis

Bleomycin is an antibiotic used widely in the treatment of malignancies, including cancer of the esophagus, lymphomas, and germ-cell tumors. In these treatment regimens, bleomycin is associated with a small but significant incidence of both an acute interstitial pneumonitis and, when more severe, life-threatening pulmonary fibrosis. As many as 10 percent of patients treated with the drug may be affected.[63] Pathologically, the disease progresses from an early stage characterized by interstitial edema with type II alveolar epithelial cell proliferation and mononuclear cell and neutrophil infiltration to a latter stage that also manifests collagen and extracellular matrix molecule deposition and tissue fibrosis. To understand the pathogenesis of this reaction, bleomycin has been used experimentally to induce interstitial pneumonitis and pulmonary fibrosis in a number of different animals. Studies of these models have implicated a variety of cytokines in the pathogenesis of this disorder. TGF-β appears to play an important role, since (1) only mice that are susceptible to bleomycin-induced injury accumulate increased amounts of TGF-β mRNA after bleomycin treatment; (2) this increase in TGF-β mRNA occurs before the increases in fibronectin and type I and type III collagen mRNA levels in the lungs of bleomycin-treated animals; and (3) antibodies against TGF-β significantly ameliorate bleomycin toxicity.[64–66] While TGF-β can be produced by a number of cells including platelets, alveolar macrophages, fibroblasts, and endothelial cells, in bleomycin-induced injury the primary site of TGF-β accumulation appears to be within alveolar macrophages. The mechanism of TGF-β induction in these cells is unknown. A direct effect has been postulated, however, since bleomycin directly stimulates TGF-β mRNA accumulation in cultured endothelial cells. IL-1 may also play an important role in bleomycin toxicity, since alveolar macrophages from bleomycin-sensitive animals release increased amounts of IL-1 compared to bleomycin-insensitive rodents and untreated animals,[67] and the IL-1-receptor antagonist diminishes bleomycin toxicity.[11] TNF has been similarly implicated because immunization with anti-TNF antibodies ameliorates bleomycin pulmonary toxicity and the administration of TNF exaggerates bleomycin-induced lung injury.[12,67] In contrast, IFN-γ[68] and GM-CSF[69] diminish collagen deposition in bleomycin-treated animals (see also Chap. 40).

Idiopathic Pulmonary Fibrosis

Idiopathic pulmonary fibrosis (IPF) is an inflammatory disease of unknown etiology. It carries a 5-year mortality of approximately 50 percent and often progresses to respiratory failure. Histologically, it is a nongranulomatous disorder characterized by a heterogeneous pattern of alveolar and interstitial inflammation and fibrosis. Initially, there is evidence of alveolar injury with exudation into the alveolar space and infiltration of the alveolar septa and epithelial areas with neutrophils, lymphocytes, macrophages, plasma cells, eosinophils, and mast cells. In its later stages, increased numbers of mast cells, fibroblasts, and connective tissue can be appreciated. Pathologists have recognized several microscopic patterns of this chronic interstitial pneumonia. They include usual interstitial pneumonia (UIP), bronchiolitis obliterans and organizing pneumonia (BOOP), and desqua-

mative interstitial pneumonia (DIP). UIP is characterized by normal lung interspersed with areas of alveolar damage, epithelial necrosis, fibrinous exudates, fibrosis, and honeycombing. This pattern is consistent with multiple and asynchronous injuries involving different areas of the lung over an extended period of time.[7] BOOP, which many now classify as a separate entity,[70] is characterized by a pattern of connective tissue proliferation within the lumina of small airways and by chronic inflammatory changes in the surrounding alveoli. Clinically, BOOP has been associated with an improved prognosis compared to the rest of the diseases in the IPF diagnostic category. DIP is characterized by a diffuse and uniform pattern of lung involvement. Lung biopsies from patients with DIP show type II pneumocyte hyperplasia, air space collections of alveolar macrophages, alveolar fibrin deposits, and interstitial inflammatory infiltrates. This pattern is more consistent with a single pulmonary insult.[7]

A variety of lines of evidence support the contention that in vivo cellular activation and cytokine production play an important role in the pathogenesis of IPF. Analysis of BAL from patients with this disorder have demonstrated elevated levels of IL-2, IFN-γ, MIP-1α, and MCP-1.[53,71–73] Alveolar macrophage, epithelial cell, and fibroblast activation are also prominent in this disorder. Alveolar macrophages from patients with IPF produce exaggerated amounts of IL-8, TGF-β, IL-1, PDGF, and insulinlike growth factors.[74–77] Similarly, epithelial cells manifest enhanced expression of TNF, TGF-β, and PDGF,[75–79] while fibroblasts from IPF lungs produce exaggerated amounts of MCP-1 after stimulation with TNF and/or IL-1.[80] The IL-1 and TNF that are produced likely play key roles in the pathogenesis of the injury and inflammation seen in this disorder. It is also likely that MIP-1α, MCP-1, and IL-8 contribute to leukocyte influx at sites of inflammation; IL-2 contributes to T-lymphocyte activation; and PDGF and IGF act as stromal-cell mitogens in this disease. The IFN-γ that is produced may contribute to the macrophage activation noted above. In addition, IFN-γ, via its known ability to inhibit stromal-cell collagen production,[37] may inhibit IPF tissue fibrosis, because high concentrations of circulating IFN-γ have been shown to correlate with increased responsiveness to corticosteroid therapy and impaired IFN-γ production is associated with tissue fibrosis.[81] (See also Chap. 111, Part I.)

Hypersensitivity Pneumonitis

Hypersensitivity pneumonitis is an inflammatory interstitial disease of the lung precipitated by inhaled antigen. In contrast to IPF, sarcoidosis, and other idiopathic pulmonary disorders, the offending agent in these disorders can often be identified in the domestic or occupational environment. Histologically, the disease is usually a granulomatous interstitial pneumonitis. Initially, the pneumonitis contains significant numbers of neutrophils. One subsequently notes a mononuclear cell infiltrate composed of macrophages and lymphocytes which are generally CD8+. BAL reveals a lymphocytic pattern consistent with the histologic findings.

Acute episodes of hypersensitivity pneumonitis often resolve with removal of the offending antigen. Chronic unchecked and/or repeated exposure can result in severe fibrotic changes of the lung and significant morbidity and mortality.

Farmer's lung is a hypersensitivity pneumonitis caused by the thermophilic actinomycetes present in moldy hay. Animal models of this disorder have been used to investigate the role that cytokines play in this process. Denis and coworkers analyzed a murine model prepared with *Micropolyspora faeni*.[25,82–86] These studies demonstrated that, in contrast to the alveolar macrophages from normals, the macrophages from the animals with hypersensitivity pneumonitis spontaneously released excessive quantities of IL-1, IL-6, and TNF, and—upon antigen stimulation—released increased amounts of IL-3, GM-CSF, and TGF-β.[82,84,85] The exact role in the pathogenesis of hypersensitivity pneumonitis that each of these cytokines plays is not clear. Studies in which the tissue levels of these molecules and/or their effector functions are modulated have, however, provided some interesting insights. TNF appears to be central in this process, since treatment with anti-TNF antibody prevented the development of hypersensitivity pneumonitis[86] and treatment with cyclosporin A decreased BAL TNF levels and tissue inflammation as defined by BAL cellularity.[85] The TGF-β that is produced may play a role in the fibrotic response seen in chronic hypersensitivity pneumonitis, since treatment with anti-TGF-β antibodies diminished the ability of alveolar macrophages from animals with hypersensitivity pneumonitis to stimulate fibroblast collagen production.[84] By contrast, IL-6 and IFN-γ appear to be important feedback cytokines since, under appropriate circumstances, both can diminish tissue responses in these murine models.[25,83]

Less information is available on human subjects with hypersensitivity pneumonitis. The information that is available appears to parallel the findings in the animal models. BAL macrophages obtained from patients with acute farmer's lung spontaneously secrete significantly greater amounts of TNF,[87] IL-1,[87] and PDGF[88] than controls. In addition, antigen avoidance or treatment with corticosteroids significantly decreased the release of these cytokines.[87] The mechanism of this stimulation of IL-1 and TNF release is poorly understood. It may, however, involve direct macrophage activation by the offending antigen, as evidenced by the ability of *M. faeni* to stimulate alveolar macrophage and blood monocyte IL-1 and TNF production.[89]

Therapeutic Implications

An optimal treatment for the interstitial pulmonary disorders would control their inflammatory and fibrotic components without preventing normal healing, inducing a state of profound immunosuppression, or generating other undesirable side effects. As a broader understanding of the mechanisms of cytokine mediation of pulmonary inflammation and fibrosis in the interstitial disorders is developed, the possibility emerges that cytokine-based treatments can accomplish these goals. Many treatments can be based on interventions that regulate the levels of bioactive cytokines. This can be accomplished by blocking cytokine production with drugs or antisense oligonucleotides, administering cytokine using recombinant protein or gene implantation, the administration of drugs or antibodies that bind to and inactivate the cytokine, or the administration of soluble blocking cytokines that bind to cytokine receptors but do not transduce biologic signals. The utility of treatment with steroids, cyclosporin A, recombinant IFN-γ, anti-TNF antibodies, anti-TGF-β antibodies, and the IL-1-receptor antagonist in animal models of the interstitial disorders[11,12,57,68,85] suggests that similar approaches eventually will be useful in humans. Many of these approaches are particularly attractive for the treatment of pulmonary disorders, since recombinant cytokines and cytokine modifiers can be applied to the lung in an organ-specific fashion via aerosol therapy.[90] Alternatively, treatment can be based on the ability to regulate target-cell response to a cytokine(s). This can be accomplished by regulating the production of cytokine receptors, inhibiting receptor signal transduction, the administration of antibodies against the cytokine receptor, or the administration of anticytokine antibodies and/or cytokine ligands coupled to cytotoxins.

Any discussion of cytokine-based therapeutics must take into account the incomplete nature of the knowledge of the role that cytokines play in the pathogenesis of the interstitial disorders. Importantly, in most cases it is still not clear whether dysregulation of a particular cytokine is a primary abnormality in the pathogenesis of the disorders, a normal healing response to a devastating insult, or an epiphenomenon. Without this information, it is possible that interventions that neutralize cytokines crucial for inflammation and scarring may improve interstitial and inflammatory disorders in the short term but have catastrophic effects if used chronically. A more detailed understanding of cytokine biology and the mechanisms of pulmonary inflammation in states of health and disease will allow appropriate targeting of the major steps in disease pathogenesis without disrupting normal healing responses. Given the current inadequate ability to treat many of these diseases with existing therapies, this represents an exciting frontier for pulmonary immunology and pharmacology.

References

1. Rochester CL, Elias JA: Cytokines and cytokine networking in the pathogenesis of interstitial and fibrotic lung disorders. *Semin Respir Med* 1993; 14:389.
2. Crystal RG, Bitterman PB, Rennard SI, et al.: Interstitial lung diseases of unknown cause: Disorders characterized by chronic inflammation of the lower respiratory tract. *N Engl J Med* 1984; 310:154.
3. Richerson HB, Seidenfeld JJ, Ratajczak HV, et al.: Models of pulmonary fibrosis: Misadventures and ramifications. *Chest* 1979; 75:267.
4. Richerson HB, Seidenfeld JJ, Ratajczak HV, et al.: Chronic experimental interstitial pneumonitis in the rabbit. *Am Rev Respir Dis* 1978; 117:5.

5. Warren JS: Intrapulmonary interleukin 1 mediates acute immune complex alveolitis in the rat. *Biochem Biophys Res Commun* 1991; 175:604.

6. Warren JS, Yabroff KR, Remick DG, et al.: Tumor necrosis factor participates in the pathogenesis of acute immune complex alveolitis in the rat. *J Clin Invest* 1989; 84:1873.

7. Crouch E: Pathobiology of pulmonary fibrosis. *Am J Physiol* 1990; 259:L159.

8. Okusawa S, Gelfand JA, Ikejima T, et al.: Interleukin 1 induces a shock-like state in rabbits. *J Clin Invest* 1988; 81:1162.

9. Leff JA, Wilke CP, Hybertson BM, et al.: Postinsult treatment with N-acetyl-L-cysteine decreases IL-1-induced neutrophil influx and lung leak in rats. *Am J Physiol* 1993; 265 (*Lung Cell Mol Physiol* 9):L501.

10. Goldblum SE, Sun WL: Tumor necrosis factor-α augments pulmonary arterial transendothelial albumin flux *in vitro*. *Am J Physiol* 1990; 258 (*Lung Cell Mol Physiol* 2):L57.

11. Piquet PF, Vesin C, Grau GE, et al.: Interleukin 1 receptor antagonist (IL-1ra) prevents or cures pulmonary fibrosis elicited in mice by bleomycin or silica. *Cytokine* 1993; 5:57.

12. Piquet PF, Collart MA, Grau GE, et al.: Tumor necrosis factor/cachectin plays a key role in bleomycin-induced pneumopathy and fibrosis. *J Exp Med* 1989; 170:655.

13. Gross TJ, Simon RH, Kelly CT, et al.: Rat alveolar epithelial cells concomitantly express plasminogen activator inhibitor-1 and urokinase. *Am J Physiol* 1991; 260:L286.

14. Chapman HA, Allen CL, Stone OL: Abnormalities in pathways of alveolar fibrin turnover among patients with interstitial lung disease. *Am Rev Respir Dis* 1986; 133:437.

15. Gerwin BI, Keski-Oja J, Seddon M, et al.: TGF-β_1 modulation of urokinase and PAI-1 expression in human bronchial epithelial cells. *Am J Physiol* 1990; 259:L262.

16. Albelda SM, Buck CA: Integrins and other cell adhesion molecules. *FASEB J* 1990; 4:2868.

17. Masinovsky B, Urdal D, Gallatin WM: IL-4 acts synergistically with IL-1β to promote lymphocyte adhesion to microvascular endothelium by induction of vascular cell adhesion molecule-1. *J Immunol* 1990; 145:2886.

18. Wolpe SD, Cerami A: Macrophage inflammatory proteins 1 and 2: Members of a novel superfamily of cytokines. *FASEB J* 1989; 3:2565.

19. Kunkel SL, Standiford T, Kashara K, et al.: Interleukin-8: The major neutrophil chemotactic factor in the lung. *Exp Lung Res* 1991; 17:17.

20. Doherty DE, Henson PM, Clark RAF: Fibronectin fragments containing the RGDS cell-binding domain mediate monocyte migration into the rabbit lung: A potential mechanism for C5 fragment-induced monocyte lung accumulation. *J Clin Invest* 1990; 86:1065.

21. Elias JA, Schreiber AD, Gustilo K, et al.: Differential interleukin-1 elaboration by unfractionated and density fractionated human alveolar macrophages and blood monocytes: Relationship to cell maturity. *J Immunol* 1985; 135:2198.

22. Kotloff RM, Little J, Elias JA: Human alveolar macrophage and blood monocyte interleukin-6 production. *Am J Respir Cell Mol Biol* 1990; 3:497.

23. Arend WP: Interleukin-1 receptor antagonist: A new member of the interleukin 1 family. *J Clin Invest* 1991; 88:1445.

24. Aderka D, Le J, Vilcek J: IL-6 inhibits lipopolysaccharide-induced tumor necrosis factor production in cultured human monocytes, U937 cells, and in mice. *J Immunol* 1989; 143:3517.

25. Denis M: Interleukin-6 in mouse hypersensitivity pneumonitis: Changes in lung free cells following depletion of endogenous IL-6 or direct administration of IL-6. *J Leuk Biol* 1992; 52:197.

26. Hance AJ, Douches S, Winchester RJ: Characterization of mononuclear phagocyte subpopulations in the human lung by using monoclonal antibodies: Changes in alveolar macrophage phenotype associated with pulmonary sarcoidosis. *J Immunol* 1985; 134:284.

27. Elias JA, Zitnik R, Ray P: Fibroblast immune-effector function, in Phipps R (ed): *Pulmonary Fibroblast Heterogeneity*. Ocala, FL, CRC Press, 1992, pp 295–322.

28. O'Garra A, Murphy K: Role of cytokines in determining T-lymphocyte function. *Curr Opin Immunol* 1994; 6:458.

29. Wahl SM: Transforming growth factor β: The good, the bad, and the ugly. *J Exp Med* 1994; 180:1587.

30. Tsunawaki S, Sporn M, Ding A, et al.: Deactivation of macrophages by transforming growth factor-β. *Nature* 1988; 334:260.

31. Roberts AB, Sporn MB, Assoian RK, et al.: Transforming growth factor type β: Rapid induction of fibrosis and angiogenesis *in vivo* and stimulation of collagen formation *in vitro*. *Proc Natl Acad Sci USA* 1986; 83:4167.

32. Hart PH, Vitti GF, Burgess DR, et al.: Potential anti-inflammatory effects of interleukin-4: Suppression of human monocyte tumor necrosis factor α, interleukin 1 and prostaglandin E$_2$. *Proc Natl Acad Sci USA* 1989; 86:3803.

33. Standiford TJ, Strieter RM, Chensue SW, et al.: IL-4 inhibits the expression of IL-8 from stimulated human monocytes. *J Immunol* 1990; 145:1435.

34. de Waal Malefyt R, Figdor CG, Huijbens R, et al.: Effects of IL-13 on phenotype, cytokine production, and cytotoxic function of human monocytes. *J Immunol* 1993; 151:6370.

35. Postlethwaite AE, Seyer JM: Fibroblast chemotaxis induction by human recombinant interleukin-4: Identification by synthetic peptide analysis of two chemotactic domains residing in amino acid sequences 70-88 and 89-122. *J Clin Invest* 1991; 87:2147.

36. Sampson PM, Rochester CL, Freundlich B, Elias JA: Cytokine regulation of human lung fibroblast hyaluronan (hyaluronic acid) production: Evidence for cytokine regulated hyaluronan (hyaluronic acid) degradation and human lung fibroblast-derived hyaluronidase. *J Clin Invest* 1992; 90:1492.

37. Kahari V-M, Chen YQ, Su MW, et al.: Tumor necrosis factor-α and interferon-γ suppress the activation of human type I collagen gene expression by transforming growth factor-β_1: Evidence for two distinct mechanisms of inhibition at the transcriptional and post-transcriptional levels. *J Clin Invest* 1990; 86:1489.

38. Elias JA, Jimenez SA, Freundlich B: Recombinant gamma, alpha, and beta interferon regulation of human lung fibroblast proliferation. *Am Rev Respir Dis* 1987; 135:62.

39. Elias JA: Tumor necrosis factor interacts with interleukin-1 and interferons to inhibit fibroblast proliferation via fibroblast prostaglandin-dependent and -independent mechanisms. *Am Rev Respir Dis* 1988; 138:652.

40. Heino J, Heinonen T: Interleukin-1-β prevents the stimulatory effect of transforming growth factor-β on collagen gene expression in human skin fibroblasts. *Biochem J* 1990; 271:827.

41. Panos RJ, Rubin JS, Aaronson SA, et al.: Keratinocyte growth factor and hepatocyte growth factor/scatter factor are heparin-binding growth factors for alveolar type II cells in fibroblast-conditioned medium. *J Clin Invest* 1993; 92:969.

42. Tanoue LT, Zitnik R, Elias JA: Systemic sarcoidosis, in Baum GL, Wolinsky E (eds): *Textbook of Pulmonary Diseases*, 5th ed. Boston: Little, Brown, 1994, pp 745–774.

43. Bitterman PB, Saltzma LE, Adelberg J, et al.: Alveolar macrophage replication: One mechanism for the expansion of the mononuclear phagocyte population in the chronically inflamed lung. *J Clin Invest* 1984; 72:460.

44. Hunninghake GW: Release of interleukin-1 by alveolar macrophages of patients with active pulmonary sarcoidosis. *Am Rev Respir Dis* 1984; 129:569.

45. Spatafora M, Merendino A, Chiappara G, et al.: Lung compartmentalization of increased TNF releasing ability by mononuclear phagocytes in pulmonary sarcoidosis. *Chest* 1989; 96:542.

46. Bost TW, Riches DWH, Schumacher B, et al.: Alveolar macrophages from patients with beryllium disease and sarcoidosis express increased levels of mRNA for tumor necrosis factor-α and interleukin-6 but not interleukin-1β. *Am J Respir Cell Mol Biol* 1994; 10:506.

47. Itoh A, Yamaguchi E, Kuzumaki N, et al.: Expression of granulocyte-macrophage colony-stimulating factor mRNA by inflammatory cells in the sarcoid lung. *Am J Respir Cell Mol Biol* 1990; 3:245.

48. Robinson BWS, McLemore TL, Crystal RG: Gamma interferon is spontaneously released by alveolar macrophages and lung T lymphocytes in patients with pulmonary sarcoidosis. *J Clin Invest* 1985; 75:1488.

49. Mornex JF, Martinet Y, Yamauchi K, et al.: Spontaneous expression of the c-sis gene and release of a platelet-derived growth factor-like molecule by human alveolar macrophages. *J Clin Invest* 1986; 78:61.

50. Rom WN, Basset P, Fells GA, et al.: Alveolar macrophages release an insulin-like growth factor 1-type molecule. *J Clin Invest* 1988; 82:1685.

51. Janson RW, King TE Jr, Hance KR, et al.: Enhanced production of IL-1 receptor antagonist by alveolar macrophages from patients with interstitial lung disease. *Am Rev Respir Dis* 1993; 148:495.

52. Standiford TJ, Rolfe MW, Kunkel SL, et al.: Macrophage inflammatory protein-1 alpha expression in interstitial lung disease. *J Immunol* 1993; 152:2852.

53. Car BD, Meloni F, Luisetti M, et al.: Elevated IL-8 and MCP-1 in the bronchoalveolar lavage fluid of patients with idiopathic pulmonary fibrosis and pulmonary sarcoidosis. *Am J Resp Crit Care Med* 1994; 149:655.

54. Steffen M, Petersen J, Oldigs M, et al.: Increased secretion of tumor necrosis factor-alpha, interleukin-1-beta, and interleukin-6 by alveolar macrophages from patients with sarcoidosis. *J Allergy Clin Immunol* 1993; 91:939.

55. Limper AH, Colby TV, Sanders MS, et al.: Immunohistochemical localization of transforming growth factor-beta 1 in the non-necrotizing granulomas of pulmonary sarcoidosis. *Am J Resp Crit Care Med* 1994; 149:197.

56. Rolfe MW, Standiford TG, Kunkel SL, et al.: Interleukin-1 receptor antagonist expression in sarcoidosis. *Am Rev Respir Dis* 1993; 148:1378.

57. Devergne O, Emilie D, Penchmaur M: Production of cytokines in sarcoid lymph nodes: Preferential expression of interleukin-1 beta and interferon gamma genes. *Human Pathol* 1992; 23:317.

58. Hyatt N, Coghill G, Morrison K, et al.: Detection of tumor necrosis factor alpha in sarcoidosis and tuberculosis granuloma using *in situ* hybridization. *J Clin Pathol* 1994; 47:423.

59. Saltini C, Spurzem JR, Lee JJ, et al.: Spontaneous release of interleukin 2 by lung T lymphocytes in active pulmonary sarcoidosis is primarily from the Leu3+DR+T cell subset. *J Clin Invest* 1986; 77:1962.

60. Homolka J, Muller-Quernheim J: Increased interleukin 6 production by bronchoalveolar lavage cells in patients with active sarcoidosis. *Lung* 1993; 171:173.

61. Itoh A, Yamaguchi E, Furuya K: Correlation of GM-CSF mRNA in bronchoalveolar fluid with indices of clinical activity in sarcoidosis. *Thorax* 1993; 48:1230.

62. Pueringer RJ, Schwartz DA, Gilbert SR, et al.: The relationship between alveolar macrophage TNF, IL-1, and PGE$_2$ release, alveolitis, and disease severity in sarcoidosis. *Chest* 1993; 103:832.

63. Schwarz MI, King TE, Rosenow EC, Martin WJ II: Drug-induced interstitial lung disease, in Schwarz MI, King TE Jr (eds): *Interstitial Lung Disease*, 2d ed. St Louis, Mosby-Year Book, 1993, pp 255–270.

64. Khalil N, Bereznay O, Sporn M, et al.: Macrophage production of transforming growth factor β and fibroblast collagen synthesis in chronic pulmonary inflammation. *J Exp Med* 1989; 170:727.

65. Hoyt DG, Lzo JS: Alterations in pulmonary mRNA encoding procollagens, fibronectin and transforming growth factor-β precede bleomycin-induced pulmonary fibrosis in mice. *J Pharmacol Exp Ther* 1988; 246:765.

66. Giri SN, Hyde DM, Hellinger MA: Effect of antibody to transforming growth factor beta on bleomycin-induced accumulation of lung collagen in mice. *Thorax* 1993; 48:959.

67. Phan SH, Kunkel SL: Inhibition of bleomycin-induced pulmonary fibrosis by nordihydroguaiaretic acid. The role of alveolar macrophage activation and mediator production. *Am J Pathol* 1986; 124:343.

68. Okada T, Sugie I, Aisaka K: Effects of gamma-interferon on collagen and histamine content in bleomycin-induced lung fibrosis in rats. *Lymph Cyt Res* 1993; 12:87.

69. Piquet PF, Grau GE, deKossodo S: Role of granulocyte-macrophage colony-stimulating factor in pulmonary fibrosis induced in mice by bleomycin. *Exp Lung Res* 1993; 19:579.

70. Wright JL, Cagle P, Churg A, et al.: Diseases of the small airways. *Am Rev Respir Dis* 1992; 146:240.

71. Meliconi R, Lalli E, Borzi RM, et al.: Idiopathic pulmonary fibrosis: Can cell mediated immunity markers predict clinical outcome? *Thorax* 1990; 45:536.

72. Robinson BWS, Rose AH: Pulmonary γ-interferon production in patients with fibrosing alveolitis. *Thorax* 1990; 45:105.

73. Standiford TJ, Rolfe MW, Kunkel SL, et al.: Macrophage inflammatory protein-1 alpha expression in interstitial lung disease. *J Immunol* 1993; 157:2852.

74. Carre PE, Mortenson RL, King TE, et al.: Increased expression of the interleukin-8 gene by alveolar macrophages in idiopathic pulmonary fibrosis. *J Clin Invest* 1991; 88:1802.

75. Khalil N, O'Connor RN, Unruh HW, et al.: Increased production and immunohistochemical localization of transforming growth factor-beta in idiopathic pulmonary fibrosis. *Am J Resp Cell Mol Biol* 1991; 5:155.

76. Antoniades HN, Bravo MA, Avila RE, et al.: Platelet-derived growth factor in idiopathic pulmonary fibrosis. *J Clin Invest* 1990; 86:1055.

77. Bitterman PB, Adelberg S, Crystal RG: Mechanisms of pulmonary fibrosis: Spontaneous release of the alveolar-macrophage-derived growth factor in the interstitial lung disorders. *J Clin Invest* 1983; 72:1801.

78. Piquet PF, Ribaux C, Karpuz V, et al.: Expression and localization of tumor necrosis factor-alpha and its mRNA in idiopathic pulmonary fibrosis. *Am J Pathol* 1993; 143:651.

79. Broekelmann TJ, Limper AH, Colby TV, et al.: Transforming growth factor beta 1 is present at sites of extracellular matrix gene expression in human pulmonary fibrosis. *Proc Natl Acad Sci USA* 1991; 88:6642.

80. Standiford TJ, Rolfe MR, Kunkel SL, et al.: Altered production and regulation of monocyte chemoattractant protein-1 from pulmonary fibroblasts isolated from patients with idiopathic pulmonary fibrosis. *Chest* 1993; 103:1215.

81. Prior C, Haslam PL: *In vivo* levels and *in vitro* production of interferon gamma in fibrosing interstitial lung diseases. *Clin Exp Immunol* 1992; 88:280.

82. Denis M, Ghadirian E: Murine hypersensitivity pneumonitis: Production and importance of colony-stimulating factors in the course of a lung inflammatory reaction. *Am J Respir Cell Mol Biol* 1992; 7:441.

83. Denis M, Ghadirian E: Murine hypersensitivity pneumonitis: Bidirectional role of interferon-gamma. *Clin Exp Allergy* 1992; 22:783.

84. Denis M, Ghadirian E: Transforming growth factor-β is gener-

ated in the course of hypersensitivity pneumonitis: Contribution to collagen synthesis. *Am J Respir Cell Mol Biol* 1992; 7:156.

85. Denis M, Cormier Y, Laviolette M: Murine hypersensitivity pneumonitis: A study of cellular infiltrates and cytokine production and its modulation by cyclosporin A. *Am J Respir Cell Mol Biol* 1992; 6:68.

86. Denis M, Cormier Y, Fournier M, et al.: Tumor necrosis factor plays an essential role in determining hypersensitivity pneumonitis in a mouse model. *Am J Respir Cell Mol Biol* 1991; 5:477.

87. Denis M, Bedard M, Laviolette M, et al.: A study of monokine release and natural killer activity in the bronchoalveolar lavage

of subjects with farmer's lung. *Am Rev Respir Dis* 1993; 147:934.

88. Shaw RJ, Clark RAF, Benedict SH, et al.: Evidence of increased platelet-derived growth factor mRNA in alveolar macrophages from some patients with interstitial lung disease. *Am Rev Respir Dis* 1989; 139:A203.

89. Denis M, Cormier Y, Tardif J, et al.: Hypersensitivity pneumonitis: Whole *Micropolyspora faeni* or antigens thereof stimulate the release of proinflammatory cytokines from macrophages. *Am J Respir Cell Mol Biol* 1991; 5:198.

90. Jaffe HA, Buhl R, Mastengeli A, et al.: Organ specific cytokine therapy. *J Clin Invest* 1991; 88:297.

Chapter 27
CHEMOKINES
KIAN FAN CHUNG

Following the characterization of several classical chemoattractants, such as N-formylmethionylleucylphenylalanine (fMLP), the complement fragment C5a, platelet-activating factor, and leukotriene B_4, an entirely new class of leukocyte chemoattractants has been discovered, and new members continue to be added to it. These cytokines have been named *chemokines* to convey their combination of *chemo*attractant and cyto*kine* properties. The chemokines constitute a superfamily of small secreted factors with little similarity in structure and function to traditional immune cytokines, such as the tumor necrosis factors (TNFs), interferons (IFNs), and interleukins (ILs). At least 18 human chemokines have been identified so far by cloning or biochemical purification and amino acid sequencing.

Chemokines have conserved sequences that indicate a common ancestral gene, and they share four conserved cysteine residues that form disulfide bonds in the tertiary structure. The chemokine superfamily has been classified into two branches according to the position of the first two cysteines in the conserved motif (Table 27-1; Fig. 27-1). The C-X-C branch (where X is an amino acid other than cysteine), also known as the α *chemokines*, is characterized by the presence of a single other amino acid between the first two cysteines in the primary structure. In the C-C branch (or β chemokines), the first two cysteines are directly adjacent to each other. In general, the biological activities of these two sub-families are somewhat distinct; most C-X-C chemokines act as chemoattractants for neutrophils, whereas most C-C chemokines act as chemoattractants for monocytes but not neutrophils. More recently, the discovery of lymphotactin, which does not attract neutrophils or monocytes but is active as a chemoattractant for lymphocytes,[1] has led to the description of another branch, the C branch. Lymphotactin lacks the first and third cysteines in the four-cysteine motif, but it shares much similarity in amino acid sequence with the C-C chemokines.

Discovery and Structure

C-X-C CHEMOKINES

One C-X-C chemokine, platelet factor 4 (PF-4), which is stored in the α granules of platelets, was described in 1955, before the chemokine superfamily had been recognized, and its amino acid sequence was published in 1977. However, IL-8, another C-X-C chemokine, is by far the most intensively studied chemokine. This substance is also called neutrophil-activating protein-1 (NAP-1), and its major actions are as a neutrophil chemoattractant and activator. The sequence of an IL-8 cDNA clone was first described in 1987, using differential hybridization to identify genes expressed in activated

TABLE 27-1   Human Chemokine Superfamily

C-X-C chemokines
    Epithelial-derived neutrophil attractant-78 (ENA-78)
    Interleukin-8 (IL-8) or neutrophil-activating protein-1 (NAP-1)
    Stromal cell-derived factor-1α and 1β (SDF-1α and 1β)
    Granulocyte chemotactic protein-2 (GCP-2)
    Melanocyte growth stimulatory activity (MGSA/GROα, β, or γ)
    Platelet factor-4 (PF-4)
    IP-10
    Monokine-induced by interferon-γ (MIG)
    Platelet basic protein
        β-thromboglobulin
        Connective tissue protein-III (CTAP-III)
        Neutrophil-activating protein-2 (NAP-2)
C-C chemokines
    RANTES (Regulated on activation, normal T-cell expressed, and secreted)
    C10
    HC-14
    I-309/T-cell activation gene 3 (TCA3)
    Macrophage inflammatory protein-1α and 1β (MIP-1α and 1β)
    Monocyte chemoattractant protein-1, 2, and 3 (MCP-1, 2, and 3)
C chemokine
    Lymphotactin

human lymphocytes.[2] This information was followed by the partial amino acid sequences of two neutrophil chemotactic factors, called *monocyte-derived neutrophil-activating peptide*[3] and *monocyte-derived neutrophil chemotactic factor*,[4] which were identical to the deduced sequence of the IL-8 cDNA clone. The gene encoding IL-8 was cloned and sequenced in 1989.[5] Several other C-X-C chemokines similar to IL-8 were discovered in rapid succession, including neutrophil-activating protein-2 (NAP-2),[6] which arises by N-terminal processing of platelet basic protein; GROα, GROβ, and GROγ[7,8]; epithelial cell-derived neutrophil-activating protein (ENA-78)[9]; and granulocyte chemotactic protein-2 (GCP-2).[10] The degree of sequence identity between IL-8 and these chemokines ranges from 24 to 46 percent. The N-terminal domain is a major determinant of the activity and potency toward neutrophils and must contain the sequence Glu-Leu-Arg (ELR) preceding the first cysteine.

The GROα/MGSA gene was identified originally from a tumorigenic Chinese hamster embryo fibroblast cell line, after which a homologous human gene was isolated.[11] The protein was purified from cultured supernatants of a human melanoma cell line and designated *melanoma growth stimulatory activity* (MGSA).[12] Two additional GRO gene products

FIGURE 27-1 Graphic representation of the amino acid sequence relationship between known human C-X-C and C-C chemokines, with the percentage identity between any two sequences shown by the position of their common branch point as measured against the scale. The target cells in the middle column are based on functional and/or binding assays. Underlined targets indicate that the mRNA for the corresponding cloned receptor is detectable. Abbreviations: for chemokines, see Table 27-1; M, monocyte/macrophage; T, T lymphocyte; N, neutrophil; Ba, basophil; Eo, eosinophil; B, B lymphocyte; MP, myeloid progenitor cells and/or precursor cell lines; IL-8RA, IL-8RB, interleukin-8 receptors types A and B. *(From Ahuja SK, Gao JL, Murphy PM: Chemokine receptors and molecular mimicry.* **Immunol Today 1994; 15:282.)**

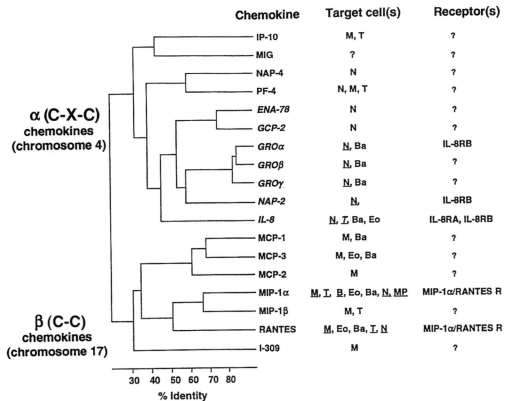

(GROβ and GROγ) later were discovered. The three GRO proteins have 90 percent sequence identity.[8] A secreted protein produced by lipopolysaccharide (LPS)-stimulated murine macrophages called macrophage inflammatory protein-2 (MIP-2) was found to be a chemoattractant for human neutrophils and to be closely related to GRO.[13] Another cDNA clone, KC, identified a transcript induced in murine fibroblasts; its amino acid sequence is similar to that of murine MIP-2.[14] Because GRO was more closely related to KC than to MIP-2, it was suggested that KC, rather than MIP-2, was the murine homolog of GRO. Another C-X-C chemokine, cytokine-induced neutrophil chemoattractant (CINC), was first purified from an epithelial clone of a normal rat kidney line stimulated by IL-1β or TNF-α and has neutrophil chemoattractant activity. Its closest reported human homolog is GRO/MGSA.[15]

C-C CHEMOKINES

Differential hybridization cloning of human tonsillar lymphocytes led to the discovery of the first human C-C chemokine gene, called LD78.[16] The cDNA isoforms of a closely related chemokine, Act-2, also were described,[17] and two similar proteins, macrophage-inflammatory protein-1α (MIP-1α) and MIP-1β, were purified from culture media of endotoxin-stimulated mouse macrophages.[18] Because the close similarity of the amino acid sequences of the murine and human proteins (75 percent sequence identity) suggested that these two molecules were homologs, the terms *human MIP-1α* and *human MIP-1β* have replaced LD78 and Act-2, respectively. The MIP-1α and MIP-1β genes can be expressed coordinately after stimulation of T cells (e.g., with anti-CD-3), of B cells, or of monocytes and macrophages (e.g., with lipopolysaccharide).[16,18–23] MIP-1α in human monocytes appears after adherence to endothelial cells and to other substrates.[24]

In murine fibroblasts, platelet-derived growth factor was shown to induce two genes: the KC gene (the murine homolog of the GRO gene) and a gene designated *JE*.[25] The human homolog of *JE* was found to encode a monocyte chemoattractant and activating factor, which led to the identification of monocyte chemoattractant protein-1 (MCP-1). MCP-1 is the best characterized C-C chemokine, having been purified and cloned from different sources.[17,26,27]

The other C-C chemokines—I-309, RANTES, and HC-14—were purified and cloned as products of activated T cells.[20,28,29] Subtractive hybridization was used to find genes expressed uniquely in T cells, and this led to the discovery of RANTES (*r*egulated on *a*ctivation, *n*ormal *T*-cell *e*xpressed, and *s*ecreted) cDNA, which encodes a 91-amino-acid polypeptide that gives rise to an 8-kDa secreted protein. The RANTES gene is expressed in IL-2–dependent T-cell lines. In peripheral blood mononuclear cells, low concentrations of RANTES transcripts can be measured in unstimulated cells, and the mRNA concentration increases 5 to 7 days after stimulation with antigen or phytohemagglutinin.[28] HC-14, discovered from IFN-γ–stimulated monocytes and now called MCP-2, has been isolated from osteosarcoma cell cultures,[30] which also yielded MCP-3.[31,32]

Sources

In general, monocytes and tissue macrophages are a rich source of C-X-C and C-C chemokines, which usually are produced by de novo synthesis. Monocytes release IL-8 in response to a large variety of proinflammatory agents, including IL-1α, IL-1β, TNF-α, GM-CSF, IL-3, lipopolysaccharide, and immune complexes. IL-8 also has been induced following adherence of monocytes to plastic and by changes in ambient oxygen concentration.[24,33,34] GROα, GROβ, and GROγ are expressed and secreted by monocytes and macrophages.[7,35,36] MCP-1 with MCP-2 is another major stimulated product of monocytes.

Lymphocytes are sources of some C-C chemokines, particularly RANTES,[20,28,37] I-309,[20,38] MIP-1α,[19,20,37] and MIP-1β,[19,21,39] but they are less prominent than mononuclear phagocytes as C-X-C chemokine producers. Neutrophils produce IL-8 in response to IL-1β, TNF-α, adherence,[40] and granulocyte/macrophage colony-stimulating factor (GM-CSF)[41]; GROα and GROβ on adherence to fibronectin[7]; and also the C-X-C chemokine MIP-1α.[42] Eosinophils release IL-8 after stimulation with the calcium ionophore A23187 but not with TNF-α or IL-1β,[43] and eosinophils of patients with hypereosinophilic syndrome express mRNA for MIP-1α.[44]

Epithelial cells stimulated with IL-1 or TNF-α produce IL-8,[45–48] GROα, GROβ, GROγ,[7,9,49] ENA-78,[9] MCP-1,[50,51] and RANTES,[52] but not MIP-1α. IL-8 expression by epithelial cells is increased by respiratory syncytial virus infections[53] and exposure to neutrophil elastase.[54] MCP-1 and RANTES immunoreactivity has been reported in human airway epithelium.[52,55] Other tissue cells, such as vascular endothelial cells and fibroblasts, also can be induced to express certain C-X-C and C-C chemokines.

Regulation

The genes for the C-C chemokines MCP-1, MIP-1α, MIP-1β, I-309, and RANTES are clustered on chromosome 17 at q11-21, while those for the C-X-C chemokines IL-8, GROα, GROβ, GROγ, IP-10, PF-4, and NAP-2 are all on chromosome 4 at q12-21. The most information is available on the transcriptional control of IL-8 gene. Several transcriptional regulatory elements can bind to the region preceding the first exon, including NF-κB, NF-IL-6, AP-1, glucocorticoid element, and an octamer-binding motif.[5] NF-IL-6 and NF-κB-like factors may act as *cis*-acting elements in IL-8 mRNA expression.[56] IL-8 mRNA expression after stimulation with IL-1 or TNF-α is rapid and results at least partly from transcriptional activation, as shown by nuclear run-off assays.[48,57–59] A secondary phase of IL-8 mRNA expression following an early rapid increase induced by IL-1 has been observed with cultured human airway epithelial cells. Enhancement of expression can be induced by cycloheximide, presumably by coinduction of inhibitors of synthesis of negative regulatory elements.[58,59] The stability of IL-8 mRNA may be influenced by RNA instability elements, AUUUA, found in the 3'-untranslated region.[60,61] IL-8 expression can be inhibited in blood monocytes[62] and in airway epithelial cells[63] by glucocorticoids, and IFN-γ, IL-4, and IL-10 can inhibit IL-8 production from blood monocytes.[62,64,65] Most of the effect of glucocorticoids on IL-8 mRNA occurs through inhibition of transcription.[63]

In the region immediately upstream from the RANTES gene there are several transcriptional consensus elements for DNA binding elements, including NF-κB, NF-IL-6, AP-1, and AP-3.[66] Many of these potential regulatory sites originally were described in promoters expressed specifically in T cells and myeloid or erythroid cells, whereas other elements were described first as consensus sites for factors responsive to specific second-messenger stimulation. This large number of potential regulatory sites raises the possibility of a wide range of transcriptional controls for RANTES expression in different tissues. For the MIP-1 genes, cis regulatory elements include GRE and CK-1.[67]

Comparison of RANTES and MIP-1α expression illustrates the differences in cellular sites and regulation of expression. For MIP-1α but not RANTES, mRNA expression and protein release can be induced in blood monocytes and alveolar macrophages by IL-1β and lipopolysaccharide.[22,68] IL-1β and LPS-induced expression and release of MIP-1α were inhibited by glucocorticoids through inhibition of transcription.[22] No GRE sites have been found upstream from the transcription initiation site of the human MIP-1α gene,[69] and it is possible that the effect of glucocorticoids could be exerted by interactions at other regulatory sites or with other transcription factors, such as AP-1. The inhibitory effect of glucocorticoids was largely reversed by cycloheximide, suggesting the intermediary effect of a protein. Part of the inhibition of MIP-1α mRNA resulted from a small increase in mRNA breakdown, which probably was related to repeating nucleotide motifs in the 3'-untranslated region of the MIP-1α mRNA.[19] In cultured human airway epithelial cells, RANTES but not MIP-1α mRNA and protein can be induced by a mixture of three cytokines—TNF-α, IL-1β, and IFN-γ—even though each of these cytokines is ineffective on its own.[52] This finding suggests that there is true synergy between these cytokines in inducing the expression of RANTES. Although there does not appear to be a GRE consensus element on the upstream region of the RANTES gene, glucocorticoids are potent inhibitors of the induced expression and release of RANTES.[52] Glucocorticoids do not inhibit all C-C chemokine expression. For example, MIP-1β gene expression induced in human monocytes by IL-7 and LPS is not inhibited by dexamethasone, although IL-4 is effective.[39]

The effect of the T_H2-derived cytokines IL-4, IL-10, and IL-13 on the induced expression of MIP-1α and RANTES also shows interesting differences. All of these cytokines inhibit the induction of MIP-1α mRNA and protein release from blood monocytes and alveolar macrophages. Blood monocytes are more sensitive than alveolar macrophages to the inhibitory effects of IL-10,[70] whereas the two cell types are similar in sensitivity to the inhibitory effects of IL-4.[68] In monocytes, the inhibition of MIP-1α mRNA induced by IL-4, IL-10, and IL-13 occurs mainly at the level of mRNA transcription. There is some additional effect on mRNA stability, particularly for IL-4 and IL-10; this effect requires de novo protein synthesis, as assessed with cycloheximide.[68,70,71] In human airway epithelial cells, on the other hand, only IL-4 exerted a significant inhibitory effect on the induction of

RANTES mRNA expression and protein release.[52] These studies suggest that endogenously released T_H2 cytokines may control the effects of chemokine expression and release.

Chemokines as Chemoattractants and Cell Activators

One of the major actions of chemokines is as chemoattractants. Migration of leukocytes from the vascular compartment into tissues involves first adhesion to the endothelial cell through the expression of integrins, then diapedesis, and then migration in response to a chemoattractant gradient. Chemokines may play a major role in activating migrating leukocytes and endothelial cells to increase adhesiveness and in establishing a chemotactic gradient. Interaction between chemokines and negatively charged proteoglycans may provide a solid phase for maintenance of a persistent chemotactic gradient following a brief burst of chemokine release.[72] The activity of IL-8 as a neutrophil chemoattractant has been shown to be potentiated by its binding to heparin sulfate, although the IL-8–activating activity is reduced.[73] MIP-1β immobilized by binding to proteoglycans binds to endothelium to trigger adhesion of T cells, particularly CD8+ T cells, to vascular cell adhesion molecule-1 (VCAM-1).[74] MIP-1β has been localized to lymph node endothelium and could act as a tethered ligand on endothelial cells. Thus, it could provide the required signals for activation of lymphocyte integrins for adhesion to endothelium and migration.

Nonchemotactic functions of chemokines that have been described relate to growth and tissue remodeling. GROα and IL-8, but not the C-C chemokines, inhibit collagen expression in synovial fibroblasts from patients with rheumatoid arthritis.[75] IL-8 is angiogenic in rat cornea and induces the migration of human umbilical-vein endothelial cells in vitro.[76] MGSA/GRO and stromal-derived factors-1α and 1β (also called pre-B cell stimulating factor) have activities as growth factors.[77] In the murine system, MIP-1α inhibits the cycling of primitive hematopoietic stem cells, while the related MIP-1β antagonizes this activity of MIP-1α.[78,79]

NEUTROPHILS

IL-8, the best studied of the C-X-C chemokines, acts on neutrophils to induce a change in shape, a transient increase in the intracellular free calcium concentration ($[Ca^{2+}]_i$), exocytosis with release of enzymes and proteins from intracellular storage organelles, and the respiratory burst through activation of NADPH-oxidase.[80] Thus, this chemokine behaves like a classical chemoattractant. IL-8 also upregulates the expression of two integrins (CD11b/CD18 and CD11c/CD18) during exocytosis of specific granules.[81,82] IL-8 activates neutrophil 5-lipoxygenase, causing the synthesis of leukotriene B_4 (LTB_4) and 5-hydroxyeicosatetraenoic acid (5-HETE),[83] and it also induces the production of platelet-activating factor.[84] Neutrophils are activated by most C-X-C cytokines, with the exception of those from platelet α granules, such as PF-4, which is virtually inactive, and interferon-γ (IFN-γ)–inducible protein (IP-10).[85] MIP-1α is the only C-C chemokine yet known to stimulate neutrophils; it causes a transient increase in $[Ca^{2+}]_i$ and a shape change.[86,87]

EOSINOPHILS

IL-8 induces an increase in $[Ca^{2+}]_i$, a shape change, and release of eosinophil peroxidase from eosinophils of patients with the hypereosinophilic syndrome,[88] and it can induce eosinophil chemotaxis of primed eosinophils.[89] However, eosinophils are more responsive to C-C than to C-X-C chemokines. RANTES is a powerful eosinophil chemoattractant, being as effective as C5a and two to three times more potent than MIP-1α.[90,91] RANTES upregulates the expression of CD11b/CD18 on eosinophils,[92] and RANTES and MIP-1α induce exocytosis of eosinophil cationic protein from cytochalasin B-treated cells, although RANTES is relatively weak in this effect.[90] When injected into the skin of dogs, RANTES induces an infiltration of eosinophils and monocytes.[93] RANTES, but not MIP-1α, also elicited a respiratory burst from eosinophils.[90] MCP-3 was found to be as effective a chemoattractant for eosinophils as RANTES.[94]

T LYMPHOCYTES

In the original description of IL-8, chemotactic activity for human T lymphocytes was described in vitro, with induction of lymphocyte infiltration on intradermal injection in rats.[95] More recent studies, however, show that IL-8 has a small chemotactic activity for either CD4+ or CD8+ T lymphocytes.[96] Intradermal injection of IL-8 in humans also does not attract lymphocytes.[97,98] RANTES is a chemoattractant for memory T cells in vitro, however.[99] Human MIP-1α and MIP-1β are also chemoattractants for distinct subpopulations of lymphocytes. MIP-1α has a predilection for CD8+ T lymphocytes, and MIP-1β, for CD4+ lymphocytes.[100] RANTES attracts both phenotypes and acts on resting and activated T lymphocytes, while MIP-1α and MIP-1β are effective on anti-CD3–stimulated cells only.[101] On the other hand, MIP-1β, but not MIP-1α, has been reported to be chemotactic for resting T cells and to enhance the adherence of CD8+ but not CD4+ cells to VCAM-1.[74]

MCP-1 induces T-cell migration.[102] Natural killer cells migrate vigorously in response to RANTES, MIP-1α, and MCP-1.[103] Human recombinant IP-10 is a chemoattractant for human monocytes and promotes T-cell adhesion to endothelial cells.[104] The C chemokine lymphotactin also has T-lymphocyte chemoattractant activity.[1] The selective chemoattractant activities for different subsets of lymphocytes suggest that specific members of the chemokine family may be involved in different immune and inflammatory responses.

BASOPHILS

IL-8 induces the release of histamine[105,106] and sulfidopeptide leukotrienes[106] from human blood basophils. Release is enhanced by pretreatment with IL3, IL5, or GM-CSF.[107] C-C chemokines are more powerful stimulants of basophils.

MCP-1 is as potent as C5a in stimulating exocytosis in human basophils[108–110] and causes the release of high concentrations of histamine. In the presence of IL-3, IL-5, or GM-CSF, there is enhanced release of histamine and production of leukotriene C_4.[108,110] RANTES and MIP-1α are less effective in causing release of histamine from basophils. MIP-1β is inactive on basophils.[111] RANTES is the most effective basophil chemoattractant,[109,111,112] while MCP-1 is more effective as an inducer of histamine and leukotriene release.[111]

MONOCYTES

In general, C-X-C chemokines have no activity toward monocytes, but IL-8 induces a small increase of $[Ca^{2+}]_i$ and a small respiratory burst.[113] By contrast, the C-C chemokines MCP-1, RANTES, I-309, HCl4 (or MCP-2), and MCP-3 attract monocytes in vitro,[30,99,114–118] and MCP-1, MCP-2, and MCP-3 induce selective infiltration of monocytes in animal skin.[30,119] All C-C chemokines stimulate an increase in $[Ca^{2+}]_i$.[87,111,118] MCP-1 also induces a respiratory burst, expression of β2-integrins (CD11b/CD18 and CD11c/CD18), and the production of IL-1 and IL-6.[116,119,120] The growth of tumor cell lines cultured in the presence of human blood lymphocytes is inhibited by the addition of MCP-1.[27]

Chemokine Receptors

The chemokine receptors form a family of structurally and functionally related proteins, being members of the superfamily of heptahelical, rhodopsin-like G-protein–coupled receptors. Thus, the responses of basophils, eosinophils, and monocytes to C-C chemokines are blocked by pretreatment of these cells with *Bordetella pertussis* toxin,[111,117] which specifically inhibits GTP-binding proteins (indicating the coupling to G proteins). The effects of C-X-C chemokines on neutrophils also induce G-protein activation.[121]

On basophils and eosinophils, in vitro studies examining the effects of cross-desensitization on $[Ca^{2+}]_i$ elevation and chemoattractant activities have revealed at least three different types of C-C chemokine receptors: (1) a receptor for MCP-1, which binds MCP-1 and MCP-3 and is expressed on basophils but not eosinophils; (2) a RANTES receptor, which binds RANTES and MCP-3 and is expressed on both basophils and eosinophils; and (3) an MIP-1α receptor, which binds MIP-1α, RANTES, and MCP-3 with lower affinity and is present on both cell types.[122] On monocytes, high-affinity binding sites have been demonstrated for MIP-1α, MIP-1β, MCP-1, and RANTES.[123–125] On the basis of competitive binding and cross-desensitization studies, a shared receptor for MIP-1α and MIP-1β; a shared receptor for RANTES, MIP-1α, and MCP-1; and a restricted, MCP-1–specific receptor have been proposed. For the C-X-C chemokine IL-8, two distinct high-affinity IL-8 receptors, one of which also binds with high affinity to the C-X-C chemokines GROα and NAP-2, have been described.[126,127]

The chemokine receptors that have been cloned can be classified into the following three general types:

1. *Specific receptors.* Specific receptors are ones that bind to only one chemokine, such as the interleukin-8 receptor A (IL-8 RA) and the MCP-1 receptor[128,129] (although the binding characteristics of the MCP-1 receptor to the closely related chemokines MCP-2 and MCP-3 are not known). IL-8 RA has been cloned from a neutrophil cDNA that was isolated from cDNA pools using its ability to confer IL-8 binding sites to COS cells,[128] and the deduced sequence is 77 percent identical to that of the IL-8 receptor B. A cDNA encoding an MCP-1 receptor has been isolated from a human cell line, and its 3-kb RNA has been found in monocytes but not in neutrophils or lymphocytes.[130]

2. *Shared receptors.* Shared receptors are ones that bind to more than one chemokine within either the C-X-C or the C-C subfamily; they are exemplified by the IL-8 receptor B (IL-8 RB) and the C-C chemokine receptor-1 (C-C CKR-1, also called the RANTES/MIP-1α receptor). IL-8 RB can be activated by C-X-C chemokines containing the sequence Glu-Leu-Arg in the N-terminal domain, including IL-8, GROα, and NAP-2, but not by C-C chemokines.[131,132] The C-C CKR-1 receptor, which binds to several C-C chemokines, has been cloned from monocyte cDNA[133,134] and has also been detected in normal neutrophils and in B and T lymphocytes.

3. *Promiscuous receptors.* Promiscuous receptors are ones that bind chemokines of both the C-X-C and the C-C subfamilies. Only one receptor of this type has been described to date, the erythrocyte chemokine receptor (ECKR).[135,136] The role of this receptor on red blood cells is unclear, but it has been suggested that it represents a mechanism by which chemokines can be removed. The ECKR has been identified as the Duffy blood group antigen expressed on red cells,[137] and it acts as a ligand through which *Plasmodium vivax* enters red blood cells.

Another class of chemokine receptors includes virally encoded receptors, such as one encoded by the cytomegalovirus open reading frame CMV US28[133] and one from herpesvirus saimiri, HSV ECRF3.[138] These probably are shared C-C and C-X-C receptors, respectively. While it is possible that these receptors have been transduced by viruses during evolution, the relevance of this is not clear.

Expression in Pulmonary Disease

PULMONARY FIBROSIS

An increased expression of IL-8 mRNA in alveolar macrophages of patients with idiopathic pulmonary fibrosis has been shown to correlate with the amount of IL-8 and the number of neutrophils recovered by bronchoalveolar lavage and the severity of the fibrosis.[139,140] In patients with idiopathic fibrosis, MCP-1 mRNA expression in lung macrophages and in lung epithelium, endothelium, and vascular smooth muscle has also been reported.[141] A similar distribution of MCP-1 protein has been observed using immunohistochemical methods in such patients.[142] Increased concentrations of IL-8, MCP-1, and MIP-1α in bronchoalveolar lavage fluid of patients with interstitial

lung disease and pulmonary sarcoidosis have been reported.[143,144] Blocking studies using anti-MIP-1α antibodies have shown that this chemokine accounts for a significant part of the monocyte chemoattractant activity observed in bronchoalveolar lavage fluid from these patients.[144] Support for such a potential role for MCP-1 has been obtained in a rat model of angiocentric granuloma, where increased MCP-1 mRNA was observed in the lung, with an increased MCP-1 concentration in bronchoalveolar lavage fluid. An anti-MCP-1 antibody blocked granuloma formation and monocyte accumulation.[145]

ACUTE LUNG INJURY

In the adult respiratory distress syndrome, high concentrations of IL-8 have been measured in the airspaces of such patients, and these correlate with the number of neutrophils recovered and with mortality.[146] Greater concentrations of IL-8 in bronchoalveolar lavage fluid were observed in patients who subsequently progressed to adult respiratory distress syndrome than in those who did not.[147] In the early stages of adult respiratory distress syndrome, the alveolar macrophage was an important source of IL-8.

In animal models of septic shock, systemic administration of LPS or IL-1 induced prolonged increase in plasma concentrations of IL-8 and IL-6,[148] while IL-8 injections in baboons led to a rapid, transient neutropenia within 1 min, followed by a rebound granulocytosis without evidence of shock.[149] Using a monoclonal antibody to IL-8, which has been shown in rabbit skin to inhibit LPS-induced accumulation of neutrophils, both lung reperfusion injury and the accompanying accumulation of neutrophils in the lung were inhibited in rabbits.[150,151]

An anti-human IL-8 antibody inhibited the recruitment of neutrophils and protected against lung injury in a rat model of IgG immune complex-induced lung injury.[152] Although a rat IL-8 has not yet been described, it is likely that this anti-human anti-IL-8 is reactive with a rat epitope on a peptide that is the homolog of human IL-8. In a similar model, increased expression of MCP-1 mRNA in alveolar macrophages has been described in association with an increased monocyte chemotactic activity of bronchoalveolar lavage fluid.[153] Neutralizing antibodies to rat MCP-1 markedly reduced monocyte/macrophage accumulation and attenuated the increased vascular permeability and hemorrhage in the lung induced by immune complexes.[154]

INFECTIONS

Pleural fluid obtained from patients with empyema contains a high concentration of IL-8, which accounts for a significant portion of the neutrophil chemotactic activity of the fluid.[155] In cystic fibrosis, increased concentrations of IL-8 have been assayed in bronchoalveolar lavage fluid and in sputum.[156,157] Neutrophil elastase, which is present in lung epithelial lining fluid and released from activated neutrophils, can stimulate IL-8 release from bronchial epithelial cells.[54] Bacterial products from *Pseudomonas* also may induce IL-8 expression in airway epithelial and bronchial glands.[158] High concentrations of IL-8 also have been reported in sputum from patients with chronic bronchitis and bronchiectasis.[157]

EXPOSURE TO IRRITANTS

In lung tissues and in alveolar macrophages of rats exposed to ozone and dust, a mineral-induced expression of MIP-2 mRNA was observed, associated with a neutrophilic inflammation.[159,160] Ozone exposure and endotoxin also induces expression of CINC mRNA as well as of the transcription factor NFκB.[161–162a] Endotoxin-induced neutrophil chemoattraction activity in bronchoalveolar lavage fluid is blocked by an anti-CINC antibody, suggesting that CINC accounts for this activity.[161] Acute pleurisy induced by intrapleural instillation of crocodilite asbestos in rabbits results from induction of IL-8 by mesothelial cells in response to a direct stimulatory effect of asbestos.[163]

ASTHMA

In allergic diseases, including asthma, there has been particular interest in the potential involvement of C-C chemokines. However, an early report has shown enhanced coexpression of IL-8 and GM-CSF in bronchial epithelial cells of patients with asthma,[164] which is of particularinterest because GM-CSF, IL-3, and IL-5 can increase the responses of basophils and eosinophils to chemokines.[89,108,110] In addition, IL-8 appears to possess chemotactic activity for primed eosinophils.[89] Human IL-8 causes accumulation of peritoneal guinea pig eosinophils in guinea pig skin,[165] and a human anti-IL-8 antibody inhibits IL-1–induced eosinophil accumulation in rat skin.[166] Expression of RANTES mRNA but not MIP-1α mRNA is increased in bronchial biopsy specimens from patients with mild asthma.[167] Although RANTES expression can be demonstrated in airway epithelium by immunohistochemistry, there does not appear to be a difference between normal subjects and asthmatics. However, the C-C chemokine MCP-1 has been shown to be overexpressed in asthmatic epithelium.[55]

A new chemokine, eotaxin, which is a major eosinophil chemoattractant, has been identified and cloned from bronchoalveolar lavage fluid of allergen-challenged sensitized guinea pigs.[168,169] Its human homolog has not been reported yet.

Conclusions

Although chemokines are structurally related, they form a diverse group of potent chemoattractants and cell activators that have effects on a wide range of cells. The central role of chemokines appears to be leukocyte trafficking, and it is likely, therefore, that chemokines are involved in immunologic and inflammatory processes as part of normal or pathologic responses. It is unclear at present why there are so many chemokines with overlapping and similar functions. Much remains unanswered about chemokines, and it is not clear how many more chemokines or chemokine receptors there are. The nature of the chemokine signal transduction also remains to be elucidated. While blocking antibodies and pharmacologic approaches will be developed to neutralize the effects of chemokines, it is not certain that specific inhibition against one or several chemokines will lead to a therapeutic effect. It is clear that chemokines have an important role in immunoregulation and inflammation.

References

1. Kelner GS, Kennedy J, Bacon KB, et al.: Lymphotactin: A cytokine that represents a new class of chemokine. *Science* 1994; 266:1395.
2. Schmid J, Weissmann C: Induction of mRNA for a serine protease and a beta-thromboglobulin-like protein in mitogen-stimulated human leukocytes. *J Immunol* 1987; 139:250.
3. Schroder JM, Mrowietz U, Morita E, Christophers E: Purification and partial biochemical characterization of a human monocyte-derived, neutrophil-activating peptide that lacks interleukin 1 activity. *J Immunol* 1987; 139:3474.
4. Yoshimura T, Matsushima K, Tanaka S, et al.: Purification of a human monocyte-derived neutrophil chemotactic factor that has peptide sequence similarity to other host defense cytokines. *Proc Natl Acad Sci USA* 1987; 84:9233.
5. Mukaida N, Shiroo M, Matsushima K: Genomic structure of the human monocyte-derived neutrophil chemotactic factor IL-8. *J Immunol* 1989; 143:1366.
6. Walz A, Baggiolini M: Generation of the neutrophil-activating peptide NAP-2 from platelet basic protein or connective tissue-activating peptide III through monocyte proteases. *J Exp Med* 1990; 171:449.
7. Haskill S, Peace A, Morris J, et al.: Identification of three related human GRO genes encoding cytokine functions. *Proc Natl Acad Sci USA* 1990; 87:7732.
8. Geiser T, Dewald B, Ehrengruber MU, et al.: The interleukin-8-related chemotactic cytokines GRO alpha, GRO beta, and GRO gamma activate human neutrophil and basophil leukocytes. *J Biol Chem* 1993; 268:15419.
9. Walz A, Burgener R, Car B, et al.: Structure and neutrophil-activating properties of a novel inflammatory peptide (ENA-78) with homology to interleukin 8. *J Exp Med* 1991; 174:1355.
10. Proost P, De Wolf-Peeters C, Conings R, et al.: Identification of a novel granulocyte chemotactic protein (GCP-2) from human tumor cells: In vitro and in vivo comparison with natural forms of GRO, IP-10, and IL-8. *J Immunol* 1993; 150:1000.
11. Anisowicz A, Bardwell L, Sager R: Constitutive overexpression of a growth-regulated gene in transformed Chinese hamster and human cells. *Proc Natl Acad Sci USA* 1987; 84:7188.
12. Richmond A, Balentien E, Thomas HG, et al.: Molecular characterization and chromosomal mapping of melanoma growth stimulatory activity, a growth factor structurally related to beta-thromboglobulin. *EMBO J* 1988; 7:2025.
13. Wolpe SD, Cerami A: Macrophage inflammatory proteins 1 and 2: members of a novel superfamily of cytokines. *FASEB J* 1989; 3:2565.
14. Oquendo P, Alberta J, Wen DZ, et al.: The platelet-derived growth factor-inducible KC gene encodes a secretory protein related to platelet alpha-granule proteins. *J Biol Chem* 1989; 264:4133.
15. Watanabe K, Kinoshita S, Nakagawa H: Purification and characterization of cytokine-induced neutrophil chemoattractant produced by epithelioid cell line of normal rat kidney (NRK-52E cell). *Biochem Biophys Res Commun* 1989; 161:1093.

16. Obaru K, Fukuda M, Maeda S, Shimada K: A cDNA clone used to study mRNA inducible in human tonsillar lymphocytes by a tumor promoter. *J Biochem* 1986; 99:885.

17. Miller MD, Krangel MS: Biology and biochemistry of the chemokines: A family of chemotactic and inflammatory cytokines. *Crit Rev Immunol* 1992; 12:17.

18. Wolpe SD, Davatelis G, Sherry B, et al.: Macrophages secrete a novel heparin-binding protein with inflammatory and neutrophil chemokinetic properties. *J Exp Med* 1988; 167:570.

19. Zipfel PF, Balke J, Irving S, et al.: Mitogenic activation of human T cells induces two closely related genes which share structural similarities with a new family of secreted factors. *J Immunol* 1989; 142:1582.

20. Miller MD, Hata S, de Waal Malefyt R, Krangel MS: A novel polypeptide secreted by activated human T lymphoctyes. *J Immunol* 1989; 143:2907.

21. Lipes MA, Napolitano M, Jeang KT, et al.: Identification, cloning, and characterization of an immune activation gene. *Proc Natl Acad Sci USA* 1988; 85:9704.

22. Berkman N, Jose P, Williams T, et al.: Dexamethasone inhibits basal, lipopolysaccharide and interleukin-1β induced expression of macrophage inflammatory protein-1α from peripheral blood monocytes and alveolar macrophages. *Am J Respir Crit Care Med* 1994; 149:A14.

23. Van Otteren GM, Standiford TJ, Kunkel SL, et al.: Expression and regulation of macrophage inflammatory protein-1α by murine alveolar and peritoneal macrophages. *Am J Respir Cell Mol Biol* 1994; 10:8.

24. Sporn SA, Eierman DF, Johnson CE, et al.: Monocyte adherence results in selective induction of novel genes sharing homology with mediators of inflammation and tissue repair. *J Immunol* 1990; 144:4434.

25. Cochran BH, Reffel AC, Stiles CD: Molecular cloning of gene sequences regulated by platelet-derived growth factor. *Cell* 1983; 33:939.

26. Yoshimura T, Yuhki N, Moore SK, et al.: Human monocyte chemoattractant protein-1 (MCP-1): Full-length cDNA cloning, expression in mitogen-stimulated blood mononuclear leukocytes, and sequence similarity to mouse competence gene JE. *FEBS Lett* 1989; 244:487.

27. Matsushima K, Larsen CG, DuBois GC, Oppenheim JJ: Purification and characterization of a novel monocyte chemotactic and activating factor produced by a human myelomonocytic cell line. *J Exp Med* 1989; 169:1485.

28. Schall TJ, Jongstra J, Dyer BJ, et al.: A human T cell-specific molecule is a member of a new gene family. *J Immunol* 1988; 141:1018.

29. Chang HC, Hsu F, Freeman GJ, et al.: Cloning and expression of a gamma-interferon-inducible gene in monocytes: A new member of a cytokine gene family. *Int Immunol* 1989; 1:388.

30. Van Damme J, Proost P, Lenaerts J-P, Opdenakker G: Structural and functional identification of two human, tumor-derived monocyte chemotactic proteins (MCP-2 and MCP-3) belonging to the chemokine family. *J Exp Med* 1992; 176:59.

31. Minty A, Chalon P, Guillemot JC, et al.: Molecular cloning of the MCP-3 chemokine gene and regulation of its expression. *Eur Cytokine Network* 1993; 4:99.

32. Opdenakker G, Froyen G, Fiten P, et al.: Human monocyte chemotactic protein-3 (MCP-3): Molecular cloning of the cDNA and comparison with other chemokines. *Biochem Biophys Res Commun* 1993; 191:535.

33. Kasahara K, Strieter RM, Chensue SW, et al.: Mononuclear cell adherence induces neutrophil chemotactic factor/interleukin-8 gene expression. *J Leukocyte Biol* 1991; 50:287.

34. Metinko AP, Kunkel SL, Standiford TJ, Strieter RM: Anoxia-

35. hyperoxia induces monocyte-derived interleukin-8. *J Clin Invest* 1992; 90:791.

35. Schroder JM, Persoon NL, Christophers E: Lipopolysaccharide-stimulated human monocytes secrete, apart from neutrophil-activating peptide 1/interleukin 8, a second neutrophil-activating protein: NH₂-terminal amino acid sequence identity with melanoma growth stimulatory activity. *J Exp Med* 1990; 171:1091.

36. Iida N, Grotendorst GR: Cloning and sequencing of a new gro transcript from activated human monocytes: Expression in leukocytes and wound tissue [published erratum appears in *Mol Cell Biol* 1990; 10:6821]. *Mol Cell Biol* 1990; 10:5596.

37. Schall TJ, O'Hehir RE, Goeddel DV, Lamb JR: Uncoupling of cytokine mRNA expression and protein secretion during the induction phase of T cell anergy. *J Immunol* 1992; 148:381.

38. Miller MD, Wilson SD, Dorf ME, et al.: Sequence and chromosomal location of the I-309 gene: Relationship to genes encoding a family of inflammatory cytokines. *J Immunol* 1990; 145:2737.

39. Ziegler SF, Tough TW, Franklin TL, et al.: Induction of macrophage inflammatory protein-1β gene expression in human monocytes by lipopolysaccharide and IL-7. *J Immunol* 1991; 147:2234.

40. Strieter RM, Kasahara K, Allen RM, et al.: Cytokine-induced neutrophil-derived interleukin-8. *Am J Pathol* 1992; 141:397.

41. Takahashi GW, Andrews DF, Lilly MB, et al.: Effect of granulocyte-macrophage colony-stimulating factor and interleukin-3 on interleukin-8 production by human neutrophils and monocytes. *Blood* 1993; 81:357.

42. Kasama T, Strieter RM, Standiford TJ, et al.: Expression and regulation of human neutrophil-derived macrophage inflammatory protein 1α. *J Exp Med* 1993; 178:63.

43. Braun RK, Franchini M, Erard F, et al.: Human peripheral blood eosinophils produce and release interleukin-8 on stimulation with calcium ionophore. *Eur J Immunol* 1993; 23:956.

44. Costa JJ, Matossian K, Resnick MB, et al.: Human eosinophils can express the cytokines tumor necrosis factor-α and macrophage inflammatory protein-1α. *J Clin Invest* 1993; 91:2673.

45. Galy AH, Spits H: IL-1, IL-4, and IFN-gamma differentially regulate cytokine production and cell surface molecule expression in cultured human thymic epithelial cells. *J Immunol* 1991; 147:3823.

46. Elner VM, Strieter RM, Elner SG, et al.: Neutrophil chemotactic factor (IL-8) gene expression by cytokine-treated retinal pigment epithelial cells. *Am J Pathol* 1990; 136:745.

47. Standiford TJ, Kunkel SL, Basha MA, et al.: Interleukin-8 gene expression by a pulmonary epithelial cell line: A model for cytokine networks in the lung. *J Clin Invest* 1990; 86:1945.

48. Kwon O, Au BT, Collins PD, et al.: Tumour necrosis factor-induced interleukin-8 expression in pulmonary cultured human airway epithelial cells. *Am J Physiol* 1994; 267:L398.

49. Anisowicz A, Zajchowski D, Stenman G, Sager R: Functional diversity of gro gene expression in human fibroblasts and mammary epithelial cells. *Proc Natl Acad Sci USA* 1988; 85:9645.

50. Standiford TJ, Kunkel SL, Phan SH, et al.: Alveolar macrophage-derived cytokines induce monocyte chemoattractant protein-1 expression from human pulmonary type II-like epithelial cells. *J Biol Chem* 1991; 266:9912.

51. Elner SG, Strieter RM, Elner VM, et al.: Monocyte chemotactic protein gene expression by cytokine-treated human retinal pigment epithelial cells. *Lab Invest* 1991; 64:819.

52. Berkman N, Robichaud A, Krishnan VL, et al.: Expression of

RANTES in human airway epithelial cells: Effects of cortioco-steroids & interleukin-4, 10 & 13. *Immunology*; in press.

53. Choi AMK, Jacoby DB: Influenza virus A infection induces interleukin-8 gene expression in human airway epithelial cells. *FEBS Lett* 1992; 309:327.

54. Nakamura H, Yoshimura K, McElvaney NG, Crystal RG: Neutrophil elastase in respiratory epithelial lining fluid of individuals with cystic fibrosis induces interleukin-8 gene expression in a human bronchial epithelial cell line. *J Clin Invest* 1992; 89:1478.

55. Sousa AR, Lane SJH, Nakhosteen JA, et al.: Increased expression of the monocyte chemoattractant protein-1 in bronchial tissues from asthmatic subjects. *Am J Respir Cell Mol Biol* 1994; 10:142.

56. Mukaida N, Mahe Y, Matsushima K: Cooperative interaction of nuclear factor-κB and cis-regulatory enhancer binding protein-like factor binding elements in activating the interleukin-8 gene by pro-inflammatory cytokines. *J Biol Chem* 1990; 265:21128.

57. Sica A, Matsushima K, Van Damme J, et al.: IL-1 transcriptionally activates the neutrophil chemotactic factor/IL-8 gene in endothelial cells. *Immunology* 1990; 69:548.

58. Mukaida N, Matsushima K: Regulation of IL-8 production and the characteristics of the receptor for IL-8. *Cytokine* 1992; 4:41.

59. Mukaida N, Harada A, Yasumoto K, Matsushima K: Properties of pro-inflammatory cell type-specific leukocyte chemotactic cytokines, interleukin 8 (IL-8) and monocyte chemotactic and activating factor (MCAF). [Review] *Microbiol Immunol* 1992; 36:773.

60. Matsushima K, Morishita K, Yoshimura T, et al.: Molecular cloning of a human monocyte-derived neutrophil chemotactic factor (MDNCF) and the induction of MDNCF mRNA by interleukin 1 and tumor necrosis factor. *J Exp Med* 1988; 167:1883.

61. Shaw G, Kamen R: A conserved AU sequence from the 3' untranslated region of GM-CSF mRNA mediates selective mRNA degradation. *Cell* 1986; 46:659.

62. Seitz M, Dewald B, Gerber N, Baggiolini M: Enhanced production of neutrophil-activating peptide-1/interleukin-8 in rheumatoid arthritis. *J Clin Invest* 1991; 87:463.

63. Kwon OJ, Au BT, Collins PD, et al.: Inhibition of interleukin-8 expression by dexamethasone in human cultured airway epithelial cells. *Immunology* 1994; 81:389.

64. Standiford TJ, Strieter RM, Chensue SW, et al.: IL-4 inhibits the expression of IL-8 from stimulated human monocytes. *J Immunol* 1990; 145:1435.

65. de Waal Malefyt R, Abrams J, Bennett B, et al.: Interleukin 10 (IL-10) inhibits cytokine synthesis by human monocytes: An autoregulatory role of IL-10 produced by monocytes. *J Exp Med* 1991; 179:1209.

66. Nelson PJ, Kim HT, Manning WC, et al.: Genomic organization and transcriptional regulation of the RANTES chemokine gene. *J Immunol* 1993; 151:2601.

67. Widmer U, Manogue KR, Cerami A, Sherry B: Genomic cloning and promoter analysis of macrophage inflammatory protein (MIP)-2, MIP-1α, and MIP-1β, members of the chemokine superfamily of proinflammatory cytokines. *J Immunol* 1993; 150:4996.

68. Standiford TJ, Kunkel SL, Liebler JM, et al.: Gene expression of macrophage inflammatory protein-1α from human blood monocytes and alveolar macrophages is inhibited by interleukin-4. *Am J Respir Cell Mol Biol* 1993; 9:192.

69. Nakao M, Nomiyama H, Shimada K: Structures of human genes coding for cytokine LD78 and their expression. *Mol Cell Biol* 1990; 10:3646.

70. Berkman N, John M, Roesems G, et al.: Inhibition of macrophage-inflammatory-protein-1α expression by interleukin-10: Differential sensitivities in human blood monocytes and alveolar macrophages. *J Immunol* 1995; 155:4412.

71. Berkman N, Roesems G, Jose PJ, et al.: Interleukin-13 (IL-13) inhibits the expression of macrophage-inflammatory-protein-1α (MIP-1α) from human blood monocytes (PBM) and alveolar macrophages (AM). *Am J Respir Crit Care Med* 1995; 151:A826.

72. Witt DP, Lander AD: Differential binding of chemokines to glycosaminoglycan subpopulations. *Curr Cell Biol* 1994; 4:394.

73. Webb LM, Ehrengruber MU, Clark-Lewis I, et al.: Binding to heparin sulfate or heparin enhances neutrophil responses to interleukin 8. *Proc Natl Acad Sci USA* 1993; 90:7158.

74. Tanaka Y, Adams DH, Hubscher S, et al.: T-cell adhesion induced by proteoglycan-immobilized cytokine MIP-1 beta [see comments] *Nature* 1993; 361:79.

75. Unemori EN, Amento EP, Bauer EA, Horuk R: Melanoma growth-stimulatory activity/GRO decreases collagen expression by human fibroblasts: Regulation by C-X-C but not C-C cytokines. *J Biol Chem* 1993; 268:1338.

76. Koch AE, Polverini PJ, Kunkel SL, et al.: Interleukin-8 as a macrophage-derived mediator of angiogenesis. *Science* 1992; 258:1798.

77. Nagasawa T, Kikutani H, Kishimoto T: Molecular cloning and structure of a pre-B-cell growth-stimulating factor. *Proc Natl Acad Sci USA* 1994; 91:2305.

78. Graham GJ, Wright EG, Hewick R, et al.: Identification and characterization of an inhibitor of haemopoietic stem cell proliferation. *Nature* 1990; 344:442.

79. Broxmeyer HE, Sherry B, Cooper S, et al.: Macrophage inflammatory protein (MIP)-1β abrogates the capacity of MIP-1α to suppress myeloid progenitor cell growth. *J Immunol* 1991; 147:2586.

80. Baggiolini M, Wymann MP: Turning on the respiratory burst. [Review] *Trends Biochem Sci* 1990; 15:69.

81. Detmers PA, Lo SK, Olsen-Egbert E, et al.: Neutrophil-activating protein 1/interleukin 8 stimulates the binding activity of the leukocyte adhesion receptor CD11b/CD18 on human neutrophils. *J Exp Med* 1990; 171:1155.

82. Detmers PA, Powell DE, Walz A, et al.: Differential effects of neutrophil-activating peptide 1/IL-8 and its homologues on leukocyte adhesion and phagocytosis. *J Immunol* 1991; 147:4211.

83. Schroder JM: The monocyte-derived neutrophil activating peptide (NAP/interleukin 8) stimulates human neutrophil arachidonate-5-lipoxygenase, but not the release of cellular arachidonate. *J Exp Med* 1989; 170:847.

84. Bussolino F, Sironi M, Bocchietto E, Mantovani A: Synthesis of platelet-activating factor by polymorphonuclear neutrophils stimulated with interleukin-8. *J Biol Chem* 1992; 267:14598.

85. Dewald B, Moser B, Barella L, et al.: IP-10, a γ-interferon-inducible protein related to interleukin-8, lacks neutrophil activating properties. *Immunol Lett* 1992; 32:81.

86. Gao J-L, Kuhns DB, Tiffany HL, et al.: Structure and functional expression of the human macrophage inflammatory protein 1α/RANTES receptor. *J Exp Med* 1993; 177:1421.

87. McColl SR, Hachicha M, Levasseur S, et al.: Uncoupling of early signal transduction events from effector function in human peripheral blood neutrophils in response to recombinant macrophage inflammatory proteins-1α and -1β. *J Immunol* 1993; 150:4550.

88. Kernen P, Wymann MP, von Tscharner V, et al.: Shape changes, exocytosis, and cytosolic free calcium changes in stimulated human eosinophils. *J Clin Invest* 1991; 87:2012.

89. Warringa RA, Koenderman L, Kok PT, et al.: Modulation and induction of eosinophil chemotaxis by granulocyte-macrophage colony-stimulating factor and interleukin-3. *Blood* 1991; 77:2694.

90. Rot A, Krieger M, Brunner T, et al.: RANTES and macrophage inhibitory protein 1α induce the migration and activation of normal human eosinophil granulocytes. *J Exp Med* 1992; 176:1489.

91. Kameyoshi Y, Dorschner A, Mallet AI, et al.: Cytokine RANTES released by thrombin-stimulated platelets is a potent attractant for human eosinophils. *J Exp Med* 1992; 176:587.

92. Alam R, Stafford S, Forsythe P, et al.: RANTES is a chemotactic and activating factor for human eosinophils. *J Immunol* 1993; 150:3442.

93. Meurer R, Van Riper G, Feeney W, et al.: Formation of eosinophilic and monocytic intradermal inflammatory sites in the dog by injection of human RANTES but not human monocyte chemoattractant protein 1, human macrophage inflammatory protein 1α, or human interleukin 8. *J Exp Med* 1993; 178:1913.

94. Dahinden CA, Geiser T, Brunner T, et al.: Monocyte chemotactic protein 3 is a most effective basophil- and eosinophil-activating chemokine. *J Exp Med* 1994; 179:751.

95. Larsen CG, Anderson AO, Appella E, et al.: The neutrophil-activating protein (NAP-1) is also chemotactic for T lymphocytes. *Science* 1989; 243:1464.

96. Bacon KB, Camp RD: Interleukin (IL)-80-induced in vitro human lymphocyte migration is inhibited by cholera and pertussis toxins and inhibitors of protein kinase C. *Biochem Biophys Res Commun* 1990; 169:1099.

97. Swensson O, Schubert C, Christophers E, Schroder JM: Inflammatory properties of neutrophil-activating protein-1/interleukin 8 (NAP-1/IL-8) in human skin: A light- and electron-microscopic study. *J Invest Dermatol* 1991; 96:682.

98. Leonard EJ, Yoshimura T, Tanaka S, Raffeld M: Neutrophil recruitment by intradermally injected neutrophil attractant/activation protein-1. *J Invest Dermatol* 1991; 96:690.

99. Schall TJ, Bacon K, Toy KJ, Goeddel DV: Selective attraction of monocytes and T lymphocytes of the memory phenotype of cytokine RANTES. *Nature* 1990; 347:669.

100. Schall TJ, Bacon K, Camp RD, et al.: Human macrophage inflammatory protein alpha (MIP-1α) and MIP-1β chemokines attract distinct populations of lymphocytes. *J Exp Med* 1993; 177:1821.

101. Taub DD, Conlon K, Lloyd AR, et al.: Preferential migration of activated CD4+ and CD8+ T cells in response to MIP-1α and MIP-1β. *Science* 1993; 260:355.

102. Carr MW, Roth SJ, Luther E, et al.: Monocyte chemoattractant protein 1 acts as a T-lymphocyte chemoattractant. *Proc Natl Acad Sci USA* 1994; 91:3652.

103. Maghazachi AA, Al Aarkaty A, Schall TJ: C-C chemokines induce the chemotaxis of NK and IL-2-activated NK cells: Role for G proteins. *J Immunol* 1994; 153:4969.

104. Taub DD, Lloyd AR, Conlon K, et al.: Recombinant human interferon-inducible protein 10 is a chemoattractant for human monocytes and T lymphocytes and promotes T cell adhesion to endothelial cells. *J Exp Med* 1993; 177:1809.

105. White MV, Yoshimura T, Hook W, et al.: Neutrophil attractant/activation protein-1 (NAP-1) causes human basophil histamine release. *Immunol Lett* 1989; 22:151.

106. Dahinden CA, Kurimoto Y, De Weck AL, et al.: The neutrophil-activating peptide NAF/NAP-1 induces histamine and leukotriene release by interleukin 3-primed basophils. *J Exp Med* 1989; 170:1787.

107. Bischoff SC, Baggiolini M, De Weck AL, Dahinden CA: Interleukin 8-inhibitor and inducer of histamine and leukotriene release in human basophils. *Biochem Biophys Res Commun* 1991; 179:628.

108. Kuna P, Reddigari SR, Rucinski D, et al.: Monocyte chemotactic and activating factor is a potent histamine-releasing factor for human basophils. *J Exp Med* 1992; 175:489.

109. Alam R, Forsythe PA, Stafford S, et al.: Macrophage inflammatory protein-1a activates basophils and mast cells. *J Exp Med* 1992; 176:781.

110. Bischoff SC, Krieger M, Brunner T, Dahinden CA: Monocyte chemotactic protein 1 is a potent activator of human basophils. *J Exp Med* 1992; 175:1271.

111. Bischoff SC, Krieger M, Brunner T, et al.: RANTES and related chemokines activate human basophil granulocytes through different G protein-coupled receptors. *Eur J Immunol* 1993; 23:761.

112. Kuna P, Reddigari SR, Schall TJ, et al.: RANTES, a monocyte and T-lymphocyte chemotactic cytokine releases histamine from human basophils. *J Immunol* 1992; 149:636.

113. Walz A, Meloni F, Clark-Lewis I, et al.: [Ca^{2+}]$_i$ changes and respiratory burst in human neutrophils and monocytes induced by NAP-1/interleukin-8, NAP-2, and gro/MGSA. *J Leukocyte Biol* 1991; 50:279.

114. Yoshimura T, Robinson EA, Tanaka S, et al.: Purification and amino acid analysis of two human monocyte chemoattractants produced by phytohemagglutinin-stimulated human blood mononuclear leukocytes. *J Immunol* 1989; 142:1956.

115. Yoshimura T, Robinson EA, Appella E, et al.: Three forms of monocyte-derived neutrophil chemotactic factor (MDNCF) distinguished by different lengths of the amino-terminal sequence. *Mol Immunol* 1989; 26:87.

116. Rollins BJ, Walz A, Baggiolini M: Recombinant human MCP-1/JE induces chemotaxis, calcium flux, and the respiratory burst in human monocytes. *Blood* 1991; 78:1112.

117. Sozzani S, Luini W, Molino M, et al.: The signal transduction pathway involved in the migration induced by a monocyte chemotactic cytokine. *J Immunol* 1991; 147:2215.

118. Miller MD, Krangel MS: The human cytokine I-309 is a monocyte chemoattractant. *Proc Natl Acad Sci USA* 1992; 89:2950.

119. Zachariae CO, Anderson AO, Thompson HL, et al.: Properties of monocyte chemotactic and activating factor (MCAF) purified from a human fibrosarcoma cell line. *J Exp Med* 1990; 171:2177.

120. Jiang Y, Beller DI, Frendl G, Graves DT: Monocyte chemoattractant protein-1 regulates adhesion molecule expression and cytokine production in human monocytes. *J Immunol* 1992; 148:2423.

121. Kupper RW, Dewald B, Jakobs KH, et al.: G-protein activation by interleukin 8 and related cytokines in human neutrophil plasma membranes. *Biochem J* 1992; 282:429.

122. Dahinden CA, Geiser T, Brunner T, et al.: Monocyte chemotactic protein 3 is a most effective basophil- and eosinophil-activating chemokine. *J Exp Med* 1994; 179:751.

123. Van Riper G, Siciliano S, Fischer PA, et al.: Characterization and species distribution of high affinity GTP-coupled receptors for human RANTES and monocyte chemoattractant protein 1. *J Exp Med* 1993; 177:851.

124. Wang JM, McVicar DW, Oppenheim JJ, Kelvin DJ: Identification of RANTES receptors on human monocytic cells: Competition for binding and desensitization by homologous chemotactic cytokines. *J Exp Med* 1993; 177:699.

125. Wang JM, Sherry B, Fivash MJ, et al.: Human recombinant macrophage inflammatory protein-1a and -b and monocyte chemotactic and activating factor utilize common and unique receptors on human monocytes. *J Immunol* 1993; 150:3022.

126. Moser B, Schumacher C, von Tscharner V, et al.: Neutrophil-activating peptide 2 and gro/melanomen growth-stimulating

activity interact with ventrophil-activating peptide 11/... interleukin 8 receptors on neutrophils. *J Biol Chem* 1991; 266:10666.

127. Schumacher C, Clark-Lewis I, Baggiolini M, Moser B: High- and low-affinity binding of GRO alpha and neutrophil-activating peptide 2 to interleukin 8 receptors on human neutrophils. *Proc Natl Acad Sci USA* 1992; 89:10542.

128. Holmes WE, Lee J, Kuang WJ, et al.: Structure and functional expression of a human interleukin-8 receptor. *Science* 1991; 253:1278.

129. Charo IF, Myers SJ, Herman A, et al.: Molecular cloning and functional expression of two monocyte chemoattractant protein 1 receptors reveals alternative splicing of the carboxyl-terminal tails. *Proc Natl Acad Sci USA* 1994; 91:2752.

130. Murphy PM: The molecular biology of leukocyte chemoattractant receptors. [Review] *Annu Rev Immunol* 1994; 12:593.

131. Murphy PM, Tiffany HL: Cloning of complementary DNA encoding a functional human interleukin-8 receptor. *Science* 1991; 253:1280.

132. Lee J, Horuk R, Rice GC, et al.: Characterization of two high affinity human interleukin-8 receptors. *J Biol Chem* 1992; 267:16283.

133. Neote K, Digregorio D, Mak JY, et al.: Molecular cloning, functional expression and signaling characteristics of a C-C chemokine receptor. *Cell* 1993; 72:415.

134. Gao JL, Kuhns DB, Tiffany HL, et al.: Structure and functional expression of the human macrophage inflammatory protein 1 alpha/RANTES receptor. *J Exp Med* 1993; 177:1421.

135. Neote K, Mak JY, Kolakowski LF Jr, Schall TJ: Functional and biochemical analysis of the cloned Duffy antigen: Identity with the red blood cell chemokine receptor. *Blood* 1994; 84:44.

136. Neote K, Darbonne W, Ogez J, et al.: Identification of a promiscuous inflammatory peptide receptor on the surface of red blood cells. *J Biol Chem* 1993; 268:12247.

137. Horuk R, Colby TJ, Darbonne WC, et al.: The human erythrocyte inflammatory peptide (chemokine) receptor: Biochemical characterization, solubilization, and development of a binding assay for the soluble receptor. *Biochemistry* 1993; 32:5733.

138. Ahuja SK, Murphy PM: Molecular piracy of mammalian interleukin-8 receptor type B by herpesvirus saimiri. *J Biol Chem* 1993; 268:20691.

139. Carre PC, Mortenson RL, King TE Jr, et al.: Increased expression of the interleukin-8 gene by alveolar macrophages in idiopathic pulmonary fibrosis: A potential mechanism for the recruitment and activation of neutrophils in lung fibrosis. *J Clin Invest* 1991; 88:1802.

140. Lynch JP, Standiford TJ, Rolfe MW, et al.: Neutrophilic alveolitis in idiopathic pulmonary fibrosis: The role of interleukin-8. *Am Rev Respir Dis* 1992; 145:1433.

141. Antoniades HN, Neville-Golden J, Galanopoulos T, et al.: Expression of monocyte chemoattractant protein 1 mRNA in human idiopathic pulmonary fibrosis. *Proc Natl Acad Sci USA* 1992; 89:5371.

142. Iyonaga K, Takeya M, Saita N, et al.: Monocyte chemoattractant protein-1 in idiopathic pulmonary fibrosis and other interstitial lung diseases. *Hum Pathol* 1994; 25:455.

143. Car BD, Meloni F, Luisetti M, et al.: Elevated IL-8 and MCP-1 in the bronchoalveolar lavage fluid of patients with idiopathic pulmonary fibrosis and pulmonary sarcoidosis. *Am J Respir Crit Care Med* 1994; 149:655.

144. Standiford TJ, Rolfe MW, Kunkel SL, et al.: Macrophage inflammatory protein-1α expression in interstitial lung disease. *J Immunol* 1993; 151:2852.

145. Jones ML, Warren JS: Monocyte chemoattractant protein 1 in a rat model of pulmonary granulomatosis. *Lab Invest* 1992; 66:498.

146. Miller EJ, Cohen AB, Nagao S, et al.: Elevated levels of NAP-1/interleukin-8 are present in the airspaces of patients with the adult respiratory distress syndrome and are associated with increased mortality. *Am Rev Respir Dis* 1992; 146:427.

147. Donnelly SC, Strieter RM, Kunkel SL, et al.: Interleukin-8 and development of adult respiratory distress syndrome in at-risk patient groups. *Lancet* 1993; 341:643.

148. Van Zee KJ, Fischer E, Hawes AS, et al.: Effects of intravenous IL-8 administration in nonhuman primates. *J Immunol* 1992; 148:1746.

149. Van Zee KJ, DeForge LE, Fischer E, et al.: IL-8 in septic shock, endotoxemia, and after IL-1 administration. *J Immunol* 1991; 146:3478.

150. Harada A, Sekido N, Kuno K, et al.: Expression of recombinant rabbit IL-8 in *Escherichia coli* and establishment of the essential involvement of IL-8 in recruiting neutrophils into lipopolysaccharide-induced inflammatory site of rabbit skin. *Int Immunol* 1993; 5:681.

151. Sekido N, Mukaida N, Harada A, et al.: Prevention of lung reperfusion injury in rabbits by a monoclonal antibody against interleukin-8. *Nature* 1993; 365:654.

152. Mulligan MS, Jones ML, Bolanowski MA, et al.: Inhibition of lung inflammatory reactions in rats by an anti-human IL-8 antibody. *J Immunol* 1993; 150:5585.

153. Brieland JK, Jones ML, Clarke SJ, et al.: Effect of acute inflammatory lung injury on the expression of monocyte chemoattractant protein-1 (MCP-1) in rat pulmonary alveolar macrophages. *Am J Respir Cell Mol Biol* 1992; 7:134.

154. Jones ML, Mulligan MS, Flory CM, et al.: Potential role of monocyte chemoattractant protein 1/JE in monocyte/macrophage-dependent IgA immune complex alveolitis in the rat. *J Immunol* 1992; 149:2147.

155. Broaddus VC, Hebert CA, Vitangcol RV, et al.: Interleukin-8 is a major neutrophil chemotactic factor in pleural liquid of patients with empyema. *Am Rev Respir Dis* 1992; 146:825.

156. Dean TP, Dai Y, Shute JK, et al.: Interleukin-8 concentrations are elevated in bronchoalveolar lavage, sputum, and sera of children with cystic fibrosis. *Pediatr Res* 1993; 34:159.

157. Richman-Eisenstat JB, Jorens PG, Herbert CA, et al.: Interleukin-8: an important chemoattractant in sputum of patients with chronic inflammatory airway diseases. *Am J Physiol* 1993; 264:L413.

158. Inoue H, Massion PP, Verki IF, et al.: Pseudomonas stimulates interleukin-8 mRNA expression selectively in airway epithelium in gland ducts, and in recruited neutrophils. *Am J Respir Cell Mol Biol* 1994; 11:651.

159. Driscoll KE, Hassenbein DG, Carter J, et al.: Macrophage inflammatory proteins 1 and 2: Expression by rat alveolar macrophages, fibroblasts, and epithelial cells and in rat lung after mineral dust exposure. *Am J Respir Cell Mol Biol* 1993; 8:311.

160. Driscoll KE, Simpson L, Carter J, et al.: Ozone inhalation stimulates expression of a neutrophil chemotactic protein, macrophage inflammatory protein 2. *Toxicol Appl Pharmacol* 1993; 119:306.

161. Blackwell TS, Holden EP, Blackwell TR, et al.: Cytokine-induced neutrophil chemoattractant mediates neutrophilic alveolity in rats in association with nuclear factor kb activation. *Am J Respir Cell Mol Biol* 1994; 11:464.

162. Haddad EB, Salmon M, Sun J, et al.: Dexamethasone inhibits ozone-induced gene expression of macrophage inflammatory protein-2 in rat lung. *FEBS Lett* 1995; 363:285.

162a. Haddad EB, Salmon M, Koto H, et al.: Ozone induction of cytokine-induced neutrophil chemoattractant and nuclear factor-κB in rat lung: Inhibition by corticosteroids. FEBBS LETT 1996; in press.

163. Boylan AM, Ruegg C, Kim KJ, et al.: Evidence of a role for mesothelial cell-derived interleukin 8 in the pathogenesis of asbestos-induced pleurisy in rabbits. *J Clin Invest* 1992; 89:1257.

164. Marini M, Vittori E, Hollemburg J, Mattoli S: Expression of the potent inflammatory cytokines granulocyte-macrophage colony stimulating factor, interleukin-6 and interleukin-8 in bronchial epithelial cells of patients with asthma. *J Allergy Clin Immunol* 1992; 82:1001.

165. Collins PD, Weg VB, Faccioli LH, et al.: Eosinophil accumulation induced by human interleukin-8 in the guinea-pig in vivo. *Immunology* 1993; 79:312.

166. Sanz MJ, Weg VB, Bolanowski MA, Nourshargh S: IL-1 is a potent inducer of eosinophil accumulation in rat skin. *J Immunol* 1995; 154:1364.

167. Berkman N, O'Connor B, Barnes PJ, Chung KF: Expression of RANTES but not macrophage-inflammatory-protein-1α (MIP-1α) mRNA from endobronchial biopsies is greater in asthmatics than in normal controls. *Eur Respir J* 1994; 7:468S.

168. Jose PJ, Griffiths-Johnson DA, Collins PD, et al.: Eotaxin: A potent eosinophil chemoattractant cytokine detected in a guinea pig model of allergic airways inflammation. *J Exp Med* 1994; 179:881.

169. Griffiths-Johnson DA, Collins PD, Rossi AG, et al.: The chemokine, eotaxin, activates guinea-pig eosinophils in vitro and causes their accumulation into the lung in vivo. *Biochem Biophys Res Commun* 1993; 197:1167.

INFLAMMATION

Chapter 28
ADHESION MOLECULES
CRAIG D. WEGNER AND KIMM J. HAMANN

With the exception of some acute lung injuries and rare cases of pulmonary vasculitis, the major focus of inflammation in lung diseases is the airspaces. Asthma and cystic fibrosis are characterized by inflammation in and around the epithelium lining the larger and more central airways. In respiratory viral infections, peribronchiolar infiltrates impair gas exchange to a greater degree, and thus are more troublesome, than the cytopathologic effects of the virus. Finally, pneumonia, acute lung injuries, and pulmonary oxygen toxicity involve an often life-threatening alveolitis. As depicted in Fig. 28-1, adhesion molecules control the retention, locomotion, and activation of leukocytes at several (at least four) phases during their transition from a quiescent state circulating in the blood to a state of effector activity at inflammatory foci.

This chapter reviews the adhesion molecules, processes, and concepts involved at each of these phases, as they have been worked out from studies performed in vitro, in situ on systemic microcirculatory beds, and in vivo in organs other than the lungs. Processes unique to the lung microvasculature and tissue will then be expounded on as well as the potential role of specific adhesion molecules in representa-

tive inflammatory lung diseases. Finally, cell-adhesion pathways in lung inflammation, approaches to the identification of inhibitors of these pathways, and the effects of such inhibitors on host defence are considered.

Microvascular Adhesion: Leukocyte Margination and Diapedesis

SYSTEMIC (BRONCHIAL) MICROVASCULATURE

By studying the adhesion of neutrophils to confluent monolayers of human umbilical vein endothelial cells (HUVECs), planar membranes containing specific purified adhesion molecule(s), or monolayers of COS cells transfected with specific adhesion molecules, followed by confirming intravital microscopy of various systemic microvascular postcapillary venules, the molecules and steps involved in neutrophil margination have been elucidated (Fig. 28-2A). At sites adjacent to foci of tissue inflammation, the expression of members of two families of adhesion molecules are upregulated on the endothelium, presumably by cytokine stimulation, to

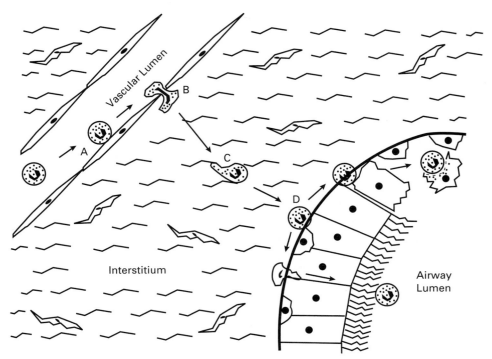

FIGURE 28-1 Four of the phases in the migration of leukocytes from the circulation to the airway lumen: (*A*) the initial "rolling" adhesion of leukocytes to the endothelium (margination), (*B*) transendothelial migration, (*C*) migration through the interstitium, and (*D*) retention and/or activation at, migration through, or leukocyte-mediated desquamation of the airway epithelium. Each of these phases uses a different set of adhesion receptors and ligands (see text and Fig. 28-2). (*From Wegner,*[240] *with permission.*)

direct leukocyte margination and eventual diapedesis at these sites. Members of the selectin family, P-selectin and E-selectin (so named because of their carbohydrate or "lectin" binding domain), cause a rapid in onset but weak adhesion, resulting in slowing or "rolling" of neutrophils along the endothelial vessel lining.[1-6] The counter-receptors for these molecules on neutrophils consist of a variety of sialylated glycoproteins, including L-selectin.[7-13]

Firm adhesion and stopping—margination—results from the slower in onset but stronger adhesion mediated by a member of the immunoglobulin supergene family, intercellular adhesion molecule-1 (ICAM-1), which is a ligand for the neutrophil β_2 integrins CD11a/CD18 (also termed LFA-1) and CD11b/CD18 (also termed Mac-1, Mo-1, or CR3).[6] Binding of these integrin receptors to their ligands requires the conversion of these receptors to an activation-specific phenotype (change in conformation?).[14,15] It is presumed that the initial slowing and rolling mediated by the selectins facilitates the conversion of a subpopulation of the neutrophil integrins to this activation-specific (increased bind-

FIGURE 28-2 (A, B) Adhesion molecules believed to regulate (*A*) The two steps of granulocyte margination and (*B*) granulocyte diapedesis in systemic microvascular beds.

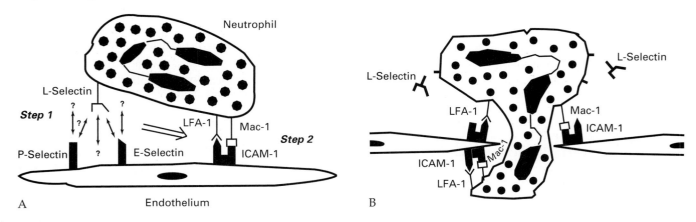

ing affinity) phenotype by stimulation of the neutrophil through (1) E-selectin–mediated adhesion,[16] (2) endothelial bound platelet-activating factor (PAF),[17,18] (3) endothelial secreted interleukin-8 (IL-8),[18] and/or (4) chemoattractants diffused from the surrounding inflamed tissue.[19] Neutrophil shedding of L-selectin[19] and translocation of CD11b/CD18 (Mac-1) from intracellular pools across the surface (from head to tail)[20] then control transendothelial migration (Fig. 28-2B).

Although the less well studied, these same molecules, steps, and processes are probably also used by other leukocyte subtypes.[8,9,21–26] The only notable addition is that, unlike the neutrophil, most other leukocyte subtypes (most notably eosinophils and lymphocytes) also express the β_1 integrin VLA-4 ($\alpha_4\beta_1$; CD49d/CD29) and the integrin $\alpha_4\beta_7$. These integrins bind to the immunoglobulin supergene family member vascular cell adhesion molecule-1 (VCAM-1) and the sialomucin MAdCAM-1, respectively, which are expressed on inflamed endothelium. In combination with Mac-1/ICAM-1 and LFA-1/ICAM-1 (CD18/ICAM-1), these interactions cause firm adhesion and initiate diapedesis.[22,26–36]

The complete dependence of neutrophils on the β_2-integrins for diapedesis in vivo is exemplified in patients with CD18 (LFA-1)-deficient leukocyte adhesion deficiency (LAD) type 1.[37,38] In severe phenotypes of this disorder, neutrophils and monocytes do not accumulate at sites of infection despite a moderate, chronic, neutrophilic leukocytosis that becomes striking during episodes of acute infection. The importance of other pathways (e.g., VLA-4/VCAM-1 and/or $\alpha_4\beta_7$/MAdCAM-1) for the diapedesis of other leukocyte subtypes is also illustrated by these patients, since eosinophils and lymphocytes do emigrate to sites of infection. Similarly, the importance of the selectin molecules in leukocyte migration is illustrated by type 2 LAD, in which patients are unable to assemble sialylated glycoproteins.[39]

PULMONARY MICROVASCULATURE

UNIQUE CAPILLARY SYSTEM: ADHESION-INDEPENDENT MARGINATION

Unlike the systemic circulation, in which margination of leukocytes occurs almost exclusively in the postcapillary venules,[40,41] the major site of margination in the pulmonary circulation is the capillary bed.[42,43] This phenomenon may be due partly to the much lower pressures and more pulsatile flow in the pulmonary circulation. However, the principal cause seems to be the smaller average diameter of the pulmonary capillaries and the large number of capillary segments (~60) that must be transversed from arteriole to venule.[44] The mean capillary diameter has been reported to be 2.0 μm in zone II and 5.8 μm in zone III.[45] The mean diameters of circulating neutrophils, monocytes, and lymphocytes have been estimated to be 7.0 μm, 6.4 μm, and 5.4 μm, respectively.[46,47] Thus, leukocytes must be deformed, in some cases substantially, to pass through the pulmonary microcirculation, and this situation produces an adhesion-independent "marginated pool." When circulating neutrophils are stimulated with any of a variety of activating agents, the increase in their retention in the lung is due initially (for the first 2 min) to an adhesion-independent

decrease in deformability,[46,48] and thereafter also to an increased CD18-dependent adhesiveness.[49]

Thus, it is interesting to speculate whether the fact that leukocytes slow in the capillaries of the pulmonary circulation owing simply to their size may make a selectin-mediated step unnecessary for their infiltration into the alveoli. In support of this theory, inhaled allergen-induced inflammation in primates has been reported to enhance ICAM-1 and E-selectin expression on blood vessels supplying the mainstem bronchus, but only ICAM-1 expression in the peripheral lung units.[50]

CD18-INDEPENDENT MIGRATION: REGULATED BY ALVEOLAR MACROPHAGES?

While the unconditional CD18 dependence of neutrophil emigration in systemic microvascular beds is universally supported by in vitro studies with HUVEC monolayers,[51,52] in vivo studies in animal models[53] and studies in patients with severe phenotypes of type 1 LAD (CD18 deficiency), infiltration of neutrophils into the alveoli through a CD18-independent pathway has been identified in animals[54] and was noted in the postmortem histologic examination of a patient with severe type 1 LAD.[53] Two sets of elegant experiments in rabbits suggest that the presence of a significant population of alveolar macrophages in normal lungs may explain the lung-specific CD18-independent pathway.

In the first study, the effect of an anti-CD18 monoclonal antibody on the accumulation of neutrophils in the alveoli and abdominal wall induced by various inflammatory stimuli was evaluated.[54] The accumulation of neutrophils in the lungs induced by the intrabronchial instillation of *Escherichia coli* endotoxin or PMA was CD18-dependent, while that induced by *Streptococcus pneumoniae* or hydrochloric acid was not. Neutrophil infiltration in the abdomen was CD18-dependent regardless of the stimulus. The CD18 independence of the *S. pneumoniae*-induced influx of neutrophils into the lung was conclusively demonstrated by showing that the influx of cells into the opposite lung caused by *E. coli* in dual-challenged animals was completely CD18-dependent.

In the second set of experiments, a CD18-independent pathway induced by *S. pneumoniae* was created in the peritoneum by the prior recruitment or injection of "primed" macrophages.[55] The *E. coli*-induced neutrophil infiltration remained CD18-dependent. Likewise, removal of these primed macrophages by washing the peritoneum restored the CD18 dependence of the *S. pneumoniae*-induced influx. The macrophage-generated product(s) elicited by *S. pneumoniae* and the adhesion molecules involved in this CD18-independent pathway remain to be identified.

More recently, the neutrophil influx and associated late-phase broncho-obstruction at 6 to 8 h after allergen inhalation in primates has been shown to be independent of ICAM-1[56] and CD18 (R.H. Gundel, personal communication). Whether this influx involves the same macrophage-generated product(s) and adhesion molecules, or E-selectin and hemorrhage,[57] also remains to be determined.

ARTERIOLES

As mentioned above, rolling, margination, and subsequent diapedesis of leukocytes in the systemic microvasculature is confined to the postcapillary venules. Observations using intravital microscopy under conditions of normal and retrograde flow at various rates have demonstrated that adherence is always much greater in the venules than the arterioles.[41] Thus, a site-specific expression of endothelial adhesion molecules in the systemic microvascular beds is indicated.

Two preliminary but convincing observations suggest that this may not be the case in lung microvascular beds. First, using intravital microscopy through pleural skin windows to examine microvascular beds of the pulmonary circulation, rolling of leukocytes along vessel walls has been observed to be common in the arterioles as well as the venules (W.W. Wagner and C.M. Doerschuk, personal communication). In addition, the expression of VCAM-1 (but not ICAM-1 or E-selectin) on arterioles of the bronchial circulation in the central airways following repeat allergen inhalations in primates has been noted (unpublished data).

Interstitial Adhesion: Migration and Priming

Maintenance of the integrity of pulmonary tissue requires the adhesion of cells to a complex of matrix molecules, including collagens, laminin, fibronectin, and glycosaminoglycans such as hyaluronic acid.[59] In addition to providing structural integrity, these molecules form the "connective tissue" through which cells must migrate after diapedesis. Once an inflammatory cell, such as an eosinophil, has traversed the endothelium, it encounters several cellular and noncellular structures, including the vascular basement membrane, the proteoglycans and glycosaminoglycans of the extracellular matrix of the lung parenchyma, and the basement membrane of the pulmonary epithelium (Fig. 28-1; Fig. 28-2C,D). Recent evidence suggests that interactions of the cells with molecules of these structures may be activating or priming events that may influence subsequent interactions with subendothelial tissue such as smooth muscle cells or the epithelial surfaces of the airways.

COMPONENTS OF THE EXTRACELLULAR MATRIX OF THE LUNG

The extracellular matrix of the lung, like interstitial matrices elsewhere in the body, contains a wide variety of proteins, proteoglycans, and glycosaminoglycans. The matrix components of the normal lung include at least eight different types of collagens, which, along with elastin, account for a large proportion of the pulmonary interstitium.[60] Of the principal interstitial collagens, type I is the most abundant collagen in the lung and is found throughout the pulmonary tissues.[61] Type IV collagen is the integral collagen of basement membrane; all basement membranes also contain laminins, various heparin sulfate proteoglycans, and nidogen/ entactin.[62,63] In addition to the collagens, lung extracellular matrix contains fibronectin, laminin, and thrombospondin, as well as glycosaminoglycans such as heparan sulfate (and associated glycoproteins) and hyaluronic acid.[60,61]

Extracellular matrix molecules are secreted primarily by

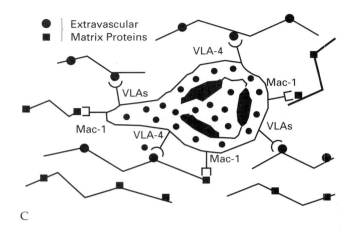

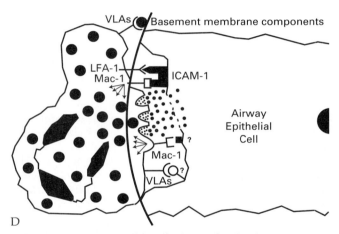

FIGURE 28-2 (C, D) Possible adhesion molecules that may regulate (C) granulocyte migration through and priming in the interstitium and (D) retention and activation of granulocytes and tissue-mediated injury proximal to the airway epithelium. (*From Wegner,*[240] *with permission.*)

cells in the matrix, especially by fibroblasts.[64] In the lung, bronchial epithelial cells also can produce fibronectin, laminin, and type IV collagen,[65] and alveolar type II cells have been shown recently to respond to transforming growth factor-β with increased production of proteoglycans.[66] In many pulmonary diseases, the production and deposition of many of the matrix molecules are altered, and these abnormalities further may complicate the cell-matrix interactions described below.

CELL RECEPTORS FOR MOLECULES OF THE EXTRACELLULAR MATRIX

The presence of cell-surface antigens has been evident for many years, but the variety of roles played by these molecules as matrix receptors is only now beginning to be understood. Table 28-1 lists the major receptors found on migrating cells in the lung and their ligands. Most known receptors for extracellular matrix proteins are members of the integrin superfamily,[67] which consist of heterodimers made up of α and β chains (Fig. 28-1). Most integrins bind

TABLE 28-1   Principal Extracellular Matrix Receptors on Inflammatory Cells

Name(s)	Integrin Subunits	CD Designation	ECM Ligands	Distribution[a]
VLA-1	$\alpha_1\beta_1$	CD49a/CD29	Collagens, laminin	Monocytes, T cells
VLA-2	$\alpha_2\beta_1$	CD49b/CD29	Collagens, laminin	Monocytes, macrophages, platelets, mast cells, T cells
VLA-3	$\alpha_3\beta_1$	CD49c/CD29	Fibronectin, collagens laminin	Monocytes, T cells, some B cells
VLA-4	$\alpha_4\beta_1$	CD49d/CD29	Fibronectin	Eosinophils, lymphocytes, monocyte, macrophages, mast cells
VLA-5	$\alpha_5\beta_1$	CD49e/CD29	Fibronectin	Monocytes, macrophages, mast cells, T cells, basophils
VLA-6	$\alpha_6\beta_1$	CD49f/CD29	Laminin	Neutrophils, monocytes, macrophages, platelets, T cells
Mac-1, CR3	$\alpha_M\beta_2$	CD11b/CD18	Fibrinogen, others?	Eosinophils, neutrophils, monocytes, macrophages, mast cells
VNR	$\alpha_V\beta_3$	CD51/CD61	Vitronectin, fibronectin, fibrinogen, collagens, thrombospondin	Platelets, macrophages, mast cells, basophils
Glycoprotein IIb/IIIa	$\alpha_{IIb}\beta_3$	CD41/CD61	Vitronectin, fibrinogen, thrombospondin	Platelets
VNR(?)	$\alpha_V\beta_5$	CD51 (α_V)	Vitronectin	Platelets, macrophages
LPAM-1	$\alpha_4\beta_7$	CD49d (α_4)	Fibronectin	Some lymphocytes
PECAM-1	nonintegrin	CD31	Heparan sulfate (HS), HS proteoglycans	Eosinophils, neutrophils, platelets, monocytes, B cells
ECMRIII, Pgp-1, Hermes AG	nonintegrin	CD44	Hyaluronic acid	Most leukocytes, including eosinophils

[a]Not exhaustive; some adhesion molecules may be expressed on quiescent or activated cells and not vice versa.

ABBREVIATIONS: VLA, very late antigen; VNR, vitronectin receptor.

only matrix proteins, but a few (like the β_2-integrins and VLA-4) also bind counter-receptors of the immunoglobulin superfamily on endothelial and other cells (see above). The integrin superfamily is subdivided on the basis of the β chains, and, of the several β families, integrins of the β_1 (very-late–activation [VLA] antigen) family seem to be the principal matrix receptors on migrating immune cells.[68] VLA integrins were first characterized on T lymphocytes[69] and have now been identified on several different myeloid cells, particularly those involved in inflammatory processes (Table 28-1). VLA receptors bind to a variety of matrix molecules, and many bind primarily through the Arg-Gly-Asp (RGD) tripeptide site (Fig. 28-3). The RGD sequence has been identified in almost all other extracellular matrix molecules, which may help to explain the multiplicity of integrin-matrix binding interactions (see Table 28-1). Nevertheless, other recognition sequences, such as the "CS-1" domain in fibronectin,[70] are important in matrix molecule interactions, and receptors do exhibit some degree of specificity and variability in affinity.[71,72]

Integrins of the β_2 (Leu-CAM) family function primarily in cell-cell adhesion and usually bind to a counter-receptor from the immunoglobulin superfamily, such as ICAM-1. However, the integrin Mac-1 ($\alpha_M\beta_2$) has been shown to bind also to the matrix protein fibrinogen[73,74] and to other unidentified matrix proteins.[75–78] The cytoadhesin (β_3) fam-

ily currently consists of two members, both of which are found on cells involved in inflammatory processes. The platelet glycoprotein IIb/IIIa, found only on platelets,[79] binds fibronectin, vitronectin, and other clotting proteins[80] and probably functions primarily during blood coagulation processes. The vitronectin receptors, $\alpha_V\beta_3$ and $\alpha_V\beta_5$, are expressed on macrophages *after* their differentiation from monocytes and mediate macrophage adhesion to vitronectin, fibrinogen, and fibronectin.[81] One of these receptors, $\alpha_V\beta_3$, also is found on human lung mast cells and some basophil cell lines,[82] but its distribution among other myeloid cells has not been studied extensively. Likewise, the distribution and binding affinities of other β families have not yet been well characterized.

There are a number of nonintegrin adhesion molecules that mediate interactions of cells with the extracellular matrix. One of these, CD44 (also known as Hermes Ag, H-CAM, ECMRIII, and Pgp-1) is related to the cartilage link proteins, and its activities have been reviewed recently.[83] Like the cartilage link proteins, CD44 binds specifically to hyaluronic acid in the extracellular matrix or on the surface of cells.[84,85] CD44 exists as a family of variants owing to alternative splicing[83] and is distributed broadly on both nonhematopoietic cells, such as epithelial cells and fibroblasts,[86] and hematopoietic cells, including macrophages and eosinophils.[87]

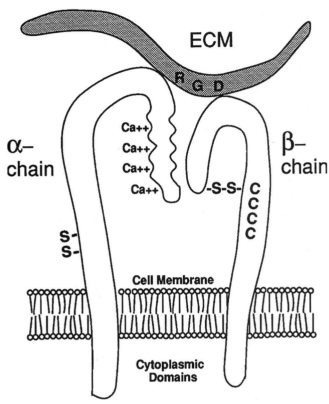

FIGURE 28-3 Schematic diagram of the basic structure of integrins. The receptor consists of two noncovalently associated transmembrane subunits, an α chain and a β chain. The β chain contains four cysteine-rich domains (C), and its "loop" is stabilized by an intrachain disulfide bond (S-S). The α chain contains three or four repeated domains that bind divalent cations (Ca^{2+} or Mg^{2+}) and are essential for integrin function. The ligand binding site is shown interacting with an RGD sequence in a putative extracellular matrix (ECM) molecule. The cytoplasmic domains link the receptor with the cytoskeleton, and regulation of integrin function may involve phosphorylation of the β-chain cytoplasmic domain.

CD31 is also a widely distributed adhesion molecule; it was named *platelet/endothelial cell adhesion molecule-1* (PECAM-1) after its discovery and function on platelets. CD31 is a member of the immunoglobulin superfamily of adhesion molecules and is found on monocytes, macrophages, some T cells, neutrophils,[88] and eosinophils,[89] as well as on endothelial cells and platelets. Like some other molecules of the immunoglobulin superfamily, CD31 can function both as a homophilic adhesion molecule interacting with itself[90] and as a heterophilic molecule interacting with heparan sulfate proteoglycans on the surface of cells or in the extracellular matrix.[91,92]

CELL ACTIVATION BY RECEPTOR INTERACTION WITH THE EXTRACELLULAR MATRIX

For many years, the regulatory actions of matrix molecules through integrins was attributed to the intracellular cytoskeletal connections possessed by these receptors.

However, recently evidence has been accumulating that both integrin and nonintegrin matrix receptors can regulate intracellular second messengers[93] and lead to so-called outside-in signals regulating the activation status of the receptor-bearing cells. Regulation of cell activation by adhesion molecules is being studied in most cell types involved in inflammatory diseases, but much of the original work was carried out in fibroblasts. In recent years, fibroblasts have been studied intensively in this regard, as well as in relation to their roles as interstitial tissue cells and synthesizers of matrix molecules. A detailed review of this information is beyond the scope of this chapter. Suffice it to say that interactions with matrix molecules such as fibronectin can significantly and rapidly alter gene expression in these cells[93] and can have important effects on the composition and architecture of lung parenchyma.

Among immune cells, lymphocytes have been studied the most extensively with regard to activation by matrix molecules. The migration and participation of lymphocytes in pulmonary diseases like asthma has been an active area of research for many years. Recently, studies of the matrix-mediated activation of T cells have revealed that the VLA receptors play important costimulatory roles. Adhesion of resting CD4+ T cells to fibronectin or laminin (but not to collagen or fibrinogen) facilitated CD3-mediated T-cell proliferation[94] and was mediated by interaction of VLA-4 and VLA-5 with fibronectin or by the binding of laminin by VLA-6. Furthermore, stimulation by fibronectin and laminin were distinct from and more potent than costimulatory signals provided by cytokines, such as IL-1β, IL-6, and IL-7.[94] VLA-5-mediated binding of T cells to fibronectin induces the DNA-binding protein AP-1, which is known to play a role in IL-2 gene regulation.[95] Cross-linking of VLA-4 ($\alpha_4\beta_1$) with antibodies led to specific phosphorylation of a 105-kDa protein,[96] while engagement of the vitronectin receptor (VNR; $\alpha_V\beta_3$) stimulated phosphorylation of a 115-kDa protein.[97] Cross-linking of the individual components of an integrin can led to differential phosphorylation as well, and stimulation with anti-α_5 monoclonal antibodies induced a different set of tyrosine-phosphorylated proteins than that induced by an anti-β_1 monoclonal antibody.[98]

Ligation of the CD44 antigen on T lymphocytes promotes T cell adhesion through the LFA-1 pathway and involves protein kinase C activation.[99] Binding of hyaluronic acid to T cells causes a rapid increase in intracellular Ca^{2+}, which is inhibited by a blocking anti-CD44 antibody.[100] Similarly, hyaluronate binding of CD44 or antibody cross-linking of CD44 on human T cell clones induced tyrosine phosphorylation typical of CD3-mediated T-cell activation and also upregulated proliferation and IL-2 production.[101,102] CD31 is found on subsets of CD4+ and CD8+ T cells, and ligation of CD31 with monoclonal antibodies can promote β-integrin adhesiveness, particularly of VLA-4.[103] This finding further suggests that cross-talk between matrix receptors is involved in lymphocyte activation and migration.

Tissue macrophages and the circulating monocytes from which they mature possess several matrix receptors through which signaling from the extracellular matrix can occur. As these cells are sources of cytokines and inflammatory mediators, activation of them in the tissues can have important effects on subsequent interactions. Adherence of monocytes to collagen matrices enhanced complement receptor expression of CR1 (CD35) and CR3 (CD11b CD18; Mac-1) and upregulated Fc-receptor–mediated phagocytosis.[104] The specific adhesion molecule(s) involved were not described in that study, but monocytes express VLA-1, VLA-2, and VLA-3, which can bind to collagen. In monocytes, adhesion to different matrix components results in selective patterns of gene expression.[105] Adhesion to fibronectin was found to regulate the expression of cytokine genes in a pattern distinct from that produced by adhesion to type IV collagen. On the other hand, while laminin is an important component of matrix structures such as basement membranes (along with type IV collagen), it was found to be relatively inefficient at stimulating expression of monocyte genes.[105] The non-integrin matrix receptors CD31 and CD44 also can signal monocytes and macrophages to regulate cell activity. Hyaluronate activation of CD44 on macrophages stimulated expression of IL-1β, tumor necrosis factor (TNF)-α, and insulin-like growth factor-1; anti-CD44 antibody blocked these effects of hyaluronate.[106] Ligation of CD31 with specific antibodies induced the generation of reactive oxygen metabolites in human monocytes, but it is not known if heparan sulfate, a putative matrix ligand for CD31,[91,92] will stimulate these cells in a similar fashion. Recently, however, macrophages were shown to respond to heparan sulfate as measured by proliferation[107] and the production of IL-1 and prostaglandin E_2.[108]

Activation of granulocytes by adherence to and migration through the pulmonary parenchyma is an important consideration in view of the proinflammatory potential of these cells and their mediators. While the role of the neutrophil in certain pulmonary diseases such as asthma remains unclear, a significant increase in the percentage of neutrophils in bronchoalveolar lavage (BAL) fluid can be a result of allergen bronchial challenge, and neutrophil mediators such as oxygen metabolites and products of arachidonate metabolism could contribute to airway responses in asthma.[109] Furthermore, a variety of stimuli, both infectious and noninfectious, can induce airways neutrophilia, and neutrophils are potent sources of toxic and proinflammatory mediators.[110] As noted above, neutrophils possess a variety of matrix receptors, including integrins as well as CD44 and CD31. Mac-1 (CD11b/CD18) on neutrophils can bind to fibrinogen and to an undetermined number of other matrix molecules. In contrast to the monocyte studies described above, cross-linking of the β2-chain (CD18) on neutrophils induced H_2O_2 production[111] and altered calcium and cAMP levels.[112,113] Neutrophils binding to laminin released specific granule constituents and were primed for subsequent superoxide release in response to formylmethionylleucylphenylalanine (fMLP).[114] Neutrophils adhering to fibronectin, vitronectin, and laminin also exhibited an augmented respiratory burst in response to TNF-α and TNF-β.[115] Both fibronectin and hyaluronic acid stimulated neutrophil function and migration in vitro.[116] In a recent study, ligation of CD31 on neutrophils (and monocytes) upregulated Mac-1 binding capacity.[117]

Mast cells and basophils also respond to matrix proteins. IL-3-dependent mast cell proliferation is augmented by vitronectin through the $α_Vβ_3$ receptor (VNR).[118] A rat basophilic cell line demonstrated enhanced $Fc_εRI$- and calcium-ionophore–mediated histamine release after binding to immobilized fibronectin; binding of these cells to fibronectin results in tyrosine phosphorylation of several proteins even in the absence of $Fc_εRI$ stimulation.[82] In another study, adhesion of mast cells to fibronectin and the resulting enhanced exocytosis of β-hexosaminidase (as an indicator of degranulation) were blocked by RGD and CS-2 peptides or by anti-VLA-4, anti-VLA-5, and anti-VNR monoclonal antibodies.[119] Similarly, augmented cytokine production by mast cells on fibronectin was inhibited by a blocking RGD peptide.[119]

As cells central to the inflammatory processes now established to exist in asthma, eosinophils have attracted much attention with regard to mechanisms of activation. Superoxide generation stimulated by fMLP was greater for human eosinophils bound to extracellular matrix components (e.g., fibronectin, laminin, collagens) than for eosinophils in suspension, although the receptors involved were not studied.[120] Furthermore, TNF and platelet-activating factor stimulated only adherent eosinophils. Cross-linking of either β1 or β2 integrins on eosinophils stimulated the respiratory burst and spreading in these cells.[121] Adhesion to fibronectin prolongs eosinophil survival by triggering autocrine generation of granulocyte/macrophage colony-stimulating factor (GM-CSF) and IL-3.[122] The effect could be blocked with antibodies to either fibronectin or the eosinophil surface antigen VLA-4. Adhesion to fibronectin also primed human eosinophils for release of mediators that may play important effector roles in respiratory diseases. Calcium-ionophore–stimulated release of leukotriene C_4 was augmented by interaction of eosinophil VLA-4 with fibronectin.[123] Likewise, adhesion of eosinophils to immobilized fibronectin for 1 to 2 h caused enhanced fMLP-stimulated release of the eosinophil granule protein eosinophil peroxidase (EPO)[124] (Fig. 28-4). Blockade with anti-VLA-4, but not anti-CD18, abrogated this augmentation (Fig. 28-4).

It seems clear that many cell-matrix interactions may occur during migration of cells through the pulmonary interstitium. Certainly, cells use the extracellular matrixes as a substratum for movement, but these interactions probably also alter the activation status of the migrating cells. These effects may include upregulation of gene expression and proliferative responses; alteration of other cell-surface receptors, which amplify the activation or augment migration; and production and release of mediators that may have similar autocrine or paracrine effects. Amplification of the inflammatory response in diseases like asthma may be one outcome of these complex interactions.

Epithelial Adhesion: the Site of Action

The epithelium lining the air spaces of the lungs plays a vital role as the first line of defence (protective barrier) against airborne particles, allergens, foreign proteins, chemicals, microbes, and viruses. In accordance with this role, the

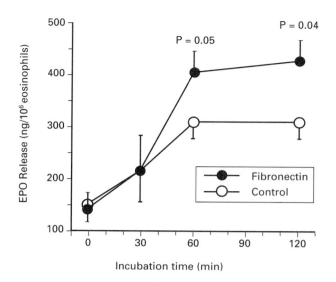

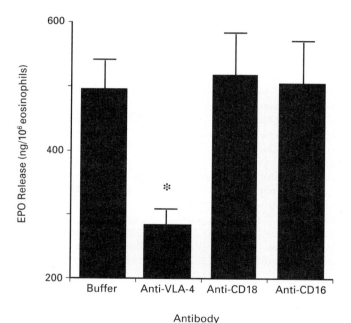

FIGURE 28-4 **Top graph: Augmentation of fMLP-stimulated release of EPO caused by exposure to fibronectin. Stimulated EPO release is augmented at 60 min and persists at 120 min** ($n = 3$). **P values represent statistical comparisons between control and fibronectin groups incubated for the same time.** *Bottom graph*: **The effect of monoclonal antibody blockade of adhesion receptors on fMLP-stimulated release of EPO from eosinophils exposed to fibronectin** ($n = 4$). **Anti-VLA-4 (HP2/1) alone blocked stimulated EPO release from eosinophils allowed to adhere to fibronectin. (*$P < 0.02$ for all comparisons)** (*From Neeley et al.,*[124] *with permission.*)

epithelium is the primary focus of most of the inflammatory responses and immune reactions in the lungs. Thus, knowledge of the expression and function(s) of the adhesion molecules found on the surface of the epithelial cells is essential to understanding host defence as well as the pathogenesis of many pulmonary diseases.

AIRWAYS

ICAM-1 EXPRESSION
Of the endothelial adhesion molecules mentioned above, only ICAM-1 is found on the surface of lung epithelial cells. ICAM-1 is expressed constitutively at a low level on airway epithelial cells cultured to a confluent monolayer in vitro, but expression can be enhanced impressively by cytokine stimulation.[58,125,126] IFN-γ is the strongest cytokine enhancer of epithelial ICAM-1 expression, and IL-1, TNF-α, and IL-4 (but not LPS) also are effective. The time course of enhanced ICAM-1 expression (onset at $\geq$ 2 h and peak at 12 to 16 h[127]) is similar to that reported for HUVECs in vitro[128] and human skin keratinocytes in vivo[129] and is indicative of the de novo protein synthesis required. In primary tracheal epithelial cells, as well as in true airway epithelial cell lines, ICAM-1 expression is not directly inhibited by corticosteroids at nontoxic concentrations.[57] However, in vivo, steroid treatment probably does minimize ICAM-1 expression by attenuating the generation of the cytokines that upregulate it.

LEUKOCYTE RETENTION AND ACTIVATION
Using immunohistochemical staining, the in vivo enhancement of airway epithelial ICAM-1 expression has been demonstrated following repeated allergen inhalation (i.e., in association with chronic inflammation) in primates.[50,58] ICAM-1 expression was most strikingly upregulated on the basolateral surface of the tracheal epithelium. Interestingly, staining for LFA-1α (CD11a/CD18), a receptor for ICAM-1 found on all leukocytes and, thus, simply a marker of leukocyte influx, revealed a marked leukocyte infiltrate just below the epithelial basement membrane and within the basolateral tracheal epithelium (i.e., just adjacent to the site of the strongest ICAM-1 staining). In similarly stained sections taken from an animal 20 min after a single allergen inhalation (i.e., representing an acute inflammation), a leukocyte emigration was also notable, but the leukocytes were not accumulated (localized) adjacent to the epithelium, which expressed ICAM-1 only weakly, if at all. Staining with nonspecific mouse serum was used to demonstrated the specificity of the enhanced ICAM-1 staining.

These results strongly suggest a role for ICAM-1 in the retention of the infiltrating leukocytes (mostly eosinophils in this case) at the focus of inflammation, the airway epithelium. Adhesion of human neutrophils to human airway epithelial cells in vitro has been shown to be enhanced and largely ICAM-1–dependent when epithelial ICAM-1 expression was induced by IL-1, TNF-α, or infection with parainfluenza virus type 2.[126,130]

In addition to contributing to leukocyte retention, epithelial ICAM-1 and other, as yet undefined epithelial ligands, by engaging CD11a (LFA-1), CD11b (Mac-1), and other leukocytes integrins (e.g., VLA-4, α₄β₇), probably also act to prime the leukocyte for enhanced mediator release and other effector functions. Adhesion via Mac-1 has been shown to enhance the respiratory burst[131] and, in separate studies, also to enhance the killing of alveolar epithelial cells[132] by neutrophils in vitro. An example of this principle is depicted in Fig. 28-2D, where adhesion, such as via Mac-1/ICAM-1, provides both a stimulatory signal for granulocyte degranulation and a protected microenvironment (pocket) between the two cells, which amplifies the direction and extracellular concentration of the mediators released while limiting their effects on bystander cells (i.e., it provides for targeted cell-mediated cytotoxicity). The basolateral-specific surface generation and expression of fibronectin by the airway epithelium[133] may act similarly to prime eosinophils[122] and/or lymphocytes[134,135] by engagement of their $\alpha_4\beta_1$ (VLA-4) or $\alpha_4\beta_7$ receptors.

Finally, lymphocyte adhesion via CD11a (LFA-1), $\alpha_4\beta_1$ or $\alpha_4\beta_7$, and/or CD28 respectively to epithelial ICAM-1, fibronectin, and/or B7 (found on dendritic cells in the airway epithelium) provides a similar costimulatory signal to both T and B lymphocytes also engaging antigen through the class II major histocompatibility complex.[25,134,136–140] When these "accessory" and costimulatory adhesions are blocked with monoclonal antibodies in vitro, 100-fold greater concentrations of antigen are required to initiate lymphocyte responses.[141,142]

ALVEOLI

Of all the organs and tissues examined to date by immunostaining, the acini of the lungs exhibit by far the highest constitutive ICAM-1 expression.[143–145] Electron microscopy and immunogold staining of normal mouse lung tissue has shown that most of this constitutive expression is on the luminal (airspace) surface of type I pneumocytes, with little if any on the subluminal surface of these cells or on type II pneumocytes or the capillary endothelium.[144] Detailed morphometric evaluation showed that ICAM-1 has a graded distribution on the luminal face of alveolar type I pneumocytes, increasing in abundance toward the interepithelial junctions. These findings suggest that, in the normal lung, constitutive alveolar ICAM-1 expression may serve an anti-inflammatory haptotactic function, directing infiltrated leukocytes out of the gas-exchange units.

Alveolar epithelial ICAM-1 expression also can be enhanced in vivo, as shown after repeated allergen inhalations in primates,[50] 48 h of pure oxygen breathing in mice,[143,146] and infection with respiratory syncytial virus[147] or *Streptococcus pneumoniae*[148] in mice. Again, using electron microscopy and immunogold staining, the increase in ICAM-1 induced by hyperoxic exposure[144] or *S. pneumoniae*[148] was found to be the result of induction of expression on the luminal surface of type II pneumocytes, which probably is a preliminary indicator of their eventual differentiation into type I pneumocytes[145] in response to these injurious insults. The total expression on the type I pneumocytes was unchanged, but the distribution gradient was lost.[144] Under these conditions, alveolar ICAM-1 seems to play a proinflammatory role similar to that on the airway epithelium described above. Evidence for this is the finding that treatment with an anti-ICAM-1 monoclonal antibody (mAb) attenuated the lung injury and dysfunction induced by hyperoxia in mice by partially (~50 percent) blocking neutrophil infiltration as well as by completely preventing degranulation of the infiltrating neutrophils (measured by

the amount of myeloperoxidase activity found in the cell-free lung lavage supernatant).[143]

Role of Specific Adhesion Molecules in Inflammatory Lung Disease

ASTHMA

Asthma is characterized by episodes of reversible airways obstruction causing chest tightness, dyspnea, and cough. In mild asthmatics, these episodes or "attacks" are relatively infrequent and can be treated effectively (reversed) with inhaled bronchodilators. However, in individuals with moderate to severe disease, the intensity of the underlying, distinctive, chronic airways inflammation is associated and seemingly linked to more frequent, intense, and prolonged attacks that are less easily reversed by bronchodilators. The reasons for this situation have become increasingly clear in recent years. The inflammation, which consists principally of an activated or primed infiltrate of T_H2 lymphocytes, eosinophils, mast cells, and possibly platelets, causes an expansion of the perivascular (interstitial) spaces and a release of mediators/growth factors, which cause thickening of the basement membrane, epithelial damage and shedding, production of viscous mucus, and hyperplasia, as well as priming and partial constriction, of airway smooth muscle.[149–156] All of these effects support an increase in airway responsiveness, which lowers the threshold for response to environmental stimuli, thus making attacks occur more frequently.[157] The presence and enhanced sensitivity (responsiveness) of the infiltrate also primes the airways for a subsequent, late-phase broncho-obstructive response elicited by the influx of additional leukocytes 4 to 6 h after an attack. Persistent late-phase responses may relate directly to the chronicity of asthma symptoms as well as to the occurrence of nighttime episodes.[158] Thus, understanding the molecules and mediators that regulate the induction and maintenance of this airways inflammation is key to the management of moderate to severe asthma.

Using mAbs to specific adhesion glycoproteins and primate models of asthma-like induced and persistent airways inflammation and responses, the expression and possible roles of specific cell-adhesion molecules in asthma have been illuminated. Below is a summary of these results in primates followed by supportive findings in atopic humans. Finally, the VLA-4/VCAM-1, IL-4, T_H2 lymphocyte hypothesis for asthma is reviewed.

PRIMATE ALLERGEN-INHALATION MODELS

Induced Airway Hyperresponsiveness

In cynomolgus monkeys with near-normal airway cell composition (> 90 percent alveolar macrophages), a single *Ascaris* inhalation induces an acute (peaking at 6 h; gone by 24 to 48 h) and variable (usually small) neutrophil infiltration, a more consistent and prolonged (6 h to 7 days) eosinophil infiltration,[127] and only rarely a small increase in airways responsiveness.[159] In contrast, three alternate-day *Ascaris* inhalations produce a more consistent (usually 10-

fold) increase in airways responsiveness (measured by the decrease in the concentration of inhaled methacholine required to produce a 100 percent increase in respiratory system resistance, PC_{100}), which was associated with a massive and essentially pure eosinophil infiltration at 3 days after the last allergen challenge.[159] The magnitude of the induced airways hyperresponsiveness was found to correlate significantly with the degree of airways epithelial desquamation induced.[127] In addition, a causal, as opposed to simply associative, role of eosinophils was indicated by the finding that the intratracheal instillation of purified eosinophil major basic protein (MBP) by itself produced an acute and marked (mean, 10-fold) increase in airways responsiveness.[160] Thus, these results suggest that repeated allergen inhalations in these monkeys induced an infiltration and activation of eosinophils that produced, possibly through the release of MBP, airway epithelial desquamation, and that this event, through a number of possible mechanisms, caused airways hyperresponsiveness.

To explore the role of specific adhesion glycoproteins in this model, mouse anti-human mAbs to ICAM-1, E-selectin, or Mac-1 (CD11b), that showed functional cross-reactivity in cynomolgus monkeys, were administered intravenously, daily beginning 1 day prior to the three alternate-day *Ascaris* inhalations. The monkeys were rested ≥ 5 weeks between each study to allow the induced airways inflammation and hyperresponsiveness to resolve, and the mAb treatment study was compared to bracketing control studies in each animal. Allergen inhalation was found to increase ICAM-1 expression on airway and alveolar endothelium and epithelium as well as inducing E-selectin expression only on airways endothelium.[50,58] Treatment with the anti-ICAM-1 mAb R6.5 attenuated both the eosinophil infiltration and the increase in airways responsiveness (60 ± 8 percent and 92 ± 34 percent, respectively).[58] By contrast, administration of the anti-E-selectin mAb CL2 did not significantly inhibit the eosinophil infiltration ($\times 10^3$ per milliliter of BAL fluid: 507 ± 118 in control animals versus 430 ± 114 in CL2⁻ treated animals) or the increase in airways responsiveness (change in log PC_{100}: −1.16 ± 0.27 in control animals versus −1.24 ± 0.29 in CL2-treated animals).[127] Finally, the anti-Mac-1 mAb LM2, while not reducing the eosinophil infiltration, significantly inhibited the activation of airway eosinophils (BAL supernatant eosinophil peroxidase activity in O.D. units: 618 ± 210 in control animals versus 185 ± 41 in LM2-treated animals) as well as the increase in airways responsiveness (change in log PC_{100}: −0.99 ± 0.16 in control animals versus −0.14 ± 0.15 in LM2-treated animals).[161]

Results with the anti-Mac-1 MAb indicate that the inhibition of induced airways hyperresponsiveness by treatment with the anti-ICAM-1 mAb may have been caused by the attenuation of an epithelial ICAM-1-binding eosinophil Mac-1 costimulatory eosinophil-activation signal in addition to the attenuation of eosinophil infiltration by blocking of endothelial ICAM-1. The importance of such a nonendothelial, ICAM-1–dependent adhesion in the induction of airways hyperresponsiveness is supported by a recent report in sensitized Brown-Norway rats. In that study, pretreatment with an mAb to ICAM-1 blocked the inhaled allergen-induced increase in airways responsiveness without reduc-

ing the eosinophil or lymphocyte infiltration.[162] To target epithelial ICAM-1 selectively and to investigate further its possible role, a placebo-controlled crossover study was used to evaluate the effects of daily inhalation administration of the anti-ICAM-1 mAb R6.5 to target epithelial ICAM-1 selectively. Of the animals that experienced greater than a half-log increase in airways responsiveness during either arm of the study, inhaled R6.5 treatment completely blocked the induced airways hyperresponsiveness in two animals, blocked it by ~50 percent in two additional animals, and was ineffective in two others.[57] However, serum concentrations of IgM anti-R6.5 antibodies (possibly neutralizing the administered R6.5) were detected in both animals in which R6.5 was ineffective and in one of the two in which it inhibited the airways hyperresponsiveness by only 50 percent. Inhaled R6.5 also attenuated eosinophil activation (BAL supernatant EPO activity) in most animals, suggesting antagonism of a costimulatory activation of eosinophils through their adhesion to epithelial ICAM-1. Interestingly, eosinophil infiltration seemed also to be attenuated. Since only small amounts of R6.5 were found to reach the airway endothelium in animals treated with inhaled R6.5 (as determined by immunostaining of frozen airway sections and biopsy specimens), the attenuation of eosinophil infiltration (biopsy results consistent with BAL-fluid results) may have been caused in part by the reduction of eosinophil activation and the consequent inflammation and desquamation proximal to the airway epithelium.

Late-Phase Response

As in atopic asthmatics, allergen inhalation in *Ascaris*-hypersensitive cynomolgus monkeys induces an immediate bronchoconstriction, which in some individuals is followed 6 to 10 h later by a second, late-phase broncho-obstruction. In these primates, dual responders (having both immediate and late-phase responses) differ from single responders (immediate response only) in having a stronger expression of ICAM-1, but not of E-selectin, on airway epithelium and endothelium; a larger number and activation (BAL supernatant EPO activity) of airway eosinophils, and ≥ 10-fold greater airway responsiveness to inhaled methacholine prior to antigen challenge.[56,163] That is, dual responders have a persisting baseline airways inflammation and hyperresponsiveness. After antigen inhalation, airway eosinophils decrease acutely, airway endothelial E-selectin expression is induced, and the severity of the late-phase airway obstruction correlates significantly with the intensity of an acute neutrophil influx and increase in airway myeloperoxidase (MPO) activity (as measured in BAL fluid at 6 h after antigen challenge).

To determine the role of ICAM-1 and E-selectin in the late-phase response, R6.5 (anti-ICAM-1) and CL2 (anti-E-selectin) were administered intravenously 1 h before *Ascaris* inhalation in dual-responder monkeys. R6.5 had little if any effect on the neutrophil influx (in BAL fluid at 6 h after the challenge) and a slight (~15 to 20 percent) but consistent attenuation of the early and late-phase airway narrowing.[56] In contrast, CL2 significantly and almost completely inhibited the neutrophil infiltration, the increase in neutrophil activation (BAL supernatant MPO activity), and the associated late-phase airways obstruction.[57]

Thus, the roles of ICAM-1 and E-selectin in the late-phase response induced by a single allergen inhalation in monkeys with preexisting airways inflammation were found to be opposite from those in the induction of airways hyperresponsiveness by multiple allergen inhalations in monkeys without baseline airways inflammation. The reasons for these different effects are not clear, but they certainly merit further investigation because of their obvious importance to the understanding of apparently distinct pathways involved in the generation of asthma-like airways inflammation and dysfunction.

The consistent, although small, attenuation of both the early and late-phase airway narrowing by treatment with the anti-ICAM-1 mAb is again consistent with a contribution of epithelial ICAM-1 to leukocyte priming and thus increased responsiveness to allergen challenge. The finding that this treatment effect was small is also compatible with the fact that eosinophils already were present and activated before anti-ICAM-1 administration, as well as with the fact that the amounts of chemoattractants released by antigen inhalation were likely so large that the costimulatory signal provided by ICAM-1–mediated adhesion was comparatively small.

Persistent Airways Eosinophilia and Hyperresponsiveness

Finally, the abilities of R6.5 (anti-ICAM-1) and CL2 (anti-E-selectin) to reverse, or to inhibit the reestablishment of, a persistent airways inflammation and hyperresponsiveness were evaluated in the above-described dual-responder monkeys.[164,165] Daily intravenous administration of R6.5 or CL2 for 7 days failed to produce a significant reversal in the persistent airways eosinophilia, eosinophil activation, or hyperresponsiveness in these animals. By contrast, daily intramuscular (systemic) dexamethasone impressively lessened all of these parameters. However, after the persistent airways inflammation and hyperresponsiveness were removed by dexamethasone treatment, the daily intravenous administration of R6.5, but not CL2, was effective in inhibiting their reestablishment. That is, and consistent with the above mentioned results and conclusions, anti-ICAM-1 treatment effectively inhibits the induction of airway eosinophilia and, more importantly, airway hyperresponsiveness. However, once established, persistent airways inflammation and hyperresponsiveness is reduced only weakly, if at all, by a short-term (≤ 1 week) antagonism with ICAM-1. Whether an antagonism of airway epithelial ICAM-1 more efficient than that achieved by intravenous R6.5, or more prolonged treatment, might be more effective requires further investigation.

Role of Lymphocytes

While the animal studies mentioned above have focused on the contribution of specific adhesion molecules to granulocyte infiltration and activation, the adhesive interactions that regulate lymphocyte infiltration, cytokine release, cytotoxic activity, and antibody production also could play a prominent role in the responses monitored. The unique and characteristic eosinophilic airways inflammation found in asthma, as well as in the primate models presented above, may be the consequence of the cytokines IL-4 and IL-5 released from selectively recruited and activated lymphocytes of the T_H2-like subtype[156] (also see below). Thus, many of the above-described effects of anti-ICAM-1 treatment attributed to the attenuation of eosinophil infiltration and activation may be instead, or also, secondary to a reduction of lymphocyte infiltration and activation. Indeed, in recent studies we have found an increase in lymphocytes that are of the CD4 phenotype and express the IL-2 receptor (CD25) in BAL fluid obtained from primates with either induced or persistent airways eosinophilia and hyperresponsiveness.[166]

SUPPORTIVE FINDINGS IN HUMANS

Using immunostaining of nasal biopsy specimens from patients with perennial allergic rhinitis and from nonatopic healthy volunteers, the following observations have been reported: (1) in the normal nasal mucosa, ICAM-1 was expressed on the endothelium more often than E-selectin, and expression of VCAM-1 was minimal or absent; (2) in perennial rhinitis, the numbers of endothelial cells expressing ICAM-1 and VCAM-1 were significantly elevated; (3) the number of vessels positive for ICAM-1 correlated with the number of infiltrated (CD11a-staining) leukocytes; and (4) the number of infiltrated neutrophils correlated with the number of E-selectin–expressing vessels.[167] Immunostaining of bronchial biopsy specimens from atopic patients with asthma, from atopic patients with rhinitis but not asthma, and from nonatopic healthy volunteers demonstrated the following: (1) ICAM-1 expression on the airway epithelium and endothelium was elevated in the asthmatics and correlated with both the number of infiltrated eosinophils and the degree of airways hyperresponsiveness; and (2) epithelial ICAM-1 expression as well as endothelial ICAM-1 and E-selectin expression were increased 6 h after allergen inhalation in the atopic nonasthmatic patients[168] (T. Fukuda, personal communication). Concentrations of circulating (shed) ICAM-1 and E-selectin, but not VCAM-1, have been found to be elevated significantly in acute exacerbations of asthma.[169] Consistent with a role of epithelial ICAM-1 in the pathogenesis of airways hyperresponsiveness, bronchial epithelial cell ICAM-1 expression was found to be significantly increased in asthmatics but not in individuals with chronic bronchitis.[170] Finally, consistent with a role of E-selectin in the late-phase response, the concentration of E-selectin in cell-free BAL supernatant was found to be increased 18 h after segmental antigen challenge in allergic subjects.[171]

VLA-4/VCAM-1, IL-4, T_H2 LYMPHOCYTE HYPOTHESIS

The chronic airways inflammation found in asthma is characterized by a strikingly selective accumulation of eosinophils and lymphocytes.[140,144] This characteristic and selective infiltrate has been hypothesized to be generated by a VLA-4/VCAM-1 emigration pathway induced by the release of IL-4 and IL-5 from T_H2 lymphocytes.[156,172,173] This hypothesis is based on the following observations: (1) VLA-4 is expressed strongly on basophils, eosinophils, and lymphocytes, but not on neutrophils and only minimally on monocytes,[28,29,174–176]; (2) endothelial VCAM-1 is upregulated selectively by stimulation or costimulation with IL-4[27,31,32,177]; (3) the principal source of IL-4 is the T_H2 lymphocyte[178]; (4) IL-4 enhances immunoglobulin production and induces class switching to IgE in B lymphocytes,[178,179] and it also upregulates ICAM-1 on airways epithelium[125]; and (5) T_H2 lymphocytes are also the major source of IL-5, an eosinophil-selective stimulator of differentiation, adhesion, and activation.[180,183]

Support for this hypothesis is found in two animal models. In guinea pigs, the eosinophil accumulation induced in a passive cutaneous anaphylaxis (PCA) reaction or by intradermal injection of platelet-activating factor (PAF), leukotriene B_4, or C5a des Arg was in all cases inhibited by an anti-VLA-4 mAb.[184] In sheep challenged with inhaled allergen, treatment with an anti-α_4 mAb prevented the late-phase broncho-obstruction and subsequent increase in airways responsiveness.[185] However, under conditions in which ICAM-1 is expressed (i.e., under most conditions, since there is a small constitutive expression of ICAM-1 on most endothelial cells in vivo), the VLA-4/VCAM-1–mediated adhesion to, and migration through, endothelial monolayers by eosinophils and/or lymphocytes is dominated by the CD18/ICAM-1 pathway.[176,186,187] That is, the VLA-4/VCAM-1–dependent pathway is notable only under conditions in which CD18/ICAM-1 is blocked or deficient (i.e., in type 1 LAD). In addition, in contrast to ICAM-1, VCAM-1 expression is not enhanced in bronchial biopsy specimens from asthmatics, even during acute exacerbations requiring emergency room attention (S. Montefort and S. T. Holgate, personal communication). Furthermore, in preliminary studies, a mouse anti-cynomolgus monkey VCAM-1 mAb failed to inhibit the eosinophil infiltration, the activation of eosinophils and lymphocytes, or the increase in airways responsiveness induced by repeated allergen inhalations in the above-mentioned primate model (C.D. Wegner, unpublished data). Finally, in the allergen-challenged sheep model, despite efficacy on functional parameters (see above), treatment with the anti-α_4 mAb had no effect on the influx of eosinophils or total leukocytes.[185] Therefore, the positive effects of the anti-α_4 mAbs in animal models may be the consequence of an α_4/fibronectin-mediated migration and/or activation of eosinophils in the interstitium (see "Cell Activation by Interaction of Receptors with the Extracellular Matrix," above, and Fig. 28-4) rather than an attenuation of a VLA-4/VCAM-1 transendothelial diapedesis pathway.

ACUTE RESPIRATORY DISTRESS SYNDROME

The acute (or adult) respiratory distress syndrome (ARDS) is a "common clinical catastrophe" following acute lung injury.[188] There are many causes of ARDS, including bypass surgery, trauma, head injuries, sepsis, emboli, pneumonia, smoke or chemical inhalation, acid aspiration, and premature birth (see Chap. 100). The most common cause, gram-negative sepsis, is estimated to cause 300,000 to 500,000 cases each year in the U.S. alone, with mortality rates equal to or exceeding 50 percent.[189] While the lungs are only one of many organs that are failing in established ARDS, they are usually the first to fail,[190] and acute lung injury remains the most common initial precipitating factor.[188] Thus, understanding the pathways involved in the pathogenesis of acute lung injury are key to future interventions into this devastating disease.

RAT COMPLEMENT-ACTIVATION MODELS

The major source of insight into the roles of various adhesion molecules in the pathogenesis of acute lung injury has come from rat models of complement activation induced by cobra venom factor (CVF), IgG immune complexes, and IgA immune complexes. A summary of the findings from these studies is shown in Table 28-2.

The neutrophil-mediated injury to the lung vasculature induced by the intravenous injection of CVF (involving increased permeability, hemorrhage and neutrophil emigration), which has an onset within minutes of injection, is apparently governed by the constitutive expression of ICAM-1 and the rapid induction of P-selectin on the pulmonary endothelium as well as by the β_2-integrins (CD11/CD18) on neutrophils.[191,192] In contrast, a similar injury after IgG immune complex deposition in the lungs is slower in onset (hours), employs the generation of cytokines (IL-1 and TNF-α) from alveolar macrophages, and is governed by the induction of E-selectin and ICAM-1 on the pulmonary endothelium as well as by leukocyte adhesions mediated by the β_1-(VLA-4) and β_2-(mostly CD11a) integrins.[193–195] Finally, in the IgA immune complex model, the acute lung injury (involving increased vascular permeability and hemorrhage) also peaks at 4 h, but it is independent of IL-1/TNF-α generation and of neutrophil-mediated vascular injury and infiltration. The ability of alveolar macrophages to complement-opsonize the IgA immune complexes via their CD11b (Mac-1, CR3) receptors, to generate oxidants (e.g., superoxide), and possibly proteases, as well as the emigration and/or activation of macrophages by adhesions dependent on CD11a, ICAM-1, and VLA-4, seem to be critical in this model.[193,196]

The induction of E-selectin on the pulmonary capillary endothelium during septic, but not traumatic/hypovolemic, shock in baboons,[197] as well as the increased serum E-selectin concentrations in patients with septic shock,[198] further indicate that this endothelial-specific adhesion molecule may have an important role in ARDS. By contrast, despite indisputable evidence of systemic neutrophil activation and heightened CD18 expression during sepsis,[199] anti-CD18 mAbs have been disappointing in their ability to confer protection against the pulmonary sequelae (e.g., permeability) in septic animal models.[200] Thus, under conditions of pronounced vascular neutrophil activation, adhesion to pulmonary microvascular endothelium through a selectin-dependent, CD18-independent mechanism may be sufficient to mediate vascular injury and neutrophil migration. Such a mechanism has also been suggested as an explanation for the E-selectin–dependent, ICAM-1–independent infiltration of neutrophils during the inhaled allergen-induced late-phase response in primates.[57]

TABLE 28-2   Contribution of Various Adhesion Molecules, Cytokines, and Leukocytes to the Lung Vascular Injury Induced by Cobra Venom Factor, IgG Immune Complexes, or IgA Immune Complexes in Rats

Factor or Parameter	FACTOR INDUCING LUNG INJURY		
	CVF	IgG IC	IgA IC
Peak injury time	20 min	4 h	4 h
Role of Alveolar Macrophages	−	++	+++
Prevention by			
Anti-CD18	+++	+++	+++
Anti-CD11a	+	++	+
Anti-CD11b	++	+	++
Anti-ICAM-1	+++	+++	++
Anti-E-selectin	ND	+++	−
Anti-P-selectin	++	ND	ND
Anti-VLA-4	−	++	+++
Anti-IL-1	−	+++	−
Anti-TNF-α	−	+++	−
Neutrophil depletion	+++	+++	−

ABBREVIATIONS: CVF, cobra venom factor; IC, immune complexes; −, no inhibition; +, significant but minimal (< 50 percent) inhibition; ++, moderate but incomplete inhibition; +++, marked (> 70 percent) inhibition; ND, no data published yet. (*Data from refs. 191 through 196.*)

REMOTE NEUTROPHIL ACTIVATION

Commonly (as in bypass and other operations, trauma, burns, hypovolemic shock, limb reattachment, and other situations involving the reestablishment of organ perfusion), acute lung injury is initiated by neutrophils that are moderately activated (and presumably therefore less deformable and expressing more CD18 than unactivated neutrophils; see "Unique Capillary System: Adhesion-Independent Margination," above) at inflammatory sites remote from the lungs. Lung injury initiated in this manner is apparently highly CD18-dependent, as increases in lung permeability induced by ischemia followed by reperfusion of the rat hind limb[201] or the rabbit intestine[202] as well as by thermal injury of rat skin[203] have been found to be almost completely prevented by anti-CD18 mAbs. Interestingly, anti-ICAM-1 mAbs were also found to be protective,[201,203] which supports a role for capillary endothelial ICAM-1 and/or alveolar epithelial ICAM-1 in this pathway of lung parenchymal injury.

PULMONARY OXYGEN TOXICITY

The impaired alveolar gas exchange in ARDS necessitates the use of increased concentrations of inhaled oxygen to achieve acceptable blood oxygen saturation. However, prolonged exposure to high concentrations of oxygen can precipitate an acute edematous lung injury in any remaining normal lung regions[204,205] and can worsen the injury in already damaged lung regions.[206–208] Initiation of hyperoxia-induced lung injury occurs through a direct increase in the intracellular production of oxygen radicals by cells located in and lining the gas-exchange units (acinis), which overwhelm the intracellular antioxidant defence mechanisms.[209,210] Once these effects are initiated, the lung injury is amplified, and morphologic changes worsen exponentially with the appearance of a marked infiltration of neutrophils after 48 to 72 h of pure oxygen breathing.[209,211]

As mentioned above, hyperoxic exposure for 48 h strikingly enhances acinar ICAM-1 expression in the lungs of mice (see "Alveoli," above).[143,144,146] In addition, daily treatment with an anti-ICAM-1 mAb attenuated the lung injury and dysfunction induced by 84 h of pure oxygen breathing in these animals.[143] This protection was congruent with the partially blocking of a small neutrophil infiltration as well as the apparent complete prevention of degranulation of the emigrated neutrophile (measured by MPO activity in cell free lung lavage fluid). These data indicate the important contribution of adhesion molecules to the activation as well as trafficking of leukocytes.

PULMONARY FIBROSIS

If the patient survives both an acute lung injury (resulting in ARDS) and the exacerbation of the damage by pulmonary oxygen toxicity, scarring or fibrosis of lung regions is common.[188,206,209] Recent studies have demonstrated that treatment of rats with anti-CD11a or anti-CD11b mAbs completely prevented the enhanced lung collagen deposition induced by silica or bleomycin.[212] Interestingly, treatment with the anti-CD11a mAb also reversed an established pulmonary fibrosis in these studies. The relevance of these observations is supported by the finding that serum concentrations of ICAM-1 (a ligand for CD11a and CD11b) appear to be increased in patients with idiopathic pulmonary fibrosis.[213]

RESPIRATORY VIRAL INFECTIONS

While in vivo pulmonary studies to date have focused on the role of adhesion molecules in granulocyte-mediated dysfunction and injury, the adhesive interactions that regulate lymphocyte infiltration, cytokine/antibody release (activation), and cytotoxic activity clearly are also prominent contributors to a variety of lung diseases. Respiratory viral infections are a major cause of hospitalization in infants, the elderly, and patients with cardiopulmonary restrictions[214] and are the most common precipitating factor for the onset or exacerbation of asthma symptoms in all age groups.[215–217] Several lines of evidence suggest that the acute morbidity associated with these infections is a consequence of the immune/inflammatory response rather than the cytopathic effects of the virus.[218–221] To investigate further the role of the inflammatory response as well as the specific adhesion molecules involved, a murine model of respiratory syncytial virus (RSV) infection has been used.

In mice, as in humans, RSV infection causes a bronchiolitis and/or pneumonia with perivascular and bronchiolar lymphocytic cuffing as well as occasional foci of alveolar lymphocytic infiltration, which peaks 6 days after inoculation. This condition is associated with a marked enhancement of ICAM-1 expression on the airways epithelium, alveolar epithelium, and/or endothelium and on the infiltrating leukocytes; an impairment of alveolar gas exchange; and an increase in airways responsiveness to inhaled methacholine.[222]

The contribution of ICAM-1 to the induced lung inflammation and dysfunction was studied using the rat monoclonal antibody to murine ICAM-1 (YN1/1.7; see refs. 143, 223, and 224) or control rat IgG administered prophylactically at 3 mg/kg intraperitoneally twice daily beginning 12 h before RSV inoculation. At day 6 after inoculation, the mice receiving YN1/1.7 (anti-ICAM-1) treatment had a significantly milder leukocyte infiltration than control animals (Fig. 28-5A) and no impairment at all of gas exchange (Fig. 28-5B). Whether this attenuation of disease was caused by the prevention of endothelial ICAM-1–mediated diapedesis or by the prevention of ICAM-1–dependent, LFA-1α–mediated lymphocyte activation and cytokine release is not known and requires further evaluations. Nevertheless, these findings, in combination with the fact that most respiratory viral infections are associated with enhanced production of IFN-γ (the most effective upregulator of epithelial ICAM-1 expression), strongly implicate ICAM-1 as a prominent contributor to the pathogenesis and morbidity of respiratory viral infections.

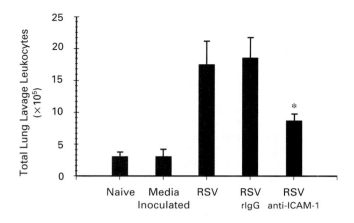

B

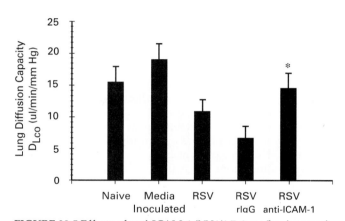

FIGURE 28-5 Effects of anti-ICAM-1 (YN1/1.7: 3 mg/kg, intraperitoneally twice a day) versus control rat IgG on (*A*) the increase in lung lavage (airspace lumen) leukocytes and (*B*) the impairment of alveolar gas exchange 6 days after inoculation with RSV or control HEp-2 media in mice. Bars represent the mean ± S.E. (*n* = 4 to 6). Asterisk (*) signifies significant protection by anti-ICAM-1 compared to RSV alone as well as RSV plus rIgG treatment (*p* < 0.05 by Student's t-test).

LUNG GRANULOMA AND TRANSPLANTATION

Likewise, lymphocytes, monocytes, and T-cell–mediated immunity are certain to have important roles in lung granulomatous diseases (such as sarcoidosis) and in transplantation. In nonpulmonary models of cell-mediated immunity/transplantation, mAbs to CD11a, ICAM-1, VLA-4, and VCAM-1 all have shown impressive immunomodulatory effects. Treatment with CD11a mAbs improves engraftment and survival after allogeneic bone marrow transplantation in mice[225] as well as after HLA-mismatched bone marrow transplantation in children with a variety of immunodeficiency and neoplastic disorders.[226] In mice, the severity of allogeneic graft-versus-host disease was reduced and survival increase by anti-CD11a and anti-ICAM-1

mAbs.[227] In a cynomolgus monkey model of allogeneic kidney transplantation, prophylactic administration of an anti-ICAM-1 mAb prolonged graft survival, while therapeutic administration of this mAb completely, and possibly permanently, reversed a pre-existing rejection produced by tapering cyclosporine to subtherapeutic levels.[228] Finally, anti-VLA-4 mAbs prevent vasculitis (but, interestingly, not lymphocyte emigration) in both rat and rabbit cardiac allografts,[229,230] and an anti-VCAM-1 mAb has been reported to attenuate murine cardiac allograft rejection.[231] Similarly, the simultaneous administration of an anti-ICAM-1 mAb, an anti-CD11a mAb, and a soluble antigen has been reported to induce T_H2 lymphocyte tolerance and to prevent IgE antibody production as well as airways eosinophil recruitment following inhalation of the same antigen in mice.[232]

Conclusion

It is now well established that the cell-surface adhesive glycoproteins that mediate cell-cell and cell-matrix interactions are principal regulators of nearly all aspects of immune/inflammatory responses (for additional information, see refs. 233–235). Many of the molecules and concepts described from studies performed in vitro and in vivo on the systemic microvasculature and nonpulmonary tissues are certainly also employed in the lungs. However, there is also convincing evidence for lung-specific pathways and properties, which are related mainly to the unique features of the pulmonary microvascular beds (including the capillaries and possibly the arterioles) and the strikingly expression of ICAM-1 on the airspace lining epithelium, the most common focus of inflammatory responses in lung disease.

Results gained from animal models with the aid of mAbs against specific adhesion molecules indicate that antagonism of but one of the many key cell-surface adhesive glycoproteins can have dramatic inhibitory effects; these results may lead to novel therapies for lung diseases. However, the dominant molecule will vary with the timing, intensity, conditions, components, and injury associated with the underlying inflammatory/immune processes. Attenuation of adhesion-mediated pathways could be achieved by (1) suppressing constitutive cell-surface expression, (2) inhibiting upregulated expression, (3) decreasing constitutive binding avidity, (4) preventing upregulated binding avidity, or (5) blocking intracellular stimulatory signals generated by ligand engagement (adhesion; for example, involving the leukocyte integrins).[25]

Currently, adhesion molecules are being used as markers of disease. Serum concentrations of soluble, presumably shed, forms of the endothelial adhesion molecules ICAM-1, E-selectin, and VCAM-1, as well as the leukocyte adhesion molecule L-selectin, are being measured as indicators of the onset of inflammation, its severity, and its reversal by therapy.[171,198,213,236,237] In addition, imaging of ICAM-1 induction in the heart following cardiac transplantation has proven an effective, non-invasive method for detecting early allograft rejection.[238]

Finally, as inhibitors of adhesion molecules are developed, their effects on host defence will need to be monitored closely. Obviously, inflammatory responses have their beneficial features, in addition to their well-documented deleterious production of tissue injury and organ dysfunction. An example of such a beneficial effect was recently reported in ozone-induced lung injury in primates.[239] Treatment with an anti-CD18 mAb markedly delayed repair of the ozone-injured bronchiolar epithelium by preventing the influx of neutrophils.

References

1. Bevilacqua MP, Stengelin S, Gimbrone MA Jr, Seed B: Endothelial leukocyte adhesion molecule 1: an inducible receptor for neutrophils related to complement regulatory proteins and lectins. *Science* 1989; 243:1160.

2. Lasky LA, Singer MS, Yednock TA, et al.: Cloning of a lymphocyte homing receptor reveals a lectin domain. *Cell* 1989; 56:1045.

3. Siegelman MH, van de Rijn M, Weissman IL: Mouse lymph node homing receptor cDNA clone encodes a glycoprotein revealing tandem interaction domains. *Science* 1989; 243:1165.

4. Geng JG, Bevilacqua MP, Moore KL, et al.: Rapid neutrophil adhesion to activated endothelium mediated by GMP-140. *Nature* 1990; 343:757.

5. Lawrence MB, Springer TA: Leukocytes roll on a selectin at physiologic flow rates: distinction from and prerequisite for adhesion through integrins. *Cell* 1991; 65:859.

6. von Andrian UH, Berger EM, Ramezani L, et al.: In vivo behavior of neutrophils from two patients with distinct inherited leukocyte adhesion deficiency syndromes. *J Clin Invest* 1993; 91:2893.

7. Kishimoto TK, Warnock RA, Jutila MA, et al.: Antibodies against human neutrophil LeCAM-1 (LAM-1/Leu-8/DREG-56 antigen) and endothelial cell ELAM-1 inhibit a common CD18-independent adhesion pathway in vitro. *Blood* 1991; 78:805.

8. Imai Y, Singer MS, Fennie C, et al.: Identification of a carbohydrate-based endothelial ligand for a lymphocyte homing receptor. *J Cell Biol* 1991; 113:1213.

9. Spertini O, Luscinskas FW, Kansas GS, et al.: Leukocyte adhesion molecule-1 (LAM-1, L-selectin) interacts with an inducible endothelial cell ligand to support leukocyte adhesion. *J Immunol* 1991; 147:2565.

10. Lowe JB, Stoolman LM, Nair RP, et al.: ELAM-1-dependent cell adhesion to vascular endothelium determined by a transfected human fucosyltransferase cDNA. *Cell* 1990; 63:475.

11. Picker LJ, Warnock RA, Burns AR, et al.: The neutrophil selectin LECAM-1 presents carbohydrate ligands to the vascular selectins ELAM-1 and GMP-140. *Cell* 1991; 66:921.

12. Ley K, Gaehtgens P, Fennie C, et al.: Lectin-like cell adhesion molecule 1 mediates leukocyte rolling in mesenteric venules in vivo. *Blood* 1991; 77:2553.

13. Erbe DV, Watson SR, Presta LG, et al.: P-Selectin and E-selectin use common sites for carbohydrate ligand recognition and cell adhesion. *J Cell Biol* 1993; 120:1227.

14. Diamond MS, Springer TA: A subpopulation of Mac-1 (CD11b/CD18) molecules mediates neutrophil adhesion to ICAM-1 and fibrinogen. *J Cell Biol* 1993; 120:545.

15. Hibbs MA, Jakes S, Stacker SA, et al.: The cytoplasmic domain of the integrin lymphocyte function-associated antigen 1 beta subunit: sites required for binding to intercellular adhesion molecule 1 and the phorbol ester-stimulated phosphorylation site. *J Exp Med* 1991; 174:1227.

16. Lo SK, Lee S, Ramos RA, Lobb R, et al.: Endothelial-leukocyte adhesion molecule 1 stimulates the adhesive activity of leukocyte integrin CR3 (CD11b/CD18, Mac-1, alpha-m, beta-2) on human neutrophils. *J Exp Med* 1991; 173:1493.

17. Casale TB, Erger RA, Little MM: Platelet-activating factor-induced human eosinophil transendothelial migration: evidence for a dynamic role of the endothelium. *Am J Respir Cell Mol Biol* 1993; 8:77.

18. Kuijpers TW, Hakkert BC, Hart MHL, Roos D: Neutrophil migration across monolayers of cytokine-prestimulated endothelial cells: a role for platelet-activating factor and IL-8. *J Cell Biol* 1992; 117:565.

19. Kishimoto TK, Jutila MA, Berg EL, Butcher EC: Neutrophil Mac-1 and MEL-14 adhesion proteins inversely regulated by chemotactic factors. *Science* 1989; 245:1238.

20. Hughes BJ, Hollers JC, Crockett-Torabi E, Smith CW: Recruitment of CD11b/CD18 to the neutrophil surface and adherence-dependent cell locomotion. *J Clin Invest* 1992; 90:1687.

21. Kansas GS, Ley K, Munro JM, Tedder TF: Regulation of leukocyte rolling and adhesion to high endothelial venules through the cytoplasmic domain of L-selectin. *J Exp Med* 1993; 177:833.

22. Shimizu Y, Newman W, Gopal TV, et al.: Four molecular pathways of T cell adhesion to endothelial cells: Roles of LFA-1, VCAM-1, and ELAM-1 and changes in pathway hierarchy under different activation conditions. *J Cell Biol* 1991; 113:1203.

23. Rosen H, Gordon S: Monoclonal antibody to the murine type 3 complement receptor inhibits adhesion of myelomonocytic cells in vitro and inflammatory cell recruitment in vivo. *J Exp Med* 1987; 166:1685.

24. Picker LJ, Kishimoto TK, Smith CW, et al.: ELAM-1 is an adhesion molecule for skin-homing T cells. *Nature* 1991; 349:796.

25. Wegner CD, Wallace RW: Adhesion molecules that regulate inflammatory cell interactions, in Chung FK, Barnes PJ (eds): *Pharmacology of the Respiratory Tract: Clinical and Experimental*. New York, Marcel Dekker, 1992:223.

26. Carlos TM, Harlan JM: Leukocyte-endothelial adhesion molecules. *Blood* 1994; 84:2068.

27. Schleimer RP, Sterbinsky SA, Kaiser J, et al.: IL-4 induces adherence of human eosinophils and basophils but not neutrophils to endothelium: association with expression of VCAM-1. *J Immunol* 1992; 148:1086.

28. Walsh GM, Mermod J-J, Hartnell A, et al.: Human eosinophil, but not neutrophil, adherence to IL-1-stimulated human umbilical vascular endothelial cells is alpha$_4$-beta$_1$ (very late antigen-4) dependent. *J Immunol* 1991; 146:3419.

29. Bochner BS, Luscinskas FW, Gimbrone MA, et al.: Adhesion of human basophils, eosinophils, and neutrophils to interleukin 1-activated human vascular endothelial cells: contribution of endothelial cell adhesion molecules. *J Exp Med* 1991; 173:1553.

30. Kyan-Aung U, Haskard DO, Lee TH: Vascular cell adhesion molecule-1 and eosinophil adhesion to cultured human umbilical vein endothelial cells in vitro. *Am J Respir Cell Mol Biol* 1991; 5:445.

31. Thornhill MH, Wellicome SM, Mahiouz DL, et al.: Tumor necrosis factor combines with IL-4 or IFN-gamma to selectively enhance endothelial cell adhesiveness for T-cells. The contribution of vascular cell adhesion-1-dependent and -independent binding mechanisms. *J Immunol* 1991; 146:592.

32. Masinovsky B, Urdal D, Gallatin WM: IL-4 acts synergistically with IL-1 beta to promote lymphocyte adhesion to microvascular endothelium by induction of vascular cell adhesion molecule-1. *J Immunol* 1990; 145:2886.

33. Berlin C, Berg EL, Briskin MJ, et al.: Alpha$_4$/Beta$_7$ integrin mediates lymphocyte binding to the mucosal vascular addressin MAdCAM-1. *Cell* 1993; 74:185.

34. Shimizu Y, Shaw S: Mucins in the mainstream. *Nature* 1993; 366:630.

35. Berg EL, McEvoy LM, Berlin C, et al.: L-selectin-mediated lymphocyte rolling on MAdCAM-1. *Nature* 1993; 366:695.

36. Briskin MJ, McEvoy LM, Butcher EC: MAdCAM-1 has homology to immunoglobulin and mucin-like adhesion receptors and to IgA1. *Nature* 1993; 363:461.

37. Anderson DC, Schmalstieg FC, Finegold MJ, et al.: The severe and moderate phenotypes of heritable Mac-1, LFA-1 deficiency: their quantitative definition and relation to leukocyte dysfunction and clinical features. *J Infect Dis* 1985; 152:668.

38. Anderson DC, Springer TA: Leukocyte adhesion deficiency: an inherited defect in the Mac-1, LFA-1 and p150,95 glycoproteins. *Annu Rev Med* 1987; 38:175.

39. Etzioni A, Frydman M, Pollack S, et al.: Brief report: recurrent severe infections caused by a novel leukocyte adhesion deficiency. *N Engl J Med* 1992; 25:1789.

40. Schmid-Schonbein GW, Usami S, Skalak R, Chien S: The interaction of leukocytes and erythrocytes in capillary and postcapillary vessels. *Microvas Res* 1980; 19:45.

41. Perry MA, Granger DN: Role of CD11/CD18 in shear rate-dependent leukocyte-endothelial cell interactions in cat mesenteric venules. *J Clin Invest* 1991; 87:1798.

42. Doerschuk CM, Allard MF, Martin BA, et al.: The marginated pool of neutrophils in the lungs of rabbits. *J Appl Physiol* 1987; 63:1806.

43. Lein DC, Wagner Jr WW, Capen RL, et al.: Physiological neutrophil sequestration in the lung: visual evidence for localization in capillaries. *J Appl Physiol* 1987; 62:1236.

44. Hogg JC: Neutrophil kinetics and lung injury. *Physiol Rev* 1987; 67:1249.

45. Glazier JB, Hughes JMB, Maloney JE, West JB: Measurement of capillary dimensions and blood volume in rapidly frozen lungs. *J Appl Physiol* 1964; 19:713.

46. Schmid-Schonbein GW, Shih YY, Chien S: Morphometry of human leukocytes. *Blood* 1985; 45:866.

47. Doerschuk CM, Downey GP, Doherty DE, et al.: Leukocyte and platelet margination within microvasculature of rabbit lungs. *J Appl Physiol* 1990; 68:1956.

48. Worthen GS, Schwab B, Elson EL, Downey GP: Mechanics of stimulated neutrophils: cell stiffening induces retention in capillaries. *Science* 1989; 245:183.

49. Doerschuk CM: The role of CD18-mediated adhesion in neutrophil sequestration induced by infusion of activated plasma in rabbits. *Am J Respir Cell Mol Biol* 1992; 7:140.

50. Wegner CD, Gundel RH, Rothlein R, Letts LG: Expression and probable roles of cell adhesion molecules in lung inflammation. *Chest* 1992; 101:34S.

51. Smith CW, Marlin SD, Rothlein R, et al.: Cooperative interactions of LFA-1 and Mac-1 with intercellular adhesion molecule-1 in facilitating adherence and transendothelial migration of human neutrophils in vitro. *J Clin Invest* 1989; 83:2008.

52. Furie MB, Tancinco MCA, Smith CW: Monoclonal antibodies to leukocyte integrins CD11a/CD18 and CD11b/CD18 or intercellular adhesion molecule-1 inhibit chemoattractant-stimulated neutrophil transendothelial migration in vitro. *Blood* 1991; 78:2089.

53. Harlan JM, Winn RK, Vedder NB: et al.: In vivo models of leukocyte adherence to endothelium, in Harlan JM, Lui DY (eds): *Adhesion: Its Role in Inflammatory Disease*. New York, Freeman 1992:117.

54. Doerschuk CM, Winn RK, Coxson HO, Harlan JM: CD18-dependent and -independent mechanisms of neutrophil emigration in the pulmonary and systemic microcirculation of rabbits. *J Immunol* 1990; 144:2327.

55. Mileski W, Harlan J, Rice C, Winn R: *Streptococcus pneumoniae*-stimulated macrophages induce neutrophils to emigrate by a CD18-independent mechanism of adherence. *Circ Shock* 1990; 31:259.

56. Gundel RH, Wegner CD, Trocellini CA, et al.: Endothelial leukocyte adhesion molecule-1 mediates antigen-induced acute airway inflammation and late-phase airway obstruction in monkeys. *J Clin Invest* 1991; 88:1407.

57. Wegner CD, Gundel RH, Churchill L, Letts LG: Adhesion glycoproteins as regulators of airway inflammation: emphasis in the role of ICAM-1, in Holgate ST, Austen KF, Lichtenstein LM, Kay AB (eds): *Asthma: Physiology, Immunopharmacology, and Treatment*, 4th ed. London, Academic Press, 1993:227.

58. Wegner CD, Gundel RH, Reilly P, et al.: Intercellular adhesion molecule-1 (ICAM-1) in the pathogenesis of asthma. *Science* 1990; 247:456.

59. Pilewski JM, Albelda SM: Adhesion molecules in the lung: an overview. *Am Rev Respir Dis* 1993; 148:S31.

60. Campa JS, Harrison NK, Laurent GJ: Regulation of matrix production in the airways, in Jolles G, Karlsson J-A, Taylor J (eds): *T-Lymphocyte and Inflammatory Cell Research in Asthma.* New York, Academic Press, 1993:221.

61. Clark JG, Kuhn C III, McDonald JA, Mecham RP: Lung connective tissue. *Int Rev Connective Tissue Res* 1983; 10:249.

62. Martin GR, Timpl R: Laminin and other basement membrane components. *Annu Rev Cell Biol* 1987; 3:57.

63. Yurchenko PD, O'Rear JJ: Basal lamina assembly. *Curr Opinion Cell Biol* 1994; 6:674.

64. Laitinen A, Laitinen LA: Airway morphology: epithelium/basement membrane. *Am J Respir Crit Care Med* 1994; 150:S14.

65. Stoner GD, Katoh Y, Foidart JM, et al.: Cultured human bronchial epithelial cells: blood group antigens, keratin, collagens, and fibronectin. *In Vitro Cell Dev Biol* 1981; 17:577.

66. Maniscalo WM, Campbell MH: Transforming growth factor-beta induces a chondroitin sulfate/dermatan sulfate proteoglycan in alveolar type II cells. *Am J Physiol* 1994; 266:L672.

67. Brown EJ, Lindberg FP: Matrix receptors of myeloid cells, in Horton MA (ed): *Blood Cell Biochemistry.* vol. 5: *Macrophages and Related Cells.* New York, Plenum Press, 1993:279.

68. Hemler ME: VLA proteins in the integrin family: structures, functions and their role on leukocytes. *Annu Rev Immunol* 1990; 8:365.

69. Hemler ME, Jacobson JG, Strominger JL: Biochemical characterization of VLA-1 and VLA-2. Cell surface heterodimers on activated T cells. *J Biol Chem* 1985; 260:15246.

70. Wayner EA, Garcia-Pardo A, Humphries MJ, et al.: Identification and characterization of the T lymphocyte adhesion receptor for an alternative cell attachment domain (CS-1) in plasma fibronectin. *J Cell Biol* 1989; 107:1881.

71. Humphries MJ, Mould AP, Yamada KM: Matrix receptors in cell migration, in McDonald JA, Mecham RP (eds): *Receptors for Extracellular Matrix.* New York, Academic Press, 1991:195.

72. Elices MJ: Leukocyte integrins, in Cheresh DA, Mecham RP (eds): *Integrins: Molecular and Biological Responses to the Extracellular Matrix.* New York, Academic Press, 1994:163.

73. Wright SD, Weitz JI, Huang AJ, et al.: Complement receptor type three (CD11b/CD18) of human polymorphonuclear leukocytes recognizes fibrinogen. *Proc Natl Acad Sci USA* 1988; 85:7734.

74. Altieri DC, Agbanyo FR, Plesia J, et al.: A unique recognition site mediates the interaction of fibrinogen with the leukocyte integrin Mac-1 (CD11b/CD18). *J Biol Chem* 1990; 265:12119.

75. Wegner CD, Smith CW, Rothlein R: CD18 dependence of primate eosinophil adherence in vitro, in Springer TA, Anderson DC, Rosenthal AS, Rothlein R (eds): *Leukocyte Adhesion Molecules: Structure, Function, and Regulation.* New York, Springer-Verlag, 1989:208.

76. Wright SD, Lo SK, Detmer PA: Specificity and regulation of CD18-dependent adhesions, in Springer TA, Anderson DC, Rosenthal AS, Rothlein R (eds): *Leukocyte Adhesion Molecules: Structure, Function, and Regulation.* New York, Springer-Verlag, 1989:190.

77. Thompson HL, Matsushima K: Human polymorphonuclear leucocytes stimulated by tumor necrosis factor-alpha show increased adherence to extracellular matrix proteins which is mediated via the CD11b/CD18 complex. *Clin Exp Immunol* 1992; 90:280.

78. Diamond MS, Garciaaguilar J, Bickford JK, et al.: The I-domain is a major recognition site on the leukocyte integrin Mac-1 (CD11b/CD18) for four distinct adhesion ligands. *J Cell Biol* 1993; 120:545.

79. Bray PF, Rosa J-P, Johnston GI, et al.: Platelet glycoprotein IIb: chromosomal localization and tissue expression. *J Clin Invest* 1987; 80:1812.

80. Albelda SM: Endothelial and epithelial cell adhesion molecules. *Am J Respir Cell Mol Biol* 1991; 4:195.

81. Krissansen GW, Elliott MJ, Lucas CM, et al.: Identification of a novel integrin β subunit expressed on cultured monocytes (macrophages): evidence that one α subunit can associate with multiple β subunits. *J Biol Chem* 1990; 265:823.

82. Hamawy MM, Mergenhagen SE, Siraganian RP: Adhesion molecules as regulators of mast-cell and basophil function. *Immunol Today* 1994; 15:62.

83. Lesley J, Hyman R, Kincade PW: CD44 and its interaction with extracellular matrix. *Adv Immunol* 1993; 54:271.

84. Aruffo A, Stamenkovic I, Melnick M, et al.: CD44 is the principal cell surface receptor for hyaluronate. *Cell* 1990; 61:1303.

85. Miyake K, Kincade PW: A new cell adhesion mechanism involving hyaluronate and CD44. *Curr Topics Microbiol Immunol* 1990; 166:87.

86. Camp RL, Kraus TA, Puré E: Variations in the cytoskeletal interaction and posttranslational modification of the CD44 homing receptor in macrophages *J Cell Biol* 1991; 115:1283.

87. Hamann KJ, Dowling TL, Neeley SP, et al.: Hyaluronic acid enhances cell proliferation during eosinopoiesis through the CD44 surface antigen. *J Immunol* 1995; 154:4073.

88. Stockinger H, Gadd SJ, Eher R, et al.: Molecular characterization and functional analysis of the leukocyte surface protein CD31. *J Immunol* 1990; 145:3889.

89. Tyler TL, Grant JA, Dowling TL, et al.: Production of developing umbilical cord blood-derived eosinophils is enhanced by heparin sulfate. Submitted, 1996.

90. DeLisser HM, Newman PJ, Albelda SM: Platelet endothelial cell adhesion molecule (CD31). *Curr Topics Microbiol Immunol* 1993; 184:37.

91. DeLisser HM, Yan HC, Newman PJ, et al.: Platelet/endothelial cell adhesion molecule-1 (CD31)-mediated cellular aggregation involves cell surface glycosaminoglycans. *J Biol Chem* 1993; 268:16037.

92. Watt SM, Williamson J, Genevier H, et al.: The heparin binding PECAM-1 adhesion molecule is expressed by CD34+ hematopoietic precursor cells with early myeloid and B-lymphoid cell phenotypes. *Blood* 1993; 82:2649.

93. Schwartz MA: Integrins as signal transducing receptors, in Cheresh DA, Mecham RP (eds): *Integrins: Molecular and Biological Responses to the Extracellular Matrix.* New York, Academic Press, 1994:33.

94. Shimizu Y, van Seventer GA, Horgan KJ, Shaw S: Costimulation of proliferative responses of resting CD4+ T cells by the interaction of VLA-4 and VLA-5 with fibronectin or VLA-6 with laminin. *J Immunol* 1990; 145:59.

95. Yamada A, Nikaido T, Nojima Y, et al.: Activation of human CD4 T lymphocytes: interaction of fibronectin with VLA-5 receptor on CD4 cells induces the AP-1 transcription factor. *J Immunol* 1991; 146:53.

96. Nojima Y, Rothstein DM, Sugita K, et al.: Ligation of VLA-4 of T cells stimulates tyrosine phosphorylation of a 105-kDa protein. *J Exp Med* 1992; 175:1045.

97. Brando C, Shevach EM: Engagement of the vitronectin receptor ($\alpha_V\beta_3$) on murine T cells stimulates tyrosine phosphorylation of a 115-kDa protein. *J Immunol* 1995; 154:2005.

98. Ticchioni M, Deckert M, Bernard G, et al.: Comitogenic effects of very late activation antigens on CD3-stimulated human thymocytes: involvement of various tyrosine kinase pathways. *J Immunol* 1995; 154:1207.

99. Koopman G, van Kooyk T, de Graaff M, et al.: Triggering of the

CD44 antigen on T lymphocytes promotes T cell adhesion through the LFA-1 pathway. *J Immunol* 1990; 145:3589.

100. Bourguignon LYW, Lokeshwar VB, Chen X, Kerrick WGL: Hyaluronic acid-induced lymphocyte signal transduction and HA receptor (GP85/CD44)-cytoskeleton interaction. *J Immunol* 1993; 151:6634.

101. Galandrini R, Albi N, Tripodi G, et al.: Antibodies to CD44 trigger effector functions of human T cell clones. *J Immunol* 1993; 150:4225.

102. Galandrini R, Galluzzo E, Albi N, et al.: Hyaluronate is costimulatory for human T cell effector functions and binds to CD44 on activated T cells. *J Immunol* 1994; 153:21.

103. Tanaka Y, Albelda SM, Horgan KJ, et al.: CD31 expressed on distinctive T cell substs is a preferential amplifier of beta 1 integrin-mediated adhesion. *J Exp Med* 1992; 176:245.

104. Newman SL, Tucci MA: Regulation of human monocyte/ macrophage function by extracellular matrix. Adherence of monocytes to collagen matrices enhances phagocytosis of opsonized bacteria by activation of complement receptors and enhancement of Fc receptor function. *J Clin Invest* 1990; 86:703.

105. Juliano RL, Haskill S: Signal transduction from the extracellular matrix *J Cell Biol* 1993; 120:577.

106. Noble PW, Lake FR, Henson PM, Riches WH: Hyaluronate activation of CD44 induces insulin-like growth factor-1 expression by a tumor necrosis factor-α-dependent mechanism in murine macrophages. *J Clin Invest* 1993; 91:2368.

107. Sorimachi K, Akimoto K, Niwa A, Yasumura Y: Induction of macrophage proliferation by heparin and heparan sulfate. *Cell Biol Int* 1993; 17:881.

108. Wrenshall LE, Cerra FB, Singh RK, Platt JL: Heparan sulfate initiates signals in murine macrophages leading to divergent biological outcomes. *J Immunol* 1995; 154:871.

109. Kay AB, Corrigan CJ: Eosinophils and neutrophils. *Br Med Bull* 1992; 48:51.

110. Abramson SL, Malech HL, Gallin JI: Neutrophils, in Crystal RG, West JB (eds): *The Lung: Scientific Foundations.* New York, Raven Press, 1991:553.

111. Nathan C, Srimal S, Farber C, et al.: Cytokine induced respiratory burst of human neutrophils: dependence on extracellular matrix proteins and CD11/CD18 integrins. *J Cell Biol* 1989; 109:1341.

112. Nathan C, Sanchez E: Tumor necrosis factor and CD11/CD18 (β_2) integrins act synergistically to lower cAMP in human neutrophils. *J Cell Biol* 1990; 109:1341.

113. Ng-Sikorski J, Andersson R, Patarroyo M, Andersson T: Calcium signaling capacity of the CD11b/CD18 integrin on human neutrophils. *Exp Cell Res* 1991; 195:504.

114. Pike MC, Wicha MS, Yoon P, et al.: Laminin promotes the oxidative burst in human neutrophils via increased chemoattractant receptor expression. *J Immunol* 1989; 142:2004.

115. Nathan CF: Neutrophil activation on biological surfaces. Massive secretion of hydrogen peroxide in response to products of macrophages and lymphocytes. *J Clin Invest* 1987; 80:1550.

116. Hakansson L, Venge P: The combined action of hyaluronic acid and fibronectin stimulates neutrophil migration. *J Immunol* 1985; 135:2735.

117. Berman ME, Muller WA: Ligation of platelet/endothelial cell adhesion molecule 1 (PECAM-1/CD31) on monocytes and neutrophils increases binding capacity of leukocyte CR3 (CD11b/CD18). *J Immunol* 1995; 154:299.

118. Bianchine PJ, Burd PR, Metcalfe DD: IL-3-dependent mast cells attach to plate-bound vitronectin. Demonstration of augmented proliferation in response to signals transduced via cell surface vitronectin receptors. *J Immunol* 1992; 149:3665.

119. Ra C, Yasuda M, Yagita H, Okumura K: Fibronectin receptor integrins are involved in mast cell activation. *J Allergy Clin Immunol* 1994; 94:625.

120. Dri P, Cramer R, Spessotto P, et al.: Eosinophil activation on biologic surfaces: production of O_2- in response to physiological soluble stimuli is differentially modulated by extracellular matrix components and endothelial cells. *J Immunol* 1991; 147:613.

121. Laudanna C, Melotti P, Bonizzato C, et al.: Ligation of members of the β_1 or the β_2 subfamilies of integrins by antibodies triggers eosinophil respiratory burst and spreading. *Immunology* 1993; 80:273.

122. Anwar ARE, Moqbel R, Walsh GM, et al.: Adhesion to fibronectin prolongs eosinophil survival. *J Exp Med* 1993; 177:839.

123. Wardlaw AJ, Walsh GM, Anwar ARE, et al.: The role of adhesion in eosinophil accumulation and activation in asthma, in Gleich GJ, Kay AB (eds): *Eosinophils in Allergy and Inflammation.* New York, Marcel Dekker, 1994:115.

124. Neeley SP, Hamann KJ, Dowling TL, et al.: Augmentation of stimulated eosinophil degranulation by VLA-4 (CD49d)-mediated adhesion to fibronectin. *Am J Respir Cell Mol Biol* 1994; 11:206.

125. Churchill L, Gundel RH, Letts LG, Wegner CD: Contribution of specific cell-adhesive glycoproteins to airway and alveolar inflammation and dysfunction. *Am Rev Respir Dis* 1993; 148:S83.

126. Tosi MF, Stark JM, Smith CW, et al.: Induction of ICAM-1 expression on human airway epithelial cells by inflammatory cytokines: effects on neutrophil-epithelial cell adhesion. *Am J Respir Cell Molecular Biol* 1992; 7:214.

127. Wegner CD, Rothlein R, Gundel RH: Adhesion molecules in the pathogenesis of asthma. *Agents Actions* [Suppl] 1991; 34:529.

128. Smith CW, Rothlein R, Hughes BJ, et al.: Recognition of an endothelial determinant for CD18-dependent human neutrophil adherence and transendothelial migration. *J Clin Invest* 1988; 82:1746.

129. Vejlsgaard GL, Ralfkiaer E, Avnstorp C, et al.: Kinetics and characterization of intercellular adhesion molecule-1 (ICAM-1) expression on keratinocytes in various inflammatory skin lesions and malignant cutaneous lymphomas. *J Am Acad Dermatol* 1989; 20:782.

130. Tosi MF, Stark JM, Hamedani A, et al.: Intercelluar adhesion molecule-1 (ICAM-1)-dependent and ICAM-1-independent adhesive interactions between polymorphonuclear leukocytes and human airway epithelial cells infected with parainfluenza virus type-2. *J Immunol* 1992; 149:3345.

131. Shappell SB, Toman C, Anderson DC, et al.: Mac-1 (CD11b/CD18) mediates adherence-dependent hydrogen peroxide production by human and canine neutrophils. *J Immunol* 1990; 144:2702.

132. Simon RH, DeHart PD, Todd RF III: Neutrophil-induced injury of rat pulmonary alveolar epithelial cells. *J Clin Invest* 1986; 78:1375.

133. Wang A, Palmer E, Cohen DS, Sheppard D: Transforming growth factor-beta induces polarized secretion of fibronectin by airway epithelial cells. (Abstract) *Am Rev Respir Dis* 1990; 141:A467.

134. Shimizu Y, van Seventer GA, Ennis E, et al.: Crosslinking of the T cell-specific accessory molecules CD7 and CD28 modulate T cell adhesion. *J Exp Med* 1992; 175:577.

135. Masumoto A, Hemler ME: Multiple activation states of VLA-4. *J Biol Chem* 1993; 268:228.

136. Koopman G, Parmentier HK, Schuurman H-J, et al.: Adhesion of human B cells to follicular dendritic cells involves both the lymphocyte function-associated antigen 1/intercellular adhesion molecule 1 and very late antigen 4/vascular cell adhesion molecule 1 pathways. *J Exp Med* 1991; 173:1297.

137. van Seventer GA, Newman W, Shimizu Y, et al.: Analysis of T cell stimulation by superantigen plus major histocompatibility complex class II molecules or by CD3 monoclonal antibody: costimulation by purified adhesion ligands VCAM-1, ICAM-1, but not ELAM-1. *J Exp Med* 1991; 174:901.

138. Dustin ML, Springer TA: T-cell receptor cross-linking transiently stimulates adhesiveness through LFA-1. *Nature* 1989; 341:619.

139. Augustin M, Dietrich A, Niedner R, et al.: Phorbol-12-myristate-13-acetate-treated human keratinocytes express B7-like molecules that serve a costimulatory role in T-cell activation. *J Invest Dermatol* 1993; 100:275.

140. Singer KH: Interactions between epithelial cells and T lymphocytes: role of adhesion molecules. *J Leukocyte Biol* 1990; 48:367.

141. Martz E: LFA-1 and other accessory molecules functioning in adhesions of T and B lymphocytes. *Hum Immunol* 1987; 18:3.

142. Regnier-Vigouroux A, Blanc D, Pont S, et al.: Accessory molecules and T cell activation I. Antigen receptor avidity differentially influences T cell sensitivity to inhibition by monoclonal antibodies to LFA-1 and L3T4. *Eur J Immunol* 1986; 16:1385.

143. Wegner CD, Wolyniec WW, LaPlante AM, et al.: Intercellular adhesion molecule-1 (ICAM-1) contributes to pulmonary oxygen toxicity in mice: role of leukocytes revised. *Lung* 1992; 170:267.

144. Kang B-H, Crapo JD, Wegner CD, et al.: Intercellular adhesion molecule-1 expression on the alveolar epithelium and its modification by hyperoxia. *Am J Respir Cell Mol Biol* 1993; 9:350.

145. Christensen PJ, Kim S, Simon RH, et al.: Differentiation-related expression of ICAM-1 by rat alveolar epithelial cells. *Am J Respir Cell Mol Biol* 1993; 8:9.

146. Welty SE, Rivera JL, Elliston JF, et al.: Increases in lung tissue expression of intercellular adhesion molecule-1 are associated with hyperoxic lung injury and inflammation in mice. *Am J Respir Cell Mol Biol* 1993; 9:393.

147. Raymond EL, McFarland ML, Van GY, et al.: Role of ICAM-1 in respiratory syncytial virus (RSV) infection in mice. (Abstract) *Am J Respir Crit Care Med* 1994; 149:A49.

148. Burns AR, Takei F, Doerschuk CM: Quantitation of ICAM-1 experssion in mouse lung during pneumonia. *J Immunol* 1994; 153:3189.

149. Laitinen LA, Heino M, Laitinen A, et al.: Damage of the airway epithelium and bronchial reactivity in patients with asthma. *Am Rev Respir Dis* 1985; 131:599.

150. Dunnill MS: The pathology of asthma with special reference to changes in the bronchial mucosa. *J Clin Pathol* 1960; 13:27.

151. Barnes PJ, Chung KF, Page CP: Inflammatory mediators and asthma. *Pharmacol Rev* 1988; 40:49.

152. Beasley R, Roche WR, Roberts JA, Holgate ST: Cellular events in the bronchi in mild asthma and after bronchial provocation. *Am Rev Respir Dis* 1989; 139:806.

153. Jeffery PK, Wardlaw AJ, Nelson FC, et al.: Bronchial biopsies in asthma. An ultrastructural, quantitative study and correlation with hyperreactivity. *Am Rev Respir Dis* 1989; 140:1745.

154. Azzawi M, Bradley B, Jeffery PK, et al.: Identification of activated T lymphocytes and eosinophils in bronchial biopsies in stable atopic asthma. *Am Rev Respir Dis* 1990; 142:1407.

155. Brewster CE, Howarth PH, Djukanovic R, et al.: Myofibroblasts and subepithelial fibrosis in bronchial asthma. *Am J Respir Cell Mol Biol* 1990; 3:507.

156. Kay AB: T lymphocytes and their products in atopic allergy and asthma. *Int Arch Allergy Appl Immunol* 1991; 94:189.

157. Boushey HA, Holtzman MJ, Sheller JR, Nadel JA: Bronchial hyperreactivity. *Am Rev Respir Dis* 1980; 121:389.

158. O'Byrne PM, Dolovich J, Hargreave FE: Late asthmatic responses: state of art. *Am Rev Respir Dis* 1987; 136:740.

159. Wegner CD, Torcellini CA, Clarke CC, et al.: Effects of single and multiple inhalations of antigen on airway responsiveness in monkeys. *J Allergy Clin Immunol* 1991; 87:835.

160. Gundel RH, Letts LG, Gleich GJ: Human eosinophil major basic protein induces airway constriction and airway hyperresponsiveness in primates. *J Clin Invest* 1991; 87:1470.

161. Wegner CD, Gundel RH, Letts LG: Efficacy of monoclonal antibodies against adhesion molecules in animal models of asthma. *Agents Actions* [Suppl] 1993; 43:151.

162. Sun J, Elwood W, Haczku A, et al.: Contribution of intercellular-adhesion molecule-1 in allergen-induced airway hyperresponsiveness and inflammation in sensitised brown-Norway rats. *Int Arch Allergy Immunol* 1994; 104:291.

163. Gundel RH, Wegner CD, Letts LG: Antigen-induced acute and late-phase responses in primates. *Am Rev Respir Dis* 1992; 146:369.

164. Gundel RH, Wegner CD, Torcellini CA, Letts LG: The role of intercellular adhesion molecule-1 in chronic airway inflammation. *Clin Exp Allergy* 1992; 22:569.

165. Letts LG, Wegner CD, Gundel RH: Adhesion molecules in acute and chronic lung inflammation. Lindley ILD (ed): *Chemotactic Cytokines. vol. 2.* New York, Plenum Press, 1993:In press.

166. Souza DJ, Gundel RH, Barton RW, et al.: Changes in T-lymphocyte subsets (CD4/CD8) and activation (IL-2R) following chronic antigen inhalations in monkeys. (Abstract) *Chest* 1993; 103:In press.

167. Montefort S, Feather IH, Wilson SJ, et al.: The expression of leukocyte-endothelial adhesion molecules is increased in perennial allergic rhinitis. *Am J Respir Cell Mol Biol* 1992; 7:393.

168. Ando N, Fukuda T, Nakajima H, Makino S: Expression of intercellular adhesion molecule-1 (ICAM-1) is upregulated in the bronchial mucosa of symptomatic asthmatics. (Abstract) *J Allergy Clin Immunol* 1992; 89:215.

169. Montefort S, Lai CKW, Kapahi P, et al.: Circulating adhesion molecules in asthma. *Am J Respir Crit Care Med* 1994; 149:1149.

170. Vignola AM, Campbell AM, Chanez P, et al.: HLA-DR and ICAM-1 expression on bronchial epithelial cells in asthma and chronic bronchitis. *Am Rev Respir Dis* 1993; 148:689.

171. Georas SN, Liu MC, Newman W, et al.: Altered adhesion molecule expression and endothelial cell activation accompany the recruitment of human granulocytes to the lung after segmental antigen challenge. *Am J Respir Cell Mol Biol* 1992; 7:261.

172. Tepper RI, Levinson DA, Stanger BZ, et al.: IL-4 induces allergic-like inflammatory disease and alters T cell development in transgenic mice. *Cell* 1990; 62:457.

173. Walker C, Virchow Jr J-C, Bruijnzeel PLB, Blaser K: T cell subsets and their soluble products regulate eosinophilia in allergic and nonallergic asthma. *J Immunol* 1991; 146:1829.

174. Weller PF, Rand TH, Goelz SE, et al.: Human eosinophil adherence to vascular endothelium mediated by binding to vascular cell adhesion molecule 1 and endothelial leukocyte adhesion molecule 1. *Proc Natl Acad Sci* 1991; 88:7430.

175. Carlos T, Kovach N, Schwartz B, et al.: Human monocytes bind to two cytokine-induced adhesive ligands on cultured endothelial cells: endothelial-leukocyte adhesion molecule-1 and vascular cell adhesion molecule-1. *Blood* 1991; 77:2266.

176. Vachula M, Vanepps DE: In vitro models of lymphocyte transendothelial migration. *Invasion Metastasis* 1992; 12:66.

177. Briscoe DM, Cotran RS, Pober JS: Effects of tumor necrosis factor, lipopolysaccharide, and IL-4 on the expression of vascular cell adhesion molecule-1 in vivo: correlation with CD3+ T cell infiltration. *J Immunol* 1992; 149:2954.

178. Paul WE: Interleukin-4: a prototypic immunoregulatory lymphokine. *Blood* 1991; 77:1859.

179. Coffman R, Ohara J, Bond MW, et al.: B cell stimulatory factor-

1 enhances the IgE response of lipopolysaccharide-activated B cells. *J Immunol* 1986; 136:4538.

180. Clutterbuck EJ, Hirst EMA, Sanderson CJ: Human interleukin-5 (IL-5) regulates the production of eosinophils in human bone marrow cultures: comparison and interaction with IL-1, IL-3, IL-6, and GMCSF. *Blood* 1989; 73:1504.

181. Walsh GM, Hartnell A, Wardlaw AJ, et al.: IL-5 enhances the in vitro adhesion of human eosinophils, but not neutrophils, in a leucocyte integrin (CD11/18)-dependent manner. *Immunology* 1990; 71:258.

182. Fujisawa T, Abu-Ghazaleh R, Kita H, et al.: Regulatory effect of cytokines on eosinophil degranulation. *J Immunol* 1990; 144:642.

183. Lopez AF, Sanderson CJ, Gamble JR, et al.: Recombinant human interleukin 5 is a selective activator of human eosinophil function. *J Exp Med* 1988; 167:219.

184. Weg VB, Williams TJ, Lobb RR, Nourshargh S: A monoclonal antibody recognizing very late activation antigen-4 inhibits eosinophil accumulation in vivo. *J Exp Med* 1993; 177:561.

185. Abraham WM, Sielczak MW, Ahmed A, et al.: Alpha$_4$-integrins mediate antigen-induced late bronchial responses and prolonged airway hyperresponsiveness in sheep. *J Clin Invest* 1994; 93:776.

186. Vankooyk Y, Vandewielvankemenade E, Weder P, et al.: Lymphocyte function-associated antigen-1 dominates very late antigen-4 in binding of activated T-cells to endothelium. *J Exp Med* 1993; 177:185.

187. Ebisawa M, Bochner BS, Georas SN, Schleimer RP: Eosinophil transendothelial migration induced by cytokines: role of endothelial and eosinophil adhesion molecules in IL-1beta-induced transendothelial migration. *J Immunol* 1992; 149:4021.

188. Petty TL: Acute respiratory distress syndrome (ARDS). *Disease-a-Month* 1990; January:1.

189. Bone RC: Corticosteroids for septic shock and adult respiratory distress syndrome, in *Second Vienna Shock Forum*. Alan R Liss, 1989:857.

190. Welbourn CRB, Young Y: Endotoxin, septic shock and acute lung injury—neutrophil, macrophages and inflammatory mediators. *Br J Sur* 1992; 79:998.

191. Mulligan MS, Polley MJ, Bayer RJ, et al.: Neutrophil-dependent acute lung injury: requirement for P-selectin (GMP-140). *J Clin Invest* 1992; 90:1600.

192. Mulligan MS, Smith CW, Anderson DC, et al.: Role of leukocyte adhesion molecules in complement-induced lung injury. *J Immunol* 1993; 150:2401.

193. Mulligan MS, Wilson GP, Todd RF, et al.: Role of beta1, beta2 integrins and ICAM-1 in lung injury after deposition of IgG and IgA immune complexes. *J Immunol* 1993; 150:2407.

194. Mulligan MS, Varani J, Dame MK, et al.: Role of endothelial-leukocyte adhesion molecule 1 (ELAM-1) in neutrophil-mediated lung injury in rats. *J Clin Invest* 1991; 88:1396.

195. Mulligan MS, Varani J, Warren JS, et al.: Role of beta2 integrins of rat neutrophils in complement- and oxygen radical-mediated acute inflammatory injury. *J Immunol* 1992; 148:1847.

196. Mulligan MS, Warren JS, Smith CW, et al.: Lung injury after deposition of IgA immune complexes: requirement for CD18 and L-arginine. *J Immunol* 1992; 148:3086.

197. Redl H, Dinges HP, Buurman WA, et al.: Expression of endothelial leukocyte adhesion molecule-1 in septic but not traumatic/hypovolemic shock in the baboon. *Am J Pathol* 1991; 139:461.

198. Newman W, Beall LD, Carson CW, et al.: Soluble E-selectin is found in supernatants of activated endothelial cells and is elevated in the serum of patients with septic shock. *J Immunol* 1993; 150:644.

199. Walsh CJ, Leeper-Woodford SK, Carey PD, et al.: CD18 adhesion receptors, tumor necrosis factor, and neutropenia during septic lung injury. *J Surg Res* 1991; 50:323.

200. Thomas JR, Harlan JM, Rice CL, Winn RK: Role of leukocyte CD11/CD18 complex in endotoxic and septic shock in rabbits. *J Appl Physiol* 1992; 73:1510.

201. Seekamp A, Mulligan MS, Till GO, et al.: Role of beta2 integrins and ICAM-1 in lung injury following ischemia-reperfusion of rat hind limbs. *Am J Pathol* 1993; 143:464.

202. Hill J, Lindsay T, Valeri CR, et al.: A CD18 antibody prevents lung injury but not hypotension after intestinal ischemia-reperfusion. *J Appl Physiol* 1993; 74:659.

203. Mulligan MS, Till GO, Smith CW, et al.: Role of leukocyte adhesion molecules in lung and dermal vascular injury after thermal trauma of skin. *Am J Pathol* 1994; 14:1008.

204. Clark JM, Lambertsen CJ: Pulmonary oxygen toxicity: A review. *Pharmacol Rev* 1971; 23:37.

205. Jackson RM: Molecular, pharmacologic, and clinical aspects of oxygen-induced lung injury. *Clin Chest Med* 1990; 11:73.

206. Witschi HR, Haschek WM, Klein-Szanto AJ, Hakkinen PJ: Potentiation of diffuse lung damage by oxygen: determining variables. *Am Rev Respir Dis* 1981; 123:98.

207. Tryka AF, Skornik WA, Godleski JJ, Brain JD: Potentiation of bleomycin-induced lung injury by exposure to 70% oxygen: morphologic assessment. *Am Rev Respir Dis* 1982; 126:1074.

208. Crouse DT, Cassell GH, Waites KB, et al.: Hyperoxia potentiates *Ureaplasma urealyticum* pneumonia in newborn mice. *Infect Immun* 1990; 58:3487.

209. Crapo JD: Morphologic changes in pulmonary oxygen toxicity. *Annu Rev Physiol* 1986; 48:721.

210. Martin WJ, Gadek JE, Hunninghake GW, Crystal RG: Oxidant injury of lung parenchymal cells. *J Clin Invest* 1981; 68:1277.

211. Crapo JD, Freeman BA, Barry BE, et al.: Mechanisms of hyperoxic injury to the pulmonary microcirculation. *Physiologist* 1983; 26:170.

212. Piguet PF, Rosen H, Vesin C, Grau GE: Effective treatment of the pulmonary fibrosis elicited in mice by bleomycin or silica with anti-CD11 antibodies. *Am Rev Respir Dis* 1993; 147:435.

213. Shijubo N, Imai K, Aoki S, et al.: Circulating intercellular adhesion molecule-1 (ICAM-1) antigen in sera of patients with idiopathic pulmonary fibrosis. *Clin Exp Immunol* 1992; 89:58.

214. Dolin R: Common viral respiratory infections, in Harrison (ed): *Harrison's Principles of Internal Medicine*. 11th ed. New York, McGraw-Hill, 1987:700.

215. Busse WW: Respiratory infections and bronchial hyperreactivity. *J Allergy Clin Immunol* 1988; 81:770.

216. Sherter CB, Polnitsky CA: The relationship of viral infections to subsequent asthma. *Clin Chest Med* 1981; 2:67.

217. McIntosh K, Ellis EF, Hoffman LS, et al.: The association of viral and bacterial respiratory infections with exacerbations of wheezing in young asthmatic children. *J Pediatr* 1973; 82:578.

218. Kim HW, Canchola JG, Brandy CD, et al.: Respiratory syncytial virus disease in infants despite prior administration of antigenic inactivated vaccine. *Am J Epidemiol* 1969; 89:422.

219. Stott EJ, Ball LA, Anderson K, et al.: Immune and histopathological responses in animals vaccinated with recombinant vaccinia viruses that express individual genes of human respiratory syncytial virus. *J Virol* 1987; 61:3855.

220. Murphy BR, Sotnidov AV, Lawrence LA, et al.: Enhanced pulmonary histopathology is observed in cotton rats immunized with formalin-inactivated respiratory syncytial virus or purified F glycoprotein and challenged with RSV 3-6 months after immunization. *Vaccine* 1990; 8:497.

221. Graham BS, Bunton LA, Wright PF, Karzon DT: Role of T lym-

phocyte subsets in the pathogenesis of primary infection and rechallenge with respiratory syncytial virus in mice. *J Clin Invest* 1991; 88:1026.

222. Raymond EL, McFarland ML, Van GY, et al.: Characterization of the lung inflammation and dysfunction induced by respiratory syncytial virus (RSV) infection in mice. (Abstract) *Am J Respir Crit Care Med* 1994; 149:A48.

223. Takei F: Inhibition of a mixed lymphocyte response by a rat monoclonal antibody to a novel murine lymphocyte activation antigen (MALA-2). *J Immunol* 1985; 134:1403.

224. Horley KJ, Carpenito C, Baker B, Takei F: Molecular cloning of murine intercellular adhesion molecule (ICAM-1). *EMBO J* 1989; 8:2889.

225. van Dijken PJ, Gharyur T, Mauch P, et al.: Evidence that anti-LFA-1 in vivo improves engraftment and survival after allogeneic bone marrow transplantation. *Transplantation* 1990; 49:882.

226. Fischer A, Griscelli C, Blanche S, et al.: Prevention of graft failure by an anti-LFA-1 monoclonal antibody in HLA-mismatched bone marrow transplantation. *Lancet* 1986; 2:1058.

227. Buyon JP, Slade SG, Reibman J, et al.: Constitutive and induced phosphorylation of the alpha- and beta-chains of the CD11/CD18 leukocyte integrin family. *J Immunol* 1990; 144:191.

228. Cosimi AB, Conti D, Delmonico FL, et al.: In vivo effects of monoclonal antibody to ICAM-1 (CD54) in nonhuman primates with renal allographs. *J Immunol* 1990; 144:4604.

229. Paul LC, Davidoff A, Paul DW, et al.: Monoclonal antibodies against LFA-1 and VLA-4 inhibit graft vasculitis in rat cardiac allografts. *Transplant Proc* 1993; 25:813.

230. Sadahiro M, McDonald TO, Allen MD: Reduction in cellular and vascular rejection by blocking leukocyte adhesion molecule receptors. *Am J Pathol* 1993; 142:675.

231. Pelletier R, Ohye R, Kincade P, et al.: Monoclonal antibody to anti-VCAM-1 interferes with murine cardiac allograft rejection. *Transplant Proc* 1993; 25:839.

232. Nakao A, Nakajima H, Tomioka H, et al.: Induction of T cell tolerance by pretreatment with anti-ICAM-1 and anti-lymphocyte function-associated antigen-1 antibodies prevents antigen-induced eosinophil recruitment into the mouse airways. *J Immunol* 1994; 153:5819.

233. Wegner CD: *The Handbook of Immunopharmacology: Adhesion Molecules*. London, Academic Press, 1994.

234. Ward PA: *Adhesion Molecules and the Lung*. New York, Marcel Dekker, 1995.

235. Harlan JM, Lui DY: *Adhesion: Its Role in Inflammatory Disease*. New York, Freeman, 1992.

236. Gearing AJH, Hemingway I, Pigott R, et al.: Soluble forms of vascular adhesion molecules, E-selectin, ICAM-1, and VCAM-1: pathological significance. *Ann NY Acad Sci* 1992; 667:324.

237. Stockenhuber F, Kramer G, Schenn G, et al.: Circulating ICAM-1—novel parameter of renal graft rejection. *Transplant Proc* 1993; 25:919.

238. Ohtani H, Strauss HW, Southern JF, et al.: Imaging of intercellular adhesion molecule-1 induction in rejecting heart—new scintigraphic approach to detect early allograft rejection. *Transplant Proc* 1993; 25:867.

239. Hyde DM, Pinkerton KE, Wegner CD, et al.: Neutrophils aid epithelial repair following short-term ozone exposure in rhesus monkeys. (Abstract) *Am J Respir Crit Care Med* 1994; 149:A231.

240. Wegner CD: Lung inflammation, in Wegner CD (ed): *The Handbook of Immunopharmacology: Adhesion Molecules*. London, Academic Press, 1994:191.

Chapter 29 _____

GRANULOMATOUS INFLAMMATORY STATES OF THE LUNG

GALEN B. TOEWS

JOSEPH P. LYNCH, III

The terms *granuloma* and *granulomatous inflammation* have been present in the medical literature since the nineteenth century. No universally accepted definition of granulomatous inflammation exists. For the purposes of this chapter, granulomatous inflammation is defined as an organized collection of lymphocytes and mononuclear phagocytes that include epithelioid cells and giant cells. Plasma cells, eosinophils, and fibroblasts also are found in most granulomas.

Granulomatous inflammation is a tissue reaction to specific antigens contained in numerous pathogenic microbes, including many species of bacteria, fungi, and parasites. Additionally, granulomatous inflammation occurs in response to inert materials typified by beryllium, lipids, and high-molecular-weight polymers. Granulomas are an important part of a number of human diseases of unknown etiology, such as sarcoidosis and Wegener granulomatosis. In these latter circumstances, an unidentified stimulus or stimuli elicit granulomatous inflammation.

The function of granulomas is to isolate a harmful agent from surrounding healthy tissues. Sequestration within a granuloma eventually may lead to the killing of a replicating microbe. Alternatively, the microbe may become metabolically dormant. Granulomatous inflammation generally subserves a beneficial effect. However, granulomatous inflammation also can lead to the serious sequela of tissue destruction and fibrosis. Cells within the granuloma release mediators that initiate and sustain progressive injury and fibrotic processes. This response likely represents an additional attempt to isolate a harmful agent from healthy tissues.

Granuloma Formation

The kinetics of granuloma formation derives almost exclusively from serial studies of experimental animal models. The time required for granuloma formation after exposure to an inciting agent varies from as little as 4 days to 2 weeks. Critical variables that account for this time span include the inciting agent for granuloma formation and the route of inoculation.[1] The assembly of a granuloma is a highly organized process.[1–3] Although inflammatory phagocytes accumulate nonspecifically at the site of microbial growth, T cells are indispensable for the formation of granulomas.[4–6] Within the forming granuloma, T cells are in close contact with mononuclear phagocytes at various stages of differentiation and activation. The granuloma has a relatively high cellular turnover. Freshly emigrant monocytes mature into epithelioid cells and multinucleated giant cells.

T LYMPHOCYTES IN GRANULOMA FORMATION

The T-cell system can be separated into three subsets according to their use of T-cell receptors and accessory molecules which interact with the major histocompatibility complex (MHC) gene product on target cells.[7] T-cell subsets include (1) CD4 α/β T cells, which recognize processed antigen pep-

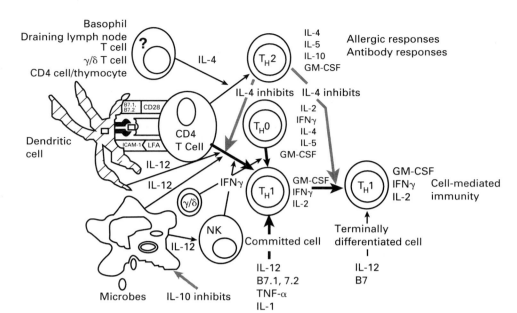

FIGURE 29-1 Cytokine-driven CD-4 lymphocyte cell development.

tides in the context of MHC class II molecules; (2) CD8 α/β T cells, which recognize antigenic peptides in the context of MHC class I molecules; and (3) γ/δ T cells, which lack both CD4 and CD8 molecules. CD4 T cells further can be separated into two subsets according to their lymphokine secretion pattern[8–15] (Fig. 29-1). T helper-1 (T_H1) cells produce IL-2 and interferon-γ but not IL-4, whereas T helper-2 (T_H2) clones produce IL-4, IL-5, and IL-10 but not interferon-γ. The existence of T-cell clones that exhibit cytokine production characteristic of both the T_H1 and T_H2 subsets of cells has also been described. This T_H0 subset of cells is considered to be a precursor T cell from which the T_H1 and T_H2 phenotype cells can differentiate.[16–18]

Class II–restricted CD4 T lymphocytes play a central role in immunity to most intracellular bacteria and fungi.[19–25] CD4 T cells from *Mycobacterium tuberculosis*–infected mice produce IL-2 and IFN-γ and hence are of the T_H1 type.[19–21] Antigen-specific CD4 T_H1 cells also have been isolated from patients suffering from tuberculosis and leprosy.[26–28] Using sensitive assays, IL-4 has been detected in mice immunized with mycobacteria. This finding raises the possibility that T_H0 cells may be an important part of the granulomatous response to this organism. At present, no evidence exists for disturbances in the T_H1/T_H2 cell balance in animal models of tuberculosis.

Class I–restricted CD8 T cells also participate in the immune response to mycobacterial and fungal pathogens.[29–34] CD8 T cells express specific cytolytic activities and produce IFN-γ.[3,35] While human class I–restricted CD8 T cells with reactivity for intracellular bacteria have been isolated less frequently, in situ analyses reveal CD8 T cells in the outer mantle surrounding granulomas.[31,36] It is presently uncertain how antigens from intracellular bacteria are introduced into the class I pathway.[37,38] Originally, it was thought that exogenous antigens remain in the endocytic compartment and hence can only be presented through the MHC class II pathway, whereas newly synthesized antigens are presented by the MHC class I pathway. Presently, no evidence exists that *M. tuberculosis* leaves the endosomal compartment and enters the cytoplasm. The endosomal compartment might, however, become leaky during persistent infection, allowing secreted proteins and/or low-molecular-weight metabolites to enter the class I pathway.

The relative contribution of T-cell subsets to acquired resistance to microbes can be investigated by adoptive transfer of T cells and by in vivo elimination of T cells by treatment with monoclonal antibodies. In murine tuberculosis and fungal infections, these two approaches have revealed a dominant role for CD4 T cells with an important contribution by CD8 T cells.[22–25,32–34,39–43] In contrast, following *Listeria monocytogenes* infection, CD8 T cells predominate with some contribution by CD4 T cells.[44–46] Differential target cell recognition is the important feature that defines subset contribution to host defenses since both T-cell subsets express similar biologic activity. *M. tuberculosis* and fungi reside in MHC class II positive mononuclear phagocytes and are highly resistant to intracellular killing. Accordingly, protection must rely on mononuclear phagocyte activation by CD4 T cells. Alternatively, *L. monocytogenes* is rapidly killed by mononuclear phagocytes but also invades MHC class II negative cells. Hence, lysis of MHC class I positive, class II negative cells is dependent on CD8 T cells.

Several lines of experimental evidence indicate an important role for γ/δ T lymphocytes in antimicrobial granulomas[47–56]: (1) γ/δ T cells from mice immunized with *M. tuberculosis* respond vigorously to *M. tuberculosis* antigens in vitro[47–49]; (2) an extraordinarily high percentage of murine, thymic, and splenic γ/δ T-cell hybridomas react with purified protein derivative (PPD)[50,51]; (3) In vitro stimulation of peripheral blood cells from normal healthy volunteers with *M. tuberculosis* results in a marked expansion of γ/δ T lymphocytes. As many as one in two γ/δ T cells from the peripheral blood of normal volunteers are stimulated by *M. tuberculosis* lysates.[54–56]

Mycobacteria likely stimulate γ/δ T cells in an antigen-specific manner. Accumulation of γ/δ T cells in murine lungs has been observed following aerosol immunization with mycobacterial antigens.[49] γ/δ T cells appear prior to α/β T cells. γ/δ T cells from *M. tuberculosis*–immunized mice respond vigorously to mycobacterial antigen preparations.[47–49] Mycobacterial-stimulated γ/δ T cells express various biologic functions relevant to defense against intracellular microbes, including lysis of mycobacteria-pulsed target cells and secretion of IFN-γ and TNF.[57,58] Taken together, these findings argue for participation of antigen-specific γ/δ T cells in antibacterial immunity in a way similar to that of α/β T cells.

CYTOKINES IN GRANULOMA FORMATION

The initiation, organization, and structural maintenance of granulomas requires communication among cells. Several animal-model systems have been used to study the role of cytokines on granuloma formation and acquired resistance against microbes.

T cell–mediated granulomatous responses are characterized by intense leukocyte recruitment to the site of antigen deposition.[59] Chemokines from the C-C supergene family (based on the homologous position of four conserved cysteine amino acids within their primary protein structure) have an important role in granulomatous inflammation. The C-C chemokine family includes macrophage inflammatory protein-1 (MIP-1, α/β), monocyte chemoattractant protein-1 (MCP-1), and RANTES (regulated on activation, normal T-cell expressed and secreted). These chemokines are chemotactic for mononuclear cells and lymphocytes.[60]

MIP-1α is produced early during *Schistosoma* egg granuloma formation. MIP-1α levels correlate both with leukocyte accumulation and the size of the developing granuloma.

Neutralization of MIP-1α in vivo significantly diminishes the granulomatous response. Granuloma macrophages appear to be the predominant cellular source of MIP-1α, but fibroblasts isolated and grown in vitro from developing granulomas also have the ability to produce MIP-1α.[61] Monocyte chemoattractant protein-1, a monocyte and lymphocyte chemotactic factor, can be isolated from T lymphocyte–dependent granulomatous responses. The production of MCP-1 also correlates with leukocyte accumulation during responses to microbes.[62]

Development of granulomas is regulated by monokines and by both T_H1 (IFN-γ) and T_H2 (IL-4) lymphokines (Fig. 29-2). Tumor necrosis factor (TNF) has been identified as an important mediator of granuloma formation since exogenous administration of TNF into *scid* mice allows granulomas to form.[63] In addition, neutralization of TNF results in decreased in vivo granuloma formation.[64] One mechanism of TNF involvement in granuloma formation is through the induction of intercellular adhesion molecule-1 (ICAM-1).[65] Blockade of TNF function inhibited the ICAM-1 expression normally noted during the development of granulomatous lesions. The presence of ICAM-1 is important to leukocyte recruitment, T-lymphocyte activation, and granuloma formation.[66–68] Tumor necrosis factor likely also regulates granuloma formation by controlling the induction of chemokine gene expression. Pulmonary fibroblasts and epithelial cells express MCP-1 mRNA after being stimulated by either TNF or IL-1.[69,70] Tumor necrosis factor thus might function in a paracrine manner to stimulate MCP production by nonimmune cells within the lung.

Interleukin-4 (IL-4) also is an important determinant of granuloma formation. Neutralization of IL-4 during an acute granulomatous response to schistosomes diminishes the leukocyte accumulation.[71,72] This effect may be related to the capacity of IL-4 to induce MCP-1 production.[73] Interleukin-

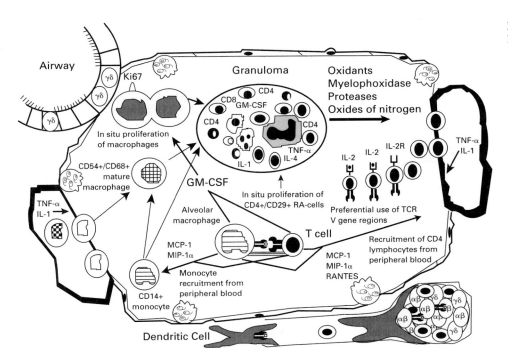

FIGURE 29-2 Mechanisms of granuloma formation.

10 (IL-10), another T_H2 cytokine, can induce MIP-1α production from granuloma fibroblasts.[74] T_H2 lymphokines appear to be important regulators of chemokine production by various cell types within the forming granuloma.[75] Interleukin-4 also is capable of activating tuberculostatic function in murine mononuclear phagocytes.[76] When given after infection, IL-4 is capable of reducing mycobacterial growth to a significant degree.

Interferon-γ (IFN-γ) plays a central role in granulomatous protection against most intracellular microbes. Interferon-γ is produced by CD4 T cells, CD8 T cells, γ/δ T cells, and natural killer cells.[35,58,76–78] Administration of recombinant IFN-γ protects mice against lethal *M. tuberculosis* infection while neutralization with anti-IFN-γ antibodies markedly exacerbates the disease.[79] Interferon-γ is a potent stimulator of tuberculostasis and fungistasis in murine mononuclear phagocytes.[80–82] Tumor necrosis factor shows marked synergy with IFN-γ in activating the tuberculostatic capacities of murine phagocytes.[80] IFN-γ-induced tuberculostasis is blocked by anti-TNF antibodies.

Granulocyte/macrophage colony-stimulating factor (GM-CSF), produced by T_H0, T_H1, and T_H2 subsets, also is a macrophage activating factor. Granulocyte/macrophage colony-stimulating factor acts either alone or in combination with other cytokines. By itself, GM-CSF activates macrophages for killing of *Candida albicans* and *Cryptococcus neoformans*.[83–85] Granulocyte/macrophage colony-stimulating factor also cooperates with IFN-γ in the induction of anticryptococcal killing mechanisms.[84] Interferon-γ and GM-CSF are not effective as an activation scheme in mycobacterial systems; however, TNF-α added to GM-CSF–treated cells induces significant intracellular destruction of mycobacteria.[86] Granulocyte/macrophage colony- stimulating factor primes macrophages for enhanced TNF-α production following stimulation by other cytokines.[87] Granulocyte/macrophage colony-stimulating factor participates in an autocrine cytokine loop to activate macrophages.

Multinucleated giant cells are a prominent feature of granulomatous inflammation. Formation of giant cells, which occurs from fusion of monocytes rather than from nuclear division without division of cytoplasm, is dependent on cytokines released by antigen-stimulated cells. Both IFN-γ and IL-4 stimulate formation of giant cells.[88,89] Both cytokines given alone are much less effective than supernatants from antigen-stimulated peripheral blood cells. Interferon-γ may stimulate formation of giant cells by enhancing expression of lymphocyte function-associated antigen-1 (LFA-1) and ICAM-1.[90] Homotypic adhesion of inflammatory macrophages might then occur through the reciprocal recognition of LFA-1 and ICAM-1 molecules on the surface of mononuclear phagocytes.

Sarcoidosis

The presence of noncaseating, epithelioid, giant cell granulomas is the pathologic hallmark of sarcoidosis. Despite the absence of an identifiable antigen, the immunohistologic pattern seen in sarcoidosis suggests that the granulomatous lesions are the result of an antigen-driven process. It seems most likely that sarcoid granulomas are the consequence of an immunologic response against an unknown antigen that has persisted at the sites of disease involvement, perhaps because of its low solubility or degradability. This hypothesis suggests that the sarcoid granuloma is "a battlefield between invading antigens and the cellular and humoral defenses of the host."[91] Considerable experimental evidence exists that formation of sarcoid granulomas is regulated by a complex interaction between T lymphocytes and accessory cells[92,93] (Fig. 29-2).

T LYMPHOCYTES IN SARCOIDOSIS

CD2+/CD3+/CD4+ lymphocytes are dramatically increased both in percentage and in absolute numbers in involved tissues from patients with sarcoidosis.[94–100] CD8+ cells are reduced at all sites of disease activity. Accordingly, the CD4/CD8 ratio is extremely high (usually greater than 10) at most sites of granuloma formation. A CD8+ T-lymphocyte predominance occurs in approximately 4 percent of patients with sarcoidosis, suggesting that variants of the disorder may exist.[101]

The T cells that accumulate in sarcoidosis are CD4+, CD29+, and CD45RO+[102–107]; this subset defines "memory" T cells.[103,104] The accumulation of memory T cells in sarcoidosis might reflect an in situ conversion from naïve to memory T cells and/or homing of memory T cells because of an ongoing immunologic response against an unknown antigen.

Lung T lymphocytes from patients with sarcoidosis proliferate at an exaggerated rate. T-helper cells from patients with active pulmonary sarcoidosis display increased expression of a cell cycle–related nuclear antigen (Ki67), a feature of proliferating cells.[108] Augmented expression of the p55 chain of the interleukin-2 receptor (IL-2R) has been noted[109,110]; this likely confers a proliferative advantage on IL-2R–bearing sarcoid T lymphocytes. Sarcoid T cells isolated from the lung strongly express additional activation antigens, such as very-late activation antigen-1 (VLA-1), transferrin receptor (CD71), and class II MHC HLA-DR antigen.[111–113] Taken together, these findings suggest that tissue lymphocytes obtained from disease sites in patients with sarcoidosis are activated lymphocytes.

ACCESSORY CELL–T-CELL INTERACTIONS

Activation of T lymphocytes is dependent on the recognition of an appropriate antigenic epitope by the T-cell receptor/CD3 complex. The T-cell receptor (TCR) can recognize antigen only when associated with cell-surface glycoproteins from the major histocompatibility complex present on an antigen-presenting cell (APC).[114] Sarcoid alveolar macrophages present antigen as efficiently as blood monocytes and three times more efficiently than alveolar macrophages obtained from normal volunteers.[115–118] Sarcoid alveolar macrophages contain large amounts of mRNA coding for class II MHC products. Sarcoid alveolar macrophages express class II MHC antigens HLA-DR, DQ, and DP.

Sarcoid alveolar macrophages also express a transferrin receptor (CD71) and ICAM-1 (CD54).[119–123] The expression of class II MHC gene determinants and accessory molecules may increase the antigen-presenting capacity of alveolar macrophages, enabling more efficient T-cell recognition of putative antigens.

Contact between the TCR and its specific antigen-MHC complex on an APC leads to internalization of the CD3 molecule.[124] T cells obtained from the respiratory tract of patients with sarcoidosis have decreased surface expression of CD3/TCR as compared with peripheral blood. Sarcoid BAL T cells show increased levels of mRNA transcripts for the β chain of TCR, which parallels the enhanced surface expression of a series of accessory molecules, including HLA-DR, VLA-1, CD29, and CD2.[125,126] These findings collectively support the hypothesis that sarcoid memory T cells are cells that have been repetitively stimulated by an unknown antigen through the α/β TCR.

To investigate whether sarcoid T lymphocytes respond to one or more antigenic stimuli, the molecular structure of the TCR gene has been investigated. Sarcoid lung T lymphocytes demonstrated a marked quantitative bias in the usage of β-chain constant region segments (Cβ1 rather than Cβ2) and variable elements (Vβ8, Vβ14, Vα2,3).[127–131] In patients with sarcoidosis, intradermal injection of Kveim-Siltzbach reagent also elicits preferential oligoclonal expression of specific Vβ genes (Vβ3, Vβ5, Vβ8) in T lymphocytes at biopsy sites when compared with paired peripheral blood T lymphocytes.[132] These findings suggest that sarcoid T lymphocytes belong to a limited number of clones (oligoclonal expansion) rather than representing a multitude of cells that are different from each other (polyclonal expansion). These data suggest that sarcoid T cells are likely proliferating in response to specific unknown antigenic pressure. Alternatively, it is possible that the preferential expression of particular V-region segments by sarcoid T cells may result from the accumulation of T-effector cells that acquire a particular homing capacity for the lung following expression of certain Vβ or Vγ genes. It recently has been established that selective use of certain V-gene regions is characteristic of lymphocytes infiltrating other organs (Vγ5, Vγ6, and Vγ7 for skin, esophagus/small intestine, and synovia, respectively).[133]

Mechanisms Accounting for Accumulation of Immunocompetent Cells in Sarcoid Granulomas

Two mechanisms likely account for the increased numbers of immunocompetent cells present in sarcoid tissues: (1) cellular recruitment from the peripheral blood to the lung; and (2) in situ proliferation. The marked increase in CD4 cells at sites of involvement is associated with a decrease in peripheral T lymphocytes.[94,95] This finding substantiates the concept that the T cell–mediated immune response is compartmentalized to the lung and other involved tissues. Increased numbers of monocytes also are recruited to the lung. An enhanced number of alveolar macrophages

obtained from patients with sarcoidosis show a monocyte-like phenotypic pattern.[134–137]

The precise molecular mechanisms responsible for cellular accumulation in sarcoidosis are unknown. The current molecular model suggests that the accumulation of inflammatory cells results from a sequential interaction of cytokines/chemokines, cell-adhesion molecules, and chemoattractants that lead to the recruitment and activation of specific leukocyte subsets.[138–140] Cell-adhesion molecules that play crucial roles in leukocyte–endothelial cell cascades include the selectins, integrins, and members of the immunoglobulin supergene family. In the first phase of leukocyte recruitment, rolling of circulating leukocytes is mediated by selectins, such as leukocytes (L) selectin on leukocytes and endothelial (E) and platelet (P) selectin on endothelial cells. Activation of lymphocyte function antigen-1 (LFA-1) or leukocyte integrin (MAC-1) leads to firm adhesion of leukocytes to the endothelial ligand ICAM-1. The binding of VLA-4 to its endothelial ligand vascular cell adhesion-1 (VCAM-1) appears to be important for lymphocytes. Firm adhesion would be followed by transmigration through endothelial cell junctions and migration along a chemoattractant gradient to an inflammatory site. A plausible schema in sarcoidosis includes antigen exposure, which leads to activation of T_H1 lymphocytes that release a number of soluble mediators including TNF-α, GM-CSF, and IFN-γ. These mediators in turn may induce endothelial cells to increase expression of E-selectin, ICAM-1, and VCAM-1. Secretion of chemoattractants subsequently might mediate the migration of leukocytes.

Several studies have demonstrated the presence of macrophage inflammatory protein-1 (MIP-1α) and monocyte chemoattractant protein-1 (MCP-1) in the lungs of patients with sarcoidosis.[141,142] Macrophage inflammatory protein-1 and MCP-1 are members of the C-C chemokine family of cytokines, which are chemotactic for monocytes and lymphocytes. C-C chemokines are produced by both alveolar macrophages and interstitial macrophages. In addition, interstitial pulmonary fibroblasts also express immunoreactive C-C chemokines. Signals for production of these chemokines are presently unknown but may include IFN-γ, which has been shown to induce these cytokines in vitro.[143]

Cytokines As Mediators of Macrophage–T-Cell Interactions

Cytokines usually are secreted transiently and locally and act in a paracrine or autocrine manner at very low concentrations by interacting with cell-membrane receptors. Cytokines act as critical mediators of cell function and cell-cell communication within granulomas.

Alveolar macrophages isolated from patients with sarcoidosis spontaneously release TNF-α, but following in vitro activation produce more than twice the amount of TNF produced by macrophages isolated from healthy subjects.[144–146] Little is known about the in vivo importance of enhanced synthesis of TNF-α in sarcoidosis. Since TNF-α is a potent inducer of C-C chemokines and ICAM-1, it likely participates in the recruitment of immunocompetent cells at sites of granuloma formation.

Both increased amounts and normal amounts of IL-1β mRNA and bioactivity have been reported from alveolar macrophages obtained from patients with sarcoidosis.[147–149] Interleukin-1 receptor antagonist has been demonstrated in sarcoid granulomas.[150]

Lung T cells obtained from patients with active sarcoidosis produce increased amounts of IL-2.[151,152] As previously mentioned, increased release of IL-2 in the lung of sarcoid patients appears to result from local chronic stimulation of pulmonary lymphocytes rather than an inherited abnormality of T cells. Interleukin-2 production occurs in a well-defined population of CD4 lymphocytes that coexpress class II MHC–restricted antigen HLA-DR.[153] Through the release of IL-2, this subset of T lymphocytes amplifies the oligoclonal T lymphocytes present at sites of disease activity.

Large amounts of IFN-γ are secreted actively and spontaneously by alveolar macrophages and pulmonary T cells from patients with sarcoidosis.[154] It is difficult to assess the relative contribution of this cytokine in the pathogenesis of sarcoidosis. Interferon-γ might be involved importantly in inducing the expression of class II MHC determinants on antigen-presenting cells, thereby enhancing their accessory function. Additionally, interferon-γ is a potent activator of macrophages. Interferon-γ can act as a negative or positive regulator of the fibroproliferative response. Interferon-γ stimulates the proliferation of quiescent human lung fibroblasts, but causes dose-dependent inhibition of the growth of TNF-α or IL-1 reactivated fibroblasts.[155]

An enhanced expression of GM-CSF mRNA has been demonstrated in inflammatory cells in the sarcoid lung.[156,157] Granulocyte/macrophage colony-stimulating factor may play an important role in the accumulation and differentiation of mononuclear phagocytes in sarcoid tissues. Granulocyte/macrophage colony-stimulating factor also induces IL-1 and TNF synthesis in mononuclear cells. Accordingly, it may play an important role in the induction of these cytokines in the lungs of sarcoid patients.

Mechanisms of Granuloma-Induced Lung Injury

The formation of granulomas within the lungs leads to deranged alveolar structures. This phenomenon leads to an attempt at repair by parenchymal cells. Macrophages obtained from patients with sarcoidosis produce increased amounts of oxidants (superoxide anion and oxygen radicals), elastase, and type IV collagenase.[158–162] It is likely that epithelioid cells, giant cells, and granuloma macrophages participate in tissue damage by the release of these injurious substances.

A fibrotic process develops in some patients, likely as a consequence of cell-mediated pulmonary injury. A variety of molecules are present in the lungs of patients with sarcoidosis, which could function as chemotactic factors for fibroblasts. Increased immunoreactive transforming growth factor-β1 (TGF-β1) and extracellular matrix proteins (fibronectin, fibronectin receptor, and decorin) have been noted in epithelioid histiocytes comprising sarcoid granulomas and the surrounding fibrous tissue.[163–167] Local accumulation of cells actively releasing these soluble mediators could cause a generalized proliferative response of cells present in the areas of tissue damage, including fibroblasts, endothelial cells, and epithelial cells.[165] Altered concentrations of eicosanoids also may play an important role in the fibrotic response. Alveolar macrophages obtained from patients with sarcoidosis release lesser amounts of E-series prostaglandins than normal macrophages.[168] The loss of this important inhibitory signal may be important in the perpetuation of both the sarcoid granulomatous lesion and the fibrotic response.

Conclusion

The initiation and maintenance of pulmonary granulomatous lesions involves leukocyte migration, leukocyte activation, and leukocyte–interstitial cell interactions (Fig. 29-2). These complex cell-cell interactions are regulated by receptor-ligand interactions between cytokines and their receptors, and cell-adhesion molecules and their various ligands. Studies of granuloma formation have identified a series of complex interrelated processes. While further studies are needed to determine the in vivo impact of various cytokines and cell-adhesion molecules and to define the genetic regulation of these molecules, it seems likely that this knowledge will facilitate rational therapeutic approaches to both enhance and suppress pulmonary granulomatous responses.

References

1. Adams DO: The granulomatous inflammatory response. A review. *Am J Pathol* 1976; 84:164–191.
2. Dannenberg AM Jr: Delayed type hypersensitivity and cell-mediated immunity in the pathogenesis of tuberculosis. *Immunol Today* 1991; 12:228–233.
3. Kaufmann SHE: CD8+ T lymphocytes in intracellular microbial infections. *Immunol Today* 1988; 9:168–174.
4. Modlin RL, Segal GP, Hofman FM, et al.: In situ localization of T lymphocytes in disseminated coccidioidomycosis. *J Infect Dis* 1985; 151(2):314–319.
5. Modlin RL, Rea TH: Immunopathology of leprosy granulomas. *Springer Semin Immunopathol* 1988; 10:359–374.
6. Moscardi-Bacchi M, Soares A, Mendes R, et al.: In situ localization of T lymphocyte subsets in human paracoccidioidomycosis. *J Med Vet Mycol* 1989; 27:149–158.
7. Janeway CA: The T cell receptor as a multicomponent signalling machine: CD4/CD8 coreceptors and CD45 in T cell activation. *Annu Rev Immunol* 1992; 10:645–674.
8. Mosmann TR, Coffman RL: TH1 and TH2 cells: Different patterns of lymphokine secretion lead to different functional properties. *Annu Rev Immunol* 1989; 7:145–173.
9. Mosmann TR, Cherwinski H, Bond MW, et al.: Two types of murine helper T cell clones: I. Definition according to profiles of lymphokine activities and secreted proteins. *J Immunol* 1986; 136:2348–2357.

10. Mosmann TR, Coffman RL: Heterogeneity of cytokine secretion patterns and functions of helper T cells. *Adv Immunol* 1989; 46:111–147.

11. Sher A, Coffman RL: Regulation of immunity to parasites by T cells and T cell–derived cytokines. *Annu Rev Immunol* 1992; 10:385–409.

12. Fernandez-Botran R, Sanders VM, Mosmann TR, Vitetta ES: Lymphokine-mediated regulation of the proliferative response of clones of T helper 1 and T helper 2 cells. *J Exp Med* 1988; 168:543–558.

13. Gajewski TF, Fitch FW: Anti-proliferative effect of IFN-γ in immune regulation: I. IFN-γ inhibits the proliferation of Th2 but not Th1 murine helper T lymphocyte clones. *J Immunol* 1988; 140:4245–4252.

14. Powrie F, Coffman R: IL-4 and IL-10 inhibit DTH and IFN-γ production. *Eur J Immunol* 1993; 23:2223–2229.

15. Powrie F, Coffman RL: Cytokine regulation of T-cell function: potential for therapeutic intervention. *Immunol Today* 1993; 14:270–274.

16. Romagnani S: Human Th1 and Th2 subsets: doubt no more. *Immunol Today* 1991; 12:256–257.

17. Kelso A, Gough NM: Coexpression of granulocyte-macrophage colony-stimulating factor γ interferon, and interleukin 3 and 4 is random in murine alloreactive T-lymphocyte clones. *Proc Natl Acad Sci U S A* 1988; 85:9189–9193.

18. Firestein GS, Roeder WD, Laxer JA, et al.: A new murine CD4+ cell subset with an unrestricted cytokine profile. *J Immunol* 1989; 143:518–525.

19. Pedrazzini T, Louis JA: Functional analysis in vitro and in vivo of *Mycobacterium bovis* strains BCG-specific T cell clones. *J Immunol* 1986; 136:1828–1834.

20. Kaufmann SHE, Fleach I: Function and antigen recognition pattern of L3T4+ T cell clones from *Mycobacterium tuberculosis*–immune mice. *Infect Immun* 1986; 54:291–296.

21. Gomez AM, Bullock WE, Taylor CL, Despa GS Jr: Role of L3T4+ T cells in host defense against *Histoplasma capsulatum*. *Infect Immun* 1988; 56:1685–1691.

22. Mody CH, Lipscomb MF, Street NE, Toews GB: Depletion of CD4+ [L3T4+] lymphocytes in vivo impairs murine host defense to *Cryptococcus neoformans*. *J Immunol* 1990; 144:1472–1477.

23. Huffnagle GB, Yates JL, Lipscomb MF: T cell–mediated immunity in the lung: a *Cryptococcus neoformans* pulmonary infection model using SCID and athymic nude mice. *Infect Immun* 1991; 59(4):1423–1432.

24. Huffnagle GB, Yates JL, Lipscomb MF: Immunity to a pulmonary *Cryptococcus neoformans* infection requires both CD4+ and CD8+ T cells. *J Exp Med* 1991; 173:793–800.

25. Huffnagle GB, Lipscomb MF, Lovchik JL, et al.: The role of CD4+ and CD8+ cells in the protective response to a pulmonary cryptococcal infection. *J Leuk Biol* 1994; 55:35–42.

26. Barnes PF, Mistry SD, Cooper CL, et al.: Compartmentalization of a CD4-sup+ T lymphocyte subpopulation in tuberculosis pleuritis. *J Immunol* 1989; 142:1114–1119.

27. Emmrich F, Kaufmann SHE: Human T cell clones with reactivity to *Mycobacterium leprae* as tools for the characterization of candidate vaccines against leprosy. *Infect Immun* 1986; 41:879–883.

28. Emmrich F, Thole J, Van Embden JDA, Kaufmann SHE: A recombinant 64 kilodalton protein of *Mycobacterium bovis* BCG specifically stimulates human T4 clones reactive to mycobacterial antigens. *J Exp Med* 1986; 163:1024–1029.

29. Singh IG, Mukherjee R, Talwar GP, Kaufmann SHE: In vitro characterization of T cells from Mycobacterium w-vaccinated mice. *Infect Immun* 1992; 60:257–263.

30. DeLibero G, Flesch I, Kaufmann SHE: Mycobacteria reactive Lyt2+ T cell lines. *Eur J Immunol* 1988; 18:59–66.

31. Rees ADM, Scoging A, Mehlert A, et al.: Specificity of proliferative response of human CD8 clones to mycobacterial antigens. *Eur J Immunol* 1988; 18:1881–1887.

32. Mody CH, Chen G-H, Jackson C, et al.: Depletion of murine CD8+ T cells in vivo decreases pulmonary clearance of a moderately virulent strain of *Cryptococcus neoformans*. *J Lab Clin Med* 1993; 121:765–773.

33. Mody CH, Paine III R, Jackson C, et al.: CD8 cells play a critical role in delayed type hypersensitivity to intact *Cryptococcus neoformans*. *J Immunol* 1994; 152(8): 3870–3879.

34. Mody CH, Chen G-H, Jackson C, et al.: Depletion of murine CD8 lymphocytes in vivo impairs survival following infection with a virulent strain of *Cryptococcus neoformans*. *Mycopathologica* 1994; 125:7–17.

35. Kaufmann SHE, Rodewald HR, Hug E, De Libero G: Cloned *Listeria monocytogenes* specific non-MHC-restricted Lyt2+ T cells with cytolytic and protective activity. *J Immunol* 1988; 140:3173–3179.

36. Cooper CL, Mueller C, Sinchaisri TA, et al.: Analysis of naturally occurring delayed type hypersensitivity reactions in leprosy by in situ hybridization. *J Exp Med* 1989; 169:1565–1581.

37. Stover CK, de la Cruz VF, Fuerst TR, et al.: New use of BCG for recombinant vaccines. *Nature* 1991; 351:456–460.

38. Aldovini A, Young RA: Humoral and cell-mediated immune responses to live recombinant BCG-HIV vaccines. *Nature* 1991; 351:479–482.

39. Hubbard RD, Flory CM, Collins FM: Memory T cell-mediated resistance to *Mycobacterium tuberculosis* infection in innately susceptible and resistant mice. *Infect Immun* 1991; 59:2012–2016.

40. Orme IM, Miller ES, Roberts AD, et al.: T lymphocytes mediating protection and cellular cytolysis during the course of *Mycobacterium tuberculosis* infection. *J Immunol* 1992; 148:189–196.

41. Muller I, Cobbold SP, Waldmann H, Kaufmann SHE: Impaired resistance against *Mycobacterium tuberculosis* infection after selective in vivo depletion of L3T4+ and Lyt2+ T cells. *Infect Immun* 1987; 55:2037–2041.

42. Orme IM: The kinetics of emergence and loss of mediator T lymphocytes acquired in response to infection with *Mycobacterium tuberculosis*. *J Immunol* 1987; 138:293–298.

43. Pedrazzini T, Hug K, Louis JA: Importance of L3T4+ and Lyt-2+ cells in the immunologic control of infection with *Mycobacterium bovis* strain bacillus Calmette-Guerin in mice. Assessment by elimination of T cell subsets in vivo. *J Immunol* 1987; 139:2032–2037.

44. Kaufmann SHE, Hug E, DeLibero G: *Listeria monocytogenes–* reactive T lymphocyte clones with cytolytic activity against infected target cells. *J Exp Med* 1986; 164:363–368.

45. DeLibero G, Kaufmann SHE: Antigen-specific Lyt2+ cytolytic T lymphocytes from mice infected with the intracellular bacterium *Listeria monocytogenes*. *J Imunol* 1986; 137:2688–2694.

46. Hardy JT, Bevan MJ: CD8+ T cells specific for a single nonamer epitope of *Listeria monocytogens* are protective in vivo. *J Exp Med* 1992; 175:1531–1538.

47. Janis EM, Kaufmann SHE, Schwartz RH, Pardoll AM: Activation of γ/δ T cells in the primary immune response to *Mycobacterium tuberculosis*. *Science* 1989; 244:713–717.

48. Inoue T, Yoshikai Y, Matsuzaki G, Nomoto K: Early appearing γ/δ-bearing T cells during infection with Calmette Guerin bacillus. *J Immunol* 1991; 146:2754–2762.

49. Augustin A, Kubo RT, Sim GK: Resident pulmonary lymphocytes expressing the γ/δ T-cell receptor. *Nature* 1989; 340:239–241.

50. O'Brien RL, Happ MP, Dallas A, et al.: Stimulation of a major subset of lymphocytes expressing T cell receptor γ/δ by an antigen derived from *Mycobacterium tuberculosis*. *Cell* 1989; 57:667–674.

51. O'Brien RL, Fu Y-X, Cranfill R, et al.: Heat shock protein hsp60-reactive γ/δ cells: a large, diversified T-lymphocyte subset with highly focused specificity. *Proc Natl Acad Sci U S A* 1992; 89:4348–4352.

52. Uyemura K, Deans RJ, Band H, et al.: Evidence for clonal selection of γ/δ T cells in response to a human pathogen. *J Exp Med* 1991; 174:683–692.

53. Modlin RL, Pirmez C, Hofmann FM, et al.: Lymphocytes bearing antigen-specific γ/δ T cell receptors accumulate in human infectious disease lesions. *Nature* 1989; 339:544–548.

54. De Libero G, Casorati G, Giachino, et al.: Selection by two powerful antigens may account for the presence of the major population of human peripheral γ/δ T cells. *J Exp Med* 1991; 173:1311–1322.

55. Kabelitz D, Bender A, Prospero T, et al.: The primary response of human γ/δ T cells to *Mycobacterium tuberculosis* is restricted to Vγ9-bearing cells. *J Exp Med* 1991; 173:1331–1338.

56. Kabelitz D, Bender A, Schondelmaier S, et al.: A large fraction of human peripheral blood γ/δ+ T cells is activated by *Mycobacterium tuberculosis* but not by its 65-kD heat shock protein. *J Exp Med* 1990; 171:667–679.

57. Barnes PF, Grisso CL, Abrams JS, et al.: γ/δ T lymphocytes in human tuberculosis. *J Infect Dis* 1992; 165:506–512.

58. Follows GA, Munk ME, Gatrill AJ, et al.: Interferon-γ and IL-2 but no detectable interleukin 4 in γ/δ T cell cultures after activation with bacteria. *Infect Immun* 1992; 60:1227–1231.

59. Curtis JL, Huffnagle GB, Chen G-H, et al.: Experimental murine pulmonary cryptococcosis: differences in pulmonary inflammation and lymphocyte recruitment induced by two encapsulated strains of *Cryptococcus neoformans*. *Lab Invest* 1994; 71:113–126.

60. Schall TJ: Biology of the RANTES/SIS cytokine family. *Cytokine* 1991; 3:165–183.

61. Lukacs NW, Kunkel SC, Strieter RM, et al.: The role of macrophage inflammatory protein 1α in *Schistosoma mansoni* IgG-induced granulomatous inflammation. *J Exp Med* 1993; 177:1551–1559.

62. Chensue SW, Warmington KS, Lukacs NW, et al.: Monocyte chemotactic protein expression during schistosome egg granuloma formation: sequence of production, localization contribution and regulation. *Am J Pathol* 1995; 146:130–138.

63. Amiri P, Locksley RM, Parslow TG, et al.: Tumor necrosis factor α restores granulomas and induces parasite egg laying schistosome-infected SCID mice. *Nature* 1992; 356:604–607.

64. Joseph AL, Boros DL: TNF plays a role in *Schistosoma mansoni* egg induced granulomatous inflammation. *J Immunol* 1993; 151:5461–5471.

65. Lukacs NW, Chensue SW, Strieter RM, et al.: Inflammatory granuloma formation is mediated by TNFα-induced intercellular adhesion molecule-I. *J Immunol* 1994; 152:5883–5889.

66. van Seventer GA, Shimona Y, Horgan KJ, Shaw S: The lymphocyte function associated antigen I ligand intracellular adhesion molecule-I provides an important costimulatory signal for T cell receptor-mediated activation of resting T cells. *J Immunol* 1990; 144:4579–4586.

67. Christensen PJ, Rolfe MW, Standiford TJ, et al.: Characterization of the production of monocyte chemoattractant protein-I and IL-8 in an allogenic immune response. *J Immunol* 1993; 151:1205–1213.

68. Robinet ED, Branellec AM, Termijtelen JY, et al.: Evidence for tumor necrosis factor-α involvement in the optimal induction of class I allospecific cytotoxic T cells. *J Immunol* 1990; 144:4555–4561.

69. Rolfe MW, Kunkel SL, Standiford TJ, et al.: Expression and regulation of human pulmonary fibroblast derived monocyte chemotactic peptide (MCP-1). *Am J Physiol (Lung Cell Mol Physiol)* 1992; 263:L536–L545.

70. Paine R III, Rolfe MW, Standiford TJ, et al.: MCP-1 expression by rat type II alveolar epithelial cells in primary culture. *J Immunol* 1993; 150:4561–4570.

71. Chensue SW, Terebuh PD, Warmington KS, et al.: Role of IL-4 and IFNγ in *Schistosoma mansoni* egg–induced hypersensitivity granuloma formation. Orchestration, relative contribution, and relationship to macrophage function. *J Immunol* 1992; 148:900–906.

72. Lukacs NW, Boros DL: Lymphokine regulation of granuloma formation in murine schistosomiasis mansoni. *Clin Immunol Immunopathol* 1993; 68:57–63.

73. Lukacs NW, Kunkel SL, Strieter RM, Chensue SW: The role of chemokines in *Schistosoma mansoni* granuloma formation. *Parasitology Today* 1994; 10(8):322–324.

74. Lukacs NW, Chensue SW, Smith RE: Production of monocyte chemoattractant protein-1 and macrophage inflammatory protein-1 alpha by inflammatory granuloma fibroblasts. *Am J Path* 1994; 144(4):711–718.

75. Chensue SW, Warmington KS, Hershey SD, et al.: Evolving T cell responses in murine schistosomiasis: TH₂ cells mediate secondary granulomatous hypersensitivity and are regulated by CD8+ cell in vivo. *J Immun* 1993; 151:1391–1400.

76. Flesch IEA, Kaufmann SHE: Activation of tuberculostatic macrophage functions by Interferon-γ, Interleukin 4 and tumor necrosis factor. *Infect Immunol* 1990; 58:2675–2677.

77. Bancroft GJ, Schreiber RD, Unanue ER: Natural immunity: a T-cell independent pathway of macrophage activation defined in the SCID mouse. *Immunol Rev* 1991; 124:5–24.

78. Kawamura I, Tsukada H, Yoshikawa H, et al.: IFN-γ producing ability as a potential marker for the protective T cells against *Mycobacterium bovis* BCG in mice. *J Immunol* 1992; 148:2887–2893.

79. Denis M: Involvement of cytokines in determining resistance and acquired immunity in murine tuberculosis. *J Leuk Biol* 1991; 50:495–501.

80. Flesch I, Kaufmann SHE: Mycobacterial growth inhibition by interferon-γ–activated bone marrow macrophages and differential susceptibility among strains of *Mycobacterium tuberculosis*. *J Immunol* 1987; 138:4408–4413.

81. Denis M: Interferon-γ–treated murine macrophages inhibit growth of tubercle bacilli via the generation of reactive nitrogen intermediates. *Cell Immunol* 1991; 132:150–157.

82. Mody CH, Tyler CL, Sitrin RG, et al.: Interferon-γ activates rat alveolar macrophages for anti-Cryptococcal activity. *Am J Respir Cell Mol Biol* 1991; 5:19–26.

83. Wang M, Friedman H, Djeu JY: Enhancement of human monocyte function against *Candida albicans* by the colony stimulating factors (CSF): IL-3 granulocyte-macrophage CSF and macrophage-CSF. *J Immunol* 1989; 143:671–677.

84. Chen G-H, Curtis JL, Mody CH: et al.: Effect of granulocyte-macrophage colony-stimulating factor (GM-CSF) on rat alveolar macrophage anti-cryptococcal activity in vitro. *J Immunol* 1994; 152:724–734.

85. Levitz SM: Activation of human peripheral blood mononuclear cells by interleukin-2 and granulocyte-macrophage colony-stimulating factor to inhibit *Cryptococcus neoformans*. *Infect Immun* 1991; 59(10):3393–3397.

86. Bermudge EL, Young CS: Recombinant granulocyte macrophage colony-stimulating factor activates human macrophages to inhibit growth or kill *Mycobacterium avium* complex. *J Leuk Biol* 1990; 48:67–73.

87. Heidenreich S, Gong J-H, Schmidt A, et al.: Macrophage activa-

tion by granulocyte/macrophage colony-stimulating factor: priming for enhanced release of tumor necrosis factor alpha and prostaglandin E$_2$. *J Immunol* 1989; 143:1198–1205.

88. Most J, Neumayer HP, Dierich MP: Cytokine-induced generation of multinucleated giant cells requires interferon-γ and expression of LFA-1. *Eur J Immunol* 1990; 20:1661–1667.

89. McInnes A, Rennick DM: Interleukin 4 induces cultured monocytes/macrophages to form giant multinucleated cells. *J Exp Med* 1988; 167:598–611.

90. Mentzer SJ, Faller DV, Burakoff SJ: Interferon-γ induction of LFA-1-mediated homotypic adhesion of human monocytes. *J Immunol* 1986; 137:108–113.

91. James DG: The battlefield called sarcoidosis (editorial). *West J Med* 1987; 147:193–194.

92. Thomas PD, Hunninghake GW: Current concepts of the pathogenesis of sarcoidosis. *Am Rev Respir Dis* 1987; 135:747–760.

93. Lynch JP III, Strieter RM: Sarcoidosis, in Lynch JP III, De Remee R (eds): *Immunologically Mediated Pulmonary Disorders*. Philadelphia, JB Lippincott, 1991:189–216.

94. Hunninghake GW, Crystal RG: Pulmonary sarcoidosis: a disorder mediated by excess helper T-lymphocyte activity at sites of disease activity. *N Engl J Med* 1981; 305:429–434.

95. Crystal RG, Roberts WC, Hunninghake GW, et al.: Pulmonary sarcoidosis: a disease characterized and perpetuated by activated lung T-lymphocytes. *Ann Intern Med* 1981; 94:73–94.

96. Semenzato G, Agostini C, Zambello R, et al.: Activated T cells with immunoregulatory functions at different sites of involvement in sarcoidosis: phenotypic and functional evaluations. *Ann N Y Acad Sci* 1986; 465:56–73.

97. Semenzato G, Pezzutto A, Chilosi M, Pizzolo G: Redistribution of T lymphocytes in the lymph nodes of patients with sarcoidosis. *N Engl J Med* 1982; 306:48–49.

98. van Maarsseveen AC, Mullink H, Alons CL, Stam J: Distribution of T-lymphocyte subsets in different portions of sarcoid granulomas: immunohistologic analysis with monoclonal antibodies. *Hum Pathol* 1986; 17:493–500.

99. Modlin RL, Hofman FM, Sharma OP, et al.: Demonstration in situ of subsets of T-lymphocytes in sarcoidosis. *Am J Dermatopathol* 1984; 6:423–427.

100. Angi MR, Forattini F, Chilosi M, et al.: Immunopathology of ocular sarcoidosis. *Int Opthalmol* 1990; 14:1–11.

101. Agostini C, Trentin L, Zambello R, et al.: CD8 alveolitis in sarcoidosis: incidence, phenotypic characteristics, and clinical features. *Am Rev Respir Dis* 1993; 95:466–472.

102. Rossi GA, Sacco O, Cosulich E, et al.: Helper T-lymphocytes in pulmonary sarcoidosis. Functional analysis of a lung T-cell subpopulation in patients with active disease. *Am Rev Respir Dis* 1986; 133:1086–1090.

103. Sanders ME, Makgoba MW, Shaw S: Human naïve and memory T cells: reinterpretation of helper inducer and suppressor inducer subsets. *Immunol Today* 1988; 9:195–198.

104. Mackay CR: T-cell memory: the connection between function, phenotype and migration pathways. *Immunol Today* 1991; 12:189–192.

105. Gerli R, Darwish S: Memory phenotype of alveolar T cells in sarcoidosis. *Chest* 1990; 98:250–251.

106. Saltini C, Kirby M, Bisetti A, Crystal RG: The lung epithelial immune system. *J Immunol Res* 1991; 3:43–48.

107. Saltini C, Kirby M, Trapnell BC, et al.: Biased accumulation of T lymphocyte with "memory"-type CD45 leukocyte common antigen gene expression on the epithelial surface of the human lung. *J Exp Med* 1990; 171:1123–1140.

108. Chilosi M, Menestrina F, Capelli PO, et al.: Immunochemical analysis of sarcoid granulomas: evaluation of Ki67+ and interleukin-2 cells. *Am J Pathol* 1988; 131:191–198.

109. Semenzato G, Agostini C, Trentin L, et al.: Evidence of cells bearing interleukin-2 receptor at sites of disease activity in sarcoid patients. *Clin Exp Immunol* 1984; 57:331–337.

110. Konishi K, Moller DR, Saltini C, et al.: Spontaneous expression of the interleukin-2 receptor gene and presence of functional interleukin-2 receptors on T lymphocytes in the blood of individuals with active pulmonary sarcoidosis. *J Clin Infect* 1988; 82:775–781.

111. Saltini C, Hemler ME, Crystal RG: T lymphocytes compartmentalized on the epithelial surface of the lower respiratory tract express the very late activation antigen complex, VLA-1. *Clin Immunol Immunopathol* 1988; 46:221–233.

112. Gerli R, Darwish S, Broccucci L, et al.: Analysis of CD4-positive T cell subpopulation in sarcoidosis. *Clin Exp Immunol* 1988; 73:226–229.

113. Costabel U, Bross KJ, Ruhle KH, et al.: Ia-like antigens on T-cells and their subpopulations in pulmonary sarcoidosis and in hypersensitivity pneumonitis: analysis of bronchoalveolar and blood lymphocytes. *Am Rev Respir Dis* 1985; 131:337–342.

114. Marrack P, Kappler JW: The T cell receptor. *Chem Immunol* 1990; 47:69–81.

115. Toews GB, Vial WC, Dunn MM, et al.: The accessory cell function of human alveolar macrophages in specific T cell proliferation. *J Immunol* 1984; 132:181–189.

116. Lem VM, Lipscomb MF, Weissler JC, et al.: Bronchoalveolar cells from sarcoid patients demonstrate enhanced antigen presentation. *J Immunol* 1985; 135:1766–1771.

117. Venet A, Hance AJ, Saltini C, et al.: Enhanced alveolar macrophage-mediated antigen-induced T-lymphocyte proliferation in sarcoidosis. *J Clin Invest* 1985; 75:293–301.

118. Toews GB, Lem VM, Weissler JC, et al.: Antigen presentation by alveolar macrophages in patients with sarcoidosis. *Ann N Y Acad Sci* 1986; 465:74–81.

119. Agostini C, Trentin L, Zambello R, et al.: Pulmonary alveolar macrophages in patients with sarcoidosis and hypersensitivity pneumonitis: characterization by monoclonal antibodies. *J Clin Immunol* 1987; 7:64–70.

120. Spurzem JR, Saltini C, Kirby M, et al.: Expression of HLA class II genes in alveolar macrophages of patients with sarcoidosis. *Am Rev Respir Dis* 1989; 140:89–94.

121. Haslam PL, Parker DJ, Townsend PJ: Increases in HLA-DQ, DP, DR, and transferrin receptors on alveolar macrophages in sarcoidosis and allergic alveolitis compared with fibrosing alveolitis. *Chest* 1990; 97:651–661.

122. Campbell DA, deBois RM, Butcher RC, Poulter LW: The density of HLA-DR antigen expression on alveolar macrophages is increased in pulmonary sarcoidosis. *Clin Exp Immunol* 1986; 65:165–171.

123. Hancock WW, Muller WA, Cotran RS: Interleukin-2 receptors are expressed by alveolar macrophages during pulmonary sarcoidosis and are inducible by lymphokine treatment of normal human lung macrophages, blood monocytes, and monocyte cell lines. *J Immunol* 1987; 138:185–191.

124. Schaffer R, Dallanegra A, Breitmayer JP, et al.: Monoclonal antibody internalization and degradation during modulation of the CD3/Ti-cell receptor complex. *Cell Immunol* 1988; 116:52–59.

125. Yamaguchi E, Okazaki N, Itoh A, et al.: Modulation of accessory molecules on lung T Cells. *Chest* 1990; 97:1393–1400.

126. Yamaguchi E, Okazaki N, Itoh A, et al.: Enhanced expression of CD2 antigen on lung T cells. *Am Rev Respir Dis* 1991; 143:829–833.

127. Moller DR, Konishi K, Kirby M, et al.: Bias toward use of a specific T cell receptor beta-chain variable region in a subgroup of individuals with sarcoidosis. *J Clin Invest* 1988; 82:1183–1191.

128. Tamura N, Moller DR, Balbi B, Crystal R: Preferential usage of the T-cell antigen receptor β-chain constant region Cβ1 element

by lung T-lymphocytes of patients with pulmonary sarcoidosis. *Ann Rev Respir Dis* 1991; 143:635–659.

129. Grunewald J, Janson CH, Eklund A, et al.: Restricted Vα 2,3 gene usage by CD4+ T lymphocytes in bronchoalveolar lavage (BAL) fluid from sarcoidosis patients correlates with HLA-DR3. *Eur J Immunol* 1992; 22:129–135.

130. Grunewald J, Olerup O, Persson M, et al.: T cell receptor V gene usage by CD4+ T cells in bronchoalveolar lavage fluid and peripheral blood of sarcoidosis patients. *Proc Natl Acad Sci U S A* 1994; 91:4965–4969.

131. Grunewald J, Shigematsu M, Nagni S, et al.: T-cell receptor V gene expression in HLA-typed Japanese patients with pulmonary sarcoidosis. *Am J Respir Crit Care Med* 1995; 151:151–156.

132. Klein JT, Horn TD, Forman JD, et al.: Selection of oligoclonal Vβ-specific T cells in the intradermal response to Kveim-Siltzbach reagent in individuals with sarcoidosis. *J Immunol* 1995; 154:1450–1460.

133. Janeway CA, Jones B, Hayday A: Specificity and function of T cells bearing γ/δ receptor. *Immunol Today* 1988; 9:73–76.

134. Hance AJ, Douches S, Winchester RJ, et al.: Characterization of mononuclear phagocyte subpopulations in the human lung by using monoclonal antibodies: changes in alveolar macrophage phenotype associated with pulmonary sarcoidosis. *J Immunol* 1985; 134:284–292.

135. Malavasi F, Funaro A, Bellone G, et al.: Definition by CB12 monoclonal antibody of a differentiation market specific for human monocytes and their bone marrow precursors. *Cell Immunol* 1986; 97:276–285.

136. Spiteri MA, Clarke SW, Poulter LW: Phenotypic and functional changes in alveolar macrophages contribute to the pathogenesis of pulmonary sarcoidosis. *Clin Exp Immunol* 1988; 74:359–364.

137. Hoogsteden HC, van Dongen JJ, van Hal PT, et al.: Phenotype of blood monocytes and alveolar macrophages in interstitial lung disease. *Chest* 1989; 95:574–577.

138. Berman JS, Beer DJ, Theodre AC, et al.: Lymphocyte recruitment to the lung. *Am Rev Respir Dis* 1990; 142:238–257.

139. Albelda SM, Smith CW, Ward DA: Adhesion molecules and inflammatory injury. *FASEB J* 1994; 8:504–512.

140. Springer TA: Adhesion receptors of the immune system. *Nature* 1990; 346:425–434.

141. Car BD, Meloni F, Luisetti M, et al.: Elevated IL-8 and MCP-1 in the bronchoalveolar lavage fluid of patients with idiopathic pulmonary fibrosis and pulmonary sarcoidosis. *Am J Respir Crit Care Med* 1994; 149:655–659.

142. Standiford TJ, Rolfe MW, Kunkel SL, et al.: Macrophage inflammatory peptide 1-α expression in interstitial lung disease. *J Immunol* 1993; 151:2852–2863.

143. Barker JN, Jones ML, Sevenson CL, et al.: Monocyte chemotaxis and activating factor production by keratinocytes in response to IFNγ. *J Immunol* 1991; 146:1192–1197.

144. Bachwich PR, Lynch JP III, Larrick J, et al.: Tumor necrosis factor production by human sarcoid alveolar macrophages. *Am J Pathol* 1986; 125:421–425.

145. Spatafora M, Merendino A, Chiappara G, et al.: Lung compartmentalization of increased TNF releasing ability by mononuclear phagocytes in pulmonary sarcoidosis. *Chest* 1989; 96:542–549.

146. Baughman RP, Strohofer SA, Buchsbaum J, Lower EE: Release of tumor necrosis factor by alveolar macrophages of patients with sarcoidosis. *J Lab Clin Med* 1990; 115:36–42.

147. Hunninghake GW: Release of interleukin-1 by alveolar macrophages of patients with active pulmonary sarcoidosis. *Am Rev Respir Dis* 1984; 129:569–572.

148. Yamaguchi E, Okazaki N, Tsuneta Y, et al.: Interleukins in pulmonary sarcoidosis: dissociation correlations of lung interleukins 1 and 2 with the intensity of alveolitis. *Am Rev Respir Dis* 1988; 138:645–651.

149. Wewers MD, Saltini C, Sellers S, et al.: Evaluation of alveolar sarcoidosis for the spontaneous expression of the interleukin-1β gene. *Cell Immunol* 1987; 107:479–488.

150. Rolfe MW, Standiford TJ, Kunkel SL, et al.: Interleukin-1 receptor antagonist expression in sarcoidosis. *Am Rev Respir Dis* 1993; 148:1378–1384.

151. Hunninghake GW, Bedell GN, Zavala DC, et al.: Role of interleukin-2 release by lung T-cells in active pulmonary sarcoidosis. *Am Rev Respir Dis* 1983; 128:634–638.

152. Pinkston P, Bitterman PB, Crystal RG: Spontaneous release of interleukin-2 by lung T lymphocytes in active pulmonary sarcoidosis. *N Engl J Med* 1983; 308:793–800.

153. Saltini C, Spurzem JR, Lee JJ, et al.: Spontaneous release of interleukin 2 by lung T lymphocytes in active pulmonary sarcoidosis is primary from the Leu3+DR+T cell subset. *J Clin Invest* 1986; 77:1962–1970.

154. Robinson RBW, McLemore TL, Crystal RG: Gamma interferon is spontaneously released by alveolar macrophages and lung T lymphocytes in patients with pulmonary sarcoidosis. *J Clin Invest* 1985; 75:1488–1495.

155. Crouch E: Pathobiology of pulmonary fibrosis. *Am J Physiol* 1990; 259:159–184.

156. Kreipe H, Radzun HJ, Heidorn K, et al.: Proliferation, macrophage colony-stimulating factor, and macrophage colony-stimulating factor–receptor expression of alveolar macrophages in active sarcoidosis. *Lab Invest* 1990; 62:697–703.

157. Itoh A, Yamaguchi E, Kuzumaki N, et al.: Expression of granulocyte-macrophage colony-stimulating factor mRNA by inflammatory cells in the sarcoid lung. *Am J Respir Cell Mol Biol* 1990; 3:245–249.

158. Cassatella MA, Berton G, Agostini C, et al.: Generation of superoxide anion by alveolar macrophages in sarcoidosis: evidence for the activation of the oxygen metabolism in patients with high-intensity alveolitis. *Immunology* 1989; 66:451–458.

159. Fels AO, Nathan CF, Cohn ZA: Hydrogen peroxide release by alveolar macrophages from sarcoid patients and by alveolar macrophages from normals after exposure to recombinant interferons alpha A, beta, and gamma and 1,25-dihdroxyvitamin D3. *J Clin Invest* 1987; 80:381–386.

160. Wallaert B, Aerts C, Voisin C: Chemiluminescence of lung macrophages and blood leukocytes in sarcoidosis. *Am Rev Respir Dis* 1986; 134:1333–1334.

161. Sibille Y, Naegel GP, Merrill WW, et al.: Neutrophil chemotactic activity produced by normal and activated human bronchoalveolar lavage cells. *J Lab Clin Med* 1987; 110:624–633.

162. Ward K, O'Connor CM, Odlum C, et al.: Pulmonary disease progression in sarcoid patients with and without bronchoalveolar lavage collagenase. *Am Rev Respir Dis* 1990; 142:636–641.

163. Okabe T, Fujisawa M, Waranabe J, Takaku F: Production of colony-stimulating factor by sarcoid granulomas in vitro. *Jpn J Med* 1987; 26:36–40.

164. Rennard SI, Hunninghake GW, Bitterman PB, Crystal RG: Production of fibronectin by the human alveolar macrophage: mechanism for the recruitment of fibroblasts to sites of tissue injury in interstitial lung diseases. *Proc Natl Acad Sci U S A* 1981; 78:7147–7151.

165. De Rochemonteix-Glave B, Dayer JM, Junod AF: Fibroblast-alveolar cell interactions in sarcoidosis and idiopathic pulmonary fibrosis: evidence for stimulatory and inhibitory cytokine production by alveolar cells. *Eur Respir J* 1990; 3:653–664.

166. Limper AH, Colby TV, Sanders MS, et al.: Immunohisto-chemical localization of transforming growth factor-β1 in the non-necrotizing granulomas of pulmonary sarcoidosis. *Am J Respir Crit Care Med* 1994; 149:197–204.

167. Hasday JD, Bachwich PB, Lynch JP III, Sitrin RB: Tissue thromboplastin and urokinase activities in bronchoalveolar fluid of patients with pulmonary sarcoidosis. *Exp Lung Research* 1988; 14:261–278.

168. Bachwich PR, Lynch JP III, Kunkel SL: Arachidonic acid metabolism is altered in sarcoid alveolar macrophages. *Clin Immunol Immunopathol* 1987; 42:27–37.

Chapter 30

REGULATION OF T CELLS IN INTERSTITIAL LUNG DISEASE

JUSSI J. SAUKKONEN AND DAVID M. CENTER

Introduction

Extrinsic Interstitial Lung Disease
  Hypersensitivity pneumonitis
  Tropical pulmonary eosinophilia
  Inorganic dust-related interstitial lung disease

Intrinsic Interstitial Lung Disease
  Sarcoidosis
  Idiopathic pulmonary fibrosis
  Connective tissue disease–associated interstitial lung disease
  Bronchiolitis obliterans organizing pneumonia
  Lymphocytic interstitial pneumonitis

Introduction

Interstitial lung diseases (ILD) comprise a heterogeneous group of lung disorders with widely varying pathogenetic mechanisms. Clinical studies of these lung disorders have been hampered by small numbers of patients and lack of dramatic objective responses to therapies utilized. In some of these diseases, helpful information has been provided by animal models in the absence of human data, and these will be discussed in this review. In most cases, therapy has consisted of immunosuppression, since immune effector cells appear to play significant roles in the pathogenesis of these diseases. Although T lymphocytes have been implicated in these clinicopathologic entities, a variety of other cell types, including alveolar macrophages, neutrophils, eosinophils, and fibroblasts, often contribute to the pulmonary interstitial lesions. It should be emphasized that although the focus of this chapter is on the role of T lymphocytes in ILD, the contribution of other cell types, whether part of the immune system or not, may be more substantial in the development of these diseases. Consequently, therapies for ILD have been directed at inhibiting the deranged function of an array of interacting cell types. Future therapies may consist of a combination of agents, each of which is a specific inhibitor of a cell type involved in a given ILD.

This chapter will focus on the pathogenesis and therapy of both extrinsic and intrinsic (autoimmune) ILD in which T lymphocytes appear to play a prominent role. The extrinsic ILD to be discussed here are hypersensitivity pneumonitis, tropical pulmonary eosinophilia, and inorganic dust–related interstitial lung disease. The intrinsic ILD discussed in this chapter are sarcoidosis, idiopathic pulmonary fibrosis, connective tissue disease–associated ILD, idiopathic bronchiolitis obliterans organizing pneumonia, and lymphocytic interstitial pneumonitis.

Extrinsic Interstitial Lung Disease

HYPERSENSITIVITY PNEUMONITIS

Hypersensitivity pneumonitis (HP), also known as extrinsic allergic alveolitis (EAA), is a chronic hypersensitivity reaction of the distal airways resulting from repeated inhalation of a specific organic antigen. Inhalational exposure to a large antigen challenge results in fever, dyspnea, cough, and chest pain within 4 to 12 h in affected individuals. Although symptoms generally resolve with antigen withdrawal, a minority of individuals with frequent or constant low-level exposures may develop symptomatic restrictive interstitial lung disease.[1]

The interstitial lesion of HP consists of lymphocytic and granulomatous interstitial infiltration with patchy areas of fibrosis.[2,3] Inhalation of specific antigen initiates mucosal immune complex formation and complement activation with ensuing recruitment of neutrophils, followed by activated macrophages and T lymphocytes.[4–6] Fibrosis may result from release of reactive oxygen intermediates, fibrogenic cytokines, and growth factors for fibroblasts.[7,8] An animal model has demonstrated the importance of the delayed-type hypersensitivity reaction in this disease. Adoptive transfer of T cells from sensitized animals to unsensitized animal recipients reproduced the pulmonary lesion of HP, while serum transfer did not.[9,10] Thus, the delayed-type hypersensitivity reaction leads to granuloma formation and release of cytokines, including interleukin-1 (IL-1) and tumor necrosis factor-alpha (TNF-α),[8] which activate further macrophages and T cells (see Figure 30-1). Although the lymphocytic alveolitis found in patients with HP, as well as in asymptomatic individuals exposed to the same specific antigen, is composed mostly of activated CD8+ cells,[1,11,12] granuloma formation and fibrosis correlate with the presence of alveolar CD4+ T cells.[1,13,14]

Alveolar CD8+ T and natural killer (NK) cells may play a role in inhibiting an exuberant immunologic and fibrotic response in antigen-sensitized individuals, i.e., in modulating granuloma formation.[1,15] Alveolar T cells from HP patients do have in vitro suppressor activity, inhibiting pokeweed mitogen–induced B-cell differentiation.[11] Similar in vitro suppressor activity was found in alveolar T cells from normal controls, but the increased absolute numbers of suppressor T cells may play a significant immunoregulatory role in individuals with HP. Pulmonary T cells from HP patients are also capable of inhibiting fibroblast proliferation in vitro.[16] Depletion of NK cells in murine HP results in increased pulmonary fibrosis in antigen-challenged mice.[17] Thus, the lymphocytic alveolitis of HP may consist largely of cells limiting an exaggerated immunologic and fibrotic response to inhaled specific antigen.

Alveolar CD8+ T cells from individuals with HP consist mostly of CD3+/CD8+/CD57+/CD56+ cytotoxic cells not restricted by major histocompatibility complex presentation of antigen. Whether release of serine proteases or other toxic secretory products by cytotoxic T lymphocytes plays a role in HP-related pulmonary injury is unknown.

Treatment of HP is centered around avoidance and reduction of antigen load. Recurrent exposure in some patients may eventually result in abatement of symptoms and may

be related to desensitization[18] a phenomenon also reported to occur in an animal model.[19] Prednisone (1 mg/kg for a 4-week trial) is utilized in patients with worsening symptoms, often alleviating symptoms rapidly but not resulting in any long-term benefit compared to untreated patients.[20] Corticosteroids suppress blood T-lymphocyte activation,[21] decrease the circulating pool of T cells,[22] may enhance suppressor T-cell function,[23] and may also suppress macrophage release of lipoxygenase products.[24] Cyclosporine has been shown to modulate murine HP, resulting in decreased proliferative ability of T cells to specific antigen and inhibition of IL-1 and TNF-α.[25] Cyclosporine blocks transcriptional activation of IL-2 and other cytokines by inhibiting the phosphatase activity of calcineurin, which regulates nuclear translocation of the transcription factor NF-AT.[26]

TROPICAL PULMONARY EOSINOPHILIA

Tropical pulmonary eosinophilia (TPE) is an interstitial lung disease resulting from hypersensitivity to antigens of the filaria *Wuchereria bancrofti* or *Brugia malayi*. An early asymptomatic phase, identifiable only by marked blood eosinophilia, is succeeded by fever, weight loss, fatigue, dyspnea, cough, wheezing, and chest discomfort.[27] ILD develops in a subset of patients despite antifilarial therapy or if the disease is left untreated for more than 6 months.

While blood and pulmonary eosinophilia characterize this disease, dysregulation of T-cell function may play a role in its pathogenesis. In endemic areas, most individuals infected with filaria have suppressed parasite-specific immune responses and few, if any, clinical manifestations of parasitic infection. Blood lymphocytes derived from these individuals have reduced in vitro proliferative responses to filarial antigens, while retaining their proliferative responses to purified

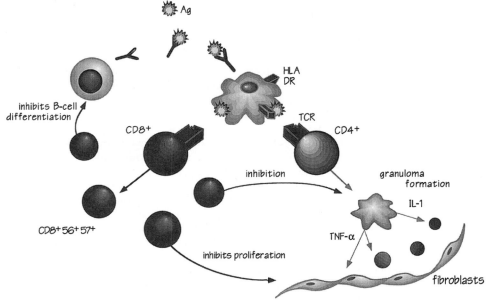

FIGURE 30-1 Immunologic events in hypersensitivity pneumonitis. Granuloma formation and fibrosis are not prominent features of HP. T cells are activated by antigen presentation and by cytokines produced by monocytoid cells. Alveolar macrophages probably are activated by cytokines produced by T cells and also by immune complexes. Granuloma formation is associated with the presence of CD4+ T cells; however, the predominant response is CD8+ pulmonary lymphocytosis. CD8+ cells inhibit granuloma formation, fibroblast proliferation, and B-cell differentiation. (*Figure used with permission of the artist, Dr. Anne Meneghetti.*)

protein derivative and streptococcal antigens.[29] However, patients afflicted with TPE have markedly enhanced parasite-specific cell-mediated and humoral responses.[27]

TPE is treated with antifilarial therapy to halt the release of microfilariae. Standard therapy with diethylcarbamazine (DEC) for 3 weeks generally is effective, but 12 to 25 percent of patients have only partial response, developing ILD or persistent symptoms.[27,30] DEC is thought to have multiple microfilaricidal effects, promoting eosinophil adherence to microfilaria and degranulation, local activation of complement, and increasing NK cell activity.[31] Single-dose ivermectin has been used to treat Bancroftian filariasis and requires further study in comparison with DEC.[32] Given the significant percentage of partial responses seen, additional therapeutic avenues need to be explored, perhaps even those suppressing the hypersensitivity response.

INORGANIC DUST–RELATED INTERSTITIAL LUNG DISEASE

Inhalation of aerosolized inorganic dusts such as silica, beryllium, asbestos, and coal-silicates may result in ILD, often after a long latency period. The mechanisms of interstitial pulmonary fibrosis in the pneumoconioses are poorly understood. Alveolar macrophages appear to have a central role, spontaneously secreting potentially injurious reactive oxygen species, IL-1, the fibrogenic cytokine TNF-α, and fibronectin. Alveolar lymphocytes are activated, perhaps by locally secreted cytokines, and produce interferon-γ (IFN-γ), which may further activate alveolar macrophages.[33]

T lymphocytes have a more prominent role in chronic beryllium disease (CBD), which is indistinguishable from sarcoidosis clinically and pathologically.[34] Inhalation of beryllium results in a chronic granulomatous inflammatory response in the lung in a small number of exposed individuals.[35] Susceptibility may rest with individuals with a glutamic acid at residue 69 of HLA-DPB1, an allele associated with autoimmune disease.[36] The disease often has high morbidity and may in some instances be fatal. It is manifested as progressive dyspnea, chest pain, and arthralgias months to years after exposure.[35]

Granulomatous inflammation and lymphoplasmacytic infiltration are thought to result from persistence of beryllium as a hapten, generating an intense cell-mediated response. Beryllium is found within the granulomas but not in normal parts of lung.[35] In nonsmoking individuals with CBD, CD4+ lymphocytic alveolitis is a prominent feature and correlates with disease severity as reflected clinically, radiologically, and in pulmonary function and exercise testing.[37,38] An increase in alveolar CD4+ Vα2+ and Vβ7+ T cells has been reported in patients with beryllium-related granulomas.[39]

In CBD, beryllium-specific CD4+ T cells accumulate in the lung[37] but are detectable in the circulation using the beryllium lymphocyte transformation test (BeLT).[40–42] This test can be used to discriminate between CBD and other granulomatous diseases and has been employed as a screening tool to identify CBD prior to the development of clinical or radiologic manifestations among exposed individuals.[40,43] More than half of individuals with positive BeLT tests have

identifiable abnormalities on exercise testing, particularly an increase in the ratio of dead space to total lung volume, indicating a defect in pulmonary vasculature.[43] The BeLT test, while specific, has variable sensitivity from one laboratory to another[40,44]; however, it is considered a crucial diagnostic test for CBD in the appropriate clinical setting.[35]

Granuloma formation in CBD is thought to proceed in a manner similar to other granulomatous inflammatory states. Beryllium is presented to alveolar lymphocytes by alveolar macrophages as a major histocompatibility gene complex (MHC) class II–restricted antigen.[37] Responding lymphocytes produce IL-2, resulting in in situ proliferation[37] and macrophage activation. Beryllium-induced proliferative responses of alveolar T lymphocytes are greater than those of blood T cells, suggesting that there is local accumulation of beryllium-specific T cells in the lungs of CBD patients.[37] Alveolar macrophages from patients with CBD and sarcoidosis express increased levels of mRNA for TNF-α and IL-6,[45] the former inducing fibroblast proliferation and collagen synthesis.[33] IL-6 further can activate and induce T-cell proliferation.[46] Granuloma formation and fibrosis are prominent features of CBD, in contrast to HP in which suppressor lymphocytes may play a significant role in modulating the local immune response.

CBD usually is responsive to treatment with corticosteroids. Since relapses are common with tapering of corticosteroids, long-term therapy is recommended.[35] Controlled trials have not been undertaken.

Intrinsic Interstitial Lung Disease

SARCOIDOSIS

Sarcoidosis is a chronic idiopathic inflammatory disease affecting multiple organ systems. Many of the clinical and pathologic findings of sarcoidosis are similar to those of chronic beryllium disease, discussed above. Clinical presentation of sarcoid is highly variable and is discussed elsewhere in this book (Chap. 112). An antigen or other inciting factor is thought to induce CD4+ T-cell and monocyte-macrophage infiltration of tissues,[47–49] with resultant formation of epithelioid cell granulomas (see Fig. 30-2).

Lymphocytic alveolitis is a common finding in active sarcoidosis, often preceding granuloma formation,[50] but does not correlate with the course of the illness.[51] The alveolitis is accounted for by increased numbers and percentages of activated CD4+/CD29+/CD45RO+ memory T cells[52–55]; in 4 percent of sarcoid patients, a CD8+ lymphocytic alveolitis is found.[56] Studies of the T-cell receptor (TCR) repertoire on bronchoalveolar T cells indicate overexpression of Cβ1,[57] Vβ8, Vβ14, and Vα2.3 genes in individuals with sarcoid.[39,58] Increased numbers of CD4+ Vα2.3+ cells[59] have been associated with HLA-DRw17 and -Dqww2 MHC haplotypes. In addition, γ/δ cell overexpression of TCR Vδ1 and Vγ9 genes has been reported.[60,61] However, data on biases in γ/δ TCR gene expression are not found consistently and may not be specific to sarcoidosis.[50,62] Overall, these data suggest that certain CD4+ T cells may proliferate to an unknown specific antigen or that T cells with specific TCR V genes preferentially migrate to the lung.[39]

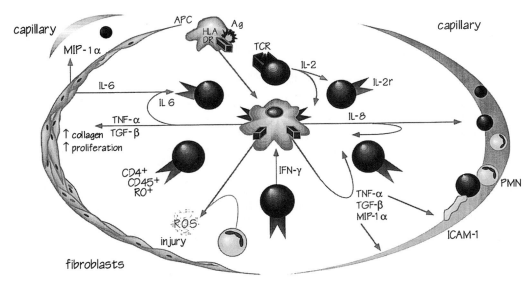

FIGURE 30-2 Immunopathogenesis of sarcoid granulomatous inflammation. Response to an unknown antigen in the lower respiratory tract is associated with mononuclear cell infiltration. Activated alveolar macrophages (AM) with enhanced antigen-presenting capacity activate CD4+/CD45/RO+ memory T cells. Local CD4+ T-cell proliferation is driven by autocrine production of IL-2 and manifested by IL-2r expression. T-cell proliferation is also enhanced by IL-6 produced by AM and fibroblasts.

Activated CD4+ T cells in turn produce IFN-γ and IL-2-activating AM. AM contribute to recruitment of mononuclear cells by elaboration of IL-2, IL-8, MIP-1α, and TNF-α through chemoattraction and modulation of adhesion molecules. Proliferation of fibroblasts and collagen synthesis is stimulated by AM production of TNF-α and by tissue injury induced by AM and neutrophils. (*Figure used with permission of the artist, Dr. Anne Meneghetti.*)

Lymphocyte accumulation within the lung in sarcoid may result from both recruitment of circulating T cells and in situ proliferation of resident CD4+ T cells. Considerable evidence indicates that in situ proliferation of T cells contributes to the lymphocytic alveolitis of sarcoidosis. Sarcoid alveolar T cells have decreased α/β TCR expression compared to blood T cells, a finding suggestive of recent alveolar T-cell activation.[63] Alveolar T cells from sarcoidosis patients spontaneously incorporate tritiated thymidine[64] and overexpress the T-cell growth factor, IL-2,[65] the IL-2 receptor,[66–68] and the proto-oncogene bcl-2.[39] However, alveolar T-cell proliferation in sarcoidosis appears to be dependent on factors within the pulmonary milieu since these cells lose their spontaneous IL-2 production and thymidine incorporation after in vitro culture.[69] Fibroblasts appear to secrete a factor inducing bcl-2 expression in T cells.[39] Overexpression of IL-6 by alveolar macrophages may be involved in maintaining T-cell proliferation in sarcoid lung.[45,70–72] Sarcoid T cells also produce IFN-γ, which may activate alveolar macrophages further.[50,73] Alveolar macrophages from sarcoidosis patients, in contrast to those from normal controls, stimulate rather than inhibit T-cell activation and proliferation.[50,74,75] However, an expanded population of alveolar macrophages with enhanced ability to downregulate T-cell responses to stimulator macrophages has been reported in sarcoid patients, suggesting that macrophage subsets may modulate local T-cell proliferation and granuloma formation.[76]

T-cell accumulation in sarcoid lung also may result from recruitment of circulating T cells. Lymphocyte extravasation is dependent on the interaction of T-cell surface adhesion

molecules with complementary receptors expressed by cytokine-activated vascular endothelial cells,[77,78] as well as on the local elaboration of T-cell chemotactic factors. The absolute CD4 count and percentage are decreased in blood of sarcoidosis patients with active disease, while the pulmonary CD4 count is increased,[79] suggesting that there is emigration of CD4+ T cells from the circulation to the lung.[39] Blood CD4+ T cells from sarcoidosis patients, when compared to T cells from normal individuals, are more predisposed to migrate across endothelium in vitro than are CD8+ T cells, in proportions correlating with bronchoalveolar lavage (BAL) CD4/CD8 ratios.[80] Cytokine activation of endothelium may play a role in promoting the adherence and subsequent transmigration of T cells across pulmonary vascular endothelium. In sarcoidosis patients with active disease, serum concentrations of soluble intercellular adhesion molecule 1 (ICAM-1), an endothelial counterreceptor for lymphocyte function-associated antigen 1 (LFA-1), are increased, correlating in one report with levels of IL-2 receptor (IL-2r) and angiotensin-converting enzyme.[39] However, since sarcoid alveolar macrophages express ICAM-1[81] and IL-2R,[82,83] it is unclear if the increased soluble adhesion and activation markers found in sarcoidosis reflect both endothelial cell and leukocyte activation.

The recruitment of CD4+ cells to the lung in sarcoidosis may be promoted further by local elaboration of T-cell chemoattractants. A variety of cytokines and chemokines have been identified in sarcoidosis tissue and BAL fluid that are chemoattractants for T cells; they include IL-1, IL-2,[50] IL-8,[39] IFN-γ,[73,84] transforming growth factor beta (TGF-β),[39]

TNF-α,[85,86] and macrophage inflammatory protein 1-alpha (MIP-1α).[87] While these T-cell chemoattractants may play a role in recruitment of lymphocytes, it is unclear what role they play in granuloma formation. Interestingly, high serum levels of IFN-γ in sarcoidosis patients prior to treatment appear to correlate with a better prognosis.[88] In summary, both T cells and macrophages are activated by the local release of cytokines implicated in T-cell proliferation and chemoattraction, endothelial cell activation, and the formation of granulomas.

Granuloma formation in sarcoidosis is thought to be related to alveolar macrophage presentation of an unknown antigen to T lymphocytes. A preparation of autologous non-viable sarcoid BAL cells was shown to be capable of inducing granuloma formation subcutaneously, indicating local production by alveolar cells of a factor or factors stimulating granuloma formation.[89] Ongoing work seeks to elucidate the factor(s) responsible for sarcoid granuloma formation.

Treatment is reserved for sarcoid patients with uveitis; cardiac, neurologic, or upper respiratory tract disease; or symptomatic pulmonary involvement. Patients with isolated bilateral hilar lymphadenopathy, erythema nodosum, hepatic granulomas, Löfgren's syndrome, or inactive fibrosis of the lung do not require treatment.[39,90] The mainstay of treatment for patients with significant disease manifestations or severe pulmonary function abnormalities[90] is corticosteroid therapy, as discussed in Chap. 112. Corticosteroids, either low dose (15 to 20 mg/day) prednisone or 1 mg/kg per day for more severe disease, hasten the resolution of symptoms but may not affect the long-term outcome of the disease.[50] Deflazacort, a calcium-sparing corticosteroid, has been used in Europe for the treatment of chronic sarcoidosis with results similar to those seen with prednisone.[91] Corticosteroids reduce spontaneous release of macrophage hydrogen peroxide and TNF-α and reduce the number of recoverable lymphocytes from BAL fluid.[92]

Corticosteroid-refractory cases, particularly those with cutaneous involvement,[93] have been treated with other immunosuppresive agents. While most patients treated with methotrexate have reported subjective improvement, only one-third with pulmonary involvement had spirometric improvement.[92,94] Methotrexate has similar effects to corticosteroids in reducing lymphocytic alveolitis and spontaneous release of hydrogen peroxide by alveolar macrophages.[92] Chlorambucil, usually in a protracted regimen, has also been used in corticosteroid-refractory cases, with moderate success.[95] Cyclosporine has been used anecdotally in the treatment of chronic refractory sarcoidosis[96] and has been used for ocular, cutaneous, and neurologic involvement.[97–99] Ketoconazole, used by several clinicians to control sarcoid-related hypercalcemia,[100–102] also has been reported to suppress T-cell proliferation through an unknown mechanism and, thus, may function also as an immunosuppressive agent (see also Chap. 112).[103]

Antimalarial agents have been used for cutaneous sarcoid but are effective in a minority of patients with pulmonary sarcoidosis.[104,105] Other experimental agents include FK-506, prostaglandin E$_2$ (which inhibits T-cell function), antibodies to leukocyte adhesion molecules (anti-CD11/CD18a and anti-ICAM-1), and IL-1R antagonist.[39]

IDIOPATHIC PULMONARY FIBROSIS

Idiopathic pulmonary fibrosis (IPF), also known as cryptogenic fibrosing alveolitis (CFA), is a progressive, inflammatory disease of the lower respiratory tract that results in fibrosis of the interstitium and alveoli. Patients usually present with worsening exertional dyspnea and dry cough, diffuse lung infiltrates, and restrictive pulmonary physiology. In the Hamman-Rich syndrome, the course is acute and fulminant and results in respiratory failure.[106] More commonly, the clinical course is chronic and relentless, resulting in a mean survival of 5 years from the time of diagnosis.[107] A variety of inciting factors have been suspected to precipitate this disease in susceptible individuals.[108,109] Circulating and pulmonary immune complexes have been reported in patients with IPF,[108,110,111] but whether these play a role in subsequent pulmonary macrophage activation is unclear. Activated macrophages release potentially injurious reactive oxygen species, recruit neutrophils that can release granule-associated proteases and collagenases, and promote fibroblast proliferation and chemotaxis (see Fig. 30-3). Ultimately, fibrosis, rather than reversible inflammation, results in progressive destruction of lung parenchyma.[108]

Prior to the development of fibrosis, a lymphoplasmacytic infiltration of the interstitium and alveolar spaces occurs, although BAL fluid may not reflect significant lymphocytosis. Lymphocyte chemoattractants, including IL-1, IL-6, IL-8, MIP-1α, and an insulin-like growth factor 1 (IGF-1)–type molecule, are produced by alveolar macrophages and activated fibroblasts, promoting T-cell recruitment and activation.[87,108]

While macrophages and neutrophils are thought to be the major mediators of lung injury in IPF, T lymphocytes may play a dual role both in contributing to lung injury and in attempting to modulate the progression of the disease. Alveolar T cells obtained from IPF patients are activated, expressing IL-2r,[112] and secreting IFN-γ,[113] which may induce local macrophage activation. Alveolar T lymphocytes from IPF patients provide excessive helper function to B cells in terms of antibody synthesis,[114,115] but whether this leads to subsequent enhanced immune complex formation relevant to this disease is unclear. Alveolar T lymphocytes from IPF patients have been reported to secrete a soluble factor inhibiting fibroblast proliferation, but alveolar T cells also induce an increase in collagen synthesis by fibroblasts.[16] While pretreatment of mice with cyclophosphamide in the bleomycin model of lung fibrosis increases pulmonary injury, transfer of splenic T cells from normal mice attenuates the injury. Thus, T cells may, to some extent, modulate the fibrotic process.[116] In humans, BAL lymphocytosis in IPF patients appears to be associated with responsiveness to treatment.[117] The histopathologic desquamative pattern, in which there is marked intraalveolar macrophage infiltration with little fibrosis, also appears to be associated with increased likelihood of response to therapy. The usual inter-

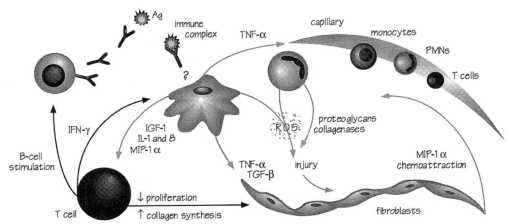

FIGURE 30-3 Immunopathogenesis of idiopathic pulmonary fibrosis. Pulmonary injury is mediated largely by alveolar macrophages (AM) and neutrophils. Activated AM release reactive oxygen species (ROS); chemoattractants for T cells, neutrophils, and monocytoid cells; fibrogenic cytokines; and cytokines activating vascular endothelium, promoting leukocyte adhesion. T cells modulate fibrosis by inhibiting proliferation of fibroblasts. T cells also stimulate antibody production. The role of immune complexes in this disease has not been elucidated fully. (*Figure used with permission of the artist, Dr. Anne Meneghetti.*)

stitial pneumonitis, in which a predominantly fibrotic picture is seen, is less likely to respond to therapy.[118,119]

Therapy for IPF includes supportive measures and immunosuppression. A trial of prednisone (1 to 2 mg/kg, up to 100 mg/day) is generally initiated and tapered after 6 weeks.[120] Low-dose prednisone is continued as maintenance therapy for 1 year if a significant response has been noted. However, only 20 to 30 percent of patients, usually those with the least fibrosis, respond. Cytotoxic therapy is reserved for patients with rapidly progressive disease or those who cannot tolerate or have failed corticosteroid therapy. While cytotoxic therapy has not been shown to be superior to corticosteroid therapy, a small long-term survival benefit appears to be afforded by cyclophosphamide or azathioprine.[121–124] Small series and anecdotal reports of the use of pulse cyclophosphamide,[92] chlorambucil, methotrexate, cyclosporine,[125,126] colchicine,[127] and antioxidant therapy[128,129] for treatment of IPF have appeared recently and await more systematic study.[121]

CONNECTIVE TISSUE DISEASE–ASSOCIATED INTERSTITIAL LUNG DISEASE

The connective tissue diseases (CTD) are chronic systemic inflammatory diseases, which may cause ILD as well as other pleuropulmonary manifestations. Detailed discussion of ILD associated with collagen-vascular disorders is beyond the scope of this chapter, but important features are summarized in Table 30-1. The CTD are idiopathic, largely autoreactive immune processes in which multiple pathogenetic mechanisms may play a role. These include immune complex–mediated injury to endothelial and epithelial cells as in the case of systemic lupus erythematosus (SLE); cell-medi-

ated cytotoxicity as in polymyositis (PM); the release of injurious reactive oxygen intermediates or proteases, as may occur in rheumatoid arthritis (RA); and smooth-muscle and fibroblast proliferation with replacement of injured tissue as in progressive systemic sclerosis (PSS). Pulmonary fibrosis appears to be associated with neutrophilic alveolitis and macrophagocytosis in the BAL fluid, while lymphocytic alveolitis often precedes the development of interstitial lung disease.[130,131]

The diagnosis of each of the CTD is based on clinical criteria. Diagnosis may be complicated further by significant overlap of clinical manifestations of CTD, such as seen with RA and mixed CTD, for example. Patients with CTD often are immunocompromised either from their disease or as a result of therapy, necessitating careful evaluation for infection or malignancy in the face of pulmonary deterioration.

Treatment is immunosuppressive, often corticosteroids and/or cytotoxic agents. Data on the efficacy of such treatment for CTD-associated ILD is not available at this time. In general, ILD in this setting is poorly responsive to therapy and is associated with significant morbidity and a poor prognosis.[132] Supportive care and treatment of infectious and other complications, including pulmonary emboli, often comprise the respiratory management of these patients.

BRONCHIOLITIS OBLITERANS ORGANIZING PNEUMONIA

Bronchiolitis obliterans organizing pneumonia (BOOP), also known as cryptogenic organizing pneumonia (COP) when idiopathic, is a clinicopathologic disorder with prominent inflammatory and fibroproliferative components. BOOP may occur in association with infections, toxic fume exposures, radiation, certain medications, CTD (SLE, RA, Sjögren's syndrome, and PM-dermatomyositis), vasculitides, chronic eosinophilic pneumonia, and HP. Most patients develop exertional dyspnea, cough, fever, and weight loss over a few months. Remission may occur spontaneously in one-quarter of patients, but the majority of patients requiring treatment respond. Relapses tend to occur in patients with BOOP associated with CTD, who may also have an accelerated clinical course.[133–135] Given the plethora of inciting factors and disease associations, the pathogenesis of this inflammatory pulmonary disorder is poorly understood.

A central role for T lymphocytes in the pathogenesis of BOOP has not been established, as multiple inflammatory cell types are prominent in BOOP. BAL fluid from patients with BOOP yields increased total leukocyte numbers, with increased neutrophilia, eosinophilia, and lymphocytosis often in excess of 40 percent of the differential count. The CD4/CD8 ratio is usually decreased.[134,136] Pathologic findings include patchy areas of granulation tissue within bronchioles, intraalveolar accumulation of foamy macrophages, lymphoplasmacytic infiltration, polypoid intraalveolar connective tissue proliferation, and rounded collections of myxomatous connective tissue.[137]

Treatment of BOOP consists of prednisone for 1 to 3 months, followed by gradual taper for a total of 6 to 12 months. High-dose intravenous methylprednisolone has been used in cases of rapidly progressive BOOP.[134] Refractory cases also have been treated with cyclophosphamide.[133,134]

LYMPHOCYTIC INTERSTITIAL PNEUMONITIS

Lymphocytic interstitial pneumonitis (LIP) may occur as an isolated clinicopathologic entity or in association with a large number of autoimmune, lymphoproliferative, and retroviral diseases.[138–142] In individuals infected with HIV-1 and human T-cell leukemia virus 1 (HTLV-I), LIP may be part of a spectrum of visceral lymphocytosis syndromes.[143–149]

Clinically, LIP generally causes fever, cough and dyspnea, and bibasilar interstitial infiltrates or consolidation, related to prominent lymphoplasmacytic infiltration of alveolar septa and spaces.[150] Some individuals are asymptomatic, while others go on to develop interstitial fibrosis,[139,143,151–155] frequent bacterial infections,[155] and bronchiectasis.[156,157]

The etiology and pathogenesis of this uncommon disease are unclear. It is likely that a variety of inciting factors and mechanisms induce LIP, reflected perhaps in significant differences in the types of predominating lymphocytes found in the lung in this disease. B-cell predominance in the lung has been reported in LIP patients.[158–160] Since polyclonal hypergammaglobulinemia is common in all LIP patients,[139,158,161] it is apparent that LIP is associated with polyclonal B-cell activation. However, other studies report T-cell predominance,[162] particularly in HIV-infected individuals. In HIV-positive adults, CD8+ T cells predominate,[143,153,163] while in HIV-infected children, both CD4+ and CD8+ T-cell predominance have been reported.[164]

CD4+ lymphocytic alveolitis was reported in patients with Sjögren's syndrome unassociated with HIV, but in those with neutrophilia there was inversion of the CD4/CD8 ratio.[165]

Lymphocytic alveolitis, unaccompanied by radiographic infiltrates, is a common finding in retroviral infection[149,166] and may represent a *forme fruste* of LIP. Understanding of the mechanisms of lymphocyte accumulation in the lungs of individuals infected with retrovirus may, in the future, provide new therapeutic avenues of the treatment of LIP. CD8+ HIV-specific cytotoxic T lymphocytes (CTL) comprise the alveolitis in early stages of HIV infection, but these are gradually supplanted by CD8+/CD57+ cells capable of suppressing CTL.[167] It is unclear whether CD8 cell accumulation in the lung in HIV-infected individuals reflects in situ proliferation or recruitment of circulating CD8+ T cells. The longitudinal changes in the phenotype of CD8 cells present in the lung may indicate that recruitment plays a significant role in the development of lymphocytic alveolitis, particularly since T-cell proliferative defects have been well described in HIV-positive individuals.[168,169]

In situ proliferation is likely to play a role in the lymphocytic alveolitis of HTLV-I infection. The transactivating protein of HTLV-I, tax, can activate genes for both IL-2 and the alpha chain of its receptor (IL-2rα),[170] which may induce the polyclonal T-cell proliferation seen in early HTLV-I infection. Increased soluble IL-2rα concentrations have been detected in BAL fluid and serum obtained from HTLV-I-infected individuals.[171] Viral protein-driven lymphocyte proliferation appears to underlie HTLV-I-related lymphoproliferative states.

An animal model of retrovirus-associated LIP may provide additional opportunities for studying the pathogenesis of LIP. Sheep infected with visna (maedi) virus, a lentivirus like HIV, develop CD8+ lymphocytic alveolitis and symptomatic LIP, eventually succumbing to opportunistic infections.[172] The severity of LIP in these animals correlates with viral load. Coinfection with common ovine respiratory pathogens is thought to contribute to the pulmonary lymphoid lesion through TNF-α-induced enhanced viral replication. Studies of lymphocyte traffic and proliferation in this model are needed. It is likely that even among retroviruses different mechanisms account for pulmonary accumulation of lymphocytes.

Although LIP is an uncommon disease, further study is needed because treatment of symptomatic patients often affords unsatisfactory results. In the pre-HIV era, approximately half of patients improved on corticosteroids, but high mortality in older patients was reported.[139,158] Anecdotal reports of treatment with chlorambucil or cyclophosphamide employed with or without corticosteroids are inconclusive.[139,173] In HIV-infected individuals, treatment of symptomatic LIP with corticosteroids usually leads to improvement of symptoms.[143,153,155] One patient was reported to improve with chlorambucil.[143] Two of three patients have been reported to improve with zidovudine treatment.[174,175] Asymptomatic individuals, rather than being treated, should be followed closely.

TABLE 30-1 Features of Interstitial Lung Disease Associated with Connective Tissue Diseases

Disease	Clinical Features	Diagnostic Findings	Pathogenesis and Immunologic Findings	Histopathology	Treatment
Rheumatoid arthritis[176-181]	Up to 70% have subclinical ILD. Usually male, smokers. Articular manifestations present. Cough, exertional dyspnea, bronchitis. Rales, clubbing.	RF: High titer. *Radiograph:* Evident in 5% of pts. Usually bibasilar interstitial infiltrates, micronodules. Pleural thickening. Eventually honeycombing. *PFT:* restrictive and/or obstructive disease, decreased D_LCO.	*BAL:* Macrophagocytosis, neutrophilia; increased neutrophil elastase, MPO, ROS, collagenase, and type III procollagen peptide. Decreased lymphocytes compared to patients without ILD. IgA immune complexes without complement deposition.	*Early:* Focal dense lymphocytic interstitial infiltration. *Late:* Alveolar septal wall fibrosis, loss of type I cells, type II hyperplasia, nodules, pleural adhesions, bronchiolitis. May have bronchiolitis obliterans with or without organizing pneumonia.	Responses disappointing. Corticosteroids, azathioprine, cyclophosphamide, or methotrexate. Bronchiolitis: Often refractory to steroids and cytotoxic agents. BOOP: Corticosteroids
Sjögren's syndrome[182,183]	May be associated with RA, SLE, PAN, PM, MCTD. Cough, dyspnea. Bibasilar rales.	+ Schirmer's test, anemia, leukopenia, cryoglobulins, + RF, + anti-ss-A/Ro, + anti-ss-B/La. *Radiograph:* Normal or reticulonodular infiltrate. *PFT:* Reduced D_LCO, restriction.	*BAL:* Lymphocytic alveolitis with reduced CD4/CD8 ratio, esp. if neutrophilia present. Macrophages: neutrophil chemotactic activity, ROS, fibronectin.	LIP, nonspecific interstitial pneumonia, BOOP, UIP. EM: ?Viral inclusions in bronchial epithelial cells.	Corticosteroids, to which LIP and BOOP anecdotally respond well.
Systemic lupus erythematosus[184-186]	Incidence unclear. Dyspnea, pleuritis, minimally productive cough. Dry rales, decreased thoracic excursion, occasional clubbing.	*Radiograph:* Atelectasis, bibasilar infiltrates, honeycombing, often with pleural effusion and cardiomegaly. *PFT:* Hypoxemia, restriction, reduced D_LCO.	?Progression from lupus pneumonitis. *BAL:* Reduced CD4/CD8 ratio. + ANA	Fibrosis, UIP, LIP reported.	Poor response to corticosteroids, cyclophosphamide, and azathioprine.
Mixed connective tissue disease[187-189]	Features of SLE, PM-DM, PSS. Dyspnea, cough, pleurisy. Often asymptomatic.	Elevated ESR, 50% have increased CPK. + High titer Ab to ENA/RNP, + anti-Sm Ab. *Radiograph:* Basilar irregular interstitial infiltrates. *PFT:* Hypoxemia, restriction, reduced D_LCO.	Circulating immune complexes, hypocomplementemia, + RF, + anti-ssDNA, + direct Coomb's hyper-γ-globulinemia.	Arterial intimal thickening and medial hypertrophy, interstitial fibrosis, lymphocytic infiltration, nonspecific interstitial pneumonitis.	Corticosteroids often ineffective. Cytotoxic agents—variable results.

| Progressive systemic sclerosis[190-195] | Up to 70% involvement; may antedate cutaneous manifestations. Exertional dyspnea, cough. End-inspiratory rales. | + ANA (speckled), + anti-centromere (CREST) *Radiograph*: Bibasilar, interstitial patterns, honeycombing, calcified granulomata in CREST, pleural disease, hilar prominence. *PFT*: Restriction, reduced D_LCO, hypoxemia, exercise desaturation. *V/Q*: Pulmonary Raynaud's phenomenon. | ?Repeated endothelial injury, interstitial inflammation, smooth-muscle proliferation, and collagen deposition. Lymphocytic alveolitis may antedate ILD. Increased macrophage-derived IL-8 chemotactic for neutrophils. Neutrophilia correlates with D_LCO and radiograph. | Endothelial and epithelial injury. Alveolar septal fibrosis, cyst formation, smooth-muscle proliferation, cuboidal epithelial cells. Bronchiectasis. Mixed interstitial inflammatory infiltrate. | Poor prognosis. Supplemental oxygen. D-penicillamine; needs further evaluation. Corticosteroids of questionable value. Cyclophosphamide promising; needs further evaluation. |
| Polymyositis/ dermatomyositis[196,197] | Dyspnea, cough; may present acutely. | + Anti-Jo-1 antibody, increased CPK, 25% + ANA. *Radiograph*: Bibasilar infiltrates, honeycombing. *PFT*: Reduced D_LCO, restriction, hypoxemia. | *BAL*: Variable cell populations. | BOOP, UIP, diffuse alveolar damage. | Corticosteroids: 40% respond. Patients with diffuse alveolar damage have poor prognosis. |

NOTE: RF = rheumatoid factor; PFT = pulmonary function tests; D_LCO = diffusion capacity; BAL = bronchoalveolar lavage; MPO = myeloperoxidase; ROS = reactive oxygen species; BOOP = bronchiolitis obliterans organizing pneumonia, RA = rheumatoid arthritis; SLE = systemic lupus erythematosus; PAN = polyarteritis nodosa; PM = polymyositis; MCTD = mixed connective tissue disease; anti-ss = anti-single stranded; LIP = lymphocytic interstitial pneumonitis; UIP = usual interstitial pneumonitis; EM = electron microscopy; DM = dermatomyositis; PSS = progressive systemic sclerosis; ESR = erythrocyte sedimentation rate; CPK = creatinine phosphokinase; ENA/RNP = extractable nuclear antigen/ribonuclear protein; anti-Sm-Ab = anti-Smith Ab; ANA = antinuclear antibody; CREST = calcinosis cutis/Raynaud's phenomenon/esophageal dysmotility/sclerodactyly/telangiectasia; V/Q = ventilation/perfusion scale.

References

1. Milburn H: Lymphocyte subsets in hypersensitivity pneumonitis. *Eur Respir J* 1992; 5:5.
2. Coleman A, Colby T: Histologic diagnosis of extrinsic allergic alveolitis. *Am J Sur Path* 1988; 12:514.
3. Richerson H, Bernstein I, Fink J, et al.: Guidelines for the clinical evaluation of hypersensitivity pneumonitis—report of the subcommittee on hypersensitivity pneumonitis. *J Allergy Clin Immunol* 1989; 84:839.
4. Pesci A, Bertorelli G, Dall'Aglio P, et al.: Evidence in bronchoalveolar lavage for third type immune reactions in hypersensitivity pneumonitis. *Eur Respir J* 1990; 3:359.
5. Yoshizawa Y, Ohdama S, Tanoue M, et al.: Analysis of bronchoalveolar lavage cells and fluids in patients with hypersensitivity pneumonitis: Sequential changes of complement components and chemotactic activities in bronchoalveolar lavage fluids. *Int Arch Allergy Appl Immunol* 1988; 87:417.
6. Salvaggio J: Immune reactions in allergic alveolitis. *Eur Respir J* 1991; 13 (suppl):S47.
7. Calhoun W: Enhanced reactive oxygen species metabolism of air space cells in hypersensitivity pneumonitis. *J Lab Clin Med* 1991; 117:443.
8. Denis M, Cormier Y, Tardif J, et al.: Hypersensitivity pneumonitis: Whole *Micropolyspora faeni* or antigens thereof stimulate the release of proinflammatory cytokines from macrophages. *Am J Respir Cell Mol Biol* 1991; 5:198.
9. Hu H, Stein-Streilein J: Hapten-immune pulmonary interstitial fibrosis (HIPIF) in mice requires both CD4+ and CD8+ T lymphocytes. *J Leukoc Biol* 1993; 54:414.
10. Bice DE, Salvaggio J, Hoffman E: Passive transfer of experimental hypersensitivity pneumonitis with lymphoid cells in the rabbit. *J Allergy Clin Immunol* 1976; 58:250.
11. Semenzato G, Agostini C, Zambello R, et al.: Lung T cells in hypersensitivity pneumonitis: Phenotypic and functional analyses. *J Immunol* 1986; 137:1164.
12. Semenzato G, Trentin L, Zambello R, et al.: Different types of cytotoxic lymphocytes recovered from the lungs of patients with hypersensitivity pneumonitis. *Am Rev Respir Dis* 1988; 137:70.
13. Murayama J, Yoshizawa Y, Ohtsuka M, Hasegawa S: Lung fibrosis in hypersensitivity pneumonitis: Association with CD4+ but not CD8+ cell dominant alveolitis and insidious onset. *Chest* 1993; 104:38.
14. Ito K, Yamasaki H, Onoue K, Ando M: Experimental hypersensitivity pneumonitis in mice induced by *Trichosporon cutaneium*: Histologic and immunologic features and effect of in vivo depletion of T cell subsets. *Exp Lung Res* 1993; 19:631.
15. Semenzato G, Trentin L: Cellular immune responses in the lung of hypersensitivity pneumonitis. *Eur Respir J* 1990; 3:357.
16. Selman M, Gonzalez G, Bravo M, et al.: Effect of lung T lymphocytes on fibroblasts in idiopathic pulmonary fibrosis and extrinsic allergic alveolitis. *Thorax* 1990; 45:451.
17. Denis M: Mouse hypersensitivity pneumonitis: Depletion of NK cells abrogates the spontaneous regression phase and leads to massive fibrosis. *Exp Lung Res* 1992; 18:761.
18. Bourke S, Banham S, Carter R, et al.: Longitudinal course of extrinsic allergic alveolitis in pigeon breeders. *Thorax* 1989; 44:415.
19. Richerson HB, Richards DW, Swanson P, et al.: Antigen-specific desensitization in a rabbit model of acute hypersensitivity pneumonitis. *J Allergy Clin Immunol* 1981; 68:226.
20. Monkare S, Haahtela T: Farmer's lung: A five-year follow-up of eighty-six patients. *Clin Allergy* 1987; 17:143.
21. McVicar D, McCrady C, Marchant R: Corticosteroids inhibit the delivery of short-term activational pulses of phorbol ester and calcium ionophore to human peripheral T cells. *Cell Immunol* 1992; 140:145.
22. Zweiman B, Atkins P, Bedard P, et al.: Corticosteroids effects on circulating lymphocyte subset levels in normal humans. *J Clin Immunol* 1984; 4:151.
23. Schatz D, Riley W, Silverstein J, Barrett D: Long-term immunoregulatory effects of therapy with corticosteroids and anti-thymocyte globulin. *Immunopharmacol Immunotoxicol* 1989; 11:269.
24. Fuller R, Kelsey C, Cole P, et al.: Dexamethasone inhibits the production of thromboxane B_2 and leukotriene B_4 by human alveolar and peritoneal macrophages in culture. *Clin Sci* 1984; 67:653.
25. Denis M, Cormier Y, Laviolette M: Murine hypersensitivity pneumonitis: A study of cellular infiltrates and cytokine production and its modulation by cyclosporin A. *Am J Respir Cell Mol Biol* 1992; 6:68.
26. Liu J: FK506 and cyclosporin, molecular probes for studying intracellular signal transduction. *Immunol Today* 1993; 14:290.
27. Ottesen E, Nutman T: Tropical pulmonary eosinophilia. *Annu Rev Med* 1992; 43:417.
28. Pinkston P, Vijayan V, Nutman T, et al.: Acute tropical pulmonary eosinophilia: Characterization of the lower respiratory tract inflammation and its response to therapy. *J Clin Invest* 1987; 80:216.
29. Ottesen E, Weller P, Heck L: Specific cellular immune unresponsiveness in human filariasis. *Immunology* 1997; 33:413.
30. Rom W, Vijayan V, Cornelius M, et al.: Persistent lower respiratory tract inflammation associated with interstitial lung disease in patients with tropical pulmonary eosinophilia following conventional treatment with diethylcarbamazine. *Am Rev Respir Dis* 1990; 142:1088.
31. Rohatgi P, Smirniotopoulos T: Tropical eosinophilia. *Semin Respir Med* 1991; 12:98.
32. Richards F, Eberhard M, Bryan R, et al.: Comparison of high dose ivermectin and diethylcarbamazine for activity against Bancroftian filariasis in Haiti. *Am J Trop Med Hyg* 1991; 44:3.
33. Donaldson K, Brown R, Brown G: Respirable industrial fibres: Mechanisms of pathogeniecity. *Thorax* 1993; 48:390.
34. Sprince N, Kazemi H, Hardy H: Current (1975) problems of differentiating between beryllium disease and sarcoidosis. *Ann NY Acad Sci* 1976; 278:654.
35. Rose C, Newman L: Hypersensitivity pneumonitis and chronic beryllium disease, in Schwartz N, King T (eds): *Interstitial Lung Disease*, 2d ed. St. Louis, Mosby, 1993; 231.
36. Richeldi L, Sorrentino R, Saltini C: HLA-DPB1 glutamate 69: A genetic marker of beryllium disease. *Science* 1993; 262:242.
37. Saltini C, Winestock K, Kirby M, et al.: Maintenance of alveolitis in patients with chronic beryllium disease by beryllium-specific helper T cells. *N Engl J Med* 1989; 320:1103.
38. Newman LS, Bobka C, Schumaker B, et al.: Compartmentalized immune response reflects clinical severity of beryllium disease. *Am J Respir Crit Care Med* 1994; 150:135.
39. Fireman E, Topilsky M: Sarcoidosis: An organized pattern of reaction from immunology to therapy. *Immunol Today* 1994; 15:199.
40. Mroz M, Kreiss K, Lezotte D, et al.: Reexamination of the blood lymphocyte transformation test in the diagnosis of chronic beryllium disease. *J Allergy Clin Immunol* 1991; 88:54.
41. Newman L, Kreiss K: Nonoccupational beryllium disease masquerading as sarcoidosis: Identification by blood lymphocyte proliferative response to beryllium. *Am Rev Respir Dis* 1992; 145:1212.
42. Kreiss K, Wasserman S, Mroz M, et al.: Beryllium disease screening in the ceramics industry: Blood lymphocyte test per-

formance and exposure-disease relations. *J Occup Med* 1993; 35:267.

43. Pappas G, Newman L: Early pulmonary physiologic abnormalities in beryllium disease. *Am Rev Respir Dis* 1993; 148:661.

44. Stokes R, Rossman M: Blood cell proliferation response to beryllium: Analysis by receiver-operating characteristics. *J Occup Med* 1991; 33:23.

45. Bost T, Riches D, Schumacher B, et al.: Alveolar macrophages from patients with beryllium disease and sarcoidosis express increased levels of mRNA for tumor necrosis factor-alpha and IL-6, but not IL-1 beta. *Am J Respir Cell Mol Biol* 1994; 10:506.

46. Lee J, Vilchek J: Interleukin-6: Multifunctional cytokine regulating immune reactions and the acute phase protein response. *Lab Invest* 1989; 61:588.

47. Hunninghake G, Fulmer J, Young R, et al.: Localization of the immune response in sarcoidosis. *Am Rev Respir Dis* 1979; 123:49.

48. Hunninghake G, Kawanami O, Ferrans V, et al.: Characterization of inflammatory and immune effector cells in the lung parenchyma of patients with interstitial lung disease. *Am Rev Respir Dis* 1981; 123:407.

49. Crystal R, Roberts W, Hunninghake G, et al.: Pulmonary sarcoidosis: A disease characterized and perpetuated by activated lung T lymphocytes. *Ann Intern Med* 1981; 94:73.

50. Weissler J: Sarcoidosis: Immunology and clinical management. *Am J Med Sci* 1994; 307:233.

51. Laviolette M, LaForge J, Tennia S, Boulet L: Prognostic value of bronchoalveolar lavage lymphocyte count in recently diagnosed pulmonary sarcoidosis. *Chest* 1991; 100:380.

52. Gerli R, Darwish S, Brocucci L, et al.: Helper inducer T cells in the lungs of sarcoidosis patients: Analysis of their pathogenic and clinical significance. *Chest* 1989; 95:811.

53. Sanders M, Makgoba M, Shaw S: Human naive and memory T cells: Reinterpretation of helper inducer and suppressor inducer subsets. *Immunol Today* 1988; 9:195.

54. Gerli R, Darwish S: Memory phenotype of alveolar T cells in sarcoidosis. *Chest* 1990; 98:250.

55. Saltini C, Kirby M, Trapnell B, et al.: Biased accumulation of T-lymphocytes with "memory"-type CD45 leukocyte common antigen gene expression on the epithelial surface of the human lung. *J Exp Med* 1990; 171:1123.

56. Agostini C, Trentin L, Zambello R, et al.: CD8 alveolitis in sarcoidosis: Incidence, phenotypic characteristics, and clinical features. *Am J Med* 1993; 95:466.

57. Tamura N, Moller D, Balbi B, et al.: Preferential usage of the T-cell antigen receptor beta-chain constant region Cbeta 1 element by lung T-lymphocytes of patients with pulmonary sarcoidosis. *Am Rev Respir Dis* 1991; 143:635.

58. Moller D, Konishi K, Kribi M, et al.: Bias toward use of a specific T-cell receptor beta-chain variable region in a subgroup of individuals with sarcoidosis. *J Clin Invest* 1988; 82:1183.

59. Grunewald J, Janson C, Eklund A, et al.: Restricted V alpha 2.3 gene usage by CD4+ T lymphocytes in bronchoalveolar lavage fluid from sarcoidosis patients correlates with HLADR3. *Eur J Immunol* 1992; 22:129.

60. Forrester J, Newman L, Wang Y, et al.: Clonal expansion of lung V delta 1+ T cells in pulmonary sarcoidosis. *J Clin Invest* 1993; 91:292.

61. Tamura N, Moller D, Balbi B, Crystal R: Diversity in junctional sequences associated with the common human V gamma 9 and V delta 2 gene segments in normal blood and lung compared with the limited diversity in a granulomatous disease. *J Exp Med* 1990; 178:121.

62. Tazi A, Fajac I, Soler P, et al.: Gamma/delta T-lymphocytes are not increased in number in granulomatous lesions of patients with tuberculosis or sarcoidosis. *Am Rev Respir Dis* 1991; 144:1373.

63. DuBois R, Kirby M, Balbi K, et al.: T-lymphocytes that accumulate in the lung in sarcoidosis have evidence of recent stimulation of the T-cell antigen receptor. *Am Rev Respir Dis* 1992; 145:1205.

64. Pinkston P, Saltini C, Muller-Quernheim J, Crystal R: Corticosteroid therapy suppresses interleukin-2 release and spontaneous proliferation of lung T-cells in active pulmonary sarcoidosis. *J Immunol* 1983; 139:755.

65. Hunninghake G, Bedell G, Zavala D, et al.: Role of interleukin-2 release in active pulmonary sarcoidosis. *Am Rev Respir Dis* 1983; 128:634.

66. Semenzato G, Agostini C, Trentin L, et al.: Evidence of cells bearing IL2 receptor at sites of disease activity in sarcoid patients. *Clin Exp Immunol* 1984; 57:331.

67. Hol B, Hintzen R, Van Lier R, et al.: Soluble and cellular markers of T cell activation in patients with pulmonary sarcoidosis. *Am Rev Respir Dis* 1993; 148:643.

68. Xaubet A, Agusti C, Roca J, et al.: BAL lymphocyte activation antigens and diffusing capacity are related to mild to moderate pulmonary sarcoidosis. *Eur Respir J* 1993; 6:715.

69. LeCossier D, Valeyre D, Loiseau A, et al.: T lymphocytes recovered by bronchoalveolar lavage from normal subjects and patients with sarcoidosis are refractory to proliferative signals. *Am Rev Respir Dis* 1988; 137:592.

70. Sahashi K, Ina Y, Takada K, et al.: Significance of interleukin 6 in patients with sarcoidosis. *Chest* 1994; 106:156.

71. Homulka J, Muller-Quernheim J: Increased interleukin 6 production by bronchoalveolar lavage cells in patients with active sarcoidosis. *Lung* 1993; 171:173.

72. Steffen M, Petersen J, Oldiga M, et al.: Increased secretion of tumor necrosis factor alpha, interleukin-1 beta, and interleukin 6 by alveolar macrophages from patients with sarcoidosis. *J Allergy Clin Immunol* 1993; 91:939.

73. Prior C, Haslam P: In vivo levels and in vitro production of interferon-gamma in fibrosing interstitial lung diseases. *Clin Exp Immunol* 1992; 88:280.

74. Venet A, Hance A, Saltini C, et al.: Enhanced alveolar macrophage-mediated antigen-induced T lymphocyte proliferation in sarcoidosis. *J Clin Invest* 1985; 75:293.

75. Lem V, Lipscomb M, Weissler J, et al.: Bronchoalveolar cells from sarcoid patients demonstrate enhanced antigen presentation. *J Immunol* 1985; 135:1766.

76. Spiteri M, Clarke S, Poulter L: Alveolar macrophages that suppress T-cell responses may be crucial to the pathogenetic outcome of pulmonary sarcoidosis. *Eur Respir J* 1992; 5:394.

77. Berman J, Beer D, Theodore A, et al.: Lymphocyte recruitment to the lung. *Am Rev Respir Dis* 1990; 142:238.

78. Furfaro S, Berman J: The relation between cell migration and activation in inflammation: Beyond adherence. *Am J Respir Cell Mol Biol* 1992; 7:248.

79. Hunninghake G, Crystal R: Pulmonary sarcoidosis: A disorder mediated by excess helper T-lymphocyte activity at sites of disease activity. *N Engl J Med* 1981; 305:429.

80. Furfaro S, Mahoney K, Saukkonen J, et al.: Preferential in vitro transendothelial migration of CD4+ lymphocytes in sarcoidosis. *Am J Respir Crit Care Med* 1994; 149:A11.

81. Melis M, Gjomarkaj M, Pace E, et al.: Increased expression of leukocyte function associated antigen-1 (LFA-1) and intercellular adhesion molecule-1 (ICAM-1) by alveolar macrophages of patients with pulmonary sarcoidosis. *Chest* 1991; 100:910.

82. Pforte A, Brunner A, Gais P, et al.: Concomitant modulation of serum-soluble interleukin-2 receptor and alveolar macrophage interleukin-2 receptor in sarcoidosis. *Am Rev Respir Dis* 1993; 147:717.

83. Hancock W, Muller W, Cotran R: Interleukin-2 receptors are expressed by alveolar macrophages during pulmonary sar-

coidosis and are inducible by lymphokine treatment of normal human lung macrophages, blood monocytes and monocyte cell lines. *J Immunol* 1987; 138:185.

84. Garlepp M, Rose A, Dench J, et al.: Clonal analysis of lung and blood T cells in patients with sarcoidosis. *Thorax* 1994; 49:577.

85. Baughman R, Strohofer S, Buchsbaum J, et al.: Release of tumor necrosis factor by alveolar macrophages of patients with sarcoidosis. *J Lab Clin Med* 1990; 115:36.

86. Bachwich P, Lynch J, Larrick J, et al.: Tumor necrosis factor production by human sarcoid alveolar macrophages. *Am J Pathol* 1986; 125:421.

87. Standiford T, Rolfe M, Kunkel S, et al.: Macrophage inflammatory protein-1 alpha expression in interstitial lung disease. *J Immunol* 1993; 151:2852.

88. Prior C, Haslam P: Increased levels of serum interferon-gamma in pulmonary sarcoidosis and relationship with response to corticosteroid therapy. *Am Rev Respir Dis* 1991; 143:53.

89. Holter J, Park H, Sjoerdsman K, et al.: Nonviable autologous bronchoalveolar lavage cell preparations induce intradermal epithelioid cell granulomas in sarcoidosis patients. *Am Rev Respir Dis* 1992; 145:864.

90. Sharma O: Pulmonary sarcoidosis and corticosteroids. *Am Rev Respir Dis* 1993; 147:1598.

91. Rizzato G, Fraioli P, Montemurro L: Long-term therapy with deflazacort in chronic sarcoidosis. *Chest* 1991; 99:301.

92. Baughman P, Lower E: The effect of corticosteroid or methotrexate therapy on lung lymphocytes and macrophages in sarcoidosis. *Am Rev Respir Dis* 1990; 142:1268.

93. Webster G, Razsi L, Sanchez M, et al.: Weekly low dose methotrexate therapy for cutaneous sarcoidosis. *J Am Acad Dermatol* 1991; 24:451.

94. Lower E, Baughman R: The use of low dose methotrexate in refractory sarcoidosis. *Am J Med Sci* 1990; 299:153.

95. Israel H, McComb B: Chlorambucil treatment of sarcoidosis. *Sarcoidosis* 1991; 8:35.

96. York E, Kovithavongs T, Man S, et al.: Cyclosporine and chronic sarcoidosis. *Chest* 1990; 98:1026.

97. Wakefield D, McCluskey P: Cyclosporine: A therapy in inflammatory eye disease. *J Ocular Pharmacol* 1991; 7:221.

98. Gupta A, Ellis C, Nickoloff B, et al.: Oral cyclosporine in the treatment of inflammatory and noninflammatory dermatoses: A clinical and immunopathologic analysis. *Arch Dermatol* 1990; 126:339.

99. Stern B, Schonfeld S, Sewell C, et al.: The treatment of neurosarcoidosis with cyclosporine. *Arch Neuro* 1992; 49:1065.

100. Glass A, Cerletty J, Elliott W, et al.: Ketoconazole reduces elevated serum levels of 1,25 dihydroxyvitamin D in hypercalcemic sarcoidosis. *J Endocrinol Invest* 1990; 13:407.

101. Adams J, Sharma O, Diz M, et al.: Ketoconazole decreases the serum 1,25 dihydroxyvitamin D and calcium concentration in sarcoidosis-associated hypercalcemia. *J Clin Endocrinol Metabol* 1990; 70:1090.

102. Bia M, Insogna K: Treatment of sarcoidosis-associated hypercalcemia with ketoconazole. *Am J Kidney Dis* 1991; 18:702.

103. Pawelec G, Ehninger G, Rehbein A, et al.: Comparison of the immunosuppressive activities of the antimycotic agents itraconazole, fluconazole, ketoconazole, and miconazole on human T-cells. *Int J Immunopharmacol* 1991; 13:299.

104. Brownstein S, Liszauer A, Carey W, et al.: Sarcoidosis of the eyelid skin. *Can J Ophthalmol* 1990; 25:256.

105. Jones E, Callen J: Hydroxychloroquine is effective therapy for control of cutaneous sarcoidal granulomas. *J Am Acad Dermatol* 1990; 23:487.

106. Olson J, Colby T, Elliott C: Hamman-Rich syndrome revisited. *Mayo Clin Proc* 1990; 65:1538.

107. Panos R, Mortenson R, Niccoli S, et al.: Clinical deterioration in patients with idiopathic pulmonary fibrosis: Causes and assessment. *Am J Med* 1990; 88:396.

108. Sheppard M, Harrison N: Lung injury, inflammatory mediators, and fibroblast activation in fibrosing alveolitis. *Thorax* 1992; 47:1064.

109. Turner-Warwick M: Interstitial lung disease of unknown etiology. *Chest* 1991; 100:232.

110. Dreisin R, Schwartz M, Theofilopoulos A, et al.: Circulating immune complexes in the idiopathic interstitial pneumonias. *N Engl J Med* 1978; 298:353.

111. Wallace W, Roberts S, Caldwell H, et al.: Circulating antibodies to lung proteins in patients with cryptogenic fibrosing alveolitis. *Thorax* 1994; 49:218.

112. Haslam P: Evaluation of alveolitis by studies of lung biopsies. *Lung* 1990; 168:984.

113. Robinson B, Rose A: Pulmonary gamma interferon production in patients with fibrosing alveolitis. *Thorax* 1990; 45:105.

114. Emura M, Nagai S, Takeuchi M, et al.: In vitro production of B cell growth factor and B cell differentiation factor by peripheral blood mononuclear cells and bronchoalveolar lavage T lymphocytes from patients with idiopathic pulmonary fibrosis. *Clin Exp Immunol* 1990; 82:133.

115. Cathcart M, Emdur L, Ahtiala-Stewart K, et al.: Excessive helper T cell function in patients with idiopathic pulmonary fibrosis: Correlation with disease activity. *Clin Immunol Immunopathol* 1987; 43:382.

116. Schrier D, Phan S: Modulation of bleomycin-induced pulmonary fibrosis in the BALB/c mouse by cyclophosphamide-sensitive T cells. *Am J Patho* 1984; 116:270.

117. Haslam P, Turton C, Lukoszek A, et al.: Bronchoalveolar lavage fluid cell counts in cryptogenic fibrosing alveolitis and their relation to therapy. *Thorax* 1980; 35:328.

118. Watters L, Schwartz M, Cherniak R, et al.: Idiopathic pulmonary fibrosis: Pretreatment bronchoalveolar lavage cell constituents and their relationships with lung histopathology and clinical response to therapy. *Am Rev Respir Dis* 1987; 135:696.

119. Turner-Warwick M, Haslam P: The value of serial bronchoalveolar lavages in assessing the clinical progress of patients with cryptogenic fibrosing alveolitis. *Am Rev Respir Dis* 1987; 135:26.

120. King T: Idiopathic pulmonary fibrosis, in Schwartz M, King T (eds): *Interstitial Lung Disease*, 2d ed. St. Louis, Mosby, 1993; 367.

121. McCune W, Vallance D, Lynch J: Immunosuppressive drug therapy. *Curr Opin Rheumatol* 1994; 6:262.

122. Winterbauer R, Hammer S, Hallman K, et al.: Diffuse interstitial pneumonitis: Clinicopathologic correlations in 20 patients treated with prednisone/azathioprine. *Am J Med* 1978; 65:661.

123. Johnson M, Kwan S, Snell N, et al.: Randomized controlled trial comparing prednisolone alone with cyclophosphamide and low dose prednisolone in combination in cryptogenic fibrosing alveolitis. *Thorax* 1989; 44:280.

124. Raghu G, Depaso W, Cain K, et al.: Azathioprine combined with prednisone in the treatment of idiopathic pulmonary fibrosis: A prospective double-blind, randomized, placebo-controlled clinical trial. *Am Rev Respir Dis* 1991; 144:291.

125. Moolman J, Bardin P, Rossouw D, et al.: Cyclosporin as a treatment for interstitial lung disease of unknown etiology. *Thorax* 1991; 46:592.

126. Venuta F, Rendina E, Ciriaco P, et al.: Efficacy of cyclosporine to reduce steroids in patients with idiopathic pulmonary fibrosis before lung transplantation. *J Heart Lung Transplant* 1993; 12:909.

127. Peters S, McDougall J, Douglas W, et al.: Colchicine in the treatment of pulmonary fibrosis. *Chest* 1993; 103:101.

128. Borok Z, Buhl R, Grimes G, et al.: Effect of glutathione aerosol on oxidant-antioxidant imbalance in idiopathic pulmonary fibrosis. *Lancet* 1991; 338:215.

129. Meyer A, Buhl R, Magnussen H: The effect of oral N-acetylcysteine on lung glutathione levels in idiopathic pulmonary fibrosis. *Eur Respir J* 1994; 7:431.

130. Edelson J, Hyland R, Ramsden M, et al.: Lung inflammation in scleroderma: Clinical, radiographic, physiologic, and cytopathological features. *J Rheumatol* 1985; 12:957.

131. Perez T, Farre J, Gossett P, et al.: Subclinical alveolar inflammation in rheumatoid arthritis: Superoxide anion, neutrophil chemotactic activity and fibronectin generation by alveolar macrophages. *Eur Respir J* 1989; 45:591.

132. Lynch J, Hunninghake G: Pulmonary complications of collagen vascular disease. *Annu Rev Med* 1992; 43:17.

133. Epler G: Bronchiolitis obliterans organizing pneumonia: Definition and clinical features. *Chest* 1992; 102:2S.

134. King T, Mortenson R: Cryptogenic organizing pneumonitis. *Chest* 1992; 102:8S.

135. Costabel U, Teschler H, Schoenfeld B, et al.: Bronchiolitis obliterans organizing pneumonia in Europe. *Chest* 1992; 102:14S.

136. Nagai S, Aung H, Tanaka S, et al.: Bronchoalveolar lavage cell findings in patients with BOOP and related diseases. *Chest* 1992; 102:32S.

137. Colby T: Pathologic aspects of bronchiolitis obliterans organizing pneumonia. *Chest* 1992; 102:38S.

138. Strimlan C, Rosenow E, Divertie M, et al.: Pulmonary manifestation of Sjögren's syndrome. *Chest* 1976; 70:354.

139. Strimlan C, Rosenow E, Weiland L, et al.: Lymphocytic interstitial pneumonitis: A review of 13 cases. *Ann Intern Med* 1978; 88:616.

140. Setoguchi Y, Takahashi G, Nokwa K: Detection of human T-cell leukemia virus-1 related antibodies in patients with lymphocytic interstitial pneumonia. *Am Rev Respir Dis* 1991; 144:1361.

141. Oleske J, Minnefor A, Cooper R, et al.: Immune deficiency syndrome in children. *JAMA* 1983; 249:2345.

142. Saldana M, Montes J, Buck B: Lymphoid interstitial pneumonia in Haitian residents of Florida (abst). *Chest* 1983; 84:347.

143. Itescu S, Brancato L, Buxbaum J, et al.: A diffuse infiltrative CD8 lymphocytosis syndrome in HIV infection: A host immune response associated with HLADR5. *Ann Intern Med* 1990; 112:3.

144. Gordon J, Golbus J, Kurtides E: Chronic lymphadenopathy and Sjögren's syndrome in a homosexual man. *N Engl J Med* 1984; 311:1441.

145. Morris J, Rosen M, Marchevsky A, et al.: Lymphocytic interstitial pneumonia in patients at risk for AIDS. *Chest* 1987; 91:63.

146. Couderc L, D'Agay M, Danon F, et al.: Sicca complex and infection with human immunodeficiency virus. *Arch Intern Med* 1987; 147:898.

147. Yoshioka M, Yamaguchi K, Yoshinaga T, et al.: Pulmonary complications in patients with adult T cell leukemia. *Cancer* 1985; 35:2491.

148. Semenzato G, Agostini C: Human retroviruses and lung involvement. *Am Rev Respir Dis* 1989; 139:1317.

149. Sugimoto M, Mita S, Tokunaga M, et al.: Pulmonary involvement in human T cell lymphotropic virus type-1 uveitis: T lymphocytosis and high proviral DNA load in bronchoalveolar lavage fluid. *Eur Respir J* 1993; 6:938.

150. Carrington C, Leibow A: Lymphocytic interstitial pneumonia (abst). *Am J Pathol* 1966; 48:36A.

151. Liebow A, Carrington C: Diffuse pulmonary lymphoreticular infiltration associated with dysproteinemia. *Med Clin North Am* 1973; 57:809.

152. McFarlane A, Davies D: Diffuse lymphoid interstitial pneumonia. *Thorax* 1973; 28:768.

153. Solal-Celigny P, Couderc L, Herman D, et al.: Lymphoid interstitial pneumonitis in acquired immunodeficiency syndrome-related complex. *Am Rev Respir Dis* 1985; 131:956.

154. Grieco M, Chinoy-Acharya P: Lymphocytic interstitial pneumonia associated with the acquired immune deficiency syndrome. *Am Rev Respir Dis* 1986; 131:952.

155. Lin R, Gruber P, Saunders R, et al.: Lymphocytic interstitial pneumonitis in adult HIV infection. *NY State J Med* 1988; 88:273.

156. Amorosa J, Miller R, Laraya-Cuasay L, et al.: Bronchiectasis in children with lymphocytic interstitial pneumonia and acquired immune deficiency syndrome: Plain film and CT observations. *Pediatr Radiol* 1992; 22:603.

157. McGuiness G, Naidich D, Garay S, et al.: AIDS associated bronchiectasis: CT features. *J Comput Assist Tomogr* 1993; 17:260.

158. Greenberg S, Haley M, Jenkins D, et al.: Lymphoplasmacytic pneumonia with accompanying dysproteinemia. *Arch Pathol* 1973; 96:73.

159. Banerjee D, Ahmed D: Malignant lymphoma complicating lymphocytic interstitial pneumonia. *Hum Pathol* 1982; 13:780.

160. Joshi V, Oleske J, Minnefor A, et al.: Pathology of suspected AIDS in children. *Pediatr Pathol* 1984; 2:71.

161. White D, Matthay R: Noninfectious pulmonary complications of infection with the human immunodeficiency virus. *Am Rev Respir Dis* 1989; 140:1763.

162. Kaufman S, Long J: Parotid mass and pulmonary nodules in a 36-year-old woman. *N Engl J Med* 1977; 297:652.

163. Guillon J, Fouret P, Mayaud C, et al.: Extensive T8+ lymphocytic visceral infiltrates in a homosexual man. *Am J Med* 1987; 82:655.

164. Broaddus C, Dake M, Stulbarg M, et al.: Bronchoalveolar lavage and transbronchial biopsy for the diagnosis of pulmonary infections in the acquired immunodeficiency syndrome. *Ann Intern Med* 1985; 102:747.

165. Wallaert B: Lymphocyte subpopulations in bronchoalveolar lavage in Sjögren's syndrome. *Chest* 1987; 92:1025.

166. Guillon J, Autran B, Denis M, et al.: Human immunodeficiency virus-related lymphocytic alveolitis. *Chest* 1988; 94:1264.

167. Sadat-Sowti B, Debre P, Idziorek T, et al.: A lectin-binding soluble factor released by CD8+CD57+ lymphocytes from AIDS patients inhibits T cell cytotoxicity. *Eur J Immunol* 1991; 21:737.

168. Pantaleo G, Koenig S, Baseler H: Defective clonogenic potential of CD8+ T lymphocytes in patients with AIDS. *J Immunol* 1990; 144:1696.

169. Clerici M, Hakim F, Venzon D, et al.: Changes in IL-2 and IL-4 production in asymptomatic HIV-infected individuals. *J Clin Invest* 1993; 91:759.

170. Yodoi J, Uchiyama T: Diseases associated with HTLV-1: virus, IL-2 receptor dysregulation, and redox regulation. *Immunol Today* 1992; 13:405.

171. Sugimoto M, Nakashima H, Matsumoto M, et al.: Pulmonary involvement in patients with HTLV-1-associated myelopathy: Increased soluble IL-2 receptors in bronchoalveolar lavage fluid. *Am Rev Respir Dis* 1989; 139:1329.

172. DeMartini J, Brodie S, Concha-Bermejillo A, et al.: Pathogenesis of lymphoid interstitial pneumonia in natural and experimental ovine lentivirus infections. *Clin Infect Dis* 1993; 17 (suppl 1):S236.

173. Essig L, Tumms E, Aancock E, et al.: Plasma cell interstitial pneumonia in macroglobulinemia: A response to corticosteroid and cyclophosphamide therapy. *Am J Med* 1974; 56:398.

174. Bach M: Zidovudine for lymphocytic interstitial pneumonia associated with AIDS. *Lancet* 1987; 2:655.

175. Helbert M: Zidovudine for lymphocytic interstitial pneumonia in AIDS (letter). Lancet 1987: 2:1390.

176. Hunninghake G, Fauci A: Pulmonary involvement in the collagen vascular diseases. *Am Rev Respir Dis* 1979; 119:471.

177. Roschman R, Rothenburg R: Pulmonary fibrosis in rheumatoid arthritis: A review of clinical features and therapy. *Semin Arthritis Rheum* 1987; 16:174.

178. Helmers R, Galvin J, Hunninghake G: Pulmonary manifestations associated with rheumatoid arthritis. *Chest* 1991; 101:235.

179. Gilligan D, O'Connor C, Wark K, et al.: Bronchoalveolar lavage in patients with mild and severe rheumatoid arthritis. *Lung* 1990; 168:221.

180. Panayi G: The pathogenesis of rheumatoid arthritis: From molecules to the whole patient. *Br J Rheumatol* 1993; 32:533.

181. Garcia J, James H, Zinkgraf S, et al.: Lower respiratory tract abnormalities in rheumatoid interstitial lung disease: Potential role of neutrophils in lung injury. *Am Rev Respir Dis* 1987; 136:811.

182. Constantopoulos S, Tsianos E, Montsopoulos H: Pulmonary and gastrointestinal manifestations of Sjögrens's syndrome. *Rheumatol Dis Clin North Am* 1992; 18:617.

183. Gardiner P, Ward C, Allison A, et al.: Pleuropulmonary abnormalities in primary Sjögren's syndrome. *J Rheumatol* 1993; 20:831.

184. Steinberg A, Klinman D: Pathogenesis of systemic lupus erythematosus. *Rheumatol Dis Clin North Am* 1988; 14:25.

185. Carette S: Cardiopulmonary manifestations of systemic lupus erythematosus. *Rheumatol Dis Clin North Am* 1988; 14:135.

186. Haupt H, Moore G, Hutchins G, et al.: The lung in systemic lupus erythematosus: Analysis of the pathologic changes in 120 patients. *Am J Med* 1981; 71:791.

187. King TE: Connective tissue disease, in Schwartz M, King T (eds): *Interstitial Lung Disease*, 2d ed. St. Louis, Mosby, 1993; 367.

188. Prakash U: Rheumatologic disease, in Murray J (ed): *Pulmonary Complications of Systemic Disease*. New York, Marcel Dekker, 1992; 385.

189. Sullivan W, Hurst D, Harmon C, et al.: A prospective evaluation emphasizing pulmonary involvement in patients with mixed connective tissue disease. *Medicine* 1984; 63:92.

190. Steen V, Lanz J, Conte C, et al.: Therapy for severe interstitial lung disease in systemic sclerosis. *Arthritis Rheum* 1994; 37:1290.

191. Akesson A, Scheja A, Lundin A, et al.: Improved pulmonary function in systemic sclerosis after treatment with cyclophosphamide. *Arthritis Rheum* 1994; 37:729.

192. Silver R, Warrick J, Kinsella M, et al.: Cyclophosphamide and low-dose prednisone therapy in patients with systemic sclerosis (scleroderma) in interstitial lung disease. *J Rheumatol* 1993; 20:838.

193. Jimenez S, Sigal S: A 15-year progressive study of treatment of rapidly progressive systemic sclerosis with *D*-penicillamine. *J Rheumatol* 1991; 18:1496.

194. Silver R, Miller K: Lung involvement in systemic sclerosis. *Rheumatol Dis Clin North Am* 1990; 16:199.

195. Lomeo R, Cornella R, Schnabel S, et al.: Progressive systemic sclerosis presenting as pulmonary interstitial fibrosis. *Am J Med* 1989; 87:525.

196. Plotz P, Dalakas M, Leff R, et al.: Current concepts in the idiopathic inflammatory myopathies: Polymyositis, dermatomyositis and related disorders. *Ann Intern Med* 1989; 111:143.

197. Salmeron G, Greenberg S, Lidsky M: Polymyositis and diffuse interstitial lung disease: A review of the pulmonary histopathologic findings. *Arch Intern Med* 1981; 141:1005.

Chapter 31

T-CELL REGULATION: ASTHMA

SOPHIE LABERGE AND DAVID M. CENTER

Introduction

Asthma is characterized by reversible airway obstruction, airway inflammation, and airway hyperresponsiveness.[1] Airway inflammation and its putative link to airway hyperresponsiveness is now recognized as a cardinal feature of asthma, contributing to the chronicity of symptoms.[2] The first histopathologic descriptions of changes associated with asthma came from postmortem studies of fatal asthma showing intense mucous plugging, bronchial smooth muscle hyperplasia, airway eosinophilia, and marked remodeling of the airway wall.[3,4] The advent of fiberoptic bronchoscopy associated with the techniques of bronchoalveolar lavage (BAL) and bronchial biopsy as a safe research tool for obtaining samples from the airways[5–7] have provided new insights in the current understanding of the pathogenesis of asthma. It now has been established that an inflammatory reaction characterized by the presence of mast cells, eosinophils, and activated lymphocytes occurs in the airways of asthmatic subjects even with clinically mild disease.[2,8–10] Although the presence of eosinophils is not exclusively specific to asthma, these cells have been implicated strongly in the pathogenesis of asthma through the release of their toxic proteins, lipid mediators, and cytokines.[11–13]

A number of lines of evidence suggest that T lymphocytes may participate in and—in some cases—orchestrate the events leading to the development of the airway inflammation observed in both atopic and nonatopic forms of asthma. First, they are capable of reacting directly with antigens and inducing a specific immune response with regulation of IgE production through interleukin (IL)-4. Secondly, T cells interact by means of secretion of other cytokines and growth factors that regulate the inflammatory response. This chapter discusses the mechanisms by which T lymphocytes may play a key role in the immune regulation of asthma. Lymphocyte activation by antigens and regulation of IgE production are discussed as pertinent to atopic asthma. The function of T lymphocyte-derived hematopoietic growth factors and chemotactic factors potentially involved in all asthmatic processes are reviewed using data from both human and animal studies.

Experimental Evidence for Lymphocyte Involvement in Asthma

HUMAN STUDIES

LYMPHOCYTE ACTIVATION IN ASTHMA
One of the major pieces of evidence for the participation of T lymphocytes in asthma came from the discovery of a subset of activated T lymphocytes both in the blood and, more specifically, in the airways of asthmatic subjects. The presence of a subset of circulating T lymphocytes in a heightened state of activation, as determined by an increased expression of HLA-DR, very late antigen (VLA)-1, and IL-2R T-cell surface activation markers, was initially described in subjects with acute asthma exacerbations.[14–16] In these studies, it was also found that the percentage of activated blood T cells and the serum concentrations of IL-2 and interferon (IFN)-γ, two T-cell derived products, decreased with clinical improvement after glucocorticoid therapy.

Increased numbers of activated T lymphocytes were also detected in the BAL fluid and bronchial mucosa of both symptomatic and asymptomatic subjects suffering from either allergic[17–19] or nonallergic asthma[20] compared to normal controls. These activated airway T lymphocytes had the memory phenotype (CD45RO), suggesting that they had previously encountered antigen.[19] In some of these studies, the numbers of activated airway lymphocytes appeared to correlate with the severity of symptoms, degree of nonspecific airway responsiveness and the extent of airway eosinophilia.[18,19,21] After inhalational antigen challenge of atopic subjects, decreased numbers of circulating blood CD4[+] T cells were associated with increased numbers of airway CD4[+] cells suggesting selective recruitment of these cells into the lung.[22,23] Further lymphocyte activation was observed after allergen inhalational challenge in sensitized subjects.[24] In contrast, a reduction in the expression of lymphocyte activation markers in BAL material together with a reduction in the number of airway eosinophils was observed after treatment with inhaled glucocorticoids.[25]

Taken together, these studies suggest that a particular subset of lymphocytes is activated in asthma and can contribute to the clinical, physiologic, and histologic manifestations which are associated with asthma.

CD4[+] T-CELL CYTOKINE PROFILES AND ASTHMA
The next major contribution to the evidence that T cells participate in the asthmatic inflammatory process comes from the identification of CD4[+] T-cell subsets, which selectively synthesize groups of cytokines.

These T-cell subsets are best defined in the murine CD4[+] T-lymphocyte population, which can be divided into functional subsets on the basis of their patterns of cytokine production.[26,27] Th1 murine T-cell clones elaborate IL-2, IFN-γ and tissue necrosis factor (TNF)-β, but not IL-4 and IL-5, whereas the Th2 T-cell clones produce IL-4, IL-5, IL-6, and IL-10, but not IL-2 and IFN-γ. Both murine Th1 and Th2 cell clones can elaborate granulocyte-macrophage colony-stimulating factor (GM-CSF), IL-3, and TNF-α. Murine Th0 clones secrete a wide variety of lymphokines that overlap Th1 and Th2 subsets. In general, Th1 cells mediate delayed-type hypersensitivity and suppress IgE synthesis, whereas Th2 cells are particularly implicated in allergic diseases by elaboration of IL-4, which regulates IgE synthesis, and IL-5, which plays a role in eosinophil hematopoiesis. Whereas in humans this classification is less distinct, in asthmatic airways IL-4 and IL-5 ("Th2") are found prominently.

ATOPIC ASTHMA

In relation to atopic asthma, the key event in the initiation of the disease process is the sensitization of the T-cell system to inhaled allergens and the subsequent reactivation of specific memory T cells after subsequent exposures.[28] Lymphocyte activation and involvement in immune responses depends on recognition of the foreign antigens by the T-cell receptor/CD3 complex.[29] Lymphocytes recognize antigen when it is presented by an antigen-presenting cell in the context of the major histocompatibility complex (MHC). Activation of the T lymphocyte is an antigen-specific event. This process involves the interaction of many cell surface receptors that strengthen the adhesion between the antigen-presenting cell and the T-cell and also provides important costimulatory signals (e.g., CD4-MHC II; CD8-MHC I; CD28-B7). In regard to the lung, the alveolar macrophages function poorly as antigen-presenting cells, whereas dendritic cells are likely to

act as the major local accessory cells.[30] Dendritic cells are distributed widely in the lung tissues but predominate within the alveolar interstitium and the airway epithelium,[31,32] being therefore ideally distributed to interact and trap the airborne antigens.

The cellular events that result from the interaction of the antigens and T lymphocytes include the activation of the lymphocyte with subsequent expression of surface immune receptors, and ultimately T-cell proliferation, generation, and secretion of hematopoietic growth factors and chemotactic factors, and B-cell activation.[33] Beyond the participation of T cells in the B-cell production of specific IgE following antigen recognition, direct activation of the T lymphocytes by antigens and subsequent release of mediators is a potential mechanism by which the asthmatic response can occur independently of the IgE pathway (Fig. 31-1).

T-LYMPHOCYTES AND REGULATION OF IgE
The production of specific IgE, a highly T cell-dependent process, requires cognate interactions between the T cells, B cells, and the antigen-presenting cells.[34,35] It is now clear that human IgE synthesis mainly and reciprocally is regulated by IL-4 and IFN-γ, two T cell-derived lymphokines. Interleukin-4, secreted by a subset of activated CD4[+] T cells ("Th2"), has a pivotal role in the isotype switching of B cells from IgG to IgE synthesis both in humans in vitro[36,37] and in mice in vivo.[38–40] In contrast, IFN-γ, a product of "Th1" T cells, downregulates IgE production.[41] A variety of other T–cell-derived cytokines, including IL-5, IL-6, and IL-10 upregulate the IL-4-dependent IgE synthesis in vitro.[42] In addition to its effect on IgE production, IL-4 is a costimulant for human B-cell proliferation in vitro[42] and induces upregulation of the low-affinity IgE receptor on human B cells[43] and monocytes[44] in vitro. Finally, lymphocytes other than

FIGURE 31-1 Postulated mechanisms of atopic asthma. Mast cells degranulate and release mediators following the reintroduction of the antigen which crosslinks the FcεRI-bound specific IgE on the surface of mast cells. Antigens may also activate Th2-like CD4[+] T cells which regulate both IgE production through the relase of IL-4 and eosinophil accumulation and activation through the release of IL-5, Il-3 and GM-CSF. (*From Corrigan CJ, Kay AB: The lymphocyte in asthma. In "Asthma and Rhinitis," William W. Busse and Stephen T. Holgate, eds, 1995, p 953. Reprinted by permission of Blackwell Science, Inc.*)

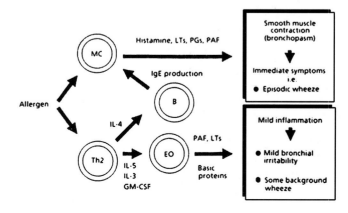

CD4$^+$ T cells are involved presumably in the regulation of IgE production. Recent studies have shown that a subset of CD4$^-$CD8$^+\gamma^+\delta^+$ have a predominant inhibitory role in the regulation of IgE production to aerosolized antigen in mice in vivo, presumably through the release of IFN-γ.[45]

Once synthesized, IgE molecules bind specifically to high-affinity receptors (FcϵRI) localized on the surface of mast cells and basophils,[46] and to low-affinity receptors (FcϵRII/CD23) on T cells, eosinophils, platelets, macrophages, and monocytes.[47] The reintroduction of the antigen, which cross-links the FcϵR-bound IgE, results in the release of an array of mast cell-derived mediators, both preformed and newly synthesized, including additional IL-4 and IL-5, which initiate and maintain the allergic response. The clinical correlate of these mast cell-initiated events[48] is the biphasic airway response in the lung characterized by an acute phase of airway obstruction that occurs within minutes following the challenge and a delayed and more prolonged phase of airway obstruction, which develops within 4 to 12 hours in a high proportion of individuals, the so-called late allergic response (Fig. 31-2). In addition, cross-linking of the low-affinity IgE receptors on the surface of monocytes, macrophages, and eosinophils with antigens results in cell activation and degranulation with subsequent release of proinflammatory mediators, which then can contribute to the allergic airway responses.[49,13]

FIGURE 31-2 Potential involvement of various mediators and cells in the development of the early and late allergic responses. Mast-cell derived mediators contribute to the onset of the immediate response which consists mainly of airway smooth muscle contraction and airway edema. The late allergic response is associated with the development of airway inflammation and airway hyperresponsiveness. The late allergic response appears to result from a complex interplay between different types of inflammatory cells and their products. ECF-A, eosinophil chemotactic factor of anaphylaxis; HETEs, hydroxyeicosatetraenoic acids; NCF-A, neutrophil chemotactic factor of anaphylaxis. *(From Sheth KK and Lemanske Jr RF: The early and late asthmatic response to allergen. In "Asthma and Rhinitis," William W. Busse and Stephen T. Holgate, eds, 1995, p 953. Reprinted by permission of Blackwell Science, Inc.)*

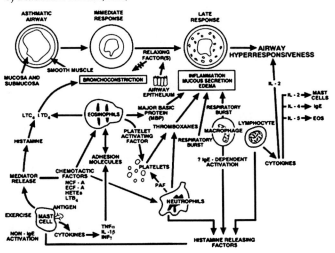

T-CELL INFLAMMATORY RESPONSE

The T-cell inflammatory response is complex and confusing because it is difficult to dissect factors that initiate the influx of CD4$^+$ T cells into the airways from the products of those infiltrating cells themselves. As noted above, much of our presumed understanding of the role of T cells in asthma comes from their identification in the airways and the identification of cytokine products with known biologic functions as chemotactic, hematopoietic growth, and activating factors for their target leukocyte.

INITIATION OF THE T-CELL INFLAMMATORY RESPONSE
Chemotactic Factors

Almost nothing is known about the earliest events in nonatopic asthma; however, some information is available following antigen activation of an atopic asthmatic response that initiates the CD4$^+$ T-cell inflammatory response. Asymptomatic asthmatics have normal bronchoalveolar T-cell differential counts and mucosal biopsies likewise are unrevealing. However, increased numbers of antigen-specific CD8$^+$ T cells can be cloned from BAL fluid, and it has been reported that there are increased numbers of CD8$^+$ T cells in the airway shortly after antigen challenge, a time when neutrophils, if any abnormal cells at all, usually are present. CD4$^+$ T cells are not seen in increased numbers in submucosa until after 24 hours, coincident with a marked increase in eosinophils. Mast cell-derived neutrophil, eosinophil, and lymphocyte chemotactic factors have been implicated in this early influx.[48]

The earliest lymphocyte chemotactic factors present in BAL fluid 4 hours following antigen challenges are the lymphocyte chemoattractant factor interleukin 16 (IL-16) and the chemokine macrophage inflammatory protein (MIP)-1α.[50] IL-16 is interesting in that it is a CD8$^+$ T-cell lymphocyte product, whose release among other chemotactic cytokines is unique after histamine challenge.[51,52] The importance of the finding that IL-16 protein and bioactivity correspond to the majority of lymphocyte chemoattractant activity found 4 hours after antigen challenge may lie in the selective chemoattractant activity of lymphocyte chemotactic factor (LCF) for CD4$^+$ cells.[53] In addition to its role as a CD4$^+$ T-lymphocyte chemotactic factor, it activates these cells to express MHC class II molecules and IL-2R, both common characteristics of airway CD4$^+$ T cells. IL-16 has similar chemotactic activity for eosinophils and monocytes by interaction with CD4 itself on all these cell types (reviewed in Ref. 53). These findings suggest that the CD8$^+$ T cells may participate in the complexion of CD4$^+$ T cells seen in asthmatic airways.

Interleukin-8 and MIP-1α also are present early after antigen challenge. Bioactivity of IL-8 appears mainly to be directed at neutrophil chemotaxis where MIP-1α is chemotactic for both CD4$^+$ and CD8$^+$ T cells. The joint selective chemoattractant activity of RANTES (regulation on activation normal T cell expressed and secreted) for CD4$^+$ T cells and eosinophils, which are present in chronic asthmatic airways, would suggest that it might play a late role because no

RANTES bioactivity or protein is detectable early after antigen challenge.

PERPETUATION AND AMPLIFICATION OF THE INFLAMMATORY RESPONSE

Hematopoietic Growth Factors

Once present, "Th-2-type" CD4[+] T cells appear to secrete a wide variety of cytokines with chemoattractant activity for all leukocyte types. In addition, many of these cytokines have the ability to stimulate the bone marrow to drive more eosinophil precursors to maturity and exit into the circulation, thereby increasing the pool of cells with potential response to locally secreted chemotactic factors. The most important of these are IL-4, IL-5, and GM-CSF.[54–59]

In addition to its major role in the regulation of IgE production, IL-4 can also contribute to the pulmonary eosinophil infiltration observed in asthma by promoting vascular cell adhesion molecule-1 (VCAM) expression on the endothelium, an adhesion molecule that may be involved in the recruitment of eosinophils.[55] IL-4, in synergy with IL-3, also is involved in the growth and differentiation of tissue mast cells in some species,[56] although its role on human lung mast cells remains to be established. Interleukin-4, in concert with IL-3, promotes the growth of human basophils and eosinophils.[57] Finally, IL-4 has a putative role in the differentiation of Th0 to Th2 cells.[42]

Interleukin-5 has been implicated particularly in the pathogenesis of asthma, as it selectively promotes the growth, differentiation, and the survival of eosinophils in culture.[58] Interleukin-5 also stimulates the antigen-dependent eosinophil activation and degranulation.[58] Interleukin-5 also can contribute to the recruitment of eosinophils into the lung by its chemoattractant activity for eosinophils[59] and its capacity to upregulate endothelial and eosinophil adhesion molecules.[60,61]

Interleukin-3 is a colony-stimulating factor for most hematopoietic cells types including the eosinophils.[13] In addition, IL-3 primes human basophils[62] and eosinophils,[13] and is also a chemoattractant for eosinophils.[63]

Granulocyte-macrophage colony-stimulating factor induces maturation and differentiation of eosinophils from bone marrow precursors[63] and increases eosinophil survival in culture.[64] It also acts as a chemoattractant factor for eosinophils.[63] In addition to its effects on hematopoiesis, GM-CSF participates in the activation of many cell types, including neutrophils and eosinophils.[65]

Evidence that a specific cytokine pattern is implicated in asthma came from a variety of sources, including in vitro studies characterizing the cytokine profile of T-cell clones derived from atopic subjects, identification of cytokine mRNA in airway biopsies and bronchoalveolar cells by the technique of in situ hybridization, and by measurement of cytokine concentrations in BAL fluid. Most randomly cloned T lymphocytes from atopic donors produced IL-2, IL-4, and IFN-γ simultaneously, thereby resembling murine Th0 cells. However, most house dust mite *Dermatophagoides pteronyssinus (Dp)*-specific T-cell clones derived from atopic patients produced IL-4 but not IFN-γ on antigen stimulation and promoted specific IgE synthesis in vitro.[66–67] In contrast, bacter-

ial antigen-specific clones derived from the same atopic subjects and *Dp*-specific clones derived from the nonatopic subjects all produced IFN-γ but not IL-4 and failed to support IgE production in vitro. In these studies, the panels of allergen-specific T-lymphocyte clones could not be distinguished on the basis of IL-2 production but resembled the murine Th2 type on the basis of IL-4 and IFN-γ.

Using the technique of in situ hybridization, Hamid and coinvestigators showed that the expression of IL-5 mRNA in mucosal bronchial biopsies obtained from atopic asthmatic subjects correlated with indices of disease severity and also the numbers of activated eosinophils and lymphocytes within the airways suggesting that IL-5, presumably released from lymphocytes, is involved in eosinophil recruitment and activation.[68] These initial observations were extended by the findings of increased numbers of bronchoalveolar cells expressing IL-2, IL-3, IL-4, IL-5, and GM-CSF mRNAs in atopic asthmatic patients in stable condition compared to normal subjects.[69] In this latter study, expression of IL-4 and IL-5 mRNAs appeared to be present predominantly in lymphocytes as assessed by the simultaneous use of the techniques of in situ hybridization and immunofluorescence microscopy. These data also showed that the pattern of cytokine mRNA expression was not exclusively a Th2-type in the sense that increased expression of IL-2 and equivalent expression of IFN-γ was found in asthmatic subjects compared to controls. Local activation of airway lymphocytes with upregulation of IL-4, IL-5 mRNA expression was similarly observed 24 hours after antigen challenge in atopic asthmatic patients.[24,70]

To determine if expression of cytokine mRNA was accompanied with in vivo translation and subsequent secretion of the corresponding proteins, Walker and coinvestigators analyzed the cytokine profile present in BAL fluid and found a characteristic Th2 cell cytokine pattern with increased IL-4 and IL-5 protein levels in allergic asthma, whereas a mixed type of cytokine pattern with both IL-2 and IL-5 predominated in nonallergic asthma.[71] Interleukin-5 was also detected in BAL fluid 48 hours after segmental antigen challenge concomitantly to the appearance of increased numbers of lavage eosinophils in subjects with allergic rhinitis.[72,73] Serum concentrations of IL-5 increased in acute exacerbations of asthma and were reduced following glucocorticoid therapy.[16] However, it cannot be concluded from these studies that other cell types, such as the mast cells[74,75] and the eosinophils,[76,77] did not participate in the elaboration of these cytokines.

In conclusion, a selective subset of activated CD4[+] T lymphocytes with a predominant Th2-like cytokine profile can be identified in asthmatic subjects and are presumably implicated in the development of the specific inflammatory reaction observed in asthma. However, the mechanisms responsible for the preferential expansion of highly polarized Th2-type lymphocytes in asthmatic subjects are still unclear. It is believed that these cells play a major role in amplifying the inflammatory response by secretion of chemotactic and activating cytokines for other leukocytes. Further, the direct or indirect effects of T-lymphocyte products on smooth muscle cell proliferation, observed in chronic asthmatic airways are just now being recognized.[78]

CD8$^+$ T CELLS AND ASTHMA

While considerable interest has focused on the role of CD4$^+$ T cells in asthma and allergic disorders, questions concerning the involvement of CD8$^+$ T cells have received less attention. A potential role for CD8$^+$ T cells was addressed above in the discussion of them as a possible airway source of an early CD4$^+$ T cell chemoattractant Il-16. Some isolated reports have documented relatively decreased numbers of circulating CD8$^+$ T cells in both allergic[79] and nonallergic asthma.[21,80] Deficient concanavalin A-induced suppressor cell activity has been reported in asthma.[81–83] Following allergen challenge, increased numbers of CD8$^+$ T cells have been retrieved in the BAL fluid from human subjects who develop isolated early airway responses as opposed to subjects who develop late allergic responses, suggesting a protective role for CD8$^+$ T cells in allergen-induced airway responses.[84] Increased numbers of CD8$^+$ T cell in BAL fluid associated with decreased numbers in the peripheral blood also suggest an active participation of these cells in nonallergic asthma.[21] Effective immunotherapy is associated with the appearance of circulating antigen-specific suppressor lymphocytes.[85–87] These studies suggest that a potential imbalance between CD4$^+$ T and CD8$^+$ T cells may contribute to the pathogenesis of asthma in some circumstances.

CD8$^+$ T cells can suppress immune responses in a variety of ways including cytolysis, release of soluble antigen-specific suppressive factors, and release of inhibitory cytokines.[88,89] Suppressor CD8$^+$ T cells downregulate antigen-induced T-cell proliferative responses in vitro[90] and regulate IgE production in vivo.[89] Although stimulated CD8$^+$ T cells secrete lymphokines, their repertoire of lymphokine production is generally more restricted compared to CD4$^+$ T cells. CD8$^+$ T cells are a major source of IFN-γ which can inhibit the proliferation of murine[91] Th2 clones in vitro and can downregulate Th2-type responses such as IgE production in vivo.[41,92] CD8$^+$ cells can also produce thyroid-binding globulin (TBG)-β when triggered by specific antigen; transforming growth factor (TGF)-β, in turn, can suppress antigen-induced T cell proliferation.[93]

Finally, recent studies have reported the potential for murine CD8$^+$ T cells to produce type-2 cytokines in vitro in response to antigen or mitogen stimulation.[94–96] These findings are consistent with the initial observations that lymphokines derived from both CD4$^+$ and CD8$^+$ lymphocytes purified from asthmatic subjects favor eosinophil survival in vitro.[97] However, the relevance of a type-2 cytokine secreting CD8$^+$ T cell subset to the pathogenesis of asthma and in humans remains to be fully investigated.[98]

EVIDENCE FOR THE ROLE OF T CELLS IN ANIMAL MODELS OF ASTHMA

Various animal studies have provided direct evidence for the participation of both CD4$^+$ and CD8$^+$ lymphocytes and their products, particularly IL-2, IL-4, IL-5, and IFN-γ in the regulation of the asthmatic responses. Research strategies have included the use of in vivo lymphocyte subset depletion, administration of recombinant cytokines, and, inversely, blocking cytokine effects using specific antibodies in animal models of asthma.

Effects of lymphocyte subset depletion on airway inflammation, airway responsiveness, and the pattern of airway obstruction after antigen challenge have been studied in different rodent models of asthma. In a mouse model of airway eosinophilia induced by ovalbumin inhalation, in vivo depletion of CD4$^+$ T cells reduced the antigen-induced eosinophil infiltration into the trachea, whereas depletion of CD8$^+$ T cells did not modify the inflammatory response to antigen.[99] Similarly, Gavett and coauthors have shown that depletion of CD4$^+$ T cells prevented the development of antigen-induced airway eosinophilia and airway hyperresponsiveness to methacholine in sensitized mice.[100] Olivenstein and coinvestigators have recently shown that depletion of CD8$^+$ T cells enhanced the production of antigen-specific IgE, the magnitude of the late allergic response, and the associated airway inflammation after antigen challenge in Sprague Dawley rats, suggesting that CD8$^+$ T cells have a immunoregulatory role in this model.[101] Consistent with these results, transfer of purified spleen CD8$^+$ T cells from ovalbumin-sensitized mice to sensitized recipients prevented the increase in airway responses to electrical field stimulation that usually occurs in sensitized animals, presumably through the production of IFN-γ by CD8$^+$ cells.[102] In the latter study, significant reduction in IgE was reported, but possible effects on the pattern of allergic inflammation were not investigated. These studies suggest that both CD4$^+$ and CD8$^+$ T cells modulate the antigen-induced airway responses.

The role of various cytokines in the airway responses to antigens also has been investigated. For example, acute single or repeated administration of IL-2 increases baseline airway responsiveness to methacholine and increases the numbers of all leukocytes retrieved in the BAL fluid, suggesting that local activation of lymphocytes and subsequent release of IL-2 may contribute to the altered airway responsiveness.[103,104] In addition, IL-2 in doses insufficient to increase airway responsiveness to inhaled methacholine substantially enhanced the airway inflammatory infiltration and also the early and late allergic responses after antigen challenge.[105] A parasite-induced murine model of pulmonary eosinophilia recently has been shown to depend on IL-4 production.[106] Similarly, a marked decrease of ovalbumin-induced airway eosinophilia associated with an absence of specific IgE was observed in IL-4 deficient mice.[107] In regard to IL-5, studies have shown that administration of anti-IL-5 monoclonal antibodies prevented airway eosinophil accumulation after a single[108–110] or repeated antigen exposure[111] in guinea pigs; reduction of lung eosinophilia was accompanied by a decrease of either in vitro[111] or in vivo[110] nonspecific airway responsiveness. Similarly, administration of anti-IL-5 antibodies decreased antigen-induced airway eosinophilia in mice.[99] On the other hand, administration of recombinant murine IFN-γ prevented the allergen-induced eosinophil infiltration in the mouse trachea, whereas anti-IFN-γ promoted eosinophil and CD4$^+$ T cell infiltration in the trachea.[112]

Taken together, these studies suggest a role for both CD4$^+$ and CD8$^+$ T cells and their products, in particular IL-4, IL-5 and IFN-γ, in the development of airway inflammation and the characteristic lung eosinophilia in various animal models of allergic asthma. However, in the majority of these studies, evaluation has been limited to the inflammatory process with some difficulties in relating changes in the inflammatory response to the airway physiology. Finally, it should be emphasized that species differences limit general application of the results to the human process.

NONALLERGIC VERSUS ALLERGIC ASTHMA

The vast majority of studies have been conducted in atopic subjects. Nonallergic or intrinsic asthma traditionally refers to asthma occurring in patients without evidence of atopy, who are negative on skin prick testing, and who have normal IgE concentrations as opposed to allergic asthma. Although both types of asthma have some distinct clinical and laboratory features, increases in numbers of circulating and airway eosinophils are found in both types of asthma. Both activated eosinophils and lymphocytes were identified in bronchial biopsies of stable subjects with either allergic or nonallergic asthma.[20] In vitro, circulating lymphocytes from both allergic and nonallergic asthmatic subjects spontaneously release factors that favor eosinophil survival, presumably GM-CSF, IL-5, and IL-3.[97]

Despite such similarities, studies comparing T-cell activation and cytokine production in peripheral blood and BAL fluid between allergic and nonallergic asthma have revealed differences in the pattern of T-cell activation. Increases in circulating $CD4^+/CD25^+$ cells are present in acute severe asthma in nonatopic asthmatic subjects and to a lesser extent in atopic asthmatic patients.[15] Determination of activated T cells, measured as the expression of IL-2 receptor and HLA-DR on T-cell subsets, showed increased numbers of $CD4^+$ $IL-2R^+$ T cells in both peripheral blood[71,113] and BAL fluid[71] of allergic asthmatic subjects in stable conditions. By contrast, nonallergic asthmatic patients exhibit a pattern of chronic activation with increased expression of IL-2R, HLA-DR, and VLA-1 surface antigens on both circulating and bronchoalveolar $CD4^+$ and $CD8^+$ T cells. The analysis of cytokine profile in the BAL fluid showed a characteristic Th2 cell cytokine pattern with increased IL-4 and IL-5 concentrations in allergic asthma, whereas a mixed type of cytokine pattern with IL-2 and IL-5 predominated in nonallergic asthma without any detectable increase in IL-4 concentration.[71] In both types of asthma, concentrations of IL-5 correlated with peripheral eosinophilia.

These studies have suggested that cell-mediated mechanisms are involved in the pathogenesis of nonallergic asthma have revealed slight basic immunologic differences in the pathogenesis of allergic and nonallergic asthma. However, the initial events that trigger the immune response still are unknown.

OTHER TYPES OF ASTHMA

Occupational asthma induced by high molecular weight compounds shares some features of allergen-induced asthma. It often is mediated by an IgE-related mechanism, and the nature of the inflammatory reaction that occurs in the airways is similar. Although not specifically studied, it is reasonable to believe that lymphocytes play a role in the

immune regulation of this type of asthma in similar ways to that of allergic asthma.[114]

Some circumstantial evidence suggests immunologic mechanisms may participate in the pathogenesis of asthma induced by low molecular weight compounds. The two best studied entities in this category are occupational exposures to toluene diisocyanates and plicatic acid (Western red cedar). Late asthmatic responses are associated with an increase in the percentage of circulating $CD8^+$ T lymphocytes by 8 hours following toluene diisocyanate exposure that persists for 24 to 48 hours.[115] An inflammatory reaction similar to that observed in allergic asthma is found in bronchial mucosa of stable subjects with occupational asthma induced by toluene isocyanate with evidence of eosinophil and lymphocyte activation.[116,117] Numbers of eosinophils also are increased in BAL fluid of subjects with occupational asthma induced by exposure to Western red cedar antigen and increased numbers of eosinophils as well as activated lymphocytes are found in bronchial biopsies.[114] Finally, late asthmatic responses and airway hyperresponsiveness induced by toluene diisocyanate are responsive to corticosteroids.[118]

In contrast to other forms of asthma, there is no evidence for an active participation of lymphocytes in the pathogenesis of exercise nor aspirin-induced asthma.

Therapeutic Implications

The recognition that chronic airway inflammation is a prominent feature in the pathology of asthma has modified the management of asthma therapy. It now is well recognized that asthma therapy must be directed to the control of the chronic airway inflammation at an early stage of the disease by means of anti-inflammatory medications. Among these anti-inflammatory drugs, the corticosteroids are the most effective drugs used in the treatment of asthma.

Although their mechanisms of action are not completely elucidated, effects of glucocorticosteroids presumably are related to their direct inhibitory effects on the inflammatory cells, including the lymphocytes. More specifically, corticosteroids can decrease lymphocyte proliferation and activation in vitro, inhibiting both IL-2 production and IL-2 receptor gene expression.[119–121] Corticosteroids also inhibit the gene transcription of several lymphocyte-derived cytokines pertinent to the pathogenesis of asthma, including IL-3, IL-5, GM-CSF.[122] In vivo, administration of corticosteroids downregulates the expression of cell activation markers on both circulating[14–16] and airway lymphocytes[25] in subjects with symptomatic atopic asthma. The improvement of nonspecific airway responsiveness and the reduction in airway eosinophilia that follow systemic corticosteroid therapy in asthmatic subjects are accompanied by a reduction in the number of bronchoalveolar cells expressing mRNA for IL-4 and IL-5.[123] Similarly, IL-4 and IL-5 gene expression in bronchoalveolar cells at sites of segmental antigen challenge is inhibitable by corticosteroids in asthmatic subjects.[124] Lastly, corticosteroids inhibit lymphocyte and eosinophil random and stimulated migration and they may have profound effect on the accumulation of these cells in the lung by preventing emigration from the blood.[125]

Although corticosteroids are potent drugs in the treatment of asthma, some individuals do not show substantial improvement of pulmonary function after corticosteroid therapy.[126,127] Some lymphocyte functional abnormalities were reported in this subgroup of corticosteroid-resistant subjects, which might represent important mechanisms of corticosteroid resistance in asthma. These abnormalities include the failure of corticosteroids to inhibit mitogen-induced lymphocyte proliferation and cytokine production in vitro,[128,129] persistent lymphocyte activation in the peripheral blood[129] as well as in the airways[130] despite intensive corticosteroid therapy, reduction of in glucocorticoid receptor binding on T cells[131] in steroid-resistant compared to steroid-sensitive asthma. Finally, Leung and coauthors showed that corticosteroid-resistant asthmatic subjects differ from corticosteroid-sensitive subjects in their pattern of cytokine gene expression in the bronchoalveolar cells.[130] In the latter study, the increase in basal IL-2 and IL-4 gene expression and the lack of inhibition of IL-4 and IL-5 gene expression following corticosteroids therapy characterized corticosteroid-resistant asthma compared to corticosteroid-sensitive asthma.

The use of cyclosporine and FK506 has been restricted to corticosteroid-dependent, severe, chronic asthma.[132,133] The mechanisms of action of these immunosuppressant agents are largely dependent of their inhibitory effects on lymphocyte proliferation and cytokine gene transcription and release.[134] However, emergence of undesirable side effects has limited the widespread use of these compounds. The efficacy of the corticosteroids implicates the T lymphocyte in the pathogenesis of asthma.

Finally, the efficacy of innovative therapies directed against cytokines using specific antagonists or drugs that act on specific cytokine receptors remains to be demonstrated.[134]

Summary

It is becoming clear that lymphocytes can regulate various aspects of the inflammatory process that occurs in asthma through their regulatory role in IgE synthesis and their capacity to generate hematopoietic growth factors and chemotactic growth factors. Collectively, the data obtained from both human and animal studies support a role for T lymphocytes in the pathogenesis of asthma and, more specifically, in the development of an eosinophil-rich airway infiltration. The relevance of T cell-mediated events must be viewed as part of a complex interplay between the lymphocytes and the other airway inflammatory cells. In this respect, lymphocyte-derived products are part of a cascade of inflammatory mediators whose interactions ultimately culminate in the characteristic histologic findings observed in asthma.

Asthma is a disease of the airways that is characterized not only by the chronic inflammation but also by the occurrence of episodic bronchoconstriction and the presence of airway hyperresponsiveness. The link between airway inflammation and the abnormal reactivity of the airway smooth muscle is not understood completely. Of interest is the recent finding that the activated T lymphocytes can interact with the airway smooth muscle cells and regulate their growth and possibly their reactivity, raising the possibility that this interaction may contribute to the airway remodeling that occurs in asthmatic subjects.[78]

References

1. Guidelines for the diagnosis and management of asthma. National Heart, Lung, and Blood Institute. National Asthma Education Program. Expert Panel Report. *J Allergy Clin Immunol* 1993; 88:425.
2. Djukanovic R, Roche WR, Wilson JW, et al.: Mucosal inflammation in asthma. *Am Rev Respir Dis* 1990; 142:434.
3. Dunnill MS: The pathology of asthma, with special reference to changes in the bronchial mucosa. *J Clin Pathol* 1960; 13:27.
4. Thurlbeck WM, Henderson JA, Fraser RG, Bates DV: Chronic obstructive lung disease: a comparison between clinical, roentgenologic, functional, and morphologic criteria in chronic bronchitis, emphysema, asthma and bronchiectasis. *Medicine* 1970; 49:81.
5. Workshop summary and guidelines: investigative use of bronchoscopy, lavage, and bronchial biopsies in asthma and other airway diseases. *J Allergy Clin Immunol* 1991; 88:808.
6. Crump JW, Pueringer RJ, Hunninghake GW: Bronchoalveolar lavage and lymphocytes in asthma. *Eur Respir* 1991; 4:39s.
7. Smith DL, Deshazo RD: Bronchoalveolar lavage in asthma: an update and perspective. *Am Rev Respir Dis* 1993; 148:523.
8. Beasley R, Roche WR, Roberts JA, Holgate ST: Cellular events in the bronchi in mild asthma and after bronchial provocation. *Am Rev Respir Dis* 1989; 139:806.
9. Jeffery PK, Wardlaw AJ, Nelson FC, et al.: Bronchial biopsies in asthma: an ultrastructural quantitative study and correlation with hyperreactivity. *Am Rev Respir Dis* 1989; 140:1745.
10. Laitinen LA, Laitinen A, Haahtela T: Airway mucosal inflammation even in patients with newly diagnosed asthma. *Am Rev Respir Dis* 1993; 147:697.
11. Gleich GJ: The eosinophil and bronchial asthma: current understanding. *J Allergy Clin Immunol* 1990; 85:422.
12. Leff AR: Inflammatory mediation of airway hyperresponsiveness by peripheral blood granulocytes: the case for the eosinophil. *Chest* 1994; 106:1202.
13. Weller PF: The immunobiology of eosinophils. *N Engl J Med* 1991; 324:1110.
14. Corrigan CJ, Hartnell A, Kay AB: T lymphocyte activation in acute severe asthma. *Lancet* 1988; i:1129.
15. Corrigan CJ, Kay AB: CD4 T-lymphocyte activation in acute severe asthma: relationship to disease severity and atopic status. *Am Rev Respir Dis* 1990; 141:970.
16. Corrigan CJ, Haczku A, Gemou-Engesaeth V, et al.: CD4 T-lymphocyte activation in asthma is accompanied by increased serum concentrations of interleukin-5: effect of glucocoticoid therapy. *Am Rev Respir Dis* 1993; 147:540.
17. Wilson JW, Djukanovic R, Howarth PH, Holgate ST: Lymphocyte activation in bronchoalveolar lavage and peripheral blood in atopic asthma. *Am Rev Respir Dis* 1992; 145:958.
18. Assawi M, Bradley B, Jeffery PK, et al.: Identification of activated T lymphocytes and eosinophils in bronchial biopsies in stable atopic asthma. *Am Rev Respir Dis* 1990; 142:1407.
19. Robinson DS, Bentley AM, Hartnell A, et al.: Activated memory T helper cells in bronchoalveolar lavage fluid from patients with atopic asthma: relation to asthma symptoms, lung function, and bronchial responsiveness. *Thorax* 1993; 48:26.

20. Bentley AM, Menz G, Storz C, et al.: Identification of T lymphocytes, macrophages, and activated eosinophils in the bronchial mucosa in intrinsic asthma: relationship to symptoms and bronchial responsiveness. *Am Rev Respir Dis* 1992; 146:500.

21. Walker C, Kaegi MK, Braun P, Blaser K: Activated T cells and eosinophilia in bronchoalveolar lavages from subjects with asthma correlated with disease severity. *J Allergy Clin Immunol* 1991; 88:935.

22. Gerblich AA, Campbell AE, Schuyler MR: Changes in T-lymphocyte subpopulations after antigenic bronchial provocation in asthmatics. *N Engl J Med* 1984; 310:1349.

23. Gerblich AA, Salik H, Schuyler MR: Dynamic T-cell changes in peripheral blood and bronchoalveolar lavage after antigen bronchoprovocation in asthmatics. *Am Rev Respir Dis* 1991; 143:533.

24. Robinson D, Hamid Q, Bentley A, et al.: Activation of CD4+ T cells, increased Th2-type cytokine mRNA expression, and eosinophil recruitment in bronchoalveolar lavage after allergen inhalation challenge in patients with atopic asthma. *J Allergy Clin Immunol* 1993; 92:313.

25. Wilson JW, Djukanovic R, Howarth PH, Holgate ST: Inhaled beclomethasone dipropionate downregulates airway lymphocyte activation in atopic asthma. *Am J Respir Crit Care Med* 1994; 149:86.

26. Mosmann TR, Coffman RL: Th1 and Th2 cells: different patterns of lymphokine secretion lead to different functional properties. *Annu Rev Immunol* 1989; 7:145.

27. Street NE, Mosmann TR: Functional diversity of T-lymphocytes due to secretion of different cytokine patterns. *FASEB J* 1991; 5:171.

28. Holt PG, McMenamin C, Shon-Hegrad MA, et al.: Immunoregulation of asthma: control of T-lymphocyte activation in the respiratory tract. *Eur Respir J* 1991; 4:6s.

29. Saltini C, Richeldi L, Holroyd KJ, et al.: Lymphocytes, in Crystal RG, West JB (eds): *The Lung: Scientific Foundations.* New York, Raven Press, 1991:459–482.

30. Hance AJ: Accessory-cell-lymphocyte interactions, in Crystal RG, West JB (eds): *The Lung: Scientific Foundations.* New York, Raven Press, 1991:483–498.

31. Holt PG, Schon-Hegrad MA, Philips MJ, McMenamin PG: Ia-positive dendritic cells form a tightly meshed network within the human airway epithelium. *Clin Exp Allergy* 1989; 19:597.

32. Sertl K, Takemura T, Tschachler E, et al.: Dendritic cells with antigen presenting capability reside in airway epithelium, lung parenchyma and visceral pleura. *J Exp Med* 1986; 163:436.

33. Kaltreider HB: Normal immune response, in Crystal RG, West JB (eds): *The Lung: Scientific Foundations.* New York, Raven Press, 1991:499–510.

34. Clark EA, Ledbetter JA: How B and T cells talk to each other. *Nature* 1994; 367:425.

35. Romagnani S: Regulation and deregulation of human IgE synthesis. *Immunol Today* 1990; 1:316.

36. Pène J, Rousset F, Brière F, et al.: IgE production by normal human lymphocytes is induced by interleukin 4 and suppressed by interferons γ and α and prostaglandin E_2. *Proc Natl Acad Sci U S A* 1988; 85:6880.

37. Del Prete G, Maggi E, Parronchi P, et al.: IL-4 is an essential factor for the IgE synthesis induced in vitro by human T cell clones and their supernatants. *J Immunol* 1988; 140:4193.

38. Finkelman FD, Katona IM, Urban JF Jr., et al.: Suppression of in vivo polyclonal IgE responses by monoclonal antibody to the lymphokine B-cell stimulatory factor 1. *Proc Natl Acad Sci U S A* 1986; 83:9675.

39. Kühn R, Rajewski K, Müller W: Generation and analysis of interleukin-4 deficient mice. *Science* 1991; 254:707.

40. Kopf M, Le Gros G, Bachmann M, et al.: Disruption of the murine IL-4 gene blocks Th2 cytokine responses. *Nature* 1993; 362:245.

41. Finkelman FD, Katona IM, Mosman TR, Coffman RL: IFN-γ regulates the isotypes of Ig secreted during in vivo humoral immune responses. *J Immunol* 1988; 140:1022.

42. Paul WE, Seder RA: Lymphocyte responses and cytokines. *Cell* 1994; 76:241.

43. Defrance T, Aubry JP, Rousset F, et al.: Human recombinant interleukin-4 induces Fcϵ receptors (CD23) on normal B lymphocytes. *J Exp Med* 1987; 165:1459.

44. Vercelli D, Jabara HH, Lee B-W, et al.: Human recombinant interleukin 4 induces FcϵR2/CD23 on normal human monocytes. *J Exp Med* 1988; 167:1406.

45. McMenamin C, Pimm C, McKersey M, Holt PG: Regulation of IgE responses to inhaled antigen in mice by antigen-specific $\gamma\delta$ T cells. *Science* 1994; 265:1869.

46. Metzger H, Alcaraz G, Hohman R, et al.: The receptor with high affinity for immunoglobulin E. *Annu Rev Immunol* 1986; 4:419.

47. Spiegelberg HL: Structure and function of Fc receptors for IgE on lymphocytes, monocytes and macrophages. *Adv Immunol* 1984; 35:61.

48. Hamann K, Gleich G: Inflammatory cells in lung disease: role of inflammatory cells in asthma.

49. Joseph M, Tonnell A-B, Torpier G, Capron A, Arnoux B, Benveniste J: Involvement of immunoglobulin E in the secretory process of alveolar macrophages from asthmatic patients. *J Clin Invest*, 1983; 71:221.

50. Cruikshank WW, Long A, Tarpy R, Kornfeld H, Carrol MP, Teran L, Holgate ST, Center DM: Early Identification of Interleukin 16 and MIPIα in Bronchoalvealor Lavage Fluid of Antigen-Challenged Asthmatics. *Am J Resp Cell Mol Biol*, 1995; 13:738.

51. Bronchial Epitheliol cells of patients with asthma release chemoattractor T factors for T lymphocytes. *J Allergy Clin Immunol* 1993; 92:412.

52. Laberge S, Cruickshank WW, Kornfeld H, Center DM: Histamine-induced secretion of lymphocyte chemoattractant factor from CD8+ and T cells is independent of transcription and translation. *J Immunol*, 1995; 155:2902.

53. Center DM, Berman JS, Kornfeld H, Theodore AC, Cruikshank WW: The Lymphocyte Chemoattractant Factor *J Lab Clin Med* 1995; 125:167.

54. Baggiolini M, Dahinden CA: CC chemokines in allergic inflammation. *Immunol Today* 1994; 15:127.

55. Schleimer RP, Sterbinsky SA, Kaiser J, et al.: Interleukin-4 induces adherence of human eosinophils and basophils but not neutrophils to endothelium: association with expression of VCAM-1. *J Immunol* 1992; 148:1086.

56. Stevens RL, Austen KF: Recent advances in the cellular and molecular biology of mast cells. *Immunol Today* 1989; 10:381.

57. Paul WE: Interleukin-4: a prototypic immunoregulatory lymphokine. *Blood* 1991; 77:1859.

58. Sanderson CJ: Interleukin-5, eosinophils and disease. *Blood* 1992; 79:3101.

59. Yamaguchi Y, Hayashi Y, Sugama Y, et al.: Highly purified murine interleukin 5 (IL-5) stimulates eosinophil function and prolongs in vitro survival. IL-5 as an eosinophil chemotactic factor. *J Exp Med* 1988; 167:1737.

60. Walsh GM, Hartnell A, Wardlaw AJ, et al.: IL-5 enhances the in vitro adhesion of human eosinophil, but not neutrophils, in a leukocyte integrin (CD11/18)-dependent manner. *Immunology* 1990; 144:642.

61. Neeley SP, Hamann KJ, White SR, et al.: Selective regulation of expression of surface adhesion molecules Mac-1, L-selectin, and

VLA-4 on human eosinophils and neutrophils. *Am J Respir Cell Mol Biol* 1993; 8:633.

62. Schleimer RP, Beneati SV, Friedman B, Bochner BS: Do cytokines play a role in leukocyte recruitment and activation in the lung? *Am Rev Respir Dis* 1991; 143:1169.

63. Resnick MB, Weller PF: Mechanisms of eosinophil recruitment. *Am J Respir Cell Mol Biol* 1993; 8:349.

64. Hallsworth MP, Litchfield TM, Lee TH: Glucocorticosteroids inhibit granulocyte-macrophage colony-stimulating factor-1 and interleukin-5 enhanced in vitro survival of human eosinophils. *Immunology* 1992; 75:382.

65. Lopez AF, Williamson DJ, Gamble JR, et al.: Recombinant human granulocyte-macrophage colony-stimulating factor stimulates in vitro mature human neutrophil and eosinophil function, surface receptor expression, and survival. *J Clin Invest* 1986; 78:1220.

66. Wierenga EA, Snoek M, De Groot C, et al.: Evidence for compartmentalization of functional subsets of CD4$^+$ T lymphocytes in atopic patients. *J Immunol* 1990; 144:4651.

67. Parronchi P, Macchia D, Piccinni M-P, et al.: Allergen- and bacterial antigen-specific T-cell clones established from atopic donors show a different profile of cytokine production. *Proc Natl Acad Sci U S A* 1991; 88:4538.

68. Hamid Q, Azzawi M, Ying S, et al.: Expression of mRNA for interleukin-5 in mucosal bronchial biopsies from asthma. *J Clin Invest* 1991; 87:1541.

69. Robinson DS, Hamid Q, Ying S, et al.: Predominant Th2-like bronchoalveolar T lymphocyte population in atopic asthma. *N Engl J Med* 1992; 326:298.

70. Krishnaswamy G, Liu MC, Su S-N, et al.: Analysis of cytokine transcripts in the bronchoalveolar lavage cells of patients with asthma. *Am J Respir Cell Mol Biol* 1993; 9:279.

71. Walker C, Bode E, Boer L, et al.: Allergic and nonallergic asthmatics have distinct patterns of T-cell activation and cytokine production in peripheral blood and bronchoalveolar lavage. *Am Rev Respir Dis* 1992; 146:109.

72. Sedgwick JB, Calhoun WJ, Gleich GJ, et al.: Immediate and late airway response of allergic rhinitis patients to segmental antigen challenge: characterization of eosinophil and mast cell mediators. *Am Rev Respir Dis* 1991; 144:1274.

73. Ohnishi T, Kita H, Weiler D, et al.: IL-5 is the predominant eosinophil-active cytokine in the antigen-induced pulmonary late-phase reaction. *Am Rev Respir Dis* 1992; 147:901.

74. Plaut M, Pierce JH, Watson CJ, et al.: Mast cell lines produce lymphokines in response to cross-linkage of FcεRI or to calcium ionophores. *Nature* 1989; 339:64.

75. Bradding P, Roberts JA, Britten KM, et al.: Interleukin-4, -5, and -6 and tumor necrosis factor-α in normal and asthmatic airways: evidence for the human mast cell as a source of these cytokines. *Am J Respir Cell Mol Biol* 1994; 10:471.

76. Broide DH, Paine MM, Firestein GS: Eosinophils express interleukin-5 and granulocyte-macrophage-colony-stimulating-factor mRNA at sites of allergic inflammation in asthmatics. *J Clin Invest* 1992; 90:1414.

77. Dubucquoi S, Desreumaux P, Janin A, et al.: Interleukin 5 synthesis by eosinophils: association with granules and immunoglobulin-dependent secretion. *J Exp Med* 1994; 179:703.

78. Lazaar AL, Albelda SM, Pilewski JM, et al.: T lymphocytes adhere to airway smooth muscle cells via integrins and CD44 and induce smooth muscle cell DNA synthesis. *J Exp Med* 1994; 180:807.

79. Engel P, Huguet J, Sanosa J, et al.: T cell subsets in allergic respiratory disease using monoclonal antibodies. *Ann Allergy* 1984; 53:337.

80. Kus J, Tse KS, Vedal S, Chan-Yeung M: Lymphocyte sub-populations in patients with allergic and non-allergic asthma. *Clin Allergy* 1985; 15:523.

81. Rola-Pleszczynski M, Blanchard R: Suppressor cell function in respiratory allergy: modulation by aminophylline and isoproterenol. *Int Arch Allergy Appl Immunol* 1981; 64:361.

82. Harper TB, Gaumer HR, Waring W et al.: A comparison of cell-mediated immunity and suppressor T-cell function in asthmatic and normal children. *Clin Allergy* 1980; 10:555.

83. Hwang K-C, Fikrig SM, Friedman HM, Gupta S: Deficient concanavalin-A-induced suppressor-cell activity in patients with bronchial asthma, allergic rhinitis and atopic dermatitis. *Clin Allergy* 1985; 15:67.

84. Gonzalez MC, Diaz P, Galleguillos FR, et al.: Allergen-induced recruitment of bronchoalveolar helper (OKT4) and suppressor (OKT8) T-cells in asthma. Relative increases in OKT8 cells in single early responders compared with those in late-phase responders. *Am Rev Respir Dis* 1987; 136:600.

85. Rocklin RE, Sheffer AL, Greineder DK, Melmon KL: Generation of antigen-specific suppressor cells during allergy desensitization. *N Engl J Med* 1980; 302:1213.

86. Nagaya H: Induction of antigen-specific suppressor cells in patients with hay fever receiving immunotherapy. *J Allergy Clin Immunol* 1985; 75:388.

87. Tamir R, Castracane JM, Rocklin RE: Generation of suppressor cells in atopic patients during immunotherapy that modulate IgE synthesis. *J Allergy Clin Immunol* 1987; 75:591.

88. Murphy DB: T cell mediated immunosuppression. *Curr Opin Immunol* 1993; 5:411.

89. Kemeny DM, Noble A, Holmes BJ, Diaz-Sanchez D: Immune regulation: a new role for the CD8$^+$ T cell. *Immunol Today* 1994; 15:107.

90. Gershon RK, Cohen P, Hensin R, Liebhaber SA: Suppressor T cells. *J Immunol* 1972; 108:586.

91. Gajewski TF, Fitch FW: Anti-proliferative effect of IFN-γ in immune regulation I. IFN-γ inhibits the proliferation of Th2 but not Th1 murine helper T lymphocyte clones. *J Immunol* 1988; 140:4245.

92. McMenamin C, Holt PG: The natural immune response to inhaled soluble protein antigens involves major histocompatility complex (MHC) class-I restricted CD8$^+$ T cell-mediated but MHC class II-restricted CD4$^+$ T cell-dependent immune deviation resulting in selective suppression of immunoglobulin E production. *J Exp Med* 1993; 178:889.

93. Miller A, Lider O, Roberts AB, et al.: Suppressor T cells generated by oral tolerization to myelin basic protein suppress both in vitro and in vivo immune response by the release of transforming growth factor β after antigen-specific triggering. *Proc Natl Acad Sci U S A* 1992; 89:421.

94. Seder RA, Boulay J-L, Finkelman F, et al.: CD8$^+$ T cells can be primed in vitro to produce IL-4. *J Immunol* 1992; 148:1652.

95. Erard F, Wild M-T, Garcia-Sanz JA, Le Gros G: Switch of CD8 T cells to noncytolytic CD8$^-$CD4$^-$ cells that make T$_H$2 cytokines and help B cells. *Science* 1993; 260:1802.

96. Croft M, Carter L, Swain SL, Dutton RW: Generation of polarized antigen-specific CD8 effector populations: reciprocal action of interleukin (IL)-4 and IL-12 in promoting type 2 versus type 1 cytokine profiles. *J Exp Med* 1994; 180:1715.

97. Walker C, Virchow J-C Jr, Bruijnzeel PLB, Blaser K: T cell subsets and their soluble products regulate eosinophilia in allergic and nonallergic asthma. *J Immunol* 1991; 146:1829.

98. LeGros G, Erard F: Non-cytotoxic, IL-4, IL-5, IL-10 producing CD8$^+$ T cells: their activation and effector functions. *Curr Opin Immunol* 1994; 6:453.

99. Nakajima H, Iwamoto I, Tomoe S, et al.: CD4$^+$ T-lymphocytes and interleukin-5 mediate antigen-induced eosinophil infiltration into the mouse trachea. *Am Rev Respir Dis* 1992; 146:374.

100. Gavett SH, Chen X, Finkelman F, Wills-Karp M: Depletion of murine CD4^p T lymphocytes prevents antigen-induced airway hyperreactivity and pulmonary eosinophilia. *Am J Respir Cell Mol Biol* 1994; 10:587.

101. Olivenstein R, Renzi PM, Yang JP, et al.: Depletion of OX-8 lymphocytes from the blood and airways using monoclonal antibodies enhances the late airway response in rats. *J Clin Invest* 1993; 92:1477.

102. Renz H, Lack G, Saloga J, et al.: Inhibition of IgE production and normalization of airways responsiveness by sensitized CD8 T cells in a mouse model of allergen-induced sensitization. *J Immunol* 1994; 152:351.

103. Renzi PM, Du T, Sapienza S, et al.: Acute effects of interleukin-2 on lung mechanics and airway responsiveness in rats. *Am Rev Respir Dis* 1991; 143:380.

104. Renzi PM, Sapienza S, Du T, et al.: Lymphokine-induced airway hyperresponsiveness in the rat. *Am Rev Respir Dis* 1991; 143:375.

105. Renzi PM, Sapienza S, Waserman S, et al.: Effect of interleukin-2 on the airway response to antigen in the rat. *Am Rev Respir Dis* 1992; 146:163.

106. Lukacs NW, Strieter RM, Chensue SW, Kundel SL: Interleukin-4-dependent pulmonary eosinophil infiltration in a murine model of asthma. *Am J Respir Cell Mol Biol* 1994; 10:526.

107. Brusselle GG, Kips JC, Tavenier JH, et al.: Attenuation of allergic airway inflammation in IL-4 deficient mice. *Clin Exp Allergy* 1994; 24:73.

108. Gulbenkian AR, Egan RW, Fernandez X, et al.: Interleukin-5 modulates eosinophil accumulation in allergic guinea pig lung. *Am Rev Respir Dis* 1992; 146:263.

109. Chand N, Harrison JE, Rooney S, et al.: Anti-IL-5 monoclonal antibody inhibits allergic late phase bronchial eosinophilia in guinea pigs: a therapeutic approach. *Eur J Pharmacol* 1992; 211:121.

110. Mauser PJ, Pitman A, Witt A, et al.: Inhibitory effect of the TRFK-5 anti-IL-5 antibody in a guinea pig model of asthma. *Am Rev Respir Dis* 1993; 148:1623.

111. Van Oosterhout AJM, Ladenius ARC, Savelkoul HFJ, et al.: Effect of anti-IL-5 and IL-5 on airway hyperreactivity and eosinophils in guinea pigs. *Am Rev Respir Dis* 1993; 147:548.

112. Iwamoto I, Nakajima H, Endo H, Yoshida S: Interferon γ regulated antigen-induced eosinophil recruitment into the mouse airways by inhibiting the infiltration of CD4$^+$ T cells. *J Exp Med* 1993; 177:573.

113. Walker C, Virchow J-C Jr, Iff T, et al.: T cells and asthma: 1. Lymphocyte subpopulations and activation in allergic and non-allergic asthma. *Int Arch Allergy Appl Immunol* 1991; 94:241.

114. Mapp CE, Saetta M, Maestrelli P, et al.: Mechanisms and pathology of occupational asthma. *Eur Respir J* 1994; 7:544.

115. Finotto S, Fabbri LM, Rado V, et al.: Increase in numbers of CD8 positive lymphocytes and eosinophils in peripheral blood of subjects with late asthmatic reactions induced by toluene diisocyanate. *Br J Indust Med* 1991; 48:116.

116. Saetta M, Di Stefano A, Maestrelli P, et al.: Airway mucosal inflammation in occupational asthma induced by toluene diisocyanate. *Am Rev Respir Dis* 1992; 145:160.

117. Bently AM, Maestrelli P, Saetta M, et al.: Activated T-lymphocytes and eosinophils in the bronchial mucosa in isocyanate-induced asthma. *J Allergy Clin Immunol* 1992; 89:821.

118. Boschetto P, Fabbri LM, Zocca E, et al.: Prednisone inhibits late asthmatic reactions and airway inflammation induced by toluene diisocyanate in sensitized subjects. *J Allergy Clin Immunol* 1987; 80:261.

119. Arya SK, Wong-Staal F, Gallo RC: Dexamethasone-mediated inhibition of human T-cell growth factor and gamma-interferon messenger RNA, *J Immunol* 1986; 133:273.

120. Reed JC, Abidi AH, Alpers JD, et al.: Effect of cyclosporin A and dexamethasone on interleukin 2 receptor gene expression. *J Immunol* 1986; 137:150.

121. Pinkson P, Saltini C, Muller-Quernheim J, Crystal RG: Corticosteroid therapy suppresses spontaneous interleukin 2 release and spontaneous proliferation of lung T-lymphocytes of patients with active pulmonary sarcoidosis. *J Immunol* 1987; 139:755.

122. Barnes PJ, Pederson S: Efficacy and safety of inhaled corticosteroids in asthma. *Am Rev Respir Dis* 1993; 148:S1.

123. Robinson D, Hamid Q, Ying S, et al.: Prednisolone treatment in asthma is associated with modulation of bronchoalveolar lavage cell interleukin-4, interleukin-5, and interferon-γ cytokine gene expression. *Am Rev Respir Dis* 1993; 148:410.

124. Liu MC, Xiao HQ, Lichtenstein LM, Huang SK: Prednisone inhibits TH2-type cytokine gene expression at sites of allergen challenge in subjects with allergic asthma. *Am J Respir Crit Care Med* 1994; 149:A944.

125. Beer DJ, Center DM: Corticosteroid modulation of lymphocyte migration. *Cell Immunol* 1980; 55:381.

126. Cypcar D, Busse WW: Steroid-resistant asthma. *J Allergy Clin Immunol* 1993; 92:362.

127. Woolcock AJ: Steroid resistant asthma: what is the clinical definition? *Eur Respir J* 1993; 6:743.

128. Corrigan CJ, Brown PH, Barnes NC, et al.: Glucocorticoid resistance in chronic asthma: glucocorticoid pharmacokinetics, glucocorticoid receptor characteristics, and inhibition of peripheral blood T cell proliferation by glucocorticoids in vitro. *Am Rev Respir Dis* 1991; 144:1016.

129. Corrigan CJ, Brown PH, Barnes NC, et al.: Glucocorticoid resistance in chronic asthma: peripheral blood T lymphocyte activation and comparison of the T lymphocyte inhibitory effects of glucocorticoids and cyclosporin A. *Am Rev Respir Dis* 1991; 144:1026.

130. Leung DYM, Martin RJ, Szefler SJ, et al.: Dysregulation of interleukin 4, interleukin 5, and interferon γ gene expression in steroid-resistant asthma. *J Exp Med* 1995; 181:33.

131. Sher ER, Leung DYM, Surs W, et al.: Steroid-resistant asthma: cellular mechanisms contributing to inadequate response to glucocorticoid therapy. *J Clin Invest* 1994; 93:33.

132. Alexander AG, Barnes NC, Kay AB: Trial of cyclosporin in corticoid-dependent chronic severe asthma. *Lancet* 1992; 339:324.

133. Gleich GT: Innovative therapy: immunosuppressive agents.

134. Schreiber SL, Crabtree GR: The mechanisms of action of cyclosporin A and FK506. *Immunol Today* 1992; 13:136.

Chapter 32 _____

INFLAMMATORY CELLS IN AIRWAYS

KIMM J. HAMANN

Asthma is a disease characterized by reversible airway obstruction usually accompanied by bronchial hyperresponsiveness. While markers of inflammation long have been used as indices of disease activity,[1] the mechanisms and cellular participants in these phenomena were less well understood until recent years. Asthma is characterized as a chronic inflammatory process in which several cell types may play key roles. Detailed descriptions of the involvement of inflammatory cells in asthma are presented throughout this book; this chapter provides an overview of the participation of inflammatory cells in the pathophysiologic processes in asthma rather than an exhaustive literature review. Because accompanying chapters are devoted to other cells involved in these inflammatory processes, this chapter will emphasize the roles of mast cells as well as of granulocytes such as basophils, neutrophils, and eosinophils. Because of the well-characterized involvement of eosinophils in asthma, a somewhat more detailed discussion of their pathophysiologic roles in this disease is presented.

Inflammation is a complex process involving many cell types, and pulmonary inflammation encompasses numerous interactions involving cell contact, adhesion, cytokine signaling, and release of a wide variety of mediators. T cells, with the initial participation of macrophages in antigen processing and presentation, are the principal activators of the chronic inflammation in asthma[2,3] (see Chap. 24). Release of proinflammatory cytokines from lymphocytes may be supplemented and amplified by release of the same or similar cytokines from monocytes and pulmonary macrophages.[4] In extrinsic asthma, mast cells with antigen-specific IgE on their surfaces also can be activated by allergens or perhaps by other stimuli in nonallergic asthma and by interleukins released by activated T cells. During the late response, recruitment of inflammatory granulocytes, such as basophils and eosinophils, plays a role in the eventual development of pathophysiologic aspects of the disease.

Mast Cells and Basophils

Mast cells develop from pluripotent stem cells under the influence of several cytokines. Although mast cells sometimes are considered the tissue counterparts of basophils, they are derived from a separate lineage through stimulation of progenitor cells with different cytokines or different combinations of cytokines (Fig. 32-1). Early progenitors of both cell lineages arise in the bone marrow, but only the basophil completes its development there.[5,6] The role of cytokines in basophil development is not fully understood; however, interleukin-3 (IL-3) appears to be a major influence during basophilopoiesis.[7] IL-5 and granulocyte/macrophage colony-stimulating factor (GM-CSF) may promote basophil development in vitro,[8] but these effects may be the result of interaction of IL-5 and GM-CSF with the IL-3 receptor owing to the fact that the receptors for these three cytokines share the same β subunit.[9,10] Mature basophils have a segmented nucleus and contain large, electron-dense cytoplasmic granules (Fig. 32-2). Preformed mediators stored in the granules include histamine and a number of less well-characterized proteases.[11] The major proteoglycan in the basophil granules is chondroitin sulfate A,[12] which may function to bind and stabilize mediators such as histamine. Basophils also contain a small amount of major basic protein,[13] a principal granule-derived mediator in eosino-phils (see below), as well as lysophospholipase,[14] and the existence of a common basophil/eosinophil precursor has been suggested.[15] Other mediators that may be released by basophils on activation include IL-4,[16–18] platelet-activating factor (PAF),[19] leukotriene C_4 (LTC$_4$),[20,21] and superoxide and free oxygen radicals.[11]

Mast cell precursors arise from a CD34+ cell lineage,[22] enter the circulation as a unique subset[22] of nongranulated mononuclear cells,[23] and eventually leave the circulation and mature in tissues. Recent studies have implicated sev-

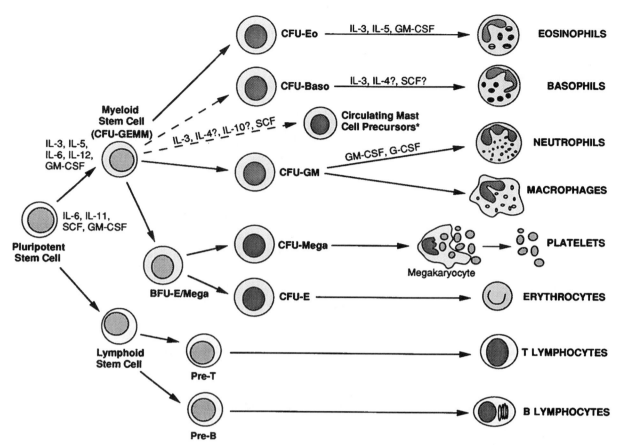

FIGURE 32-1 Simplified scheme of hematopoiesis. BFU = burst-forming unit (producing multiple colonies); CFU = colony-forming unit; GEMM = granulocyte, erythrocyte, monocyte, megakaryocyte. Only the major cytokines for the granulocyte lineages (known to date) are shown. Other cytokines may be involved. Dotted lines indicate uncertain lineage derivations. For example, some schemes suggest that CFU-Baso originate directly from BFU-E/Mega progenitors.* Mast cell precursors are released into the circulation as nongranular mononuclear cells, which migrate to the tissues, where they mature into granule-containing mature cells. (Cells are not drawn to scale.)

eral cytokines in the development of mast cell precursors. IL-3 induces the proliferation and differentiation of mast cell progenitors in vitro[24] or in vivo,[25] and the combination of IL-3 and IL-10 can promote the growth of mast cell progenitors.[26] More recently, the c-*kit* ligand stem-cell factor (SCF), also known as mast cell growth factor,[27] has been shown to have a potent mast cell colony-forming activity when combined with IL-4 and IL-10, and cells produced in these cultures contain high concentrations of histamine.[28] In addition to histamine, the granules contain a number of preformed mast cell mediators as well as chondroitin sulfate E (Fig. 32-2). Several mediators, such as LTC_4 and PAF, as well as prostaglandin D_2 (PGD_2), also are synthesized on cell activation.

Basophils and mast cells express a wide range of surface receptors and antigens (Fig. 32-2).[8] Both cell types express high-affinity IgE receptors (FcεRI). The binding of IgE to these surface receptors causes the release of important preformed mediators, such as histamine, as well as of newly generated products, such as leukotrienes and prostaglandins.[29] Basophils also express the CD11/CD18 (β_2) inte-

grins Mac-1, LFA-1, and pl50,95, while mast cells apparently do not have detectable $\beta2$-integrins on their surface. IgE cross-linking upregulates these integrins on the surface of basophils.[30] Both mast cells and basophils possess $\beta1$-(CD29/CD49) integrins; the expression of VLA-4 on basophils and the adhesion of basophils to endothelium is mediated, at least in part, by VLA-4/VCAM-1 interaction.[31] Human lung mast cells express VLA-2, a receptor for collagens and laminin,[32] as well as the $\beta3$-vitronectin receptor CD41/CD61.[33] Adhesion of mast cells and basophils to other cells or to the extracellular matrix through these receptors can regulate not only cell migration and cytoskeletal reorganization but also through intracellular signaling pathways, proliferation and cell secretion.[34] Among several other receptors, one important receptor that both mast cells and basophils possess is the H_2-receptor (H_2-R) for histamine.[8] Studies suggest that mast cell- or basophil-derived histamine may act on H_2-receptors on these cells to limit the inflammatory process by inhibiting further histamine and cytokine release.[35,36] Similarly, engagement of the prostaglandin D_2 receptor on basophils by PGD_2 released by mast cells or

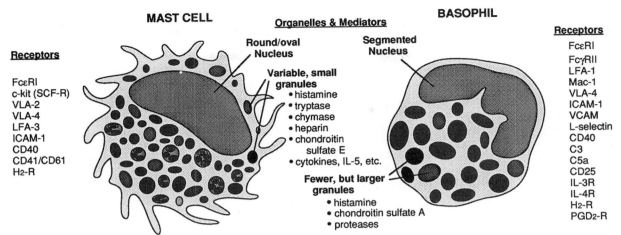

FIGURE 32-2 Schematic diagram of major human mast cell and basophil morphologic features, preformed (stored) mediators, and receptor/surface antigens (see text). Human mast cell membranes have multiple surface folds, and their granules show a variety of substructural patterns such as "scrolls" and "lattices." Peripheral blood basophils do not show the surface projections of the mast cells, and their granules are larger, fewer, and more homogenously electron dense. According to current information, the basophil receptor repertoire appears to be more diverse than that of the tissue-dwelling mast cell and to more closely resemble that of other circulating granulocytes.

other cells[37] may inhibit histamine release.[38] Basophils also express complement receptors, such as that for C5a, which is a strong chemotactic factor for human basophils.[39] Cytokine receptors on basophils are likely important during maturation in the bone marrow, but they may also play a role in activation of basophil migration by means of priming effects and the regulation of adhesion molecules.[11,21]

Mast cells are numerous in the human lung and have been considered for many years to be central to the immunologic processes involved in asthma.[40] The bronchoalveolar lavage (BAL) fluid of asthmatics contains more mast cells than that of normal subjects,[41,42] and mast cell degranulation occurs in the mucosa of asthmatic subjects.[43,44] A number of studies have found the degree of bronchial hyperresponsiveness in asthmatics to be correlated with both the number of mast cells and the histamine concentration in BAL fluid.[42,45,46] Studies of mast cells isolated from patients with asthma also have demonstrated greater mediator release than in mast cells from normal control subjects.[42,47] Histamine and PGD$_2$ are potent bronchoconstrictors and are associated with the early-phase bronchoconstrictor response to allergen challenge in extrinsic asthma patients. The importance of mast cells to this early response is underscored by the fact that the bronchoconstriction during this phase can be inhibited almost entirely by administering a combination of antagonists to prostaglandin and histamine.[48,49] The importance of mast cells to the late asthmatic response is less clear, however, and it has been suggested that, when considering FcεRI+, histamine-containing cells, the mast cell is responsible for the acute response to antigen challenge, while the basophil is characteristic of the late-phase response.[50]

Basophils have been described in the sputum of symptomatic asthmatics,[51] and large numbers appear in the BAL fluid during the late-phase response.[52] Spontaneous histamine release is increased in circulating basophils from atopic asthmatics[53] and from food-allergic subjects[54] and, as with mast cells, has been correlated with bronchial reactivity.[55,56] In addition, basophils from patients with occupational asthma due to western red cedar released histamine when challenged directly with the causative agent of this disease, plicatic acid.[57] While histamine is found in both mast cells and basophils, tryptase and PGD$_2$ are found only in mast cells. It has been suggested, therefore, that the disproportionate increase of histamine over tryptase[52,58] is indirect evidence that some BAL-fluid histamine comes from basophils.[59] Moreover, while the immediate response to antigen is associated with the mast-cell-derived PGD$_2$, increases in histamine release during the late response are not associated with an increase in PGD$_2$ release.[50,60]

Both mast cells and basophils produce cytokines, which may be important in cell migration and activation in asthmatic processes. Mast cells appear to generate a larger number of these mediators.[18] Basophils can produce IL-4 on activation,[16] but this cytokine seems not to be stored in the granules.[18] Immunohistochemical examination of mast cells, however, demonstrates the presence of IL-4, IL-5, IL-6, and tumor necrosis factor-α (TNF-α) in their granules.[61,62] These cytokines can be produced and/or released following IgE binding, although unlike basophils, the amount of IL-4 released by mast cells is insufficient to regulate IgE production by B cells.[63] The production and release of cytokines by these cells has important implications for the regulation of inflammatory processes in asthma and other diseases, and the details of these interactions await further studies.

Neutrophils

While eosinophils appear to be the predominant infiltrating granulocyte in asthma (see discussion below), neutrophils have been primarily associated with chronic inflammatory lung disease such as chronic obstructive pulmonary disease (COPD). Nevertheless, a role for neutrophils in asthma has been suggested,[64] although the details of their contribution to asthma are still unclear.[65] Neutrophils originate in the bone marrow from the myeloid progenitor cell called CFU-GEMM, which is common to granulocytes, erythrocytes, monocytes, and megakaryocytes (Fig. 32-1). IL-3 and GM-CSF are important growth factors for multipotent progenitors, while granulocyte colony-stimulating factor (G-CSF) appears to direct the differentiation of more committed cells to neutrophils.[66] Mature neutrophils are characterized by a multilobed nucleus and a cytoplasm containing about 200 granules[67] (Fig. 32-3). Roughly two-thirds of these granules are termed *specific* or *secondary granules*, and the remaining third are the *azurophilic* or *primary granules*, which are more electron-dense than the secondary granules.[67] The azurophilic granules contain a large number of stored proteins, primarily enzymes, such as elastase; lysozyme; cathepsins B, D, and G; proteinase 3; and myeloperoxidase, which are discharged into endocytic vesicles or into the extracellular space upon degranulation.[68] Recently, *bactericidal/permeability increasing protein* (BPI) and a group of bactericidal proteins called *defensins* also were described in azurophilic granules.[69,70] The secondary or "specific" granules also contain lysozyme, collagenase, and bactericidal proteins like lactoferrin, which are not found in the azurophilic granules.[71] Neutrophils also elaborate lipid mediators, such as LTB$_4$, and substantial amounts of several reactive oxygen metabolites during the respiratory burst.[71]

There are several classes of receptors on the surface of human neutrophils, including complement receptors for C3b and C5a[71] and the immunoglobulin receptors FcγRII, FcγRIIIB, and FcαR, which have been implicated in the activation and recruitment of neutrophils in inflammatory processes in the lung.[72] While neutrophils do not possess either the high-affinity or the low-affinity receptor for IgE (FcεRI and FcεRII, respectively), they do possess the Mac-2/ε-binding protein on their surface, which permits interaction/activation of neutrophils with IgE, leading to the respiratory burst.[73] In addition to the hematopoietic cytokine receptors for GM-CSF and G-CSF,[74] neutrophils possess receptors for the activating chemotactic factors LTB$_4$ and PAF and for the chemokine IL-8.[75–77] Adhesion molecules, which may be involved in the recruitment of neutrophils in the lung, include the β2-(CD11/CD18) integrins Mac-1, LFA-1, and p150,95, as well as L-selectin.[78]

While neutrophil products have the potential for altering airway function and causing tissue damage, the evidence that neutrophils play an important role in asthma remains controversial.[79,80] Nevertheless, neutrophil mediators such as oxygen metabolites and histamine-releasing factor may play amplifying roles in asthmatic reactions in the lung.[81] Neutrophil elastase is a potent secretagogue for cultured serous cells or airway submucosal glands[82,83] and may play a role in the development of airway hypersecretion in asthma. The epithelial cell detachment seen in asthma has been reproduced by culturing neutrophils with human epithelial cell/basement membrane preparations and was shown to be mediated by proteases released by the neutrophils.[84] A number of neutrophil chemotactic factors, such as C5a, LTB4, and IL-8, are associated with asthma,[85] and some studies find increased numbers of activated neutrophils in BAL fluids after challenge in atopic[86] and occupational[65] asthmatics. Other studies have demonstrated similar numbers of neutrophils in bronchial biopsy samples or BAL fluid from asthmatic and normal individuals.[80] In canine models, bronchial hyperresponsiveness induced by ozone has been associated with neutrophil accumulation.[87] Inhibition of neutrophil migration into the airways, however, does not prevent ozone-induced hyperreactivity,[88] and the prevention of hyperresponsiveness is not associated with a decrease in airway neutrophilia.[89] It has been suggested that neutrophils, because they are recruited between 2 and 4 h after antigen challenge (the "transition phase"), could play a transient role subsequent to early-phase mast cell involvement but before eosinophil and basophil involvement during the late-phase reactions.[64] The role(s) of neu-

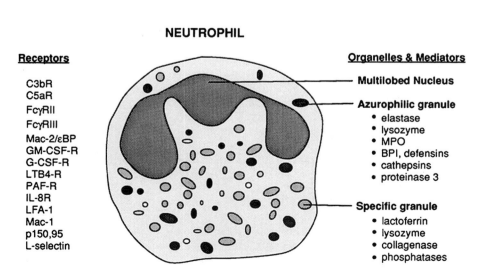

NEUTROPHIL

Receptors

C3bR
C5aR
FcγRII
FcγRIII
Mac-2/εBP
GM-CSF-R
G-CSF-R
LTB4-R
PAF-R
IL-8R
LFA-1
Mac-1
p150,95
L-selectin

Organelles & Mediators

Multilobed Nucleus

Azurophilic granule
- elastase
- lysozyme
- MPO
- BPI, defensins
- cathepsins
- proteinase 3

Specific granule
- lactoferrin
- lysozyme
- collagenase
- phosphatases

FIGURE 32-3 Diagram of the major morphologic features and receptors of the human neutrophil. The two major granule types—azurophilic (or primary) and specific (or secondary)—contain several enzymatic mediators. There are also other, less prominent granule types, and azurophilic granules themselves have been divided into at least two subtypes possessing different peroxidases. Lactoferrin may be increased in asthmatic sputum, and elastase has recently attracted attention as a potential mediator of pathophysiologic features of asthma, such as airway hypersecretion and epithelial desquamation.

trophils in asthma remain obscure, and further investigation is needed to clarify the participation of these inflammatory cells in the complex processes involved in asthma.

Eosinophils

Although eosinophils have been associated with asthma and other respiratory diseases since the early 1900s,[90,91] strong evidence has emerged recently suggesting that eosinophils are not only participants but key effector cells in allergy and asthma.[92–95] Eosinophils and their mediators may play additional roles in the lung in tissue repair/remodeling and antigen presentation.[96] In human asthma, eosinophils are the distinctive infiltrating cells,[97–99] and it is the bioactivity of the mediators of these cells that may be critical to major pathophysiologic events in asthma.[100] Accordingly, this section will examine the roles of eosinophils in asthma primarily through discussion of the cell products that, once released by eosinophils, mediate these functions.

Eosinophils differentiate from an eosinophil colony-forming unit (CFU-Eo) under the direction of at least three different cytokines, GM-CSF, IL-3, and I-5[101, 102] (Fig. 32-1). Mature human eosinophils are slightly larger than neutrophils and have bilobed nuclei (Fig. 32-4). The intense staining of the cytoplasmic granules of these cells given by acid dyes such as eosin led Paul Ehrlich to name the cells *eosinophils*. As viewed by transmission electron microscopy, it is possible to discern three major types of granules.[103] The first consists of large, crystalloid-containing *specific* or *secondary granules*. Most of the granules in normal human eosinophils are of this type. They contain the four principal basic proteins—major basic protein (MBP), eosinophil peroxidase (EPO), eosinophil cationic protein (ECP), and eosinophil-derived neurotoxin (EDN) (Table 32-1).[104,105] These basic proteins give eosinophils their avidity for acid dyes. The second population consists of granules that are similar in size to those of the first type but lack a crystalloid.[106] These are sometimes called primary granules. They may contain Charcot-Leyden crystal (CLC) protein. The third population consists of dense *small granules*, which are positive for enzymes such as acid phosphatase and arylsulfatase (Fig. 32-4). A possible fourth population of "granules" has been described as vesiculotubular structures or "microgranules."[103] Lipid bodies are also prominent organelles in eosinophils and serve as sites for arachidonic acid (fatty acid) storage and metabolism. In addition to the major granule proteins, eosinophils synthesize de novo and release a wide variety of mediators, which may be involved in the pathophysiologic processes in asthma[105,107] (Table 32-2). These include a number of arachidonate-derived lipids, particularly LTC$_4$,[108] and another important lipid mediator, PAF. It is now known that eosinophils can also produce and release a variety of cytokines as well,[109] and that these cytokines may be important mediators in human asthma.[110]

The expression and function of a large number of eosinophil receptors and surface markers has been an area of intense research in the last few years. Eosinophils express a

TABLE 32-1   Some Properties of Human Eosinophil Granule Proteins and Their cDNAs and Genes

Protein	Site	Molecular mass (kDa)	pI[a]	Activities	MOLECULAR BIOLOGY		
					cDNA	Gene	Chromosome
MBP	Core	14	10.9	(1) Causes histamine release from basophils and rat mast cells; (2) causes bronchial constriction and hyperreactivity; (3) neutralizes heparin; (4) potent helminthotoxin and cytotoxin; (5) bactericidal	~900 NT (prepro-MBP)	3.3kb 5 introns	11
ECP	Matrix	21	10.8	(1) Causes histamine release from rat mast cells; (2) potent neurotoxin; (3) potent helminthotoxin; (4) inhibits cultures of peripheral blood lymphocytes; (5) weak RNase activity; (6) bactericidal	~725 NT (pre-ECP)	~1.2 kb 1 intron in UTR	14
EDN	Matrix	18–19	8.9	(1) Potent neurotoxin; (2) inhibits cultures of peripheral-blood lymphocytes; (3) potent RNase activity; (4) weak helminthotoxin	~725 NT (pre-EDN)	~1.2 kb 1 intron in UTR	14
EPO	Matrix	71–77	10.8	In the presence of H_2O_2 + halide: (1) kills microorganisms and tumor cells; (2) causes histamine release from rat mast cells; (3) inactivates leukotrienes; (4) can damage respiratory epithelium ($\pm H_2O_2$); (5) may contribute to bronchial hyperreactivity	~2,500 NT (2,106-NT ORF)	12 kb 11 introns	17

[a] Calculated from amino acid sequences deduced from the cDNAs.
ABBREVIATIONS: NT, nucleotides; ORF, open reading frame; UTR, untranslated region.
SOURCE: Modified from Hamann et al.[104]

TABLE 32-2 Human Eosinophil Mediators Generated de Novo and Their Major Bioactivities

Mediator	Bioactivity in Pulmonary Tissue
Oxygen metabolites	
Superoxide anion	Toxic for microorganisms and cells; may act synergistically with granule proteins
Hydrogen peroxide	Toxic for microorganisms and cells; can cause contraction of airway smooth muscle
Singlet oxygen	Toxic for microorganisms and cells; may cause pulmonary tissue damage
Lipids	
Leukotriene C_4	Bronchial and vascular constrictor; causes increase in vascular permeability
Platelet activating factor	Bronchial and vascular constrictor; causes bronchial edema, mucus secretion, and platelet aggregation, and can activate mast cells, neutrophils, and eosinophils
Prostaglandin E_2	Vasodilator, causes mucus secretion; can inhibit inflammatory cell function
Prostaglandin D_2	Bronchoconstrictor; causes pulmonary vasoconstriction, increase in vascular permeability, and platelet aggregation
Prostaglandin $F_{2\alpha}$	Bronchoconstrictor; causes platelet aggregation
Thromboxane A_2	Bronchial and vascular constrictor; causes platelet aggregation
Cytokines	
TGF-β_1	Regulates cell proliferation; can inhibit TH2 cytokines, but cooperates with IL-2 and IL-5 in isotype-switching to upregulate B-cell production of IgA
TGF-α	Similar to epidermal growth factor; promotes cell proliferation and angiogenesis
TNF-α	Promotes fibroblast and lymphocyte proliferation, but may suppress myeloid growth
MIP-1α	"C-C" chemokine; chemoattractant for B cells, eosinophils, and some T cells
IL-3, IL-5, GM-CSF	Promote priming and activation of inflammatory cells and granulocyte differentiation; enhance survival of granulocytes
IL-6	Multiple effects on T cells, B cells, and hematopoiesis
IL-8	"C-X-C" chemokine; neutrophil activator and chemoattractant
Neuropeptides	
Substance P	Bronchoconstrictor; causes vascular edema, vasodilation; stimulates mucus secretion and degranulation of mast cells
Vasoactive intestinal peptide	Bronchoconstrictor and vasodilator

ABBREVIATIONS: TGF, transforming growth factor; TNF, tumor necrosis factor; MIP, macrophage inflammatory protein; IL, interleukin; GM-CSF, granulocyte/macrophage colony-stimulating factor.

variety of adhesion molecules and receptors for complement proteins, immunoglobulins, cytokines, and lipid mediators[107] (Fig. 32-4). Because the integrin adhesion molecules on eosinophils are involved in the recruitment and migration of these cells, as well as in their activation, they have been the subject of especially active research recently. The β2-integrins Mac-1 and LFA-1 can be upregulated on activated eosinophils and can mediate the adhesion of these cells to endothelial ICAM-1 or ICAM-2.[111] Eosinophils, but not neutrophils, express the β1-integrin VLA-4, which binds to VCAM-1 on activated endothelium and may be one factor involved in the selective recruitment of eosinophils in asthma.[111] Furthermore, interaction of eosinophil VLA-4 with its other ligand, fibronectin, can activate eosinophils and augment the release of bioactive eosinophil mediators.[112]

EOSINOPHIL GRANULE PROTEINS IN ASTHMA

MAJOR BASIC PROTEIN

The potent toxicity of major basic protein (MBP) to several cell types and the known association of eosinophils with asthma led to studies of the role of MBP in damaging cells and tissues of the respiratory system. Early studies of cultures of the epithelial cell layer of guinea pig tracheal rings or human bronchial rings with MBP produced changes that mimicked the pathology of asthma,[113] and did so at or below MBP concentrations actually found in sputum from asthmatic patients.[114] Complementing these in vitro studies, immunofluorescent localization of MBP in the respiratory tissues of allergic and asthmatic patients has revealed large numbers of intact eosinophils in asthmatic lung tissue lamina propria in association with areas of damage.[115] MBP was

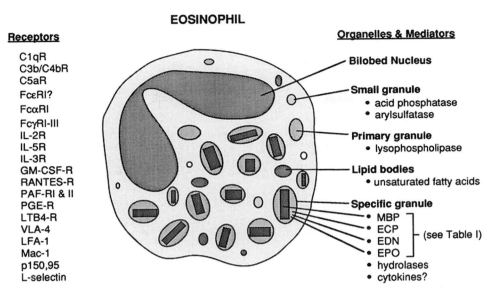

EOSINOPHIL

Receptors

C1qR
C3b/C4bR
C5aR
FcεRI?
FcαRI
FcγRI-III
IL-2R
IL-5R
IL-3R
GM-CSF-R
RANTES-R
PAF-RI & II
PGE-R
LTB4-R
VLA-4
LFA-1
Mac-1
p150,95
L-selectin

Organelles & Mediators

Bilobed Nucleus

Small granule
• acid phosphatase
• arylsulfatase

Primary granule
• lysophospholipase

Lipid bodies
• unsaturated fatty acids

Specific granule
• MBP
• ECP   (see Table I)
• EDN
• EPO
• hydrolases
• cytokines?

FIGURE 32-4 Schematic diagram of a mature human eosinophil illustrating major features, including the bilobed nucleus and the distinctive core-containing specific (secondary) granules (see also Table 32-1). Eosinophils have several classes of receptors, including those for complement proteins, immunoglobulins (IgA, IgG, and perhaps IgE), cytokines/chemokines, and several types of lipid mediators. Major adhesion molecules include the β1- and β2-integrins as well as selectins.

also localized to obstructive mucous plugs and the desquamated clumps of epithelial cells known as Creola bodies.[115] A similar study of paranasal sinus tissue from patients with asthma or allergic rhinitis showed few eosinophils and little or no extracellular MBP where epithelium was intact; however, areas of damage were clearly associated with eosinophil infiltration and extracellular release of MBP into tissues.[116] In recent years, studies of the roles of eosinophil granule MBP in respiratory diseases have led to hypotheses that the protein has noncytotoxic, stimulatory effects. We have recently reviewed some of the evidence for the participation of eosinophils in the induction of airway hyperreactivity.[93] Briefly, this evidence comes from a variety of sources, ranging from in vitro stimulatory effects of purified MBP on isolated airway smooth muscle[117] to correlative observations of eosinophil counts and airway responsiveness in patients with asthma.[118,119] Animal models have been used extensively in examining these effects. For example, the in vitro hyperreactivity of isolated lung strips from Sephadex-treated rats correlated with the number of blood eosinophils.[120] Direct application of MBP onto canine tracheal segments augments the subsequent response to acetylcholine.[121] In a guinea pig model, MBP elicited a dose-dependent direct contraction of tracheal smooth muscle, in addition to a shift in the dose-response relationship for acetylcholine like that seen in the canine model.[122] Human MBP also has been recently tested in an intact primate model of asthma.[123] As in guinea pigs, instillation of MBP directly into the trachea induced an immediate, transient bronchoconstriction and a dose-related increase in airway responsiveness to inhaled methacholine.[124] In subsequent studies, acid polyamino acids, such as polyglutamic and polyaspartic acids, inhibited MBP toxicity in a charge-depen-

dent manner and prevented MBP-induced increases in airway responses to methacholine.[125]

Eosinophil MBP also may have direct effects on other inflammatory cells. Incubation of purified human basophils[126] or rat peritoneal mast cells[127] with MBP results in a noncytotoxic, dose-dependent release of histamine from the target cells. This action could potentially amplify pathophysiologic processes in inflamed tissues. The results of studies on activities of guinea pig eosinophil MBP and synthetic oligopeptides derived from MBP sequences[128] suggest that this histamine-releasing property may depend not only on the basicity of MBP but also on the arrangement of the basic and hydrophobic amino acids.[129]

EOSINOPHIL PEROXIDASE
Eosinophil peroxidase (EPO) is an abundant protein in the matrix of the human eosinophil specific granule.[130] It has a mass of about 75 kDa,[131] is rich in arginine and leucine, and has a calculated pI of 10.9. A combination of EPO, H_2O_2, and halide can induce rat mast cell degranulation and histamine release,[132] and EPO bound to mast cell granules catalyzes the iodination of proteins and the killing of microorganisms.[132] This enzyme can also interact with other inflammatory cells, and it can potentiate the killing of microorganisms by mononuclear phagocytes.[133,134] While EPO-neutrophil interactions can result in decreased EPO catalytic activity, neutrophils to which the protein has bound show increased adhesiveness to endothelial cells.[135] EPO also binds to the extracellular matrix constituents collagen and elastin,[136] but the effects, if any, of these phenomena on inflammatory cell migration have not been elucidated. EPO may play a role in the pathophysiology of a number of diseases, including asthma. EPO can be a marker of eosinophil involvement,

and late-phase responses have been associated with increases in EPO in BAL fluids from primates.[137] Direct intratracheal instillation of EPO in cynomolgus monkeys induced an immediate, transient bronchoconstriction, although, unlike MBP, neither EPO alone nor EPO in combination with H_2O_2 and KI significantly increased airway responsiveness to inhaled methacholine.[124] In vivo, inhibition of EPO activity attenuates eosinophil-induced increases in microvascular permeability; this attenuation occurred without a concomitant reduction in $\cdot O_2^-$ production[138] and suggests a role for the EPO + H_2O_2 + halide system in this type of lung injury.

EOSINOPHIL-DERIVED NEUROTOXIN AND EOSINOPHIL CATIONIC PROTEIN

The proteins eosinophil-derived neurotoxin (EDN, also known as EPX) and eosinophil cationic protein (ECP) are closely related immunologically and are localized to the specific granule matrix.[104,139] ECP is a potent cellular toxin and EDN a less potent one; however, both can inhibit T-lymphocyte proliferation in a noncytotoxic fashion, although the mechanisms involved are unclear.[140] ECP-mediated toxicity may involve the formation of transmembrane channels similar to those formed during membrane-complement interactions.[141] Both molecules demonstrate similar neurotoxic properties in their ability to provoke the Gordon phenomenon in rabbits.[142,143] The roles of EDN and ECP in human disease are still rather speculative; however, these molecules may be partly responsible for neurologic abnormalities in patients with hypereosinophilic syndrome (HES) and other eosinophilic diseases.[144–146] Increased serum concentrations of ECP occur in allergen-provoked asthma,[147] and the concentrations of ECP and EDN/EPX were increased in groups of asthmatics.[148,149] The number of eosinophils and the extracellular concentration of ECP in the BAL fluid were found to be increased in asthmatics and to correlate with pulmonary function and the clinical severity of the disease.[98] BAL fluid from allergic rhinitis patients showed a marked increase in eosinophil granule proteins, including EDN and ECP, after segmental antigen challenge.[58] In patients with obstructive airway disease, increased ECP concentrations in the sputum were correlated with the change in FEV_1 and airway resistance.[150] In a guinea pig model, ECP causes dose-dependent damage to tracheal epithelium in vitro, while EDN lacked toxicity.[151] However, neither EDN nor ECP had any effect on bronchoconstriction or airway responsiveness in a recent study on the effects of eosinophil granule proteins directly applied to the trachea of cynomolgus monkeys.[124] Therefore, while the toxicities of these proteins may be important in the pathology of human disease, their ability to stimulate physiologic parameters in a manner similar to MBP has not been unequivocally demonstrated. On the other hand, a recent pathologic association of eosinophilia with fibrosis[152,153] has led to the examination of the effects of these granule proteins on fibroblasts. The effects of purified granule proteins on human fibroblast viability and mitogenicity were examined. ECP, MBP, and EPO were cytotoxic, whereas EDN acted as a mitogen and induced a dose-depen-

dent increase in [^3H]thymidine incorporation by cultured fibroblasts.[153]

LIPID MEDIATORS

Eosinophils produce two principal lipid mediators involved in asthma and allergic diseases—platelet-activating factor (PAF) and leukotriene C_4 (LTC_4). PAF is produced by several inflammatory cell types, including eosinophils, and its role as a mediator in inflammatory processes has been reviewed recently.[154,155] Acetyltransferase activity is present in many cells, including human eosinophils, and its activity appears to be the rate-limiting step for the production of PAF[156] in low-density (hypodense) eosinophils.[157–159] Eosinophils contain a large amount of the stored PAF precursor alkylacyl glycerophosphocholine[157] and, of all blood cell types, eosinophils are probably the richest source of PAF.[156] PAF production can be enhanced in vitro by activation of peripheral blood eosinophils with stimulants such as formylmethionylleucylphenylalanine (fMLP), A23187, or the eosinophil chemotactic factor of anaphylaxis (ECF-A) tetrapeptides Ala (Val)-Gly-Ser-Glu.[156,160,161] PAF is named for its biologic effect on platelets, but it has a wide variety of activities on other cells and tissues. Indeed, PAF is capable of eliciting many of the characteristics of allergic reaction and asthma.[155] In humans, bronchial hyperresponsiveness is a key feature of asthma, and inhalation of PAF induces increased bronchial reactivity in normal and asthmatic subjects,[162,163] in addition to rapid direct bronchoconstriction.[162] Eosinophils possess PAF receptors,[164] and PAF-eosinophil interactions have generated considerable attention regarding their role in asthma and allergic diseases.[155] PAF has been shown to be a potent in vitro chemotactic factor for eosinophils derived from either eosinophilic[165] or normal[166] donors. Inhalation of PAF in baboons and guinea pigs elicits a rapid and significant increase in eosinophil numbers in bronchoalveolar lavage fluid.[167,168] PAF may act as an eosinophil "activating" factor, and PAF-activated eosinophils are cytotoxic to guinea pig tracheal segments in vitro.[169] PAF induces LTC_4 synthesis and release by purified human eosinophils,[170] as well as eosinophil degranulation and release of preformed mediators such as EPO, ECP, β-glucuronidase, and arylsulfatase B.[171,172] Furthermore, at greater concentrations, PAF activates human eosinophils to release superoxide anion.[172]

Eosinophils possess the metabolic machinery to process phospholipids along several eicosanoid pathways, but the predominant product of arachidonic acid oxygenation in human eosinophils may be LTC_4.[108] Human eosinophils produce LTC_4 when stimulated by calcium ionophore or when incubated with exogenous arachidonic acid, which also may induce a fast, transient increase in cytosolic calcium.[173–176] Interaction of eosinophils with IgG-coated particles may lead to LTC_4 formation and release and may involve the eosinophil IgG receptors FcγRII[177] and/or FcγRIII.[178] Eosinophils can be activated in vitro by monocyte supernatants to generate enhanced levels of LTC_4.[179] Priming of eosinophils for enhanced LTC_4 release by alveolar macrophage supernatants has been attributed to GM-CSF,[180] and both IL-3 and IL-5 have been shown to prime normal human eosinophils to produce LTC$_4$ in response to fMLP, C5a, and PAF.[181,182] In addition to these hematopoietic factors, TNF-α may potentiate LTC$_4$ synthesis by normal human eosinophils stimulated by fMLP.[182] There is an increased proportion of hypodense eosinophils in asthmatics,[183,184] and these cells produce more of LTC$_4$.[185,186] Nedocromil sodium, an anti-asthma medication that inhibits the late asthma response to inhaled antigen and controls chronic asthmatic symptoms, also inhibits the in vitro reduction in eosinophil density and the secretion of LTC$_4$ from eosinophils induced by A23187 or opsonized zymosan.[187] Another anti-inflammatory drug, prednisone, suppresses eosinophil (and basophil) influx and LTC$_4$ production in skin chambers during the late-phase responses of atopic subjects.[188]

Additional evidence for the involvement of leukotrienes in asthma and allergy has been reviewed recently.[189,190] Recent work with animal models supports a role for eosinophil-produced leukotrienes in the development of airway hyperresponsiveness. Inhibitors of LTC$_4$ production can suppress airway eosinophilia and hyperresponsiveness induced by Sephadex particles in rats.[191] Preincubation of eosinophils derived from either cord blood or peripheral blood with a leukotriene inhibitor attenuated LTC$_4$ production and blocked the ability of eosinophils applied to the tracheal epithelium to cause direct contraction and to augment the response to methacholine.[192,193] It seems clear that eosinophil-derived eicosanoids have the potential to contribute to the pathophysiologic features of asthma and allergic disease. Further clarification of the details and extent to which specific mediators are involved in vivo await further tests and therapeutic trials.

OTHER MEDIATORS

Eosinophils can generate and release oxygen metabolites in response to most of the agonists that cause degranulation and/or production of lipid mediators as discussed above. For example, in a recent study of asthmatic children, eosinophils from asthmatic patients released more $\dot{O}_2{}^-$ than eosinophils or neutrophils from healthy control subjects.[194] However, preincubation with GM-CSF or PAF resulted in augmented $\dot{O}_2{}^-$ production by control eosinophils only; $\dot{O}_2{}^-$ generation by eosinophils from asthmatic children was refractory to enhancement by these factors, suggesting in-vivo priming of the cells in asthmatics.[194] Other microenvironmental factors can affect the eosinophil respiratory burst,[195] and differential modulation of eosinophil $\dot{O}_2{}^-$ production by endothelial cells and extracellular matrix components has been demonstrated.[195] Oxygen radicals likely are involved in the pathogenesis of asthma, but their specific effects in this disease are still unclear, and in vitro studies have sometimes yielded contradictory results.[196,197] Much work remains to be done on the generation of oxygen radicals in eosinophils and their possible roles in the pathophysiology of asthma.

A new field of eosinophil research has emerged in the last few years following the discovery that eosinophils are capable of synthesizing, perhaps storing,[109] and releasing cytokines with major activities in the pulmonary tissues. Table 32-2 lists the cytokines that have been shown to be produced by human eosinophils. Some of these cytokines, like

ASTHMA: THE EOSINOPHIL HYPOTHESIS

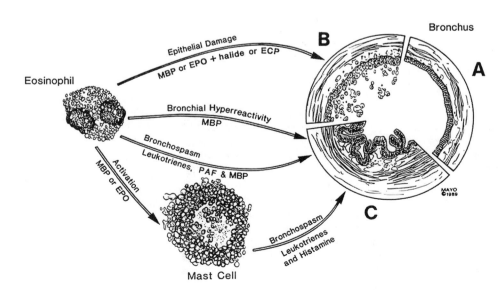

FIGURE 32-5 A schematic summary of the proposed roles of eosinophils in asthma. The effects of eosinophil mediators (e.g., MBP, PAF, and LTC$_4$) on the airways are illustrated by comparing a section of normal bronchus (*A*) with a section damaged by MBP, ECP, or EPO (*B*), showing epithelial desquamation, and with a bronchial section (*C*) showing smooth muscle hypertrophy, constriction, and edema of the lamina propria, resulting in reduction in the caliber of the airway. (See text for abbreviations.) (From *Hamann et al.,*[93] with permission.)

IL-5 or MIP-1α, may act to amplify the eosinophilic inflammation during asthma. Others, like IL-3 and GM-CSF, may act not only on eosinophils but on other inflammatory granulocytes as well; IL-8 has a specific neutrophil chemotactic activity.[198] Still others, such as TGF-β1, may have a critical role in chronic inflammation by promoting fibroblast activation and growth.[109] It is likely that research over the next few years will reveal additional cytokines produced by eosinophils and an increased complexity of eosinophil interactions with other cells in the lung.

Conclusion

It seems clear that inflammation in the lung during asthma is a complex event and that several cell types are involved, from T cells and mast cells during early responses to perhaps neutrophils during transitional events and basophils and eosinophils during late-phase responses. Furthermore, it is likely that these cells are not restricted entirely to these "phases," and that considerable overlap exists with respect to the release of some mediators and, consequently, the functions of these cells in the chronic inflammation of asthma. Nevertheless, recent compelling evidence has led to hypotheses that place the eosinophil as an effector cell central to the pathophysiologic events of asthma (Fig. 32-5). Other cells, of course, have critical roles in this disease; indeed, research must continue to examine the entire process of asthmatic inflammation if significant advances in the therapeutic treatment of asthma are to be made.

References

1. Holgate ST, Howarth PH, Wilson J, Djukanovic R: Bronchoalveolar lavage and bronchial biopsy in asthma, in Kobayashi S, Bellanti JA (eds): *Advances in Asthmology*. New York, Excerpta Medica, 1991:3.
2. Corrigan CJ, Kay AB: The lymphocyte in asthma, in Busse WW, Holgate ST (eds): *Asthma and Rhinitis*. Cambridge, Blackwell Scientific, 1995:450.
3. Corrigan CJ: Immunological aspects of asthma: implications for future treatment. *Clin Immunother* 1994; 1:31.
4. Lohmann-Matthes M-L, Steinmüller C, Franke-Ullmann G: Pulmonary macrophages. *Eur Respir J* 1994; 7:1678.
5. Dvorak AM: Biology and morphology of basophilic leukocytes, in BACH MK (ed): *Immediate Hypersensitivity—Modern Concepts and Developments*. Immunology Series, vol. 7. New York, Marcel Dekker, 1978:369–405.
6. Dvorak AM: Morphologic and immunologic characterization of human basophils, 1879 to 1985. *Riv Immunol Immunofarmacol* 1988; 8:50.
7. Saito H, Hatake K, Dvorak AM, et al.: Selective differentiation and proliferation of hematopoietic cells induced by recombinant human interleukins. *Proc Natl Acad Sci USA* 1988; 85:2288.
8. Warner JA, Kroegel C: Pulmonary immune cells in health and disease: mast cells and basophils. *Eur Respir J* 1994; 7:1326.
9. Lopez AF, Eglington JM, Lyons AB, et al.: Human interleukin-3 inhibits the binding of granulocyte macrophage colony-stimulating factor and interleukin-5 to basophils and strongly enhances their functional activity. *J Cell Physiol* 1990; 145:69.
10. Kitamura T, Sato N, Arai K, Miyajima A: Expression cloning of the human IL-3 receptor cDNA reveals a shared beta subunit for the human IL-3 and GM-CSF receptors. *Cell* 1991; 66:1165.
11. Alam R, Grant JA: Basophils: biology and function in airway disease, in Busse WW, Holgate ST (eds): *Asthma and Rhinitis*. Cambridge, Blackwell Scientific, 1995:242.
12. Metcalf DD, Blande CE, Wasserman SI: Biochemical and functional characterization of proteoglycans isolated from basophils of patients with chronic myelogenous leukemia. *J Immunol* 1984; 132:1943.
13. Ackerman SJ, Kephart GM, Habermann TM, et al.: Localization of eosinophil granule major basic protein in human basophils. *J Exp Med* 1983; 158:946.
14. Dvorak AM, Ackerman SJ: Ultrastructural localization of Charcot-Leyden crystal protein (lysophospholipase) to granules and intragranular crystals in mature human basophils. *Lab Invest* 1989; 60:557.
15. Denburg JA, Richardson M, Telizyn S, Bienenstock J: Basophil/mast cell precursors of human peripheral blood. *Blood* 1990; 61:775.
16. Brunner T, Heusser CH, Dahinden CA: Human peripheral blood basophils primed by interleukin-3 (IL-3) produce IL-4 in response to immunoglobulin E receptor stimulation. *J Exp Med* 1993; 177:605.
17. MacGlashan DM Jr, White JM, Huang S-K, et al.: Secretion of interleukin-4 from human basophils: the relationship between IL-4 mRNA and protein in resting and stimulated basophils. *J Immunol* 1994; 152:3006.
18. Schroeder JT, MacGlashan DM Jr, Kagey-Sobotka A, et al.: Cytokine generation by human basophils. *J Allergy Clin Immunol* 1994; 94:1189.
19. Triggiani M, Schleimer RP, Warner JA, Chilton FH: Differential synthesis of 1-acyl-2-acetyl-*sn*-glycero-3-phosphocholine and platelet-activating factor by human inflammatory cells. *J Immunol* 1991; 147:660.
20. Grant JA, Lichtenstein LM: Release of slow reacting substance of anaphylaxis from human leukocytes. *J Immunol* 1974; 112:897.
21. Kurimoto Y, de Weck AL, Dahinden CA: Interleukin 3-dependent mediator release in basophils triggered by C5a. *J Exp Med* 1989; 170:467.
22. Agis H, Willheim M, Sperr WR, et al.: Monocytes do not make mast cells when cultured in the presence of SCF: Characterization of the circulating mast cell progenitor as a c-kit+, CD34+, Ly-, CD14-, CD17-, colony-forming cell. *J Immunol* 1993; 151:4221.
23. Dvorak Am, Furitsu T, Ishizaka T: Ultrastructural morphology of human mast cell progenitors in sequential cocultures of cord blood cells and fibroblasts. *Int Arch Allergy Immunol* 1993; 100:219.
24. Tsuji T, Sugimoto K, Yanai T, et al.: Induction of granulocyte-macrophage colony-stimulating factor (GM-CSF) and granulocyte colony-stimulating factor (G-CSF) expression in bone marrow and fractionated marrow cell populations by interleukin 3 (IL-3): IL-3-mediated positive feedback mechanisms of granulopoiesis. *Growth Factors* 1994; 11:71.
25. Mayer P, Valent P, Schmidt G, et al.: The in vivo effects of recombinant human interleukin-3: demonstration of basophil differentiation factor, histamine-producing activity and priming of GM-CSF-responsive progenitors in nonhuman primates. *Blood* 1989; 74:613.
26. Rennick D, Hunte B, Dang W, et al.: Interleukin-10 promotes the growth of megakaryocyte, mast cell, and multilineage colonies: analysis with committed progenitors and Thy1 lo Sca1+ stem cells. *Exp Hematol* 1994; 22:136.

27. Anderson DM, Lyman SD, Baird A, et al.: Molecular cloning of mast cell growth factor, a hematopoietin that is active in both membrane bound and soluble forms. *Cell* 1990; 63:235.

28. Rennick D, Hunte B, Holland G, Thompson-Snipes L: Cofactors are essential for stem cell factor-dependent growth and maturation of mast cell progenitors: comparative effects of interleukin-3 (IL-3), IL-4, IL-10, and fibroblasts. *Blood* 1995; 85:57.

29. Dvorak AM: Basophils and mast cells: piecemeal degranulation in situ and in vivo: a possible mechanisms for cytokine-induced function in disease, in Coffey RG (ed): *Granulocyte Responses to Cytokines*. New York, Marcel Dekker, 1992:169.

30. Bochner BS, McGlashan DW, Marcotte GV, Schleimer RP: IgE-dependent regulation of human basophil adherence to vascular endothelium. *J Immunol* 1989; 142:3180.

31. Bochner BS, Luscinskas FW, Gimbrone MA, et al.: Adhesion of human basophils, eosinophils, and neutrophils to interleukin-1 activated human vascular endothelial cells: contributions of endothelial cell adhesion molecules. *J Exp Med* 1991; 173:1553.

32. Pilewski JM, Albelda SM: Adhesion molecules in the lung: an overview. *Am Rev Respir Dis* 1993; 148:S31.

33. Guo C-B, Kagey-Sobotka A, Lichtenstein LM, Bochner BS: Immunotyping and functional analysis of purified human uterine mast cells. *Blood* 1992; 79:708.

34. Hamawy MM, Mergenhagen SE, Siraganian RP: Adhesion molecules as regulators of mast-cell and basophil function. *Immunol Today* 1994; 15:62.

35. Lichtenstein LM, Gillespie E: Inhibition of histamine release controlled by H_2 receptor. *Nature* 1973; 244:287.

36. Vannier E, Miller LC, Dinarello CA: Histamine suppresses gene expression and synthesis of TNFα via histamine H_2 receptors. *J Exp Med* 1991; 174:281.

37. Harvima RJ, Schwartz LB: Mast cell-derived mediators, in Foreman JC (ed): *Immunopharmacology of Mast Cells and Basophils*. New York, Academic Press, 1993:115.

38. Virgolini I, Li S, Sillaber C, Majdic O, et al.: Characterization of prostaglandin binding sites on human basophils: Evidence for a prostaglandin E_1, I_2 and D_2 receptor. *J Biol Chem* 1992; 267:12700.

39. Lett-Brown MA, Boetcher DA, Leonard EJ: Chemotactic responses of normal basophils to C5a and to a lymphocyte-derived chemotactic factor. *J Immunol* 1976; 117:246.

40. Marom ZM: The role of mast cells in bronchial asthma: mechanisms and possible therapeutic implications. *Mount Sinai J Med* 1991; 58:472.

41. Tomioka M, Ida S, Yuriko D, et al.: Mast cells in bronchoalveolar lumen of patients with bronchial asthma. *Am Rev Respir Dis* 1984; 129:1000.

42. Wardlaw AJ, Dunnette S, Gleich GJ, et al.: Eosinophils and mast cells in bronchoalveolar lavage fluid in mild asthma: relationship to bronchial hyperreactivity. *Am Rev Respir Dis* 1988; 137:62.

43. Beasley R, Roche WR, Roberts JA, Holgate ST: Cellular events in the bronchi in mild asthma and after bronchial provocation. *Am Rev Respir Dis* 1989; 139:806.

44. Pesci A, Foresi A, Bertorelli G, et al.: Histochemical characteristics and degranulation of mast cells in epithelial and lamina propria from asthmatics and normal subjects. *Am Rev Respir Dis* 1993; 147:684.

45. Kirby JG, Hargreave FE, Gleich GJ, O'Bynre PM: Bronchoalveolar cell profiles of asthmatics and non-asthmatic subjects. *Am Rev Respir Dis* 1987; 136:379.

46. Casale TB, Wood D, Richerson HB, et al.: Elevated bronchoalveolar lavage fluid histamine levels in allergic asthmatics are associated with methacholine bronchial hyperreactivity. *J Clin Invest* 1987; 79:1197.

47. Flint KC, Leung KBP, Hudspith BN, et al.: Bronchoalveolar mast cells in extrinsic asthma: a mechanism for the initiation of allergen-specific bronchoconstriction. *Br Med J Clin Res* 1985; 291:923.

48. Beasley R, Varley J, Robinson C, Holgate ST: Cholinergic-mediated bronchoconstriction induced by prostanglandin D_2, its initial metabolite 9α,11β-prostaglandin F_2 and prostaglandin $F_{2\alpha}$ in asthma. *Am Rev Respir Dis* 1987; 136:1140.

49. Holgate ST, Emanuel MB, Howarth PH: Astemizole and other H_1 antihistamine drug treatments of asthma. *J Allergy Clin Immunol* 1985; 76:375.

50. Lichtenstein LM, Bochner BS: The role of basophils in asthma. *Ann NY Acad Sci* 1991; 629:48.

51. Kimura I, Tanizaki Y, Saito K, et al.: Appearance of basophils in the sputum of patients with bronchial asthma. *Clin Allergy* 1975; 1:95.

52. Liu, MC, Hubbard WC, Proud D, et al.: Immediate and late inflammatory responses to ragweed antigen challenge of the peripheral airway in allergic asthmatics. *Am Rev Respir Dis* 1991; 144:51.

53. Akagi K, Townley RG: Spontaneous histamine release and histamine content in normal subjects and subjects with asthma. *J Allergy Clin Immunol* 1989; 83:742.

54. Djukanovic R, Mann M, Rimmer J, Spackman D, et al.: The effect of inhaled allergen on circulating basophils in atopic asthma. *J Allergy Clin Immunol* 1992; 90:175.

55. Neijins HJ, Raatgeep HC, Degenhart HJ, Kerrebijn KF: Release of histamine from leucocytes and its determinants in vitro in relation to bronchial responsiveness to inhaled histamine and exercise in vivo. *Clin Allergy* 1982; 12:577.

56. Maruyama N, Tamura G, Aizawa T, et al.: Accumulation of basophils and their chemotactic activity in the airways during natural airway narrowing in asthmatic individuals. *Am J Respir Crit Care Med* 1994; 150:1086.

57. Chan-Yeung M: Mechanism of occupational asthma due to western red cedar (*Thuja plicata*). *Am J Ind Med* 1994; 25:13.

58. Sedgwick J, Calhoun WJ, Gleich GJ, et al.: Immediate and late airway response of allergic rhinitis patients to segmental antigen challenge: characterization of eosinophil and mast cell mediators. *Am Rev Respir Dis* 1991; 144:1274.

59. Calhoun WJ, Liu MC: Bronchoalveolar lavage and bronchial biopsy in asthma, in Busse WW, Holgate ST (eds): *Asthma and Rhinitis*. Cambridge, Blackwell Scientific, 1995:130–144.

60. Naclerio RM, Proud D, Togia AG, et al.: Inflammatory mediators in late antigen-induced rhinitis. *N Engl J Med* 1985; 313:65.

61. Walsh LJ, Trinchieri G, Waldorf HA, et al.: Human dermal cells contain and release tumor necrosis factor-α, which induces endothelial leukocyte adhesion molecule-1. *Proc Natl Acad Sci USA* 1991; 88:4220.

62. Bradding P, Feather IH, Howarth PH, et al.: Interleukin-4 is localized to and released from human lung mast cells. *J Exp Med* 1992; 176:1381.

63. Gauchat J-F, Henchoz S, Mazzei G, et al.: Induction of human IgE synthesis in B-cells by mast cells and basophils. *Nature* 1993; 365:340.

64. Williams TJ, Das A, von Uexkull, Nourshargh S: Neutrophils in asthma. *Ann NY Acad Sci* 1991; 629:73.

65. Fabbri LM, Boschetto P, Zocco E, et al.: Bronchoalveolar neutrophilia during the late asthmatic reactions induced by toluene diisocyanate. *Am Rev Respir Dis* 1987; 136:36.

66. Demetri GD, Griffin JD: Granulocyte colony-stimulating factor and its receptor. *Blood* 1991; 78:2791.

67. Marmont AM, Damasio E, Zucker-Franklin D: Neutrophils, in Zucker-Franklin D, Greaves MF, Grossi CE, Marmont AM (eds): *Atlas of Blood Cells: Function and Pathology*, 2d ed. Philadelphia, Lea & Febiger, 1988:157.

68. Doherty NS, Janusz MJ: Neutrophil proteases: their physiological and pathological roles, in Hellewell PG, Williams TJ (eds): *Immunopharmacology of Neutrophils.* New York, Academic Press, 1994:55.

69. Lehrer RI, Ganz T, Selsted ME, et al.: Neutrophils and host defense. *Ann Intern Med* 1988; 109:127.

70. Spitznagel JK: Antibiotic proteins of human neutrophils. *J Clin Invest* 1990; 86:1381.

71. Sibille Y, Marchandise F-X: Pulmonary immune cells in health and disease: polymorphonuclear neutrophils. *Eur Respir J* 1993; 6:1529.

72. Reynolds HY: Mechanisms of inflammation in the lungs. *Am Rev Med* 1987; 38:295.

73. Truong MJ, Gruart V, Kusnierz JP, et al.: Human neutrophils express immunoglobulin E (IgE)-binding proteins (Mac2/εBP) of the S-type lectin family: role in IgE-dependent activation. *J Exp Med* 1993; 177:243.

74. Dispersio J, Billing P, Kaufman S, et al.: Characterization of the human granulocyte-macrophage colony-stimulating factor (GM-CSF) receptor. *J Biol Chem* 1988; 263:1834.

75. Martin TR, Pistorese BP, Chi EY, et al.: Effects of leukotriene B_4 in the human lung: Recruitment of neutrophils into the alveolar spaces without a change in protein permeability. *J Clin Invest* 1989; 84:1609.

76. Dent G, Ukena D, Chanez P, et al.: Characterization of PAF receptors on human neutrophils using the specific antagonist, WEB 2086: correlation between receptor binding and function. *FEBS Lett* 1989; 244:365.

77. Moser B, Schumacher C, von Tscharner V, et al.: Neutrophil-activating peptide 2 and gro/melanoma growth-stimulatory activity interact with neutrophil activating peptide-1/interleukin-8 receptors on human neutrophils. *J Biol Chem* 1991; 266:10666.

78. Pardi R, Inverardi L, Bender JR: Regulatory mechanisms in leukocyte adhesion: flexible receptors for sophisticated travellers. *Immunol Today* 1992; 13:224.

79. Kay AB, Corrigan CJ: Eosinophils and neutrophils. *Br Med Bull* 1992; 48:51.

80. Fabbri LM, Papi A, Boschetto P, Ciaccia A: Neutrophils in asthma, in Busse WW, Holgate ST (eds): *Asthma and Rhinitis.* Cambridge, Blackwell Scientific, 1995:383.

81. Busse WW, Calhoun WF, Sedgwick JD: Mechanism of airway inflammation in asthma. *Am Rev Respir Dis* 1993; 147:S20.

82. Breuer R, Christensen TG, Niles RM, et al.: Human neutrophil elastase causes glycoconjugate release from the epithelial cell surface of hamster trachea in organ culture. *Am Rev Respir Dis* 1989; 139:779.

83. Sommerhoff CP, Krell RD, Williams JL, et al.: Inhibition of human neutrophil elastase by ICI 200,355. *Eur J Pharmacol* 1991; 193:153.

84. Venaille TJ, Mendis AHW, Phillips MJ, et al.: Role of neutrophils in mediating human epithelial cell detachment from native basement membrane. *J Allergy Clin Immunol* 1995; 95:597.

85. Teran LM, Montefort S, Douglass J, Holgate ST: Neutrophil and eosinophil chemotaxins in asthma. *Q J Med* 1993; 86:761.

86. Pradalier A: Late phase reaction in asthma: basic mechanisms. *Int Arch Allergy Immunol* 1993; 101:322.

87. Fabbri LM, Aizawa H, Alpert SE, et al.: Airway hyperresponsiveness and changes in cell counts in bronchoalveolar lavage after ozone exposure in dogs. *Am Rev Respir Dis* 1984; 129:288.

88. Li ZY, O'Byrne PM, Lane CG, et al.: The effect of an anti-CD11b/CD18 monoclonal antibody on ozone-induced neutrophil influx and airway hyperresponsiveness in dogs. *Am Rev Respir Dis* 1991; 143:43A.

89. O'Byrne PM, Walters EH, Aizawa H, et al.: Indomethacin inhibits the airway hyperresponsiveness but not the neutrophil influx induced by ozone in dogs. *Am Rev Respir Dis* 1984; 130:220.

90. Ellis AG: The pathological anatomy of bronchial asthma. *Am J Med Sci* 1908; 136:407.

91. Huber HL, Koessler KK: The pathology of bronchial asthma. *Arch Intern Med* 1922; 30:689.

92. Holgate ST, Roche WR, Church MK: The role of the eosinophil in asthma. *Am Rev Respir Dis* 1991; 143:566.

93. Hamann KJ, White SR, Gundel RH, Gleich GJ: Interactions between respiratory epithelium and eosinophil granule proteins in asthma: the eosinophil hypothesis, in Farmer SG, Hay DWP (eds): *The Airway Epithelium: Structure and Function in Health and Disease.* New York, Marcel Dekker, 1991:255.

94. Calhoun WJ, Sedgwick J, Busse WW: The role of eosinophils in the pathophysiology of asthma. *Ann NY Acad Sci* 1991; 629:62.

95. Reed CE: The importance of eosinophils in the immunology of asthma and allergic disease. *Ann Allergy* 1994; 72:376.

96. Weller PF: The immunobiology of eosinophils. *N Engl J Med* 1991; 324:1110.

97. Horn BR, Robin ED, Theodore J, Van Kessel A: Total eosinophil counts in the management of asthma. *N Engl J Med* 1975; 292:1152.

98. Bousquet J, Chanez P, Lacoste JY, et al.: Eosinophilic inflammation in asthma. *N Engl J Med* 1990; 323:1033.

99. Griffin E, Håkansson L, Formgren H, et al.: Blood eosinophil number and activity in relation to lung function in patients with asthma and eosinophilia. *J Allergy Clin Immunol* 1991; 87:548.

100. Leff AR, Hamann KJ, Wegner CD: Inflammation and cell-cell interactions in airway hyperresponsiveness. *Am J Physiol* 1991; 260:L189.

101. Clutterbuck EJ, Hirst EMA, Sanderson CJ: Human interleukin-5 (IL-5) regulates the production of eosinophils in human bone marrow cultures: comparison and interaction with IL-1, IL-3, IL-6 and GM-CSF. *Blood* 1989; 73:1504.

102. Weller PF: Cytokine regulation of eosinophil function. *Clin Immunol Immunopathol* 1992; 1:2.

103. Dvorak AM, Ackerman SJ, Weller PF: Subcellular morphology and biochemistry of eosinophils, in Harris JR (ed): *Blood Cell Biochemistry,* vol. 2. New York, Plenum Press, 1991:237–344.

104. Hamann KJ, Barker RL, Ten RM, Gleich GJ: The molecular biology of eosinophil granule proteins. *Int Arch Allergy Appl Immunol* 1991; 94:202.

105. Hamann KJ: Eosinophil mediators, in Busse WW, Holgate ST (eds): *Asthma and Rhinitis.* Cambridge, Blackwell Scientific, 1995:298.

106. Dvorak AM, Letourneau L, Login GR, et al.: Ultrastructural localization of the Charcot-Leyden crystal protein (lysophospholipase) to a distinct crystalloid-free granule population in mature human eosinophils. *Blood* 1988; 72:150.

107. Kroegel C, Virchow J-C Jr, Luttmann W, et al.: Pulmonary immune cells in health and disease: the eosinophil leukocyte (part I). *Eur Respir J* 1994; 7:519.

108. Weller PF, Lee CW, Foster DW, et al.: Generation and metabolism of 5-lipoxygenase pathway leukotrienes by human eosinophils: predominant production of leukotriene C_4. *Proc Natl Acad Sci USA* 1983; 80:7626.

109. Moqbel R, Levi-Scaffer F, Kay AB: Cytokine generation by eosinophils. *J Allergy Clin Immunol* 1994; 94:1183.

110. Yousefi S, Hemmann S, Weber M, et al.: IL-8 is expressed by human peripheral blood eosinophils: Evidence for increased secretion in asthma. *J Immunol* 1995; 154:5481.

111. Bochner BS, Undem BJ, Lichtenstein LM: Immunological aspects of allergic asthma. *Ann Rev Immunol* 1994; 12:295.

112. Neeley SP, Hamann KJ, Dowling TL, et al.: Augmentation of stimulated eosinophil degranulation by VLA-4 (CD49d)-mediated adhesion to fibronectin. *Am J Respir Cell Mol Biol* 1994; 11:206.

113. Frigas E, Loegering DA, Solley GO, et al.: Elevated levels of the eosinophil granule major basic protein in the sputum of patients with bronchial asthma. *Mayo Clinic Proc* 1981; 56:345.

114. Gleich GJ, Frigas E, Loegering DA, et al.: Cytotoxic properties of the eosinophil major basic protein. *J Immunol* 1979; 123:2925.

115. Filley WV, Holley KE, Kephart GM, Gleich GJ: Identification by immunofluorescence of eosinophil granule major basic protein in lung tissues of patients with bronchial asthma. *Lancet* 1982; 2:11.

116. Harlin SL, Ansel DG, Lane SR, et al.: A clinical and pathologic study of chronic sinusitis: the role of the eosinophil. *J Allergy Clin Immunol* 1988; 81:867.

117. Flavahan NA, Slifman NR, Gleich GJ, Vanhoutte PM: Human eosinophil major basic protein causes hyperreactivity of respiratory smooth muscle: Role of the epithelium. *Am Rev Respir Dis* 1988; 138:685.

118. Durham SR, Kay AB: Eosinophils, bronchial hyperreactivity and late-phase asthmatic reactions. *Clin Allergy* 1985; 15:411.

119. Ferguson AC, Wong FWM: Bronchial hyperresponsiveness in asthmatic children: Correlation with macrophages and eosinophils in broncholavage fluid. *Chest* 1989; 96:988.

120. Spicer BA, Baker R, Laycock SM, Smith H: Correlation between blood eosinophilia and airways hyperresponsiveness in rats. *Agents Actions* 1989; 26:63.

121. Brofman JD, White SR, Blake JS, et al.: Epithelial augmentation of trachealis contraction caused by MBP of eosinophils. *J Appl Physiol* 1989; 66:1867.

122. White SR, Munoz NM, Gleich GJ, et al.: Epithelial-dependent contraction of airway smooth muscle caused by eosinophil MBP. *Am J Physiol Lung Cell Mol Physiol* 1990; 259:L294.

123. Gundel RH, Gerritsen ME, Gleich GJ, Wegner CD: Repeated antigen inhalation results in a prolonged airway eosinophilia and airway hyperresponsiveness in primates. *J Appl Physiol* 1990; 68:779.

124. Gundel RH, Letts LG, Gleich GJ: Human eosinophil major basic protein induces airway constriction and airway hyperresponsiveness in primates. *J Clin Invest* 1991; 87:1470.

125. Barker RL, Gundel RH, Gleich GJ, et al.: Acidic polyamino acids inhibit human eosinophil granule major basic protein toxicity: Evidence of a functional role for pro MBP. *J Clin Invest* 1991; 88:798.

126. O'Donnell MC, Ackerman SJ, Gleich GJ, Thomas LL: Activation of basophil and mast cell histamine release by eosinophil granule major basic protein. *J Exp Med* 1983; 157:1981.

127. Zheutlin LM, Ackerman SJ, Gleich GJ, Thomas LL: Stimulation of basophil and rat mast cell histamine release by eosinophil granule-derived proteins. *J Immunol* 1984; 133:2180.

128. Tasaka K, Mio M, Aoki I, Saito T: Guinea pig eosinophil major basic protein (GMBP) as a potent histamine releaser: I. Histamine releasing activity of GMBP and its chemical structure. *Agents Actions* [Special Conference Issue] 1992; C242.

129. Tasaka K, Mio M, Nakai S, Aoki I: Guinea pig eosinophil major basic protein as a potent histamine releaser: II. Structure-activity relationships of GMBP₁ and GMPB₂. *Agents Actions* [Special Conference Issue] 1992; C246.

130. Enomoto T, Kitani T: Electron microscopic studies on peroxidase and acid phosphatase reaction in human leukocytes in normal and leukemic cells and on phagocytosis. *Acta Haematol Jpn* 1986; 29:554.

131. Carlson MG, Peterson CG, Venge P: Human eosinophil peroxidase: purification and characterization. *J Immunol* 1989; 134:1875.

132. Henderson WR, Jong EC, Klebanoff SJ: Binding of eosinophil peroxidase to mast cell granules with retention of peroxidactic activity. *J Immunol* 1980; 124:1383.

133. Ramsey PG, Martin T, Chi E, Klebanoff SJ. Arming of mononuclear phagocytes by eosinophil peroxidase bound to *Staphylococcus aureus*. *J Immunol* 1982; 128:415.

134. Nogueira NM, Klebanoff SF, Cohn ZA: *Trypanosoma cruzi*: sensitization to macrophage killing by eosinophil peroxidase. *J Immunol* 1982; 128:1705.

135. Zabucchi G, Menegazzi R, Cramer R, et al.: Mutual influence between eosinophil peroxidase (EPO) and neutrophils: neutrophils reversibly inhibit EPO enzymatic activity and EPO increases neutrophil adhesiveness. *Immunology* 1990; 69:580.

136. Zabucchi G, Soranzo MR, Menegazzi R, et al.: Uptake of human eosinophil peroxidase and myeloperoxidase by cells involved in the inflammatory process. *J Histochem Cytochem* 1989; 37:499.

137. Gundel RH, Wegner CD, Torcellini CA, Letts LG: Airway inflammation and late-phase responses in primates. *Am Rev Respir Dis* 1992; 145:A33.

138. Yoshikawa S, Parker JS, Seibert AF, Kays SG: The peroxide-H_2O_2-halide system contributes to eosinophil-induced injury in isolated perfused rat lungs. *FASEB J* 1992; 6:A1058.

139. Gleich GJ, Loegering DA, Bell MP, Checkel JL: Biochemical and functional similarities between human eosinophil-derived neurotoxin and eosinophil cationic protein: homology with ribonuclease. *Proc Natl Acad Sci USA* 1986; 83:3146.

140. Peterson CGB, Skoog V, Venge P. Human eosinophil cationic proteins (ECP and EPX) and their suppressive effects on lymphocyte proliferation. *Immunobiology* 1986; 171:1.

141. Young JDE, Peterson CGB, Venge P, Cohn ZA: Mechanisms of membrane damage mediated by human eosinophil cationic protein. *Nature* 1986; 321:613.

142. Durack DT, Sumi SM, Klebanoff SJ: Neurotoxicity of human eosinophils. *Proc Natl Acad Sci USA* 1979; 76:1443.

143. Fredens K, Dahl R, Venge P: The Gordon phenomenon induced by the eosinophil cationic protein and eosinophil protein X. *J Allergy Clin Immunol* 1982; 70:361.

144. Chusid MJ, Dale DC, West BC, Wolff SM: The hypereosinophilic syndrome: analysis of fourteen cases with review of the literature. *Medicine (Baltimore)* 1975; 54:1.

145. Martin RW, Duffy J, Engel AG, et al.: The clinical spectrum of the eosinophilia-myalgia syndrome associated with L-tryptophan ingestion. *Ann Intern Med* 1990; 113:124.

146. Fredens K, Tottrup A, Kirstensen IB, et al.: Severe destruction of esophageal nerves in a patient with achalasia secondary to gastric cancer: A possible role of eosinophilic neurotoxic proteins. *Dig Dis Sci* 1989; 34:297.

147. Dahl R, Venge P, Olsson I: Variations of blood eosinophils and eosinophil cationic protein in serum in patients with bronchial asthma: studies during inhalation challenge tests. *Allergy* 1978; 33:211.

148. Venge P, Dahl R, Peterson CGB: Eosinophil granule proteins in serum after allergen challenge of asthmatic patients and the effects of anti-asthmatic medication. *Int Arch Allergy Appl Immunol* 1988; 87:306.

149. Adelroth E, Rosenhall L, Johansson SA, et al.: Inflammatory cells and eosinophilic activity in asthmatics investigated by bronchoalveolar lavage: The effects of antiasthmatic treatment with budesonide or terbutaline. *Am Rev Respir Dis* 1990; 142:91.

150. Virchow JC, Holscher U, Virchow C Sr: Sputum ECP levels correlate with parameters of airflow obstruction. *Am Rev Respir Dis* 1992; 146:604.

151. Motojima S, Frigas E, Loegering DA, Gleich GJ: Toxicity of eosinophil cationic proteins for guinea pig tracheal epithelium in vitro. *Am Rev Respir Dis* 1989; 139:801.

152. Peterson MW, Hunninghake GW: Prognostic role of eosinophils in pulmonary fibrosis. *Chest* 1987; 92:51.

153. Noguchi H, Kephart GM, Colby TV, Gleich GJ: Tissue eosinophilia and eosinophil degranulation in syndromes associated with fibrosis. *Am J Pathol* 1992; 140:521.

154. Barnes PJ, Chung KF, Page CP: Platelet-activating factor as a mediator of allergic disease. *J Allergy Clin Immunol* 1988; 81:919.

155. Chung KF, Barnes PJ: Platelet-activating factor and asthma, in Kaliner MA, Barnes PJ, Persson CGA (eds): *Asthma: Its Pathology and Treatment*. New York: Marcel Dekker, 1991:267.

156. Lee TC, Lenihan DJ, Malone B, et al.: Increased biosynthesis of platelet activating factor in activated human eosinophils. *J Biol Chem* 1984; 259:5526.

157. Ojima-Uchiyama A, Masazawa Y, Sugiura T, et al.: Phospholipid analysis of human eosinophils: high levels of alkylacylglycerophosphocholine (PAF precursor). *Lipids* 1988; 23:815.

158. Ojima-Uchiyama A, Masuzawa Y, Sugiura T, et al.: Production of platelet-activating factor by human normodense and hypodense eosinophils. *Lipids* 1991; 26:1200.

159. Cromwell O, Wardlaw AJ, Champion A, et al.: IgG-dependent generation of platelet-activating factor by normal and low density human eosinophils. *J Immunol* 1990; 145:3862.

160. Burke LA, Crea AEG, Wilkinson JRW, et al.: Comparison of the generation of platelet-activating factor and leukotriene C_4 in human eosinophils stimulated by unopsonized zymosan and by the calcium ionophore A23187: the effects of nedocromil sodium. *J Allergy Clin Immunol* 1990; 85:26.

161. Capron M, Benveniste J, Braquet P, Capron A: Role of PAF-acether in IgE-dependent activation of eosinophils, in Braquet P (ed): *New Trends in Lipid Mediators Research: The Role of Platelet-Activating Factor in Immune Disorders*. Basel, Karger, 1988:10.

162. Cuss FM, Dixon CMS, Barnes PJ: Effects of inhaled platelet activating factor on pulmonary function and bronchial responsiveness in man. *Lancet* 1986; 2:189.

163. Chung KF, Dent G, McCusker M, et al.: Effect of a ginkgolide mixture (BN 52063) in antagonising skin and platelet responses to platelet activating factor in man. *Lancet* 1987; 1:248.

164. Ukena D, Krugel C, Dent G, et al.: PAF-receptors on eosinophils: identification with a novel ligand, [^{3}H]WEB 2086. *Biochem Pharmacol* 1989; 38:1702.

165. Wardlaw AJ, Moqbel R, Cromwell O, Kay AB: Platelet-activating factor: A potent chemotactic and chemokinetic factor for human eosinophils. *J Clin Invest* 1986; 78:1701.

166. Tamura N, Agrawal DK, Swiaman FA, Towley RG: Effects of platelet activating factor on the chemotaxis of normodense eosinophils from normal subjects. *Biochem Biophys Res Commun* 1987; 142:638.

167. Arnoux B, Denjean A, Page CP, et al.: Accumulation of platelets and eosinophils in baboon lung after PAF-acether challenge: inhibition by ketotifen. *Am Rev Respir Dis* 1988; 137:855.

168. Coyle AJ, Unwin SC, Page CP, et al.: The effect of the selective antagonist BN 52021 on PAF and antigen-induced bronchial hyperreactivity and eosinophil accumulation. *Eur J Pharmacol* 1988; 148:51.

169. Yukawa T, Read RC, Kroegel C, et al.: The effects of activated eosinophils and neutrophils on guinea pig airway epithelium in vitro. *Am J Respir Cell Mol Biol* 1990; 2:341.

170. Bruijnzeel PLB, Kok PTM, Hamelink ML, et al.: Platelet-activating factor induces leukotriene C_4 synthesis by purified human eosinophils. *Prostaglandins* 1987; 34:205.

171. Kroegel C, Yukawa T, Dent G, et al.: Stimulation of degranulation from human eosinophils by platelet activating factor. *J Immunol* 1989; 142:3518.

172. Kroegel C, Yukawa T, Dent G, et al.: Platelet activating factor induces eosinophil perioxidase release from purified human eosinophils. *Immunology* 1988; 64:559.

173. Shaw RJ, Walsh GM, Cromwell O, et al.: Activated human eosinophils generate SRS-A leukotrienes following IgG-dependent stimulation. *Nature* 1985; 316:150.

174. Tamura N, Agrawal DK, Townley R: A specific radioreceptor assay for leukotriene C_4 and the measurement of calcium ionophore-induced leukotriene C_4 production from human leukocytes. *J Pharmacol Methods* 1987; 18:327.

175. Owen WF Jr, Soberman RJ, Yoshimoto T, et al.: Synthesis and release of leukotriene C_4 by human eosinophils. *J Immunol* 1987; 138:532.

176. Kok PTM, Hamelink ML, Kijne Am, et al.: Arachidonic acid can induce leukotriene C_4 formation by purified human eosinophils in the absence of other stimuli. *Biochem Biophys Res Commun* 1988; 153:676.

177. deAndres B, del Pozo V, Cardaba B, et al.: Phosphoinositide breakdown is associated with Fcγ-RII-mediated activation of 5'-lipoxygenase in murine eosinophils. *J Immunol* 1991; 146:1566.

178. Hartnell A, Kay AB, Wardlaw AJ: IFN-γ induces expression of FcγRIII (CD16) on human eosinophils. *J Immunol* 1992; 148:1471.

179. Elsas P, Lee TH, Lenzl HL, Dessein AJ: Monocytes activate eosinophils for enhanced helminthotoxicity and increased generation of leukotriene C_4. *Ann Inst Pasteur/Immunol* 1987; 138:97.

180. Howell CJ, Pujol J-L, Crea AEG, et al.: Identification of an alveolar macrophage-derived activity in bronchial asthma that enhances leukotriene C_4 generation by human eosinophils stimulated by ionophore A23187 as a granulocyte-macrophage colony-stimulating factor. *Am Rev Respir Dis* 1989; 140:1340.

181. Fabian I, Kletter Y, Mor S, et al.: Activation of human eosinophil and neutrophil functions by haematopoietic growth factors: comparisons of IL-1, IL-3, IL-5 and GM-CSF. *Br J Haematol* 1992; 80:137.

182. Takafuji S, Bischoff SC, de Weck AL, Dahinden CA: IL-3 and IL-5 prime normal human eosinophils to produce leukotriene C_4 in response to soluble agonists. *J Immunol* 1991; 147:3855.

183. Prin L, Capron M, Tonnel AB, et al.: Heterogeneity of human peripheral blood eosinophils: variability in cell density and cytotoxic ability in relation to the level and the origin of hypereosinophilia. *Int Arch Allergy Appl Immunol* 1983; 72:336.

184. Fukuda T, Dunnette SL, Reed CE, et al.: Increased numbers of hypodense eosinophils in the blood of patients with bronchial asthma. *Am Rev Respir Dis* 1985; 132:981.

185. Wang SR, Yang CM, Wang SSM, et al.: Enhancement of A23187-induced production of the slow-reacting substance on peripheral leukocytes from subjects with asthma. *J Allergy Clin Immunol* 1986; 77:465.

186. Kauffman HF, van der Belt B, deMonchy JGR, et al.: Leukotriene C_4 production by normal-density and low-density eosinophils of atopic individuals and other patients with eosinophilia. *J Allergy Clin Immunol* 1987; 79:611.

187. Sedgwick JB, Bjornsdottir U, Geiger KM, Busse WW: Inhibition of eosinophil density change and leukotriene C_4 generation by nedocromil sodium. *J Allergy Clin Immunol* 1992; 90:202.

188. Charlesworth EN, Kagey-Sobotka A, Schleimer RP, et al.: Prednisone inhibits the appearance of inflammatory mediators and the influx of eosinophils and basophils associated with the cutaneous late-phase response to allergen. *J Immunol* 1991; 146:671.

189. Piacentini GL, Kaliner MA: The potential roles of leukotrienes in bronchial asthma. *Am Rev Respir Dis* 1991; 143:596.

190. Naclerio RM, Baroody RM, Togias AG: The role of leukotrienes in allergic rhinitis: a review. *Am Rev Respir Dis* 1991; 143:591.

191. Asano M, Inamura N, Nakahara K, et al.: A 5-lipoxygenase inhibitor, FR110302, suppresses airway hyperresponsiveness and lung eosinophilia induced by Sephadex particles in rats. *Agents Actions* 1992; 36:215.

192. Hamann KJ, Strek ME, Baranowski SL, et al.: Physiological

effects of activated eosinophils cultured from human umbilical cord blood on guinea pig treachealis in situ. *Am J Physiol* 1993; 265:L301.

193. Strek ME, White SR, Hsiue TR, et al.: Effect of mode of activation of human eosinophils on tracheal smooth muscle contraction in guinea pigs. *Am J Physiol* 1993; 264:L475.

194. Schauer U, Leinhaas C, Jager R, Rieger CHL: Enhanced superoxide generation by eosinophils from asthmatic children. *Int Arch Allergy Appl Immunol* 1991; 96:317.

195. Dri P, Cramer R, Spessotto P, et al.: Eosinophil activation on biologic surfaces: Production of O_2^- in response to physiologic sol-

uble stimuli is differentially modulated by extracellular matrix components and endothelial cells. *J Immunol* 1991; 147:163.

196. Davis WB, Falls GA, Sun X-H, et al.: Eosinophil-mediated injury to lung parenchymal cells and interstitial matrix. *J Clin Invest* 1984; 74:269.

197. Ayars GH, Altman LC, Gleich GJ, et al.: Eosinophil- and eosinophil granule-mediated pneumocyte injury. *J Allergy Clin Immunol* 1985; 76:595.

198. Kunkel SL, Standiford T, Kasahara K, Strieter RM: Interleukin-8 (IL-8): the major chemotactic factor in the lung. *Exp Lung Res* 1991; 17:17.

Chapter 33

MACROPHAGES

GALEN B. TOEWS

Macrophages can influence almost every aspect of acute and chronic inflammatory responses. Macrophages are involved from the first breaching of the epithelium to its repair. Without phagocytosis by macrophages, invading microbes would multiply in tissues, senescent cells would accumulate, and wounds would go unmended. Macrophages secrete more than 100 substances, the biologic effects of which vary from induction of cell growth to induction of cell death. Furthermore, macrophages can be activated to carry out their various functions more effectively. Macrophages are a monotypic, dispersed, differentiating cell population that can react to soluble and particulate stimuli derived from both mammalian tissues and microbes. Macrophages in the bone marrow, circulation, and tissue compose the mononuclear phagocyte system. These cells are a "system" because of their common origin, similar morphology, and shared functions.

Life History

Macrophages originate from the granulocyte-macrophage colony-forming unit (GM-CFU), a common progenitor cell for both granulocytes and monocyte/macrophages.[1,2] The production of monocytes in vivo is controlled by various glycoprotein growth factors. Interleukin-3 (IL-3), granulocyte/macrophage colony-stimulating factor (GM-CSF), and macrophage colony-stimulating factor (M-CSF) stimulate the mitotic activity of monocyte precursors.[3–5] These colony-stimulating factors induce differentiation of the GM-CFU into a monoblast, which differentiates into promonocytes, the earliest morphologically identifiable cell in this series. The bone marrow transit time from the first monocytic precursor to mature monocytes is approximately 6 days. Newly formed monocytes remain in the marrow for only a short time (less than 24 h) and then migrate to the peripheral blood.[6] No marrow reserve comparable to that for granulocytes exists. Circulating human monocytes have a half-life of approximately 3 days.[7] The total pool of blood monocytes is composed of a circulating pool (25 to 40 percent) and a marginating pool (adherent to the endothelium of blood vessels; 60 to 75 percent).[8] Monocytes in the circulation are heterogeneous in size, cell density, and surface markers.

Migration of monocytes into different tissues appears to be a random phenomenon in the absence of localized inflammation. Once in tissues, monocytes probably do not reenter the circulation.

ALVEOLAR MACROPHAGES

Alveolar macrophages (AMs) are derived from blood monocytes. Studies of patients undergoing bone marrow or lung transplants suggests that AMs have a life-span of months and perhaps years.[9,10] The AM population is maintained by movement of blood monocytes into the lung and by local proliferation. Movement of cells is the predominant mechanism. It is unknown which, if any, monocyte chemoattractants, receptors, and ligands modulate monocyte traffic to the normal human lung. Approximately 1 percent of the AM population in the normal human lung is proliferating at any one time.[11]

Functional Attributes of Macrophages

Four critical attributes allow macrophages to accomplish a broad group of biologic functions (Fig. 33-1). Macrophages (1) recognize signals from the environment, (2) phagocytose particulate material, (3) produce and secrete large numbers of mediators, and (4) migrate in response to various stimuli. These attributes can be integrated to produce complex macrophage functions.

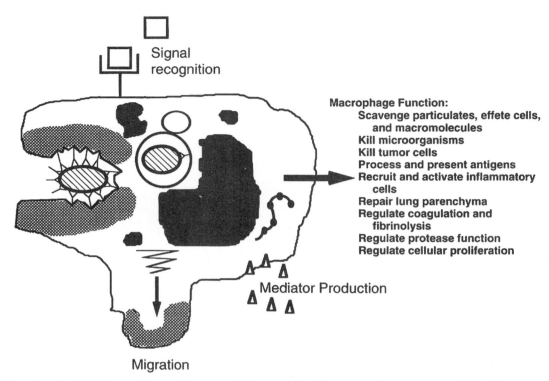

Signal
recognition

Macrophage Function:
   Scavenge particulates, effete cells,
      and macromolecules
   Kill microorganisms
   Kill tumor cells
   Process and present antigens
   Recruit and activate inflammatory
      cells
   Repair lung parenchyma
   Regulate coagulation and
      fibrinolysis
   Regulate protease function
   Regulate cellular proliferation

Mediator Production

Migration

FIGURE 33-1 Four functional attributes of macrophages can be integrated to allow macrophages to accomplish a diverse group of complex biologic functions.

RECOGNITION OF SIGNALS

Macrophages constantly sample the environment and respond to environmental stimuli. Macrophages, like virtually every cell except mature erythrocytes, ingest soluble and particulate materials from their surroundings by absorptive endocytosis or pinocytosis. Receptor-mediated endocytosis allows materials less than 1 μm in diameter to be ingested (lipoproteins and viruses, for example). Most endocytosed particles are taken up in clathrin-coated vesicles. Actin filaments have little or no role in this process.

The ability of macrophages to interact with their environment is mediated by surface receptors capable of binding specific ligands, including immunoglobulins,[12–16] complement proteins, cytokines, toxins, polysaccharides, lipids, and hormones (Table 33-1). Receptor-ligand interactions allow the macrophage to take up microorganisms and respond to cytokines and proteins. The response to stimuli that bind to the macrophage membrane is usually twofold. First, the macrophage internalizes the stimulus and subjects it to endocytic processing and digestion. Second, the macrophage secretes bioactive molecules into the surrounding environment. These two basic processes allow macrophages to participate in inflammatory and immune reactions.

This section will focus primarily on the activities of IgG and complement receptors, the most comprehensively studied of macrophage receptors.[17–19] The rate of uptake of an opsonized particle can be increased several hundredfold by the synergistic action of Fc receptors (FcR) and the receptor for the third component of complement (CR3). FcR and CR3 are key surface molecules for the clearance of microorganisms and for antibody-dependent cell cytotoxicity (ADCC).

FCγ RECEPTORS

Three sets of Fcγ receptors recognize the Fc domain of immunoglobulin G: FcγRI, FcγRII, and FcγRIII. Each of the three classes of FcγR is represented by at least two transcripts. The transcripts differ mainly in their cytoplasmic domain. All of the transcripts have closely related extracellular and transmembrane regions. The FcγRs are membrane glycoproteins having two to three extracellular domains with Ig-like features. They act as signal-transducing molecules. Generation of superoxide anions and prostaglandins, as well as membrane depolarization, can be induced via these receptors.[17] The molecular biology of the FcγR family and the intracellular signals delivered by FcγRs have recently been reviewed.[20,21]

FcγRI

FcγRI is a heavily glycosylated 72-kDa protein that is expressed principally on monocytes and macrophages.[22] Unstimulated human monocytes express approximately 10,000 to 40,000 molecules on their surface; this expression is enhanced by interferon-γ, glucocorticoids, and complement component C5a.[23,24] FcγRI binds to soluble monomeric IgG,

TABLE 33-1   Macrophage Membrane Receptors and/or Molecules Binding to Macrophage Membranes

Immunoglobulins	**Hormones and proteins**
IgG1	α_1-Antiprotease-protease complexes
IgG2	α_1-Antithrombin
IgG3	α_2-Macroglobulin-protease complexes
IgG4	Ceruloplasmin
IgE	Coagulation factor VIIa
IgA	Estrogen
Complement components	Fibrin
C1q	Fibrinogen products
C3b	Fibronectin
C3bi	Insulin
C3d	Lactoferrin
C5a	Laminin
Glycoproteins and carbohydrates	Maleylated proteins (multiple receptors)
Mannose/fucose terminal glycoproteins	Parathormone
Mannose-6-phosphate terminal glycoproteins	Progesterone
Galactose terminal glycoproteins	Transferrin
Heparin	**Peptides and small molecules**
Glycosylative protein end-products	Adenosine
Regulatory proteins and cytokines	Bombesin
M-CSF	Bradykinin
GM-CSF	Calcitonin
TFN-α	Dexamethasone
Il-1	Epinephrine
Il-2	Glucagon
Il-3	Glucocorticosteroids
Il-4	Histamine (H_1 and H_2 receptors)
IL-6	N-formylated peptides
IFN-$\alpha\beta$	Platelet-activating factor
IFN-γ	Serotonin
MCP-1	Somatomedin
MIP-1α	Somatotropin
MIP-1β	Substance P
RANTES	Tuftsin
Lipids and lipoproteins	Vasoactive intestinal peptide
LDL	1,2,5-Dihydroxyvitamin D_3
β-VLDL	**Pharmacologic agents**
Modified LDL (e.g., acetylated LDL)	Muscarinic and nicotinic cholinergic agonists
Leukotriene C	α_1/α_2-Adrenergic agonists
Leukotriene D_4	β_1/β_2-Adrenergic agonists
Leukotriene B_4	
Prostaglandin E_2	
Adhesion molecules	
LFA-1 (integrin $\alpha L\beta_2$)	
MAC-1 (integrin $\alpha M\beta_2$)	
p150/95 (integrin $\alpha X\beta_2$)	
ICAM-1	
GPIV (binds to thrombospondin)	

exhibiting a subclass specificity of IgGI > IgGIII > IgGIV > IgGII. FcγRI mediates both the binding of IgG-coated particles and the triggering of phagocytosis and cytolytic responses.[25]

FcγRII

FcγRII is a 40-kDa glycoprotein that is present on phagocytes, B lymphocytes, and platelets.[26] Surface expression of FcγRII varies from 30,000 receptors on neutrophils to 260,000 receptors on human alveolar macrophages.[27] FcγRII binds

monomeric IgG with relatively low affinity, but it effectively mediates the phagocytosis of IgG-coated particles and antibody-dependent cytotoxic reactions.[21] Binding of IgG occurs with a subclass specificity of IgGIII > IgGI > IgGIV $\gg$ IgGII.

FcγRIII

FcγRIII is a heterogeneous population of molecules (50 to 80 kDa) that are expressed on mature macrophages, neutrophils, and natural killer cells but not on blood monocytes.[21] FcγRIII mediates phagocytosis and antibody-dependent cytotoxicity in mononuclear cells, where it is expressed as a transmembrane protein.[25] FcγRIII recognizes IgG with a subclass specificity of IgGI = IgGIII ≫ IgGII = IgGIV.

The three FcγRs appear to have substantially similar functions. This redundancy may confer a selective advantage, as illustrated by patients who lack FcγRI on their monocytes.[28] These patients showed no increased susceptibility to infectious diseases, suggesting that FcγRII and FcγRIII can substitute for functions normally performed by FcγRI.

COMPLEMENT RECEPTORS

Macrophages express two distinct receptors for the third component of complement: complement receptor 1 (CR1) and complement receptor 3 (CR3). These receptors mediate binding and phagocytosis of complement-coated microorganisms and other particles.[29]

Complement Receptor 1

CR1 is a glycosylated protein that preferentially binds C3b but also recognizes C3bi and C4b. There are four allelic forms, with molecular weights of 160, 190, 220, and 250 kDa, respectively. CR1 is found on all phagocytic leukocytes, on erythrocytes, on a subpopulation of lymphocytes, and on glomerular podocytes.[30]

Complement Receptor 3

CR3 (Mo-1, Mac-1, CD11b/18), the receptor for C3bi, is a member of the β_2 integrin family that includes the lymphocyte functional antigen-1 (LFA-1) and p150,95. The integrins are all heterodimers made up of a common β subunit of about 90 kDa and distinct α subunits of 150 kDa. CR3 is found on monocytes, macrophages, granulocytes, and some lymphocytes.[31] CR3 clearly recognizes proteins in addition to C3bi. CR3 recognizes a sequence in the γ chain of fibrinogen, which is similar to the ARG-GLY-ASP (RGD) sequence recognized in C3bi. This sequence is present in both fibrinogen and fibrin and may enable phagocytes to adhere to clots.[32–35] CR3 also recognizes lipopolysaccharide (LPS) by using a binding site on CR3 distinct from that used for proteins.[36–38] The portion of LPS that is recognized is in the lipid A region. CR3 may also have the capacity to bind directly to *Histoplasma capsulatum*.[39] The capacity of CR3 to bind directly to microbes without the intervention of antibody or complement might represent an opsonin-independent mechanism by which macrophages can recognize potential pathogens before the onset of immunity.

Several observations suggest that CR3 functions in cell-cell and cell-substrate adhesion. CR3 also participates in the adhesion of phagocytic cells to endothelial cells.[40–45] Finally, evidence for a role of CR3 in adhesion phenomenon also comes from observations of patients that exhibit a genetic deficiency in the CD18 complex known as leukocyte adhesion deficiency. These patients present with recurrent life-threatening infections; phagocytes from these patients fail to bind C3bi-coated particles and show defective cytocidal activity in vitro. All patients exhibit a failure to form exudates at sites of infection.[46,47] Thus, CR3, LFA-1, and p150,95 appear to be essential for immigration of leukocytes from the vasculature and for defense against infectious agents.

MANNOSE RECEPTOR

Macrophages are capable of ingesting microorganisms in the absence of complement or immunoglobulin. Nonopsonic phagocytosis is mediated principally by oligosaccharide-containing moieties on the surface of microorganisms.[48,49] The ability to recognize surface lectins on foreign cells may represent a primitive mechanism of host defense that evolved before the appearance of immunoglobulins and complement. The best characterized of these receptors is the mannose receptor, a 162-kDa membrane glycoprotein that binds mannose and fucose-BSA with high affinity.[50,51] Alveolar macrophages and mouse inflammatory macrophages express this receptor.[52] COS cells infected with cDNA for the human mannose receptor acquire the capacity to ingest yeast, zymosan particles, and *Pneumocystis carinii*, indicating that this receptor mediates phagocytosis.[53,54]

SECRETORY PRODUCTS OF MACROPHAGES

Macrophages are highly secretory cells.[12,15,55–61] Much of the functional capacity of macrophages depends on their ability to produce and release secretory products into phagolysosomes or into the extracellular space (Table 33-2). Most of the macrophage-secreted molecules are released following stimulation and activation of the cell. Bacterial products and cytokines are the primary activation stimuli. The amount of secreted molecules varies among macrophages from different tissue compartments, depending in part on the state of differentiation of the cells. Determining the precise role of macrophage-secreted products during a physiologic or pathologic process is difficult. The spectrum of molecules released at any time during most of these processes is not known. Single macrophage products can have diverse activities, and a single activity can reflect the action of many macrophage products. Finally, few of the products listed in Table 33-2 arise solely from macrophages. Evaluation of the importance of macrophages as a source of secretory products requires a consideration of the anatomic and pathophysiologic circumstances.

In spite of these complexities, macrophage secretory products can be grouped into several categories. The cytokines released by macrophages fall into three categories. The first category includes those cytokines that promote or mediate the acute inflammatory response as well as the early responses of lymphocytes. Tissue macrophages rapidly release these cytokines following the uptake of bacteria and viruses. These cytokines include IL-1, TNF, IL-6, C-C and C-X-C chemokines, and IL-12.[62–64] These macrophage products critically influence the early local and systemic responses. A second category of cytokines includes those that inhibit inflammation. These cytokines, including IL-10, TGF-β, and IL-1 receptor antagonist, tend to be released late after stimulation and serve to dampen the response.[65–67] Finally, macrophages release cytokines that promote tissue repair following inflammation. These include platelet-derived growth factor and fibroblast growth factor, both of which induce growth of fibroblasts and angiogenesis.[58]

Numerous secretory products are involved in host defense processes. Macrophages generate at least 10 components of

TABLE 33-2   Secretory Products of Macrophages

Cytokines, growth factors, and hormones
  Growth factors
    GM-GSF
    M-CSF
    G-CSF
    Erythropoietin
    Erythroid colony potentiating factor
    Factor increasing monocytopoiesis (FIM)
  Proteins involved in host defense and inflammation
    C1
    C4
    C2
    C3
    C5
    Factor B
    Factor D
    C3b inactivation
    βIH
    Lysozyme
    Interferon-γ
    Fibronectin
    Lactoferrin
  Cytokines that promote acute inflammation and regulate lymphocytes
    TNF
    IL-1α/β
    IL-6
    IL-8
    IL-12
    GROα/β/γ
    CTAPIII
    β-Thromboglobulin
    IP-10
    MCP-1
    MIP-1α
    MIP-1β
  Cytokines that inhibit acute inflammation and lymphocyte responses
    IL-10
    TGF-β1,2,3
    IL-1 receptor antagonist
  Factors that promote tissue repair
    Platelet-derived growth factor (PDGF)
    Fibroblast growth factor (FGF)
    Angiogenesis factor
  Hormones
    1α-dehydroxyvitamin D_3
    Insulin-like activity
Reactive oxygen intermediates
  O_2^-
  H_2O_2
  OH·
Reactive nitrogen intermediates
  NO·
  NO_2
  NO_3
Enzymes that affect connective tissues and serum proteins
  Acid hydrolases
  Acid phosphatases
  Amyloid proteinase

  Amylase
  β-Galactosidase
  β-Glucuronidase
  Cathepsins
  Collagenases (types I, II, III, and IV)
  Cytolytic proteinase
  Elastase
  Hyaluronidase
  Lipoprotein lipase
  Lysozyme
  Nucleases
  Phospholipase A_2
  Plasminogen activator
  Ribonucleases
  Sulfatases
Inhibitors of enzymes
  α_1-Antichymotrypsin
  α_1-Antiprotease
  α_2-Macroglobulin
  Inhibitors of plasminogen
  Inhibitors of plasminogen activator
  Lipomodulin
Matrix proteins
  Chondroitin sulfate proteoglycans
  Fibronectin
  Gelatin-binding protein
  Thrombospondin
Lipids
  PGE_2
  $PGF_{2\alpha}$
  Prostacylin
  Thromboxane A_2
  Leukotrienes B, C, D, and E
  Mono-HETES
  Di-HETES
  PAF
  Lysophospholipids
Coagulation factors
  Factor X
  Factor IX
  Factor V
  Thromboplastin
  Prothrombin
  Thrombospondin
  Fibrinolysis inhibitor
  Tissue factor
  Factor VII/VIIA
  Factor X activator
  Prothrombinase
Small molecules
  Purines
  Pyrimidines
  Glutathione
  Thymidine
  Uracil
  Uric acid
  Deoxycytidine
  Neopterin
  cAMP

the complement cascade, which are crucial for the recognition and ingestion of microbes. Macrophages produce reactive oxygen intermediates, reactive nitrogen intermediates, and lysosomes, all of which are crucial for the killing of intracellular pathogenic microorganisms.[68–70]

Macrophages also release enzymes that affect connective tissue proteins. Enzymes that degrade connective tissue include elastase, collagenases, and plasminogen activators. Inhibitors of proteolytic enzymes include α_1-antiprotease, α_2-macroglobulin, and plasminogen activator inhibitor.

Macrophage Functions

Macrophages can complete complex biologic tasks by virtue of their capacity to recognize and take up a wide range of exogenous materials and then respond by releasing biologi-

cally relevant molecules. Macrophages can (1) initiate cell-mediated immune responses, (2) dampen immune responses, (3) participate in the wound healing and repair process that follows inflammation, and (4) destroy microorganisms. Antigen presentation and microbicidal function will be discussed in more detail later.

The ability of macrophages to degrade complex antigens and to present small fragments of the antigen to T lymphocytes in the context of class I and class II major histocompatibility (MHC) antigens forms the basis for the initiation of cell-mediated immunity. Antigen presentation requires endocytosis and degradation of the protein; transport of the immunogenic peptide to the membrane surface via MHC antigens; membrane expression of class I or class II MHC antigens; expression of adhesion molecules, including ICAM and LFA-1; expression of costimulatory molecules, including B7; and secretion of soluble cytokines (Fig. 33-2).

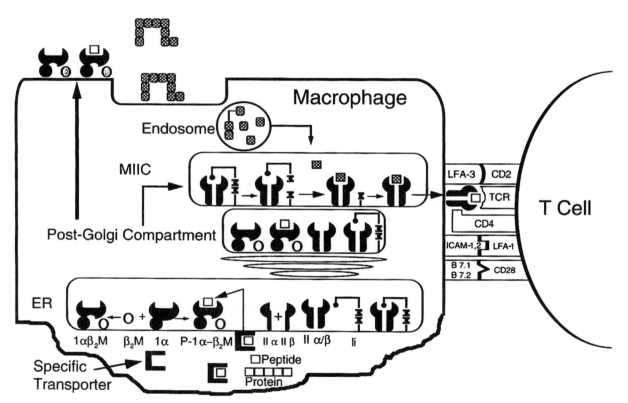

FIGURE 33-2 Pathways for antigen processing and presentation by macrophages. *MHC II:* MHC IIα and MHC IIβ chains assemble in the endoplasmic reticulum (ER). The class II invariant chain (li) binds to MHC II to inhibit binding of endogenous peptides to MHC II in the ER. The MHC II-li complex is transported to a post-Golgi compartment and then to a late endosome, referred to as the MIIC. In the MIIC, li is cleaved, and the processed antigen binds to MHC II. The peptides that bind to MHC II are derived from exogenous proteins that are proteolytically processed in the endosome. Peptide binding to MHC II signals the egress of the MHC II-peptide molecule to the cell surface. *MHC I:* The 45-kDa class I heavy chain and the 15-kDa β_2-microglobulin chain associate in the ER. Proteins present in

the cytoplasm or ER (endogenous or viral peptides) are the primary source of class I peptides. Endogenous peptides bind to class I and are transported to the cell surface. Cell-surface molecules on macrophages have the ability to interact with cell-surface molecules on T lymphocytes. Antigen-induced stimulation results from interaction of MHC II-peptide with the TCR. Accessory molecules contribute by (1) functioning as adhesion molecules strengthening the interaction between the macrophage and the T cell (LFA-1/ICAM, CD2/LFA-3), (2) modifying the TCR-mediated transmembrane signal (CD4), or (3) initiating distinct costimulatory signals required to activate resting T cells (B7.1, B7.2/CD28).

Macrophages also are a major effector cell for the destruction of microorganisms. Destruction of a microorganism requires recognition and binding of the microbe; phagocytosis; formation of a phagolysosome; initiation of a respiratory burst; and release of the products of the respiratory burst enzymes and cationic proteins into the phagosome to destroy the microbe. The destruction of a tumor cell requires a similar sequence of events.

ACTIVATION OF LYMPHOCYTES BY MACROPHAGES

The activation of T lymphocytes is a central event in the development of immune responses. This event is antigen-specific, depending on the recognition of the appropriate antigenic epitope by the T-cell receptor/CD3 complex.[71,72] The T-cell receptor (TCR) recognizes partially digested (processed) peptides (11 to 30 amino acids long).[73,74] The antigen can only be recognized when it is associated with cell-surface MHC glycoproteins on another cell.[75,76] Thus, activation of lymphocytes requires the participation of an antigen-presenting cell (APC).[77–82]

ANTIGEN PROCESSING
An immunogenic determinant can be expressed on the surface of the antigen-presenting cell in association with an MHC molecule 30 to 60 min after internalization.[83–85] Several distinct antigen processing pathways have been defined. The pathway used depends on whether the antigen is an exogenous protein that has been internalized by the cell or an endogenously synthesized protein, such as a viral antigen produced in an infected cell. The type of antigen-presenting cell involved is also a critical determinant. Two distinct forms of MHC molecules exist. Exogenous antigens are usually presented in association with class II MHC molecules (HLA-DP, -DQ, -DR in humans), while endogenous antigens are presented in association with class I molecules (HLA-A, -B, -C in humans)[86–93] (Fig. 33-2). This discussion is limited to the processing and presentation of exogenous proteins.

Most exogenous protein antigens are internalized by standard endocytic or phagocytic processes. The great bulk of internalized proteins are transported to acidic compartments, where they are degraded to amino acids or small peptides. Processing consists of both the fragmentation of proteins to peptides and the unfolding of the protein antigen.[94–97] The denatured peptides have the conformational structure required to associate with and bind to class II MHC molecules. The length of peptides isolated from class II molecules is 11 to 30 residues.[98–101] Class II MHC molecules not only select the peptide but also save it from complete degradation. The interaction between MHC molecules and processed antigen likely takes place in a distinct free lysosomal vesicle termed the MIIC.[102–111] The association of the processed antigen and the class II MHC dimer results in a stable molecule which is expressed on the cell surface of the antigen-presenting cell.

ANTIGEN-PRESENTING CELL/T LYMPHOCYTE INTERACTION
A central event in the interaction between an antigen-presenting cell and a T lymphocyte is the recognition of the anti-genic epitope presented in association with the MHC molecule by the TCR/CD3 complex. Thus, the expression of class II MHC on the macrophage membrane is necessary for the cell to function as an APC. Macrophage class II MHC expression is regulated. Human monocytes and macrophages express a basal level of class II MHC proteins, but the level of expression increases markedly after exposure to IFN-γ.[112,113] Upregulation of class II MHC expression in vivo is particularly striking after infection with microorganisms.[114]

While the binding of the T-cell receptor to the MHC peptide complex of the APC provides specificity for T-cell activation, T-cell activation requires other complementary interactions. Several receptor-ligand interactions occur that are believed to promote cell-to-cell contact as well as to provide important transmembrane signaling.[115,116] LFA-1 molecules on the T cell interact with ICAM-1 molecules on the APC, and CD2 interacts with LFA-3. CD4 interacts with class II MHC molecules. Engagement of the T-cell receptor promotes cell-to-cell contact. Engagement of the T-cell receptor changes the affinity of the LFA-1 molecule without increasing the number of molecules on the T-cell surface. Similar mechanisms appear to operate for CD4 and CD2. The expression of ICAM-1 also is upregulated during this response; ICAM-1 increases in response to IL-1 and IFN-γ and after macrophages bind to substrates.[117–123]

Antigen-presenting cells also express membrane molecules that regulate the response, growth, and differentiation of T cells. B7 is an important costimulatory molecule that is expressed on APCs. B7 is a member of the immunoglobulin superfamily; it binds to its counter-receptor (CD28 or CTLA-4) on CD4+ T cells.[124–128] Engagement of CD28 by B7 enhances transcription of cytokine genes, particularly through the expression of an enhancer protein that binds to the IL-2 gene.[129,130] Anti-B7 monoclonal antibodies block antigen presentation and the mixed leukocyte response (MLR), indicating their important costimulatory role.[131,132]

Other cytokines are also released during antigen-presenting T-cell interactions. While IL-1 originally was believed to be a major costimulatory molecule, its role as a stimulatory molecule for T-cell activation is more limited than initially proposed. The expression of IL-1 by macrophages is influenced profoundly during antigen presentation. CD4-macrophage contact induces transcription of IL-1 mRNA. The expression and eventual secretion of IL-1 likely importantly affects the local microenvironment in which antigen presentation takes place.[133]

The presence of costimulatory molecules may be an important determinant of the outcome of an APC-T-cell interaction. Anergy rather than activation results when murine T cells recognize antigen bound to class II MHC molecules in the absence of costimulators.[134–136] While the exact molecular basis of these interactions is unclear, it is certain that the early cascade of macrophage-T-cell interactions is important in determining the outcome of in vivo antigen presentation.

The interplay between macrophages and lymphocytes is a critical process that is central to the development and maintenance of an immune response. The interplay between macrophages and T cells is reciprocal and symbiotic. The interaction results in the activation of both cells, and both cells have obligate requirements for each other for their function. CD4+ cells cannot recognize antigens unless an APC processes the protein antigen and exhibits the peptide/class II MHC complex to the TCR/CD3 complex. Macrophages require cytokines secreted by activated CD4+ T cells to express their full spectrum of functions. Thus, innate immunity and specific immunity are tightly interrelated.

ROLE OF PULMONARY MACROPHAGES IN ANTIGEN PRESENTATION

Alveolar macrophages are less effective than blood monocytes in inducing proliferation of blood T lymphocytes in response to soluble "recall" antigens.[137–144] Alveolar macrophages are also less effective than other accessory cells in activating T lymphocytes necessary for antibody production.[145,146] In contrast, alveolar macrophages are as effective as accessory cells in the induction of proliferation of blood T lymphocytes by mitogenic lectins.[137–139,143,147,148] Furthermore, alveolar macrophages effectively stimulate the proliferation of T-lymphocyte lines and clones in response to soluble antigens.[141,142,149] These findings suggest that alveolar macrophages restimulate recently activated T cells effectively but are ineffective in stimulating the proliferation of naive T lymphocytes or resting memory cells.

Alveolar macrophages produce a variety of mediators that inhibit lymphocyte proliferation, including prostaglandin E_2, superoxide anion, and vitamin D metabolites.[146,148,150,151] While this effect appears to be dominant when macrophages outnumber the target T lymphocytes, suppressive influences do not entirely explain the inability of these cells to serve efficiently as accessory cells for antigen-induced responses.[137,139] Alveolar macrophages might excessively degrade intracellular antigens.[152,153] The capacity of alveolar macrophages to bind with T lymphocytes also is less than that of monocytes.[142]

Resident alveolar macrophages may be an important means by which the lung disposes of potentially antigenic inhaled substances without initiating an immune response. In fact, depletion of alveolar macrophages in vivo dramatically enhances the capacity of experimental animals to generate immune responses against inhaled antigens.[154] However, the role of alveolar macrophages likely changes once an inflammatory response against foreign antigens is occurring in the lung. Alveolar macrophages from patients with sarcoidosis function better as antigen-presenting cells for antigen-induced lymphocyte proliferation than do monocytes.[140,155] This change in alveolar macrophage function may represent the recruitment of less mature macrophages,[156] cytokine-induced expression of greater amounts of class II MHC antigens,[157] or release of greater amounts of cytokines.[158,159] Additionally, an influx of T lymphocytes may foster productive alveolar macrophage-lymphocyte interactions. Thus, alveolar macrophages appear to play an important role in locally amplifying a developing pulmonary immune response.

MICROBIAL KILLING

Macrophages represent a major defense against invasion of the host by a wide variety of microorganisms, including bacteria, fungi, viruses, and protozoa. Failure to kill microbes can result from a failure at the stage of recognition, disposition, or killing. Failure to kill a microbe may result from abnormalities in the macrophage or from active subversion of the destructive process by the microorganism.

MICROBIAL RECOGNITION

Macrophages recognize microbes primarily through the action of opsonins—molecules that bind to specific sites on both the macrophage and the microbe. IgG and complement are the most extensively studied opsonins. These opsonins bind to Fcγ receptors and complement receptors, respectively, on the surface of macrophages. Fcγ receptors and mannose receptors on macrophages are constitutively active. These receptors bind ligands on microbes and induce the phagocytosis of the bound particles. CRI and CRIII constitutively mediate binding of complement-coated particles. When appropriately activated, they also mediate phagocytosis.[160–162] However, ligation of CRI and CRIII does not initiate certain cellular activities that follow Fc receptor ligation. Stimulation of CRI and CRIII does not stimulate release of arachidonate metabolites and does not promote secretion of H_2O_2 by these cells.[163,164] It is of interest that several microbes that multiply inside macrophages, such as *Mycobacterium tuberculosis*, *Legionella pneumophila*, *Histoplasma capsulatum*, and *Mycobacterium leprae*, all are ingested by way of CR3 on the surface of macrophages. The inability of CRIII to activate the respiratory burst might allow these organisms to be engulfed without oxidant injury.

PHAGOCYTOSIS

The nature of the intracellular signal(s) that mediates the movement of pseudopods around ligand-coated microbes is unknown. The response of macrophages to ligation of phagocytosis-promoting receptors is highly localized in the cytoplasm.[165] Accordingly, it is likely that ligated receptors present binding sites for cytoskeletal proteins rather than generating signals through soluble molecules. In most instances, FcγR and complement receptors must diffuse in the plane of the macrophage plasma membrane to engage the immobile opsonins bound to the capsules of microbes. Both receptors exhibit great lateral mobility and aggregate in zones in which ligands are concentrated.[166,167] Particle engulfment requires engagement of specific receptors and the generation of transmembrane signals. Movement of the phagocyte plasma membrane over a ligand-coated particle is governed by the availability of unbound receptors on the surface of the phagocyte and of ligands on the surface of the particle (zipper hypothesis).[168,169] Thus, particle engulfment requires the sequential and circumferential interaction of phagocyte surface receptors with complementary ligands on the surface of the particle.

While sequential interactions between ligands on a particle and receptors on a phagocyte are necessary conditions, they are not sufficient. Receptor ligation initiates transmembrane signals that promote metabolic changes and cytoskeletal rearrangements in the underlying cytoplasm. The intracellular signals generated by these receptors and the mechanisms by which they regulate cytoskeletal activities remain uncertain.

Actin appears to play a central role in the movement of the cell membrane around the particle.[170–174] The assembly and cross-linking of F-actin filaments leads to the formation of a scaffolding of actin filaments in the zone of cytoplasm adjacent to a particle undergoing engulfment. The formation of this stiff gel, which increases in volume as actin is progressively recruited, and the protrusion of this gel against a relatively compliant plasma membrane is believed to cause pseudopod extension and additional plasma membrane contact with the surface of the particle.[175,176] CR3 may also be linked to the cytoskeleton.

SECRETION OF LYTIC EFFECTOR SUBSTANCES

The term *macrophage* covers a continuum of cellular alteration beginning with blood marrow precursors and continuing through the blood monocyte to the fully developed tissue macrophage. The transformation of monocytes to macrophages in culture results in a marked decline in antimicrobial activity. Monocytes most nearly resemble neutrophils in their antimicrobial systems.

Monocytes respond to stimulation with a brisk respiratory burst resulting in the production of a variety of oxygen radicals, such as superoxide anion, hydrogen peroxide, hydroxyl radical, and singlet oxygen.[177] However, this respiratory burst is weaker than that produced by an equivalent number of neutrophils. Monocytes contain a peroxidase in cytoplasmic granules that is identical to the myeloperoxidase (MPO) of neutrophils.[178] After particle ingestion, the MPO of monocytes is released into the phagosome, where it can react with H_2O_2 and a halide to form a microbicidal system. Stimulated monocytes form a chlorinated species, presumably ClOH.[179,180] The MPO-H_2O_2-halide system has been implicated in the killing of *Candida albicans* and *Aspergillus fumigatus* by human monocytes.[179,181,182]

Transformation of human monocytes to macrophages in culture results in a marked decline in antimicrobial activity against a variety of pathogens, including *Cryptococcus neoformans*, *Toxoplasma gondii*, and *Leishmania donovani*.[183–185] This decrease in potency is related to a decrease in the magnitude of the respiratory burst and the loss of the granule peroxidase over time. As monocytes mature into tissue macrophages in vivo or in vitro, the granule peroxidase is lost.[186,187]

The respiratory burst of resident macrophages in response to stimulation is increased severalfold when macrophages are activated in vivo.[188,189] Activation of macrophages can be induced in vitro by the addition of GM-CSF, TNF-α, and interferon-γ.[190–192] The oxygen-dependent microbicidal activity of mature, activated macrophages may be due to the formation of H_2O_2, hydroxyl radical, and/or nitrogen oxides.

Activated macrophages form nitrite (NO_2), nitrate (NO_3), and nitric oxide (NO·) by the oxidation of the guanidine nitrogen of L-arginine with the formation of L-citrulline.[193–196] Nitrogen oxide formation by macrophages appears to contribute to tumor cell injury, fungistasis, and antiparasitic activity.[197–200] Nitrogen oxides may produce their injurious effect in part by causing iron loss from the target cell by an attack on iron-sulfur centers, with associated inhibition of DNA synthesis and mitochondrial respiration.

Macrophages also use nonoxidative mechanisms to kill microbes, including proteases, lysozyme, acid hydrolases, and defensins.[201] Defensins are present in the alveolar macrophages of some species. The defensins exist as multiple members of a closely related family of broad-spectrum cytotoxic peptides. Defensins kill many gram-positive organisms (*Staphylococcus epidermidis*, *Staphylococcus aureus*, *Streptococcus*, and *Listeria monocytogenes*). They also kill gram-negative bacterial species (*E. coli*, *Pseudomonas aeruginosa*, *Klebsiella pneumoniae*), but less effectively than gram-positive organisms. Defensins also kill fungi and inactivate certain viruses.[202,203]

Summary

Macrophages are multifaceted, versatile cells. They are admirably equipped to recognize and destroy rapidly replicating prokaryotic and eukaryotic invaders. By virtue of their enormous array of membrane-bound receptors and secretory products, macrophages also regulate the proliferation and function of other cells, such as lymphocytes. Macrophage functions can be upregulated profoundly by exposure to a wide variety of extracellular stimuli. The functions exhibited by a given macrophage population likely depend on the precise inductive and suppressive signals that have been received. The appropriate regulation of macrophage function is essential to the well-being of the host. An inability to activate macrophages can lead to an inability to destroy microbes and may have profoundly deleterious consequences for the host. Alternatively, exuberant stimulation or insufficient suppression can lead to extensive tissue injury. An understanding of the molecular mechanisms involved in the control of macrophage development and activation are likely to provide critical points for pharmacologic intervention.

References

1. Ersle VAJ, Lichtman MA: Structure and function of the marrow, in Williams WJ, Beutler E, Ersle VAJ, Lichtman MA (eds): *Hematology.* New York, McGraw-Hill, 1990: 37.
2. Lambertesen RH, Weiss L: A model of intramedullary hematopoietic microenvironments based on stereologic study of the distribution of endocloned marrow colonies. *Blood* 1984; 63:287.
3. Sieff CA: Hematopoietic growth factors. *J Clin Invest* 1987; 79:1549.
4. Metcalf D: Haematopoietic growth factors: 1. *Lancet* 1989; 1:825.

5. Metcalf D: The molecular control of normal and leukemic granulocyte and macrophages. *Proc R Soc Lond [Biol]* 1987; 230:389.

6. Whitelaw DM: The intravascular life span of monocytes. *Blood* 1966; 28:445.

7. Whitelaw DM: Observations on human monocyte kinetics after pulse labeling. *Cell Tissue Kinet* 1972; 5:311.

8. Meuret G, Hoffmann G: Monocyte kinetic studies in normal and disease states. *Br J Haematol* 1973; 24:275.

9. Thomas ED, Rambegh RE, Sale GE, et al.: Direct evidence for bone marrow origin of the alveolar macrophage in man. *Science* 1976; 192:1016.

10. Winston DJ, Territo MC, Ho WG, et al.: Alveolar macrophage dysfunction in human bone marrow transplant recipients. *Am J Med* 1982; 73:859.

11. Bitterman PB, Saltzman LE, Adelberg S, et al.: Alveolar macrophage replication: one mechanism for the expansion of the mononuclear phagocyte population in the chronically inflamed lung. *J Clin Invest* 1984; 74:460.

12. Adams, DO, Hamilton TA: The cell biology of macrophage activation. *Annu Rev Immunol* 1984; 2:283.

13. Springer TA: Adhesion receptors of the immune system. *Nature* 1990; 346:425.

14. Gordon S, Perry UH, Rabinowitz S, et al.: Plasma membrane receptors of the mononuclear phagocyte system. *J Cell Sci [Suppl]* 1988; 9:1.

15. Adams DO, Hamilton TA: Macrophages as destructive cells, in Gallin JI, Goldstein IM, Snyderman R (eds): *Host Defenses in Inflammation: Basic Principles and Clinical Correlates*, 2nd ed. New York, Raven Press, 1992; 637.

16. Uquccioni M, D'Apuzzo M, Loetscher M, et al.: Actions of the chemotactic cytokines MCP-1, MCP-2, RANTES, MIP-1δ, MIP-1β on human monocytes. *Eur J Immunol* 1995; 25:64.

17. Ravetch JV, Kinet J: Fc receptors. *Annu Rev Immunol* 1991; 9:457.

18. Brown EJ: Complement receptors and phagocytosis. *Curr Opin Immunol* 1991; 3:76.

19. Rosen H, Law SKA: The leukocyte cell surface receptor(s) for the iC3b product of complement. *Curr Top Microbiol Immunol* 1989; 99.

20. Mellman I: Relationships between structure and function in the Fc receptor family. *Curr Opin Immunol* 1988; 1:16.

21. Funger MW, Shen L, Graziano RF, Guyre PM: Cytotoxicity mediated by human Fc receptors for IgG. *Immunol Today* 1989; 111:97.

22. Peltz G, Frederick K, Anderson CL, Peterlin BM: Characterization of the human monocyte high affinity Fc receptor (huFcRI). *Mol Immunol* 1988; 25:243.

23. Perussia B, Dayton ET, Lazarus R, et al.: Immune interferon induces the receptor for monomeric IgGI on human monocytic and myeloid cells. *J Exp Med* 1983; 158:1092.

24. Kurlander RJ, Batker J: The binding of human immunoglobulin G1 monomer and small, covalently cross-linked polymers of immunoglobulin G1 to human peripheral blood monocytes and polymorphonuclear leukocytes. *J Clin Invest* 1982; 69:1.

25. Anderson CL, Shen L, Eicher DM, et al.: Phagocytosis mediated by three distinct Fc receptor classes on human leukocytes. *J Exp Med* 1990; 171:1333.

26. Unkless JC, Scigliano E, Freedman VH: Structure and function of human and murine receptors for IgG. *Annu Rev Immunol* 1988; 6:251.

27. Rossman MD, Chen E, Chien P, et al.: Fc receptor recognition of IgG ligand by human monocytes and macrophages. *Am J Respir Cell Mol Biol* 1989; 1:211.

28. Ceuppens JL, Baroja ML, Van Vaeck F, Anderson CL: Defect in the membrane expression of high affinity 72-kD Fcγ receptors on phagocytic cells in four healthy subjects. *J Clin Invest* 1988; 82:571.

29. Ehlenberger AG, Nussenzweig V: The role of membrane receptors for C3b and C3d in phagocytosis. *J Exp Med* 1977; 145:357.

30. Ahearn JM, Fearon DT: Structure and function of the complement receptors CR1 (CD35) and CR2 (CD21). *Adv Immunol* 1989; 46:183.

31. Hynes RO: Integrins: versatility, modulation, and signaling in cell adhesion. *Cell* 1992; 69:11.

32. Wright SD, Reddy PA, Jong MTC, Erickson BW: C3b1 receptor (complement receptor type 3) recognizes a region of complement protein C3 containing the sequence Arg-Gly-Asp. *Proc Natl Acad Sci USA* 1987; 84:1965.

33. Wright SD, Weitz JI, Huang AJ, et al.: Complement receptor type three (CD11b/CD18) of human polymorphonuclear leukocytes recognizes fibrogen. *Proc Natl Acad Sci USA* 1988; 85:7734.

34. Altieri DC, Bader R, Mannucci PM, Edgington TS: Oligospecificity of the cellular adhesion receptor MAC-1 encompasses an inducible recognition specificity for fibrinogen. *J Cell Biol* 1988; 107:1893.

35. Wright SD, Lo SK, Detmers PA: Specificity and regulation of CD18-dependent adhesions, in Springer TA, Anderson DC, Rothlein R, Rosenthal AS, (eds): *Leukocyte Adhesion Molecules: Structure, Function, and Regulation*. New York, Springer-Verlag, 1989; 190.

36. Wright SD, Jong MTC: Adhesion-promoting receptors on human macrophages recognize *E. coli* by binding to lipopolysaccharide. *J Exp Med* 1986; 164:1876.

37. Wright SD, Levin SM, Jong MTC, et al.: CR3 (CD11b/CD18) expresses one binding site for Arg-Gly-Asp-containing peptides, and a second site for bacterial lipopolysaccharide. *J Exp Med* 1989; 169:175.

38. Dana N, Styrt B, Griffin JD, et al.: Two functional domains in the phagocyte membrane glycoprotein Mol identified with monoclonal antibodies. *J Immunol* 1986; 137:3259.

39. Bullock WE, Wright SD: The role of adherence-promoting receptors, CR3, LFA-1, and p150.95 in binding of *Histoplasma capsulatum* by human macrophages. *J Exp Med* 1987; 165:195.

40. Rosen H, Gordon S: Monoclonal antibody to the murine type 3 complement receptor inhibits adhesion of myelomonocytic cells in vitro and inflammatory cell recruitment in vivo. *J Exp Med* 1987; 166:1685.

41. Tuomanen El, Saukkonen K, Sande S, et al.: Reduction of inflammation, tissue damage, and mortality in bacterial meningitis in rabbits treated with monoclonal antibodies against adhesion-promoting receptors of leukocytes. *J Exp Med* 1988; 170:959.

42. Wallis WJ, Hickstein DD, Schwartz BR, et al.: Monoclonal antibody-defined functional epitopes on the adhesion-promoting glycoprotein complex (CDw18) of human neutrophils. *Blood* 1986; 67:1007.

43. Lo SK, van Seventer GA, Levin SM, Wright SD: Two leukocyte receptors (CD11a/CD18 and CD11b/CD18) mediate transient adhesion to endothelium by binding to different ligands. *J Immunol* 1989; 143:3325.

44. Lo SK, Detmers PA, Levin SM, Wright SD: Transient adhesion of neutrophils to endothelium. *J Exp Med* 1989; 169:1779.

45. Wright SD, Detmers PA: Adhesion-promoting receptors on phagocytes. *J Cell Sci [Suppl]* 1988; 9:99.

46. Anderson DC, Springer TA: Leukocyte adhesion deficiency: an inherited defect in the Mac-1, LFA-1, and p150,95 glycoproteins. *Annu Rev Med* 1987; 38:175.

47. Todd RF III, Freyer DR: The CD11/CD18 leukocyte glycoprotein deficiency. *Hematol/Oncol Clin North Am* 1988; 2:13.

48. Sharon N: Surface carbohydrates and surface lectins are recognition determinants in phagocytosis. *Immunol Today* 1984; 5:143.

49. Ofek I, Sharon N: Lectinophagocytosis: a molecular mechanism of recognition between cell surface sugars and lectins in the phagocytosis of bacteria. *Infect Immun* 1988; 56:539.

50. Ezekowitz RAB: The mannose receptor and phagocytosis, In van Furth R (ed): *Mononuclear Phagocytes: Biology of Monocytes and Macrophages*. Dordrecht, Kluwer, 1992: 208.

51. Taylor ME, Conary JT, Lennartz MR, et al.: Primary structure of the mannose receptor contains multiple motifs resembling carbohydrate-recognition domains. *J Biol Chem* 1990; 265:12156.

52. Shepherd VL, Campbell EJ, Senior RM, Stahl PD: Characterization of the mannose/fucose receptor on human mononuclear phagocytes. *J Retic Soc* 1982; 32:423.

53. Ezekowitz RA, Williams DJ, Koziel H, et al.: Uptake of *Pneumocystis carinii* mediated by the macrophage mannose receptor. *Nature* 1991; 351:155.

54. Ezekowitz RA, Sastry K, Bailly P, Warner A: Molecular characterization of the human macrophage mannose receptor: demonstration of multiple carbohydrate recognition-like domains and phagocytosis of yeasts in Cos-1 cells. *J Exp Med* 1990; 172:1785.

55. Gordon S: Biology of the macrophage. *J Cell Sci [Suppl]* 1986; 4:267.

56. Nathan CF: Secretory products of macrophages. *J Clin Invest* 1987; 79:319.

57. Helin EH: Macrophage procoagulant factors—mediators of inflammatory and neoplastic tissue lesions. *Med Biol* 1986; 64:167.

58. Rappolee DA, Werb Z: Macrophage derived growth factors. *Curr Top Microbiol Immunol* 1992; 181:87.

59. Unanue ER: Macrophages, antigen presenting cells and the phenomena of antigen handling and presentation, in Paul WE (ed): *Fundamental Immunology*, 3rd ed. New York, Raven Press, 1993; 111.

60. Takemura R, Werb Z: Secretory products of macrophages and their physiological function. *Am J Physiol* 1984; 246:C1.

61. Auger MJ, Ross JA: The biology of the macrophage, in Lewis CE, McGee JO'D (eds): *The Macrophage*. Oxford, Oxford University Press, 1992; 1.

62. Wolpe SD, Cerami A: Macrophage inflammatory proteins 1 and 2: members of a novel superfamily of cytokines. *FASEB J* 1989; 3:2565.

63. Oppenheim JJ, Zachariae COC, Mukaida N, Matsushima K: Properties of the novel proinflammatory supergene intercrine cytokine family. *Annu Rev Immunol* 1991; 9:617.

64. Wolf SF, Temple PA, Kobayashi M, et al.: Cloning of cDNA for natural killer cell stimulatory factor. *J Immunol* 1991; 146:3074.

65. de Vries JE: Interleukin 10 (IL-10) inhibits cytokine synthesis by human monocytes: an autoregulatory role of IL-10 produced by monocytes. *J Exp Med* 1991; 174:1209.

66. Assoian AK, Fleurodelys BE, Stevenson HC, et al.: Expression and secretion of type-β transforming growth factor by activated human macrophages. *Proc Natl Acad Sci USA* 1987; 84:6020.

67. Arend WP, Welgus HG, Thompson RC, Eisenberg SP: Biological properties of recombinant human monocyte-derived interleukin-1 receptor antagonist. *J Clin Invest* 1990; 85:1694.

68. Nathan CF, Tsunawaki S: Secretion of toxic oxygen products by macrophages: regulatory cytokines and their effects on the oxidase, in Evered D, Nugent J, O'Connor M (eds): *Biochemistry of Macrophages*. Ciba Foundation Symposium 118. London, Pitman, 1986; 211.

69. Hibbs JB, Taintor RR, Vavrin Z, Rachlin EM: Nitric oxide: a cytotoxic activated macrophage effector molecule. *Biochem Biophys Res Commun* 1988; 157:87.

70. Green SJ, Nacy CA, Meltzer MS: Cytokine-induced synthesis of nitrogen oxide in macrophages. *J Leukocyte Biol* 1991; 50:93.

71. Clevers H, Alarcon B, Wileman T, Terhorst C: The T cell receptor/CD3 complex: a dynamic protein ensemble. *Annu Rev Immunol* 1988; 6:629.

72. Davis MM, Bjorkman PJ: T-cell antigen receptor genes and T-cell recognition. *Nature* 1988; 334:395.

73. Bevan MJ: Class discrimination in the world of immunology. *Nature* 1987; 325:192.

74. Sette A, Buus S, Colon S, et al.: Structural characteristics of an antigen required for its interaction with Ia and recognition by T cells. *Nature* 1987; 328:395.

75. Rosenthal AS, Shevach EM: Function of macrophages in antigen recognition by guinea pig T lymphocytes: I. Requirement for histocompatible macrophages and lymphocytes. *J Exp Med* 1973; 138:1194.

76. Shevach EM, Rosenthal AS: Function of macrophages in antigen recognition by guinea pig T lymphocytes: II. Role of the macrophage in the regulation of genetic control of the immune response. *J Exp Med* 1973; 138:1213.

77. Babbit BP, Allen PM, Matsueda G, et al.: Binding of immunogenic peptides to Ia histocompatibility molecules. *Nature* 1985; 317:359.

78. Buus S, Colon S, Smith C, et al.: Interaction between a "processed" ovalbumin peptide and Ia molecules. *Proc Natl Acad Sci USA* 1986; 83:3968.

79. Bjorkman PJ, Saper MA, Samraoui B, et al.: Structure of the human class I histocompatibility antigen, HLA-A2. *Nature* 1987; 329:506.

80. Bjorkman PJ, Saper MA, Samraoui B, et al.: The foreign antigen binding site and T cell recognition regions of class I histocompatibility antigens. *Nature* 1987; 329:506.

81. Unanue ER: The regulatory role of macrophages in antigenic stimulation: II. Symbiotic relationship between lymphocytes and macrophages. *Adv Immunol* 1981; 31:1.

82. Vitetta ES, Fernandez-Botran R, Myers CD, Sanders VM: Cellular interactions in the humoral immune response. *Adv Immunol* 1989; 45:1.

83. Lanzavecchia A: Receptor-mediated antigen uptake and its effect on antigen presentation to class II-restricted T lymphocytes. *Annu Rev Immunol* 1990; 8:773.

84. Ziegler K, Unanue ER: Identification of a macrophage antigen-processing event required for I-region-restricted antigen presentation to lymphocytes. *J Immunol* 1981; 127:1869.

85. Harding CV, Unanue ER: Antigen processing and intracellular Ia: possible roles of endocytosis and protein synthesis in Ia function. *J Immunol* 1989; 142:12.

86. Buus S, Sette A, Colon SM, et al.: The relation between major histocompatibility complex (MHC) restriction and the capacity of Ia to bind immunogenic peptides. *Science* 1987; 235:1353.

87. Germain RN: The ins and outs of antigen processing and presentation. *Nature* 1986; 322:687.

88. Townsend A, Ohlen C, Bastin J, et al.: Association of class I major histocompatibility heavy and light chains induced by viral peptides. *Nature* 1989; 340:443.

89. Sweetser MT, Morrison LA, Braciale VL, Braciale TJ: Recognition of preprocessed endogenous antigen by class I but not class II MHC-restricted T cells. *Nature* 1989; 342:180.

90. Staerz UD, Karasuyama H, Garner AM: Cytotoxic T lymphocytes against a soluble protein. *Nature* 1987; 329:449.

91. Nuchtern JG, Biddison WE, Klausner RD: Class II MHC molecules can use the endogenous pathway of antigen presentation. *Nature* 1990; 343:74.

92. Schwartz RH: Fugue in T-lymphocyte recognition. *Nature* 1987; 326:738.

93. Braciale T, Braciale U: Antigen presentation: structural themes and functional variations. *Immunol Today* 1991; 12:124.

94. Chestnut R, Colon S, Grey HM: Requirement for the processing of antigens by antigen presenting B cells: I. Functional comparison of B cell tumors and macrophages. *J Immunol* 1982; 129:2382.

95. Kovac Z, Schwartz RH: The molecular basis of the requirement

for antigen processing of pigeon cytochrome c prior to T cell activation. *J Immunol* 1985; 134:3233.

96. Streicher HZ, Berkower IJ, Busch M, et al.: Antigen conformation determines processing requirements for T cell activation. *Proc Natl Scad Sci USA* 1984; 81:6831.

97. Allen PM, Strydom DJ, Unanue ER: Processing of lysozyme by macrophages: identification of the determinant recognized by two T cell hybridomas. *Proc Natl Acad Sci USA* 1984; 81:2489.

98. Rudensky AY, Preston-Hurlburt P, Hong S-C, et al.: Sequence analysis of peptides bound to MHC class II molecules. *Nature* 1991; 353:622.

99. Hunt DF, Michel H, Dickinson TA, et al.: Peptides presented to the immune system by the murine class II major histocompatibility complex molecule I-A^d. *Science* 1992; 256:1817.

100. Chicz RM, Urban RG, Lane WS, et al.: Predominant naturally processed peptides bound to HLA-DR1 are derived from MHC-related molecules and are homogeneous in size. *Nature* 1992; 358:764.

101. Nelson CA, Roof RW, McCourt DW, Unanue ER: Identification of the naturally processed form of hen egg white lysozyme bound to the murine major histocompatibility complex class II molecules 1-A^k. *Proc Natl Acad Sci USA* 1992; 89:7380.

102. Brodsky FM, Guagliardi L: The cell biology of antigen processing and presentation: *Annu Rev Immunol* 1991; 9:707.

103. Harding CV, Collins DS, Slot JW, et al.: Liposome-encapsulated antigens are processed in lysosomes, recycled and presented to T cells. *Cell* 1991; 64:393.

104. Harding CV, Collins DS, Kanagawa O, et al.: Liposome-encapsulated antigens engender lysosomal processing for class II MHC presentation and cytosolic processing for class I presentation. *J Immunol* 1991; 147:2860.

105. Bretscher MS, Lutter R: A new method for detecting endocytosed proteins. *EMBO J* 1988; 7:4087.

106. Pisoni RL, Acker TL, Lisowski KM, et al.: A cysteine-specific lysosomal transport system provides a major route for the delivery of thiols to human fibroblast lysosomes: possible role in supporting lysosomal proteolysis. *J Cell Biol* 1990; 110:327.

107. Harding CV, Unanue ER, Slot JM, et al.: Functional and ultrastructural evidence for intracellular formation of major histocompatibility complex class II-peptide complexes during antigen processing. *Proc Natl Acad Sci USA* 1990; 87:5553.

108. Guagliardi LE, Koppelman B, Blum JS, et al.: Colocalization of molecules involved in antigen processing and presentation in an early endocytic compartment. *Nature* 1990; 343:133.

109. Pieters J, Hortsmann H, Bakke O, et al.: Intracellular transport and localization of major histocompatibility complex class II molecules and associated invariant chain. *J Cell Biol* 1991; 115:1213.

110. Peters PJ, Neefjes JJ, Oorschot V, et al.: Segregation of MHC class II molecules from MHC class I molecules in the Golgi complex for transport to lysosomal compartments. *Nature* 1991; 349:669.

111. Neefjes JJ, Stollorz V, Peters PJ, et al.: The biosynthetic pathway of MHC class II but not class I molecules intersects the endocytic route. *Cell* 1990; 61:171.

112. Smith BR, Ault KA: Increase of surface Ia-like antigen expression on human monocytes independent of antigen stimuli. *J Immunol* 1981; 127:2020.

113. Sztein MB, Steeg PS, Johnson HM, Oppenheim J: Regulation of human peripheral blood monocyte DR antigen expression by lymphokines and recombinant interferons. *J Clin Invest* 1984; 73:556.

114. Beller DI, Kiely J-M, Unanue ER: Regulation of macrophage populations: I. Preferential induction of Ia-rich peritoneal exudates by immunological stimuli. *J Immunol* 1980; 124:1426.

115. van Seventer GA, Shimizu Y, Shaw S: Roles of multiple accessory molecules in T-cell activation. *Curr Opin Immunol* 1991; 3:294.

116. Liu Y, Linsley PS: Costimulation of T-cell growth. *Curr Opin Immunol* 1992; 4:265.

117. Dustin ML, Springer TA: role of lymphocyte adhesion receptors in transient interactions and cell locomotion. *Annu Rev Immunol* 1991; 9:27.

118. Dustin ML, Springer TA: Adhesion receptor in the immune system. *Nature* 1989; 341:619.

119. Harding CV, Unanue ER: Modulation of antigen presentation and peptide-MHC-specific, LFA-1-dependent T cell-macrophage adhesion. *J Immunol* 1991; 147:767.

120. Dougherty GJ, Murdoch S, Hogg N: The function of human intercellular adhesion molecule-1 (ICAM-1) in the generation of an immune response. *Eur J Immunol* 1988; 18:35.

121. Dang LH, Michalek MT, Takei F, et al.: Role of ICAM-1 in antigen presentation demonstrated by ICAM-1 defective mutants. *J Immunol* 1990; 144:4082.

122. Siu G, Hedrick SM, Brian AA: Isolation of the murine intracellular adhesion molecule-1 (ICAM-1) gene. ICAM-1 enhances antigen-specific T cell activation. *J Immunol* 1989; 143:3813.

123. van Seventer GA, Shimizu Y, Horgan KJ, Shaw S: The LFA-1 ligand ICAM-1 provides an important costimulatory signal for T cell receptor mediated activation of resting T cells. *J Immunol* 1990; 144:4579.

124. Freeman GJ, Freedman AS, Segil JM, et al.: B7, a new member of the Ig superfamily with unique expression on activated and neoplastic B cells. *J Immunol* 1989; 143:2714.

125. Linsley PS, Clark E, Ledbetter JA: T-cell antigen CD28 mediates adhesion with B cells by interacting with activation antigen B7/B8-1. *Proc Natl Acad Sci USA* 1990; 87:5031.

126. Gimmi CD, Freeman GJ, Gribben JG, et al.: B-cell surface antigen B7 provides a costimulatory signal that induces T cells to proliferate and secrete interleukin 2. *Proc Natl Acad Sci USA* 1991; 88:6575.

127. Linsley PS, Brady W, Grasmaire L, et al.: Binding of the B cell activation antigen B7 to CD28 costimulates T cell proliferation and IL-2 mRNA accumulation *J Exp Med* 1991; 173:721.

128. Kohno K, Shibata Y, Matsuo Y, Minowada J: CD28 molecule as a receptor-like function for accessory signals in cell mediated augmentation of IL-2 production. *Cell Immunol* 1990; 131:1.

129. Fraser JD, Irving BA, Crabtree GR, Weiss A: Regulation of interleukin-2 gene enhancer activity by the T cell accessory molecule CD28. *Science* 1991; 251:313.

130. Verweij CL, Geerts M, Aarden LA: Activation of interleukin-2 gene transcription via the T cell surface molecule CD28 is mediated through a NFkB-like response element. *J Biol Chem* 1991; 266:14179.

131. Razi-Wolf Z, Freeman GJ, Galvin F, et al.: Expression and function of the murine B7 antigen: the major costimulatory molecule expressed by peritoneal exudate cells. *Proc Natl Acad Sci USA* 1992; 89:4210.

132. Koulova L, Clark EA, Shu G, Dupont B: The CD28 ligand B7/BB1 provides costimulatory signal for alloactivation of CD4+ T cells. *J Exp Med* 1991; 173:759.

133. Weaver CT, Unaune ER: The costimulatory function of antigen-presenting cells. *Immunol Today* 1990; 11:49.

134. Lamb JR, Feldmann M: Essential requirement for major histocompatibility complex recognition in T cell tolerance induction. *Nature* 1984; 308:72.

135. Jenkins MK, Schwartz RH: Antigen presentation by chemically modified splenocytes induces antigen-specific T cell unresponsiveness in vitro and in vivo. *J Exp Med* 1987; 165:302.

136. Mueller DL, Jenkins MK, Schwartz RH: Clonal expression vs. functional clonal inactivation. *Annu Rev Immunol* 1987; 7:445.

137. Mayernik DG, Ul-Haq A, Rinehart JJ: Differentiation-associated alternation in human monocyte-macrophage accessory cell function. *J Immunol* 1983; 130:2156.

138. Ettensohn DB, Roberts NJ Jr: Human alveolar macrophage support of lymphocyte responses to mitogens and antigens. Analysis and comparison with autologous peripheral-blood-derived monocytes and macrophages. *Am Rev Respir Dis* 1983; 128:516.

139. Toews GB, Vial WC, Dunn MM, et al.: The accessory cell function of human alveolar macrophages in specific T cell proliferation. *J Immunol* 1984; 132:181.

140. Venet A, Hance AJ, Saltini C, et al.: Enhanced alveolar macrophage-mediated antigen-induced T lymphocyte proliferation in sarcoidosis. *J Clin Invest* 1985; 75:293.

141. Lipscomb MF, Lyons CR, Nunez G, et al.: Human alveolar macrophages: HLA-DR-positive macrophages that are poor stimulators of a primary mixed leukocyte reaction. *J Immunol* 1986; 136:497.

142. Lyons CR, Ball EJ, Toews GB, et al.: Inability of human alveolar macrophages to stimulate resting T cells correlates with decreased antigen-specific T cell-macrophage binding. *J Immunol* 1986; 137:1173.

143. Ettensohn DB, Lalor PA, Roberts NJ Jr: Human alveolar macrophage regulation of lymphocyte proliferation *Am Rev Respir Dis* 1986; 133;1091.

144. Holt, PG, Schon-Hegrad MA, Oliver J: MHC class II antigen-bearing dendritic cells in pulmonary tissues of the rat. *J Exp Med* 1988; 167:262.

145. Lawrence EC, Theodore BJ, Martin RR: Modulation of poke-weed-mitogen-induced immunoglobulin secretion by human bronchoalveolar cells. *Am Rev Respir Dis* 1982; 126:248.

146. Kaltreider HB, Caldwell JL, Byrd PK: The capacity of normal murine alveolar macrophages to function as antigen-presenting cells for the initiation of primary antibody-forming cell responses to sheep erythrocytes in vitro. *Am Rev Respir Dis* 1986; 133:1097.

147. Schuyler MR, Todd LS: Accessory cell function of rabbit alveolar macrophages. *Am Rev Respir Dis* 1981; 123:53.

148. Liu MC, Proud D, Schleimer RP, Plaut M: Human lung macrophages enhance and inhibit lymphocyte proliferation. *J Immunol* 1984; 132:2895.

149. Holt PG: Down-regulation of immune responses in the lower respiratory tract: the role of alveolar macrophages. *Clin Exp Immunol* 1986; 63:261.

150. Rich EA, Tweardy DJ, Fujiwara W, Ellner JJ: Spectrum of immunoregulatory functions and properties of human alveolar macrophages. *Am Rev Respir Dis* 1987; 136:258.

151. deShazo RD, Banks DE, Diem JE, et al.: Bronchoalveolar lavage cell-lymphocyte interactions in normal nonsmokers and smokers. *Am Rev Respir Dis* 1983; 127:545.

152. Weinberg DS, Unanue ER: Antigen-presenting function of alveolar macrophages: uptake and presentation of *Listeria monocytogenes*. *J Immunol* 1981; 126:794.

153. Ullrich SE, Herscowitz HB: Immunological function of alveolar macrophages: interaction with a soluble protein antigen and the immunogenicity of alveolar macrophage-associated antigen. *J Reticuloendothel Soc* 1980; 28:111.

154. Thepen T, VanRooijen N, Kraal G: Alveolar macrophage elimination in vivo is associated with an increase in pulmonary immune response in mice. *J Exp Med* 1989; 170:499.

155. Lem VM, Lipscomb MF, Weissler JC, et al.: Bronchoalveolar cells from sarcoid patients demonstrate enhanced antigen presentation. *J Immunol* 1985; 135:1766.

156. Hance AJ, Douches S, Winchester RJ, et al.: Characterization of mononuclear phagocyte subpopulations in the human lung by using monoclonal antibodies: changes in alveolar macrophage phenotype associated with pulmonary sarcoidosis. *J Immunol* 1985; 134:284.

157. Razma AG, Lynch JP III, Wilson BS, et al.: Expression of Ia-like (DR) antigen on human alveolar macrophages isolated by bronchoalveolar lavage. *Am Rev Respir Dis* 1984; 129:419.

158. Wewers MD, Saltini C, Sellers S, et al.: Evaluation of alveolar macrophages in normals and individuals with active pulmonary sarcoidosis for the spontaneous expression of the interleukin 1β gene. *Cell Immunol* 1987; 107:479.

159. Hunninghake GW: Release of interleukin-I by alveolar macrophages of patients with active sarcoidosis. *Am Rev Respir Dis* 1984; 129:569.

160. Wright SD, Silverstein SC: Tumor-promoting phorbol esters stimulate C3b and C3b' receptor-mediated phagocytosis in cultured human monocyte. *J Exp Med* 1982; 156:1149.

161. Pommier CG, Inada S, Fries LF, et al.: Plasma fibronectin enhances phagocytosis of opsonized particles by human peripheral blood monocytes. *J Exp Med* 1983; 157:1844.

162. Bohnsack JF, Kleinman HK, Takahashi T, et al.: Connective tissue proteins and phagocyte cell function. Laminin enhances complement and Fc-mediated phagocytosis by cultured human phagocytes. *J Exp Med* 1985; 161:912.

163. Yamamoto K, Johnson RB Jr: Dissociation of phagocytosis from stimulation of the oxidative metabolic burst in macrophages. *J Exp Med* 1984; 159:405.

164. Aderem AA, Wright SD, Silverstein SC, Cohn ZA: Ligated complement receptors do not activate the arachidonic acid cascade in resident peritoneal macrophages. *J Exp Med* 1985; 161:617.

165. Griffin FM Jr, Silverstein SC: Segmental response of the macrophage plasma membrane to a phagocytic stimulus. *J Exp Med* 1974; 139:323.

166. Michl J, Unkeless JC, Pieczonka MM, Silverstein SC: Modulation of Fc receptors of mononuclear phagocytes by immobilized antigen-antibody complexes. Quantitative analysis of the relationship between ligand number and Fc receptor response. *J Exp Med* 1983; 157:1746.

167. Michl J, Pieczonka MM, Unkeless JC, et al.: Fc receptor modulation in mononuclear phagocytes maintained on immobilized immune complexes occurs by diffusion of the receptor molecule. *J Exp Med* 1983; 157:2121.

168. Griffin FM Jr, Griffin JA, Leider JE, Silverstein SC: Studies on the mechanism of phagocytosis: I. Requirements for circumferential attachment of particle-bound ligands to specific receptors on the macrophage plasma membrane. *J Exp Med* 1975; 142:1263.

169. Griffin FM Jr, Griffin JA, Silverstein SC: Studies on the mechanism of phagocytosis: II. The interaction of macrophages with anti-immunoglobulin IgG-coated bone marrow-derived lymphocytes. *J Exp Med* 1976; 144:788.

170. Boxer LA, Hedley-Whyte ET, Stossel TP: Neutrophil actin dysfunction and abnormal neutrophil behavior. *N Engl J Med* 1974; 291:1093.

171. Wang E, Michl J, Pfeffer LM, et al.: Interferon suppresses pinocytosis but stimulates phagocytosis in mouse peritoneal macrophages: related changes in cytoskeletal organization. *J Cell Biol* 1984; 98:1328.

172. Axline SG, Resven EP: Inhibition of phagocytosis and plasma membrane mobility of the cultivated macrophage by cytochalasin B. Role of subplasmalemmal microfilaments. *J Cell Biol* 1974; 62:647.

173. Sheterline P, Hopkins CR: Transmembrane linkage between

surface glycoproteins and components of the cytoplasm in neutrophil leucocytes. *J Cell Biol* 1981; 90:743.

174. Greenberg S, Di Virgillo F, El-Khoury J, Silverstein SC: F-actin dynamics in phagocytosing macrophages. *J Cell Biol* 1988; 107:453a.

175. Cooper J: The role of actin polymerization in cell motility. *Annu Rev Physiol* 1991; 53:585.

176. Oster G, Perelson AS: The physics of cell motility. *J Cell Sci [Suppl]* 1987; 8:35.

177. Reiss M, Roos D: Differences in oxygen metabolism of phagocytosing monocytes and neutrophils. *J Clin Invest* 1978; 61:480.

178. Box A, Wever R, Roos D: Characterization and quantification of the peroxidase in human monocytes. *Biochim Biophys Acta* 1978; 525:37.

179. Lehrer RI: The fungicidal mechanisms of human monocytes: I. Evidence for myeloperoxidase-linked and myeloperoxidase-independent candidacidal mechanisms. *J Clin Invest* 1975; 55:338.

180. Lamper MB, Weiss SJ: The chlorinating potential of the human monocyte. *Blood* 1983; 62:645.

181. Diamond RD, Haudenschild CC: Monocyte-mediated serum-independent damage to hyphal and pseudohyphal forms of *Candida albicans in vitro*. *J Clin Invest* 1981; 67:173.

182. Washburn RG, Gallin JI, Bennett JE: Oxidative killing of *Aspergillus fumigatus* proceeds by parallel myeloperoxidase-dependent and independent pathways. *Infect Immun* 1987; 55:2088.

183. Diamond RD, Root RK, Bennett JE: Factors influencing killing of *Cryptococcus neoformans* by human leukocytes in vitro. *J Infect Dis* 1972; 125:367.

184. Wilson CB, Tsai V, Remington JS: Failure to trigger the oxidative metabolic burst by normal macrophages. Possible mechanism for survival of intracellular pathogens. *J Exp Med* 1980; 151:328.

185. Murray HW, Cartelli DM: Killing of intracellular *Leishmania donovani* by human mononuclear phagocytes. Evidence for oxygen-dependent and -independent leishmanicidal activity. *J Clin Invest* 1983; 72:32.

186. van Furth R, Hirsch JG, Fedorko ME: Morphology and peroxidase cytochemistry of mouse promonocytes, monocytes and macrophages. *J Exp Med* 1970; 132:794.

187. Johnson WD Jr, Mei B, Cohn ZA: The separation, long-term cultivation and maturation of the human monocyte. *J Exp Med* 1977; 146:1613.

188. Johnston RB Jr, Godzik CA, Cohn ZA: Increased superoxide anion production by immunologically activated and chemically elicited macrophages. *J Exp Med* 1978; 148:115.

189. Nathan CF, Root RK: Hydrogen peroxide release from mouse peritoneal macrophages. Dependent on sequential activation and triggering. *J Exp Med* 1977; 146:1648.

190. Bermudez LEM, Young LS: Recombinant granulocyte-macrophage colony-stimulating factor activates human macrophages to inhibit growth or kill *Myobacterium avium* complex. *J Leukocyte Biol* 1990; 48:67.

191. De Titto EH, Catterall JR, Remington JS: Activity of recombinant tumor necrosis factor on *Toxoplasma gondii* and *Tyrpanosoma cruzi*. *J Immunol* 1986; 137:1342.

192. Nathan CF, Murray HW, Wieve ME, Rubin BY: Identification of interferon-γ as the lymphokine that activates human macrophage oxidative metabolism and antimicrobial activity. *J Exp Med* 1983; 158:670.

193. Stuehr DJ, Marletta MA: Mammalian nitrate biosynthesis: mouse macrophages produce nitrite and nitrate in response to *Escherichia coli* lipopolysaccharide. *Proc Natl Acad Sci USA* 1985; 82:7738.

194. Stuehr JD, Marletta MA: Induction of nitrite/nitrate synthesis in murine macrophages by BCG infection, lymphokines, or interferon-g. *J Immunol* 1987; 139:518.

195. Stuehr DR, Gross SS, Sakuma I, et al.: Activated murine macrophages secrete a metabolite of arginine with the bioactivity of endothelium-derived relaxing factor and the chemical reactivity of nitric oxide. *J Exp Med* 1989; 1690:1011.

196. Marletta MA, Yoon PS, Lyengar R, et al.: Macrophage oxidation of L-arginine to nitrite and nitrate: nitric oxide is an intermediate. *Biochemistry* 1988; 27:8706.

197. Stuehr DJ, Nathan CF: Nitric oxide. A macrophage product responsible for cytostasis and respiratory inhibition in tumor target cells. *J Exp Med* 1989; 169:1543.

198. Granger DL, Hibbs HB Jr, Perfect JR, Durack DT: Specific amino acid (L-arginine) requirement for the microbiostatic activity of murine macrophages. *J Clin Invest* 1988; 81:1129.

199. Granger DL, Hibbs HB Jr, Perfect JR, Durack DT: Metabolic fate of L-arginine in relation to microbiostatic capability of murine macrophages. *J Clin Invest* 1990; 85:264.

200. Green SJ, Meltzer MS, Hibbs JB Jr, Nacy CA: Activated macrophages destroy intracellular *Leishmania major* amastigotes by an L-arginine-dependent killing mechanism. *J Immunol* 1990; 144:278.

201. Elsbach P, Weiss J: Oxygen independent antimicrobial systems of phagocytes, in Gallin JI, Goldstein IM, Snyderman R (eds): *Inflammation: Basic Principles and Clinical Correlates*, 2nd ed. New York, Raven Press, 1990; 603.

202. Lehrer RI, Ganz T, Selsted ME: Defensins: endogenous antibiotic peptides of animal cells. *Cell* 1991; 64:229.

203. Ganz T, Selsted ME, Lehrer RI: Defensins. *Eur J Hematol* 1990; 44:1.

Chapter 34 _____
PRINCIPLES OF IMMUNOTHERAPY IN ALLERGIC RHINITIS

HEMALINI MEHTA, APARNA KUMAR,
AND WILLIAM W. BUSSE

The use of pollen extracts to treat hay fever first was attempted by Noon at St. Mary's Hospital in London in 1911.[1] These initial approaches were based on the idea that pollen produced a toxin, and that immunization with pollen extracts would result in the formation of protective "antitoxin." Empirical protocols evolved in which therapy was started with lower doses and gradually increased over a period of weeks to years. This seemed to reduce the rate of side effects, including anaphylaxis.

Since the 1960s, a number of double-blind, placebo-controlled trials have established the efficacy of immunotherapy in the management of allergic rhinitis when high-quality extracts are used at optimal dosage.[2] In the last decade, a number of well-designed studies have shown a beneficial effect in asthma for specific allergens.[3] This is discussed in more detail in the following chapter. The use of immunotherapy remains controversial, since the mechanism of action remains unclear, treatment protocols often are poorly defined, and there remains the possibility of rare life-threatening reactions. Its use further is limited, since many allergens are incompletely characterized and standardized extracts are available for only a limited number of allergens.

Mechanism of Action (Table 34-1)

For many years, immunotherapy was thought to work by producing "blocking antibodies" that could bind and neutralize antigen, thus preventing the triggering of cell-surface IgE. An increase in serum IgG concentrations can be demonstrated with immunotherapy, although IgG titers do not necessarily correlate with clinical response.[4] A switch from predominantly IgG$_1$ to IgG$_4$ occurs as therapy continues, but the significance of this is also unclear.[5] Blood IgE concentrations tend to increase initially and later decline with continued therapy.[6] There is also a modest increase in secretory IgA and IgG with immunotherapy.[7] The onset of clinical improvement precedes these changes.

Current interest has focused on the role of T lymphocytes in the response to allergens. The late-phase reaction, which occurs 3 to 24 h after antigen exposure, is thought to be mediated in part by proinflammatory cytokines produced by T cells. T-helper type 1 (Th1) cells secrete interleukin-2 (IL-2) and interferon γ (IFN-γ). Th2 cells, however, generate a cytokine profile that includes IL-4 and IL-5. IL-4 appears to be a major signal in switching B cells to IgE production,

TABLE 34-1   Immunologic Changes Associated with Specific Immunotherapy

1. Increased specific IgG
2. initial increase in IgG_1
3. Later increase in IgG_4
4. Initial increase in IgE
5. Later decrease in specific IgE
6. Increase in secretory IgA and IgG
7. Decreased eosinophil migration
8. Increased IL-2 and INF-γ (?Th1-type response)

while IL-5 is important in the terminal differentiation and activation of eosinophils.[8] There is evidence that the T cells, which respond to antigen challenge in atopic individuals, have a Th2 cytokine profile.[9] In patients treated for grass-pollen hay fever, skin biopsy specimens were examined 24 h after an intradermal challenge. Decreased numbers of eosinophils were noted, as well as an increase in levels of IL-2 and IFN-γ, suggesting a shift in cytokine expression towards a Th1 type response associated with immunotherapy.[10]

Safety of Immunotherapy

Side effects of immunotherapy are generally immediate or delayed local reactions or systemic reactions. Systemic reactions are any reactions occurring distant to the site of injection. These may include itchy eyes or skin, urticaria, sense of constriction in the throat, wheezing, hypotension, and angioedema of the airways.

In 1986, the Committee on the Safety of Medicines published a report recommending tight constraints on the use of immunotherapy in the United Kingdom, prompted by the occurrence of 5 deaths in the preceding 18 months and a total of 26 deaths since 1957.[11] Concern was expressed about the lack of evidence for long-term benefits and lack of standardized dosages. As a result, specific immunotherapy is no longer used in the United Kingdom and Scandinavia, but still has wide acceptance in other European countries and the United States.

Lockey et al. reported 46 fatalities during a 42-year period from the use of immunotherapy and skin testing combined, based on a retrospective survey.[12] The Food and Drug Administration (FDA) received a total of 35 reports of deaths following allergen immunotherapy from 1985 to 1993. There were no reports of deaths from allergen skin testing during this period.[13] The majority of reported patients (83 percent) had a prior history of asthma, and most (22 out of 29) could be described as having moderate to severe asthma requiring corticosteroids, hospitalization, emergency room visits or having a history of respiratory arrest. Other risk factors included a high degree of sensitivity by skin testing or in vitro studies, history of prior systemic reactions, immunotherapy given during allergy season, dosing error, patient leaving clinic immediately after injection, patient being symptomatic from environmental exposure at the time of injection, and immunization being done at home. There also seemed to be increased risk during the initial buildup phase

of therapy. The FDA estimates an annual death rate of 0.7 deaths per million exposures, based on 52.3 million uses of allergen extracts during the same time period.

The use of new high-potency standardized extracts has improved the efficacy of immunotherapy but may also have resulted in an increase in the number of life-threatening reactions.[14] The frequency of systemic reactions is reported to be higher with the use of "rush protocols," in which the buildup doses are given over a 1- to 3-day period.[15] The majority of systemic reactions occur 15 to 45 min after immunization, with the most severe reactions occurring in the first 30 min.[17]

The risk of serious side effects can be reduced by premedication with antihistamines or corticosteroids[16,17] and by stopping the protocol when large local reactions (>10 cm) are observed.[17] Caution should also be exercised when freshly prepared vials of extract are used, as potency may vary between manufacturers and between batches, resulting in inadvertent dosing errors.

Contraindications (Table 34-2)

In certain patients, immunotherapy should be avoided or used cautiously after careful consideration of the risk/benefit ratio.

In patients taking beta–adrenoceptor antagonists, anaphylaxis is more severe and refractory to therapy. The concomitant use of beta-adrenergic blocking agents and allergen immunotherapy should be avoided when possible.[18] Skin testing with allergen extracts should be done with caution; and RAST testing may be a safer alternative in patients receiving beta-adrenoceptor antagonists. Immunotherapy also should be avoided in patients with other diseases that preclude the use of epinephrine, such as unstable angina or severe hypertension.

During pregnancy, immunotherapy appears to be safe, and there is no evidence of teratogenicity.[19] However, precautions should be taken to minimize the risk of anaphylaxis and subsequent possible spontaneous abortion of the fetus. Immunotherapy should not be initiated during pregnancy because of the increased risk during the buildup phase. Maintenance doses can be continued or reduced slightly.

Immunotherapy should be avoided in active autoimmune disease and malignancy. Although circulating immune complexes have not been demonstrated in patients receiving immunotherapy,[20] caution should be used until mechanisms are understood more clearly.

Immunotherapy should not be initiated or should be performed with extreme caution in unstable asthmatics with an FEV_1 persistently below 70 percent of predicted values or for those continuously using systemic corticosteroids.[21,22]

TABLE 34-2   Contraindications for Specific Immunotherapy

1. Use of beta blocker or contraindication to epinephrine use.
2. Active autoimmune disease or malignancy
3. Pregnancy (maintenance therapy can be continued)
4. FEV_1 less than 70% of predicted in unstable asthmatics

Dosage and Duration of Therapy

Conventional high-dose immunotherapy is usually started with one to two subcutaneous injections per week with increasing doses until a maintenance dose is reached, at which point the interval is increased to every 2 to 4 weeks. Very low dose therapy (Rinkle immunotherapy) has been shown to be no more effective than placebo[23] and is not recommended.

In the 1940s, protein nitrogen units (PNU) were introduced in an effort to standardize dosage. Weight of pollen per volume of extracting solution (w/v) has also been used. Neither of these units reflects the biologic activity of the extract. In the United States, allergy units (AU) have been introduced. These are determined by a variety of techniques including skin testing in an allergic population, ability of specific components of the extract to bind human IgE, and quantity of individual major antigenic determinants. International reference preparations have been prepared under the auspices of the World Health Organization for a number of extracts.

The recommended duration of therapy usually is 3 to 5 years. Recent data suggest that therapy for < 3 years results in high relapse rates, and that one-third of patients who receive immunotherapy for ≥ 3 years will have a prolonged effect.[24]

Alternative Therapy

Immunotherapy has been attempted by routes other than subcutaneous injection, but none have been sufficiently documented to be recommended for clinical use at this time. Nasal immunotherapy has been studied and probably does produce some reduction in rhinitis symptoms during the pollen season.[25] This benefit is offset by the induction of clinical symptoms during treatment. Chemical modification of allergens to reduce side effects while retaining immunogenicity may prove to be a solution to this problem.

Oral immunotherapy with birch pollen extract in enteric-coated capsules has been shown to reduce clinical symptoms, increase IgG concentrations, and decrease IgE response during pollen season.[26] The dose required to produce this effect is 100 to 300 times greater than for subcutaneous therapy and would be economically unfeasible. This approach will need further evaluation.

Sublingual immunotherapy has been reported with both low- and high-dose protocols. The theory behind this form of treatment remains unclear. It is likely that a large portion of allergen introduced by this route will be digested in the stomach or the intestine. Studies on sublingual therapy have lacked objective evidence for efficacy. This form of immunotherapy cannot be recommended for clinical use at this time.

Future Directions

Continued effort will be made in the future to identify major allergens and produce high-quality standardized extracts for commercial use. With the recognition of the role of T cells in promoting allergic inflammation, new therapeutic modalities are possible. Identification of peptides (epitopes) on antigens that are recognized by specific T cells but do not bind IgE may allow induction of T-cell tolerance.

Conventional high-dose immunotherapy is effective in reducing clinical symptoms related to specific allergen exposure in sensitive individuals. It does have certain risks, including the possibility of life-threatening anaphylactic reactions. The risk can be minimized by the selection of appropriate patients, use of high-quality extracts, and the employment of a slow buildup phase. Premedication with antihistamines can be used to reduce the risk of local or systemic reactions. Patients should be observed for a minimum of 30 minutes following injection, and their protocol should be adjusted according to the severity of side effects.

Allergic Rhinitis

Allergic rhinitis, or hay fever, is a common medical problem for patient and physician alike. The estimated frequency of allergic rhinitis in the general U.S. population ranges from 15 to 20 percent. About 3 million workdays and 2 million days of school are lost each year because of allergic and other forms of chronic rhinitis. Allergic rhinitis can begin at any age, but it usually appears before age 20; most commonly, symptoms occur between the ages of 12 and 15 years. It rarely presents before 18 months of age. Usually an individual requires 2 or more years of exposure to the offending allergen before symptoms develop. Allergic rhinitis appears equally in males and males and females, with no apparent racial or ethnic predilection.

Allergic rhinitis may be seasonal or perennial, depending on the sensitizing allergen. Plant pollens typically produce symptoms in the spring, summer, or fall, while perennial exposure to nonseasonal allergens such as animal dander and dust mites leads to symptoms year round. The most common allergens include pollens from grasses, tress, and weeds, molds, dust mites, and animal dander. Pollens from weeds, grasses and trees vary from one geographic location to another. To identify the offending allergen, the clinician must become familiar with the individual plant pollination seasons in his or her area.

Allergic rhinitis is an IgE-mediated reaction, with release of mediators and recruitment of inflammatory cells. The immune reaction to a sensitizing allergen is characterized by IgE antibody production with its binding firmly to receptors on circulating basophils and tissue mast cells. The bridging of two IgE antibodies by multivalent antigen triggers release of mediators from the mast cell and basophil. With this property, the mast cell assumes a pivotal role in the immediate phase of the allergic reaction. It releases several inflammatory mediators, such as histamine, prostaglandin D_2, leukotrienes C_4, D_4, and E_4, and kininogens, which are capable of inducing acute symptoms. Histamine is probably the most important of these mediators to the production of acute allergic rhinitis. Histamine causes vascular engorgement, producing nasal congestion; it stimulates secretion of mucus through a direct action and increases plasma protein extravasation, causing tissue edema; and by an indirect reflex mechanism, it increases glandular secretion.[27] Sneezing can also be provoked by challenging the nasal mucosa directly with histamine.[28] In addition, mast-cell-derived chemotactic factors may contribute to the recruitment of neutrophils, basophils and eosinophils to the nasal mucosa.[29] These cells account for the appearance of the late-phase response to antigen, which develops 3 to 11 h after the initial exposure.[30] The late-phase reaction becomes important in establishing the chronic nature of allergic rhinitis and acts to sensitize, or prime, the nasal tissue. This priming effect means that the concentration of allergen required to produce allergic symptoms is reduced.

Typically, patients with allergic rhinitis suffer from paroxysms of sneezing, nasal pruritus, clear rhinorrhea, and congestion that fluctuate from side to side as well as in level of intensity. Frequently, allergic individuals will also complain of symptoms of fatigue. On physical examination, the nasal mucosa is congested and classically pale blue in color, with secretions that are clear and watery. Excessive nasal itching may lead to nose rubbing and the so-called *allergic salute*, a characteristic gesture of pushing the tip of the nose upward with the palm of the hand. Prolonged nose rubbing in children may lead to the formation of a transverse crease across the bulbar portion of the nose.[31] The conjunctiva show vascular engorgement with a clear discharge. The periorbital skin may show allergic "shiners," which are caused by venous engorgement. Last, on examination of the ears, a middle-ear effusion may be detected.

The diagnosis of allergic rhinitis is usually straightforward. An accurate, detailed history and physical examination can be helpful in patients who have a temporal association between symptoms and exposure to seasonal allergens. Demonstrating the presence of eosinophils on a nasal smear may be effective in initial screening; however, this is not diagnostic for allergic rhinitis.[32] An increase of total serum IgE concentrations is found in 30 to 40 percent of patients with allergic rhinitis. Because of wide variations, this test is of limited value in this disease. Carefully performed allergen skin testing using potent preparations with positive and negative controls is the diagnostic procedure of choice for identifying the offending allergen in individual patients.

Treatment Modalities (Fig. 34-1)

AVOIDANCE

Once specific allergens are identified, the patient should avoid further exposure. Allergen avoidance is the most effective therapy for allergic rhinitis when exposure can be avoided. Exposure to seasonal pollens can be reduced by closing windows and doors and running an air conditioner both in the house and car.[33] Although effective, this approach has limitations, which are of both practical and environmental relevance. Specific control measures for the reduction of house dust mites and animal dander are, in contrast, practical and effective and include covers for bedding, changes in household cleaning practices, the use of acari-

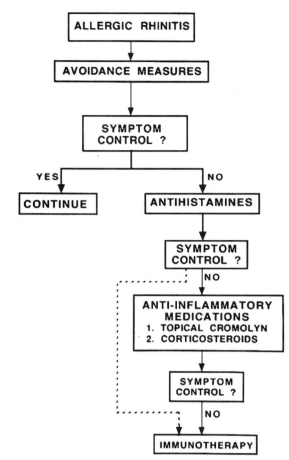

FIGURE 34-1 Flowchart for the treatment of allergic rhinitis.

cides and filters. Most common aeroallergens, however, cannot be avoided completely. This is especially true for patients with multiple sensitivities that result in constant exposure to airborne allergens, causing continuous symptoms.

MEDICATIONS

For patients who cannot avoid allergen exposure totally, medications are necessary for symptom control.[34] The usual first-line medication for individuals with allergic rhinitis is antihistamines. Traditional H_1-antihistamines are sedating, but when they are given on a regular basis at bedtime, they often are tolerated. Second-generation nonsedating antihistamines—such as terfenadine, loratadine, and astemizole—are in most cases as potent as traditional antihistamines. Antihistamines are best at reducing sneezing, nasal itching, and rhinorrhea but have little effect on nasal congestion.

Topical disodium cromoglycate may be effective for patients who do not respond to antihistamines. Intranasal disodium cromoglycate, which prevents the release of certain inflammatory mediators and has few side effects, has little decongestant activity and does not give prompt symptomatic relief. Intranasal corticosteroids (beclamethasone, budesonide, triamcinolone, fluticasone, and flunisolide) are the most potent medications available for allergic rhinitis. When used for more than 4 to 7 days, these corticosteroid sprays prevent the allergen-provoked pathophysiology of both the early and late phases of allergic rhinitis.[35] Since immune responses to allergens are the cause of allergic rhinitis, therapy to modify this reaction is potentially important. Furthermore, it is proposed that immunotherapy for allergic rhinitis both improves symptom control and has disease-modifying properties. In this sense, the consideration of immunotherapy is of interest and importance in the treatment of allergic rhinitis.

Immunotherapy in Allergic Rhinitis

PATIENT SELECTION

Factors to be considered in patient selection before immunotherapy is initiated are listed in Chap. 35 and in Table 34-3. The relationship of the symptoms to exposure to the allergen should be confirmed by history of worsening of symptoms during certain seasons of the year or on contact with the allergen. Specific IgE antibody should be demonstrated by skin-test reactivity or radioallergosorbent testing (RAST). In addition, the magnitude of the skin reaction provides a semiquantitative assessment of the patient's relative skin hypersensitivity. This helps assess the initial starting dose of allergen to be injected but does not necessarily indicate the level of clinical sensitivity. Although some have proposed that patients with the greatest degree of sensitivity based on skin-test reactivity or allergen challenge are most likely to benefit from immunotherapy, this needs further confirmation.[36] Indications for immunotherapy include classic seasonal rhinitis symptoms during two or more consecutive seasons with an inability to control symptoms by avoiding the aeroallergen and/or by use of well-tolerated pharmacotherapy.[37] Immunotherapy also may be indicated for patients who have had one season of rhinitis with unusually severe symptoms or intolerable side effects from medications. Exposure to animal dander is avoidable for most

patients, but animal-sensitive veterinarians, animal handlers, and technicians may appropriately be considered for immunotherapy.

Data showing the effectiveness of immunotherapy in children < 6 years of age are incomplete. Untreated, mild allergic rhinitis in children remits spontaneously in 10 percent of cases within 5 years and improves in an additional 33 percent.[38] As a consequence, immunotherapy in this age group should be individualized. It is seldom necessary to initiate immunotherapy in patients over 50 years of age, since symptoms tend to decrease with age. Older adults also rarely develop new sensitivities.

Finally, patients on immunotherapy should be able to comply with the treatment program and give informed consent after a discussion of the relative risks and benefits of the treatment. Because the possibility for an acute allergic reaction to immunotherapy exists, the physician should be in attendance and have the facilities, equipment, and experience required to treat adverse reactions, including severe anaphylaxis.

ANTIGEN SELECTION

GRASS POLLEN

Grass pollens are among the most frequent cause of allergic rhinitis worldwide, with an estimated 10 to 30 percent of allergic patients showing sensitivity. Grass pollen allergens stem from several important species and are extensively cross-reactive.

The first documentation of immunotherapy, by Noon and Cantab, appeared in Lancet in 1911.[1] In those early trials, 13 of 20 patients treated with timothy pollen extracts had fewer symptoms during the pollen season. This was followed several years later by a randomized blinded placebo-controlled study in 1954 of 200 individuals with grass pollen rhinitis. Of the 100 patients treated with active extracts, 78 had good to excellent control of their symptoms during the pollen season, whereas only 33 of 100 patients receiving placebo had

TABLE 34-3   Studies of Efficacy of Immunotherapy in Allergic Rhinitis

Reference	Allergen	Age Group	NO. IMPROVED/NO. TREATED		Significant Difference
			Extract	Placebo	
Frankland[39]	Grass	Adult	78/99	33/99	Yes
McAllen[40]	Grass	Adult/Child	68/94	31/94	Yes
Norman[43]	Ragweed	Adult	14/18	7/18	Yes
Fontana[44]	Ragweed	Child	17/35	15/35	No
Pence[46]	Mountain cedar	Adult	13/17	6/15	Yes
Horst[48]	*Alternaria*	Adult/Child	10/13	3/11	Yes
Ohman[50]	Cat	Adult	5/9	2/8	Yes
Valvovirta[51]	Dog	Child	11/15	2/12	Yes
McHugh[4]	Dust mite	Adult	20/30	6/30	Yes

SOURCE: Modified from Bush et al.,[56] with permission.

any symptom control.[39] McAllen reported a double-blind, randomized, placebo-controlled study of 94 patients ranging from 12 to 60 years of age, who were treated with either grass pollen or placebo.[40] Successful control of symptoms was reported by 72 percent of those receiving grass pollen extract, while only 33 percent of those receiving placebo showed improvement. Grammer et al.[41] studied rush injection therapy with polymerized extracts of timothy, orchard, and Bermuda grass in 40 patients. Symptom scores and medication use were reduced significantly during the grass pollen season in the actively treated group compared to placebo.

Grass pollen allergens are well characterized, and high-quality commercial extracts are available. The studies cited above indicate that selected individuals with allergic rhinitis and grass pollen sensitivity are suitable candidates for immunotherapy and receive benefit. Trials have not compared the response to antihistamine therapy or inhaled nasal corticosteroids. Nor have studies begun to address the influence of immunotherapy on long-term cost-effective control.

WEED POLLEN

Most allergenic weeds belong to the family Asteraceae and are a major cause of allergic symptoms. Of the members of this family, ragweed has been studied most extensively.

In 1963, Lowell and Franklin randomized adults and children to receive injections of ragweed extracts or a histamine-containing placebo.[42] In this 3-year study, treated patients had significantly lower symptom scores and used fewer medications during the ragweed season. A 4-year trial, by Norman et al. comparing the effects of immunotherapy with Amb a I (a major short ragweed antigen), crude ragweed extract, and placebo, showed a dose-dependent improvement in symptoms in the treated group during the pollen season.[43] Although other ragweed immunotherapy studies in children have shown fewer rhinitis symptoms compared to controls, a study of 92 children failed to detect a difference in symptoms or medication use between the group treated for 1 year and controls.[44] This may be due in part to the low doses used in the treatment.

Standardized ragweed extracts are available in the United States with sufficient data to support data to support the use of ragweed immunotherapy in individuals with allergic rhinitis.

TREE POLLEN

There are limited reports of immunotherapy for rhinitis with tree pollen. These have usually included studies with birch or mountain cedar pollen extracts.

Nuchel-Petersen et al. compared treatment with a partially purified, standardized extract of birch pollen to a combination of alder, birch, and hazel extract. In this double-blind study of 45 patients, both groups showed a reduction in symptoms and medication use following 3 years of treatment.[45] Additionally, both groups demonstrated a significant decline in nasal response to provocative challenge after 2 and 3 years of therapy. Treated patients tolerated 30 times more pollen exposure than prior to the start of treatment. Pence et al. conducted a double-blind study of 40 individu-

als showing lower daily symptom scores in subjects receiving mountain cedar allergen extracts.[46]

Tree pollen extracts currently available in the United States are quite variable. Further blinded controlled studies are needed to confirm the usefulness of tree pollen immunotherapy in allergic rhinitis.

FUNGI

Many fungi have been reported as allergens. *Cladosporium* and *Alternaria* are the best studied of this group.

Dreborg et al. studied 30 children, ages 5–17, over 10 months in a double blind placebo-controlled trial with a purified and standardized extract of *Cladosporium herbarum*.[47] Although the treated patients showed no difference in nasal and ocular symptoms, those who received therapy showed a reduction in conjunctival sensitivity in allergen challenge. Treated patients also required less medication during the two week peak in *Cladosporium* counts. A recent study using *Alternaria* extract involved 24 patients, ages 5–56 years, examined over 12 months.[48] Treated patients had lower symptom scores on exposure to *Alternaria* spores and a decrease in response to nasal provocation.

Adequate controlled immunotherapy studies with fungal extracts are lacking. Fungal allergenic extracts are highly variable and complex with no readily available standardized extracts. For these reasons, fungal immunotherapy is not strongly recommended for the treatment of allergic rhinitis.

ANIMAL DANDER

Sensitivity to domestic animals is a significant cause of allergic rhinitis. Additionally, 10 to 30 percent of individuals exposed to laboratory animals develop allergic reactions.[49]

In a double-blind randomized study of cat-induced rhinitis, treated subjects were able to tolerate a longer period of exposure to cats before developing symptoms.[50] Actively treated patients also had a decrease in intensity of ocular and nasal symptoms.

A number of commercial cat extracts available in the United States have been standardized for content of *Fel d I*. The *Fel d I* protein is the major cat allergen and is found primarily in the epithelium of the animal. Although cat immunotherapy can decrease allergic symptoms in patients exposed to the animal, in most instances symptoms return given sufficient exposure. Therefore, this form of immunotherapy is usually reserved for individuals who have short periods of exposure that is unavoidable, such as veterinarians and laboratory assistants.

The major allergens responsible for dog allergies are less well characterized. Valovirta et al. reported on 27 children, 5–18 years of age, with allergic rhinitis on exposure to dogs.[51] The treated group had no difference in symptoms, but did show a decrease in conjunctival response compared to placebo.

Despite the prevalence of sensitivity to laboratory animals, few studies have been done in this group. Wahn et al., studied 11 subjects with symptoms on exposure to laboratory animals.[52] Individuals selected for treatment were given injections of one or more commercial animal extracts (mouse, rat, or rabbit) with secondary improvement in nine subjects. The major source of allergen for mice and rats is urinary protein. Commercially available extracts for rodents are variable.

HOUSE DUST MITES

House dust, containing primarily house dust mites, has long been known to trigger allergic rhinitis. The two mites primarily responsible for producing allergen and causing symptoms in the United States are *Dermatophagoides pteronyssinus and Dermatophagoides farinae*. The major allergens have been identified as proteins termed *Der p* I(from *D. pteronyssinus*) and *Der f* I(from *D. farinae*), which are dust mite digestive enzymes.

Gabriel et al. enrolled 66 individuals with positive skin tests to *D. pteronyssinus* and a history of 3 or more consecutive years of rhinitis in a double-blinded, placebo-controlled study.[53] After 1 year of treatment, there was no significant difference in skin test reactivity, nasal challenge, or specific IgE concentrations. Patients' diaries and physicians' assessments, however, suggested symptomatic improvement in the treated group. In a double-blinded, placebo-controlled trial with 30 patients, a high content of Der p I was used.[54] Additional patients received conventional mite extract and histamine control. High-dose immunotherapy patients had improvement in clinical scores and nasal challenge.

Several well-characterized and standardized dust mite extracts currently are available. Some evidence supports the use of mite immunotherapy for allergic rhinitis. Individuals with moderate disease appear to improve the most. Environmental control measures to minimize exposure to dust mites should be attempted before beginning immunotherapy.

Allergic rhinitis is a common medical problem for the patient and the physician. Many individuals experience an improvement in symptoms with avoidance measures and/or the use of pharmacologic therapy. For those patients who are unresponsive to therapy, who have unusually severe symptoms or intolerable medication side effects, or for whom avoidance of long-term medical treatment is of importance, immunotherapy should be considered. Immunotherapy is not necessarily a cure and is not effective in all patients. However, when given properly, it can be successful in up to 80 to 90 percent of patients.[54] The duration of improvement after cessation of treatment is not known. In one study, the positive effects of immunotherapy lasted for several years after its cessation.[55] In general, immunotherapy with pollen extracts and dust mites appears to be effective. Fungal and animal dander immunotherapy need further controlled trials.

References

1. Noon L: Prophylactic vaccination against hay fever. *Lancet* 1911; 1:1572.
2. Ohman JL: Allergen immunotherapy: Review of efficacy and current practice. *Med Clin North Am* 1992; 76:977.91.
3. Bousquet J, Michel FB: Specific immunotherapy in asthma: Is it effective? *J Allergy Clin Immunol* 1994; 94:1.
4. McHugh SM, Lavelle B, Kemeny DM, et al.: A placebo-controlled trial of immunotherapy with two extracts of *D. pteronyssinus* in allergic rhinitis comparing clinical outcome with changes in antigen-specific IgE, IgG and IgG subclasses. *J Allergy Clin Immunol* 1990; 86:521.
5. Nakagawa T: The role of IgG subclass antibodies in the clinical response to immunotherapy in allergic disease. *Clin Exp Allergy* 1991; 21:289.
6. Creticos PS, Van Metre TE Jr, Mardiney MR, et al.: Dose response of IgE and IgG antibodies during ragweed immunotherapy. *J Allergy Clin Immunol* 1984; 73:94.
7. Platts-Mills TAE, von Maur RK, Ishizaka K: IgA and IgG antiragweed antibodies in nasal secretions. *J Clin Invest* 1976; 57:1041.
8. Norman PS: Modern concepts of immunotherapy. *Curr Opin Immunol* 1993; 5:968.
9. Ricci M, Rossi O, Bertoni M, Matucci A: The importance of Th2-like cells in the pathogenesis of airway allergic inflammation. *Clin Exp Allergy* 1993; 23:360.
10. Varney V, Hamid QA, Gaga M, et al.: Influence of grass pollen immunotherapy on cellular infiltration and cytokine mRNA expression during allergen-induced late phase cutaneous responses. *J Clin Invest* 1993; 92:644.
11. Committee on Safety of Medicine. Desensitizing vaccines. *Br Med J* 1986; 293:948.
12. Lockey RF, Benedict LM, Turkeltaub PC, Bukantz SC: Fatalities from immunotherapy (IT) and skin testing. *J Allergy Clin Immunol* 1987; 79:660.
13. Turkeltaub PC: Deaths associated with allergenic extracts. *FDA Med Bull* May 1994; 7.
14. Bousquet J, Michel FB: Safety considerations in assessing the role of immunotherapy in allergic disorders. *Drug Safety* 1994; 10:5.
15. Bousquet J, Hejjaoui A, Dhivert H, et al.: Immunotherapy with a standard *Dermatophagoides pteronyssinus* extract: III. Systemic reactions during rush protocols in patients suffering from asthma. *J Allergy Clin Immunol* 1989; 83:797.
16. Hejjaoui A, Ferrando R, Dhivert H, et al.: Systemic reactions occurring during immunotherapy with standardized pollen extracts. *J Allergy Clin Immunol* 1992; 89:925.
17. Hejjaoui A, Dhivert H, Michel FB, Bousquet J: Immunotherapy with a standardized *Dermatophagoides pteronyssinus* extract: IV. Systemic reactions according to the immunotherapy schedule. *J Allergy Clin Immunol* 1990; 85:473.
18. Executive Committee, American Academy of Allergy and Immunology. Position statement, beta-adrenergic blockers, immunotherapy, and skin testing. *J Allergy Clin Immunol* 1989; 84:129.
19. Metzger WJ, Turner E, Patterson R: The safety of immunotherapy during pregnancy. *J Allergy Clin Immunol* 1978; 61:268.
20. Yang WH, Dorvla G, Osterland CK, Gilmore NJ: Circulating immune complexes during immunotherapy. *J Allergy Clin Immunol* 1979; 63:300.
21. Malling HJ, Weeke B: Position paper of the European Academy of Allergy and Clinical Immunology: Immunotherapy. *Allergy* 1993; 48(suppl 14):9.
22. International Consensus Report on the Diagnosis and Management of Asthma. *Allergy* 1992; 47(suppl 1):1.
23. Van Metre TE, Adkinson NF Jr, Amodio FJ, et al.: A controlled study of the effectiveness of the Rinkel method of immunotherapy for ragweed pollen hay fever. *J Allergy Clin Immunol* 1980; 65:288.
24. Hejjaoui A, Knani J, Dhivert H, et al.: Duration of specific immunotherapy with a standardized mite extract after its cessation (abstract). *J Allergy Clin Immunol* 1992; 89:319.

25. Bjorksten B: Local immunotherapy is not documented for clinical use (editorial). *Allergy* 1994; 49:299.

26. Taudorf E, Laursen L, Lanner A, et al.: Specific IgE, IgG, and IgA antibody response to oral immunotherapy in birch pollinosis. *J Allergy Clin Immunol* 1989; 83:589.

27. Despot JE: Inflammatory mediators in allergic rhinitis. *Immunol Allergy Clin North Am* 1987; 7:37.

28. Doyle WJ: Physiologic responses to intranasal dose-response challenges with histamine, methacholine, bradykinin and prostaglandin in adult volunteers with and without nasal allergy. *J Allergy Clin Immunol* 1990; 86:924.

29. Nagakura T, Onda T, Iikura Y, et al.: In vitro and in vivo antigen-induced release of high-molecular-weight neutrophil chemotactic activity from human nasal tissue. *Am J Rhinol* 1988; 2:7.

30. Dvoracek JE: Induction of nasal late-phase reactions by insufflation of ragweed-pollen extract. *J Allergy Clin Immunol* 1984; 73:363.

31. Myers MA: The "nasal crease": A physical sign of allergic rhinitis. *JAMA* 1960; 174:1204.

32. Zeiger RS: Allergic and non-allergic rhinitis: Classification and pathogenesis: Part II. Non-allergic rhinitis. *Am J Rhinol* 1989; 3:113.

33. Solomon WR: Exclusion of particulate allergens by window air conditioners. *J Allergy Clin Immunol* 1980; 65:305.

34. Smith JM: Epidemiology and natural history of asthma, allergic rhinitis, and atopic dermatitis, in Middleton E Jr, Reed CE, Ellis EF, et al. (eds): *Allergy Principles and Practice*, 4th ed. St. Louis: Mosby, 1993:1109.

35. Pipkorn U, Proud D, Lichtenstein LM, et al.: Inhibition of mediator release in allergic rhinitis by pretreatment with topical glucocorticosteroids. *N Engl J Med* 1987; 316:1506.

36. Osterballe O: Immunotherapy in hayfever with two major allergens 19,25 and partially purified extract of timothy grass pollen: A controlled double-blind study. In vivo variables, season 1. *Allergy* 1980; 35:473.

37. Rocklin RE: Clinical and immunologic aspects of allergen-specific immunotherapy in patients with seasonal allergic rhinitis and/or allergic asthma. *J Allergy Clin Immunol* 1983; 72:323.

38. Osterballe O: Specific immunotherapy with purified grass pollen extracts. *Dan Med Bull* 1984; 31:207.

39. Frankland AW, Augustin R: Prophylaxis of summer hayfever and asthma: A controlled trial comparing crude grass-pollen extracts with the isolated main protein component. *Lancet* 1954; 1:1055.

40. McAllen NK: Hyposensitization in grass pollen hay fever. *Acta Allergol* 1969; 24:421.

41. Grammer LC, Shaughnessy MA, Finkle AM, et al.: A double-blind placebo controlled trial of polymerized whole grass administered in an accelerated dosage schedule for immunotherapy of grass pollinosis. *J Allergy Clin Immunol* 1986; 78:1180.

42. Lowell FC, Franklin W: A "double-blind" study of the effectiveness and specificity of injection therapy in ragweed hayfever. *N Engl J Med* 1965; 273:675.

43. Norman PS, Winkenwerder WL, Lichtenstein LM: Immunotherapy of hayfever with ragweed antigen E: Comparisons with whole pollen extracts and placebos. *J Allergy* 1968; 42:93.

44. Fontana VJ, Holt LE Jr, Mainland D: Effectiveness of hyposensitization therapy in ragweed hayfever in children. *JAMA* 1969; 195:985.

45. Nuchel-Peterson B, Janniche H, Munch EP, et al.: Immunotherapy with partially purified and standardized tree pollen extracts: I. Clinical studies from a three-year double-blind study of patients treated with pollen extracts either of birch or combination of alder, birch and hazel. *Allergy* 1988; 43:353.

46. Pence HL, Mitchel DQ, Greeley RI, et al.: Immunotherapy for mountain cedar pollinosis: a double-blind controlled study. *J Allergy Clin Immunol* 1976; 58:39.

47. Dreborg S, Agrell B, Foucard T, et al.: A double-blind, multicenter immunotherapy trial in children using a purified and standardized *Cladosporium herbarum* preparation: I. Clinical results. *Allergy* 1986; 41:131.

48. Horst M, Hejjaoui A, Horst V, et al.: Double-blind placebo-controlled rush immunotherapy with a standardized *Alternaria* extract. *J Allergy Clin Immunol* 1990; 85:460.

49. Knysak D: Animal aeroallergens. *Immunol Allergy Clin North Am* 1989; 9:357.

50. Ohman JL Jr, Findlay SR, Leitermann KM: Immunotherapy in cat-induced asthma: Double-blind trial with evaluation of in vivo and in vitro responses. *J Allergy Clin Immunol* 1984; 74:230.

51. Valovirta E, Koivikko A, Vanto T, et al.: Immunotherapy in allergy to dog: A double-blind study. *Ann Allergy* 1984; 53:85.

52. Wahn U, Siriginian RP: Efficacy and specificity of immunotherapy with laboratory animal allergen extracts. *J Allergy Clin Immunol* 1980; 65:413.

53. Gabriel M, Ng HK, Allan WGL, et al.: Study of prolonged hyposensitization with *D. pteronyssinus* extract in allergic rhinitis. *Clin Allergy* 1977; 7:325.

54. Fireman P: Overview of management of allergic rhinitis/congestion. *J Respir Dis* 1992; 13:s15.

55. Mosbech H, Osterballe O: Does the effect of immunotherapy last after termination of treatment? *Allergy* 1988; 43:523.

56. Bush RK, Huftel MA, Busse WW: Patient selection, in Lockey RF, Bukantz SC (eds): *Allergen Immunotherapy*. New York: Marcel Dekker, 1991:25–49.

Chapter 35

IMMUNOTHERAPY AND ASTHMA

BINA JOSEPH

WILLIAM W. BUSSE

Allergy is a significant component of asthma in many patients. Although current pharmacologic therapy is effective in treating asthma, the suppression of bronchial inflammation occurs only when therapy is administered. Therefore, a "therapeutic" approach that acts to modulate the immune response to allergen is appealing and, in theory, may provide lasting improvement. Furthermore, it also is appealing to consider therapy that reduces the need for regular use of medication. It is on the basis of these premises that "immunotherapy" has attracted interest and offers a potentially unique appeal, complementing current concepts of asthma.

Since immune responses to sensitizing antigen are a central factor in the propagation of airway inflammation, the methods to modify this response are of critical interest. The principal therapeutic approach to this end presently available is allergen immunotherapy. The principles of immunotherapy are discussed in the preceding chapter. Despite evidence to indicate that immunotherapy may be beneficial in selected patients, there remains concerns about this approach. This section reviews the importance of allergens in asthma and evidence that immunotherapy may be effective treatment in selected patients.

Role of Allergens in Asthma

Although the precise mechanisms and overall contribution of allergens to asthma remains to be established, 75 to 85 percent of asthma patients have positive immediate skin tests to common aeroallergens. This association and other more direct evidence from epidemiologic studies and bronchoprovocation suggest that airborne allergens are important in chronic asthma.

In infants, aeroallergens have a small role in triggering asthma, and viral respiratory infections are the primary precipitants of wheezing. This association may relate to the lack of allergen exposure and sensitization. In children over 5 years of age, in contrast, allergens play a major role in asthma. Furthermore, the severity of childhood asthma has been found to be directly proportional to the number of positive skin tests.[8,9] Children with multiple positive skin tests are more likely to have daily rather than intermittent asthma symptoms.[9] There are also data to suggest that early exposure to allergen in children is an important factor in the subsequent development of asthma.

In adults with asthma, the contribution of allergies to airway disease is more diverse and age-dependent. Adults with an onset of asthma before age 30 continue to show a significant association with allergen sensitivity and asthma. In contrast, allergens do not appear to play a significant role in adults over 50 years of age. These associations are important in determining individuals who are candidates for allergen immunotherapy.

The Contribution of Allergen Exposure to the Onset of Asthma

In the past decade, an increasing emphasis has been placed on the role of inflammatory factors in asthma. Allergen exposure activates the airway allergic process, including mast cells and begins the recruitment of inflammatory cells. This process initiates an inflammatory cascade that results in recruitment and activation of other cells, including eosinophils, basophils, neutrophils, and lymphocytes, to produce the late-phase allergic response. The late allergic response is a laboratory model that is felt to represent mechanisms associated with the development of chronic inflammation.

There is also clinical evidence that the late allergic reaction is relevant to asthma. Crimi et al.[12] have demonstrated that bronchoprovocation with allergen primes the airway of the asthma patient and promotes the late-phase response. These observations suggest that allergen exposure can enhance the inflammatory response in asthma. Furthermore, seasonal exposure to allergen causes increased airway responsiveness on postseasonal bronchial challenge with allergen.[13] Seasonal allergen exposure also leads to increased bronchial reactivity to nonspecific stimuli such as histamine and methacholine.

Allergen sensitivity also appears to dictate the level of asthma severity. In a study of 11 patients who experienced respiratory arrest, O'Hollaren et al. found increased skin test reactivity to *Alternaria* and increased specific IgE concentrations.[14] All of the severe episodes of asthma occurred during times of *Alternaria* exposure. Pollart et al.[15] found an increased frequency of grass pollen-specific IgE in 54 of 59 patients treated in an emergency room with acute asthma during grass pollination season. Interestingly, samples of dust taken from the residences of 15 of these patients contained very high concentrations of grass pollen. Pollart et al.[5] studied 102 asthma patients seen in an emergency room with acute asthma and found that the prevalence of specific IgE antibodies to dust mites, cockroach, cat dander, grass, and ragweed pollen was four times greater than that among nonasthma controls. Burrows et al.[16] found a direct correlation between the presence of asthma and serum IgE concentrations. In the same study, however, no association was found between positive skin test responses to aeroallergens and incidence of asthma.

Recognition of the Allergic Component of Asthma

To ascertain the relevance of allergens to asthma, a detailed history is helpful in detecting association with occupation, the home environment, and animal exposure. Clues from this information should be corroborated by the documentation of objective IgE sensitivity by skin testing with appropriate extracts, or, alternately, the use of RAST testing that assesses the concentration if IgE antibody in the serum to be tested.[17] However, skin testing is more accurate in the diagnosis of immediate hypersensitivity to allergens. Positive tests for IgE antibody to allergens should be evaluated in conjunction with the clinical history in establishing the importance of particular allergens to asthma.

Evidence for presence of IgE antibody alone, without clinical correlation, is insufficient to diagnose and treat allergic disease. However, with certain allergens, i.e., house dust mite and molds, the association of antigen sensitivity to

asthma may be less evident than that with animal danders or pollens.

Management of Allergic Asthma

The basic principles of therapy are similar in allergic and nonallergic asthma: use of bronchodilators to control the bronchospastic component of the disease and anti-inflammatory drugs, i.e., corticosteroids and/or nedocromil or cromolyn (particularly in children), to modulate the inflammatory component of the disease. For patients in whom an IgE-mediated component to their asthma exists, antigen avoidance or control is a reasonable and effective form of therapy. For example, in dust mite allergy, avoidance measures are available—i.e. encasement of mattresses and pillows, washing bedding with hot water, and removal of carpeting and furry toys (where feasible) can lead to a reduction in symptoms[18] Moreover, regular use of a dehumidifier to maintain humidity at less that 50 percent reduces the dust mites as well as molds in the environment. Fungicides can destroy molds on which dust mites feed and acracides such as benzoic acid can kill the dust mites.[18] Spraying tannic acid solution on carpeting and upholstered furniture inactivates dust mite and cat allergens.

In patients with asthma caused by exposure to pets, elimination of animals from the living area is best; however, this is not always acceptable to the patient or family. For asthma patients with an allergy to cat, bathing the animal and using an indoor air filter system or removing carpeting may reduce allergen concentrations.[19] However, it is important that the patient be aware that cat dander can remain in the environment for 6 months after removal of the animal.

Although allergen avoidance is central in asthma therapy in the allergic subject, this approach is not always practical, is highly restrictive to an individual's lifestyle, and does not always lead to antigen avoidance.

Patient Selection for Immunotherapy

There are no clearly established guidelines for patient selection for immunotherapy. Some physicians consider immunotherapy only when all other forms of therapy have failed. Others recommend immunotherapy early in the course of the disease and treatment to reduce the need for medication and hopefully modify disease severity. Despite this lack of guidelines, several factors must be taken into consideration before initiating immunotherapy, including the potential intensity of the reaction to an allergen, previous experience of immunotherapy with a particular allergen, cost and duration of each type of treatment, and the potential risk to the patient.

To minimize risk and improve efficacy, the International Consensus for the Diagnosis and Management of Asthma[42] has made the following recommendations:

1. Immunotherapy must be prescribed by specialists and administered by physicians who are capable of managing acute, severe allergic reactions such as anaphylaxis.

2. Patients with multiple sensitivities may not benefit from immunotherapy.
3. Immunotherapy is most effective in children and young adults.
4. The patient should not have labile asthma at the time of immunotherapy.
5. FEV_1 values should be at least 70 percent of the predicted value at the time of immunotherapy.

As discussed, the confirmation of an IgE-mediated component to asthma should be established by appropriate testing *and* clinical correlation of symptoms to allergen exposure. Individuals who demonstrate a sensitivity by skin test reaction are more likely to benefit from immunotherapy.[20] The severity and duration of the patient's symptoms should be considered when initiating immunotherapy; patients with mild asthma who are well controlled with pharmacologic therapy may not be candidates for immunotherapy. In contrast, patients with severe asthma, i.e. an FEV_1 <70 percent predicted, also are unlikely to be good candidates for immunotherapy even though they are most in need of assistance.

To assess the potential efficacy of immunotherapy in individual patients, one should consider the frequency of beta$_2$-adrenergic agonist use, exacerbations with acute asthma, frequency of nocturnal awakening with asthma, and time lost from work. Measures of pulmonary function, as with peak flow meters (at home) and spirometry, provide excellent objective evidence for disease severity and assessment of therapeutic intervention.

Availability of well-characterized, standardized extracts is also crucial to success with immunotherapy. Extracts that are of low potency or contain nonspecific allergens are usually of limited benefit. Immunotherapy is most effective in children over the age of 6 years and adults over 50 years of age. Sociologic and logistic factors are also important. As with all forms of treatment, patient compliance is vital. The patient should be committed to a regular schedule for immunotherapy injections. Prolonged duration between injections often increases the likelihood of serious adverse reactions. To improve safety for patients, it is important for them to remain in the clinic for at least 30 min after the injection and have available a self-injection of epinephrine. If a systemic reaction occurs after the patient leaves the clinic, prompt administration of epinephrine and treatment in an acute care facility are important. Factors that must be taken into account in initiating immunotherapy are summarized in Table 35-1. Adverse reactions and contraindications to immunotherapy are discussed in the preceding chapter and must be considered before the embarking on this form of therapy. Table 35-2 outlines guidelines for the safe administration of immunotherapy.

Effectiveness of Allergen Immunotherapy in Asthma

HOUSE DUST MITE

Allergens derived from house dust have been recognized as important factors in rhinitis and asthma. Prior to 1960, aller-

TABLE 35-1   Considerations for Initiating Immunotherapy

1. **Presence of an IgE-mediated disease amenable to immunotherapy**
   a. Allergic rhinitis
   b. Asthma with allergic triggers
2. **Documentation of specific sensitivity**
   a. Exposure to putative allergen, related to appearance of symptoms
   b. Presence of specific IgE antibody
      (1) Skin tests
      (2) In vitro assays (RAST)
      (3) Provocative challenge
3. **Severity and duration of symptoms**
   a. Subjective symptoms
   b. Objective parameters: time lost from work, emergency room visits, pulmonary function tests
   c. Response to allergen avoidance
   d. Response to conventional medication
4. **Availability of quality allergenic extracts**
5. **Age of patient**
   a. Children over 6
   b. Adults less than 50
6. **Sociologic and logistic factors**
   a. Ability of patient to comply
   b. Cost
   c. Discussion of risks versus benefits
   d. Availability of facilities to treat untoward reactions
   e. Occupation of candidate
7. **Objective evidence of efficacy of immunotherapy (controlled clinical trials)**

SOURCE: Adapted from Bush et al.,[1] with permission.

TABLE 35-2   Rules for the Safe Administration of Allergen Immunotherapy

1. Implement stringent measure to prevent errors in dosage.
2. Reduce the dosage when patients have symptoms from current allergen exposure (during allergy season).
3. Avoid allergy injections in patients with unstable or moderately symptomatic asthma especially those with low baseline lung function (i.e., FEV_1 <70% predicted).
4. Reduce dosage of extracts during dose escalation if the interval between shots is greater than 2 weeks or if maintenance doses are delayed.
5. Escalate dose more slowly in highly sensitivity patients (i.e., patients with large skin test reactions or very high RAST IgE levels).
6. Avoid allergen immunotherapy in patients receiving beta adrenergic blocking agents.
7. Have patients wait in the office for at least 30 min after an injection to avoid the occurrence of a systemic reaction after leaving.
8. Have subcutaneous epinephrine available, as well as medications (such as nebulized beta$_2$-adrenergic agonist) to treat asthmatic reaction.

SOURCE: Adapted from Ohman Jr.,[7] with permission.

genic components in house dust material were identified and extracts of whole dust were taken from the residences of persons with dust mite hypersensitivity to be used for skin testing as well as immunotherapy. This created obvious problems; the quality of the house dust extract was not representative of a particular geographic area and often contained contaminants such as animal dander and mold. In 1964, Voorhorst et al.[23] identified the genus *Dermatophygoides* as the main allergenic component of house dust. Since then, standardized extracts containing *D. pteronyssinus* and/or *D. farinae* have been used for skin testing and immunotherapy.

House dust mite hypersensitivity in early childhood is a significant risk factor in the development of asthma.[20,24] In a study of 67 children, Sporik et al.[20] found that the age of onset of wheezing was inversely proportional to the extent of dust mite exposure at the age of 1 year. Furthermore, there are an increasing number of studies showing conclusively that house dust mite avoidance is an effective form of therapy. In addition, there are data to suggest that immunotherapy with house dust mite is associated with a relief of asthma symptoms. D'Souza et al.[25] used immunotherapy in 96 patients with house dust mite allergy. Immunotherapy was associated with a significant improvement in asthma symptoms, reduction in medication use and tolerance to allergen exposure. Improvement was apparent in individuals with a high degree of skin test reactivity to allergen prior to immunotherapy.

Warner et al.[26] observed that *D. pteronyssinus* immunotherapy improved lung function and reduced medication use in children with moderately severe perennial asthma and positive skin tests as well as bronchial provocation to *D. pteronyssinus*. Patients treated by Warner et al.[26] had a docu-

mented reduction in wheezing and nocturnal symptoms and improvements in their activity level as compared with the placebo treatment group. Although bronchial provocation to house dust mite allergen following immunotherapy did cause changes in the immediate response to *D. pteronyssinus*, there was a significant reduction in late response.

Bousquet et al.[27] have attempted to identify those individuals allergic to the house dust mite who would most likely benefit from immunotherapy. In a prospective study of 215 patients with positive skin tests to *D. pteronyssinus*, they observed that children and adults with mild asthma benefited from immunotherapy when outcomes were assessed by a reduction in symptoms and medication scores. Patients with chronic sinusitis, aspirin sensitivity, and more severe asthma—defined as FEV_1 <70 percent predicted prior to initiation of immunotherapy—derived little or no benefit from this form of therapy. Patients with allergies in addition to house dust mite sensitivity also derived little benefit from immunotherapy.

Newton et al.[28] conducted a double-blind, placebo-controlled study of 14 asthma patients with positive skin tests to house dust mite and found that immunotherapy did not result in significant improvement of symptoms. However, there was a statistically significant reduction in bronchial responsiveness to house dust mite antigen on rechallenge after immunotherapy. These data should be interpreted with caution, as the study group was small.

Gaddie et al.[29] noted no improvement in pulmonary function, symptom scores, or skin test reactivity in a group of perennial asthmatics who were also allergic to house dust mites and who were treated with extracts of *D. pteronyssinus*. The authors do note that the low dosage of their extract may explain the lack of response.

TABLE 35-3   Selected Placebo Controlled Studies of Allergen Immunotherapy in Asthma

Antigen	Reference	Duration of Study, months	No. Active	Subjects Placebo	Age Group	Type of Study	Significant Difference
Mixed grasses	Ortolani et al.[32]	10	8	7	Adult	Double blind	yes
Bermuda grass pollen	Armentia Medina et al.[33]	2	19	11	Child/Adult	Double blind	yes
D. pteronyssinus	Warner et al.[26]	12	27	24	Child	Double blind	yes
D. pteronyssinus	Gaddie et al.[29]	12	26	29	Child/Adult	Double blind	no
Cat	Ohman et al.[40]	4–5	9	8	Adult	Double blind	yes
Cat and dog	Sundin et al.[39]	12	22	17	Child/Adult	Double	yes
Cladosporium herbarium	Dreborg et al.[36]	10	16	14	Child	Double blind	yes
Alternaria	Horst et al.[38]	12	13	11	Child/Adult	Double blind	yes

SOURCES: Adapted from Bush et al.[1] and Ohman Jr.,[4] with permission.

POLLENS

An estimated 10 to 30 percent of allergic individuals have grass pollen allergy. Although the role of airborne pollens in asthma exacerbations is not as clear as with house dust mites or animal dander, they can contribute to airway disease. Crimi et al.[13] evaluated 11 patients with birch pollen sensitivity. The early and late bronchial response to inhaled birch pollen extract was increased after the birch pollen season; the change in airway responsiveness correlated with an increase in serum IgE concentrations. This increased responsiveness was not seen in patients who were treated with either inhaled or systemic corticosteroids. These observations show that allergen exposure of sensitized individuals increases postseasonal bronchial responsiveness. Although the precise mechanism for this effect on the airway is not established, the increase in IgE concentration indicates an immune effect that can be regulated by corticosteroids.

Ortolani et al.[31] treated 15 individuals who were sensitive to grass pollen with immunotherapy and found a statistically significant improvement in symptom scores—i.e. for wheeze, shortness of breath, and cough—but no change in serum IgE concentrations or airway reactivity to grass pollen. Armentia-Medini et al.[32] conducted a double-blind, placebo controlled study of 30 patients with Bermuda grass pollen sensitivity. In contrast to the findings of Ortolani et al.[31] this group found a statistically significant decrease in the bronchial reactivity to Bermuda grass pollen as well as a reduction in nonspecific reactivity to methacholine following immunotherapy.

Although there are numerous studies to show the benefit of ragweed immunotherapy in allergic rhinitis (see previous chapter), few studies have evaluated the efficacy of ragweed immunotherapy in asthma. In 1957, Johnstone et al.[33] found that high-dose ragweed immunotherapy led to a complete loss of asthma symptoms. If low-dose immunotherapy was used, symptom reduction did not occur. Twenty years later, Bruce et al.[34] evaluated 29 ragweed-sensitive asthma patients who were treated for 8 months with ragweed pollen extract. There was no change in medication scores, symptom scores, or bronchial provocation to ragweed. However, Bruce et al.[34] did suggest that the lack of observed response to therapy may have resulted from the low concentrations of ragweed extract used.

Creticos et al.[35] observed a reduction in skin test sensitivity and bronchial challenge to ragweed following immunotherapy. Although both the active and placebo-treated group had a similar reduction in asthma symptoms, the actively treated group demonstrated improvement in peak flow values during ragweed season. The placebo-treated group continued to show reduced peak flow values with increased use of medication.

MOLDS

The report by O'Hollaren et al.[14] strongly suggested that some *Alternaria*-sensitive patients are at increased risk for severe attacks of asthma. Such observations raise the possibility that this particular mold may be very important to the pathogenesis of asthma and that early intervention in management of mold hypersensitivity could result in an improved outcome. There are also data to suggest that immunotherapy with *Alternaria* may alleviate asthma symptoms in both children and adults. Dreborg et al.[36] conducted a double-blind, placebo-controlled study of 30 children, all of whom had positive skin tests and RAST tests to *Cladosporium*. Immunotherapy was administered for 10 months. After 6 months, medication scores—e.g., frequency of asthma medication use—were decreased, but no improvement was noted in symptom score or in peak expiratory flow rates. However, after 10 months of treatment, there was a reduction in both the medication scores and bronchial response to *Cladosporium* extract.

Malling et al.[37] conducted a study of 22 adult asthma patients who were treated with *Cladosporium* extract. Eight percent of the treated group showed either an improvement or a lack of change in symptoms when compared to the control group. Of the treated group, approximately 70 percent experienced large local reactions and all had an increase in asthma during the buildup period when the dose of extract was increased. Horst et al.[38] administered immunotherapy by a rush technique (rapid escalation in dose) in individuals with an allergy only to *Alternaria*. There was a statistically significant reduction in symptom scores and medication use as well as reduction in skin test reactivity in the treated group.

ANIMAL DANDER

Patients with animal dander hypersensitivity are especially suitable for study since their history of exposure to the allergen—as opposed to plant antigens—is easier to verify. Usually, the patient gives a clear history of animal exposure that causes asthma. Allergy to cat dander, as confirmed by skin testing in young children (3 years of age), carries an increased risk of promoting the development of asthma later in life.[24] Sundin et al.[39] conducted a study of 41 patients, some of whom were treated with cat immunotherapy and others with a dog extract. In the patients treated with the cat extract, there was reduction in the bronchial reactivity to both cat allergen and histamine. The airway response to cat allergen was reduced 11-fold. There were no significant changes in the group treated with dog extract.

Ohman et al.[40] found a reduction in the skin test response as well as bronchial sensitivity to cat allergen in subjects treated with cat extract. This group also found a delay in time required to cause an onset of pulmonary and ocular symptoms in immunotherapy-treated patients when they were exposed to cats. Van Metre et al.[41] also observed reduction in skin sensitivity to cat extract with reduction in specific bronchial reactivity in patients undergoing cat immunotherapy with allergens.

Summary

Immunotherapy should be considered in selected patients in whom appropriate avoidance measures and pharmacologic therapy have been ineffective. Although immunotherapy is not proven to be first-line therapy for all patients with asthma, there is a considerable body of evidence suggesting that immunotherapy has a role in the management of asthma and remains the only immunomodulating technique available at this time for management of allergic asthma.

References

1. Bush RK, Huftel MA, Busse WW: Patient selection, in Lockey RF, Bukantz SC (eds): Allergen Immunotherapy. New York: Marcel Dekker, 1991; 25.
2. Brown JE, Greenberger PA: Immunotherapy and asthma. *Immunol Allergy Clin North Ame* 1993; 13:939.
3. Bousquet J, Michel FB: Specific immunotherapy in asthma: Is it effective? *J Allergy Clin Immunol* 1994; 94:1.
4. Ohman JL Jr: Allergen immunotherapy in asthma: Evidence for efficacy. *J Allergy Clin Immunol* 1989; 84:133.
5. Pollart SM, Chapman MD, Fiocco GP, et al.: Epidemiology of acute asthma: IgE antibodies to common inhalant allergens as a risk factor for emergency room visits. *J Allergy Clin Immunol* 1989; 83:875.
6. Bush RK: The role of allergens in asthma. *Chest* 1992; 101:378S.
7. Ohman JL Jr: Allergen immunotherapy: Review of efficacy and current practice. 1992; 76:977.
8. Zimmerman B, Feanny S, Reisman J, et al.: Allergy in asthma: I, The dose relationship of allergy to severity of childhood asthma. *J Allergy Clin Immunol* 1988; 81:63.
9. Zimmerman B, Chambers C, Forsyth L: Allergy in asthma: II, The highly atopic infant and chronic asthma. *J Allergy Clin Immunol* 1988; 81:71.
10. Martin AJ, Landau LI, Phelan PD: Natural history of allergy in asthmatic children followed to adult life. *Med J Aust* 1981; 2:470.
11. Inouye T, Tarlo S, Border I, et al.: Severity of asthma in skin test negative and skin test positive patients. *J Allergy Clin Immunol* 1985; 75: 313.
12. Crimi E, Gianiorio P, Orengo G, et al.: Late asthmatic reaction to perennial and seasonal allergens. *J Allergy Clin Immunol* 1990; 85:885.
13. Crimi E, Voltolini S, Gianiorio P, et al.: Effect of seasonal exposure to pollen on specific bronchial sensitivity in allergic patients. *J Allergy Clin Immunol* 1990; 85:1014.
14. O'Hollaren MT, Yunginger JW, Oxford KP, et al.: Exposure to an aeroallergen as a possible precipitating factor in respiratory arrest in young patients with asthma. *N Engl J Med* 1991; 324:359.
15. Pollart SM, Reid MJ, Fling JA, et al.: Epidemiology of emergency room asthma in northern California: Association with IgE antibody to rye grass pollen. *J Allergy Clin Immunol* 1988; 82:224.
15. Pollart SM, Chapman MD, Fiooco GP, et al.: Epidemiology of acute asthma: IgE antibodies to common inhalant allergens as a risk factor for emergency room visits. *J Allergy Clin Immunol* 1989; 83:875.
16. Burrows B, Martinez FD, Halonen MM, et al.: Association of asthma with serum IgE levels and skin-test reactivity to allergens. *N Engl J Med* 1989; 320:271.
17. VanArsdel PP Jr, Larson EB: Diagnostic tests for patients with suspected allergic disease. *Ann Intern Med* 1989; 110:304.
18. Nelson HS, Hirsch R, Ohman JL Jr, et al.: Recommendations for the use of residential air-cleaning devices in the treatment of allergic respiratory diseases. *J Allergy Clin Immunol* 1988; 82:661.
19. Middleton E Jr: Asthma, inhaled allergens, and washing the cat. *Am Rev Respir Dis* 1991; 143:1209.
20. Sporik R, Holgate ST, Platts-Mills TAE, et al.: Exposure to house dust mite allergen (Der pI) and the development of asthma in children. *N Engl J Med* 1990; 323:502.
21. Osterballe O: Immunotherapy in hayfever with 2 major allergens 19, 25 and partially purified extract of timothy grass pollen. A controlled double-blind study: In vivo variable, season 1. *Allergy* 1980; 35:473.
22. Smith JM: Epidmeiology and natural history of asthma, allergic rhinitis, and atopic dermatitis (eczema), in, Middleton E Jr, Reed CE, Ellis EF, et al. (eds): *Allergy Principles and Practice*, 3d ed. St Louis: Mosby, 1988:891.
23. Voorhorst R, Spieksma-Boezeman MIA, Spieksma FThM: Is a mite (Dermatophygoides) the producer of house dust mite allergen? *Allergy Asthma* 1964; 10:329.
24. Sears MR, Herbison GP, Holdaway MD, et al.: The relative risks of sensitivity to grass pollen, house dust mite and cat dander in the development of childhood asthma. *Clin Exp Allergy* 1989; 19:419.
25. D'Souza, Pepys J, Wells ID, et al.: Hyposensitization with dermatophygoides pteronyssinus in house dust allergy: A controlled study of clinical and immunological effects. *Clin Allergy* 1973; 3:177.
26. Warner JO, Price JF, Soothill JF, Hey EN: Controlled trial of hyposensitization to *Dermatophygoides pteronyssinus* in children with asthma. *Lancet* 1978; 2:912.
27. Bousquet J, Hejjaoui A, Clauzel AM, et al.: Specific immunotherapy with a standardized *Dermatophagoides pteronyssinus* extract: Prediction of efficacy of immunotherapy. *J Allergy Clin Immunol* 1988; 82:971.
28. Newton DAG, Maberly DJ, Wilson R: House dust mite hyposensitization. *Br J Dis Chest* 1978; 72:21.
29. Gaddie J, Skinner C, Palmer KNV: Hyposensitization with house dust mite vaccine in bronchial asthma. *Br Med J* 1976; 2:561.
30. Ford AW, Platts-Mills TAE: Standardized extracts, dust mite, and other arthropods (inhalants). *Clin Rev Allergy* 1987; 5:49.
31. Ortolani C, Pastorello E, Moss RB, et al.: Grass pollen immunotherapy: A single year double-blind, placebo-controlled study in patients with grass pollen-induced asthma and rhinitis. *J Allergy Clin Immunol* 1984; 73:283.
32. Armentia-Medina A, Blanco-Quiros A, Martin-Santos JM, et al.: Rush immunotherapy with a standardized bermuda grass pollen extract. *Ann Allergy* 1989; 63:127.
33. Johnstone DE: Study of the role of antigen dosage in the treatment of pollenosis and pollen asthma. *AMA J Dis Child* 1957; 94:1.
34. Bruce CA, Norman PS, Rosenthal RR, et al.: The role of ragweed pollen in autumnal asthma. *J Allergy Clin Immunol* 1977; 59:449.
35. Creticos SP, Reed CE, Norman PS, et al.: The NIAID cooperative study of the role of immunotherapy in seasonal ragweed-induced adult asthma. *J Allergy Clin Immunol* 1993; 91:226.
36. Dreborg S, Agrell B, Foucard T et al.: A double- blind, multicentre immunotherapy trial in children, using a purified and standardized cladosporium herbarum preparation. *Allergy* 1986; 41:131.
37. Malling HJ, Dreborg S, Weeke B: Diagnosis and immunotherapy of mold allergy: Clinical efficacy and side effects of immunotherapy with cladosporium herbarum. *Allergy* 1986; 41:507.
38. Horst M, Hejjaoui A, Horst V, et al.: Double-blind, placebo-controlled rush immunotherapy with a standardized alternaria extract. *J Allergy Clin Immunol* 1990; 85:460.
39. Sundin B, Lilja G, Graff-Lonnevig, et al.: Immunotherapy with partially purified and standardized animal dander extracts: Clinical results from a double-blind study on patients with animal dander asthma. *J Allergy Clin Immunol* 1986; 77:478.
40. Ohman JL, Findlay SR, Leiterman SB: Immunotherapy in cat-induced asthma: Double blind trial with evaluation of in vivo and in vitro responses. *J Allergy Clin Immunol* 1984; 74:230.
41. Van Metre TE Jr, Marsh DG, Adkinson NF: Immunotherapy decreases skin sensitivity to cat extract. *J Allergy Clin Immuno* 1989; 83:888.
42. International Consensus Report on the Diagnosis and Management of Asthma: *Allergy* 1992; 47(suppl 1):1.

TOXICOLOGY AND ENVIRONMENTAL FACTORS

Chapter 36

OCCUPATIONAL ASTHMA

LESLIE C. GRAMMER, III

Definition

A generally accepted definition of asthma is the one proposed by the National Heart, Lung, and Blood Institute (NHLBI) expert panel report: a lung disease with the following characteristics: (1) airway obstruction that is reversible either with treatment or spontaneously, (2) airway hyperresponsiveness, and (3) airway inflammation.[1] Asthma due to a specific sensitizing exposure in the workplace environment is occupational asthma. The onset of occupational asthma is generally preceded by a latent period of weeks, months, or years during which the worker is asymptomatic. Then, specific immunologic sensitization to a workplace agent occurs, resulting in asthma upon exposure to that agent. Essentially, the same scenario occurs in the nonoccupational setting and results in allergen-induced asthma—for example, cat asthma.

Other lung diseases associated with variable airway obstruction and/or airway hyperresponsiveness do not fit the above definition of occupational asthma. Whether reactive airways dysfunction syndrome (RADS) should be classified as occupational asthma is a matter of some debate.[2–4] The criteria for the diagnosis of RADS are reviewed in Table 36-1 (see also Chap. 38).

Byssinosis, or reversible airway obstruction caused by textile dust exposure, is not generally considered to be occupational asthma.[3] Workers who have asthma prior to a given employment and whose asthma is exacerbated by workplace exposures or conditions such as cold air, exercise, or irritants in the workplace would not be categorized as having occupational asthma.

Medicolegal Aspects

Most sensitizing agents that have been reported to cause occupational asthma are proteins of plant, animal, or microorganism derivation and are not specifically regulated

TABLE 36-1　Criteria for the Diagnosis of Reactive Airways Dysfunction Syndrome

1. Absence of prior respiratory symptoms
2. Onset of symptoms after a single exposure
3. Symptoms simulating asthma (cough, wheeze, dyspnea) begin within 24 h of exposure and persist for at least 3 months
4. Positive methacholine bronchoprovocation challenge
5. Exclusion of other pulmonary diseases

by the Occupational Safety and Health Administration (OSHA). Some of the low-molecular-weight sensitizing agents such as isocyanates, anhydrides, and platinum are regulated by OSHA, and there are published standards for airborne exposure in the Code of Federal Regulations (CFR 29.1910.1000).[5] A division of the U.S. Department of Labor, OSHA is responsible for determining and enforcing these legal standards. The National Institute of Occupational Health and Safety (NIOSH), a division of the U.S. Department of Health and Human Services, is responsible for reviewing available data on exposure to hazardous agents and providing recommendations to OSHA relative to airborne exposure limits to hazardous agents. However, NIOSH has no regulatory or enforcement authority.

More than 200 different substances have been reported to act as respiratory sensitizing agents and causes of occupational asthma.[6,7] In many industrialized nations—for instance, the United Kingdom and France—occupational asthma due to well-recognized sensitizing agents such as flour dust, colophony, isocyanates, and platinum is legally defined, and there are explicit protocols for compensation. This is not the case in the United States, where worker's compensation is administered individually by each state. Occupational asthma is generally recognized as a compensable work-related disease under worker's compensation legislation. However, no state currently has explicit legal criteria for the diagnosis of occupational asthma; therefore, adjudication of compensation is not a simple matter.

Physicians who diagnose and treat occupational asthma should be familiar with OSHA's Hazard Communication Standard (CFR29.1910.1200).[5] Often referred to as "workers' right to know" legislation, this standard has made it mandatory that workers exposed to hazardous substances such as respiratory sensitizing agents be informed of the hazards and be trained in proper handling of the substance. In addition, material safety data sheets (MSDS) on all hazardous substances in the workplace must be available to employees. The MSDS is a compendium of information on a hazardous substance. One section lists reported adverse health effects, such as whether the substance is a known respiratory sensitizer. Obtaining MSDS is often a useful endeavor for a physician caring for a patient in whom the diagnosis of occupational asthma is being considered.

Etiologic Agents

Most of the 200 agents that have been described to cause occupational asthma are high-molecular-mass ($\geq$ 3kDa) heterologous proteins of plant, animal, or microorganism origin.[8–10] Low-molecular-weight chemicals can act as irritants and aggravate preexisting asthma. They may also act as allergens if they are capable of haptenizing autologous proteins in the respiratory tract.[11–13] Numerous reviews of occupational asthma include information on etiologic agents.[6,7,14–17] A representative list of agents and industries associated with occupational asthma can be found in Table 36-2.

A useful rubric for the classification of agents causing occupational asthma is to divide them into high-molecular-weight (heterologous proteins) or low-molecular-weight (chemicals capable of conjugating to autologous proteins in the respiratory tract) types. High-molecular-weight agents are generally complete antigens, while low-molecular-weight agents act as haptens and must therefore link with a carrier protein to be immunogenic. Most low-molecular-weight chemicals are not capable of causing occupational asthma because they cannot react with autologous proteins; substances with molecular masses less than 1 kDa are not recognized by the human immunologic system.

Chloramine T, a highly reactive derivative of chlorine with potent bactericidal properties, is used as a disinfectant in many industries and is a recognized cause of occupational asthma.[18] Numerous pharmaceutical products, especially beta-lactam antibiotics, have been reported to induce occupational asthma in health-care personnel and manufacturing employees.[19] Nickel[20] and platinum salts[21] are well-recognized causes of occupational asthma.

Among the chemical compounds known to cause occupational asthma are ethylenediamine, diisocyanates, and the acid anhydrides. Formaldehyde, a respiratory irritant at ambient concentrations $\geq$ 1 ppm, is often cited as a cause of occupational asthma; however, documented instances of formaldehyde-induced IgE-mediated asthma are extremely rare.[22–24] A bifunctional aldehyde, glutaraldehyde has been reported to cause occupational asthma.[25] Ethylenediamine, a chemical used in the shellac and photographic developing industries, has been reported to cause occupational asthma.[26] Reactive azo dyes,[27] piperazine and dimethyl ethanolamine are other chemicals that have also been reported to be associated with occupational asthma.[28]

Isocyanates are required catalysts in the production of a variety of products including polyurethane foam, vehicle spray paint, and protective surface coatings. Approximately 5 to 10 percent of isocyanate workers develop asthma from exposure to subtoxic levels after a variable period of latency.[29] Among the isocyanates that have been described to cause occupational asthma are toluene diisocyanate (TDI), hexamethylene diisocyanate (HDI), diphenylmethyl diisocyanate (MDI), and isoperone diisocyanate (IPDI).[29] The histology of bronchial biopsies from workers with isocyanate asthma is very suggestive of an immunologic mechanism.[30,31] Compared to those with negative bronchial challenges, isocyanate workers with positive challenges have a higher incidence and level of antibody against isocyanate protein conjugates.[32] However, most isocyanate workers with positive challenges do not have detectable specific IgE in their serum; in short, the immunologic mechanism(s) underlying isocyanate asthma are currently unknown. Hypersensitivity pneumonitis[33] and hemorrhagic pneumonitis[34] have also been reported to be caused by immunologic reactions to isocyanates.

Acid anhydrides are curing agents used in the manufacture of epoxy resins that result in anticorrosive coating materials. Occupational asthma is one of three types of immunologic respiratory disease that may result from anhydride exposure.[35] Among the acid anhydrides that have been

TABLE 36-2   Examples of Allergens Causing Occupational Asthma

Etiologic Agent	Manufacturing or Industry Use
Low molecular weight	
Chemicals capable of reacting with autologous proteins	
Chloramine T	Food industry disinfectant, processing plants
Antibiotic agents	Hospitals, pharmaceutical plants
Other drugs—piperazine hydrochloride, α-methyldopa, amprolium hydrochloride, sulfone chloramide	Hospitals, pharmaceutical plants
Reactive azo dyes	Dye manufacturing
Platinum salts	Platinum processing plants
Nickel	Nickel-plating processes
Ethylenediamine	Shellac/lacquer industry
Plicatic acid	Western red cedar lumber industry
Isocyanates (TDI, MDI, HDI, IPDI)	Production of paints, surface coatings, insulation, polyurethane foam
Anhydrides (TMA, PA, TCPA, HHPA, MA, PMDA)	Manufacture of curing agents, plasticizers, anticorrosive coatings
High molecular weight	
Proteolytic enzymes	Plastic polymer resin manufacturing, detergent industry, pharmaceutical industry, meat tenderizer manufacturing, beer clearing
Animal proteins	
Mammalian proteins	Lab research, veterinarians, grooms, breeders, pet shops
Egg proteins	Egg processing and confectionery industry
Avian proteins	Poultry breeding, bird fanciers
Insect scales	Beekeepers, insect control, bait handlers, entomologists
Vegetable proteins	
Latex	Health care industry
Flour	Baking industry
Green coffee beans, carob beans, tea, garlic, soybeans	Workers in food processing plants
Castor beans	Fertilizer plants
Vegetable gums	Printing industry
Wood dusts—maple, mahogany, oak, walnut	Carpenters, sawyers, wood pulp workers, foresters, cabinetmakers
Orris root, rice flour	Hairdressing salons
Microorganism proteins	
Penicillium casei	Cheese manufacturing
Thermophilic molds	Mushroom farms

reported to cause occupational asthma are trimellitic anhydride (TMA), maleic anhydride (MA), phthalic anhydride (PA), tetrachlorophthalic anhydride (TCPA), pyromellitic anhydride (PMDA), and hexahydrophthalic anhydride (HHPA).[36]

High-molecular-weight protein agents that cause occupational asthma may be of animal, plant, or microorganism origin. Proteolytic enzymes of plant microorganism or animal source are potent sensitizing agent.[37,38] Animal proteins derived from urine, dander, or saliva can result in occupational asthma in a variety of workplace settings.[39,40] Avian proteins, including egg proteins such as lysozyme,[41] have been reported to cause occupational asthma.[42,43] Just as insect proteins from house dust mite and cockroach can

induce asthma in the domestic setting, insect proteins in the workplace are potent sensitizers.[44–47] In terms of plant protein antigens, exposure to latex antigens, particularly that dispersed by powder in gloves, is becoming an important cause of occupational asthma in health-care workers.[48–50] In the baking industry, flour proteins are well recognized to cause occupational asthma.[51–54] Numerous other plant foodstuff proteins have been described to cause occupational asthma with inhalational exposure—tea,[55] garlic,[56] coffee beans,[57] and soybeans.[58] Other plant protein sources causing occupational asthma include castor beans,[59] vegetable gums,[60] wood dusts,[61] and dried flowers.[62,63] Wood dust from western red cedar is well recognized to cause occupational asthma, but the antigen appears to be the low-molecular-weight chemical plicatic acid and not a high-molecular-weight plant protein.[64,65]

A variety of microorganisms have been reported to be sensitizing agents in occupational asthma. Among these are molds[66–68] and thermophilic actinomycetes.[6]

Pathophysiology

The pathogenesis of asthma is unknown. The major pathophysiologic abnormalities of asthma, occupational or otherwise, are bronchoconstriction, excess mucus production, and edema and inflammatory infiltration—including activated T cells and eosinophils—of the bronchial walls.[69] There is evidence that these abnormalities may be at least in part explained by neurogenic mechanisms and release of chemical mediators and cytokines. Type I hypersensitivity involving cross-linking IgE on the surface of mast cells and basophils resulting in release of mediators such as histamine and leukotrienes and cytokines such as interleukin 4 (IL-4) and IL-5 is believed to be the triggering mechanism in most types of immediate-onset asthma. There is increasing evidence that cellular mechanisms may be very important in asthma.[70,71]

Irrespective of the precise immunologic mechanism(s) involved, there are a number of characteristic patterns of asthma that can occur after a single inhalation challenge. (Table 36-3). The immediate reaction occurs within minutes of challenge, is IgE-mediated, lasts several hours, and is preventable with bronchodilators or cromolyn sodium. The late asthmatic response occurs 4 to 6 h after exposure to allergen; it is preventable with cromolyn or corticosteroids but not bronchodilators. Approximately half of patients with an immediate response also have a late response, and these patients are described as having a dual response. Another pattern that has been described after a single challenge with agents such as diisocyanates and western red cedar is the repetitive pattern in which a worker has repetitive asthmatic responses occurring over a period of several days. The mechanism is unknown but is generally reversible with a bronchodilator. Other atypical patterns—square wave, progressive, and prolonged immediate—have been described with diisocyanate challenges; the mechanisms resulting in these patterns have not been elucidated.[72] There is an increasingly large body of literature implicating immunologic mechanisms, in particular cellular mechanisms, in the pathophysiology of asthmatic responses to isocyanates.[73–75]

Epidemiology

The epidemiology of occupational asthma has not been well defined. Most studies have several limitations. First, there is a relatively high turnover in jobs associated with asthma, in effect selecting those workers who are not sensitized, known as the "well-worker effect." Second, occupational diseases in general are underreported.[14] Finally, the incidence of occupational asthma appears to depend on the agent and level of exposure.[76] The incidence in rat-exposed workers is 6 percent[77]; in isocyanate workers, 5 to 10 percent[29]; in proteolytic enzyme workers, 45 percent[8]; and in platinum workers, > 50 percent.[21] In studies from the United Kingdom, the greatest number of occupational asthma cases are reported from exposure to isocyanates, flour, and colophony.[78,79] In the United States, it has been estimated that approximately 2 percent of asthma is occupational.[80] In a U.S. Social Security Disability survey, approximately 15 percent of asthma cases were classified as occupational in origin.[81]

Host Factors

There are no studies reporting gender, race, or age as risk factors for the development of occupational asthma. In a limited study of 57 workers exposed to HHPA, neither race nor age was a risk factor.[82] Two risk factors that have been evaluated in several studies are atopy and cigarette smoking.

Atopy, the predilection to develop specific IgE to common allergens, is generally defined by positive skin tests to common aeroallergens such as ragweed pollen, house dust mite, and cat dander. Atopy has been reported to be a risk factor for development of occupational asthma due to high-molecular-weight allergens such as insect protein,[83] flour,[84] and detergent enzymes.[85] While there is a report of platinum asthma being associated with atopy,[86] asthma due to other low-molecular-weight chemicals such as isocyanates,[87] anhydrides,[37,88] and western red cedar[64] is not associated with atopic diathesis.

It is not clear whether cigarette smoking is a risk factor for occupational asthma. In a study of platinum salts[89,90] and an anhydride,[91] positive associations were reported. However, in reports of occupational asthma caused by animal dander,[92] a proteolytic enzyme,[93] and colophony,[94] no such association could be demonstrated.

HLA class II alleles have been studied in isocyanate asthma[95]; a positive association was reported with DQB1*0503 and DQB1*0201/0301.

TABLE 36-3 Types of Respiratory Response to Single Inhalation Challenge

	Immediate	Late	Dual	Repetitive	Atypical[a]
Asthma onset	10–30 min	4–6 h	10–30 min then 4–6 h	Periodic after initial attack	10–30 min
Duration	1–2 h	2–6 h	6–12 h	Days	6–10 h
Immune mechanism	IgE	IgE (IgG)	IgE, others?	? T cell	Unknown

[a] Atypical patterns: progressive, square-waved, prolonged immediate.

TABLE 36-4   Historical Information Useful in the Diagnosis of Occupational Asthma

1. Circumstances of onset of asthma
2. Sensitizers in the workplace
3. Temporal relationship between workplace exposure to sensitizers and disease occurrence or exacerbation
4. Clinical course of asthma and current disease severity

Diagnosis

HISTORY AND PHYSICAL

The history and physical examination of a patient with possible occupational asthma are very similar to those of a patient with asthma possibly related to a nonoccupational allergen. An overview of useful historical information is listed in Table 36-4. First, it is important to understand the circumstances and exposures at the onset of the disease. In particular, it is important to determine whether there are sensitizers in the workplace and what exposures to those substances were at the disease onset. In addition to information the patient provides, review of MSDS and available industrial hygiene data may prove useful. The nature of the temporal relationship between workplace exposure to sensitizers and disease occurrence and exacerbation should be explored. In addition to interviewing the patient, review of medical records—inpatient, outpatient, and occupational health—may provide additional corroborative data. Finally, in conjunction with physical examination and pulmonary function tests, the clinical course of the asthma and the current disease severity should be ascertained.

WORKPLACE AND EXPOSURE ASSESSMENT

In addition to patient interview and review of MSDS and available industrial hygiene data, it may be useful to gather additional information relative to exposure to sensitizers in the workplace. This generally requires contact with the employer, which should only be done with the patient's full knowledge and consent. Speaking with medical personnel, toxicologists, and industrial hygienists can often result in useful information. Occasionally a work-site visit to view the processes and exposures can be of value.

IMMUNOLOGIC ASSESSMENT

Immunologically mediated inflammation of the bronchial wall is associated with occupational asthma. The pathogenetic mechanisms of the immunologic hypersensitivity are essentially the same as those described for nonoccupational asthma. The primary immune response results from a series of cognate and noncognate interactions between antigen presenting cells—macrophages, B cells, and Langerhans cells—and T cells.[96] Both humoral and cellular immunologic responses may occur; the former are currently most implicated in the pathogenesis of occupational asthma. Specifically, the immunoglobulin isotype responsible for occupational asthma is IgE. Other immunoglobulin classes

such as IgG and IgA have been reported to be elevated in occupational asthma, but their role in the disease pathogenesis appears minor.

Specific IgE can be demonstrated by in vivo or in vitro techniques.[96,97] In either case, the preparation and characterization of the test reagents is key, because the reliability of both cutaneous tests and serologic assays is dependent on the potency of the allergenic reagents employed.[98] Standard methods for performing cutaneous tests[99] and serologic assays for specific IgE[100] are necessary. It is important to recognize that a positive immunologic test is corroborative, not diagnostic, since a small proportion of asymptomatic individuals will also have a positive serologic test. It is also important to recognize that specific IgE cannot be demonstrated in most cases of occupational asthma due to isocyanates and western red cedar. However, in individuals with occupational asthma due to most other allergens, specific IgE can be demonstrated if tests are properly performed with well-characterized reagents.

PULMONARY FUNCTION TESTS

Pulmonary function tests are useful to define objectively the relationship between asthma and the workplace.[3] A variety of methods have been proposed to evaluate that relationship. The gold standard is specific inhalation challenge provided that the putative allergen is known, the challenge method is established, and the worker is symptomatic.[3,72] Few physicians have access to such facilities and thus other methods have been reported.

Single cross-shift measures of pulmonary function are not necessarily helpful, because not all challenge-positive workers demonstrate positive results.[3] Serial cross-shift pulmonary function studies before and after a period of time off work have been reported to provide useful confirmatory data. Serial monitoring of peak expiratory flow rate (PEFR) was first reported as a diagnostically useful tool by Burge and colleagues[101]; subsequently, the utility of monitoring PEFR has been reported by a number of other investigators.[102–106] In studies comparing specific inhalation challenge and serial PEFR at work and off work, the sensitivity and specificity of PEFR was reported to be better than 80 percent.[104,105] Serial measurements of nonspecific bronchial hyperresponsiveness have also been reported to be useful both alone[107] and in combination with PEFR monitoring.[108]

Prognosis

It is clear that many workers with occupational asthma do not completely recover even though they have been removed from exposure to a sensitizing agent. Prognostic factors that have been examined include specific IgE, duration of symptoms, pulmonary function tests, and nonspecific bronchial hyperreactivity (BHR). An unfavorable prognosis was reported to be associated with a persistent high level of specific IgE,[109] long duration of symptoms (> 1 to 2 years), abnormal pulmonary function tests, and a high degree of BHR.[110–112] From these studies, the obvious conclusion is that early diagnosis and removal from exposure are requisite for the goal of complete recovery. In workers who remain exposed after a diagnosis of occupational asthma is made, further deterioration of lung function and increase in BHR are to be expected.[113] It should be appreciated that life-threatening attacks and even deaths have been reported.[114,115]

Treatment

Occupational asthma is best managed by avoidance of the offending etiologic agent. This avoidance can be accomplished in a variety of ways. An employee could be moved to another job that entailed no exposure to the sensitizing agent. Other possibilities include improved ventilation, enclosing the process, or use of personal protective equipment such as respirators. Because the latter are often poorly tolerated, their utility is primarily as a temporary protection. Ideally, the workplace environment should be designed to limit the concentration of respiratory sensitizers to very low levels.

Acutely, occupational asthma can be treated with the same drugs used to treat other types of asthma: β-adrenergic agonists and corticosteroids. However, chronic pharmacologic management of occupational asthma is ill advised in the presence of continued exposure. As noted above, continued deterioration and even death may ensue.

Allergen immunotherapy has been reported to be efficacious in the treatment of a few cases of occupational asthma caused by animal allergens,[116] flour dust,[117] and platinum.[118] In general, however, immunotherapy is not a practical approach, since avoidance is clearly the treatment of choice.

Prevention

Prevention of occupational asthma is clearly the goal. Minimizing exposure to respiratory sensitizing agents is obviously important. Engineering controls such as improved ventilation or enclosing processes are often useful. Industrial hygiene monitoring and explicit safety procedures, such as use of respirators during accidental spills, are important. Worker and management education about symptoms of occupational asthma and minimizing exposure to respiratory sensitizers are also important.

Thus far, no preemployment screening criteria have been reported to be highly predictive of development of occupational asthma in an individual worker. Currently the most practical approach is the development of medical surveillance programs to identify workers with occupational asthma at an early stage when removal is most likely to result in complete recovery.[119] In prospective studies of TMA-exposed employees, serial questionnaires and serologic studies have proved useful in predicting which individuals are likely to develop an immunologic respiratory disease due to TMA.[120,121] After identifying individuals at risk, a number of options including increased frequency of surveillance or job relocation can be considered. Medical sur-

veillance programs, early detection, and removal are currently the best means of preventing permanent asthma due to occupational allergens.

References

1. *Guidelines for the Diagnosis and Management of Asthma*: National Heart, Lung, and Blood Institute, National Asthma Education Program expert panel report. Publication No 91-3042A, June 1991.
2. Smith DD: Medical-legal definition of occupational asthma. *Chest* 1990; 98:1007.
3. Chan-Yeung M: A clinician's approach to determine the diagnosis, prognosis, and therapy of occupational asthma. *Med Clin North Am* 1990; 74:811.
4. Gautrin D, Boulet LP, Boutet M, et al.: Is reactive airways dysfunction syndrome a variant of occupational asthma? *J Allergy Clin Immunol* 1994; 93:12.
5. Office of the Federal Register National Archives and Records Administration: *Code of Federal Regulations 1900-1910*. Washington, DC: Federal Register, 1993.
6. Brooks SM: Occupational and environmental asthma, in Rom WN (ed): *Environmental and Occupational Medicine*, 2d ed. Boston: Little, Brown, 1992: 393–446.
7. Chan-Yeung M, Malo JL: Aetiological agents in occupational asthma. *Eur Respir J* 1994; 7:346.
8. Brooks SM: The evaluation of occupational airways disease in the laboratory and workplace. *J Allergy Clin Immunol* 1982; 70:56.
9. Murphy RLH Jr: Industrial diseases with asthma, in Weiss EB, Segal MS (eds): *Bronchial Asthma: Mechanisms and Therapeutics*. Boston: Little, Brown, 1976:517.
10. Bush RK, Kagen SL: Guidelines for the preparation and characterization of high molecular weight allergens used for the diagnosis of occupational lung disease. *J Allergy Clin Immunol* 1989; 84:814.
11. Agius RM, Nee J, McGovern B, Robertson A: Structure activity hypotheses in occupational asthma caused by low molecular weight substances. *Ann Occup Hygiene* 1991; 35:129.
12. Gauggel DL, Sarlo K, Asquith TN: A proposed screen for evaluating low-molecular-weight chemicals as potential respiratory allergens. *J Appl Toxicol* 1993; 13:307.
13. Aguis RM, Elton RA, Sawyer L, Taylor P: Occupational asthma and the chemical properties of low molecular weight organic substances. *Occup Med* 1994; 44:34.
14. Bernstein IL: Occupational asthma. *Clin Chest Med* 1981; 2:255.
15. Grammer LC: Occupational immunologic lung disease, in Patterson R, Zeiss CR, Grammer LC, Greenberger PA (eds): *Allergic Diseases: Diagnosis and Management*, 4th ed. Philadelphia: J Lippincott, 1993:745–762.
16. Bernstein DI, Bernstein IL: Occupational asthma, in Middleton E Jr, Reed CE, Ellis EF, et al (eds): *Allergy: Principles and Practice*, 4th ed. St. Louis: Mosby-Year Book, 1993:1369–1393.
17. Cockcroft D: Occupational asthma. *Ann Allergy* 1990; 65:169.
18. Blasco A, Joral A, Fuente R, et al.: Bronchial asthma due to sensitization to chloramine T. *J Invest Allergol Clin Immunol* 1992; 2:167.
19. Chida T: A study on dose-response relationship of occupational allergy in a pharmaceutical plant. *Jpn J Ind Health* 1986; 28:77.
20. Malo JL, Cartier A, Doepner M, et al.: Occupational asthma caused by nickel sulfate. *J Allergy Clin Immunol* 1982; 69:55.
21. Cromwell O, Pepys J, Parish WE, Hughes EG: Specific IgE antibodies to platinum salts in sensitized workers. *Clin Allergy* 1979; 9:109.

22. Hendrick DJ, Lane DJ: Occupational formalin asthma. *Br J Ind Med* 1977; 34:11.

23. Dykewicz MS, Patterson R, Cugell DW, et al.: Serum IgE and IgG to formaldehyde-human serum albumin: Lack of relation to gaseous formaldehyde exposure and symptoms. *J Allergy Clin Immunol* 1991; 87:48.

24. Grammer LC, Harris KE, Cugell DW, Patterson R: Evaluation of a worker with possible formaldehyde-induced asthma. *J Allergy Clin Immunol* 1993; 92:29.

25. Chan-Yeung M, McMurren T, Catonio-Begley F, Lam S: Clinical aspects of allergic disease: Occupational asthma in a technologist exposed to glutaraldehyde. *J Allergy Clin Immunol* 1993; 91:974.

26. Lam S, Chan-Yeung M: Ethylenediamine-induced asthma. *Am Rev Respir Dis* 1980; 121:151.

27. Nilsson R, Nordlinder R, Wass U, et al.: Asthma, rhinitis, and dermatitis in workers exposed to reactive dyes. *Br J Ind Med* 1993; 50:65.

28. Vallieres M, Cockcroft DW, Taylor DM, et al.: Dimethyl ethanolamine-induced asthma. *Am Rev Respir Dis* 1977; 115:867.

29. Balaan MR, Banks DE: The respiratory effects of isocyanates, in Rom WN (ed): *Environmental and Occupational Medicine*, 2d ed. Boston: Little, Brown, 1992:967.

30. Saetta M, di Stefano A, Maestrelli P, et al.: Airway mucosal inflammation in occupational asthma induced by toluene diisocyanate. *Am Rev Respir Dis* 1992; 145:160.

31. Saetta M, Maestrelli P, di Stefano A, et al.: Effect of cessation of exposure to toluene diisocyanate (TDI) on bronchial mucosa of subjects with TDI-induced asthma. *Am Rev Respir Dis* 1992; 145:169.

32. Grammer LC, Harris KE, Malo JL, et al.: The use of an immunoassay index for antibodies against isocyanate human protein conjugates and application to human isocyanate disease. *J Allergy Clin Immunol* 1990; 86:94.

33. Walker CL, Grammer LC, Shaughnessy MA, et al.: Diphenylmethane diisocyanate hypersensitivity pneumonitis: A serologic evaluation. *J Occup Med* 1989; 31:315.

34. Patterson R, Nugent KM, Harris KE, Eberle ME: Case reports: Immunologic hemorrhagic pneumonia caused by isocyanates. *Am Rev Respir Dis* 1990; 141:226.

35. Zeiss CR, Wolkonsky P, Pruzansky JJ, Patterson R: Clinical and immunologic evaluation of trimellitic anhydride workers in multiple industrial settings. *J Allergy Clin Immunol* 1982; 70:15.

36. Grammer LC, Patterson R: Trimellitic anhydride, in Rom WN (ed): *Environmental and Occupational Medicine*, 2nd ed. Boston: Little, Brown, 1992: 987–991.

37. Novey HS, Keenan WJ, Fairshter RD, et al.: Pulmonary disease in workers exposed to papain: Clinico-physiological and immunologic studies. *Clin Allergy* 1980; 10:721.

38. Hayes JP, Newman Taylor AJ: Bronchial asthma in a paediatric nurse caused by inhaled pancreatic extracts. *Br J Ind Med* 1991; 48:355.

39. Gross NJ: Allergy to laboratory animals: Epidemiologic, clinical and physiologic aspects and a trial of cromolyn in its management. *J Allergy Clin Immunol* 1980; 66:158.

40. Lincoln TA, Boltan NE, Garrett AS: Occupational allergy to animal dander and sera. *J Occup Med* 1974; 16:465.

41. Bernstein JA, Kraut A, Bernstein DI, et al.: Occupational asthma induced by inhaled egg lysozyme. *Chest* 1993; 103:532.

42. Blanco Carmona JG, Juste Picon S, Garces Sotillos M, Rodriguez Gaston P: Occupational asthma in the confectionery industry caused by sensitivity to egg. *Allergy* 1992; 47:190.

43. Hargreave FE, Pepys J: Allergic respiratory reactions in bird fanciers provoked by allergen inhalation provocation tests. *J Allergy Clin Immunol* 1972; 50:157.

44. Siracusa A, Bettini P, Bacoccoli R, et al.: Asthma caused by live fish bait. *J Allergy Clin Immunol* 1994; 93:424.

45. Lunn JA: Millworkers' asthma: Allergic responses to the grain weevil (*Sitophilus granarius*). *Br J Ind Med* 1966; 23:149.

46. Gibbons HL, Dillie JR, Cauley RG: Inhalant allergy to the screw worm fly. *Arch Environ Health* 1965; 10:424.

47. Bernstein DI, Gallagher JS, Bernstein IL: Meal worm asthma: Clinical and immunologic studies. *J Allergy Clin Immunol* 1983; 72:475.

48. DeZotti R, Larese F, Fiorito A: Asthma and contact urticaria from latex gloves in a hospital nurse. *Br J Ind Med* 1992; 49:596.

49. Caruso B, Caputo M, Senna G, Andri L: Immunoblotting study of specific antibody patterns against latex and banana. *Allergie Immunol* 1993; 25:187.

50. Slater JE: Continuing medical education: Latex allergy. *J Allergy Clin Immunol* 1994; 94:139.

51. Blanco Carmona JG, Juste Picon S, Garces Sotillos M: Occupational asthma in bakeries caused by sensitivity to alpha-amylase. *Allergy* 1991; 46:274.

52. Walker CL, Grammer LC, Shaughnessy MA, Patterson R: Baker's asthma: Report of an unusual case. *J Occup Med* 1989; 31:439.

53. Wilber RD, Ward GW: Immunologic studies in a case of baker's asthma. *J Allergy Clin Immunol* 1976; 58:366.

54. van der Brempt X, Ledent C, Mairesse M: Rhinitis and asthma caused by occupational exposure to carob bean flour. *J Allergy Clin Immunol* 1992; 90:1008.

55. Cartier A, Malo JL: Occupational asthma due to tea dust. *Thorax* 1990; 45:203.

56. Falleroni AF, Zeiss CR, Levitz D: Occupational asthma secondary to inhalation of garlic dust. *J Allergy Clin Immunol* 1981; 68:156.

57. Lehrer SB: Bean hypersensitivity in coffee workers' asthma: A clinical and immunological appraisal. *Allergy Proc* 1990; 11:65.

58. Ferrer A, Torres A, Roca J, et al.: Characteristics of patients with soybean dust-induced acute severe asthma requiring mechanical ventilation. *Eur Respir J* 1990; 3:429.

59. Coombs RR, Hunter A, Jonas WE, et al.: Detection of IgE (IgND) specific antibody (probably reagin) to castor bean allergen by the red cell linked antigen antiglobulin reaction. *Lancet* 1968; 1:1115.

60. Lagier F, Cartier A, Somer J, et al.: Occupational asthma caused by guar gum. *J Allergy Clin Immunol* 1990; 85:785.

61. Godnic-Cvar J, Gomzi M: Case report of occupational asthma due to palisander wood dust and bronchoprovocation challenge by inhalation of pure wood dust from a capsule. *Am J Ind Med* 1990; 18:541.

62. Quirce S, Garcia-Figueroa B, Olaguibel JM, et al.: Occupational asthma and contact urticaria from dried flowers of *Limonium tataricum*. *Allergy* 1993; 48:285.

63. Schroeckenstein DC, Meier-Davis S, Yunginger JW, Bush RK: Allergens involved in occupational asthma caused by baby's breath (*Gypsophila paniculata*). *J Allergy Clin Immunol* 1990; 86:189.

64. Chan-Yeung M, Barton GM, MacLean L, Grzybowski S: Occupational asthma and rhinitis due to western red cedar (*Thuja plicata*). *Am Rev Respir Dis* 1973; 108:1094.

65. Chan-Yeung M: Immunologic and non-immunologic mechanisms in asthma due to western red cedar (*Thuja plicata*). *J Allergy Clin Immunol* 1982; 70:32.

66. Gottlieb SJ, Garibaldi E, Hutcheson PS, Slavin RG: Occupational asthma to the slime mold *Dictyostelium discoideum*. *J Occup Med* 1993; 35:1231.

67. Cullinan P, Cannon J, Sheril D, Newman Taylor A: Asthma following occupational exposure to *Lycopodium clavatum* in condom manufacturers. *Thorax* 1993; 48:774.

68. Côté J, Chan H, Brochu G, Chan-Yeung M: Occupational asthma caused by exposure to neurospora in a plywood factory worker. *Br J Ind Med* 1991; 48:279.

69. Glassroth J, Smith LJ: Asthma-pathophysiology, in Patterson R, Zeiss CR, Grammer LC, Greenberger PA (eds): *Allergic Diseases: Diagnosis and Management*, 4th ed. Philadelphia: Lippincott, 1993: 611–633.

70. Gratziou C, Carroll M, Walls A, et al.: Early changes in T lymphocytes recovered by bronchoalveolar lavage after local allergen challenge of asthmatic airways. *Am Rev Respir Dis* 1992; 145:1259.

71. Azzawi, Johnston PW, Majundar S, et al.: T lymphocytes and activated eosinophils in airway mucosa in fatal asthma and cystic fibrosis. *Am Rev Respir Dis* 1992; 145:1477.

72. Cartier A, Malo JL: Occupational challenge tests, in Bernstein IL, Chan-Yeung M, Malo JL, Bernstein DI (eds): *Asthma in the Workplace*. New York: Marcel Dekker, 1993: 215–247.

73. Vandenplas O, Malo JL, Saetta M, et al.: Occupational asthma and extrinsic alveolitis due to isocyanates: Current status and perspectives. *Br J Ind Med* 1993; 50:213.

74. Di Stefano A, Saetta M, Maestrelli P, et al.: Mast cells in the airway mucosa and rapid development of occupational asthma induced by toluene diisocyanate. *Am Rev Respir Dis* 1993; 147:1005.

75. Maestrelli P, Calcagni PG, Saetta M, et al.: Sputum eosinophilia after asthmatic responses induced by isocyanates in sensitized subjects. *Clin Exp Allergy* 1994; 24:29.

76. Burge PS: New developments in occupational asthma. *Br Med Bull* 1992; 48:221.

77. Carroll KB, Pepys J, Longbottom JL, et al.: Extrinsic allergic alveolitis due to rat serum proteins. *Clin Allergy* 1975; 5:443.

78. Meredith S: Reported incidence of occupational asthma in the United Kingdom, 1989–90. *J Epidemiol Commun Health* 1993; 47:459.

79. Gannon PF, Burge PS: The SHIELD scheme in the West Midlands Region, United Kingdom: Midland Thoracic Society Research Group. *Br J Ind Med* 1993; 50:791.

80. NIAID Task Force Report: *Asthma and Other Allergic Diseases*. NIH Publication No. 79-387:330. Washington, DC: Department of Health, Education and Welfare, 1979.

81. Blanc P: Occupational asthma in a national disability survey. *Chest* 1987; 92:613.

82. Grammer LC, Shaughnessy MA, Lowenthal M, Yarnold PR: Risk factors for immunologically mediated respiratory disease from hexahydrophthalic anhydride. *J Occup Med* 1994; 36:642.

83. Burge PS, Edge G, O'Brien IM, et al.: Occupational asthma, rhinitis and urticaria in a research establishment breeding locusts. *Thorax* 1979; 34:415.

84. Herxheimer H: The skin sensitivity to flour of baker's apprentices: A final report of long-term investigation. *Acta Allergol* 1967; 28:42.

85. Newhouse ML, Tagg B, Pocock SJ: An epidemiological study of workers producing enzyme washing powders. *Lancet* 1970; 1:689.

86. Pepys J, Pickering CAC, Hughes EG: Asthma due to inhaled chemical agents: Complex salts of platinum. *Clin Allergy* 1972; 2:391.

87. Moller D, Brooks SM, McKay R, et al.: Chronic asthma due to toluene diisocyanate. *Chest* 1986; 90:494.

88. Zeiss CR, Patterson R, Pruzansky JJ, et al.: Trimellitic anhydride-induced airway syndromes: Clinical and immunologic studies. *J Allergy Clin Immunol* 1977; 60:96.

89. Brooks S, Baker DB, Gann PH, et al.: Cold air challenge and platinum skin reactivity in platinum refinery workers. *Chest* 1990; 97:1401.

90. Venables K, Dally MB, Nunn AJ, et al.: Smoking and occupational allergy in workers in a platinum refinery. *Br Med J* 1989; 299:939.

91. Venables K, Topping M, Howe W, et al.: Interaction of smoking and atopy in producing specific IgE antibody against a hapten-protein conjugate. *Br Med J* 1985; 290:201.

92. Slovak A, Hill R: Laboratory animal allergy: A clinical survey of an exposed population. *Br J Ind Med* 1981; 38:38.

93. Mitchell CA, Gandevia B: Respiratory symptoms and skin reactivity in workers exposed to proteolytic enzymes in the detergent industry. *Am Rev Respir Dis* 1971; 104:1.

94. Burge P, Perks W, O'Brien I, et al.: Occupational asthma in an electronics factory: A case-control study to evaluate aetiological factors. *Thorax* 1979; 34:300.

95. Bignon JS, Aron Y, Ju LY, et al.: HLA class II alleles in isocyanate-induced asthma. *Am J Respir Crit Care Med* 1994; 149:71.

96. Abhas AK, Lichtman AH, Pober JS: *Cellular and Molecular Immunology*. Philadelphia: Saunders, 1991.

97. Grammer LC, Patterson R, Zeiss CR: Guidelines for the immunologic evaluation of occupational lung disease: Report of the subcommittee on immunologic evaluation of occupational immunologic lung disease. *J Allergy Clin Immunol* 1989; 84:805.

98. Grammer LC, Patterson R: Immunologic evaluation of occupational asthma, in Bernstein IL, Chan-Yeung M, Malo JL, Bernstein DI (eds): *Asthma in the Workplace*. New York: Marcel Dekker, 1993: 125–143.

99. Norman PS: Skin testing, in Rose NR, DeMacario EC, Fahey JL, (eds): *Manual of Clinical Laboratory Immunology*, 4th ed. Washington, DC: American Society for Microbiology, 1992: 685–688.

100. Hamilton RG, Adkinson NF: Measurement of total serum immunoglobulin E and allergen specific immunoglobulin E antibody, in Rose NR, DeMacario EC, Fahey JL, et al. (eds): *Manual of Clinical Laboratory Immunology*, 4th ed. Washington, DC: American Society for Microbiology, 1992: 689–701.

101. Burge PS, O'Brien IM, Haris MG: Peak flow rate records in the diagnosis of occupational asthma due to isocyanates. *Thorax* 1979; 34:317.

102. Venables KM, Burge PS, Davison AG, Newman-Taylor AJ: Peak flow rate records in surveys: Reproducibility of observers' reports. *Thorax* 1984; 39:828.

103. Liss GM, Tarlo SM: Peak expiratory flow rates in possible occupational asthma. *Chest* 1991; 100:63.

104. Côté J, Kennedy S, Chan-Yeung M: Sensitivity and specificity of PC_{20} and peak expiratory flow rate in cedar asthma. *J Allergy Clin Immunol* 1990; 85:592.

105. Perrin B, Lagier F, L'Archevêque J, et al.: Occupational asthma: Validity of monitoring of peak expiratory flow rates and nonallergic bronchial responsiveness as compared to specific inhalation challenge. *Eur Respir J* 1992; 5:40.

106. Hennenberger PK, Stanbury MJ, Trimbath LS, Kipen HM: The use of portable peak flowmeters in the surveillance of occupational asthma. *Chest* 1991; 100:1515.

107. Hargreave FE, Dolovich J, Boulet LP: Inhalation provocation tests. *Semin Resp Med* 1983; 4:224.

108. Cartier A, Pineau L, Malo JL: Monitoring of maximum expiratory peak flow rates and histamine inhalation test in the investigation of occupational asthma. *Clin Allergy* 1984; 14:193.

109. Grammer LC, Shaughnessy MA, Henderson J, et al.: A clinical and immunologic study of workers with trimellitic-anhydride-induced immunologic lung disease after transfer to low exposure jobs. *Am Rev Respir Dis* 1993; 148:54.

110. Lam S, Wong R, Chan-Yeung M: Nonspecific bronchial reactivity in occupational asthma. *J Allergy Clin Immunol* 1979; 63:28.

111. Hudson P, Cartier A, Pineau L, et al.: Follow-up of occupational asthma caused by crab and various agents. *J Allergy Clin Immunol* 1985; 76:682.

112. Pisati G, Baruffini A, Zedda S: Toluene diisocyanate induced asthma: Outcome according to persistence on cessation of exposure. *Br J Ind Med* 1993; 50:60.

113. Marabini A, Dimich-Ward H, Kwan SY, et al.: Clinical and socioeconomic features of subjects with red cedar asthma: A follow-up study. *Chest* 1993; 104:821.

114. Chan-Yeung M, Lam S: State of the art-occupational asthma. *Am Rev Respir Dis* 1986; 137:686.

115. Anonymous: Incident reports: Car paint death. *Toxic Subst Bull* 1985; 4:7.

116. Wahn U, Siraganian RP: Efficacy and specificity of immunother-apy with laboratory animal allergen extracts. *J Allergy Clin Immunol* 1980; 65:413.

117. Thiel H, Ulmer WT: Baker's asthma: Development and possibility for treatment. *Chest* 1978; 78:400.

118. Levene GM, Calnan CD: Platinum sensitivity treatment by specific hyposensitization. *Clin Allergy* 1971; 1:75.

119. Balmes J: Surveillance for occupational asthma. *J Occup Med* 1991; 6:101.

120. Boxer MB, Grammer LC, Harris KE, et al.: Six-year clinical and immunologic follow-up of workers exposed to trimellitic anhydride. *J Allergy Clin Immunol* 1987; 80:147.

121. Grammer LC, Harris KE, Sonenthal KR, et al.: A cross-sectional survey of 46 employees exposed to trimellitic anhydride. *Allergy Proc* 1992; 13:139.

Chapter 37

OZONE, NITROGEN DIOXIDE, AND SULFUR DIOXIDE

HELGO MAGNUSSEN AND RUDOLF JÖRRES

Within the past few decades there has been increasing concern about the potential effects of air pollution on human health. This chapter summarizes the evidence gained from different approaches indicating that the gaseous air pollutants ozone, nitrogen dioxide, and sulfur dioxide contribute to respiratory health risks.

Ozone

FORMATION AND EXPOSURE LEVELS

Within the lower atmosphere, ozone is produced primarily by photochemical reactions, which require hydrocarbons, nitrogen dioxide, and UV radiation from the sun. The daily variation of ozone levels, usually with peaks in the afternoon, is superimposed onto a seasonal cycle that shows a minimum during winter, an increase during springtime, and a maximum in the summer. Furthermore, considerable spatial variation in ozone levels is observed. In urban areas, daily variation of ozone levels may be greater than in rural areas due to rapid destruction of ozone by nitric oxide during the night. Downtransport of ozone from the upper atmosphere appears to be of minor importance. Significant primary sources of ozone can be found indoors or in the workplace, for example, produced by electrostatic devices such as xerographic copy machines.

Background concentrations of ozone have increased steadily within this century. In most areas of industrialized countries, background concentrations averaged over a year are in the range of 20 to 40 parts per billion (ppb). However, due to annual cycles in ozone levels and differences between regions, part of the population is exposed to higher levels of ozone. For the 1980s it has been estimated that about half of the U.S. population was living in areas where peak concentrations of more than 120 ppb were encountered. In many parts of Europe, exposure conditions appear to be not grossly different from most areas of the United States.

EPIDEMIOLOGIC STUDIES

Most of the epidemiologic evidence for adverse effects of ozone arises from studies on acute effects in children. Studies were designed as summer camp studies or were matched to air pollution episodes.[1-3] Symptoms and lung function parameters were monitored, and their relationship to variations in ambient levels of ozone was studied. These studies demonstrated a negative association between the level of ozone and symptoms or spirometric lung function indices, even for short-term exposures.[4] The consistency of the results is striking in view of the fact that studies differed largely in duration and intensity of exposure, exercise levels, and study populations. The magnitude of the ozone-associated decrements in FVC and FEV_1 in children ranges between 0.1 and 1.3 ml per ppb ozone.[2] Effects were transient, however, although one study presented evidence that the effects of ozone could persist over several weeks.[1]

The acute effect of ozone on morbidity and mortality in subjects with preexisting respiratory diseases is less clear. Some studies demonstrated an association between ozone concentration and hospital admissions for asthma[5]; others did not detect a significant correlation between ozone levels and the rate of hospitalization for respiratory disorders.[6]

To assess the ozone-related risk for chronic respiratory morbidity, populations exposed to different levels of ozone have been compared. Symptoms of chronic respiratory disease,[7] lung function impairment,[8,9] and the rate of annual decline of FEV_1[10] have been found to be associated with increased levels of ozone. Naturally, the analysis of such studies is confounded by the difficult task of separating the specific effects of ozone from those of concomitantly occurring air pollutants.[8,10]

In summary, the database is consistent in demonstrating short-term detrimental effects of ozone on symptoms and lung function. Possibly due to the presence of confounding factors, there is no conclusive evidence for adverse effects of ozone on asthma exacerbations or for long-term effects of ozone on respiratory morbidity and mortality.

EXPOSURE STUDIES

SYMPTOMS

The effects of ozone in experimental exposure studies have been studied extensively during the past two decades. Inhalation of ozone causes symptoms such as cough, sore throat, chest pain, pain on deep inspiration, and shortness of breath.[11] Symptoms appear not to be closely related to changes in lung function,[12] although some of them are linked to the maneuvers required for spirometric lung function measurement.

LUNG FUNCTION

Many studies have demonstrated that exposure to low levels of ozone causes significant changes in lung function characterized by a decrease in spirometric lung volumes caused by inhibition of deep inspiration.[11,13] Compared to the impairment in FEV_1 or FVC, increases in airway resistance produced by ozone are low and less consistently observed. Deterioration of lung function has been shown even at ozone concentrations as low as 80 ppb, if exposures were prolonged over 6.6 h of nearly continuous exercise.[14] The ozone response appears to be a function of the total inhaled dose and exposure rate (concentration times ventilation per hour).[15] Therefore, the concentration versus time pattern significantly influences the lung function response.[16] On average, the lung function response to ozone declines with age.[17,18] Interindividual variability is large[17–19] (Fig. 37-1), and strong predictors have not been found. The lung func-

tion response to ozone does not depend markedly on the degree of nonspecific airway responsiveness, although individuals with mild asthma have been reported to show slightly greater responses to ozone on average than normoreactive individuals.[12,20] Furthermore, patients with chronic obstructive pulmonary disease (COPD) do not show responses significantly different from those of healthy individuals.[21]

Adaptation or tolerance has been described for repeated exposures to ozone.[22–24] The time period over which adaptation persisted was shortest in those who were most sensitive to ozone.[22] On average, adaptation is lost within a 7-day interval.[23] To date, neither the physiologic basis of adaptation is known nor has it been revealed what role adaptation could play in ambient air exposures to ozone.

NONSPECIFIC AIRWAY RESPONSIVENESS

Bronchial responsiveness to nonspecific stimuli such as histamine or methacholine is enhanced after ozone exposure.[14,24–26] On average, the increase in nonspecific airway responsiveness disappears within 1 day after exposure.[25] It is reduced in subsequent exposures; however, baseline responsiveness is not completely restored.[24] In this sense, tolerance to ozone is less pronounced regarding methacholine responsiveness. As far as can be deduced from published data, the effects of ozone on methacholine responsiveness and lung function appear not to be closely associated.[12] In contrast to methacholine responsiveness, exercise-induced airway obstruction is not exaggerated or facilitated by ozone exposure.[27]

ALLERGEN RESPONSIVENESS

There are few data regarding the possible impact of ozone on allergen responsiveness in humans. Acute nasal responses to allergen were not altered after ozone exposure compared to filtered air exposure,[28] whereas bronchial allergen responsiveness was reported to be enhanced after exposure to an ozone concentration as low as 120 ppb for 1 h at rest.[29] Unfortunately, this study comprised only a small group of individuals with allergic asthma. A recent study showed a significant and nearly homogeneous increase in bronchial allergen responsiveness in a larger group with allergic asthma, after a 3-h exposure to 250 ppb ozone during moderate exercise[12] (Fig. 37-2). In addition, individuals with allergic rhinitis but without asthma demonstrated a marginal bronchial allergen response after ozone exposure.

MECHANISMS OF ACTION

Due to its low solubility in water, ozone is able to penetrate into deeper regions of the lung. About 40 percent of inhaled ozone is absorbed in the extrathoracic airways and another 55 percent in the intrathoracic airways. There is slight dependence on the ventilatory pattern, and large variability between individuals.[30] The local uptake is determined by the relationship between concentration, flow, area, and tissue properties and is maximal in the region of the terminal bronchioles.[31]

Ozone-induced damage involves lipid peroxidation and loss of functional groups of biomolecules, especially within

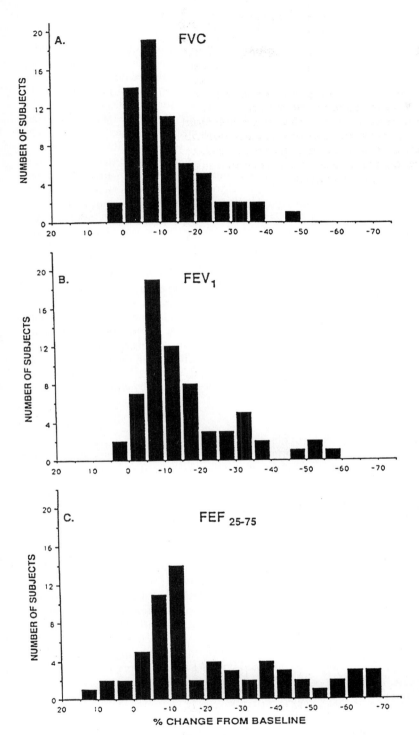

FIGURE 37-1 Frequency distribution of percent changes in lung function parameters following short-term exposure to 350 ppb ozone in healthy subjects (n = 64). (*From Weinmann et al.,*[19] *with permission.*)

cell membranes.[32] Several compounds produced by degradation of fatty acids have been detected that are capable of activating eicosanoid metabolism.[33] The cellular and biochemical effects caused by ozone are thought to be due directly to oxidation and peroxidation or indirectly to activation of inflammatory cells that are recruited into the airways.

INFLAMMATORY PROCESSES

It is not known in detail which mechanisms are responsible for the ozone-induced changes in lung function and airway responsiveness. Apparently, these effects are linked to the inflammatory processes induced by ozone. Airway inflammation has been demonstrated using the technique of bronchoalveolar lavage (BAL).[26,34–37] As the dominating cellular

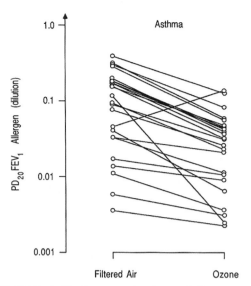

FIGURE 37-2 Individual provocative doses of allergen necessary to cause a 20 percent fall in FEV$_1$ after exposure to filtered air or 250 ppb ozone (n = 24). (*Jörres et al.,*[12] *with permission.*)

event, ozone causes an influx of neutrophils into the airways. However, the role of neutrophils is not understood fully because responses to ozone such as an increase in airway responsiveness have been observed preceding the neutrophil influx.[38] Ozone causes an increase in the levels of various inflammatory mediators within the BAL fluid. The concentrations of cyclooxygenase products of arachidonic acid such as prostaglandins PGE$_2$ and PGF$_{2\alpha}$ and thromboxane B$_2$ (TXB$_2$) are routinely increased after ozone exposure, whereas leukotrienes seem not to be markedly affected. Levels of interleukins IL-6 and IL-8 as well as granulocyte-macrophage colony-stimulating factor (GM-CSF) were increased after ozone exposure. Simultaneous use of the methods of isolated airway lavage and BAL demonstrated that ozone-induced airway inflammation occurs in the upper as well as in the lower airways.[37] It has been suggested that the functional impairment induced by ozone, which is characterized by a decrease in inspiratory capacity, is caused by stimulation of nonmyelinated C fibers.[11] Cyclooxygenase products are involved in these processes as indicated by the fact that the decrease in spirometric volumes could be reduced by the cyclooxygenase inhibitor indomethacin.[39,40] In contrast, the ozone-induced increase in methacholine responsiveness appears not to be mediated by cyclooxygenase products.[40]

To explain the increase in airway responsiveness after ozone exposure, release of neuropeptides has been proposed as one contributing mechanism.[41,42] Increased levels of substance P have been detected in the BAL fluid of humans exposed to ozone.[36] These findings suggest that neutral endopeptidase (NEP) could be involved, as shown directly in experimental animals.[43] So far, however, there are no data that demonstrate directly the contribution of neuropeptides to the ozone response in humans.

CELL DAMAGE AND PERMEABILITY

Studies utilizing BAL consistently demonstrate increased concentrations of various indicators of cell damage and of increased epithelial and vascular permeability, such as lactate dehydrogenase (LDH), total protein, fibronectin, and albumin.[34,35,37] The increase in epithelial permeability also has been assessed directly in humans.[44] It could be hypothesized that the effects observed after ozone inhalation are partially linked to this phenomenon. Increased epithelial permeability could be associated with facilitated penetration of inhaled agents such as methacholine and histamine or allergens, thus leading to an increased airway response. How-ever, it is not clear whether alterations in permeability exert differential effects on these different endpoints.

The cellular damage within the respiratory tract has been studied in animals. In accordance with the data on ozone uptake, primary damage was found to be localized to respiratory bronchioles and proximal alveolar ducts.[45,46] Whereas ciliated cells lose their cilia and their number as well as that of type I pneumocytes decrease after ozone exposure, nonciliated cells may show hypertrophy and hyperplasia. The changes induced by ozone appear to be reversible partially when ambient or near-ambient ozone concentrations are involved. Prolonged exposure to high concentrations of ozone can induce interstitial fibrosis in the region of respiratory bronchioles and alveolar ducts.[46] However, these observations have yet to be substantiated by clinical observations in humans.

DRUG EFFECTS

Several approaches have been followed to modulate the airway responses to ozone. Whereas β$_2$-adrenoreceptor agonists[47,48] and atropine[47] appear to prevent only ozone-induced increases in airway resistance, indomethacin has been reported to reduce the decrements in spirometric volumes caused by ozone[39] without major effect on nonspecific airway responsiveness.[40] In dogs, pretreatment with inhaled corticosteroids attenuated the increase in pulmonary resistance and neutrophil influx caused by ozone but did not affect the increase in airway responsiveness.[49] Taken together, it could be speculated that the mechanism governing the ozone-induced increase in airway responsiveness is not linked to cell-mediated airway inflammation induced by ozone, in contrast to the lung function response. On the other hand, the individual lung function response appears not to be correlated with the inflammatory response.

IN VITRO STUDIES

Recently, human bronchial epithelial cell lines and primary cells have been exposed to ozone in vitro. Ozone caused release of (1) the arachidonic acid products TXB$_2$, PGE$_2$, and leukotrienes C$_4$, D$_4$, and E$_4$[50]; and (2) platelet-activating factor (PAF),[51] IL-6 and IL-8,[52] fibronectin, and LDH.[52] These data are consistent with the hypothesis that the airway epithelium is the primary source of the products that can be detected in bronchoalveolar lavage fluid after in vivo exposure.

Nitrogen Dioxide

FORMATION AND EXPOSURE LEVELS

Nitrogen oxides are produced in combustion processes, the major component being nitric oxide, which may be oxidized to form nitrogen dioxide. Due to the continuous production of nitric oxide, its concentrations in urban areas are often higher than those of nitrogen dioxide. Urban nitrogen dioxide comes predominantly from motor vehicles; other sources such as power stations may play a role outside areas of significant traffic. Elevated concentrations of nitrogen dioxide also may be encountered in the workplace, in bus garages, during welding, and in ice-skating arenas. In homes with gas cooking and heating, it can form a major part of indoor air pollution.

On average, concentrations of nitrogen dioxide are below 50 ppb, even in urban areas. However, there may be sites, especially those exposed to heavy traffic, where peak values are > 100 ppb—as great as 400 ppb during severe air pollution episodes. In kitchens where gas stoves are used for cooking, short-term exposures to concentrations exceeding 500 ppb [0.5 ppm (parts per million)] have been described. Because of the different usage of gas stoves in different countries, the relevance of this source of nitrogen dioxide exposure varies from country to country.

EPIDEMIOLOGIC STUDIES

Several studies have provided evidence of an association between nitrogen dioxide levels and the frequency[53,54] or duration[55] of respiratory illness and lung function impairment.[53] This applies to outdoor as well as to indoor exposures. The effects are especially well analyzed in children, showing that long-term exposure even to slightly increased concentrations of nitrogen dioxide significantly increases the odds of respiratory illness.[56]

For patients with asthma, significant associations between nitrogen dioxide concentrations and respiratory symptoms as well as peak flow have been reported.[57] The majority of cross-sectional and longitudinal studies, however, did not find significant associations between the outdoor concentrations of nitrogen dioxide and several measures of respiratory illness, including hospital admissions. However, most analyses were severely handicapped by the strong associations between nitrogen dioxide and other air pollutants.[58]

In summary, although there is evidence for short-term effects of nitrogen dioxide, especially in children, its long-term effects cannot be considered to be established.

EXPOSURE STUDIES

SYMPTOMS

Nitrogen dioxide is capable of inducing symptoms by causing mucous membrane irritation, although very high concentrations are needed to elicit these effects. During exposure to lower concentrations of nitrogen dioxide, most studies did not find significant increases in symptom scores.

LUNG FUNCTION

The majority of studies indicate that nitrogen dioxide exerts only minimal or negligible effect on lung function[59] except at high concentrations, which can be encountered, for example, in the workplace. Older individuals are not more susceptible to nitrogen dioxide than young adults.[60] It has been demonstrated that threshold concentrations necessary to increase airway resistance in short-term exposures are about 1.5 ppm in patients with chronic bronchitis and that these patients showed impaired gas exchange at higher concentrations of nitrogen dioxide.[61] Increased susceptibility to nitrogen dioxide in patients with chronic obstructive pulmonary disease (COPD) has also been suggested by other investigators, the response being markedly heterogeneous between patients.[62] In view of the small effects on lung function, however, it is difficult to assess with certainty the risk due to nitrogen dioxide in patients with COPD.[63]

NONSPECIFIC AIRWAY RESPONSIVENESS

Healthy individuals can show increased nonspecific responsiveness after breathing nitrogen dioxide.[64,65] This has also been demonstrated in patients with asthma, in whom short-term exposure to nitrogen dioxide enhanced airway responsiveness to histamine[66] and methacholine.[67] Other studies, however, were not able to confirm these findings.[68,69] Furthermore, nitrogen dioxide exposure potentiated exercise-induced bronchoconstriction and the airway response to hyperventilation of cold air[70] as well as bronchoconstriction elicited by hyperventilation of air containing a fixed concentration of sulfur dioxide.[71] The increase in sulfur dioxide responsiveness appears not to be specific for sulfur dioxide but linked to the hyperventilation response.[72] Studies suggest that the effects of nitrogen dioxide depend crucially on the participants chosen and on the type of exposure protocol. A meta-analysis of published data showed that in patients with asthma the increase in nonspecific airway responsiveness occurred at significantly lower concentrations of nitrogen dioxide compared to those in healthy individuals.[73] Furthermore, short exposures at rest produced larger effects than prolonged exposures involving exercise.

ALLERGEN RESPONSIVENESS

Nitrogen dioxide has been reported to enhance both early and late phase bronchial responsiveness to inhaled allergens in patients with asthma,[74] although other authors could not substantiate a significant effect of nitrogen dioxide exposure alone.[75]

MECHANISMS OF ACTION

Nitrogen dioxide shows only limited solubility in water. It is mostly retained within the large and small airways, with low absorption in the alveolar region.[76] The percentage of total deposition depends slightly on the ventilation rate and ranges between about 70 and 90 percent.[70] The uptake of nitrogen dioxide within the bronchial system probably is governed by chemical reactions within the epithelial lining fluid and not simply determined by its physical solubility.[77]

Nitrogen dioxide is a nitrogen-centered free radical with oxidative properties similar to those of ozone, although less reactive.[78] As for ozone, nitrogen dioxide may cause damage by lipid peroxidation[79] and by generation of various reaction products with epithelial surface constituents,[80] which, in turn, can cause cell activation.

INFLAMMATORY PROCESSES

Several authors utilized the technique of BAL to study the effects of experimental exposures to nitrogen dioxide. Healthy individuals showed a reduction in their functional activity of α_1-protease inhibitor after exposure to high concentrations of nitrogen dioxide.[81] There was no such change after continuous exposure to a lower concentration or discontinuous exposure with higher peak values of nitrogen dioxide.[82] In addition, the concentration of the antiprotease α_2-macroglobulin was increased after breathing nitrogen dioxide.[83] After exposure to high concentrations of nitrogen dioxide, a concentration-dependent increase in the number of mast cells and increased numbers of lymphocytes and lysozyme-positive alveolar macrophages were reported (Fig. 37-3).[84] The levels of angiotensin-converting enzyme (ACE) and β_2-microglobulin, as markers of cell activiation, and the ratio of CD4+/CD8+ T lymphocytes were not changed. The increase in the number of mast cells and lymphocytes persisted up to 1 day after exposure and the increase in the percentage of lysozyme-positive macrophages persisted up to 3 days.[85] Smokers showed a response different from that of nonsmokers,[86] and patients with asthma had a response different from that of healthy participants.[59] In the asthma patients, exposure to nitrogen dioxide induced increased concentrations of TXB$_2$ and PGD$_2$ and decreased concentrations of 6-keto PGF$_{1\alpha}$ (a metabolite of PGI$_2$). After repeated exposures of healthy individuals to high concentrations of nitrogen dioxide,[87] the increase in the numbers of mast cells

and lymphocytes was abolished, but the ratio of CD4+ and CD8+ cells was slightly increased and the number of B cells and natural killer (NK) cells reduced. These data contrast to another study, which found no changes in CD4+/CD8+ subpopulations and an increase in NK cells.[88]

CELL DAMAGE AND PERMEABILITY

Apparently, nitrogen dioxide at ambient concentrations does not change epithelial permeability. This has been concluded from the fact that concentrations of total protein, albumin, leukocyte elastase, and LDH were not significantly altered by nitrogen dioxide exposure in lavage studies. However, it has to be taken into account that changes in alveolar permeability have been shown to occur with a delay of several hours after exposure[89] and could have been missed by other investigators.

Information on cell damage from nitrogen dioxide has been derived from animal exposure experiments. Most studies showed that maximum cell damage occurred at the transition between terminal bronchioles and alveolar ducts,[78] although major changes were observed also in the large bronchi.[90] Prolonged exposure to extremely high concentrations of nitrogen dioxide may result in centriacinar emphysema.[91] On the other hand, signs of mild interstitial fibrosis[92] as well as the development of bronchiolitis obliterans[93] have been reported. The latter findings correspond to what is known from inhalation accidents in humans involving high concentrations of nitrogen dioxide.

DRUG EFFECTS

There are very few data on the pharmacologic modulation of nitrogen dioxide responses. Antihistamines appear to attenuate the bronchoconstrictor response, which has been observed in patients with chronic bronchitis after short-term inhalation of nitrogen dioxide;[94] atropine or β_2-adrenoreceptor agonists are ineffective. Pretreatment with vitamin C prevented the increase in airway responsiveness caused by previous exposure to a high concentration of nitrogen dioxide.[65] These findings are compatible with the hypothesis that nitrogen dioxide acts in vivo at least partially through alteration of the prostaglandin and histamine metabolism within the airways. Furthermore, pretreatment with vitamins C and E diminished the amount of lipid peroxidation in BAL fluid, thus demonstrating the role of oxidant stress caused by nitrogen dioxide.[79]

IN VITRO STUDIES

When human bronchial epithelial cells grown as explant cultures were exposed to a low concentration of nitrogen dioxide, ciliary beat frequency decreased significantly.[95] Furthermore, there was a significant release of GM-CSF, IL-8, tumor necrosis factor α (TNF-α), leukotriene C$_4$, and of indicators of cell membrane damage.[95,96] In addition, the generation of reactive oxygen intermediates in human alveolar macrophages was increased in a concentration-dependent manner after short-term exposures to nitrogen dioxide.[97]

FIGURE 37-3 Relative changes in total cell counts for mast cells (squares), lymphocytes (triangles), and alveolar macrophages (circles) 24 h after short-term exposure to different concentrations of nitrogen dioxide. (*Sandström et al.,*[84] *with permission.*)

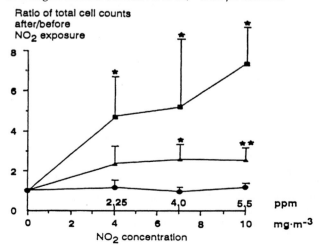

Sulfur Dioxide

FORMATION AND EXPOSURE LEVELS

In contrast to ozone, sulfur dioxide is a direct product of combustion processes, especially from fossil fuels containing a high percentage of sulfur. In recent decades, the distribution of sources has changed, because the large number of small sources from coal burning in individual households has been drastically reduced in many areas of the industrialized world. Instead, the smaller number of large emission sources related mainly to power plants has become more important. Furthermore, high concentrations of sulfur dioxide can be found in some workplaces, for example, in paper manufacturing and oil refining.

Due to the shift in sources and the use of filter devices, distribution characteristics and levels of sulfur dioxide have changed over time. Sulfur dioxide concentrations are linked to weather conditions. During winter, heating can lead to increased emission of sulfur dioxide, and atmospheric conditions of low air exchange can lead to increased concentrations of ambient sulfur dioxide over prolonged periods of time. By contrast, unstable air convection conditions in summertime could favor short-term peak values. The daily variation of sulfur dioxide shows different patterns in different areas. Therefore, individual exposures to sulfur dioxide are often difficult to predict. Current average annual concentrations in most areas are < 20 ppb. During air pollution episodes, concentrations > 100 ppb can occur for several hours, with peak concentrations well exceeding 200 ppb. In some places, especially in eastern European countries, much higher concentrations have been reported. For example, in some areas of East Germany, peak concentrations > 500 ppb have been recorded regularly during the 1980s.

EPIDEMIOLOGIC STUDIES

Various indices of lung function have been investigated to detect potential acute effects of sulfur dioxide. Overall, small and transient deteriorations of FEV_1 and FVC were revealed in children[98] as well as in adult patients with airway obstruction.[99] These studies showed the close association of black smoke and total suspended particulates with levels of sulfur dioxide, thus making it difficult to attribute specific effects to sulfur dioxide alone.

Epidemiologic studies have suggested that high levels of sulfur dioxide are linked to increased daily mortality,[100,101] with delay over several days, and to respiratory morbidity due to asthma[102] or bronchitis.[103] This is in accordance with those studies analyzing the well-known London smog episode in December, 1952. Patients with preexisting respiratory diseases appear to be especially at risk from sulfur dioxide. Again, a major outcome of most studies was that these acute effects of sulfur dioxide had to be considered within the whole pollutant mixture, which constitutes (winter) smog and generally contains high levels of suspended particulates. In the analysis of the Six Cities Study, it was found that mortality was more closely related to the levels of particulate matter than to sulfur dioxide.[104]

There are several studies on the association between long-term exposure to sulfur dioxide and chronic respiratory disease. Symptoms such as persistent cough or phlegm have been reported to be associated with long-term exposure to sulfur dioxide.[105] Other studies reported that total suspended particulate matter was of greater importance than sulfur dioxide with respect to symptom scores[106] and that intermittent exposure to sulfur dioxide and particles caused symptoms of bronchial irritation but no chronic deterioration.[107] Recent data from reunified Germany suggest that the highly elevated levels of sulfur dioxide and particulate matter in the eastern part of Germany were not associated with increased prevalences of hayfever and asthma.[108]

In summary, there is evidence for short-term effects of sulfur dioxide. However, data on long-term effects do not give conclusive support to the hypothesis of adverse health effects from sulfur dioxide.

EXPOSURE STUDIES

SYMPTOMS

Symptoms caused by inhalation of sulfur dioxide comprise cough, chest tightness, and wheezing[109,110] and are closely linked to the obstructive airway response caused by this stimulus.

LUNG FUNCTION

The airway response to low levels of sulfur dioxide has been studied by many authors in healthy individuals as well as in patients with bronchial asthma. The prominent feature of the lung function response induced by sulfur dioxide is bronchoconstriction. In healthy individuals, sulfur dioxide caused airway obstruction only when inhaled in a concentration of 5 ppm during short-term exposures at rest.[109] In contrast, patients with asthma showed airway obstruction at 1 ppm sulfur dioxide. Furthermore, these patients can develop bronchoconstriction after short-term exposure to 250 to 600 ppb sulfur dioxide when ventilation rates are increased by hyperventilation or exercise,[110,111] and individual patients may show a response at even lesser concentrations.[111] The rate of ventilation and the route of inhalation modulate the degree of bronchoconstriction caused by sulfur dioxide.[112] This can be attributed to its high absorption in the upper respiratory tract, which differs between mouth and nose, depending on flow rates.[113] When sulfur dioxide was contained in dry or dry and cold air, significantly stronger responses were observed when compared to a mixture with partially humidified air.[114] The degree of bronchial responsiveness to sulfur dioxide does not correlate with the airway responsiveness to methacholine[115] or histamine.[116] Furthermore, asthma patients develop tolerance to the bronchoconstrictor response to sulfur dioxide within repeated short-term exposures,[117] though it appears to persist only over short periods.

NONSPECIFIC AIRWAY RESPONSIVENESS

A few investigators have studied the effect of ambient concentrations of sulfur dioxide on airway responsiveness. They did not observe a change in histamine[117] or methacholine[118] responsiveness induced by sulfur dioxide exposure.

ALLERGEN RESPONSIVENESS

Bronchial responsiveness to inhaled allergens in patients with asthma was not increased after breathing sulfur dioxide alone.[75] The bronchial allergen response was significantly enhanced after simultaneous exposure to nitrogen dioxide and sulfur dioxide for a prolonged period at rest, despite the facts that nitrogen dioxide alone did not exert a significant effect and that under these exposure conditions sulfur dioxide is largely absorbed in the upper respiratory tract.[112,113]

MECHANISMS OF ACTION

Sulfur dioxide readily dissolves in the surface fluid layer of airway epithelium. The site of absorption depends on several factors, amongst which nasal anatomy, the relationship between nasal and oral breathing, and inspiratory flow rates are most important.[113] Increased flow rates reduce the percentage of sulfur dioxide absorbed in the upper airways, a mechanism that occurs during exercise.[111,112]

Partially depending on pH, sulfur dioxide can undergo a number of reactions with water, oxygen, or ammonia to yield hydrogen ions, sulfuric acid, sulfites or bisulfites, and sulfates. These products, as well as sulfur dioxide itself, are dissolved within the epithelial fluid layer or may be absorbed onto particulate matter, thus offering the potential for additional reactions and transport mechanisms. It is known that sulfites produced from sulfur dioxide can react with disulfide bonds in a variety of biologic macromolecules such as albumin and glutathione. It has not been clarified, however, which mechanisms ultimately lead to cell damage or cell activation in humans under ambient (nontoxic) exposure conditions.

INFLAMMATORY PROCESSES

There is scarce information on the cellular and biochemical events underlying the airway response to sulfur dioxide in human beings. When healthy individuals were exposed to high levels of sulfur dioxide for short periods of time, an acute inflammatory response was observed in the BAL fluid.[119,120] Total cell number, total and relative numbers of mast cells and lymphocytes, and total numbers of macrophages and lysozyme-positive macrophages increased significantly with increasing concentrations of sulfur dioxide, showing a plateau at about 11 ppm sulfur dioxide.[119] Changes in the numbers of mast cells, lymphocytes, and lysozyme-positive macrophages occurred 4 h after exposure. Cell numbers reached their maximum 24 h after exposure and had returned to baseline values 3 days after the end of exposure.[120] There was no detectable shift in the relative numbers of CD4+ and CD8+ lymphocytes.

The response to sulfur dioxide is thought to be controlled by two potential mechanisms: (1) stimulation of sensory nerves,[121,122] and (2) cell influx[119,120,123] and cell activation resulting in a variety of inflammatory mediators. In recent years, inhalation of metabisulfite aerosols has been recognized as mimicking some effects of sulfur dioxide,[124,125] although responses appear not to correlate well.[126] Metabisulfite aerosols are able to liberate sulfur dioxide, depending on pH, and to circumvent the loss of sulfur dioxide due to absorption in the upper respiratory tract. The inflammatory mediators released after sulfur dioxide exposure could cause mucus secretion and alterations of airway walls similar to those observed in chronic bronchitis. In addition, some are capable of stimulating sensory nerve endings, hence a potential link to neurogenic inflammation. The sensory nerve endings responsible for bronchoconstriction after sulfur dioxide inhalation are generally identified with C-fiber and irritant receptors,[122] and cholinergic reflex mechanisms have been proposed to elicit the acute sulfur dioxide response.[127] However, data are not quite consistent,[128,129] and direct evidence in humans is not available.

CELLULAR DAMAGE AND PERMEABILITY

Lavage studies performed in humans did not show altered levels of albumin in BAL fluid after short-term exposures to high levels of sulfur dioxide.[119,120] Therefore, alveolar permeability appears not to be changed by this type of exposure.

The cellular damage induced by high levels of sulfur dioxide has been studied in a variety of animal species. High levels of sulfur dioxide can result in alterations similar to those in chronic bronchitis.[123] Short exposures caused loss of tracheal epithelium, while longer exposures led to epithelial thickening and increased volume of mucous glands.[130] Changes were partially or totally reversible, depending on sulfur dioxide concentration. Interestingly, airway responsiveness to methacholine decreased after sulfur dioxide exposure, in contrast to the action of other air pollutants. Because of high absorption of sulfur dioxide and different anatomy, animal studies show large differences between species and between the outcomes for different exposure regimes.

DRUG EFFECTS

It has been shown that β_2-adrenoreceptor agonists,[131] disodium cromoglycate[132,133] (Fig. 37-4), nedocromil sodium,[134] and theophylline[135] are able to block or to attenuate the sulfur dioxide–induced bronchoconstriction. In contrast, inhaled steroids appear to inhibit the sulfur dioxide response only partially,[136] and ipratropium bromide has no protective effect.[137] These data suggest that both bronchial smooth-muscle relaxation and blocking effects on C fibers of neural pathways can lead to a reduction of sulfur dioxide–induced bronchoconstriction.

Mixtures of Different Air Pollutants

The potential synergy between the actions of different air pollutants has been studied within experimental exposure settings, either by subsequent or by simultaneous exposure to the different compounds. Whereas the response to ozone was not amplified by previous exposure to peroxyacetyl nitrate[138] or nitric acid fog,[139] a recent study suggested that

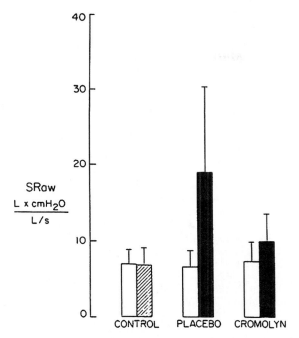

FIGURE 37-4 Protective effect of disodium cromoglycate on sulfur dioxide–induced bronchoconstriction. Mean values of specific airway resistance before exercise while breathing air or sulfur dioxide (control, open bars), after exercise alone (cross-hatched bar), and after exercise while breathing sulfur dioxide (full bars). (*Sheppard et al.,*[132] *with permission.*)

preexposure to nitrogen dioxide could exert a delayed effect on the spirometric airway response to ozone.[140] Healthy individuals did not demonstrate significant synergy between the effects of ozone and sulfur dioxide.[141] Conversely, in patients with asthma, sulfur dioxide–induced bronchoconstriction could be elicited after preexposure to a low dose of ozone,[142] whereas simultaneous exposure to sulfur dioxide and nitrogen dioxide did not indicate synergistic lung function effects.[143] These results illustrate that the types of air pollutants, their concentrations, and the characteristics of the participants are essential factors in the outcome of the studies. Furthermore, the time pattern of combined exposures may play a more important role than previously recognized.

References

1. Lioy PJ, Vollmuth TA, Lippmann M: Persistence of peak flow decrement in children following ozone exposures exceeding the National Ambient Air Quality Standard. *J Air Pollut Control Assoc* 1985; 35:1068.
2. Kinney PL, Ware JH, Spengler JD: A critical evaluation of acute ozone epidemiology results. *Arch Environ Health* 1988; 43:168.
3. Castillejos M, Gold DR, Dockery D, et al.: Effects of ambient ozone on respiratory function and symptoms in Mexico City schoolchildren. *Am Rev Respir Dis* 1992; 145:276.
4. Braun-Fahrländer C, Künzli N, Domenighetti G, et al.: Acute effects of ambient ozone on respiratory function of Swiss schoolchildren after a 10-minute heavy exercise. *Pediatr Pulmonol* 1994; 17:169.
5. Cody RP, Weisel CP, Birnbaum G, Lioy PJ: The effect of ozone associated with summertime photochemical smog on the frequency of asthma visits to hospital emergency departments. *Environ Res* 1992; 58:184.
6. Bates D, Baker-Anderson M, Sizto R: Asthma attack periodicity: A study of hospital emergency visits in Vancouver. *Environ Res* 1990; 51:51.
7. Euler G, Abbey D, Hodgkin J, Magie A: Chronic obstructive pulmonary disease symptom effects of long-term cumulative exposure to ambient levels of total oxidants and nitrogen dioxide in California Seventh-Day Adventists Residents. *Arch Environ Health* 1988; 43:279.
8. Detels R, Sayre J, Coulson A, et al.: The UCLA population studies of chronic obstructive respiratory disease: IV. Respiratory effect of long-term exposure to photochemical oxidants, nitrogen dioxide, and sulphates on current and never smokers. *Am Rev Respir Dis* 1981; 124:673.
9. Schwartz J: Lung function and chronic exposure to air pollution: A cross-sectional analysis of NHANES II. *Environ Res* 1989; 50:309.
10. Detels R, Tashkin DP, Sayre JW, et al.: The UCLA population studies of chronic obstructive respiratory disease: IX. Lung function changes associated with chronic exposure to photochemical oxidants: A cohort study of never smokers. *Chest* 1987; 92:594.
11. Hazucha MJ, Bates DV, Bromberg PA: Mechanisms of action of ozone on the human lung. *J Appl Physiol* 1989; 67:1535.
12. Jörres R, Nowak D, Magnussen H: The effect of ozone exposure on allergen responsiveness in subjects with asthma or rhinitis. Accepted for publication in: *Am J Respir Crit Care Med* 1996.
13. Hazucha MJ: Relationship between ozone exposure and pulmonary function changes. *J Appl Physiol* 1987; 62:1671.
14. Horstman DH, Folinsbee LJ, Ives PJ, et al.: Ozone concentration and pulmonary response relationships for 6.6-hour exposures with five hours of moderate exercise to 0.08, 0.10, and 0.12 ppm. *Am Rev Respir Dis* 1990; 142:1158.
15. McDonnell WF, Smith MV: Description of acute ozone response as a function of exposure rate and total inhaled dose. *J Appl Physiol* 1994; 76:2776.
16. Hazucha MJ, Folinsbee LJ, Seal E Jr: Effects of steady-state and variable ozone concentration profiles on pulmonary function. *Am Rev Respir Dis* 1992; 146:1487.
17. Drechsler-Parks DM, Bedi JF, Horvath SM: Pulmonary function responses of older men and women to ozone exposure. *Exp Gerontol* 1987; 22:91.
18. McDonnell WF, Muller KE, Bromberg PA, Shy CM: Predictors of individual differences in acute response to ozone exposure. *Am Rev Respir Dis* 1993; 147:818.
19. Weinmann GG, Bowes SM, Gerbase MW, et al.: Response to acute ozone exposure in healthy men. *Am J Respir Crit Care Med* 1995; 151:33.
20. Kreit JW, Gross KB, Moore TB, et al.: Ozone-induced changes in pulmonary function and bronchial responsiveness in asthmatics. *J Appl Physiol* 1989; 66:217.
21. Kehrl HR, Hazucha MJ, Solic JJ, Bromberg PA: Responses of subjects with chronic obstructive pulmonary disease after exposures to 0.3 ppm ozone. *Am Rev Respir Dis* 1985; 131:719.
22. Horvath SM, Gliner JA, Folinsbee LJ: Adaptation to ozone: Duration of effect. *Am Rev Respir Dis* 1981; 123:496.
23. Linn WS, Medway DA, Anzar UT, et al.: Persistence of adaptation to ozone in volunteers exposed repeatedly for six weeks. *Am Rev Respir Dis* 1982; 125:491.
24. Folinsbee LJ, Horstman DH, Kehrl HR, et al.: Respiratory responses to repeated prolonged exposure to 0.12 ppm ozone. *Am J Respir Crit Care Med* 1994; 149:98.

25. Golden JA, Nadel JA, Boushey HA: Bronchial hyperirritability in healthy subjects after exposure to ozone. *Am Rev Respir Dis* 1978; 118:287.

26. Seltzer J, Bigby BG, Stulbarg M, et al.: O$_3$-induced change in bronchial reactivity to methacholine and airway inflammation in humans. *J Appl Physiol* 1986; 60:1321.

27. Weymer AR, Gong H Jr, Lyness A, Linn WS: Pre-exposure to ozone does not enhance or produce exercise-induced asthma. *Am J Respir Crit Care Med* 1994; 149:1413.

28. Bascom R, Naclerio RM, Fitzgerald TK, et al.: Effect of ozone inhalation on the response to nasal challenge with antigen of allergic subjects. *Am Rev Respir Dis* 1990; 142:594.

29. Molfino NA, Wright SC, Katz I, et al.: Effect of low concentrations of ozone on inhaled allergen responses in asthmatic subjects. *Lancet* 1991; 338:199.

30. Gerrity TR, Weaver RA, Bernsten J, et al.: Extrathoracic and intrathoracic removal of O$_3$ in tidal-breathing humans. *J Appl Physiol* 1988; 65:393.

31. Hu, SC, Ben-Jebria A, Ultman JS: Simulation of ozone uptake distribution in the human airways by orthogonal collocation on finite elements. *Comput Biomed Res* 1992; 25:264.

32. Mustafa MG: Biochemical basis of ozone toxicity. *Free Radic Biol Med* 1990; 9:245.

33. Leikauf GD, Zhao Q, Zhou S, Santrock J: Ozonolysis products of membrane fatty acids activate eicosanoid metabolism in human airway epithelial cells. *Am J Respir Cell Mol Biol* 1993; 9:594.

34. Koren HS, Devlin RB, Graham DE, et al.: Ozone-induced inflammation in the lower airways of human subjects. *Am Rev Respir Dis* 1989; 139:407.

35. Devlin RB, McDonnell WF, Mann R, et al.: Exposure of humans to ambient levels of ozone for 6.6 hours causes cellular and biochemical changes in the lungs. *Am J Respir Cell Mol Biol* 1991; 4:72.

36. Hazbun ME, Hamilton R, Holian A, Eschenbacher WL: Ozone-induced increases in substance P and 8-epi-prostaglandin F$_{2\alpha}$ in the airways of human subjects. *Am J Respir Cell Mol Biol* 1993; 9:568.

37. Aris RM, Christian D, Hearne PQ, et al.: Ozone-induced airway inflammation in human subjects as determined by airway lavage and biopsy. *Am Rev Respir Dis* 1993; 148:1363.

38. Murlas C, Roum JH: Sequence of pathologic changes in the airway mucosa of guinea pigs during ozone-induced bronchial hyperreactivity. *Am Rev Respir Dis* 1985; 131:314.

39. Schelegle ES, Adams WC, Siefkin AD: Indomethacin pretreatment reduces ozone-induced pulmonary function decrements in human subjects. *Am Rev Respir Dis* 1987; 136:1350.

40. Ying RL, Gross KB, Terzo TS, Eschenbacher WL: Indomethacin does not inhibit the ozone-induced increase in bronchial responsiveness in human subjects. *Am Rev Respir Dis* 1990; 142:817.

41. Murlas CG, Murphy TP, Chodimella V: O$_3$-induced mucosa-linked airway muscle hyperresponsiveness in the guinea pig. *J Appl Physiol* 1990; 69:7.

42. Tepper JS, Costa DL, Fitzgerald S, et al.: Role of tachykinins in ozone-induced acute lung injury in guinea pigs. *J Appl Physiol* 1993; 75:1404.

43. Murlas CG, Lang Z, Williams GJ, Chodimella V: Aerosolized neutral endopeptidase reverses ozone-induced airway hyperreactivity to substance P. *J Appl Physiol* 1992; 72:1133.

44. Kehrl HR, Vincent LM, Kowalsky RJ, et al.: Ozone exposure increases respiratory epithelial permeability in humans. *Am Rev Respir Dis* 1987; 135:1124.

45. Moffat RK, Hyde DM, Plopper CG, et al.: Ozone-induced adaptive and reactive cellular changes in respiratory bronchioles of bonnet monkeys. *Exp Lung Res* 1987; 12:57.

46. Barr BC, Hyde DM, Plopper CG, Dungworth DL: Distal airway remodelling in rats chronically exposed to ozone. *Am Rev Respir Dis* 1988; 137:924.

47. Beckett WS, McDonnell WF, Horstman DH, House DE: Role of the parasympathetic nervous system in acute lung response to ozone. *J Appl Physiol* 1985; 59:1879.

48. Gong H, Bedi JF, Horvath SM: Inhaled albuterol does not protect against ozone toxicity in non-asthmatic athletes. *Arch Environ Health* 1988; 43:46.

49. Stevens WHM, Ädelroth E, Wattie J, et al.: Effect of inhaled budesonide on ozone-induced airway hyperresponsiveness and bronchoalveolar lavage cells in dogs. *J Appl Physiol* 1994; 77:2578.

50. McKinnon K, Madden MC, Noah TL, Devlin RB: In vitro ozone exposure increases release of arachidonic acid products from a human bronchial epithelial cell line. *Toxicol Appl Pharmacol* 1993; 118:215.

51. Samet JM, Noah TL, Devlin RB, et al.: Effect of ozone on platelet-activiating factor production in phorbol-differentiated HL-60 cells, a human bronchial epithelial cell line (BEAS S6), and primary human bronchial epithelial cells. *Am J Respir Cell Mol Biol* 1992; 7;514.

52. Devlin RB, McKinnon KP, Noah T, et al.: Ozone-induced release of cytokines and fibronectin by alveolar macrophages and airway epithelial cells. *Am J Physiol* 1994; 266:L612.

53. Speizer FE, Ferris B Jr, Bishop YMM, Spengler JD: Respiratory disease rates and pulmonary function in children associated with NO$_2$ exposure. *Am Rev Respir Dis* 1980; 121:3.

54. Neas LM, Dockery DW, Ware JH, et al.: Association of indoor nitrogen dioxide with respiratory symptoms and lung function in children. *Am J Epidemiol* 1991; 134:204.

55. Braun-Fahrländer C, Ackermann-Liebrich U, Schwartz J, et al.: Air pollution and respiratory symptoms in preschool children. *Am Rev Respir Dis* 1992; 145:42.

56. Hasselblad V, Eddy DM, Kotchmar DJ: Synthesis of environmental evidence: Nitrogen dioxide epidemiology studies. *J Air Waste Manage Assoc* 1992; 42:662.

57. Lebowitz MD, Collins L, Holberg CJ: Time series analyses of respiratory responses to indoor and outdoor environmental phenomena. *Environ Res* 1987; 43:332.

58. Bates DV, Sizto R: Air pollution and hospital admissions in Southern Ontario: The acid summer haze effect. *Environ Res* 1987; 43:317.

59. Jörres R, Nowak D, Grimminger F, et al.: The effect of 1 ppm nitrogen dioxide on bronchoalveolar lavage cells in normal and asthmatic subjects. *Eur Respir J* 1995; 8:416.

60. Drechsler-Parks DM, Bedi JF, Horvath SM: Pulmonary function responses of older men and women to NO$_2$. *Environ Res* 1987; 44:206.

61. von Nieding G, Wagner HM, Krekeler H, et al.: Grenzwertbestimmung der akuten NO$_2$-Wirkung auf den respiratorischen Gasaustausch und die Atemwegswiderstände des chronisch lungenkranken Menschen. *Int Arch Arbeitsmed* 1971; 27:338.

62. Morrow PE, Utell MJ, Bauer MA, et al.: Pulmonary performance of elderly normal subjects and subjects with chronic obstructive pulmonary disease exposed to 0.3 ppm nitrogen dioxide. *Am Rev Respir Dis* 1992; 145:291.

63. Hackney JD, Linn WS, Avol EL, et al.: Exposures of older adults with chronic respiratory illness to nitrogen dioxide: A combined laboratory and field study. *Am Rev Respir Dis* 1992; 146:1480.

64. Mohsenin V: Airway responses to 2.0 ppm nitrogen dioxide in normal subjects. *Arch Environ Health* 1988; 43:242.

65. Mohsenin V: Effect of vitamin C on NO$_2$-induced airway hyperresponsiveness in normal subjects: A randomized double-blind experiment. *Am Rev Respir Dis* 1987; 136:1408.

66. Bylin G, Hedenstierna G, Lindvall T, Sundin B: Ambient nitrogen dioxide concentrations increase bronchial responsiveness in subjects with mild asthma. *Eur Respir J* 1988; 1:606.

67. Mohsenin V: Airway responses to nitrogen dioxide in asthmatic subjects. *J Toxicol Environ Health* 1987; 22:371.

68. Hazucha MJ, Ginsberg JF, McDonnell WF, et al.: Effects of 0.1 ppm nitrogen dioxide on airways of normal and asthmatic subjects. *J Appl Physiol* 1983; 54:730.

69. Jörres R, Magnussen H: Effect of 0.25 ppm nitrogen dioxide on the airway response to methacholine in asymptomatic asthmatic patients. *Lung* 1991; 169:77.

70. Bauer MA, Utell MJ, Morrow PE, et al.: Inhalation of 0.30 ppm nitrogen dioxide potentiates exercise-induced bronchospasm in asthmatics. *Am Rev Respir Dis* 1986; 134:1203.

71. Jörres R, Magnussen H: Airways response of asthmatics after a 30 min exposure, at resting ventilation, to 0.25 ppm NO_2 or 0.5 ppm SO_2. *Eur Respir J* 1990; 3:132.

72. Rubinstein I, Bigby BG, Reiss TF, Boushey HA Jr: Short-term exposure to 0.3 ppm nitrogen dioxide does not potentiate airway responsiveness to sulfur dioxide in asthmatic subjects. *Am Rev Respir Dis* 1990; 141:381.

73. Folinsbee LJ: Does nitrogen dioxide exposure increase airways responsiveness? *Toxicol Indust Health* 1992; 8:273.

74. Tunnicliffe WS, Burge PS, Ayres JG: Effect of domestic concentrations of nitrogen dioxide on airway responses to inhaled allergen in asthmatic patients. *Lancet* 1994; 344:1733.

75. Devalia JL, Rusznak C, Herdman MJ, et al.: Effect of nitrogen dioxide and sulphur dioxide on airway response of mild asthmatic patients to allergen inhalation. *Lancet* 1994; 344:1668.

76. Miller FJ, Overton JH, Myers ET, Graham JA: Pulmonary dosimetry of nitrogen dioxide in animals and man, in Schneider T, Grant L (eds): *Air Pollution by Nitrogen Oxides.* New York, Elsevier Scientific, 1982; 376–386.

77. Postlethwait EM, Bidani A: Reactive uptake governs the pulmonary air space removal of inhaled nitrogen dioxide. *J Appl Physiol* 1990; 68:594.

78. Mustafa MG, Tierney DF: Biochemical and metabolic changes in the lung with oxygen, ozone, and nitrogen dioxide toxicity. *Am Rev Respir Dis* 1978; 118:1061.

79. Mohsenin V: Lipid peroxidation and antielastase activity in the lung under oxidant stress: Role of antioxidant defenses. *J Appl Physiol* 1991; 70:1456.

80. Postlethwait EM, Langford SD, Bidani A: Transfer of NO_2 through pulmonary epithelial lining fluid. *Toxicol Appl Pharmacol* 1991; 109:464.

81. Mohsenin V, Gee JBL: Acute effect of nitrogen dioxide exposure on the functional activity of α_1-protease inhibitor in bronchoalveolar lavage fluid of normal subjects. *Am Rev Respir Dis* 1987; 136:646.

82. Johnson DA, Frampton MW, Winters RS, et al.: Inhalation of nitrogen dioxide fails to reduce the activity of human lung alpha-1-proteinase inhibitor. *Am Rev Respir Dis* 1990; 142:758.

83. Frampton MW, Finkelstein JN, Roberts NJ Jr, et al.: Effects of nitrogen dioxide exposure on bronchoalveolar lavage proteins in humans. *Am J Respir Cell Mol Biol* 1989; 1:499.

84. Sandström T, Stjernberg N, Eklund A, et al.: Inflammatory cell response in bronchoalveolar lavage fluid after nitrogen dioxide exposure of healthy subjects: A dose-response study. *Eur Respir J* 1991; 3:332.

85. Sandström T, Andersson MC, Kolmodin-Hedman B, et al.: Bronchoalveolar mastocytosis and lymphocytosis after nitrogen dioxide exposure in man: A time-kinetic study. *Eur Respir J* 1990; 3:138.

86. Helleday R, Sandström T, Stjernberg N: Differences in bronchoalveolar cell response to nitrogen dioxide exposure between smokers and nonsmokers. *Eur Respir J* 1994; 7:1213.

87. Sandström T, Helleday R, Bjermer L, Stjernberg N: Effects of repeated exposure to 4 ppm nitrogen dioxide on bronchoalveolar lymphocyte subsets and macrophages in healthy men. *Eur Respir J* 1992; 5:1092.

88. Rubinstein I, Reiss TF, Bigby BG, et al.: Effects of 0.60 ppm nitrogen dioxide on circulating and bronchoalveolar lavage lymphocyte phenotypes in healthy subjects. *Environ Res* 1991; 55:18.

89. Rasmussen TR, Kjaergaard SK, Tarp U, Pedersen OF: Delayed effects of NO_2 exposure on alveolar permeability and glutathione peroxidase in healthy humans. *Am Rev Respir Dis* 1992; 146:654.

90. Kawakami M, Yasui S, Yamawaki I, et al.: Structural changes in airways of rats exposed to nitrogen dioxide intermittently for seven days: Comparison between major bronchi and terminal bronchioles. *Am Rev Respir Dis* 1989; 140:1754.

91. Blank J, Glasgow JE, Pietra GG, et al.: Nitrogen dioxide-induced emphysema in rats: Lack of worsening by beta-aminopropionitrile treatment. *Am Rev Respir Dis* 1988; 137:376.

92. Glasgow JE, Pietra GG, Abrams WR, et al.: Neutrophil recruitment and degranulation during induction of emphysema in the rat by nitrogen dioxide. *Am Rev Respir Dis* 1987; 135:1129.

93. Guidotti TL: The higher oxides of nitrogen: Inhalation toxicology. *Environ Res* 1978; 14:443.

94. von Nieding G, Krekeler H: Pharmakologische Beeinflussung der akuton NO_2-Wirkung auf die Lungenfunktion von Gesunden und Kranken mit einer chronischen Bronchitis. *Int Arch Arbeitsmed* 1971; 29:55.

95. Devalia JL, Sapsford RJ, Cundell DR, et al.: Human bronchial epithelial cell dysfunction following *in vitro* exposure to nitrogen dioxide. *Eur Respir J* 1993; 6:1308.

96. Devalia JL, Campbell AM, Sapsford RJ, et al.: Effect of nitrogen dioxide on synthesis of inflammatory cytokines expressed by human bronchial epithelial cells *in vitro*. *Am J Respir Cell Mol Biol* 1993; 9:271.

97. Kienast K, Knorst M, Lubjuhn S, et al.: Nitrogen dioxide-induced reactive oxygen intermediates production by human alveolar macrophages and peripheral blood mononuclear cells. *Arch Environ Health* 1994; 49:246.

98. Brunekreef B, Lumens M, Hoek G, et al.: Pulmonary function changes associated with an air pollution episode in January 1987. *JAPCA* 1989; 39:1444.

99. Wichmann HE, Sugiri D, Islam MS, et al.: Pulmonary function and carboxyhaemoglobin during the smog episode in January 1987. *Zentralbl Bakteriol Mikrobiol Hyg Ser B* 1988; 187:31.

100. Wichmann HE, Müller W, Allhoff P, et al.: Health effects during a smog episode in West Germany in 1985. *Environ Health Perspect* 1989; 79:89.

101. Derriennic F, Richardson S, Mollie A, Lellouch J: Short-term effects of sulphur dioxide pollution on mortality in two French cities. *Int J Epidemiol* 1989; 18:186.

102. Walters S, Griffiths RK, Ayres JG: Temporal association between hospital admissions for asthma in Birmingham and ambient levels of sulphur dioxide and smoke. *Thorax* 1994; 49:133.

103. Sunyer J, Saez M, Murillo C, et al.: Air pollution and emergency room admissions for chronic obstructive pulmonary disease: A 5-year study. *Am J Epidemiol* 1993; 137:710.

104. Dockery DW, Pope CA, Xiping X, et al.: An association between air pollution and mortality in six U.S. cities. *New Engl J Med* 1993; 329:1753.

105. Chapman RS, Calafiore DC, Hasselblad V: Prevalence of persistent cough and phlegm in young adults in relation to long-term sulfur dioxide exposure. *Am Rev Respir Dis* 1985; 132:261.

106. Euler G, Abbey D, Hodgkin J, Magie A: Chronic obstructive pulmonary disease symptom effects of long-term cumulative exposure to ambient levels of total suspended particulates and

sulfur dioxide in California Seventh-Day Adventists residents. *Arch Environ Health* 1987; 42:213.

107. Dodge R, Solomon P, Moyers J, Hayes C: A longitudinal study of children exposed to sulfur oxides. *Am J Epidemiol* 1985; 121:720.

108. von Mutius E, Martinez FD, Fritzsch C, et al.: Prevalence of asthma and atopy in two areas of West and East Germany. *Am J Respir Crit Care Med* 1994; 149:358.

109. Sheppard D, Wong WS, Uehara CF, et al.: Lower threshold and greater bronchomotor responsiveness of asthmatic subjects to sulfur dioxide. *Am Rev Respir Dis* 1980; 122:873.

110. Linn WS, Venet TG, Shamoo DA, et al.: Respiratory effects of sulfur dioxide in heavily exercising asthmatics: A dose-response study. *Am Rev Respir Dis* 1983; 127:278.

111. Sheppard D, Saisho A, Nadel JA, Boushey HA: Exercise increases sulfur dioxide-induced bronchoconstriction in asthmatic subjects. *Am Rev Respir Dis* 1981; 123:486.

112. Bethel RA, Erle DJ, Epstein J, et al.: Effect of exercise rate and route of inhalation on sulfur dioxide-induced bronchoconstriction in asthmatic subjects. *Am Rev Respir Dis* 1983; 128:592.

113. Frank NR, Yoder RE, Brain JD, Yokoyama E: $SO_2(^{35}S$ labeled) absorption by the nose and mouth under conditions of varying concentrations and flow. *Arch Environ Health* 1969; 18:315.

114. Sheppard D, Eschenbacher WL, Boushey HA, Bethel RA: Magnitude of the interaction between the bronchomotor effects of sulfur dioxide and those of dry (cold) air. *Am Rev Respir Dis* 1984; 130:52.

115. Horstman DH, Roger LJ, Kehrl H, Hazucha M: Airway sensitivity of asthmatics to sulfur dioxide. *Toxicol Environ Health* 1986; 2:289.

116. Magnussen H, Jörres R, Wagner HM, von Nieding G: Relationship between the airway response to inhaled sulfur dioxide, isocapnic hyperventilation, and histamine in asthmatic subjects. *Int Arch Occup Environ Health* 1990; 62:485.

117. Sheppard D, Epstein J, Bethel RA, et al.: Tolerance to sulfur dioxide-induced bronchoconstriction in subjects with asthma. *Environ Res* 1983; 30:412.

118. Hazucha MJ, Kehrl HR, Roger LJ, Horstman DH: Airway responsiveness to methacholine of asthmatics exposed to 0.25, 0.5 and 1.0 ppm SO_2 (abstract). *Am Rev Respir Dis* 1984; 129(suppl 2):A145.

119. Sandström T, Stjernberg N, Andersson MC, et al.: Cell response in bronchoalveolar lavage fluid after sulfur dioxide exposure. *Scand J Work Environ Health* 1989; 15:142.

120. Sandström T, Stjernberg N, Andersson MC, et al.: Cell response in bronchoalveolar lavage fluid after exposure to sulfur dioxide: A time-response study. *Am Rev Respir Dis,* 1989; 140:1828.

121. Sant'Ambrogio G: Nervous receptors in the tracheobronchial tree. *Annu Rev Physiol* 1987; 49:611.

122. Coleridge HM, Coleridge JGC: Reflexes evoked from the tracheobroncheal tree and lungs, in Cherniack NS, Widdicombe JG (eds): *Handbook of Physiology. The Respiratory System II.* Bethesda, American Physiological Society, 1986; 395–429.

123. Shore SA, Kariya ST, Anderson K, et al.: Sulfur-dioxide induced bronchitis in dogs: Effects on airway responsiveness to inhaled and intravenously administered methacholine. *Am Rev Respir Dis* 1987; 135:840.

124. Schwartz HJ, Chester EH: Bronchospastic responses to aerosolized metabisulfite in asthmatic subjects: Potential mechanisms and clinical implications. *J Allergy Clin Immunol* 1984; 74:511.

125. Fine JM, Gordon T, Sheppard D: The roles of pH and ionic species in sulfur dioxide- and sulfite-induced bronchoconstriction. *Am Rev Respir Dis* 1987; 136:1122.

126. Field PI, McClean M, Simmul R, Berend N: Comparison of sulphur dioxide and metabisulphite airway reactivity in patients with asthma. *Thorax* 1994; 49:250.

127. Mansour E, Ahmed A, Cortes A, et al.: Mechanisms of metabisulfite-induced bronchoconstriction: Evidence for bradykinin B_2-receptor stimulation. *J Appl Physiol* 1992; 72:1831.

128. Lötvall JO, Skoogh BE, Lemen RJ, et al.: Bronchoconstriction induced by inhaled sodium metabisulfite in the guinea pig: Effect of capsaicin pretreatment and of neutral endopeptidase inhibition. *Am Rev Respir Dis* 1990; 142:1390.

129. Sakamoto T, Tsukagoshi H, Barnes PJ, Chung KF: Involvement of tachykinin receptors (NK_1 and NK_2) in sodium metabisulfite-induced airway effects. *Am J Respir Crit Care Med* 1994; 149:387.

130. Scanlon PD, Seltzer J, Ingram RH Jr, et al.: Chronic exposure to sulfur dioxide: Physiologic and histologic evaluation of dogs exposed to 50 or 15 ppm. *Am Rev Respir Dis* 1987; 135:831.

131. Koenig JQ, Marshall SG, Horike M, et al.: The effects of albuterol on SO_2-induced bronchoconstriction in allergic adolescents. *J Allergy Clin Immunol* 1987; 79:54.

132. Sheppard D, Natel JA, Boushey HA: Inhibition of sulfur dioxide-induced bronchoconstriction by disodium cromoglycate in asthmatic subjects. *Am Rev Respir Dis* 1981; 124:257.

133. Myers DJ, Bigby BG, Boushey HA: The inhibition of sulfur dioxide-induced bronchoconstriction in asthmatic subjects by cromolyn is dose-dependent. *Am Rev Respir Dis* 1986; 133:1150.

134. Bigby B, Boushey H: Effects of nedocromil sodium on the bronchomotor response to sulfur dioxide. *J Allergy Clin Immunol* 1993; 92:195.

135. Koenig JQ, Dumler K, Rebolledo V, et al.: Theophylline mitigates the bronchoconstrictor effects of sulfur dioxide in subjects with asthma. *J Allergy Clin Immunol* 1992; 89:789.

136. Wiebicke W, Jörres R, Magnussen H: Comparison of the effects of inhaled corticosteroids on the airway response to histamine, methacholine, hyperventilation, and sulfur dioxide in subjects with asthma. *J Allergy Clin Immunol* 1990; 86:915.

137. McManus MS, Koenig JQ, Altman LC, Pierson WE: Pulmonary effects of sulfur dioxide exposure and ipratropium bromide pretreatment in adults with nonallergic asthma. *J Allergy Clin Immunol* 1989; 83:619.

138. Drechsler-Parks DM, Bedi JF, Horvath SM: Interaction of peroxyacetyl nitrate and ozone on pulmonary functions. *Am Rev Respir Dis* 1984; 130:1033.

139. Aris R, Christian D, Sheppard D, Balmes JR: The effects of sequential exposure to acidic fog and ozone on pulmonary function in exercising subjects. *Am Rev Respir Dis* 1991; 143:85.

140. Hazucha MJ, Folinsbee LJ, Seal E, Bromberg PA: Lung function response of healthy women after sequential exposures to NO_2 and O_3. *Am J Respir Crit Care Med* 1994; 150:642.

141. Folinsbee LJ, Bedi JF, Horvath SM: Pulmonary response to threshold levels of sulfur dioxide (1.0 ppm) and ozone (0.3 ppm). *J Appl Physiol* 1985; 58:1783.

142. Koenig JQ, Covert DS, Hanley QS, et al.: Prior exposure to ozone potentiates subsequent response to sulfur dioxide in adolescent asthmatic subjects. *Am Rev Respir Dis* 1990; 141:377.

143. Linn WS, Jones MP, Bailey RM, et al.: Respiratory effects of mixed nitrogen dioxide and sulfur dioxide in human volunteers under simulated ambient exposure conditions. *Environ Res* 1980; 22:431.

Chapter 38 _____

REACTIVE AIRWAYS DYSFUNCTION SYNDROME: OCCUPATIONAL ASTHMA WITHOUT LATENCY

STUART M. BROOKS

Definition

Reactive Airways Dysfunction Syndrome

Factors of Importance in Pathogenesis

Hypothetical Model for RADS

Diagnosis

Management and Prevention

Definitions

BROAD DEFINITION

Occupational asthma is an important occupational respiratory ailment, both in terms of morbidity and disability and in the total number of cases.[1] A fundamental problem involves a consensus definition of occupational asthma. This dilemma may arise because the definition of occupational asthma may vary in different countries, may be modified by clinical criteria, and may be more appropriate for certain circumstances than others. For example, a definition used in the context of a surveillance system for triggering a public health investigation or intervention may be less restrictive than a definition that is appropriate for workers' compensation purposes or legal purposes.[2]

A broad definition of occupational asthma is that it is a disorder characterized by episodes of reversible airflow limitation caused by the inhalation of a substance or material that a worker manufactures or uses directly or that is incidentally present at the work site.[3] Chan-Yeung qualified the definition as "variable air flow limitation caused by a specific agent in the workplace."[4] This latter definition limits the scope of occupational asthma because it necessitates incriminating a specific substance in the workplace. This theme has been echoed by compensation boards, which accept a diagnosis of occupational asthma only for a finite number of specific agents. In the United Kingdom, the Industrial Injuries Advisory Council defined occupational asthma as "asthma that develops after a variable period of symptomless expo-

sure to a sensitizing agent at work."[5] To qualify, asthma must be caused by a predetermined and limited number of agents (platinum salts, isocyanates, epoxy resins, acid anhydrides, colophony fumes, proteolytic enzymes, laboratory animals and insects, and grain dust).

Definitions that insist on sensitization exclude nonallergic causes for consideration as occupational asthma. This restriction negates the concept that nonallergic factors can cause occupational asthma, which seems contrary to what is generally appreciated about the pathogenesis of asthma in the general population (i.e., extrinsic-allergic versus intrinsic-nonallergic asthma). Gandevia[6] was one of the first to describe an asthmatic condition of nonallergic basis, which he termed *inflammatory*, but later, Brooks et al.[7] coined the term *reactive airways dysfunction syndrome* (RADS). Newman-Taylor[8] classified agents into two groups: (1) nonspecific stimuli (inciters) that provoke airway narrowing but do not themselves increase airway responsiveness, and (2) specific stimuli (inducers) that provoke both airway narrowing and increase nonspecific bronchial responsiveness. According to this classification, occupational asthma falls into the second category. The stimuli are able to "induce" or "switch on," asthma and nonspecific bronchial hyperresponsiveness, either on an allergic or nonallergic basis.

Thus, it is appropriate to consider occupational asthma as evolving by an allergic and/or a nonallergic mechanism. In this context, *occupational asthma with latency* is analogous to allergic occupational asthma, or a condition occurring after a preceding latent period of exposure when allergic sensitization to a substance or material present in the workplace occurs; it is characterized physiologically by variable and work-related airflow limitation and the presence of both specific and nonspecific airway hyperresponsiveness. At present, there are at least 200 agents that have been documented to cause allergic occupational asthma.[3] In contrast, *occu-pational asthma without latency* is essentially nonallergic occu-pational asthma, or an airways condition that develops without a preceding latent period, occurring after an inordinate workplace irritant exposure; it is distinguished physiologically by persistent nonspecific airway hyperresponsiveness. The two distinguishing clinical features pertinent to these definitions are *latency* and *specific airway hyperresponsiveness*, but both types of asthma demonstrate nonspecific airway hyperresponsiveness. Additionally, in both allergic and nonallergic asthma, pathologic changes depict bronchial mucosal injury and inflammation.[9]

NONSPECIFIC AIRWAY HYPERRESPONSIVENESS

The inclusion of nonspecific airway hyperresponsiveness as a key feature of occupational asthma seems justified. First, certain airway conditions can simulate occupational asthma but are better considered as "occupational airways disorders" rather than as asthma.[3] For example, exposures to cotton dust (byssinosis) and grain dust produce airways disorder with variable air flow limitation but usually without nonspecific airway hyperresponsiveness.[10,11] Occasionally, the term *airways hyperresponsiveness* has been used to describe important features of asthma, such as variable airflow limitation, bronchodilator responsiveness, and exercise-induced bronchospasm. Whether these latter features of asthma equate with pharmacologic reactivity is not discerned; however, each feature is an acknowledged characteristic of asthma and present in a high proportion of asthmatic individuals.[12–19] The requirement of methacholine/histamine hyperresponsiveness as a criterion for "active" occupational asthma seems sound considering the fact that the vast majority of asthmatic persons are reported to show this phenomenon.[20–23] In this chapter, nonspecific airway hyperresponsiveness is equated with a physiologically enhanced response to inhaled bronchoconstricting pharmacologic agents (methacholine, histamine, carbachol, etc.). Of course, persons who recover from occupational asthma with latency because of a significant time away from the inciting (sensitizing) agent (for example, toluene diisocyanante) may lose both their specific and nonspecific airway hyperresponsiveness.

BRONCHIAL IRRITABILITY

The physiologic feature of enhanced methacholine and histamine responsiveness translates clinically as "bronchial irritability." Mortagy et al. utilized the term *bronchial irritability* to describe the response, to a self-administered questionnaire, of two populations to 12 "environments," including

cold air; smoky atmospheres; traffic fumes; and common household chemicals, such as hair sprays, perfumes, bleaches, etc.[24] The designation *bronchial irritability syndrome* applied to persons with both bronchial symptoms to the irritants and histamine hyperreactivity; 27 percent of persons with this designation had a physician's diagnosis of asthma. Bronchial irritability symptoms and methacholine reactivity have also been linked by other investigators.[25]

The vast majority of clinically active asthmatic patients manifest airway hyperresponsiveness to pharmacologic bronchoconstrictors. Clinically active asthma is characterized by both symptoms of bronchial irritability and methacholine/histamine airway hyperresponsiveness. The degree of methacholine/histamine sensitivity that equates best with the presence of occupational asthma is important to note, and data suggest that a PC_{20} value ≤ 8 mg/ml is a good predictor of asthmatic airway responsiveness.[26–30] While methacholine hyperresponsiveness can be present in individuals without bronchial irritability symptoms,[15,31–37] when such symptoms are present, the prevalence of methacholine/histamine hyperreactivity is great.[25,38,39]

AIRWAY REACTIVITY SCORE

The relationship between airway reactivity and disease severity was examined in a study of 24 subjects with stable chronic bronchial asthma.[25] Disease severity was assessed by assigning a disease severity score (DSS), representing six clinical and therapeutic parameters. Airway hyperresponsiveness was assessed by an airway reactivity score (ARS), based on the number of positive responses to a questionnaire concerning exposure to 22 nonspecific inhaled irritants, and methacholine challenge testing and determining (Table 38-1). Significant negative correlations were noted between DSS, ARS, and cumulative dose of methacholine causing a 20 percent reduction in FEV_1 (CMD_{20}). In other words, the higher the clinical scores, the less the methacholine CMD_{20}. Significant correlations between ARS and CMD_{20} ($r = 0.60$, $p < 0.002$) suggested the consistency with which the ARS estimated methacholine hyperresponsiveness. It appears that there is value in using clinical information for assessing airway hyperresponsiveness.

Reactive Airways Dysfunction Syndrome

ROLE OF HIGH-LEVEL EXPOSURES

Prior to the description of RADS in 1985, there were published reports of individuals developing a chronic respiratory disorder after a high-level irritant gas exposure. Harkonen et al. followed seven mine workers involved in a pyrite dust explosion who sustained SO_2-induced lung injury.[40] Four years after the accident, an asthmalike condition characterized by reversible airway obstruction was observed in three persons, four workers showed positive histamine challenges, but two subjects responded neither to histamine or bronchodilators. The authors concluded that nonspecific airway hyperresponsiveness was a frequent sequela of high-level SO_2 exposure and could persist for years. In another report, Charan and coworkers described

TABLE 38-1   Airway Reactivity Questionnaire[a]

Is your asthma worsened by or do any of the following produce wheezing, chest tightness, and/or coughing?

	Yes	No
1. Heat		
2. Cold		
3. Rain or dampness		
4. Sudden change in temperature		
5. Dust		
6. Tobacco smoke		
7. Cooking or frying odors		
8. Fumes		
9. Perfume		
10. Household spray		
11. Soap powders		
12. Antiperspirants		
13. Cut grass		
14. Varnish		
15. Household cleaners		
16. Respiratory infections		
17. Cosmetics (including aftershave lotion)		
18. Ammonia (Lysol or Clorox)		
19. Solvents (including alcohol and nail polish remover)		
20. Crude oil		
21. Sawdust		
22. Periods of high air pollution		

[a] The number of positive responses is recorded as a percentage of the total, providing an airway reactivity score (ARS). A score of zero is given if all responses are negative, and a score of 100 is given if all responses are positive.

five cases of accidental exposure to high levels of SO_2, with three survivors developing severe, and another mild, airway obstruction.[41] Flury et al. described a 50-year-old man, who inhaled substantial quantities of concentrated ammonia vapors; over the next 5 years, serial pulmonary function testing documented the development of an obstructive lung disorder.[42] Although methacholine challenges were not performed, the authors indicated that hyperreactive airways were present and likely the direct result of the inhalation injury. Donham et al. described an acute toxic exposure to high concentrations of hydrogen sulfide after agitation of liquid manure.[43] One survivor had respiratory symptoms persisting for > 2 months after the incident. Other reports of persistent obstructive airways disease after high-level irritant exposures include the study of Murphy et al. on a subject who inhaled vapors liberated from mixing several drain cleaning agents; and the studies of Hasan et al., Kennedy et al., and Kaufman and Bukon reporting on subjects with chlorine gas exposures.[44–47] Some individuals exposed to a single heavy exposure of toluene diisocyanate (TDI) develop respiratory symptoms within 24 h that persist for years.[48,49]

CLINICAL PICTURE

RADS was first designated in 1985.[7] Ten individuals developed a persistent asthmalike illness after a single exposure to high concentrations of an irritant vapor, fume, gas, or smoke.

Respiratory symptoms and continued presence of nonspecific airway hyperresponsiveness were documented in all patients, who were followed for about 3 years' mean duration. In one person, the persistence of disease was documented to persist for $\geq$ 12 years. Generally, the causative exposure was short-lived, often lasting just a few minutes, but, on occasion, was as long as 12 h. There usually was a time interval between the exposure and development of symptoms; this time period was immediate in three patients but several hours in the other seven (mean was approximately 9 h). In almost all instances, the exposure was caused by an accident or a situation where there were very poor ventilation and limited air exchange in the area. When tested, all patients displayed a positive methacholine challenge test. Pulmonary function was normal in three of 10 and showed airflow limitation in seven. There was no identifiable evidence of preexisting respiratory complaints in any patient studied; two were found to be atopic, but in all others no evidence of an allergy was identified.

Although the incriminating etiologic agents varied in each case, all were irritants in nature and included uranium hexafluoride gas, floor sealant, spray paint containing significant concentrations of ammonia, heated acid, 35% hydrazine, fumigating fog, metal coating remover, and smoke inhalation. In two cases, bronchial biopsies documented bronchial epithelial cell injury and bronchial wall inflammation. There were lymphocytes and plasma cells present, but no eosinophilia was observed. Desquamation of respiratory epithelium was seen in one biopsy, and goblet cell hyperplasia in another. There was no evidence of mucous gland hyperplasia, basement membrane thickening, or smooth-muscle hypertrophy.

OTHER EXAMPLES OF RADS

Since the 1985 description of RADS, there have been a number of subsequent reports of RADS-like disorders from irritant exposures.[50–57] Other case examples reported as RADS include three Philadelphia police officers exposed to "toxic fumes" from a roadside truck accident[54]; a female computer operator exposed to a floor sealant[53]; and workers exposed to TDI,[48] possibly acetic acid,[58] and isocyanate fumes.[59] Moisan described RADS-like illnesses after smoke inhalation in three patients.[60]

RADS WITH ATYPICAL FEATURES

Among published cases of RADS, some displayed atypical features compared to the original RADS description, such as a longer duration of exposure before an onset, different physiologic manifestations, less massive exposure, or influences of host factors, which had not been described in the original report.[58,61–70] Tarlo provided a retrospective review of the files of 154 consecutive workers assessed for "occupational asthma."[68] Of 59 individuals considered as having occupational asthma, a subset of 10 (and possibly an additional 15) with asthma symptoms for an average of 5 years was characterized by disease initiated by an exposure to high concentrations of an irritant. The RADS clinical criteria were modified in the study, and exposure was not limited to just a single accident or incident at work. It was concluded that "irritant-induced" occupational asthma is common in a population referred for assessment of possible occupational asthma. The prevalence was estimated to be 6 percent for definite irritant-induced asthma, and there were another 10 percent with a possible diagnosis. Boulet implied there was prolonged induction of increased airway hyperresponsiveness after the inhalation of high concentrations of irritants in four "normal" individuals and aggravation of airway hyperresponsiveness in another with "mild" preexisting asthma.[63] Two individuals were believed to have developed sensitization after only an intense short-term exposure. Gilbert and Auchincloss reported a case of RADS manifested by a restrictive rather than an obstructive lung function defect, presumably on the basis of constriction of bronchioles or alveolar ducts.[65] The ensuing clinical reports on RADS suggest that many investigators were modifying the benchmarks for RADS so that the designation of RADS did not always follow the original diagnostic criteria; some cases could best be termed as *variants of RADS*.

In a recent investigation, two clinical presentations of occupational asthma without latency were observed.[61] In one type of occupational asthma, there was the sudden-onset presentation, which is epitomized by RADS; characteristically, there was sudden-onset asthma (within 24 h), usually following an accidental and excessive exposure to high-level irritant gases, vapors, or fumes. Because of the extreme magnitude of the exposure, the affected individual became immediately ill (within 24 h) and usually required prompt medical care. Atopy did not contribute to the pathogenesis of RADS.[7] The second type of occupational asthma without latency appeared to be less sudden in onset and had features that contrasted with RADS. The causative exposure was not always brief and, in some cases, lasted > 24 h; the subsequent onset of asthma was, therefore, not so sudden. In cases with a more prolonged exposure, there was a longer time interval before asthma symptoms developed (> 24 h) and a delay in instituting medical care. Exposures lasting > 24 h were characteristically not a single accident or spills but rather were often intermittent exposure events in nature. However, these intermittent exposures were always persistent and, very importantly, there was never a delay of > 24 h between complete cessation of exposure and the onset of active asthma symptoms. In contrast to RADS, where atopy played no major role in development, it appeared that atopy or a preexisting "allergic potential" was consequential in the pathogenesis of the not-so-sudden type (i.e., onset > 24 h).

PROGNOSIS

Individuals with RADS generally continue to report bronchial irritability symptoms and demonstrate evidence of nonspecific airways hyperresponsiveness for years after the inciting incident. The persistent symptoms are analogous to persons with allergic asthma who leave an industry and no longer have exposure. A number of studies have also documented the poor outcome of patients with allergic occupational asthma.[71–75] For allergic asthma, a more favorable prognostic outcome is associated with a shorter duration of

symptoms before diagnosis, relatively normal pulmonary function, and a lesser degree of bronchial responsiveness.[76] Continued occupational exposure appears to lead to persistent symptoms and permanent bronchial hyperresponsiveness.[76,77]

Factors of Importance in Pathogenesis (Table 38-2)

REFLEX

Patients with RADS have an increased sensitivity to irritants and physical and chemical stimuli because of their nonspecific airway hyperresponsiveness.[7] A number of dusts, gases, fumes, and vapors, if present in sufficient concentrations, cause bronchoconstriction by a direct effect on bronchial irritant receptors. Individuals with occupational asthma/RADS develop bronchoconstriction following exposure to many and varied airborne irritants at concentrations not affecting "normal" individuals and will react to the stimuli in a more vigorous manner. Thus, workplace exposure can be an important source for exacerbating preexisting asthma.

AIRWAY SITE OF DAMAGE

The site at which irritant exposures come into contact with responding tissue may be an important determinant of the nature and severity of the bronchospastic reaction. Because the number of mast cells is greatest in the terminal bronchioles, irritant interaction in this area may be more likely to cause mast cell degranulation and an asthmatic reaction than responses in larger airways. In occupational asthma, the site of deposition of inhaled particles also depends on the degree of airway obstruction present at any time. In the presence of bronchospasm, airway radius decreases and the deposition occurs more by impaction. The net effect is a more central deposition of inhaled material. As bronchial constriction subsides, the particles can reach more peripheral airways. The normal pulmonary defenses may be impaired by environmental and occupational agents indigenous to a workplace, including cigarette smoke, air pollution, chemicals, and dust, which may impair lung defense mechanisms and lead to a worsened response to an irritant exposure.

Another mechanism may be connected to the location of the airway injury from the irritant. By partitioning the cen-

TABLE 38-2   Possible Mechanisms in Nonallergic Occupational Asthma

Reflex
Alteration in deposition and clearance of particles
Airway inflammation
Bronchial smooth-muscle hyperresponsiveness
Adrenergic influences
Neuropeptides
Epithelial damage
Microvascular leakage
Pharmacologic
Immunologic?

tral and peripheral airway resistance using a catheter-tip micromanometer, Ohrui and colleagues concluded that both central and peripheral airway hyperresponsiveness occur in patients with clinically active bronchial asthma; however, during remission of asthma, considerably greater change resides in the peripheral airways.[78] The site of airway smooth-muscle thickening also may be important.[79] Since a majority of irritants are soluble in nature and are more likely absorbed within the central airways, a more central airway injury perhaps evolves pathophysiologically into increased central/larger airway inflammation and smooth-muscle hyperplasia and translates clinically into initiation of active asthma.

AIRWAY INFLAMMATION

Airway inflammation is critical in the pathogenesis of nonspecific airway hyperresponsiveness and leads to many of the manifestations of RADS. Pathologic investigations have documented airway inflammation in RADS.[7] Almost all inflammatory cells present in the bronchial wall and lumen have been implicated in the pathogenesis of asthma but, presently, none can be singled out as the most important.[4,80–83] In the original description of RADS, eosinophilic inflammation was limited and most of the cells were mononuclear.[7] The eosinophil is likely a proinflammatory cell, rather than an anti-inflammatory cell, and has the capacity to be recruited selectively from the circulation in response to IgE-dependent signals.[84] The eosinophil secretes mediators that cause damage to the bronchial epithelium and lead to bronchoconstriction and airway hyperresponsiveness. Eosinophils in asthma patients are likely "activated" and display enhanced release of toxic oxygen radicals.[85] Other cells present in the bronchial mucosa may be important. The main role of the mast cell appears to be initiation of allergen-induced responses. During the acute stage, neutrophilic inflammation may predominate; neutrophils have the potential to cause tissue damage through the elaboration of granule-derived proteases, oxygen metabolites, and lipid-derived mediators, including prostaglandins, leukotriene B_4, and platelet-activating factor (PAF).[86] Macrophages have low-affinity receptors for IgE, but whether they act as proinflammatory cells or have an ability to regulate immunologic responses is not known. Platelets may be important, but their exact role is also not clear. Lymphocytes may act as immunoregulators and possibly by releasing chemotactic cytokines. Lymphokines may also play a role in attracting granulocytes to the lung.[87]

CELLULAR DEFECTS IN BRONCHIAL SMOOTH MUSCLE

These have been postulated in asthma, but this observation has not been shown for RADS. Mechanisms to explain an exaggerated smooth-muscle contraction response in occupational asthma without latency may include: (1) a decrease in baseline airway caliber, (2) increased responsiveness of the smooth muscle itself, (3) component(s) of inflammation, (4) an abnormality in the autonomic and/or cholinergic nervous control of the smooth muscle, (5) an increase in the accessibility of the stimuli to target cells, and (6) effects of various peptide neurotransmitters.[88–90]

NEUROPEPTIDES

Neuropeptides conceivably are important in the pathogenesis of occupational asthma without latency, especially following inordinate exposure to irritants. The roles of neuropeptides have been elucidated for occupational asthma caused by TDI.[91] Vasoactive intestinal peptide (VIP) is a 28-amino acid peptide, nonadrenergic bronchodilator and is 100-fold more potent than isoproterenol; it has potent anti-inflammatory activity in the lung, including inhibiting inflammatory cell function, antagonizing major humoral mediators of inflammation, and attenuating acute edema.[90] It is possible that, in severe lung airway injury with inflammation, a defect in VIP-inhibiting control of airway smooth muscle can cause airways hyperresponsiveness. Inflammatory cells (mast cells, neutrophils, eosinophils) release numerous peptidases (e.g., mast cells release trypase) that rapidly degrade VIP.[90] This effect may be like "taking the brakes off" cholinergic nerves, resulting in an exaggerated reflex cholinergic bronchoconstriction, and may contribute to the bronchial hyperresponsiveness.[90] Excitatory neuropeptides, including substance P, neurokinin A, and calcitonin gene–related peptide, are characterized by rapid-onset smooth-muscle contractile effects; these substances are secreted from unmyelinated sensory nerves (C-fibers) and display inflammatory effects.[90] Substance P causes airway smooth-muscle contraction, stimulates mucus secretion, increases microvascular permeability and exudation of plasma into the airway lumen, degranulates mast cells and possibly has chemotactic properties.

EPITHELIAL DAMAGE

Damage to the airway epithelium may represent a critical step in the pathogenesis of RADS. Once injured, an airway epithelium is capable of generating products of the 15-lipoxygenase pathway of arachidonate metabolism, including 8,15-diHETE metabolites, the chemotactic agents for neutrophils, which may augment the airway inflammatory response.[92,93] Mattoli et al. reported that in vitro exposure of bronchial epithelial cells to TDI results in a dose-dependent release of 15-HETE that is inhibited by nedocromil sodium.[92] Injury to the epithelium also may lead to production of leukotriene B_4, a potent chemotactic agent, which can attract granulocytes but also may cause smooth-muscle contraction and, possibly, influence airway responsiveness.[89,93] Airway epithelium also modulates the bronchoconstrictor effects of many spasmogens, possibly by releasing a relaxant substance.[94,95] Damage to the airway epithelium may result in exposure of afferent nerve endings. Stimulation of unmyelinated vagal afferent may introduce axon reflexes and release of tachykinins; this can cause bronchoconstriction, increase vascular permeability, and potentiate vagally mediated airway smooth-muscle contraction.[96,97] Bradykinin, for example, may be an inflammatory mediator, which selectively can stimulate C-fiber nerve endings and cause release of sensory neuropeptides by an axon reflex.[90] Direct epithelial cell damage caused by high-level irritant exposure may produce "neurogenic inflammation" and subsequent changes similar to allergic occupational asthma. The airway inflammation induced by high-level irritating inhalants may stimulate tachykinin release, destroy local enzymes that metabolize tachykinins and thereby amplify their effects, or simply expose nerve endings and enhance their triggering.[83] It is conceivable that, once injured, permanent changes may develop in a nerve ending. For example, it has been reported that interruption of conduction in some fibers of a cutaneous nerve can evoke an induction or upregulation of α_2-adrenergic receptors (or their actions) in otherwise normal sensory nerve terminals and lead to causalgia.[98] Thus, following an injury to an airway, partial nerve injury may initiate an enhancement of the responsiveness of a proportion of C-fiber sensory units, which may translate into an altered release of various neuropeptides or changes in receptor numbers.

Shedding of an epithelium is augmented by eosinophil products, such as the cationic major basic protein (MBP). Epithelial removal also accentuates the bronchoconstrictor effects of tachykinins, in part, because of the lack of metabolism of tachykinins by neutral endopeptidase (NEP).[95,99–102] NEP is bound to the membranes of selected airway cells with receptors for tachykinins, which allows the enzyme to cleave tachykinins at the cell surface.[101] Decreased NEP activity occurs with epithelial removal, causing an exaggeration of neurogenic inflammation and bronchoconstrictor response. An example of the potential importance of the downregulation of NEP by a chemical insult is exemplified by the studies of Sheppard et al.[91] In guinea pigs exposed to TDI, bronchomotor tone response to inhaled substance P increased and was associated with a decrease in airway tissue NEP activity. Once damage to an airway epithelium has occurred, epithelial repair may be delayed by continued exposure to the environmental agent or for other unexplained reasons. Thus, altered epithelial function may persist even after termination of exposure, resulting in continued airways hyperreactivity to nonspecific irritants (such as cold air, fumes, odors, and dusts) and asthma symptoms.

Alterations in the "tight junctions" between bronchial epithelial cells from irritating and toxic substances may facilitate immunologic mechanisms by allowing easier access to the submucosal area of the airways where greater numbers of mast cells are located or by facilitating formation of hapten-protein conjugates.[103] These structural alterations may become permanent and help to explain how persistent symptoms may be induced by a single high-level or even a repetitive lower-level exposure.

MICROVASCULAR LEAKAGE

Microvascular leakage may be an important factor in the pathogenesis of RADS.[104] The studies of Van De Graaf et al. and others demonstrated an increased plasma exudation into the airways of asthmatic individuals.[105] The leakage occurs at the level of the postcapillary venules, possibly as a consequence of mediators (i.e., histamine, bradykinin, leukotrienes, PAF) on vascular endothelium, allowing

extravasation to occur. Neuropeptides also greatly enhance microvascular leakage.[90,104] Microvascular leakage causes submucosal edema and airway narrowing; it may also contribute to epithelial shedding and may be important in stimulating mucous secretion and lead to plugging of bronchioles. There can be an effect on mucociliary clearance, and leakage may act as a source of inflammatory mediators, including complement fragments (C3a, C5a, or anaphylatoxins), and kininogen-precursor of bradykinin.[90,104]

ATOPY AND ALLERGY

The observation that the preexisting atopic state precedes delayed irritant-induced asthma (> 24 h) may be clarified in several ways. First, more prolonged irritant exposure in an atopic individual may cause bronchial mucosal damage and increased bronchial mucosal permeability; this alteration permits airway mucosal entrance of greater amounts of environmental aeroallergens.[61] If the atopic person were previously sensitized to the aeroallergens, then the increased allergen absorption could cause interaction with specific IgE on mast cells and a more pronounced allergic response, and hence, new-onset asthma. A modified theory suggests that antigen sensitivity is enhanced by irritant exposure, a scenario supported by the work of Molfino et al., who demonstrated enhanced specific bronchial responsiveness to aeroallergen after preexposure to low levels of ozone.[105]

Perhaps there are "sensitive" or "susceptible" persons in the general population who are at increased risk for asthma development from irritant exposures, owing to a predisposition for manifesting an exaggerated response to irritants. In fact, there may be a constellation of inherent airway physiologic and pathologic changes among some segments of the population that makes this subset more susceptible to irritant-induced airway injury and the potential for developing asthma. Atopy or allergic potential can be considered a risk factor, since atopic individuals are at an increased risk for developing asthma and more often show accelerated decreases in lung function measurements or exaggerated responses to irritants.[106–114] There is a complex interplay between a new asthma onset, airway injury from various causes, airway inflammation, and IgE-mediated hypersensitivity.[115]

It may be that persons who develop not-so-sudden irritant-induced asthma already have preexisting damaged airway mucosa. An irritant injury to an already damaged bronchial mucosa may accelerate pathophysiologic processes causing clinical asthma. The "preexisting damaged airway theory" is supported by a variety of evidence. Nonspecific airway hyperresponsiveness is a common finding among atopic individuals with rhinitis, asymptomatic asthmatics, and also normal persons in the general population.[116–120] Persons with nonspecific airway hyperresponsiveness respond more unfavorably to irritant exposures than do normal persons[85,86]; irritant exposures may further influence bronchial reactivity.[109,121–123] Importantly, such individuals may show distinct pathologic changes in their airways, whether they are symptomatic or not.[124–127] In such a scenario, a likely inaugural event for irritant-induced asthma initiation is further bronchial mucosal injury from repeated and/or prolonged irritant exposures. Another consideration is that the presence of an atopic state translates clinically as greater concentrations of IgE antibodies binding to bronchial epithelial cells.[128] Such an occurrence influences intracellular responsiveness of bronchial epithelial cells to agonists and antagonists and results in an abnormal response to consequent irritant exposures.[129] What actually transpires is not completely understood, but it can be inferred that such an irritant injury in some way impairs respiratory epithelium function and leads to the cascade of biochemical, physiologic, and pathologic events, that is associated with the onset of clinical asthma.

Exposure factors including chemical type and reactivity, chemical sources, and concentration can be consequential. Intense high-level exposure is significant in the pathogenesis of RADS and allergic occupational asthma. Heavy exposures also have been implicated in the pathogenesis of TDI-asthma.[9,49] For TDI, workers with exposures to frequent spills are more likely to report asthma symptoms or show changes in lung function tests.[130,131] An unmistakable relationship exists between the magnitude of exposure and the prevalence of allergic sensitization. This association has been reported for western red cedar,[132, 133] isocyanates,[134] colophony,[135,136] baking products,[137] and acid anhydrides.[138]

Industrial factors include procedures inherent to industrial operations and processes, unique working conditions of the plant or industry, industrial hygiene practices employed in the industry or plant operation, and engineering features of the industrial site. For example, TDI-asthma is reported more commonly among workers employed in polyurethane processing than in TDI manufacturing, and a "mill effect" or plant effect has been described to explain noted differences in byssinosis and, possibly, TDI-asthma frequency among workers with similar exposures.[139–141] HDI and TDI have the same vapor pressures and are volatile at room temperature. MDI, with a very low vapor pressure at room temperature, becomes volatile when heated and can lead to asthma; this is noted in industrial processes such as foundry work.[142,143]

Job type or activity can influence disease initiation. Spray painting, for example, is an especially hazardous type of exposure. In such circumstances with the diisocyanates, high levels of vapors (HDI, TDI) and particulates (MDI) are airborne.[144] Other potentially dangerous job activities may include pouring, grinding, blasting, sanding, sawing, and heating. Unsafe working practices can lead to spills or accidents and resultant high-level exposures.

Geographic and climatic factors such as wind direction and humidity may be influential. Accidental spills involving irritant chemicals may only affect persons downwind from the spill. Meteorologic conditions have been incriminated in allergic asthma epidemics, such as in Barcelona, Spain, where unloading of soybeans caused asthma outbreaks.[145]

Economic factors could conceivably influence the prevalence of RADS by increasing the utilization of a product or accelerating work activity that might more likely lead to an accident. Ishizaki and associates demonstrated an association between the numbers of reported cases of allergic symptoms in workers exposed to western red cedar dust and the quantity of western red cedar imported into Japan.[146] Coincidentally with greater imports and a wider distribution of wood, cases of western red cedar asthma were reported from all over Japan.

Cigarette smoking is said to influence some atopic workers for occupational allergic sensitization but may also cause bronchial injury and inflammation and put subjects exposed to irritants at greater risk for adverse outcomes. An association between atopy, cigarette smoking, and allergic sensitization is reported for workers exposed to green coffee beans, tetrachlorophthalic anhydride, and platinum salts.[147–150] This relationship does not hold for detergent enzymes, laboratory animals, and colophony.[151–153]

A mechanism postulated to explain the connection between cigarette smoking and allergic sensitization proclaims that the inhalation of cigarette smoke produces an injury to the bronchial epithelium. Possibly it causes widening of the tight junctions between epithelial cells. This occurrence then enhances bronchial epithelial permeability and leads to heightened penetration of an antigen through the epithelial layer.[154,155]

Workplace irritants may provoke consequences similar to cigarette smoking. Both cigarette smoke and many workplace exposures seem to share equal irritant potential. The manifestations of increased permeability from irritant gases may be related to the initiation of bronchial inflammation. Bronchial inflammation has been noted for a single low-level exposure to ozone, SO_2, and NO_2.[156,157] Exposure leads to bronchial mucosal injury and increased permeability. Industrial operations utilizing irritant agents are, therefore, doubly dangerous because of the risk of heavy exposures and because of occurrence of spills and accidents, which may both lead to an allergic- (through increased antigen penetration due to increased bronchial permeability) or nonallergic-induced asthmatic condition. Irritant gases such as chlorine and ammonia are indigenous to the platinum refining industry, where sensitization is frequent. Their presence may inaugurate bronchial epithelial injury. Biagini and associates postulated that platinum salt allergic sensitization in monkeys required a concomitant exposure to ozone before allergic sensitization to platinum salts could be invoked.[158] Other animal studies have documented that an antecedent exposure to an airborne irritant enhances allergic sensitization to an allergen. Exposure to low concentrations of SO_2 promotes allergic sensitization in guinea pigs[159] and leads to increased epithelial permeability.[160] Similar increased allergic sensitization has also been reported to occur after ozone exposure.[161]

Hypothetical Model for RADS

The genesis of nonallergic occupational asthma embodies the culmination of many complex successions and aftermaths.[155] In the beginning, there is *homeostasis*, or a balance between the cellular and biochemical affectors and effectors of the airway status. The airway steadfastness can be likened to a pendulum, maintaining a relative constancy of the regulation of bronchomotor tone and cellular and biochemical balance through interactions among (1) respiratory epithelium, (2) smooth-muscle cell tone, (3) neural activity, (4) vascular integrity, (5) indigenous leukocyte and monocyte cellular constituents, and (6) endogenous humoral components. Cholinergic mechanisms dominate the neural bronchial smooth-muscle excitatory (bronchoconstrictor) pathway, while nonadrenergic, noncholinergic (NANC) nerves and neuropeptides, such as VIP, appear to represent the major bronchial inhibitory (bronchodilator) smooth-muscle control. There are fine tuning and modulation by such elements as sensory afferent neural activators (i.e., C-fibers, cough receptors, and rapidly and slowly adapting stretch receptors), adrenergic mechanisms (i.e., alpha- and beta-receptor activity), and other NANC nerves and neuropeptides (i.e., tachykinins). Other modulators of airway homeostasis include epithelial smooth-muscle inhibitory mechanisms [i.e., an epithelial-derived relaxant factor (E_pDRF)], the state of microvascular leakage, circulation of endogenous hormone (i.e., catecholamines), circulatory mediator (i.e., histamine) influences, other neuropeptides, and indigenous bronchial mucosal and luminal cells (i.e., macrophage, mast cells, etc.)

RADS is a "big bang" affair. The initial massive epithelial damage and disruption are followed by direct activation of NANC pathways (axon reflexes) and institution of neurogenic inflammation. High-level irritant exposure *initiates* massive airway injury. There is mast cell degranulation and macrophage activation. Chemotactic factors are released, and mucosal inflammation ensues. Epithelial cell destruction is substantial. Mast cell contents are released, while epithelial cells and vascular exudates introduce more chemotactic factors and further the recruitment of inflammatory cells, including eosinophils. Lung cells are activated. The severe epithelial injury leads to a reduced capacity for recovery. There may result compensatory up- and/or down-regulation of receptors and possibly genetic cellular alterations.

The important inaugural event involves initiation of *bronchial epithelial injury*. What exactly transpires is not completely understood, but the injury in some way impairs respiratory epithelium function (e.g., loss of ciliary activity, reduced NEP activity, possibly decreased release of E_pDRF) and initiates epithelial cell release of inflammatory mediators (i.e., leukotriene B_4, 15-lipoxygenase products). There is activation of NANC nerves (neurokinin A, substance P, etc.), which induces changes in microvascular permeability and causes mucous cell secretion. Mast cells release their contents (chemotactic factors and possibly cyclo- and lipoxygenase products).

The accompanying inflammation leads to cellular *activation* of the important effector cells: alveolar macrophages, eosinophils, and mast cells. Activated alveolar macrophages release increased amounts of mediators, such as thromboxanes, prostaglandins, and PAF. PAF attracts human eosinophils and causes eosinophil infiltration of the airways. Induction of new antigenic determinants may lead to "self-antigens," which enhance the inflammatory response and perpetuate the event. As activated eosinophil numbers increase, the degree and extent of epithelial damage increases. The activated eosinophils show enhanced killing properties, enhanced toxic oxygen radical production, and enhanced leukotriene production. Activated eosinophils also may display enhanced release of eosinophil cationic protein,

peroxidase, or eicosanoids. Nervous stimulation promotes mast cell degranulation, possibly through axon reflexes. Mononuclear cell activation results in T-cell activation and the release of various cytokines. Secretion of a granulocyte chemotactic activator by activated T lymphocytes and monocytes might be a mechanism whereby granulocytes are attracted to sites of inflammation. The presence of many activated cells will lead to exaggerated cellular responses and boosts nonspecific bronchial hyperresponsiveness. A vicious cycle may ensue: the presence of eosinophils introduces more widespread and diffuse airway epithelial injury (i.e., macro-injury) and desquamation.

Eventually, there is an attempt for *recovery*, which is characterized by resolution of inflammation, epithelial cell repair, neural activity inhibition, and improvement of vascular integrity. The greater the degree and extent of the injury, the more unlikely will be complete recovery. There may be laying down of submucosal collagen and other repair processes occurring. Irreversible changes in the airways' mechanical and biochemical status may result. There may be down- or upregulation of various receptors in response to persistent stimuli. There may be changes at the gene level, with transformation in gene coding.

The *sequela*, or new state of homeostasis, of the foregoing represents the culmination of the initiation, evolutionary, and repair processes. Depending on the degree of bronchial injury and the completeness of recovery, the sequela represents the residuum of cumulative injuries to the airways. The sequela may be one of complete recovery or may manifest as a chronic persistent asthmatic condition with nonspecific airway hyperresponsiveness.

Diagnosis

CLINICAL EVIDENCE

The criteria for confirming a diagnosis of RADS are listed in Table 38-3. The major requirement for the diagnosis of RADS is the appropriate medical history. The patient often describes the accident very clearly, usually because of the psychologically traumatic nature of the experience. In fact, the patient may be able to ascertain the exact day and time that the asthma onset occurred. This is in contrast to allergic occupational asthma, where the onset may be more difficult to discern and the history is not as specific. Malo et al. investigated 162 patients to assess the value of a clinical history (taken by an open medical questionnaire) in predicting the accuracy of the diagnosis of allergic occupational asthma as subsequently confirmed by inhalation challenges.[162] It was estimated that the history alone had a positive predictive value of 63 percent and a negative predictive value of 83 percent. There was agreement between the physician's initial assessment and the confirmed diagnosis in only 84 of the 162 cases (52 percent).

It is important to note that there have been no similar comparisons of the accuracy of the history in predicting documented RADS cases. There is no question that for both RADS and not-so-sudden irritant asthma the history is crucial. In allergic occupational asthma, the exact onset of the ill-

TABLE 38-3   Clinical Criteria for Diagnosis of Reactive Airways Dysfunction Syndrome

Absence of previous respiratory complaints or disease.

High-level exposure that almost always is due to an accident or spill.

Exposure is to an irritant agent, usually a gas, vapor, or fume.

Onset of asthma symptom is immediate, usually within minutes or hours, and always within 24 h.

Exposure incident is of such a magnitude that patient requires immediate medical treatment by a physician.

Symptoms are typical of asthma, with cough, dyspnea, and wheezing predominating.

Atopy does not appear to be a predisposing host factor.

Pulmonary function testing may show airflow limitation.

Methacholine challenge is positive in a range seen in asthmatics ($PC_{20} \leq 8$ mg/ml). Nonspecific airway hyperresponsiveness persists for years or indefinitely.

Other respiratory disorders are excluded.

Bronchial biopsy shows evidence of inflammation, often without eosinophilia.

---

ness cannot be precisely determined; usually, the onset is recalled only to within a season, year, or month. RADS, however, can be dated specifically. As indicated previously, the patient may even be able to identify the exact time of the day that the illness began. The reason for this clear-cut time discrimination is because RADS is a dramatic event, generally following an accident or unusual precipitous incident. The details become clear in the patient's mind. The exposure is always an irritant in nature and usually a vapor or gas. It is rare for a high-level dust exposure to be etiologic.

Symptoms of cough, dyspnea, and wheezing suggest asthma as a diagnosis. In RADS, a cough is a predominant symptom and may lead to an incorrect diagnosis of "chronic bronchitis" or recurrent bouts of "acute bronchitis." Some patients have such an intractable cough that it frequently interrupts an interview with the physician or makes spirometric testing difficult to complete.

The response of symptoms to being away from work is not as significant for RADS as for allergic occupational asthma. Burge suggested that asking two questions will identify the majority of patients with allergic occupational asthma[163]: Are your symptoms improved on days off? Are your symptoms improved on vacation? Persons with RADS (or irritant-induced asthma) may also note improvement away from work because their induced nonspecific airway hyperresponsiveness makes them more sensitive to varied low-level irritants and physical factors in their workplace. Symptoms may not improve over a 2-day weekend or occasional days off but might within a period of weeks.

An important differentiating clinical designation for RADS and allergic occupational asthma is the temporal relationship between exposure and disease onset. As much knowledge as possible of the incriminated etiologic agent is essential for diagnosis. Allergic occupational asthma rarely develops after a single exposure. Sensitization takes time and requires some latent period. The latent period criterion is of critical importance in establishing a medical-legal probability of causation.[2] This latent period is variable for allergic

occupational asthma and may range from months to years. Allergic sensitization from laboratory animals and complex salts of platinum can lead to sensitization within a few months. It has been reported that isocyanate-sensitization requires a mean period of 2 years; for colophony, 4 years is required, and up to 10 years or longer for other agents.[164]

The physician considers allergic occupational asthma when a patient has been exposed to a known sensitizing agent and has documented asthma.[165]

OBJECTIVE EVIDENCE OF WORK RELATIONSHIP

Pulmonary function measured on a day away from work may be normal in RADS patients but also in up to 50 percent of persons with allergic occupational asthma.[163] Many persons with RADS will not demonstrate airflow reversibility. Serial measurements of spirometry in different environments, such as when the patient has been away from work for a time and then again when the patient returns to work, may be necessary to induce a change in air flow limitation.[4] However, in both types of occupational asthma (latency and no latency), the bronchospasm at work results from different mechanisms (e.g., irritant-induced versus allergen-induced).

It is likely that two simple measurements of spirometry, one before and one after a work shift, might establish a work-related irritant response. Burge, however, found that only 22 percent of patients with allergic occupational asthma caused by colophony demonstrated a significant decrease in FEV_1 over a work shift; 11 percent of fellow workers who did not have occupational asthma had similar changes in FEV_1.[73] Furthermore, if the process is allergic in nature, conceivably occurrence of a late asthmatic response could be missed. This may explain the low incidence of significant reductions in FEV_1 for the colophony-induced asthmatic group.

Attention must be addressed to normal diurnal variation of pulmonary function testing. Spirometric values are lower in the early morning and higher in the late afternoon. Diurnal variation is much greater in asthmatic patients, particularly those with poorly controlled disease. Therefore, the diurnal improvement in FEV_1 over a usual daytime work could negate or minimize results, leading to a false-negative or inconclusive interpretation study.[163] For an allergic etiology, a "stop-resume" work test with measurement of serial PEFR values may be helpful.[165–167] Combining PEFR with a positive clinical history increases the sensitivity but reduces the specificity of diagnostic reliability.[71]

Serial measurement of nonspecific bronchial responsiveness in conjunction with prolonged recording of PEFR may provide additional evidence for allergic occupational asthma.[167] Significant decreases in methacholine PC_{20} away from work with appropriate reductions in PEFR suggest an allergic occupational association. In the case of nonallergic occupational asthma, testing for the presence of nonspecific bronchial hyperresponsiveness is very important.[168,169] A finding of increased nonspecific bronchial reactivity may be the only objective finding discerned. A positive challenge test supports the presence of an asthma syndrome when pulmonary function tests are normal. A negative methacholine challenge test usually excludes allergic asthma but will always exclude RADS. Persons showing only immediate-onset allergic asthmatic reactions may have absence of nonspecific airway hyperresponsiveness. There are case reports of patients with TDI-asthma without bronchial hyperresponsiveness.[170] Possibly, methacholine hyperresponsiveness wanes after the patient with allergic asthma has been away from a sensitizing exposure for a significant period of time.[171] In this case, the diagnosis of occupational asthma will be very difficult to confirm.

Skin tests and serology using common allergens such as house dust, danders, and grass and tree pollens may be useful in determining the presence of an atopic status. Although serologic testing is highly specific, it is often a less-sensitive indicator of sensitization than skin testing.[172] It must be remembered that both skin testing and serologic testing document exposure and sensitization but may not necessarily be associated with symptoms of asthma.

Specific inhalation challenge rarely is indicated to differentiate between allergic and nonallergic occupational asthma. It may be used to establish an allergic diagnosis where this is in doubt, to determine the precise etiologic agent in a complex working environment, and to confirm the diagnosis for medicolegal purposes.[4] There are ethical considerations for performing specific bronchial challenge tests for medicolegal reasons. A negative specific bronchial inhalation challenge test must be interpreted in context. A patient who has been away from the exposure for a period of time can lose sensitivity.[173] Challenge testing may be falsely negative if the incorrect substance is used for testing or if there is a circumstance where a combination of substances is necessary to produce a response. The method of challenge testing may not provide the correct exposure. Although laboratory exposure may be controlled, it is nevertheless artificial.

Management and Prevention

OVERVIEW

Smith attempted to dissect categories of occupational asthma for compensation purposes.[2] While these distinctions may be important for compensation purposes, they are not essential for medical management. The management of occupational asthma is no different from that of any type of asthma, regardless of etiology. Optimal management of any patient with occupational asthma (allergic or nonallergic) requires cooperation of both the employer and employee and often of compensation authorities as well.[4] The primary goal of management is to keep the patient symptom-free without progressive loss of pulmonary function, while at the same time minimizing any adverse effects from therapy.

ENVIRONMENTAL CONTROL

Environmental control is essential. Because sensitization is not an issue, patients with RADS may be able to work, as long as the levels of irritant exposure do not exceed the symptom threshold for the individual patient.

DRUG THERAPY

Medical therapy usually is required for management but should not be an alternative to environmental control. Cromolyn and inhaled corticosteroids are useful in reducing the degree of airway hyperreactivity.[174,175] For RADS, inhaled bronchodilators can be used for acute bronchospastic responses to irritants. The use of systemic corticosteroids should be avoided and restricted to only the initial acute phase, most proximate to the initial injury. Corticosteroids can be given (1 mg/kg) within the first 48 h after the exposure and perhaps for the first few weeks after the injury. The prompt treatment of the inhalation injury may limit the degree of airway injury in some cases. Once the acute stage has passed, systemic corticosteroids should not be used, but inhaled steroids are recommended. The pathology and pathogenesis of RADS are different from allergic occupational asthma where eosinophils predominate and corticosteroids may be effective. In cases of the atypical, not-so-sudden irritant-induced asthma, oral corticosteroids might be appropriate, but even in these cases systemic corticosteroid use should be minimized. In all types of occupational asthma without latency, inhaled steroids are the mainstay of drug treatment.

PREVENTION

The identification of one or several cases of asthma associated with the workplace often provides an opportunity to prevent future problems. A single suspected case is a sentinel event that should lead to investigation and confirmation. Education of primary care physicians is helpful in order to stress the need and importance of reporting and/or referring cases of potential occupational asthma.[176] Worker education concerning safety measures involved in handling procedures and avoidance of spills may be beneficial.[3] Product formulation changes have been successful in the detergent industry where encapsulation of the enzyme portion of the product has reduced the exposure to workers and lessened allergic occupational asthma prevalence. It has been suggested that preemployment screening could theoretically detect and eliminate prospective employees with high-risk or susceptibility factors.[177] At this time, hiring practices based on preemployment screening is not yet medically defensible and would likely run into problems with discrimination and violation of individual workers' rights.

IMPAIRMENT AND DISABILITY

The American Thoracic Society has defined impairment as "a medical condition resulting from functional abnormality that may be temporary or permanent and that may preclude gainful employment."[178,179] Disability awards must take into account not only the degree of impairment but also the job description. There currently are inadequate guidelines for assessing impairment or disability in patients with allergic and nonallergic occupational asthma.[180] It seems reasonable to consider the degree of nonspecific bronchial responsiveness, determined by inhalation testing, as well as the clinical assessment. Clinical outcomes for asthma are being developed and may be appropriate for occupational asthma. Quality-of-life questionnaires also may be appropriate for assessment. In the assessment of patients with RADS, spirometry is often normal, so American Medical Association guidelines based on FEV_1 are inappropriate.

References

1. Malo J-L: Compensation for occupational asthma in Quebec. *Chest* (suppl) 1990; 98:236S.
2. Smith D: Medical-legal definition of occupational asthma. *Chest* 1990; 98:1007.
3. Brooks S: Occupational asthma, in EG W (ed): *Bronchial Asthma. Mechanisms and Therapeutics.* Boston, Little, Brown, 1985; 461.
4. Chan-Yeung M: Occupational asthma. *Chest* 1990; 98:148S.
5. Industrial IAC: *Occupational Asthma.* London, Her Majesty's Stationery Office, 1981.
6. Gandevia B: Occupational asthma, part I. *Med J Aust* 1970; 2:332.
7. Brooks S, Weiss MA, Il B: Reactive airways dysfunction syndrome: Persistent asthma syndrome after high-level irritant exposure. *Chest* 1985; 88:376.
8. Newman-Taylor A: Occupational asthma. *Postgrad Med J* 1988; 64:505.
9. Brooks S: Occupational and environmental asthma, in Rom WN (ed): *Environmental and Occupational Medicine.* Boston, Little, Brown, 1992; 393.
10. Zuskin E, Wolfson R, Harpel G, et al.: Byssinosis in carding and spinning workers. *Arch Environ Health* 1969; 19:666.
11. Chan-Yeung M, Enarson D, Gryzbowski S: Grain dust and respiratory health. *Can Med Assoc J* 1985; 133:969.
12. Burney P, Britton J, Chinn S, et al.: Descriptive epidemiology of bronchial reactivity in adult population: Results from a community study. *Thorax* 1987; 42:38.
13. MacDowell KF, Beauchamp HD: in Weiss E, Stein M (eds): *Bronchial Asthma: Mechanisms and Therapeutics,* 3d ed. Boston, Little, Brown, 1993; 459.
14. Joseph I, Gregg I, Mullee M, et al.: A longitudinal study of nonspecific bronchial responsiveness in asthma. *Thorax* 1987; 42:711.
15. Hopp R, Townley R, Biven R, et al.: The presence of airway reactivity before the development of asthma. *Am Rev Respir Dis* 1990; 141:2.
16. Pattermore P, Asher M, Harrison A, et al.: The interrelationship among bronchial hyperresponsiveness, the diagnosis of asthma and asthma symptoms. *Am Rev Respir Dis* 1990; 142:549.
17. Stanescu D, Frans A: Bronchial asthma without increased airways reactivity. *Eur J Respir Dis* 1982; 63:5.
18. Britton J, Tattersfield A: Does measurement of bronchial hyperreactivity help in the clinical diagnosis of asthma. *Eur J Respir Dis* 1986; 68:233.
19. Chhabra S, Shailendra N, Gaur M, Khanna A: Clinical significance of nonspecific hyperresponsiveness in asthma. *Chest* 1989; 96:596.
20. Moser K: Definition of asthma, in Weiss E, Stein M (eds): *Bronchial Asthma: Mechanisms and Therapeutics,* 3d ed. Boston, Little, Brown, 1993; 11.
21. American Thoracic Society: Definition and classification of chronic bronchitis, asthma and pulmonary emphysema. *Am Rev Respir Dis* 1962; 85:762.
22. Woolcock A: Asthma, in Murray J, Nadel J (eds): *Textbook of Respiratory Medicine.* Philadelphia, Saunders, 1988; 1030.
23. Toelle B, Peat J, Salome C, et al.: Toward a definition of asthma for epidemiology. *Am Rev Respir Dis* 1992; 146:633.
24. Mortagy A, Howell J, Waters W: Respiratory symptoms and bronchial reactivity: Identification of a syndrome and its relation to asthma. *Br Med J* 1986; 293:525.
25. Brooks SM, Bernstein IL, Raghuprasad PK, et al.: Assessment of airway hyperresponsiveness in chronic stable asthma. *J Allergy Clin Immunol* 1990; 85:17.
26. ATS Ad Hoc Committee: Guidelines for the evaluation of impairment/disability in patients with asthma. *Am Rev Respir Dis* 1993; 147:1056.
27. Chan-Yeung M, Vedal S, Kus J, et al.: Symptoms, pulmonary function and airway hyperreactivity in western red cedar compared to those in the office workers. *Am Rev Respir Dis* 1984; 130:1038.
28. Chan-Yeung M, MacLean L, Paggiaro P: A follow-up of 232 patients with occupational asthma due to western red cedar. *J Allergy Clin Immunol* 1987; 79:792.
29. Chan-Yeung M: Evaluation of impairment/disability in patients with occupational asthma. *Am Rev Respir Dis* 1987; 135:950.
30. Hargreave F, Ryan G, Thompson N, et al.: Bronchial responsiveness to histamine or methacholine in asthma: Measurement and clinical significance. *J Allergy Clin Immunol* 1981; 68:347.
31. Bakke P, Baste V, Gulsvik A: Bronchial responsiveness in a Norwegian community. *Am Rev Respir Dis* 1991; 143:317.
32. Casale T, et al.: Airway response to methacholine in asymptomatic nonatopic cigarette smokers. *J Appl Physiol* 1987; 62:1888.
33. Burney P, Britton J, Chinn S, et al.: Descriptive epidemiology of bronchial reactivity in adult population: Results from a community study. *Thorax* 1987; 42:38.
34. Rijcken B, Schouten J, Weiss S, et al.: The relationship of nonspecific bronchial responsiveness to respiratory symptoms in a random population sample. *Am Rev Respir Dis* 1987; 136:62.
35. Rice S, Bierman C, Shapiro G, et al.: Identification of exercise-induced asthma among intercollegiate athletes. *Ann Allergy* 1985; 55:790.
36. Weiler J, Metzger W, Donnelly A, et al.: Prevalence of bronchial hyperresponsiveness in highly trained athletes. *Chest* 1986; 90:23.
37. Gerrard J. Cockcroft D, Mink J, et al.: Increased nonspecific bronchial reactivity in cigarette smokers with normal lung function. *Am Rev Respir Dis* 1980; 122:577.
38. Cockcroft D, Killian D, Mellon J, Hargreave F: Bronchial reactivity to inhaled histamine: A method and clinical survey. *Clin Allergy* 1977; 7:235.
39. Cockcroft D: Bronchial inhalation tests: I. Measurement of nonallergic bronchial responsiveness. *Ann Allergy* 1985; 55:527.
40. Harkonen H, Nordman H, Korhonen O, et al.: Long-term effects from exposure to sulfur dioxide: Lung function four years after a pyrite dust explosion. *Am Rev Respir Dis* 1983; 128:840.
41. Charan N, Meyers C, Lakshminarayan S, et al.: Pulmonary injuries associated with acute sulfur dioxide inhalation. *Am Rev Respir Dis* 1979; 119:555.
42. Flury K, Ames D, Rodarte J, et al.: Airway obstruction due to ammonia. *Mayo Clin Proc* 1983; 58:389.
43. Donham K, Knapp L, Monson R, et al.: Acute toxic exposure to gases from liquid manure. *J Occup Med* 1982; 24:142.
44. Murphy D, Fairman R, Lapp N, et al.: Severe airways disease due to the inhalation of fumes from cleaning agents. *Chest* 1976; 69:372.
45. Hasan F, Gehshan A, Fulechan F: Resolution of pulmonary dysfunction following acute chlorine exposures. *Arch Environ Health* 1983; 38:76.

46. Kennedy S, Enarson D, Janssen R, et al.: Lung health consequences of reported accidental chlorine gas exposure among pulpmill workers. *Am Rev Respir Dis* 1991; 143:74.

47. Kaufman J, Burkons D: Clinical, roentgenologic and physiologic effects of acute chlorine exposure. *Arch Environ Health* 1971; 23:29.

48. Luo J-L, Nelsen K, Fischbein A: Persistent reactive airway dysfunction after exposure to toluene diisocyanate. *Br J Ind Med* 1988; 47:239.

49. Moller D, RT M, Il B, et al.: Persistent airways disease caused by toluene diisocyanate. *Am Rev Respir Dis* 1986; 134:175.

50. Alford P, McLees B, Case L: Reactive airways dysfunction syndrome (RADS) in workers post exposure to sulfur dioxide (SO$_2$). *Chest* 1988; 94:87S.

51. Angelillo V: Reactive airway dysfunction syndrome (RADS): A report of three cases. *Respir Care* 1992; 37:254.

52. Donnelly S, FitzGerald M: Reactive airways dysfunction syndrome (RADS) due to chlorine gas exposure. *Irish J Med Sci* 1990; 159:275.

53. Lerman S, Kipen H: Reactive airways dysfunction syndrome. *Am Fam Physician* 1988; 38:135.

54. Promisloff R, Phan A, Lenchner G, Chachelli A: Reactive airways dysfunction syndrome in three police officers following a roadside chemical spill. *Chest* 1990; 98:928.

55. Gautrin D, Boulet L-P, Boutet M, et al.: Is reactive airways dysfunction syndrome a variant of occupational asthma? *J Allergy Clin Immunol* 1994; 93:12.

56. Kennedy S: Acquired airway hyperresponsiveness from nonimmune irritant exposures. *Occup Med* 1992; 7:287.

57. Kern DG: Outbreak of the reactive airways dysfunction syndrome after a spill of glacial acetic acid. *Am Rev Respir Dis* 1991; 144:1058.

58. Rajan K, Davies B: Reversible airways obstruction and interstitial pneumonitis due to acetic acid. *Br J Ind Med* 1989; 46:67.

59. Axford A, McKerrow C, Jones A, et al.: Accidental exposure to isocyanate fumes on a group of firemen. *Br J Ind Med* 1976; 33:65.

60. Moisan T: Prolonged asthma after smoke inhalation: A report of three cases and a review of previous reports. *J Occup Med* 1991; 33:458.

61. Brooks S, Fox R, Giovinco-Barbas J, et al.: Irritant-induced asthma: Role of allergic diathesis in pathogenesis. *Am Rev Respir Dis* 1993; 147:A378.

62. Bernstein I, Bernstein D, Weiss M, Campbell G: Reactive airways disease syndrome (RADS) after exposure to toxic ammonia fumes. *J Allergy Clin Immunol* 1989; 83:173.

63. Boulet L-P: Increase in airway responsiveness following acute exposure to respiratory irritants: Reactive airways dysfunction syndrome or occupational asthma? *Chest* 1988; 94:476.

64. Deschamps D, Rosenberg N, Soler P, et al.: Persistent asthma after accidental exposure to ethylene oxide. *Br J Ind Med* 1992; 49:523.

65. Gilbert R, Auchincloss Jr J: Reactive airways dysfunction syndrome presenting as a reversible restrictive defect. *Lung* 1989; 167:55.

66. Chan-Yeung M, Lam S, Kennedy SM, Frew AJ: Persistent asthma after repeated exposure to high concentrations of gases in pulpmills. *Am J Respir Crit Care Med* 1994; 149:1676.

67. Moore B, Sherman M: Chronic reactive airways disease following acute chlorine gas exposure in an asymptomatic atopic patient. *Chest* 1991; 100:855.

68. Tarlo S, I B: Irritant-induced occupational asthma. *Chest* 1989; 96:297.

69. Wade J III, Newman L: Diesel asthma: Reactive airways disease following overexposure to locomotive exhaust. *J Occup Med* 1993; 35:149.

70. Demeter SL, Cordasco EM: Reactive airways dysfunction syndrome: A subset of occupational asthma. *J Disability* 1990; 1:25.

71. Cote J, Kennedy S, Chan-Yeung M: Outcome of patients with cedar asthma with continuous exposure. *Am Rev Respir Dis* 1990; 141:373.

72. Paggiaro P, Loi A, Rossi O, et al.: Follow-up study of patients with respiratory disease due to toluene diisocyanate (TDI). *Clin Allergy* 1984; 14:463.

73. Burge P: Occupational asthma in electronic workers caused by colophony fumes: Follow-up of affected workers. *Thorax* 1982; 37:348.

74. Malo J-L, Cartier A, Ghezzo H, et al.: Patterns of improvement in spirometry, bronchial hyperresponsiveness and specific IgE antibody levels after cessation of exposure in occupational asthma caused by snowcrab processing. *Am Rev Respir Dis* 1988; 138:807.

75. Hudson P, Cartier A, Pineau L, et al.: Follow-up of occupational asthma caused by crab and various agents. *J Allergy Clin Immunol* 1985; 76:262.

76. Chan-Yeung M, MacLean L, Paggiaro P: A follow-up of 232 patients with occupational asthma due to western red cedar. *J Allergy Clin Immunol* 1987; 79:792.

77. Chan-Yeung M: Immunologic and nonimmunologic mechanisms in asthma due to western red cedar (*Thuja plicata*). *J Allergy Clin Immunol* 1982; 70:32.

78. Ohrui T, Sekizawa K, Yanai M, et al.: Partitioning of pulmonary responses to inhaled methacholine in subjects with asymptomatic asthma. *Am Rev Respir Dis* 1992; 146:1501.

79. Ebina M, Takahashi T, Chiba T, Motomiya M: Cellular hypertrophy and hyerplasia of airway smooth muscle underlying bronchial asthma. *Am Rev Respir Dis* 1993; 148:720.

80. Chan-Yeung M, et al.: Evidence for mucosal inflammation in occupational asthma. *Clin Exper Allergy* 1990; 20:1.

81. DeMonchy J, Kauffman H, Venge P, et al.: Bronchoalveolar eosinophilia during allergen-induced late asthmatic reactions *Am Rev Respir Dis* 1985; 31:373.

82. Diaz P, Gonzales M, Galleguillos F, et al.: Leukocytes and mediators in bronchoalveolar lavage during allergen-induced late phase asthmatic reactions. *Am Rev Respir Dis* 1989; 139:1383.

83. Fine M, Balmes J: Airway inflammation and occupational asthma. *Clin Chest Med* 1988; 9:577.

84. Djukanmovic R, Roche W, Wilson J, et al.: State of the art: Mucosal inflammation in asthma. *Am Rev Respir Dis* 1990; 142:434.

85. Cerasoli F Jr, Tocker J, Selig W: Airway eosinophils from actively sensitized guinea pigs exhibit enhanced superoxide anion release in response to antigen challenge. *Am J Respir Cell Mol Biol* 1991; 4:355.

86. Beasley R, Roche W, Roberts J, et al.: Cellular events in the bronchi in mild asthma and after bronchial provocation. *Am Rev Respir Dis* 1989; 139:806.

87. Corrigan C, Collard P, Nagy L, et al.: Cultured peripheral blood mononuclear cells derived from patients with acute severe asthma ("status asthmaticus") spontaneously elaborate a neutrophil chemotactic activity distinct from interleukin-8. *Am Rev Respir Dis* 1991; 143:538.

88. Boushey HA, et al.: State of the art: Bronchial hyperreactivity. *Am Rev Respir Dis* 1980; 121:389.

89. Leff A: State of the art: Endogenous regulation of bronchomotor tone. *Am Rev Respir Dis* 1988; 137:1198.

90. Barnes P: Neuropeptides and asthma. *Am Rev Respir Dis* (suppl) 1991; 143:28S.

91. Sheppard D, Thompson J, Scypinski L, et al.: Toluene diisocyanate increases airway responsiveness to substance P and decreases airway enkephalinase. *J Clin Invest* 1988; 81:2647.

92. Mattoli S, Mezzetti M, Patalano F, et al.: Nedocromil sodium

prevents the release of 15-hydroxyeicosatetraenoic acid from human bronchial epithelial cells exposed to toluene diisocyanate in vitro. *Int Arch Appl Immunol* 1990; 92:16.

93. Daniel E, O'Byrne P: Autonomic nerves and airway smooth muscle: Effects of inflammatory mediators on airway nerves and muscle. *Am Rev Respir Dis* 1991; 143:3S.

94. Cuss F, Barnes P: Epithelial mediators. *Am Rev Respir Dis* 1987; 136:32S.

95. Flavahan N, Aarhus L, Rimele T, et al.: Respiratory epithelium inhibits bronchial smooth muscle tone. *J Appl Physiol* 1985; 58:834.

96. Barnes P: Asthma as an axon reflex. *Lancet* 1986; 1:242.

97. Lundberg J, Brodin E, Saira A: Effects and distribution of vagal capsaicin-sensitive substance P neurons with special reference to the trachea and lungs. *Acta Physiol Scand* 1983; 119:243.

98. Sato J, Perl E: Adrenergic excitation of cutaneous pain receptors induced by peripheral nerve injury. *Science* 1991; 251:1606.

99. Frossard N, Rhoden K, Barnes P: Influence of epithelium on guinea pig airway in response to tachykinins: Role of endopeptidases and cyclooxygenases. *J Pharmacol Exp Ther* 1989; 248:292.

100. Tschirhart E, Landry Y: Epithelium releases a relaxant factor: Demonstration of substance P. *Eur J Pharmacol* 1986; 132:103.

101. Nadel J, Borson B: Modulation of neurogenic inflammation by neutral endopeptidase. *Am Rev Respir Dis* (suppl) 1991; 143:33S.

102. Grandordy B, Frossard N, Rhoden K, et al.: Tachykinin-induced phosphoinositide breakdown in airway smooth muscle and epithelium: Relationship to contraction. *Mol Pharmacol* 1988; 33:515.

103. Hogg J, Pare P, Boucher R, et al.: The pathophysiology of asthma. *Can Med Assoc J* 1979; 121:409.

104. Barnes P: New concepts in the pathogenesis of bronchial hyperresponsiveness and asthma. *J Allergy Clin Immunol* 1989; 83:1013.

105. Molfino N, Wright S, Katz I, et al.: Effect of low concentrations of ozone on inhaled allergen responses in asthmatic subjects. *Lancet* 1991; 338:199.

106. Annesi I, Oryszczyn M-P, Frette C, et al.: Total circulating IgE and FEV$_1$ in adult men: An epidemiologic longitudinal study. *Chest* 1992; 101:642.

107. Frew A, Kennedy S, Chan-Yeung M: Methacholine responsiveness, smoking, and atopy as risk factors for accelerated FEV$_1$ decline in male working populations. *Am Rev Respir Dis* 1992; 146:878.

108. Braman S, Barrows A, DeCotiis B, et al.: Airway hyperresponsiveness in allergic rhinitis. *Chest* 1987; 91:671.

109. Harving H, Dahl R, Molhave L: Lung function and bronchial reactivity in asthmatics during exposure to volatile organic compounds. *Am Rev Respir Dis* 1991; 143:751.

110. Holtzman M, Cunningham J, Sheller J, et al.: Effect of ozone on bronchial reactivity in atopic and nonatopic subjects. *Am Rev Respir Dis* 199; 120:1059.

111. Kagamimori S, Katoh T, Naruse Y, et al.: The changing prevalence of respiratory symptoms in atopic children in response to air pollution *Clin Allergy* 1986; 16:299.

112. McBride D, Koenig J, Luchtel D, et al.: Inflammatory effects of ozone in the upper airways of subjects with asthma. *Am J Respir Crit Care Med* 1994; 149:1192.

113. Bascom R, Naclerio R, Fitzgerald T, et al.: Effect of ozone inhalation on the response to nasal challenge with antigen of allergic subjects. *Am Rev Respir Dis* 1990; 142:594.

114. Horstman D, Folinsbee J, Ives P, et al.: Ozone concentration and pulmonary response relationships for 6.6-hour exposures with five hours of moderate exercise to 0.08, 0.10, and 0.12 ppm. *Am Rev Respir Dis* 1990; 142:1158.

115. Yano T, Ichikawa Y, Komatu S, et al.: Association of *Mycoplasma pneumoniae* antigen with initial onset of bronchial asthma. *Am J Respir Crit Care Med* 1994; 149:1348.

116. Kawasaki A, Mizushima Y, Hoshino K, et al.: Bronchial hypersensitivity in asthmatics in long-term symptom-free states. *Chest* 1993; 103:370.

117. Radford P, Hopp R, Rus D, et al.: Longitudinal changes in bronchial hyperresponsiveness in asthmatic and previously asthmatic children. *Chest* 1992; 101:624.

118. Burrows B, Sears M, Flannery E, et al.: Relationship of bronchial responsiveness assessed by methacholine to serum IgE, lung functions, symptoms and diagnoses in 11-year-old New Zealand children. *J Allergy Clin Immunol* 1992; 90:376.

119. Godden D, Ross S, Abdalla M, et al.: Outcome of wheeze in childhood: Symptoms and pulmonary function 25 years later. *Am J Respir Crit Care Med* 1994; 149:106.

120. Zwick H, Popp W, Budick G, et al.: Increased sensitization to aeroallergens in competitive swimmers. *Lung* 1990; 168:111.

121. Forastiere F, Agabiti N, Corbo G, et al.: Passive smoking as a determinant of bronchial responsiveness in children. *Am J Respir Crit Care Med* 1994; 149:365.

122. Chai K, Jeyaratnam J, Chan T, Lim T: Airway responsiveness of firefighters after smoke exposure. *Br J Ind Med* 1990; 47:524.

123. Gaddy J, Busse W: Enhanced IgE-dependent basophil histamine release and airway reactivity in asthma. *Am Rev Respir Dis* 1986; 134:969.

124. Laitinen L, Laitinen A, Haahtela T: Airway mucosal inflammation even in patients with newly diagnosed asthma. *Am Rev Respir Dis* 1993; 147:697.

125. Laitinen L, Heino M, Laitinen A, et al.: Damage of the airway epithelium and bronchial reactivity in patients with asthma. *Am Rev Respir Dis* 1985; 131:599.

126. Roche W, Beasley R, Williams J, Holgate S: Subepithelial fibrosis in the bronchi of asthmatics. *Lancet* 1989; 1:520.

127. Campbell A, Chanez P, Vignola A, et al.: Functional characteristics of bronchial epithelium obtained by brushing from asthmatics and normal subjects. *Am Rev Respir Dis* 1993; 147:529.

128. Campbell AM, Chanez P, Vignola M, et al.: Expression of IgE and the high affinity receptor for IgE (FceRI) by bronchial epithelial cells of asthmatics. *J Allergy Clin Immunol* 1994; 93:197.

129. Ali K, Calderon EG, Brooks SM, et al.: Adrenergic effects of immunoglobulin E (IgE) on A549 human pulmonary epithelial cells. *Am Rev Respir Dis* 1993; 147:A.

130. Brooks SM, et al.: *Epidemiologic Study of Workers Exposed to Isocyanate.* NIOSH Health Hazard Evaluation Report, 1980.

131. Karol M: Survey of industrial workers for antibodies to toluene diisocyanate. *J Occup Med* 1981; 23:741.

132. Vedal S, Enarson D, Kus J, et al.: Symptoms and pulmonary function in western red cedar workers related to duration of employment and dust exposure. *Arch Environ Health* 1986; 41:179.

133. Brooks SM, et al.: An epidemiologic study of workers exposed to western red cedar and other wood dusts. *Chest* 1981; 80:30.

134. Wegman DH, et al.: A dose-response relationship in TDI workers. *J Occup Med* 1974; 16:258.

135. Burge PS, et al.: Respiratory disease in workers exposed to solder flux fumes containing colophony (pine resin). *Clin Allergy* 1978:8:1.

136. Burge P, Edge G, Hawkins R, et al.: Occupational asthma in a factory making flux-colored solder containing colophony. *Thorax* 1981; 36:828.

137. Musk A, Venables K, Crook B, et al.: Respiratory symptoms, lung function and sensitization to flour in a British bakery. *Br J Ind Med* 1989; 46:636.

138. Venables K: Low molecular weight chemicals, hypersensitivity, and direct toxicity to the acid anhydrides. *Br J Ind Med* 1989; 46:222.

139. Jones RN, et al.: Mill effect and dose response relationships in byssinosis. *Br J Ind Med* 1979; 36:305.

140. Weill H, et al.: *Respiratory and Immunologic Evaluation of Isocyanate Exposure in a New Manufacturing Plant.* Washington, DC, NIOSH, US Government Printing Office, 1981.

141. Diem JE, et al.: Five-year longitudinal study of workers employed in a new toluene diisocyanate manufacturing plant. *Am Rev Respir Dis* 1982; 126:420.

142. Johnson A, Chan-Yeung M, MacLean L, et al.: Respiratory abnormalities among workers in an iron and steel foundry in Vancouver. *Br J Ind Med* 1985; 42:94.

143. Zammit-Tabona M, Sherkin M, Kijek K, et al.: Asthma caused by dimethyl methane diisocyanate in foundry workers: Clinical bronchoprovocation and immunologic studies. *Am Rev Respir Dis* 1983; 128:226.

144. Seguin P, Allard A, et al.: Prevalence of occupational asthma in spray painters exposed to several types of isocyanates, including polymethylene polyphenylisocyanate. *J Occup Med* 1987; 29:340.

145. Anto J, Sunyer J, Rodriguez-Roisin R, et al.: Community outbreaks of asthma associated with inhalation of soybean dust. *N Engl J Med* 1989; 320:1097.

146. Ishizaki T, et al.: Occupational asthma from western red cedar dust (*Thuja plicata*) in furniture factory workers. *J Occup Med* 1973; 15:580.

147. Venables K, Topping M, Howe W, et al.: Interaction of smoking and atopy in producing specific IgE antibody against a hapten protein conjugate. *Br Med J* 1985; 290:201.

148. Zetterstrom I, Osterman K, Machado L, et al.: Another smoking hazard: Revised serum IgE concentration and increased risk of occupational allergy. *Br Med J* 1981; 283:1215.

149. Brooks S, Baker DB, Gann PH, et al.: Cold air challenge and platinum skin reactivity in platinum refinery workers. *Chest* 1990;

150. Venables K et al.: Smoking and occupational allergy in workers in a platinum refinery. *Br Med J* 1989; 299:939.

151. Mitchell CA, Gandevia B: Respiratory symptoms and skin reactivity in workers exposed to proteolytic enzymes in the detergent industry. *Am Rev Respir Dis* 1971; 104:1.

152. Slovak A, Hill R: Laboratory animal allergy: A clinical survey of an exposed population. *Br J Ind Med* 1981; 38:38.

153. Burge P, Perks W, O'Brien I, et al.: Occupational asthma in an electronics factory: A case control study to evaluate aetiological factors. *Thorax* 1979; 34:300.

154. Simani AS, Inoue S, Hogg JC: Penetration of the respiratory epithelium of guinea pigs following exposure to cigarette smoke. *Lab Invest* 1974; 31:75.

155. Alberts M, Brooks S: Advances in occupational medicine. *Clin Chest Med* 1992; 13:281.

156. Koren H, Devlin R, Graham D, et al.: Ozone-induced inflammation in the lower airways of human subjects. *Am Rev Respir Dis* 1989; 139:407.

157. Sandstrom T, Stjernberg N, Andersson M-C, et al.: Cell response in bronchoalveolar lavage fluid after sulfur dioxide exposure. *Scand J Work Environ Health* 1989; 15:142.

158. Biagini R, Moorman W, Lewis T, et al.: Ozone enhancement of platinum asthma in a primate model. *Am Rev Respir Dis* 1986; 134:719.

159. Reidel F, Kramer M, Scheibenbogen C, et al.: Effects of SO_2 exposure on allergic sensitization in the guinea pig. *J Allergy Clin Immunol* 1988; 82:527.

160. Vai F, et al.: SO_2-induced bronchopathy in rat: Abnormal permeability of the bronchial epithelium in vivo and in vitro after anatomic recovery. *Am Rev Respir Dis* 1980; 121:851.

161. Osebold J, Gershwin L, Zee Y: Studies on the enhancement of allergic lung sensitization by inhalation of ozone and sulfuric acid aerosol. *J Environ Pathol Toxicol Oncol* 1990; 3:221.

162. Malo J, Ghezzo H, L'archeveque J, et al.: Is the clinical history a satisfactory means of diagnosing occupational asthma? *Am Rev Respir Dis* 1991; 143:528.

163. Burge P: Problems in the diagnosis of occupational asthma. *Br J Dis Chest* 1987; 81:105.

164. Burge P: Diagnosis of occupational asthma. *Clin Exp Allergy* 1989; 19:649.

165. Canadian Thoracic Society: Occupational asthma: Recommendations for diagnosis, management, and assessment of impairment. *Can Med Assoc J* 1989; 140:1029.

166. Burge P: Single and serial measurements of lung function in the diagnosis of occupational asthma. *Eur J Respir Dis* (suppl 123) 1982; 63:47.

167. Cartier A, Pineau L, J-L M: Monitoring of maximum expiratory peak flow rates and histamine inhalation tests in the investigation of occupational asthma. *Clin Allergy* 1984; 14:193.

168. Cockcroft D: Bronchial inhalation tests: I. Measurement of nonallergic bronchial responsiveness. *Ann Allergy* 1985; 55:527.

169. Cartier A, Bernstein I, Burge P, et al.: Guidelines for bronchoprovocation in the investigation of occupational asthma. *J Allergy Clin Immunol* 1989; 84:823.

170. Smith A, Brooks S: Absence of airway hyperreactivity to methacholine in workers sensitized to toluene diisocyanate (TDI). *J Occup Med* 1980; 22:327.

171. Lam S, Wong R, Chan-Yeung M: Nonspecific bronchial reactivity in occupational asthma. *J Allergy Clin Immunol* 1979; 63:28.

172. Bernstein D, Bernstein I: Occupational asthma, in Middleton EJ, Reed C, Ellis E (eds): *Allergy: Principles and Practice.* St Louis, Mosby, 1988; 1197.

173. Banks D, Sastre J, Butcher B, et al.: Role of inhalation challenge testing in the diagnosis of isocyanate-induced asthma. *Chest* 1989; 95:414.

174. Cockcroft D, Murdock K: Comparative effects of inhaled salbutamol, sodium cromogycate and beclomethasone on allergeninduced early asthmatic response, late asthmatic response and increased bronchial responsiveness to histamine. *J Allergy Clin Immunol* 1987; 79:734.

175. Mapp C, Boschetto P, dal Vecchio L, et al.: Protective effects of antiasthma drugs in late asthmatic reactions and increased airway responsiveness induced by toluene diisocyanate in sensitized subjects. *Am Rev Respir Dis* 1987; 136:1403.

176. Rosenstock L: Role of physician in environmental and occupational asthma. *Chest* 1990; 98:162S.

177. Venables K: Epidemiology and the prevention of occupational asthma. *Br J Ind Med* 1987; 44:73.

178. American Thoracic Society: Evaluation of impairment (disability secondary to respiratory disease). *Am Rev Respir Dis* 1982; 126:945.

179. American Thoracic Society: Evaluation of impairment and disability. *Am Rev Respir Dis* 1986; 133:1205.

180. Chan-Yeung M: Evaluation of impairment/disability in patients with occupational asthma. *Am Rev Respir Dis* 1987; 135:950.

Chapter 39

THERAPY OF OCCUPATIONALLY INDUCED COPD

W.K.C. MORGAN

There is little doubt that certain occupational and environmental exposures lead to the development of chronic airflow limitation; however, there is little agreement as to the prevalence of occupationally induced airway obstruction, the pathophysiologic mechanisms involved, or how often it leads to significant impairment and disability. There exists an overly facile urge to lump all airway obstruction that occurs in workers under the all-embracing term, chronic obstructive pulmonary disease (COPD),[1] thereby implying that no matter the type of exposure, the pathophysiology is similar, the symptoms the same, the effects permanent, and a recommended treatment of bronchodilators and corticosteroids. Although occupational asthma is included by some as part of occupational COPD, most authorities are eclectic enough to treat the former as a separate entity.

Factors Influencing the Effects of Inhaled Agents[2]

The effects on the respiratory system of particles, gases, vapors, and fumes depend on the physical and chemical characteristics of the inhaled material and also on various host factors.

Dealing first with the physical factors, the effects depend on the site of deposition or the point of contact of the inhaled agent. In this context, it is helpful to divide the respiratory tract into three regions: (1) the nose and upper respiratory tract as far as the larynx; (2) the larynx, trachea, and conducting airways as far down as the terminal bronchioles; and (3) the lung parenchyma or gas-exchanging surface of the lung.

During quiet breathing, which under normal circumstances is entirely nasal, the nose filters out the majority of particles larger than 3 μm and virtually all particles > 6 μm. Irritant gases, when inhaled, likewise first come in contact with the nose and those that are soluble dissolve in the respiratory mucus and secretions present in the nose and nasopharynx. Only a small volume of such soluble gases reaches the larynx and beyond unless exposure has been heavy.

During normal breathing the majority of particles will be deposited in the trachea and conducting airways. These for the most part are between 4 and 10 μm and are deposited mainly as a result of inertial impaction. A significant number of particles below 5 μm will settle in the alveoli as a result of sedimentation. The likelihood of gravitational settling is determined by Stokes' law. Those particles most likely to undergo deposition by sedimentation are between 1 and 3 μm in size. Many smaller particles below 1 μm reach the alveoli and are deposited owing to brownian motion (diffusion); however, a fair number of such small particles are breathed back out into the atmosphere.

Changes in respiratory rate, in flow rates in the airways, tidal volume, body position, and when the subject starts to mouth breathe can greatly influence the site, number, and proportion of particles deposited and can similarly influence the point of contact in the respiratory tract of inhaled gases and vapors.

Certain other physical characteristics may be important, such as the shape and penetrability of the inhaled agent. These are of major importance when it comes to the deposition of mineral fibers and in particular, asbestos. In this context, the length of the fiber greatly influences the likelihood of interception. The latter is also influenced by whether the fiber is serpentine or needle shaped. The solubility of irritant gases is of great importance and those that are readily soluble, such as chlorine and ammonia, produce instant cough and upper airway irritation with the result that the affected subject removes himself from contact as quickly as possible. Thus, the main effects of soluble gases are exerted on the nose, nasopharynx, larynx, trachea, and larger bronchi. Less soluble gases, such as the oxides of nitrogen, are less irritant and can penetrate more deeply into the lungs without causing much in the way of immediate response such as coughing. As such, should they reach the smaller airways and alveoli, they induce bronchiolitis and pulmonary edema.

The chemical properties of inhaled particles or gas, and in this regard, the acidity and alkalinity of the agent, are likewise important. The propensity of the inhaled agent to combine with substances in the lung (e.g., carbon monoxide, manganese, hydrogen cyanide, etc.) may lead to systemic effects. Fibrogenicity also varies and depends partly on the chemical and physical structure of the inhaled agent. Thus, whereas coal dust leads to only limited fibrosis, inhaled asbestos is markedly fibrogenic.

Finally, genetic, environmental, and acquired host factors also influence the deposition site and effects of inhaled substances. The clearing mechanisms of the lungs and airways vary significantly among subjects of the same age, height, and sex. Some individuals can clear particles from the airways rapidly yet others are slow clearers. This ability appears to be inherited and does not change over time. Narcotics, cold, alcohol, viral infections, and the like influence clearance as, more importantly, does cigarette smoking. Airways geometry likewise influences the side of deposition and the presence of the allergic diathesis (atopy) may uncommonly be important.

Pathophysiologic Responses of the Respiratory Tract to Particles, Gases, Vapors, and Fumes[2]

The site of deposition varies according to the factors described above. It is useful to consider the type of response in the three main regions of the respiratory tract, that is, the nose and nasopharynx, the trachea and conducting airways, and the lung parenchyma. The deposition of particles, gases, and vapors in the nasopharynx is not associated with the development of COPD and so no further mention will be made of this region. Airway responses characterized by reversible airflow limitation will likewise be omitted, and attention will be directed at the type of irreversible airway obstruction that is somewhat imprecisely referred to as COPD or chronic airflow limitation (CAL). The obstruction that characterizes CAL may be produced by chronic bronchitis, emphysema of the centrilobular (centriacinar) and panlobular (panacinar) types, and bronchiolitis.

CHRONIC BRONCHITIS

Although formerly chronic bronchitis and emphysema were lumped together as part of the effects of cigarette smoking, it now is clear that they are separate responses to a variety of agents. Both, for example, are produced by cigarette smoking, although the relative frequency of the two conditions in smokers differs significantly. Some degree of chronic bronchitis is invariably seen in moderate or heavy smokers of more than 5 years' duration. The same is not true for emphysema, which affects only about 14 to 15 percent of smokers.[3]

The conducting airways of the lung, when insulted by various more or less irritating agents, respond in a nonspecific manner. Such insults include inert dusts, cigarette smoke, various fumes, and irritant gases. No matter the agent, provided the dose is limited and not immediately overwhelming, the response is the same, namely, an increase in the secretion of mucus associated with some nonspecific bronchial hyperresponsiveness and a minor degree of airway obstruction that can only be detected in a minority. The latter predominantly affects the large airways but also produces some effect on the smaller airways.[4] Histologic examination of the mucosa of the large airways will show mucous gland hypertrophy while the smaller airways show an increased number of goblet cells. At least in cigarette smokers, the cessation of smoking is associated with a complete or almost complete reversion to normality of the histologic changes seen in the mucosa of chronic bronchitics. This is associated with a concomitant decline in cough and sputum production as well.

EMPHYSEMA

Emphysema is best defined as the disruption of the alveolar-capillary surface associated with an increase in the residual volume. The most common form of emphysema, the centrilobular (centriacinar) variety, occurs in about 13 to 15 percent of smokers and is preceded by small airways disease. Breathlessness occurs only when a large proportion of the small airways are narrowed. In persistent smokers, histologic examination of the small airways shows a bronchiolitis and narrowing of the lumina of the respiratory and terminal bronchioles. Nevertheless, it is clear that centrilobular emphysema, or at least the emphysema that tends to occur in the center of the lobule, can be present in the absence of small airways disease and may be seen in the lungs of nonsmokers, be they coal miners, tin workers with stannosis, or dwellers of cities that were formerly heavily polluted such as London, Pittsburgh, Manchester, and St. Louis.[5,6] The emphysema that is seen in such circumstances is located in the center of a macule similar to that seen in coal workers' pneumoconiosis. The macule seen in the lungs of subjects exposed to pollution is composed of soot rather than coal dust. The focal emphysema that characterizes coal workers' pneumoconiosis, stannosis, and the inhabitants of polluted cities is not accompanied by bronchiolitis unless the individual is or has been a smoker. Once emphysema is present, it is impossible for it to regress or improve, and the same is true for the hyperinflation and obstruction, which for the most part, are a consequence of the lung's loss of elastic recoil and the presence of small airways disease.

The second common type of emphysema is panlobular or panacinar emphysema. This type of emphysema is often found in the lungs of older persons who are not smokers. It also is seen when there is extensive scarring of the lungs such as occurs in conglomerate coal workers' pneumoconiosis (progressive massive fibrosis) and in chronic sarcoidosis and chronic fibrotic tuberculosis. It tends to be located subpleurally. It is also seen in certain subjects with chronic extrinsic allergic alveolitis (e.g., farmers' lung).

A less common cause of panlobular emphysema is α_1-antiprotease deficiency. Significant and disabling emphysema is more common in cigarette smoking persons with α_1-antiprotease deficiency than in nonsmokers and, in general, smokers develop the condition earlier than do nonsmokers. Indeed, some nonsmokers with α_1-antiprotease deficiency never develop emphysema. In subjects with α_1-antiprotease deficiency, bronchitis occurs less often and frequently appears later than the emphysema does. This tends to be true, whether those afflicted are smokers or not. Moreover, loss of elastic recoil often develops before there is evidence of significant airway obstruction.

Panlobular emphysema also is seen when there is bronchial and bronchiolar obliteration associated with obstruction. In general, its relationship to occupational exposures is poorly documented and by no means convincing. It has been suggested that the type of emphysema that occurs after acute cadmium exposure is panlobular, but this is by no means generally accepted.

BRONCHIOLITIS

Bronchiolitis is seen in a variety of occupationally related diseases and conditions, including the extrinsic allergic alveolitides, particularly farmers' lung, after exposure to irritant gases such as the oxides of nitrogen, sulfur dioxide, and chlorine, after the inhalation of cadmium fumes, and in persons who have been exposed to asbestos, particularly when there has been sufficient exposure to induce asbestosis. Bronchiolitis is also seen after prolonged exposure to a variety of silicates (e.g., talc, kaolin). In general, occupationally induced bronchiolitis does not lead to the development of disabling airway obstruction except in those who develop chronic farmers' lung and certain other extrinsic allergic alveolitides. It is also an uncommon sequel to the inhalation of nitrogen dioxide.

Management and Therapy of Occupationally Induced COPD

In the majority of instances, the treatment of occupationally induced COPD is initiated automatically. Thus, a repetitive ritual has evolved in the absence of proven efficacy, and for which there is little, if any, scientific basis. The presence of breathlessness, whatever the cause, invariably demands the exhibition of at least bronchodilators, including one or more β-adrenergic agonists, which are often prescribed both orally and by inhalation, ipratropium or similar agents by inhalation, mast cell stabilizers such as a cromoglycate and its derivatives, various theophylline and similar xanthine preparations, both oral and inhaled steroids, and often sundry mucolytics, not to mention intermittent positive pressure breathing and vigorous chest vibration administered either manually or mechanically. Success is variously measured by nonsignificant and often clinically undetectable increases in the forced expiratory volume in 1 s (FEV_1) or the forced expiratory flow between 25 and 75 percent of the vital capacity (FEF_{25-75}). The latter is an extraordinarily variable and nonspecific test of ventilatory capacity. Alternatively, diaphragmatic function and mucociliary clearance have been measured, often rather less than more accurately. It is claimed that theophylline and β-adrenergic agonists hasten mucociliary clearance and improve diaphragmatic strength and endurance. Most such minor pathophysiologic changes that have been demonstrated have not been accompanied by a significant or sustained sense of well-being or a reduction of breathlessness. Their effects could equally well be attributed to suggestion or a placebo effect.

In any consideration of the treatment of COPD, whether occupationally related or not, it is essential to decide on the pathophysiology of the airway obstruction before embarking on a therapeutic regimen. This requires an understanding of the morphologic and cellular basis of airflow limitation. One must ask the question whether CAL is a consequence of bronchitis, emphysema, and if the latter, what type of emphysema, or of bronchiolitis or another type of pathophysiologic effect of the inhaled agent. It is essential to know the mechanisms that produce the airway obstruction that is present.[5]

MANAGEMENT OF BRONCHITIS

Bronchitis in itself is characterized by the presence of cough, sputum, and some minor airway obstruction that predominantly affects the large airways and does not lead to cor pulmonale. Bronchial hyperresponsiveness also may occur. Individuals with bronchitis, especially if concomitant small airways disease and emphysema are present, often show more severe and prolonged morbidity after an upper respiratory tract infection such as influenza. Following such infections the bronchitic subject's sputum often becomes purulent and contains a number of bacteria. Under such circumstances, *Haemophilus influenzae* and *Streptococcus pneumoniae* frequently are isolated from the sputum. Provided the subject is producing mucoid sputum and has no such infection, the sputum tends to contain fewer organisms. Nevertheless, during the acute episode, organisms other than *H. influenzae* and *S. pneumoniae* may frequently be isolated and these include *Escherichia coli*, *Serratia marcescens*, *B proteus*, *Staphylcoccus aureus*, *Pseudomonas*, and various anaerobes.

Bronchitis unaccompanied by emphysema seldom, if ever, causes significant breathlessness and the standard tests of ventilatory capacity seldom fall outside the normal range. Nonetheless, when a group of nonsmoking bronchitics is compared to a comparable reference group without bronchitis, those with bronchitis often have a slightly lower FEV_1 and an increased residual volume along with some impairment of forced expiratory flows at high lung volumes. As such, no one has demonstrated conclusively that any form of treatment in such subjects is of benefit.

The most effective way of eliminating or ameliorating irritant-induced bronchitis is to curtail or limit exposure to the offending dust, gas, or fume. This can be effected by controlling exposure to the agent responsible through industrial hygiene measures or by ensuring that the subject regularly wears respiratory protection. A second, but less practical method, is to substitute a less irritant agent; however, this is frequently not feasible with the substitute often being more expensive or less effective. In general, unless there is permanent damage, the mucous gland hypertrophy and goblet cell hyperplasia that characterize bronchitis slowly regress over 6 to 9 months. The persistence of cough and sputum, especially if the latter is purulent, suggests permanent anatomic damage such as is seen in heavy cigarette smokers, but not in those exposed to dust alone. Under such circumstances, the epithelium loses its cilia and is often replaced by pseudosquamous or overtly squamous epithelium as is seen in bronchiectasis and in heavy smokers.

Should a nonsmoking, heavily dust-exposed worker complain of cough and sputum, and should he also have evidence of sufficient airway obstruction to cause breathlessness, then it can be assured that the industrial bronchitis is not responsible for the dyspnea. Some other cause such as bronchiectasis, asthma, or bronchiolitis should be sought. It is rare, indeed, for a nonsmoker with industrial bronchitis to request treatment for his cough and sputum, but should this be the case it is probably worthwhile providing him with an ipratropium inhaler and suggesting he take two puffs two to three times a day. An attempt should also be made to lessen dust exposure either through better dust control or the wearing of respiratory protection such as masks.

MANAGEMENT OF EMPHYSEMA

By definition, the term emphysema indicates alveolar-capillary destruction. Such tissue loss is permanent, and a major therapeutic goal is to prevent further loss of the gas-exchanging surface and to avert or limit further small airways disease and their associated decline in the FEV_1.

In subjects who have centrilobular emphysema and extensive progressive small airways disease with a bronchiolitis of the respiratory and terminal bronchioles, the cessation of smoking is of paramount importance. Within a few months of stopping smoking, the FEV_1 of the affected subject, having previously been declining at an excess rate, levels off so that the annual decrement reverts to that of a nonsmoking person of the same age, height, and sex.[3] The decline is that due to aging alone. Because the mild focal dust emphysema that occurs in nonsmoking coal miners, tin workers, and former

nonsmoking dwellers in heavily polluted cities, is not associated with bronchiolitis and progressive small airways disease,[6,7] and, furthermore, because such subjects have a virtually normal ventilatory capacity and FEV_1, no specific treatment is required. A dust-exposed worker who develops sufficient airway obstruction to cause symptoms is virtually always a smoker. If the individual has severe enough airways obstruction to cause symptoms, then the administration of bronchodilators, systemic and inhaled steroids, along with xanthine derivatives constitute the usual therapeutic regimen. Although salbutamol and ipratropium by inhalation often alleviate symptoms such as cough and early morning breathlessness, and in addition, produce a temporary improvement in ventilatory capacity, there is no evidence that they permanently improve the ventilatory capacity or lessen the rate of decline of the FEV_1.[8] There is little doubt, however, that many subjects feel better after the use of inhaled β-adrenergic agonists and ipratropium.

Should the subject still be smoking, it could be argued that the administration of inhaled corticosteroids is worth trying. It has been suggested that this form of therapy would in theory limit the inflammatory response in the respiratory and terminal bronchioles thereby slowing down and limiting the development of further small airways disease. There can, however, be no justification for inhaled steroids in afflicted workers who have given up smoking because smoking cessation leads to a reversion to the normal rate of decline of the FEV_1.[3] This always, of course, assumes that the person has truly given up smoking, and this is by no means always the case. As such, if there is any doubt a carboxyhemoglobin level should be obtained.

There is little, if any, justification for using xanthine derivatives as a means of improving diaphragmatic function and mucociliary clearance. Many of the same limitations apply to the use of oral corticosteroids, and these have been reported to lead to an increase in muscle weakness when used in respiratory failure associated with chronic airflow obstruction.

MANAGEMENT OF BRONCHIOLITIS

The type of bronchiolitis arising from irritant gases such as the oxides of nitrogen, chlorine, and sulfur dioxide is usually an acute phenomenon that is often associated with pulmonary edema and concomitant bronchopneumonia. Silo-fillers' disease is the most common occupational cause of bronchiolitis and is due to the inadvertent inhalation of certain oxides of nitrogen (NO_2 and N_2O_4).

In a significant exposure the subject usually notices a brown gas being emitted from the silage. This may precipitate coughing and some irritation of the eyes and nose at which time the person promptly leaves the silo. Even though the subject has left the silo, this does not guarantee that pulmonary edema will not develop within the next 2 to 6 hours. This manifests itself with the sudden onset of shortness of breath, cyanosis, and the classical features of noncardiogenic pulmonary edema. Such onset requires prompt treatment with oxygen, antibiotics, and sometimes mechanical ventilation. Should the patient recover, in about 10 days more than 50 percent of subjects will develop fever and have further episodes of severe shortness of breath; the chest radiograph will show the presence of multiple small nodules throughout both lungs; a finding is pathognomic of bronchiolitis obliterans.

Both the bronchioles and alveoli undergo injury at the time the gases are inhaled; however, the response on the alveoli to the insult occurs more rapidly and the alveolar-capillary membrane becomes hyperpermeable within a few hours. In contrast, the response, which affects the bronchioles, evolves more gradually and presumably, there is a delay in the appearance of the bronchiolitis as collagen and elastin are laid down in the lumina of the bronchioles. Only if a large number of lumina are occluded, will the symptoms of shortness of breath and fever appear.

It has been suggested that the prompt administration of corticosteroids within hours of exposure may avert the development of bronchiolitis obliterans. This is an assumption, and no clinical trial has been carried out to confirm this hypothesis nor is such a trial likely to take place. If it is decided to use corticosteroids—and there are enough anecdotal reports to suggest that they should be tried—then an oral dose of 40 mg prednisone daily for 1 week with the dose gradually decreasing to 20 mg daily over the second week is probably sufficient. If the subject cannot take the corticosteroids by mouth, an equivalent intravenous dose should be given. Greater doses of corticosteroids increase the risk of pneumonia and are likely to lead to other side effects.

Although some subjects die from respiratory failure after the development of bronchiolitis obliterans, those who recover are often left with respiratory impairment. This is obstructive in some, but in others the impairment has been in gas transfer often associated with some restriction.

The effects of the inhalation of other irritant gases such as sulfur dioxide and chlorine should be treated in the same fashion as those of nitrogen dioxide. Bronchiolitis obliterans, however, is a much less common sequel following exposure to other gases than it is in silo-fillers' disease and the other occupations, for example, welding in which the oxides of nitrogen may be inhaled.

Summary

There is little specific about occupationally induced COPD other than the fact that it seldom, if ever, produces disabling impairment. When severe COPD is found in dust-exposed subjects, they are virtually always smokers or have complicated pneumoconiosis. The airway obstruction of complicated coal workers' pneumoconiosis and silicosis is often accompanied by panlobular emphysema. Although symptomatic treatment with bronchodilators is often used, no measurable improvement has been documented. This fact should not be taken as an indication that dust exposure is not important. Because many dusts will induce specific pneumoconioses leading to severe impairment and occasionally death, the best and most effective approach is to reduce exposure to dust, fumes, vapors, and irritant gases to the lowest level that is feasible.

References

1. Burge PS: Occupation and chronic obstructive pulmonary disease (COPD). *Eur Respir J* 1994; 7:1032.
2. Morgan WKC: The deposition and clearance of dust from the lungs, in Morgan WKC, Seaton, A (eds): *Occupational Lung Diseases*, 3d ed. Philadelphia, WB Saunders, 1995: 111–126.
3. Fletcher CM, Peto R, Tinker C, Speizer F: *The Natural History of Chronic Bronchitis*. Oxford, Oxford University Press, 1976.
4. Hankinson JL, Reger RB, Morgan WKC: Maximal expiratory flows in coal miners. *Am Rev Respir Dis* 1977; 116:175.
5. Decramer M, Lacquer LM, Fagard R, Rogiers P: Corticosteroids contribute to muscle weakness in chronic respiratory failure. *Am Rev Respir Dis* 1994; 150:11.
6. Gough J: The pathogenesis of emphysema, in Liebow A, Smith DF (eds): *The Lung*. Baltimore, Williams and Wilkins, 1968:109.
7. Morgan WKC: Bronchitis, airways obstruction and occupation, in Parkes WR (ed): *Occupational Lung Disorders*. London, Butterworth Heinemann, 1994:
8. Anthonisen NR, Connett JE, Kiley JP, et al: Effects of smoking intervention and the use of an inhaled anticholinergic bronchodilator on the rate of decline of FEV_1. *JAMA* 1994; 272:1497.

Chapter 40

TOXIC INJURY OF THE LUNG PARENCHYMA

WILLIAM J. MARTIN II AND STANLEY REHM

Inhalation injury to the lung parenchyma results from exposure to a wide variety of gases, vapors, fumes, and particulate material.[1] This chapter will focus on those characteristics of gaseous inhalants that are associated with injury to the lower respiratory tract, the underlying mechanisms of injury, and a general overview of current and future therapeutic approaches.

Acute injury to the lung parenchyma typically results in noncardiac pulmonary edema. The integrity of the alveolar-capillary barrier is maintained by both the alveolar epithelium (type I and type II alveolar epithelial cells) and the pulmonary capillary endothelium (Table 40-1), with the former contributing the majority of the barrier function.[2] Noxious gases that successfully reach the alveoli may injure these cellular components or alter a critical constituent of alveolar lining material, such as surfactant. The end result of either process is identical; loss of integrity of the alveolar-capillary barrier results in edema that impairs gas exchange and may lead to progressive respiratory distress and death.

Factors Related to Pulmonary Parenchymal Injury

Three important determinants of whether the inhaled material will injure the lower respiratory tract and alveolar structures are the size of particulates, solubility of gas, and biologic reactivity (Table 40-2). The role of particulate material in facilitating lung parenchymal injury associated with toxic gases often is neglected. Inhaled particles characteristically generate fibrotic lung diseases, but when particles are interspersed with toxic gases, as in the smoke generated by cigarettes or other fires, the particles may serve as a vehicle for transporting adsorbed gases and other noxious material to the alveolar level.

The site of deposition is determined, at least in part, by the size of the particle.[3] For example, particles of 10- to 15-μm diameter typically will be deposited in the oronasal and upper airway mucosa; as particle size diminishes there is a pattern of increasing deposition at more distal sites, so that particles in the 5- to 10-μm range may produce injury to the airways of the lower respiratory tract. In aerodynamic terms, particles between 2 and 5 μm in diameter are suited ideally for deposition in the alveoli. By contrast, when particles are smaller than 1 μm, their movement is akin to Brownian motion, and although inhaled particles may reach the alveoli, they are likely to be exhaled again without deposition in the lung.

For gases inhaled in the absence of admixed particulate material, the key determinant of the site of injury is the water solubility of the gas (Table 40-3). To reach alveolar tissue, inhaled gases must traverse 20 generations of bifurcating airways; turbulence in these airways ensures extensive contact with mucosal surfaces, which absorb water-soluble components of the inspired gases. Gases that are highly water solu-

Table 40-1   Cellular Sites of Pulmonary Parenchymal Injury

Capillary endothelial cells
Type I alveolar epithelial cells
Type II alveolar epithelial cells

TABLE 40-2   Toxic Inhalation and Parenchymal Injury

Factors that determine pulmonary parenchymal injury
   Properties of gas or inhaled material
      size of particulates
      solubility
      reactivity

ble, such as ammonia, hydrochloric acid, and sulfur dioxide, are filtered effectively out in the tracheobronchial tree; this may result in substantial injury to the airways, but the alveolar tissue typically is spared. Gases of intermediate solubility, such as chlorine, can cause damage along the entire respiratory tract from the glottis to the alveolus. Those gases that have low water solubility, such as ozone, phosgene, and the oxides of nitrogen (NO$_x$), are the most likely to generate substantial injury to the alveolar-capillary barrier, resulting in life-threatening pulmonary edema.

Once the gas reaches the alveolar level, the nature and degree of acute injury is determined by the reactivity of the gas. Those that are biologically nonreactive, such as methane, cause asphyxia by displacement of ambient oxygen, but do not result in lung parenchymal injury. These inert gases must be present in high concentrations for their dilutive effect on inhaled oxygen to be clinically meaningful; in contrast, the chemical asphyxiants cyanide and carbon monoxide interfere with oxygen transport within cells, and may result in significant tissue asphyxia at minute concentrations measured as parts per million. As with the inert gases, however, the alveolar tissue itself is not typically injured, so that pulmonary edema is not encountered.

Sometimes the nature of the inhaled substance is clearly documented, as occurs with industrial accidents involving ammonia or chlorine; in these cases, the site and type of injury can reasonably be predicted. On the other hand, inhalation occurring in the setting of combustion of plastics and organic materials typically involves a mixture of toxic gases, with mixed patterns of injury involving multiple areas of the respiratory tract. Nonetheless, efforts at identifying and characterizing the material inhaled can provide important clinical information for guiding therapeutic interven-

tions, as well as prognostic implications regarding the clinical course and possible sequelae of the injury.

Spectrum of Toxic Inhalation Injury

Injury to the lower respiratory tract may occur from a wide variety of different exposures. Occupational exposures represent the greatest hazard for significant injury. For example, accidental chlorine gas exposure can occur among pulp-mill workers because chlorine is an important component of the bleaching process in the manufacture of paper.[4] Similarly, a dairy farmer may be exposed to life-threatening amounts of nitrogen dioxide if he or she enters a silo where the heavy reddish-brown gas has accumulated just above the silage.[5,6] During oxyacetylene welding, exposure to cadmium fumes can result in noncardiac pulmonary edema and the acute respiratory distress syndrome (ARDS).[7] Obviously, both industry and workers share a desire to minimize risk of exposure to toxic gases in the workplace. However, the risk of occupational exposure remains high, and a substantial number of toxic gas inhalations occur every year. The memory of the events in Bhopal, India, serves to underscore the importance of toxic inhalation as a risk both to workers and to residents of neighboring communities.

Smoke inhalation is probably the most common form of toxic inhalation.[8] Again, the nature of the combustible material dictates the site of injury. Heat alone may damage the upper airways; this invariably is accompanied by evidence for direct thermal injury to the face and oral mucosa. Water-soluble acids and aldehydes are common by-products of fires and contribute substantially to upper airway injury and laryngeal edema. Extensive injury to the upper airways may, in fact, diminish exposure of the lower respiratory tract to the noxious by-products of combustion. Common by-products found in severe smoke inhalation may include asphyxiants such as cyanide and carbon monoxide as well as directly injurious agents such as ammonia and phosgene. Recognition of the type of material burned and its potential combustive products may predict whether inhalation injury will be predominantly in the upper or lower airways.

Finally, a common form of toxic inhalation is neither an accidental nor an occupational exposure; rather, it is a consequence of a therapeutic intervention. Supplemental oxygen for patients who are developing progressive hypoxemia is an appropriate and expected therapeutic intervention. However, when oxygen concentrations exceed the protective threshold afforded by antioxidant defense mechanisms of the lung, progressive injury can occur to capillary endothelial and to alveolar epithelial cells.[9] Oxygen toxicity is a major contributing factor to the high mortality associated with ARDS.

Although the spectrum of toxic inhalation is wide, the mechanisms underlying these injuries are remarkably similar. Of the gases that result in lung injury, the best studied is clearly oxygen; some insights gained from this predictable exposure can be extrapolated to other types of toxic inhalations that have not been as well studied. An improved understanding of possible underlying mechanisms may suggest common therapeutic strategies that could mitigate the

TABLE 40-3   Examples of Gas Solubility and Site of Injury to Respiratory Tract

H$_2$O Solubility	Gas	Site of Injury
High	NH$_3$	Upper
	HCl	
	SO$_2$	
Intermediate	Cl$_2$	Upper and lower
Low	O$_3$	Lower
	Phosgene (COCl$_2$)	
	Nitrogen oxides (NO$_x$)	

injurious effects of various inhalants on the alveolar capillary unit.

Mechanisms of Injury at the Alveolar Level

The simplicity of the alveolar capillary unit is a wonder. The lungs contain more than 300 million alveoli where gas exchange occurs by diffusion across type I alveolar epithelial cells and capillary endothelial cells, which share a common basement membrane. The type II alveolar epithelial cell is thought to serve as progenitor of the type I cell, which is an end-mitotic cell with a large surface area covering most of the alveolar space.[10] When the type I cell is injured or dies, the type II cell undergoes division; one daughter cell differentiates into a type I cell, while the other daughter cell retains its type II cell characteristics. In addition to its parenting function, the type II cell is as critical to the functional integrity of the alveolar capillary unit as it is the major producer of pulmonary surfactant. Surfactant is a mixture of proteins and unsaturated phospholipids, which reduces surface tension within the alveoli. If surfactant is decreased or its function is impaired, alveolar collapse rapidly ensues and gas exchange is impaired. The absence of functional pulmonary surfactant in the lungs is the recognized cause for the respiratory distress syndrome of premature infants; in adults, functional inactivity of surfactant in subjects with ARDS is just now receiving increasing attention. Thus, toxic inhalations, which result in damage to the alveolar capillary unit, may do so by injuring either key cellular constituents, or inactivating the alveolar-lining surfactant material.

It is reasonable to assume that inhalation of toxic or noxious material will result in direct injury to cells lining the respiratory tract. Certainly, highly reactive gases or acid aerosols will result in immediate disruption of cell membrane and loss of integrity of the cell. However, many injuries that occur at the alveolar level are sublethal, and gas exchange can continue to occur, albeit impaired. Then, 48 to 72 h later, evidence for a further deterioration in gas exchange or worsening of pulmonary edema may occur. This results from a delayed cytotoxic effect caused by the inhaled substance or may reflect a second mechanism of injury. Increasing evidence suggests that secondary inflammatory responses contribute to clinical deterioration in many types of toxic inhalations. Thus, acute injury at the alveolar level frequently is characterized by both direct and indirect mechanisms of injury (Table 40-4).

TABLE 40-4   Mechanisms of Injury to Alveolar-Capillary Barrier

Direct toxic effect
  Parent compound or chemical
  Metabolite or by-product
Indirect toxic effect
  Inflammatory mediators
  Inflammatory cells

DIRECT INJURY

The prototype for direct injury to alveolar epithelium and capillary endothelium is oxidant-mediated injury. The lung is especially vulnerable to oxidant injury because, of all internal organs, the lung receives the highest concentration of oxygen, and it has a large surface area vulnerable to membrane attack. The site of injury mediated by oxygen-derived radicals, however, may not be easily predictable from the type of exposure. For example, inhalation of high concentrations of oxygen results in an initial injury not to the alveolar epithelial cells, but predominantly to the capillary endothelium.[11,12] Conversely, ingestion of the herbicide paraquat also results in oxidant injury to the lung; however, this occurs following gastrointestinal absorption into the bloodstream and concentration within the type I and type II cells, which results in an irreversible injury and sloughing of the alveolar epithelium.[13] Thus, paraquat, which is bloodborne, results in injury to the alveolar epithelium, while oxygen, which is airborne, results in injury to the capillary endothelium. The consequence, however, is the same with disruption of the integrity of the alveolar capillary unit and the development of noncardiac pulmonary edema.

A schema for generation of O_2-derived radicals is shown in Fig. 40-1. Oxygen, as a ubiquitous electron acceptor, accepts electrons either singly or in pairs. The cytochrome oxidase system of the mitochondria ensures that divalent electron transfers occur, avoiding the risk of radical generation from single electron transfers. Nonetheless, single electron transfers occur frequently, and cells living in aerobic environments have evolved antioxidant defense mechanisms, including superoxide dismutase, catalase, and the glutathione peroxidase/reductase system. When these antioxidant defenses are overwhelmed, single electron transfers may be propagated and, in the presence of suitable catalysts such as iron, result in the formation of highly toxic products like the hydroxyl radical (•OH). These cascades are well described elsewhere and are beyond the scope of this chapter.

Many reactive gases and combustion products result in oxygen radical generation. Phosgene, which is used in chemical warfare and in the synthesis of plastics and chemicals, causes noncardiac pulmonary edema; it is directly toxic to cells, but also is capable of generating O_2-derived radicals by facilitating single electron transfers.[14] The therapeutic challenge in dealing with hypoxemia in a phosgene-injured subject may be similar to the difficulties encountered in subjects with paraquat toxicity.[15] The toxic substance results in oxidant injury to the alveolar capillary unit, impairing gas exchange and inducing hypoxemia. Use of supplemental oxygen to correct the hypoxemia, however, may result in further oxidant injury and contribute to progressive respiratory deterioration. Thus, the initial skirmish line for survival often relates to the ability or inability to control a direct toxic injury to one of the key cellular constituents of the alveolar capillary unit.

Surfactant also is susceptible to injury. The functional properties of surfactant likely are related both to protein constituents (surfactant proteins A, B, C, and possibly D) and to unsaturated phospholipids. Pulmonary surfactant functions

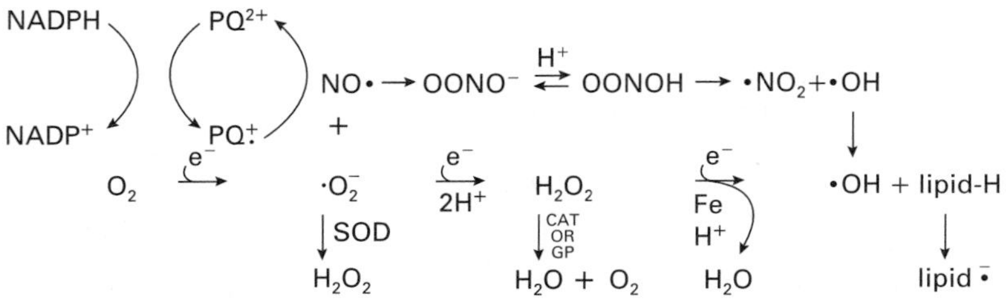

FIGURE 40-1 Mechanisms of O_2-derived radical generation. PQ = paraquat, example of toxin that facilitates single electron (e^-) transfers; SOD = superoxide dismutase; CAT = catalase; GP = glutathione peroxidase; Fe = iron; $\cdot O_2^-$ = superoxide; NO$\cdot$ = nitric oxide; OONO$^-$ = peroxynitrite; H_2O_2 = hydrogen peroxide; $\cdot$OH = hydroxyl radical; lipid$\cdot$ = lipid peroxide.

as a detergent to reduce the surface tension of the alveolar spaces, thereby permitting retained inflation of the alveoli during exhalation. Many factors are known to disrupt surfactant function and contribute to alveolar collapse.[16–18] Furthermore, surfactant synthesis and turnover are likely altered with exposure to toxic gases. New approaches to correction of functional surfactant deficiencies are being proposed, such as instillation of exogenous surfactant into the airways.[19]

INDIRECT INJURY

It is well recognized that an inflammation response in the lung may impair gas exchange and contribute to lung injury. Inflammation is a normal host response to substances entering the airways, which require neutralization or clearance from the lungs. Under normal circumstances, this inflammation response occurs on a continuing basis to maintain the alveolar structures free of invading microorganisms and particulate matter. However, if inhalation of noxious material is sufficient to induce a massive inflammation response, gas exchange may be impaired and cell injury can occur.

The alveolar macrophage is predominantly responsible for controlling the inflammation response within the alveoli. Alveolar epithelial cells and endothelial cells can release mediators of inflammation, but the macrophage is ultimately the conductor of this orchestrated response. The ability to recruit and activate polymorphonuclear leukocytes, lymphocytes, and monocyte-derived cells allows macrophages to coordinate a graduated and appropriate response to any perceived dangers or injuries within the alveoli. In cases of widespread injury or massive deposition of material in the alveoli, the inflammation response may become exaggerated, placing the alveolar-capillary unit at risk.

Polymorphonuclear leukocytes, including neutrophils and eosinophils, are potent mediators of injury. An important aspect of the armamentarium of these inflammatory cells is the ability to generate toxic O_2-derived species, hypohalite anions, and proteases.[20] Major basic protein released by eosinophils also can be directly cytotoxic. When activated within the confines of the alveolar spaces, these inflammatory cells may injure normal parenchymal cells as "innocent bystanders."

For example, oxygen toxicity is characterized by both direct and indirect mechanisms of injury. Oxygen is directly toxic to lung parenchymal cells,[21] and studies utilizing neutrophil depletion have demonstrated that the inflammation response also is a major factor contributing to oxygen toxicity.[22] A similar observation has been made with phosgene inhalation, demonstrating the importance of the neutrophil in the causation of noncardiac pulmonary edema.[23]

Thus, therapeutic strategies that attempt to control toxic injury to the lower respiratory tract must focus on reducing both the direct and indirect mechanisms of injury. Failure to do so may result in continued injury to the alveolar capillary unit with evolution of the injury into ARDS and the eventual death of the patient.

Gases that Produce Injury at the Alveolar Level

The toxic gases with the best-characterized patterns and mechanisms of alveolar injury include chlorine, the nitrogen oxides, and oxygen. Many of the clinical and mechanistic features of the gas-mediated injuries are shared by other toxic inhalations. Although less studied, some of the data and information to be described are equally applicable to these other gases.

CHLORINE

Chlorine is the prototype for gases of intermediate water solubility, which are capable of producing extensive damage to the entire respiratory tract.[4,24] Commonly encountered in swimming pools, water and sewage treatment facilities, and as a bleaching agent in the manufacture of paper, chlorine can cause widespread injury to epithelial cells[24]; with massive exposures, pulmonary edema may be evident within minutes. Although the reaction of chlorine with water results in the generation of hydrogen chloride, chlorine itself is many times more toxic than hydrogen chloride. One explanation for this enhanced toxicity is that the hydration of chlorine results in the generation of O_2-derived radicals, which exacerbate the injury.[25]

OXIDES OF NITROGEN

Ozone, phosgene, and the oxides of nitrogen are poorly soluble in water and thus bypass most of the airway epithelium to exert effects primarily at the alveolar level. However, in terms of clinically important lung injury, the most commonly encountered gases in this category of low water solubility are the oxides of nitrogen, consisting of nitrogen dioxide (NO_2), nitrogen tetroxide (N_2O_4), and nitric oxide (NO).

Nitrogen dioxide and nitrogen tetroxide are functionally interchangeable; the former is responsible for silo-filler's lung disease, and is encountered in a variety of industrial settings including welding, production of explosives, and combustion of fuels. Inhalation results in pulmonary edema secondary to diffuse capillary endothelial damage[26] with a contributing injury from secondary recruitment of inflammatory cells.[27] Following exposure, a typical triphasic response may occur. During the initial phase, cough, dyspnea, wheezing, chest pain, and fever may be present despite a normal chest x-ray.[28] In the second phase, chest radiographic evidence of noncardiac pulmonary edema results, and ARDS may be clinically evident. The final phase is an obliterative bronchiolitis, which occurs as a sequel to extensive damage of the terminal bronchioles.

In contrast to the other nitrogen oxides, NO also is an endogenous biologic product that can have both beneficial and deleterious effects. Seldom encountered in toxic gas exposures, NO is an endogenous mediator of cell function, including a role as the endothelium-derived relaxing factor that induces smooth muscle relaxation.[29] In the cellular environment, NO is enzymatically generated by nitric oxide synthase (NOS) in both constitutive and inducible forms. For this reaction, nitrogen is derived from arginine, the oxygen from molecular oxygen, and a free electron is generated from nicotine adenine dinucleotide phosphate (NADPH). Nitric oxide can be a physiologic mediator or signal, or in the case of alveolar macrophages,[30] can be used to mediate toxicity. Uncontrolled generation of nitric oxide has been implicated in systemic vasodilatation associated with sepsis.[31] Recent studies also suggest that NO is a critical mediator of lung injury following exposure to paraquat. Although paraquat is a potent generator of toxic O_2-derived radicals, injury to the lung is substantially reduced when NOS is inhibited,[32] suggesting that NO is the mediator of the lung injury. Nitric oxide is being considered as a therapeutic agent for pulmonary disorders such as pulmonary hypertension and ARDS. However, it is clearly a two-edged sword. Further studies will likely examine the threshold of toxicity of the lung parenchyma to NO to determine its potential safety as a novel therapeutic agent.

OXYGEN

The dangers of excessive oxygen were recognized virtually from the time of its discovery. Joseph Priestly, the codiscoverer of oxygen, prophetically stated that "the air which nature has provided for us is as good as we deserve," while across the English Channel, Lavoisier also warned against the use of high concentrations of oxygen, which might "burn the candle of life too quickly."

Oxygen toxicity is well recognized clinically.[9] From a practical standpoint the use of oxygen in concentrations of 50 percent or less in mechanically ventilated patients is thought to be safe for almost indefinite periods. By contrast, when oxygen concentrations exceed 60 percent, the risk of toxicity increases, and every effort must be made to reduce the concentration to a safer level. The first site of histopathologic

injury is the capillary endothelium.[11,12] Of interest, capillary endothelial cells in vitro appear to have a threshold for toxicity at approximately 60 percent O_2,[33] the same range observed for clinical evidence of toxicity. The presumed mechanism is that oxygen facilitates the generation of single-electron transfers (Fig. 40-1) to a degree that overwhelms endogenous antioxidant defense mechanisms. Although the type I and type II alveolar epithelial cells are also susceptible to oxygen toxicity, it appears that the capillary endothelial cells may be the weakest component of the alveolar-capillary barrier. Additionally, oxygen appears to interfere with surfactant function.[34] Together with the loss of the alveolar-capillary barrier and outpouring of serum into the alveoli, surfactant dysfunction is likely an important contributor to the clinical presentation of oxygen toxicity.

Therapeutic Approaches

Following a significant toxic inhalation, direct injury to the lung parenchymal cells and surfactant is almost instantaneous; therapeutic interventions are therefore focused primarily on replacing the injured surfactant and limiting the extent of the indirect injuries mediated by inflammatory cells.

As noted earlier, most injuries to the lung parenchyma are generated by oxygen-derived radicals. Unfortunately there is at present little available for treatment to augment the antioxidant defense mechanisms of the lower respiratory tract. Recent studies in experimental animal models have shown that liposome-encapsulated antioxidant enzymes may afford some protection,[35] and aerosolization of other agents, such as glutathione-containing compounds, may prove efficacious in smoke inhalation injuries where byproducts such as acrolein are likely to be present. To date, however, such interventions have not been used to any significant degree in humans.

For those situations in which toxic gases injure alveolar surfactant, replacement with human or artificial surfactant soon may become feasible. Recently, phosgene toxicity to the lung has been substantially reduced by the use of exogenous surfactant[36]; therapeutic trials are currently under way to assess the feasibility of such replacement in patients with ARDS, including that caused by toxic gases.

The most widely available pharmacologic intervention for controlling indirect injuries mediated by inflammatory cells is the use of corticosteroids. It is possible that corticosteroids significantly reduce the inflammation response associated with the second or third phase following acute inhalation injury, but although corticosteroids have been associated anecdotally with recovery from inhalation injury, no prospective studies have yet validated their role.

In the face of such a limited therapeutic armamentarium, it is of critical importance to avoid exacerbating the lung injury by well-intentioned but deleterious administration of excessive oxygen. Most clinically significant toxic gas exposures require supplemental oxygen to overcome the attendant hypoxemia, but the concentration of oxygen required may be minimized if atelectasis is alleviated through the judicious use of mechanical ventilation or facemask-applied positive airway pressure. Efforts are currently under way to develop intravascular gas-exchange devices that can absorb carbon dioxide and release oxygen directly into the vasculature, allowing the lung to recover from oxidant-induced or other acute injury.

Even in cases of severe noncardiac pulmonary edema, improvement can be amazingly quick and complete. However, depending on the nature of the toxic inhalation, delayed sequelae such as pulmonary fibrosis or bronchiolitis obliterans may occur. Further studies examining the underlying mechanisms of lung injury and repair may provide better therapeutic approaches for the management of acute injury and the prevention of irreversible late sequelae.

References

1. Wald PH, Balmes JR: Respiratory effects of short-term, high-intensity toxic inhalations: Smoke, gases, and fumes. *Intensive Care Med* 1987; 2:260–278.

2. Wangensteen OD, Wittmers LE Jr, Johnson JA: Permeability of the mammalian blood-gas barrier and its components. *Am J Physiol* 1969; 214(4):719–727.

3. Lippmann M, Albert RE: The effect of particle size on the regional deposition of inhaled aerosols in the human respiratory tract. *Am Ind Hyg Assoc J* 1969; 30:257–275.

4. Kennedy SM, Enarson DA, Janssen RG, Chan-Yeung M: Lung health consequences of reported accidental chlorine gas exposures among pulpmill workers. *Am Rev Respir Dis* 1991; 143:74–79.

5. Grayson RR: Silage gas poisoning: nitrogen dioxide pneumonia, a new disease in agricultural workers. *Ann Intern Med* 1956; 45:398–408.

6. Moskowitz RL, Lyons JA, Cottle HR: Silofiller's disease. *Am J Med* 1964; 36:457–462.

7. Beton DC, Andrews GS, Davies HJ, et al.: Acute cadmium fume poisoning. *Br J Ind Med* 1966; 23:292–301.

8. Haponik EF: Clinical smoke inhalation injury: Pulmonary effects. *Occup Med* 1993; 8(3):431–468.

9. Jenkinson SG: Pulmonary oxygen toxicity. *Clin Chest Med* 1982; 3:109.

10. Adamson IYR, Bowden DH: The type 2 cell as progenitor of alveolar epithelial regeneration. *Lab Invest* 1974; 30(1):35–42.

11. Kistler GS, Caldwell PRB, Weibel ER: Development of fine structural damage to alveolar and capillary lining cells in oxygen poisoned rat lungs. *J Cell Biol* 1967; 32:605–628.

12. Crapo JD, Peters-Golden M, Marsh-Salin J, Shelburne JS: Pathologic changes in the lungs of oxygen-adapted rats: a morphometric analysis. *Lab Invest* 1978; 39:640.

13. Sykes BI, Purchase IFH, Smith LL: Pulmonary ultrastructure after oral and intravenous dosage of paraquat to rats. *J Pathol* 1977; 121:233–241.

14. Babad H, Zeiler AG: The chemistry of phosgene. *Chem Rev* 1973; 73:75–91.

15. Fisher KH, Clements JA, Wright RR: Enhancement of oxygen toxicity by the herbicide paraquat. *Am Rev Respir Dis* 1973; 107:246–252.

16. Tierney DF, Johnson RP: Altered surface tension of lung extracts and lung mechanics. *J Appl Physiol* 1965; 20:1253–1260.

17. Holm BA, Enhorning G, Notter RH: A mechanism by which plasma proteins inhibit surfactant function. *Chem Phys Lipids* 1988; 49:49–55.

18. Matalon S, Holm BA, Loewen G, et al.: Sublethal hyperoxic injury to alveolar epithelium and the pulmonary surfactant system. *Exp Lung Res* 1988; 14:1021–1033.

19. Holm BA: Surfactant replacement therapy. *Am Rev Respir Dis* 1993; 148:834–836.

20. Babior BM: Oxygen-dependent microbial killing by phagocytes (two parts). *N Engl J Med* 1978; 298:659–668; 721–725.

21. Martin WJ II, Gadek JE, Hunninghake GW, Crystal RG: Oxidant injury of lung parenchymal cells. *J Clin Invest* 1981; 68:1277–1288.

22. Shasby DM, VanBenthuysen KM, Tate RM, et al.: Granulocytes mediate acute edematous lung injury in rabbits and in isolated rabbit lungs perfused with phorbol myristate acetate: role of oxygen radicals. *Am Rev Respir Dis* 1982; 125:443–447.

23. Ghio AJ, Kennedy TP, Hatch GE, Tepper JS: Reduction of neutrophil influx diminishes lung injury and mortality following phosgene inhalation. *J Appl Physiol* 1991; 71(2):657–665.

24. Adelson L, Kaufman J: Fatal chlorine poisoning: report of two cases with clinicopathologic correlation. *Am J Clin Pathol* 1971; 56:430–442.

25. Charan NB, Lakshminarayan S, Meyers GC, Smith DD: Effects of accidental chlorine inhalation in pulmonary function. *West J Med* 1985; 143:333–336.

26. Guidotti TL: Toxic inhalation of nitrogen dioxide: morphologic and functional changes. *Exp Mol Pathol* 1980; 33:90–103.

27. DeNicola DB, Rebar AH, Henderson RF: Early indicators of lung damage: V. Biochemical and cytological response to NO_2 inhalation. *Toxicol Appl Pharmacol* 1981; 60:301–312.

28. Summer W, Haponik E: Inhalation of irritant gases. *Clin Chest Med* 1980; 2:273–387.

29. Palmer RMJ, Ferrige AG, Moncada S: Nitric oxide release accounts for the biological activity of endothelium-derived relaxing factor. *Nature* 1987; 327:524–526.

30. Hibbs JB, Vavrin Z, Taintor RR: L-arginine is required for expression of the activated macrophage effector mechanism causing selective metabolic inhibition in target cells. *J Immunol* 1987; 138:550–565.

31. Petros A, Bennett D, Vallance P: Effect of nitric oxide synthase inhibitors on hypotension inpatients with septic shock. *Lancet* 1991; 338:1557–1558.

32. Berisha HI, Hedayatollah P, Absood A, Said SI: Nitric oxide as a mediator of oxidant lung injury due to paraquat. *Proc Natl Acad Sci U S A* 1994; 91:7445–7449.

33. Martin WJ II, Kachel DL: Oxygen-mediated impairment of human pulmonary endothelial cell growth: evidence for a specific threshold of toxicity. *J Lab Clin Med* 1989; 113(4):413–421.

34. Matalon S, Holm B, Notter R: Modulation of pulmonary hyperoxic injury by administration of exogenous surfactant. *J Appl Physiol* 1987; 62:756–761.

35. Barnard ML, Baker RR, Matalon S: Mitigation of oxidant injury to lung microvasculature by intratracheal instillation of antioxidant enzymes. *Am J Physiol* 1993; 265(4 pt 1):L340–L345.

36. Currie WD, Pearlstein RD, Sanders RL, Frosolono MF: Attenuation of phosgene toxicity by surfactant replacement therapy. *Am J Respir Crit Care Med* 1994; 149:A160.

PART 2

PHARMACOLOGY OF CONDUCTING AIRWAYS

BETA-ADRENERGIC AGONISTS

Chapter 41

INTRODUCTION: BETA-ADRENERGIC RECEPTORS

JOHN W. JENNE

Introduction
Role and Subtypes of Beta-Adrenergic Receptors

Introduction

While asthma is increasingly recognized as an inflammatory disease and it is assumed that anti-inflammatory therapy will retard its progression, there is little question that residual bronchospasm, whatever its cause, also must be treated. A lifestyle limited by bronchospasm is a poor lifestyle.

For decades, β-adrenergic agonists have been central in the treatment of bronchospasm, and yet controversy continues around them today. Patients have been subjected to this controversy through the media, and physicians are left to answer questions without definitive answers from existing data. Is the slight increase in bronchial responsiveness while on β$_2$-adrenergic agonists really harmful or simply a minor concomitant of therapy, easily overridden by the bronchodilator? How much of the increased asthma mortality in heavy users of inhaled β-adrenergic agonists is cause and how much effect? Most unfortunately, there is controversy regarding the wisdom of using the new long-acting β-adrenergic agonists at a time when these new drugs are able to stabilize the airways at higher levels throughout the day and night.

In this section (Chaps. 41 to 48), the following topics are outlined: receptor-drug interactions, mechanisms of action and subsensitivity, the evolution of β-adrenergic agonists, the pharmacokinetics and dynamics of various treatment modes, actions and potential toxicities of the drugs, issues of the prevailing controversies, and a perspective combining two modalities, which is the middle ground at this time. Specific approaches to treatment situations are considered in later chapters.

Role and Subtypes of Beta-Adrenergic Receptors

In the airways, the proportion of β$_1$- and β$_2$-adrenoreceptor subtypes in any species depends upon the density of the adrenergic nervous supply for that species and the generation of bronchus. In the densely innervated cat trachea, β$_1$-adrenoreceptors predominate. In the guinea pig and dog trachea, β$_2$-adrenergic receptors predominate, particularly distally. In the guinea pig, below the carina, adrenergic receptors are entirely β$_2$; in the pig, airway receptors are β$_1$-adrenoreceptors.

Relaxation of isolated human bronchial smooth muscle is mediated by the β$_2$-adrenoreceptor subtype.[1,2] Thus, the β$_1$-selective agonist prenalterol has no bronchodilating action in vivo.[3] Beta-adrenergic agonists act both directly and indirectly in relaxing smooth muscle indirectly inhibiting acetylcholine release at prejunctional β$_2$-adrenergic receptors.[4] Physiologic concentrations of plasma epinephrine at 0.2 to 0.4 nM/L provide low-level, but probably important, relaxation of airways[5] and some inhibition of mast cell mediator discharge. Systemically administered β-adrenergic agonists are effective in a range of 5 to 100 nM, or 1 to 20 ng/mL of the current β$_2$-adrenergic compounds. Both systemic and inhaled β$_2$-adrenergic agonists inhibit the release of mediators into the blood after antigen challenge.[6]

Mast cell adrenoreceptors are β$_2$-adrenergic. In vitro, β$_2$-adrenergic agonists inhibit release of histamine and leukotrienes from passively sensitized human lung fragments and dispersed mast cells in the same concentrations

449

required to relax bronchial smooth muscle.[7,8] Mononuclear and polymorphonuclear leukocytes and eosinophils also have β_2-adrenergic receptors,[9,9a,10] and β_2-adrenergic agonists inhibit secretion of bronchoactive substances. Human alveolar macrophages have β_2-adrenergic receptors[11] but respond rather weakly to isoproterenol compared to forskolin. There may be long-term downregulation of β_2-adrenergic receptors on mononuclear leukocytes and lung membranes, as their numbers bear a reciprocal relationship to plasma catecholamines.[12] Human submucosal glands are predominantly β_2, and β_2-adrenergic agonists stimulate mucous secretion in vitro.[13]

Vasoconstriction in the lung is mediated by α-adrenergic receptors, and vasodilation by β-adrenergic receptors; these are exclusively β_2 in humans.[14,15] Animal studies show that topical application of β-adrenergic agonists enhances mucosal blood flow and yet reduces leakiness of the microvasculature caused by various mediators,[16] perhaps through relaxation of contractile elements in the postcapillary venules, thus restoring pore size.[17]

With the current usage of greater doses of β_2-adrenergic agonists by nebulization and occasionally parenterally, their cardiac ramifications are assuming new importance. In most species, cardiac β_2-selective receptors coexist with β_1-adrenergic receptors, but they are in the substantial minority. However, radioligand studies with highly specific β-adrenoreceptor antagonists show that human hearts have a higher proportion of β_2-adrenergic receptors than other mammalian species (from 20 to 60 percent of the total[18,19]; SA node > atrium > ventricle).[20] Right atrial β_1- and β_2-adrenoreceptors are primarily associated with heart rate rather than inotropicity; left atrial adrenoreceptors influence force, as do left ventricular β_1 and β_2 receptors. Variable responses of the left ventricle to β_2-adrenergic agonists can be explained in terms of both affinity and efficacy, now measurable with modern techniques.

Work with selective agonists and antagonists has established that other systemic effects—lipolysis, hypokalemia, hypomagnesemia, and tremor—are also β_2-adrenoreceptor mediated. Further work is establishing that tachyphylaxis develops in these and other responses.

Finally, a role for corticosteroids in maximizing β_2-adrenoreceptor responsiveness is being demonstrated in some systems, thus adding further rationale to its anti-inflammatory role in combination with β_2-adrenergic agonists in all but the mildest asthmatics. The interplay between inflammatory mediators and β_2-adrenergic receptor desensitization suspected from in vitro studies adds further rationale for their combined use.

References

1. Goldie RG, Paterson JW, Spina D, Wale JL: Classification of beta-receptors in human isolated bronchus. *Br J Pharmacol* 1984; 81:611.
2. Zaagsma J, Van Der Heijden PJCM, van der Schaar MWG, Blank CMC: Comparison of functional beta-adrenoceptor heterogeneity in central and peripheral airway smooth muscle of guinea pig and man. *J Recept Res* 1991; 3:89.
3. Lofdahl C-G, Svedmyr N: Effects of prenalterol in asthmatic patients. *Eur J Clin Pharmacol* 1982; 23:297.
4. Rhoden KJ, Meldrum LA, Barnes PJ: Inhibition of cholinergic neurotransmission in human airways by β-2 adrenoceptors. *J Appl Physiol* 1988; 65:700.
5. Barnes PJ, Fitzgerald GA, Dollery CT: Circadian variation in adrenergic responses in asthmatic subjects. *Clin Sci* 1982; 62:349.
6. Howarth PH, Durham SR, Lee TH, et al.: Influence of albuterol, cromolyn sodium and ipratropium bromide on the airway circulating mediator response to allergen bronchial provocation in asthma. *Am Rev Respir Dis* 1985; 132:986.
7. Skidmore IF: Beta-agonists as mast cell stabilizers, in Kay, AB (ed) *Asthma: Clinical Pharmacology and Therapeutic Progress.* Blackwell Scientific Publications, Oxford, London, Boston 1986:173.
8. Church MK, Hiroi J: Inhibition of IgE-dependent histamine release from human dispersed lung mast cells by anti-allergic drugs and salbutamol. *Br J Pharmacol* 1987; 90:421.
9. Davis C, Conolly ME, Greenacre JK: β adrenoceptors in human lung bronchus and lymphocytes. *Br J Clin Pharmacol* 1980; 10:425.
9a. Tatsou Y, Ukena D, Kroegel C, et al.: Beta$_2$-adrenergic receptors on eosinophils: Binding and functional studies. *Am Rev Respir Dis* 1990; 141:1446.
10. Munoz NM, Vita AJ, Neeley SP, et al.: Beta adrenergic modulation of formyl-methionine-phenylalanine-stimulated secretions of eosinophil peroxidase and leukotriene C_4. *J Pharmacol Exp Ther* 1994; 268:139.
11. Liggett SB: Identification and characterization of a homogeneous population of β_2-adrenergic receptors on human alveolar macrophages. *Am Rev Respir Dis* 1989; 139:552.
12. Liggett SB, Marker JC, Shah SD, et al.: Direct relationship between mononuclear leukocyte and lung β-adrenergic receptors and apparent reciprocal regulation of extravascular, but not intravascular α- and β-adrenergic receptors by the sympathochromaffin systems in humans. *J Clin Invest* 1988; 82:48.
13. Phipps RJ, Williams IP, Richardson PS, et al.: Sympathetic drugs stimulate the output of secretory glycoprotein from human bronchi in vitro. *Clin Sci* 1982; 63:23.
14. Carstairs JR, Nimmo AJ, Barnes PJ: Autoradiographic visualization of beta-adrenoceptor subtypes in human lung. *Am Rev Respir Dis* 1985; 132:541.
15. Godden DJ: Reflex and nervous control of the tracheobronchial circulation. *Eur J Clin Pharmacol* 1990; 3(suppl 12):602s.
16. Persson CGA, Erjefalt I, Andersson P: Leakage of macromolecules from guinea pig tracheobronchial microcirculation: Effects of allergen, leukotrienes, tachykinins and antihistamine drugs. *Acta Physiol Scand* 1986; 127:95.
17. Persson CGA: Plasma exudation in tracheobronchial and nasal airways: A mucosal defense mechanism becomes pathogenic in asthma and rhinitis. *Eur J Respir Dis* 1990; 3(suppl 12):652s.
18. Hedberg A, Minneman KP, Molinoff PB: Differential distribution of beta$_1$- and beta$_2$-adrenergic receptors in cat and guinea pig heart. *J Pharmacol Exp Ther* 1980; 213:503.
19. Hall JA, Kaumann AJ, Brown MJ: Selective beta$_1$-adrenoceptor blockade enhances positive inotropic responses to endogenous catecholamines mediated through beta$_2$-adrenoceptors in human atrial myocardium. *Circ Res* 1990; 66:1610.
20. Kaumann AJ: Is there a third heart beta-adrenoceptor? *Trends Pharmacol Sci* 1989; 10:316.

BETA₂-ADRENERGIC RECEPTOR-AGONIST INTERACTION

JOHN W. JENNE

The Receptor

An understanding of β-adrenergic receptors in some depth is necessary to understand developments in β₂-adrenergic drugs. Beta₂-adrenergic receptors activate the enzyme adenylyl cyclase with production of cyclic adenosine monophosphate (cAMP), which is generally thought to be responsible for the bulk of the activity of these drugs through protein phosphorylation by cAMP-dependent kinases. Figure 42-1 shows the components of this system. Adenylyl cyclase is in juxtaposition with a stimulatory (beta) and inhibitory receptor, each with their respective guanine nucleotide-binding proteins (G proteins). Receptors acting through G proteins have an alpha helix containing seven membrane-spanning domains. Figure 42-1 shows the extracellular terminus, the hydrophilic loops, the hydrophobic core in the lipid bilayer cell membrane, and the cytoplasm terminal carboxyl group.

Using site-directed mutagenesis, regions of the receptor have been identified that are crucial to ligand binding, G-protein coupling, and the development of agonist-induced subsensitivity. Much work has been done with hamster β₂-adrenergic receptor, which consists of 418 amino acids. The ligand-binding domain, or "pocket," lies 30 to 40 percent of the way into the bilayer (Fig. 42-2). At tissue pH, ligand amines are partially protonated, and the receptor binding site contains an acidic counter ion (Fig. 42-2). Substitution for Asp[113] in the third transmembrane domain greatly reduces the affinity of both agonist and antagonist. The catechol hydroxy groups of the agonist interact with the hydroxyl side chains of the serine residues at positions 204 and 207 of the fifth transmembrane domain, which is necessary for activation, and the aromatic ring undergoes hydrophobic reactions with the Phe[290] in the sixth domain.[1] As reviewed by Jasper and Insel,[2] other amino acids play important roles. Treatment of the receptor with sulfhydryl reducing agents activates it and is synergistic with agonists, lending support to the idea that activation of the receptor involves sulfhydryl bond rearrangement (see below).

The human receptor has been cloned and studied.[3]

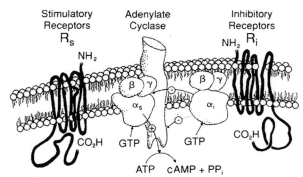

Figure 42-1 Receptor control of adenylyl cyclase system. The stimulatory receptor (R_s; β-adrenergic receptor) and the inhibitory receptor (R_i; α_2-adrenergic receptor, M_2 receptor) each possess the classic membrane-receptor structure (seven transmembrane α-helices), and each is coupled to the enzyme through a coupling regulatory protein (G protein), which is either stimulatory (G_s) or inhibitory (G_i) and consists of three subunits. The complexing of GTP with the α_s subunit activates adenylyl cyclase. Its release as GDP (not shown) terminates activation but increases the affinity of the β-adrenergic receptor for the agonist. The coupling of G_s protein to adenylyl cyclase has not been well studied. The β-agonist binding site is estimated to be located about 30% within the cell membrane. (*Modified from Levitzki A: Transmembrane signaling to adenylate cyclase in mammalian cells and in* Saccromyces cervisiae. *Trends Biol Sci 1988; 13:298, with permission.*)

Despite some differences in amino acid composition and a total of 413 rather than 418, the structures in the "pocket" and protein coupling regions are the same.

G Proteins

G proteins are crucial elements in the coupling of agonists to their effector enzyme or channel and figure prominently in their regulation and some mechanisms of desensitization (See also Chap. 43). Whether stimulatory or inhibitory, they are heterotrimers of α, β, and γ subunits. The GDP-GTP exchange takes places in the α fragment, and the β and γ fragments anchor the G proteins to the membrane bilayer while the exchange takes place.

Binding of the β-adrenergic agonist to the β-adrenergic receptor in its high-affinity state for ligand causes a conformational change involving certain residues of the third intracellular loop (222 to 229 in the hamster receptor), resulting in the following events: (1) binding of GTP to the α fragment with simultaneous release of GDP, and a change in receptor-ligand affinity to a low-affinity state; (2) dissociation of the α-GTP fragment from the β and γ fragments; (3) activation of adenylyl cyclase by combination of the α-GTP fragment with the catalytic fragment; and (4) termination of enzyme activation by hydrolysis of GTP by enzyme-bound GTPase, and resumption of the high-affinity state.[4]

Figure 42-2 Three-dimensional barrel structure of the β-adrenergic receptor. Epinephrine is shown binding inside the "barrel" composed of seven transmembrane-spanning α-helices. The critical residues for ligand binding, Asp^{113} and Ser^{204} and Ser^{207}, are within the transmembrane-spanning region (Asp^{79} in transmem-brane helix II not shown for clarity). The inset shows a view from above the receptor indicating a hypothetical orientation of epinephrine with key residues from helices III and V. (*From Jasper and Insel,[2] with permission.*)

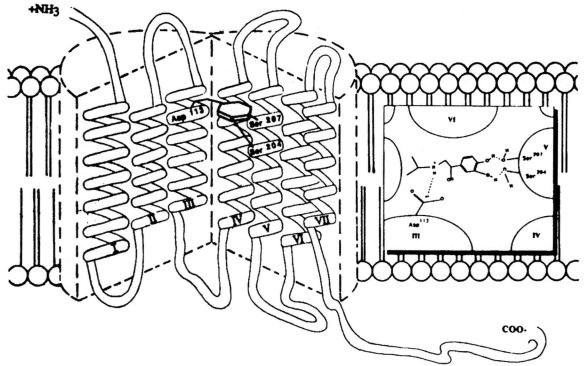

Various agonists are inhibitory to adenylyl cyclase through the action of the α subunit of the G$_i$ protein. Among these are α$_2$-adrenergic receptors for adrenergic agonists, the M$_2$-muscarinic receptor, the A$_1$-adenosine receptor, and the somatostatin receptor.

The β-adrenergic receptor alternates between the high- and low-affinity states for its agonist, characterized by the dissociation constants K$_H$ and K$_L$, respectively. Figure 42-3 shows the reduction in agonist affinity occurring when GTP combines with the G$_{s\alpha}$ fragment. The computer-derived curves represent competition between the antagonist (^{3}H) dihydroalprenolol (DHA) and isoproterenol-binding sites at various concentrations of the latter. With addition of GTP, the curve becomes steeper and shifts to the right, coinciding with a shift in percentage of low-affinity sites from 23 percent to 100 percent of the total[5] (Fig. 42-3). This phenomen is important in understanding the concept of full and partial agonists, since partial agonists bind less avidly to the high-affinity form. Using the same techniques, it is possible to show that corticosteroids produce a greater proportion of high-affinity receptor sites.[6]

Guanylyl 5-yl-imidophosphate (GppNHp), a nonhydrolyzable form of GTP, and sodium fluoride (NaF) both act directly on the G$_s$ stimulatory protein, causing maximum activation of adenylyl cyclase. Hence, they are useful in testing competency of the system beyond this point, while forskolin bypasses the G protein and directly activates adenylyl cyclase.

Figure 42-3 Computer-modeled curves for inhibition of (−)(^{3}H) dihydroalprenolol binding to frog erythrocyte membranes by (−) isoproterenol in the presence and absence of GTP. K$_H$ is the high-affinity dissociation constant for isoproterenol, and K$_L$ the low-affinity constant, while %R$_H$ and %R$_L$ are the percentage of receptors in each state. Addition of GTP to the receptor-nucleotide binding protein complex causes the high-affinity state for isoproterenol to be altered to a low-affinity state, but in the cell there is now an enhanced ability of the GTP-nucleotide binding protein (G$_{GTP}$) to interact with adenylate cyclase. (*From Kent et al.,[5] with permission.*)

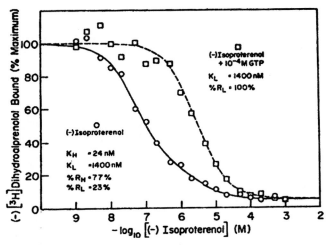

CHOLERA AND PERTUSSIS TOXIN EFFECTS ON G PROTEINS

Cholera and pertussis toxin are used to identify mechanisms involving the G$_s$ and G$_i$ proteins, respectively. Both toxins, by ribosylating the α subunit, interfere with its function, but in different ways. Ribosylation of the G$_s$ α fragment by cholera toxin prevents hydrolysis of GTP, once combined with adenylyl cyclase, causing persistent stimulation. This effect is instrumental in the persistent diarrhea of that disease. Ribosylation of the G$_i$ α fragment by pertussis toxin inactivates the G$_i$ α fragment with increased activity of adenylyl cyclase. Thus, use of pertussis toxin is an experimental tool to identify a mechanism functioning through the G$_i$ protein if its action is blocked by the toxin. These tools have been useful in dissecting mechanisms of desensitization to β-adrenergic agonists.

Drug-Receptor Interaction

FULL AND PARTIAL AGONISTS

Pharmacologic action of a drug results from the temporary occupancy of a variable proportion of its receptors. Distinction is made between *affinity* of a drug and its *efficacy*, or ability to activate the receptor. Compounds possessing both affinity and efficacy are termed *agonists*, and drugs lacking efficacy but possessing affinity are termed *antagonists*, which compete with the agonist for the receptor. *Full agonists* such as the catecholamines are well coupled and require occupancy of only a fraction of the total receptor population to exert their maximum effect, E_{max}, or *intrinsic activity*. They have high efficacy. The remaining receptors are termed *spare receptors*. *Partial agonists*, such as albuterol, (salbutamol), fenoterol, and terbutaline, are less well coupled. Although they affect all or nearly all receptors at their E_{max}, their E_{max} is generally lower.[7,8] In the presence of a functional antagonist, a larger proportion of receptor occupation is required to produce the same response.

Catecholamines interact with Ser^{204} and Ser^{207} and are anchored by their aliphatic hydroxyl and the amino group to produce maximum stimulation. Propranolol or atenolol are unable to interact with Ser^{204} and Ser^{207} but are sufficiently anchored by their aliphatic structures to compete nevertheless. Pindalol forms a hydrogen bond with its indole nitrogen group to only one Ser site and therefore is a partial agonist, able to produce some activation.

Figure 42-4 shows the cAMP accumulation in CHO (Chinese Hamster Ovary) cells transfected with human β$_2$-adrenergic receptors as a function of receptor occupancy by (-) isoproterenol (full agonist), requiring 0.62 percent of the receptors for 50 percent maximum cAMP, and the partial agonists (-) trimetoquinol (TMQ) and 3',5'-diiodo-TMQ, requiring 8.4 percent and 100 percent occupancy, respectively.[9]

THE "TWO-STATE" MODEL OF DRUG-RECEPTOR INTERACTION

Jasper and Insel[1] propose a "two-state" model of the β$_2$-adrenergic receptor in which the active state is a high-affin-

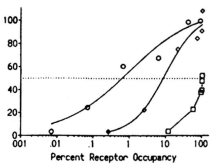

Figure 42-4 Cyclic adenocine monophosphate (cAMP) accumulation in CHO β_2-adrenergic receptor cells as a function of receptor occupancy induced by (−) isoproterenol, (−) trimetoquinol (TMQ), and 3′,5′-diiodo-TMQ. Isoproterenol represents a full agonist, and only 0.62 percent receptor occupancy is required to produce 50 percent maximum cAMP. TMQ is a partial agonist (in relaxation studies) and requires 8.4 percent occupancy for 50 percent maximum cAMP. 3′,5′-diiodo-TMQ requires 100 percent occupancy to produce 50 percent of maximum cAMP. Key: ○ = (−) isoproterenol; ◇ = (− TMQ; □ = 3′,5′-diiodo-TMQ. (*From Fraundorfer et al.,[9] with permission.*)

ity (agonist-receptor-G_s) ternary complex, stabilized by disulfide linkage between receptor and G_s protein. These bonds are broken when the G_s union is terminated with the arrival of GTP, using the model described in Fig. 42-3. When a series of full and partial agonists was examined, there was a correlation between their intrinsic activity and the ratio of K_L/K_H.[5] Their affinity for receptor was proportional to their efficacy. Intrinsic activity was correlated with that fraction of receptors occupied in the high-affinity active state. Partial agonists gave intermediate values, proportional to their efficacy. Full agonists were visualized as "pulling" the receptor into the active state, and partial agonists spent less time in the active state since they were less completely coupled. The agonist must surmount an energy barrier to arrive in a ternary complex.[10]

FUNCTIONAL ANTAGONISM

In isolated respiratory muscle, relaxation by β-adrenergic agonists bears a reciprocal relationship to the concentration of the contractile agonist, varying with each constrictant and, to some degree, with the relaxant. As one drug is increased, the effect of the other decreases. When both agonists operate through separate receptors, this is termed *functional antagonism*. While the principle of functional antagonism seems intuitively simple, there are great variations depending upon the particular constrictant, the relaxant, and the species. In canine bronchi, Torphy et al. showed that relaxation by isoproterenol and its generation of cAMP and protein kinase A is strongly inhibited by methacholine.[11] However, relaxation caused by isoproterenol was much less antagonized by histamine or leukotriene D_4, despite similar degrees of constriction. Indeed, the effect of varying leukotriene D_4 was very slight.[11] Not only is the type of constrictant important, but also the type of relaxant (and species). At the same target tension, whether produced by

histamine, acetylcholine, KC1, or 5-HT (serotonin), relaxation varies between isoproterenol, forskolin, and the xanthine isobutyl methylxanthine (IBMX) but not dibutryl cAMP, and is different for each contractile agonist as well.[12]

An inverse correlation was noted between the ability of isoproterenol to relax guinea pig trachea contracted by various muscarinic agonists (methacholine, oxotremorine, McN-A343, or histamine) and their ability to generate 1,4,5-triphosphate (IP_3) in bovine trachea in the absence of relaxant.[13] The same relationship was shown in human bronchi,[14] but, surprisingly, histamine and methacholine showed similar degrees of functional antagonism to isoproterenol in this tissue (Fig. 42-5), with respect to both contraction and the simultaneous generation of IP_3. These investigators postulated that protein kinase C (PKC) exerts negative feedback at the receptor coupling or at adenylyl cyclase itself. Conversely, generation of IP_3 by phospholipase C (PLC) is one potential site of action of β-adrenergic agonists. In bovine trachea, salbutamol, forskolin, and dibutyryl cAMP are poor inhibitors of generation of IP_3 caused by 1 μM carbachol but are good inhibitors of its generation by 100 μM histamine.[15] The same applies to isoproterenol in canine trachea.[16] Why such distinctions occur is unclear. Carbacholine and acetylcholine are full agonists with large receptor reserves, which they draw upon as their concentration increases. Isoproterenol is also a full agonist and must draw upon its receptor reserve to resist contraction.[17] In canine trachea, the contractile action of histamine and McN-A-343, both partial agonists, is more susceptible to isoproterenol than the contractile action of full agonists.[18,19]

MECHANISMS OF FUNCTIONAL ANTAGONISM

What mechanisms can be invoked to explain functional antagonism between contractants and β-agonist action? At least four loci of interaction can be offered.

1. Muscarinic agonists inhibit adenylyl cyclase at the M_2 inhibitory receptor, operating through G_i, consistent with earlier data by Sakary et al.[20]; cAMP production by cul-

Figure 42-5 Relaxation of human bronchial smooth muscle by isoproterenol after contraction by increasing concentrations of methacholine (*left panel*) and histamine (*right panel*) at 0.1, 1.0, 10, 100, and 1000 μM, respectively. Contraction levels are expressed as percentages of the response to 0.1 mM methacholine in each experiment. It is significant that in human bronchi, the degree of functional antagonism is relatively similar. (*From van Amsterdam et al.,[14] with permission.*)

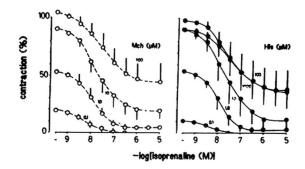

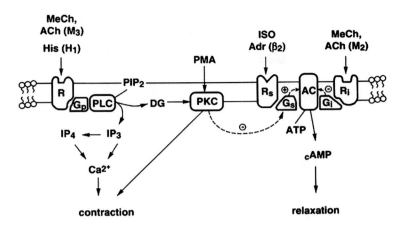

Figure 42-6 Membrane components involved in smooth-muscle contraction and relaxation showing their possible interactions. Metacholine (MeCh) and acetylcholine (ACh) act on the M_3 receptor, and histamine (His) at the H_1 receptor, and acting through the putative G protein (G_p) on phospholipase C (PLC) to produce inositol triphosphate (IP_3) and diacylglycerol (DG) with contraction. Relaxation by isoproterenol (ISO) or adrenaline (Adr) occurs through stimulation of adenylyl cyclase (AC) by way of stimulatory G protein (G_s). Inhibition of AC by muscarinic agonists occurs at the M_2 receptor through the inhibitory G protein (G_i), and PKC is postulated to inhibit AC at G_s. Both are possible mechanisms of functional antagonism. Not shown is a postulated negative feedback of PKC on the action of phospholipase C, as well as its inhibition by cAMP as discussed in the text. (*Adapted from Meurs et al.,*[23] *with permission.*)

tured human tracheal smooth-muscle cells stimulated by 1 μM isoproterenol is inhibited 60 percent by 1 μM carbachol, operating through the M_2-receptor.[21,22]

2. Conversely, β-adrenergic agonists antagonize the activity of PLC responding to various constrictants, as discussed in more detail later.

3. Since the ability of various agonists to exert functional antagonism correlates with their ability to produce IP_3, one or more products of this cascade, very possibly PKC, is suspected as the active feedback agent. PKC is able, through phosphorylation, to uncouple the $β_2$-adrenergic receptor and adenylyl cyclase (Fig. 42-6).[23]

4. Beta-adrenergic agonists and muscarinic agonists exert opposite effects on the K_{Ca} channel in smooth muscle, promoting relaxation and contractility, respectively, as the channel is stimulated or inhibited (see below).

From a clinical perspective, the question really is whether functional antagonism is anything more than an in vitro phenomenon, which may not be applicable to the patient, particularly in the range of agonist concentrations involved. A fourfold increase in either methacholine or histamine by inhalation causes an approximate tripling of airway resistance *and* a roughly 50 percent reduction in the protection by infused isoproterenol in dogs.[23a] It seems likely that the variation in cholinergic drive or histamine release, and other mediators, should be equally susceptible. Of course, factors of airway geometry and inflammatory obstruction complicate interpretations. More isoproterenol is required to reach E_{max} for specific airway conductance in the asthmatic patient than in normal individuals. This is also related to the severity of asthma, and hence is consistent with functional antagonism.[24]

Desensitization of Beta-Adrenergic Receptors

ACUTE (0 TO 24 h) AGONIST-INDUCED DESENSITIZATION

The current understanding of agonist-induced desensitization is the result of research over two decades, mostly from

in vitro systems. Transfer of this information to in vivo systems is still very fragmentary and is easier when dealing with structures obtainable in a homogeneous living state, such as blood cellular elements, rather than tissue fixed in place, such as respiratory smooth muscle.

A classic paper of Su et al. demonstrated the sequence of desensitization over time to 1 μM isoproterenol using astrocytoma 1321N1 cells[25] (Fig. 42-7). Within minutes, cells underwent a 50 to 60 percent reduction in adenylyl cyclase activity, and a 10-fold increase in the K_d, the dissociation rate constant for binding of isoproterenol to the receptor. This constituted an "uncoupling" of receptor to the enzyme. It involved no loss of receptors and, if agonist was removed, the original activity returned with a $t_{1/2}$ of 7 min. Partial agonists caused only partial uncoupling. Continued exposure to agonists resulted also in a loss of receptors over a 2 to 6 h incubation, with 80 to 90 percent loss by 24 h (downregulation). This was termed *long-term* desensitization. These

Figure 42-7 Time-course of decrease in β-adrenergic receptor density, isoproterenol-stimulated adenylyl cyclase activity, and isoproterenol-stimulating cAMP accumulation during incubation of 1321N1 astrocytoma cells with 1 μM isoproterenol. The slide illustrates the more rapid loss of adenylyl cyclase function than receptor number, contrasting uncoupling with downregulation as two distinct processes. (*From Su et al.,*[25] *with permission.*)

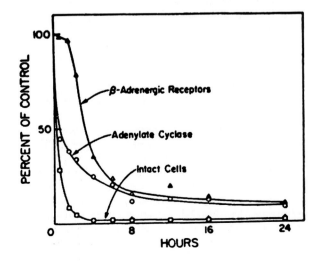

receptors were not easily renewed. Return of activity required synthesis of new protein. Thus, desensitization was envisioned as at least a two-stage process, uncoupling followed by downregulation.

Further studies revealed a concentration factor. The uncoupling process could occur at a much lower concentration of agonist, with little or no loss of receptor number. Human lymphocytes exposed to only 0.01 nM isoproterenol rapidly lost the ability to generate cAMP, with no loss of receptor number. However, exposure to 1 μM isoproterenol resulted in receptor loss beginning at 10 min.[26]

RECEPTOR PHOSPHORYLATION AND UNCOUPLING

Short-term desensitization, occurring within minutes, involves phosphorylation of specific sites of the β-adrenergic receptor with resulting uncoupling from adenylyl cyclase.[27] The same low-affinity state for ligand occurs upon addition of GTP (Fig. 42-3). Almost simultaneously with uncoupling is a sequestration of the receptor into numerous vesicles, removing it from the cell membrane. The two processes are evidently independent, however. Sequestered receptors have lost their coupling to G_s protein, as none is present. If the β-adrenergic agonist is removed, sequestered receptors rapidly return to their membrane location, apparently none the worse for wear. G_s protein is also restored, even before their arrival at the membrane site. Rapid sequestration has been duplicated in an in vivo system. Rats given 5 mg/kg isoproterenol intraperitoneally undergo a 40 percent sequestration of uncoupled lung receptors into a vesicular fraction, which is maximum at 10 min; the number returns to baseline over the next 3 h.[28]

Long-term desensitization results from the continued presence of agonist beyond a critical point, maintaining receptors in their sequestered state, whence a process of degradation commences (downregulation). When agonist is removed, restoration occurs with synthesis of new protein and return of receptors to their membrane site.

The short-term desensitization process can be further characterized as "low-agonist" (nanomolar) and "high-agonist" (micromolar) desensitization.[27] Low-agonist exposure is believed to activate only the cAMP-dependent protein kinase A (PKA), disrupting coupling to G_s, while high-agonist exposure activates both PKA and the agonist-specific β-adrenergic receptor kinase (β-ARK), further disrupting coupling. β-ARK is a cytoplasmic enzyme[29] that apparently migrates to the cell membrane to phosphorylate the receptor, once the receptor is occupied.[30] Its action is thought to depend upon a conformational change, which exposes certain receptor sites in the last 7 kDA of the cytoplasmic "tail." This action is believed to be facilitated by "β-arrestin."[27]

Figure 42-8 is a summary of these processes as depicted by Hausdorff et al.[27] The further interaction with β-arrestin is not shown but occurs at the cytoplasmic tail of the receptor and depends on the presence of β-ARK; β-arrestin actually "chokes off" adrenergic receptor activity. Phosphorylation by PKA apparently takes place at two regions in the third cytoplasmic loop critical for coupling. Only low-agonist desensitization would be expected at the plasma catecholamine levels found physiologically or even after the systemic administration of β-adrenergic agonists in treating

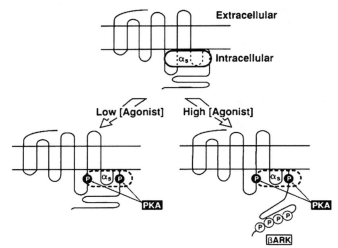

Figure 42-8 Model of postulated mechanisms for agonist-induced phosphorylation and desensitization of the β-adrenoreceptor. At low (nanomolar) agonist concentrations (as with circulating drugs), the cAMP-dependent protein kinase A produced by β-adrenergic agonist stimulation phosphorylates one or both of two sites of the receptor adjacent to the α_s subunit of the G_s protein, disrupting coupling. At high (micromolar) concentrations of agonist, β-ARK, is also activated, phosphorylating sites on the distal portion of the carboxyl termination of the β-adrenoceptor, further disrupting coupling. It has also been postulated that a 48-kDa protein, β-arrestin, facilitates the phosphorylation process. (From Hausdorff et al.: FASEBJ 1990; 4:2881, with permission.)

asthma. One can only speculate on the concentrations achieved by aerosolization. Concentration of catecholamines required for high-agonist desensitization have thus been found only at adrenergic synaptic sites in the nervous system.[31]

HOMOLOGOUS AND HETEROLOGOUS DESENSITIZATION

Homologous desensitization refers to desensitization only of receptors specific for a β-adrenergic agonist; heterologous desensitization refers to desensitization of a variety of receptor utilizing adenylyl cyclase, such as β-adrenergic receptors or prostaglandin $E_2(PGE_2)$. Heterologous desensitization is mediated by cAMP and involves phosphorylation by PKA. Cyclic AMP is the operative factor. Homologous desensitization originates from agonist activation of the β-ARK acting upon the β-adrenergic receptor as it is deformed by agonist.

REGULATION OF mRNA FOR BETA-ADRENERGIC RECEPTOR

In DDT₁ MF-2 hamster vas deferens muscle cells, β-adrenergic receptor mRNA levels are downregulated by β-adrenergic agonists and upregulated by corticosteroids. Hadcock et al. followed levels of mRNA for the receptor and the generation of new mRNA over 36 h in cultured cells.[32] Stimulation by 10 μM isoproterenol caused a reduction in mRNA "stability," with a decrease in its $t_{1/2}$ from 12 to 5 h, but had no effect on mRNA transcription rate. Dexamethasone increased transcription of new mRNA sharply, about fourfold, but had no effect on mRNA stability. When both were

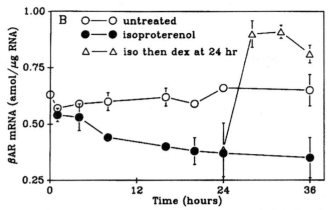

Figure 42-9 Interplay of agonist and glucocorticoid-induced modulation of β-adrenergic receptor mRNA concentrations. DDT_1 MF-2 cells (vas deferens smooth muscle) were treated with vehicle (○) or 10 μM isoproterenol alone (●) or with 500 nM dexamethasone added (△). RNA was extracted, and DNA-excess solution hybridization performed. Isoproterenol by itself resulted in a decrease in steady state levels of mRNA, while corticosteroid resulted in rapid synthesis, providing a net increase in mRNA levels. (*From Hadcock et al.,[32] with permission.*)

present, net mRNA levels were maintained at about 30 percent over basal levels (Fig. 42-9).

REGULATION AT THE LEVEL OF G PROTEINS

In S49 mouse lymphoma cells stimulated by isoproterenol or forskolin for 24 h, the steady-state level of $G_{i\alpha}$ increases threefold due to an increased rate of synthesis.[33] Synthesis of mRNA for $G_{s\alpha}$ also increases by 70 percent, but its $t_{1/2}$ decreases from 55 to 34 h, producing a net decrease of 25 percent in its steady-state level. Both the effects of G_i and G_s require cAMP, as mutant cells lacking PKA activity do not respond.

LONG-TERM AGONIST-INDUCED DESENSITIZATION (TOLERANCE)

Short-term in vitro studies are poor models for long-term administration during therapy of asthma, and brief application in vivo or subcutaneously of very large doses of isoproterenol, such as the 5 mg/kg applied intraperitoneally to rats producing rapid sequestration of receptors, is not particularly relevant.[28] Doses only one-hundredth of this or less were administered over a 7-day period to guinea pigs using a mini-infusion pump to produce a situation somewhat more akin to actual treatment conditions, with rather surprising results.[34] At a rate of 60 ng/kg/h, isoproterenol achieved superphysiologic concentrations in plasma, averaging 40 nM. As assessed by (^{3}H) DHA binding, there was an 80 percent reduction in receptor density (B_{max}) in lung membranes, little change in K_d for (^{3}H) DHA, but changes in the G_s protein, as revealed by its inability to undergo ADP ribosylation with cholera toxin and a 50 percent reduction in the maximum ability of isoproterenol to protect lung parenchymal strips against histamine contraction. Similar changes in G_s have been proposed when rat adiposites were exposed to 21 days of isoproterenol infusion.[35]

The loss of β-adrenergic receptors after long-term exposure was confirmed in a study of lung receptors in guinea pigs following a 7-day exposure to norepinephrine.[36] Beta₂-adrenergic receptors in airway smooth muscle were reduced in number by a mean value of 46 percent, and the mRNA by 75 percent, with a smaller decrease in the functional response to albuterol. Beta₂-adrenergic receptors in other lung tissues were downregulated similarly, more so those in the alveoli. The disparity between receptor loss and function loss was considered possibly indicative of the presence of spare receptors. Receptor coupling was not examined.

Whether causally related or not, a study of human β₂-adrenergic receptor polymorphism in asthmatic and normal individuals detected one fairly common mutation, Arg16 → Gly. This was more prevalent in those patients requiring oral corticosteroids but not in the asthma population as a whole.[37] This could be a very significant finding, because in vitro fibroblasts transfected with this mutation showed a markedly greater tendency to downregulation.[38] This study illustrates the sophistication with which the β-adrenergic system must be explored in asthma and asthma treatment.

AGONIST-INDUCED DESENSITIZATION OF THE ISOLATED BRONCHUS AND REVERSAL BY CORTICOSTEROIDS

In 1972, Fleish and Titus showed that rat tracheal smooth muscle exposed to high concentrations of isoproterenol developed subsensitivity to isoproterenol relaxation.[39] One study reported that incubation of guinea pig trachea with 0.24 μM isoproterenol for 20 min caused tachyphylaxis to subsequent relaxation against histamine. Preincubation with indomethacin prevented isoproterenol-induced desensitization.[39a] Rat trachea exposed to 5 μM isoproterenol for 30 min resulted in a 180-fold loss of affinity for this ligand but a sufficient number of remaining receptors to prevent any lowering of E_{max}, no loss of sensitivity to aminophylline, and negligible prevention of desensitization by incubation with 40 μM methylprednisolone.[40]

Beta-adrenergic receptors in normal human bronchial smooth muscle are no less susceptible to desensitization in vitro than rat or guinea pig trachea. Exposure of the isolated human bronchus for 25 min to a concentration of isoproterenol or terbutaline only 10-fold greater than their EC_{50} caused a 50-fold shift to the right in the dose-response curve and cross-desensitization between the two (Fig. 42-10).[41] (EC_{50} is the concentration required to produce half maximum effect.) Much the same result was reported by Davis and Conolly with exposure of human bronchi to 1.0 μM isoproterenol for 60 min, but they recorded a 21 percent reduction in E_{max}.[42] These investigators reported a "wide and significant variation" in the susceptibility of bronchi to desensitization between individual lungs but little variation within the same lung. They further reported a 60 percent recovery from 400 μM isoproterenol over 150 min, hastened by 150 μM hydrocortisone and prevented by the presence of as little as 1 nM isoproterenol. Cyclohexamide had virtually no effect on recovery. Bronchial wall generation of cAMP paralleled the relaxation in its susceptibility to desensitization. Human bronchial spirals exposed to isoproterenol con-

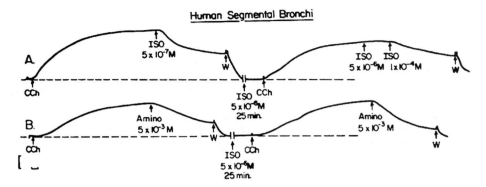

Figure 42-10 Human segemental bronchus desensitized by exposure to 10^{-6}M isoproterenol for 25 min. The desensitized bronchus now showed cross-resistance to terbutaline as well, but not aminophylline (not shown). (*From Avner and Jenne,*[41] *with permission.*)

centrations 100 times greater than their EC_{50} produced a similar shift. In neither study did indomethacin alter desensitization.

A detailed study of the time and concentration factors and the effect of corticosteroid has been done using pig bronchus, with its predominantly β_1-adrenoreceptor subtype.[43] Exposure to 1 μM isoproterenol caused a 21.9- and 35.5-fold increase in the EC_{50} at 3 and 6 h. Desensitization was related to only the l-form and was significantly reduced by only 5 μM cortisol to 7.6- and 5.0-fold changes, respectively. Treatment with 5 or 25 μM indomethacin or 25 or 100 μM mepacrine (an inhibitor of PLA_2) did not alter desensitization. The authors felt that their low concentration of corticosteroid was consistent with therapeutic concentrations in patients, whereas the high concentrations employed by others might have interfered in the amine uptake process, complicating interpretation.

One concludes from these and other studies that agonist-induced desensitization of smooth muscle is a general phenomenon, although mechanisms may depend on the species to some extent, and that corticosteroids probably have some inhibitory effect. The extension of these findings to patients during both acute and chronic exposure awaits better information on actual levels encountered by smooth muscle during high- and low-intensity treatment and the effects over time, perhaps with improved animal models.

Beta-Adrenergic Desensitization Secondary to Inflammation

An impressive literature has documented the ability of a variety of inflammatory products to alter β-adrenergic function, particularly as studied in vitro. This suggests the possibility that β-adrenoreceptor dysfunction can be acquired during inflammatory events leading to the asthmatic crisis and hamper the response to treatment.

ANTIGEN CHALLENGE

Antigen challenge of intact guinea pigs or of their tissues has provided most of the information and grounds for speculation. Figure 42-11 shows the effect of in vitro challenge of sensitized guinea pig trachea by antigen on its subsequent dose-response curve 1 h after administration of epineph-

rine.[44] There was a marked decrease in relaxation paralleled by a 50 percent reduction in receptor number. Significantly, desensitization was specific for the β-adrenergic system, since relaxation by vasoactive intestinal peptide (VIP) was not significantly altered. Desensitization was prevented by 30 μg/ml hydrocortisone or by 5 μg/ml indomethacin, consistent with a role of PLA_2 and its products.

There are several prominent hypotheses for various inflammatory mechanisms affecting β-adrenergic function.

PHOSPHOLIPASE A_2 AND ITS PRODUCTS

Phosphatidylcholine breakdown occurs through a localized increase in PLA_2 in the receptor domain of the cell bilayer, a process also occurring with mechanical trauma, antigen challenge, and histamine stimulation.[45] It also occurs with β-agonist presentation. Thus, incubation of guinea pig trachea with isoproterenol or albuterol causes release of PGE_2 into the medium.[46] Preincubation with 15 μM indomethacin prevents desensitization and PGE_2 release. However, if 0.3 nM to 0.3 μM PGE_2 is added back to indomethacin-treated trachea exposed to isoproterenol, desensitization is reestablished. The desensitization process is believed principally due to uncoupling. Taki et al. have proposed that increased levels of PLA_2 could have a deleterious direct effect on the lipoprotein membrane supporting the receptor, affecting its function.[47]

CYTOKINES

By repeated antigen challenge of guinea pig trachea and with exposure to interleukin 1β (IL-1β), Wills-Karp et al. found that heterologous desensitization occurred and that synthesis of $G_{i\alpha}$ inhibitory protein was increased, since exposure to pertussis toxin prevented desensitization.[48]

PLATELET-ACTIVATING FACTOR

Platelet-activating factor (PAF) impairs the ability of isoproterenol to relax both guinea pig and human trachea. Agrawal et al.[49] hypothesized that PAF desensitizes through a non-specific, postreceptor effect. There is also persistence of in vivo hyperactivity after PAF exposure through an unknown mechanism.

PROTEIN KINASE C

There is increasing evidence that PKC causes desensitization of the β-adrenergic system. The chief proponents of this view are Meurs et al., who studied peripheral lymphocytes

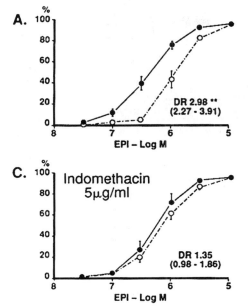

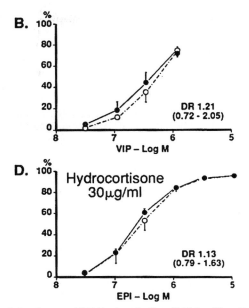

Figure 42-11 Effect of antigen challenge on the sensitivity to relaxation by epinephrine (*A.*) and VIP (*B.*). Control (●) and sensitized (○) guinea pig trachea were contracted maximally with pilocarpine, and relaxation curves plotted 1 h after ovalbumin challenge. Note that anaphylaxis produced desensitization to epi-

nephrine but not VIP. Preincubation (1 h) to either 5 µg/ml indomethacin (*C.*) or 30 µg/ml hydrocortisone (*D.*) prevented desensitization to epinephrine. (*From Daffonchio et al.,[44] with permission.*)

obtained from stable asthmatics before and 24 h after inhalational challenge by house dust mite.[50] Before challenge, cAMP production and ligand-binding characteristics were indistinguishable from those of normal cells. After challenge, there was a loss of receptor binding of (^{3}H) DHA and significant uncoupling from adenylyl cyclase. Desensitization was heterologous, or nonspecific. Both histamine (H_2) and isoproterenol responses were impaired. Stimulation by GppNHp and NaF, both acting on the G_s nucleotide binding protein, was impaired also, indicating that uncoupling was taking place beyond this point, i.e., between G_s and adenylyl cyclase or beyond.[50,51] Incubation of lymphocytes with phorbal myristate acetate (PMA), an activator of PKC, produced similar desensitization, leading the authors to hypothesize that PKC activation by receptor-mediated turnover of phosphoinositiol diphosphate occurs during anaphylaxis to produce uncoupling.[52] Heterologous desensitization of rabbit bronchial epithelial cells in culture is achieved upon exposure to bradykinin and can be mimicked by exposure to diactanoyl glyceride (DAG) and PMA, suggesting that bradykinin production of PKC is responsible.[53]

INFECTIOUS PRODUCTS

Infectious states caused by viruses and bacteria must also be considered as altering β-adrenergic function. The variety of inflammatory products that affect such function has been reviewed.[54] A direct suggestion of the effect of activated defense cells is the strong correlation between reactive oxygen species production and diminished β-adrenergic function when macrophages are incubated in contact with guinea pig trachea, an effect ameliorated by oxygen scavengers.[55]

Corticosteroid "Reversal" of Desensitization

Since corticosteroids decrease the inflammatory components of an obstructed airway, much of the improved bronchodilator response subsequent to their use must be explained simply on physical grounds as inflammation lessens. However, at the cellular level, there are also potential mechanisms for an improved response. These can be classified as (1) enhancement of the normal responses, and (2) reversal of any desensitization present. These are dependent on the tissue, species, duration of contact, and dose of a particular corticosteroid.

1. *Corticosteroids increase the proportion of receptors in their high-affinity state* towards ligand, as illustrated with peripheral polymorphonuclear leukocytes exposed to 0.5 µM unbound hydrocortisone,[6] and human lymphocytes desensitized by oral terbutaline following 100 mg oral prednisone.[56]
2. *Corticosteroids exert a two- to threefold increase in receptor number,* as first shown in rat lung[57] and human lung cells[58] and hamster DDT I MF-2 smooth-muscle cells.[32]
3. *Corticosteroids induce synthesis of lipocortins,* a family of phospholipase-inhibiting proteins typified by lipocortin-1, which inhibit degradation of lipid precursors to lyso-PAF and arachidonic acid in a variety of cells. However, in contrast to mast cells from mouse, rat, and guinea pig lung, Schleimer noted that "physiologically relevant concentrations of glucocorticoids do not inhibit leukotriene release from human lung tissue, or purified human lung mast cells."[59]

Relative Tissue Susceptibility to Tachyphylaxis: Airway versus Inflammatory Cells.

Judging from clinical studies, β-adrenergic receptors from airway smooth muscle are relatively resistant to tachyphylaxis compared to peripheral leukocytes. Lung cell homogenates also appear more resistant. When collected from patients undergoing lung resection who had received at least 1.0 mg terbutaline subcutaneously during the preceding 24 h, peripheral mononuclear cells already showed downregulation of receptors while lung cells did not.[60] In vitro exposure of the lung cells for 36 h showed a severalfold greater requirement for terbutaline concentrations to desensitize than calculated to be present during systemic application in patients, but this could occur over a longer period.[61]

In an animal model, preexposure of guinea pig trachea to 1 μM of the β$_2$-adrenergic agonist clenbuterol for 15 min had no effect on isoproterenol relaxation of methacholine contraction. However, the same treatment of ovalbumin-sensitized trachea resulted in significant desensitization of the ability of 10 nM isoproterenol to inhibit anaphylactic release of histamine or anaphylactic contraction.[62]

Tashkin et al. found that peripheral lymphocytes of asthmatic patients had impaired ability to generate cAMP despite a normal receptor number and had susceptibility to downregulation during oral therapy.[63] Downregulation was corrected by a single dose of hydrocortisone.[64] While a preceding course of oral terbutaline did not alter the histamine threshold of the airways nor the protective ability of subcutaneous terbutaline against histamine, it did reduce tolerance for antigen challenge and the protective ability of terbutaline in 2 of 3 asthmatic patients.[63] Apparently, anti-inflammatory responses were more easily desensitized. More documentation in this area is urgently needed.

In Vitro Studies of Excised Asthmatic Airways

From the preceding material, a strong case can be made that the airways in the patient with severe asthma develop some impairment of β-adrenergic responses during the acute attack. Two groups of investigators have described extensive studies from asthmatic airways studied post mortem after fatal attacks. Goldie et al. studied bronchial spirals from seven such patients and found a four to fivefold reduction in sensitivity to isoproterenol, compared to nonasthmatic airways, but no changes in the response to theophylline.[65] Subsequently, these authors reported detailed studies of bronchial β$_2$-adrenergic receptor populations and functions from a single asthmatic lung removed 7.5 h post mortem compared to bronchi from nonasthmatic lungs.[66] Autoradiographs in conjunction with β$_2$-specific [125] iodocyanopindolol (ICYP) binding revealed a fourfold *increase* of receptors overlying smooth muscle in the asthmatic bronchus, but a 10- and 13-fold *reduction* in sensitivity to

isoproterenol- and fenoterol-induced relaxation, respectively. The authors postulated that a defect in receptor coupling (or beyond) was responsible.

Bai et al. studied tissues from seven patients with fatal asthma attacks, selected from a larger number for retention of their contractile response to acetylcholine and electrical field stimulation (EFS). These tissues were compared to tissues from 14 normal individuals, matched for an equal postmortem delay.[67,68] The maximum tension developed (T_{max}) to EFS, histamine, and acetylcholine was 60 to 70 percent greater in the asthmatic trachea, but EFS-stimulated nonadrenergic, noncholinergic relaxation was the same. Sensitivity to isoproterenol was an average of 4.5-fold less in trachea (mean IC_{50} = 61.3 nM versus 12.6 nM in controls, p = .01) and marginally less to theophylline (37 μM vs. 5.7 μM, p = .04). In fourth-generation bronchi, contractile responses to acetylcholine, histamine, and EFS did not differ from those in normal individuals, but there was a 9.4-fold reduction in sensitivity to isoproterenol and negligible reduction to theophylline. The density of β$_2$-adrenergic receptors in smooth muscle from both trachea and bronchi showed no relationship to sensitivity to isoproterenol. In fact, receptor density was increased. Receptor autoradiograph data on four of the previous seven fatal asthma cases and two new cases compared to four matched controls revealed a surprising two- to threefold increase in β-adrenergic receptor expression in asthmatic bronchi and trachea, as well as increased agonist affinity for isoproteronol as demonstrated by competitive binding experiments. Yet, there was a very significant 13-fold decrease in relaxant potency in trachea (p = .003) and a 17-fold decrease in bronchi (p < .001), leading the authors to assume that the impairment to isoproterenol relaxation lies distal to the receptor, perhaps in coupling to adenylyl cyclase.[69]

These postmortem results in fatal asthma contrast with the majority of results from mild to moderate asthma studied incidental to lung surgery. Whicker et al. found no change in sensitivity to isoproterenol or theophylline but a decreased sensitivity to histamine and carbachol.[70] The only other study with comparable numbers of asthma patients came to a different conclusion, however. Cerrina et al. studied bronchial spirals from tissues removed at thoracotomy and compared preoperative PC$_{40}$ (concentration producing 40% reduction in SGaw) to histamine with the tissue pD$_2$ ($-\log_{10}EC_{50}$) to histamine, finding no relationship. However, asthmatic tissues were relatively unresponsive to isoproterenol, and the tissues of four asthma patients, seven bronchitis patients, and five normal individuals showed a significant negative correlation between preoperative histamine reactivity and in vitro isoproterenol sensitivity (p < .001).[71] The issue of β$_2$-adrenergic dysfunction in asthma has been discussed in a recent review.[72] Obviously postmortem tissue, or any excised tissue then studied in vitro, may not accurately reflect the circumstances existing in vivo, and in the postmortem studies, controls could particularly be a problem. Even now, in vitro knowledge supports the routine use of corticosteroids or other anti-inflammatory agents in all but mild cases of asthma and early, vigorous use of them in the impending asthma crisis. Corticosteroids should act to sustain receptor sensitivity to β-adrenergic drugs of both inflammatory cells and smooth muscle in the airways. Obviously, much more needs to be known about receptor behavior under these circumstances. Most recently, an extensive "State of the Art" summary has been published which provides more detail on beta₂-adrenergic receptors, their regulation, and the interaction of beta₂ agonists and corticosteroids at the cellular genome level.[73,74]

References

1. Strader CD, Sigal IS, Dixon RAF: Mapping the functional domains of the β-adrenergic receptor. *Am J Respir Cell Mol Biol* 1989; 1:81.

2. Jasper JR, Insel PA: Evolving concepts of partial agonism. The β-adrenergic receptor as a paradigm. *Biochem Pharmacol* 1992; 43:119.

3. Fraser CM, Venter JC: Beta-adrenergic receptors: Relationship of primary structure, receptor function, and regulation. *Am Rev Respir Dis* 1990; 141 (suppl):522.

4. Lefkowitz RJ, Kobilka BK, Caron MG: The new biology of drug receptors. *Biochem Pharmacol* 1989; 38:2941.

5. Kent RS, DeLean A, Lefkowitz RJ: A quantitative analysis of beta-adrenergic receptor interaction: Resolution of the high and low affinity states of the receptor by computer modelling of ligand binding data. *Mol Pharmacol* 1980; 17:14.

6. Davies AO, Lefkowitz RJ: In vitro and in vivo desensitization of beta-adrenergic receptors in human neutrophils. Attenuation by corticosteroids. *J Clin Invest* 1983; 71:565.

7. Kenakin TP, Ferris RM: Effects of in vivo β-adrenoceptor downregulation on cardiac responses to prenalterol and pirbuterol. *J Cardiovasc Res* 1983; 5:90.

8. Delhaye M, Teton G, Camus JC, et al.: Effects of full and partial β-adrenergic agonists and antagonists on human lung adenylate cyclase. *Biochem Pharmacol* 1983; 32:1831.

9. Frandorfer PF, Fertel RH, Miller DD, Feller DR: Biochemical and pharmacological characterization of high affinity trimetoquinol analogues on guinea pig and human beta adrenergic receptor subtypes: Evidence for partial agonism. *J Pharmacol Exp Ther* 1994; 270:665.

10. Jack D: A way of looking at agonism and antagonism: Lessons from albuterol, salmeterol, and other β-adrenoceptor agonists. *Br J Clin Pharmacol* 1991; 31:501.

11. Torphy, TJ, Burman M, Schartz LW, Wasserman MA: Differential effects of methacholine and leukotriene D₄ on cyclic nucleotide content and isoproterenol-induced relaxation in the opossum trachea. *J Pharmacol Exp Ther* 1986; 237:332.

12. Koenig SM, Mitchell RW, Kelly E, et al.: β-adrenergic relaxation of dog trachealis: Contractile agonist-specific interaction. *J Appl Physiol* 1989; 67:181.

13. van Amsterdam RGM, Meurs H, Brouwer F, et al.: Role of phosphoinositide metabolism in functional antagonism of airway smooth muscle contraction by beta-adrenoreceptor agonists. *Eur J Pharmacol (Mol Pharmacol Sect)* 1989; 172:175.

14. van Amsterdam RGM, Meurs H, TenBerge EJ, et al.: Role of phosphoinositide metabolism in human bronchial smooth muscle contraction and in functional antagonism by beta-adrenoceptor agonists. *Am Rev Respir Dis* 1990; 142:1124.

15. Hall IP, Chilvers ER: Inositol phosphates and airway smooth muscle. *Pulm Pharmacol* 1989; 2:113.

16. Madison JM, Brown JK: Differential inhibitory effects of forskolin, isoproterenol and dibutyryl cyclic AMP in canine tracheal smooth muscle. *J Clin Invest* 1988; 82:1462.

17. Lemoine H, Overluck C, Kohl A, et al.: Formoterol, fenoterol, and salbutamol as partial agonists for relaxation of maximally contracted guinea pig trachea: Comparison of relaxation with receptor binding. *Lung* 1992; 170:164.

18. Gunst SJ, Stropp JQ, Flavahan NA: Analysis of receptor reserves in canine tracheal smooth muscle. *J Appl Physiol* 1987; 62(4):1755.

19. Madison JM: Muscarinic receptor reserve of airway smooth muscle and the response to isoproterenol. *J Appl Physiol* 1990; 68:1017.

20. Sankary RM, Jones CA, Madison JM, Brown JK: Muscarinic cholinergic inhibition of cyclic AMP accumulation in airway smooth muscle. Role of a pertussis toxin-sensitive protein. *Am Rev Respir Dis* 1988; 13:145.

21. Hall IP, Widdop S, Townsend P, Daykin K: Control of cyclic AMP levels in primary cultures of human tracheal smooth muscle cells. *Br J Pharmacol* 1992; 107:422.

22. Hall IP, Widdop S, Saykin K: Muscarinic receptors coupling in cultured human airway smooth muscle. *Am Rev Respir Dis* 1993; 147:A173.

23. Meurs H, Roffel AF, Elzinga CRS, et al.: Muscarinic receptor-mediated inhibition of adenylyl cyclase and its role in the functional antagonism of cholinergic airway smooth muscle contraction by β-agonists. *Am Rev Respir Dis* 1992; 45:A438.

23a. Jenne JW, Shaughnessy TK, Druz WS, Manfredi CJ, Vestal RE: In vivo functional antagonism between isoproterenol and bronchoconstrictants in the dog. *J Appl Physiol* 1987; 63(2):812.

24. Barnes PJ, Pride NB: Dose-response curves to inhaled β-adrenoceptor agonists in normal and asthmatic subjects. *Br J Clin Pharmacol* 1983; 15:677.

25. Su YF, Harden TK, Perkens JP: Catecholamine-specific desensitization of adenylate cyclase. Evidence for a multistep process. *J Biol Chem* 1980; 255:7410.

26. Krall JF, Connelly M, Tuck ML: Acute regulation of beta adrenergic catecholamine sensitivity in human lymphocytes. *J Pharmacol Exp Ther* 1980; 214:554.

27. Hausdorff WP, Caron MG, Lefkowitz RJ: Turning off the signal: Desensitization of β-adrenergic receptor function. *FASEB* 1990; 4:2881.

28. Strasser RH, Stiles GL, Lefkowitz RJ: Translocation and uncoupling of the β-adrenergic receptor in rat lung after catecholamine-promoted desensitization in vivo. *Endocrinology* 1984; 115:1392.

29. Benovic JL, Strasser RH, Caron MG, Lefkowitz RJ: β-Adrenergic receptor kinase: Identification of a novel protein kinase that phosphorylates the agonist-occupied form of the receptor. *Proc Natl Acad Sci USA* 1986; 83:2797.

30. Strasser RH, Benovic JL, Caron MG, Lefkowitz RH: β-Agonist and prostaglandin E₁-induced translocation of the β-adrenergic receptor kinase: Evidence that the kinase may act on multiple adenylate cyclase-coupled receptors. *Proc Natl Acad Sci USA* 1986; 83:6362.

31. Bevan JA, Su C: Variation of intra- and perisynaptic adrenergic transmitter concentrations with width of synaptic cleft in vascular tissue. *J Pharmacol Exp Ther* 1974; 190:30.

32. Hadcock JR, Wang H-Y, Malbon CC: Agonist-induced destabilization of β-adrenergic receptor mRNA. *J Biol Chem* 1989; 264:19928.

33. Hadcock JR, Ros M, Watkins DC, Malbon CC: Cross regulation between G-protein-mediated pathways. Stimulation of adenylyl cyclase increases expression of the inhibitory G-protein, G$_{iα2}$. *J Biol Chem* 1990; 265:14784.

34. Nerme V, Abrahamsson J, Vauquelin G: Chronic isoproterenol administration causes altered beta adrenoceptor-G$_s$ coupling in guinea pig lung. *J Pharmacol Exp Ther* 1990; 252:1341.

35. Izawa T, Komabayashi T, Suda K, et al.: Some characteristics of the β-adrenergic system in rat adipocyte membranes after the

chronic administration of isoproterenol. *Res Commun Chem Pathol Pharmacol* 1988; 60:253.

36. Nishikawa M, Mak JCW, Shirasaki H, et al.: Long-term exposure to norephinephrine results in down-regulation and reduced mRNA expression of pulmonary β-adrenergic receptors in guinea pigs. *Am J Resp Cell Mol Biol* 1994; 10:91.

37. Reihsaus E, Innis M, MacIntyre N, Liggett S: Mutations in the gene encoding for the β₂ adrenergic receptor in normal and asthmatic subjects. *Am J Resp Cell Mol Biol* 1993; 8:334.

38. Green SA, Jacinto MT, Liggett SB: Genetic determinants of altered β₂-adrenergic receptor agonist promoted down-regulation in asthma. *Crit Care Med* 1984; 149:A849.

39. Fleisch JH, Titus E: The prevention of isoproterenol desensitization and isoproterenol reversal. *J Pharmacol Exp Ther* 1972; 181:425.

39a. Douglas JS, Lewis AJ, Ridgeway, P, Brink C, Bouhuys A: Tachyphylaxis to β-adrenoceptor agonists in guinea pig airway smooth muscle in vivo and in vitro. *Eur J Pharmacol* 1977; 42:195.

40. Lin CS, Hurwitz L, Jenne JW, Avner BP: Mechanisms of isoproterenol-induced desensitization of tracheal smooth muscle. *J Pharmacol Exp Ther* 1977; 203:12.

41. Avner BP, Jenne JW: Desensitization of isolated human bronchial smooth muscle to beta receptor agonists. *J Allergy Clin Immunol* 1981; 68:51.

42. Davis C, Conolly ME: Tachyphylaxis to beta-adrenoceptor agonists in human bronchial smooth muscle. Studies in vitro. *Br J Pharmacol* 1980; 10:417.

43. Goldie RG, Spino D, Paterson JW: Beta agonist-induced desensitization of pig bronchus. *J Pharmacol Exp Ther* 1986; 237:275.

44. Daffonchio L, Abbracchio MP, DiLuca M, et al.: β-Adrenoceptor desensitization induced by antigen challenge in guinea-pig trachea. *Eur J Pharmacol* 1990; 1778:21.

45. Blackwell GJ, Flower RJ, Nijkamp FP, Vane JB: Phospholipase A₂ activity of guinea pig isolated perfused lungs: Stimulation and inhibition by anti-inflammatory steroids. *Br J Pharmacol* 1978; 62:79.

46. Omini C, Abbracchio MP, Daffonchio L, et al.: Beta-adrenoceptor desensitization in the lung. A phenomenon related to prostanoids. *Prog Biochem Pharmacol* 1985; 20:63.

47. Taki F, Takasi K, Sataki T, et al.: The role of phospholipase in reducing β-adrenergic responsiveness in experimental asthma. *Am Rev Respir Dis* 1986; 133:362.

48. Wills-Karp M, Uchida Y, Lee JY, et al.: Organ culture with pro-inflammatory cytokines reproduces impairment of the β-adrenoceptor-mediated relaxation in trachease of a guinea pig antigen model. *Am J Respir Cell Mol Biol* 1993; 38:153.

49. Agrawal DK, Bergren DR, Byorth PJ, Townley RG: Platelet-activating factor induces nonspecific desensitization to bronchodilators in guinea pig. *J Pharmacol Exp Ther* 1991; 259:1.

50. Meurs H, Koeter GH, de Vries K, Kauffman HF: The beta-adrenergic system and allergic bronchial asthma: Changes in lymphocyte beta-adrenergic receptor number and adenylate cyclase activity after an allergen-induced attack. *J Allergy Clin Immunol* 1982; 70:272.

51. Zaagsma J, Van Der Heijden PJCM, van der Schaar MWG, Blank CMC: Comparison of functional beta-adrenoceptor heterogeneity in central and peripheral airway smooth muscle of guinea pig and man. *J Recept Res* 1991; 3:89.

52. Meurs H, Kauffman HF, Timmerman A, et al.: Phorbol 12-myristate 13-acetate induces beta adrenergic receptor uncoupling in and non-specific desensitization of adenylate cyclase in human mononuclear lymphocytes. *Biochem Pharmacol* 1986; 35:4217.

53. Mardini IA, Higgins NC, Zhou S, et al.: Functional behavior of the β-adrenergic receptor adenylyl cyclase system in rabbit airway epithelium. *Am J Respir Cell Mol Biol* 1994; 11:287.

54. Nijkamp FP, Henricks PAJ: Receptors in airway disease. Beta-adrenoceptors in lung inflammation. *Am Rev Respir Dis* 1990; 141:5145.

55. Loesberg C, Henricks PAJ, Nijkamp FP: Inverse relationship between superoxide anion production of guinea pig alveolar macrophages and tracheal β-adrenergic receptor function: Influence of dietary polyunsaturated fatty acids. *Int J Immunopharmacol* 1989; 11:165.

56. Brodde O-E, Brinkman M, Schemuth R, et al.: Terbutaline-induced desensitization of human lymphocyte β₂-adrenoceptors. *J Clin Invest* 1985; 76:1096.

57. Mano K, Akbarzadek A, Townley RG: Effect of hydrocortisone on beta-adrenoceptor receptors of lung membranes. *Life Sci* 1979; 25:1925.

58. Frazer CM, Venter JC: The synthesis of beta-adrenergic receptors in cultured human lung cells. Induction by glucocorticoids. *Biochem Biophys Res Commun* 1980; 94:390.

59. Schleimer RP: Effects of glucocorticosteroids on inflammatory cells relevant to their therapeutic applications in asthma. *Am Rev Respir Dis* 1991; 141 (suppl):S59.

60. Hauck RW, Bohm M, Gengenbach S, et al.: Beta₂ adrenoceptors in human lung and peripheral mononuclear leukocytes of untreated and terbutaline-treated patients. *Chest* 1990; 98:375.

61. Bohm M, Gengenbach S, Hauck RW, et al.: Beta-adrenergic receptors and m-cholinergic receptors in human lung. Findings following in vivo and in vitro exposure to the β-adrenergic agonist, terbutaline. *Chest* 1991; 100:1246.

62. Van Der Heijden PJCM, van Amsterdam JGC, Zaagsma J: Desensitization of smooth muscle and mast cell β-adrenoceptors in the airways of the guinea pig. *Eur J Respir Dis* 1984; 65:128.

63. Tashkin DP, Conolly ME, Deutsch RI, et al.: Subsensitization of beta-adrenoreceptors in airways and lymphocyte of healthy and asthmatic subjects. *Am Rev Respir Dis* 1982; 125:185.

64. Hui KK, Conolly ME, Tashkin DP: Methylprednisolone reverses the beta agonist-induced decrease in beta receptor number in human lymphocytes. *Clin Pharmacol Ther* 1982; 32:566.

65. Goldie RG, Spino S, Henry PJ, et al.: In vitro responsiveness of human asthmatic bronchus to carbachol, histamine, beta-adrenoceptor agonists and theophylline. *Br J Pharmacol* 1986; 22:669.

66. Spina D, Rigby PJ, Paterson JW, Goldie RG: Autoradiographic localization of β-adrenoceptors in asthmatic human lung. *Am Rev Respir Dis* 1989; 140:1410.

67. Bai TR, Prasad FW: Abnormalities in airway smooth muscle in fatal asthma. *Am Rev Respir Dis* 1990; 141:552.

68. Bai TR: Abnormality of airway smooth muscle in fatal asthma. A comparison between trachea and bronchus. *Am Rev Respir Dis* 1991; 143:441.

69. Bai TR, Mak JCW, Barnes PJ: A comparison of beta-adrenergic receptor density and in vitro relaxant responses to isoproterenol in asthmatic airway smooth muscle. *Am J Respir Cell Mol Biol* 1992; 6:647.

70. Whicker SD, Armour CL, Black JL: Responsiveness of bronchial smooth muscle from asthmatic patients to relaxant and contractant agents. *Pulm Pharmacol* 1988; 1:25.

71. Cerrina J, LeRoy LM, Labat C, et al.: Comparison of human bronchial muscle responses to histamine in vivo with histamine and isoproterenol agonists in vitro. *Am Rev Respir Dis* 1986; 134:57.

72. Bai TR: β-Adrenergic receptors in asthma: A current perspective. *Lung* 1992; 170:125.

73. Barnes, PJ: Beta-adrenergic receptors and their regulation. State of the Art. *Am J Respir Crit Care Med* 1995; 152:838.

74. Peters MJ, Adcock IM, Brown CR, Barnes PJ: β-agonist inhibition of steroid-receptor DNA binding activity in human lung. *Am Rev Resp Dis* 1993; No. 4, part 2: A772.

Chapter 43

BETA-ADRENERGIC PHARMACEUTICALS

JOHN W. JENNE

The Evolution of Present Day Beta$_2$-Adrenergic Agonists (Fig. 43-1)

Epinephrine was first extracted and shortly thereafter synthesized in the early 1900s. It was found to be extremely valuable in acute asthma, but it had undesirable pressor and cardiovascular effects. Its action was rather brief, due to the rapid methylation of the 3,4 OH catechol group by catechol-O-methyltransferase (COMT), in situ ("uptake 2") as well as by reuptake in nerve endings ("uptake 1").

By replacing the terminal methyl group of adrenaline with an isopropyl group to produce *isoproterenol* (isoprenaline), the pressor effects were eliminated, and this led to the concept of dual α- and β-adrenergic receptors. Use of isoproterenol by metered-dose inhaler (MDI) and nebulization was popular from 1950 to 1970, but its cardiac stimulation was the major drawback.

Ephedrine, the active ingredient of the ephedra plant used for centuries for its antiasthmatic properties, was synthesized and introduced in the 1930s. Through inhibition reuptake of norepinephrine into nerve endings, this compound mimicked norepinephrine's α- and β-adrenergic properties, which included mild bronchodilation, cardiovascular effects, and central nervous system (CNS) stimulation. When combined with a fixed quantity of theophylline to enhance bronchodilation and a barbiturate to counteract the CNS effects, it was very popular for single and multiple dosing prior to 1970; its use rapidly declined with the introduction of individualized dosing for theophylline and the new β$_2$-adrenergic agonists.

In 1967, Lands proposed that there were distinct β$_1$ and β$_2$ subtypes, the former in heart, adipose tissue, and small intestine, and the latter in smooth muscle of bronchi, vasculature, and uterus.[1] We now know a third adrenoreceptor subtype, β$_3$, in adipose tissue and heart.[2] Many compounds were empirically synthesized in an attempt to accentuate β$_2$-adrenergic properties, the foremost of which was *isoetharine*, which is related to isoproterenol but possesses an ethyl group in the side chain. While somewhat β$_2$-selective, its duration of action is short, since it has a catechol nucleus.

Replacement of the catechol nucleus with a resorcinol group causes considerable prolongation of action (e.g., metaproterenol). However, there is weak β$_2$-selectivity and full agonist activity on cardiac receptors, since metaproterenol otherwise resembles isoproterenol.

Greater β$_2$-adrenergic selectivity was achieved by lengthening the side chain at the 1-position. This has led to development of four new compounds: (1) *albuterol* (salbutamol) is created by adding a *t*-butyl group on the terminal N and a hydroxymethyl group at one of the catechol OH groups forming a saligenin; (2) *terbutaline* is created by adding a *t*-butyl group at the N and forming a 3,5 OH ring grouping (resorcinol) as for metaproterenol; (3) *fenoterol* is created by adding a hydroxyphenyl group on the ring N ("feno" = phenyl) and the 3,5 OH group; and (4) *pirbuterol* is created by inserting an N in the ring but is otherwise similar to albuterol. The racemic mixture of optical enantiomer (+) (−) is used in both inhaled and oral forms.

A more recent development has been the introduction of "pro-drugs," namely *bitolterol*, which is hydrolyzed locally into the active *colterol*, and *bambuterol*, which is hydrolyzed locally to terbutaline. *Tulobuterol* has metabolites that are even more active.

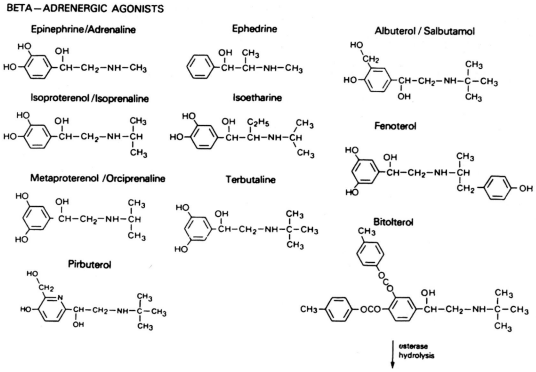

BETA—ADRENERGIC AGONISTS

FIGURE 43-1 Beta-adrenergic agonists and their evolution toward more β_2-selective compounds, with alterations to the N-terminal group of isoproterenol (nonselective) and changes in the catechol ring structure producing more prolonged activity.

Only fenoterol is not available in the United States. In some cases, the two names shown represent U.S. and European nomenclature. Bitolterol is hydrolyzed to colterol.

Most recently, slow-acting, highly β_2-selective compounds have been developed by increasing lipophilicity through bulky additions to the side chain. Such lipophilicity retains the compounds in the vicinity of the receptor through their solubility in the membrane lipid bilayer (see Fig. 43-2). *Formoterol* (formoterol fumarate) and *salmeterol* (salmeterol xinofoate) now are being marketed and will receive detailed attention in this chapter. Previously termed *long-acting* compounds such as albuterol or tertbutaline are now termed *short-acting*.

Modes of Action of Beta₂-Adrenergic Compounds

ELECTRICAL POLARITY AND ION CHANNELS

In its relaxed quiescent state, human airway smooth muscle maintains a net negative voltage (E_m), about -45 mV, across the cell membrane directed internally, principally determined by the equilibrium concentration of K^+ according to the Nernst equation. Human smooth muscle is relatively

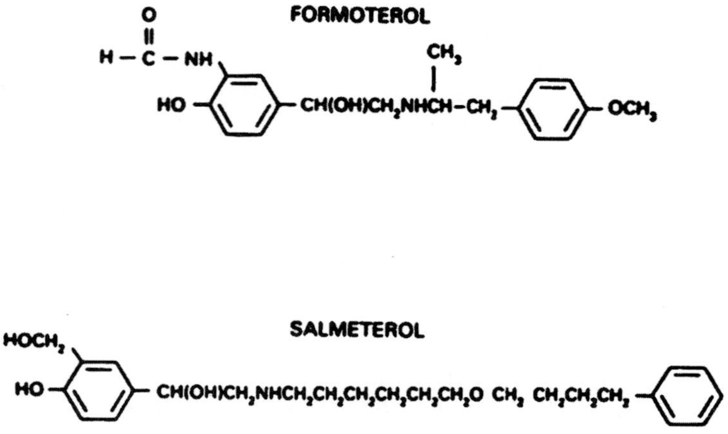

FIGURE 43-2 Structure of new long-acting β_2 adrenergic agonists, formoterol and salmeterol. Note the addition of lipophilic groupings.

quiescent compared to that of other species, but with depolarization, electrical activity increases and contraction is more readily induced by contractile agonists or electrical field stimulation. Conversely, as the E_m becomes more negative, such as from exposure to a bronchodilator, slow waves diminish, and the cell becomes more resistant to contractile influences.

Movement of calcium, potassium, and sodium through the cell membrane takes place through highly selective ion channels. These are relatively impermeable until "opened" by some necessary condition. They can be studied by isolating a very small patch of membrane containing a few channels at the end of a finely tapered pipette ("patch clamp") and measuring their conductivity toward a particular ion as conditions are altered. Thus, any voltage dependency can be studied.

A 10,000-fold gradient exists for calcium between the extracellular concentrations (1 to 2 mM) and the intracellular levels (100 to 700 μM). Airway smooth muscle, like vascular smooth muscle, has voltage-dependent gates that open as the cell becomes depolarized, but, unlike the latter, these channels are not blocked by dipyridine calcium channel blockers, nor do they provide the calcium for the acute phase of agonist contraction.

CONTRACTILE "MACHINERY" OF SMOOTH MUSCLE AND THE EFFECTS OF BETA-ADRENERGIC DRUGS

The inositol phospholipid system (cascade) is an important means of signal transduction in a wide variety of cells, including smooth muscle. Stimulating agonists are linked by their receptor through G proteins to phospholipase C (PLC), a membrane phosphodiesterase whose substrate is phosphoinositol diphosphate (PIP_2). Two products result: (1) water soluble inositol (1,3,4) triphosphate (IP_3) and its related compounds, whose function is to release a sharp spike of calcium from the endoplasmic reticulum, thus initiating cell function; and (2) diactinoyl glycerol (DAG), a lipid-soluble compound remaining in the cell membrane, which sensitizes protein kinase C (PKC) to the lower levels of calcium that follow the initial spike (Fig. 43-3). Once activated, PKC phosphorylates various cell proteins with additional effects. Figure 43-3 shows these processes in smooth muscle.

By forming a complex with calmodulin (Ca_4M), calcium activates myosin light chain kinase (MLC-K), which then initiates the so-called rapid cycling phase of smooth-muscle contraction by phosphorylating MLC at the Ser^{19} residue (Fig. 43-3). As PKC becomes activated, phosporylation of additional contractile proteins occurs, the so-called actin intermediate proteins, which contribute to the sustained ("latched bridge") phase. Calcium concentrations in the sustained state depend upon an external supply.[3] Beta-adrenergic agonists cause an abrupt decrease in unbound calcium through the action of cAMP[4,5] (Fig. 43-4). Two other mechanisms of relaxation involving cAMP are reasonably certain: (1) activation of protein kinase A (PKA), which converts MLC-K to a less active form[6]; and (2) inhibition of PLC hydrolysis of PIP_2, which easily is demonstrated with histamine-contracted respiratory smooth muscle.[7,8]

POTASSIUM CHANNEL ACTIVATION BY BETA-ADRENERGIC DRUGS

Simultaneously with depolarization of a cell during agonist-induced contraction, there commences an increase in the outward K^+ current whose effect is to limit depolarization, rendering the cell more stable. This resistance to depolarization is termed *rectification*. The cell attempts to maintain its negative membrane voltage.

The K channel with the greatest conductivity is the K_{ca} channel, activated by an increase in unbound Ca^{2+} and in the presence of depolarization. This channel is also activated by β-adrenergic drugs. There are two mechanisms. One is through cAMP activation of PKA and subsequent phosphorylation of K-channel proteins. The other is directly through the recombinant G_s alpha protein fragment (α_s-GTP[γS]) not involving cAMP. K-channel activation is now being recognized as a major means of action of β-adrenergic agonists.[9,10]

Figure 43-5 shows the effect of isoproterenol and methacholine on K-channel currents, or "open channel probability" (nP^o) of outside-out patches of porcine tracheal myocytes.[9] Note that isoproterenol and methacholine have opposite actions. This is an example of functional antagonism.

While addition of 0.5 μg/mL cAMP-dependent PKA increased K^+ conduction to its near maximum value compared to control, a further ninefold increase over control was contributed by the addition of the activated α subunit (α_s-GTP[γS]) of the G_s protein. In other experiments, isoproterenol caused as much relaxation as forskolin, with only half the generation of cAMP. Both observations provide strong evidence that an additional, non-cAMP mechanism is involved. This has been an important recent development.

In Vitro Characterization of Bronchodilators

DOSE-RESPONSE TERMINOLOGY

Determination of prospective β$_2$-selective compounds entails the testing of hundreds or thousands of analogs on animal tissues representative of β$_1$- and β$_2$-actions, using isoproterenol as the nonselective reference compound. Thus, Brittain studied metaproterenol (orciprenaline), albuterol (salbutamol), and trimetoquinol on force production by the electrically driven guinea pig left ventrical (β$_1$), the spontaneous rate of the right ventrical (mostly β$_1$), and trachea relaxation (β$_2$).[11] As shown in Fig. 43-6, isoproterenol and metaproterenol are full agonists on right and left atrium, but metaproterenol is considerably less potent. Its EC_{50} [the concentration producing 50 percent of maximum (E_{max}) effect] is shifted several logs to the right. The others are partial agonists. Their E_{max} is clearly less. They have less efficacy, and their intrinsic activity is less than half that of the two full agonists. Against trachea (not shown), all except trimetoquinol are full agonists under these conditions, the latter being a very potent partial agonist with a compound curve suggesting more than one mechanism of action.

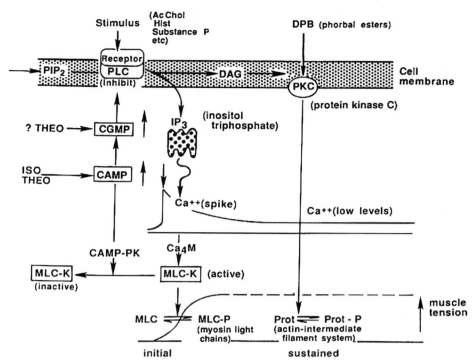

FIGURE 43-3 Two postulated modes of activation of smooth muscle contraction—the calmodulin mode and the protein kinase C (PKC) mode, each activating (phosphorylating) their own set of contractile proteins. Upon receptor stimulation, phosphatidylinositol 4,5-biphosphate (PIP_2) is hydrolyzed by phospholipase C (PLC) to the water-soluble myoinositol 1,4,5-triphosphate (IP_3), which releases calcium from the sarcoplasmic reticulum to produce a calcium spike. This forms a complex with calmodulin (Ca_4M) to activate myosin light chain kinase (MLC-K), thus catalyzing the phosphorylation of myosin light chains in the initial, rapid-cycling phase of muscle contraction. MLC-K (active) is in equilibrium with MLC-K (inactive), and cAMP generation favors the less active form (through cAMP-dependent protein kinase). Cyclic AMP appears to inhibit sharply the action of PLC and hence the breakdown of PIP_2. This is one mechanism of protection against contractile agonists acting at this receptor site. The lipid-soluble diacylglycerol (DAG) sensitizes PKC to low levels of calcium with gradual activation (phosphorylation) of a different set of contractile proteins, the actin-intermediate system, which functions during the sustained phase, along with some contribution from MLC-P. Calcium also continues to trickle in through the cell membrane. The action of cAMP generated by β-adrenergic agonists (ISO) or theophylline (THEO) in inhibiting PLC is indicated, as well as the possible action of cGMP. [*From Jenne JW, Tashkin DP, in Spector SL (ed): Provocative Challenge Procedures: Background and Methodology. Mount Kisco, NY: Futura, 1989; 461, with permission.*]

In an informative and entertaining Lilly Prize Lecture, Dr. David Jack described the development of selective β₂-agonists and the evolving concepts behind them, which culminated in the development of salmeterol.[12] They used guinea pig left atrium and trachea and rat left atrial and lung membranes, using the nonselective beta blocker (I^{125})-(−) diiodopindalol to determine relative affinities. Salbutamol was shown to have a potency at β₂-receptors ≥ 500 times that for β₁-receptors, but an affinity only threefold greater. Therefore, the main cause of selectivity was a *much greater efficacy at the β₂-adrenergic receptor despite appreciable binding to both β₂ and β₁*. This is a most important concept and explains the greater potency of fenoterol on β₂-adrenergic receptors in the left human ventricle compared to albuterol (see below). Potency is a reflection of effective receptor coupling and differs from affinity, which only represents binding per se.

Against inherent tone of superfused human bronchi, the rank order of potency was formoterol, salmeterol, isoproterenol, and albuterol,[13] similar to that seen using electrically contracted guinea pig trachea.[14] A similar order of potency has been found using human bronchi under inherent tone by another group using a conventional immersion bath.[15] Against relaxation by theophylline (assumed to be 100 percent), isoproterenol and formoterol are full agonists, but salbutamol and salmeterol are partial agonists (Fig. 43-7).

EFFECTIVE CONCENTRATIONS, ONSET AND OFFSET OF ACTION

The large differences between compounds in their equieffective concentrations, range of EC_{50}, and the mean onset and recovery times are shown in Table 43-1.[13] One clinical rami-

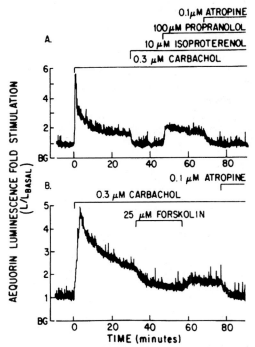

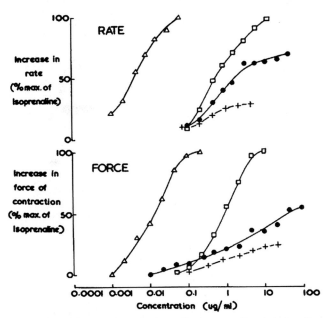

FIGURE 43-4 Effect of isoproterenol and forskolin on the intracellular (Ca^{2+}) response to carbacholine in bovine trachea. While isoproterenol stimulates adenylyl cyclase through its β-adrenergic receptor to produce cAMP, forskolin stimulates the enzyme directly. (*From Takuwa et al.,[4] with permission.*)

FIGURE 43-6 Dose-response curves for isoprenaline (–△–), salbutamol (–●–), orciprenaline (–□–), and trimetoquinol (–+–) in increasing force and rate of contractions of isolated left and right atrial strips, respectively. Each dose-response curve is the mean of four or more individual experiments. (*From Brittain,[11] with permission.*)

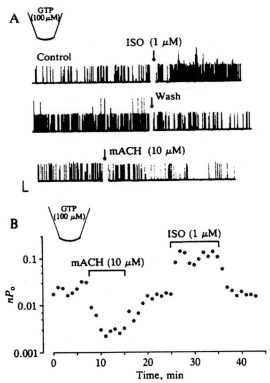

FIGURE 43-5 Stimulation by isoproterenol and inhibition by methacholine of K_{Ca} channel activity in an outside-out patch of a porcine tracheal myocyte. (*A*) The tracing shows current deflections responding to these agonists. (*B*) The currents have been filtered and digitized, expressed as the probability (nP°) of channel opening. The agonists are functionally antagonistic. (*From Kume et al.,[9] with permission.*)

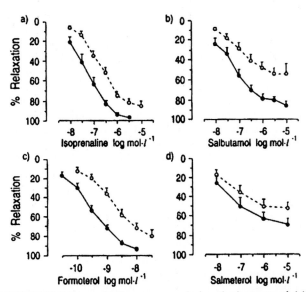

FIGURE 43-7 Concentration-response (relaxation) curves of: (a) isoprenaline; (b) salbutamol; (c) formoterol; and (d) salmeterol on isolated human bronchi, expressed as a percentage of maximal theophylline relaxation (3×10^{-3}mol/L). Experiments were performed on preparations at resting tone (●) or precontracted with acetylcholine 10^{-3}mol/L (○). Values are mean ± SEM. (*From Naline AT et al.: Eur J Pharmacol 1994; 251:127, with permission.*)

TABLE 43-1 Human Isolated Bronchus: Relaxant Potencies, Onset, and Offset of β-Adrenoreceptor Agonists

Agonist	Equieffective Concentration, nM (Isoprenaline = 1)	Onset $t_{1/2}$, min	Recovery $t_{1/2}$, min	n
Isoprenaline	1.0 [EC_{50} = 26.6 (18.9–36.4)]	1.5 (± 0.1)	2.2 (± 0.3)	14
Clenbuterol	0.2 (0.02–1.36)	2.3 (± 0.9)	12.7 (± 5.4)	5
Fenoterol	0.9 (0.1–11.3)	2.1 (± 0.4)	4.6 (± 0.9)	4
Formoterol	0.05 (0.02–0.10)	5.3 (± 1.4)	6.6 (± 1.3)	5
Quinprenaline	141 (55–235)	—	≥20 (20–>180)	3
Salbutamol	9 (2–44)	3.3 (± 0.3)	6.8 (± 1.3)	5
Salmeterol	0.09 (0.06–0.13)	35.6 (± 4.6)	>275	8
Terbutaline	5.4 (3.9–7.6)	3.0 (± 0.4)	6.9 (± 1.9)	4

NOTE: Potency values are expressed as geometric means (with 95% confidence limits) or range, in parentheses; onset and duration values are expressed as arithmetic means (± SEM) or range.
SOURCE: From Nials et al.[13]

fication of this is that while even formoterol itself could suffice as a "rescue" bronchodilator when bronchospasm is "breaking through," salmeterol is inadequate because of its long onset time. A short-acting drug is needed and is a crucial concomitant to the use of salmeterol.

The realization that lipophilicity increases duration of action spawned many new compounds, only two of which, formoterol and salmeterol, have reached the market. Yet despite similar q 12 h dosing patterns, there are several fundamental differences between these two in their in vitro behavior:

1. The recovery half-life for formoterol is very sensitive to the initial concentration, while that from salmeterol is relatively insensitive. Figure 43-8 illustrates this.[16] When drug-free buffer is introduced following varying concentrations and relaxation, recovery half-life is surprisingly short for formoterol, little more than for albuterol, but dependent on the concentration that was present. No concentration dependency is seen with salmeterol.

2. Another difference between formoterol and salmeterol is the phenomenon of "delayed activation" for the latter. Despite the removal of salmeterol from the muscle bath, the receptor continues to be slowly loaded up during a prolonged period. This is related to its slow onset of relaxation, seen in vitro and in vivo. It is as if the lipid depot becomes charged rapidly but is not easily discharged and continues to load the receptor in a rate-limiting process, as seen in Fig. 43-9.[17]

3. Finally, there is a difference in the "reassertion" of drug temporarily displaced by a β-adrenoreceptor antagonist. While exposure to a β-adrenoreceptor antagonist quickly terminates the smooth muscle relaxing effect of salmeterol in vitro, its removal by washing is rapidly accompanied by reassertion of its action. This is not the case for formoterol, as the action does not resume to the same degree with repeated washing and soon is gone. Figure 43-10 shows the phenomenon of reassertion of salmeterol on electrically pulsed guinea pig trachea in vitro.[14] Sotalol, a water-soluble β-adrenergic antagonist, easily blocks relaxing activity (i.e., the active site is readily accessible to a hydrophilic antagonist), but, once removed with washing,

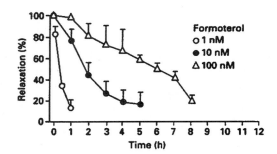

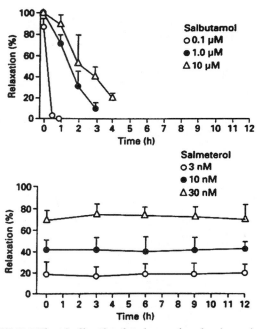

FIGURE 43-8 Electrically stimulated superfused guinea pig trachea. The relationship between the concentration of β-adrenoreceptor agonist and the duration of inhibitory action for: *upper panel:* formoterol (1 nM, ○; 10 nM, ●; 100 nM, △); *middle panel:* salbutamol (0.1 μM, ○; 1.0 μM, ●; 10 μM, △); and *lower panel:* salmeterol (3 nM, ○; 10 nM, ●; 30 nM, △). Values are arithmetic means of at least four experiments. Vertical bars represent SEM. (*From Johnson et al.,[16] with permission.*)

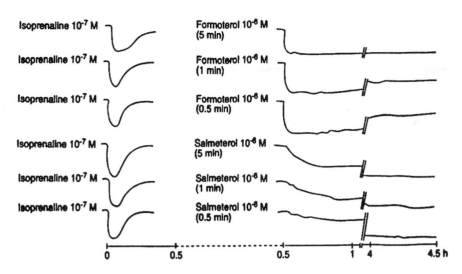

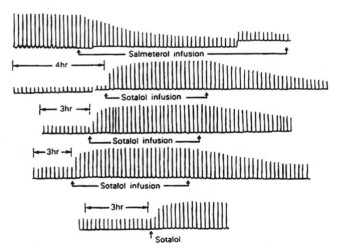

FIGURE 43-9 Relaxation of continually superfused airway smooth muscle with drug exposure for the indicated times. This illustrates the principle that while the rate of onset of activity of salmeterol is related to the duration of exposure, the maximal effect is independent of contact time and continues to build up despite removal of drug. Apparently the drug is "charging" a reservoir from which drug continues to diffuse into the active configuration despite removal from surrounding medium. (*From Anderson et al.,*[17] *with permission.*)

the original activity returns at the same level. This behavior is best visualized as due to the movement of the "head" portion of salmeterol in and out of position while the rest of the molecule, or "tail," remains firmly anchored in another (inactive) part of the β-adrenoreceptor (or a membrane site close to the active site). The length of the molecule is consistent with either of these possibilities.

Studies using artificial lipid bilayer membranes show that, despite its great lipophilicity, salmeterol leaves the bilayer into an aqueous media with a half-life of only 25 min. This is inadequate to explain its long duration of effect.[18] Indeed, the ability of salmeterol to maintain its original activity in guinea pig trachea despite continuing perfusion by buffer suggests that salmeterol is so firmly fixed in place at the receptor that its eventual loss of activity after hours may be due to receptor turnover and renewal.

FIGURE 43-10 Transient reversal of salmeterol-induced relaxant response in the superfused, electrically stimulated guinea pig trachea by sotalol. Note the reassertion of salmeterol inhibition when the sotalol infusion is terminated. The "tail" of salmeterol apparently remains firmly at the active site, while the "head" is temporarily displaced. (*From Nials et al.,*[14] *with permission.*)

THE CONCEPT OF PLASMALEMMA MICROKINETIC DIFFUSION

A concept has been developed to explain these behaviors by Anderson et al., as diagrammed in Fig. 43-11.[17] Hydrophilic, short-acting bronchodilators such as salbutamol remain in the aqueous biophase and are applied directly to the receptor. Their onset of action is diffusion-limited, and their effectiveness over several hours most likely due to drug held in the adjacent tissues. Formoterol, a lipophilic agonist, is rapidly taken up (1 min) by the "lipid depot" of the lipid bilayer, whence it is slowly released to the receptor via the aqueous phase as long as drug is still in the depot. The long duration of action after an administration by MDI is due to the very high concentrations presented and stored. Salmeterol, which is even more lipophilic than formoterol, is also rapidly taken up by the lipid depot, but its transfer to the receptor occurs at an extremely slow rate-limiting process, possibly directly through the membrane to receptor, and is less concentration-dependent. This process may be slowed as well due to an unfavorable energy of activation (E_a) before becoming effectively coupled to the active site.

ADVERSE EFFECTS OF SALMETEROL ON BETA$_2$-ADRENERGIC RECEPTOR?

A perplexing feature of salmeterol is its ability at greater than usual concentrations to mimic β$_2$-adrenergic agonist actions by some mechanism not susceptible to β-adrenoreceptor blockade. Thus, while failing itself to inhibit leukotriene D$_4$ (LTD$_4$)–induced H$_2$O$_2$ generation by guinea pig and human eosinophils, 10 μM competitively antagonizes the ability of formoterol to do so.[19] While 1 μM salmeterol itself relaxes guinea pig trachea, an action sensitive to a β-adrenoreceptor antagonism, at 10 μM, salmeterol blocks the action of formoterol, and this action is not sensitive to a β-adrenoreceptor blockade.[20] While salmeterol itself relaxes human bronchi by a β$_2$-adrenergic receptor, 1 μM salmeterol mediates action, decreasing the efficacy of epinephrine by 1.7 logs.[15]

As a partial agonist, salmeterol could in theory be expected to inhibit the action of a full agonist in a competi-

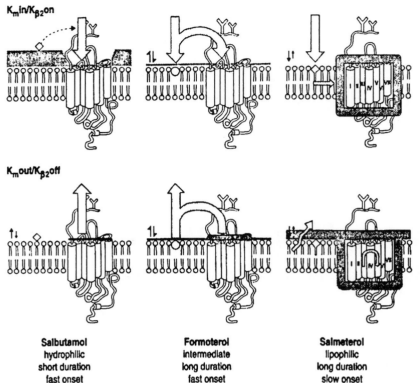

FIGURE 43-11 Diffusion microkinetic model contrasting movement on and off receptor of salbutamol, formoterol, and salmeterol. The thick shaded areas represent energetically unfavorable barriers to drug passage, and the large arrows major drug movement. Salbutamol, due to its high hydrophilicity, associates rapidly with the receptor but also diffuses from the tissue rapidly, causing a short duration of action. Formoterol, which is more lipophilic than salbutamol, associates with both lipid membrane and receptor rapidly, but is released from the lipid membrane over an extended period of time while it continues to keep the receptor charged. Salmeterol, even more lipophilic, associates predominantly with the lipid membrane and its interaction with the receptor is energetically unfavorable, causing a slow onset of action but avid retention and long duration of activity. (*From Anderson et al.,[17] with permission.*)

tive manner, if present in an adequate concentration, and this has now been demonstrated in vitro with those β_2 agonists (with higher efficacy including albuterol).[20a] Could this become clinically relevant? There are at least two reports that suggest this. In one, three young asthma patients were placed on salmeterol in addition to other therapy which, for two of these patients, included oral corticosteroids and nebulized albuterol. Another patient with more mild disease with exercise-induced bronchospasm, received oral terbutaline. Between 1 and 4 weeks later, each experienced the rapid progression of an attack, poorly responsive to nebulized β-adrenergic agonist. The patient with mild disease developed severe exercise-induced asthma after vigorous exertion. While the temporal relation to salmeterol may have been coincidental, the authors note that each patient from the outset did not have the expected improvement on salmeterol. They felt compelled to publish the cases with the advice that patients not responding to salmeterol should not be continued on it.[21]

A second report describes an asthma patient who responded appropriately to salbutamol and to formoterol when used alone but did not when these were preceded by salmeterol; nor did he respond to salmeterol alone. The case is well documented with pulmonary function.[22] It may be that a rare asthma patient idiosyncratically fails to respond to salmeterol, perhaps because of an altered receptor, but the presence of the drug prevents normal responses to endogenous and/or exogenous β_2-adrenergic stimulation. What still are needed are systematic studies of the effect of underlying long-acting β-adrenergic agonists on the dose-response

curves to conventional β_2-adrenergic agonists, both initially in the treatment and later when tachyphylaxis or other receptor changes may have occurred. The first such study has appeared showing a 2.5-fold shift to the right on the dose-response curve to albuterol, (ΔFEV_1) in patients on salmeterol.[23] However, the subsensitivity claimed seems to depend on a slight inequality of the initial baseline values, and would disappear if absolute values of FEV_1 were used. Clearly, more studies are needed on this crucial issue.

References

1. Lands AM, Arnold A, McAuliff JP, et al.: Differentiation of receptor systems activated by sympathomimetic amines. *Nature* 1967; 214:597.
2. Kaumann AJ: Is there a third heart beta-adrenoceptor. *Trends Pharmacol Sci* 1989; 10:316.
3. Rasmussen H: The calcium messenger system (pt II). *N Engl J Med* 1986; 314:1164.
4. Takuwa Y, Takuwa N, Rasmussen H: The effect of isoproterenol on intracellular calcium concentration. *J Biol Chem* 1988; 263:762.
5. Rasmussen H, Kelly G, Douglas JS: Interactions between Ca^{2+} and cAMP messenger muscle contraction. *Am J Physiol* 1990; 258:L279.
6. de Lanerolle P, Paul RJ: Myosin phosphorylation/dephosphorylation and regulation of airway smooth muscle contractility. *Am J Physiol* 1991; 261:L1.
7. van Amsterdam RGM, Meurs H, TenBerge EJ, et al.: Role of phosphoinositide metabolism in human bronchial smooth muscle contraction and in functional antagonism by beta-adrenoceptor agonists. *Am Rev Respir Dis* 1990; 142:1124.

Salbutamol
hydrophilic
short duration
fast onset

Formoterol
intermediate
long duration
fast onset

Salmeterol
lipophilic
long duration
slow onset

$K_m in/K_{\beta 2} on$

$K_m out/K_{\beta 2} off$

8. Hall IP, Hill SJ: β-Adrenoceptor stimulation inhibits histamine-stimulated inositol phospholipid hydrolysis in bovine tracheal smooth muscle. *Br J Pharmacol* 1988; 95:1204.

9. Kume H, Graziano MP, Kotlikoff MI: Stimulatory and inhibitory regulation of calcium-activated potassium channels by guanine nucleotide-binding protein. *Proc Natl Acad Sci USA* 1992; 89:11051.

10. Kume H, Hall IP, Washabau RJ, et al.: β-Adrenergic agonists regulate K_{Ca} channels in airway smooth muscle by cAMP-dependent and -independent mechanisms. *J Clin Invest* 1994; 93:371.

11. Brittain RT: A comparison of the pharmacology profile of salbutamol with that of isoproterenol, orciprenaline (metaproterenol) and trimetoquinol. *Postgrad Med J* 1971; 47:11.

12. Jack D: A way of looking at agonism and antagonism: Lessons from albuterol, salmeterol, and other β-adrenoceptor agonists. *Br J Clin Pharmacol* 1991; 31:501.

13. Nials AT, Coleman RA, Johnson M, et al.: Effect of beta-adrenoceptor agonists in human bronchial smooth muscle. *Br J Pharmacol* 1993; 110:1112.

14. Nials AT, Sumner MT, Johnson M, Coleman RA: Investigation into factors determining the duration of action of the β_2-adrenoceptor agonist, salmeterol. *Br J Pharmacol* 1993; 108:507.

15. Naline E, Zhang Y, Qian Y, et al.: Relaxant effects and durations of action of formoterol and salmeterol on the isolated human bronchus. *Eur Respir J* 1994; 7:914.

16. Johnson M, Butchers PR, Coleman RA, et al.: The pharmacology of salmeterol. *Life Sci* 1993; 52:2131.

17. Anderson GP, Linden A, Rabe KF: Why are long-acting beta-adrenergic agonists long-acting? *Eur Respir J* 1994; 7:569.

18. Rhodes DB, Newton R, Butler R, Herbette L: Equilibrium and kinetic studies of the interactions of salmeterol with membrane bilayers. *Mol Pharmacol* 1992; 42:596.

19. Rabe KF, Giembycz MA, Dent G, et al.: Salmeterol is a competitive antagonist at beta-adrenoceptors mediating inhibition of respiratory burst in guinea pig eosinophils. *Eur J Pharmacol* 1993; 231:305.

20. Jeppsson AB, Kallstrom RL, Waldeck B: Studies on the interaction between formoterol and salmeterol in guinea pig trachea in vitro. *Pharmacol Toxicol* 1992; 71:272.

20a. Källström B-L, Sjöberg J, Waldeck B: The interaction between salmeterol and β_2-adrenoceptor agonists with higher efficacy on guinea-pig trachea and human bronchus in vitro. *Br J Pharmacol* 1994; 113:687.

21. Clark CE, Ferguson AD, Siddorn JA: Respiratory arrests in young asthmatics on salmeterol. *Respir Med* 1993; 87:227.

22. Ulrik CS, Kok-Jensen A: Different bronchodilating effect of salmeterol and formoterol in an adult asthmatic. *Eur Respir J* 1994; 7:1003.

23. Grove A, Lipworth BJ: Bronchodilator subsensitivity to salbutamol after twice daily salmeterol in asthmatic patients. *Lancet* 1995; 346:201.

Chapter 44

PHYSIOLOGIC ACTIONS OF BETA-ADRENERGIC AGONISTS

JOHN W. JENNE

An excellent discussion of recent work on the actions of β_2-adrenergic agonists is that of Kendall and Haffner.[1] Table 44-1 lists these actions, and the emphasis in this chapter is on those actions important to pulmonary clinicians.

Mucociliary Transport

The actions of β_2-adrenergic agonists on mucociliary behavior in humans are still conjectural. The velocity of mucus transport is highly dependent on the rheologic properties and quantity of mucus and underlying periciliary fluid. The bronchial epithelium absorbs salt and water from the surface fluid and thus regulates the depth of mucus, which normally is 2 to 5 μM. In some species, both β-adrenergic and cholinergic agonists increase basal chloride secretion and slow sodium absorption and hence slow or reverse water flow.[2] On human epithelium, β_2-adrenergic agonists appear to have little effect on chloride secretion.[3]

Respiratory mucus is constituted from secretions from many cell types but primarily from submucus glands. During abnormal states, many chemical entities alter its character. Information gained from animal tissues is not necessarily transferable to humans.[4] Sampling of submucosal gland ducts with micropipettes established that α-adrenergic agonists cause a thin secretion arising from serous cells, while β-adrenergic agonists produce a scanty fluid of high protein content, presumably from mucus cells. Muscarinic agonists stimulate both cell types.[5] In human airways, in vitro α-adrenergic agonists increase mucus secretion, but β-adrenergic agonists have no effect.[6] Another group, however, has reported glycoprotein synthesis and secretion by both α- and β-adrenergic stimulation.[7]

Beta$_2$-adrenergic agonists increase ciliary beat frequency. Inhalation of 1000 μg terbutaline by metered-dose inhaler (MDI) actually doubles whole lung clearance of labeled albumen aerosols, as revealed by scintigraphy.[8] The response to an allergen includes an increased ciliary beat frequency, but mucus transport is slowed. Prior inhalation of disodium cromoglycate, FPL 55712, or terbutaline prevents the slowing, and it must be considered that some of this action by terbutaline is caused by inhibition of mast cell discharge.[9]

The concentration of a β-adrenergic agonist that is achieved in the surface layer of a bronchus is not known. It has been calculated that if 5 percent of an inhaled dose of albuterol were contained in the fluid layer of the human trachea and main bronchi, with a calculated volume of 1.4 mL, the concentration would be 30 μM.[10] Using cultured rabbit epithelial cells, these authors found that such a concentration, if sustained, "shut down" the generation of cyclic adenosine monophosphate (cAMP) through tachyphylaxis. Bradykinin also depressed the system, presumably because of negative feedback by generated protein kinase C. Thus,

TABLE 44-1   Actions of Beta$_2$-Adrenergic Agonists

HEART		LUNG	
Tachycardia	S A node, right atrium	Bronchodilation	Large, small airways
Increased CO	Peripheral vasodilation	Mucociliary	↑ Ciliary beat frequency, glycoprotein synthesis
Inotropism	Left ventricle (β_1,β_2)		↑ Cl$^-$, H$_2$O, epithelium
			↑ Surfactant secretion
ECG	↑ QT$_c$, ↓ QS$_2$ index, T wave		
Myocardial necrosis	Proportional β_1, animals, ? humans	Pulmonary vasodilation	↓ P$_{O_2}$ ($\dot{V}/\dot{Q}$)
Arrhythmias	Most asymptomatic, concern when heart disease	Anti-inflammatory	Mast cells, PMN ↓ Capillary permeability

SYSTEMIC			
Effect	Cause	Effect	Cause
Hypokalemia	Insulin release Muscle Na$^+$, K$^+$-ATPase	↑ Pulse pressure Tremor	↓ Peripheral resistance ↑ Force, fast twitch fib. ↓ Force, slow twitch fib.
Hyperglycemia	Glycogenolysis Gluconeogenesis	↑ Lactate	
Increased FFA	Lipolysis ($\beta_2>\beta_1,?\beta_3$)	↑ cAMP	Various tissues ($\beta_2>\beta_1$)
Hypomagnesemia		↑ renin	
Thermogenesis	↑ O$_2$, CO$_2$ R.Q.=k	Uterine relaxation Detrusor relaxation	

there is a risk in generalizing from results obtained acutely to chronic effects.

Anti-Inflammatory Actions of Beta$_2$-Adrenergic Agonists

Several lines of experimental evidence suggest that β_2-adrenergic agonists have an anti-inflammatory effect, but this has been difficult to translate clinically. The most striking evidence was the demonstration that 2 puffs of either salbutamol or sodium cromoglycate inhibited the increase in serum histamine or neutrophil chemotactic factor that ensued upon inhalational allergen challenge.[11] Albuterol also inhibits discharge of mediators from mast cells in sensitized human lung fragments at appropriately low concentrations[12] as well as the release of histamine, leukotriene C$_4$, and prostaglandin D$_2$ (PGD$_2$).[13] In the latter study, formoterol and salmeterol also inhibited mediator discharge at suitably lower concentrations, with sensitivities in the order formoterol > isoproterenol > salmeterol > albuterol.

Beta$_2$-adrenergic agonists readily inhibit the respiratory burst of human peripheral neutrophils, but tachyphylaxis soon develops[14] and, in concentrations $\leq 10^{-8}$ M, albuterol inhibits peroxidase release from sensitized eosinophils.[15] Rabe et al. found that, whereas albuterol and formoterol inhibited the release of H$_2$O$_2$ from sensitized guinea pig eosinophils, salmeterol did not. Yet salmeterol had the ability to block the others competitively.[16]

Beta$_2$-adrenergic agonists have also been shown to possess antipermeability actions in animal models whose mucous membranes are irritated by toxic substances. Considerable work on the mechanism of their protective action has led to the proposal that relaxation of contractile elements in the endothelium of postcapillary venules reduces pore size and closes gap junctions between cells.[17] The intact guinea pig has been very useful to demonstrate the relative efficacy of β_2-adrenergic agonists in reducing airway permeability caused by inhaled irritants such as histamine or bradykinin. Thus, Advenier et al. showed that formoterol and salbutamol inhaled prior to inhaled bradykinin inhibited microvascular leakage into airways.[18] Salmeterol, 100 μg/mL, strongly inhibited the appearance of histamine-induced labeled plasma protein into bronchial lavage fluids for at least 8 h, while 1.0 mg/mL albuterol inhibited extravasation for 2 h.[19]

In the latter study, both drugs also inhibited the accumulation of neutrophils induced by an aerosol of lipopolysaccharide. Both anti-inflammatory effects of β_2-adrenergic agonists were blocked by propranolol. For guinea pigs receiving 10 μg/mL nebulized formoterol for 2 min (15 minutes preceding challenge) the late-phase response was inhibited completely, and the cellular influx (macrophages, eosinophils, neutrophils, lymphocytes) obtained by bronchoalveolar lavage (BAL) 24 h after antigen challenge also was blocked.[20] Aerosolization of 2 mg/mL albuterol before the 4 h after antigen challenge reduced the neutrophils in bronchial lavage fluid collected 24 h later and tended to reduce eosinophils.[21] Hutson et al. published results showing an effect principally on neutrophils, but the dose was only 0.1 mg/mL nebulized albuterol.[22]

PATIENT STUDIES

With the advent of formoterol and salmeterol, the question of an anti-inflammatory effect assumed prime importance. In a sufficient dose, albuterol was shown to block the airway obstruction of the late-phase response completely,[23] as did usual doses of salmeterol[24] and formoterol.[25] This was surprising in view of the inflammatory genesis of this obstruction.

Further studies using more controls suggested that the inherent bronchodilation of the β_2-adrenergic agonist accounted for all the reversal of obstruction in the late phase. Weersink et al. gave a single dose of 50 μg salmeterol by MDI to asthmatic patients challenged with house dust mite. Serum markers for eosinophilic degranulation, eosinophil cationic protein (ECP) and eosinophil-derived neurotoxin (EDN), with the allergic response, were unaffected by salmeterol.[26] A similar study was done with 24 μg formoterol, again with no effect on the rise in serum ECP, nor the lymphocyte CD25 marker [interleukin 2R (IL-2R)], nor eosinophils in blood and sputum.[27]

Using BAL in stable asthma patients, Adelroth et al. compared 600 μg budesonide bid and 500 μg terbutaline qid, sampling serum ECP before and after 4 weeks.[28] There was a definite decrease in ECP levels for patients receiving budesonide, a suggestive reduction (decrease in four, increase in one) in the patients receiving terbutaline, and no changes in the cell populations on either regimen. The authors felt the results were inconclusive. Laitinen et al. placed patients with mild asthma on either 600 mg budesonide bid or 2 puffs of terbutaline bid. Bronchial biopsies before and after 12 weeks of therapy revealed a normalization of epithelium in the corticosteroid-treated patients, but no change in the damaged epithelium of the terbutaline-treated patients. Several cell types in the epithelium were reduced in the corticosteroid-treated group (eosinophils, neutrophils, lymphocytes, plasma cells), but only lymphocytes were reduced in the patients treated with terbutaline.[29]

Asthma patients on 6 to 8 weeks of salmeterol or placebo have shown no changes by BAL in lymphocytes with CD4, CD8, HLA-DR, and CD25 markers[30]; biopsy counts for mast cells (Aal), eosinophils (ES-2), CD3, CD4, and CD8; nor in BAL assays for albumin, histamine, PGD, and ECP.[31]

Heart and Vasculature

Systemic administration of a β_2-adrenergic agonist, or inhalation of a sufficiently large dose, produces an increase in heart rate, a slight increase in contractile force, a decrease in peripheral vascular resistance, and an increase in cardiac output. The increase in rate is primarily caused by action on peripheral β_2-adrenergic receptors but also is a consequence of direct stimulation of rate-determining tissues in the right atrium.

RECEPTORS

In the hearts of most species, β_2-adrenergic receptors coexist with β_1-adrenergic receptors but are in the minority. Human hearts contain a higher proportion than other mammals, from 25 to 60 percent of the total by various estimates[32,33] and highest in the order sinoatrial node > right atrium > ventricle.[34] Radioligand-binding studies indicate a β_1-/β_2-adrenergic receptor ratio of approximately 65:35 in human left atrium and left ventricle and 50:50 in human right atrium as determined in different laboratories.[35,36] In the canine left ventricle, 80 to 90 percent of β-adrenoreceptors are β_1, as are the majority in coronary arteries, while β_2-adrenergic receptors predominate in arterioles.[37]

Beta$_2$-adrenergic receptors in the heart are believed to be more tightly coupled than β_1-adrenoreceptors[38] and are more likely to activate adenylyl cyclase at lower concentrations compared to β_1-adrenoreceptors.[39] However, if β_1-adrenergic receptors are regulated neuronally, and β_2-adrenergic receptors through the circulation,[40] then β_1-adrenergic receptors would be exposed to greater concentrations of catecholamines (micromolar) than would β_2-adrenergic receptors (nanomolar).[41] Thus, experiments done in these tissue baths do not necessarily duplicate the physiologic situation. The described effect of stimulating either adrenoreceptor subtype depends upon its location and on the efficacy of the particular agonists. In the right atrium, both subtypes produce a rate increase, while in the left atrium and left ventricle, either subtype increases force.[42] Using guinea pig atrium, Brittain showed that isoproterenol and metaproterenol were full agonists on both right and left atrium, while albuterol and trimetoquinol were partial agonists whose dose-response curves did not reach the same maximum effect (E_{max}) at any concentration (see Fig. 43-6).[43] Terbutaline and salmeterol are also partial agonists, while fenoterol is a full agonist.[44]

While both albuterol and fenoterol have affinity for either adrenoreceptor subtype, only fenoterol has efficacy for both in the left ventricle of humans. Albuterol has efficacy for only β_2-adrenergic receptors and is still a partial agonist. Its intrinsic activity (E_{max}) is far less than for fenoterol on left ventricular force, 11 percent compared to 130 percent, respectively.[42,45,46] These studies provide an adequate explanation for the greater cardiac effects of fenoterol in vivo.

The effect of fenoterol exceeds that of albuterol. Figures 44-1 and 44-2 and Tables 44-2 and 44-3 document the effect of large doses by MDI and nebulization.[47–50]

LEFT VENTRICULAR CONTRACTILITY

Albuterol and terbutaline cause minimal inotropism compared to isoproterenol. Graded doses of isoproterenol and albuterol were administered intravenously to six patients during cardiac catheterization studies of mitral stenosis.[51] At the maximum dosages used, the results shown in Table 44-4 were found. Both drugs caused an increase in whole body oxygen uptake and central blood volume and a decrease in peripheral resistance. Despite equal effects in decreasing

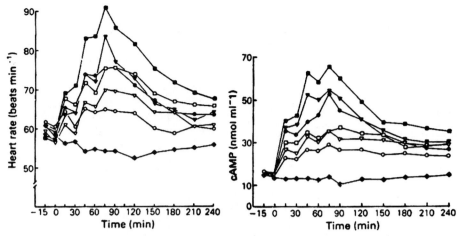

FIGURE 44-1 Effects of cumulative applications of inhaled fenoterol and salbutamol by metered-dose inhaler on heart rate and plasma cyclic AMP in normal individuals; (◆) placebo, (○) 1200 μg albuterol, (▽) 1800 μg albuterol, (□) 2400 μg albuterol, (●) 1200 μg fenoterol, (▼) 1800 μg fenoterol, and (■) 2400 μg

fenoterol. Note that 1200 μg fenoterol gives about the same increase in heart rate as 2400 μg albuterol but more cAMP, the latter being a β_2-adrenergic response. (*Adapted from Scheinin et al.,*[47] *with permission.*)

FIGURE 44-2 The effects of treatment (mean ± SEM) with nebulized drugs on heart rate (HR), electromechanical systole (QS_2I), plasma potassium (K^+), and forced expiratory volume in 1 s (FEV_1) in the four subjects who received two consecutive doses

of drug. (◇) Ipratropium bromide, 0.5 mg, and (■) fenoterol; (□) salbutamol, each at 5.0 mg. (*From Bremner P et al.,* Respir Med *1992; 86:419, with permission.*)

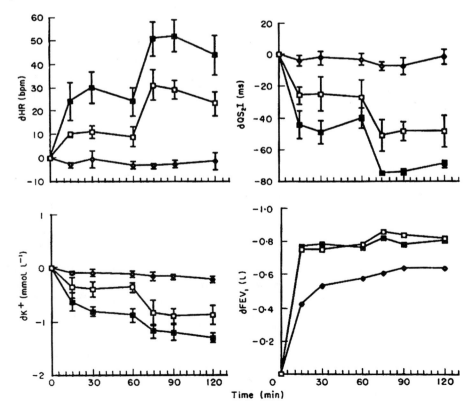

TABLE 44-2   Cumulative Effect 5 min after 400, 600, and 800 μg of Beta-Adrenergic Agonists Given Consecutively by MDI at 15-min Intervals on Cardiovascular Parameters (the 600 μg Data are Omitted)[a]

Parameter	Time	Dose	Placebo	Isoproterenol	Fenoterol	Albuterol
Heart rate	5	400	−2.2	5	4.5	3.4
	35	800	−3.0	6.9	16.9	4.1
QS_2 index[b]	5	400	1.8	−14.4	−6.9	−6.3
	35	800	9.1	−31	−30	−13.2
QT_c	5	400	−7	8	8	10
	35	800	0	20	30	20
Systolic blood pressure	5	400	2.4	6.3	5.6	0.9
	35	800	0.8	14.0	16.7	8.8
Diastolic blood pressure	5	400	−2.3	−7.7	−7.3	−9.4
	35	800	0.9	−11.9	−11.2	−11.1

[a] Mean values only.
[b] The QS_2 index is the QS_2 interval corrected for heart rate. The QS_2 interval is the duration of electromechanical systole. A decrease in QS_2 index is a measure of positive inotropic effect.
SOURCE: Adapted from Crane J, Burgess C, Beasley R, *Thorax* 1989; 44:136–140 with permission.

TABLE 44-3   Successive MDI Dosing (in μg) in Patients with Asthma

	SALBUTAMOL		FENOTEROL		ISOPROTERENOL	
	400	1600	400	1600	400	1600
FEV_1 (L)	0.4	0.6	0.6	0.7	0.4	0.6
QS_2 index (ms)[a]	0.3	−6.1	−5.7	−16.1	−21.5	−36.4
K^+ (mM/L)	−0.1	−0.5	−0.2	−0.8	−0.2	−0.4

[a] For definition of QS_2 index, see footnote to Table 44-2.
SOURCE: From Nials AT, Coleman RA, Johnson M, et al: *Br J Pharmacol* 1993; 110:1112, with permission.

TABLE 44-4   Effects of Intravenous Isoproterenol and Salbutamol in Humans (Mean Values in Six Patients with Mitral Valve Disease, ± SD)

	ISOPROTERENOL		SALBUTAMOL	
	Control	0.1 μg/kg	Control	2.0 lg/kg
Heart rate (beats/min)	70 ± 7.8	+10.6 ± 5.0	78 ± 13.0	+25.5 ± 7.5
Cardiac output (L/min)	2.8 ± 0.5	+1.05 ± 0.35	3.0 ± 0.65	+1.1 ± 7.5
Peripheral resistance (units)	38.0 ± 2.0	−12.5 ± 3.8	37.0 ± 7.4	−14.4 ± 4.1
Ejection time (ms)	280 ± 250	−48.0 ± 30.0	250 ± 150	−15.0 ± 8.3
Ejection rate (mL/s)	135 ± 20	+62 ± 27.0	160 ± 24.0	+8.0 ± 11.2
Stroke volume	39.0 ± 4.5	+7.6 ± 2.6	38.0 ± 5.5	+0.7 ± 2.1

SOURCE: From Gibson and Coltart,[51] with permission.

peripheral resistance, the minimal increase in ejection rate and stroke volume from albuterol contrasted sharply with the stimulatory effect of isoproterenol on myocardial contractility.

The increase in heart rate induced by intravenous infusion of albuterol in normal adults can be increased further by hypoxemia and further still by a combination of hypoxemia and hypercapnea induced by breathing decreased concentrations of O_2 and increased concentrations of CO_2.[52]

In severe left ventricular dysfunction, β_2-selective agonists have been shown to exert both afterload reduction and positive inotropism without energy cost to the myocardium.[53] Thus, in 10 patients with severe arteriosclerotic heart disease, an oral dose of 20 mg pirbuterol was compared to 6 mg albuterol. These two drugs had indistinguishable effects, consisting of a decrease in systemic vascular resistance from 23 to 19 units, an increase in cardiac output from 3.7 to 4.5 L/min; an increase in maximum left ventricular dp/dt from 821 to 1411 mmHg/s; but no change in myocardial O_2 uptake or extraction of lactate, glucose, and free fatty acids. Similar results are shown with intravenous terbutaline.[54] The authors concluded that positive inotropism occurred without cost to the myocardium. In intact dogs, relatively high doses of albuterol enhanced left ventricular function with increased coronary flow but, in contrast to metaproterenol and isoproterenol, did not deplete high-energy stores of the myocardium, while consuming much less oxygen.[55]

HEART RATE AND PERIPHERAL VASCULAR RESISTANCE

While usual doses of albuterol or terbutaline by MDI have little or no effect on heart rate, a large dose, such as the 10 puffs of albuterol given over 10 min by MDI to nonmedicated patients with mild asthma, produced a surprising widening of pulse pressure and a mean increase in heart rate of 23 percent, maximal after 5 min and detectable up to 150 min.[56] An increase in insulin paralleled these changes. Yet, when 2 puffs of albuterol were administered at 25-min intervals (up to 13 puffs), there was no increase in heart rate as there was with fenoterol.[57] Fenoterol is clearly more potent than albuterol on heart rate, cAMP elevation, and in causing decrease in serum potassium when cumulative doses by MDI ≤ 2400 µg are compared[47] (Fig. 44-1).

Although 2 puffs, or 400 µg, fenoterol produced only small effects on heart rate and blood pressure in normal adults, mean cardiac output was increased 26 percent 15 min later and was accompanied by an 18 percent mean decrease in peripheral vascular resistance, a 16 percent increase in stroke volume, and an 18 percent increase in velocity of circumferential shortening of the left ventricle.[41] Surprisingly, there was no demonstrable tolerance to these effects after 2 weeks of regular therapy. The authors emphasized that mere observance of pulse rate and blood pressure can underestimate the effects of metered dose inhalers on the cardiovascular system.

Changes in cardiac output following the initial dose of a systemic β_2-adrenergic agonist are not trivial. Subcutaneous injection of only 0.25 mg terbutaline to normal adults increased heart rate by 17 beats/min at 60 min, increased cardiac output 48 percent at 30 to 60 min, and increased stroke volume 14 percent at 15 min. Systolic blood pressure increased from 130 to 140 mmHg at 30 and 60 min, while diastolic pressure decreased from 81 to 66 mmHg at 15 min. Systemic vascular resistance decreased by 36 percent at 30 min.[58]

In pulmonary hypertension secondary to chronic obstructive pulmonary disease (COPD), subcutaneous injection of terbutaline increases right ventricular ejection fraction as well as left, undoubtedly secondary to reduced pulmonary vascular resistance.[59]

There are host-factor variables in the pulse response. Increases in pulse rate in patients with asthma or COPD have been substantially less than those elicited by β-adrenergic agonists in normal individuals, possibly because of tolerance induced by prior therapy with β-adrenergic agonists[58] and/or inherently less β-adrenergic responsiveness in patients with asthma.[60] Some investigators have found little evidence of induction of tolerance to cardiovascular effects by usual doses of β_2-adrenergic agonists, however.[61,62]

EFFECT OF SYMPATHETIC STIMULATION AND HYPOKALEMIA ON PACEMAKER CELLS

The normal potential across a myocardial cell during its resting, polarized state is -80 to -90 mV directed internally, primarily dependent on the potassium gradient, in a resting equilibrium maintained by an Na^+, K^+-ATPase in the cell membrane in a pumping mechanism, which slowly moves Na^+ out of the cell and feeds K^+ into the cell. The action potential sequence of pacemaker cells (S-A node, A-V junction, ventricular conduction system) differs from the myocardial working cells in that, during phase 4, there is a gradual decrease of the negative potential until a threshold is reached at which the cell spontaneously depolarizes. Sympathetic stimulation or β-adrenergic agonists increase this slope, as does a drop in serum K^+, increasing automaticity. Hypokalemia then becomes an adverse effect of β_2-adrenergic agonists with a potential for arrhythmia production that is augmented by any preexisting hypokalemia (diuretics, corticosteroids, alkalosis).[63]

Metabolic Actions

Beta$_2$-adrenergic agonists decrease serum K^+ by two mechanisms: (1) direct stimulation of the Na^+, K^+-ATPase, principally in muscle and red blood cells; and (2) stimulation of insulin release with its stimulation of the Na^+, K^+-ATPase, principally in muscles, liver, and adipose tissue. Each mechanism is operative with a sufficient dose, and the decrease in serum K^+ can be prompt and substantial, particularly following a subcutaneous injection, since insulin concentrations clearly mirror serum drug concentrations,[56] as do elevations in cAMP.[64] With subcutaneous injection of 0.25 mg terbutaline, there was a mean decrease of 0.6 meq/L within 30 min.[65] Nebulization of albuterol has even been advocated as an emergency measure to reduce K^+ concentrations in patients on dialysis; 10 and 20 mg of nebulized albuterol cause decreases in serum K^+ of 0.62 and 0.92 meq, respectively.[66]

Beta$_2$-adrenergic agonists also cause an increase in glucose and lactate, both presumably as the result of glycogenolysis. An increase in free fatty acids caused by lipolysis now appears to be more of a β$_2$-adrenergic receptor–mediated phenomenon, although β$_3$-receptors may also be involved in adipose tissues.[34]

Lipworth have utilized these responses in an elegant series of studies of metabolic, airway, cardiovascular, and tremor responses, employing dose-response curves to cumulative doses of albuterol by MDI up to 4000 μg.[67–69] They find that metabolic responses show some evidence of tachyphylaxis for both low-dose (800 μg/24 h) and high-dose (4000 μg/24 h) albuterol. There is some effect on tremor and heart rate as well, but no effect on bronchodilation (Table 44-5).

Oral β$_2$-adrenergic agonists produce very significant metabolic responses, but these develop appreciable tachyphylaxis (cAMP, lactate, glucose) compared to the small degree seen in the peak bronchodilator response.[70] In a later study, focusing on tremor (see below), 5.0 mg oral terbutaline and 4.0 mg oral albuterol were compared.[71] The cAMP response to an initial dose of terbutaline was twice that of albuterol, and the lactate-response differential was even greater, despite equivalent effects on the airways. On a thrice-daily dosing schedule, cAMP and lactate responses were equal, the intensity of the terbutaline response showing relative tachyphylaxis. These drugs evidently distribute somewhat differently into their effector compartments. They remain there for hours after drug cessation, as indicated by persisting tremor even 16 h after the last dose.[71] Finally, a 25 percent increase in O$_2$ consumption and CO$_2$ production results from normal adults inhaling 800 μg albuterol by MDI, again peaking at 5 min. Theophylline will add to this. Remarkably, the β$_2$-adrenergic response becomes nearly flat after a few weeks of inhaled therapy—truly an amazing demonstration of tachyphylaxis.[72] This effect on O$_2$ consumption also has been noted by others.[73,74]

Skeletal Muscle

Skeletal muscle consists of fast- and slow-contracting motor units in varying proportions, depending on the muscle. Beta$_2$-adrenergic agonists and circulating catecholamines stimulate only the β$_2$-adrenergic receptors on slow-contracting fibers, reducing the amplitude of their subtetanic fusion and prolonging relaxation such that tremor is produced.[75,76]

Patients vary widely in their tremor responses to oral or inhaled β$_2$-adrenergic agonists.[77,78] For example, in an elderly population of COPD patients taken off all sympathomimetics for 2 weeks, an oral dose of a β$_2$-adrenergic agonist, terbutaline or metaproterenol, produced a 20-fold increase in tremor. The overall response was proportional to the baseline physiologic tremor, amounting to an average twofold increase, which was perceptible to most patients and uncomfortable to some.[78] In a later study, the initial response to 5.0 mg of terbutaline exceeded that to 4.0 mg of albuterol by a factor of three, yet the bronchodilator response was equivalent,[71] and this phenomenon was independently confirmed by others[79]; cAMP and lactate responses also were greater. Later, on a maintenance dose, baseline tremor increased to the same degree on either drug; however, the response to an acute dose still showed tachyphylaxis in absolute terms.

Hypoxemia

Following inhalation of isoproterenol, about 50 percent of asthma patients will have a decrease in arterial P$_{O_2}$ ≤ 15 mmHg. This reaches a maximum in 5 min and resolves over the next 15 min.[80,81] With currently used inhaled β$_2$-adrenergic agonists, the decrease in Pa$_{O_2}$ is minimal.[82] Decrease in Pa$_{O_2}$ has been attributed to increased perfusion caused by β$_2$-adrenergic dilation of pulmonary blood vessels in poorly ventilated areas of the lung. Part of the increased perfusion may also occur from the increase in cardiac output being preferentially distributed to these areas as they open up.[81] Since the smooth muscle of pulmonary vessels contains exclusively β$_2$-adrenergic receptors,[83] relaxation of vasoconstriction should occur with either isoproterenol or β$_2$-specific agents.

These changes have been studied precisely using the multiple inert-gas technique.[80] In six patients with mild asthma and one with severe obstruction, there was clearly a bimodal distribution of $\dot{V}/\dot{Q}$ ratios, with the minor mode involving ratios near 0.1 and containing 20 percent of the cardiac output but little ventilation. Following isoproterenol, perfusion to this low $\dot{V}/\dot{Q}$ mode doubled, resulting in an average decrease of 10 mmHg in the P$_{O_2}$ patients with mild asthma, but no change in the severely obstructed patient (Fig. 44-3).

In general, the largest decreases in Pa$_{O_2}$ occur in those patients with greater initial oxyhemoglobin saturation and therefore are of little consequence. However, a study in

TABLE 44-5 Mean Systemic Responses to Cumulative Dosing of 40 Puffs (4000 μg) Albuterol after 14 Days of Preceding Placebo, Low, and High Dose by MDI

2 weeks Premedication	Δ Pulse beats/min	Δ K$^+$ meq/L	Δ Glucose, M/L	Δ Tremor, % acceleration
Placebo	+28	−0.92	+1.23	+688
LD (800 μg/24 h)	+24	−0.74	+1.15	+498
HD (4000 μg/24 h)	+15	−0.45	+0.58	+509

MDI = metered-dose inhaler; LD = low dose; HD = high dose.
SOURCE: From Lipworth et al.,[68] with permission.

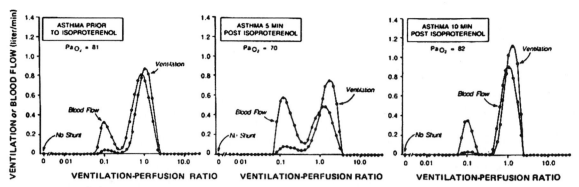

FIGURE 44-3 Sequence of $\dot{V}/\dot{Q}$ ratios at baseline, 5, and 10 min postinhalation of isoproterenol determined by the six inert-gas technique. Note that there is nearly twice the perfusion through the low $\dot{V}/\dot{Q}$ mode. (*Adapted from Wagner et al.,[79] with permission.*)

acutely asthmatic children employing noninvasive oximetry recorded a fall in Sa_{O_2} of 5 percent in half of the patients after liquid aerosols of salbutamol; this corresponded to significant decrease in P_{O_2}.[84] Therefore, a significant decrease in Pa_{O_2} is possible even with selective β_2-adrenergic agonists. During the hypoxemia of a severe attack, any further decrease in P_{O_2} could be deleterious.

References

1. Kendall MJ, Haffner C: The acute unwanted effects of beta$_2$ receptor agonist therapy, in Beasley R, Pearce NE (eds): *The Role of Beta Receptor Agonist Therapy in Asthma Mortality*. Boca Raton, FL, CRC Press, 1993:163.
2. Al-Bazzaz FJ, Cheng E: Effect of catecholamines on ion transport in dog tracheal epithelium. *J Appl Physiol* 1979; 47:397.
3. Knowles MR, Murray GF, Shallal JA, et al.: Ion transport in excised human bronchi and its neurohumeral control. *Chest* 1982; 81:11S.
4. Chediak AJ, Wanner A: Mucociliary function, in Weiss EB, Stein M (eds): *Bronchial Asthma. Mechanisms and Therapeutics*. Boston, Little, Brown, 1993:371.
5. Basbaum CB, Vekn I, Brezina L, Nadel JA: Tracheal submucosal gland cells stimulated in vitro with adrenergic and cholinergic agonists. *Cell Tissue Res* 1981; 220:481.
6. Shelhamer JH, Maron Z, Kaliner M: Immunological and neurophysiologic stimulation of mucus glycoprotein from human airways. *J Clin Invest* 1980; 66:1400.
7. Phipps RJ, Williams IP, Richardson, PS, et al.: Sympathetic drugs stimulate the output of secretory glycoprotein from human bronchi in vitro. *Clin Sci* 1982; 63:23.
8. Mortenson J, Groth S, Lange P, Hermansen F: Effect of terbutaline on mucociliary clearance in asthmatic and healthy subjects after inhalation from a pressurized inhaled and dry powder inhaler. *Thorax* 1991; 46:817.
9. Weissberger D, Oliver W Jr, Abraham WM, Wanner A: Impaired tracheal mucus transport in allergic bronchoconstriction. Effect of terbutaline pre-treatment. *J Allergy Clin Immunol* 1981; 67:357–362.
10. Mardini IA, Higgins NC, Zhou S, et al.: Functional behavior of the β-adrenergic receptor adenylyl cyclase system in rabbit airway epithelium. *Am J Respir Cell Mol Biol* 1994; 11:287.
11. Howarth PH, Durham SR, Lee TH: Influence of albuterol, cro-molyn sodium and ipratropium bromide on the airway circulating mediator response to allergen bronchial provocation in asthma. *Am Rev Respir Dis* 1985; 132:986.
12. Church MK, Hiroi J: Inhibition of IgE-dependent histamine release from human dispersed lung mast cells by anti-allergic drugs and salbutamol. *Br J Pharmacol* 1987; 90:421.
13. Butcher PR, Cousins SA, Vardey CJ: Salmeterol: A potent and long-acting inhibitor of the release of inflammatory and spasmogenic mediators from human lung. *Br J Pharmacol* 1987; 92:745P.
14. Nielson CP: β-Adrenergic modulation of the polymorphonuclear leukocyte respiratory burst is dependent upon the mechanism of cell activation. *J Immunol* 1987; 139:2392.
15. Munoz NM, Vita AJ, Neeley SP, et al.: Beta adrenergic modulation of formyl-methionine-phenylalanine-stimulated secretions of eosinophil peroxidase and leukotriene C$_4$. *J Pharmacol Exp Ther* 1994; 268:139.
16. Rabe KF, Giembycz MA, Dent G, et al.: Salmeterol is a competitive antagonist at beta-adrenoceptors mediating inhibition of respiratory burst in guinea pig eosinophils. *Eur J Pharmacol* 1993; 231:305.
17. Erjefalt I, Persson CGA: Pharmacological control of plasma exudation in the tracheobronchial airways. *Am Rev Respir Dis* 1991; 143:1008.
18. Advenier C, Qian Y, Koune JD, et al.: Formoterol and salbutamol inhibit bradykinin- and histamine-induced airway microvascular leakage in guinea pig. *Br J Pharmacol* 1992; 105:792.
19. Whelan CJ, Johnson M: Inhibition by salmeterol of increased vascular permeability and granulocyte accumulation in guinea pig lung and skin. *Br J Pharmacol* 1992; 105:831.
20. Sugiyama H, Okada C, Bewtra AK, et al.: The effect of formoterol on the late asthmatic phenomenon in guinea pigs. *J Allergy Clin Immunol* 1992; 89:858.
21. Matsumoto T, Ashida Y, Tsukusa R: Pharmacological modulation of immediate and late airway response and leukocyte infiltration in the guinea pig. *J Pharmacol Exp Ther* 1994; 269:1236.
22. Hutson PA, Holgate ST, Church MK: The site of cromolyn sodium and albuterol on early and late phase bronchoconstriction and airway leukocyte infiltration after allergen challenge on non-anesthetized guinea pigs. *Am Rev Respir Dis* 1988; 138:1157.
23. Twentyman OP, Finnerty JP, Holgate ST: The inhibitory effect of nebulized albuterol on the early and late asthmatic reactions and increase in airway responsiveness provoked by inhaled allergen in asthma. *Am Rev Respir Dis* 1991; 14:782.
24. Twentyman OP, Finnerty JP, Harris A, et al.: Protection against allergen-induced asthma by salmeterol. *Lancet* 1990; 336:1338.

25. Palmqvist M, Balder B, Lowhagen D, et al.: Late asthmatic reaction decreased after treatment with salbutamol and formoterol, a new long-acting beta-2 agonist. *J Allergy Clin Immunol* 1992; 89:844.

26. Weersink EJM, Albers R, Koeter GH, et al.: Partial inhibition of the early and late asthmatic response by a single dose of salmeterol. *Am J Respir Crit Care Med* 1994; 150:1262.

27. Wong BJ, Dolovich J, Ramsdale EH, et al.: Formoterol compared with beclomethasone and placebo on allergen-induced asthmatic responses. *Am Rev Respir Dis* 1992; 146:1156.

28. Adelroth E, Rosenhall L, Johansson S, et al.: Inflammatory cells and eosinophilic activity in asthmatics investigated by bronchoalveolar lavage. *Am Rev Respir Dis* 1990; 143:423.

29. Laitinen LA, Laitinen A, Haahtela T: A comparative study of the effects of an inhaled corticosteroid, budenoside, and a beta$_2$-agonist, terbutaline, on airway inflammation in newly diagnosed asthma: A randomized, double blind, parallel-group controlled trial. *J Allergy Clin Immunol* 1992; 90:32.

30. Gratziou C, Roberts JA, Bradding P, Holgate PH: The influence of the long-acting beta-agonist salmeterol xinofoate on T-lymphocyte lavage populations and activation status in asthma. *Am Rev Respir Dis* 1992; 145:A67.

31. Roberts JA, Bradding P, Walls AF, et al.: The effect of salmeterol xinofoate therapy on lavage findings in asthma. *Am Rev Respir Dis* 1992; 145:A418.

32. Hedberg A, Minneman KP, Molinoff PB: Differential distribution of beta$_1$- and beta$_2$-adrenergic receptors in cat and guinea pig heart. *J Pharmacol Exp Ther* 1980; 213:503.

33. Hall JA, Kaumann AJ, Brown MJ: Selective beta$_1$-adrenoceptor blockade enhances positive inotropic responses to endogenous catecholamines mediated through beta$_2$-adrenoceptors in human atrial myocardium. *Circ Res* 1990; 66:1610.

34. Kaumann AJ: Is there a third heart beta-adrenoceptor? *Trends Pharmacol Sci* 1989; 10:316.

35. Burton BF, Jones CR, Molenaar P, Summers, RT: Characterization and autoradiographic localization of beta-adrenoceptor subtypes in human cardiac tissues. *Br J Pharmacol* 1987; 92:299.

36. Robberecht P, Delhaye M, Taton G, et al.: The human heart beta-adrenergic receptors: I. Heterogeneity of the binding sites: Presence of 50% beta$_1$ and 50% beta$_2$ adrenergic receptors. *Mol Pharmacol* 1983; 24:169.

37. Cooke L, Muntz KH: Differences in beta adrenergic receptor agonist affinity between cardiac myocytes and coronary arterioles in canine heart. *J Pharmacol Exp Ther* 1994; 269:351.

38. Brodde O: β$_1$- and β$_2$-adrenoceptors in the human heart. Properties, functions and alterations in chronic heart failure. *Pharmacol Rev* 1991; 43:203.

39. Green SA, Holt BD, Liggett SB: β$_1$ and β$_2$ adrenergic receptors display subtype-selective coupling to G$_s$. *Mol Pharmacol* 1992; 41:889.

40. Minneman KP, Hegstrand LR, Molinoff PB: The pharmacological specificity of β$_1$- and β$_2$-adrenergic receptors in rat heart and lung in vitro. *Mol Pharmacol* 1979; 16:21.

41. Chapman KR, Smith DL, Rebuck AS, Leenan FHH: Hemodynamic effects of an inhaled beta$_2$ agonist. *Clin Pharmacol Ther* 1984; 35:762.

42. Kaumann AJ, Hall JA, Murray KJ, et al.: A comparison of the effect of adrenaline and noradrenaline in human heart. The role of beta$_1$ and beta$_2$ adrenoceptors in the stimulation of adenylate cyclase and contractile force. *Eur Heart J* 1989; 10:29.

43. Brittain RT: A comparison of the pharmacology profile of salbutamol with that of isoproterenol, orciprenaline (metaproterenol) and trimetoquinol. *Postgrad Med J* 1971; 47:11.

44. Ball DI, Brittain RT, Coleman RA, et al.: Salmeterol, a novel, long-action β$_2$-adrenoceptor agonist: Characterization of pharmaco-

logical activity in vitro and in vivo. *Br J Pharmacol* 1991; 104:665.

45. O'Donnell SR: An examination of some beta-adrenoceptor stimulants for selectivity using the trachea and atria of the guinea pig. *Eur J Pharmacol* 1972; 19:371.

46. Brodde OE, Daul A, Wellstrein A, et al.: Differentiation of beta$_1$ and beta$_2$ adrenoceptor mediated effects in humans. *Am J Physiol* 1988; 251:H119.

47. Scheinin M, Kaulus MM, Laurikainen E, Allonen H: Hypokalemia and other non-bronchial effects of inhaled fenoterol and salbutamol: A placebo controlled dose-response study in healthy volunteers. *Br J Clin Pharmacol* 1987; 24:645.

48. Windom HH, Burgess CD, Siebers RWL, et al.: The pulmonary and extrapulmonary effects of inhaled β-agonists in patients with asthma. *Clin Pharmacol Ther* 1990; 48:296.

49. Crane J, Burgess C, Beasely R: Cardiovascular and hypokalemic effects of inhaled salbutamol, fenoterol, and isoprenaline. *Thorax* 1989; 44:136.

50. Bremner P, Burgess C, Beasley R, et al.: Nebulized fenoterol causes greater cardiovascular effects than equivalent bronchodilator doses of salbutamol in asthmatics. *Respir Med* 1992; 86:419.

51. Gibson DG, Coltart DJ: Hemodynamic effects of intravenous salbutamol in patients with mitral valve disease: Comparison with isoproterenol and atropine. *Postgrad Medicine* 1971; 47:40.

52. Leitch AG, Clancy LJ, Costello JF, Flenley DC: Effect of intravenous infusions of salbutamol on ventilatory response to carbon dioxide and hypoxia on heart rate and plasma potassium in normal men. *Br Med J* 1976; 1:365.

53. Timmis AD, Bergman G, Monoghan M, Jewitt DE: Potential value of oral beta$_2$ adrenoceptor agonists in left ventricular failure. *Am J Cardiol* 1981; 47:427.

54. Wang RY, Lee PK, Yu DY, et al.: Myocardial metabolic effects of I.V. terbutaline in patients with severe heart failure. *J Clin Pharmacol* 1983; 23:362.

55. Naylor WG, McInnes I: Salbutamol and orciprenaline-induced changes in myocardial function. *Cardiovasc Res* 1972; 6:725.

56. Kung M, Croley SW, Phillips BA: Systemic cardiovascular and metabolic effects associated with the inhalation of an increased dose of albuterol: Influence of mouth rinsing and gargling. *Chest* 1987; 91:382.

57. Tandon MK: Cardiopulmonary effects of fenoterol and salbutamol aerosols. *Chest* 1980; 77:429.

58. Sackner MA, et al.: Hemodynamic effects of epinephrine and terbutaline in normal man. *Chest* 1975; 68:616.

59. Matthay RA, Langor R, Brent BN, et al.: Cardiovascular effects of terbutaline in patients with COPD, pulmonary hypertension and decreased RV function. *Am Rev Respir Dis* 1981; 123:16.

60. Shelhamer JH, et al.: Abnormal adrenergic responsiveness in allergic subjects: Analysis of isoproterenol-induced cardiovascular and plasma cyclic adenosine monophosphate responses. *J Allergy Clin Immunol* 1980; 66:52.

61. Lipworth BJ, Clark RA, Dhillon DP, McDevitt DG: Comparison of the effects of prolonged treatment with low and high doses of inhaled terbutaline on beta-adrenoceptor responsiveness in patients with chronic obstructive pulmonary disease. *Am Rev Respir Dis* 1990; 142:33.

62. Lipworth BJ, Struthers AD, McDevitt DG: Tachyphylaxis to systemic but not to airway responses during prolonged therapy with high dose inhaled salbutamol in asthmatics. *Am Rev Respir Dis* 1989; 140:586.

63. Lipworth BJ, McDevitt DG, Struthers AD: Electrocardiographic changes induced by inhaled salbutamol after treatment with bendrofluazide: Effects of replacement therapy with potassium, magnesium, and triamterene. *Clin Sci* 1990; 78:255.

64. Fairfax AJ, Rehahn M, Jones D, O'Malley BO: Comparison between the effects of inhaled isoprenaline and fenoterol on plasma cyclic AMP and heart rate in normal subjects. *Br J Clin Pharmacol* 1984; 17:165.

65. Kung M, White JR, Burki NK: The effect of subcutaneously administered terbutaline on serum potassium of asymptomatic adult asthmatics. *Am Rev Respir Dis* 1984; 129:329.

66. Allon M, Dunlay R, Copkney C: Nebulized albuterol for acute hyperkalemia in patients on dialysis. *Ann Intern Med* 1989; 110:426.

67. Lipworth BJ, Tregaskis BF, McDevitt DG: β-Adrenoceptor responses to inhaled salbutamol in the elderly. *Br J Clin Pharmacol* 1989; 28:725.

68. Lipworth BJ, Struthers AD, McDevitt DG: Tachphylaxis to systemic but not to airway responses during prolonged therapy with high dose inhaled salbutamol in asthmatics. *Am Rev Respir Dis* 1989; 140:586.

69. Lipworth BJ, Clark RA, Dhillon DP, McDevitt DG: Subsensitivity of beta-adrenoceptor responses in asthmatic patients taking regular low dose inhaled salbutamol. *Eur J Clin Pharmacol* 1990; 380:203.

70. Jenne JW, Chick W, Strickland RD, Wall FJ: Subsensitivity of beta responses during therapy with long-acting beta-2 preparation. *J Allergy Clin Immunol* 1977; 59:383.

71. Jenne JW, Valcarenghi G, Druz WS, et al.: Comparison of tremor responses to orally administered albuterol and terbutaline. *Am Rev Respir Dis* 1986; 134:708.

72. Wilson SR, Amoroso P, Moxham J, Ponte J: Modification of the thermogenic effect of acutely inhaled salbutamol by chronic inhalation in normal subjects. *Thorax* 1993; 48:886.

73. Newth CJL, Amsler B, Anderson GP, Morley J: The ventilatory and oxygen costs in the anesthetized Rhesus monkey of inhaling drugs used in therapy and diagnosis of asthma. *Am Rev Respir Dis* 1991; 143:766.

74. Vaisman N, Levy LD, Pencharz PB: Effect of salbutamol on resting energy expenditure in patients with cystic fibrosis. *J Pediatr* 1987; 111:137.

75. Marsden CD, Meadows J: The effect of adrenaline on the contraction of human muscle. *J Physiol (Lond)* 1970; 207:429.

76. Bowman WC, Nott MW: Actions of sympathomimetic amines and their antagonists in skeletal muscle. *Pharmacol Rev* 1964; 21:27.

77. Thiringer G, Svedmyr N: Re-evaluation of skeletal muscle tremor due to bronchodilator agents. *Scand J Respir Dis* 1975; 56:93.

78. Jenne JW, Ridley DF, Marcucci R, et al.: Objective and subjective tremor responses to oral beta-2 agents on first exposure. *Am Rev Respir Dis* 1982; 126:607.

79. Levy S, Mallett S, Levinem S: Comparison of the effects of two beta$_2$ agonists with respect to bronchodilator and skeletal muscle tremor response. *Am Rev Respir Dis* 1986; 133(4):A63.

80. Ingram RH Jr: Ventilation-perfusion changes after aerosolized isoproterenol in asthma. *Am Rev Respir Dis* 1970; 101:364.

81. Wagner PD, Dantzker DR, Iacovoni VE, et al.: Ventilation-perfusion inequality in asymptomatic asthma. *Am Rev Respir Dis* 1978; 118:511.

82. Palmer NKV, Legge JS, Hamilton WFD, Diament ML: Comparison of effect of salbutamol and isoprenaline on spirometry, blood gas tensions in bronchial asthma. *Br Med J* 1970; 2:23.

83. Carstairs JR, Nimmo AJ, Barnes PJ: Autoradiographic visualization of beta-adrenoceptor subtypes in human lung. *Am Rev Respir Dis* 1985; 132:541.

84. Tal A, Pasterkamp H, Leahy A: Arterial oxygen desaturation following salbutamol inhalation in acute asthma. *Chest* 1984; 86:868.

Chapter 45

PHARMACOKINETICS OF BETA-ADRENERGIC AGONISTS

JOHN W. JENNE

Introduction

Serum Drug Concentrations with Various Dosing Modalities
    Oral dosing
    Inhalation by metered-dose inhaler
    Nebulization
    Subcutaneous administration
    Intravenous
    Pharmacokinetic/dynamic modeling

Introduction

Beta$_2$-adrenergic agonists are supplied as salts of racemic mixtures. The ($-$), or (l), form is several hundred times more effective at β-adrenergic receptors than the ($+$), or (d), form. Catecholamines such as epinephrine and isoproterenol are rapidly metabolized by catechol-O-methyltransferase (COMT) and also conjugated with glucoronide. The phenolic ring hydroxyl group of the noncatechols is sulfated by at least one of two phenol sulfotranferases found particularly in gut mucosa and liver but also in other tissues, even including bronchial epithelial cells. The compounds undergo first-pass metabolism, as indicated by a higher proportion of the drug remaining unconjugated when given IV than by mouth. When added to their incomplete oral absorption, this results in relatively low bioavailability. Thus, 0.5 mg terbutaline subcutaneously is roughly equivalent to 5.0 mg by mouth in its bronchodilator activity.

We now are becoming aware that the processes involved in the pharmacokinetics of these β$_2$-adrenergic agonists are stereoselective. This affects albuterol and terbutaline, but in different ways. The ($-$) enantiomer of albuterol is sulfated about 10 times more efficiently as the ($+$) form, and this should result in a much higher proportion of the ($+$) form in serum.[1] By contrast, the ($+$) form of terbutaline is metabolized about twice as efficiently as the ($-$) form, and their proportion in serum is about 1:2, respectively.[2] Heretofore, serum measurements have not been stereoselective, although such methods now are appearing, and the values in the literature cannot be used to compare one drug with another.

The short-acting β$_2$-adrenergic agents such as albuterol, fenoterol, and terbutaline possess a phenolic hydroxyl group and an aliphatic amine. The latter has a pK_a of about 10, so that these compounds are completely ionized at physiologic pH and are therefore water soluble. They are only slightly protein bound and have large distribution volumes. The lipophilic compounds such as salmeterol are highly protein bound.

The kinetic parameters of albuterol and terbutaline are shown in Table 45-1.

At steady state, assuming first-order kinetics, the concentration of drug in plasma, C_{pss}, is

$$C_{pss} = \frac{D \cdot f}{\tau \cdot Cl_{tot}}$$

where
D = dose
f = fractional absorption
τ = dosing interval
Cl_{tot} is overall clearance

Serum Drug Levels with Various Dosing Modalities

ORAL DOSING

When albuterol is given orally in its rapidly absorbed form, 4 mg (as base) q 6 h, mean concentrations at steady state average about 12 ng/mL,[3] and a therapeutic range is considered to be 10 to 20 ng/mL. In contrast, terbutaline, 5 mg q 6 h, gives serum concentrations of 4 to 5 ng/mL.[4] Figures 45-1A and 1B show plasma concentrations and the corresponding FEV$_1$ changes when using albuterol syrup, 5.2 mg q 8 h, and sustained action preparations, 8 mg q 12 h, the latter being a sustained-release preparation.[5] Note the close correlation between concentrations and the FEV$_1$ in this midtherapeutic range. The $t_{1/2}$ for albuterol is 5 to 6 h measured from steady state. By contrast, terbutaline, with its

TABLE 45-1 **Pharmacokinetic Parameters of Racemates and Emantiomers**

	Protein Binding, %	Cl_{tot}, L/h/kg	CL_R, L/h/kg	V_D, L/kg	$t_{1/2}$ h	F_{abs}	F_{avail}
(±) Albuterol	8	0.46	0.28	2.5	5–6	75	50
(±) Terbutaline	15	0.20	0.1	4.0	13	40	15
(+) Terbutaline	—	0.19	0.16	3.5	12.7	—	—
(−) Terbutaline	—	0.13	0.09	2.6	15.3	—	—

NOTE: Cl_{tot} = total clearance; Cl_R = renal clearance; V_D = distribution volume; $t_{1/2}$ = half-life; F_{abs} = fractional absorption; F_{avail} = fractional available unchanged drug.
SOURCE: From Morgan,[7] with permission.

longer mean $t_{1/2} \geq 13$ h,[6] gives smaller peak-trough differences, apparently unloading more slowly from a larger distribution volume[7] (Table 45-1).

INHALATION BY METERED-DOSE INHALER

In the nonintubated patient, there are important differences in pattern of deposition between metered-dose inhaler (MDI) or dry particle inhaler (DPI) and nebulization.[8]

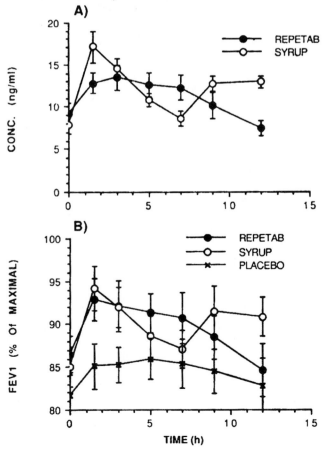

FIGURE 45-1 Albuterol plasma concentration (*A*) and effects on FEV_1 (*B*) after administration of sustained-action preparation (8 mg q 12 h) and albuterol syrup (5.2 mg q 8 h). Standard deviations are expressed as SEM. *B* also shows placebo data. (*From Hochhaus et al.,[5] with permission.*)

Zainudin et al. found that while all three routes delivered approximately 10 percent of 400 μg of labeled albuterol to the lung, the MDI delivery to the gastrointestinal tract (swallowed drug) constituted about 80 percent of the dose, compared to only 2 to 3 percent of the dose by nebulization. It is noteworthy that the FEV_1 response was 35.6 percent for MDI, compared to 25.2 percent for DPI and 25.8 percent for nebulization.[8]

Following inhalation, there is a wave of drug absorption, which undoubtedly represents drug passing rapidly through the alveolar-capillary interface and probably into mucosal and submucosal vessels as well. Concentrations peak at about 5 min and decline rapidly thereafter.[9] When 1000 μg (10 puffs) of albuterol was administered by MDI to normal adults, mean serum concentration reached about 6 ng/mL, while 4000 μg produced a peak of about 21 ng/mL at 5 min (Fig. 45-2). Fenoterol concentrations at these doses were only one-seventh as great. In a preliminary report, 6 puffs of albuterol inhaled by normal adults by MDI with a cylindrical spacer over 3 min produced a mean serum peak concentration of 7.5 ng/mL at 10 min, but concentrations were already one-half this by 3 min.[9a] When 10 puffs were given to mechanically ventilated patients by these authors into the inspiratory line through a holding chamber, mean maximal concentration was 9.9 ng/mL (range 4.5 to 14.7), again peaking at 10 min. As judged by the absorbed drug, the efficiency per puff in these two situations was surprisingly similar. In both cases, levels decreased to about 40 percent of the peak at 30 min consistent with the alpha phase of distribution from the central compartment. Such levels are only an index of drug deposition, although they undoubtedly will exert some bronchodilation through systemic distribution. However the kinetics of bronchodilation, the onset and offset at the bronchial smooth-muscle receptors, follow a different time scale with a much slower decay. Thus, when 10 puffs of albuterol were given to ventilated patients with chronic obstructive pulmonary disease in the same manner as above, bronchodilation had nearly maximized at 5 min and continued unabated at 60 min (see below).[10]

Serum concentrations can be used to substantiate and compare delivery efficiency by different devices and techniques. For example, it would be useful to document the extremely poor efficacy shown for one commercial MDI-adaptor device applied at the endotracheal tube in mechanically ventilated patients, as opposed to the very efficient wet nebulization into the inspiratory line.[11] Unchanged drug appearing in the urine in the first 30 min has also been used

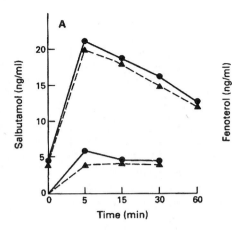
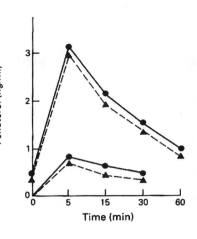

FIGURE 45-2 (*A*) Mean plasma concentrations (ng/mL) of salbutamol and fenoterol at 5, 15, and 30 min after inhalation of 1 mg, and 5, 15, 30, and 60 min after inhalation of 4 mg following pretreatment with placebo (▲) or atenolol 25 mg (●). (*From Newnham et al.,[9] with permission.*)

to monitor lung deposition and has been cleverly employed to optimize inhaler technique.[12] The sulfated portion appears soon thereafter, arising from gut absorption.[13]

NEBULIZATION

When 0.15 mg/kg albuterol was nebulized as a single dose to 12 adults with acute asthma, peak levels averaged 30 nM/L (about 7.2 ng/mL), ranging from 11 to 76 nM/L (2.6 to 18 ng/mL), and the area under the curve of serum levels varied 10-fold.[14] Thus, single-dose nebulization of 5 mg albuterol provides mean concentration below the therapeutic range, but concentrations vary widely between individuals. During continuous nebulization, serum concentrations accumulate to a steady state, which can reach toxic concentrations at a sufficient dosing rate. Lin et al. nebulized 0.4 mg/kg/h of albuterol to adults for 4 h. Concentrations exceeded the 10 to 20 ng/mL range and, in one patient, reached 61.6 ng/mL, producing a supraventricular tachycardia.[15] Yet a mean rate of 0.67 mg/kg/h has been administered to children for a mean duration of 37 h without adverse effect.[16] Obviously, children are more robust than adults. In adults, the rates should not exceed 0.2 mg/kg/h, and close monitoring of heart rate and rhythm is mandatory.

SUBCUTANEOUS ADMINISTRATION

Subcutaneous injection of terbutaline or epinephrine produces almost immediate action and ensures delivery. It can supplement the inhaled route and be used in an emergency, for example, for patients with severe asthma away from medical facilities. When 0.5 mg of terbutaline is administered subcutaneously, significant concentrations are present within a few minutes and peak at 20 min, averaging 7.4 ng/mL in adults.[17] Figure 45-3 shows that concentrations achieved by 0.75 mg of subcutaneous terbutaline peak at about 11 ng/mL, and lasts for several hours. Concentration following more conventional doses would be one-third of this, but still in the therapeutic range as used in oral dosing.[18] Epinephrine, 0.3 mg subcutaneously, has about the same bronchodilating effect as 0.25 mg of terbutaline and the same duration of action.[19]

FIGURE 45-3 Mean FEV₁ data (*above*) and serum K⁺ concentration (*below*) fitted to an effect-compartment model (dotted lines) following subcutaneous injection of 0.75 mg terbutaline, an unusually large dose. Note the shallower decay of FEV_1 due to the nonlinearity of the dose-response relationship, and the precipitous decrease in K^+. The effect compartment is the compartment in which the receptors are assumed to be localized, using pharmacokinetic/dynamic modeling (*From Osterhuis B, et al.,[26] with permission.*)

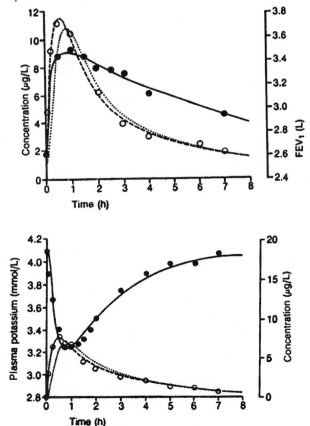

INTRAVENOUS

When terbutaline is injected IV as a loading dose, its concentration disappears in an initial (alpha) phase with a $t_{1/2}$ of 8 to 12 min, a second (beta) phase of 3 to 4 h, and a terminal (gamma) phase of 17 to 20 h.[20] Table 45-1 shows its pharmacokinetic parameters. When 250 μg of terbutaline IV was administered as a loading dose, it produced a mean peak concentration of 7.7 ng/mL,[20] and 5 μg/kg albuterol caused a mean peak of 14 ng/mL.[14] But 0.133 μg/kg/min of albuterol infused into adults for 5 h plateaued at concentrations averaging 20 ng/mL.[21] Accordingly, a loading dose of 10 μg/kg albuterol over 10 min followed by a maintenance of 0.1 to 2.0 μg/kg/min administered by syringe pump should provide high therapeutic levels. The terbutaline maintenance rates advocated by Uden range from 0.1 to 0.5 μg/kg/min.[22] Higher rates than these are seen in the literature, at least in children, and there is a lack of needed data on serum concentrations in these situations.

PHARMACOKINETIC/DYNAMIC MODELING

A complete drug evaluation requires a pharmacokinetic/dynamic (PK/PD) evaluation. This has been facilitated using a model based upon the standard E_{max} relationship,[23] in which E is the particular effect being measured, E_{max} is the known maximum effect obtainable for that drug, E_0 is the effect at zero time or on placebo, EC_{50} is the concentration (Conc) required to produce half maximum effect, and N is the Hill slope factor, which is an arbitrary exponent that relates to the slope of the linear portion of the log-dose curve. Thus

$$E = E_0 + \frac{E_{max} \cdot Conc^N}{Conc^N + EC_{50}^{\ N}}$$

This equation describes a typical sigmoid curve relating effect to the log of the drug concentration. Figure 45-4 shows the relationships obtained in two studies with oral albuterol; Table 45-2 lists the EC_{50}'s of several physiologic parameters from the model.[5]

The PK/PD model can be used to show that the peak serum fenoterol concentration following inhalation of 400 μg by MDI (0.3 ng/mL at 10 min) is able to account for only a small fraction of the decrease in airway resistance that

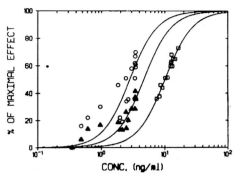

FIGURE 45-4 Relationship between albuterol plasma concentration and the effects on FEV_1 for group 1 (□) and group 2 (▲) and peak expiratory flow rate (○) of group 2. The lines show the model-predicted concentration-effect relationship. (*From Hochhaus et al.,*[24] *with permission.*)

results. This indicates that the bulk of the effect is caused by its topical action[24] and confirms earlier work in this area.[25]

Another use of modeling is to calculate the drug concentration in the "effect" compartment; these are slightly delayed from drug concentrations in the central compartment of a patient receiving 0.75 mg terbutaline subcutaneously (Fig. 45-3).[26] The response of the FEV_1 decreases less rapidly than the serum drug concentrations, caused by its markedly nonlinear relationship to them (Fig. 45-3).

References

1. Walle UK, Pesola Gr, Walle T: Stereoselective sulphate conjugation of salbutamol in humans: Comparison of hepatic, intestinal and platelet activity. *Br J Clin Pharmacol* 1993; 35:413.
2. Borgstrom L, Nyberg L, Jonsson S, et al.: Pharmacokinetic evaluation in man of terbutaline as separate enantiomers and as the racemate. *Br J Clin Pharmacol* 1989; 27:49.
3. Powell ML, Chung M, Weisberger M, et al.: Multiple dose albuterol kinetics. *J Clin Pharmacol* 1986; 26:643.
4. Bengtsson B, Fagerstrom P: Extrapulmonary affects of terbutaline during prolonged administration. *Clin Pharmacol Ther* 1982; 31:726.

TABLE 45-2   Pharmacokinetic/Dynamic Parameters for Albuterol, Terbutaline, and Fenoterol

	Albuterol EC_{50}, ng/mL	Terbutaline EC_{50}, ng/mL	Fenoterol EC_{50} ng/mL
↑ FEV_1	5, 10 (o)	2.3 (sc)	—
↑ PEFR	2.8 (o)	4.5 (IV)	—
↓ RAW	—	3.7 (sc)	0.38 (IV)
↑ HR	18 (IV)	13.0 (IV)	1.04 (IV)
↓ K^+	—	8, 8.9 (sc)	—

NOTE: FEV_1 = forced expiratory volume in 1 s; PEFR = peak expiratory flow rate; RAW = airway resistance; HR = heart rate; K^+ = serum potassium; o = oral; IV = intravenous; sc = subcutaneous; EC_{50} = concentration required for half maximum effect.
SOURCE: From Hochhaus and Möllman,[23] with permission.

5. Hochhaus G, Hendeles L, Harmon E, Möllman H: PK/PD analysis of albuterol action: Application to a comparative assessment of β_2-adrenergic drugs. *Eur J Pharm Sci* 1993; 1:73.

6. Fagerstrom PO: Pharmacokinetics of terbutaline after parenteral administration. *Eur J Respir Dis* 1984; 54 (suppl 134):101.

7. Morgan DJ: Clinical pharmacokinetics of β-agonists. *Clin Pharmacokinet* 1990; 18:270.

8. Zainudin BMZ, Biddiscombi M, Tolfree SEJ, et al.: Comparison of bronchodilator responses and deposition patterns of salbutamol inhaled from a pressurized metered dose inhaler, as a dry powder, and as a nebulized solution. *Thorax* 1990; 45:569.

9. Newnham DM, Wheeldon NM, Lipworth BJ, McDevitt DG: Single dosing comparison of the β_1/β_2 activity of inhaled fenoterol and salbutamol in normal subjects. *Thorax* 1993; 48:656.

9a. Duarte A, Dhand R, Reid R, et al.: Serum albuterol levels after metered-dose inhaler administration to ventilated patients and healthy controls. *Am J Respir Crit Care Med* 1995; 151:A430.

10. Dhand R, Jubran A, Tobin MJ: Bronchodilator delivery by metered-dose inhaler in ventilator supported patients. *Am J Respir Crit Care Med* 1995; 151:1827.

11. Manthous CA, Hall JB, Schmidt GA, Wood LDH: Metered dose inhaler versus nebulized albuterol in mechanically ventilated patients. *Am Rev Respir Dis* 1993; 148:1567.

12. Hindle M, Newton DAG, Chrystyn H: Investigations of an optimal inhaler technique with the use of urinary salbutamol excretion as a measure of relative bioavailability to the lung. *Thorax* 1993; 48:607.

13. Hindle M, Chrystyn H: Determination of the relative bioavailability of salbutamol to the lung following inhalation. *Br J Clin Pharmacol* 1992; 34:311.

14. Janson C: Plasma levels and effects of salbutamol after inhaled or I.V. administration in stable asthma. *Eur Respir J* 1991; 4:544.

15. Lin RY, Smith AJ, Hergenroeder P: High serum albuterol levels and tachycardia in adult asthmatics treated with high-dose continuously aerosolized albuterol. *Chest* 1993; 103:221.

16. Katz RW, Kelly HW, Crowley MR: Safety of continuous nebulized albuterol for bronchospasm in infants and children. *Pediatrics* 1993; 92:666.

17. Van den Berg W, Leferink JG, Maes RAA, et al.: Correlation between terbutaline serum levels, cAMP plasma levels and FEV$_1$ in normals and asthmatics after subcutaneous administration. *Ann Allergy* 1980; 44:233.

18. Van den Berg W, Leferink JG, Maes RAA, et al.: The effects of oral and subcutaneous terbutaline in asthmatic patients. *Eur J Respir Dis* 1984; 65:181.

19. Sackner MA, Greeneitch N, Silva G, Wanner A: Bronchodilator effects of terbutaline and epinephrine in obstructive lung disease. *Clin Pharmacol Ther* 1974; 16:499.

20. Leferink JG, Van den Berg W, Wagemaker-Engels J, et al.: Pharmacokinetics of terbutaline, a β_2-sympathomimetic, in healthy volunteers and asthmatic patients. *Arzneimittel Forschung* 1982; 32:159.

21. Fairfax AJ, McNabb WR, Davis HJ, Spiro SG: Slow-release oral salbutamol and aminophylline in nocturnal asthma: Relation of overnight changes in lung function and plasma drug levels. *Thorax* 1980; 35:526.

22. Uden DL: Guidelines for intravenous terbutaline use in status asthmaticus, in Weiss EB, Stein M (eds): *Bronchial Asthma: Mechanisms and Therapeutics*, 3d ed. Boston, Little, Brown, 1993; 1221.

23. Hochhaus G, Möllman H: Pharmacokinetic/pharmacodynamic characteristics of the β-2-agonists terbutaline, salbutamol and fenoterol. *Pharmacol Ther Toxicol* 1992; 30:342.

24. Hochhaus G, Schmidt E, Rominger KL, Möllman H: Pharmacokinetic/dynamic correlation of pulmonary and cardiac effects of fenoterol in asthmatic patients after different routes of administration. *Pharm Res* 1992; 9:291.

25. Thiringer G, Svedmyr N: Comparison of infused and inhaled terbutaline in patients with asthma. *Scand J Respir Dis* 1975; 57:17.

26. Osterhuis B, Braat MCP, Roos CM, et al.: Pharmacokinetic/pharmacodynamic modeling of terbutaline bronchodilation in asthma. *Clin Pharmacol Ther* 1986; 40:469.

Chapter 46 _____

PHARMACODYNAMICS AND CLINICAL MANAGEMENT

JOHN W. JENNE

Individual Variability of Dose-Response Curves

Single and Multiple Dosing by MDI: Short- and Long-Acting Agents

The Distinction Between Bronchodilation and Protection Against Challenge

Effect of Corticosteroids on Airway Caliber and Relaxation by Beta-Adrenergic Agonist

Intermittent versus Continuous Nebulization

Nebulization versus High-Intensity Metered-Dose Inhalation

Parenteral Beta-Adrenergic Agonists

Inhaled Route in Mechanically Ventilated Patients

Individual Variability of Dose-Response Curves

Individual patients require different amounts of a bronchodilator for a therapeutic response, even when they share the same baseline of FEV_1. However, there are few formal presentations of this in the literature. Barnes and Pride performed full cumulative dose-response curves until responses had plateaued using albuterol by metered-dose inhaler (MDI) in eight patients with stable asthma and also isoproterenol in four of them.[1] Figure 46-1 shows the considerable variability with only these eight patients, but there is an important trend. Those whose baseline FEV_1 exceeded 1.5 L generally required only 100 to 200 µg albuterol to reach their plateau value, while those beginning at a baseline below 1.5 L generally required a total dose in the neighborhood of 1000 µg. The plateau FEV_1 also was lower, perhaps indicative of some fixed obstruction. In a sense, this relationship between dose and severity of obstruction suggests functional antagonism, although other components of obstruction, such as inflammation, certainly confuse the question.

An early study by Williams and Kane demonstrated the extreme sensitivity of the patient with asthma to small amounts of isoproterenol, but it is the ultimate plateauing of the FEV_1 that is more relevant to clinical management.[2]

Single and Multiple Dosing by MDI: Short- and Long-Acting Agents

Figure 46-2 shows the dose-response relationship in a series of patients for 50 µg salmeterol compared to 200 µg salbutamol.[3] Note that the salmeterol has a slower onset; one study found that 90 percent of the peak drug effect of this dose of salbutamol is reached by 4.8 min, while 50 µg salmeterol requires 9.6 min.[4]

The onset of action of 24 µg of formoterol is nearly as rapid as that of salbutamol. A minute after inhalation, 200 µg salbutamol reached 63 percent of its maximum response, but formoterol was not substantially different at 47 percent.[5] A 12-µg dose of formoterol has a slower onset. At a dose of 24 µg, formoterol is satisfactory for both rescue and twice daily maintenance therapy.

Multiple dosing, both initially and 12 weeks into the course of treatment, has been compared between albuterol and salmeterol (Fig. 46-3).[6,7] The large peak-trough swings with the short-acting agent are evident. There is no reduction in the peak FEV_1 on either regimen after 12 weeks. This long duration of activity with salmeterol avoids peak-trough effects that occur with albuterol and increased patient comfort. For patients with persistent bronchospasm, it is useful to consider drugs that are administered twice daily, e.g.,

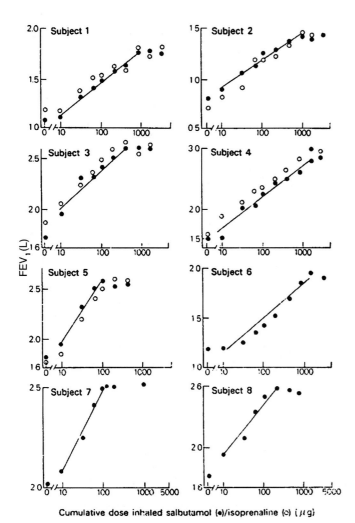

FIGURE 46-1 Cumulative dose-response curves for salbutamol by MDI in eight patients with stable asthma with varying degrees of impaired FEV_1. Dosing was continued until a plateau was reached. The figure illustrates that the principle of functional antagonism applies in human asthma. [*From Barnes and Pride,*[1] *with permission.*]

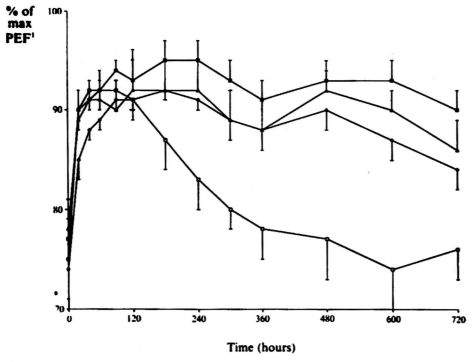

FIGURE 46-2 Peak flow (PEF) after inhalation of salbutamol 200 μg (□) and salmeterol 50 μg (◆), 100 μg (▲), and 200 μg (■). PEF is expressed as mean (SEM) percentage of the best individual registration over the four test days. [*From Ullman and Svedmyr,*[3] *with permission.*]

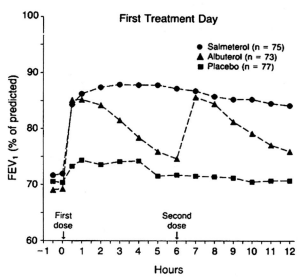

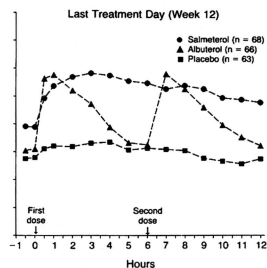

FIGURE 46-3 Mean FEV$_1$ in the treatment groups (salbutamol 200 μg, q 6 h, and salmeterol 50 μg, q 12 h) as a percentage of the predicted value on the first and last days of treatment. For the second dose, placebo was given to the salmeterol and placebo groups, and albuterol to the albuterol group. [*From Pearlman et al.,[6] with permission.*]

either salmeterol or formoterol. Rather than increasing the standard dose of inhaled corticosteroids, substitution of salmeterol for albuterol provides far more bronchodilation and patient satisfaction.[8] Salmeterol has been effectively and satisfactorily dosed at twice the standard dose for patients with more severe but stable asthma.[9] Another option is to combine the β-adrenergic agonist with either theophylline or ipratropium bromide to increase the general level of bronchodilation and to minimize the trough effects. Nevertheless, worsening of unstable asthma requires adjustment of the corticosteroid dose rather than an increase in bronchodilators.

The Distinction Between Bronchodilation and Protection Against Challenge

A rather startling development was the observation by Ahrens et al. that the time-course differs between bronchodilation and protection against bronchial challenge using histamine or methacholine, the protective effect declining more rapidly[10] (Fig. 46-4).

The same principle has been shown with exercise.[11] The reasons for this difference are unknown. For equal degrees of bronchoconstriction by methacholine and adenosine monophosphate (AMP), it has also been shown that the response to a β$_2$-adrenergic agonist is greater with the inflammatory agent, presumably because of added nonbronchodilator actions such as inhibition of mediator release.[12]

FIGURE 46-4 *A.* Activity ratio versus time of 1 (△) and 4 puffs (■) of metaproterenol, along with placebo (●). The "activity ratios" represent the PC$_{20}$ for histamine after drug divided by the PC$_{20}$ before drug. *B.* The effect on FEV$_1$ of the same doses. Note that the maximum bronchodilator effect is sustained out to at least 2 h, while the activity ratio is falling. [*From Ahrens et al.,[10] with permission.*]

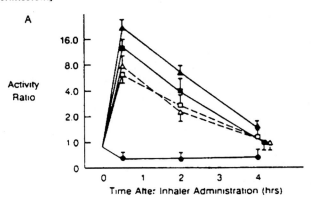

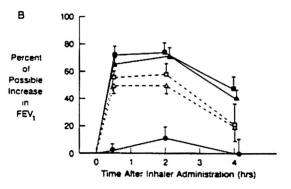

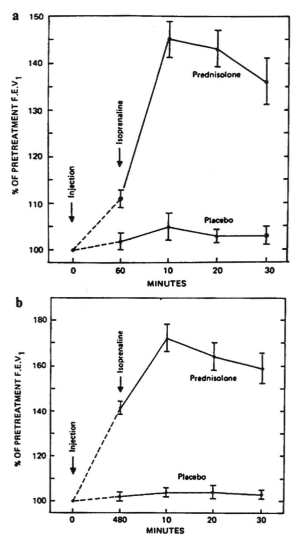

FIGURE 46-5 Restoration of adrenergic responsiveness by corticosteroids in asthma. Changes in FEV$_1$ after inhalation of 200 μg isoproterenol (isoprenaline) sulfate from a pressurized aerosol (A) 1 h and (B) 8 h after a single intravenous injection of placebo or 40 mg prednisolone. Group mean values ± SEM for eight patients. [From Ellul-Micallef and Fenech,[14] with permission.]

Effect of Corticosteroids on Airway Caliber and Relaxation by Beta-Adrenergic Agonist

In the 1970s, Ellul-Micallef published reports of a marked effect of a single dose of corticosteroids [whether administered intravenously (IV), orally, or topically] on bronchial caliber in stable asthma.[13] The FEV$_1$ was noticeably better even by 1 h and peaked at 6 to 8 h. Even more interesting was the effect of the IV corticosteroid on the action of inhaled isoproterenol, i.e., there was marked amplification of its effect in those with diminished adrenergic responsiveness[14] (Fig. 46-5). This series of papers is very provocative because

it shows corticosteroid effects in isolation under controlled conditions. Certainly there is the suggestion that corticosteroids may even enhance the effect of endogenous catecholamines.

The topical application of corticosteroids in less severe asthma has also been shown to enhance the peak flow. Possibly enhanced action of β-adrenergic agonists also is involved here.

Intermittent versus Continuous Nebulization

In the life-threatening attacks of pediatric asthma, a fair amount of experience has been gained with continuous nebulization.[15–17] Papo et al. compared continuous nebulization of 0.3 mg/kg/h of albuterol to the same total dose applied every 20 min through the same apparatus.[17] Figure 46-6 shows the superiority of the continuous approach. One can only wonder why this occurs, but it may be that the airways narrow slightly between intermittent doses, somewhat limiting distribution of inhaled drug.

Nebulization versus High-Intensity Metered-Dose Inhalation

The use of high-intensity treatment by MDI for the acute attack is being advocated by some as a replacement for wet nebulization, despite the fact that the latter is certainly effective and advocated in the recent recommendations of the National Heart, Lung, and Blood Institute.[18] In that report, it was recommended that 2.5 mg albuterol be nebulized every 20 min during the first hour as needed and then followed at hourly intervals over the next 3 h. The MDI alternative in one scheme is to titrate the MDI dose, first applying 4 puffs, each separated by about 30 s, waiting 5 min, and then giving

FIGURE 46-6 Mean asthma scores compared with baseline for both continuous and intermittent nebulization of albuterol during the first 4 h of treatment (mean ± SEM). [From Papo et al.,[17] with permission.]

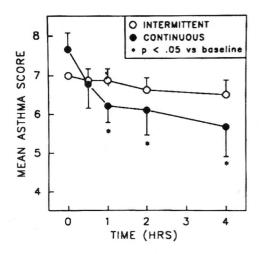

TABLE 46-1   Ratios of Equivalent Dose (MDI/Neb) in Various Studies using Dose-Response Curves

Authors	Ratio MDI:Neb	Drug	Spacer	Nebulizer
Cushley et al.[36]	1:1	Terbutaline	With and without	Dose leaving neb; face mask
Mestitz et al.[37]	1:2	Terbutaline	No	2.0 mL, face mask
Blake et al.[21]	1:2.5	Albuterol	Yes	2.0 mL, mouthpiece PC_{20} endpoint
Madsen et al.[38]	1:4	Terbutaline	Yes	2.0 mL, face mask
Weber et al.[39]	1:7	Terbutaline	No	1.0 mL, IPPB, Y tube
Harrison et al.[40]	1:12.5	Albuterol	No	2.0 mL

PC_{20} is the concentration of *histamine* producing a 20% drop in FEV_1; IPPB represents intermittent postivie pressure nebulized by Bennett apparatus, commonly used at that time.

1 puff every minute to a maximum of 12 puffs or as limited by side effects, usually tremor (J. Fink, personal communication). If this is not successful, nebulization should then commence. The necessary MDI dose can then be repeated in 1 h and then given, 4 to 6 puffs, at intervals of 2 to 4 h thereafter. Experience with this schedule, or versions of it, has been good but limited.[19] Advantages are claimed from the standpoint of cost, convenience, and better individualization of treatment. A valved spacer has advantage for some patients.[20]

The question of equivalence between a series of MDI puffs and wet nebulization, using a suitable dose-response approach, has been approached by at least six groups (Table 46-1). Unfortunately, the results are surprisingly disparate, and as many as 10 puffs may be needed to equal 2.5 mg albuterol by nebulization.[21] Nevertheless, in the acute crisis, 4 puffs with holding chamber, every 30 min, performs equally well.[21a]

Parenteral Beta-Adrenergic Agonists

The subcutaneous route, using either 0.25 to 0.5 mg terbutaline or 0.3 mg epinephrine, is especially valuable in those acutely ill patients who are responding only sluggishly to the inhaled medication. Appel et al. have published an impressive series in which the subcutaneous administration of epinephrine worked remarkably well in those who had not responded by 90 min to several nebulizations of metaproterenol.[22] They speculate that such patients have too much plugging of their airways to respond adequately to inhaled agents. The question of IV administration of β_2-adrenergic agonists in acute asthma has been studied over the years, with mixed results. A recent multicenter study compared 5.0 mg nebulized albuterol $\times$ 2 with 500 μg albuterol IV over 60 min in 47 acute, hypercapnic asthma patients.[23] Results were clearly superior at 60 min with nebulization. Mean serum albuterol concentrations were 10.0 ng/mL in the group receiving IV treatment and 7.8 ng/mL in the group treated by nebulization, proving systemic absorption of significant amounts. The authors provide a review of the literature to date on this contested issue (IV

approach usually inferior) but do not rule out a later role for cases refractory to nebulization.

Such cases have been published in pediatric status asthmaticus. They employ a loading dose followed by a maintenance dose. Dietrich et al. loaded patients with 10 μg/kg terbutaline, repeated in 30 min, and then maintained at 0.5 μg/kg/min for an average of 44 h.[24] Bohn et al. used a 10 μg/kg loading dose of albuterol followed by a maintenance dose beginning at 0.3 μg/kg/min and increasing to a mean rate of 1.7 μg/kg/min, with no toxicity.[25] An aggressive terbutaline loading and maintenance scheme, based upon considerable practical experience, has been published along with nomograms.[26] A loading dose, given over 10 minutes, is desirable to reach therapeutic concentration quickly. Since concentrations at first decline rather rapidly in the alpha phase of rapid distribution, the loading dose should be followed soon by a maintenance dose. If the patient has been receiving large doses by nebulization, concentrations are likely to be already substantial. Dosing is obviously very empirical, and careful monitoring and measurement of CPK-MB levels are necessary.

Inhaled Route in Mechanically Ventilated Patients

For years, small-volume nebulization was the standard in mechanically ventilated patients, and this was effective. With increased interest in the MDI, a profusion of devices was presented, adapted to the elbow connector of the endotrachial tube, directly to the inspiratory line, or to a holding chamber in the line. However, there has been no proof of efficacy for most of these, nor comparisons between them.

With the aid of bench models, it now has been established that the in-line reservoir system is most efficient,[27,28] and, using lung scans, this seems to be the case in vivo as well.[29] But deposition in the lung, 5 to 6 percent, is only about half that (10 percent) in the nonintubated patient.[30] Deposition by small-volume nebulization is even less.[30,31] It is efficacy, however, that must be the final arbiter of any comparison; with a variety of drugs, doses, and techniques, investigators have not been very successful in demonstrating efficacy.[32,33]

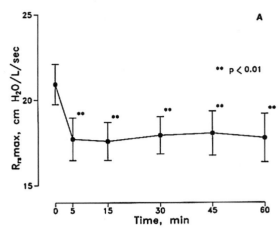

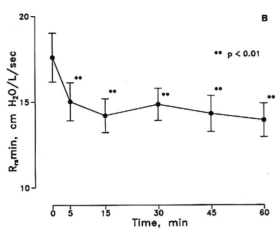

FIGURE 46-7 Effect of albuterol on maximal inspiratory resistance (R$_{rs}$ max; *panel A*) and minimal airway resistance (R$_{rs}$ min; *panel B*). Significant decreases in R$_{rs}$ max and R$_{rs}$ min were observed 5 min after albuterol administration, which were sustained for 60 min ($p < .01$). Bars represent SE. [*From Dhand et al.,*[35] *with permission.*]

Using a popular commercial swivel adaptor to the endotracheal tube for cumulative dosing of albuterol over 60 min to a total of 100 puffs, Manthous et al. showed no efficacy as determined by the effect on inspiratory pressure on mechanically ventilated patients; however, nebulization of 2.5 mg albuterol produced a significant reduction in inspiratory pressure. A total of 7.5 mg albuterol by nebulization was slightly more effective but caused mild toxicity (heart rate, premature atrial contractions), while 15.0 mg caused more toxicity (premature ventricular contractions).[34] There also is evidence that 10 puffs of albuterol, given at 20-s intervals through an in-line cylindrical reservoir to patients with chronic obstructive pulmonary disease, produces a significant decrease in inspiratory resistance[35] (Fig. 46-7).

References

1. Barnes PJ, Pride NB: Dose-response curves to inhaled β-adrenoceptor agonists in normal and asthmatic subjects. *Br J Clin Pharmacol* 1983; 15:677.
2. Williams MH, Kane C: Dose-response of patients with asthma to inhaled isoproterenol. *Am Rev Respir Dis* 1975; 111:321.
3. Ullman A, Svedmyr N: Salmeterol, a long acting inhaled β$_2$ adrenoceptor agonist: Comparison with salbutamol in adult asthmatic patients. *Thorax* 1988; 43:674.
4. Beach Jr, Young CL, Stenton SC, et al.: A comparison of the speeds of action of salmeterol and salbutamol in reversing methacholine-induced bronchoconstriction. *Pulm Pharmacol* 1992; 5:133.
5. Derom EY, Pauwels R: Time course of bronchodilating effect of inhaled formoterol, a potent and long-acting sympathomimetic. *Thorax* 1992; 47:3.
6. Pearlman DS, Chervinsky P, LaForce C, et al.: A comparison of salmeterol with albuterol in the treatment of mild to moderate asthma. *N Engl J Med* 1992; 327:1420.
7. D'Alonza GE, Nathan RA, Henochowicz S, et al.: Salmeterol xinofoate as maintenance therapy compared with albuterol in patients with asthma. *JAMA* 1994; 271:1412.
8. Greening AP, Ind PW, Northfield M, Shaw G: Added salmeterol versus higher-dose corticosteroid in asthma patients with symptoms on existing inhaled corticosteroid. *Lancet* 1994; 344:219.
9. Palmer JR, Stuart AM, Shepherd GL, Viskum K: Inhaled salmeterol in the treatment of patients with moderate to severe reversible obstructive airways disease—a 3 month comparison of the efficacy and safety of twice-daily salmeterol (100 micrograms) with salmeterol (50 micrograms). *Respir Med* 1992; 86:409.
10. Ahrens RC, Harris JB, Milavetz G, et al.: Use of bronchial provocation with histamine to compare the pharmacodynamics of inhaled albuterol and metaproterenol in patients with asthma. *J Allergy Clin Immunol* 1987; 79:876.
11. Konig P, Hordvik NL, Serby CW: Fenoterol in exercise-induced asthma. Effect of dose on efficacy and duration of action. *Chest* 1984; 85:462.
12. O'Connor BJ, Aikman SL, Barnes PJ: Tolerance to the nonbronchodilator effects of inhaled β$_2$-agonists in asthma. *N Engl J Med* 1992; 327:1204.
13. Ellul-Micallef R, Borthwick RC, McHardy GJR: The time-course of response to prednisolone in chronic bronchial asthma. *Clin Sci* 1974; 47:105.
14. Ellul-Micallef R, Fenech FF: Effect of intravenous prednisolone in asthmatics with diminished adrenergic responsiveness. *Lancet* 1975; 2:1269.
15. Katz RW, Kelly HW, Crowley MR: Safety of continuous nebulized albuterol for bronchospasm in infants and children. *Pediatrics* 1993; 92:666.
16. Moler FW, Hurwitz ME, Custer JR: Improvement in clinical asthma score and PaCO$_2$ in children with severe asthma treated with continuously nebulized terbutaline. *J Allergy Clin Immunol* 1988; 81:1101.
17. Papo MC, Frank JA, Thompson AE: A prospective randomized study of continuous versus intermittent nebulized albuterol for severe status asthmaticus in children. *Crit Car Med* 1993; 21:1479.
18. National Heart and Lung Institute: *Guidelines for the Diagnosis and Management of Asthma*. Bethesda, MD, NHLBI Information Center, 1991.
19. Newhouse MT: Emergency department management of life-threatening asthma. *Chest* 1993; 103:661.

20. Dolovitch MB, Ruffin R, Corr D, Newhouse MT: Clinical evaluation of a simple demand inhalation aerosol delivery device. *Chest* 1983; 84:37.
21. Blake K, Hoppe M, Harmon E, Hendeles L: Relative amount of albuterol delivered to lung receptors from a metered dose inhaler and nebulizer solution; bioassay by histamine provocation. *Chest* 1991; 101:309.
21a. Idris AH, McDermott MF, Raucci JC, et al.: Emergency department treatment of severe asthma. *Chest* 1993; 103:665.
22. Appel DW, Karpel JP, Sherman M: Epinephrine improves expiratory flow rates in patients with asthma who do not respond to inhaled metaproterenol sulfate. *J Allergy Clin Immunol* 1989; 84:90.
23. Salmeron S, Brochard L, Mal H: Nebulized versus intravenous albuterol in hypercapnic acute asthma. A multicenter, double-blind randomized study. *Am J Respir Crit Care Med* 1994; 149:1466.
24. Dietrich KA, Conrad SA, Romero MD: Creatine kinase (CK) isoenzymes in pediatric status asthmaticus treated with intravenous terbutline. *Crit Care Med* 1991; 19:539.
25. Bohn D, Kalloghian A, Jenkins J, et al.: Intravenous salbutamol in the treatment of status asthmaticus in children. *Crit Care Med* 1984; 12:392.
26. Uden DL: Guidelines for intravenous terbutaline use in status asthmaticus, in Weiss EB, Stein M (eds): *Bronchial Asthma. Mechanisms and Therapeutics* (3d ed). Boston, Little, Brown, 1993; 1221.
27. Rau JL, Harwood RJ, Groff JL: Evaluation of a reservoir device for metered-dose bronchodilator delivery to intubated adults. An in vitro study. *Chest* 1992; 102:924.
28. Ebert J, Adams AA, Green-Eide B: An evaluation of spacers and adaptors: Their effect on the respirable volume of medication. *Respir Care* 1992; 37:862.
29. Fuller HD, Dolovitch MB, Turpie FH, Newhouse MT: Efficiency of bronchodilator aerosol delivery to the lungs from the metered dose inhaled in mechanically ventilated patients. A study comparing four different actuator devices. *Chest* 1994; 105:214.
30. Fuller HD, Dolovich MB, Posmituck G, et al.: Pressurized aerosol versus jet aerosol delivery to mechanically ventilated patients. Comparison of dose to the lungs. *Am Rev Respir Dis* 1990; 141:440.
31. MacIntyre NR, Silver RM, Miller CW, et al.: Aerosol delivery in intubated, mechanically ventilated patients. *Crit Care Med* 1985; 13:81.
32. Gross NJ, Jenne JW, Hess D: Bronchodilator therapy, in Tobin MJ (ed): *Principles and Practice of Mechanical Ventilation* 1994; New York, McGraw-Hill, 1994; 1077–1123.
33. Manthous CA, Hall JB: Administration of therapeutic aerosols to mechanically ventilated patients. *Chest* 1994; 106:560.
34. Manthous CA, Hall JB, Schmidt GA, Wood LDH: Metered dose inhaler versus nebulized albuterol in mechanically ventilated patients. *Am Rev Respir Dis* 1993; 148:1567.
35. Dhand R, Jubran A, Tobin MJ: Bronchodilator delivery by metered-dose inhaler in ventilator supported patients. *Am J Respir Crit Care Med* 1995; 151:1827–1833.
36. Cushley MJ, Lewis RA, Tattersfield AE: Comparison of three techniques of inhalation on the airway response to terbutaline. *Thorax* 1983; 38:90.
37. Mestitz H, Copeland JM, McDonald CF: Comparison of outpatient nebulized vs metered dose inhaled terbutaline in chronic air flow obstruction. *Chest* 1989; 96:1237–1240.
38. Madsen ED, Bundgaard A, Hidlinger KC: Cumulative dose-response study comparing terbutaline pressurized aerosol administered via a pear shaped spacer and terbutaline in a nebulized solution. *Eur J Clin Pharmacol* 1982; 23:271.
39. Weber RW, Petty WE, Nelson HS: Aerosolized terbutaline in asthmatics, comparison of dosage strength, schedule and method of delivery. *J Allergy Clin Immunol* 1979: 63:116.
40. Harrison BA, Pierce RJ: Comparison of wet and dry salbutamol. *Aust N Z J Med* 1983; 13:29.

Chapter 47

ADVERSE EFFECTS OF BETA-ADRENERGIC AGONISTS

JOHN W. JENNE

The "asthma paradox"—the increasing incidence of asthma and asthma mortality despite advances in drug therapy—continues to drive investigators to examine any potential deleterious role of β-adrenergic agonists. The issue is difficult and has polarized expert opinion into two camps: those who emphasize early use of inhaled corticosteroids and constantly warn against reliance on β$_2$-adrenergic agonists, and those who, while acknowledging the importance of corticosteroids, feel that treatment of residual bronchospasm is of prime importance. Finding the proper balance in this issue is important, especially now that long-acting β$_2$-adrenergic agonists, salmeterol and formoterol, are available and have so much to offer in stabilizing the airways.

The available evidence bearing on possible adverse effects is of two types: (1) relatively short-term studies examining the effects of inhaled β$_2$-adrenergic agonists on a number of airway properties, from which long-term speculations are made; and (2) retrospective epidemiologic studies of death and near-death episodes seeking clues that might implicate certain drug therapies.

Adverse Effects on the Airways

1971 TO 1989

These studies can be divided into two periods. The earliest, from 1971 to the late 1980s, began with a proposal by Conolly et al. that tachyphylaxis induced by inhaled isoproterenol was responsible for excessive asthma deaths.[1] This was based upon studies with guinea pigs, in which tachyphylaxis induction by isoproterenol reduced their ability to survive histamine challenge. Animal studies also alerted the profession to the possibility that large doses of inhaled isoproterenol combined with hypoxia, possibly further aggravated by chlorofluorohydrocarbons in the mixture, could sensitize the heart to fatal arrhythmias or lead to bradycardia and asystole.[2]

With the introduction of selective β$_2$-adrenergic agonists in the mid-1970s, studies appeared showing the production of a degree of airway tachyphylaxis by oral regimens.[3–5] Others found no evidence of this.[6] Tachyphylaxis of systemic β$_2$-adrenergic receptor-mediated responses [decrease in eosinophils, rise in lactate, rise in plasma cyclic adenosine monophosphate (cAMP)] was more pronounced than the effect on airways.[3] Some negative studies had not employed a preliminary washout period to remove possible preexisting tachyphylaxis.[7]

An important advance was the demonstration by Holgate et al., using a dose-response curve to inhaled albuterol, that tachyphylaxis could be readily produced in normal individuals with a progressive dosing increase to 400 μg qid over a 4-week period[8] but not in atopic normal individuals or atopic asthma patients.[9] Such tachyphylaxis could be reversed by an intravenous dose of 200 mg hydrocortisone applied 6 h previously. Systemic responses were also affected. Why atopy should render subjects less susceptible to tachyphylaxis remains a mystery, unless some subsensitivity already exists in such patients. Using the entire response curve over time, Weber et al. showed slight tachyphylaxis development over 12 weeks in asthma patients on 500 μg qid terbutaline by metered-dose inhaler (MDI).[10] This also was shown in a large multicenter study that lacked controls but that was nevertheless convincing.[11] There was

497

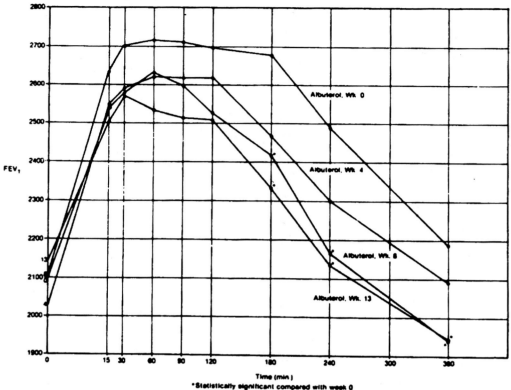

FIGURE 47-1 Absolute values of mean FEV_1 after inhalation of albuterol by MDI at study weeks 0, 4, 8, and 13 on a maintenance schedule four times daily. There was no significant difference in peak values, but the duration of effect was significantly less at weeks 8 and 13. Despite the lack of a placebo control, the data are highly suggestive of some degree of tachyphylaxis development. (*From Repsher et al.,[11] with permission.*)

about a 50 percent reduction in the area under the curve by the 8-week point, at which it stabilized (Fig. 47-1). The peak response was not as sensitive an indicator of tachyphylaxis. With this reduction in duration, the trough discomfort between doses is obviously accentuated.

The issue of tachyphylaxis has been extensively studied by Lipworth et al. by comparing the slope of the cumulative dose-response to a total of 4000 μg albuterol.[12,13] None was found in the FEV_1 response following either low- (800 μg/day) or high-dose (4000 μg/day) albuterol, but there was tachyphylaxis in the response of heart rate increase, decrease in serum K^+, increase in blood glucose, and increased tremor, especially at the higher dose. Nevertheless, six years later, in more severe asthmatics on 24 μg bid of the longer acting formoterol by dry powder inhaler (DPI), and despite inhaled corticosteroids, this group did find tachyphylaxis of both peak and duration of bronchodilation and systemic responses to cumulative doses.[13a]

Tachyphylaxis of the protective ability of the β₂-adrenergic agonists against bronchodilator challenge was next studied. A reduced ability was shown to develop against exercise-induced bronchospasm[14] but not against histamine challenge.[15] In three asthma patients studied, Tashkin et al. also found no loss in protective ability of subcutaneous terbutaline against histamine while on oral terbutaline but, in two of them, reduced ability to protect against allergen challenge, restored by administering 40 mg prednisone 16 h before challenge.[16] Coupled with in vitro studies showing differ-

ences in susceptibility to tachyphylaxis between mast cell receptors and those in airway smooth muscle,[17] these studies foretold the current studies showing greater tachyphylaxis of protection from an inflammatory challenge.

1989 TO PRESENT

Attention once again focused on adverse effects of β₂-adrenergic agonists, arising out of New Zealand mortality data. Analysis of therapy preceding a fatal outcome led to concerns over the powerful 200 μg/puff fenoterol and subsequent analysis of its systemic effects in comparison with albuterol. Studies also resumed on possible adverse effects of chronic β₂-adrenergic agonist use on the airways, beginning with several papers documenting a small increase in airway hyperresponsiveness.[18,19]

Perhaps the studies with the greatest impact were those by Sears et al.[20] and Taylor et al.,[21] in which 66 patients with mild to moderate asthma (mean FEV_1 77 percent, most on inhaled corticosteroids, were begun on either 400 μg fenoterol qid by dry powder inhaler (DPI) or only "as needed" medication. After 24 weeks, they were crossed over. There was a significant fall in mean FEV_1 of 0.15 L, and a reduction in morning peak flow but increased evening flow (Fig. 47-2). Bronchial responsiveness to methacholine increased significantly on the regular regimen, the PC_{20} (concentration producing a 20% reduction in FEV_1) falling from 1.63 to 1.15 doubling doses (DD).

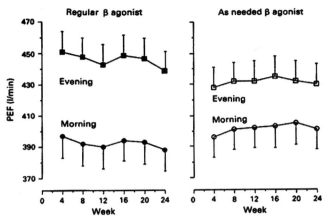

FIGURE 47-2 Mean morning and evening peak flow rates (with standard error bars) during regular and as needed β-adrenergic agonist treatment, averaged over each 4-week period. (*From Taylor et al.,*[21] *with permission.*)

Patients on the regular regimen experienced a more frequent need for emergency medication and judged control of their asthma to be worse (p = .003). The slightly reduced 8:00 A.M. peak flow might be considered "rebound bronchospasm" from the dose the evening before, but more correctly it should be considered a temporary inability of the airway to maintain its caliber, which persists following bronchodilator withdrawal. This is probably similar to the temporary 10 percent reduction in FEV_1 and 6.5 percent reduction in peak flow found by Wahedna et al. after withdrawal from a 21-day course of albuterol.[22] In that study, patients with mild asthma underwent a preliminary washout for 14 days to remove any preexisting tachyphylaxis, and then post- and predrug values were compared. The PC_{20} also showed a decrease of 1.47 DD to methacholine and a loss of protective ability by albuterol ranging from 1.1 to 1.65 DD over at least a 59-h period while the FEV_1 was returning to normal.

O'Connor et al. compared tachyphylaxis development of terbutaline protection against methacholine and against AMP challenge. The latter is considered to be "inflammatory" provocation.[23] Following a 7-day washout, patients with mild asthma (mean FEV_1 97 percent) commenced terbutaline, 500 µg qid by DPI. After 7 days, there was reduced protection against methacholine (PC_{20} reduced by 0.5 DD) but a greater loss against AMP (PC_{20} reduced by 2.1 DD) (Fig. 47-3).

Perhaps the most revealing study regarding this dichotomy compared the tachyphylaxis development in protection against methacholine and allergen challenge.[24] After a 30-day washout, patients with mild asthma commenced a 14-day period on albuterol, 200 µg qid. In contrast to the other studies, there was no change in 8:00 A.M. flows or in basal sensitivity to methacholine, but there was an increased sensitivity to graded challenges by allergen (fall in PC_{20} of 0.91 DD) and a greater loss of protection against allergen (fall of 1.2 DD) compared to methacholine (fall of 0.7 DD) (Fig. 47-4).

Continuously inhaled salmeterol also appears to lose some of its own protective ability against methacholine. Patients with mild asthma on 50 µg bid sustained loss of effect at 28 and 56 days, with reduced increase in PC_{20} after drug (from 3.3 to 1.0 DD)[25] and this has very recently been confirmed by a different group.[25a] Yet an earlier study failed to demonstrate this loss of protection but most of these asthmatics were also on inhaled corticosteroids.[25b] A loss of effect against exercise-induced asthma also has been observed, the decrease in placebo of 34.8 percent FEV_1 being only 11.9 percent on salmeterol initially but, when studied at 4 weeks, 32.9 and 24 percent, respectively.[26]

These studies suggest some degree of inherent instability of bronchi while on continuous use of a bronchodilator and in the bronchodilator's ability to protect against a challenge, especially an inflammatory one. The apparent lack of any effect on bronchodilator response is suspect because the degree of asthma in the patients studied was so mild in relation to the dose. Is the instability due to tachyphylaxis of $β_2$-adrenergic receptors affecting inherent airway caliber homeostatic mechanisms, or are the contractile properties per se of the airway being enhanced? The phenomenon still defies explanation and is of great concern to many concerned with asthma demographics.[27] The amelioration of the risk with corticosteroids and the true risk when adequately bronchodilated await definition.

An intriguing new line of animal investigation has begun with an approach using large doses of fenoterol nebulized to guinea pigs, examining their airways in detail both in vivo and in vitro.[28] Another batch of animals received repeated ovalbumin challenge to their airways (chronic allergen expo-

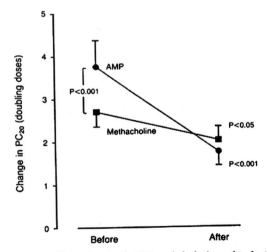

FIGURE 47-3 Effect of a single 500-µg inhalation of terbutaline on airway responsiveness to methacholine and AMP. The effect is shown as the mean (±SEM) change in PC_{20}, expressed in doubling doses, after the inhalation of terbutaline as compared with placebo before and after 7 days of treatment with terbutaline. After the 7-day period, there was significantly reduced protection against AMP (p < .001) and methacholine (p < .05) as compared with the values before treatment. The difference in the changes in PC_{20} for AMP and methacholine was significant before treatment (p < .001) but it was abolished after treatment. (*From O'Connor et al.,*[23] *with permission.*)

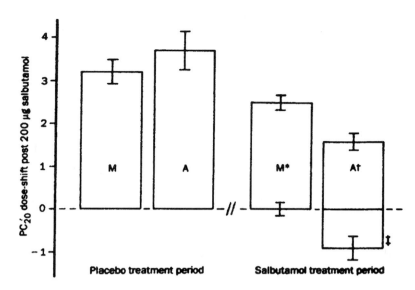

FIGURE 47-4 Methacholine PC_{20} and allergen PC_{20} before and after 200 µg salbutamol during the two treatment periods. Results ($n = 12$) are expressed as the dose shift (mean ± SEM), as doubling doses of each, calculated as $\Delta log_{10}PC_{20} \div 0.3$. Baseline PC_{20} values during placebo treatment period are arbitrarily defined as 0. SE bars at bottom of two salbutamol treatment period bars represent dose-shift compared with placebo period (M = methacholine; A = allergen; *p = .026; †p = .025; ‡p = .0009). (*From Cockcroft et al.*,[24] *with permission.*)

sure), with and without concurrent fenoterol. At 72 h following fenoterol, both in vivo and in vitro airway responses to acetylcholine were still accentuated, with a twofold increase in maximum tension produced by acetylcholine but no evidence of reduced bronchodilator efficacy. The effect with chronic exposure to allergen was grossly similar. The question is whether this hyperresponsiveness is specific to a muscarinic stimulus or is a general contractility phenomenon, and whether other β_2-adrenergic agonists will behave similarly. Wills-Karp et al. have shown that chronic allergen exposure increases muscarinic responsiveness, and this appears as bronchodilator insensitivity.[29]

A second intriguing and still-evolving line of investigation is the hypothesis that bronchial hyperresponsiveness is caused by accumulation of the (+) enantiomer of the inhaled racemic mixtures of β_2-adrenergic agonists, as based upon a guinea pig model.[30,31]

Adverse Effects on the Heart

The current emphasis on high-dose inhaled therapy in the acute attack and the concerns arising over β_2-adrenergic agonists from epidemiologic studies have prompted careful study of the potential toxic effects of β_2-adrenergic agonists.

ARRHYTHMIAS

In the late stages of life-threatening asthma, it is primarily asphyxia rather than arrhythmias that is responsible for death. In an analysis of 10 asthma patients first seen in respiratory arrest (no apparent respirations), only two had arrhythmias other than sinus tachycardia (one with atrial fibrillation and the other sinus bradycardia). Both of these arrhythmias responded rapidly to manual ventilation with oxygen.[32]

By far the greatest problem in life-threatening asthma is undertreatment. However, there remain questions as to whether β_2-adrenergic agonists cause deaths and whether these deaths are avoidable. Arrhythmias have not been

noted in large overdoses of β_2-adrenergic agonists. However, by analogy to the malignant ventricular arrhythmias of several acquired or congenital entities with prolonged QT_c intervals (the QT interval for corrected heart rate), the argument has been made that such prolongation by β_2-adrenergic agonists combined with hypoxemia and hypokalemia could be responsible for fatal arrhythmias.[33] QT_c prolongation is a predictor of sudden death in acute myocardial infarction, and the incidence of ventricular tachycardia or fibrillation is highly correlated with hypokalemia.[34]

Various authors have concluded that fenoterol is "less beta₂-selective" than albuterol, based upon its similarity to isoproterenol in effect on heart rate and prolongation of QT_c when cumulatively dosed to 26 puffs.[35] The dangers of high-dose fenoterol (200 µg/puff) prompted a reduction to 100 µg/puff and caution in dosing recommendation.

Does fenoterol have less beta₂ selectivity than albuterol? When dosed equally up to 1200, 1800, and 2400 µg in normal individuals, there was a larger peak effect on heart rate, cAMP elevation, decrease in serum K^+, and T-wave depression (see Fig. 44-2).[36] When fenoterol, albuterol, and formoterol were given by MDI at 400 µg every 30 min for five doses, the effect on heart rate, QT_c interval, serum K^+, and FEV_1 was more pronounced for fenoterol than albuterol.[37] When fenoterol, albuterol, and isoproterenol were given at 400 µg at 0, 30, 40, and 45 min and responses followed to 60 min, fenoterol and isoproterenol produced greater inotropic stimulation (QS_2 interval shortening) than albuterol, and fenoterol produced an earlier effect on FEV_1 (see Table 44-4).[38] When either 5.0 mg nebulized fenoterol or albuterol were administered to stable asthma patients and the dose repeated in 1 h (in those judged able to tolerate it), a similar pattern was seen (see Fig. 44-2). Bremner et al. concluded that "the observed differences between fenoterol and albuterol in severe asthma provide a plausible mechanism, which may explain the increased risk of death associated with fenoterol in severe asthma."[39]

It is unclear whether fenoterol is less beta₂-selective than albuterol, or if fenoterol has greater efficacy for the β_1-

adrenoreceptor. In New Zealand, the drug has been withdrawn from use and this has coincided with a reduction in asthma mortality. In other countries, where its use is retained, fenoterol is administered at a reduced dose of 100 μg/puff.

It it has been difficult to identify malignant arrhythmias caused by β_2-adrenergic agonists in clinical circumstances, and it is unethical to attempt to duplicate experimentally the degree of hypoxemia and stress for such studies. Mild hypoxemia (90% O_2 saturation) adds to prolongation of the QT_c caused by fenoterol,[40] but addition of theophylline does not, although it potentiates the inotropic and chronotropic effects.[41] Several studies have monitored heart rhythm using substantial doses of β_2-adrenergic agonists. No abnormalities were seen in young asthma patients when 0.25 mg terbutaline was given subcutaneously and repeated in 30 min, despite the fact that serum K^+ decreased from 4.3 to 3.2 meq/L. The QT_c changes exactly mirrored the decrease in K^+.[42] Arrhythmias were not seen in 10 acute asthmatics followed over 120 min after multiple nebulized 2.5 mg doses of albuterol (avg. 2.7 doses, range 1 to 6) while serum K^+ concentrations steadily decreased from a mean of 4.5 to 3.7 meq/L.[43]

Older patients with chronic obstructive pulmonary disease (COPD) are prone to asymptomatic rhythm disturbances. In acute exacerbations treated with 5.0 mg terbutaline nebulized four times daily, there was no increase in serious arrhythmias immediately and for 60 min following each treatment compared to the interim periods. Abnormalities improved somewhat as patients improved.[44]

Perhaps the most informative study was done by Higgins et al. in 19 stable COPD patients who were monitored while receiving either 5.0 mg nebulized albuterol or 4.0 mg terbutaline every 4 h delivered with room air.[45] Two patients experienced arrhythmias only with nebulization (short runs of ventricular tachycardia in one; two episodes of paroxysmal atrial tachycardia in the other), and in three others, there were more frequent runs of atrial fibrillation or increased ventricular bigeminy or trigeminy. In all cases, the patients remained asymptomatic. The authors concluded that "nebulization in older patients with severe COPD cannot be considered completely safe."

Two case reports of acutely ill patients with underlying heart disease are particularly instructive. In one, a 60-year-old man with mild hypertension was admitted to the hospital with acute asthma. His electrocardiogram showed left axis deviation and minimum T-wave inversion in lateral leads. He received 5.0 mg albuterol by nebulization every 4 h and oxygen, with improved breathing. However, on the third, fourth, and fifth treatment, he noted chest pain radiating to the neck and finally developed a myocardial infarction.[46] The authors recommend 2.5 mg rather than 5.0 mg when risk factors for a history of ischemic heart disease exist. A second case was a 58-year-old man with severe COPD who was admitted for a myocardial infarction. Initially, he had a 6-beat salvo of ventricular tachycardia and isolated ventricular premature contractions. On the tenth day, he received his first 5.0-mg tablet of terbutaline, and 2 h later began having 20 to 30 unifocal ventricular premature contractions per minute; these diminished gradually over sev-

eral hours. Three months later he was "rechallenged," but with 2.5 mg terbutoline first, and 1 h later with a second 2.5-mg dose; the ectopic events recurred as intensely as before. He remained asymptomatic throughout.[47] There are also reports of patients with ischemic heart disease who develop angina with nebulization of 5.0 mg albuterol.

These cases illustrate the potential danger of modest systemic levels of β_2-adrenergic agonists in the elderly, when underlying heart disease exists—especially in patients with COPD. The current trend to use tailored doses by MDI is a good one from this standpoint, and monitoring and adequate oxygenation during their use in an emergent situation are imperative. If nebulization is used, doses should not routinely exceed 2.5 mg of albuterol.

MYOCARDIAL DEPRESSION. SYNERGISM WITH HYPOXEMIA

Isoproterenol, administered progressively to dogs from 0.1 to 500 μg/kg at 5- to 10-min intervals or given as six injections of 2.5 μg/kg at 5-min intervals, causes increased heart rate and stroke volume and decreased peripheral resistance but does not affect survival.[2] However, on 12% O_2, which causes a Pa_{O_2} of 35 to 40 mmHg, 10 to 50 μg/kg isoproterenol caused severe hypotension and idioventricular rhythm, slowing to asystole.[2] The same outcome occurred with metaproterenol and albuterol, only at somewhat larger doses. Adverse effects were blocked with propranolol, but subtype-specificity was not examined. In one report, myocardial depression was related to intravenous albuterol administration in a young woman.[48] The message is clear. High doses of even albuterol are more toxic under severely hypoxemic conditions.

MYOCARDIAL NECROSIS

For years, pharmacologists have studied the occurrence of myocardial necrosis, arrhythmias, and death following administration of β-adrenergic drugs, particularly isoproterenol, to animals[49] and have been aware of similar lesions in humans. In humans, the best documented examples of catecholamine-induced myocardial necrosis are seen at autopsy of patients with pheochromocytomas of the adrenal gland and frequent "adrenal storms." These consist of individual focal lesions of myocardial necrosis with a lymphocytic and histiocytic infiltrate, but only rare neutrophils, involving primarily the endocardial zone of the left ventricle.[49,50] These lesions have also been observed in intracranial hemorrhage and were reported in four fatal asthma attacks in children, two of whom had received no intravenous sympathomimetic drugs.[48] In these cases, myocardial necrosis is believed to be caused by excessive endogenous sympathetic stimulation, some of which may be mediated through nervous discharge.

ANIMAL STUDIES

Isoproterenol causes focal myocardial necrosis in various animal species over a wide dosage range. The apex and papillary muscle are the sites of predilection, and lesions occur subendocardially in both ventricles and occasionally in the atrium. Lesions are distinct from those seen in myocardial infarction. Necrotic muscle cells show a loss of the normal pattern of cross-striation with prominent "contraction bands" (agglomerated masses of contractile protein) in their cytoplasm. The arrhythmias that may occur concurrently consist of premature contractions, ventricular tachycardia, and fibrillation. Doses producing these lesions in rats vary enormously and depend on weight and age; fat rats being substantially more susceptible. Dogs are more susceptible than rats, and rabbits are relatively resistant.[51] Isoproterenol-induced arrhythmias and necrosis are potentiated by corticosteroids, thyroxine, and, most importantly, ≥ 40 μg/mL plasma concentrations of theophylline.

Studies comparing salbutamol, terbutaline, and metaproterenol demonstrated that only metaproterenol had similar myocardial toxicity to isoproterenol.[52] The data suggest that the more beta$_1$-stimulating action a compound has, the more likely it is to cause myocardial necrosis. The β$_1$-adrenergic antagonist, practolol, is able to block all myocardial changes without affecting the decrease in blood pressure from either drug, indicating again that the beta$_1$ actions of salbutamol are responsible for myocardial toxicity and that the hypoperfusion is not the cause of damage.

The heart has a curious but fortunate ability to develop resistance to insults such as the necrosis produced by isoproterenol.[53] Once a heart is damaged, and survives, it is relatively resistant to the next dose for a period of at least several months. Small daily doses will also produce resistance. In some cases, this phenomenon might be helpful to the asthma patient. As the result of extensive animal studies exploring the conditions and drug combinations producing this injury and these arrhythmias,[50,51,54] some of their findings are already applicable to human use. More detail is available in the review by Sly et al.[55]

RELEVANCE OF ANIMAL TOXICITY STUDIES TO HUMANS

Due to differences in species, body fat, age, previous drug exposure, and mode of administration, it is impossible to translate the myocardial toxicity data in experimental animals directly to the human case. Furthermore, the disparity between fatal dosage of isoproterenol and the dosage producing microscopic lesions means that damage that is occurring in humans may be missed. There is now evidence that this is the case. Cardiac-specific serum creatine phosphokinase (CPK-MB) isozyme concentrations indicative of injury increased in 15 of 19 children being treated with intravenous isoproterenol, methylprednisolone, and aminophylline for life-threatening asthma. These CPK-MB concentrations returned to normal when isoproterenol was stopped, while the other drugs were continued.[56] A more serious result was in an 18-year-old woman with plasma theophylline concentrations of 25 to 30 μg/mL who received isoproterenol in doses ≤ 0.32 μg/kg/min for over 24 h and who then developed cardiac arrest. The myocardium contained necrotic lesions.[57]

On the other hand, in 20 children treated with intravenous terbutaline and methylprednisolone, but not aminophylline,

there was no increase in CPK-MB concentrations at mean infusion rates of 0.9 μg/kg/min for doses ≤ 3.0 μg/kg/min following a loading dose of 10 μg/kg.[58] Similarly, in seven children with a terbutaline maintenance dose averaging 0.5 μg/kg/min over 44 h, no change in CPK-MB concentration was observed.[59] In the children treated by Katz et al. with continuous nebulized terbutaline, one-third of whom were receiving aminophylline, there was no significant increase in serum CPK-MB.[60] With selective β$_2$-adrenergic agonists, the danger to the myocardium is reduced greatly.

Epidemiologic Studies

The following account does not do justice to these studies. More detail can be found in a recent excellent monograph on the β$_2$-agonist controversy[61] and by others discussing the questions surrounding their use.[62]

An increase in asthma deaths in Great Britain has been attributed to the introduction of a "forte" strength of isoproterenol (0.4 mg/puff compared to 0.08 mg/puff previously used). Increased mortality was not observed in countries not using "forte" isoproterenol. Fenoterol was studied extensively in New Zealand asthma during the late 1970s and early 1980s. Three case-control studies have been published,[63–65] all of them analyzing mortality retrospectively. The use of fenoterol was associated with an approximate fourfold increase in mortality compared to albuterol. Since the dose per puff of fenoterol was twice that of albuterol and it is more potent systemically, it was suggested that fenoterol use was relatively more dangerous for patients. Other, behavioristic explanations were also considered. Patients with more severe asthma may have required a stronger preparation or sought one ("confounding by severity"). Patients with such a strong medication may have been deluded into waiting too long to seek medical assistance. At any rate, the epidemic subsided coincident with the declining market share for fenoterol and its withdrawal. This also coincided with increased attention to asthma management.

The Saskatchewan studies, covering 8 years of experience, arose from retrospective analyses of 12,301 asthma patients. In the first study, 129 asthma patients using β$_2$-adrenergic agonists and hospitalized for severe asthma were matched with 665 controls who were also hospitalized that year but not previously using β$_2$-adrenergic agonists. The incidence of death or near-death episodes was greater in the group receiving β$_2$-adrenergic agonists particularly in those using fenoterol. While the initial publication emphasized the danger of fenoterol, the indictment became a class indictment of β$_2$-adrenergic agonists when, in order to meet the criticism that the controls were not matched, a subsequent publication examined each hospitalization in detail and the physicians involved with the case.[66] With further matching of severity factors, there was little difference in the outcome. Correcting for the difference in dose per puff between fenoterol and albuterol, the mean odds ratio now became 2.5 for fenoterol and 2.0 for albuterol, an insignificant difference. The authors concluded that β$_2$-adrenergic agonists are "independently associated with asthma death or near-death" and "not seriously confounded by severity." Thus, the implication was

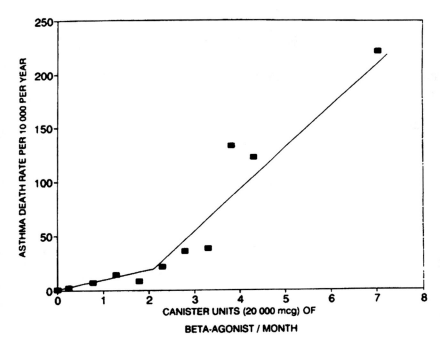

FIGURE 47-5 Observed and fitted change-point dose-response curve of asthma death rate versus amount of combined inhaled β-adrenergic agonist use in canister units of 20,000 µg per month. This model allows risk increases at low doses. (*From Suissa et al.,*[57] *with permission.*)

that their use was harmful. However, the problem in such a study is that retrospective controls for asthmatic death or near-death, picked from nonfatal cases, must remain clearly suspect.

A final publication has looked at mortality from asthma using the entire cohort of 12,301 cases as controls, again beginning with those cases on fenoterol and/or albuterol.[67] When corrected to the same dose (µg/µg), the mortality rate as a function of number of canisters used (corrected to albuterol dose and size) takes an abrupt upwards slope above 2.0 canister units per month (Fig. 47-5). At greatest doses, the curve for fenoterol is steeper than that for albuterol, but there are too few cases to reach statistical significance. Nevertheless, this fact again raises the specter that fenoterol could be more harmful than albuterol. However, as the authors admit, fenoterol might have been prescribed specifically because the asthma was more severe. Also noted is that there was no increase in cardiac deaths on the autopsy reports for those patients receiving β₂-adrenergic agonists. The authors now favor the interpretation that β₂-adrenergic agonists are a "marker of severe, poorly controlled asthma, itself the cause of high risks observed."

To fulfill Koch's postulates for the hypothesis that β₂-agonist use worsens asthma,[68] one must prospectively show that their reduction improves asthma, assuming that use of corticosteroids is not excessive. This will be a difficult task. Patient comfort must be considered, as well as steroid side effects. These studies are very important and will be awaited with great interest.

Miscellaneous Safety Concerns

1. In a 16-week comparison of 14,113 patients receiving 50 µg bid salmeterol and 7082 patients on albuterol (two puffs four times daily), there were fewer withdrawals due to asthma for patients treated with salmeterol (2.7 percent versus 3.9 percent, p = .0002).[69] However, the number of respiratory deaths due to asthma numbered 12 (0.007 percent on salmeterol and 2 (0.02 percent on albuterol (p = .105). Independent reviewers concluded that 10 of the deaths on salmeterol could have been managed with more adroit corticosteroid use. The information packets have been strengthened.

2. Multiple dosing by MDI again raises the issue of myocardial toxicity due to chlorofluorohydrocarbons (CFCs) under hypoxic conditions. Studies in the early 1970s revealed that the half-life of the F-11 and F-12 CFCs were 20 to 30 s and that it would require continuous inhalations over 2 min to reach toxic levels.[70] Nevertheless, it is prudent to build some interruptions into a high-intensity MDI dosing regimen in view of the limited information that is available.

3. Only mention can be made of these circumstances that can enhance the arrhythmic potential of sympathomimetics. These include ischemic heart disease, hyperthyroidism, monoamine oxidase inhibitors, tricyclic antidepressants, and the presence of halogenated anesthetics. Epinephrine and β₂-adrenergic agonists can increase blood pressure, and, with its α-adrenergic component, epinephrine may cause precipitous and dangerous increases in blood pressure in hypertensive patients or those taking β-adrenoreceptor antagonists. Diabetes and wide-angle glaucoma can also be aggravated by large doses of β₂-adrenergic agonists.[71]

A PERSPECTIVE ON SAFETY VERSUS EFFICACY OF BETA₂-ADRENERGIC AGONISTS

JOHN W. JENNE

Summary

1. In two epidemics, epidemiologists have incriminated a potent β-adrenergic agonist then in use, isoproterenol "forte" (400 μg/puff) in Great Britain and fenoterol (200 μg/puff) in New Zealand. Their use coincided with excess asthma mortality. A compelling conclusion is that *metered-dose inhaler* (MDI) *use may cause delay in seeking needed medical attention.*

2. In the retrospective case-control Saskatchewan study, asthma mortality has been correlated with β₂-adrenergic agonist use as a class. While earlier papers tended to incriminate β₂-adrenergic agonists as causative, a recent position is that heavy use (over 2 canisters/month) is a *marker of severe asthma* and warrants careful management and optimal corticosteroid use.

3. Beta₂-adrenergic agonists administered by MDI probably produce some ongoing *increase in airway hyperresponsiveness,* the mechanisms and prognostic implications of which are poorly understood. Considerable opposition to their regular use remains in some quarters, based upon this phenomenon. Some *drug tolerance develops,* more evident in their anti-bronchoconstrictive that bronchodilating action, and most apparent against inflammatory (mast-cell discharging) stimuli.

4. Salmeterol xinofoate, 50 μg (42 μg at dispenser), and formoterol fumarate, 12 or 24 μg, each every 12 h, are an enormous improvement in patient comfort over a 24-h period. Their long action depends on their lipophilic properties, but their *receptor behavior differs.* These are safe provided the following are observed:
   a. Patients using the slow-onset salmeterol should carry a rapid-acting β₂-adrenergic agonist with them for occasional breakthrough bronchospasm.
   b. Rarely, patients commencing salmeterol note no improvement. According to isolated case reports documenting subsequent severe attacks, these patients *should not continue on the drug.*
   c. Worsening control of asthma warrants immediate attention to corticosteroid management rather than increasing the dose of bronchodilators.

5. In the emergency management of the acute severe attack, the following minimize toxicity of β₂-adrenergic agonists:
   a. *Avoid hypoxemia* at all costs and monitor cardiac rhythm.
   b. Larger doses of β₂-adrenergic agonists produce *hypokalemia.* This should be countered with supplemental potassium.
   c. The inhaled route of administration of β-adrenergic agonists minimizes toxicity, particularly using a promising MDI-spacer protocol titrated to severity. If nebulization is used repeatedly or continuously, serum concentrations accumulate. One should attempt to limit albuterol dosing in older patients and those with suspected heart disease.
   d. Failure to respond to aggressive inhaled (and subcutaneous) use of β-adrenergic agonists may warrant an intravenous protocol. *Isoproterenol should be avoided if possible.* Serial determination of CPK-MB are indicated.

6. Beta₂-adrenergic agonists are indispensable in treating residual bronchospasm, once anti-inflammatory drugs are in place at conventional levels. Heavy corticosteroid use also carries a price. New long-acting β₂-adrenergic agonists offer great promise provided appropriate precautions are followed.

References for Chapters 47 and 48

1. Conolly ME, et al.: Resistance to beta adrenoceptor stimulants (a possible explanation for the rise in asthma deaths). *Br J Pharmacol* 1971; 43:380.
2. McDevitt DG, Shanks RG, Swaton JG: Further observation on the cardiotoxicity of isoprenaline during hypoxia. *Br J Pharmacol* 1974; 50:335.
3. Jenne JW, Chick W, Strickland RD, Wall FJ: Subsensitivity of beta responses during therapy with long-acting beta-2 preparation. *J Allergy Clin Immunol* 1977; 59:383.
4. Nelson HS, Raine D Jr, Donner C, Posey WC: Subsensitivity to the bronchodilator action of albuterol produced by chronic administration. *Am Rev Respir Dis* 1977; 116:871.

5. Plummer AL: The development of tolerance to beta$_2$-adrenergic agents. *Chest* 1978; 73:949.

6. Larsson S, Svedmyr N, Thiringer G: Lack of bronchial beta-adrenoreceptor resistance in asthmatics during long-term treatment with terbutaline. *J Allergy Clin Immunol* 1976; 59:93.

7. Jenne JW: Whither beta adrenergic tachyphylaxis? *J Allergy Clin Immunol* 1982; 70:413.

8. Holgate ST, Baldwin CJ, Tattersfield AE: Beta-adrenergic resistance in normal human airways. *Lancet* 1977; 2:375.

9. Harvey JE, Tattersfield AE: Airway response to salbutamol. Effect of regular salbutamol inhalations in normal, atopic and asthmatic subjects. *Thorax* 1982; 37:280.

10. Weber RW, Smith KA, Nelson HS: Aerosolized terbutaline in asthmatics: Development of subsensitivity with long-term administration. *J Allergy Clin Immunol* 1982; 70:417.

11. Repsher LH, Anderson JA, Bush RK, et al.: Assessment of tachyphylaxis following prolonged therapy of asthma with inhaled albuterol aerosol. *Chest* 1984; 85:34.

12. Lipworth BJ, Struthers AD, McDevitt DG: Tachyphylaxis to systemic but not to airway responses during prolonged therapy with high dose inhaled salbutamol in asthmatics. *Am Rev Respir Dis* 1989; 140:586.

13. Lipworth BJ, Clark RA, Dhillon DP, McDevitt DG: Comparison of the effects of prolonged treatment with low and high doses of inhaled terbutaline on beta-adrenoceptor responsiveness in patients with chronic obstructive pulmonary disease. *Am Rev Respir Dis* 1990; 142:338.

13a. Newnham DM, Grove A, McDevitt DG, Lipworth BJ: Subsensitivity of bronchodilator and systemic β_2-adrenoceptor responses after regular twice daily treatment with eformoterol dry powder in asthmatic patients. *Thorax* 1995; 50:497.

14. Gibson GJ, Greenacre JK, Konig P, et al.: Use of exercise challenge to investigate possible tolerance to beta adrenoceptor stimulation in asthma. *Br J Dis Chest* 1978; 72:199.

15. Peel ET, Gibson GJ: Effects of long-term inhaled salbutamol therapy on the provocation of asthma by histamine. *Am Rev Respir Dis* 1980; 121:973.

16. Tashkin DP, Conolly ME, Deutsch RI, et al.: Subsensitization of beta-adrenoreceptors in airways and lymphocyte of healthy and asthmatic subjects. *Am Rev Respir Dis* 1982; 125:185.

17. Bruynzeel PLB: Changes in the β-adrenergic system due to β-adrenergic therapy: Clinical consequences. *Eur J Respir Dis* 1984; 135:62.

18. Kraan J, Koeter GH, van der Mark THW, et al.: Changes in bronchial hyperactivity induced by 4 weeks of treatment with anti-asthmatic drugs in patients with allergic asthma: A comparison between budesonide and terbutaline. *J Allergy Clin Immunol* 1985; 76:628.

19. van Schayck CP, Graffsma SJ, Visch MB, et al.: Increased bronchial hyperresponsiveness after inhaling salbutamol during one year is not caused by subsensitization to salbutamol. *J Allergy Clin Immunol* 1990; 86:793.

20. Sears MR, Taylor DR, Print CG, et al.: Regular inhaled beta-agonist treatment in bronchial asthma. *Lancet* 1990; 336:1391.

21. Taylor DR, Sears MR, Herbison GP, et al.: Regular inhaled beta agonists in asthma: Effects on exacerbation and lung function. *Thorax* 1993; 48:134.

22. Wahedna I, Wong CS, Wisniewski AFZ, et al.: Asthma control during and after cessation of regular beta$_2$ agonist treatment. *Am Rev Respir Dis* 1993; 148:707.

23. O'Connor BJ, Aikman SL, Barnes PJ: Tolerance to the nonbronchodilator effects of inhaled β_2-agonists in asthma. *N Engl J Med* 1992; 327:1204.

24. Cockcroft DW, McParland CP, Britto SA, et al.: Regular induced salbutamol and airways responsiveness to allergen. *Lancet* 1993; 342:833.

25. Cheung D, Timmers MD, Zwinderman AH, et al.: Long-term effects of a long-acting beta-2 adrenoreceptor agonist, salmeterol, on airway hyperresponsiveness in patients with mild asthma. *N Engl J Med* 1992; 327:1198.

25a. Bhaget R, Kalva S, Swystun VA, Cockcroft DW: Rapid onset of tolerance to the bronchoprotective effect of salmeterol. *Chest* 1995; 108:1235.

25b. Booth H, Fishwick K, Harkawat R, et al.: Changes in methacholine induced bronchoconstriction with the long-acting β_2 agonist salmeterol in mild to moderate asthmatic patients. *Thorax* 1993; 48:1121.

26. Ramage L, Lipworth BJ, Ingram CG, et al.: Reduced protection against exercise induced bronchoconstriction after chronic dosing with salmeterol. *Respir Med* 1994; 88:363.

27. Britton J: Tolerance to beta-agonists in asthma. *Lancet* 1993; 342:818.

28. Wang Z, Bramley AM, McNamara A, et al.: Chronic fenoterol exposure increases in vivo and in vitro airway responses in guinea pigs. *Am J Respir Crit Care Med* 1994; 149:960.

29. Wills-Karp M, Gilmour MI: Increased cholinergic antagonism underlies impaired β-adrenergic response in ovalbumin-sensitized guinea pigs. *J Appl Physiol* 1993; 74:2729.

30. Sanjar S, Kristersson A, Mazzoni L, et al.: Increased airway reactivity in the guinea-pig follows exposure to intravenous isoprenaline. *J Physiol* 1990; 425:43.

31. Morley J, Chapman ID, Foster A, et al.: Effects of (+) and racemic salbutamol in airway responses in the guinea pig. *Br J Pharmcol* 1991; 104:295P.

32. Mullen M, Mullen B, Carey M: The association between β-agonist use and death from asthma. *JAMA* 1993; 270:1842.

33. Robin ED: Sudden death in bronchial asthma, and inhaled beta-adrenergic agonists. *Chest* 1992; 101:1699.

34. Kendall MJ, Haffner C: The acute unwanted effects of beta$_2$ receptor agonist therapy, in Beasley R, Pearce NE (eds): *The Role of Beta Receptor Agonist Therapy in Asthma Mortality*. Boca Raton, FL, CRC press, 1993; 163.

35. Wong CS, Pavord ID, Williams J, et al.: Bronchodilator cardiovascular and hypokalemic effects of fenoterol, salbutamol, and terbutaline in asthma. *Lancet* 1990; 3536:1396.

36. Scheinin M, Kaulus MM, Laurikainen E, Allonen H: Hypokalemia and other non-bronchial effects of inhaled fenoterol and salbutamol. A placebo controlled dose-response study in healthy volunteers. *Br J Clin Pharmacol* 1987; 24:645.

37. Bremner P, Woodman K, Burgess C, et al.: A comparison of the cardiovascular and metabolic effects of formoterol, salbutamol and fenoterol. *Eur Respir* 1993; 6:204.

38. Windom HH, Burgess CD, Siebers RWL, et al.: The pulmonary and extrapulmonary effects of inhaled β-agonists in patients with asthma. *Clin Pharmacol Ther* 1990; 48:296.

39. Bremner P, Burgess C, Beasley R, et al.: Nebulized fenoterol causes greater cardiovascular and hypokalemic effects than equivalent bronchodilator doses of salbutamol in asthmatics. *Respir Med* 1992; 86:419.

40. Bremner P, Burgess C, Crane J, et al.: Cardiovascular effects of fenoterol under conditions of hypoxemia. *Thorax* 1992; 47:814.

41. Flatt A, Burgess C, Windom H, Beasley R: The cardiovascular effects of inhaled fenoterol alone and during treatment with oral theophylline. *Chest* 1989; 96:1317.

42. Clifton GD, Hunt BA, Patel R, Burki NK: Effects of sequential doses of parenteral terbutaline on plasma levels of potassium and related cardiopulmonary responses. *Am Rev Respir Dis* 1990; 141:575.

43. Dickens GR, Randall AM, West R, et al.: Effect of nebulized albuterol on serum potassium and cardiac rhythm in patients with asthma or chronic obstructive pulmonary disease. *Pharmacotherapy* 1994; 4:729.

44. Lim R, Walshaw MJ, Saltissi S, Hind CRK: Cardiac arrhythmias during acute exacerbations of chronic airflow limitation: Effect of fall in plasma potassium concentration induced by nebulized beta$_2$ agonist therapy. *Postgrad Med J* 1989; 65:449.

45. Higgins RM, Cookson WOCM, Lane DJ, et al.: Cardiac arrhythmias caused by nebulized beta-agonist therapy. *Lancet* 1987; 11:863.

46. Shovlin CL, Tam FWK: Salbutamol nebulizer and precipitation of critical cardiac ischemia. *Lancet* 1990; 335:258.

47. Kinney EL, Trautlein JJ, Harbaugh CV, et al.: Ventricular tachycardia after terbutaline. *JAMA* 1978; 240:2247.

48. Raper R, Fisher M, Bihari D: Profound, reversible myocardial depression in acute asthma treated with high-dose catecholamines. *Crit Care Med* 1992; 20:710.

49. Kahn DS, Rona G, Chappel CI: Isoproterenol induced cardiac necrosis. *Ann N Y Acad Sci* 1969; 156:285.

50. Balazs T, Bloom S: Cardiotoxicity of adrenergic bronchodilators and vasodilating antihypertensive drugs, in van Stee EW (ed): *Cardiovascular Toxicology*. New York, Raven Press, 1982;

51. Whitehurst VE, Joseph X, Hohmann JR, et al.: Cardiotoxic effects in rats and rabbits treated with terbutaline alone and in combination with aminophylline. *J Am Coll Toxicol* 1983; 2:147.

52. Magnussen G, Hansson E: Myocardial necrosis in the rat: A comparison between isoprenaline, orciprenaline, salbutamol and terbutaline. *Cardiology* 1973; 58:174.

53. Balazs T, Otake S, Noble JF: The development of resistance to the ischemic cardiopathic effect of isoproterenol. *Toxicol Appl Pharmacol* 1972; 21:200.

54. Joseph X, Whitehurst VE, Bloom S, Balazs T: Enhancement of cardiotoxic effects of beta-adrenergic bronchodilators by aminophylline in experimental animals. *Fund appl Toxicol* 1981; 1:443.

55. Sly RM, Jenne JW, Cohn J: Toxicity of beta-adrenergic drugs, in Jenne JW, Murphy S (eds): *Drug Therapy for Asthma Research and Clinical Practice*. Vol. 31, *Lung Biology in Health and Disease*. New York, Marcel Dekker, 1987; 953.

56. Maguire JF, Geha RS, Umetsu DJ: Myocardial specific creatinine phosphokinase isozyme elevation in children with asthma treated with intravenous isoproterenol. *J Allergy Clin Immunol* 1986; 78:631.

57. Kurland G, Williams J, Lewiston NW: Fatal myocardial toxicity during continuous infusion intravenous isoproterenol therapy of asthma. *J Allergy Clin Immunol* 1979; 63:407.

58. Moore J, Claud D, Driscoll D, et al.: Intravenous terbutaline control of severe pediatric asthma. *Am Rev Respir Dis* 1992; 145:A740.

59. Dietrich KA, Conrad SA, Romero MD: Creatine kinase (CK) isoenzymes in pediatric status asthmaticus treated with intravenous terbutaline. *Crit Care Med* 1991; 19:539.

60. Katz RW, Kelly HW, Crowley MR: Safety of continuous nebulized albuterol for bronchospasm in infants and children. *Pediatrics* 1993; 92:666.

61. Beasley R, Pearce NE: *The Role of Beta Receptor Agonist Therapy in Asthma Mortality*. Boca Raton, FL, CRC Press, 1993.

62. Barnes PJ, Chung KF: Questions about inhaled β$_2$-adrenoceptor agonists in asthma. *Trends Pharmacol Sci* 1992; 13:20.

63. Crane J, Pearce NE, Flatt A, et al.: Prescribed fenoterol and death from asthma in New Zealand. 1980–1983: A case-control study. *Lancet* 1989; 1:917.

64. Pearce N et al.: Case-control study of prescribed fenoterol and death from asthma in New Zealand, 1977–1981. *Thorax* 1990; 45:170.

65. Grainger J, Woodman K, Pearce N, et al.: Prescribed fenoterol and death from asthma in New Zealand, 1981–1987: A further case control study. *Thorax* 1991; 46:105.

66. Ernst P, Habbick B, Suissa S, et al.: Is the association between inhaled beta$_2$-agonist use and life-threatening asthma because of confounding by severity? *Am Rev Respir Dis* 1993; 148:75.

67. Suissa S, Ernst P, Bolvin J, et al.: A cohort analysis of excess mortality in asthma and the use of inhaled β-agonists. *Am J Respir Crit Care Med* 1994; 149:604.

68. Taylor DR, Sears MR: Regular beta-adrenergic agonists. Evidence, not reassurance, is what is needed. *Chest* 1994; 106:552.

69. Castle W, Fuller R, Hall J, Palmer J: Serevent nationwide surveillance study: Comparison of salmeterol with salbutamol in asthmatic patients who require regular bronchodilator treatment. *Br Med J* 1993; 306:1034.

70. Dollery CT, Williams FM, Draffan GH, et al.: Arterial blood levels of fluorohydrocarbons in asthmatic patients following use of pressurized aerosols. *Clin Pharmacol Ther* 1974; 15:59.

71. Hoffman BB, Lefkowitz RJ: Catecholamines and sympathomimetic drugs, in Gilman AG (ed): *Goodman and Gilman's The Pharmacological Basis of Therapeutics*, 8th ed. New York, McGraw-Hill, 1993; 187.

DRUGS THAT INHIBIT PHOSPHODIESTERASE

Chapter 49

CHEMISTRY, EFFICACY, AND TOXICITY

KLAUS F. RABE
GORDON DENT

Introduction

Phosphodiesterase (3′,5′-cyclic nucleotide 5′-nucleotidohydrolase; EC 3.1.4.17; PDE) is the name of the group of enzymes that catalyze the degradation of the 3′,5′-cyclic nucleotides cyclic AMP (adenosine 3′,5′-cyclic monophosphate) and cyclic GMP (guanosine 3′,5′-cyclic monophosphate). Cyclic AMP and cyclic GMP are intracellular "second messengers" that mediate the actions of several neurotransmitters, hormones, and autacoids; they are of interest in pulmonary pharmacology because increased intracellular concentrations of cyclic AMP and cyclic GMP are associated with both relaxation of airway smooth muscle (Chap. 50) and suppression of the function of a range of immune cells that may participate in inflammatory lung diseases (Chap. 61).[1]

Phosphodiesterase enzymes have been classified according to the scheme shown in Table 49-1. Most of these families have been demonstrated to comprise several isoenzymes

and, to date, 16 distinct gene products—several exhibiting a number of alternative splice variants—have been identified.[2] This multiplicity of PDE enzymes has pharmacological implications, as the potential exists to inhibit selectively the isoenzymes of a particular cell type to exert highly precise actions in a specific disease.[3] The development of agents capable of such specific actions will rely on a detailed understanding of the biochemistry of individual isoenzymes and their physiological roles, the study of which is still in its early stages. At present, the PDE inhibitors available for therapeutic use include the methylxanthines—nonselective inhibitors of all PDE isoenzymes—and a small number of "second generation" inhibitors with varying selectivity for specific families of isoenzymes.

Since theophylline is by far the most widely used PDE inhibitor in pulmonary therapeutics, this chapter and Chaps. 50 and 51 will concentrate on the chemistry, efficacy, and toxicity, the bronchodilator and smooth muscle relaxant

TABLE 49-1 Isoenzymes of Cyclic Nucleotide Phosphodiesterase (PDE)[a]

Type	Family	Characteristics
1	Ca^{2+}/CaM-dependent PDE family	Hydrolyzes cAMP and cGMP with similar efficiency. Enzymatic activity dependent on calcium ions and calmodulin. Many inhibitors of CaM activation available (e.g., trifluoroperazine), few selective inhibitors of catalytic site.
2	cGMP-stimulated PDE family	Low affinity for cAMP and cGMP. cAMP hydrolysis stimulated by cGMP. Inhibited by EHNA.
3	cGMP-inhibited PDE family	High affinity for cAMP and cGMP. cAMP hydrolysis inhibited by cGMP. Some members inhibited by cAMP or insulin-dependent phosphorylation. Many selective inhibitors (e.g., milrinone, cilostamide, sulmazole, siguazodan, enoximone).
4	cAMP-specific PDE family	Preferentially hydrolyzes cAMP. Selectively inhibited by Ro 20-1724. Other inhibitors include rolipram, denbufylline, and tibenelast.
5	cGMP-specific PDE family	High affinity for cGMP. Inhibited by dipyridamole and M & B 22-948 (zaprinast).
6	Photoreceptor PDE family	High affinity for cGMP. Activated by photoreceptor transducin. Consist of three or four subunits, including regulatory γ-subunit. Inhibited by dipyridamole and zaprinast.
7	High affinity, cAMP-specific PDE	High affinity for cAMP. Not inhibited by cGMP, milrinone, or Ro 20-1724.

[a] Abbreviations: CaM, calmodulin; cAMP, cyclic AMP; cGMP, cyclic GMP; EHNA, erythro-9-(2-hydroxyl-3-nonyl)-adenine; M & B 22-948 (zaprinast), 2-o-propoxyphenyl-8-azapurin-6-one (see Fig. 49-3); Ro 20-1724, 4-(3-butoxy-4-methoxybenzyl)-2-imidazoline.

properties, and the clinical applications, respectively, of theophylline. However, where appropriate, isoenzyme-selective drugs that are either in clinical use or undergoing clinical trials also will be discussed.

Chemistry

METHYLXANTHINES

The plant alkaloids theophylline (from the tea bush, *Thea sinensis*), caffeine (from the coffee bean, *Coffea arabica*), and theobromine (from the cocoa bean, *Theobroma cacao*) are closely related in structure, belonging to the class of methylxanthines (Fig. 49-1). Xanthine (2,6-dioxypurine) is itself a derivative of the purine portion of the cyclic purine nucleotides, which are substrates for PDE. A series of synthetic structural analogues of cyclic AMP and cyclic GMP has been derived from xanthine and the opiate alkaloid papaverine. Extensive structure-activity studies of these derivatives have given some indication of the effects of substitution (at various positions of the molecules) on the potency of the various pharmacological actions of the drugs (Fig. 49-2).[4] In particular, the in vitro and in vivo bronchial relaxant properties of methylxanthines appear to be influenced greatly by the substituents at the 3- and 7-nitrogen atoms, while substitution at the 1-nitrogen and 8-carbon atoms affects the ability of the methylxanthine to act as an antagonist at adenosine receptors.[4] Thus, theophylline (1,3-dimethylxanthine; Fig. 49-1) is effective as a bronchodilator and as an adenosine antagonist while enprofylline (3-propylxanthine) lacks a methyl group at the N-1 position and is a poor antagonist at most classes of adenosine receptors, but retains a bronchodilator potency greater than that of theophylline.[5] Substitution at the C-8 position renders the methylxanthine more stable by reducing its susceptibility to hydroxylation to 1,3-dimethyluric acid, but this advantage may be offset by other disadvantages, possibly accruing from the increased potency of the methylxanthine as an antagonist of adenosine.[6] Trisubstitution at the N-1, N-3, and N-9 positions leads to isomerization of the imidazyl ring in the purine group of the methylxanthine; the 8–9 double bond localizes to the 7–8 position (Fig. 49-2), and pharmacological activity is lost.[6]

Synthetic compounds based on the xanthine molecule have formed the basis for studies of the relationship of chemical structure to the ability of a drug to inhibit PDE, and these studies have led to the identification of 3-isobutyl-1-methylxanthine (IBMX; Fig. 49-3) and a theobromine derivative, 1-(5-oxohexyl)-3,7-dimethylxanthine (pentoxifylline), as PDE inhibitors of greater potency than the plant alkaloids,[7,8] which are also more potent as in vitro relaxants of airway smooth muscle preparations.[8,9] Like theophylline, IBMX and pentoxifylline inhibit all PDE isoenzymes with roughly equal potency.[8,10] Other compounds identified by these means include zaprinast (Fig. 49-3), which is of interest in view of its

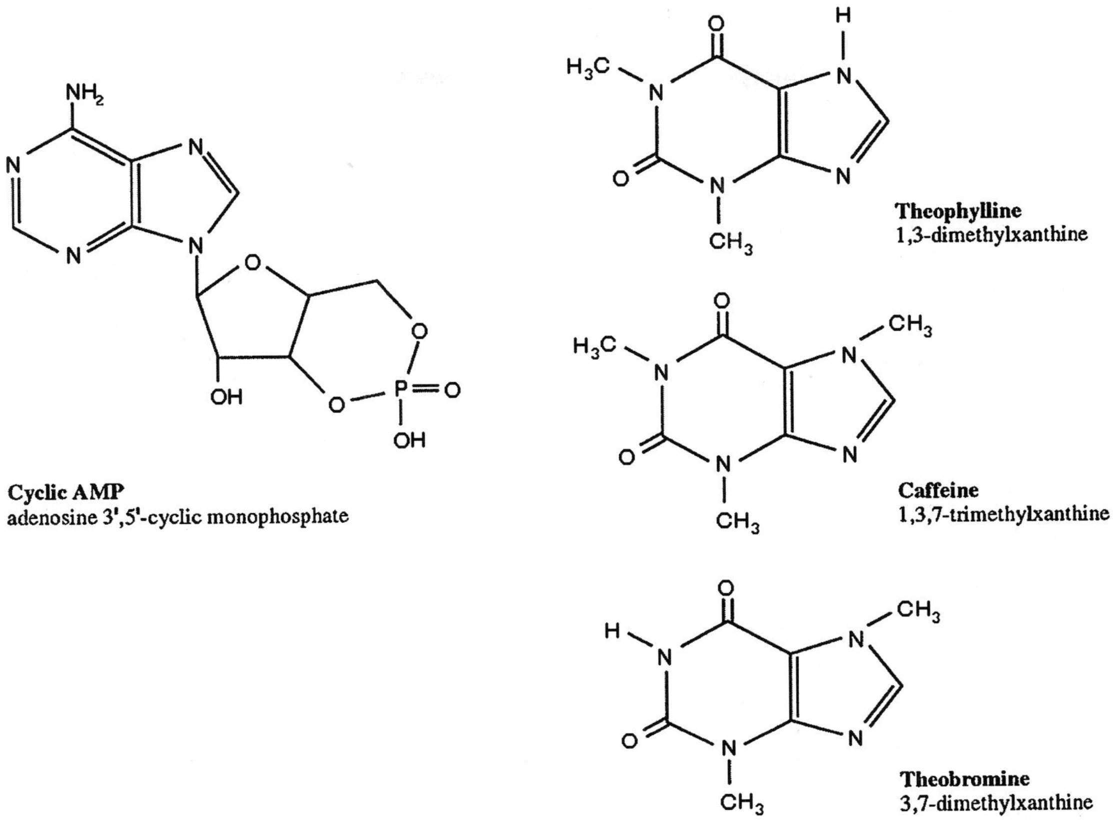

FIGURE 49-1 Chemical structures of cyclic AMP, theophylline, caffeine, and theobromine.

high potency in inhibiting the PDE5 and, to a lesser extent PDE1 families and its very low potency against the other isoenzymes; and denbufylline (1,3-di-*n*-butyl-7-[2′-oxo-propyl]-xanthine), which selectively inhibits the PDE4 family of isoenzymes.[10]

SELECTIVE PHOSPHODIESTERASE INHIBITORS

A vigorous research program occurring in recent years has identified a large number of nonxanthine compounds with

selectivity as inhibitors of specific PDE isoenzymes. The prototypic PDE3 and PDE4 inhibitors, milrinone and rolipram (Fig. 49-3), have generated a series of molecules with related structures which exhibit high potency and marked selectivity for the type 3 or type 4 enzymes over that of other families.[7,11] Little advantage has resulted from development of selective PDE5 inhibitors, while selective inhibitors of PDE1 are commonly antagonists of calmodulin binding. The only selective inhibitor of PDE2 so far identified is also an inhibitor of adenosine deaminase. Most studies of isoenzyme-selective

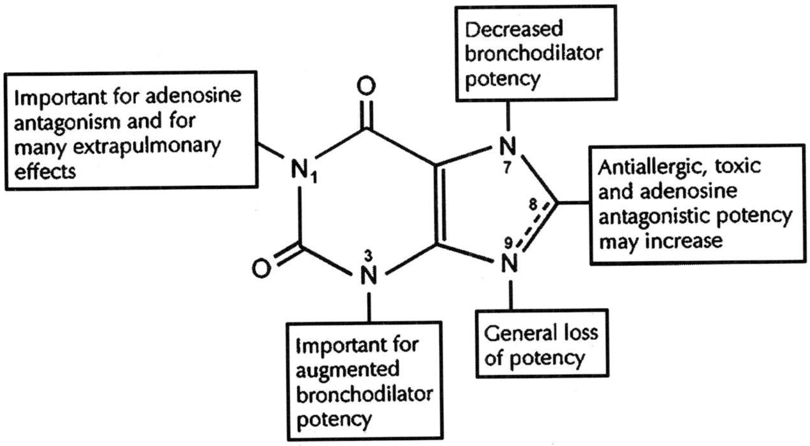

FIGURE 49-2 Some features of alkyl substitution at various positions of the xanthine molecule. When the 9-nitrogen is substituted, the 8–9 double bond is moved to the 7–8 position. (From Persson and Karlsson.[4])

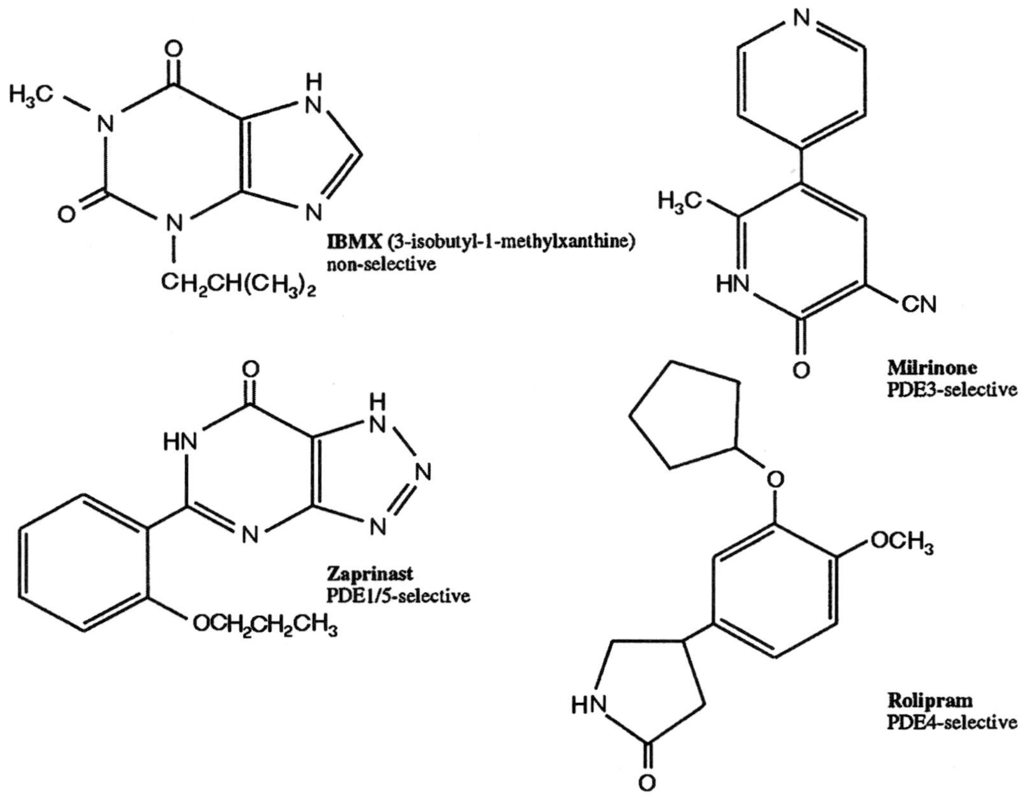

IBMX (3-isobutyl-1-methylxanthine) non-selective

Milrinone PDE3-selective

Zaprinast PDE1/5-selective

Rolipram PDE4-selective

FIGURE 49-3 Chemical structures of IBMX (nonselective PDE inhibitor), zaprinast (selective inhibitor of PDE1 and PDE5), mil- rinone (selective PDE3 inhibitor), and rolipram (selective PDE4 inhibitor).

PDE inhibitors have, therefore, concentrated on inhibitors of PDE3 and PDE4, and structure–activity relationships have been identified that may facilitate the development of more selective drugs in the future.[7,11]

The selective PDE3 inhibitors already have found a clinical application in the treatment of congestive heart failure, owing to their positive inotropic action; these drugs have also excited interest as a result of their potency as relaxants of airway smooth muscle (Chap. 50). Selective PDE4 inhibitors have been developed in the search for agents effective in the treatment of depression and dementia, but their apparent anti-inflammatory actions have also led to interest in their potential for the treatment of such diseases as bronchial asthma.[12,13]

Efficacy

Within the range of 5 to 20 μg/ml (28 to 110 μM), serum theophylline concentration exhibits a log-linear relationship to the bronchodilator effect of the drug (Fig. 49-4).[14] In severe asthma, the maintenance of serum theophylline concentrations at the upper end of this range causes maximal improvement in lung function.[15] At lower serum concentrations, however, theophylline is effective against both exercise-induced bronchoconstriction and late asthmatic responses while causing little direct bronchodilation, as determined by improvement in baseline lung function.

Theophylline may be administered enterally—by which route it is well absorbed—or parenterally (usually as intravenous aminophylline) and is cleared by either excretion in the urine or metabolism to monomethyl and dimethyl uric acids in the liver[15]; these metabolites are very rapidly excreted, suggesting that they may be actively secreted by the renal tubules.[15] The serum half-life of theophylline is approximately 8 h in adults and 3.6 h in children, but considerable variation is observed both between and within individuals.

FIGURE 49-4 The relationship between serum theophylline concentration and bronchodilation in six asthmatic patients. (Adapted from Mitenko and Ogilvie.[14])

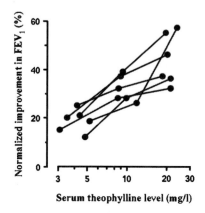

Changes in the rate of clearance of the drug frequently underlie the occurrence of toxicity (see below).

The ability of theophylline to exert toxic effects at concentrations only slightly above the therapeutic range has led to great interest in the pharmacokinetics of the drug. The kinetics of theophylline clearance generally are linear, as a result of the balance between the diuretic action of high concentrations. This causes increased excretion of unmetabolized drug and the rapid excretion of the methyl uric acid metabolites, which are a greater proportion of the excreted product at lower theophylline serum concentrations.[15] Tolerance to the diuretic action of theophylline can occur after multiple doses, however, leading to a loss of first-order kinetics in clearance and an increase in the serum half-life. The development of sustained-release formulations of theophylline has allowed improved maintenance of serum concentrations with a single evening dose (or a one-third morning dose and a two-thirds evening dose). Serum concentrations thus remain within the therapeutic range throughout the day and at their highest during the early hours of the morning, when the risk of nocturnal attacks in severe asthmatics is greatest (Chap. 51).[16]

A range of N-7 substituted theophylline derivatives, including 7-(2,3-dihydroxypropyl)-theophylline (also known as dyphylline, diprophylline, or glyphylline) and 7-(2-hydroxypropyl)theophylline (proxyphylline), have been developed and marketed for use in asthma therapy. These drugs, however, have the disadvantages of low bioavailability after oral dosing, rapid clearance, and low bronchodilator potency.[5,15] Effects apart from bronchodilation are probably also reduced. The addition of 300 mg each of proxyphylline and diprophylline to an intravenous dose of 200 mg theophylline caused a markedly smaller increase in protection against bronchoconstriction than was effected by elevating the theophylline dose by 150 mg (Chap. 51).

A nonmethyl substituted xanthine, 3-propylxanthine (enprofylline), is a more potent bronchodilator than theophylline but is very rapidly cleared, so that maintenance of adequate serum levels is more difficult. The bronchodilator of action enprofylline is interesting because it is more potent than the-ophylline in inhibiting PDE[17] but is a poor antagonist of most adenosine receptors.[5,18] This suggests that the adenosine antagonism of xanthine derivatives does not alone account for their bronchodilator properties. It is also interesting to note that enprofylline has an efficacy similar to theophylline in suppressing late asthmatic responses to allergen inhalation, although a fourfold lower steady-state serum concentration results in a lesser inhibitory effect against the immediate bronchoconstrictor response to allergen.[18]

Toxicity

Theophylline and other methylxanthines have numerous extrapulmonary actions that complicate their use in the treatment of obstructive lung disease.[5,19] After enteral administration, methylxanthines are absorbed rapidly and distributed throughout all body compartments,[5] where their nonselective PDE inhibitory action, along with other actions such as adenosine receptor antagonism, leads to a broad range of effects. In addition to side effects at serum concentrations

within the therapeutic range, there are several toxic effects of theophylline that are exhibited at serum concentrations above this range.

Acute toxicity is rare and is almost always associated with very high serum concentrations of theophylline (>40 μg/ml),[20] well above the range of effective bronchodilator concentrations (5 to 20 μg/ml).[19] Within the therapeutic concentration range, an average of 56 percent of theophylline is bound to plasma proteins. At greater concentrations, the protein binding is saturated, resulting in disproportionate increases in free-drug concentrations and increased risk of toxicity.[5] Chronic overdosing is a more common cause of adverse effects, although severe toxicity is infrequent, and the mortality rate is higher in acute overdosing.[20] The severity of toxicity in acute overdosing correlates closely with serum concentration, and most deaths in these cases occur while serum concentrations still are very high (>100 μg/ml); the correlation of toxicity with serum concentrations is less clear in chronic overmedication.[20]

Theophylline toxicity can result from a variety of causes, including patient or practitioner error,[20] impaired drug metabolism resulting from infection or liver disease (which also reduces theophylline binding to plasma proteins),[5] and heart failure or drug interactions,[19] which may reduce the clearance of theophylline.[5,15,20,21] It is particularly important to note that theophylline exhibits interactions with erythromycin and certain histamine H_2-receptor antagonists; use of both of these drugs may be indicated in asthma and chronic obstructive pulmonary disease, where upper respiratory tract infection is common and where corticosteroid use is often associated with gastric ulceration. The most common manifestations of theophylline toxicity are cardiovascular and gastrointestinal reactions, although a small number of patients may exhibit central nervous system effects, which more often are associated with chronic rather than acute overdosing. Electrolyte imbalances are frequently observed in acute overdose but are less common in cases of chronic overdose.

CARDIOVASCULAR EFFECTS

The most common cardiovascular effects of theophylline are sinus tachycardia and runs of premature ventricular beats. Arrhythmias also have been noted less frequently, although acute toxicity resulting from rapid intravenous administration of the soluble theophylline salt aminophylline (theophylline ethylenediamine) has resulted in sudden death from cardiac arrhythmias.[5] Therapeutic serum concentrations of theophylline rarely induce tachycardia or ectopic beats, even in patients with chronic ventricular arrhythmia.[15]

The adverse effects of high concentrations of theophylline on cardiac rhythm appear to result directly from its PDE-inhibitory action. Since cyclic AMP itself has demonstrable arrhythmogenic properties, resulting from increased cytosolic calcium concentrations in the cardiac muscle,[22] the reduced survival observed in groups of patients treated for congestive heart failure with the selective PDE3 inhibitor milrinone may be the result of cyclic AMP-dependent arrhythmias, particularly fast atrial fibrillation.[23–25] In view of this phenomenon, it would appear that PDE inhibitors acting on cardiac cyclic AMP-hydrolyzing enzymes inevitably must induce tachycardia as a side effect,[22] and it is interesting to note that derivatives of theophylline containing a large alkyl substituent at the N-3 position (such as enprofylline) exhibit both increased bronchodilator potency and increased risk of tachycardia.[6]

GASTROINTESTINAL EFFECTS

Nausea and emesis are frequent side effects in the early stages of theophylline treatment; gastric discomfort and diarrhea also may occur. These effects are poorly correlated with serum theophylline concentration and often diminish during long-term therapy.[15] Gastrointestinal effects occur most frequently in patients receiving high theophylline dosages for severe asthma but also can be associated with relatively low doses in chronic treatment. In animal studies, the emetic side effects of xanthine bronchodilators correlate closely with their potency as PDE inhibitors, but only weakly with their adenosine antagonistic activity,[26] suggesting that this adverse effect is also an inherent feature of PDE inhibitory drugs. Since nausea and vomiting are recognized side effects of selective inhibitors of PDE4,[11] inhibition of this isoenzyme in particular may mediate the emetic actions of methylxanthines.

Theophylline and caffeine stimulate gastric secretion (acid and pepsin) and may induce discomfort or (rarely) gastric bleeding. Relaxation of the lower esophageal sphincter also may occur, and the two conditions together can favor gastroesophageal reflux.[6] The stimulation of gastric secretion is likely to be mediated by adenosine antagonism, since this action is not exhibited by enprofylline, while relaxation of the sphincter is a property shared by theophylline and enprofylline and probably results from PDE inhibition.

CENTRAL NERVOUS SYSTEM EFFECTS

In addition to headache and dizziness, central nervous system stimulation leading to tension, anxiety, restlessness, and dysphoria are induced by ingestion of high doses of caffeine or theophylline.[5] Seizures can occur in patients with no previous indication of neurological disorder with high serum concentrations of theophylline (usually >50 µg/ml).[20,27] This severe and life-threatening toxic effect has been observed in the absence of minor adverse effects and can only be predicted by measurement of serum theophylline concentration.[15] Theophylline-induced seizures occasionally are resistant to treatment with conventional anticonvulsants,[5] and the mechanism through which the seizures occur remains unclear, although the ability of theophylline to cause significant reductions in cerebral blood flow and oxygenation may be important.[28] The induction of seizures has been proposed to result from adenosine receptor antagonism, but a recent report has shown no beneficial effects of adenosine A_1 receptor agonists against convulsions induced by toxic concentrations of theophylline in mice.[29]

ELECTROLYTE EFFECTS

Hypokalemia is exhibited in most cases of acute theophylline toxicity[30] and is probably due to a direct effect on the renal tubules.[31] Severe hypokalemia is less common in chronic theophylline overdosing, although increased risk of electrolyte disturbances, including hypokalemia, hyponatremia, and hypophosphatemia, has been demonstrated for a therapeutic range of serum theophylline concentrations from 5.5 to 110 µM (approximately 1 to 20 µg/ml) after oral theophylline dosing.[32] Intravenous theophylline administration in patients suffering from recurrent asthmatic attacks leads to increased excretion of magnesium, calcium, and sodium, and depresses serum potassium concentrations.[33] These side effects may be mediated by PDE inhibition, since the selective PDE4 inhibitor, rolipram, also induces acute reductions in plasma osmolality and sodium concentration; concentrations nonetheless return to normal within 1 week of regular rolipram use.[34] While enprofylline is commonly reported to lack the diuretic action of theophylline,[6] diminished adenosine antagonism may not abolish the electrolyte disturbances caused by PDE-inhibiting methylxanthines. Further research is required in this area.

Summary

Although the mechanism by which theophylline exerts its beneficial effects in obstructive airways disease remains controversial (Chaps. 50 and 51), the relationship between the chemistry of theophylline and other xanthine derivatives and their pharmacological and toxicological effects is fairly well understood. Similar investigations are under way with isoenzyme-selective PDE inhibitors and it should, in time, become clear which actions are mediated by PDE inhibition and, more precisely, which PDE isoenzymes are involved in these particular responses.

The development of enprofylline, which has a narrower range of molecular actions than theophylline, may assist in the understanding of methylxanthine pharmacology and of the efficacy and safety of these drugs in chronic therapy. A recent study of long-term treatment of 348 asthmatic patients with oral theophylline or enprofylline revealed both drugs to be effective in controlling asthma symptoms, with enprofylline being slightly more effective than theophylline in limiting the requirement for additional inhaled corticosteroids.[35] Both drugs are generally well tolerated and, assuming careful monitoring of serum levels and optimization of daily dosing to individual patients, the safety profile of theophylline is good. The beneficial effects of theophylline in asthma and chronic airways obstruction (Chap. 51) suggest that theophylline remains a useful drug in pulmonary therapeutics.

References

1. Dent G, Magnussen H, Rabe KF. Cyclic nucleotide phosphodiesterases in the human lung. *Lung* 1994; 72:129.

2. Beavo JA, Conti M, Heaslip RJ. ASPET Meeting Report: Multiple cyclic nucleotide phosphodiesterases. *Mol Pharmacol* 1994; 46:399.

3. Beavo J. Multiple phosphodiesterase isoenzymes: background, nomenclature and implications. In: Beavo J, Houslay MD, editors. *Cyclic nucleotide phosphodiesterases: structure, regulation and drug action*. Chichester: Wiley, 1990: 3–15.

4. Persson CGA, Karlsson J-A. In vitro responses to bronchodilator drugs. In: Jenne JW, Murphy S, editors. *Drug therapy for asthma: research and clinical practice. Lung biology in health and disease*, vol 31. New York: Marcel Dekker, 1987: 129–176.

5. Rall TW. Drugs used in the treatment of asthma: the methylxanthines, cromolyn sodium, and other agents. In: Gilman AG, Rall TW, Nies AS, Taylor P, editors. *Goodman & Gilman's The pharmacological basis of therapeutics*. 8th ed. New York: Pergamon, 1990: 618–637.

6. Persson CGA. Development of safer xanthine drugs for treatment of obstructive airways disease. *J Allergy Clin Immunol* 1980; 78:817.

7. Erhardt PW. Second-generation phosphodiesterase inhibitors: structure–activity relationships and receptor models. In: Beavo J, Houslay MD, editors. *Cyclic nucleotide phosphodiesterases: structure, regulation and drug action*. Chichester: Wiley, 1990: 317–332.

8. Cortijo J, Bou J, Beleta J, Cardelús I, Llenas J, Morcillo E, Gristwood RW. Investigation into the role of phosphodiesterase IV in bronchorelaxation, including studies with human bronchus. *Br J Pharmacol* 1993; 108:562.

9. Rabe KF, Tenor H, Dent G, Schudt C, Liebig S, Magnussen H. Phosphodiesterase isoenzymes modulating inherent tone in human airways: identification and characterization. *Am J Physiol* 1993; 264 (*Lung Cell Mol Physiol* 8):L458.

10. Nicholson CD, Challiss RAJ, Shahid M. Differential modulation of tissue function and therapeutic potential of selective inhibitors of cyclic nucleotide phosphodiesterase isoenzymes. *Trends Pharmacol Sci* 1991; 12:19.

11. Lowe JA III, Cheng JB. The PDE IV family of calcium-independent phosphodiesterase enzymes. *Drugs Fut* 1992; 17:799.

12. Torphy TJ, Undem BJ. Phosphodiesterase inhibitors: new opportunities for the treatment of asthma. *Thorax* 1991; 46:512.

13. Dent G, Giembycz MA. Selective phosphodiesterase inhibitors in the therapy of asthma. *Clin Immunother* 1995; 3:423.

14. Mitenko PA, Ogilvie RI. Rational intravenous doses of theophylline. *N Engl J Med* 1973; 289:600.

15. Hendeles L, Weinberger M. Theophylline: a "state of the art" review. *Pharmacotherapy* 1983; 3:2.

16. Steinijans VW, Trautmann H, Johnson E, Beier W. Theophylline steady-state pharmacokinetics: recent concepts and their application in chronotherapy of reactive airway diseases. *Chronobiol Int* 1987; 4:331.

17. Toll JBC, Andersson RGG. Effects of enprofylline and theophylline on purified human basophils. *Allergy* 1984; 39:515.

18. Pauwels R, van Renterghem D, van der Straeten M, Johannesson N, Persson CGA. The effect of theophylline and enprofylline on allergen-induced bronchoconstriction. *J Allergy Clin Immunol* 1985; 76:583.

19. Milgrom H, Bender B. Current issues in the use of theophylline. *Am Rev Respir Dis* 1993; 147:S33.

20. Sessler CN. Theophylline toxicity: clinical features of 116 consecutive cases. *Am J Med* 1990; 88:567.

21. Greenberger PA, Cranberg JA, Ganz MA, Hubler GL. A prospective evaluation of elevated serum theophylline concentrations to determine if high concentrations are predictable. *Am J Med* 1991; 91:67.

22. Lubbe WF, Podzuweit T, Opie LH. Potential arrhythmogenic role of cyclic adenosine monophosphate (AMP) and cytosolic calcium overload: implications for prophylactic effects of beta-blockers in myocardial infarction and proarrhythmic effects of phosphodiesterase inhibitors. *J Am Coll Cardiol* 1992; 19:1622.

23. Cruickshank JM. Phosphodiesterase III inhibitors: long-term risks and short-term benefits. *Cardiovasc Drugs Ther* 1993; 7:655.

24. Feneck RO. The European Milrinone Multicentre Trial Group: Intravenous milrinone following cardiac surgery: I. Effects of bolus infusion followed by variable dose maintenance infusion. *J Cardiothorac Vasc Anesth* 1992; 6:554.

25. Varriale P, Ramaprasad S. Aminophylline induced atrial fibrillation. *Pacing Clin Electrophysiol* 1993; 16:1953.

26. Howell RE, Muehsam WT, Kinnier WJ. Mechanism for the emetic side effect of xanthine bronchodilators. *Life Sci* 1990; 46:563.

27. Zwillich CW, Sutton FD, Neff TA, Cohn WM, Matthay RA, Weinberger MM. Theophylline-induced seizures in adults: correlation with serum concentrations. *Ann Intern Med* 1975; 82:784.

28. Nishimura M, Yoshioka A, Yamamoto M, Akiyama Y, Miyamoto K, Kawakami Y. Effect of theophylline on brain tissue oxygenation during normoxia and hypoxia in humans. *J Appl Physiol* 1993; 74:2724.

29. Hornfeldt CS, Larson AA. Adenosine receptors are not involved in theophylline-induced seizures. *J Toxicol Clin Toxicol* 1994; 32:257.

30. Shannon M: Hypokalemia, hyperglycemia and plasma catecholamine activity after severe theophylline intoxication. *J Toxicol Clin Toxicol* 1994; 32:41.

31. Bowman WC, Rand MJ. *Textbook of pharmacology*. 2nd ed. Oxford: Blackwell, 1980.

32. Flack JM, Ryder KW, Strickland D, Whang R. Metabolic correlates of theophylline therapy: a concentration-related phenomenon. *Ann Pharmacother* 1994; 28:175.

33. Knutsen R, Bohmer T, Falch J. Intravenous theophylline-induced excretion of calcium, magnesium and sodium in patients with recurrent asthmatic attacks. *Scand J Clin Lab Invest* 1994; 54:119.

34. Sturgess I, Searle GF. The acute toxic effect of the phosphodiesterase inhibitor rolipram on plasma osmolality. *Br J Clin Pharmacol* 1990; 29:369.

35. Chapman KR, Ljungholm K, Kallen A. The International Enprofylline Study Group. Long-term xanthine therapy of asthma: enprofylline and theophylline compared. *Chest* 1994; 106:1407.

Chapter 50 _____

BRONCHODILATION AND SMOOTH MUSCLE RELAXATION

KLAUS F. RABE
GORDON DENT

Introduction

Theophylline has bronchodilator action, which can improve baseline lung function, and some inhibitory effect on early asthmatic reactions, both of which confer a protective effect against exercise-induced bronchoconstriction and late asthmatic reactions (see Chap. 49). In addition, theophylline has beneficial hemodynamic effects in conditions of pulmonary hypertension that are associated with chronic obstructive pulmonary disease (COPD) or severe asthma. The clinical effectiveness of theophylline, including its therapeutic application in asthma, is the subject of (Chap. 51). Here the ability of theophylline and inhibitors of specific phosphodiesterase (PDE) isoenzymes to relax the smooth muscle of airways and pul-monary arteries, thereby effecting bronchodilation and reduction in pulmonary blood pressure, is discussed. Evidence that theophylline could exert its beneficial effects in asthma through an immunomodulatory action leading to a reduction of airway inflammation is presented elsewhere (Chap. 61).

Putative Mechanisms for Theophylline-Induced Bronchodilation

The mechanism by which theophylline causes bronchodilation has been a source of controversy for many years. As described in Chap. 49, theophylline is known to be both an inhibitor of PDE and an antagonist at adenosine receptors. In addition, theophylline has been reported to increase extracellular concentrations of catecholamines by inhibiting their cellular reuptake or metabolism,[1] although the relevance of this action to the clinical effects of the drug remains unclear.[2] The evidence for the involvement of PDE inhibition and adenosine antagonism in the bronchodilator action of theophylline is briefly discussed below. The relationship of PDE inhibition to airway smooth muscle relaxation is discussed in greater depth in subsequent sections of this chapter.

PHOSPHODIESTERASE INHIBITION

There is a general correlation between PDE inhibitor potency (measured in lung homogenates) of a range of methylxan-

517

thines and their ability to relax rat tracheal smooth muscle in vitro (see Chap. 49). A comparison of the methylxanthines IBMX and pentoxifylline with theophylline also reveals that the drugs with the greater potency in inhibiting airway PDE enzyme activity have greater potency in relaxing bronchial smooth muscle (see below). The relevance of this relationship to the effectiveness of methylxanthines as bronchodilators has been questioned frequently, since concentrations of the drugs that lie within the therapeutic range exert only slight inhibitory actions on lung PDE activity.[3] However, as demonstrated below, the concentration-dependencies of inhibition of cyclic AMP–PDE activity and relaxation of bronchial smooth muscle in vitro are similar, and adenosine antagonism does not appear to be involved in the relaxant action. Theophylline is a relatively weak bronchodilator compared with β-adrenoceptor agonists,[4,5] and the small degree of PDE inhibition by therapeutic theophylline concentrations may be reflected in this small degree of bronchodilation. Since airway resistance is inversely proportional to the fourth power of the radius, the small reductions in airway smooth muscle tone caused by the PDE-inhibitory action of theophylline may be sufficient to account for the apparent increase in airway caliber in vivo. Increased PDE inhibitory potency in vivo is related to increased bronchodilation (see Chap. 49). This suggests that the importance of PDE inhibition in the bronchodilator response to theophylline may outweigh that of adenosine antagonism.

Investigations have begun to demonstrate the effectiveness of some selective PDE inhibitors as bronchodilators (see below), but direct comparisons of the concentration dependencies of the drugs for PDE inhibition and in vivo bronchodilation are still awaited.

ADENOSINE RECEPTOR ANTAGONISM

Theophylline is an antagonist at adenosine receptors (Chap. 49), and, since adenosine causes bronchoconstriction in patients with asthma[6] or COPD,[7] this antagonist action has been proposed as the cause of bronchodilation by theophylline. Since a significant degree of adenosine antagonism is caused by the-ophylline at concentrations within the therapeutic range, this action of the drug has been assumed to be of greater relevance than PDE inhibition to its clinical effects. In fact, investigation of structure–activity relationships reveals the airway relaxant activity of xanthine derivatives to be unrelated to their potency as adenosine antagonists.[3] Since no definite role has yet been demonstrated for adenosine in asthmatic bronchoconstriction, the likelihood of adenosine antagonism being a therapeutically relevant action of the-ophylline remains difficult to assess.

Adenosine enhances allergic mediator release from lung mast cells, and antagonism of adenosine receptors may be expected to suppress asthmatic reactions to allergen. However, enprofylline—which is a less potent adenosine antagonist than theophylline—exerts only slightly lesser inhibition of early asthmatic responses and slightly greater inhibition of late responses than a fourfold greater serum concentration of theophylline.[8] Thus, while adenosine receptor blockade may be involved to some extent in the ability of theophylline to protect against bronchoconstriction, it is probably not a major factor in this effect.

Role of Cyclic Nucleotides in Smooth Muscle Tone

Cyclic AMP and cyclic GMP concentrations within cells are increased in response to a variety of agents (see Chap. 49).[9] Within the cell, the cyclic nucleotides activate two protein kinases, known as cyclic AMP–dependent protein kinase (protein kinase A) and cyclic GMP–dependent protein kinase (protein kinase G). These enzymes catalyze the phosphorylation of a variety of proteins that are involved in the induction and maintenance of smooth muscle contraction.[10] A significant biochemical consequence of the phosphorylation events resulting from activation of the kinases in smooth muscle is the lowering of intracellular calcium ion concentrations by inhibition of calcium channel opening and stimulation of calcium "pump" activity.[11] In addition, opening of the large conductance Ca^{2+}-activated potassium channel (BK_{Ca}), which appears to be involved in termination of excitatory processes mediated by calcium ions and/or membrane depolarization,[12] is stimulated by both protein kinase A and protein kinase G.[11] This latter mechanism of smooth muscle relaxation is interesting because opening of BK_{Ca} is also evoked by β-adrenoceptor agonists through both cyclic AMP–dependent and cyclic AMP–independent pathways.[13]

That cyclic AMP plays a role in mediating airway smooth muscle relaxation has been demonstrated by its fullfilment of six well defined criteria, as described in the following list (from Torphy, 1994)[11]:

1. Adenylyl cyclase activity is stimulated by β-adrenoceptor agonists (which relax airway smooth muscle) in cell-free systems.
2. β-Adrenoceptor agonists increase cyclic AMP content in airway smooth muscle with concentration- and time-dependencies consistent with those of the relaxant response.
3. Phosphodiesterase inhibitors both mimic and potentiate the response to β-adrenoceptor agonists.
4. Cyclic AMP analogs mimic the relaxant effects of β-adrenoceptor agonists.
5. Protein kinase A is present in airway smooth muscle and is regulated by β-adrenoceptor agonists in a manner consistent with its mediating relaxation.
6. Several potential substrates for protein kinase A have been identified that are likely to be involved in the regulation of airway smooth muscle tone.

Evidence is accumulating that cyclic AMP can activate both protein kinases A and G and that, in fact, protein kinase G may predominate in mediating the decrease in intracellular calcium concentrations.[11] Since airway smooth muscle also relaxes in response to agents that act through increasing intracellular cyclic GMP (e.g., nitroprusside), this cyclic nucleotide may be of similar importance to cyclic AMP in the regulation of smooth muscle tone.

Actions of Phosphodiesterase Inhibitors on Airway Smooth Muscle

IN VITRO PROPERTIES

Early studies of the PDE activity of crude lung homogenates revealed human lung to contain enzymes corresponding to PDEs 1, 2, 3, 4, and 5 (see Chap. 49 for classification).[9] Further investigations of the isoenzyme profiles of isolated airways have demonstrated the presence of PDEs 1 through 5 in both human bronchus (where the type 3, 4, and 5 isoenzymes predominate) and human trachea, which apparently differs from bronchus, in exhibiting greater PDE1 activity.[14]

Theophylline relaxes the inherent tone of human bronchial rings in vitro at concentrations similar to those that inhibit cyclic AMP hydrolysis by PDE in homogenates of the same tissue (Fig. 50-1). The EC_{50} value (for relaxation) is approximately 80 μM[15]; this corresponds to roughly 14 $\mu g/ml$. Theophylline displays no selectivity for particular isoenzyme families in human bronchus, exhibiting IC_{50} values (concentrations inhibiting by 50 percent the rate of hydrolysis of 0.25 μM cyclic AMP) of approximately 250 μM for each purified isoenzyme.[15] Two other nonselective methylxanthine PDE inhibitors, IBMX and pentoxifylline, also relax bronchial smooth muscle with potencies similar to those exhibited for PDE inhibition.[15,16]

In human bronchial smooth muscle preparations studied in vitro, 8-phenyltheophylline (a methylxanthine adenosine receptor antagonist of greater potency than theophylline and with minimal PDE inhibitory actions) has no effect on inherent tone at concentrations at which theophylline is an effective relaxant.[14] This suggests that adenosine antagonism in vitro does not contribute to the airway-relaxing effects of theophylline.

When isoenzyme-selective PDE inhibitors are studied, more complicated results are obtained. While zardaverine, a mixed inhibitor of PDE3 and PDE4, is similar to theophylline in relaxing bronchial rings and inhibiting PDE in the same range of concentrations,[16] selective inhibitors of PDE3 and PDE4 behave differently (Fig. 50-2). Selective PDE3 inhibitors are effective in vitro relaxants of inherent muscle tone in human bronchi,[16,17] but selective PDE4 inhibitors relax these tissue preparations very weakly,[16,17] even though PDE4 constitutes a greater proportion of the bronchial PDE activity than PDE3. In small bronchi (internal diameter <2 mm), however, PDE3 inhibitors also are ineffective relaxants.[18] This correlation of relaxation effect to airway diameter (generation) is not observed with theophylline.[19]

The situation is even more complex for bronchi precontracted with muscarinic cholinoceptor agonists (methacholine or carbachol), histamine, or leukotriene (LT)D_4. Under these conditions, a selective PDE4 inhibitor, rolipram, has been reported to relax bronchial smooth muscle by some workers[17,20] but not by others.[18] Interestingly, PDE3 inhibitors exhibit differential relaxant effects depending on the contractile stimulus. Thus, although rolipram displays no distinction in its relaxant action between methacholine- and histamine-contracted tissues, the PDE3 inhibitor Org 9935 is severalfold more potent in relaxing bronchial contractions caused by histamine than by methacholine (Fig. 50-3).[20] A less-marked difference also can be observed with IBMX, which relaxes histamine-contracted bronchial rings

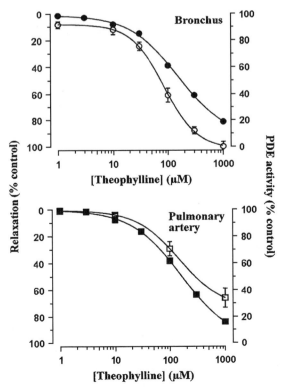

FIGURE 50-1 Inhibition of cyclic AMP phosphodiesterase activity (solid symbols) and relaxation of smooth muscle (open symbols) of human bronchus (*upper panel*) and pulmonary artery (*lower panel*) by theophylline.

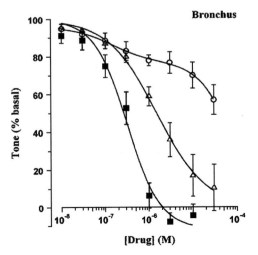

FIGURE 50-2 Effects of the mixed PDE3–PDE4 inhibitor zardaverine (■), the selective PDE3 inhibitor motapizone (Δ), and the selective PDE4 inhibitor rolipram (○) on inherent tone in human bronchus. (Data taken from Rabe et al.[16])

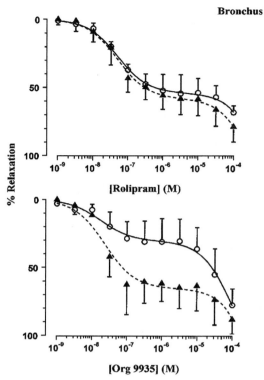

FIGURE 50-3 Relaxation of histamine- (▲) and methacholine-precontracted (○) human bronchial rings by the selective PDE4 inhibitor rolipram (*upper panel*) and the selective PDE3 inhibitor Org 9935 (*lower panel*). (From de Boer et al.[20])

tracted by muscarinic cholinoceptor agonists. By contrast, isoproterenol-induced relaxation of LTD_4-precontracted bronchi is profoundly potentiated by siguazodan (Fig. 50-4),[18] reaffirming the potency of PDE3 inhibitors in reversing non-cholinoceptor–mediated contractions of human airway smooth muscle.

Human bronchial smooth muscle also relaxes in vitro in response to the nitric oxide donor, sodium nitroprusside, an effect that is thought to be mediated by the activation of soluble guanylyl cyclase, which causes production of cyclic GMP. This relaxant response is potentiated in LTD_4-precontracted bronchial rings by an inhibitor of cyclic GMP–specific PDE5, zaprinast,[18] while the nitroprusside-induced relaxation of acetylcholine-contracted tissues is enhanced only very slightly by rolipram, which acts predominately through cyclic AMP.[17] Siguazodan—the target enzyme of which, PDE3, is inhibited by cyclic GMP (see Chap. 49)—does not enhance relaxant responses to nitroprusside.[17,18]

Under conditions of basal- or carbachol-induced tone, there is synergy between inhibitors of PDE3 and PDE4 in relaxing human bronchial smooth muscle (Fig. 50-4).[16,18] In fact, the inhibition of PDE3 with micromolar concentrations of siguazodan can unveil relaxant effects of rolipram under conditions where they are not apparent in the absence of PDE3 inhibition.[18] This finding, along with the recognition that PDE4 inhibitors suppress the proinflammatory actions of several immune cells,[9] has led to a growing interest in mixed inhibitors of PDE3 and PDE4 as potential anti-asthma drugs.[9,21]

IN VIVO PROPERTIES

Theophylline causes measurable bronchodilation after oral or intravenous administration in patients with airways obstruction (see Chap. 49), while intravenous administration also improves lung function in normal subjects.[4] This basal bronchospasmolytic action of the drug is less pronounced than its antibronchospastic effect; theophylline protects against the bronchoconstriction induced by histamine or methacholine with significant effects against histamine-induced constriction at serum concentrations less than 5 μg/ml (see Chap. 51).[22] Whether the protective effects of theophylline involve physiological actions in addition

with greater potency than rings contracted with methacholine.[20] This phenomenon has an interesting in vivo correlate; namely, the greater potency of theophylline against histamine-induced, compared with methacholine-induced, bronchoconstriction (see Chap. 51).

In acetylcholine- or carbachol-precontracted bronchi, the relaxation induced by the β-adrenoceptor agonist isoproterenol is enhanced by rolipram but not by the selective PDE3 inhibitor siguazodan,[17,18] again demonstrating the relative lack of efficacy of PDE3 inhibitors in airways con-

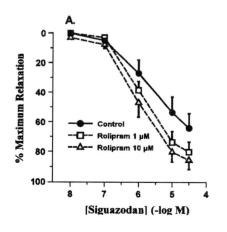

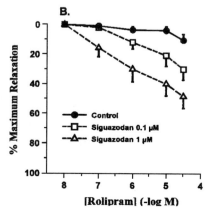

FIGURE 50-4 Interaction between PDE3 and PDE4 inhibitors in relaxation of human bronchus. Relaxation of carbachol-precontracted bronchial rings by the selective PDE3 inhibitor siguazodan (*left panel*) and the selective PDE4 inhibitor rolipram (*right panel*) alone (●) or in the presence of the complementary drug (□, Δ). (From Torphy et al.[18])

to bronchodilation remains a subject for further investigation.

Animal studies have demonstrated the bronchodilator effects of intravenously administered, nonselective PDE inhibitors (theophylline and enprofylline) and selective inhibitors of PDE3 and PDE4.[23] It is interesting to note that both nonselective and PDE3-selective drugs induce cardiac dysrhythmias in anesthetized dogs, suggesting that this side effect of methylxanthines probably is caused by their inhibition of PDE3.[24] Intravenous administration of a selective PDE3 inhibitor, CI 930, also protects against LTD$_4$- and allergen-induced bronchoconstriction in sensitized guinea pigs, while the selective PDE4 inhibitor, rolipram, is effective only against allergen.[25] The latter finding implies that PDE4 inhibition is effective in allergen responses as a result of suppression of IgE-dependent mediator release from inflammatory cells, rather than through a direct action on airway smooth muscle. In cynomolgus monkeys, rolipram is ineffective against the acute bronchoconstriction induced by allergen inhalation; however, it decreases airway hyperresponsiveness occurring after repeated allergen exposure.[26] Again, this finding points toward a suppression of inflammatory reactions in the airways, rather than an action on smooth muscle contraction.

Actions of Phosphodiesterase Inhibitors on Pulmonary Vascular Smooth Muscle

One of the areas of therapeutics in which isoenzyme-selective PDE inhibitors are already in use is in the treatment of congestive heart failure. PDE3 inhibitors such as milrinone are used for their cardiotonic and vasodilator actions,[27] which ensue from the ability of cyclic AMP and cyclic GMP to increase ventricular contractility and to relax vascular smooth muscle. While both the PDE isoenzyme profiles and the responses of systemic blood vessels to PDE inhibitors have been widely studied, information about PDEs in the pulmonary circulation is scarce. Since pulmonary hypertension can accompany chronic obstructive pulmonary disease (COPD) and acute asthma, it is worthwhile to investigate the actions on the pulmonary vasculature of drugs intended for use in these conditions. In fact, milrinone and theophylline decrease mean pulmonary blood pressure in patients exhibiting pulmonary hypertension,[28,29] and this property of theophylline has been proposed to contribute to its clinical effectiveness in the treatment of COPD.

Biochemical studies have revealed the presence of PDEs of the 1, 3, 4, and 5 families in human pulmonary arteries, with PDE3 and PDE5 being the predominant isoenzymes.[30] This profile corresponds closely with that observed in systemic blood vessels and aortic smooth muscle cells.

Theophylline relaxes pulmonary artery rings that have been contracted with prostaglandin (PG)F$_{2\alpha}$ in vitro. As described above for bronchus, this relaxant action is exerted in the same range of concentrations that inhibits cyclic AMP hydrolysis by PDE from pulmonary artery homogenates (Fig. 50-1). To date, no comparison has been made with inhibition of PDE-catalyzed cyclic GMP breakdown, although,

in view of the lack of isoenzyme selectivity of theophylline, this is assumed to occur at similar drug concentrations. Pulmonary artery also resembles bronchus in both relaxing to IBMX and in its failure to relax in response to 8-phenyltheophylline, suggesting that this vasodilator action of theophylline also is mediated by PDE inhibition rather than by adenosine antagonism.[30]

Theophylline is both less potent and less efficacious in relaxing pulmonary artery rings in vitro than in relaxing bronchial rings at a similar initial muscle tone. This difference may reflect differences in the nature of the musculature and that the total PDE activity in pulmonary artery homogenates is approximately double that in bronchi.[30]

Inhibitors of PDE3 and PDE5, as well as mixed PDE3–PDE4 inhibitors, also relax human pulmonary artery in vitro. PDE4 inhibitors, however, are very poor relaxants and this may reflect the relative lack of PDE4 in this tissue. Marked synergy is observed between the relaxant effects of PDE3 and PDE5 inhibitors, and this may point to the importance of cyclic GMP in the regulation of vascular tone.[30] The ability of theophylline to inhibit both PDE3 and PDE5 may, therefore, account for its effectiveness in alleviating pulmonary hypertension, although the actions of PDE5 inhibitors and of a combination of selective inhibitors of PDE3 and PDE5 in vivo remain to be investigated.

Clinical Studies of Selective Phosphodiesterase Inhibitors

To date, isoenzyme-selective PDE inhibitors have been studied only acutely for their effects in human airways in vivo. The results of these studies largely have been disappointing because only brief bronchodilation is observed with mixed PDE3/PDE4 inhibitors, while side effects, particularly nausea and vomiting, are pronounced.[31,32] One such drug, AH 21-132 (benafentrine), is ineffective when administered orally, but it reverses methacholine-induced bronchoconstriction in healthy volunteers when administered intravenously or by inhalation.[31] Zardaverine produces improvement in baseline lung function when administered by inhalation to asthmatic patients.[32] In both cases, however, the bronchodilation is very short-lived, and, in the case of zardaverine, repeated inhalation at 15 min intervals produces significant bronchodilation only during the first hour. A selective PDE3 inhibitor, enoximone, has exhibited some bronchodilating capacity in patients with COPD,[33] and a PDE4 inhibitor, tibenelast, causes some bronchodilation in severe asthmatics.[34] However, much research remains to be conducted into the possible effectiveness of such drugs in disease control. Several other inhibitors of PDE3, PDE4, or both are undergoing clinical trials for effectiveness in experimental asthmatic responses or in clinical asthma,[22] and the results of these studies may indicate the therapeutic potential of drugs of this type.

As stated above, selective PDE3 inhibitors already have found a clinical application in the treatment of congestive heart failure, but their potential for decreasing pulmonary hypertension in lung disease is largely unexplored. A PDE3 inhibitor, milrinone, decreases pulmonary capillary wedge pressure and also mean pulmonary artery pressure and pulmonary vascular resistance when administered intravenously to patients with heart failure following cardiac surgery.[9] Whether such drugs have a beneficial effect in pulmonary hypertension accompanying COPD or severe asthma remains to be investigated. Unfortunately, treatment with PDE3 inhibitors often is associated with tachycardia,[27,35] and it may be advisable to seek to regulate pulmonary hemodynamics with drugs that have less pronounced cardiac actions.

Summary

Theophylline exerts a direct relaxant effect on airway smooth muscle, which may underlie its clinical bronchodilator properties. In vitro, this relaxant effect appears to be mediated by PDE inhibition and not by adenosine antagonism, although this finding cannot necessarily be extrapolated to the in vivo situation. Similarly, theophylline causes an adenosine-independent relaxation of pulmonary arteries in vitro. The concentrations of theophylline required to relax human bronchus in vitro lie within the range of therapeutic serum concentrations (the EC_{50} for relaxation of bronchial rings is approximately 80 μM, corresponding to 14 $\mu g/ml$). Because lower serum concentrations of theophylline exert significant protective effects against bronchoconstriction induced by exercise or allergen, evidence for the immunomodulatory and potential anti-inflammatory actions of theophylline (Chap. 51) must be taken into account when interpreting these findings.

References

1. Bowman WC, Rand MJ. *Textbook of pharmacology.* 2nd ed. Oxford: Blackwell, 1980.
2. Persson CGA. Overview of effects of theophylline. *J Allergy Clin Immunol* 1986; 78:780.
3. Persson CGA, Karlsson J-A. In vitro responses to bronchodilator drugs. In: Jenne JW, Murphy S, editors. *Drug therapy for asthma: research and clinical practice (Lung Biology in Health and Disease,* vol 31). New York: Marcel Dekker, 1987: 129–176.
4. Schultze-Werninghaus G, Debelić M. *Asthma: Grundlagen—Diagnostik—Therapie.* Berlin: Springer-Verlag, 1988.
5. Magnussen H, Jörres R, Hartmann V. Bronchodilator effect of theophylline preparations and aerosol fenoterol in stable asthma. *Chest* 1986; 90:722.
6. Cushley MJ, Tattersfield AE, Holgate ST. Inhaled adenosine and guanosine on airway resistance in normal and asthmatic subjects. *Br J Clin Pharmacol* 1983; 15:161.
7. Oosterhoff Y, de Jong JW, Jansen MA, Koeter GH, Postma DS. Airway responsiveness to adenosine 5'-monophosphate in chronic obstructive pulmonary disease is determined by smoking. *Am Rev Respir Dis* 1993; 147:553.
8. Pauwels R, van Renterghem D, van der Straeten M, Johannesson N, Persson CGA. The effect of theophylline and enprofylline on allergen-induced bronchoconstriction. *J Allergy Clin Immunol* 1985; 76:583.
9. Dent G, Magnussen H, Rabe KF. Cyclic nucleotide phosphodiesterases in the human lung. *Lung* 1994; 72:129.
10. Giembycz MA, Raeburn D. Current concepts on mechanisms of force generation and maintenance in airways smooth muscle. *Pulm Pharmacol* 1992; 5:279.
11. Torphy TJ: β-Adrenoceptors, cAMP and airway smooth muscle relaxation: challenges to the dogma. *Trends Pharmacol Sci* 1994; 15:370.
12. Edwards G, Weston AH. Potassium channel openers and vascular smooth muscle relaxation. *Pharmac Ther* 1990; 48:237.
13. Small RC, Chiu P, Cook SJ, Foster RW, Isaac L. β-Adrenoceptor agonists in bronchial asthma: role of K^+-channel opening in mediating their bronchodilator effects. *Clin Exp Allergy* 1993; 23:802.
14. Rabe KF, Magnussen H, Dent G. Theophylline and selective PDE inhibitors as bronchodilators and smooth muscle relaxants. *Eur Respir J* 1995; 8:637.
15. Cortijo J, Bou J, Beleta J, Cardelús I, Llenas J, Morcillo E, Gristwood RW. Investigation into the role of phosphodiesterase IV in bronchorelaxation, including studies with human bronchus. *Br J Pharmacol* 1993; 108:562.
16. Rabe KF, Tenor H, Dent G, Schudt C, Liebig S, Magnussen H. Phosphodiesterase isoenzymes modulating inherent tone in human airways: identification and characterization. *Am J Physiol: Lung Cell Mol Physiol* 264; 1993; L458.
17. Qian Y, Naline E, Karlsson J-A, Raeburn D, Advenier C. Effects of rolipram and siguazodan on the human isolated bronchus and their interaction with isoprenaline and sodium nitroprusside. *Br J Pharmacol* 1993; 109:774.
18. Torphy TJ, Undem BJ, Cieslinski LB, Luttmann MA, Reeves ML, Hay DWP. Identification, characterization and functional role of phosphodiesterase isozymes in human airway smooth muscle. *J Pharmacol Exp Ther* 1993; 265:1213.
19. Finney MJB, Karlsson J-A, Persson CGA. Effects of bronchoconstriction and bronchodilation on a novel human small airway preparation. *Br J Pharmacol* 1985; 85:29.
20. de Boer J, Philpott AJ, van Amsterdam GM, Shahid M, Zaagsma J, Nicholson CD. Human bronchial cyclic nucleotide phosphodiesterase isoenzymes: biochemical and pharmacological analysis using selective inhibitors. *Br J Pharmacol* 1993; 106:1028.
21. Torphy TJ, Undem BJ. Phosphodiesterase inhibitors: new opportunities for the treatment of asthma. *Thorax* 1991; 46:512.
22. Magnussen H, Reuss G, Jörres R. Theophylline has a dose-related effect on the airway response to inhaled histamine and methacholine in asthmatics. *Am Rev Respir Dis* 1987; 136:1163.
23. Dent G, Giembycz MA. Selective phosphodiesterase inhibitors in the therapy of asthma. *Clin Immunother* 1995 3:423.
24. Heaslip RJ, Buckley SK, Sickels BD, Grimes D. Bronchial vs. cardiovascular activities of selective phosphodiesterase inhibitors in the anesthetized beta-blocked dog. *J Pharmacol Exp Ther* 1991; 257:741.
25. Howell RE, Sickels BD, Woeppel SL. Pulmonary antiallergic and bronchodilator effects of isozyme-selective phosphodiesterase inhibitors in guinea-pigs. *J Pharmacol Exp Ther* 1993; 264:609.
26. Turner CR, Andreson CJ, Smith WB, Watson JW. Effects of rolipram on responses to acute and chronic antigen exposure in monkeys. *Am J Respir Crit Care Med* 1994; 149:1153.
27. Cruickshank JM. Phosphodiesterase III inhibitors: long-term risks and short-term benefits. *Cardiovasc Drugs Ther* 1993; 7:655.
28. Harris MN, Daborn AK, O'Dwyer JP. Milrinone and the pulmonary vascular system. *Eur J Anaesthesiol Suppl* 1992; 5:27.
29. Grützmacher J, Schicht R, Schlaeger R, Sill V. Plasma level-dependent hemodynamic effects of theophylline in patients with chronic obstructive lung disease and pulmonary hypertension. *Semin Respir Med* 1985; 7:171.

30. Rabe KF, Tenor H, Dent G, Schudt C, Nakashima M, Magnussen H. Identification of PDE isozymes in human pulmonary artery and the effect of selective PDE inhibitors. *Am J Physio*l: (*Lung Cell Mol Physiol* 266; 1994; L536.

31. Foster RW, Rakshi K, Carpenter JR, Small RC. Trials of the bronchodilator activity of the isoenzyme-selective phosphodiesterase inhibitor AH 21-132 in healthy volunteers during a methacholine challenge test. *Br J Clin Pharmacol* 1992; 34:527.

32. Brunnée T, Engelstätter R, Steinijans VW, Kunkel G. Bronchodilatory effect of inhaled zardaverine, a phosphodiesterase III and IV inhibitor, in patients with asthma. *Eur Respir J* 1992; 5:982.

33. Leeman M, Lejeune P, Melot C, Naeije R. Reduction in pulmonary hypertension and in airway resistances by enoximone (MDL 17,043) in decompensated COPD. *Chest* 1987; 91:662.

34. Israel E, Mthur PN, Tashkin D, Drazen JM. LY186655 prevents bronchospasm in asthma of moderate severity. *Chest* 1988; 94:71S.

35. Lubbe WF, Podzuweit T, Opie LH. Potential arrhythmogenic role of cyclic adenosine monophosphate (AMP) and cytosolic calcium overload: implications for prophylactic effects of beta-blockers in myocardial infarction and proarrhythmic effects of phosphodiesterase inhibitors. *J Am Coll Cardiol* 1992; 19:1622.

Chapter 51 _____

THEOPHYLLINE IN THE TREATMENT OF BRONCHIAL ASTHMA AND CHRONIC OBSTRUCTIVE PULMONARY DISEASE

KLAUS F. RABE
GORDON DENT
HELGO MAGNUSSEN

Introduction

Theophylline first was synthesized by Albert Kossel in 1889,[1] and, for this achievement, along with his work on purines, he was awarded the Nobel Prize in 1910. In 1922, Samson Raphael Hirsch first described the bronchodilator effects of theophylline in human airway smooth muscle,[2] confirming the detailed observations made by Henry Hyde Salter in 1859 on the clinical effects of coffee in patients with bronchial asthma.[3] These observations added to the two recognized effects of theophylline as a diuretic and cardiotonic drug,[4,5] but it was not until 1937 that theophylline was used for the treatment of obstructive airways disease, following the description by George Hermann of its beneficial effect in severe asthma.[6]

During the last 25 years, the use of theophylline has become worldwide. The introduction of sustained-release formulations,[7,8] improved availability of drug monitoring techniques,[9] and standardized dosing strategies[10,11] have resulted in increased efficacy with clinically acceptable toxicity profiles, making theophylline one of the most prescribed therapies for asthma and chronic obstructive airways disease.[12,13]

National and international asthma guidelines recommend the use of theophylline in some cases as second-line, and in most cases as third-line, treatment for patients who are not adequately controlled with corticosteroids and β-adrenoceptor agonists, although it is recognized that patients with nocturnal symptoms may especially benefit from this form of treatment.[14–17] It may be speculated, however, that the introduction of long-acting β₂-adrenoceptor agonists,[18,19] which also have been shown to be clinically effective in nocturnal asthma, will influence this clinical attitude (see Chaps. 42 and 46). The well-accepted concept that asthma is primarily an inflammatory disease of the airways, along with the development and broad use of inhaled corticosteroids, has further removed emphasis from the use of theophylline in mild forms of asthma.[12,14] The recognition that theophylline may itself have clinically significant anti-asthma activities apart from bronchodilation (see Chap. 50) has recently prompted a large research effort and has led to speculation on the reappraisal of the drug as an immunomodulator, which may change its position in future guidelines.[13]

The role of theophylline in treatment of chronic obstructive pulmonary disease (COPD) has been a subject of debate and controversy.[20,21] In clinical practice, theophylline is widely used for this disease, although the individual responses of patients can be unpredictable; compared with its use in asthma, the effects of theophylline on airway dimensions in COPD are invariably much more subtle and may, in many cases of severe COPD, be absent. These phenomena have obscured the rationale for use of theophylline in COPD, and the numerous accounts of its effects on pulmonary and cardiovascular function,[22,23] dyspnea,[24,25] diaphragmatic[26–29] and skeletal muscle contractility,[30] respiratory drive,[31,32] exercise capacity,[33,34] and mucociliary clearance[35–38] have not led to a general consensus on either how theophylline works or how it should be used in these cases. Not until quite recently have the results of clinical withdrawal studies indicated that the beneficial effects of theophylline treatment in patients with severe COPD are best evaluated through standardized symptom assessment and quantification of exercise capacity, rather than through classical lung function parameters.[24,25,39]

Theophylline in the Treatment of Bronchial Asthma

ACTIONS OF THEOPHYLLINE IN EXPERIMENTAL ASTHMATIC REACTIONS

In addition to its acute bronchodilator action (see Chap. 50), theophylline has been demonstrated to exert significant protective effects against bronchoconstriction induced by recognized asthma triggers, including exercise and allergens, and by experimental bronchoconstrictor agents such as histamine and methacholine. These experimental studies are useful in indicating the effectiveness of theophylline against particular types of bronchial reactivity.

HISTAMINE AND METHACHOLINE

Several demonstrations have been made of the inhibition of histamine- and methacholine-induced bronchoconstriction by theophylline, administered either orally or intravenously. A single oral dose of theophylline—producing a mean serum theophylline concentration of 13 μg/ml and a small bronchodilation (7.6 percent increase in FEV_1)—has been shown to protect asthmatic children against these reactions. In these studies, the dose of inhaled constrictor required to reduce FEV_1 by 20 percent ($PD_{20}FEV_1$) increased threefold for methacholine and twofold for histamine, although no correlation could be observed in these experiments between serum theophylline concentration and bronchoprotective effects.[40] A 1.3-fold increase in $PD_{20}FEV_1$ to histamine also has been observed in adult asthmatics at a mean serum theophylline concentration of 13 μg/ml after several days of oral administration of a sustained-release theophylline preparation.[41] In another study of asthmatic adults, in which histamine and methacholine reactivity were measured after each of three intravenous doses of aminophylline, a clear relationship was observed between serum theophylline concentration and protection against both methacholine and histamine bronchial provocation (Fig. 51-1). A significant degree of protection against histamine-induced bronchoconstriction (measured as dose causing 100 percent increase in specific airways resistance, $PD_{100}sR_{aw}$) occurred at serum theophylline concentrations as low as 3.2 μg/ml.[42] In this study, theophylline protected more effectively against histamine- than against methacholine-induced bronchoconstric-

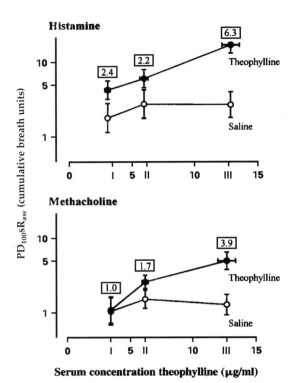

FIGURE 51-1 Theophylline protects against histamine- and methacholine-induced bronchoconstriction in asthmatics. Effects of intravenous saline (○) or theophylline (●) on bronchial reactivity to inhaled histamine (*upper panel*) or methacholine (*lower panel*). I, II, and III indicate the serum theophylline concentrations attained after intravenous administration of 100 mg aminophylline prior to the first provocation challenge, 100 mg aminophylline prior to a second challenge, and 200 mg aminophylline prior to a third challenge, respectively. (Data from Magnussen et al.[42])

tion, a finding that intriguingly correlates with in vitro data showing nonselective PDE inhibitors to more effectively relax human bronchi contracted with histamine than those contracted with methacholine (Chap. 50), although there are insufficient data at present to propose a definite relation between these phenomena.

EXERCISE

Theophylline also exerts a concentration-dependent protective effect against exercise-induced bronchoconstriction in asthmatic subjects. Following administration of a single oral dose of theophylline to asthmatic children, a diminishing protection is observed over time, paralleling the decrease in mean serum theophylline concentration to 16, 13, and 10 μg/ml at 2, 4, and 6 h, respectively, after administration.[43] In mildly asthmatic adults treated with intravenous aminophylline (equivalent to 200 or 351 mg anhydrous theophylline), protection against exercise-induced bronchoconstriction (measured as decrease in FEV_1 or increase in sR_{aw}) is related to the dose and to serum concentration of theophylline; significant protection was observed after a dose resulting in a mean serum concentration of 6.7 μg/ml,

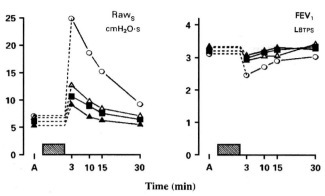

FIGURE 51-2 Theophylline protects against exercise-induced bronchoconstriction. Mean airway responses to cold-air breathing during exercise in patients receiving saline (○), aminophylline containing 200 mg (△) or 351 mg theophylline (▲), or 200 mg theophylline + 300 mg proxyphylline + 300 mg diprophylline (■) by intravenous infusion. Points represent baseline lung function values (*A*) 15 min after drug infusion and values measured at 3, 10, 15, and 30 min after exercise. (From Magnussen et al.[44])

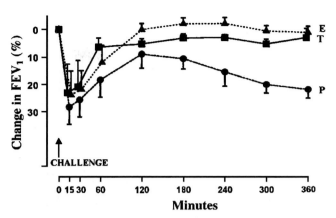

FIGURE 51-3 Theophylline and enprofylline protect against early and late asthmatic reactions to allergen inhalation. The percentage change in FEV_1 following allergen inhalation in asthmatic patients treated with placebo (P), theophylline (T), or enprofylline (E) is illustrated. (Adapted from Pauwels et al.[45])

and significantly greater protection occurred after a dose resulting in a mean serum concentration of 10 μg/ml (Fig. 51-2).[44] The addition of 300 mg each of diprophylline and proxyphylline to the lower dose of theophylline increases the protective action only slightly, paralleling the poor bronchodilator action of these drugs (see Chap. 49), but the degree of protection against exercise-induced bronchoconstriction by aminophylline does not correlate with the magnitude of acute bronchodilation, suggesting a difference in the mechanisms through which these actions are mediated.[44]

ALLERGENS

An important report published in 1985 illustrated the effectiveness of theophylline against bronchial reactions induced by inhalation of specific allergen in asthmatic subjects (Fig. 51-3). In this study, the intravenous infusion of theophylline (7.2 mg/kg loading dose followed by a maintenance infusion of 74 mg/h, leading to steady mean serum concentrations of approximately 10.5 μg/ml) or enprofylline (2.7 mg/kg followed by 71 mg/h, leading to steady mean serum concentrations of 2.7 μg/ml) caused a minor initial bronchodilation and a significant protection against both the immediate and late bronchoconstrictor responses (measured as decrease in FEV_1 and as decrease in specific airways conductance, sG_{aw}) to inhaled allergen.[45] Despite the fourfold lower serum concentration of enprofylline (associated with a slightly smaller initial bronchodilation), this drug exerted a greater protective effect against the late asthmatic reaction to inhaled allergen. The greater potency of enprofylline confirms the importance of PDE inhibition relative to adenosine antagonism in protection against bronchial reactions in an experimental asthmatic response.

Toluene diisocyanate (TDI), a trigger of occupational asthma in persons sensitized through exposure in the workplace, causes a typical asthmatic dual reaction of immediate and delayed bronchoconstriction after inhalation. Treatment

of sensitized persons for 7 days with oral sustained-release theophylline (6.5 mg/kg twice daily, producing mean serum concentrations of 18 μg/ml) causes significant protection against both the early and late asthmatic bronchoconstriction responses to inhaled TDI (Fig. 51-4).[46] In an interesting comparison, an inhaled corticosteroid (beclomethasone; 1 mg twice daily for 7 days prior to TDI exposure) did not suppress the immediate reaction, while significantly inhibiting the late response.[46] In spite of its protective effect against TDI-induced bronchoconstriction, theophylline does not prevent the induction of bronchial hyperresponsiveness to inhaled methacholine following TDI exposure (Fig. 51-4, right panels)—a finding reproduced in later studies with allergen[47,48]—while beclomethasone abolishes the increase in responsiveness. In a more recent study of allergen-induced bronchial hyperresponsiveness, however, the increase in methacholine reactivity 8 h after allergen inhalation was shown to be partially blocked by treatment with oral sustained-release theophylline (individually optimized to give mean serum theophylline concentrations of 13 μg/ml).[49] While it remains to be determined, therefore, whether theophylline has an effect on airways hyperresponsiveness, it is clear that this will not be substantial. In asthmatic patients, airways responsiveness to inhaled histamine is reduced during a 3-week period of treatment with beclomethasone (800 μg/day) but no improvement is observed in patients receiving theophylline doses producing steady serum concentrations of 55 to 100 μM (10 to 20 μg/ml); when treatments are crossed over, patients receiving theophylline in place of the corticosteroid exhibit an increase in bronchial responsiveness, while those receiving beclomethasone in place of theophylline show a decrease.[50]

Acknowledging the ability of theophylline at serum concentrations less than 10 μg/ml to protect against histamine- and exercise-induced bronchoconstriction,[42,44] a study of the effects of low doses of theophylline on allergic asthmatic

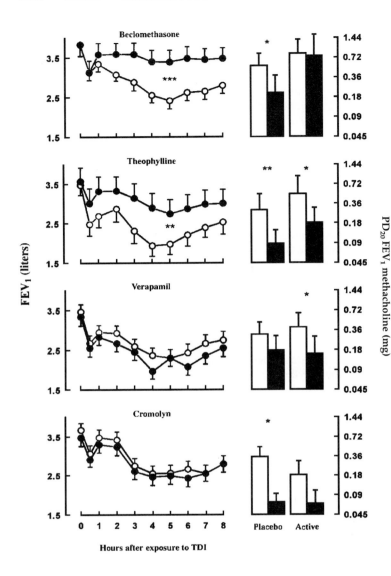

FIGURE 51-4 Theophylline protects against early and late asthmatic reactions to a common occupational asthma trigger but does not reduce airway reactivity. Shown are changes in FEV_1 and bronchial reactivity to methacholine following inhalation of toluene diisocyanate by sensitized subjects treated with placebo (○) or the following drugs (●): an inhaled corticosteroid (beclomethasone); oral slow-release theophylline; a calcium antagonist (verapamil); disodium cromoglycate (Cromolyn). The right panel shows PD_{20} FEV_1 methacholine before (□) and after (■) TDI Exposure. * = p < 0.05; ** = p < 0.01; *** = p < 0.001. (From Mapp et al.[46])

reactions recently has been undertaken. In this study, patients receiving oral sustained-release theophylline (200 mg twice daily) attained mean steady serum theophylline concentrations of 7.8 μg/ml and exhibited significant inhibition of late asthmatic reactions following inhalation of house dust mite extract.[48] This observation demonstrates a protective effect against asthmatic reactions for a concentration at the lower end of the "therapeutic range" of bronchodilator serum concentrations. Analysis of the data for individual subjects in this study, however, revealed no statistically significant correlation between serum theophylline concentration and inhibition of late responses. Thus, more data must be collected to determine whether low doses of theophylline can consistently protect against allergic asthmatic reactions.

Although the acute bronchodilator action of theophylline may be fairly weak compared with that of β-adrenoceptor agonists (see Chap. 50), the drug possesses some potentially important bronchoprotective properties that are likely to be of therapeutic benefit in asthmatic patients. Recent reports of suppressed airway inflammation after allergen inhalation in asthmatic subjects treated with low doses of theophylline (see Chap. 61) suggest that some of the beneficial effects of theophylline may be observable at lower serum concentrtions than the current target concentrations in clinical application of the drug. Since protection against exercise-induced asthmatic bronchoconstriction and the late asthmatic response to allergen is conferred by relatively low serum theophylline concentrations, it will be interesting to see the effects of long-term treatment with low theophylline doses in clinical asthma. It is conceivable, however, that the protective effects of theophylline ensue from a prolonged relaxant action on the airway smooth muscle. Recognizing this possibility, and notwithstanding the suggestion that they themselves may possess anti-inflammatory properties, the ability of long-acting β-adrenoceptor agonists, such as salmeterol and formoterol, to mimic the protective actions of theophylline also should be investigated thoroughly.

CLINICAL USE OF THEOPHYLLINE IN ASTHMA

Setting aside its demonstrated effectiveness against experimental asthmatic responses, theophylline has been used in the clinical treatment of asthma for several decades and remains the most widely prescribed anti-asthma drug in the world.[13] Although theophylline has been relegated to a second- or third-line treatment in asthma therapy, often regarded as useful only when inhaled corticosteroids and inhaled β_2-adrenoceptor agonists fail to achieve therapeutic goals,[16] the availability of sustained-release preparations and improved drug monitoring techniques have allowed more reliable maintenance of serum theophylline concentrations, thereby permitting more precise control of drug actions and facilitating avoidance of toxic effects associated with excessive serum drug concentrations.

ACUTE ASTHMA

The bronchodilator action of theophylline underlies the use of intravenous aminophylline in the management of acute severe asthma, a condition in which it has been used effectively for over 50 years.[13] Since theophylline (even by the intravenous route) is less effective than inhaled β_2-adrenoceptor agonists in causing bronchodilation,[15] this treatment is generally reserved for patients who fail to respond to β-adrenoceptor agonists. Although coadministration of a β-adrenoceptor agonist and theophylline can produce additive, or even synergic, acute bronchodilation,[5,51] no long-term benefit for symptom control has been demonstrated to result from administering intravenous aminophylline in conjunction with nebulized β-adrenergic agonists to patients who respond to the latter drug alone.[5,13] In fact, the addition of aminophylline to the treatment regimen can increase the incidence of side effects without producing any significant additional therapeutic benefit.[52]

Patients undergoing acute asthma exacerbations who fail to exhibit satisfactory improvement in FEV_1 or PEFR after treatment with inhaled β-adrenoceptor agonist may benefit from intravenous aminophylline. Rapid infusion of aminophylline can cause severe cardiac arrhythmias (see Chap. 49), and, if the drug is to be used in acute asthma, it should be administered by slow infusion (recommended rate is 0.6 mg/kg lean body weight per h)[15] with careful monitoring of serum concentrations.

CHRONIC ASTHMA

In view of the weak acute bronchodilator action of theophylline relative to β-adrenoceptor agonists, the ability of the drug to prevent the symptoms of chronic asthma and to reduce the need for emergency medication appears more important from a clinical perspective.[5] Therapeutic doses of theophylline that sustain a serum concentration above 10 μg/ml cause an increased frequency of asymptomatic days and a prolonged improvement of lung function in asthmatic patients[53] and reduce the need for repeated short courses of daily corticosteroids.[54]

In patients whose asthma is uncontrollable by bronchodilators alone and who, therefore, require chronic corticosteroid therapy, the addition of theophylline to a treatment regimen including inhaled beclomethasone or alternate-day oral prednisolone causes a reduction in the frequency of nocturnal symptoms, decreased use of inhaled β-adrenoceptor agonists, and increased exercise tolerance,[54] demonstrating that theophylline can exert therapeutic effects in addition to those conferred by regular corticosteroid use. Withdrawal of theophylline from a treatment regimen of oral and inhaled corticosteroids, inhaled β_2-adrenoceptor agonists, inhaled muscarine antagonists drugs, cromoglycate, and regular oral the-ophylline in a group of young severe asthmatics has been demonstrated to cause a substantial deterioration in symptom control that cannot be rectified by increased corticosteroid doses, but responds to reintroduction of theophylline.[55] Further studies of patients with severe chronic asthma have shown deterioration in lung function and symptom control in corticosteroid-dependent asthmatics after theophylline withdrawal,[13] and this deterioration appears to be accompanied by increased signs of airway inflammation. Theophylline appears, therefore, to have a role in the management of chronic asthma which is independent of its bronchodilator capacity. In particular, a set of severe asthmatics appear to benefit particularly from symptom control by theophylline that is not achievable with corticosteroids.[55] The reason why some patients exhibit this requirement for theophylline remains unclear and requires further investigation.[13] Since many bronchoprotective actions of theophylline are observed at serum concentrations below the bronchodilator range (see above), it is feasible that theophylline at lower doses than those commonly prescribed may be of use in chronic asthma therapy, although research in this area is just beginning, and a reevaluation of the role and appropriate dosages of the-ophylline must await the results of well-controlled studies.

NOCTURNAL ASTHMA

Patients with asthma exhibit circadian variations in airway tone and airway responsiveness such that, in more severe cases, the decreased caliber and increased responsiveness occurring during the night are manifested as nocturnal asthma attacks.[56] Theophylline may be effective in the treatment of this condition, since administration of a sustained-release formulation of the drug at night controls nocturnal symptoms.[57] Slow-release oral β_2-adrenoceptor agonists are less effective than theophylline against nocturnal asthma,[58] but inhalation of the long-acting β_2-adrenoceptor agonists salmeterol and formoterol improves lung function and decreases methacholine responsiveness over a 24-hour period in asthmatic patients,[19] while regular use of inhaled salmeterol attenuates the early morning decrease in peak expiratory flow rate in patients with nocturnal asthma symptoms.[18] It remains unclear whether the actions of these drugs in nocturnal asthma reflect prolonged bronchodilation or a suppression of cyclical inflammatory processes in the airway wall.[56]

Theophylline in the Treatment of Chronic Obstructive Pulmonary Disease

While there is much evidence for the efficacy of theophylline in controlling the symptoms of reversible airways obstruc-

TABLE 51-1   Bronchodilator Effects of Theophylline in Patients with COPD

Study Design	Intervention	Results
PC, DB, CO $n = 10$, $FEV_1 = 0.7$ <15% BD response	Oral theophylline high and low dose (single dose Rx)	a. 21.3% increase in FEV_1 b. No significant change in dyspnea c. Theophylline levels = 9–12.5 μg/ml and 17–22 μg/ml
DB, CO $n = 20$, $FEV_1 = 2.0$	Theophylline withdrawal (S/P 6 months of Rx)	a. 20.8% decrease in FEV_1 b. Nocturnal dyspnea increased by 46.7% c. Theophylline levels = 65.5 mmol/liter (11.8 μg/ml)
PC, SB $n = 30$, $FEV_1 = 2.1$	Oral bamyphylline (60 days of Rx)	a. ≈ 20% increase in FEV_1 b. ≈ 19% increase in Pa_{O_2} c. Bamyphylline levels = 1.2–1.25 μg/ml
PC, DB, CO $n = 60$, $FEV_1 = 31\%$ <15% BD response	Oral theophylline (2 months of Rx)	a. 13% increase in FEV_1; significantly decreased dyspnea b. 9% increase in Pa_{O_2} c. 9% increase in Pa_{CO_2} d. 19% increase in VE (due to increase in VT) e. 29% decrease in Ppl/Ppl_{max} f. Theophylline levels = 14.8 μg/ml
PC, DB, CO $n = 14$, $FEV_1 = 0.7$ <25% BD response	Oral theophylline high and low dose (1 week of Rx)	a. 14.6% increase in FEV_1 b. No significant change in dyspnea c. Theophylline levels = 8.7–13 μg/ml and 16–23.6 μg/ml
PC, DB, CO $n = 12$, $FEV_1 = 1.36$ <15% BD response	Oral theophylline (4 weeks of Rx)	a. No significant changes in FEV_1, ABG, and 12-minute walk test b. Significant improvement in dyspnea rating c. Theophylline levels = 12–19 μg/ml
PC, DB, CO $n = 19$, $FEV_1 = 1.0$ <25% BD response	Oral aminophylline and/or inhaled salbutamol (2 weeks of Rx)	a. Significant improvements in FEV_1, 6-minute walk test, and symptoms b. Aminophylline and salbutamol were additive c. Theophylline levels = 12.3 ± 2.9 μg/ml
PC, DB, CO $n = 40$, $FEV_1 = 1.0$ "no fluctuations in past"	Oral theophylline (4 weeks of Rx)	a. 15% increase in FEV_1 b. 3.3% increase in Pa_{O_2} c. 2.4% decrease in Pa_{CO_2} d. No significant change in symptoms e. Theophylline levels = 15.1 ± 4.22 μg/ml
PC, DB, CO $n = 10$, $FEV_1 = 0.7$ <25% BD response	Oral theophylline and/or inhaled metaproterenol (1 week of Rx)	a. No significant changes with theophylline b. Significant effects with additive Rx but only in dyspnea c. Theophylline levels = 11.6 ± 1 and 12.8 ± 1.3 μg/ml
PC, DB $n = 30$, $FEV_1 = 0.6$ <30% BD response	IV aminophylline (72 h of Rx)	a. No significant improvements in FEV_1, ABG, or symptoms b. Theophylline levels = 46–75 μmol/liter (8.3–13.5 μg/ml)
PC, SB, CO $n = 38$, $FEV_1 = 29\%$ <15% BD response	Oral theophylline (2 months of Rx) (low, medium, and high dosing)	a. Significant improvements in FEV_1, trapped gas, 6-minute walk test, and dyspnea b. Theophylline levels = 6.3, 12.1, and 18.3 μg/ml
PC, DB, CO $n = 25$, $FEV_1 = 39\%$	Oral theophylline and/or salbutamol (3 weeks of Rx)	a. Significant increase in FEV_1 with theophylline (not salbutamol) b. Significant additive effects for FEV_1 + FVC, no symptomatic improvement c. Treatment failures: placebo, salbutamol > theophylline > combination d. Theophylline levels = 13.1 ± 1 μg/ml
SB, CO $n = 16$, $FEV_1 < 2.0$	IV aminophylline and salbutamol (single dose Rx)	a. 17% increase in FEV_1 with theophylline; 24% increase with salbutamol b. Salbutamol > theophylline in increasing sG_{aw} c. Additive effects with combined therapy d. Theophylline levels = 24.5 μg/ml
PC, DB, CO $n = 12$, $FEV_1 ≤ 1.6$ ≤ 15% BD response	Oral aminophylline and/or salbutamol (2 weeks of Rx)	a. Significant increases in FEV_1: 14% for theophylline; 16% for salbutamol b. Significant additive spirometric effect with combination therapy; reduced dyspnea and wheeze approached significance c. Theophylline levels = 12.9 ± 2.8 μg/ml and 15.3 ± 2.9 μg/ml

SOURCE: from Vaz Fragoso and Miller.[59]

Abbreviations: ABG, arterial blood gas measurements; BD, inhaled bronchodilator response (inclusion criterion); CO, crossover; DB, double-blind; FEV_1, forced expiratory volume in 1 s (mean baseline value in liters or percent predicted); Pa_{CO_2}, arterial partial pressure of carbon dioxide; Pa_{O_2}, arterial partial pressure of oxygen; PC, placebo controlled; Ppl, pleural pressure; Rx, therapy; SB, single-blind; sG_{aw}, specific airways conductance; VE, expiratory ventilation; VT, tidal volume.

tion in asthma, controversy has surrounded the use of the drug in the treatment of diseases characterized by chronic obstruction of the airways. Theophylline has a number of demonstrable actions that may be of clinical benefit in chronic airways obstruction, and which should be considered in decisions on individual treatment programs. The lack of short-term bronchodilation does not necessarily indicate that no benefit can be gained by the patient from regular long-term use of theophylline. Recent investigations of the effects of withdrawal of theophylline from COPD patients receiving optimized bronchodilator therapy suggest that theophylline is important in the control of symptoms in a substantial proportion of patients and that individual responses need to be assessed in order to determine a patient's requirement for theophylline treatment.[24,25]

BRONCHODILATION

Although bronchodilation often may be unobservable after theophylline administration in patients with COPD,[5] several studies have demonstrated varying degrees of improvement in lung function resulting from theophylline treatment (Table 51-1), where a bronchodilating effect of theophylline most often is associated with prolonged therapy in patients with chronic, stable COPD.[59] Additive bronchodilation can be achieved by combining theophylline and β_2-adrenoceptor agonists, although such studies have utilized doses that may have been suboptimal.[25] Thus, a unique contribution of theophylline is not clear, and prediction of a benefit to be gained from the use of theophylline, alone or in combination with a β-adrenoceptor agonist, cannot be made confidently on the basis of the patient's acute bronchodilator response to inhaled β-adrenoceptor agonist.[25,59–61]

RELIEF OF DYSPNEA

The predominant complaint of COPD patients is dyspnea accompanied by reduced exercise tolerance,[62] and these symptoms also have been shown in some studies to be controlled by theophylline (Table 51-1). Improvement in dyspnea ratings can be observed in the absence of significant measurable bronchodilation;[24,25,59,60] the ability to demonstrate effectiveness of theophylline in relieving dyspnea depends to some extent on the sensitivity of the dyspnea index used for assessment.[62] Studying changes in symptom score (indicating cough, sputum production, and dyspnea) and transition dyspnea index in COPD patients upon theophylline withdrawal or continuance, reveals significant worsening of dyspnea in a majority of patients after withdrawal of long-term theophylline treatment (Table 51-2).[25] An accompanying decrease in exercise tolerance (measured by the 6-minute walking test) is observed after theophylline withdrawal,[25] while exercise tolerance also has been shown to be increased by the introduction of theophylline to the treatment schedule of COPD patients.[63,64] The increased respiratory muscle performance that may underlie improved exercise tolerance in patients treated with theophylline (see below)[59,65] appears to be associated with reduction in trapped gas volume;[64] the reduction in hyperinflation and increased muscle performance might account, at least in part, for the improvement in lung function conferred by theophylline.[59]

IMPROVEMENT OF RESPIRATORY AND CARDIOVASCULAR PERFORMANCE

Theophylline has a well-characterized ability to increase diaphragmatic contractility, and this is more pronounced in

TABLE 51-2   Effects of Theophylline Withdrawal on Symptoms in Severe COPD[a]

	PLACEBO GROUP WITHDRAWN		THEOPHYLLINE GROUP CONTINUED	
	Days 1 & 2	Days 5 & 6	Days 1 & 2	Days 5 & 6
6-minute walking distance (m)	357 ± 124	227 ± 116	419 ± 145	446 ± 139‡
CRQ	97.9 ± 11.4	95.4 ± 16.6	101.7 ± 18.1	103.1 ± 20.8
BDI	4.4 ± 2.2	—	4.5 ± 2.7	—
TDI	—	−0.9 ± 1.9	—	0.4 ± 2.6‡
OCD	53.0 ± 15.6	52.9 ± 15.4	49.2 ± 16.3	51.2 ± 18.1
MRC scale	1.9 ± 1.0	2.1 ± 1.1	2.1 ± 1.0	1.9 ± 1.1
Symptom score	3.4 ± 1.7	4.2 ± 1.7†	2.8 ± 1.6	2.8 ± 1.9
Auscultation score	5.8 ± 2.8	6.7 ± 3.5†	5.9 ± 2.0	5.6 ± 1.8

SOURCE: from Kirsten et al.[25]

[a] Six-minute walking distance, results of the chronic respiratory disease questionnaire, clinical ratings of overall dyspnea and clinical scoring of symptoms and auscultation findings before and 2 days after withdrawal of theophylline. Values are mean ± standard deviation. † $p < .05$, compared with days 1 and 2; ‡ $p < .05$, compared with placebo group.

Abbreviations: BDI, baseline dyspnea index; CRQ, chronic respiratory disease questionnaire; MRC, Medical Research Council; OCD, oxygen cost diagram; TDI, transitional dyspnea index.

fatigued (hypoxic) diaphragm than under normal conditions.[59] This action leads to pronounced increases in maximal transdiaphragmatic or pleural pressure and in ventilatory endurance in COPD patients with marked hypoxia/hypercapnia,[29,65] while increases are insignificant in patients with mild hypoxia.[27,66] Hypoventilation in some COPD patients, which is thought to result from depressed central nervous system respiratory drive, also may be overcome by theophylline,[31] although the importance of this mechanism is not fully understood.

As stated in Chap. 50, theophylline decreases pulmonary arterial pressure and pulmonary vascular resistance as a result of pulmonary vasodilation and, partly, as a result of the positive inotropic action of the drug. Hypoxia in severe COPD is associated with reflex pulmonary vasoconstriction and increased pulmonary arterial resistance, and these symptoms have been shown to be diminished by oral (sustained-release) or intravenous theophylline in COPD patients without cor pulmonale, who have increased cardiac output, oxygen consumption, and oxygen saturation.[67] Patients with cor pulmonale—a possible complication of COPD—appear to receive much less hemodynamic benefit from theophylline. While improvements in pulmonary hemodynamics may account for some of the improvements in dyspnea and exercise tolerance, this remains to be confirmed; the lack of hemodynamic improvement in patients exhibiting cor pulmonale does not necessarily imply that no improvement in lung function or relief of dyspnea can be achieved with theophylline treatment.

Summary

Despite the reservations expressed in international therapy guidelines, theophylline is used worldwide in the treatment of asthma (in conjuction with an increased use of inhaled corticosteroids) and COPD. The reason for this broad acceptance may be that theophylline has a wide range of actions that serve the needs of both patient groups, and that practitioners are aware that many aspects of the diseases may not be understood by assessment of simple functional parameters. Despite the well-recognized problem of a narrow therapeutic window and the risk of side effects and toxicity, modern theophylline preparations—in conjunction with efficient drug monitoring—render the drug well-tolerated and safe in long-term treatment.

There is considerable evidence that theophylline provides a therapeutic benefit to patients with COPD if the treatment is individualized and clinically documented through therapy withdrawal under monitoring of the patient's physiological status. Theophylline also is a major component of some asthma therapy, and this is not likely to change in the foreseeable future. Several reports in the literature describe the effects of theophylline at serum concentrations less than 10 μg/ml, and 75 percent maximal bronchodilator effects have been demonstrated in asthmatic patients at 10 μg/ml, although these findings have not been confirmed in all subsequent investigations. At present, it seems speculative and uncertain whether recent findings regarding the immunomodulatory role of the drug, or the introduction of long-acting β_2-adrenoceptor agonists, will substantially influence the therapeutic role of theophylline in clinical practice.

References

1. Kossel A. Über das Theophyllin, einen neuen Bestandteil des Thees. *Z Physiol Chemie* 1889; 13:298.
2. Hirsch S. Klinischer und experimenteller Beitrag zur krampflösenden Wirkung der Purinderivate. *Klin Wochschr* 1922; 1:615.
3. Salter H. On some points in the treatment and clinical history of asthma. *Edinburgh Med J* 1859; 4:1109.
4. Persson CGA. Overview of effects of theophylline. *J Allergy Clin Immunol* 1986; 78:780.
5. Hendeles L, Weinberger M. Theophylline: a "state of the art" review. *Pharmacotherapy* 1983; 3:2.
6. Hermann G, Aynesworth MB. Successful treatment of persistent extreme dyspnea "status asthmaticus": use of theophylline diethylamine (aminophylline) intravenously. *J Lab Clin Med* 1937; 23:135.
7. Hendeles L, Amarshi N, Weinberger M. A clinical and pharmacokinetic basis for the selection and use of slow release theophylline products. *Clin Pharmacokinet* 1984; 9:95.
8. Götz J, Sauter R, Steinijans VW, Jonkman JHG. Steady-state pharmacokinetics of a once-daily theophylline formulation (Euphylong) when given twice daily. *Int J Clin Pharmacol Ther Toxicol* 1994; 32:168.
9. David-Wang AS, Scarth B, Freeman D, Chapman KR. A rapid monoclonal antibody blood theophylline assay: lack of cross-reactivity with enprofylline. *Ther Drug Monit* 1994; 16:323.
10. Steinijans VW, Schulz H-U, Beier W, Radtke HW. Once daily theophylline: multiple-dose comparison of an encapsulated micro-osmotic system (Euphylong) with a tablet (Uniphyllin). *Int J Clin Pharmacol Ther Toxicol* 1986; 24:438.
11. Steinijans VW, Trautmann H, Johnson E, Beier W. Theophylline steady-state pharmacokinetics: recent concepts and their application in chronotherapy of reactive airway diseases. *Chronobiol Int* 1987; 4:331.
12. Barnes PJ. New drugs for asthma. *Eur Respir J* 1992; 5:1126.
13. Barnes PJ, Pauwels R. Theophylline in the management of asthma: time for reappraisal? *Eur Respir J* 1994; 7:579.
14. British Thoracic Society. Guidelines on management of asthma. *Thorax* 1993; 48(suppl):S1.
15. National Heart, Lung and Blood Institute National Asthma Education Program Expert Panel. Guidelines for the diagnosis and management of asthma. *J Allergy Clin Immunol* 1991; 88:425.
16. International Asthma Project. International consensus report on diagnosis and management of asthma. *Eur Respir J* 1992; 5:601.
17. Hargreave FE, Dolovich J, Newhouse MT. The assessment and treatment of asthma: a conference report. *J Allergy Clin Immunol* 1990; 85:1098.
18. Fitzpatrick MF, Mackay T, Driver H, Douglas NJ. Salmeterol in nocturnal asthma: a double-blind, placebo-controlled trial of a long acting inhaled β_2-agonist. *Br Med J* 1990; 301:1365.
19. Rabe KF, Jörres R, Nowak D, Behr N, Magnussen H. Comparison of the effects of salmeterol and formoterol on airway tone and responsiveness over 24 hours in bronchial asthma. *Am Rev Respir Dis* 1993; 147:1436.
20. Lam A, Newhouse MT. Management of asthma and chronic airflow limitation: are methylxanthines obsolete? *Chest* 1990; 98:44.
21. McFadden ER Jr. Methylxanthines in the treatment of asthma: the rise, the fall, and the possible rise again. *Ann Intern Med* 1991; 115:323.

22. Matthay RA, Berger HJ, Loke J, Gottschalk A, Zaret BL. Effects of aminophylline upon right and left ventricular performance in chronic obstructive pulmonary disease. *Am J Med* 1978; 65:903.

23. Matthay RA, Berger HJ, Davies R, Loke J, Gottschalk A, Zaret BL. Improvement in cardiac performance by oral long-acting theophylline in chronic obstructive pulmonary disease. *Am Heart J* 1982; 104:1022.

24. Mahler DA, Matthay RA, Snyder PE, Wells CK, Loke J. Sustained-release theophylline reduces dyspnea in nonreversible obstructive airway disease. *Am Rev Respir Dis* 1985; 131:22.

25. Kirsten DK, Wegner RE, Jörres RA, Magnussen H. Effects of theophylline withdrawal in severe chronic obstructive pulmonary disease. *Chest* 1993; 104:1101.

26. Aubier M, De Troyer A, Sampson M, Macklem PT, Roussos C. Aminophylline improves diaphragmatic contractility. *N Engl J Med* 1981; 305:249.

27. Foxworth JW, Reisz GR, Knudson SM, Cuddy PG, Pyszcznski DR, Emory CE. Theophylline and diaphragmatic contractility. *Am Rev Respir Dis* 1988; 138:1532.

28. Moxham J, Miller J, Wiles CM, Morris AJR, Green M. The effect of aminophylline on the human diaphragm. *Thorax* 1985; 40:288.

29. Murciano D, Aubier M, Lecocguic Y, Pariente R. Effects of theophylline on diaphragmatic strength in patients with chronic obstructive pulmonary disease. *N Engl J Med* 1984; 311:349.

30. Brophy C, Mier A, Moxham J, Green M. The effect of aminophylline on respiratory and limb muscle contractility in man. *Eur Respir J* 1989; 2:652.

31. Aubier M, Murciano D, Fournier M, Milic-Emili J, Pariente R, Derenne JP. Central respiratory drive in acute respiratory failure of patients with chronic obstructive pulmonary disease. *Am Rev Respir Dis* 1980; 122:191.

32. Saunders JS, Berman TM, Bertlett MM, Kronenberg RS. Increased hypoxic ventilatory drive due to administration of aminophylline in normal men. *Chest* 1980; 78:279.

33. Eaton ML, MacDonald FM, Church TR, Niewoehner DE. Effects of theophylline on breathlessness and exercise tolerance in patients with chronic airflow obstruction. *Chest* 1982; 82:538.

34. Belman MJ, Sieck GC, Mazar A. Aminophylline and its influence on ventilatory endurance in humans. *Am Rev Respir Dis* 1985; 131:226.

35. Matthys H, Wastag E, Daikeler G, Kohler D. The influence of aminophylline and pindolol on the mucociliary clearance in patients with chronic bronchitis. *Br J Clin Pract* 1983; 23S:10.

36. Iravani J, Melville GN. Theophylline and mucociliary function. *Chest* 1987; 92:38S.

37. Pearson MG, Ahmad D, Chamberlain MJ, Morgan WKC, Vinitski S. Aminophylline and mucociliary clearance in patients with irreversible airflow limitation. *Br J Clin Pharmacol* 1985; 20:688.

38. Sutton PP, Pavia D, Bateman JRM, Clarke SW. The effect of oral aminophylline on lung mucociliary clearance in man. *Chest* 1981; 80:889S.

39. Aamodt T, Dahle R, Horgen O. Effects of withdrawal of sustained-release theophylline in patients with chronic obstructive lung disease. *Allergy* 1988; 43:411.

40. McWilliams BC, Menendez R, Kelly WH, Howick J. Effects of theophylline on inhaled methacholine and histamine in asthmatic children. *Am Rev Respir Dis* 1984; 130:193.

41. Cartier A, Lemire I, L'Archeveque J, Ghezzo H, Martin RR, Malo J-L. Theophylline partially inhibits bronchoconstriction caused by inhaled histamine in subjects with asthma. *J Allergy Clin Immunol* 1986; 77:570.

42. Magnussen H, Reuss G, Jörres R. Theophylline has a dose-related effect on the airway response to inhaled histamine and methacholine in asthmatics. *Am Rev Respir Dis* 1987; 136:1163.

43. Pollock J, Kiechel F, Cooper D, Weinberger M. Relationship of serum theophylline concentration to inhibition of exercise-induced bronchospasm and comparison with cromolyn. *Pediatrics* 1977; 60:840.

44. Magnussen H, Reuss G, Jörres R. Methylxanthines inhibit exercise-induced bronchoconstriction at low serum theophylline concentration and in a dose-dependent fashion. *J Allergy Clin Immunol* 1988; 81:531.

45. Pauwels R, van Renterghem D, van der Straeten M, Johannesson N, Persson CGA. The effect of theophylline and enprofylline on allergen-induced bronchoconstriction. *J Allergy Clin Immunol* 1985; 76:583.

46. Mapp C, Boschetto P, Dal Vecchio L, Crespoli S, de Marzo N, Paleari D, Fabbri LM. Protective effect of antiasthma drugs on late asthmatic reactions and increased airway responsiveness induced by toluene diisocyanate in sensitized subjects. *Am Rev Respir Dis* 1987; 136:1403.

47. Cockcroft DW, Murdock KY, Gore BP, O'Byrne PM, Manning P. Theophylline does not inhibit allergen-induced increase in airway responsiveness to methacholine. *J Allergy Clin Immunol* 1989; 83:913.

48. Ward AJM, McKenniff M, Evans JM, Page CP, Costello JF. Theophylline—an immunomodulatory role in asthma? *Am Rev Respir Dis* 1993; 147:518.

49. Crescioli S, Spinnazzi A, Plebani M, Pozzani M, Mapp CE, Boschetto P, Fabbri LM. Theophylline inhibits early and late asthmatic reactions induced by allergens in asthmatic subjects. *Ann Allergy* 1991; 66:245.

50. Dutoit JI, Salome CM, Woolcock AJ. Inhaled corticosteroids reduce the severity of bronchial hyperresponsiveness in asthma but oral theophylline does not. *Am Rev Respir Dis* 1987; 136:1174.

51. Jenne JW. Physiology and pharmacology of the xanthines. In: Jenne JW, Murphy S, editors. *Drug therapy for asthma: research and clinical practice.* (Lung Biology in Health and Disease, vol 31.) New York: Marcel Dekker, 1987: 297–334.

52. Siegel D, Sheppard D, Gelb A, Weinberg PF. Aminophylline increases the toxicity but not the efficacy of an inhaled β-adrenergic agonist in the treatment of acute exacerbations of asthma. *Am Rev Respir Dis* 1985; 132:283.

53. Hambleton G, Weinberger M, Taylor J, Cavanaugh M, Ginchansky E, Godfrey S, Tooley M, Bell T, Greenberg S. Comparison of cromoglycate (cromolyn) and theophylline in controlling symptoms of chronic asthma: a collaborative study. *Lancet* 1977; i:381.

54. Nassif EG, Weinberger M, Thompson R, Huntley W. The value of maintenance theophylline in steroid-dependent asthma. *N Engl J Med* 1981; 304:71.

55. Brenner M, Berkowitz R, Marshall N, Strunk RC. Need for theophylline in severe steroid-requiring asthmatics. *Clin Allergy* 1988; 18:143.

56. Busse WW. Pathogenesis and pathophysiology of nocturnal asthma. *Am J Med* 1988; 85(suppl. 1B):24.

57. Barnes PJ, Greening AP, Neville L, Timmers J, Poole GW. Single dose slow-release aminophylline at night prevents nocturnal asthma. *Lancet* 1982; i:299.

58. Heins M, Kurtin L, Oellerich M, Maes R, Sybrecht GW. Nocturnal asthma: slow-release terbutaline versus slow-release theophylline therapy. *Eur Respir J* 1988; 1:306.

59. Vaz Fragoso CA, Miller MA. Review of the clinical efficacy of theophylline in the treatment of chronic obstructive pulmonary disease. *Am Rev Respir Dis* 1993; 147:S40.

60. Dullinger D, Kronenberg R, Niewoehner DE. Efficacy of inhaled metaproterenol and orally-administered theophylline in patients with chronic airflow obstruction. *Chest* 1986; 89:171.

61. Thomas P, Pugsley JA, Stewart JH. Theophylline and salbutamol improve pulmonary function in patients with irreversible chronic obstructive pulmonary disease. *Chest* 1992; 101:160.

62. Wegner RE, Jörres RA, Kirsten DK, Magnussen H. Factor analy-

sis of exercise capacity, dyspnoea ratings and lung function in patients with severe COPD. *Eur Respir J* 1994; 7:725.

63. Guyatt GH, Townsend M, Pugsley SO, Keller JL, Short HD, Taylor DW, Newhouse MT. Bronchodilators in chronic air-flow limitation. *Am Rev Respir Dis* 1987; 135:1069.

64. Chrystyn H, Mulley BA, Peake MD. Dose response relation to oral theophylline in severe chronic obstructive airways disease. *Br Med J* 1988; 297:1506.

65. Murciano D, Auclair M-H, Pariente R, Aubier M. A randomized, controlled trial of theophylline in patients with severe chronic obstructive pulmonary disease. *N Engl J Med* 1989; 320:1521.

66. Kongragunta VR, Druz WS, Sharp JT. Dyspnea and diaphragmatic fatigue in patients with chronic obstructive pulmonary disease. *Am Rev Respir Dis* 1988; 137:662.

67. Parker JO, Ashekian PB, Di Giorgi S, West RO. Hemodynamic effects of aminophylline in chronic obstructive pulmonary disease. *Circulation* 1967; 35:365.

ANTICHOLINERGIC AGENTS

Chapter 52
MODE OF ACTION
NICHOLAS J. GROSS

Anatomy of the Cholinergic Parasympathetic System

Tonic and Phasic Activity of the Cholinergic System

Muscarinic Receptor Subtypes

Muscarinic Receptors in Lungs

Muscarinic Receptor Subtype Damage in Airway Diseases

Actions of Anticholinergic Agents

Cholinergic mechanisms account for a substantial proportion of airway tone or narrowing in normal and abnormal airways. They are also responsible, to a substantial degree, for phasic increases in airway resistance in response to various stimuli. The simplest statement of the mode of action of anticholinergic agents, therefore, is that they counteract these tonic and phasic actions of the cholinergic branch of the autonomic nervous system.

Anatomy of the Cholinergic Parasympathetic System

Efferent nerves of the cholinergic parasympathetic system arise in the vagal nuclei in the brainstem and travel through the vagus nerve to the lungs, entering at the hila and branching with the airways (Fig. 52-1).[1] These (preganglionic) fibers terminate in the peribronchial ganglia on the cell bodies of the postganglionic nerves of the parasympathetic system (see also Chap. 6). From these ganglia, short fibers of the postganglionic nerves travel to airway smooth muscle and submucosal glands, supplying these structures with a mediator, acetylcholine, not from typical neuromuscular junctions but rather from varicosities along the postganglionic axon. Release of acetylcholine results in immediate contraction of smooth muscle, bronchoconstriction, and release of mucus from submucosal glands via muscarinic acetylcholine receptors on these structures. Physiologic evidence suggests that mucosal ciliary activity is also cholinergically stimulated; however, parasympathetic neural innervation of ciliated epithelial cells has not been convincingly demonstrated.

Peribronchial ganglia and muscarinic receptors are concentrated in the larger, central airways and are sparse in smaller, peripheral airways.[1-3] Physiologic studies also suggest that anticholinergic agents preferentially dilate the central airways, in contrast to other bronchodilators,[4] findings that suggest that the cholinergic system acts preferentially on central airways.

Because there are important interactions between the vagal parasympathetic system and other branches of the autonomic system that oppose the cholinergic system, the latter also will be described in outline here. A more complete description is provided in Chap. 54.

FIGURE 52-1 Diagrammatic representation of vagal afferent and efferent pathways.

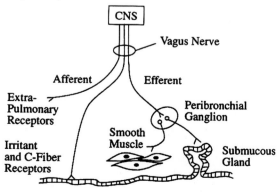

Branches of the adrenergic arm of the autonomic nervous system also enter the lung through the hila and travel along the airways but are very sparse in humans in comparison with parasympathetic nerves.[1] Neither α- nor β-adrenergic endings are found in proximity with smooth-muscle cells. Instead, β-adrenergic terminals are found on the bodies of the parasympathetic postganglionic cells in the peribronchial ganglia, where they are believed to inhibit transmission of cholinergic drive through the parasympathetic system. In addition, β-adrenergic receptors are present on bronchial smooth-muscle cells and can presumably respond to circulating catecholamines as well as exogenous β-adrenergic agents. Beta-adrenergic activation thus could result in smooth-muscle relaxation either by inhibiting ongoing cholinergic traffic at the cholinergic postganglionic cell or by stimulating β-adrenergic receptors on airway smooth muscle. Beta-adrenergic receptors on airway structures are found throughout the airways, suggesting bronchodilator action on small as well as large airways.[3]

An additional autonomic arm is known, by analogy with the gastrointestinal tract, as the third nervous system, or nonadrenergic, noncholinergic (NANC) system.[5] Its action, like that of the sympathetic nervous system, is bronchodilatory and is felt to be the principal physiologic opposition to parasympathetic bronchoconstriction. The anatomy of this system in the respiratory tract still is obscure; its pre- and postganglionic fibers may be shared with the parasympathetic system as its mediators, vasoactive intestinal peptide (VIP), peptide histidine methionine (PHM), and possibly other peptides, appear to be located in secretory vesicles in the varicosities of the parasympathetic postganglionic fibers and released along with acetylcholine. Nitric oxide is released from the same sites, but whether it is the principal mediator of the NANC system,[6] or whether its generation is stimulated by VIP[7] is unclear.

Tonic and Phasic Activity of the Cholinergic System

Tonic activity of the parasympathetic system provides a continuous low level of release of acetylcholine, which is the main component of bronchomotor tone, from postganglionic fibers. This tone may be altered in disease states.[8] In addition, cholinergic activity may be increased acutely by neural reflexes. Irritant and C-fiber receptors in the airways and elsewhere can be activated by a wide variety of stimuli—mechanical stimulation, irritant aerosols, some inflammatory mediators, allergens, and cold, dry air.[9] Activation of these receptors results in afferent and efferent vagal traffic and rapid bronchoconstriction that can be blocked by vagal transection, vagal cooling, ganglion blocking agents, or anticholinergic agents such as atropine. Acetylcholine release can be detected following the above stimuli. The evidence for vagal reflex bronchoconstriction is thus strong, at least in animals. However, it is thought to be responsible for only a portion of the bronchoconstriction in clinical airway obstruction, as anticholinergic agents rarely reverse the obstruction completely in humans.[9]

Muscarinic Receptor Subtypes

Atropine and related agents are anticholinergic by virtue of the fact that they compete with the cholinergic agonist, acetylcholine, for the ligand-binding site of muscarinic receptors. In this chapter, current notions of this area will be presented in summary; for a more detailed account, see Chap. 7. Five muscarinic receptor subtypes, M_1 to M_5, have been revealed by molecular cloning techniques.[10] Sequence analysis shows them to belong to the superfamily of plasma membrane receptors whose intracellular actions are transduced through coupling to G proteins. (Beta-adrenergic receptors and rhodopsin are some of the other numerous members; see also Chap. 1.) In common with other receptors of this superfamily, they consist of a single polypeptide, of approximately 550 to 600 amino acid residues, that contains 7 membrane-spanning helices that separate 4 extracellular and 4 intra-cellular domains. The membrane-spanning domains are thought to be arranged in a ringlike pocket, or pore, that contains the agonist-binding site. The sequence of transmembrane domains is distinct for muscarinic receptor proteins and highly conserved among them, presumably conferring specificity for the acetylcholine ligand. In contrast to other members of the superfamily, all muscarinic receptors also contain a large third cytoplasmic loop, but its sequence is different for each muscarinic subtype, presumably conferring specificity for their intracellular actions. Ligand-receptor binding is presumed to result in conformational changes in the intracellular domain(s) that result in intracellular events. These events are mediated through G proteins, the form of the response being determined by the type of G protein(s) with which it is able to interact.

Cloning and expression of receptor subtypes into *Xenopus* oocytes and mammalian cells have revealed two generic types of response (presumably others will be revealed by further studies). Activation of M_1, M_3, or M_5 receptors is coupled via G_p/G_{11} proteins and phospholipase C to hydrolysis of phosphoinositide 4,5 biphosphate (PIP_2) to inositol 1,4,5 triphosphate (IP_3), which promotes the release of calcium ions from intracellular stores and, hence, smooth-muscle contraction. Activation of M_2 or M_4 receptors is coupled via G_i/G_0 proteins to inhibition of adenylyl cyclase. This has the effect of inhibiting the conversion of ATP to cyclic AMP, thus counteracting the bronchodilator effect of endogenous or pharmacologic β-adrenergic agonists, which promote the formation of cyclic AMP.

Muscarinic Receptors in Lungs

Molecular techniques have revealed the presence of three muscarinic receptor subtypes in airway structures: M_1, M_2, and M_3. These, together with physiologic studies using more-or-less selective muscarinic subtype inhibitors, have yielded a picture of the muscarinic system of the airways (Fig. 52-2).[11] M_1-receptors are found in the peribronchial ganglia, where their function is unknown. It is speculated that they amplify vagal cholinergic drive in a collateral manner to adjacent postganglionic cells of the cholinergic system.

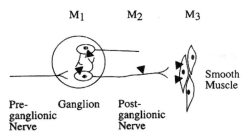

FIGURE 52-2 Scheme of muscarinic receptor subtypes (filled triangles) in the airways. The precise location of M_1 receptors within the peribronchial ganglion is speculative.

M_2-receptors are present on postganglionic prejunctional nerves, where they appear to be "autoreceptors" that respond to local acetylcholine concentration by inhibiting further acetylcholine release from the varicosities and terminals of these nerves (feedback inhibition). M_3-receptors are present on smooth muscle and mucous glands. Their activation results in contraction of smooth muscle and release of mucus. According to this scheme, activation of M_1- and M_3-receptors would promote airway obstruction, whereas activation of M_2-receptors would modulate airway obstruction.

Muscarinic Receptor Subtype Damage in Airway Diseases

From the above picture, any process that selectively inactivated M_2-receptors would tend to promote airway obstruction both by contraction of smooth muscle and by mucus release. Recently, it has been shown that parainfluenza virus may damage M_2 autoreceptors selectively,[12,13] which would provide an explanation for the transient bronchoconstriction associated with acute respiratory infections commonly seen in children. M_2-receptors also may be damaged selectively by major basic protein of eosinophils or reactive oxygen species released by allergic responses.[14] A fuller elucidation of the function of muscarinic receptor subtypes in the airways in health and disease is needed.

Actions of Anticholinergic Drugs

All anticholinergic agents presently available for clinical use are nonselective with regard to muscarinic receptor subtype. They inhibit both the receptor subtype that limits airway obstruction (M_2) as well as those that promote it (M_1 and M_3). Their overall action on airway function can be seen as a summation of these opposing effects, which is both a disadvantage of current therapies and a potential direction for the development of future therapies. An anticholinergic agent that selectively inhibited M_1- and M_3-muscarinic subtypes

and that stimulated the M_2-subtype would seem to be ideal for the treatment of obstructive airway diseases. An analogy for this concept exists in the adrenergic nervous system, where treatment of hypertension by a nonselective α-adrenergic antagonist (e.g., phentolamine) is much less effective in controlling blood pressure than a selective α_1-adrenergic antagonist (e.g., prazosin). The development of anticholinergic agents with selective actions on muscarinic receptor subtypes is underway, and some promising agents have been synthesized.[15]

References

1. Richardson JB: Nerve supply to the lungs. *Am Rev Respir Dis* 1979; 119:785.
2. Barnes PJ: Cholinergic control of airway smooth muscle. *Am Rev Respir Dis* 1987; 136:542.
3. Barnes PJ, Basbaum CB, Nadel JA: Autoradiographic localization of autonomic receptors in airway smooth muscle: Marked differences between large and small airways. *Am Rev Respir Dis* 1983; 127:758.
4. Ingram RH, Wellman JJ, McFadden ER, Mead J: Relative contribution of large and small airways to flow limitation in normal subjects before and after atropine and isoproterenol. *J Clin Invest* 1977; 59:696.
5. Barnes PJ: The third nervous system in the lungs: Physiology and clinical perspectives. *Thorax* 1984; 39:561.
6. Ward JK, Belvisi MG, Fox AJ, et al.: Modulation of cholinergic neural bronchoconstriction by endogenous nitric oxide and vasoactive intestinal peptide in human airways in vitro. *J Clin Invest* 1993; 92:736.
7. Lilly CM, Stamler JS, Gaston B, et al.: Modulation of vasoactive intestinal peptide pulmonary relaxation by NO in tracheally perfused guinea pig lungs. *Am J Physiol* 1993; 265:L410.
8. Gross NJ, Co E, Skorodin MS: Cholinergic bronchomotor tone in COPD: Estimates of its amount in comparison to normal. *Chest* 1989; 96:984.
9. Gross NJ: Cholinergic control, in Barnes PJ, Rodger IW, Thomson NC (eds): *Asthma: Basic Mechanisms and Clinical Management.* London, Academic Press, 1988; p 381.
10. Wess J: Molecular basis of muscarinic acetylcholine receptor function. *Trends Pharmacol Sci* 1993; 141:308.
11. Gross NJ, Barnes PJ: A short tour around the muscarinic receptor. *Am Rev Respir Dis* 1988; 138:765.
12. Fryer AD, Fakahany EE, Jacoby DB: Parainfluenza virus type I reduces the affinity of agonists for muscarinic receptors in guinea-pig lung and heart. *Eur J Pharmacol* 1990; 181:51.
13. Fryer AD, Jacoby DB: Parainfluenza virus infection damages inhibitory M_2-muscarinic receptors on pulmonary parasympathetic nerves in the guinea pig. *Br J Pharmacol* 1991; 102:267.
14. Jacoby DB, Gleich GJ, Fryer AD: Human eosinophil major basic protein is an endogenous allosteric antagonist at the inhibitory muscarinic M_2 receptor. *Am Rev Respir Dis* 1992; 145:A436.
15. Cereda E, Ezhaya A, Bellora E, et al.: New pyrrolidin-, piperidin- and azepin-2-oxocarboxylic acid esters are preferential M_1, M_3 muscarinic antagonists. *Eur J Med Chem* 1994; 29:411.

CLINICAL APPLICATION

NICHOLAS J. GROSS

Available Agents

Atropine is a naturally occurring alkaloid found in many plants, particularly of the *Datura* genus. In former times, the leaves and other parts of the plant were smoked or made into fuming powders. Atropine base as extracted and purified from these sources exists in two isomeric forms in approximately equal amounts, only one of which is physiologically active in humans. As the base is relatively insoluble, the sulfate is the form used in clinical practice. Several closely related alkaloids with very similar actions are also found in plants—scopolamine and hyoscine. All naturally occurring agents of this class are tertiary ammonium compounds, by reference to the 3-valent nitrogen atom in the tropane ring (Fig. 53-1). They are freely absorbed from mucosal surfaces and widely distributed throughout the body, including the brain. This drawback has led to the development of quaternary ammonium congeners in which the nitrogen atom is 5-valent. All are synthetic, some resemble atropine closely, others are quite different. They are relatively poorly absorbed.

Ipratropium bromide is the only quaternary agent of this class currently approved for respiratory use in the United States.[1] It is available in metered-dose inhaler (MDI) and as a solution for nebulization. The current MDI contains a suspension of the drug in vehicle with propellants. A newer powder formulation that contains no freon propellants is under development in the United States and is available in some other countries. Oxitropium bromide is quite similar structurally to ipratropium. In vitro studies suggest it is more potent and longer-lasting in effect. An MDI formulation has been studied in the United States[2] and is available in Europe. Several other closely related agents are under development (e.g., flutropium, tiotropium, and atropine methylnitrate). In addition, some quaternary alkaloids that do not resemble the atropine/scopolamine compounds structurally, but which possess anticholinergic properties, also have been studied for their respiratory uses (e.g., glycopyrrolate and thiazinamium). Glycopyrrolate was developed many years ago as a gastric spasmolytic agent and is consequently available for general use in the United States; however, it has not been approved for respiratory use. Some of these agents possess antihistaminic and antiallergic properties.

Pharmacologic Considerations

PHARMACOKINETICS AND PHARMACODYNAMICS

The pharmacologic properties of atropine and related tertiary ammonium compounds have been well-studied and are fully described in standard texts.[3] In brief, atropine relaxes smooth muscle in the gastrointestinal and biliary tracts, the airways, the iris, and the peripheral vasculature, and decreases the tone of the bladder and urethra. On the heart, small doses cause mild bradycardia, but doses in the usual therapeutic range cause a dose-dependent increase in heart rate. Atropine also reduces the rate of apocrine and salivary secretions and inhibits mucociliary clearance in the respiratory tract. Atropine crosses the blood-brain barrier and causes mild central stimulation in usual doses. At higher doses, it can cause excitement, disorientation, hallucinations

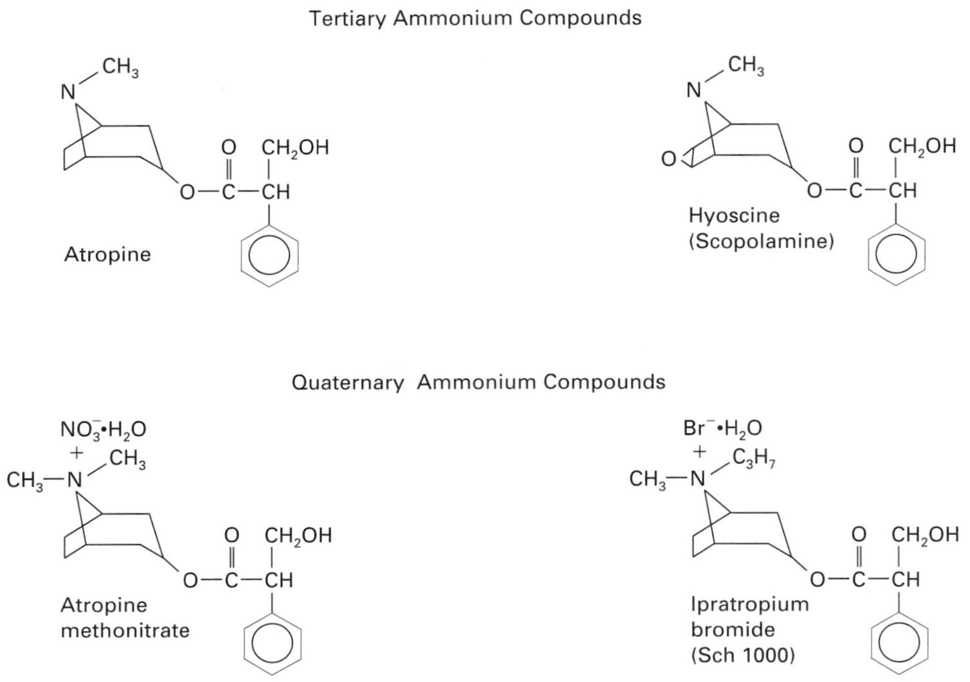

Tertiary Ammonium Compounds

Atropine

Hyoscine
(Scopolamine)

Quaternary Ammonium Compounds

Atropine
methonitrate

Ipratropium
bromide
(Sch 1000)

FIGURE 53-1 Structures of some anticholinergic bronchodilators. (*Reprinted with permission from Am Rev Respir Dis 1984; 129:856.*)

and coma (see Chap. 54). As atropine is well absorbed from mucosal surfaces, the above effects are seen following oral or inhalational administration, as well as parenteral administration.

In contrast, ipratropium, because of poor absorption, only acts locally. When delivered to the eye, for example, it dilates the pupil, but is not significantly absorbed. When delivered to the respiratory tract, it results in bronchodilatation, but blood concentrations are too low to measure even following large doses. Thus, in common with other quaternary agents, it has functional selectivity solely due to this property. If injected intravenously (for experimental purposes only), it causes most of the systemic effects of atropine; however, even by this route CNS effects are absent because of the blood-brain barrier.

The half-life of atropine in the circulation is about 3 h; that for ipratropium is similar. However, the effect of ipratropium following inhalation is longer than that of atropine by 1 to 2 h, presumably because ipratropium is not removed from the respiratory tract by absorption. The duration of effect of oxitropium is longer by a few hours, and those of glycopyrrolate and tiotropium may be as long as 12 h or more.

DOSE RESPONSE

The recommended dose of atropine for respiratory use is 0.015 to 0.04 mg/kg; namely, 1.0 to 2.5 mg for adults. At

these doses, mild anticholinergic effects are common. At only slightly higher doses, more severe side effects are seen.

Dose-response studies of ipratropium by MDI suggest maximal effect following 40 to 80 µg.[4-8] However, it is likely that even the higher dose is suboptimal in patients with severe airways disease as the penetration of particles into the lower respiratory tract is impaired by airways obstruction.[9,10] One study in patients with moderate chronic obstructive pulmonary disease (COPD) suggest that optimal effect may require 160 µg by MDI.[11] The currently recommended dose of ipratropium by MDI in the United States is 36 µg (two puffs) up to every 6 h, which is probably suboptimal in most patients. In other countries, a double-strength form is available. A 6 month study (uncontrolled) in which the dose of ipratropium was quadrupled showed that this dose was effective and safe.[12] The optimal dose of oxitropium by MDI in patients with COPD is 100 to 200 µg.[2]

Dose-response studies of ipratropium nebulized solution vary widely, presumably reflecting the differences among studies in patient population and nebulizer technique, to which responses are highly sensitive. The optimal dose has been variously reported to be between 50 to 125 µg[8,13] and 400 µg.[11] Again, patients with more severe airways appear to require higher doses. The currently recommended dose is 500 µg.

Tolerance (subsensitivity or tachyphylaxis) to anticholinergic agents has not been found, with one exception.[14] This is in keeping with the general rule that antagonists do not down-regulate the target receptor, and may indeed up-regulate it,[15] as has been found to be the case in one study using ipratropium.[16]

Clinical Efficacy

EFFICACY AGAINST STIMULATED BRONCHOCONSTRICTION

Numerous studies have examined the ability of an anticholinergic agent to protect against the effects of a variety of bronchospastic stimuli in the laboratory.[17] The results of some of these studies are summarized in Table 53-1. As expected, anticholinergic agents are very effective in preventing bronchoconstriction caused by inhalation of cholinergic agents such as methacholine, acetylcholine, or carbachol. They were less effective against the inhalation of inflammatory mediators such as histamine, bradykinin, prostaglandin F_{2a}, serotonin, or leukotrienes. Their protective effect against nonspecific irritants such as sulfur dioxide, ozone, nebulized distilled water or dilute citric acid, carbon dust, or cigarette smoke varies from more-or-less complete protection in normal subjects to partial protection at best in subjects with airways disease. Against allergen-induced bronchoconstriction, some protection is often seen, but this is never complete, presumably indicating that such bronchoconstriction is mediated to only a minor extent by vagal reflexes.

Against the bronchoconstriction induced in many asthmatics by the inhalation of cold, dry air or by exercise, anticholinergic agents are only poorly protective. Alternative agents such as β-adrenergic agonists or cromolyn-like drugs are more effective. Protection against nocturnal bronchospasm varies greatly among subjects and is only partial.[18,19] Thus for many of the stimuli that are thought to be important causes of bronchospastic attacks, anticholinergic agents provide only partial and inconsistent protection.

However, there are two situations in which clinically important bronchospastic stimuli may be more effectively treated with an anticholinergic agent than with alternative therapy. These are bronchospasm induced by psychogenic stimuli and by β2-adrenergic blockade. Subjects whose asthma was believed to be psychogenic in origin responded better to ipratropium than subjects whose asthma was not considered to be psychogenic.[20] In two controlled studies, bronchospasm induced by the suggestion to the subjects that they were inhaling an agent to which they were allergic was blocked effectively by an anticholinergic agent.[21,22] β2-adrenergic blocking agents can precipitate acute bronchospasm in asthmatics, presumably by inhibiting adrenergic opposition to cholinergic tone. When these agents have been used inadvertently, treatment of the resulting attack with an adrenergic bronchodilator is ineffective because the β2-adrenergic receptors are blocked. Anticholinergic agents can not only prevent such bronchospasm, but can reverse it once it has occurred.[23,24]

EFFICACY IN STABLE ASTHMA

There is a very large number of short- and long-term studies that have compared the efficacy of an anticholinergic agent with an alternative bronchodilator in patients with stable asthma. These have been reviewed in more detail elsewhere.[1,25–27] As the findings are quite consistent, they are presented in summary form. The typical short-term response of stable asthmatic patients to an anticholinergic agent is shown in Fig. 53-2. The onset of bronchodilatation occurs within minutes but proceeds more slowly than following an adrenergic agent; peak bronchodilatation occurs typically 1 to 2 h after inhalation rather than 10 to 30 min after an adrenergic agent. At peak, the increase in airflow is significantly less than that achieved with an adrenergic bronchodilator. The duration of action varies with the agents, and ipratropium is not noticeably different from conventional β-

TABLE 53-1   Summary of Efficacy of Anticholinergic Agents Against Specific Bronchospastic Stimuli

Stimulus	Efficacy of Anticholinergic Agents	Efficacy of Adrenergic Agents Relative to Anticholinergic Agents
Cholinergic agents	Fully protective	Less effective
Histamine	Partially protective	More effective
Mediators, $PGF_{2\alpha}$, serotonin	Partially protective	More effective
β-Blockade	Protective	Ineffective
Gases, dusts, irritants	Usually protective	—
Antigens	Variable	More effective
Exercise, hyperventilation	Modestly protective	More effective
Psychogenic factors	Good protection	Less effective

SOURCE: *Reprinted with permission from Am Rev Respir Dis* 1984; 129:856.

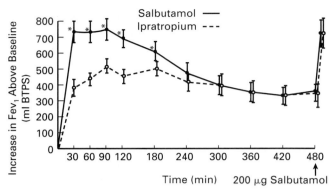

FIGURE 53-2 Increase in FEV$_1$ in 25 asthmatic patients following inhalation of 200 μg albuterol by metered-dose inhaler (MDI) or 40 μg ipratropium by MDI on separate days. All patients received an additional dose of albuterol at the end of the study. Asterisks denote significant difference between agents ($p < .05$). (Reprinted with permission from J Allergy Clin Immunol 1982; 69:60.)

adrenergic agents in this population. However, there is considerable variation among subjects; some respond almost as well to the anticholinergic agent as to the β-adrenergic; others respond very poorly.

Attempts to identify subgroups of asthmatics who respond better to anticholinergic agents have not been very successful. It has been suggested that asthmatics age > 40 y may respond better than younger ones,[28] although there are reports of children who responded well.[29] Intrinsic asthmatics and those with longer duration of asthma may respond better.[30] Again, these findings are statistical and do not identify responders. At present, an individual trial remains the only way to identify responders.[31]

For the above reasons, anticholinergic agents are not regarded as first-line treatment for chronic stable asthma. In very mild asthmatics, who are troubled by the side effects of an adrenergic agent, they may suffice, and in very severe asthma that is already being treated with all alternative therapy, they may provide an increment of bronchodilatation that will enable the patient to function better. No anticholinergic agents currently are approved by the Food and Drug Administration of the United States for treatment of asthma.

EFFICACY IN ACUTE SEVERE ASTHMA

In the United States and a number of other countries, β-adrenergic bronchodilator in repeated and sufficient dosage is the standard of care for this life-threatening condition. However, several studies have examined the role of nebulized ipratropium either alone or in combination with a β-adrenergic agent in acute severe asthma.[32] Many of these studies present problems with interpretation, because they included insufficient numbers of subjects to ensure adequate statistical power. Two studies overcome these problems—a large multicenter study by Rebuck and colleagues that includes sufficient patients,[33] and a meta-analysis by Ward of nine published studies.[32]

Rebuck and colleagues randomized 148 patients with

acute severe asthma to receive either 0.5 mg of ipratropium, 1.25 mg fenoterol, or the combination of both treatments by nebulization as the sole initial bronchodilator treatment for 90 min.[33] Fenoterol, a β$_2$-selective adrenergic agent, caused significantly greater bronchodilatation than ipratropium. The combination of fenoterol and ipratropium was significantly more effective than either drug alone (Fig. 53-3).

Ward performed meta-analysis of seven studies that compared ipratropium alone with a β$_2$-adrenergic agonist alone in acute severe asthma and showed that the β$_2$-adrenergic agonist caused significantly greater bronchodilatation.[32] He performed a similar meta-analysis for the effect of a β$_2$-adrenergic agonist alone versus a β$_2$-agonist plus ipratropium. This showed a greater and more significant benefit from the combination than from a β$_2$-adrenergic agonist alone (Fig. 53-4).

These results suggest that an anticholinergic agent used alone is not as effective as a β$_2$-adrenergic agonist in acute severe asthma, but that the addition of the anticholinergic agent ipratropium adds significantly to the bronchodilatation achieved by a β$_2$-adrenergic agonist alone in the immediate management of acute severe (status) asthma.

EFFICACY IN STABLE COPD

Several hundred published studies have compared the short- and long-term effects of anticholinergics with alternative bronchodilators in patients with COPD.[1,25] Although patients with COPD rarely exhibit as much improvement of airways obstruction with a bronchodilator as do those subjects with asthma, most are capable of some bronchodilation.[34] With few exceptions, studies show that an anticholinergic agent provides improvement in airflow that is as great and as prolonged as that due to any other agent.

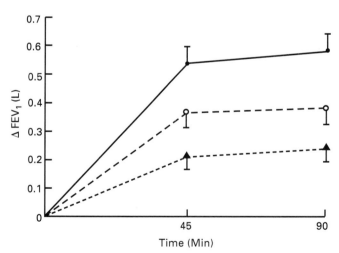

FIGURE 53-3 Bronchodilator treatment of acute severe asthma in 148 patients. Patients received either ipratropium 0.5 mg, or fenoterol 1.25 mg, or the combination by wet nebulization as the sole initial bronchodilator. Bars are ± SE. Differences between treatments were significant, $p < .05$. (Reprinted with permission from Am J Med 1987; 82:59–64.)

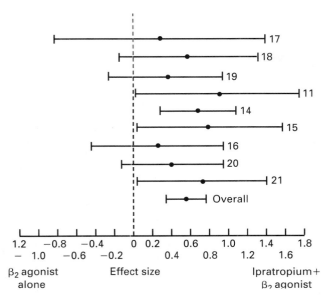

FIGURE 53-4 Meta-analysis of nine studies comparing the effect of a β₂-adrenergic agonist alone with that of a β₂-agonist plus ipratropium in acute severe asthma. Bars show 95 percent confidence limits. The pooled result, "overall," is shown. Numbers adjacent to bars refer to individual studies in the original publication. (*Reprinted with permission from Ward MJ: in Anticholinergic Therapy in Obstructive Airways Disease. Franklin Scientific Publications, London*).

Figure 53-5 provides an example.[35] As in asthma, the time to peak effect is longer, 30 to 120 min, but at peak the effect is significantly greater than that following an adrenergic agent. The duration of action also is longer by 1 to 2 h.

Most such studies compare recommended doses of each class of agent which, as stated above, may not be optimal doses. In studies that have employed cumulative dosing to reach optimal bronchodilatation, the anticholinergic agent has generally been found to cause maximal obtainable bron-

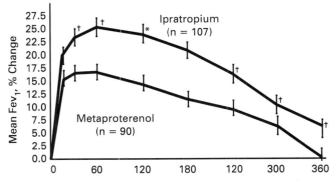

FIGURE 53-5 Bronchodilator response in stable COPD. Patients received 36 μg ipratropium or 1.5 mg metaproterenol by metered-dose inhaler (MDI). Symbols denote significant differences between treatments. (*Reprinted with permission from Am J Med 1985; 81(suppl 5A):81–86.*)

chodilatation in patients with COPD, whereas that caused by use of a β-adrenergic agent could be augmented by subsequent anticholinergic use.[36]

In confirming that the response to anticholinergic and β-adrenergic agents is different in asthma and COPD, a few studies have examined the responses to these two classes of agents in patients with either asthma or COPD.[37,38] All show a consistent pattern. An example is shown in Fig. 53-6; asthmatic patients responded better to a β-adrenergic agent than to an anticholinergic agent, but patients with COPD responded better to the anticholinergic agent. There appears to be, therefore, a qualitative difference in the response to bronchodilator class that is related to the diagnosis; patients with asthma respond better to adrenergic agents while patients with COPD respond better to an anticholinergic agent. This difference may be due to the fact that airways obstruction in asthma has many mechanisms, including all those due to airways inflammation, resulting in mucosal edema and inflammatory exudates in the airways lumen that are not amenable to anticholinergic activity, while the obstructive mechanisms in COPD are largely due to structural damage to airway walls and tethering of small airways.[36] Consequently, abrogation of cholinergic activity has a relatively minor effect on airways caliber in asthma while the reversal of cholinergic tone may be the only means of increasing airflow in COPD. Anticholinergic agents thus achieve all the available bronchodilatation in COPD, unlike in asthma.

EFFICACY IN ACUTE EXACERBATIONS OF COPD

A number of studies have compared the effects of anticholinergics with β-adrenergic agonists in acute exacerbations of COPD.[39–42] In summary, patients with acute exacerbations of COPD tended to be less responsive to any bronchodilator; an anticholinergic bronchodilator alone was as effective as a β-adrenergic bronchodilator alone or as a methylxanthine alone; combinations of bronchodilators did not substantially augment the bronchodilatation achieved by a single agent. Thus, present evidence suggests that the choice of bronchodilator has little effect on the improvement in airflow during the initial treatment of acute COPD. However, an anticholinergic agent has no tendency to produce hypoxemia as is sometimes seen with β-adrenergic agents,[41,43] and other side effects are less.

EFFICACY IN PEDIATRIC USE

The dose-response to ipratropium solution in children has been studied.[44,45] Doses of 100 to 250 μg were considered to be optimal; namely, about one-half the adult dose. However, the authors point out that the dose-response relationship is not strong, and these doses were well-tolerated.

The efficacy of ipratropium in the treatment of acute severe asthma was studied in two trials in Toronto, Canada.[46,47] In view of the results of similar trials in adults that tended to show that an anticholinergic alone was not as effective as a β-adrenergic agent alone (above), the pediatric trials concentrated on the question of whether the addition

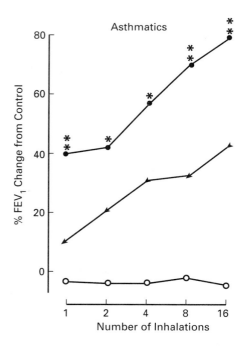

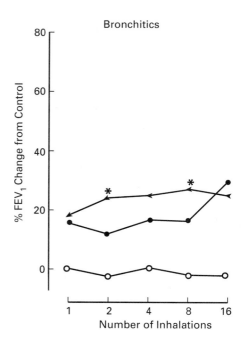

FIGURE 53-6 Response of six patients with asthma and six patients with chronic bronchitis to cumulative inhalations of fenoterol (200 μg per inhalation, squares) versus ipratropium (20 μg per inhalation, triangles), versus placebo. Baseline FEV_1 values were comparable in the two groups. Significant differences between active agents are indicated by a single asterisk ($p < .05$) or double asterisk ($p < .01$). (*Reprinted with permission from Br J Clin Pharmacol 1978; 6:547–49.*)

of ipratropium to a β-adrenergic agent significantly augmented the magnitude of bronchodilatation. The studies included patients aged 5 to 15 years whose presenting FEV_1 was < 50 percent of predicted. In the first study,[46] all subjects received nebulized salbutamol inhalations every 20 min for 2 h. At 1 h, one-half of the subjects received nebulized ipratropium in addition to salbutamol, and the other one-half received placebo in addition to salbutamol. While the responses of the two groups were identical during the first hour, the group that received ipratropium experienced significant further bronchodilatation during the second hour. In the second Toronto study,[47] a similar protocol was used except that the ipratropium group received nebulized ipratropium at onset and every 40 min in addition to salbutamol treatments, while the control group received placebo plus salbutamol. The group that received ipratropium experienced significantly greater bronchodilatation at all times from 20 to 150 min after the initial treatment. These results, therefore, support the notion that the addition of ipratropium to a β-adrenergic agent improves the response of children with acute severe asthma. However, two other studies found no benefit from the addition of ipratropium.[48,49]

Ipratropium by MDI has been used to treat chronic childhood asthma in several studies.[50–52] Again the protocol usually has compared an adrenergic agent alone with a β-adrenergic agent plus ipratropium. In summary, these trials have shown only moderate benefit at most from the addition of ipratropium. A consensus report[53] is that ipratropium is safe in pediatric asthma and can be added to optimal first-line agents, but that its efficacy in this condition is still undetermined.

The potential role of anticholinergic agents has been studied in a variety of other pediatric conditions, such as exercise-induced bronchospasm, viral bronchiolitis, bron-chopulmonary dysplasia, and cystic fibrosis. The results of these studies do not suggest clear benefit from the use of an anticholinergic bronchodilator. These and similar topics have recently been extensively reviewed.[54]

Combination with Other Agents

Inhalers or tablets that combine more than one bronchodilator have not been available in the United States for many years; however, a similar effect is achieved *de facto* by the use of two inhalers, for example, and this practice is widespread. A previous review of such combinations[55] suggests that greater bronchodilatation often can be achieved. However, this could result simply from the fact that more bronchodilator is given with combinations. It well may be that optimal doses of a single agent, which are usually substantially more than the recommended doses, can achieve all the possible bronchodilatation, as has been shown for COPD.[36,56] However, there are many factors other than the magnitude of bronchodilatation that suggest combination therapy may have advantages.

Combinations of a β-adrenergic and an anticholinergic agent provide the rapid onset of the former with the more prolonged action of the latter, plus augmented bronchodilatation at all points between. Side effects are not increased, as might occur if large doses of the β-adrenergic agonist alone were used. If both agents were combined in the same MDI, the combination would probably be less expensive than two single-agent inhalers, and compliance would likely be enhanced.

When two MDIs are used in sequence, there is little evidence to suggest that the order of their use is important; commonly, the β-adrenergic agonist is used first because of its more rapid onset of action. Unfavorable interactions between anticholinergic and β-adrenergic agents have not been reported.

Combination MDIs that contain both ipratropium and fenoterol are very widely used outside the United States. Currently in the United States, however, a combination MDI that contains ipratropium and albuterol is approaching the final stages of development.[57]

References

1. Gross NJ: Ipratropium bromide. *N Engl J Med* 1988; 319:486–94.
2. Skorodin MS, Gross NJ, Moritz T, et al.: Oxitropium bromide: a new anticholinergic bronchodilator. *Ann Allergy* 1985; 56:229–32.
3. Brown JH: Atropine, scopolamine, and related antimuscarinic drugs, in Gilman AG, Rall TW, Nies AS, Taylor P (eds): *The Pharmacological Basis of Therapeutics*, 8th ed. New York, Pergamon Press, 1990:150–165.
4. Storms WW, DoPico GA, Reed CE: Aerosol Sch 1000: an anticholinergic bronchodilator. *Am Rev Respir Dis* 1975; 111:419–22.
5. Gross NJ: Sch 1000: a new anticholinergic bronchodilator. *Am Rev Respir Dis* 1975; 112:823–28.
6. Yeager Jr H, Weinberg RM, Kaufman LV, Katz S: Asthma: comparative bronchodilator effects of ipratropium bromide and isoproterenol. *J Clin Pharmacol* 1976; 16:198–204.
7. Allen CJ, Campbell AH: Dose response of ipratropium bromide assessed by two methods. *Thorax* 1980; 35:137–39.
8. Gomm SA, Keaney NP, Hunt LP, et al.: Dose-response comparison of ipratropium bromide from a metered-dose inhaler and by jet nebulization. *Thorax* 1983; 38:297–301.
9. Dolovich MB, Sanchis J, Rossman C, Newhouse MT: Aerosol penetrance: a sensitive index of peripheral airways obstruction. *J Appl Physiol* 1976; 40:468–71.
10. Pavia D, Thomson ML, Clark SW, Shannon HS: Effect of lung function and mode of inhalation on penetration of aerosol into the human lung. *Thorax* 1977; 32:194–97.
11. Gross NJ, Petty TL, Friedman M, Skorodin MS, et al.: Dose-response to ipratropium nebulized solution in COPD, a 3-center study. *Am Rev Respir Dis* 1989; 139:1188–91.
12. Leak A, O'Connor T: High dose ipratropium, is it safe? *Practitioner* 1988; 232:9–10.
13. Jenkins CR, Chow CM, Fisher BL, Marlin GE: Comparison of ipratropium bromide and salbutamol by aerosolized solution. *Aust NJ J Med* 1981; 11:513–16.
14. Vaughan TR, Bowen RE, Goodman DL, et al.: The development of subsensitivity to atropine methylnitrate, a double-blind, placebo-controlled crossover study. *Am Rev Respir Dis* 1988; 138:771–74.
15. Shifrin GS, Klein WL: Regulation of muscarinic acetylcholine receptor concentration in cloned neuroblastoma cells. *J Neurochem* 1980; 34:993–99.
16. Newcomb R, Tashkin DP, Hui KK, et al.: Rebound hyperresponsiveness to muscarinic stimulation after chronic therapy with an inhaled antimuscarinic antagonist. *Am Rev Respir Dis* 1985; 132:12–15.
17. Gross NJ, Skorodin MS: Anticholinergic, antimuscarinic bronchodilators. *Am Rev Respir Dis* 1984; 129:856–70.
18. Cox ID, Hughes DTD, McDonnell KA: Ipratropium bromide in patients with nocturnal asthma. *Postgrad Med J* 1984; 60:526–28.
19. Coe CI, Barnes PJ: Reduction in nocturnal asthma by an inhaled anticholinergic drug. *Chest* 1986; 90:485–88.
20. Rebuck AS, Marcus HI: SCH 1000 in psychogenic asthma. *Scand J Respir Dis* 1979; 103(suppl):186–91.
21. McFadden Jr ER, Luparello T, Lyons HA, Bleeker E: The mechanism of action of suggestion in the induction of acute asthma attacks. *J Psychosom Med* 1969; 31:134–43.
22. Nield JE, Cameron IR: Bronchoconstriction in response to suggestion, its prevention by an inhaled anticholinergic agent. *Br Med J* 1985; 290:674.
23. Grieco MH, Pierson Jr RN: Mechanism of bronchoconstriction due to beta-adrenergic blockade. *J Allergy Clin Immunol* 1971; 48:143–52.
24. Ind PW, Dixon CMS, Fuller RW, Barnes PJ: Anticholinergic blockade of propanolol induced bronchoconstriction (abstract). *Thorax* 1986; 41:718.
25. Gross NJ: Anticholinergic bronchodilators, in Barnes PJ, Roger IW, Thomson NC (eds): *Asthma: Basic Mechanisms and Clinical Management*, 2nd ed. New York, Academic Press, 1992: 555–67.
26. Sterling GM: Anticholinergic therapy in chronic asthma. *Postgrad Med J* 1987; 63(suppl):41–46.
27. Wolstenholme RJ: The role of anticholinergic drugs in chronic asthma, in Gross NJ (ed): *Anticholinergic Therapy in Obstructive Airways Disease*. London, Eng, Franklin Scientific Publications, 1993:163–68.
28. Ullah MI, Newman GB, Saunders KB: Influence of age on ipratropium and salbutamol in asthma. *Thorax* 1981; 36:523–29.
29. Vichyanond P, Sladek WA, Syr S, et al.: Efficacy of atropine methylnitrate alone and in combination with albuterol in children with asthma. *Chest* 1990; 98:637–42.
30. Jolobe OMP: Asthma versus non-specific reversible airflow obstruction, clinical features and responsiveness to anticholinergic drugs. *Respiration* 1984; 45:237–42.
31. Brown IG, Chan CS, Kelley CA, et al.: Assessment of the clinical usefulness of nebulized ipratropium bromide in patients with chronic airflow limitation. *Thorax* 1984; 39:272–76.
32. Ward MJ: The role of anticholinergic agents in acute asthma, in Gross NJ (ed): *Anticholinergic Therapy in Obstructive Airways Disease*. London, Eng, Franklin Scientific Publications, 1993: 155–162.
33. Rebuck AS, Chapman KR, Abboud R, et al.: Nebulized anticholinergic and sympathomimetic treatment of asthma and chronic obstructive airways disease in the emergency room. *Am J Med* 1987; 82:59–64.
34. Gross NJ: COPD, a disease of reversible airways obstruction. *Am Rev Respir Dis* 1986; 133:725–36.
35. Tashkin DP, Ashutosh K, Bleeker E, et al.: Comparison of the anticholinergic ipratropium bromide with metaproterenol in chronic obstructive pulmonary disease, a 90-day multicenter study. *Am J Med* 1986; 81(suppl 5A):81–86.
36. Gross NJ, Skorodin MS: Role of the parasympathetic in airway obstruction due to emphysema. *N Engl J Med* 1984; 311:421–25.
37. Marlin GE, Bush DE, Berend N: Comparison of ipratropium bromide and fenoterol in asthma and chronic bronchitis. *Br J Pharmacol* 1978; 6:547–49.
38. Lefcoe NM, Toogood JH, Blennerhassett G, et al.: The addition of an aerosol anticholinergic to an oral beta agonist plus theophylline in asthma and bronchitis: a double-blind single-dose study. *Chest* 1982; 82:300–05.
39. O'Driscoll BR, Taylor RJ, Horsley MG, et al.: Nebulized salbutamol with and without ipratropium bromide in acute airflow obstruction. *Lancet* 1989; i:1418–20.
40. Lloberes P, Ramis L, Montserrat JM, et al.: Effect of 3 different bronchodilators during an exacerbation of chronic obstructive pulmonary disease. *Eur Respir J* 1988; 1:536–39.

41. Karpel JP, Pesin J, Greenberg D, Gentry E: A comparison of the effects of ipratropium bromide and metaproterenol sulfate in acute exacerbations of COPD. 1990; 98:835–39.

42. Karpel JP: Bronchodilator responses to anticholinergic and beta-adrenergic agents in acute and stable COPD. *Chest* 1991; 99: 871–76.

43. Gross NJ, Bankwala Z: Effects of an anticholinergic bronchodilator on arterial blood gases of hypoxemic patients with chronic obstructive pulmonary disease. *Am Rev Respir Dis* 1987; 136: 1091–94.

44. Davis A, Vickerson F, Worsley G, et al.: Determination of dose-response relationship for ipratropium in asthmatic children. *J Pediatr* 1984; 105:1002–05.

45. Friberg S, Graff-Lonnevig V: Ipratropium bromide (Atrovent) in childhood asthma: a cumulative dose-response study. *Ann Allergy* 1989; 62:131–34.

46. Beck R, Robertson C, Galdes-Sebaldt M, Levison H: Combined salbutamol and ipratropium bromide by inhalation in the treatment of severe acute asthma. *J Pediatr* 1985; 107:605–08.

47. Reisman J, Galdes-Sebaldt M, Kazim F, et al.: Frequent administration by inhalation of salbutamol and ipratropium bromide in the initial management of severe acute asthma in children. *J Allergy Clin Immunol* 1988; 81:16–20.

48. Storr J, Lenney W: Nebulized ipratropium and salbutamol in asthma. *Arch Dis Child* 1986; 61:602–03.

49. Boner AL, De Stefano G, Niero E, et al.: Salbutamol and ipratropium bromide solution in the treatment of bronchospasm in asthmatic children. *Ann Allergy* 1987; 58:54–58.

50. Mann NP, Hiller EJ: Ipratropium bromide in children with asthma. *Thorax* 1982; 37:72–74.

51. Sly PD, Landau LI, Olinsky A: Failure of ipratropium bromide to modify diurnal variation of asthma in asthmatic children. *Thorax* 1987; 42:357–60.

52. Freeman J, Landaw LI: The effects of ipratropium bromide and fenoterol nebulizer solutions in children with asthma. *Clin Pediatr* 1989; 28:556–60.

53. Warner JO, Getz M, Landaw LI, et al.: Management of asthma: a consensus statement. *Arch Dis Child* 1989; 64:1065–79.

54. Reisman JJ, Canny GJ, Levison H: The role of anticholinergic drugs in paediatric airways disease, in Gross NJ (ed): *Anticholinergic Therapy in Obstructive Airways Disease*. London, Eng, Franklin Scientific Publications, 1993:169–180.

55. Chervinsky P: Concomitant bronchodilator therapy and ipratropium bromide: a clinical review. *Am J Med* 1986; 81(suppl 5A):67–72.

56. Easton PA, Jadue C, Dhingra S, Anthonisen NR: A comparison of bronchodilating effects of a beta-2 adrenergic agent (salbutamol) and an anticholinergic agent (ipratropium bromide) given by aerosol alone or in combination. *N Engl J Med* 1986; 325:753–59.

57. Combivent Inhalation Aerosol Study Group. In chronic obstructive pulmonary disease, a combination of ipratropium and albuterol is more effective than either agent alone, an 85-day multicenter trial. *Chest* 1994; 105:1411–19.

Chapter 54

SIDE EFFECTS AND TOXICITY
NICHOLAS J. GROSS

Anticholinergic drugs can be divided into two categories according to the valency of the nitrogen atom in the tropane ring: the 3-valent, tertiary ammonium alkaloids, which include all the natural agents such as atropine and its congeners; and the 5-valent, quaternary ammonium alkaloids, which are synthetic (see Chap. 53). The most striking result of this difference has to do with the absorbability from mucosal surfaces, the former agents being well-absorbed and the latter agents being exceedingly poorly absorbed. Although both groups may produce similar effects in vitro, the poor absorption of quaternary agents when delivered to the respiratory tract, for example, results in a high degree of functional selectivity that can be exploited for clinical purposes. The adverse-effect profiles of the two groups differ markedly and will be discussed separately. None of the agents currently approved for respiratory use are selective for muscarinic receptor subtypes.

Tertiary Ammonium Compounds

Atropine is the principal member of this group, which includes scopolamine, hyoscine, and homatropine, among other naturally occurring agents. The side effects and toxicity of atropine and its congeners have been known for many years and are described in detail in standard texts[1,2]; they will be summarized herein. These effects are dose-related. As atropine is more-or-less quantitatively absorbed from mucosal surfaces (and to an extent from the skin as well), side effects can occur whenever sufficient amounts of atropine are administered by whatever route. Atropine has a very small therapeutic margin, and many of the side effects described in the sections that follow occur at usual clinical doses.

RESPIRATORY TRACT

In addition to relaxation of airways smooth muscle, atropine has important side effects on the mucociliary apparatus. These are of particular relevance because, when delivered by inhalation, the local concentration of atropine will be highest at the mucosal surface. Furthermore, dysfunction of mucosal secretions and their clearance is almost always a feature of airways diseases,[3] even without treatment effects.

Atropine reduces the volume of mucus that is released from mucosal explants from the human lower respiratory tract.[4,5] In animals, it appears not to affect basal rates of secretion as much as it reduces stimulated hypersecretion.[3,6–8] A similar effect is seen in human nasal mucosa in vivo, where atropine does not alter basal secretion but inhibits stimulated secretion.[9] Mucous rheology, a difficult field of investigation, appears not to be greatly altered by atropine.[10] However, ciliary beat frequency is impaired in human respiratory tissue by atropine and hyoscine.[11,12]

As overall effects on mucociliary clearance, rather than its components, are the most relevant concern in human disease, these have been extensively studied. A variety of models and methods have indeed shown that atropine impairs mucociliary clearance in human airways.[13–16] This might be expected to delay clearance of secretions from the respiratory tract, possibly contributing to airways obstruction and infection. Although such effects mainly have been observed in healthy tissue, retention of secretions and mucous plugging are features of severe asthma. The possibility that they might be aggravated by atropine makes it highly questionable whether atropine ever should be used in status asthmaticus.

CENTRAL NERVOUS SYSTEM

Tertiary ammonium compounds cross the blood-brain barrier and affect mental function (effects that have been exploited for recreational purposes for centuries). In small doses (0.5 to 1.0 mg), they may cause mild excitement, restlessness, and irritability. These effects appear to be more common in the elderly, possibly because of underlying cerebrovascular disease, poor nutrition, intercurrent diseases, and concomitant medications. Central nervous system depression also can occur and may take the form of drowsiness, fatigue, amnesia, and an altered sleep pattern. With increasing dosage, a variety of more serious acute effects may be seen, including disorientation, hallucinations, and coma. Death is unusual even following a substantial dosage.[1,2]

Unusual idiosyncratic reactions occasionally have been reported following even small or conventional doses. An acute psychosis has been reported following inhalation of atropine for respiratory purposes.[17] This is uncommon, but by no means rare, particularly in older patients. A similar reaction has been reported in children[18] and in association with hyperpyrexia.[19]

Atropine-like agents do not cause tremor; indeed they are sometimes used to treat the tremor of parkinsonism. However, they are contraindicated in myasthenia gravis except to counteract excess anticholinesterase treatment.

EYE

Anticholinergic agents cause blurred vision and raise intraocular tension by inhibiting sphincteric contraction of the iris and the ciliary muscle of the lens. These effects can be quite long-lasting, and can be seen after conventional doses of atropine given via the respiratory route. Because of the effect on intraocular tension, atropine and similar agents by any route are contraindicated in patients with narrow-angle glaucoma, although not in wide-angle glaucoma. As undiagnosed glaucoma is not uncommon in older subjects, symptoms of acute glaucoma following atropine treatment should

be carefully heeded. The ocular effects can be readily reversed by topical pilocarpine or physostigmine.

CARDIOVASCULAR SYSTEM

The effect of atropine on heart rate is biphasic; small doses produce a minor slowing of heart rate, while larger doses result in tachycardia without significant effects on blood pressure or cardiac output. In large doses, atrial arrhythmias and atrioventricular dissociation may occur. Anticholinergic agents have rather trivial effects on either the systemic or pulmonary vasculature.

GASTROINTESTINAL SYSTEM

Atropine-like agents inhibit the release of secretions from the salivary glands and commonly cause dryness of the mouth in clinical doses. With larger doses, dysphagia and dysphonia can occur. These agents may relax the lower esophageal sphincter,[20,21] a consideration in patients with asthma in whom reflux may contribute to bronchospasm. In the stomach, atropine-like agents reduce the volume and solute content of both basal and stimulated secretions. They inhibit gastric motility and delay gastric emptying, an effect that has been demonstrated following conventional doses administered by aerosol to asthmatic subjects.[22]

GENITOURINARY SYSTEM

The urinary sphincter is under parasympathetic control, relaxing in response to cholinergic stimulation. Thus, anticholinergic agents can inhibit its relaxation. In subjects without bladder-neck obstruction, this rarely causes symptoms, but in older men with prostatic hypertrophy, even usual doses of atropine can precipitate acute urinary retention. Atropine-like agents also may impair male potency. For these patients, anticholinergic agents thus are contraindicated.

OTHER EFFECTS

Atropine commonly causes hotness and dryness of the skin at usual doses, but this is rarely troublesome except in hot climates, where body temperature may rise. Atropine has negligible effects on uterine contraction. It crosses the placenta and is secreted in breast milk, but adverse effects on the fetus and newborn are believed not to occur.[1]

IDIOSYNCRASY, TACHYPHYLAXIS, AND DRUG INTERACTIONS

Most of the above effects of atropine-like agents are dose related, and idiosyncratic reactions are unusual. The acute psychosis and hyperpyrexial reactions mentioned above are idiosyncratic. Patients with Down's syndrome are reported to be unusually sensitive to anticholinergic agents.[2] Tolerance has not been reported after prolonged use.

Interactions between atropine and other drugs are quite uncommon; an extensive review of the literature reveals only two.[2] Atropine, and presumably its congeners, potentiate the effect of suxamethonium, and atropine interacts with pralidoxime, an agent that activates cholinesterases following organophosphorus poisoning.

Quaternary Ammonium Compounds

These agents—ipratropium, oxitropium, atropine methylnitrate, glycopyrrolate, and so on—have a relatively wide therapeutic margin when administered by inhalation for the reasons discussed above. If given parenterally, for example, for experimental purposes, they produce systemic effects that are similar to the tertiary ammonium compounds; however, they are unable to cross the blood-brain barrier and so do not produce CNS effects. Among these agents, the effects of ipratropium and oxitropium have been most studied.

RESPIRATORY TRACT

Because of the potentially deleterious effects of atropine on mucociliary clearance (above), the effects of ipratropium have been examined carefully.[23,24] Despite extensive searches for similar effects, ipratropium has been found to have negligible effects on mucociliary clearance,[15,25–27] mucus composition,[28] or histology of the mucosa.[29] A small decrease in the volume of mucus secreted was found after seven weeks continuous treatment with ipratropium.[30] Oxitropium has been studied similarly and has been found to resemble ipratropium in its lack of effects on the mucociliary apparatus.[31] It is not clear why these agents lack effects on the physiology of mucus, yet are potent relaxants of airways smooth muscle. Presumably, they must traverse the mucosal layer to reach smooth muscles in the submucosa. These agents are not selective for muscarinic receptor subtypes. Their lack of effect, therefore, although welcome, is unexplained.

A different effect is found in the nasal passages where ipratropium causes a significant reduction in stimulated hypersecretion without affecting basal secretion rates.[32] This might be due either to differences in physiologic control of secretions between the upper and lower respiratory tracts or to the fact that larger concentrations of the drug on the mucosal surface occur following nasal administration. Whatever the mechanism, it can result in some nasal discomfort.

EYE

Extensive, although short-term, studies have examined the effect on intraocular pressure following inhalation of ipratropium. These studies show that in both normal subjects and patients with narrow-angle glaucoma no effects on intraocular tension, pupil diameter or accommodation occurred following inhalation of ipratropium, even in doses up to four times the recommended dosage.[26,33,34] The drug probably can be safely used in patients with glaucoma provided the precaution stated in the next paragraph is carefully observed.

Caution should be observed that the drug is not inadvertently sprayed into the eye. Prolonged pupillary dilatation and blurred vision will occur in this event,[35] which could precipitate acute glaucoma in a susceptible subject. The addition of salbutamol appears to intensify this effect.[36,37] The metered-dose inhaler (MDI) should never be pointed toward the eye. The current recommendation is that the mouthpiece be placed directly in the patient's mouth. Otherwise, it is probably advisable for the patient to close the eyes before activating the MDI. When ipratropium is nebulized with a face mask, the eyes should be protected as leakage can occur around the upper portion of the mask. When nebulized ipratropium is taken through a mouthpiece, an extension may be placed on the T-piece to ensure that excess ipratropium is vented away from the patient.

GENITOURINARY SYSTEM

In a double-blind crossover study, ipratropium was given to men 50 to 70 years of age, with no effect on urinary flow characteristics or cytostometric indices.[38] Unlike atropine, therefore, ipratropium can be safely given to these patients who are most at risk for urinary retention.

CARDIOVASCULAR SYSTEM

Studies with inhaled ipratropium show (unlike β-adrenergic bronchodilators) that it has trivial effects on heart rate and hemodynamics,[39,40] even when given in doses eightfold in excess of the recommended dosage.[41]

GAS EXCHANGE

β-adrenergic bronchodilators, by any route, may reduce the arterial oxygen tension of patients with airways disease. This effect has been attributed to reversal of endogenous mechanisms that modulate perfusion to poorly ventilated regions, thus increasing ventilation-perfusion inequality. Atropine methonitrate had no such effect either in normal subject[42] or in patients with chronic obstructive pulmonary disease (COPD) who were hypoxemic at rest[43] (Fig. 54-1). Similarly, ipratropium did not affect adversely Pa_{O_2} in patients with acute exacerbations of COPD.[44]

PARADOXICAL BRONCHOCONSTRICTION

Several short reports from the United Kingdom have documented the unusual occurrence of paradoxical bronchoconstriction; this reaction immediately follows the use of ipratropium, usually by nebulization and takes the form of increased symptoms and a rapid decrease in FEV_1. It has been attributed to various causes, including hypotonicity of the nebulizer solution,[45,46] sensitivity to bromide ions,[47] and preservatives in the solution.[48,49] However, alteration of the tonicity and preservative of the solution has not eliminated entirely the phenomenon, including reports of occurrence in preterm infants,[50,51] raising the possibility that it is an

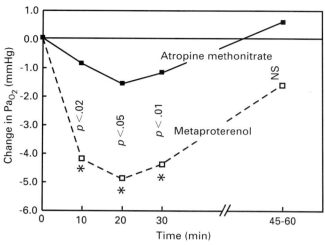

FIGURE 54-1 Serial measurements of arterial P_{O_2} in 12 subjects with COPD and hypoxemia at rest and following inhalation of atropine methonitrate or metaproterenol on separate days. Symbols denote significant differences between treatments. (Reprinted by permission from Am Rev Respir Disease 1987; 136:1091–94.)

idiosyncratic reaction to the drug itself. There are also anecdotal accounts of paradoxical bronchoconstriction following oxitropium use. Although it is estimated in Europe that the frequency of this unusual reaction is perhaps 1–3/1000 patients, there are no reports of its occurrence in the United States. However, it would be appropriate to promptly withdraw the drug if the patient's symptoms increased immediately after using it, particularly if this occurred upon instituting the drug for the first time to a patient.

TACHYPHYLAXIS

Tachyphylaxis to ipratropium has been examined in several large-scale, long-term studies and has not been found. There is one report of tachyphylaxis to atropine methonitrate.[52] The clinical significance of this is unknown.

OTHER EFFECTS

The safety of quaternary ammonium compounds in pregnancy and lactation has not been systematically studied. Because of their poor ability to cross membranes, significant delivery from the mother to the fetus or to breast milk seem extremely unlikely. Animal studies with ipratropium and oxitropium show no evidence of teratogenicity in the embryo.

Ipratropium has been used in patients with cystic fibrosis.[53] Meconium ileus occurred for the first time in an adult patient on two occasions following the use of nebulized ipratropium.[54] This was attributed to the effect of swallowed drug on intestinal motility.

THERAPEUTIC MARGIN AND LONG-TERM STUDIES

An indication of the wide therapeutic margin of quaternary compounds is provided by a case report in which a patient with COPD who was enrolled in a study of atropine methonitrate was inadvertently given approximately 1000 times the intended dose and about 10 times the toxic dose of atropine sulfate. The patient experienced no effects other than dry mouth and headache.[55]

The typical incidence of side effects from conventional use of ipratropium MDI is provided by two large, multicenter, three-month studies: one in 164 patients with asthma,[56] and one in 261 patients with COPD.[57] A short paroxysm of coughing was the commonest adverse effect in both studies. This and the very large clinical experience obtained since ipratropium became available for general use in most European countries in the mid-1970s and in the United States in 1987 suggest that ipratropium is remarkably safe.

Management of Anticholinergic Toxicity

The most common side effects of anticholinergic drugs are mild—dryness of the mouth or cough—and require no treatment or change in management. More serious side effects and toxicity (e.g., following atropine) can usually be promptly reversed by a cholinersterase inhibitor (e.g., physostigmine or neostigmine). Ocular toxicity can be treated with topical physostigmine. Atropine psychosis and other rare effects of anticholinergic toxicity can be rapidly reversed by parenteral administration of 1 to 2 mg physostigmine. This should be administered cautiously as the effects of unopposed cholinergic activity (e.g., bronchospasm) can occur. Further, anticholinesterases are rapidly metabolized and the toxic effects of the anticholinergic drug can recur. Phenothiazines should be avoided as they have some anticholinergic activity.

References

1. Brown JH: Atropine, scopolamine, and related antimuscarinic drugs, in Gilman AG, Rall TW, Nies AS, Taylor P (eds): *The Pharmacological Basis of Therapeutics*, 8th ed. New York, Pergamon Press, 1990:150–165.
2. Anonymous: Antimuscarinic agents, in Reynolds JEF (ed): *Martindale: The Extra Pharmacopoeia*, 29th ed. London, Eng, Pharmaceutical Press, 1989:522–45.
3. Wanner A: Clinical aspects of mucociliary transport. *Am Rev Respir Dis* 1977; 116:73–125.
4. Sturgess J, Reid L: An organ culture study of the effect of drugs on the secretory activity of the human bronchial submucosal gland. *Clin Sci* 1972; 43:533–43.
5. Boat TF, Kleinerman JI: Human respiratory tract secretions. 2. Effect of cholinergic and adrenergic agents on in vitro release of protein and mucous glycoproteins. *Chest* 1975; 67(suppl):32–34.
6. Ueki I, German VF, Nadel JA: Micropipette measurement of airway submucosal gland secretion; autonomic effects. *Am Rev Respir Dis* 1980; 121:351–57.
7. Marin MG, Davis B, Nadel JA: Effect of acetylcholine on Cl⁻ and

Na$^+$ fluxes across dog tracheal epithelium in vitro. *Am J Physiol* 1976; 231:1546–49.

8. King M, Angus GE: Effect of aerosolized bronchodilators on viscoelastic properties of canine tracheal mucus. *Chest* 1981; 80(suppl):852–54.

9. Borum P: Nasal disorders and anticholinergic therapy. *Postgrad Med J* 1987; 63(suppl 1):61–68.

10. Lopez-Vidriero MT, Costello J, Clark TJH, et al.: Effect of atropine on sputum production. *Thorax* 1975; 30:543–47.

11. Corssen G, Allen CR: Acetylcholine: Its significance in controlling ciliary activity of human respiratory epithelium in vitro. *J Appl Physiol* 1959; 14:901–04.

12. Yeates DB, Aspin N, Levison H, et al.: Mucociliary tracheal transport rates in man. *J Appl Physiol* 1975; 39:487–95.

13. Foster WM, Bergofsky EH: Airway mucus membrane: effects of beta-adrenergic and anticholinergic stimulation. *Am J Med* 1986; 81(suppl 5A):28–35.

14. Berger J, Albert RE, Sanborn K, Lippman M: Effects of atropine and methacholine on deposition and clearance of inhaled particles in the donkey. *J Toxicol Environ Health* 1978; 4:587–604.

15. Sackner MA, Chapman GA, Dougherty RD: Effects of nebulized ipratropium bromide and atropine sulfate on tracheal mucus velocity and lung mechanics in anesthetized dogs. *Respiration* 1977; 34:181–85.

16. Groth ML, Langenback EG, Foster WM: Influence of inhaled atropine on lung mucociliary function in humans. *Am Rev Respir Dis* 1991; 144:1042–47.

17. Bergman KR, Pearson C, Waltz GW, Evans R: Atropine-induced psychosis, an unusual complication of therapy with inhaled atropine sulfate. *Chest* 1980; 78:891–93.

18. Herschman ZL, Silverstein J, Blumberg G, Lehrfield A: Central nervous system toxicity from nebulized atropine sulfate. *J Toxicol Clin Toxicol* 1991; 29:273–77.

19. Torline RL: Extreme hyperpyrexia associated with central anticholinergic syndrome. *Anesthesiology* 1992; 76:470–71.

20. Cotton BR, Smith G: Single and combined effects of atropine and metaclopramide on the lower oesophageal sphincter pressure. *Br J Anaesthesia* 1981; 53:869–74.

21. Hey VMF, Phillips K, Woods I: Pethidine, atropine, metaclopramide and the lower oesophageal sphincter. *Anaesthesia* 1983; 38:650–53.

22. Botts LD, Pingleton SK, Schroeder CE, et al.: Prolongation of gastric emptying by aerosolized atropine. *Am Rev Respir Dis* 1985; 131:725–26.

23. Wanner A: Effect of ipratropium on airway mucociliary function. *Am J Med* 1986; 81(suppl 5A):23–27.

24. Gross NJ: Ipratropium bromide. *N Engl J Med* 1988; 319:486–94.

25. Francis RA, Thomson ML, Pavia D, Douglas RB: Ipratropium bromide: mucociliary clearance rate and airway resistance in normal subjects. *Br J Dis Chest* 1977; 71:173–78.

26. Ruffin RE, Wolff RK, Dolovich MB, et al.: Aerosol therapy with Sch 1000: short-term mucociliary clearance in normal and bronchitic subjects and toxicology in normal subjects. *Chest* 1978; 73:510–06.

27. Pavia D, Bateman JR, Sheahan NF, Clarke SW: Clearance of lung secretions in patients with chronic bronchitis: effect of terbutaline and ipratropium bromide aerosols. *Eur J Respir Dis* 1980; 61:245–253.

28. Chervinsky P: Double-blind study of ipratropium bromide, a new anticholinergic bronchodilator. *J Allergy Clin Immunol* 1977; 59:22–30.

29. Fasske E, Jungst G, Themann H: Light and electron microscopy studies of human bronchial epithelium following treatment with

Sch 1000 metered dose inhaler (MDI) (abstract). *Postgrad Med J* 1975:51(suppl 7):107.

30. Ghafouri MA, Patil KD, Kass I: Sputum changes associated with use of ipratropium bromide. *Chest* 1984; 86:387–93.

31. Pavia D, Lopez-Vidriero MT, Agnew JE, et al.: Effect of four-week treatment with oxitropium on lung mucociliary clearance in patients with chronic bronchitis or asthma. *Respiration* 1989; 55:33–43.

32. Meltzer EO: Anticholinergic treatment of nasal disorders. *Immunol Allergy Clin N Am* 1991; 11:31–44.

33. Scheuffler G: Ophthalmotonometry, pupil diameter and visual accommodation following repeated administration of Sch1000 MDI in patients with glaucoma (abstract). *Postgrad Med J* 1975; 51(suppl 7):132.

34. Thumm HW: Ophthalmic effects of high doses of Sch 1000 MDI in healthy volunteers and patients with glaucoma (abstract). *Postgrad Med J* 1975; 51(suppl 7):132–33.

35. Samaniego F, Newman LS: Migratory anisocoria: a novel clinical entity. *Am Rev Respir Dis* 1986; 143:844.

36. Kalra L, Bone M: The effect of nebulized bronchodilator therapy on intraocular pressure in patients with glaucoma. *Chest* 1988; 93:739–41.

37. Shah P, Dhurjon L, Metcalfe T, Gibson JM: Acute angle closure glaucoma associated with nebulized ipratropium bromide and salbutamol. *Br Med J* 1992; 304:40–41.

38. Molkenboer JFWM, Lardenoye JG: The effect of Atrovent on micturition function, double-blind cross-over study. *Scand J Respir Dis* 1979; 103(suppl):154–58.

39. Anderson WM: Hemodynamic and non-bronchial effects of ipratropium bromide. *Am J Med* 1986; 81(suppl 5A):45–52.

40. Chapman KR, Smith DL, Rebuck AS, Leenen FH: Hemodynamic effects of inhaled ipratropium bromide, alone and combined with an inhaled beta2-agonist. *Am Rev Respir Dis* 1985; 132: 845–47.

41. Sackner MA, Friedman M, Silva G, Fernandez R: The pulmonary hemodynamic effects of aerosols of isoproterenol and ipratropium in normal subjects and patients with reversible airways obstruction. *Am Rev Respir Dis* 1977; 116:1013–22.

42. Field GB: The effects of posture, oxygen, isoproterenol, and atropine on ventilation-perfusion relationships in the lung in asthma. *Clin Sci* 1967; 32:279–88.

43. Gross NJ, Bankwala Z: Effects of an anticholinergic bronchodilator on arterial blood gases of hypoxemic patients with chronic obstructive pulmonary disease. *Am Rev Respir Dis* 1987; 136: 1091–94.

44. Karpel JP, Pesin J, Greenberg D, Gentry E: A comparison of the effects of ipratropium bromide and metaproterenol sulfate in acute exacerbations of COPD. 1990; 98:835–39.

45. Connolly CK: Adverse reaction to ipratropium bromide. *Br Med J* 1982; 285:934–35.

46. Mann JS, Howarth PH, Holgate ST: Bronchoconstriction induced by ipratropium bromide in asthma: relation to hypotonicity. *Br Med J* 1984; 289:469.

47. Patel KR, Tullett WM: Bronchoconstriction in response to ipratropium bromide. *Br Med J* 1983; 286:1318.

48. Miszkiel KA, Beasley R, Holgate ST: The influence of ipratropium bromide and sodium cromoglycate on benzalkonium-induced bronchoconstriction in asthma. *Br J Clin Pharmacol* 1988; 26:295–301.

49. Rafferty P, Beasley R, Holgate ST: Comparison of the efficacy of preservative free ipratropium bromide and Atrovent nebulizer solution. *Thorax* 1988; 43:446–50.

50. O'Callaghan C, Milner AD, Swarbrick A: Paradoxical bron-

choconstriction in wheezing infants after nebulized preservative free iso-osmolar ipratropium bromide. *Br Med J* 1989; 299: 1433–34.

51. Yuksel B, Greenough A, Green S: Paradoxical response to nebulized ipratropium bromide in preterm infants asymptomatic at follow up. *Respir Med* 1991; 85:189–94.

52. Vaughan TR, Bowen RE, Goodman DL, et al.: The development of subsensitivity to atropine methylnitrate: a double-blind, placebo-controlled, crossover study. *Am Rev Respir Dis* 1988; 138:771–74.

53. Kattan M, Mansell A, Levison H, et al.: Response to aerosol salbutamol, SCH 1000 and placebo in cystic fibrosis. *Thorax* 1980; 35:531–35.

54. Mulherin D, Fitzgerald MX: Meconium ileus equivalent in association with nebulized ipratropium bromide in cystic fibrosis. *Lancet* 1990; 335:552.

55. Gross NJ, Skorodin MS: Massive overdose of atropine methonitrate with only slight untoward effects. *Lancet* 1985; ii:386.

56. Storms WW, Bodman SF, Nathan RA, et al.: Use of ipratropium bromide in asthma: results of a multi-clinic study. *Am J Med* 1986; 81(suppl 5A):61–65.

57. Tashkin DP, Ashutosh K, Bleeker ER, et al.: Comparison of the anticholinergic bronchodilator ipratropium bromide with metaproterenol in chronic obstructive pulmonary disease: a 90-day multi-center study. *Am J Med* 1986; 81(suppl 5A):81–89.

CORTICOSTEROIDS

Chapter 55
CHEMISTRY AND MODE OF ACTION
STEPHEN J. LANE AND TAK H. LEE

General Pharmacology of the Glucocorticoids

Structure-Function Relationship

Bioavailability

The Glucocorticoid Receptor

Interaction of the GR with Transcriptionally Active Molecules

Interaction of the GR with DNA

Synthetic glucocorticoids are the mainstay of treatment for many inflammatory diseases, including bronchial asthma. In recent years more potent and topically active glucocorticoids have been developed by manipulation of the basic structure of the hydrocortisone molecule. The current model of glucocorticoid action proposes binding to a specific cytoplasmic receptor that, when activated, translocates to the nucleus where it interacts with other transcriptionally active molecules at protein-protein and at protein-DNA levels. The specifically ligand-activated glucocorticoid receptor (GR) then binds to sequences of DNA in a manner allowing it to directly suppress or induce gene transcription.

General Pharmacology of the Glucocorticoids

Corticosteroids are hormones that are synthesized in the adrenal cortex. They may be classified in relation to their pharmacologic effects as *glucocorticoids* and *mineralocorticoids*. The glucocorticoids are synthesized in the zona reticularis and fasciculata, and they play a central role in carbohydrate, protein, and lipid homeostasis, as well as exerting anti-inflammatory effects.[1] They are secreted in response to pituitary-derived adrenocorticotropic hormone (ACTH) and hypothalamic corticotropin-releasing hormone (CRH), respectively. The mineralocorticoids (e.g., aldosterone) synthesized in the zona glomerulosa and influence electrolyte and water balance under the control of the renin-angiotensin-aldosterone system independent of pituitary control. Mineralocorticoid receptors have an equal affinity for aldosterone and the physiologic glucocorticoids cortisol and corticosterone, which circulate at concentrations higher than those of aldosterone. In mineralocorticoid target tissues, the glucocorticoids are selectively converted by the 11-β-hydroxysteroid dehydrogenase into their 11-keto analogs, which do not bind to the mineralocorticoid receptor.[2] Although it is feasible to develop synthetic agents that have more potent glucocorticoid effects than mineralocorticoid effects, it is not possible to separate the anti-inflammatory effects and the metabolic effects.

The most important determinant of response to a particular glucocorticoid agent is the structural component of the administered agent.[3] Although certain features are essential for the pharmacologic effect of the glucocorticoids, additional structural modifications increase their potency and the duration of their effects. Another important determinant of response to glucocorticoid therapy relates to the systemic deposition of the individual compounds, which is integrally related to molecular structure, as this will affect the rate of elimination and distribution of the glucocorticoid. The potency of a particular glucocorticoid is related to the binding affinity of the steroid molecule to the cytoplasmic glucocorticoid receptor. The pharmacologic action of a drug depends on the dose administered and the conditions that affect the disposition of the drug. These conditions ultimately determine the concentration-time profile and the availability of the drug at the cellular site of action.

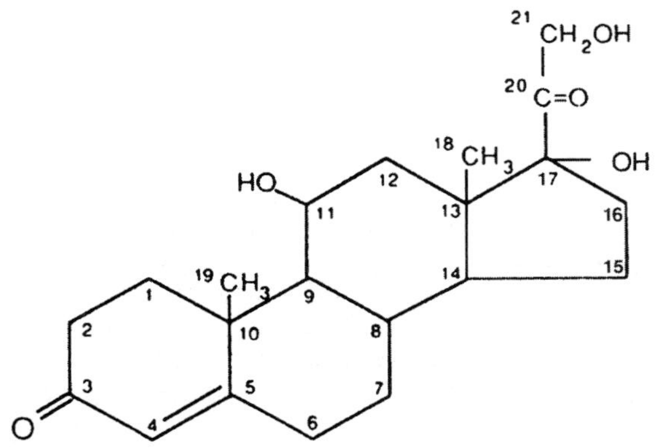

FIGURE 55-1 Basic chemical structure of glucocorticoids.

Structure-Function Relationship

The basic chemical structure of the glucocorticoids (Fig. 55-1) consists of 21 carbon atoms with a total of four rings comprising three 6-carbon rings and a single 5-carbon ring. The anti-inflammatory glucocorticoids additionally have (1) an unsaturated double bond at C-4=C-5, (2) a 2-carbon side chain at C-17, (3) a hydroxyl (—OH) radical group at C-11, (4) a methyl (—CH$_3$) group at C-18 and C-19, and (5) a ketone radical (=O) at C-3 and C-20. Synthetic analogs are made by substitution at sites on the basic cortisol molecule to enhance anti-inflammatory activity and reduce mineralocorticoid activity with respect to cortisol. The values for the relative glucocorticoid and mineralocorticoid potencies are presented in Table 55-1 and are approximations based on several sources.[1]

The introduction of an unsaturated C-1=C-2 double bond on cortisol results in the molecule prednisolone, which has reduced mineralocorticoid side effects and a fourfold increase in glucocorticoid activity as compared with cortisol. The biologic half-life of prednisolone is extended to 12 to

36 h whereas for cortisol it is 8 to 12 h. The biologic half-lives of the glucocorticoids are characterized as short-, intermediate-, or long-acting based on the duration of ACTH suppression following a single dose of glucocorticoid (Table 55-1). The addition of a methyl group at the 6α position of prednisolone forms methylprednisolone. Methylprednisolone is slightly more potent in glucocorticoid activity than prednisolone, and, because of the structural modification, there is a significant difference between the two in relation to protein binding. The addition of halogen atoms greatly increases the potencies and the half-lives of glucocorticoids by increasing binding affinity and decreasing hepatic breakdown. Dexamethasone is a synthetic analog with 25-fold the glucocorticoid potency of cortisol with minimal mineralocorticoid effect. It is a modification of prednisolone with a fluorine atom at the 9α position (enhanced glucocorticoid activity) and a methyl group at the 16α position (decreased mineralocorticoid activity). Its biologic half-life is increased to 36 to 54 h. Most steroids are poorly water-soluble and must be conjugated to improve water solubility. Conjugation also affects the rate of absorption and the duration of action. The phosphate and hemisuccinate conjugates at C-21 increase the water solubility of prednisolone, hydrocortisone, and methylprednisolone, allowing for their parenteral administration. Further alterations at the C-17 and C-21 positions result in glucocorticoids with enhanced topical activity and minimal systemic adverse effects. Two methods can be used to develop topical steroids. A steroid can be conjugated with a poorly soluble acetonide group that facilitates the delivery of a relatively large glucocorticoid dose with minimal systemic absorption (e.g., triamcinolone acetonide). Another method is to increase the potency of a weak glucocorticoid by conjugation with an ester group (e.g., beclomethasone dipropionate, the 17,21-dipropionate form of 9α-chloro-16β-methylprednisolone). Aerosolized administration results in a potent topical effect on the lung with subsequent metabolism, removal of the propionate groups, and systemic absorption of the relatively weak glucocorticoid beclomethasone.

TABLE 55-1   Relative Potencies of the Glucocorticoids

	GCS[a] Potency	Equivalent GCS Dose (mg)	MCS[b] Potency	Plasma $t_{1/2}$ (min)	Biologic $t_{1/2}$ (h)
Short-acting					
Cortisol	1	25	1	90	8–12
Intermediate-acting					
Prednisolone	4	5	0	200	12–36
Methylprednisolone	5	4	0	200	12–36
Triamcinolone	5	4	0	200	12–36
Long-acting					
Betamethasone	25	0.60	0	300	36–54
Dexamethasone	30	0.75	0	300	36–54
Mineralocorticoids					
Corticosterone	0.3	—	15	—	—
Fludrocortisone	10	—	125	—	—

[a]GCS, glucocorticosteroid; [b]MCS, mineralocorticoids.

Bioavailability

The most commonly used glucocorticoid for oral administration in the United Kingdom is prednisolone. Its absorption has been demonstrated to be both extensive and rapid.[4] In addition, it does not require hepatic interconversion to an active form as does prednisone, and, therefore, its bioavailability is more predictable and independent of hepatic disease states. Little is known about the distribution characteristics of the glucocorticoids. It is assumed that only the unbound or free fraction of the hydrophobic glucocorticoid molecule is available for passive distribution to target cells. The naturally occurring glucocorticoids, in addition to prednisolone, exhibit unusual plasma protein–binding in that they bind with low affinity and high capacity to serum albumin, and, conversely, with high affinity and low capacity to the α_1-globulin transcortin. This results in a concentration-dependent variation in the total protein fraction that is bound, resulting in dose-dependent, nonlinear kinetics of deposition. Since the elimination of the glucocorticoid is dependent on drug metabolism, which in turn is dependent on the free fraction of the drug available to the cell, the clearance of these glucocorticoids increases with the dose administered.

After a single dose of orally administered prednisolone peak serum concentrations are achieved between 1 to 2 h.[4] Its serum half-life is 2 to 3 h and its biologic half-life is 24 to 36 h. Elimination is primarily by reduction of the C-4═C-5 unsaturated double bond and of the ketone moiety at C-3, forming tetrahydro forms that then are conjugated to water-soluble sulfate esters and subsequently excreted in the bile. Thirty percent of the administered drug can be excreted unchanged in the urine. There are many factors that influence prednisolone deposition.[3] Higher plasma concentrations of prednisolone were observed following early morning rather than evening dosing, and deposition was shown to be more rapid in females as compared with males. Rifampicin and the anticonvulsants phenytoin and phenobarbitone can enhance clearance by accelerating metabolic breakdowns by inducing hepatic microsomal enzymes. Oral estrogen contraceptives reduced clearance by increasing transcortin levels. The macrolide antibiotics, specifically troleandromycin and erythromycin, reduced the hepatic clearance of methylprednisolone with no effect on prednisolone elimination.

Several studies have shown similar pharmacokinetic profiles in asthmatic adults and children as compared with nonasthmatic subjects.[5] Georgitis and colleagues examined the bioavailability of a single dose of 20 mg prednisolone orally in 12 healthy subjects using high-performance liquid chromatography (HPLC).[4,6] Serum prednisolone demonstrated peak concentrations at 1.23 ± 0.063 h (mean ± SEM), a mean residence time of 5.1 ± 0.49 h, and an absolute bioavailability of 97.5 percent when compared with an equal dose of intravenous prednisolone phosphate.

Interest also has focused on whether impaired bioavailability of glucocorticoids can account for the differences in therapeutic responses in corticosteroid-dependent and corticosteroid-resistant asthma. May and co-workers measured the pharmacokinetic profile of a single dose of 15 mg oral prednisolone in 12 corticosteroid-dependent asthmatic subjects by radioimmunoassay (RIA) and found no interindividual differences in these subjects with respect to C_{max}, plasma half-life, or area under the concentration-time curve, and concluded that differences in prednisolone bioavailability is not a factor in determining the dose required to control asthma.[7] Rose and colleagues compared the bioavailability of a single dose of 40 mg prednisolone intravenously in 7 severe corticosteroid-dependent asthmatic subjects and 13 healthy nonasthmatic volunteers.[8] Plasma prednisolone was measured by HPLC over an 8-h test period. They found no differences in plasma half-lives, apparent volumes of distribution, or concentration-dependent protein binding between the two groups. The apparent plasma clearances were 201 ± 54 and 198 ± 38 mL/min per 1.73 m^2 for the asthmatic and the normal groups, respectively. They concluded that the plasma protein binding, distribution, and clearance of prednisolone are not responsible for the large prednisolone requirement of corticosteroid-dependent asthmatics. Rose extended the above studies to corticosteroid-dependent and corticosteroid-resistant asthmatic children and again found no differences in bioavailability parameters.[5] Lane et al. have examined the pharmacokinetic profile of an oral dose of 40 mg prednisolone in asthmatics who were corticosteroid-sensitive (CS) or corticosteroid-resistant (CR) and nonasthmatic control subjects. Peak prednisolone concentrations (C_{max}) in plasma occurred at 1 h after the oral prednisolone dose.[9] The area under the concentration-time curve (AUC) in the CS group was 2778 ± 374 h/ng per mL (mean ± SEM) and 2510 ± 206 h/ng per mL (mean ± SEM) in the CR group ($p = .92$). Estimated clearance values were 155 ± 8 mL/min per 1.73 m^2 (mean SEM) in the CS group and 157 ± 17 mL/min per 1.73 m^2 (mean ± SEM) in the CR group ($P = .9$). There was no significant difference in AUC, C_{max}, and estimated clearance values between the normal group studied (2089 ± 124 h/ng per mL, 595 ± 15 ng/mL and 188 ± 7 mL/min per 1.73 m^2, respectively) and each of the asthmatic groups. Clinical corticosteroid resistance in asthmatic subjects thus is not reflected in any gross abnormality of the absorption or elimination of prednisolone. These data are consistent with pharmacokinetic studies carried out in CR asthma by other groups, which observed no differences in estimated clearance values of a single dose of oral prednisolone between well-characterized CR and CS asthmatic subjects.[10,11]

The Glucocorticoid Receptor

Glucocorticoids mediate their effects through soluble receptor proteins that act by transcriptionally regulating a small number of target genes.[12] In vivo binding to ligand is the only known event that converts the glucocorticoid receptor (GR) to a transcriptionally competent factor. The GR receptor complex is a 300 kDa phosphoprotein complex that has been shown by immunocytochemical techniques to be located mainly in the cytoplasm in nearly all human cell types, including macrophages, lymphocytes, eosinophils, and neutrophils, and so can be considered an essential housekeeping protein. It has a receptor density (R_o) of 2000 to 30,000 binding sites per cell.[13,14] The R_o for monocytes and lymphocytes have been reported to range from 1 to 9×10^3 receptor sites per cell and the dexamethasone binding affinity (K_d) from 2 to 8 nmol/L.[15–17] Maximal specific saturation of nuclear translocated GRs occurs at 15 min and is maintained over a 60-min period in human monocytes. Lane and Lee showed that the dexamethasone K_d is 2.45 ± 0.58 nM (mean $\pm$ SEM) in CS asthmatics and 1.6 ± 0.35 nM (mean $\pm$ SEM) in the CR asthmatics (P = .14).[18] On this same study, the R_o was 3605 ± 984 (mean $\pm$ SEM) and 4757 ± 692 (mean $\pm$ SEM) binding sites per nucleus in the CS and CR groups, respectively.[18]

Knowledge of the nature of these receptors has increased following purification of the receptor protein by chromatographic and antibody isolation, identification of specific DNA recognition sites for the receptor, cloning of the cDNA for the receptor protein, and determination of its genomic structure.[19–21] Glucocorticoids enter the cell by passive diffusion where they bind the GR noncovalently by hydrophobic and hydrogen ion interactions. This results in a conformational change in the GR described as *activation.* This process modifies the receptor structure allosterically, whereupon the GR undergoes dephosphorylation, dissociates two 90-kDa–associated heat-shock proteins (HSP), forms dimers, and translocates to the nucleus in a temperature-dependent fashion (Fig. 55-2). In the nucleus the GR interacts with other transcriptionally active molecules and binds finally to sequences of DNA known as glucocorticoid response elements (GREs) in the promoter region of the glucocorticoid-responsive genes.

The GR belongs to a highly conserved superfamily of hormone-receptor proteins characterized by a remarkable overall structural unity with impressive functional diversity[12] (Fig. 55-3). The gene coding for the GR lies on chromosome 2 and contains a total of 10 exons and has a minimum size of 80 kb.[20] Exon 1 contains only an untranslated sequence, and the amino terminal residues are found in exon 2. The DNA-binding domain is encoded by exons 3 and 4 and the ligand-binding domain is formed from exons 5–9. The use of GR cDNA expression vectors has revealed that these hormone receptors are organized structurally into five homologous domains, each responsible for different functions and each with different degrees of conservation within the superfamily.[22,23] These are ligand and HSP90 binding, receptor dimerization, nuclear localization, DNA binding, and *trans*-activation of gene expression[24] (Fig. 55-3).

Deoxyribonucleic acid–binding is encoded by a central domain, which is the most highly conserved region of the receptor.[25] This is a cysteine-rich 70-amino-acid sequence that folds into two zinc finger motifs, each of them with a zinc atom tetrahedrically coordinated to four cysteines.[26,27] It corresponds to base-pair cDNA sequence 1333–1542. A Gly–Ser–Val sequence in the root of the N-terminal zinc finger determines hormone response specificity and binds as dimers to the major groove on the GRE.[28,29] The GR subfamily, which includes the androgen and progesterone receptors, has this amino acid sequence whereas the estrogen receptor subfamily has not. The C-terminal finger binds to a sugar-phosphate flanking sequence of the GRE and is possibly involved in receptor dimerization.

The corticosteroid-binding domain of the GR is located at the C-terminal end and is the next most-conserved region within the superfamily. It corresponds to base-pair cDNA sequence 1675–2466.[28] This region binds the ligand in a hydrophobic pocket and participates in several other functions including dimerization and nuclear translocation, and is the binding site for the two heat-shock proteins. It also contains a 30-amino-acid region that is involved in hormone-dependent transcriptional activation. The major *trans*-activating domain of the hGR has been identified at the N-terminal domain, which is independent of hormone binding.[29] The N-terminal domain is the least conserved within the superfamily and possesses a marked cell-type and promoter specificity. It also is the immunogenic site of the receptor. In the GR it corresponds to base-pair cDNA sequence 133–1333. The nuclear translocation domain is a short sequence resembling that of the SV40 tumor antigen.[30]

Interaction of the GR with Transcriptionally Active Molecules

When in the nucleus the GR interacts with other transcriptionally active molecules by direct protein interaction in order to affect gene transcription, after which the GR binds to (GREs) in the promoter regions of the glucocorticoid-responsive genes, resulting in enhancement or suppression of gene transcription.[31–33] A well-characterized transcription factor interaction with the GR is with the proinflammatory AP-1.[34,35] AP-1 is the heterodimeric product of Fos and Jun proteins and is formed in activated cells by overexpression of the c-*fos* proto-oncogene. AP-1 binds to its DNA binding site (the TRE or TPA responsive element, TGACTCA) in order to effect gene transcription of certain proinflammatory peptides (e.g., collagenase or alphafetoprotein). The induction of AP-1 is enhanced by the cytokines IL-2, TNF-α, TGF-β, FGF, and IDGF; PMA, anti-CD3, LTB$_4$, and A23187. Its induction in human monocytes is suppressed by IL-4 and IFN-γ at the transcriptional and posttranscriptional levels, respectively[36,37] (Fig. 55-4). AP-1 and GR mutually repress each others DNA-binding and transactivating functions by (1) direct protein-protein interaction between amino acid residues GR$_{440–553}$ and Fos$_{40–110}$ independently of DNA binding, and (2) by Fos-GR competition at mutually exclusive or overlapping DNA binding sites ("composite GRE").[38] It is interesting that AP-1, a central proinflammatory peptide, and GR, an central ligand-activated anti-inflammatory peptide, interact directly at these levels in order to reciprocally affect gene transcription. AP-1 is one of an increasing number of transcription factors that interfere with the GR at protein-protein and protein-DNA levels (e.g., NF$_K$B, CREB, and calreticulin.[33–35] It therefore is likely that eventual gene transcription by the GR is affected by the ratio of interacting proinflammatory and anti-inflammatory transcription factors present in the nucleii of inflamed cells. Glucocorticoids have been shown to have different actions in different cell types and depend on the presence of tissue specific steroid-responsive genes, on the presence or absence of inflammation in the tissue, and on the state of cellular differentiation.

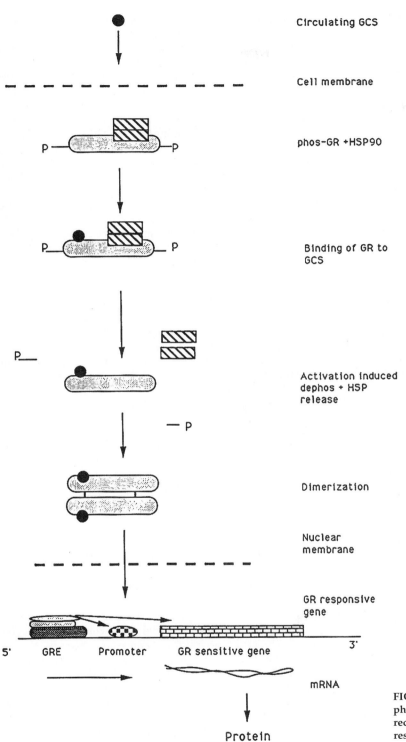

Circulating GCS

Cell membrane

phos-GR +HSP90

Binding of GR to GCS

Activation induced dephos + HSP release

Dimerization

Nuclear membrane

GR responsive gene

5'   GRE   Promoter   GR sensitive gene   3'

mRNA

Protein

FIGURE 55-2 Mechanism of glucocorticoid action. P, phosphate; HSP, heat-shock protein; GR, glucocorticoid receptor; GCS, glucocorticosteroid; GRE, glucocorticoid response element.

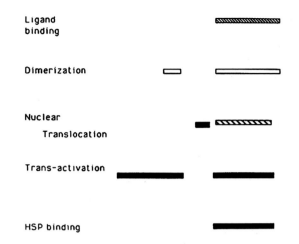

FIGURE 55-3 Structure-function of the glucocorticoid receptor.

Interaction of the GR with DNA

Based on the sequence of their DNA-binding motifs, two groups of steroid receptors can be distinguished: *group I receptors* recognize the motif 5'-TGACCT-3' as the 3' palindrome (estrogen, thyroid hormone, retinoic acid, and vitamin D receptors), whereas *group II receptors* (GR, mineralocorticoid, progesterone, and androgen receptors) bind to 5'-TGTCCT-3'.[39] Most GREs consist of two half-site hexamers separated by three base pairs, with a sequence resembling the consensus sequence GGTACA*nnn*TGTYCT (where *n* is any nucleotide and where Y = T or C).[40] In fact T is found in 65 percent of GREs. The 3' half-site of the con-

sensus GRE is more conserved among the various GREs than is the 5' counterpart, and a palindromic GRE maintained activated GRE-dependent transcription as well as did a consensus GRE. A systematic study on the effects of point mutations in the GRE revealed that changes of the T in position 3 are not tolerated, and that position 6 must be occupied by a pyrimidine.[41] GREs have been detected as close as 39 base pairs and as far away as 2.6 kb pairs downstream of the transcription initiation site. Binding of the GR to this sequence in vitro results in promoter enhancement or repression of subsequent gene transcription. GREs can modulate the expression of heterologous promoters in a distance- and orientation-independent manner.[42] The regulatory diversity of this single hGR-GRE interaction, however, is limited. These DNA recognition sites may be denoted "simple" GREs to distinguish them from the recently characterized "composite" GREs. Composite GREs do not contain the above consensus sequence and depend on protein-protein interactions between the GR and other transcription factors to achieve a combinatorial regulation on gene expression. Diamond has shown that the activity of composite GREs depends not only on the binding of GR but also on the binding of other nonreceptor transcription factors (e.g., the AP-1 complex).[31] The GR-GRE receptor complex was inactive in inducing in vitro transcription in the absence of AP-1 activity. The presence of the Jun/Jun homodimer conferred promoter enhancement while the Fos/Jun hetero-dimer conferred promoter repression. It is therefore fascinating that the Fos and Jun nonreceptor products conferred glucocorticoid responsiveness by novel protein-GRE binding in in vitro assays. Because of their regulatory versatility, composite GREs may prove to be the prevalent mode by which steroids regulate cytokine gene expression.

The effects of the GR on gene transcription depend critically on tissue-specific and activator-dependent interaction with *cis*-elements present in the promoter regions of these genes. For example, IL-8 gene transcription is enhanced by PMA, IL-1β, and TNF-α by interaction with its minimal enhancer region at –94 to –71 base-pair (bp) of the IL-8 promoter.[43–45] Dexamethasone directly suppresses this activation through its GRE (–330 to –325 bp) in a fibrosarcoma cell line but by transcriptional interference with the NF$_K$B recognition site (–80 to –69 bp) in a glioblastoma cell line independently of the GRE. Several mechanisms have been shown to result in direct *cis*-repression of genes by the GR.[39,40] First, the GR can neutralize the binding of a basal tissue specific enhancer. Second, the GR can interfere transcriptionally with other transcription factors, and vice versa, at a protein-protein level. Third, the GR can displace other transcription factors at overlapping DNA binding sites. Glucocorticoids also regulate cytokine gene expression at posttranscriptional levels. They can alter the stability of steady-state levels of specific cytokine mRNAs. Kern and colleagues have demonstrated that IL-1β gene transcription was unaffected by 10 μM dexamethasone in lipopolysaccharide-(LPS) stimulated human adhered monocytes using nuclear transcription run-off assays.[46] Posttranscriptionally, dexamethasone prolonged the IL-1β half-life, moderately inhibited the translation of its precursors, and profoundly inhibited its release into the extracellular fluid. The GR also

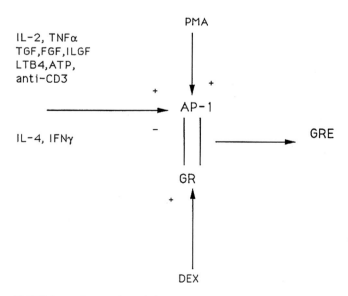

FIGURE 55-4 Interaction of the GR with AP-1 at the protein level. The GR becomes active transcriptionally in the presence of dexamethasone only. AP-1 is activated nonspecifically by PMA in addition to various cytokines and mediators. GR and the Fos component of AP-1 interact to influence reciprocally the effect of each other on gene transcription.

can regulate gene expression in a *trans* fashion (e.g., by the generation of lipocortins).[47] Glucocorticoids upregulate lipocortin expression at the transcriptional and posttranscriptional levels. In some in vitro systems lipocortins appear to mediate glucocorticoid-induced suppression of eicosanoid and prostanoid generation from arachidonic acid breakdown by noncompetitive inhibition of phospholipase A_2 (PLA_2) activity.[48] It has been shown, however, that although mitogen-driven lymphocyte proliferation was inhibited by the dexamethasone, this effect was independent of arachidonic acid breakdown, suggesting that the anti-inflammatory mechanism of the lipocortins is distinct from PLA_2 inhibition.[49] In addition, work by Davidson and Dennis has demonstrated that the effect of the lipocortins on PLA_2 inhibition in vitro can be overcome by increasing the concentration of phospholipid substrate.[50] Lipocortin has been shown to bind to the phospholipid substrate, indicating that the effects of lipocortin on PLA_2 inhibition may result from substrate depletion by lipocortin rather than by noncompetitive inhibition of PLA_2 and indeed suggests its effects may be artifactual.[50]

It therefore is evident that positive or negative regulation of gene expression is a complex and versatile system. Its efficiency is governed by (1) in vivo hormone binding to GR, which alters the kinetics of the subsequent GR-GRE interaction[51]; (2) protein-protein interaction of the GR with other nonreceptor transcriptional factors[34,52]; (3) GR-DNA interactions, which depend on the nature and quantity of GRE response elements[31]; (4) dimerization of the GR[53]; and (5) as yet undefined GRE-chromatin interactions, which determine the tissue and cell specificities of the glucocorticoids.[54]

References

1. Goodman S, Gilman A (eds): *The Pharmacological Basis of Therapeutics*, 4th ed. New York, Macmillan 1970:1604–42.
2. Funder JW, Pearce PT, Smith PT, Smith AI: Mineralocorticoid action: target tissue specificity is enzyme, not receptor, induced. *Science* 1988; 242:583–585.
3. Szefler SJ: General pharmacology of glucocorticoids, in Anti-inflammatory steroid action; basic and clinical aspects, New York Academic Press 1989:353–376.
4. Georgitis JW, Flesher KA, Szefler SJ. Bioavailability of a liquid prednisolone preparation. *J Allergy Clin Immunol* 1982; (70)4:243–247.
5. Rose JQ, Nickelson JA, Ellis EF, et al.: Prednisolone disposition in steroid-dependant asthmatic children. *J Allergy Clin Immunol* 1981; 67:188–193.
6. Rose JQ, Jusko WJ: Corticosteroid analysis in biological fluids by high performance liquid chromatography. *J Chromatogr* 1979; 162:273–280.
7. May CS, Caffin JA, Halliday JW, Bochner F: Prednisolone pharmacokinetics in asthmatic patients. *Br J Dis Chest* 1980; 74:91–92.
8. Rose RQ, Nickelson JA, Yurchak AM, et al.: Prednisolone disposition in steroid dependent asthmatics. *J Allergy Clin Immunol* 1980; 66:366–373.
9. Lane SJ, Palmer JBD, Skidmore IF, Lee TH: Corticosteroid pharmakokinetics in asthma. *Lancet* 1991; 336:1265.
10. Corrigan CJ, Brown PH, Barnes NC, et al.: Glucocorticoid pharmacokinetics, glucocorticoid receptor characteristics, and inhibition of peripheral blood T cell proliferation by glucocorticoids in vitro. *Am Rev Respir Dis* 1991; 144:1016–1025.
11. Alvarez J, Surs W, Leung DYM, et al.: Steroid resistant asthma: immunologic and pharmacologic features. *J Allergy Clin Immunol* 1992; 89:714–721.
12. Evans RE: The steroid and thyroid hormone receptor superfamily. *Science* 1988; 240:889–895.
13. Munck A, Mendel DB, Smith LI, Orti E: Glucocorticoid receptors and actions. *Am Rev Respir Dis* 1990; 141(suppl. part 2):S2–S10.
14. Miesfeld RL: The structure and function of steroid receptor proteins. *Crit Rev Biochem Mol Biol* 1989; 24(2):101–117.
15. Chrousos GP, Vingerhoeds A, Brandon D, et al.: Primary cortisol resistance in man. A glucocorticoid receptor-mediated disease. *J Clin Invest* 1982; 69:1261–1269.
16. Werb ZR, Foley R, Munck A: Interaction of glucocorticoids with macrophages: identification of glucocorticoid receptors in monocytes and macrophages. *J Exp Med* 1978; 147:1684–1694.
17. Lippman M, Barr R: Glucocorticoid receptors in purified subpopulations of human peripheral blood lymphocytes. *J Immunol* 1977; 118:1977–1981.
18. Lane SJ, Lee TH: Glucocorticoid receptor characteristics in monocytes of patients with corticosteroid resistant bronchial asthma. *Am Rev Respir Dis* 1991; 143:1020–1024.
19. Hollenberg SM, Weinberger C, Ong ES, et al.: Primary structure and expression of a functional human glucocorticoid receptor cDNA. *Nature* 1985; 318:635–641.
20. Encio IJ, Detera-Wadleigh SD: The genomic structure of the human glucocorticoid receptor. *J Biol Chem* 1991; 266(11):7182–7188.
21. Leclerc S, Xie B, Roy RN, Govindan MV: Purification of a human glucocorticoid receptor gene promoter-binding protein: production of polyclonal antibodies against the purified factor. *J Biol Chem* 1991: 266:8711–8719.
22. Carlstedt-Duke J, Stromstedt PE, Wrange O, et al.: Domain structure of the glucocorticoid receptor protein. *Proc Natl Acad Sci U S A* 1988; 84:4437–4440.
23. Giguere V, Hollenberg SM, Rosenfeld MG, Evans RM: Functional domains of the glucocorticoid receptor. *Cell* 1986; 46:645–652.
24. Wahli W, Martinez E: Superfamily of steroid nuclear receptors: positive and negative regulators of gene expression. *FASEB J* 1991; 5:2243–2249.
25. Archer TK, Hager GL, Omichinski JG: Sequence-specific DNA binding by glucocorticoid "zinc-finger peptides". *Proc Natl Acad Sci U S A*; 1990; 87(19):7560–7564.
26. Green S, Kumar V, Thenlaz I, et al.: The N-terminal DNA binding zinc finger of the estrogen and glucocorticoid receptors determines target gene specificity. *EMBO J* 1988; 7:3037–3044.
27. Luisi BF, Xu WX, Otwinowski Z, et al.: Crystallographic analysis of the interaction of the glucocorticoid receptor with DNA. *Nature* 1991; 352:497–505.
28. Carlstedt-Duke J, Stromstedt PE, Persson B, et al.: Identification of hormone interacting amino acid residues within the steroid binding domain of the glucocorticoid in relation to other steroid hormone receptors. *J Biol Chem* 1988; 263;6842–6846.
29. Hollenberg SM, Evans RM: Multiple and cooperative trans-activation domains of the human glucocorticoid receptor. *Cell* 1988; 55;899–906.
30. Kaderon D, Richardson W, Markham AF, Smith AE: Sequence requirements for nuclear localization of SV40 large T-antigen. *Nature* 1984; 311:33–38.
31. Diamond MI, Miner JN, Yoshinaga SK, Yamamoto KR: Transcription factor interactions: selectors of positive or negative regulation from a single DNA element. *Science* 1990; 249:1266–1272.
32. Yang-Yen HF, Chambard JC, Sun YL, et al.: Transcriptional interference between c-Jun and the glucocorticoid receptor: mutual inhibition of DNA binding due to direct protein-protein interaction. *Cell* 1990; 62:1205–1214.
33. Burns K, Duggan B, Atkinson BA, et al.: Modulation of gene

expression by calreticulin binding to the glucocorticoid receptor. *Nature* 1994; 367:476–480.

34. Kerrpola TK, Luk D, Curran T: Fos is a preferential target of glucocorticoid receptor inhibition of AP-1 activity in vitro. *Mol Cell Biol* 1993; 13:3782–3790.

35. Jonat J, Rahmsdorf HF, Park KK, et al.: Antitumor promotion and anti-inflammation: down modulation of AP-1 (fox/jun) activity by glucocorticoid hormone. *Cell* 1990; 62:1189–1204.

36. Dokter WHA, Esselink MT, Halie MR, Vellenga E: Interleukin-4 inhibits the liposaccaride-induced expression of c-*jun* and c-*fos* mRNA and AP-1 binding activity in human monocytes. Blood 1993; 81:337–343.

37. Radzioch D, Varesio L: c-*fos* mRNA expression in macrophages is downregulated by interferon-γ at the post-transcriptional level. *Mol Cell Biol* 1991; 11(5):2718–2722.

38. Tsai SY, Srinivasan G, Allan GF, et al.: Recombinant human glucocorticoid receptor induces transcription of human response genes in vitro. *J Biol Chem* 1990; 265:17055–17061.

39. Gronemeyer H: Control of transcription activation by steroid hormone receptors. *FASEB J* 1992; 2524–2529.

40. Beato M: Gene regulation by steroid hormones. Cell 1989; 56:335–344.

41. Martinez E, Givel F, Wahli W: A common ancestor DNA motif for invertebrate and vertebrate hormone response elements. *EMBO J* 1991; 10:263–268.

42. Venkatesh VC, Ballard PL: Glucocorticoids and gene expression. *Am J Respir Cell Mol Biol* 1991; 4:301–303.

43. Mukaido N, Morita M, Ishikawa Y, et al.: Novel mechanism of glucocorticoid-mediated gene repression; NF$_K$B is target for glucocorticoid-mediated gene IL-8 gene repression. *J Biol Chem* 1994; 269:13289–13295.

44. Mukaido N, Mahe Y and Matsushima K: Cooperative interaction of NF$_K$B and *cis*-regulatory enhancer binding protein-like factor binding elements in activating the IL-8 gene by pro-inflammatory cytokines. *J Biol Chem* 1990; 265:21128–21133.

45. Mukaido N, Gussella GL, Kasahara T, et al.: Molecular analysis of the inhibition of IL-8 production by dexamethasone in a human fibrosarcoma cell line. *Immunology* 1992; 75:674–679.

46. Kern JA, Lamb RJ, Reed JC, et al.: Dexamethasone inhibition of interleukin 1 beta production by human monocytes. *J Clin Invest* 1988; 81:237–244.

47. Flower RJ: Lipocortin and the mechanism of action of glucocorticoids. *Br J Pharmacol* 1988; 94:987–1015.

48. Wallner BP, Mattaliano RJ, Hession C, et al.: Cloning and expression of human lipocortin-1, a phospholipase A2 inhibitor with potential anti-inflammatory activity. *Nature* 1986; 320:77–81.

49. Almawi WY, Sewell KL, Zanker B, et al.: Mode of action of the glucocorticosteroids as immunosuppressive agents. *Prog Leukocyte Biol* 1990; 10A:321–326.

50. Davidson FF, Dennis EA: Biological relevance of lipocortins and related proteins as inhibitors of phospholipase A2. *Biochem Pharmacol* 1989; 38:3645–3651.

51. Schauer M, Chalepakis G, Willman T, Beato M: Binding of hormone accelerates the kinetics of glucocorticoid and progesterone receptor binding to DNA. *Proc Natl Acad Sci U S A* 1989; 86(4):1123–1127.

52. Ptashne M: How eukaryotic transcriptional activators work. *Nature* 1988; 335:683–689.

53. Kumar V, Chambron P: The estrogen receptor bind tightly to its responsive element as a ligand induced homodimer. *Cell* 1988; 55:145–156.

54. Yamamoto KR: Steroid receptor regulated transcription of specific genes and specific gene networks. *Ann Rev Genet* 1985; 19:209–232.

Chapter 56

PHARMACOKINETICS/ ROUTE OF ADMINISTRATION

P. M. O'BYRNE

Glucocorticosteroids have been used to treat a variety of airway diseases since the early 1950s, following an initial study of Carryer and colleagues,[1] who reported the benefits of oral cortisone on ragweed pollen-induced hay fever and asthma. This was followed by a report by Gelfand,[2] who demonstrated clinical benefit from inhaled cortisone in a small group of patients with allergic or nonallergic asthma. Subsequently, a multicenter trial by the Medical Research Council in the United Kingdom in 1956 demonstrated improvement in acute severe asthma in a placebo-controlled trial,[3] and reports at that time described benefit in chronic asthma,[4] demonstrating the unequivocal benefit of glucocorticosteroids in asthma. Subsequently, both oral and inhaled corticosteroids have evolved into the most important and useful drugs currently available to treat asthma. They also have been used to treat a number of other airway diseases, including chronic obstructive pulmonary disease (COPD), sarcoidosis, allergic bronchopulmonary aspergillosis, and croup; however, because the most widespread, and best studied, use of glucocorticosteroids in the treatment of airway diseases is in the treatment of asthma, much of this chapter focuses on their application in that disease.

Pharmacokinetics of Glucocorticosteroids

Most of the actions of glucocorticosteroids—and almost certainly their anti-inflammatory activity—occur through activation of the glucocorticosteroid receptor (GCSr),[5] which is found in virtually all of the body's cells. Only one receptor type has been identified. The receptor, in the resting state, is bound to two molecules of heat shock protein (HSP)90, and one molecule of the immunophilin p59.[5] Binding of the glucocorticosteroid to the receptor disassociates the receptor from HSP90, resulting in a conformational change of the receptor complex. The steroid-receptor complex then binds to the promoter-enhancer regions of target genes, glucocorticosteroid response elements (GRE), resulting in upregulation or downregulation of the gene, and thereby of the gene product (Fig. 56-1). (See Chap. 55.)

The steroid-receptor complex can regulate gene product in at least four other ways (see Fig. 56-1)[6] [see Chap. 55]. First, the complex can bind directly, by protein-protein interaction, with the transcription factor, activator protein-1 (AP-1), which is unregulated during inflammation, thereby inhibiting the proinflammatory effects of a variety of

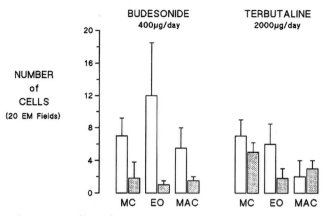

FIGURE 56-1 Effect of treatment with the inhaled glucocorticosteroid, budesonide, or the inhaled β₂-adrenergic agonist, terbutaline, on numbers of mast cells (MC), eosinophils (EO), and macrophages (MAC) in airway biopsies from asthmatic subjects. Budesonide, but not terbutaline, reduced the numbers of inflammatory cells in the airway biopsies. *(From Jeffery et al.,[56] with permission).*

cytokines.[7] Second, the complex can bind to a GRE that overlaps the upregulatory site for another proinflammatory product (i.e., a cytokine).[8] Third, the complex is known to reduce the availability of another important transcription factor for cytokine production, NFkB.[9] Lastly, glucocorticosteroids can increase the levels of cell ribonucleases, thereby reducing the levels of mRNA.[10]

ABSORPTION AND FATE OF GLUCOCORTICOSTEROIDS

Cortisone was the first glucocorticosteroid developed for clinical application in the early 1950s. Before the end of that decade, hydrocortisone, prednisolone, methylprednisolone, prednisone, triamcinolone, and dexamethasone were developed and were in clinical use. Cortisone and prednisone are prodrugs, which require hydroxylation in the liver to the active compounds hydrocortisone and prednisolone. All of these glucocorticosteroids were advances over the parent compound, either with less affinity for the mineralocorticosteroid receptor, or with enhanced affinity for the GCSr, or improved uptake and metabolism. For example, the unsaturation of the 1-2 bond of the hydrocortisone skeleton produced prednisolone, which improved the stability in the liver and doubled its half-life ($T_{1/2}$). The binding affinity for the GCSr for prednisolone also is 12 times greater and for dexamethasone 25 times greater compared to hydrocortisone.[6] Most of these compounds still are widely used as the systemic glucocorticosteroids of choice in a variety of inflammatory diseases.

All of these compounds are absorbed readily across epithelial lining by diffusion. No active transport systems are required for glucocorticosteroid absorption. The oral bioavailability of the systemic glucocorticosteroids ranges from 60 percent for hydrocortisone to 90 percent for methylprednisolone. This difference does not reflect the ability of the drug to be absorbed across the gut epithelium, but rather the efficiency of the first-pass metabolism through the liver. All the systemically available glucocorticosteroids are metabolized by p450 systems in the liver, and their clearance rates can be altered by severe liver diseases and liver cirrhosis. The systemic $T_{1/2}$ also varies from 1.9 h for hydrocortisone to 4.4 h for dexamethasone.

In the 1960s, modification of the hydrocortisone skeleton produced glucocorticosteroids with topical selectivity for dermal application and the treatment of skin diseases. These were betamethasone valerate and beclomethasone dipropionate (BDP), which are highly lipophilic compounds, as indeed are dexamethasone and triamcinolone. These compounds were tried by inhalation in the treatment of asthma in the early 1970s.[11] Since then, BDP has been a mainstay of asthma treatment. Later, other lipophilic glucocorticosteroids—flunisolide, budesonide, and fluticasone propionate (FP)—were developed for the treatment of asthma and allergic rhinitis. The lipophilic glucocorticosteroids have two main advantages for topical use in the airways. They have a very high binding affinity for the GCSr, being at least 100 times greater than hydrocortisone. They also have a very efficient first-pass hepatic metabolism, resulting in very low oral bioavailability. The clearance rates for budesonide and fluticasone, for example, are very close to maximal hepatic clearance, and thus entirely limited by hepatic blood flow (approximately 1.5 L/min), and the resulting *oral bioavailability* resulting from gut absorption for budesonide is 11 percent[12] and for fluticasone is 1 percent.[13] This also means that the *systemic bioavailability* of these compounds results almost entirely from absorption across the lung epithelium, rather than from the gut epithelium.

CURRENTLY AVAILABLE INHALED CORTICOSTEROIDS

Currently, five topically active glucocorticosteroids are available by the inhaled route for the treatment of asthma. These are BDP, triamcinalone, flunisolide, budesonide, and FP (Figure 56-2). Their pharmacologic properties are shown in Table 56-1.

Beclomethasone 17α,21-dipropionate has been available by inhalation for the treatment of asthma since 1972.[11] It has all of the properties of the other lipophilic glucocorticosteroids; however, because of its early development, there is little pharmacokinetic information available on this compound. It is biotransformed to its active metabolite, beclomethasone monopropionate (BMP), in the liver, and the further metabolism of BMP appears to be slower than the newer topically active glucocorticosteroids, budesonide and FP.

Triamcinolone has also not been fully characterized with regard to its pharmacokinetics, and its oral bioavailability is not known. One study[14] has reported plasma levels after maximal plasma concentrations of (C_{max}) of 1.2, 2.3, and 4.5 nmoles/L after single inhaled doses of 400, 800, and 1600 µg, respectively. These are similar to the C_{max} achieved with budesonide and FP. Its plasma $T_{1/2}$ is 1.5 h after intravenous administration.[15] Triamcinalone has a moderate affinity for the GCSr.

Flunisolide has an oral bioavailability of 21 percent, indicating high first-pass liver metabolism. It has, however, a

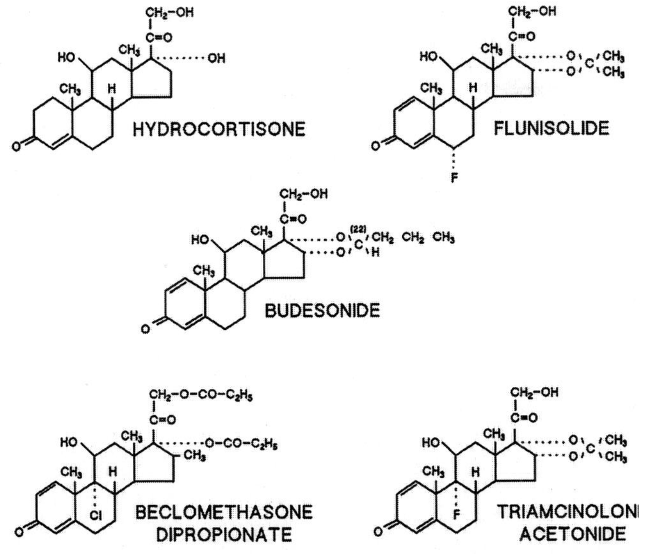

FIGURE 56-2 Structure of four inhaled glucocorticosteroids compared to the parent compound, hydrocortisone.

lower affinity for the GCSr, being 5 times lower than budesonide and 10 times lower than FP in human lung tissues. Its plasma $T_{1/2}$ after intravenous administration is 1.6 h, which is almost identical to the $T_{1/2}$ after inhalation of a single dose, indicating no lung metabolism.[16]

Budesonide has been the most extensively studied inhaled glucocorticosteroid for its pharmacokinetics.[17] Its oral bioavailability is 11 percent, indicating excellent first-pass liver metabolism; plasma clearance is 1.4 L/min, which is close to the maximal liver clearance. The plasma $T_{1/2}$ after intravenous administration is 3 h. After a single inhaled dose of 500 μg, the peak plasma levels achieved are within 30 min, and the $T_{1/2}$ is 2 h,[18] which suggests that there is little lung metabolism. Budesonide has a high binding affinity for the GCSr, which is 10 times that of dexamethasone.

Fluticasone propionate is the newest inhaled glucocorticosteroid available to treat asthma. Its oral bioavailability is 1 percent, which is the lowest of the available inhaled glucocorticosteroids. This is not only because of rapid first-pass liver metabolism, which is 0.87 L/min/1.73m^2, but also

because of poor absorption across the gut epithelium. The plasma $T_{1/2}$ after intravenous administration is 3 h.[19] To date, there is no information available about the pharmacokinetics after inhaled dosing. It has the highest binding affinity to the GCSr yet measured, being 18 times that of dexamethasone.

DOSE-RESPONSE CHARACTERISTICS OF INHALED GLUCOCORTICOSTEROIDS

Establishing the dose-response characteristics of the glucocorticosteroids in asthma has been difficult. This is mainly because the dose-response characteristics vary greatly among patients, and even vary in the same patient when the disease is mild and more severe. There also has been no general agreement about which outcome variable to measure or how long to wait after initiating treatment at any specific dose before measuring a response. This is quite different from, for example, examining the dose-response of an inhaled β$_2$-adrenergic agonist, where the outcome variable of improvement in forced expiratory volume in 1s (FEV$_1$) or peak expiratory flow (PEF) is standardized, and the response can be measured over minutes to hours. The maximal clinical benefit for an inhaled glucocorticosteroid can take 6 to 8 weeks to be achieved,[20] and for some physiologic parameters, such as improvements in airway hyperresponsiveness, can continue for 1 to 2 years.[21,22] For these reasons, there still is considerable debate as to whether a dose-response effect exists for inhaled glucocorticosteroids. Some studies have demonstrated a clinically useful benefit from increasing the inhaled doses twofold or fourfold,[23-26] whereas others have not.[27,28] It appears, from examining these studies, that patients with relatively mild asthma have a steep dose-response effect, achieving maximal benefit from doses of inhaled glucocorticosteroids, such as budesonide or BDP as low as 200 to 400 μg/day. By contrast, patients with more severe asthma often get clinical benefit from greater inhaled doses of 800 to 1600 μg/day. Several recent studies have also identified that, in both children and adults, once asthma control is achieved, the doses of inhaled glucocorticosteroids needed to maintain control are less.[29,30] Lastly, there are less common patients with very severe asthma, who do not achieve asthma control, even with inhaled doses of glucocorticosteroids greater than 2000 μg/day.

TABLE 56-1   Comparison of the Currently Available Inhaled Glucocorticosteroids to the Reference Glucocorticosteroid, Dexamethasone

	Relative Binding Affinity for Human GCSr	Topical Skin Blanching Potency	Clearance (L/min)	Half life (h)	Oral Bioavailability (%)
Dexamethasone	1	1	0.2	4.4	65
Beclomethasone	0.4/13	600	NA	NA	NA
Triamcinolone	3.6	330	1.4	1.5	NA
Flunisolide	1.8	330	1.8	1.6	21
Budesonide	9.4	980	4.3	2.8	11
Fluticasone	18.0	1200	3.5	3.1	1

ABBREVIATIONS: GCSr, glucocorticosteroid receptor; NA, information not available.
SOURCE: Adapted from Brattsand and Selroos.[6]

The dose frequency of inhaled glucocorticosteroids has been addressed in several studies. These studies have demonstrated that, in patients with moderate to severe asthma, four times daily administration of the inhaled glucocorticosteroids is better than the same total dose administered twice daily[31,32]; however, this benefit is less obvious in patients with milder asthma. An additional factor that must be considered is the compliance of the patient with four times daily dosing. For these reasons, twice daily dosing, morning and evening, generally is recommended for most asthmatics; however, if this does not achieve optimal asthma control, the same total dose delivered over four treatments may provide better control. In patients with mild asthma, once daily dosing, preferably in the evening, has been demonstrated to be effective.[33]

Routes of Administration

Glucocorticosteroids are administered either systemically (orally or intravenously) or topically (inhaled) to treat airway diseases. Systemic administration generally is reserved for patients with severe asthma, or as a trial of therapy to attempt to optimize lung function in patients thought to have a component of fixed airflow obstruction, or in patients with a mainly peripheral lung disease such as sarcoidosis. Glucocorticosteroids, such as prednisone or methylprednisolone, are rapidly and completely absorbed across the gastrointestinal tract and have a very high oral bioavailability. Therefore, intravenous glucocorticosteroids need only be used to treat airway diseases in exceptional circumstances, such as patients who cannot swallow or who are vomiting. Despite this, large doses of intravenous methylprednisolone (e.g., 125 mg intravenously three times daily) are recommended by most consensus documents on the treatment of acute, severe asthma in the emergency room.[34,35] The majority of severe exacerbations of asthma, however, can be adequately treated with oral prednisone (0.5 to 1 mg/kg/day, or its equivalent).

Inhaled glucocorticosteroids are the preferred route to treat airway diseases. This is because of the availability of topically potent glucocorticosteroids, which are very effective and have many fewer systemic unwanted effects than systemically administered glucocorticosteroids. This has been shown best in the studies of Toogood and colleagues,[36,37] who compared clinical equivalent doses of inhaled and oral glucocorticosteroids. These studies suggest that, in patients with moderate to severe asthma, inhaled glucocorticosteroids, such as BDP or budesonide, are as effective as much greater doses of oral glucocorticosteroids, with much less risk of systemic side effects. Indeed, one study suggested that inhaled budesonide 1000 μg/day is as effective at maintaining asthma control as 50 mg/day oral prednisone, but it has the potential risk of adverse events of 9 mg/day prednisone.[37]

Inhaled glucocorticosteroids can be delivered to the airways by a wide variety of inhaler systems, each of which has inherent advantages and disadvantages. These must be considered when making a choice of inhaler systems for a specific clinical circumstance because no currently available inhaler system is ideal in every clinical situation. Three main types of systems currently exist. These are pressurized metered-dose inhalers (pMDI), which has been the main delivery system in the past 20 years, dry powder systems, and wet nebulizers. The main advantages of pMDIs are their portability, ease of use (in a properly instructed and coordinated patient), low cost of manufacture, and low inspired flow rates needed to achieve lung dosing. The pMDIs also have a number of disadvantages, such as oropharyngeal deposition of drug, which results in up to 70 percent of the dose delivered from the pMDI being deposited in the oropharynx and 10 to 15 percent deposited in the lungs.[38] This oropharyngeal deposition greatly increases the risks of the development of oropharyngeal candidiasis. Also improper use by an uncoordinated patient is a major cause of lack of efficacy of the medications. These disadvantages can, however, be minimized by the use of a large volume spacer device. These devices greatly reduce oropharyngeal deposition,[39] and therefore total body dose of the inhaled glucocorticosteroid, and almost completely eliminates the risk of oral candidiasis.[40] Also, spacer devices reduce the need for coordination between activating the device and inspiration. For these reasons, patients using inhaled glucocorticosteroids delivered by a pMDI should always do so together with a spacer device. The contents of the pMDI for the different inhaled glucocorticosteroids contain different additives as propellants and stabilizers. Some pMDIs use oleic acid, which can cause bronchoconstriction when inhaled by some asthmatic subjects.[41] Another disadvantage of pMDIs that cannot be easily overcome, however, is the possibility that chlorofluorocarbons (CFCs), which are used as propellants in all pMDIs, will be proscribed by law in the future.

An advantage of the dry powder devices is that they do not use CFCs, but rather have just the drug being inhaled (in the case of the turbuhaler), or drug plus a filler, such as lactose. Many dry powder devices can be cumbersome to load and use and are single-dose devices or have few doses of drug without refilling. The exception is the budesonide turbuhaler, which comes with up to 200 doses in each device, is portable, and easy to use.[42] A potential disadvantage of dry powder systems is that patients need to generate inspired flow rates of ≥ 30 L/min to obtain optimal lung delivery. This is feasible in almost all patients, even those with very severe airflow obstruction.

Wet nebulizer devices have been used extensively to deliver bronchodilators to treat acute, severe asthma. There are solutions of some of the inhaled glucocorticosteroids, especially budesonide, which has been delivered by wet nebulizer, with clinical benefit in infants or very young children to treat asthma[43] and, more recently, croup.[44]

Clinical Use of Glucocorticosteroids

The vast majority of studies examining the efficacy and safety of glucocorticosteroids in airway diseases have been conducted in patients with asthma, and these drugs have the best established place in asthma therapy. For this reason, most of the information in this chapter focuses on asthma, but their usefulness in other airway diseases is also considered.

Asthma is a disease characterized by the presence of dyspnea, wheezing, chest tightness, and cough. These are usually caused by airflow obstruction, which is characteristically variable. Asthmatics also are known to have airway hyperresponsiveness to a variety of chemical bronchoconstrictor stimuli and physical stimuli, such as exercise and hyperventilation of cold dry air.[45] More recently, it has been recognized that asthma symptoms, variable airflow obstruction, and airway hyperresponsiveness occur as a consequence of a characteristic form of cellular inflammation and structural changes in the airway wall.[46] The inflammation consists of the presence of activated eosinophils, lymphocytes, and an increased number of mast cells, which have been described both in bronchoalveolar lavage fluid and airway biopsies from patients with mild stable asthma,[47–49] as well as asthmatic subjects with much more severe disease.[50] There also are characteristic structural changes described in asthmatic airways, which appear to be characteristic of the disease and which are likely caused by persisting airway inflammation.[50] These changes include patchy desquamation of the airway epithelium, thickening of the reticular collagen layer of the basement membrane,[51] and airway smooth muscle hypertrophy.[50]

Airway inflammation has been known to be present in asthmatic airways for more than 100 years[52]; however, only recently has an emphasis been placed on treating airway inflammation[53] rather than the consequences of the inflammation, which are bronchoconstriction and asthma symptoms.[54] The only anti-asthma medications that have been demonstrated to improve airway inflammation[55,56] (Fig. 56-3), airway hyperresponsiveness[57,58] (Fig. 56-4), airflow obstruction, and symptoms[59] in asthmatics are corticosteroids. This evidence provides a rationale for using inhaled corticosteroids much earlier in the treatment of asthma than

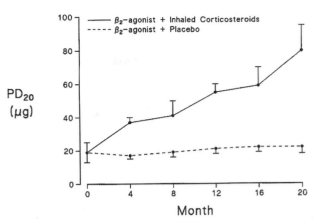

FIGURE 56-4 Effects of treatment with an inhaled β2-adrenergic agonist alone or together with an inhaled glucocorticosteroid on airway responsiveness in asthmatic children. Only treatment with the inhaled glucocorticosteroid improved airway responsiveness, and this effect continued over 22 months. (*From van Essen-Zandvliet et al,[21] with permission.*)

previously when they were often reserved as third- or fourth-line therapy for patients in whom bronchodilators were not providing control of asthma.[54] However, more recent evidence indicates that inhaled corticosteroids should be used early in managing asthma as the initial regular treatment in patients with daily symptoms.

OBJECTIVES OF ASTHMA MANAGEMENT

There have been several recent published consensus statements from a variety of countries on asthma management.[53,60–62] These documents have been remarkably consistent in identifying the goals and objectives of asthma treatment. These are:

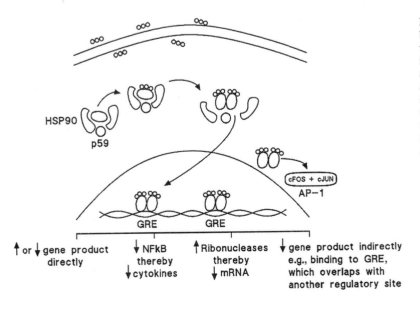

FIGURE 56-3 Diagrammatic representation of the binding of glucocorticosteroids to the GCSr complex, which disassociates into two molecules of HSP90, the immunophilin p59, and the activated GCSr, which attaches to the GRE, the DNA binding domains. The activated GCSr can also bind directly to the transcription factor AP-1, which prevents AP-1 binding to its recognition site on target genes. The activated GCSr can also upregulate or downregulate protein transcription through at least four other mechanisms, as demonstrated (also see text).

1. To minimize or eliminate asthma symptoms
2. To achieve the best possible lung function
3. To prevent asthma exacerbations
4. To do the above with the fewest possible medications
5. To educate the patient about the disease and the goals of management

One objective, which is implied but not explicitly stated, is the prevention of the decline in lung function and the development of fixed airflow obstruction, which occurs in some asthmatic patients.

In addition to these goals and objectives, each of these documents has identified what is meant by the term *asthma control*. This includes the above objectives of minimal or no symptoms and best lung function, but it also includes minimizing the need for rescue medications, such as inhaled β_2-adrenergic agonists to less than daily use, minimizing the variability of flow rates that is characteristic of asthma, as well as having normal activities of daily living. Achieving this level of asthma control should be an objective from the first visit of the patient to the treating physician.

Unfortunately, many studies suggest that this does not happen. This may be, in part, because the patient has learned to live with daily asthma symptoms and limitations in daily activities, and minimizes these to the physician. Alternatively, the idea of asthma control may not be widely accepted or understood by many physicians who see patients with asthma. This means that many (perhaps even most) patients with diagnosed asthma are not optimally controlled.

REASONS FOR EARLY INTERVENTION WITH INHALED GLUCOCORTICOSTEROIDS

Early intervention with inhaled corticosteroids in asthma means beginning this treatment as the first regular treatment used after a diagnosis is established. An argument for early intervention with inhaled corticosteroids could be made if one or more of the following conditions were met:

1. Inhaled corticosteroids were *more effective* than other regular treatment to achieve optimal asthma control and meet the other treatment objectives.
2. Inhaled corticosteroids prevented the decline in lung function over time that occurs in asthmatics.
3. Inhaled corticosteroids were safer than an *equally effective* treatment modality.
4. Inhaled corticosteroids were cost beneficial as an initial treatment of asthma, as measured by a benefit to the patient or to society by reducing the morbidity of asthma, which was not available by using any other medication.

Studies using inhaled corticosteroids have addressed all of these issues and these will be considered below.

Efficacy of Early Intervention with Inhaled Glucocorticosteroids

There is little debate in the literature that corticosteroids are the most effective treatment for asthma[63] or that the inhaled route is preferable to minimize unwanted effects. There is,

however, considerable debate over the early use of inhaled corticosteroids in asthmatic patients considered to have mild asthma.[64] These patients are usually treated with regular inhaled β_2-adrenergic agonists or oral theophylline or with drugs considered to be less clinically effective than inhaled corticosteroids, such as cromoglycate or nedocromil sodium. In a study of newly diagnosed asthmatics seen in specialty clinics, early intervention with the inhaled corticosteroid, budesonide, was shown to be an effective first-line treatment, when compared with an inhaled β_2-adrenergic agonist, as indicated by reduced symptoms, improvements in lung function, and improvements in methacholine airway hyperresponsiveness.[59] However, many patients considered to have mild asthma are not seen in specialty clinics but are managed in primary care practices. It is possible that these patients are, in fact, ideally controlled without the use of inhaled corticosteroids. To address this issue, the efficacy and cost benefit of inhaled corticosteroids, supplemented with bronchodilators as needed, has been compared to bronchodilators alone as first-line treatment of asthma in primary care practice.[20] This double-blind study compared budesonide 400 µg/day, budesonide 800 µg/day, and placebo in patients considered by their primary care physician to have such mild asthma that they would not derive any clinical benefit from inhaled corticosteroids. In this patient population in whom self-reported symptoms were mild at the start of the study, 40 to 60 percent of the patients were experiencing nocturnal or early morning symptoms in the month before entering the study. These symptoms suggest that asthma control was not optimal. The study demonstrated that inhaled budesonide 400 µg/day provided better asthma control and was cost beneficial when compared to bronchodilators alone in the management of these patients with mild asthma and that no differences could be demonstrated between 400 µg/day and 800 µg/day of budesonide; however, the study had insufficient power to detect differences between dosages, had they been present. The percentage of patients experiencing daily symptoms decreased to less than 10 percent over the course of the study in the budesonide treatment groups. There also was a mean 60 to 70 L/min increase in morning and evening peak expired flow rates, and an elimination of exacerbations of asthma requiring emergency room management, indicating that a clinically useful improvement was achieved in this patient population with a dose of budesonide as low as 400 µg/day. This study supports the early intervention with inhaled corticosteroids for adult patients with regular daily symptoms of asthma and suggests that low doses (budesonide 400 µg/day or possibly less) are effective in the management of asthmatic patients with mild to moderate asthma. In addition, the study reinforces the need to strive for optimal control of asthma and, once control is achieved, to identify the minimum amounts of medication needed to maintain control. Lastly, this study has demonstrated that inhaled corticosteroid treatment is more cost beneficial than asthma therapy with bronchodilators alone.

Another reason for recommending low doses of inhaled corticosteroids as first-line therapy for asthma is the recent concern about the safety of regularly administered inhaled

β_2-adrenergic agonists. Sears and coworkers[65] have demonstrated deterioration in a number of parameters of asthma control and reduced the time to an asthma exacerbation[66] when the inhaled β_2-adrenergic agonist, fenoterol, was used on a regular rather than intermittent basis. Retrospective studies have associated increased risk of asthma mortality with increased use of the β_2-adrenergic agonist, fenoterol,[67,68] and salbutamol.[68] Regular use of inhaled β_2-adrenergic agonists has been demonstrated to increase airway responsiveness in asthmatics[69,70] and to result in loss of functional antagonism to the bronchoconstrictor effects of inhaled methacholine[71] and adenosine monophosphate (AMP).[72]

Effects of Inhaled Glucocorticosteroids on Lung Function over Time

Asthmatics lose lung function more rapidly than nonasthmatics, although less rapidly than cigarette smokers. In occasional asthmatics, this leads to severe, permanent, fixed airflow obstruction, with all of the attendant disability and handicap associated with this condition. A number of recent studies in both adults and children have demonstrated that inhaled steroids provide a protective effect against the deterioration in lung function seen with prolonged regular use of inhaled bronchodilator therapy alone. In one study, patients with asthma and patients with COPD, previously treated with regular inhaled bronchodilators, were treated with inhaled beclomethasone 800 µg/day or placebo for 2 years.[73] Before the addition of inhaled corticosteroids, FEV_1 had been declining at a rate of 160 mL/year. In the first 6 months of corticosteroid therapy, the FEV_1 *increased* by 460 mL and then continued to decline at a rate of 100 mL/year (significantly less than with bronchodilators alone). This protective effect of inhaled corticosteroids was most marked in the asthmatic patients and was associated with significant improvement in methacholine-elicited airway hyperresponsiveness in the asthmatic patients only and with decreased asthma symptoms and exacerbations.

A second, recently reported study[30] has addressed this issue in a different way. These investigators had previously reported that the treatment of newly diagnosed asthmatics with inhaled budesonide 1200 µg/day for 2 years improved asthma control as indicated by reduced symptoms, improvements in lung function, and improvements in methacholine airway hyperresponsiveness, when compared to inhaled β_2-adrenergic agonists.[59] The subjects receiving budesonide were subsequently randomly allocated to continuing for a third year on a lower dose of inhaled budesonide (400 µg/day) or placebo. The improvements in all parameters were maintained on the lower dose of budesonide but were lost on placebo. The subjects who had previously been treated with inhaled β_2-adrenergic agonists only were treated with the greater dose of inhaled budesonide for the third year, and while they improved in all parameters when compared to the first 2 years of treatment, the improvement in lung function or methacholine airway hyperresponsiveness was significantly less than that achieved by the subjects treated for the first year of the study with inhaled budesonide (Fig. 56-5). This suggests that these asthmatics had lost lung func-

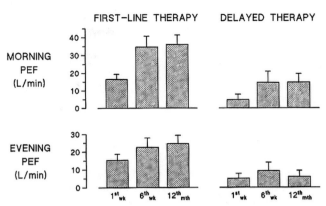

FIGURE 56-5 Comparison of the improvements in morning and evening peak expired flow (PEF) rates in asthmatic children treated with budesonide as first-line therapy within 1 year of diagnosis of asthma and patients treated more than 2 years after diagnosis. (*From Agertoft and Pedersen,[29] with permission.*)

tion that might have been preserved with the early use of inhaled corticosteroids.

A final study that supports these observations has been reported by Agertoft and Pedersen,[29] who studied two cohorts of asthmatic children for up to 7 years. One cohort was treated with inhaled corticosteroids shortly after diagnosis, whereas the other received a variety of other antiasthma medications, including cromones, theophylline, and regular inhaled β_2-adrenergic agonists, but not inhaled corticosteroids. Some children in the second cohort were converted to inhaled corticosteroids, but on average 5 years after an initial diagnosis. These children in whom treatment with inhaled corticosteroids was started later did not achieve the level of lung function of the children treated early, even after 3 years of treatment with inhaled corticosteroids. The study also measured growth velocity in these children and concluded that doses of inhaled budesonide up to 400 µg/day were not associated with a reduction in growth velocity.

These studies, taken together, indicate that inhaled corticosteroids can diminish the decline in lung function that occurs in asthmatics and suggest that early intervention with inhaled corticosteroids can optimize lung function in asthmatics.

Cost Benefit of Inhaled Glucocorticosteroids in Asthma

Until recently, few studies have examined the cost benefit of early intervention with inhaled corticosteroids. However, several recent studies have demonstrated that inhaled corticosteroids are cost beneficial when compared to other antiasthma treatments. For example, Ädelroth and Thompson,[74] have shown that the costs to the Swedish health-care system declined when patients were treated with inhaled corticosteroids because of a reduction in hospital utilization and physician visits when asthma control was optimized. In the study by Cuddy and associates,[20] a cost-effectiveness analysis of the use of inhaled corticosteroids in patients thought to have very mild asthma in primary care practice, demonstrated an advantage with inhaled corticosteroids; again, this resulted mainly from keeping patients out of hospital emergency rooms as asthma control improved.

INHALED GLUCOCORTICOSTEROIDS IN PREGNANCY

Asthma symptoms often improve during pregnancy, but in many patients asthma persists and can even worsen. Good asthma control is essential to achieve during pregnancy because the hypoxia of acute severe asthma is a great risk to the fetus. There are many years of experience of using inhaled glucocorticosteroids during pregnancy to treat asthma, and studies that have examined the incidence of prematurity or congenital malformations have shown no evidence of increased risk with the use of inhaled glucocorticosteroids.[75,76] Therefore, inhaled glucocorticosteroids should be used as clinically indicated to treat asthma during pregnancy.

INHALED GLUCOCORTICOSTEROIDS IN COPD

Patients with stable COPD vary greatly in their responses to systemic glucocorticosteroids. Most studies that have examined their effects in placebo-controlled trials have identified a small benefit, with some patients having a large, clinically useful improvement in lung function, whereas others obtain no benefit at all.[77,78] This means that all patients with newly diagnosed COPD should have a therapeutic trial with ingested glucocorticosteroids to establish whether they are in the "steroid-responsive" group.

The effects of inhaled glucocorticosteroids on improving or maintaining lung function in patients with COPD is even less clear. Studies have shown conflicting results, with some demonstrating no improvement in lung function[79,80]; others have shown improvements in some patients, but not others,[81,82] and one investigation demonstrated a reduction in the decline in FEV$_1$ with the use of inhaled glucocorticosteroids when compared to placebo.[73] Part of this confusion likely resulted because of the inclusion, in some studies, of patients with both asthma and COPD. However, taken together, the studies suggest that, as with the use of systemic glucocorticosteroids, some patients with COPD will benefit from inhaled glucocorticosteroids, whereas others will not, and it is not possible to distinguish the two groups of patients without an empirical therapeutic trial.

INHALED GLUCOCORTICOSTEROIDS IN SARCOIDOSIS [SEE ALSO CHAP. 112]

Sarcoidosis usually improves with treatment with systemic glucocorticosteroids, and they are the treatment of choice for patients with symptomatic lung disease, or pulmonary infiltrated or fibrosis, or for systemic manifestations of sarcoidosis.[83] Early efforts to treat pulmonary sarcoidosis with inhaled BDP were not successful. More recently, several placebo controlled studies have demonstrated that inhaled budesonide in doses from 1200 to 2400 μg/day were effective in maintaining improvements in symptoms and lung function that were achieved with systemic glucocorticosteroids used for 2 to 4 months.[84] Inhaled budesonide used

initially does not appear to achieve the rapidity of improvements seen with systemic glucocorticosteroids. Therefore, there is a role for inhaled glucocorticosteroids in maintaining improvements achieved with systemic glucocorticosteroids, thereby reducing the risks of systemic side effects of glucocorticosteroids. However, inhaled glucocorticosteroids cannot be used to treat the systemic manifestations of sarcoidosis, nor in patients with severe life-threatening disease.

INHALED GLUCOCORTICOSTEROIDS IN CROUP

Systemic glucocorticosteroids are effective in reducing the duration of intubation, and risk of reintubation, in children with severe croup.[88] More recently, nebulized budesonide has been demonstrated, in a double-blind, placebo-controlled trial, to improve stridor and cough in children with less severe disease.[44,89]

Side Effects of Glucocorticosteroids

Inhaled glucocorticosteroids are absorbed across the lung into the systemic circulation and have effects beyond the lungs. Concerns about their systemic unwanted effects have greatly limited their use, especially in children. There are anti-asthma medications, such as the cromones, which have virtually no systemic unwanted effects. However, these drugs are, in general, not as effective in achieving optimal asthma control as are inhaled glucocorticosteroids, nor have they been shown to prevent the decline in lung function in asthmatics.

The side effects of inhaled glucocorticosteroids are dose-related, with little or no evidence of clinically relevant systemic unwanted effects at doses of less than 400 μg/day of beclomethasone or budesonide in children and of less than 1000 μg/day in adults.[63] Fortunately, optimal asthma control can be achieved with these or lesser doses in the majority of asthmatics. Indeed, the studies of Haahtela and colleagues,[30] and Agertoft and Pedersen[29] have demonstrated that once optimal control is achieved by inhaled glucocorticosteroids, it can be maintained by much lower doses. Therefore, drugs that are as effective as inhaled glucocorticosteroids as first-line therapy of asthma and have fewer side effects do not currently exist.

LOCAL SIDE EFFECTS

The main side effects that occur with lower doses of inhaled glucocorticosteroids are oral candidiasis, because of the oropharyngeal deposition of the inhaled glucocorticosteroid, and dysphonia. Clinically obvious oral candidiasis occurs in 5 to 10 percent of adult asthmatics treated with inhaled glucocorticosteroids,[90] but in only 1 percent of children.[91] However, positive oropharyngeal cultures for Candida have been demonstrated in up to 45 percent of children and 70 percent of adults using glucocorticosteroids.[90] The risk of clinically obvious oral candidiasis is increased by the concomitant use of antibiotics and inhaled glucocorticosteroids and is greatly reduced by the use of a large volume spacer to deliver the inhaled glucocorticosteroid,[40] and by mouth rinsing after use. Clinically obvious candidiasis is easily treated by swishing and swallowing the antifungal agent, nystatin, twice daily for 3 to 5 days.

Dysphonia is a more common topical side effect of inhaled glucocorticosteroids, which has been reported to occur in up to 30 percent of patients.[90] It is more common in patients who use their voices a lot, is sometimes temporary, and is only really troublesome in patients who are using their voice to earn their income. The incidence can also be reduced by the use of a spacer device.[92]

Glucocorticosteroids applied topically to the skin cause skin thinning and atrophy. This is because the glucocorticosteroid remains on the skin for several hours. By contrast, inhaled corticosteroids are rapidly absorbed across the airway mucosa and are unlikely to have this effect on the airway mucosa. Indeed, several investigations have studied airway biopsies of asthmatics who have been using inhaled glucocorticosteroids for months or years and have not demonstrated evidence of airway mucosal atrophy,[93] but rather repair of the epithelial damage that is a characteristic feature of asthma.[94]

SYSTEMIC SIDE EFFECTS

Doses of inhaled glucocorticosteroids of greater than 400 μg/day of beclomethasone or budesonide in children and greater than 1000 μg/day in adults result in unwanted systemic side effects, such as changes in growth velocity in children, and biochemical changes indicating effects on bones and the adrenal glands in adults. All physicians who treat asthmatics should be conscious of the potential for the development of the types of adverse effects that occur in patients who use ingested glucocorticosteroids to treat asthma or other diseases. These adverse effects of ingested glucocorticosteroids are discussed below.

EFFECTS OF THE HYPOTHALAMIC-PITUITARY-ADRENAL (HPA) AXIS   The effects of glucocorticosteroids on the HPA axis can be measured in a number of different ways. The most common used, easiest to obtain, but least sensitive method has been the measurement of early morning serum cortisol levels. Much more sensitive measurements to the effects of excess glucocorticosteroids on the HPA axis are 24-h urinary cortisol or the short tetracosactrin (ACTH) stimulation test.[95]

The different inhaled glucocorticosteroids are not equal in their effect on the HPA axis. For example, in children, a dose-dependent effect on urinary cortisol concentration has been demonstrated with doses of BDP from 200 to 800 μg/day.[96] By contrast, 400 μg/day budesonide does not cause any effect on urinary cortisol, even when used for up to 1 year.[97] In adults, many studies have examined the effects of inhaled glucocorticosteroids on HPA axis function, and there is no convincing evidence that doses of BDP < 500 μg/day or budesonide < 600 μg/day have any measurable effect on the HPA axis[98–100] (Fig. 56-6). The measurable effects seen with greater doses clearly indicate systemic activity of the inhaled glucocorticosteroid, but are of questionable clinical

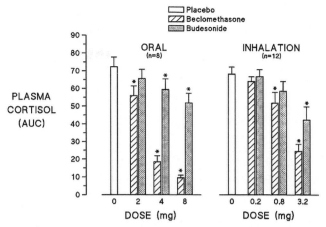

FIGURE 56-6 Effects of treatment with increasing doses of either oral or inhaled beclomethasone or budesonide on adrenal function in normal volunteers. Equivalent doses of budesonide had less effect on plasma cortisol concentrations than beclomethasone. (*From Johansson et al.,*[99] *with permission.*)

significance. There are only two case reports of clinically evident adrenal insufficiency in patients who have been treated with only inhaled glucocorticosteroids after the inhaled glucocorticosteroid has been withdrawn. These were an adult, who was treated with a very high dose of inhaled budesonide (6400 μg/day)[101] and a child who was using much lower doses (250 μg/day).[102]

OSTEOPOROSIS   This is an important complication of the use of ingested glucocorticosteroids, particularly in high-risk patients, such as postmenopausal women.[103] This occurs through an increase in bone resorption and a decrease in bone formation and results in increased risk of bone fractures, especially hip and spine. Inhaled corticosteroids have been demonstrated to have effects on bone metabolism, although there is little evidence that, at the conventional doses, they cause osteoporosis and no evidence that they cause increased risk of fractures.

The effects of inhaled glucocorticosteroids on bone metabolism have been demonstrated by measuring serum osteocalcin, which measures changes in bone formation, and urinary hydroxyproline, measured after a 12-h fast, which is increased with increased bone resorption. Pyridium cross-links in urine is another measure of bone resorption and has the advantage over urinary hydroxyproline of not being dietary dependent; however, to date, the effects of inhaled glucocorticosteroids on this measure of bone resorption have not been reported.

The effects of BDP and budesonide on serum osteocalcin and urinary hydroxyproline have been studied in adults. Both have been shown to influence serum osteocalcin concentration in a dose-dependent manner,[104,105] but only BDP increases urinary hydroxyproline excretion at doses up to 2000 μg/day.[104] In children, doses of budesonide up to 800 μg/day[106] and of fluticasone of up to 200 μg/day[107] have no effect on any biochemical marker of bone turnover.

Bone densitometry has been measured in adult asthmatics over a 2-year period while these patients were taking varying doses of inhaled BDP (mean dose 630 μg/day).[108] This study suggested that these patients had no increase in bone loss. To date, there also are no studies that have demonstrated that these biochemical markers of bone turnover are associated with increased risk of bone fracture.

POSTERIOR SUBCAPSULAR CATARACTS   These occur more frequently in patients taking oral glucocorticosteroids, and this greatly complicates the issue of whether they occur with greater frequency in patients using inhaled glucocorticosteroids. The available studies in adults[109] and children[110] suggest that once the confounding effect of ingested glucocorticosteroids is removed, there is no evidence that inhaled glucocorticosteroids increase the risk of developing posterior subcapsular cataracts.

GROWTH RETARDATION IN CHILDREN   Growth retardation with the use of inhaled glucocorticosteroids is a major reason that these drugs are used sparingly, perhaps even underused, to treat asthma in children. There is little doubt that systemic glucocorticosteroids can stunt growth in children and that this effect is usually permanent.[111] Resolving this issue for inhaled glucocorticosteroids in asthmatic children has been exceedingly difficult. This is in part because asthmatic children do not have the same growth patterns as nonasthmatic children. Many asthmatic children have delayed onset of puberty, and this effect appears more severe in children with severe asthma.[112] However, these children eventually catch up with their nonasthmatic peers and achieve normal height.[112,113] Thus, studying asthmatic children and comparing them to nonasthmatic controls may not be appropriate. Studies examining growth in children also need to be continued over several years because individual children have very different growth patterns. Almost all longitudinal studies of growth in asthmatic children treated with inhaled glucocorticosteroids indicate that daily doses of BDP or budesonide ≤ 800 μg/day do not stunt growth.[112–114]

A surrogate method for measuring growth in children is knemometry, which measures short-term linear growth in the lower leg in children. This method is extremely sensitive to the systemic effects of glucocorticosteroids. Daily doses of 2.5 mg prednisone can totally inhibit lower leg growth (Fig. 56-7).[115] By contrast, 400 μg/day inhaled budesonide has no effect on knemometry measurements,[116] whereas daily doses of 800 μg/day of budesonide,[116] 400 μg/day of BDP, or 200 μg/day fluticasone cause significant inhibition[117] (see Fig. 56-7). The clinical correlation of these measurements is not known; however, this very sensitive marker of systemic glucocorticosteroid activity may be useful for establishing the largest dose of inhaled glucocorticosteroids that has no systemic activity in children.

METABOLIC EFFECTS   Altered glucose and lipid metabolism occurs with ingested glucocorticosteroids, but clinically relevant effects have not been demonstrated with doses of BDP or budesonide ≤ 2000 μg/day.[105,118]

STEROID PSYCHOSIS   This may occur in as many as 2 percent of patients treated with systemic glucocorticosteroids and has been reported to occur very occasionally in patients taking inhaled glucocorticosteroids. Data on eight patients have been reported thus far; they developed symptoms within days of being treated with either inhaled BDP or budesonide.[119,120] The psychosis resolved promptly after stopping the inhaled glucocorticosteroid.

RISKS OF LUNG INFECTION   These are not increased in patients using inhaled glucocorticosteroids.[121] Inhaled glucocorticosteroids also do not increase the risks of reactivation of pulmonary tuberculosis, and therefore prophylactic isoniazid treatment is not needed in patients with inactive pulmonary tuberculosis, who receive inhaled glucocorticoids.

SKIN BRUISING   Bruising occurs as a dose-dependent side effect of inhaled glucocorticosteroid use. It is rare at daily

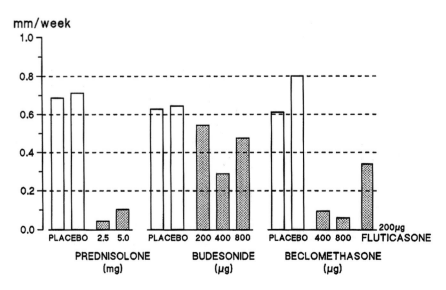

FIGURE 56-7 Effect of inhaled glucocorticosteroids on growth in children. Lower leg growth (mm/week) assessed by knemometry in three different studies. In one study, daily doses of 2.5 and 5 mg prednisolone by mouth were compared to placebo. In a second study, 200, 400, and 800 μg budesonide daily were compared with placebo. In a third study, 200 μg fluticasone propionate was compared with 400 and 800 μg beclomethasone dipropionate daily. (*From Barnes and Pedersen,*[63] *with permission.*)

doses of less than 1000 μg/day, and its incidence increases with age and duration of treatment. In one study of older patients receiving large doses of BDP, the prevalence of easy bruising was 47 percent for those on inhaled glucocortico-steroids versus 22 percent for those who were not.[122]

Conclusions

Inhaled corticosteroids are the most effective medications currently available to treat symptomatic asthma, and are, fortunately, free of clinically relevant unwanted effects, when used in the doses needed to provide optimal control in most asthmatic patients. Inhaled corticosteroids also improve the physiologic abnormalities of variable airflow obstruction and airway hyperresponsiveness that character-ize asthma, as well as reducing the decline in lung function over time that occurs in asthmatics. Inhaled corticosteroids are also cost beneficial when compared to other treatments, even in patients with milder asthma, treated in primary care settings. For these reasons, inhaled corticosteroids should be considered the first-line therapy for patients with regular, daily asthma symptoms and should be started early after a diagnosis is made, rather than delaying until all other treat-ment options have been tried and not provided optimal con-trol of asthma.

Inhaled glucocorticosteroids also have a role in the man-agement of other airway diseases, such as COPD in some patients, in the maintenance treatment of sarcoidosis, and in the management of croup.

There are, however, several issues about the early inter-vention with inhaled corticosteroids that have not yet been resolved. One such issue is whether inhaled corticosteroids should be used in asthmatic patients who have very mild and infrequent symptoms, or who develop symptoms only after being exposed to an inciting stimulus, such as exercise or cold air, and who have normal airway caliber most of the time. The current consensus statements do not recommend regular treatment in such patients, and this recommendation should remain until more information is available about the natural history of asthma in such patients. These very mild asthmatics do have evidence of airway inflammation and structural changes in airway biopsies[47–49]; however, it is not yet known whether they lose lung function more rapidly than nonasthmatics, or whether the morbidity of having very mild asthma warrants the use of regular treatment. The long-term effects of small doses of inhaled corticosteroids also is not fully defined. Although the studies of Agertoft and Pedersen[29] have provided details of up to 7 years of treatment on some of the potential unwanted effects in chil-dren, these studies will need to be extended further before the concerns and fears of using inhaled corticosteroids very early in asthma can be allayed.

References

1. Carryer HM, Koelsche GA, Prickman LE, et al.: The effect of cortisone on bronchial asthma and hay fever occurring in sub-jects sensitive to ragweed pollen. *J Allergy* 1950; 21:282.

2. Gelfand ML: Administration of cortisone by the aerosol method in the treatment of bronchial asthma. *N Engl J Med* 1951; 245:293.

3. Medical Research Council: Controlled trial of effects of corti-sone acetate in status asthmaticus. *Lancet* 1956; ii:803.

4. Foulds WS, Greaves DP, Herxheimer H, Kingdom LG: Hydrocortisone in treatment of allergic conjunctivitis, allergic rhinitis, and bronchial asthma. *Lancet* 1955; i:234.

5. Muller M, Renkawitz R: The glucocorticoid receptor. *Biochem Biophys Acta* 1991; 1088:171.

6. Brattsand R, Selroos O: Glucocorticosteroids, in Page CP, Metzger WK (eds): *Drugs and the Lung*. New York, Raven, 1994:101–220.

7. Schule R, Rangarajan P, Kliewers S, et al: Functional antagonism between oncogene c-*jun* and the glucocorticoid receptor. *Cell* 1990; 62:1217.

8. Ray A, Laforge KS, Sehgal PB: On the mechanisms of efficient repression of the interleukin-6 promoter by glucocorticoids: enhancer TATA box and RNA start site occlusion. *Mol Cell Biol* 1990; 10:5736.

9. Adcock IM, Gelder CM, Shirasaki H, et al.: Effects of steroids on transcription factors in human lung. *Am Rev Respir Dis* 1992; 145:A834.

10. Tobler A, Meier R, Seitz M, et al.: Glucocorticoids down-regu-late gene expression of GM-CSF, NAP-1/IL-8 and IL-6, but not M-csf in human fibroblasts. *Blood* 1992; 79:45.

11. Morrow-Brown H: The introduction and early development of inhaled steroid therapy, in Myging N, Clark TJH (eds): *Topical Steroid Treatment for Asthma and Rhinitis*. London, Balliere Tindall, 1980:66–76.

12. Ryffeldt A, Andersson P, Edsbacker S, et al.: Parmacokinetics and metabolism of budesonide, a selective glucocorticoid. *Eur J Respir Dis* 1982; 63:86.

13. Harding S: The human pharmacology of fluticasone propi-onate. *Respir Med* 1990; 84:25.

14. Zaborny BA, Lukacsko P, Barinov-Colligon I, Ziemniak JA: Inhaled corticosteroids in asthma: a dose-proportionality study with triamcinolone acetonide aerosol. *J Clin Pharmacol* 1992; 32:463.

15. Mollman H, Rohdewald P, Schmidt EW, et al.: Pharmaco-kinetics of triamcinolone acetonide and its phosphate ester. *Eur J Clin Pharmacol* 1985; 29:85.

16. Chaplin MD, Rooks W, Svenson EW, et al.: Flunisolide metabo-lism and dynamics of a metabolite. *Clin Pharmacol Ther* 1980; 27:402.

17. Brogden RN, McTavish D: Budesonide: An updated review of its pharmacological properties and therapeutic efficacy in asthma and rhinitis. *Drugs* 1992; 44:375.

18. Pedersen S, Steffensen G, Ekman I, et al.: Pharmacokinetics of budesonide in children with asthma. *Eur J Clin Pharmacol* 1987; 31:579.

19. Harding SM: The human pharmacology of fluticasone dipropi-onate. *Respir Med* 1990; 84:25.

20. Cuddy L, Taylor DW, Birch S, et al.: The clinical efficacy of inhaled corticosteroids as first line therapy for asthma in pri-mary care practice. *Am Rev Respir Dis* 1992; 145:A420.

21. van Essen-Zandvliet EE, Hughes MD, Waalkens HJ, et al.: Effects of 22 months of treatment with inhaled corticosteroids and/or beta2-agonists on lung function, airway responsiveness and symptoms in children with asthma. *Am Rev Respir Dis* 1992; 146:547.

22. Juniper EF, Kline PA, Vanzieleghem MA, et al.: Effect of long-term treatment with inhaled corticosteroids on airway hyperre-sponsiveness and clinical asthma in nonsteroid dependent asthmatics. *Am Rev Respir Dis* 1990; 142:832.

23. Gaddie J, Petrie GR, Reid IW, et al.: Aerosol beclomethasone

dipropionate: a dose-response study in chronic bronchial asthma. *Lancet* 1973; ii:280.

24. Costello JF, Clark TJH: Responses of patients receiving high doses of beclomethasone dipropionate. *Thorax* 1974; 29:571.

25. Toogood JH, Lefcoe NM, Haines DSM, et al.: A graded dose assessment of the efficacy of beclomethasone dipropionate aerosol for severe chronic asthma. *J Allergy Clin Immunol* 1977; 59:298.

26. Ellul-Micallef R, Johansson SA: Acute dose-response studies in bronchial asthma with a new corticosteroid, budesonide. *Br J Clin Pharmacol* 1983; 15:419.

27. Brompton Hospital/Medical Research Council: Double blind trial comparing two dosage schedules of beclomethasone dipropionate aerosol with placebo in chronic bronchial asthma. *Br J Dis Chest* 1979; 73:121.

28. Boe J, Rosenhall L, Alton M, et al.: Comparison of dose-response effects of inhaled beclomethasone dipropionate and budesonide in the management of asthma. *Allergy* 1989; 44:349.

29. Agertoft L, Pedersen S: Effects of long-term treatment with an inhaled corticosteroid on growth and pulmonary function in asthmatic children. *Respir Med* 1994; 88:373.

30. Haahtela TH, Jarvinen M, Kava T, et al.: Effects of reducing or discontinuing inhaled budesonide in patients with mild asthma. *N Engl J Med* 1994; 331:700.

31. Malo JL, Cartier A, Merland N, et al.: Four times-a-day dosing frequency is better than twice-a-day regimes in subjects requiring a high dose inhaled steroid, budesonide, to control moderate to severe asthma. *Am Rev Respir Dis* 1989; 140:624.

32. Toogood JH: An appraisal of the influence of dose frequency on the antiasthmatic activity of inhaled corticosteroids. *Ann Allergy* 1985; 55:49.

33. Campbell LM, Watson DG, Venables TL, et al.: Once daily budesonide turbuhaler compared to placebo as initial prophylactic therapy for asthma. *Br J Clin Res* 1991; 2:111.

34. British Thoracic Society: Guidelines for management of asthma in adults: acute severe asthma. *BMJ* 1990; 301:797.

35. Hargreave FE, Dolovich J, Newhouse MT, et al.: The assessment and treatment of asthma: a conference report. *J Allergy Clin Immunol* 1990; 85:1098.

36. Toogood JH, Baskerville JC, Errington N, et al.: Determinants of the response to beclomethasone aerosol at various dosage levels: a multiple regression analysis to identify clinically useful predictors. *J Allergy Clin Immunol* 1977; 60:367.

37. Toogood JH, Baskerville JC, Jennings B, et al.: Bioequivalent doses of budesonide and prednisone in moderate and severe asthma. *J Allergy Clin Immunol* 1989; 84:688.

38. Newman SP, Pavia D, Morem F, et al.: Deposition of pressurized aerosols in the human respiratory tract. *Thorax* 1981; 36:52.

39. Toogood JH, Baskerville JC, Jennings B, et al.: Use of spacers to facilitate inhaled corticosteroid treatment of asthma. *Eur J Respir Dis* 1984; 129:723.

40. Salzman GA, Pyszcynski DR: Oropharyngeal candidiasis in patients treated with beclomethasone dipropionate delivered by metered-dose inhaler alone and with Aerochamber. *J Allergy Clin Immunol* 1988; 81:424.

41. Engel T: Patient related side-effects of CFC propellants. *J Aerosol Med* 1991; 4:163.

42. Engel T, Heinig JH, Malling HJ, et al.: Clinical comparison of inhaled budesonide delivered either via pressurized metered dose inhaler or turbuhaler. *Allergy* 1989; 44:220.

43. Lodrup Carlsen KC, Nikander K, Carlsen K-H: How much nebulized budesonide reaches infants and toddlers? *Arch Dis Child* 1992; 67:1077.

44. Klassen TP, Feldman ME, Watters LK, et al.: Nebulized budesonide for children with mild-to-moderate croup. *N Engl J Med* 1994; 331:285.

45. Hargreave FE, Ryan G, Thomson NC, et al.: Bronchial responsiveness to histamine or methacholine in asthma: measurement and clinical significance. *J Allergy Clin Immunol* 1981; 68:347.

46. Djukanovic R, Roche WR, Wilson JW, et al.: State of the art: mucosal inflammation in asthma. *Am Rev Respir Dis* 1990; 142:434.

47. Kirby JG, Hargreave FE, Gleich GJ, O'Byrne PM: Bronchoalveolar cell profiles of asthmatic and nonasthmatic subject. *Am Rev Respir Dis* 1987; 136:379.

48. Beasley R, Roche WR, Roberts JA, Holgate ST: Cellular events in the bronchi in mild asthma and after bronchial provocation. *Am Rev Respir Dis* 1989; 139:806.

49. Jeffery PK, Wardlaw AJ, Nelson FC, et al.: Bronchial biopsies in asthma: An ultrastructural, quantitative study and correlation with hyperreactivity. *Am Rev Respir Dis* 1989; 140:1745.

50. Dunnill MS, Massarell GR, Anderson JA: A comparison of the quantitive anatomy of the bronchi in normal subjects, in status asthmaticus, in chronic bronchitis and in emphysema. *Thorax* 1969; 24:176.

51. Roche WR, Beasley R, Williams JH, Holgate ST: Subepithelial fibrosis in the bronchi of mild asthmatics. *Lancet* 1989; i:520.

52. Osler W: *The Principals and Practice of Medicine.* New York, Appleton, 1892:497.

53. National Heart, Lung, and Blood Institute, National Institutes of Health: Guidelines for the diagnosis and management of asthma. US Department of Health and Human Services Publication No. 91-3042, 1991.

54. Rebuck AS, Chapman KR: Asthma: II. Trends in pharmacologic therapy. *Can Med Assoc J* 1987; 136:483.

55. Ädelroth E, Rosenhall L, Johansson S-A, et al.: Inflammatory cells and eosinophil activity in asthmatics investigated by bronchoalveolar lavage: The effects of antiasthmatic treatment with budesonide or terbutaline. *Am Rev Respir Dis* 1990; 142:91.

56. Jeffery PK, Godfrey RW, Ädelroth E, et al.: Effects of treatment on airway inflammation and thickening of the basement membrane reticular collagen in asthma: A quantitative light and electron microscopic study. *Am Rev Respir Dis* 1992; 145:890.

57. Juniper E, Kline P, Vanzieleghem M, Hargreave F: Reduction of budesonide after a year of increased use: a randomized controlled trial to evaluate whether improvements in airway responsiveness and clinical asthma are maintained. *J Allergy Clin Immunol* 1991; 87:483.

58. Krahn J, Koeter GH, van der Mark TW, et al.: Changes in bronchial hyperreactivity induced by 4 weeks of treatment with anti-asthmatic drugs in patients with asthma: a comparison between budesonide and terbutaline. *J Allergy Clin Immunol* 1985; 76:628.

59. Haahtela TH, Jarvinen M, Kava T, et al.: Comparison of a β_2-agonist, terbutaline, with an inhaled corticosteroid, budesonide, in newly detected asthma. *N Engl J Med* 1991; 325:388.

60. Woolcock AJ, Rubinfeld A, Seale P, et al.: The Australian asthma management plan. *Med J Aust* 1989; 151:650.

61. Hargreave FE, Dolovich J, Newhouse MT: The assessment and treatment of asthma: a conference report. *J Allergy Clin Immunol* 1990; 85:1098.

62. British Thoracic Society, Research Unit of the Royal College of Physicians of London, King's Fund Center, National Asthma Campaign: Guidelines for management of asthma in adults: I. chronic persistent asthma. *BMJ* 1990; 301:651.

63. Barnes PJ, Pedersen S: Efficacy and safety of inhaled corticosteroids in asthma. *Am Rev Respir Dis* 1993; 148:S1.

64. Drazen J, Israel E: Treating mild asthma, when are inhaled steroids indicated? *N Engl J Med* 1994; 331:737.

65. Sears MR, Taylor DR, Print CG, et al.: Regular inhaled beta-agonist treatment in bronchial asthma. *Lancet* 1990; 336:1391.

66. Taylor DR, Sears MR, Herbison GP, et al.: Regular inhaled β-agonists in asthma: effects on exacerbations and lung function. *Thorax* 1993; 48:134.

67. Crane J, Pearce N, Flatt A, et al.: Prescribed fenoterol and death from asthma in New Zealand, 1981–83: case-control study. *Lancet* 1989; i:917.

68. Spitzer WO, Suissa S, Ernst P, et al.: The use of β-agonists and the risk of death and near death from asthma. *N Engl J Med* 1992; 326:501.

69. Krahn J, Koeter GH, van der Mark TW, et al.: Changes in bronchial hyperreactivity induced by 4 weeks of treatment with anti-asthmatic drugs in patients with asthma: a comparison between budesonide and terbutaline. *J Allergy Clin Immunol* 1985; 76:628.

70. Vanthenen AS, Knox AJ, Higgins BG, et al.: Rebound increase in bronchial responsiveness after treatment with inhaled terbutaline. *Lancet* 1988; i:554.

71. Cheung D, Timmers MC, Zwinderman AH, et al.: Long-term effects of a long acting β₂-adrenoceptor agonist, salmeterol, on airway hyperresponsiveness in patients with mild asthma. *N Engl J Med* 1992; 327:1198.

72. O'Connor BJ, Aikman SL, Barnes PJ: Tolerance to the nonbronchodilator effects of inhaled β₂-agonists in asthma. *N Engl J Med* 1992; 327:1204.

73. Dompeling E, Van Schayk CP, Van Grunsven PM, et al.: Slowing the deterioration of asthma and chronic obstructive pulmonary disease during bronchodilator therapy by adding inhaled corticosteroids. *Ann Intern Med* 1993; 118:770.

74. Ädelroth E, Thompson S: Advantages of high dose budesonide (letter). *Lancet* 1988; i:476.

75. Stenius-Aarniala B, Piirila P, Teramo K: Asthma and pregnancy: a prospective study of 198 pregnancies. *Thorax* 1988; 43:12.

76. Greenberger PA: Asthma in pregnancy. *Clin Chest Med* 1992; 13:597.

77. Postma DS, Peters I, Steenhuis EJ, Sluiter HJ: Moderately severe airflow obstruction: Can corticosteroids slow down obstruction? *Eur Respir J* 1988; 1:22.

78. Postma DS, Steenhuis EJ, van der Weele, Sluiter HJ: Severe airflow obstruction: Can corticosteroids slow down progression? *Eur J Respir Dis* 1985; 67:56.

79. Engel T, Heinig JH, Madsen O, et al.: A trial of inhaled budesonide on airway responsiveness in smokers with chronic bronchitis. *Eur Respir J* 1989; 2:935.

80. Weir DC, Gove RI, Robertson AS, Burge PS: Corticosteroid trials in non-asthmatic chronic airflow obstruction: a comparison of oral prednisolone and inhaled beclomethasone dipropionate. *Thorax* 1990; 45:112.

81. Renkema TEJ, Sluiter HJ, Koeter GH, Postma DS: A two-year prospective study on the effect of inhaled and inhaled plus oral corticosteroid therapy for obstructive airways disease. *Am Rev Respir Dis* 1990; 141:A504.

82. Kerstjens HAM, Brand PLP, Hughes MD, et al.: A comparison of bronchodilator therapy with and without inhaled corticosteroid therapy for obstructive airway disease. *N Engl J Med* 1992; 327:1413.

83. Israel HL, Fronts DW, Beggs RA: A controlled trial of prednisone treatment of sarcoidosis. *Am Rev Respir Dis* 1973; 107:609.

84. Williams MH: Beclomethasone dipropionate. *Ann Intern Med* 1981; 95:464.

85. Selroos O: Further experiences with inhaled budesonide in the treatment of pulmonary sarcoidosis, in Grassi C, Rizzato G, Pozzi E (eds): *Sarcoidosis and Other Granulomatous Disorders.* Amsterdam, Elsevier Science, 1988:637–640.

86. Vieira L, Mendes B, Barbara C, et al.: Oral and inhaled corticosteroids in the treatment of pulmonary sarcoidosis. *Eur Respir J* 1990; 3:423A.

87. Zych D, Pawlicka L, Zielinski J: Inhaled budesonide in the treatment of pulmonary sarcoidosis. *Sarcoidosis* 1993; 10:56.

88. Kairys SW, Olmstead EM, O'Connor GT: Steroid treatment in laryngotracheitis: a meta-analysis of the evidence from randomized trials. *Pediatrics* 1989; 83:683.

89. Husby S, Agertoft L, Mortensen S, Pedersen S: Treatment of croup with nebulized steroid (budesonide): a double blind, placebo controlled study. *Arch Dis Child* 1993; 68:352.

90. Toogood JH, Jennings B, Greenway RW, Chuang L: Candidiasis and dysphonia complicating beclomethasone treatment of asthma. *J Allergy Clin Immunol* 1980; 65:145.

91. Shaw NJ, Edmunds AT: Inhaled beclomethasone and oral candidiasis. *Arch Dis Child* 1986; 61:788.

92. Toogood JH, Baskerville J, Jennings B, et al.: Use of spacers to facilitate inhaled corticosteroid treatment of asthma. *Am Rev Respir Dis* 1984; 129:723.

93. Broder I, Tarlo SM, Davies GM, et al.: Safety and efficacy of long-term treatment with inhaled beclomethasone dipropionate in steroid-dependent asthma. *Can Med Assoc J* 1987; 136:129.

94. Laitinen LA, Laitinen A, Haartela T: A comparative study of the effects of an inhaled corticosteroid, budesonide, and of an inhaled β₂-agonist, terbutaline, on airway inflammation in newly diagnosed asthma. *J Allergy Clin Immunol* 1992; 90:32.

95. Brown PH, Blundell G, Greening AP, Crompton GK: Screening for hypothalamo-pituitary-adrenal axis suppression in asthmatics taking high dose inhaled corticosteroids. *Respir Med* 1991; 85:511.

96. Bisgaard H, Damkjaer Nilsen M, Andersen B, et al.: Adrenal function in children with bronchial asthma treated with beclomethasone dipropionate or budesonide. *J Allergy Clin Immunol* 1988; 81:1088.

97. Bisgaard H, Pedersen S, Damkjaer Nilsen M, Osterballe O: Adrenal function in asthmatic children treated with inhaled budesonide. *Acta Paediatr Scand* 1991; 80:213.

98. Lofdahl C-G, Mellstrand T, Svedmyr N: Glucocorticoids and asthma. Studies of resistance and systemic effects of glucocorticoids. *Eur J Respir Dis* 1984; 65:69.

99. Johansson SA, Andersson KE, Brattsand R, et al.: Topical and systemic glucocorticoid potencies of budesonide and beclomethasone dipropionate in man. *Eur J Clin Pharmacol* 1982; 22:523.

100. Ebden P, Jenkins A, Houston G, Davies BH: Comparison of two high dose corticosteroid aerosol treatments, beclomethasone dipropionate (1500 μg/day) and budesonide (1600 μg/day) for chronic asthma. *Thorax* 1986; 41:869.

101. Wong J, Black P: Acute adrenal insufficiency associated with high dose inhaled steroids. *BMJ* 1992; 340:1289.

102. Zwaan CM, Odink RJH, Delemarre-van de Waal HA, et al.: Acute adrenal insufficiency after discontinuation of inhaled corticosteroid therapy. *Lancet* 1992; 340:1415.

103. Reid DM, Nicholl JJ, Smith MA, et al.: Corticosteroids and bone mass in asthma: comparisons with rheumatoid arthritis and polymyalgia rheumatica. *BMJ* 1986; 293:1463.

104. Puolijoki H, Liippo K, Herrala J, et al.: Does high dose inhaled beclomethasone (BDP) affect calcium metabolism? *Eur Respir J* 1991; 4:483s.

105. Jennings BH, Larsson B, Andersson K-E, Johannsson S-A: The assessment of systemic effects of inhaled glucocorticosteroids: a comparison of budesonide and beclomethasone dipropionate in healthy volunteers, in Jennings BH (ed): *Assessment of Systemic Effects of Inhaled Glucocorticosteroids.* Thesis, University of Lund, 1990; VII:1–14.

106. Wolthers OD, Juul Riis B, Pedersen S: Bone turnover in asthmatic children treated with inhaled budesonide. *Eur Respir J* 1992; 5:311s.

107. Wolthers OD, Karpessen-Nielsen H, Pedersen S: Bone turnover

in asthmatic children treated with inhaled fluticasone propionate and beclomethasone dipropionate. *Paediatr Respir Dis* 1994; (in press).

108. Luengo M, Del Rio L, Guanabens N, Picado C: Long-term effect of oral and inhaled glucocorticosteroids on bone mass in chronic asthma. A two year follow up study. *Eur Respir J* 1991; 4:342s.

109. Toogood JH, Markov AE, Baskerville J, Dyson C: Association of ocular cataracts with inhaled and oral steroid therapy during long-term treatment of asthma. *J Allergy Clin Immunol* 1993; 91:571.

110. Simons FE, Persaud MP, Gillespie CA, et al.: Absence of posterior subcapsular cataracts in young patients treated with inhaled corticosteroids. *Lancet* 1993; 342:776.

111. Oberger E, Engstrom I, Karlberg J: Long term treatment with inhaled glucocorticosteroids/ACTH in asthmatic children. *Acta Paediatr Scand* 1990; 79:77.

112. Balfour-Lynn L: Effect of asthma on growth and puberty. *Pediatrician* 1987; 24:237.

113. Martin AJ, Landau LI, Phelan PD: The effects on growth of childhood asthma. *Acta Paediatr Scand* 1981; 70:683.

114. Hiller EJ, Groggins RC, Lenney W, et al.: Beclomethasone dipropionate powder inhalation treatment in chronic childhood asthma. *Progr Respir Res* 1981; 17:285.

115. Wolthers OD, Pedersen S: Short term linear growth in asthmatic children during treatment with prednisolone. *BMJ* 1990; 301:145.

116. Wolthers OD, Pedersen S: Growth of asthmatic children during treatment with budesonide: a double blind trial. *BMJ* 1991; 303:163.

117. Wolthers OD, Pedersen S: Short term growth during treatment with inhaled fluticasone propionate and beclomethasone dipropionate. *Arch Dis Child* 1993; 90:517.

118. Ebden P, McNally P, Samanta A, Fancourt GJ: The effects of high dose inhaled beclomethasone dipropionate on carbohydrate and lipid metabolism in normal and diet controlled diabetic subjects. *Respir Med* 1989; 83:289.

119. Phelan MC: Beclomethasone mania. *Br J Psychiatry* 1989; 155:871.

120. Connett G, Lenney W: Inhaled budesonide and behavioural disturbances. *Lancet* 1991; 338:634.

121. Brompton Hospital/Medical Research Council: Double blind trial comparing two dosage schedules of beclomethasone dipropionate aerosol with placebo in chronic bronchila asthma. *Br J Dis Chest* 1979; 73:121.

122. Mak VHF, Melcor R, Spiro SG: Easy bruising as a side-effect of inhaled corticosteroids. *Eur Respir J* 1992; 5:1068.

ANTI-INFLAMMATORY THERAPIES OTHER THAN CORTICOSTEROIDS

Chapter 57 _____

ANTIHISTAMINES

NICHOLAS J. WITHERS, ANOOP J. CHAUHAN, AND STEPHEN
T. HOLGATE

In 1911, Dale and Laidlaw's experiments on the airways of sensitized guinea pigs showed that histamine, a naturally occurring biogenic amine, acts as a bronchoconstrictor.[1] Riley and West later confirmed that, in both the skin and the airways, histamine was located almost entirely in mast cells.[2] Since these early discoveries, a diversity of biologic activities have been attributed to histamine (Table 57-1). These are mediated through activation of specific cell-surface receptors, and the use of agents that selectively antagonize the pharmacologic action of histamine has led to the classification of histamine receptors into subtypes H_1, H_2, and, more recently, H_3.[3,4]

The major allergic responses are mediated through the H_1-receptor. In addition to causing airway smooth muscle to contract, histamine has a powerful effect on the pulmonary vasculature, eliciting dilation of the precapillary arterioles and increased leakage from the postcapillary venules and fenestrated capillaries.[5] This microvascular effect is seen in asthma, anaphylaxis, and allergic rhinitis and also occurs in the skin in urticaria and in the histamine-induced skin wheal.

The major clinical effects of histamine are summarized in Table 57-2. H_2 effects include esophageal contraction, gastric acid secretion, and increased lower airway secretion. H_3 receptors, located presynaptically in the central nervous system, inhibit the synthesis and release of histamine from neural tissue.[6] Although the main function of the H_3 receptor may be to turn off histamine secretion, its exact physiologic role is currently not known.

As noted above, it is principally through the H_1 receptor that histamine exerts its effects in allergic disease. The neurogenic inflammatory process seen in allergic disease involves bronchoconstriction and increased microvascular leakage, which are in part H_3-mediated responses. In the

TABLE 57-1   Receptor-Mediated Biologic Activities of Histamine in Humans

Target Tissue	Effect	Receptor Type
Leukocytes		
Lymphocytes	↓ Lymphocyte production	H_2
	↓ Lymphokine production	
	↓ Ig production	
	Activates suppressor cells	
Basophils	↓ Chemotaxis	H_2
	↓ Histamine secretion	
	↓ IgE-dependent degranulation	
Eosinophils	Activates chemotaxis	H_1/H_2
	Stimulates cAMP	H_2
Neutrophils	Activates chemotaxis	H_2
	↓ Lysosome secretion	
Upper airways	Rhinorrhea (muscarinic reflex)	H_1
	Mucosal edema	
Lower airways		
Bronchiolar smooth muscle	Contraction/relaxation	H_1
		$H_2(?)$
Bronchial epithelium	↑ Permeability	H_2
Secretory glands/goblet cells	↑ Glycoprotein secretion	H_1/H_2
	Mucus secretion	H_1
	Activation of cough receptors	
General	Probably inhibits histamine synthesis and secretion	H_3
Adrenal medulla	Adrenalin secretion	H_1
Gastrointestinal		
Oxyntic mucosa	↑ Acid and pepsin secretion	H_2
Gastrointestinal smooth muscle	Relaxation/contraction	H_1
Cardiovascular		
Smooth muscle arteries and veins	Contraction	H_1
Pulmonary artery	Constriction	H_1
	Dilation	H_2
Basilar artery	Constriction	H_1
Carotid artery	Dilation	H_2
Postcapillary venules	Dilation	H_1
Facial cutaneous	Dilation	H_2
Vascular endothelium	↑ Permeability	H_1/H_2
	Prostaglandin I_2 release	H_1
Cardiac	↑ Sinoatrial activity	H_2
	↑ Force of contraction	
	↑ Atrial and ventricular automaticity	
Nervous system		
Central nervous system	Inhibition of histamine metabolism	H_3
	Neural regulation	$H_1/H_2/H_3$
Peripheral nervous system	Stimulates sensory nerves (pain and itching), "flare" of triple response	H_1

SOURCE: From Chauhan and Holgate,[74] with permission.

future, H_3-receptors may prove to be therapeutic targets for the treatment of asthma, but this chapter will concentrate on the pharmacology of H_1-receptor antagonists.

The older, first-generation antihistamines, such as diphenhydramine, pyrilamine, and phenbenzamine, have been used in the treatment of asthma and allergic disease since they were introduced more than 50 years ago. However, their use has been greatly limited by a combination of narrow therapeutic indices and numerous unwanted side effects, produced both by antagonism of the histamine receptor itself and by blockade of other receptors, notably muscarinic-cholinergic, serotoninergic, and α-adrenergic receptors. The introduction of the newer, second-generation antihistamines, such as terfenadine, astemizole, cetirizine, and loratadine, with their much more favorable adverse effect profile, has led to a reappraisal of the role of this family of drugs in the management of asthma and allied allergic disorders.

General Pharmacokinetics of Antihistamines

ABSORPTION

Most antihistamines are well absorbed following oral administration. The first-generation compounds are small

TABLE 57-2   Clinical Effects and Ligands of Histamine Receptors in Humans

Characteristic	H_1	H_2	H_3
Locations	Brain; gastrointestinal and bronchial smooth muscle	Brain, stomach, uterine smooth muscle	Brain, bronchial smooth muscle, sensory nerve endings
Functions	↑ Vascular permeability	↓ gastric acid secretion	?reduces cholinergic neurotransmission in human airways
	Smooth muscle contraction	↑ esophageal motility	?Cerebral vasodilation
	Pruritus	↑ lower airways mucous secretion	
	Atrioventricular node conduction		
	Stimulation of vagal afferent nerves of airways		
Typical agonist	Na-methylhistamine	4,5-methylhistamine	(R)a-methylhistamine
Typical antagonist	First-generation: chlorpheniramine	Cimetidine, ranitidine	Thioperamide
	Second-generation: cetirizine		

SOURCE: From Chauhan and Holgate,[74] with permission.

and lipophilic and in consequence cross the blood-brain barrier relatively easily. Second-generation antihistamines are larger and have charged side chains (Fig. 57-1). They are thus more lipophobic than the first-generation compounds and less readily enter the central nervous system.

METABOLISM AND EXCRETION

Most antihistamines, including all first-generation compounds, are metabolized in the liver via the cytochrome P-450 system. Terfenadine undergoes extensive first-pass metabolism, in which 99 percent of the drug is transformed to two major metabolites. Cetirizine, now an antihistamine agent in its own right, is a metabolite of hydroxyzine via the same hepatic pathway.

Once absorbed, the antihistamines are excreted by the renal route (cetirizine, ketotifen), the fecal route (astemizole), or both (terfenadine). In the case of terfenadine, fecal excretion accounts for 60 percent of the dose, and renal for 40 percent. Fecal excretion does not represent lack of absorption, but is primarily a result of biliary excretion. Antihistamines are also excreted in breast milk in a concentration comparable to that in serum.

The half-lives of antihistamines vary greatly, from 1.5 h for acrivastine to 10 days for astemizole. The half-lives of all antihistamines are shorter in children and longer in the elderly than in healthy middle-aged adults, which accounts for the higher incidence of sedation in the elderly.[7]

Pharmacology of Antihistamines

IN VITRO PHARMACOLOGY

COMPETITIVE INHIBITION OF H_1 RECEPTORS IN THE LUNG

Pulmonary Circulation

In the lungs, histamine elicits both vascular and smooth muscle effects through the H_1-receptors. The principal actions of histamine on the pulmonary circulation are to cause vasoconstriction and to increase microvascular permeability, leading to pulmonary edema. In vitro studies show that histamine causes just such an increase in vascular resistance in the isolated guinea pig pulmonary circulation. This change is not seen in the presence of the H_1-antagonist mepyramine,[8] and, indeed, some vasodilation may be seen, which is mediated by H_2-receptors.[9]

In addition to the change in vascular tone, histamine also increases pulmonary microvascular permeability, causing increased lymph flow, extravasation of protein, and an increased water content, resulting in edema.[10] This increase in lymph flow and the increased water content of the lung can be inhibited by the H_1-receptor antagonist, diphenhydramine, but not by the H_2-receptor antagonist, metiamide.[11]

Respiratory Smooth Muscle

There is considerable interspecies variation in the response of respiratory smooth muscle to histamine. The guinea pig respiratory tract appears to resemble human tissue most closely both in its response and its sensitivity to histamine.[12] In general, histamine causes contraction of respiratory smooth muscle. However, in preparations with either spontaneous or induced tone, histamine also can cause relaxation. Histamine-induced contraction of respiratory smooth muscle is inhibited by H_1-receptor antagonists, a finding that forms a fundamental part of the definition of the H_1-receptor.[13]

OTHER EFFECTS OF ANTIHISTAMINES

Mediator Release

It has been known for many years that antihistamines can inhibit anaphylactic mediator release from rat and guinea pig mast cells.[14,15] These studies also confirmed that, at higher concentrations, these drugs can induce histamine release. Subsequent workers have repeated these in vitro findings using rat mast cells, human basophils, and human lung fragments with several different second-generation antihistamine compounds.[16–18] It has been shown that these effects are not related to the antagonism of histamine at H_1-receptors[19] but result, rather, either from direct "stabiliza-

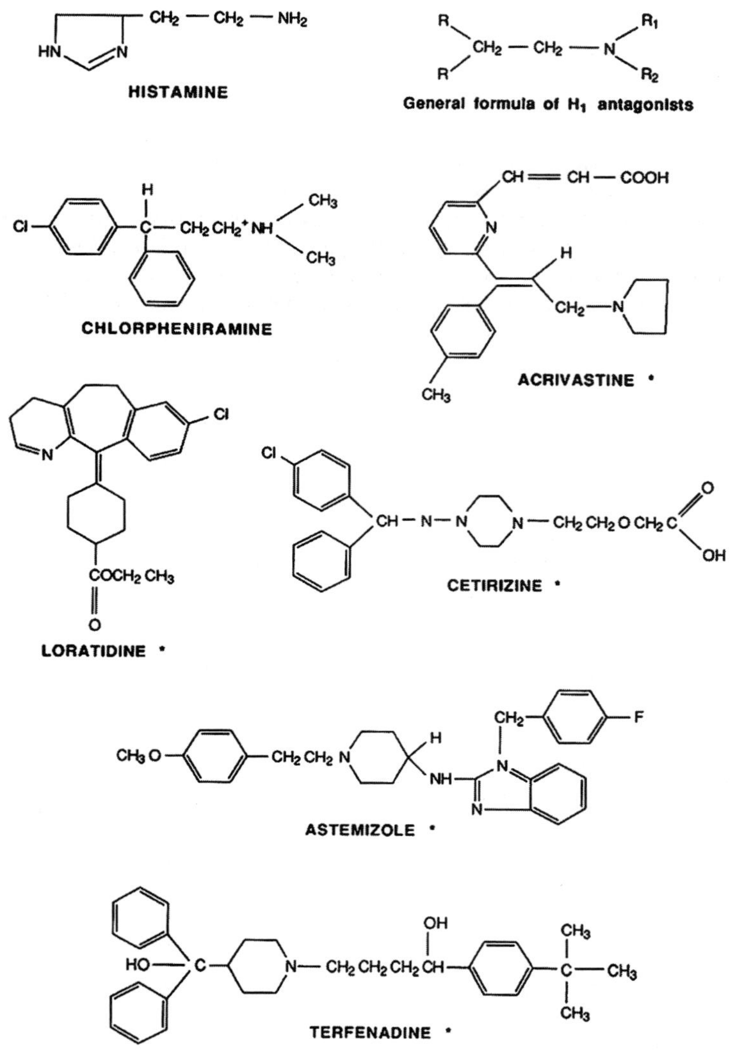

FIGURE 57-1 Structural formulas of H$_1$-receptor antagonists * = Second-generation antihistamines. (*From Chauhan and Holgate,*[74] *with permission.*)

tion" of the mast cell membrane, from competitive inhibition of the binding of calcium to membrane phospholipids,[20] or from binding of the drug to calmodulin and preventing calcium from activating it.[21]

Anti-Inflammatory Effects

Some of the antihistamines are known to have effects on inflammatory cells in humans. Cetirizine decreases eosinophil chemotaxis and activation at sites of mast cell activation.[22] Ketotifen also inhibits platelet migration and medi-ator release.[23]

Effects on β$_2$-Adrenergic Receptors

Ketotifen has been reported to prevent the downregulation of β$_2$-adrenergic receptors, which has been demonstrated in asthmatic subjects treated with β$_2$-adrenergic agonists.[24] This effect has been shown in guinea pig lung and spleen and can itself be blocked by the presence of specific β$_2$-adrenergic antagonists.[25]

IN VIVO PHARMACOLOGY

INHIBITION OF BRONCHOCONSTRICTION

Histamine Provocation

Given that they block the H$_1$ receptor, antihistamines should be effective in inhibiting or decreasing the direct bronchoconstricting effect of histamine, which forms the basis of the histamine provocation test that is used widely as a diagnostic and investigative tool to assess bronchial hyperresponsiveness in asthma. In vivo studies demonstrate the ability of all of the newer-generation antihistamines to afford substantial protection against histamine-induced bronchoconstriction in asthmatic subjects, amounting to a ≥30- to 50-fold shift of the bronchoconstrictor dose-response curve.[26–31]

Bronchoconstriction Induced by Other Factors

In addition to their ability to block histamine-induced bronchoconstriction, several antihistamines inhibit bronchospasm caused by other provoking factors, implying that histamine has a causal role in these mechanisms of bronchoconstriction. In exercise-induced asthma, a number of studies have demonstrated an increase in circulating histamine concentrations,[32] and there is some evidence that antihistamines can attenuate exercise-induced bronchoconstriction.[33] Similarly, antihistamines can inhibit bronchoconstriction induced by isocapneic hyperventilation,[34] hypertonic saline,[35] adenosine and adenosine-5'-monophosphate (AMP), [36,37] benzalkonium chloride,[38] and fog.[39] However, antihistamines have only a limited effect on bradykinin-induced bronchoconstriction and have no effect on that induced by sulfur dioxide or sodium metabisulfite.

ANTIHISTAMINES AS BRONCHODILATORS

As early as 1949, it was demonstrated that chlorpheniramine could cause bronchodilation in asthmatic subjects,[40] a fact subsequently confirmed in other studies.[41] Other first-generation antihistamines also have been shown to have bronchodilatory properties,[42] but these compounds have anticholinergic, serotoninergic, and α-adrenergic properties that may have contributed to the observed effect. Several of the newer-generation antihistamines cause bronchodilation in asthma, suggesting the existence of increased histamine tone in this disease. Azelastine[43] and terfenadine[33,44] both cause bronchodilation in asthmatic patients, presumably owing to blockade of the effects of 'basal' histamine released from activated mast cells and basophils.[45]

Clinical Efficacy

ASTHMA

EARLY STUDIES

Following the discovery that histamine has potent actions as a vasoactive agent and a bronchoconstrictor and the development of compounds to block the H_1-receptor, studies were carried out to examine the efficacy of these drugs in the treatment of asthma in humans. These early studies were not blinded and did not have adequate placebo control. Results were inconclusive, showing that diphenhydramine caused subjective improvement in 50 percent,[46] 33 percent,[47] and 12 percent[48] of asthmatic patients. Similarly, pyribenzamine caused improvement in only 28 percent of those treated.[48] Further trials concentrated on parameters of lung function and found little or nor evidence of benefit. Karlin reviewed all of this earlier literature and reported that only about 10 to 12 percent of asthmatic patients felt any subjective improvement on antihistamine treatment and that there was very scarce evidence for any objective improvements.[49]

Few further studies were carried out until the demonstration that an intravenous injection of 10 mg of chlorpheniramine produced significant improvement in the FEV_1 of asthmatic patients, with the more severely ill patients demonstrating a greater benefit.[41] Subsequent studies using inhaled antihistamines demonstrated significant bronchodilation in both adult[42] and child[50] asthmatics but did not show any clinical benefit when antihistamines were added in childhood asthma.[51] Problems such as their unpleasant

sedative and anticholinergic effects meant that these relatively weak antihistamines could be given only in rather low doses, and, thus, they proved disappointing in the management of asthma.

SECOND-GENERATION ANTIHISTAMINES

The development of more potent second-generation antihistamines with fewer adverse effects has led to a re-examination of their role in allergic disease, in particular asthma. Most studies have concentrated on mild atopic asthma, but several have examined the efficacy of these newer compounds in chronic perennial asthma.

In a double-blind placebo-controlled study of 17 chronic asthmatics, loratadine attenuated the bronchial response to histamine but was no different from placebo in its effect on lung function, use of rescue medication, or patient symptom scores.[52] An earlier trial using terfenadine showed significantly less symptoms and β_2-adrenergic agonist use in patients receiving active treatment than in those receiving placebo.[53] Terfenadine also produced a small improvement in FEV_1, which was not thought to be of clinical significance.

In atopic asthmatics, astemizole was more effective than placebo in preventing allergen-induced bronchoconstriction but had no effect on symptom control or use of β_2-adrenergic agonists.[54] In children, treatment with astemizole did not make any difference in reported symptoms or peak expiratory flow. However, children on active treatment were able to tolerate significantly greater concentrations of histamine during bronchial challenge.[55]

Azelastine has been shown to be superior to placebo in the control of asthmatic symptoms in adults.[56] These improvements only reached statistical significance with larger doses of the drug (6 mg daily), and side effects, including dry mouth and drowsiness, were common. In pollen-sensitive asthmatics, azelastine improved symptoms of rhinitis but had no effect on bronchial hyperresponsiveness or asthmatic symptoms.[56]

Ketotifen has a mode of action similar to the anti-inflammatory agent sodium cromoglycate (SCG) and has been studied extensively both in adults and—because, unlike SCG, it can be administered orally—especially in children. An improvement in daytime symptoms was demonstrated in a double-blind placebo-controlled study of ketotifen in 50 adult asthmatics,[57] but these improvements were only seen in those patients not already taking corticosteroids, and the dose of 2 mg twice daily caused frequent episodes of drowsiness. Interestingly, a further trial using smaller doses of ketotifen has shown the compound to have a mild corticosteroid-sparing effect in corticosteroid-dependent asthmatics.[58] In a long-term multicenter study of childhood asthma, ketotifen proved to be better than placebo,[59] while other studies have shown that the maximum benefit from treatment with this drug may not appear until 6 months after the start of treatment.[60]

OTHER ALLERGIC DISORDERS

ALLERGIC RHINITIS

Histamine is an important mediator in allergic rhinitis, and, thus, both the older and the newer-generation antihistamines have been used in the management of this disorder. Randomized double-blind placebo-controlled studies have shown that most of the newer-generation antihistamines are better than placebo in the management of seasonal and perennial rhinitis, with little difference between the drugs in terms of efficacy or side effects.[61–66]

URTICARIA AND ANGIOEDEMA

All of the cardinal features of urticaria—vasodilation, vascular permeability, pruritus, wheals, and flares—are mediated either partly or wholly by histamine release, and it is known that patients with urticaria have elevated concentrations of histamine in their skin.[67] Antihistamines are particularly useful in the relief of pruritus, and the sedative effects of the older-generation drugs can be clinically beneficial in this disorder. Often patients with recurrent urticaria or angioedema find benefit from prophylactic antihistamines, and it is in this setting that the new, nonsedative drugs have found particular use.

Safety, Toxicity, and Adverse Events

CENTRAL NERVOUS SYSTEM SEDATION

The major barrier to the clinical use of the first-generation antihistamines is their unfavorable side effects. One property of all first-generation compounds is that they cause central nervous system (CNS) sedation. The mechanism by which CNS sedation occurs still is not understood fully, but may result from H_1-receptor blockade[68] or, more likely, to interference with cholinergic receptors.[19] A further important CNS interaction of the antihistamines is that they potentiate the sedative effects of tranquilizers and alcohol.[69]

The second generation antihistamines cause far less CNS sedation, with a reported incidence of <10 percent. The main reason is the presence of large side chains and a generally higher molecular weight, which increases lipophobicity of the compounds and thereby decreases their CNS penetration. Sedation is therefore usually dose-related and may correlate with higher concentrations of the drug in the lung.[70,71] In some disorders, notably insomnia, urticaria (with pruritus), and motion sickness, the CNS-sedative properties of antihistamines may be advantageous.

INTERACTION WITH OTHER RECEPTORS

Earlier generation antihistamines are less specific for H_1-receptors than newer ones, and their interaction with other receptors causes unwanted side effects. These include dry mouth, urinary hesitancy, and blurred vision (from the antimuscarinic effect) as well as hypotension (from the α-adrenergic blockade seen with promethazine). The newer compounds are more specific in their binding, with cetirizine showing no other receptor effects[72] and terfenadine only displaying weak binding to serotoninergic receptors.[73]

CARDIAC ARRHYTHMIAS

A more recent, and somewhat worrying, discovery is the potential arrhythmogenic properties of the newer antihista-

mines terfenadine and astemizole. Both drugs may prolong the QT interval of the electrocardiogram and predispose to potentially fatal torsade des pointes ventricular tachycardias. This adverse event is related to increased serum concentrations, as may be caused by an overdose. The use of excessive doses of these compounds therapeutically is no longer recommended. Their use should also be avoided in patients with known prolongation of the QT interval. Also, concurrent prescription of macrolides antibiotics (erythromycin) or antifungal agents (ketoconazole), which inhibit the hepatic metabolism of the antihistamines, is absolutely contraindicated.

Conclusion

The evidence for the role of histamine as a major mediator in allergic disease is now well established. The recognition that the major allergic properties of histamine are mediated by the H_1-receptor has led to the development of a large number of H_1-receptor blocking drugs, and the subsequent discovery of the newer-generation antihistamines has made it possible to achieve blockade of this receptor with a satisfactory side effect profile. However, despite their proven pharmacologic potency, the clinical experience with the antihistamine family as a whole in asthma has not been successful. Their role in the management of this important allergic disorder is not proven, and at present they cannot be recommended for this use.

References

1. Dale H, Laidlaw P: The physiologic action of B-imidazoylethylamine. *J Physiol* 1910; 41:318.
2. Riley J, West G: The presence of histamine in mast cells. *J Physiol* 1953; 120;528.
3. Black J, Duncan W, Durant C, et al.: Definition and antagonism of histamine H_2 receptors. *Nature* 1972; 236:385.
4. Arrang J, Garbag M, Lancelot J, et al.: Highly potent and selective ligands for histamine H_3-receptors. *Nature* 1987; 327:117.
5. White M, Slater J, Kaliner M: Histamine and asthma. *Am Rev Respir Dis* 1987; 135:1165.
6. Schwartz J, Arrang J, Garbag M, Pollard H: A third histamine receptor sub-type: characterization, localization and functions of the H_3 receptor. *Agents Actions* 1990; 30:13.
7. Simons F: H_1-receptor antagonists: clinical pharmacology and therapeutics. *J Allergy Clin Immunol* 1989; 84:845.
8. Goadby P, Phillips E: Some effects of burimamide on isolated perfused pulmonary circulation of the guinea pig. *Br J Pharmacol* 1973; 49:368.
9. Turker R: Presence of H_2-receptors in the guinea pig pulmonary vascular bed. *Pharmacology* 1973; 9:306.
10. Brigham K, Owen P: Increased sheep lung vascular permeability caused by histamine. *Circ Res* 1975; 37:647.
11. Brigham K, Bowers R, Owen P: Effects of antihistamines on the lung vascular response to histamine in unanaesthetised sheep. *J Clin Invest* 1976; 58:391.
12. Muccitelli R, Tucker S, Hay D: Is the guinea pig trachea a good in vitro model of human large and central airways? Comparison on leukotriene, methacholine, histamine and antigen induced contractions. *J Pharmacol Exp Ther* 1987; 243:473.

13. Ash A, Schild H: Receptors mediating some actions of histamine. *Br J Pharmacol* 1966; 27:427.

14. Arunlakshana O, Schild H: Histamine release by antihistamines. *J Physiol* 1953; 119:47P.

15. Mota I, Dias Da Silva W: The anti-anaphylactic and histamine releasing properties of the antihistamines: their effect on mast cells. *Br J Pharmacol* 1960; 15:396.

16. Guschin I, Deryugin I, Kaminka M: Histamine liberating action of antihistamines on isolated rat mast cells. *Bull Exp Biol Med* 1978; 85:352.

17. Lichtenstein L, Gillespie E: The effects of the H_1- and H_2-antihistamines on "allergic" histamine release and its inhibition by histamine. *J Pharmacol Exp Ther* 1972; 192:441.

18. Church M, Gradidge C: Inhibition of histamine release from human lung *in vitro* by antihistamines and related drugs. *Br J Pharmacol* 1980; 69:663.

19. Rimmer S, Church M: The pharmacology and mechanisms of action of histamine H_1 antagonists. *Clin Exp Allergy* 1990; 20:3.

20. Church M, Young K: The characteristics of inhibition of histamine release from human lung fragments by sodium cromoglycate, salbutamol and chlorpromazine. *Br J Pharmacol* 1983; 78:671.

21. Peachell P, Pearce F: Effects of calmodulin on histamine secretion from mast cells. *Agents Actions* 1985; 16:43.

22. van Epps D, Kutvirt S, Potter J: In vitro effects of cetrizine and histamine on human neutrophil function. *Annals Allergy* 1987; 59:13.

23. Page C, Tomiak R, Morley J, Saunders R: Susceptibility of platelet dependent bronchoconstriction by antihistamine drugs. *Am Rev Respir Dis* 1984; 129:A24.

24. de Vos C: Pharmacologic modulation of allergic cutaneous inflammation. Berlin; *Proc XIV Congress Eur Acad Allergol Clin Immunol* 1989; 149.

25. Koshimo T, Agrawal D, Townley R: Effect of ketotifen on the down regulation of beta adrenoreceptors in guinea pig lung and spleen. *Am Rev Respir Dis* 1988; 137:855–860.

26. Holgate S, Emmanuel M, Howarth P: Astemizole and other H_1-antihistamine drug treatment of asthma. *J Allergy Clin Immunol* 1985; 76:375.

27. Town G, Holgate S: Comparison of the effect of loratadine on the airway and skin responses to histamine, methacholine and allergen in asthmatic patients. *J Allergy Clin Immunol* 1990; 86:886.

28. Raffery P, Holgate S: Terfenadene (Seldane) is a potent and selective H1 receptor antagonist in asthmatic airways. *Am Rev Respir Dis* 1987; 135:181.

29. Mattson D, Poppins H, Nikander-Hurme R: Preventative effect of ketotifen, a new antiallergic agent on histamine-induced bronchoconstriction in asthmatics. *Clin Allergy* 1979; 9:411.

30. Brik A, Tashkin D, Gong Jr H, et al.: Effect of cetirizine, a new antihistamine H_1-receptor antagonist, on airway dynamics and responsiveness to inhaled histamine in mild asthma. *J Allergy Clin Immunol* 1987; 80:51.

31. Magnussen H, Alba A, Bohatiuk G, et al.: The inhibitory effect of azelastine and ketotifen on histamine-induced bronchoconstriction in asthmatic patients. *Chest* 1987; 91:855.

32. Lee T, Brown M, Nagy L, et al.: Exercise induced release of histamine and neutrophil chemotaxis factors in atopic asthmatics. *J Allergy Clin Immunol* 1982; 70:73.

33. Patel J: Terfenadine in exercise induced asthma. *Br Med J* 1984; 288:1496.

34. Badier M, Beaumont D, Urehek J: Attenuation of hyperventilation induced bronchospasm by terfenadine: a new antihistamine. *J Allergy Clin Immunol* 1988; 81:437.

35. Wilmot C: Role of histamine and prostaglandins in the bronchial response to inhaled hypertonic saline. *Thorax* 1988; 43:865.

36. Phillips G, Rafferty P, Beasley C, et al.: The contribution of mast cell mediators to AMP induced bronchoconstriction in intrinsic asthma. *Thorax* 1987; 42:939.

37. Rafferty P, Beasley C, Holgate ST: The contribution of histamine to bronchoconstriction produced by inhaled allergen and adenosine 5′-monophosphate in asthma. *Am Rev Respir Dis* 1987; 136:369.

38. Miszkiel K, Beasley R, Rafferty P, et al.: The contribution of histamine release to bronchoconstriction provoked by inhaled benzalkonium chloride in asthma. *Br J Clin Pharmacol* 1988; 25:157.

39. Hopp R, Bewtra A, Nair N, et al.: Effect of terfenadine on the bronchoconstriction induced by ultrasonically nebulised distilled water. *Allergy* 1988; 61:13.

40. Hirxheimer H: Antihistamines in bronchial asthma. *Br Med J* 1949; 2:901.

41. Popa V: Bronchodilating activity of an H_1 blocker, chlorpheniramine. *J Allergy Clin Immunol* 1977; 59:54.

42. Nogrady S, Hartley J, Handslip P, et al.: Bronchodilation after inhalation of the antihistamine clemastine. *Thorax* 1978; 33:479.

43. Kemp J, Meltzer E, Orge H: A dose-response study of the bronchodilator action of azelastine in asthma. *J Allergy Clin Immunol* 1987; 79:893.

44. Cookson W, Higgins R, Chadwick G, et al.: A clinical trial of the H_1-antihistamine terfenadine in atopic asthma. *Am Rev Respir Dis* 1987; 135:A387.

45. White J, Eiser N: The role of histamine and its receptors in the pathogenesis of asthma. *Br J Dis Chest* 1983; 77:215.

46. Eyermann C: Clinical experience with a new antihistamine drug. *J Allergy* 1946; 17:210.

47. Kailsche G, Prickman L, Carryer H: The symptomatic treatment of bronchial asthma and hay fever with Benadryl. *Proc Staff Meeting Mayo Clin* 1945; 20:432.

48. Bernstein T, Rose J, Feinberg S: New antihistamine drugs in hay fever and other allergic conditions. *Illinois Med J* 1947; 92:90.

49. Karlin J: The use of antihistamines in asthma. *Ann Allergy* 1972; 30:342.

50. Groggins R, Milner A, Stokes G: The bronchodilator effects of chlorpheniramine in childhood asthma. *Br J Dis Chest* 1979; 73:297.

51. Henry R, Hodges I, Milner A: Bronchodilating effects of the H_1-receptor antagonist clemastine. *Arch Dis Child* 1983; 58:304.

52. Dirksen A, Engel T, Frolund L, et al.: Effect of a non-sedative antihistamine (loratadine) in moderate asthma. *Allergy* 1989; 44:566.

53. Taytard A, Beaumont D, Pujet J, et al.: Treatment of bronchial asthma with terfenadine: a randomised controlled trial. *Br J Clin Pharmacol* 1987; 30:229.

54. Cistero A, Abadias M, Lleonart R, et al.: Effect of astemizole on allergic asthma. *Ann Allergy* 1992; 69:123.

55. Backer V, Bach-Mortensen N, Becker U, et al.: Bronchial hyperresponsiveness and exercise-induced asthma in children. *Allergy* 1989; 44:209.

56. Tinkelman D, Bucholtz G, Kemp J, et al.: Evaluation of the safety and efficacy of multiple doses of azelastine to adult patients with bronchial asthma over time. *Am Rev Respir Dis* 1990; 141:569.

57. Dyson A, Mackay A: Ketotifen in adult asthma. *Br Med J* 1980; 280:360.

58. Lane D: A steroid sparing effect of ketotifen in steroid-dependent asthmatics. *Clin Allergy* 1980; 10:519.

59. Rackham A, Brown C, Chandra R, et al.: A Canadian multi-centre study with Zadifen (ketotifen) in the treatment of bronchial asthma in children aged 5–17 years. *J Allergy Clin Immunol* 1989; 84:286.

60. Guybout P, Choffel C, Constans P, et al.: Efficacy of ketotifen in adult asthmatic patients: a six month double-blind versus placebo study. *Respiration* 1984; 46(Suppl 1):20.

61. Kemp J, Buckley C, Gershwin M, et al.: Multi-centre, double-blind, placebo-controlled trial of terfenadine in seasonal allergic rhinitis and conjunctivitis. *Ann Allergy* 1984; 54:502.

62. Weler J, Donnelly A, Campbell B, et al.: Multi-centre, double-blind, multiple dose, parallel groups efficacy and safety trial of azelastine, chlorpheniramine and placebo in the treatment of spring allergic rhinitis. *J Allergy Clin Immunol* 1988; 82:801.

63. Frolund L, Etholm B, Irland K, et al.: A multicentre study of loratadine, clemastine and placebo in perennial allergic rhinitis. *Allergy* 1990; 45:254.

64. Rijntes E, Ghys L, Rihoux J: Astemizole and cetirizine in the treatment of seasonal allergic rhinitis: a comparative, double-blind multi-centre study. *J Int Med Res* 1990; 18:219.

65. Reed C, Aaronson D, Bahna S, et al.: Comparison of cetirizine and astemizole treatment of seasonal allergic rhinitis. (Abstract) *Ann Allergy* 1991; 66:104.

66. Lockley R, Findley S, Mitchell D, et al.: Effect of cetirizine versus terfenadine in seasonal allergic rhinitis. *Ann Allergy* 1993; 70:311.

67. Shalit M, Schwartz L, von Allmen C, et al.: Release of histamine and tryptase during continuous and interrupted cutaneous challenge with allergen in humans. *J Allergy Clin Immunol* 1990; 86:117.

68. Diffley D, Tran V, Snyder S: Histamine H_1 receptors labelled in vivo: antidepressant and antihistamine interactions. *Eur J Pharmacol* 1980; 64:177.

69. Cohen A, Hamilton M, Peek A: The effect of acravistine (BW825C), diphenhydramine and terfenadine in combination with alcohol on human CNS performance. *Eur J Clin Pharmacol* 1987; 32:279.

70. Friedman H: Loratadine: a potent, non-sedating and long-acting H_1 antagonist. *Am J Rhinol* 1986; 1:95.

71. Simons F, Simons K: H_1 receptor antagonist treatment of chronic rhinitis. *J Allergy Clin Immunol* 1988; 81:975.

72. Snyder S, Snowman A: Receptor effects of cetirizine? *Ann Allergy* 1987; 59:4–8.

73. Cheng C, Woodward JK: Antihistaminic effect of terfenadine: a new piperidine-type antihistamine. *Drug Rev Resp* 1982; 2:181.

74. Chauhan A, Holgate ST: Histamine and histamine receptors, in Townley RG, Grawal DA (eds): *Immunopharmacology of Allergic Diseases*. New York, Marcel Dekker, 1996 (in press).

Chapter 58

DISODIUM CROMOGLYCATE

NICHOLAS J. WITHERS AND STEPHEN T. HOLGATE

First discovered in 1965 as a result of earlier investigations with the naturally occurring antispasmodic khellin,[1] disodium cromoglycate (SCG) is an anti-allergic, anti-inflammatory drug, which is used principally as a prophylactic agent in asthma. It is a derivative of chromone-2-carboxylic acid and consists of two chromone rings with two carboxylic acid groups, joined by a flexible linking chain (Fig. 58-1). SCG is a white, odorless powder, which is very soluble in water and is totally ionized at physiologic pH. It is chemically and pharmacologically distinct from other compounds used in the treatment of asthma.

Pharmacokinetics of Disodium Cromoglycate

ABSORPTION

SCG is poorly absorbed from the gastrointestinal tract, and thus its main routes of administration are by inhalation to the lungs or topically to the eyes and nose. Approximately 10 percent of an inhaled dose enters the lungs and is absorbed systemically. Clearance from the lungs is rapid, 75 percent of the dose being removed at 2 hours and more than 98 percent at 24 hours. After inhalation of a single 20-mg dose of SCG, the compound appears rapidly in the blood, with a maximum systemic concentration of 9.2 ng/mL after 15 min.[2] Mean plasma half life is about 80 min.

METABOLISM AND EXCRETION

SCG does not undergo systemic or presystemic metabolism in humans, and unchanged drug is excreted in the urine (50 percent after intravenous administration and 10 percent after inhalation) and the bile (50 percent and 87 percent).[2] The larger fraction that appears in the bile following inhalation is due to the high proportion of an inhaled dose that is swallowed. The amount of SCG absorbed after inhalation depends on both the delivery system and the dose of drug.[3]

There is no known accumulation in any organs other than the liver and kidney prior to excretion. SCG binds weakly to plasma albumin in a nonspecific way owing to its highly polar nature. It therefore does not displace other protein-bound drugs from albumin and, thus, the incidence of drug interactions is low. SCG is not excreted in human breast milk and does not cross the blood-brain barrier.

Experimental Pharmacology of Disodium Cromoglycate

IN VITRO PHARMACOLOGY

IMMUNOLOGIC EFFECTS

Mast Cell Stabilization
Early experimental work demonstrated that SCG inhibited the release of biologically active chemicals following antigen

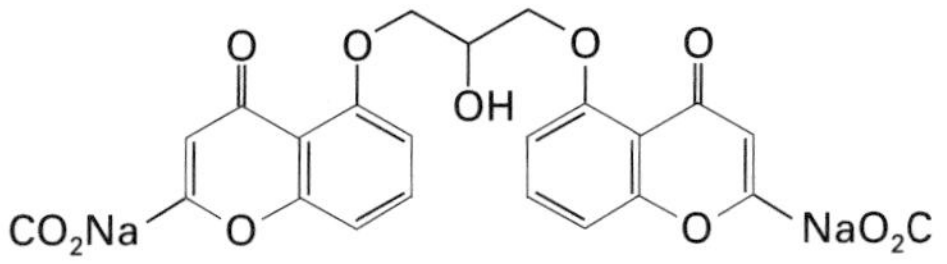

FIGURE 58-1 Chemical structure of disodium cromoglycate.

challenge in tissues presensitized with reaginic (IgE) antibodies.[4] Initial in vitro work in animals demonstrated an inhibitory effect of SCG on histamine release from rat peritoneal mast cells following challenge with anti-IgE.[5,6] Further studies have shown similar findings in these cells following exposure to nonimmunologic stimuli, including phospholipase A, compound 48/80, and calcium ionophore.[7] More recently, inhibition of the release of tumor necrosis factor-α (TNF-α) from rat peritoneal mast cells challenged with anti-IgE has been shown.[8]

In humans, SCG has no effect on skin mast cells, but it has been shown to inhibit histamine release from intestinal mast cells with greater efficacy than for any other mast cell type.[9] In the lung, histamine release from lavage mast cells is inhibited in a dose-dependent manner, while release from parenchymal cells is only partially blocked.[10] The inhibition of histamine release from lavage mast cells may well be significant, as they reside on the mucosal surface and are likely to encounter antigen in the airways.[11]

SCG has also been shown to inhibit Prostaglandin D_2 (PGD_2) release from human mast cells. Its effect on PGD_2 is similar in efficacy to its effect on histamine release, and, as with histamine release, no effect is seen on skin mast cells.

Effects on Other Inflammatory Cells

Although the mast cell is the key cell type affected by SCG, this agent has been shown also to inhibit the activation of other cell types. In vitro chamber studies have demonstrated that SCG can inhibit the chemotaxis of eosinophils to zymosan-activated serum.[12] This is a dose-related reaction, with a IC_{50} of approximately $2 \times 10^{-7} M$ (100 ng/mL). SCG also blocks chemotaxis of and mediator release from neutrophils, the inhibition of neutrophil chemotaxis induced by platelet-activating factor being dose-related with a IC_{50} of $2 \times 10^{-8} M$ (10 ng/mL). Furthermore, SCG has been shown to suppress the release of cytotoxic mediators from eosinophils and neutrophils coated with complement[13] or antibody.[14]

More recently, further in-vitro properties of SCG have been described involving mononuclear cells. Stimulation with interleukin-4 (IL-4) promotes release of IgE antibody from tonsillar mixed mononuclear cells of nonatopic subjects. SCG inhibits this release in a dose-related manner, also causing an increase in IgG_4 release.[15] SCG also inhibits T-cell-driven IgE synthesis by human B cells by inhibiting IL-4–driven switching to IgE.[16]

NONIMMUNOLOGIC EFFECTS

The discovery that SCG can protect against exercise-induced bronchoconstriction has prompted research into nonim-

munologic effects of this compound. The activity of afferent C fibers in dog lungs following stimulation with capsaicin is inhibited by SCG.[17] This finding may explain the ability of the drug to inhibit reflex bronchoconstriction induced by cigarette smoke, metabisulfite, and cold air (see below). SCG also inhibits neurogenic inflammation in the rat trachea after vagal stimulation[18] and in guinea pig trachea stimulated by capsaicin.[19] It has been proposed that these effects may be explained in part by a direct action of this compound on vascular endothelial cells to reduce permeability.[20] It also has been shown in rats that SCG blocks bronchospasm caused by the neuropeptide neurokinin A.[21] However, this effect may be explained, in part, by blockade of neurokinin A activation of mast cells and of mast-cell mediator release.

Most recently, clear evidence has shown that SCG possesses tachykinin antagonist properties and can cause a dose-dependent inhibition of edema induced by substance P and neurokinin in human skin without affecting the flare response.[22] This effect may help to explain some of the nonimmunologic clinical properties of this compound and also may lead to its broader use in the future for other conditions, such as hyperalgesia, in which tachykinin-containing nerves are thought to be important.

IN VIVO PHARMACOLOGY

ANIMAL MODELS

The effects of SCG on several animal models of the inflammatory response in asthma have been investigated. In sheep sensitive to *ascaris suum*, pretreatment with SCG (via aerosol) protects against the increased lung resistance seen with both early and late reactions following antigen challenge.[23] A similar effect has been shown on the early and late bronchoconstrictor response to antigen in guinea pig models.[24] Lavage studies on this guinea pig model demonstrate that SCG decreases eosinophil and neutrophil infiltration following antigen challenge by 54 percent and 68 percent, respectively.

TRIALS IN HUMANS

In humans, single doses of inhaled SCG have been shown to exert a protective effect against a wide variety of stimuli. Antigen challenge studies have demonstrated the ability of SCG to reduce the severity of the early asthmatic reaction and decrease the amount of mediator release.[25,26] In the late reaction, the influx of neutrophils and eosinophils is inhibited by SCG, as is the increase in bronchial hyperreactivity.[27] As mentioned above, SCG also can block exercise-induced asthma and, in addition, has an effect on the activation of eosinophils[28] and platelets[29] that often is seen in this form of asthma. Pretreatment with SCG attenuates asthmatic reactions caused by various other stimuli, including cold air,[30] fog,[31] sulfur dioxide,[32] and sodium metabisulfite.[33] Several studies have demonstrated that short-term treatment (< 6 weeks) with SCG can provide protection against increases in bronchial reactivity in the pollen season,[34,35] while longer-term use reduces bronchial reactivity in asthmatic patients.[36,37]

EVIDENCE FOR ANTI-INFLAMMATORY ACTION

Several studies have demonstrated that SCG has an anti-inflammatory effect on the airways in vivo. Treatment with SCG in allergic asthmatics also has been shown to reduce the number of eosinophils found in sputum.[38] The number of eosinophils in peripheral blood has been shown to correlate with the severity of asthma,[39] and subsequent studies with SCG have demonstrated its ability to decrease plasma eosinophil numbers in symptomatic, allergic asthmatics.[40]

Asthmatics have been shown to have increased concentrations of albumin in their sputum, suggesting a leakage of plasma from inflamed airways. After 2 days of treatment with SCG, the sputum concentration of albumin in asthmatics have been shown to decrease to those of normal control subjects, further suggesting that this compound has a clinical anti-inflammatory effect.[41]

The increasing use of bronchoscopy and bronchoalveolar lavage as investigative tools in asthmatics have made possible more direct assessment of the anti-inflammatory effects of SCG in recent years. Diaz and colleagues examined bronchoalveolar lavage fluid from allergic asthmatics before and after 8 weeks of treatment with either SCG or placebo. The percentage of eosinophils in the treated group was significantly less than either the percentage in the placebo group or the baseline values.[42] A study of bronchoscopic biopsy samples from children receiving long-term treatment with SCG showed two with moderate inflammation, six with mild inflammation, and nine with no evidence of inflammation.[43]

EFFECTS ON SMOOTH MUSCLE

Animal studies have not shown any evidence that SCG has smooth muscle relaxant properties either in vitro or in vivo. However, several studies have demonstrated a bronchodilator effect of the drug in humans. Chung and colleagues found that, in stable asthmatic children, nebulized SCG was an effective bronchodilator, giving a duration and degree of bronchodilation similar to those achieved with salbutamol.[44] Further studies have demonstrated some evidence of bronchodilation as measured by peak expiratory flow both at rest[45] and following exercise.[46]

MECHANISM OF ACTION

The antigen-induced release of histamine and other mediators from mast cells is initiated by aggregation of Fc receptors bound to mast cell membranes,[47] and, like many other secretory systems, it requires extracellular calcium. Following this trigger, a series of biochemical events results in a transient increase in the permeability of the mast cell plasma membrane to calcium ions. Electrophysiologic studies in rat peritoneal mast cells have shown that mast cell degranulation is dependent on a sustained increase of intracellular calcium following a transient increase of calcium release from intracellular stores. The sustained phase of free calcium results from the opening of a chloride channel, which, in turn, activates a membrane calcium channel, allowing calcium to enter the cell from outside.[48]

Incubation of mast cells with SCG abolishes or inhibits the calcium channel conductance that follows cross-linking of membrane-bound IgE by antigen.[49] Further studies have shown that SCG inhibits uptake of radioactive calcium into purified rat mast cells following stimulation with compound 48/80[50] and antigen.[51] More recently, Reinsprecht and colleagues have demonstrated the ability of SCG to block intermediate-conductance channels in both mucosal-type mast cells and colonic carcinoma cells.[52] Blockade of Cl^- channel activity is sufficient to inhibit antigen-induced mediator secretion from rat mucosal-type mast cells and may represent a new mode of action for SCG and other anti-inflammatory drugs.[53]

Interest has surrounded the ability of SCG to induce phosphorylation of a 78,000 dalton protein in rat peritoneal mast cells. This phosphorylation occurs 30 to 60 s after stimulation of the cells and is associated with the inhibitory effects of SCG on calcium influx and degranulation.[54,55] This ability to transfer phosphate groups may ultimately explain the ability of SCG to block calcium-dependent degranulation. By acting on events occurring after activation of the mast cell, SCG would have no effect on nonactivated cells, explaining its favorable side effect profile. It has been postulated, but not proved, that similar activity-modulating mechanisms explain the effects of SCG on other inflammatory cells.

Clinical Efficacy

ASTHMA

Numerous studies of the use and efficacy of SCG in asthma have been published (Table 58-1). When reviewing the earlier studies, several points must be taken into account. First, many of the early trials lacked a placebo group. Second, many of the trials in the UK used SCG in combination with 0.1 mg isoprotenerol, so that results must be interpreted with some caution.

One early study of 252 adult and child asthmatics that did employ a placebo arm demonstrated that, after 4 weeks, 72 percent of patients on active SCG treatment showed some symptomatic improvement as evaluated by their physicians.[56] The Brompton Hospital/Medical Research Council long-term study of SCG examined the efficacy of the compound on 100 patients with severe asthma. Four treatment regimens (SCG + isoproterenol; SCG alone; isoproterenol alone; and placebo) were used, with the end-point being withdrawal from the trial prior to its end because of poor control of asthma. At the end of 1 year, the percentages of patients remaining well in the four groups were 80 percent, 67 percent, 25 percent, and 16 percent respectively.[57]

In childhood asthma, early placebo-controlled studies demonstrated significantly less respiratory symptoms following SCG treatment,[58,59] while 60 percent of patients expressed a preference for SCG because of fewer exacerbations and less frequent nocturnal symptoms.[60]

These early studies employed SCG delivered as a dry powder aerosol. The subsequent development of nebulizer and metered-dose inhaler delivery systems for the com-

TABLE 58-1   Major Early Clinical Trials of the Efficacy of Disodium Cromoglycate in the Treatment of Asthma

Authors	Protocol	Outcomes
Brompton Hospital/MRC (1972)[57]	1 year double-blind placebo trial of SCG in adults with severe asthma	SCG statistically better than placebo after 4 weeks
Hyde et al. (1973)[58]	8-week double-blind placebo followed by 12 months unblinded SCG treatment in 33 asthmatic children	26 of 33 showed a decreased frequency of asthma attacks 25 of 33 had a decreased need for bronchodilators
Hiller et al. (1977)[62]	Double-blind placebo-controlled crossover trial of nebulized 1% SCG in 17 asthmatic children	11 of 17 showed improvement in symptom scores
Geller-Bernstein and Levin (1982)[63]	12-week double-blind crossover trial of SCG via aerosolized MDI in 46 severely asthmatic children aged 4–13 years	Significant improvement in peak expiratory flow, asthma severity, and pulmonary function
Rubin et al. (1983)[67]	12-week double-blind crossover trial of treatment with aerosolized SCG in 31 adult asthmatics	Patients on SCG showed improved breathlessness at rest and morning PEF and significant decrease in the use of bronchodilators

ABBREVIATIONS: SCG, disodium cromoglycate; MDI, metered-dose inhaler; PEF, peak expiratory flow.

pound prompted further trials using these methods of administration. Nebulized SCG was superior to terbutaline in the treatment of mild asthma in children 6 to 12 years old,[61] while a further study of this mode of delivery showed that 11 out of 17 children receiving SCG treatment showed significant improvement in respiratory scores when compared to a placebo group.[62] In a study of nebulized SCG in children aged 3 months to 2 years, Geller-Bernstein and colleagues recorded improvements in respiratory symptom scores in 24 children 1 year old or older but not in 20 children younger than 1 year.[63] Several trials have compared the efficacy of metered-dose inhaler administration of SCG to that of dry powder administration. In most cases, both modes of administration have proved equally effective and superior to placebo.[64–67]

COMPARISON WITH THEOPHYLLINE
Several studies have compared SCG with other established asthma medications (Table 58-2). One such double-blind crossover study compared nebulized cromoglycate with liquid theophylline in the control of symptoms in preschool children with chronic asthma. Patients receiving theophylline, averaged 46.5 percent symptom-free days, whereas among those receiving SCG, the average increased to 61 per-

cent.[68] Perhaps more significant, no adverse effects were reported in the SCG arm, whereas in the theophylline arm side effects were numerous despite careful monitoring of plasma concentrations. An earlier study of shorter duration in adults found no significant difference between theophylline and SCG treatment using peak expiratory flow and use of other medications as judgment criteria.[69] However, SCG treatment again resulted in significantly more symptom-free days. Further studies have shown little difference in efficacy between the two treatments in the short-term management of chronic asthma. However, most studies show theophylline to be associated with a much greater frequency of adverse events. For long-term use, SCG has the added benefit of its ability to decrease bronchial hyperreactivity.

CORTICOSTEROID-SPARING EFFECTS
Early clinical trials with SCG reported that treatment with this compound could lead to reduction of corticosteroid usage in some patients.[70,71] On this basis, SCG received its first license in the USA for use as a corticosteroid-sparing drug. Subsequent clinical trials continued to examine this property of the drug. In one such study of 23 steroid-dependent asthmatic children, 18 managed to complete a 12-month open-ended treatment regimen with SCG. Of these, 7 dis-

TABLE 58-2   Major Trials Comparing Disodium Cromoglycate to Theophyllines and Examining Corticosteroid-Sparing Effects

Author	Protocol	Outcomes
Newth et al. (1982)[68]	Double-blind crossover comparison of SCG and theophylline in preschool children	More symptom-free days on SCG; more adverse events with theophylline
Hambleton et al. (1977)[69]	Short-term comparison of SCG and theophylline in adult asthmatics	No significant differences in efficacy; significantly more adverse events with theophyllines
Friday et al. (1973)[72]	23 steroid-dependent asthmatic children treated openly with SCG for 12 months	Of 18 who finished trial, 7 discontinued corticosteroids, and 10 reduced corticosteroid dosage
Toogood et al. (1981)[73]	6-month study of effect of SCG introduction in 36 stable asthmatic children already taking inhaled corticosteroids	No corticosteroid-sparing effect was demonstrated

continued corticosteroids, 10 decreased their dosage, and 1 increased his dosage.[72]

In a study of 30 patients over a 6-month period, the addition of SCG did not show any beclomethasone-sparing effect or any other clinical advantage.[73] Two further studies have not shown any additional benefit from combined corticosteroid and SCG treatment[74,75] implying that the corticosteroid-sparing effect of SCG may not be as great as once thought.

OTHER ALLERGIC DISORDERS

SCG has also been shown to have some clinical efficacy in several allied allergic and inflammatory disorders. In both allergic and nonallergic perennial rhinitis, controlled trials have shown SCG to be superior to placebo.[76,77] However, patient selection appears important, with a further study showing no benefit in those patients with nasal eosinophilia or large nasal polyps.[78] Furthermore, although SCG has been shown to inhibit antigen-induced nasal blockage in 70 percent of patients with hayfever, most adult patients with seasonal rhinitis, do not derive a clinically significant degree of symptom relief from SCG.[79,80]

When taken by mouth, SCG can be effective in the management of food allergy in patients proved to have definite sensitization to antigens in food.[81] SCG also reduces symptoms in acute seasonal conjunctivitis,[82] chronic allergic conjunctivitis,[83] and vernal keratoconjunctivitis.[84]

Safety, Toxicity, and Adverse Events

SCG has extremely low toxicity in various species regardless of its route of administration. It has proved impossible to achieve toxic levels SCG by inhalation in a range of mammalian species. High-dose parenteral administration has produced renal tubular toxicity in rats, but at lower doses no lesions were seen.[85] No evidence of chromosomal damage has been seen, and long-term animal studies have shown no neoplastic effect.[86] SCG appears to be safe in pregnancy, with very low rates of placental transfer. A study of its use in 296 pregnant asthmatic women found a lower rate of fetal abnormalities than that reported for the population at large.[87]

The many long-term clinical trials of SCG have reported a very low incidence of adverse events. In one prospective study of 375 patients, the incidence of side effects, all of which were minor and reversible, was 2 percent.[88] The most commonly reported adverse event is cough following inhalation of the dry powder, which seldom necessitates a change in management.

Conclusion

Originally described as a novel anti-allergic drug acting by mast cell stabilization, SCG now is recognized as a compound having many actions. Its anti-inflammatory properties and excellent long-term safety record make it a useful prophylactic agent in the management of chronic asthma. In particular, it is of most use in those forms of asthma with an obvious provoking factor (e.g. exercise, cold air, pollens, animal fur), in reflex-induced bronchoconstriction, and in the management of childhood asthma, in which the introduction of inhaled corticosteroids as a first-line prophylactic therapy is not always desirable.

References

1. Proctor R: Cromolyn sodium (drug evaluation data). *Drug Intell Clin Pharm* 1974; 8:20.
2. Walker S, Evans M, Richards A, Paterson J: The fate of (^{14}C)disodium cromoglycate in man. *J Pharm Pharmacol* 1972; 24:525.
3. Fuller R, Collier J: The pharmacokinetic assessment of sodium cromoglycate. *J Pharm Pharmacol* 1983; 35:289.
4. Cox J: Disodium cromoglycate (FPL670) (Intal): A specific inhibitor of reaginic antibody/antigen mechanisms. *Nature* 1967; 216:1328.
5. Goose J, Blair A: Passive cutaneous anaphylaxis in the rat, induced with two homologous regin-like antibodies sera and its specific inhibition with disodium cromoglycate. *Immunology* 1969; 16:749.
6. Wells E, Jackson C, Harper S, et al.: Characterization of primate bronchoalveolar mast cells II. Inhibition of histamine, LTC4 and PGD2 release from primate bronchoalveolar mast cells and comparison with rat peritoneal mast cells. *J Immunol* 1986; 137:3941.
7. Johnson H, Bach N: Prevention of calcium ionophore-induced release of histamine in rat mast cells by disodium cromoglycate. *J Immunol* 1975; 114:514.
8. Bissonnette E, Befus D: Modulation of mast cell function in the GI tract, in Wallace JL (ed.); *Handbook of Immunopharmacology: Gastrointestinal System.* New York, Academic Press, 1993:95.
9. Okayama Y, Benyon R, Rees P, et al.: Inhibition profiles of sodium cromoglycate and nedocromil sodium on mediator release from mast cells of human skin, lung, tonsil, adenoid, and intestine. *Clin Exp Allergy* 1992; 22:401.
10. Leung K, Flint K, Brostoff J, et al.: Effects of sodium cromoglycate and nedocromil sodium on histamine secretion from human lung mast cells. *Thorax* 1989; 43:756.
11. Flint K, Leung K, Pearce F, et al.: Human mast cells recovered by bronchoalveolar lavage: their morphology, histamine release and the effects of sodium cromoglycate. *Clin Sci* 1985; 68:427.
12. Bruijnzeel P, Warring, R, Kok P, Kreukniet J: Inhibition of neutrophil and eosinophil induced chemotaxis by nedocromil sodium and sodium cromoglycate. *Br J Pharmacol* 1990; 99:798.
13. Kay A, Walsh G, Moqbel R, et al.: Disodium cromoglycate inhibits activation of human inflammatory cells in vitro. *J Allergy Clin Immunol* 1987; 80:1.
14. Rand T, Lopez A, Gamble J, Vadas M: Nedocromil sodium and cromolyn (sodium cromoglycate) selectively inhibit antibody-dependent granulocyte-mediated cytotoxicity. *Int Arch Allergy Appl Immunol* 1988; 87:151.
15. Kimata H, Yoshida A, Ishioka C, Mikawa H: Disodium cromoglycate (DSCG) selectively inhibits IgE production and enhances IgG4 production by human B cells in vitro. *Clin Exp Immunol* 1991; 84:395.
16. Loh R, Jabara H, Geha R: Disodium cromoglycate inhibits Sµ-Sε deletional switch recombination and IgE synthesis in human B cells. *J Exp Med* 1994; 180:663.
17. Dixon M, Jackson D, Richards I: The action of sodium cromoglycate on 'C' fibre endings in the dog lung. *Br J Pharmacol* 1980; 70:11.
18. Norris A, Leeson M, Jackson D, Holroyde M: Modulation of neurogenic inflammation in rat trachea. *Pulm Pharm* 1990; 3:180.

19. Erjefalt I, Persson C: Anti-asthma drugs attenuate inflammatory leakage of plasma into airway lumen. *Acta Physiol Scand* 1986; 128:653.

20. Persson C: Cromoglycate, plasma exudation and asthma. *Trends Pharmacol Sci* 1987; 8:202.

21. Joos G, Pauwels R, van der Straeten M: The mechanism of tachykinin-induced bronchoconstriction in the rat. *Am Rev Respir Dis* 1988; 137:1038.

22. Crossman D, Dashwood M, Taylor G, et al.: Sodium cromoglycate: evidence of tachykinin antagonist activity in the human skin. *J Appl Physiol* 1993; 75:167.

23. Abraham W, Stevenson J, Chapman G, et al.: The effects of nedocromil sodium and cromolyn sodium on antigen-induced responses in allergic sheep in vivo and in vitro. *Chest* 1987; 92:913.

24. Hutson P, Holgate S, Church M: The effect of cromolyn sodium and albuterol on early and late phase bronchoconstriction and airway leukocyte infiltration after allergen challenge of non-anaesthetised guinea-pigs. *Am Rev Respir Dis* 1988; 138:1157.

25. Altounyan R: Inhibition of experimental asthma by a new compound, disodium cromoglycate 'INTAL.' *Acta Allergol* 1967; 22:487.

26. Pepys J, Hargreave F, Chan M, McCarthy D: Inhibitory effects of disodium cromoglycate on allergen-inhalation tests. *Lancet* 1986; 2:134.

27. Twentyman O, Varley J, Holgate S: Effect of beclomethasone and cromoglycate on late phase bronchoconstriction and increased hyperresponsiveness. *J Allergy Clin Immunol* 1989; 83:245.

28. Venge P, Henrikson J, Dahl R: Eosinophils in exercise-induced asthma. *J Allergy Clin Immunol* 1991; 88:699.

29. Johnson C, Belfield P, Davis S, et al.: Platelet activation during exercise induced asthma: effort of prophylaxis with cromoglycate and salbutamol. *Thorax* 1986; 41:290.

30. Juniper E, Latimer K, Morris M, et al.: Airway responses to hyperventilation of cold dry air: duration of protection by cromolyn sodium. *J Allergy Clin Immunol* 1986; 78:387.

31. Black J, Smith C, Anderson S: Cromolyn sodium inhibits the increased responsiveness to metacholine that follows ultrasonically nebulised water challenge in patients with asthma. *J Allergy Clin Immunol* 1987; 80:39.

32. Sheppard D, Nadel J, Boushey H: Inhibition of sulfur dioxide-induced bronchoconstriction by disodium cromoglycate in asthmatic patients. *Am Rev Respir Dis* 1981; 124:257.

33. Dixon C, Ind P: Inhaled sodium metabisulphate induced bronchoconstriction: inhibition by nedocromil sodium and sodium cromoglycate. *Br J Clin Pharmacol* 1990; 30:371.

34. Bleecker E, Britt E, Mason P: The effect of cromolyn on antigen and metacholine airways reactivity during ragweed season in allergic asthma. *Chest* 1982; 82:227.

35. Lowhagen O, Rak S: Modification of bronchial hyperreactivity after treatment with sodium cromoglycate during pollen season. *J Allergy Clin Immunol* 1985; 75:460.

36. Chabra S, Gaur S: Effect of long-term treatment with sodium cromoglycate on nonspecific bronchial hyperresponsiveness in asthma. *Chest* 1989; 95:1235.

37. Orefice U, Struzzo P, Dorigo R, Peratoner A: Long term treatment with sodium cromoglycate, nedocromil sodium and beclomethasone dipropionate reduces bronchial hyperresponsiveness in asthmatic subjects. *Respiration* 1992; 59:97.

38. Kennedy M: Disodium cromoglycate in the control of asthma. *Br J Dis Chest* 1969; 63:96.

39. Bousquet J, Chanez P, Lacoste J: Eosinophilic inflammation in asthma. *N Engl J Med* 1990; 323:1033.

40. Easton J: Effect of cromolyn sodium (disodium cromoglycate) on the peripheral eosinophilia of asthmatic children. *Ann Allergy* 1973; 31:134.

41. Heilpern S, Rebuck A: Effect of disodium cromoglycate (INTAL) on sputum protein composition. *Thorax* 1972; 27:726.

42. Diaz P, Galleguillos F, Gonzalez MC, et al.: Bronchoal-veolar lavage in asthma: the effect of disodium cromoglycate (cromolyn) on leukocyte counts, immunoglobulins, and complement. *J Allergy Clin Immunol* 1984; 74:41.

43. Backman A, Finnila M-J, Holopainen E, et al.: Observation of bronchial mucosa following long-term disodium cromoglycate therapy, in Pepys J, Yamamura Y, (eds): *Proceedings of the 8th International Congress on Allergology.* Tokyo, Fisons plc, 1973:45.

44. Chung J, Jones R: Bronchodilator effects of sodium cromoglycate and its clinical implications. *Br Med J* 1979; 11:1033.

45. Hughes D, Mindorff C, Levison H: The immediate effect of sodium cromoglycate on the airways. *Ann Allergy* 1982; 48:6.

46. Weiner P, Greif J, Fireman E: Bronchodilating effect of cromolyn sodium in asthmatic patients at rest and following exercise. *Ann Allergy* 1984; 53:186.

47. Fewtrell C, Metzger H: Large oligomers of IgE are more effective than dimers in stimulating rat basophilic leukemic cells. *J Immunol* 1980; 125:701.

48. Penner R, Matthews G, Neher E: Regulation of calcium influx by secondary messengers in rat mast cells. *Nature* 1988; 334:499.

49. Mazurek N, Schindler H, Schurholz T, Pecht I: the cromolyn binding protein constitutes the Ca^{2+} channels of basophils opening upon immunological stimulus. *Proc Natl Acad Sci* 1984; 81:6841.

50. Spataro A, Bosman H: Mechanisms of action of disodium cromoglycate–mast cell calcium ion influx after histamine releasing stimulus. *Biochem Pharmacol* 1976; 25:505.

51. Foreman JC, Garlano LG: Cromoglycate and other antiallergic drugs: a possible mechanism of action. *Br Med J* 1976; 1:820.

52. Reinsprecht M, Pecht I, Schindler H, Romanin C: Potent block of Cl^- channels by antiallergic drugs. *Biochem Biophys Res Commun* 1992; 188:957.

53. Romanin C, Reinsprecht M, Pecht I, Schindler H: Immunologically activated chloride channels involved in degranulation of rat mucosal mast cells. *EMBO J* 1991; 10:3606.

54. Theoharides T, Sieghart W, Greengard P, Douglas W: Antiallergic drug cromolyn may inhibit histamine secretion by regulating phosphorylation of a mast cell protein. *Science* 1980; 207:80.

55. Wells E, Mann J: Phosphorylation of a mast cell protein in response to treatment with anti-allergic compounds. *Biochem Pharmacol* 1983; 32:837.

56. Bernstein I, Siegel S, Brandon M, et al.: A controlled study of cromolyn sodium sponsored by the Drug Committee of the American Academy of Allergy. *J Allergy Clin Immunol* 1972; 50:235.

57. Brompton Hospital/Medical Research Collaborative Trial: Long-term study of disodium cromoglycate in treatment of severe extrinsic or intrinsic bronchial asthma in adults. *Br Med J* 1972; 3:378.

58. Hyde J, Isenberg P, Flora L: Short- and long-term prophylaxis with cromolyn sodium in chronic asthma. *Chest* 1973; 63:875.

59. McLean W, Lozano J, Hannaway P, et al.: Cromolyn treatment of asthmatic children. *Am J Dis Child* 1973; 125:332.

60. Berman B, Fenton M, Girsh L: Cromolyn sodium in the treatment of children with severe, perennial asthma. *J Pediatr* 1975; 55:621.

61. Shapiro G, Furukawa C, Pierson W, et al.: Double-blind evaluation of nebulised cromolyn, terbutaline and the combination in childhood asthma. *J Allergy Clin Immunol* 1988; 81:449.

62. Hiller E, Milner A, Lenney W: Nebulised sodium cromoglycate in young asthmatic children. *Arch Dis Child* 1977; 52:875.

63. Geller-Bernstein C, Levin S: Nebulised sodium cromoglycate in the treatment of wheezy bronchitis in infants and young children. *Respiration* 1982; 43:294.

64. Losewicz S, Robertson C, Costello J, Price J: Delivery of sodium cromoglycate by pressurised aerosol. *Clin Allergy* 1984; 14:187.

65. So S, Yu D: Sodium cromoglycate delivered by pressurised aerosol in the treatment of asthma. *Clin Allergy* 1981: 12:479.

66. Robson R, Taylor B, Taylor B: Sodium cromoglycate: Spincaps or metered dose aerosol. *Br J Clin Pharmacol* 1981; 11:383.

67. Rubin A, Alroy G, Spitzer S: The treatment of asthma in adults using sodium cromoglycate pressurised aerosol: a double-blind controlled trial. *Curr Med Res Opin* 1983; 8:553.

68. Newth C, Newth C, Turner J: Comparison of nebulised cromoglycate and oral theophylline in controlling symptoms of chronic asthma in pre-school children: a double blind study. *Aust NZ J Med* 1982; 12:197.

69. Hambleton G, Weinberger M, Taylor J, et al.: Comparison of cromoglycate (cromolyn) and theophylline in controlling symptoms of chronic asthma. A collaborative study. *Lancet* 1977; 1:381.

70. Smith J, Devey C: Clinical trial of disodium cromoglycate in the treatment of asthma in children. *Br Med J* 1968; 2:340.

71. Moran F, Bankier J, Boyd G: Disodium cromoglycate in the treatment of allergic bronchial asthma. *Lancet* 1968; 2:137.

72. Friday G, Faktor M, Bernstein R, Fireman P: Cromolyn therapy for severe asthma in children. *J Paediatr* 1973; 83:299.

73. Toogood J, Jennings B, Lefcoi N: A clinical trial of combined cromolyn/beclomethasone treatment for asthma. *J Paediatr* 1981; 67:317.

74. Dawood A, Hendry A, Walker S: The combined use of betamethasone valerate and sodium cromoglycate in the treatment of asthma. *Clin Allergy* 1977; 7:161.

75. Hiller E, Milner A: Betamethasone 17 valerate aerosol and disodium cromoglycate in the treatment of asthma. *Br J Dis Chest* 1975; 69:103.

76. Hopper I, Dawson J: The effect of disodium cromoglycate in perennial rhinitis. *J Laryngol Otol* 1972; 86:725.

77. Brain D, Singh K, Trotter C, Viner A: Sodium cromoglycate 2% solution in perennial rhinitis. *J Laryngol Otol* 1974; 88:1001.

78. Mygind N, Hansen I, Jorgensen M: Disodium cromoglycate nasal spray in adult patients with perennial rhinitis. *Acta Allergol* 1972; 27:372.

79. Frankland A, Walker S: A comparison of intranasal betamethasone valerate and sodium cromoglycate in seasonal allergic rhinitis. *Clin Allergy* 1975; 5:295.

80. Holopainen E, Backman A, Salo O: Effect of disodium cromoglycate on seasonal allergic rhinitis. *Lancet* 1971; 1:55.

81. Ortolani C, Pastorello E, Zanussi C: Prophylaxis of adverse reactions in foods. A double-blind study of oral sodium cromoglycate for the prophylaxis of adverse reactions to foods and additives. *Ann Allergy* 1983; 50:105.

82. Lindsay-Miller A: Group comparative trial of 2% sodium cromoglycate (Opticrom) with placebo in the treatment of seasonal allergic conjunctivitis. *Clin Allergy* 1979; 9:271.

83. van Bijsterveld O: A double-blind, crossover trial comparing sodium cromoglycate eyedrops with placebo in the treatment of chronic conjunctivitis. *Acta Opthalmol* 1984; 69:479.

84. Henawi M: Clinical trial with 2% sodium cromoglycate (Opticrom) in vernal keratoconjunctivitis. *Br J Ophthalmol* 1980; 64:483.

85. Brogden R, Speight T, Avery G: Sodium cromoglycate (cromolyn sodium): A review of its mode of action, pharmacology, therapeutic efficacy and use. *Drugs* 1974; 7:164.

86. Cox J: Review of chemistry, pharmacology, toxicity, metabolism, side-effects, anti-allergic properties in vitro and in vivo of disodium cromoglycate, in Pepys J, Frankland A (eds): *Disodium Cromoglycate in Allergic Airway Disease.* London, Butterworth, 1970:13.

87. Wilson J: Use of sodium cromoglycate during pregnancy. *J Pharm Med* 1982; 8(Suppl):45.

88. Settipane G, Klein D, Boyd G, et al.: Adverse reactions to cromolyn. *JAMA* 1979; 23:811.

NEDOCROMIL SODIUM

NICHOLAS J. WITHERS, STEPHEN T. HOLGATE

Introduction

Pharmacokinetics of Nedocromil Sodium

Pharmacology of Nedocromil Sodium

Clinical Efficacy

Safety, Toxicity, and Adverse Events

Conclusion

Nedocromil sodium (NS) is a novel chemical entity, the disodium salt of pyraquinoline dicarboxylic acid (Fig. 59-1) and the first of a new series of compounds designed specifically to treat airways inflammation in asthma. It is chemically distinct from all other drugs currently used in asthma management.

Nedocromil was selected as a potential improvement on the established anti-inflammatory agent sodium cromoglycate (SCG) because of its activity in models of immediate hypersensitivity, and subsequent experimental data have shown it to have anti-inflammatory properties in vitro, in animal models, and in patients with asthma.[1] Clinical trials have demonstrated its efficacy and possible superiority to SCG in the management of chronic asthma.

Pharmacokinetics of Nedocromil Sodium

ABSORPTION

With its unique physical and chemical properties, nedocromil is suited ideally for topical delivery to the airways. It undergoes rapid, complete absorption through lung tissue but shows negligible absorption through the tight epithelial junctions of the gastrointestinal tract. Thus, following administration of a 4 mg dose from a metered dose inhaler, approximately 10 percent enters the lung and is able to interact with inflammatory cells, while the remaining 90 percent enters the gastrointestinal tract, undergoes minimal absorption, and is excreted for the most part in the feces.[2]

FIGURE 59-1 Chemical structure of nedocromil sodium.

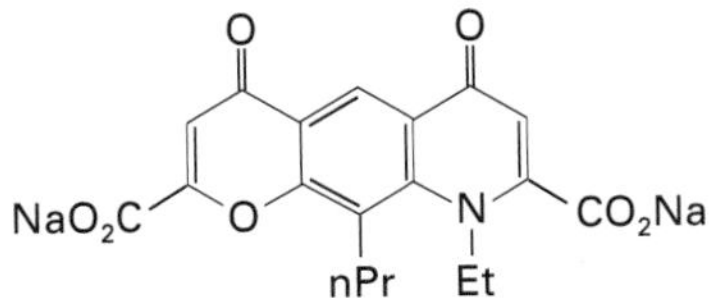

Systemic concentrations of nedocromil are relatively low and result mainly from absorption through the lung. Early studies show bioavailability of NS to be 6 to 9 percent after inhalation of 4 mg,[3] with peak plasma concentrations (approximately 2.8 ng/mL) occurring at 15 min. Systemic drug is associated predominantly with the plasma phase. Absorption of NS may be increased by exercise, FEV_1 and the two together.[4]

METABOLISM AND EXCRETION

There is no detectable metabolism of NS following intravenous administration. Using radiolabeled NS, it has been shown that 55 percent of an intravenous dose is recovered in the urine after 2 hours, and that the full dose is recovered by 96 hours (64 percent in the urine and 36 percent in the feces).[3] Tissue accumulation is minimal because of the poor lipid solubility of the drug, and relatively low levels of protein binding ensure that it does not interact with other pharmacologically active agents via displacement.

Pharmacology of Nedocromil Sodium

IN VITRO PHARMACOLOGY

IMMUNOLOGIC EFFECTS

Effects on Inflammatory Cells
Like sodium cromoglycate, nedocromil has been shown to have many different actions on the principal cells involved in the underlying airway inflammation of asthma. Table 59-1 outlines the major anti-inflammatory actions of nedocromil, comparing them to those of sodium cromoglycate.

EOSINOPHIL CHEMOTAXIS   The influx of eosinophils into the lung and the subsequent release of potent inflammatory mediators is an important step in the pathogenesis of airway inflammation in asthma. Many different proinflammatory

TABLE 59-1   Comparison of the Effects of Nedocromil Sodium and Sodium Cromoglycate on Inflammatory Cells In Vitro

Cell Type	Response Inhibited	Nedocromil Sodium	Sodium Cromoglycate	Reference
Human alveolar macrophage	IgE-dependent enzyme	+++	++ and —	22
Human blood platelet (ASA)	Aspirin-induced cytotoxic mediator release	+++	—	32
Human blood eosinophil/ neutrophil	fMLP-induced activation	+++	++	13
		+++	++	13
Human blood neutrophil	Chemotaxis induced by ZAS/PAF/fMLP/ LTB$_4$	+++	+++	5, 12
Human blood eosinophil	Chemotaxis induced by ZAS,	—	+++	5
	PAF/LTB$_4$	+++	—	5

ABBREVIATIONS: ASA; aspirin-sensitive asthmatic; +, slightly active; ++, moderately active; +++, very active; —, no activity. See text for explanation for other abbreviations.
SOURCE: Courtesy of Dr. A A Norris. Scientific Support Manager, Fisons plc, UK.

mediators, including platelet activating factor (PAF), leukotriene B$_4$ (LTB$_4$), zymosan-activated serum (ZAS), N-formyl methionyl leucylphenylalanine (fMLP), interleukin-5 (IL-5), and IL-8, act as eosinophil chemoattractants.

Nedocromil has been shown to block the chemotactic response of eosinophils to LTB$_4$, PAF,[5] and IL-5,[6] but not ZAS.[5] The first of these studies also demonstrated that sodium cromoglycate did not inhibit eosinophil chemotaxis caused by LTB$_4$ or PAF but did inhibit ZAS-induced migration, indicating different modes of action for these two anti-inflammatory drugs. The action of IL-5 and IL-8 on eosinophils is potentiated in the presence of granulocyte macrophage colony stimulating factor (GM-CSF) and IL-3. Nedocromil-induced inhibition of IL-8 chemotaxis of eosinophils primed with IL-3 and GM-CSF also has been demonstrated in vitro.[7]

MEDIATOR RELEASE AND EFFECTS ON EPITHELIAL CELLS
Leukotriene C$_4$ is released by eosinophils following stimulation with calcium ionophore and with zymosan. Nedocromil has been shown to inhibit these reactions in some studies,[8,9] while others have failed to confirm this result.[10] Activated eosinophils and their products have been shown to impair ciliary beating activity in cultured airway epithelial cells, an effect that can be inhibited by incubating eosinophils with nedocromil.[11]

Neutrophils

Nedocromil inhibits neutrophil chemotaxis caused by PAF, LTB$_4$, fMLP, and ZAS in a manner similar to that of disodium cromoglycate.[5,12] However, Carolan and colleagues reported no inhibitory effect of nedocromil on chemoattractant-stimulated neutrophil migration through cellular and noncellular barriers.[13] In one study, the release of LTB$_4$ from neutrophils was inhibited by nedocromil only in cells taken from asthmatics,[14] whereas another study showed no inhibitory effect at all.[9]

Mast Cells

Like sodium cromoglycate, nedocromil inhibits the release of a wide range of inflammatory mediators from animal and human lung mast cells. Release of histamine,[15] heparin,[16] protease,[17] and tumor necrosis factor-α[18] following immunologic stimulation is blocked by nedocromil, as is the release of prostaglandins (PGD$_2$)[19] and leukotrienes (LTC$_4$). Nedocromil shows a greater inhibitory effect than sodium cromoglycate on the release of histamine from mast cells in lavage fluid both of normal volunteers and asthmatic patients.[15,20] Nedocromil also inhibits release of histamine and PGD$_2$ from human intestinal mast cells, but it has no action on skin mast cells.[20]

Macrophages

Anti-IgE or antigen will trigger blood monocytes and airway macrophages to release preformed and newly synthesized mediators that contribute to airway inflammation.[21] Release of lysosomal enzyme from human alveolar macrophages following stimulation by anti-IgE can be inhibited by nedocromil, as can the anti-IgE-induced release of oxygen free radicals from peripheral monocytes.[22] In vitro, nedocromil inhibits both the release of TNF-α from rat peritoneal macrophages that is seen 4 h after stimulation with lipopolysaccharide and the late (16-h) antigen-induced release of IL-6 from human asthmatic alveolar macrophages.[23]

Bronchial Epithelial Cells

Bronchial epithelial cells, which once were thought to act only as a physical barrier between the external environment and underlying lung tissue, now are known to play an active role in the processes of asthma. Evidence now exists for epithelial cell production and release of many of the cytokines and other inflammatory mediators central to the underlying inflammatory response in asthma.

Toluene diisocyanate, a cause of occupational asthma, causes the release of the arachidonic acid metabolite 15-HETE from cultured bronchial epithelial cells; nedocromil reduces this response by 50 percent.[24] The bronchial epithelium of asthmatic patients shows increased synthesis and release of GM-CSF.[25] Pretreatment of cultured epithelial cells with nedocromil inhibits the production of GM-CSF and of IL-8, which is seen in untreated cells following stimulation with IL-1.[26]

Platelets

Recent studies have suggested an important role for platelets in the inflammatory process in asthma.[27–29] Platelet "shape change," aggregation, release of thromboxane A_2, and formation of inositol trisphosphate (ITP_3) all can be stimulated in vitro by PAF. Further in vitro studies have demonstrated that nedocromil can inhibit all of these responses.[30] It also can inhibit IgE-mediated platelet activation[22] and IgE-dependent antiparasitic functions of platelets[31] and prevent the abnormal platelet response to aspirin seen in aspirin-sensitive asthmatics.[32] Interestingly, the shape change and IP_3 formation induced by calcium ionophore is not blocked by nedocromil, which suggests an action of nedocromil at the cell membrane.[30]

B Cells

In the presence of T lymphocytes, IL-4 stimulates production of immunoglobulins by mononuclear cells in both atopic and nonatopic individuals. Nedocromil inhibits IL-4-induced production of IgE and IgG_4, but has no effect on IL-4–stimulated production of IgM, IgA, and IgG_{1-3} or on spontaneous IgE and IgG_4 release from mononuclear cells in atopic subjects.[33]

NONIMMUNOLOGIC EFFECTS

As well as its many immunologic actions, nedocromil also has been shown in vitro to have other neuromodulatory properties, which may have some relevance to its efficacy in asthma. It can inhibit a nonadrenergic, noncholinergic bronchoconstricting response in guinea-pig bronchi.[34] This effect is achieved through inhibition of neuropeptide release rather than end organ antagonism and is not demonstrated by sodium cromoglycate. Nedocromil also will inhibit substance-P–induced potentiation of the cholinergic response in the isolated innervated rabbit trachea[35] and substance-P–induced release of histamine from human lung mast cells.[36]

IN VIVO PHARMACOLOGY

ANIMAL MODELS

Animal models have been employed extensively to examine both the immunologic and the nonimmunologic properties of nedocromil. In several species, nedocromil has been shown to inhibit the cellular infiltration in the lungs associated with the response to antigen and noxious agents.[37–40] It also inhibits bronchospasm and the late-phase bronchoconstrictor response in animal models.[38,41] It inhibits the late-phase reaction to antigen even when administered after the early phase, which implies that it prevents the recruitment of eosinophils characteristic of this phase.[41]

Nedocromil also has been shown to inhibit the hyperresponsiveness to PAF seen in sensitized guinea pigs following intratracheal instillation of IL-5.[42] Hyperresponsiveness and migration of eosinophils into the airways only was prevented when nedocromil was administered in vivo, which implies that the drug interferes with the development of lung inflammation by inhibiting the recruitment into the lung of a target on which PAF and IL-5 interact.

Nedocromil has been shown to inhibit cough induced by citric acid in dogs through a nonimmunologic mechanism.[43] This cough response is a result of activation of neuronal mechanisms and is not inhibited by sodium cromoglycate.

TRIALS IN HUMANS

When nedocromil is administered 30 min before antigen challenge in allergic asthmatic patients, it can inhibit both the early asthmatic reaction[44] and the late-phase response.[45] In contrast to its action in animal models, it does not inhibit the late response when administered after the early reaction.[45] In asthmatics, nedocromil inhibits the bronchoconstrictor response to a wide variety of stimuli, including cold dry air,[47] fog (ultrasonically nebulized distilled water),[48] sodium metabisulfite,[49,50] substance P,[51] neurokinin A,[52,53] sulfur dioxide,[54] bradykinin,[55] capsaicin,[56] and adenosine monophosphate.[57,58] In general, the trials that compared the efficacy of nedocromil to that of sodium cromoglycate found the former to be superior in its inhibition of the bronchoconstrictor response.[49–51,57,58] Nedocromil also is more effective than placebo in protecting against exercise-induced asthma both in children[59,60] and in adults.[61–63] A dose of 4 mg of nedocromil had an effect on exercise-induced bronchoconstriction similar to that of a 20 mg dose of sodium cromoglycate,[60,62] but cromoglycate appears to have a longer duration of action.[62]

MECHANISM OF ACTION

Although the mechanism of action of nedocromil sodium still is not understood fully, it probably will be found to be similar to that of sodium cromoglycate (see Chap. 58). Like SCG, nedocromil is highly water soluble, has negligible fat solubility, and, at physiologic pH values, is ionized totally. It is unlikely, therefore, that the compound enters cells, suggesting that its many actions are via an as yet undiscovered cell-surface binding site.

Nedocromil has also been shown to initiate phosphorylation of a 78,000-dalton protein in rat peritoneal mast cells,[64] and more recent studies show that it is able to open a chloride channel in isolated rabbit vagus nerve, causing a slow depolarization of the nerve prior to blocking the channel.[65] By contrast, SCG can block chloride channel opening but cannot open the channel, and this difference in potency in vitro may explain the superiority of nedocromil over SCG in many clinical studies.

Clinical Efficacy

ASTHMA

ADDITION TO BRONCHODILATOR THERAPY

Since the first introduction of nedocromil in the United Kingdom in 1986, many studies have examined the clinical efficacy of the drug in the management of asthma. Several of these have examined the effect of adding nedocromil or placebo to the treatment regimen of moderate asthmatics already maintained on either inhaled or oral bronchodilators.[66–72] Most such studies have shown an improvement in total symptom scores, a significant increase in peak expiratory flow and FEV_1, and a decrease in β_2-adrenergic agonist use in patients following treatment with nedocromil as compared with placebo. One study revealed a significant decrease in β_2-adrenergic agonist use during nedocromil treatment but, interestingly, also found a large decrease in use in the placebo arm.[69] No significant difference between the effects of 8 mg and 16 mg daily doses has been shown.[67]

REPLACEMENT OF BRONCHODILATORS

Several clinical trials have examined the efficacy of nedocromil administered as a substitute for either inhaled bronchodilators[73,74] or oral theophylline.[68,72] When used in place of inhaled bronchodilators, nedocromil caused a significant decrease in symptom scores and diurnal peak expiratory flow variation. Patients treated with salbutamol deteriorated from their baseline values and had a significant increase in plasma eosinophilia.[73]

In one large study, a daily dose of 16 mg of nedocromil was significantly more effective than placebo in controlling asthma symptoms following withdrawal of theophylline.[72] When nedocromil was added to maintenance therapy and then substituted for theophylline, the severity of symptoms and the twice-daily peak expiratory flow rates improved significantly within 2 weeks. A direct comparison of nedocromil and theophylline in a double-blind trial in 73 asthmatics showed no difference in patient symptom scores, inhaled bronchodilator use, or spirometry findings.[75]

CORTICOSTEROIDS AND CORTICOSTEROID-SPARING EFFECTS

Because of the laboratory evidence indicating that nedocromil has anti-inflammatory properties, numerous studies have been carried out to examine its efficacy both as an alternative to inhaled corticosteroids and as an agent that can reduce corticosteroid dosages in steroid-dependent patients (Table 59-2). Two double-blind, placebo-controlled studies demonstrated that both nedocromil and beclomethasone dipropionate gave significantly better symptom scores than placebo.[76,77] Improvements were also seen in spirometry results, but these were significantly greater in the corticosteroid-treated group. Several crossover studies also have shown improvements over baseline in most parameters with both nedocromil and corticosteroid treatment, but, once again, beclomethasone proved to be significantly more effective than nedocromil in several areas, including response to histamine provocation.[78–80]

Some studies have found that nedocromil has a significant corticosteroid-sparing effect in steroid-dependent asthmatics. In a 12 week double-blind, placebo-controlled study of asthmatics taking inhaled corticosteroids plus a mean daily oral dose of 8 mg prednisone, Boulet and colleagues found

TABLE 59-2   Major Trials Comparing Nedocromil Sodium and Other Treatments in the Management of Asthma

Trial	Drug Compared	Protocol	Outcomes
de Jong et al. (1992)[73]	Salbutamol	Double-blind crossover study in allergic asthmatics	Decreased symptom scores and peak flow variability on nedocromil
Crimi et al. (1991)[75]	Theophylline	Double-blind trial	No significant difference in symptom scores or spirometry
Bergmann et al. (1990)[76]	Beclomethasone dipropionate	Placebo-controlled blinded comparison	Improvements in symptom scores with both treatments BDP caused significantly greater improvement in spirometry
Harper et al. (1990)[79]	Beclomethasone dipropionate	Comparison as additional therapy in unstable asthmatics	BDP superior to nedocromil
Lal et al. (1993)[96]	Sodium cromoglycate	Comparison as additional therapy in patients receiving corticosteroids	Nedocromil superior to SCG in control of symptoms

ABBREVIATIONS: BDP, beclomethasone dipropionate; SCG, sodium cromoglycate.

that the dosage of oral corticosteroids could be reduced in significantly more patients on nedocromil than on placebo.[81] Patients showed no changes in symptom score or spirometry but they did show a significant increase in use of β_2-adrenergic agonists. In a further study, asthmatics were rendered unstable by a 50 percent reduction in inhaled corticosteroid dosage. Subsequent introduction of nedocromil significantly improved the symptom scores and peak expiratory flow as compared to placebo.[82] Similar results were seen following reduction of inhaled corticosteroids by Bone and colleagues.[83]

The corticosteroid-sparing effects of nedocromil have not been demonstrated universally. In patients maintained on high dosages of inhaled corticosteroids (1000 to 2000 μg per day of beclomethasone), nedocromil only made possible a minor overall reduction in dosage. In a group of corticosteroid-dependent asthmatics taking at least 8 mg per day of prednisolone, nedocromil showed no difference from placebo in reduction of corticosteroid dosage.[84]

The benefit of adding nedocromil to the regimen of patients already receiving corticosteroids has been examined in several studies. In general, nedocromil is better than placebo at improving peak expiratory flow values and symptom scores and at reducing use of β_2-adrenergic agonists.[85–88]

COMPARISON WITH SODIUM CROMOGLYCATE

Some early studies in humans suggested that nedocromil was better than SCG at inhibiting several bronchoconstrictor responses[49–51,57,58] (see also above). Several studies have compared the clinical efficacy of nedocromil to that of the older, more established anti-inflammatory SCG. In one such trial, nedocromil proved to be better than SCG at controlling nocturnal and daytime symptoms in asthmatics already controlled with β_2-adrenergic agonists and inhaled corticosteroids. A second study, albeit unblinded, confirmed this difference,[89] although Boldy and Ayres could find no difference in efficacy between therapeutic doses of the two compounds in 69 asthmatics more than 50 years old.[90]

Safety, Toxicity, and Adverse Events

Nedocromil does not interact with any metabolic processes and is rapidly cleared from the plasma. It is unable to cross either the blood-brain or the placental barrier and does not accumulate in any body compartment. Therefore, it would be predicted to be an extremely safe drug. Numerous safety evaluation studies have been undertaken in a broad range of animal species using several routes of administration with doses many times greater than used clinically. All the species used were found to handle nedocromil in a manner similar to humans, and no significant toxicity was revealed.[91]

In both bronchial challenge studies and therapeutic studies, nedocromil has been well tolerated by asthmatics and healthy volunteers.[92,93] Long-term studies lasting more than 12 months show that the most common adverse events are unpleasant taste (12 percent), nausea (4 percent), cough (7 percent), headache (6 percent), sore throat (5.7 percent), and vomiting (1.7 percent).[94,95] Nedocromil causes fewer adverse events than theophylline and has a profile of adverse effects similar to that of SCG.[90,96] Adverse effects are usually mild and transient, and the most common one, unpleasant taste, has caused cessation of nedocromil treatment in less than 1 percent of patients who experienced it. Data from children are more limited, but nedocromil appears to have an adverse-effect profile similar to that of placebo and is on the whole well tolerated.[97,98]

Conclusion

Nedocromil sodium has been shown to be an anti-inflammatory agent with actions on many different immunologic and nonimmunologic events relevant to asthma. Like SCG, it appears to have an excellent side effect profile, and laboratory and clinical studies suggest it is better than SCG in the management of many bronchoconstrictor responses. These properties make it a useful prophylactic, anti-inflammatory agent in the treatment of chronic asthma, with particular advantages, as seen with SCG, in childhood asthma and in certain forms of asthma with an obvious provoking factor.

References

1. Abraham R, Kauffman H, Groen H, et al.: The effect of nedocromil sodium on the early and late reaction and allergen-induced bronchial hyperresponsiveness. *J Allergy Clin Immunol* 1991; 87:993.
2. Auty R, Clarke A: Kinetics and disposition of nedocromil sodium in man: a preliminary report. *Eur J Respir Dis* 1986; 69(Suppl 147):246.
3. Neale M, Brown K, Foulds R, et al.: The pharmacokinetics of nedocromil sodium, a new drug for the treatment of reversible obstructive airways disease, in human volunteers and patients with reversible obstructive airways disease. *Br J Clin Pharmacol* 1987; 24:493.
4. Ghosh S, Neale M, McIlroy I, Patel K: Effect of physiological manoeuvres on the absorption of inhaled nedocromil sodium. *Thorax* 1989; 44:888P.
5. Bruijnzeel P, Warring R, Kok P, Kreukniet J: Inhibition of neutrophil and eosinophil induced chemotaxis by nedocromil sodium and sodium cromoglycate. *Br J Pharmacol* 1990; 99:798.
6. Resler B, Sedgewick J, Busse W: Inhibition of interleukin-5 effects on human eosinophils by nedocromil sodium. *J Allergy Clin Immunol* 1992; 89:235.
7. Warringa R, Mengelers H, Maikoe T, et al.: Inhibition of cytokine-primed eosinophil chemotaxis by nedocromil sodium. *J Allergy Clin Immunol* 1993; 91:802.
8. Sedgewick J, Bjornsdottir U, Geiger K, Busse W: Inhibition of eosinophil density change and leukotriene C4 generation by nedocromil sodium. *J Allergy Clin Immunol* 1992; 90:202.
9. Bruijnzeel P, Warringa R, Kok P, Kreukniet J: Nedocromil sodium inhibits the A23187 and opsonised zymosan-induced leukotriene formation by human eosinophils but not by human neutrophils. *Br J Pharmacol* 1989; 96:631.
10. Burke A, Crea A, Wilkinson J, et al.: Comparison of the generation of platelet-activating factor and leukotriene C4 in human eosinophils stimulated by unopsonised zymosan and by the calcium ionophore A23187: the effects of nedocromil sodium. *J Allergy Clin Immunol* 1990; 85:26.
11. Devalia J, Sapsford R, Rusznak C, Davies R: The effect of human

eosinophils on cultured human nasal epithelial cell activity and the influence of nedocromil sodium. *Am J Respir Cell Mol Biol* 1992; 7:270–277.

12. Bruijnzeel P, Warringa R, Kok P: Inhibition of platelet activating factor- and zymosan-activated serum-induced chemotaxis of human neutrophils by nedocromil sodium, BN 52021 and sodium cromoglycate. *Br J Pharmacol* 1989; 97:1251.

13. Carolan E, Casale T: Effects of nedocromil sodium and WEB 2086 on chemoattractant-stimulated neutrophil migration through cellular and noncellular barriers. *Ann Allergy* 1992; 69:323.

14. Radeau T, Chavis C, Godard P, et al.: Arachidonate 5-lipoxygenase metabolism in human neutrophils from patients with asthma: in vitro effects of nedocromil sodium. *Int Arch Allergy Appl Immunol* 1992; 97:209.

15. Leung K, Flint K, Brostoff J, et al.: Effects of sodium cromoglycate and nedocromil sodium on histamine secretion from human lung mast cells. *Thorax* 1989; 43:756.

16. Energack L, Bergstrom S: Effect of nedocromil sodium on the compound exocytosis of mast cells. *Drugs* 1989; 37(Suppl 1):44.

17. Wilsoncroft P, Reynia S, Brain S: Nedocromil sodium modulates the ability of rat peritoneal mast cells to degrade neuropeptides. *Br J Pharmacol* 1991; 104(Suppl 5):404.

18. Bissonnette E, Befus AD: Modulation of mast cell function in the GI tract, In Wallace JL (ed); *Handbook of Immunopharmacology: Gastrointestinal System.* New York, Academic Press, 1993; 95

19. Lebel B, Bousquet J, Chanez P, et al.: Spontaneous and non-specific release of histamine and PGD$_2$ by bronchoalveolar lavage cells from asthmatic and normal subjects: effect of nedocromil sodium. *Clin Allergy* 1988; 18:605.

20. Okayama Y, Benyon R, Rees P, et al.: Inhibition profiles of sodium cromogycate and nedocromil sodium on mediator release from mast cells of human skin, lung, tonsil, adenoid, and intestine. *Clin Exp Allergy* 1992; 22:401.

21. Capron A, Dessaint J, Capron M, et al.: From parasites to allergy: the second receptor for IgE (FcERII). *Immunol Today* 1992; 7:15.

22. Thorel T, Joseph M, Tsicopoulos A, et al.: Inhibition by nedocromil sodium of IgE-mediated activation of human mononuclear phagocytes and platelets in allergy. *Int Arch Allergy Appl Immunol* 1988; 85:232.

23. Borish L, Williams J, Johnson S, et al.: Anti-inflammatory effects of nedocromil sodium: inhibition of mononuclear phagocytic cell function. *Clin Exp Allergy* 1992; 22:984.

24. Allegra L, Masiero M, Calabro F, et al.: Nedocromil sodium partially prevents 15-HETE release from bronchial epithelial cells exposed to isocyanates in vitro. *Am Rev Respir Dis* 1990; 141:A118.

25. Mattoli S, Mattoso V, Soloperto M, et al.: Cellular and biochemical characteristics of bronchoalveolar lavage fluid in symptomatic nonallergic asthma. *J Allergy Clin Immunol* 1991; 87:794.

26. Marini M, Soloperto M, Zheng Y, et al.: protective effect of nedocromil sodium on the IL-1-induced release of GM-CSF from cultured human epithelial cells. *Pulm Pharmacol* 1992; 5:61.

27. Knauer K, Lichenstein L, Adkinson NJ, Fish J: Platelet activation during antigen-induced airway reaction in asthmatic patients. *N Engl J Med* 1981; 304:1404.

28. Kay A: Inflammatory cells in bronchial asthma. *J Asthma* 1989; 23:335.

29. Durham S, Dawes J, Kay A: Platelets in asthma [Letter]. *Lancet* 1985; 2:36.

30. Roth M, Soler M, Lefkowitz H, et al.: Inhibition of receptor-mediated platelet activation by nedocromil sodium. *J Allergy Clin Immunol* 1993; 91:1217.

31. Thorel T, Joseph M, Vorng H, Capron A: Regulation of IgE-dependent antiparasite functions of rat macrophages and

platelets by nedocromil sodium. *Int Arch Allergy Appl Immunol* 1988; 85:227.

32. Marquette C, Joseph M, Tonnell A: The abnormal in vitro responses of platelets from aspirin-sensitive asthmatics is inhibited after inhalation of nedocromil sodium but not of sodium cromoglycate. *Br J Clin Pharmacol* 1990; 29:525.

33. Kimata H, Mikawa H: Nedocromil sodium selectively inhibits IgE and IgG4 production in human B cells stimulated with IL-4. *J Immunol* 1993; 151:6723.

34. Verleden G, Belvisi M, Stretton C, Barnes P: Nedocromil sodium modulates nonadrenergic, noncholinergic bronchoconstrictor nerves in guinea-pig airways in vitro. *Am Rev Respir Dis* 1991; 143:114.

35. Armour C, Johnson P, Black J: Nedocromil sodium inhibits substance-P-induced potentiation of cholinergic neural responses in the isolated innervated rabbit trachea. *J Auton Pharmacol* 1991; 11:167.

36. Louis R, Radermecker M: Substance P-induced histamine release from human basophils, skin and lung fragments: effect of nedocromil sodium and theophylline. *Int Arch Allergy Appl Immunol* 1990; 92:329.

37. Abraham W, Sielczak M, Wanner A, et al.: Cellular markers of inflammation in the airways of allergic sheep with and without allergen-induced late responses. *Am Rev Respir Dis* 1988; 138:1565.

38. Hutson P, Holgate S, Church M: Inhibition by nedocromil sodium of early and late phase bronchoconstriction and airway cellular infiltration provoked by ovalbumin in conscious sensitised guinea-pigs. *Br J Pharmacol* 1988; 94:6.

39. Jackson D, Eady R: Acute transient SO$_2$-induced airway hyperreactivity: effects of nedocromil sodium. *J Appl Physiol* 1988; 65:1119.

40. Schellenberg R, Ishida K, Thomson R: Nedocromil sodium inhibits airway hyperresponsiveness and eosinophilic infiltration induced by repeated antigen challenge in guinea-pigs. *Br J Pharmacol* 1991; 103:1842.

41. Abraham W, Stevenson J, Eldridge M, et al.: Nedocromil sodium in allergen-induced bronchial responses and airway hyperresponsiveness in allergic sheep. *J Appl Physiol* 1988; 65:1062.

42. Pretolani M, Lefort J, Vargaftig B: Inhibition by nedocromil sodium of recombinant human interleukin-5-induced lung hyperresponsiveness to platelet-activating factor in actively sensitised guinea pigs. *J Allergy Clin Immunol* 1993; 91:809.

43. Jackson D: The effect of nedocromil sodium, sodium cromoglycate and codeine phosphate on citric acid-induced cough in dogs. *Br J Pharmacol* 1988; 93:609.

44. Svendsen U, Nielsen N, Frolund L, Madsen F, Weeke B: Effects of nedocromil sodium and placebo delivered by pressurised aerosol in bronchial antigen challenge. *Allergy* 1986; 41:468.

45. Crimi E, Brusasco V, Crimi P: Effect of nedocromil sodium on the late asthmatic reaction to bronchial antigen challenge. *J Clin Allergy Immunol* 1989; 83:985.

46. Herdman M, Davies R: Effect of inhaled nedocromil sodium delivered by metered dose inhaler and the breath actuated Autohaler on allergen induced bronchospasm. *Thorax* 1991; 46:294P.

47. Juniper E, Kline P, Morris M, Hargreave F: Airway constriction by isocapnic hyperventilation of cold, dry air: comparison of magnitude and duration of protection by nedocromil sodium and sodium cromoglycate. *Clin Allergy* 1987; 17:523.

48. del Bufalo C, Fasono L, Patalano F, Gunella G: Inhibition of fog-induced bronchoconstriction by nedocromil sodium and sodium cromoglycate in intrinsic asthma. *Respiration* 1989; 55:181.

49. Dixon C, Ind P: Inhaled sodium metabisulphate induced bron-

choconstriction: inhibition by nedocromil sodium and sodium cromoglycate. *Br J Clin Pharmacol* 1990; 30:371.

50. Wright W, Zhang Y, Salome C, Woolcock A: Effect of inhaled preservatives on asthmatic patients. 1. Sodium metabisulphite. *Am Rev Respir Dis* 1990; 141:1400.

51. Crimi N, Palermo F, Oliveri R, et al.: Effect of nedocromil on bronchospasm induced by inhalation of substance P in asthmatic subjects. *Clin Allergy* 1988; 18:375.

52. Crimi N, Palermo F, Oliveri R, et al.: Protection of nedocromil sodium on bronchoconstriction induced by inhaled neurokinin A (NKA) in asthmatic patients. *Clin Exp Allergy* 1992; 22:75.

53. Joos G, Pauwels R, van der Straeten M: The effect of nedocromil sodium on the bronchoconstrictor effect of neurokinin A in subjects with asthma. *J Allergy Clin Immunol* 1989; 83:663.

54. Dixon C, Fuller R, Barnes P: Effect of nedocromil sodium on sulphur dioxide induced bronchoconstriction. *Thorax* 1987; 42:462.

55. Dixon C, Barnes P: Bradykinin-induced bronchoconstriction: inhibition by nedocromil sodium and sodium cromoglycate. *Br J Clin Pharmacol* 1989; 27:831.

56. Hansson L, Choudry N, Fuller R, Pride N: Effect of nedocromil sodium on the airway response to inhaled capsaicin in normal subjects. *Thorax* 1988; 43:935.

57. Phillips G, Scott V, Richards R, Holgate ST: Effect of nedocromil sodium and sodium cromoglycate against bronchoconstriction induced by inhaled adenosine 5'-monophosphate. *Eur Respir J* 1989; 2:210.

58. Richards R, Phillips G, Holgate S, et al.: Nedocromil sodium is more potent than sodium cromoglycate against AMP-induced bronchoconstriction in atopic asthmatic subjects. *Clin Exp Allergy* 1989; 19:285.

59. Boner A, Vallone G, Bennati D: Nedocromil sodium in exercise-induced bronchoconstriction in children. *Ann Allergy* 1989; 62:38.

60. Cavagni G, Caffarelli C, Bertolini P, Giordano S: Comparison of sodium cromoglycate (SCG) with nedocromil (N) in exercise-induced bronchospasm (EIB) in children. *Ann Allergy* 1992; 68:95.

61. Albazzaz M, Neale M, Patel K: Dose-response study of nebulised nedocromil sodium in exercise induced asthma. *Thorax* 1989; 44:816.

62. Konig P, Hordvik N, Kreutz C: The preventive effect and duration of action of nedocromil sodium and cromolyn sodium on exercise-induced asthma (EIA) in adults. *J Allergy Clin Immunol* 1987; 79:64.

63. Morton A, Ogle S, Fitch K: Effects of nedocromil sodium, cromolyn sodium and a placebo in exercise-induced asthma. *Ann Allergy* 1992; 68:143.

64. Wells E, Jackson C, Harper S, et al.: Characterisation of primate bronchoalveolar mast cells II. Inhibition of histamine, LTC$_4$ and PGD$_2$ release from primate bronchoalveolar mast cells and comparison with rat peritoneal mast cells. *J Immunol* 1986; 137:3941.

65. Jackson D, Pollard C, Roberts S: The effect of nedocromil sodium on the isolated rabbit vagus nerve. *Eur J Pharmacol* 1992; 221:175.

66. Cua-Lim F, Agbayani B, Lachica D: A double-blind comparative trial of nedocromil sodium and placebo in the management of bronchial asthma. *Phil J Int Med* 1985; 23(4):181.

67. van As A, Chick T, Bodman S, et al.: A group comparative study of the safety and efficacy of nedocromil sodium (Tilade) in reversible airways disease. *Eur J Respir Dis* 1986; 69(Suppl 147):143.

68. Callaghan B, Teo N, Clancy L: Effects of the addition of nedocromil sodium to maintenance bronchodilator therapy in the management of chronic asthma. *Chest* 1992; 101:787.

69. Williams H: Multi-centre clinical trial of nedocromil sodium in reversible airways disease in adults: a general practitioner collaborative study. *Curr Med Res Opin* 1989; 11:417.

70. Greif J, Fink G, Smorzik Y, et al.: Nedocromil sodium and placebo in the treatment of bronchial asthma. *Chest* 1989; 96:583.

71. Bianco S, Del Bono N, Grassi V, Orefice U: Effectiveness of nedocromil sodium versus placebo as additions to routine asthma therapy: a multicentre double-blind, group comparative trial. *Respiration* 1989; 56:204.

72. Cherniack, Wasserman S, Ramsdell J, et al.: A double-blind multicenter group comparative study of the efficacy and safety of nedocromil sodium in the management of asthma. *Chest* 1990; 97:1299.

73. de Jong J, Teengs J, Postma D, et al.: Double blind, crossover study comparing the efficacy of nedocromil sodium and salbutamol on airway reactivity and symptoms in allergic asthma [Abstract]. *Eur Respir J* 1992; 5(Suppl 15):83.

74. Marcoux J, Findlay S, Furukawa C, et al.: A placebo-controlled comparison of nedocromil sodium (Tilade) and salbutamol in mild to moderate asthma [Abstract]. *Eur Respir J* 1992; 5(Suppl 15):83.

75. Crimi E, De Benedetto F, Grassi V, et al.: Nedocromil sodium versus theophylline in the treatment of bronchial asthma. *Allergy Clin Immunol News* 1991; (Suppl 1):328.

76. Bergmann K, Bauer C, Overlavk A: A placebo-controlled blinded comparison of nedocromil sodium and beclomethasone dipropionate in bronchial asthma. *Lung* 1990; 168(Suppl):230.

77. Bel E, Timmers C, Hermans J, et al.: The long-term effects of nedocromil sodium and beclomethasone dipropionate on bronchial responsiveness to methacholine in nonatopic asthmatics. *Am Rev Respir Dis* 1990; 141:21.

78. Svendsen U, Frolund L, Madsen F, Nielsen N: A comparison of the effects of nedocromil sodium and beclomethasone dipropionate on pulmonary function, symptoms and bronchial responsiveness in patients with asthma. *J Allergy* 1989; 84:224.

79. Harper G, Neill P, Vathenen A, et al.: A comparison of inhaled beclomethasone dipropionate and nedocromil sodium as additional therapy in asthma. *Respir Med* 1990; 84:463.

80. Groot C, Lammers J, Molema J, et al.: Effects of inhaled beclomethasone and nedocromil sodium on bronchial hyperresponsiveness to histamine and distilled water. *Eur Respir J* 1992; 5:1075.

81. Boulet L, Cartier A, Cockcroft D, et al.: Tolerance to reduction of oral steroid dosage in severely asthmatic patients receiving nedocromil sodium. *Respir Med* 1990; 84:317.

82. Ruffin R, Alpers J, Koremer D, et al.: A 4 week Australian multicentre study of nedocromil sodium in asthmatics. *Eur J Respir Dis* 1986; 69(Suppl. 147):336.

83. Bone M, Kubik M, Keaney N, et al.: Nedocromil sodium in adults with asthma dependent on inhaled corticosteroids: a double-blind placebo-controlled study. *Thorax* 1989; 44:654.

84. Goldin J, Bateman E: Does nedocromil sodium have a steroid sparing effect in adult asthmatic patients requiring maintenance oral corticosteroids? *Thorax* 1988; 43:982.

85. Lal S, Malhotra S, Gribben D, Hodder D: Nedocromil sodium: a new drug for the management of bronchial asthma. *Thorax* 1984; 39:809.

86. Fyans P, Chatterjee P, Chatterjee S: Effects of adding nedocromil sodium (Tilade) to the routine therapy of patients with bronchial asthma. *Clin Exp Allergy* 1989; 19:521.

87. Wells A, Drennan C, Holst P, et al.: Comparison of nedocromil sodium at two dosage frequencies with placebo in the management of chronic asthma. *Respir Med* 1992; 86:311.

88. Williams A, Stableforth D: The addition of nedocromil sodium to maintenance therapy in the management of patients with bronchial asthma. *Eur J Respir Med* 1986; 69(Suppl 147):340.

89. Orefice U, Struzzo P, Dorigo R, Peratoner A: Long-term treat-

ment with sodium cromoglycate, nedocromil sodium and beclomethasone dipropionate reduces bronchial hyperresponsiveness study in asthmatic patients. *Respiration* 1992; 59:97.

90. Boldy D, Ayres J: Nedocromil sodium and sodium cromoglycate in patients over 50 years of age with reversible airflow obstruction. *Thorax* 1989; 44:362P.

91. Clark B, Clarke A: Nedocromil sodium preclinical safety evaluation studies: a preliminary report. *Eur J Respir Dis* 1986; 69(Suppl 147):246.

92. Gonzalez J, Brogden R: Nedocromil sodium. A preliminary review of its pharmacodynamic and pharmacokinetic properties and therapeutic efficacy in the treatment of reversible obstructive airways disease. *Drugs* 1987; 34:560.

93. Brogden R, Sorkin E: Nedocromil sodium. An updated review of its pharmacological properties and therapeutic efficacy in asthma. *Drugs* 1993; 45:693.

94. Lal S: Correspondence. *Respir Med* 1991; 85:85.

95. Carrasco E, Sepulveda R: The acceptability, safety and efficacy of nedocromil sodium in long-term clinical use in patients with perennial asthma. *J Int Med Res* 1988; 16:394.

96. Lal S, Dorow P, Vehno K, Chatterjee S: Nedocromil sodium is more effective than cromolyn sodium in the treatment of chronic reversible airways disease. *Chest* 1993;.

97. Armenio L, Baldini G, Bardare M, et al.: Double blind, placebo controlled study of nedocromil sodium in asthma. *Arch Dis Child* 1993; 8:193.

98. Buscino L, Cantani A, Di Fazio AL: A double-blind, placebo-controlled study to assess the efficacy of nedocromil sodium in the management of childhood grass-pollen asthma. *Clin Exp Allergy* 1990; 20:683.

Chapter 60

NEUROGENIC INFLAMMATION

PETER J. BARNES

In rodents, there is now considerable evidence for neurogenic inflammation in the airways due to the antidromic release of neuropeptides from nociceptive nerves or C fibers through an axon reflex,[1-3] and it is possible that it may contribute to the inflammatory response in asthma and chronic bronchitis.[4,5] This has suggested that suppression or prevention of neurogenic inflammation may have therapeutic benefit in the treatment of asthma and other airway diseases.

Neurogenic Inflammation in Airway Diseases

It was proposed several years ago that neurogenic inflammation and peptides released from sensory nerves might be important as an amplifying mechanism in asthmatic inflammation[4] (Fig. 60-1). Despite the extensive evidence for neurogenic inflammation in rodent airways,[3] the relevance of neurogenic inflammation in human airways is far less certain. This is partly because it has proved difficult to apply the same experimental approaches used in animal studies to patients with airway disease.[6]

SENSORY NERVES IN HUMAN AIRWAYS

In comparison with rodent airways, substance P (SP)- and calcitonin gene-related peptide (CGRP)-immunoreactive nerves are very sparse in human airways. Quantitative studies indicate that SP-immunoreactive fibers constitute only 1 percent of the total number of intraepithelial fibers, whereas in guinea pig they make up to 60 percent of the fibers.[7] This raises the possibility that sensory nerves in humans may

contain some unidentified transmitter, which may be involved in neurogenic inflammation. Chronic inflammation may cause changes in the pattern of innervation, through the release of neurotrophic factors from inflammatory cells. Thus, in chronic arthritis and inflammatory bowel disease there is an increase in the density of SP-immunoreactive nerves.[8,9] A striking increase in SP-like immunoreactive nerves has been reported in the airway of patients with fatal asthma.[10] This increased density of nerves is particularly noticeable in the submucosa. Whether this apparent increase is due to proliferation of sensory nerves or is due to increased synthesis of tachykinins has not yet been established. Recently, increased concentrations of SP in bronchoalveolar lavage fluid of patients with asthma have been reported, with a further rise after allergen challenge,[11] suggesting that there may be an increase in SP in the airways of asthmatic patients. Similarly SP has been detected in the sputum of asthmatic patients after hypertonic saline inhalation.[12] Substance P also increases in the bronchoalveolar lavage of normal volunteers exposed to ozone, possibly because of a reduction in neutral endopeptidase (NEP) activity.[13]

Cultured sensory neurons are stimulated by nerve growth factor (NGF), which markedly increases the transcription of preprotachykinin A (PPT-A) gene, the major precursor peptide for tachykinins.[14] Similarly adjuvant-induced inflammation in rate spinal cord increases the gene expression of PPT-A.[15] Preliminary studies suggest that allergen challenge is associated with a doubling in PPT-A mRNA-positive neurons in nodose ganglia of guinea pigs and an increase in SP immunoreactivity in the lungs.[16] However, bronchial biopsies of patients with mild asthma have not revealed any evidence of increased SP-immunoreactive nerves.[17] This may

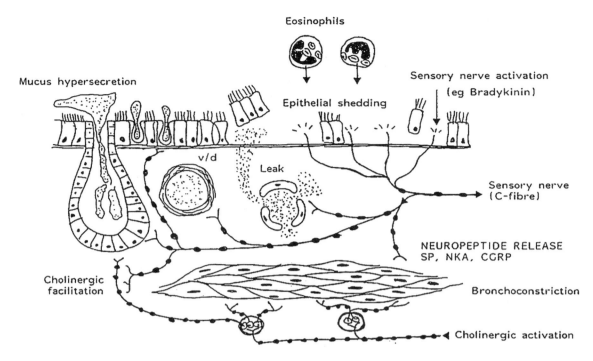

FIGURE 60-1 Possible neurogenic inflammation in asthmatic airways via retrograde release of peptides from sensory nerves through an axon reflex. Substance P (SP) causes vasodilatation, plasma exudation, and mucous secretion, whereas neurokinin A (NKA) causes bronchoconstriction and enhanced cholinergic reflexes and calcitonin gene-related peptide (CGRP) vasodilatation.

indicate that the increased innervation[10] may be a feature of either prolonged or severe asthma and indicates the need for more studies.

SENSORY NERVE ACTIVATION

Sensory nerves may be activated in airways disease. In asthmatic airways the epithelium is often shed, thereby exposing sensory nerve endings. Sensory nerves in asthmatic airways may be "hyperalgesic" as a result of exposure to inflammatory mediators such as prostaglandins and certain cytokines (such as interleukin-1β and tumor necrosis factor [TNF]-α).[18] Hyperalgesic nerves may then be activated more readily by other mediators, such as kinins.

Capsaicin induces bronchoconstriction and plasma exudation in guinea pigs[19] and increases airway blood flow in pigs.[20] In humans, capsaicin inhalation causes cough and a *transient* bronchoconstriction that is inhibited by cholinergic blockade and is probably caused by a laryngeal reflex.[21,22] This suggests that neuropeptide release does not occur in human airways, although it is possible that insufficient capsaicin reaches the lower respiratory tract because the dose is limited by coughing. In patients with asthma, there is no evidence that capsaicin induces a greater degree of bronchoconstriction than in normal individuals.[21]

Bradykinin is a potent bronchoconstrictor in asthmatic patients and also induces coughing and a sensation of chest tightness, which closely mimics a naturally occurring asthma attack.[23,24] Yet, it is a weak constrictor of human airways in vitro, suggesting that its potent constrictor effect is mediated indirectly. Bradykinin is a potent activator of bronchial C fibers in dogs[25] and releases sensory neuropeptides from perfused rodent lungs.[26] In guinea pigs, bradykinin instilled into the airways causes bronchoconstriction, which is reduced significantly by a cholinergic antagonist (as in asthmatic patients[24]) and also by capsaicin pretreatment.[27] The plasma leakage induced by inhaled bradykinin is inhibited by a neurokinin (NK)₁-antagonist and bronchoconstriction by an NK₂-antagonist.[28,29] This indicates that bradykinin activates sensory nerves in the airways and that part of the airway response is mediated by release of constrictor peptides from capsaicin-sensitive nerves. In asthmatic patients, an inhaled nonselective tachykinin antagonist, FK 224, reduces the bronchoconstrictor response to inhaled bradykinin and also blocks the cough response in those subjects who coughed in response to bradykinin.[30]

STUDIES WITH NEP INHIBITORS

In rodents, inhibition of NEP with thiorphan or phosphoramidon results in striking potentiation of tachykinin and sensory nerve-induced effects and has been used as an approach to explore the potential for neurogenic inflammation in disease.[31] Several factors relevant to exacerbations of asthma appear to impair NEP activity and therefore increase neurogenic inflammation (Fig. 60-2). Intravenous acetorphan, which is hydrolyzed to thiorphan, was administered to asthmatic subjects and although there was potentiation of the wheal and flare response to intradermal SP, there was no

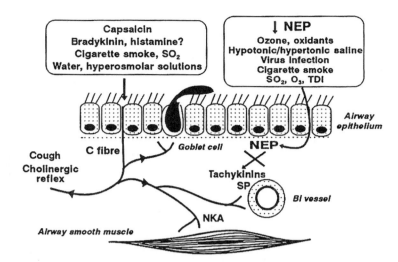

FIGURE 60-2 Neutral endopeptidase (NEP) breaks down tachykinins in the airways. Several factors reduce NEP activity in the airways and may thereby enhance neurogenic inflammation. TDI, tolulene = 2,4 = diisocyanate.

effect on baseline airway caliber or on bronchoconstriction induced by a "neurogenic" trigger sodium metabisulfite.[32] The lack of effect could be due to inadequate inhibition of NEP in the airways, particularly at the level of the epithelium. Nebulized thiorphan has been shown to potentiate the bronchoconstrictor response to inhaled NKA in normal and asthmatic subjects,[33,34] but there was no effect on baseline lung function in asthmatic patients,[34] indicating that there is unlikely to be any basal release of tachykinins. NEP is expressed strongly in the human airway,[35] but there is no evidence based on immunocytochemical staining or in situ hybridization that it is defective in asthmatic airways (J Baraniuk, PJ Barnes, unpublished observations) and the fact that after inhaled thiorphan, the bronchoconstrictor response to inhaled NKA is enhanced further in asthmatic subjects provides supportive functional data that NEP function may not be impaired, at least in mild asthma.[34] Of course, it is possible that NEP may become dysfunctional after viral infections or exposure to oxidants and thus contribute to asthma exacerbations.

TACHYKININ RESPONSES

In inflammatory bowel disease, there is evidence for a marked upregulation of tachykinin receptors, particularly in the vasculature, suggesting that chronic inflammation may cause changes in tachykinin receptor expression.[36,37] In patients with allergic rhinitis an increased vascular response to nasally applied SP is observed.[38] Evidence indicates that NK_1-receptor gene expression may be increased in the lungs of asthmatic patients.[39] This might be due to increased transcription in response to activation of transcription factors, such as activator protein-1 (AP-1), which are activated in human lung by cytokines such as TNF-a.[40] A consensus sequence both for AP-1 binding has been identified upstream of the NK_1-receptor gene.[41] Corticosteroids conversely reduce NK_1-receptor gene expression,[42] presumably through an inhibitory effect on AP-1 activation.

Modulation of Neurogenic Inflammation

Neurogenic inflammation may be modulated in several ways[43] (Fig. 60-3), and these may provide novel approaches to anti-inflammatory therapy of airways disease in the future.

INHIBITION OF SENSORY NEUROPEPTIDE EFFECTS

Antagonists of tachykinin or CGRP receptors should be effective. An NK_1-antagonist would be particularly useful because this receptor mediates most of the mucosal inflammatory effects of tachykinins, including vasodilatation, mucous secretion, and plasma exudation. Several highly potent and stable peptide and nonpeptide tachykinin agonists recently have been developed, which are highly selec-

FIGURE 60-3 Modulation of neurogenic inflammation in airway sensory nerves.

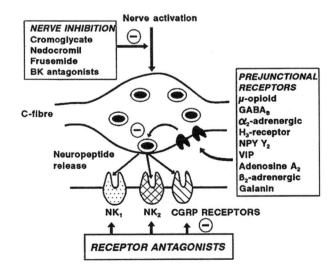

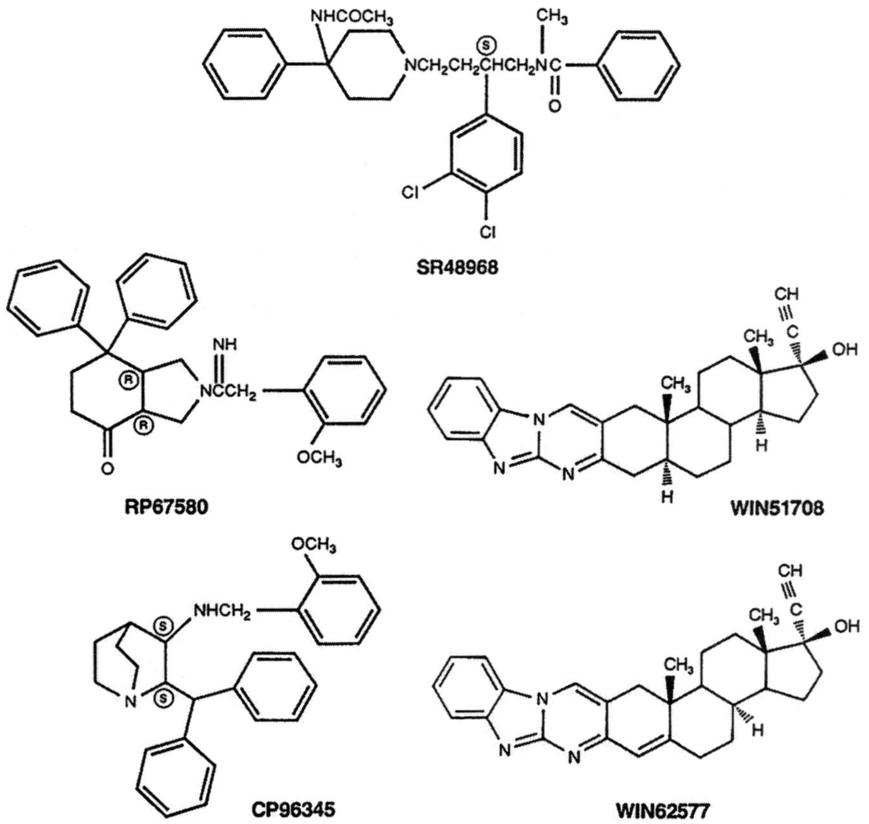

FIGURE 60-4 Structures of nonpeptide tachykinin antagonists.

tive for either NK_1- or NK_2-receptors[44] (Fig. 60-4). The NK_1-receptor antagonist CP 96,345 is effective in blocking the plasma exudation response to vagus nerve stimulation and to cigarette smoke in guinea pig airways,[45,46] without affecting the bronchoconstrictor response, which is blocked by the NK_2-antagonist SR 48,968.[47] Similar results have been obtained with the very potent NK_2-selective antagonist FK 888.[48] CP 96,345 also blocks hyperpnea-, metabisulfite- and bradykinin-induced plasma exudation in guinea pigs,[28,49,50] but it has no effect on the acute plasma exudation induced by allergen in sensitized animals.[28] These specific antagonists are useful new tools in probing the involvement of tachykinins in disease and several clinical trials are underway.

Bradykinin appears to release tachykinins from sensory nerves in the airways and capsaicin pretreatment or tachykinin antagonists markedly attenuate bradykinin-induced bronchoconstriction in guinea pigs.[27,28] Similar results also have been reported in humans. The nonselective peptide tachykinin antagonist, FK 224, has a significant inhibitory effect on bradykinin-induced bronchoconstriction in asthmatic airways.[30] Whether tachykinin antagonists are effective in other challenges or in the clinical control of asthma is currently under investigation using more potent nonpeptide antagonists. It is unlikely that such drugs would have a major clinical effect, at least in mild asthma, because there are many other inflammatory mechanisms in asthma. Furthermore, the effects mediated by tachykinins, such as plasma exudation and mucous secretion may be difficult to measure. Preliminary evidence indicates that FK 224 given for 4 weeks to patients with chronic bronchitis results in a significant decrement in mucous production and improves symptoms, particularly cough.[51]

Glucocorticosteroids may also be effective in neurogenic inflammation. Glucocorticoids inhibit the increased expression of NK_1-receptors in asthmatic lung and this effect is probably mediated via interaction with the transcription factor AP-1.[39]

INHIBITION OF SENSORY NEUROPEPTIDE RELEASE

Because multiple peptides are released from sensory nerves (and there is no evidence for selective release), it is likely that antagonism of a single peptide may not be entirely effective in controlling neurogenic inflammation. A more attractive approach may be to inhibit the release of all peptides. Several different agonists act on prejunctional receptors on sensory nerves in airways to inhibit the release of sensory neuropeptides, thus inhibiting neurogenic inflammation[43,52] (see Fig. 60-3). Opioids are the most effective agonists in this respect, and perhaps this is not surprising because they inhibit the release of SP from nociceptive fibers in the central nervous system.[53] Opioids inhibit ϵ-nonadrenergic, noncholinergic (ϵ-NANC) bronchoconstriction in guinea pig bronchi in vitro[54–56] and in vivo,[57,58] while having no effect on matched tachykinin-induced bronchoconstriction, thereby indicating an effect on the release of tachykinins. This has now been confirmed because SP release from rat airways is potently inhibited by opioids.[59] The effects of opioids are mediated by opioid receptors because they are inhibited by naloxone. A μ-opioid receptor is involved because μ-selective agonists are effective, whereas δ- and κ-agonists are not.[54,56,57] A μ-opioid agonist also modulates cholinergic neurotransmission in guinea pig airways, but this is largely via an inhibitory effect on the facilitatory action of ∈-NANC nerves.[56] Opioids also inhibit neurogenic microvascular leak in guinea pig airways[57,58] (Fig. 60-5), mucous secretion from human bronchi in vitro,[60] and cigarette smoke-induced goblet cell discharge from guinea pig airways in vivo.[61] Opioids also inhibit ozone-induced hyperreactivity in guinea pigs, which appears to be mediated via sensory nerves.[62]

Several other agonists are also effective. These include the inhibitory central neurotransmitter gamma-amino butyric acid (GABA), which acts via a GABA$_B$-receptor,[63] neuropeptide Y,[64,65] α$_2$-agonists,[64,66] galanin,[67,68] corticotrophin-releasing factor,[69,70] β$_2$-agonists,[71] adenosine A$_2$-receptors,[72] and histamine through an H$_3$-receptor.[73,74] The fact that so many different receptors have an inhibitory effect raises the question of whether there is a common inhibitory mechanism. In the central nervous system, several of the agonists that are inhibitory to neuropeptide release have been found to open a common K+ channel.[75] The K+ channel activator, cromakalim, and its active stereoisomer, levacromakalim, are effective in inhibiting ∈-NANC bronchoconstriction in guinea pigs in vivo and in vitro. Their effects are inhibited by blockers of adenosine triphosphate (ATP)-sensitive channels.[76–78] Levacromakalim also blocks neurogenic plasma exudation in airways[78] and cigarette smoke-induced goblet cell secretion in guinea pigs.[79] However, a potent ATP-sensitive channel blocker completely inhibits the effect of levacromakalim but has no effect against the inhibitory actions of an opioid or α$_2$-agonists. By contrast, charybdotoxin, an inhibitor of large conductance Ca^{2+}-activated K+-channels, is extremely effective in inhibiting these inhibitory actions, indicating that a common Ca^{2+}-activated K+ channel may be involved, which hyperpolarizes the sensory nerve and inhibits neuropeptide release.[77]

FIGURE 60-5 Inhibitory effect of an opioid on vagus nerve-induced plasma leakage, measured by Evans blue (EB) dye extravasation in guinea pig trachea. The lack of effect of morphine on substance P (SP)-induced extravasation suggests that this is mediated via opioid receptors on sensory nerves. (*Adapted, with permission.*[58])

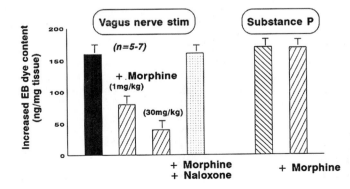

Another agent that inhibits neuropeptide release from sensory nerves in airways is the red dye, ruthenium red. Ruthenium red is a selective inhibitor of capsaicin-induced contraction of guinea pig airways in vitro, but has no effect against ∈-NANC bronchoconstriction induced by electrical field stimulation or bradykinin.[80] A synthetic analog of capsaicin, capsazepine, is also a competitive blocker of capsaicin effects on peripheral sensory nerves, but it has no effect on electrically induced neuropeptide release.[81] Capsazepine inhibits capsaicin-induced bronchoconstriction in guinea pig bronchi in vitro, although it has no effect on ∈-NANC contraction induced by electrical field stimulation.[82] Recently capsazepine has been found to inhibit cough induced in guinea pigs by capsaicin and citric acid aerosols,[83] indicating that protons (H$^+$) may release an endogenous capsaicin-like agonist.

There have been few clinical studies of potential prejunctional modulators of neuropeptide release in asthma, although in the last century opioids were often used in the treatment of severe asthma. An inhaled μ-opioid agonist, the pentapeptide BW 443C, was ineffective in inhibiting metabisulfite-induced bronchoconstriction, which is believed to act through neural mechanisms.[84] One problem with BW 443C is that it may be degraded by NEP in the airway epithelium and may not therefore reach a high enough concentration in the vicinity of the airway sensory nerves. Another agent that has a prejunctional modulatory effect in guinea pigs is the H$_3$-receptor agonist α-methyl histamine.[74] However, inhalation of α-methyl histamine had no effect on either resting tone or metabisulfite-induced bronchoconstriction in asthmatic patients.[85] The GABA$_B$ agonist, baclofen, which is effective in modulating ∈-NANC responses in guinea pig airways,[63] has recently been found to have some beneficial effect in asthma.[86]

INHIBITION OF SENSORY NERVE ACTIVATION

Activation of sensory nerves may be inhibited by local anesthetics, but it has been difficult to achieve adequate local anesthesia of the respiratory tract. Inhalation of local anesthetics, such as lidocaine, has not had consistent inhibitory effects on various airway challenges, and indeed may even promote bronchoconstriction in some patients with asthma.[87] This paradoxical bronchoconstriction may be due to the greater anesthesia of laryngeal afferents, which are linked to a tonic nonadrenergic bronchodilator reflex.[88,89] Other drugs may inhibit the activation of airway sensory nerves. Cromolyn sodium and nedocromil sodium may have direct effects on airway C fibers,[90,91] and this might contribute to their anti-asthma effect. Nedocromil sodium is highly effective against bradykinin-induced and sulfur dioxide-induced bronchoconstriction in asthmatic patients,[90,92] which are believed to be mediated by activation of sensory nerves in the airways. In addition, nedocromil sodium, and to a lesser extent, cromolyn sodium, inhibit ∈-NANC bronchoconstriction in guinea pig bronchi in vitro, indicating an effect on release of sensory neuropeptides as well as on activation.[93] The loop diuretic, furosemide (frusemide), given by nebulization, behaves in a similar fashion to nedocromil sodium and inhibits metabisulfite-induced bronchoconstriction in asthmatic patients[94] and also ε-NANC and cholinergic bronchoconstriction in guinea pig airways in vitro.[95] In addition, nebulized furosemide also inhibits certain types of cough[96] and has a direct inhibitory effect on the activation of single afferent fibers in the airways,[97] providing further evidence for an effect on sensory nerves.[98] Furosemide and cromones have very similar actions in inhibiting indirect, but not direct, airway challenges, suggesting a common mechanism of action. There is some evidence that furosemide and cromones act through inhibition of certain types of chloride channels[99,100], and more potent inhibitors of these channels may be developed in the future as potential anti-asthma treatments.

Bradykinin is a potent activator of airway C fibers[101] and enhances ε-NANC responses in the airways.[102] These effects are mediated via B$_2$-receptors. Bradykinin B$_2$-receptor antagonists, such as icatibant (HOE 140), may therefore have inhibitory effects on neurogenic inflammation in the airways. Icatibant itself is a peptide, and although it is potent and has long-lasting effects in the airways,[103,104] there may be problems in delivering a peptide to the respiratory tract. Nonpeptide bradykinin antagonists now in development may be more suitable.

REPLACEMENT OF NEP

Because defective function of NEP may be critical in amplifying neurogenic inflammation another strategy would be to replace the enzyme. Indeed, recombinant human NEP inhibits cough induced by tachykinins in guinea pig.[105] It also may be possible to increase the activity of NEP in the airways. Thus, corticosteroids have been reported to increase the activity of NEP in airways, and this may be at the level of gene expression in epithelial cells,[106] although this has not been confirmed in other studies.[107]

SENSORY DENERVATION

Exposure of adult animals to high concentrations of capsaicin depletes sensory neuropeptides, which are only slowly repleted. Topical application of capsaicin might therefore be a useful approach to controlling neurogenic inflammation in the respiratory tract. Although this may be difficult to achieve in the lower airways, it appears to be feasible in the nose. Nasal application of capsaicin is reported to be effective in controlling nonallergic vasomotor rhinitis for periods of over a year.[108]

Conclusions

Although neurogenic inflammation in the airways has been documented clearly in rodent airways in association with many of the triggers that are relevant in asthma and chronic obstructive airways disease, the role of neurogenic inflammation in human airway disease has not yet been defined. Strategies to inhibit neurogenic inflammation may be worthy of consideration, but it is unlikely that neurogenic inflammation is the sole mechanism contributing to the

inflammation of the airways in these diseases. This implies that modulators of neurogenic inflammation would not be as effective as corticosteroids. It remains a possibility that patients with certain types of asthma (e.g., brittle unstable asthma) may have a more prominent neurogenic inflammatory component, although it is likely that glucocorticosteroids would have some inhibitory effect on this neurogenic component. In chronic obstructive pulmonary disease, which is resistant to the action of corticosteroids, neurogenic inflammation may be more important and may play a role in the regulation of the chronic mucous hypersecretion, stimulated by cigarette smoke, in chronic bronchitis. A more promising approach may be the development of drugs that inhibit sensory nerve activation because such drugs may have a suppressive effect on symptoms such as cough and chest tightness, in addition to inhibition of cholinergic reflex effects and inhibition of neurogenic inflammation.

References

1. Barnes PJ: Neurogenic inflammation in airways and its modulation. *Arch Int Pharmacodyn* 1990; 303:67.
2. McDonald DM: Neurogenic inflammation in the respiratory tract: actions of sensory nerve mediators on blood vessels and epithelium of the airway mucosa. *Am Rev Respir Dis* 1987; 136:S65.
3. Solway J, Leff AR: Sensory neuropeptides and airway function. *J Appl Physiol* 1991; 71:2077.
4. Barnes PJ: Asthma as an axon reflex. *Lancet* 1986; i:242.
5. Barnes PJ: Sensory nerves, neuropeptides and asthma. *Ann N Y Acad Sci* 1991; 629:359.
6. Barnes PJ: Neuropeptides and asthma, in Kaliner MA, Barnes PJ, Kunkel GHM, Baraniuk J (eds): *Neuropeptides in Respiratory Medicine.* New York, Dekker, 1994:285–311.
7. Bowden J, Gibbins IL: Relative density of substance P-immunoreactive nerve fibres in the tracheal epithelium of a range of species. *FASEB J* 1992; 6:A1276.
8. Levine JD, Dardick SJ, Roizan MF, et al.: Contribution of sensory afferents and sympathetic efferents to joint injury in experimental arthritis. *J Neurosci* 1986; 6:3423.
9. Holzer P: Local effector functions of capsaicin-sensitive sensory nerve endings: involvement of tachykinins, calcitonin gene related peptide, and other neuropeptides. *Neuroscience* 1988; 24:739.
10. Ollerenshaw SL, Jarvis D, Sullivan CE, Woolcock AJ: Substance P immunoreactive nerves in airways from asthmatics and non-asthmatics. *Eur Respir J* 1991; 4:673.
11. Nieber K, Baumgarten CR, Rathsack R, et al.: Substance P and β-endorphin-like immunoreactivity in lavage fluids of subjects with and without asthma. *J Allergy Clin Immunol* 1992; 90:646.
12. Tomaki M, Ichinose M, Nakajima N, et al.: Elevated substance P concentration in sputum after hypertonic saline inhalation in asthma and chronic bronchitis patients. *Am Rev Respir Dis* 1993; 147:A478.
13. Hazgun ME, Hamilton R, Holian A, Eschenbacher WL: Ozone-induced increases in substance P and 8 epi-prostaglandin F2$_\alpha$ in the airways of human subjects. *Am J Respir Cell Mol Biol* 1993; 9:568.
14. Lindsay RM, Harmar AJ: Nerve growth factor regulates expression of neuropeptide genes in sensory neurons. *Nature* 1989; 337:362.
15. Minami M, Kuraishi Y, Kawamura M, et al.: Enhancement of

preprotachykinin A gene expression by adjuvant-induced inflammation in the rat spinal cord: possible inducement of substance P-containing spinal neurons in nociceptor. *Neurosci Lett* 1989; 98:105.

16. Fischer A, Philippin B, Saria A, et al.: Neuronal plasticity in sensitized and challenged guinea pigs: neuropeptides and neuropeptide gene expression. *Am J Respir Crit Care Med* 1994; 149:A890.

17. Howarth PH, Djukanovic R, Wilson JW, et al.: Mucosal nerves in endobronchial biopsies in asthma and non-asthma. *Int Arch Allergy Appl Immunol* 1991; 94:330.

18. Cunha FQ, Poole S, Lorenzetti BB, Ferreira SH: The pivotal role of tumour necrosis factor α in the development of inflammatory hyperalgesia. *Br J Pharmacol* 1992; 107:660.

19. Lundberg JM, Saria A, Lundblad L, et al.: Bioactive peptides in capsaicin-sensitive C-fiber afferents of the airways: functional and pathyphysiological implications. New York, Marcel Dekker, 1987.

20. Alving K, Matran R, Lacroix JS, Lundberg JM: Allergen challenge induces vasodilation in pig bronchial circulation via a capsaicin sensitive mechanism. *Acta Physiol Scand* 1988; 134:571.

21. Fuller RW, Dixon CMS, Barnes PJ: The bronchoconstrictor response to inhaled capsaicin in humans. *J Appl Physiol* 1985; 85:1080.

22. Midgren B, Hansson L, Karlsson JA, et al.: Capsaicin-induced cough in humans. *Am Rev Respir Dis* 1992; 146:347.

23. Barnes PJ: Bradykinin and asthma. *Thorax* 1992; 47:979.

24. Fuller RW, Dixon CMS, Cuss FMC, Barnes PJ: Bradykinin-induced bronchoconstriction in man: mode of action. *Am Rev Respir Dis* 1987; 135:176.

25. Kaufman MP, Coleridge HM, Coleridge JCG, Baker DG: Bradykinin stimulates afferent vagal C-fibres in intrapulmonary airways of dogs. *J Appl Physiol* 1980; 48:511.

26. Saria A, Martling CR, Yan Z, et al.: Release of multiple tachykinins from capsaicin-sensitive nerves in the lung by bradykinin, histamine, dimethylphenylpiperainium, and vagal nerve stimulation. *Am Rev Respir Dis* 1988; 137:1330.

27. Ichinose M, Belvisi MG, Barnes PJ: Bradykinin-induced bronchoconstriction in guinea-pig in vivo: role of neural mechanisms. *J Pharmacol Exp Ther* 1990; 253:1207.

28. Sakamoto T, Barnes PJ, Chung KF: Effect of CP-96,345, a nonpeptide NK$_1$-receptor antagonist against substance P-, bradykinin-, and allergen-induced airway microvascular leak and bronchoconstriction in the guinea pig. *Eur J Pharmacol* 1993; 231:31.

29. Sakamoto T, Tsukagoshi H, Barnes PJ, Chung KF: Role played by NK$_2$-receptors and cyclooxygenase activation in bradykinin B$_2$ receptor-mediated airway effects in guinea pigs. *Agents Actions* 1993; 111:117.

30. Ichinose M, Nakajima N, Takahashi T, et al.: Protection against bradykinin-induced bronchoconstriction in asthmatic patients by a neurokinin receptor antagonist. Lancet 340:1248, 1992.

31. Nadel JA: Neutral endopeptidase modulates neurogenic inflammation. *Eur Respir J* 1991; 4:745.

32. Nichol GM, O'Connor BJ, Le Compte JM, et al.: Effect of neutral endopeptidase inhibitor on airway function and bronchial responsiveness in asthmatic subjects. *Eur J Clin Pharmacol* 1992; 42:495.

33. Cheung D, Bel EH, den Hartigh J, et al.: An effect of an inhaled neutral endopeptidase inhibitor, thiorphan, on airway responses to neurokinin A in normal humans in vivo. *Am Rev Respir Dis* 1992; 145:1275.

34. Cheung D, Timmers MC, Bel EH, et al.: An isolated neutral endopeptidase inhibitor, thiorphan, enhances airway narrowing to neurokin A in asthmatic subjects in vivo. *Am Rev Respir Dis* 1992; 195:A682.

35. Baraniuk JN, Mak J, Letarte M, et al.: Neutral endopeptidase mRNA expression in airways. *Am Rev Respir Dis* 1991; 143:A40.

36. Mantyh CR, Gates TS, Zimmerman RP, et al.: Receptor binding sites for substance P but not substance K or neuromedin K are expressed in high concentrations by arterioles, venules and lymph nodes in surgical specimens obtained from patients with ulcerative colitis and Crohn's disease. *Proc Natl Acad Sci USA* 1988; 85:3235.

37. Mantyh PW: Substance P and the inflammatory and immune response. *Ann N Y Acad Sci* 1991; 632:263.

38. Devillier P, Dessanges JF, Rakotashanaka F, et al.: Nasal response to substance P and methacholine with and without allergic rhinitis. *Eur Respir J* 1988; 1:356.

39. Adcock IM, Peters M, Gelder C, et al.: Increased tachykinin receptor gene expression in asthmatic lung and its modulation by steroids. *J Mol Endocrinol* 1993; 11:1.

40. Adcock IM, Shirasaki H, Gelder CM, et al.: The effects of glucocorticoids on phorbol ester and cytokine stimulated transcription factor activation in human lung. *Life Sci* 1994; 55:1147.

41. Nakanishi S: Mammalian tachykinin receptors. *Annu Rev Neurosci* 1991; 14:123.

42. Ihara H, Nakanishi S: Selective inhibition of expression of the substance P receptor mRNA in pancreatic acinar AR42J cells by glucocorticoids. *J Biol Chem* 1990; 36:22,441.

43. Barnes PJ, Belvisi MG, Rogers DF: Modulation of neurogenic inflammation: novel approaches to inflammatory diseases. *Trends Pharmacol Sci* 1990; 11:185.

44. Watling KJ: Nonpeptide antagonists heralded a new era in tachykinin research. *Trends Pharmacol Sci* 1992; 13:266.

45. Lei Y-H, Barnes PJ, Rogers DF: Inhibition of neurogenic plasma exudation in guinea pig airways by CP-96,345, a new non-peptide NK$_1$-receptor antagonist. *Br J Pharmacol* 1992; 105:261.

46. Delay-Goyet P, Lundberg JM: Cigarette smoke-induced airway oedema is blocked by the NK$_1$-antagonist CP-96,345. *Eur J Pharmacol* 1991; 203:157.

47. Advenier C, Naline E, Toty L, et al.: Effects on the isolated human bronchus of SR 48968, a potent and selective nonpeptide antagonist of the neurokinin A (NK$_2$) receptors. *Am Rev Respir Dis* 1992; 146:1177.

48. Hirayama Y, Lei YH, Barnes PJ, Rogers DF: Effects of two novel tachykinin antagonists FK 224 and FK 888 on neurogenic plasma exudation, bronchoconstriction and systemic hypotension in guinea pigs in vivo. *Br J Pharmacol* 1993; 108:844.

49. Solway J, Kao BM, Jordan JE, et al.: Tachykinin receptor antagonists inhibit hypernea-induced bronchoconstriction in guinea pigs. *J Clin Invest* 1993; 92:315.

50. Sakamoto T, Tsukagoshi H, Barnes PJ, Chung KF: Involvement of tachykinin receptors (NK1 and NK2) in saline metabisulfite-induced airway effects. *Am J Resp Crit Care Med* 1994; 149:387.

51. Ichinose M, Katsumata U, Kikuchi R, et al.: Effect of tachykinin receptor antagonist on chronic bronchitis patients. *Am Rev Respir Dis* 1993; 147:A318.

52. Barnes PJ: Modulation of neurotransmission in airways. *Physiol Rev* 1992; 72:699.

53. Jessel TM, Iversen LL: Opiate analgesics inhibit substance P release from rat trigeminal nucleus. *Nature* 1977; 268:549.

54. Frossard N, Barnes PJ: μ-Opioid receptors modulate noncholinergic constrictor nerves in guinea-pig airways. *Eur J Pharmacol* 1987; 141:519.

55. Bartho L, Amann R, Saria A, et al.: Peripheral effects of opioid drugs in capsaicin-sensitive neurones of the guinea pig bronchus and rabbit ear. *Naunyn Schmiedeberg Arch Pharm* 1987; 336:316.

56. Belvisi MG, Stretton CD, Barnes PJ: Modulation of cholinergic neutrotransmission in guinea-pig airways by opioids. *Br J Pharmacol* 1990; 100:131.

57. Belvisi MG, Rogers DF, Barnes PJ: Neurogenic plasma extravasation: inhibition by morphine in guinea pig airways in vivo. *J Appl Physiol* 1989; 66:268.

58. Belvisi MG, Chung KF, Jackson DM, Barnes PJ: Opioid modulation of non-cholinergic neural bronchoconstriction in guinea-pig in in vivo. *Br J Pharmacol* 1988; 95:413.

59. Ray NJ, Jones AJ, Keen P: The effect of morphine and sodium cromoglycate on the release of substance P from capsaicin sensitive neurones in rat trachea. *Br J Pharmacol* 1989; 98:864P.

60. Rogers DF, Barnes PJ: Opioid inhibition of neurally mediated mucus secretion in human bronchi: implications for chronic bronchitis therapy. *Lancet* 1989; i:930.

61. Kuo H-P, Rohde J, Barnes PJ, Rogers DF: Differential effects of opioids on cigarette smoke, capsaicin and electrically-induced goblet cell secretion in guinea pig trachea. *Br J Pharmacol* 1992; 105:361.

62. Yeadon M, Wilkinson D, Darley-Usmar V, et al.: Mechanisms contributing to ozone-induced bronchial hyperreactivity in guinea pigs. *Pulm Pharmacol* 1992; 5:39.

63. Belvisi MG, Ichinose M, Barnes PJ: Modulation of non-adrenergic non-cholinergic neural bronchoconstriction in guinea-pig airways via GABA$_B$ receptors. *Br J Pharmacol* 1989; 97:1125.

64. Matran R, Martling C-R, Lundberg JM: Inhibition of cholinergic and nonadrenergic, noncholinergic bronchoconstriction in the guinea-pig mediatd by neuropeptide Y and alpha$_2$-adrenoceptors and opiate receptors. *Eur J Pharmacol* 1989; 163:15.

65. Stretton CD, Belvisi MG, Barnes PJ: Neuropeptide Y modulates non-adrenergic non-cholinergic neural bronchoconstriction in vivo and in vitro. *Neuropeptides* 1990; 17:163.

66. Grundstrom N, Andersson RGG: In vivo demonstration of alpha$_2$-adrenoceptor mediated inhibition of the excitatory non-cholinergic neurotransmission in guinea pig airways. *Naunyn Schmiedeberg Arch Pharm* 1985; 328:236.

67. Giuliani S, Ammann R, Papini AM, et al.: Modulatory action of galanin on responses due to antidromic activation of peripheral terminals of capsaicin-sensitive sensory nerves. *Eur J Pharmacol* 1989; 163:91.

68. Takahashi T, Belvisi MG, Barnes PJ: Modulation of neurotransmission in guinea-pig airways by galanin and the effect of a new antagonist galantide. *Neuropeptides* 1994; 26:245.

69. Wei ET, Kiang JC: Inhibition of protein exudation from the trachea by corticotropin releasing factor. *Eur J Pharmacol* 1987; 140:63.

70. Rogers DF, Lei Y-H, Barnes PJ: Corticotrophin-releasing factor intubation of neurogenic plasma exudation and bronchoconstriction in guinea pigs in vivo. *Am Rev Respir Dis* 1993; 147:A814.

71. Verleden GM, Belvisi MG, Rabe K, et al.: β$_2$-Adrenoceptors inhibit NANC neural bronchoconstrictor responses in vitro. *J Appl Physiol* 1993; 74:1195.

72. Kamikawa Y, Shimo Y: Adenosine selectively inhibits non-cholinergic transmission in guinea pig bronchi. *J Appl Physiol* 1991; 66:2084.

73. Ichinose M, Barnes PJ: Histamine H$_3$-receptors modulate non-adrenergic non-cholinergic bronchoconstriction in guinea pig in vivo. *Eur J Pharmacol* 1989; 174:49.

74. Ichinose M, Belvisi MG, Barnes PJ: Histamine H$_3$-receptors inhibit neurogenic microvascular leakage in airways. *J Appl Physiol* 1990; 68:21.

75. Christie MJ, North RA: Agonists at μ-opioid, M$_2$-muscarinic, and GABA$_B$-receptors increase the ionic potassium conductance in rat lateral paratracheal nerves. *Br J Pharmacol* 1988; 95:896.

76. Ichinose M, Barnes PJ: A potassium channel activator modulates both noncholinergic and cholinergic neurotransmission in guinea pig airways. *J Pharmacol Exp Ther* 1990; 252:1207.

77. Stretton CD, Miura M, Belvisi MG, Barnes PJ: Calcium-activated potassium channels mediate prejunctional inhibition of peripheral sensory nerves. *Proc Natl Acad Sci U S A* 1992; 89:1325.

78. Lei Y-H, Barnes PJ, Rogers DF: Inhibition of neurogenic plasma exudation and bronchoconstriction by K+ channel activator BRL 38227 in guinea pig airways in vivo. *Eur J Pharmacol* 1993; 239:257.

79. Kuo H-P, Rohde JAL, Barnes PJ, Rogers DF: K+ channel activator inhibition of neurogenic goblet cell secretion in guinea pig trachea. *Eur J Pharmacol* 1992; 221:385.

80. Maggi CA, Patacchini R, Santicioli P, et al.: The "efferent" function of capsaicin-sensitive nerves: ruthenium red discriminates between different mechanisms of activation. *Eur J Pharmacol* 1989; 170:167.

81. Dray A, Campbell EA, Hughes GA, et al.: Antagonism of capsaicin-induced activation of C-fibres by a selective capsaicin antagonist, capsazepine (abstract). *Br J Pharmacol* 1991.

82. Belvisi MG, Miura M, Stretton D, Barnes PJ: Capsazepine as a selective antagonist of capsaicin-induced activation of C-fibres in guinea pig bronchi. *Eur J Pharmacol* 1992; 215:341.

83. Lalloo UG, Belvisi MG, Fox AJ, et al.: Capsazepine, a selective capsaicin antagonist, inhibits capsaicin and citric acid-induced cough in guinea pigs (abstract). *Am J Respir Crit Care Med* 1995;

84. O'Connor BJ, Chen-Wordsell M, Barnes PJ, Chung KF: Effect of an inhaled opioid peptide on airway responses to sodium metabisulphite in asthma. *Thorax* 1991;

85. O'Connor BJ, Lecomte JM, Barnes PJ: Effect of an inhaled H$_3$-receptor agonist on airway responses to sodium metabisulphite in asthma. *Br J Clin Pharmacol* 1993; 35:55.

86. Dicpinigaitis PV, Spungev AM, Bauman WA, et al.: Inhibition of bronchial hyperresponsiveness by the GABA-agonist baclofen. *Chest* 1994; 106:758.

87. McAlpine LG, Thomson NC: Lidocaine-induced bronchoconstriction in asthmatic patients. Relation to histamine airway responsiveness and effect of preservative. *Chest* 1989; 96:1012.

88. Lammers J-WJ, Minette P, McCusker M, et al.: Nonadrenergic bronchodilator mechanisms in normal human subjects in vivo. *J Appl Physiol* 1988; 64:1817.

89. Lammers J-WJ, Minette P, McCusker M, et al.: Capsaicin-induced bronchodilatation in mild asthmatic subjects: possible role of nonadrenergic inhibitory system. *J Appl Physiol* 1989; 67:856.

90. Dixon N, Jackson DM, Richard IM: The effect of sodium cromoglycate on lung irritant receptors and left ventricular receptors in anasthetized dogs. *Br J Pharmacol* 1979; 67:569.

91. Jackson DM, Norris AA, Eady RP: Nedocromil sodium and sensory nerves in the dog lung. *Pulm Pharmacol* 1989; 2:179.

92. Dixon CMS, Fuller RW, Barnes PJ: The effect of nedocromil sodium on sulphur dioxide induced bronchoconstriction. *Thorax* 1987; 42:462.

93. Verleden GM, Belvisi MG, Stretton CD, Barnes PJ: Nedocromil sodium modulates non-adrenergic non-cholinergic bronchoconstrictor nerves in guinea-pig airways in vitro. *Am Rev Respir Dis* 1991; 143:114.

94. Nichol GM, Alton EWFW, Nix A, et al.: Effect of inhaled furosemide on metabisulfite- and methacholine-induced bronchoconstriction and nasal potential difference in asthmatic subjects. *Am Rev Respir Dis* 1990; 142:576.

95. Elwood W, Lötvall JO, Barnes PJ, Chung KF: Loop diuretics inhibit cholinergic and non-cholinergic nerves in guinea pig airways. *Am Rev Respir Dis* 1991; 143:1340.

96. Ventresca GP, Nichol GM, Barnes PJ, Chung KF: Inhaled furosemide inhibits cough induced by low chloride content solutions but not by capsaicin. *Am Rev Respir Dis* 1990; 142:143.

97. Fox AJ, Barnes PJ, Dray A: Stimulation of afferent fibres in the

guinea pig trachea by non-isoosmotic and low chloride solutions and its modulation by frusemide. *J Physiol* 1995;

98. Barnes PJ: Diuretics and asthma. *Thorax* 1993; 48:195.

99. Perkins R, Dent G, Chung KF, Barnes PJ: Effect of anion transport inhibitors and extracellular Cl⁻ concentrations of eosinophil respiratory burst activity. *Biochem Pharmacol* 1992; 43:2480.

100. Jackson DM, Pollard CE, Roberts SM: The effect of nedocromil sodium on the isolated rabbit vagus nerve. *Eur J Pharmacol* 1992; 221:175.

101. Fox AJ, Barnes PJ, Urban L, Dray A: An in vitro study of the properties of single vagal afferents innervating guinea-pig airways. *J Physiol* 1993; 469:21.

102. Miura M, Belvisi MG, Barnes PJ: Effect of bradykinin in airway neural responses in vitro. *J Appl Physiol* 1992; 73:1537.

103. Höck FJ, Wirth K, Albus U, et al.: HOE 140 a new potent and long acting bradykinin-antagonist: in vitro studies. *Br J Pharmacol* 1991; 102:769.

104. Sakamoto T, Sun J, Barnes PJ, Chung KF: Effect of a bradykinin receptor antagonist HOE 140 against bradykinin and vagal stimulation-induced airway responses in guinea pig. *Eur J Pharmacol* 1994; 251:137.

105. Kohrogi H, Nadel JA, Malfroy B, et al.: Recombinant human enkephalinase (neutral endopeptidase) prevents cough induced by tachykinins in awake guinea pigs. *J Clin Invest* 1989; 84:781.

106. Borson DB, Jew S, Gruenert DC: Glucocorticoids induce neutral endopeptidase in transformed human trachea epithelial cells. *Am J Physiol* 1991; 260:L83.

107. Proud D, Subauste MC, Ward RE: Glucocorticoids do not alter peptidase expression on a human bronchial epithelial cell line. *Am J Respir Cell Mol Biol* 1994; 11:57.

108. Lacroix J-S, Buvelot JM, Polla BS, Lundberg JM: Improvement of symptoms of non-allergic chronic rhinitis by local treatment with capsaicin. *Clin Exp Allergy* 1991; 21:595.

THEOPHYLLINE: ANTI-INFLAMMATORY EFFECTS

JAN-ANDERS KARLSSON

Theophylline has been the most widely used antiasthma drug worldwide for the past 10 to 20 years despite the introduction of novel agents like β_2 adrenergic agonists, sodium cromoglycate, and inhaled glucocorticoids. This position reflects the important acute and long-term beneficial effects of theophylline in asthma patients, which would appear to be all the more significant in view of the well-recognized limitations with theophylline therapy—very variable pharmacokinetics in different patients, a narrow therapeutic margin, and potentially severe adverse reactions. Although most studies have been unable to demonstrate a clear advantage with theophylline over β_2 adrenergic agonists and inhaled steroids in mild asthma, theophylline seems to have unique pharmacologic properties in a population of severely ill patients.[1]

Theophylline long has been used in the treatment of asthma. In the last century strong coffee (owing to its high content of caffeine) was suggested by Dr. H. H. Salter as an effective remedy for acute shortness of breath,[2] but it was not until the middle of the Twentieth Century that methylxan-

thine pharmacology had been delineated and its use widely accepted in asthma therapy.[2] Numerous studies have demonstrated a relaxant effect in isolated airway tissue and a bronchodilator response after intravenous infusions in animals and man.[3] Theophylline thus has been regarded generally as a bronchodilator agent.

In man, the anti-inflammatory effects of theophylline have been demonstrated in vitro in isolated cell and tissue preparations and in animal studies in vivo. Accumulating evidence from clinical studies supports the view that theophylline could have such an effect also in the bronchial tree of patients with airways obstruction, and potent anti-inflammatory and immunomodulatory effects have indeed been demonstrated already in doses lower than those normally recommended for "bronchodilation" in asthma patients. Wider confirmation of such anti-inflammatory effects in asthma patients could lead to the use of theophylline as a prophylactic agent. An altered dosing regimen would also improve the therapeutic margin and reduce the risk of severe adverse reactions. In the light of these recent findings, it is now timely to reappraise the pharmacodynamic effects of theophylline and to reevaluate its role in asthma therapy.

Theophylline as a Cyclic Nucleotide–phosphodiesterase Inhibitor

Methylxanthines, like theophylline and caffeine, are widely known for their inhibitory effects on cyclic nucleotide phosphodiesterases (PDEs). These enzymes hydrolyze the purine cyclic nucleotides (cyclic adenosine monophosphate, cyclic AMP, and cyclic guanosine monophosphate, cyclic GMP) to their respective 5′-mononucleotides (5′-AMP, 5′-GMP), which do not activate cyclic nucleotide protein kinases. Multiple PDE isoenzymes with differing cell and tissue distribution have been identified and categorized into families.[4] It is clear from sequencing data that further isoenzymes and splicing variants exist within each family,[5] and entirely new families, such as the type VII, also have been proposed.[6] Theophylline is a nonspecific inhibitor of the five traditional enzyme families. However, its low potency [> 100 μM is required for 50 percent inhibition of enzyme activity[7]] on isolated PDE enzyme preparations in vitro is notable. Indeed, many of its pharmacologic effects are exerted at concentrations below those needed for PDE inhibition, and consequently it has been argued that this mechanism of action cannot account for the biologic effects of theophylline. For example, a significant relaxation of tracheal smooth muscle is obtained at concentrations that do not produce a change in intracellular cyclic nucleotide levels.[8,9]

The recommended therapeutic range (plasma concentration between 10 to 20 mg/L = 55 to 110 μM) thus seems to be below the concentration range in which theophylline inhibits cyclic nucleotide–PDE activity in vitro. However, it has been reported that therapeutic concentrations of theophylline inhibited the respiratory burst in neutrophils and that the ex vivo response to isoprenaline was potentiated in blood cells from theophylline-treated patients.[10] The authors suggested that this effect most likely was due to cyclic nucleotide–PDE inhibition. This observation raises the possibility that a small enzyme inhibition leads to a disproportionately large functional response or that whole cell responses are produced by inhibition of PDE activity in a subcellular compartment. In this latter situation, whole cell cyclic AMP levels would not reflect such a subtle change.

It also is possible that isoforms of the PDE isoenzyme families have an increased sensitivity to theophylline.[11] These questions are still unresolved and the obvious discrepancies between cell responses and PDE inhibition have stimulated the search for other mechanisms of action.

IS PDE ACTIVITY INCREASED IN INFLAMMATORY CELLS FROM ATOPIC INDIVIDUALS?

Cyclic AMP–PDE activity has been reported to be increased in mononuclear leukocytes obtained from atopic individuals, with the most marked differences being in the monocyte population.[12,13,14] Hanafin and colleagues[11,15] have sug-

gested the existence of two immunochemically distinct cyclic AMP–PDE in monocytes from patients with atopic dermatitis and that this unique PDE resembles the PDE IV in that it is inhibited by rolipram.[11] Interestingly, theophylline is almost 10 times more potent on this enzyme than on the "normal" PDE IV isolated from monocytes of healthy subjects.[11] This is consistent with PDE inhibition as a mechanism by theophylline in asthma. However, the possible role of this novel isoenzyme is as yet uncertain since not all studies have been able to reproduce these findings.[16,17]

It has been speculated that this increased cyclic AMP–PDE activity in monocytes from atopic subjects results in decreased intracellular cyclic AMP concentrations and, therefore, enhanced PGE$_2$ generation, which, in turn, would inhibit IFNγ production from T helper-1 cells. Interferon-γ is considered one of the endogenous inhibitors of T helper-2 cells, so inhibition of this cytokine would potentially aggravate the allergic reaction. However, this theory is contradicted by the observation that cyclic AMP–PDE inhibitors are much more potent suppressors of cytokine release from T helper-1 than T helper-2 cells.[18]

At this point in time it is pertinent to conclude that there still is insufficient evidence to support the hypothesis that cyclic AMP–PDE activity is increased in atopy and that this could explain onset and progression of the disease.

Adenosine-Receptor Antagonism and Other Proposed Mechanisms of Action

Theophylline is an adenosine-receptor antagonist at concentrations 10 to 100 times less than those generally required for PDE inhibition. This mechanism thus occurs at therapeutic concentrations and it has been suggested that adenosine-receptor antagonism could explain its antiasthma actions.[19,20] Theophylline has been shown to increase mediator release from human basophils by antagonism of adenosine[21] (see section Basophils and mast cells). Adenosine has virtually no effect on smooth muscle tone in human nonasthmatic bronchi[22] but has been reported to contract asthmatic bronchi in vitro.[23] In asthmatics, but not healthy subjects, inhalation of adenosine or 5′-AMP (also acting through adenosine receptors) causes bronchospasm, supporting a potential role for adenosine as a mediator of asthma.

Although attractive, considerable evidence has now accumulated to refute this theory. First, adenosine is at best only a very weak bronchoconstrictor and, second, theophylline-like compounds that are not adenosine-receptor antagonists can still produce bronchodilation. For example, enprofylline, 3-propylxanthine, which is devoid of adenosine-receptor antagonism[24] is about three times more potent than theophylline as a relaxant of airways smooth muscle in vitro[22,24] and is as efficacious as theophylline in asthma patients.[25–27] Isbufylline, another xanthine derivative that seems to lack adenosine-receptor antagonism, retains theophylline-like bronchodilator and anti-inflammatory effects in preclinical studies.[28]

Even though adenosine-receptor antagonism cannot explain the anti-asthma actions of theophylline, this mechanism is of importance for many of theophylline's extrapulmonary effects. In the CNS, kidney, gastrointestinal tract, and adipose tissue, adenosine plays an important physiologic role. Antagonism of this inhibitory or suppressive effect can explain the CNS-excitatory effect (eventually culminating in seizures), acid secretion, diuresis and lipolysis readily observed in patients treated with theophylline. Proof of concept was obtained in enprofylline-treated patients in which these actions could not be observed.[26]

Other mechanisms that have been proposed include enhanced release of adrenaline from the adrenal medulla, increased uptake of cytoplasmic Ca^{2+} into intracellular organelles, and selective antagonism of prostaglandin-mediated responses.[29,30] There is little experimental evidence to support any of these mechanisms as being important at therapeutically relevant concentrations of theophylline.

Thus, despite the many reported discrepancies between concentrations necessary for pharmacologic effects in in vitro and in vivo studies and those attained with clinical doses of theophylline, PDE inhibition remains the most likely explanation for the pulmonary effects of theophylline. Interestingly, enprofylline is about three times more potent than theophylline as a PDE inhibitor and it is likewise some three times more potent as an antiasthma agent in patients.[25,26] However, in addition to PDE inhibition, other as yet unidentified cellular mechanisms may well contribute to the desirable anti-inflammatory and bronchodilatory effects of theophylline.

Use of Theophylline in Acute and Chronic Asthma

Theophylline generally is regarded as a bronchodilator agent, which is one of the reasons for its widespread use in acute asthma. Slow, intravenous infusions of aminophylline are commonly used in acute severe asthma even though it seems to be less effective than a nebulized β_2-receptor agonist.[31] Some studies have indicated that there may be no additional benefits from adding theophylline to nebulized β_2-adrenergic agonist[32] but that it may rather increase the frequency of adverse reactions.[33,34] Theophylline should therefore be used primarily in patients not responding well to β_2-adrenergic agonists.

Theophylline has a moderate bronchodilator effect in asthmatic, but not in healthy, subjects, although it is generally less efficacious than a β_2 adrenoceptor agonist. Theophylline and sodium cromoglycate are both effective in young asthmatics,[35] but in clinical studies directly comparing theophylline with inhaled glucocorticoids, the latter seems to provide significantly better symptom control.[36] Furthermore, a narrow therapeutic window, variable pharmacokinetics[37] and potentially severe adverse reactions[38] have relegated theophylline to third- or fourth-line therapy after β_2-adrenergic agonists and inhaled corticosteroids.[39,40]

Theophylline, however, seems to have additional beneficial effects over and above airways smooth muscle relaxation in a subgroup of patients also taking inhaled glucocorticoids.[41,42] This was particularly noticeable in a study by Brenner and co-workers[1] in severe asthmatics controlled by inhaled and oral steroids, nebulized β_2-adrenergic agonist, an anticholinergic, sodium cromoglycate, and theophylline. When they attempted to withdraw theophylline, the patients deteriorated in spite of increased doses of corticosteroids, and the investigators had to reintroduce theophylline (Fig. 61-1).

Other studies also have examined the controlled withdrawal of theophylline in patients with asthma. Discontinuation was associated with increases in symptoms and a decline in lung function, particularly during nighttime. There was a parallel increase in T lymphocytes and inflammatory cells in the airways, suggesting that theophylline has immunomodulatory effects.[43,44]

Taken together, these data demonstrate the beneficial effects of theophylline, particularly in chronic, severe asthma. Interestingly, in this category of patients, theophylline seemed to have unique properties not possessed by high-dose glucocorticoids.

Bronchodilator Effects

RELAXATION OF AIRWAYS SMOOTH MUSCLE

Theophylline produces a concentration-dependent relaxation of isolated airway preparations. In spite of its relatively low potency, theophylline has the ability to completely relax smooth muscle tone in vitro. Compared with β_2-adrenoceptor agonists, it produces a more complete relaxation, and this difference becomes more apparent the more highly contracted is the tissue[45] (Fig. 61-2). Similar observations have been made in human bronchi in vitro.[22] Theophylline, like β_2-adrenergic agonists, relaxes airways tissue from human large bronchi down to bronchioles and irrespective of the mediator used to cause the contraction (functional antagonism). Theophylline also is an effective relaxant of bronchial tissue from asthmatic subjects, even though the same preparations may sometimes show a reduced responsiveness to β_2-adrenergic agonists.[46,47] It is tempting to speculate that this could at least partly explain the beneficial effects of theophylline in some patients not responding well to β-adrenergic therapy.

It has been postulated that the smooth muscle relaxant effect is due to the opening of large conductance Ca^{2+} activated K^+-channels, since it can be inhibited by charybdotoxin.[48,49] These ion channels are opened by increases in intracellular cyclic AMP (for example by β_2-adrenergic receptor agonists), so inhibition of PDE activity may still be involved.

IN VIVO EFFECTS

The bronchodilator effect of theophylline can be observed in conscious and anesthetized animals, although most studies have demonstrated that pretreatment with systemic theophylline dose-dependently inhibits mediator-induced bronchospasm.[50] Few studies have been able to demonstrate reversal of tone in anesthetized animals due to the difficulty in maintaining a sustained increase in tone for a sufficiently

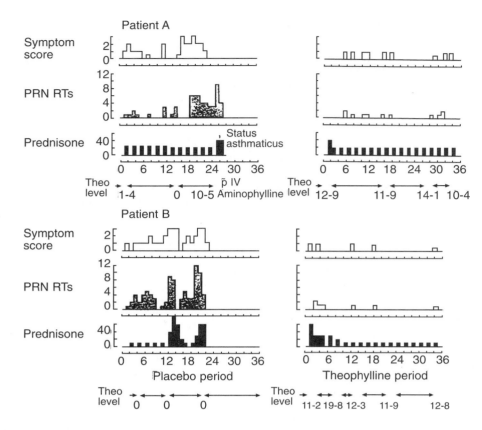

FIGURE 61-1 Effect of withdrawal of theophylline in two severely ill asthmatics. When theophylline was replaced by placebo treatment (left panel), the symptom score increased as did the use of bronchodilator (PRN RTs) and of prednisone. Patient A went into status asthmaticus and received IV theophylline as indicated. Both patients were well-controlled during the theophylline period (right-hand panel). (*From Ref. 1.*)

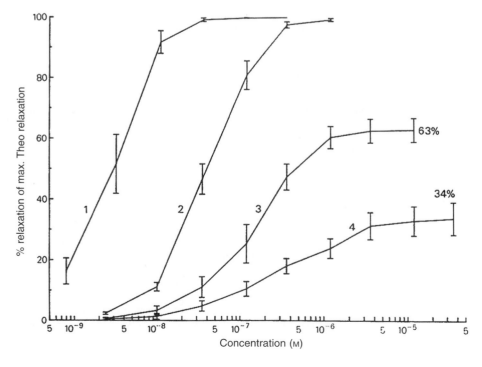

FIGURE 61-2 An increase in airways tone reduced the efficacy of isoprenaline more than that of theophylline. Cumulative concentration-response curves for isoprenaline-induced relaxation of guinea-pig isolated, spontaneously contracted (*1*) trachea or contracted by carbachol (*2*) 0.54 μM, (*3*) 5.4 μM, (*4*) 54 μM. Mean results are shown and vertical bars indicate SEM. (*From Ref. 45.*)

long period of time. It generally is accepted, however, that inhibition of induced bronchospasm in animals translates into protective and bronchodilator effects in man.

EFFECTS ON HUMAN BRONCHIAL TONE

Administration of theophylline to asthma patients is associated with a rapid improvement in airway function.[3] This effect is more pronounced in subjects with a low predicted FEV_1; that is, the more obstructive is the patient. Paradoxically, healthy subjects may have an increase rather than a decrease in airway smooth muscle tone. It generally is held that the acute improvement in lung function caused by a high dose is mainly a bronchodilator response, although an anti-inflammatory effect may well contribute. Theophylline has a protective effect against inhaled challenges with histamine, exercise, cold air, and distilled water,[51-55] although there is not always a clear relationship to the bronchodilator response. Theophylline inhibits exercise-induced airways obstruction[56] at plasma concentrations below those necessary for antagonism of histamine and methacholine,[52] further supporting the view that theophylline has effects other than bronchodilation.

Effects of Theophylline on Inflammatory Cells in Vitro

Cyclic AMP is an important intracellular second messenger involved in cell differentiation, maturation, and activation, as well as in secretory and other processes. Consequently, inhibition of cyclic AMP PDE activity by theophylline suppresses a range of functions in many different types of inflammatory cells.

BASOPHILS AND MAST CELLS

Histamine and leukotriene release from human mast cells and basophils is inhibited by high concentrations of theophylline.[57,58] When anti-IgE was used as a stimulant of histamine release from human leukocytes or passively sensitized human lung fragments, theophylline produced a 50 percent inhibition at a concentration of about 300 μM.[58] This concentration is three to six times above the recommended therapeutic interval, and it is therefore unlikely that theophylline exerts this effect in asthma patients. It is of interest to note that adenosine can suppress histamine release from human isolated basophils and that theophylline potently inhibited adenosine in these experiments.[21] Theophylline antagonized adenosine at a concentration (10 μM) that did not affect histamine release. Accordingly, adenosine-receptor antagonism has been suggested as an explanation for the antiasthmatic effects of theophylline (as discussed above).[21] Whether inhibition of histamine release by this mechanism could contribute to the effect of theophylline in acute asthma and to its partial inhibition of the immediate bronchospasm produced by antigen-challenge remains unknown.

MONOCYTES AND MACROPHAGES

Human alveolar macrophages have few β_2-adrenergic receptors on their surface and, consequently, β_2-adrenergic agonists and other agents that act through the cyclic AMP pathway have little effect on intracellular cyclic AMP concentrations and mediator release. Theophylline inhibits the production of reactive oxygen species from monocytes and macrophages, albeit at high concentrations.[59,60] This inhibitory effect seems to be caused by cyclic AMP–PDE inhibition.[60] Tumor necrosis factor-α and IL-1β are major proinflammatory cytokines produced by these cells when stimulated with lipopolysaccharide (LPS). Agents that increase intracellular cyclic AMP, such as theophylline, reduce mRNA levels for TNF-α and protein release from human monocytes.[61] Interleukin-1β release, on the other hand, is not inhibited by theophylline.

In apparent contrast to these in vitro findings, alveolar macrophages from patients treated with theophylline have a reduced bactericidal function.[62] These experimental data suggest that at therapeutic concentrations, theophylline has little effect on human monocytes and alveolar macrophages. However, some functions performed by the macrophage (e.g., bactericidal and phagocytic activities) seem to be sensitive to lesser concentrations of PDE inhibitors.

EOSINOPHILS

Guinea-pig eosinophils contain primarily a tightly membrane-bound cyclic AMP–specific PDE (type IV), which is inhibited by theophylline with an IC_{50} value (concentration causing 50% inhibition of PDE IV) of 124 μM.[63] The PDE isoenzyme(s) in human eosinophils has not yet been characterized, but theophylline inhibits degranulation (release of eosinophil-derived neurotoxin; EDN) induced by exposure to serum immunoglobulin A and serum immunoglobulin G.[64] The half-maximal effect was produced at concentrations between 100 and 1000 μM, which is similar to that needed to inhibit PDE IV in guinea-pig eosinophils.

In contrast to the study by Kita and colleagues,[64] a high concentration of theophylline (1 mM) was necessary to cause partial inhibition of superoxide generation from zymosan-stimulated human eosinophils, and lesser concentrations even enhanced mediator production.[65] These authors demonstrated that this enhancement was caused by adenosine-receptor antagonism, suggesting that perhaps at higher concentrations PDE inhibition mediated the reduced superoxide generation. Whether the different effects on EDN and oxygen radicals are caused by the use of different mediators (perhaps with separate second messenger pathways) is not known.

In contrast to these in vitro data, one year treatment of patients with theophylline has been reported to reduce plasma concentrations of major basic protein (MBP) in asthmatics,[66] and a recent study by Sullivan and co-workers[67] found that theophylline therapy downregulated the activation-marker EG2 on eosinophils (Fig. 61-3). Considering the presumed central role of the eosinophil in asthma pathology, these in vivo effects of theophylline may help to explain its antiasthmatic effects.

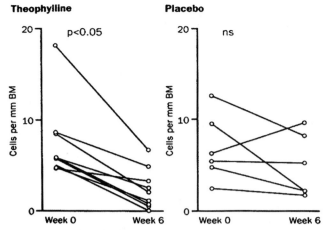

FIGURE 61-3 Theophylline treatment for 6 weeks reduced the number of EG2-positive (activated) eosinophils in the basement membrane (Bμ) as assessed in bronchial biopsies. The number of EG2-positive eosinophils per millimeter of basement membrane was counted before and after treatment. Theophylline and placebo groups were not significantly different prior to treatment. (*From Ref. 67.*)

NEUTROPHILS

Even though the neutrophil is transiently activated early in the acute allergic response, it is not considered to be of major importance in asthma pathology. Nevertheless, theophylline (at a concentration of 100 μM) suppressed calcium-ionophore (A23187) and fMLP-induced respiratory burst.[68] In a separate study, the inhibitory effect of isoproterenol on the respiratory burst was significantly potentiated in whole blood from theophylline-treated patients.[10] The ex vivo chemotactic response of neutrophils and monocytes obtained from asthmatic children treated with theophylline also was reduced as compared with that from control children.[69]

These data suggest that the function of neutrophils is downregulated during theophylline therapy, although the importance of this finding remains obscure.

T-LYMPHOCYTES

Several in vitro studies in asthmatic subjects have shown that theophylline has potent effects on T lymphocytes. Theophylline inhibits the proliferation of several T cell clones[70–72] whereas suppressor cell (CD8+) activity is increased by theophylline.[73–75] Natural killer (NK) cell activity can be reduced by theophylline in vitro and in vivo,[76] and NK cells obtained from the blood of theophylline-treated asthmatics also have reduced cytotoxicity, most likely from inhibition of PDE activity.[77]

Interleukin-2 (IL-2) release triggered by T-cell receptor activation is sensitive to agents that stimulate cyclic AMP accumulation[78] and phytohemagglutinin (PHA)-induced IL-2 production also is inhibited.[71]

T helper-2 cells secreting cytokines (IL-4, IL-5, and IL-10) are proposed to be of major importance in the pathogenesis of asthma[79] although these cytokines possibly could be pro-

duced by other T cells. It is conceivable that potent effects on T lymphocyte proliferation and cytokine release could explain some of the anti-inflammatory and immunomodulatory effects of theophylline.

Anti-Inflammatory Effects of Theophylline in Animal Models

PRECLINICAL STUDIES IN EXPERIMENTAL ANIMALS

Theophylline has been shown to attenuate inflammation in animal models of asthma. Antigen challenge in sensitized animals produces acute bronchospasm followed by an increase in the number of inflammatory cells infiltrating the airway wall, mediator release, enhancement of microvascular leakage of macromolecules, late-phase bronchoconstrictor responses, and airways hyperresponsiveness.

The acute bronchospasm induced by exposure to an antigen aerosol is caused by the release of preformed and newly synthesized bronchoactive mediators such as histamine and the peptidoleukotrienes. It has repeatedly been demonstrated that when theophylline is given before antigen challenge, this immediate bronchoconstrictor response can be almost completely prevented. The marked relaxant effect of theophylline on airways smooth muscle in vitro could explain this inhibitory effect, although alternative mechanisms have been proposed. A study in anesthetized guinea-pigs by Andersson and colleagues[50] suggested that theophylline may act as an antiinflammatory drug rather than as a bronchodilator in this species; intravenous administration of theophylline (0.1 to 0.5 mg/kg) inhibited the antigen-induced acute and late-phase constrictor responses in anesthetized, sensitized animals[50] at a dose well below that required to antagonize the bronchospasm produced by histamine (2 to 18 mg/kg).[50] Theophylline also has been shown to suppress histamine and leukotriene release from mast cells and basophils in vitro[21,57,58] and from anti-IgE–stimulated human lung fragments.[58] Interestingly, the late-phase airways obstruction in these animals could be inhibited by administration of the drug 90 min after challenge, indicating that inhibition of the immediate response is not necessary for attenuation of the late-phase response. Theophylline has similarly been shown to inhibit the antigen-induced early- and late-phase reactions in sensitized sheep.[80]

Antigen-challenge of sensitized guinea-pigs characteristically results in the airways eosinophilia that occurs 12 to 24 h after exposure. The eosinophilia is preceded by a neutrophilia, and sometimes is concomitant with an increase in the number of macrophages and lymphocytes. The number of eosinophils is increased both in airways tissue and in BAL (bronchoalveolar lavage) fluid, and there is clear evidence of activation since increased concentrations of MBP can be detected in BAL fluid.[81,82] In lung tissue, deposits of immunoreactive MBP were associated with epithelial damage and edema formation.[82] Administration of oral theophylline before antigen challenge significantly reduced the eosinophilia in guinea-pigs.[83,84] Likewise in the rat, theophylline reduced the anaphylactic bronchospasm.[85,86] This inhibitory effect in the rat may have been due primarily to inhibition of leukotriene release from the rat lung, since 5-hydroxytryptamine (5-HT; serotonin) release was not affected.[86]

Acute administration of theophylline also has been shown to attenuate nonallergic pulmonary inflammation such as that induced by acetaldehyde[87] and bacillus calmette guerre (BCG).[88] Most interestingly, however, was the inhibition of the BCG-induced granuloma formation, which supports the view that theophylline can suppress the activity of the immune system.

Pulmonary inflammation and airway hyperresponsiveness also can be produced in certain rat strains by exposure to an endotoxin aerosol.[89] At least part of this response is due to production of TNF-α since this agent on its own has been shown to produce similar effects as the endotoxin inhalation.[90] When given IP 30 min before the endotoxin exposure, therapeutic concentrations of theophylline inhibited the neutrophil sequestration into BAL fluid and reduced the ensuing airways hyperresponsiveness to serotonin.[91] Theophylline inhibited lipopolysaccharide-induced TNF-α production from human monocytes,[61] which perhaps could explain some of its anti-inflammatory effects in this rat model. Injection of *Escherichia coli* causes sepsis and multiorgan failure as a result of plasma protein extravasation in guinea-pigs and this is attenuated by theophylline.[92]

It is obvious from animal experiments that theophylline has wide-ranging anti-inflammatory effects that include inhibition of allergic bronchospasm and eosinophilia and, in some models, inhibition of airways hyperresponsiveness.

MICROVASCULAR LEAKAGE

Plasma protein extravasation is one of the characteristics of an inflammatory reaction, and it has been proposed to be an important pathogenetic mechanism in asthma.[93] In the airways, the endothelium in the postcapillary venules loses its barrier function and allows the paracellular penetration of plasma macromolecules into surrounding tissue. These proteins and their proteolytic degradation products display potent proinflammatory properties.

Mediator- or antigen-induced increases in microvascular leakage in the guinea-pig or rat was attenuated by theophylline.[94–96] Local intratracheal infusion of theophylline had a protective effect, suggesting that theophylline was acting directly on the venular endothelium.[94,96]

When platelet-activating factor (PAF) was used to promote extravasation, locally administered theophylline (200 μg IT) was more effective in attenuating leakage into the bronchi and lavage fluid than in the trachea. Although theophylline is a nonselective PDE inhibitor, previous studies with isozyme-selective inhibitors have suggested that PDE types IV and V are involved in microvascular leak in the guinea-pig tracheobronchial tree.[96]

EXTRAPULMONARY IMMUNOMODULATORY EFFECTS

Theophylline has been examined in various models of autoimmune disease. Diabetes-prone Bio-Breeding rats were treated with oral theophylline when they were between 30 and 125 days old. Theophylline (serum concentrations 10 to 30 mg/L) significantly decreased the incidence of diabetes in these rats, as assessed by serum and urinary glucose levels. Pancreatic β-cell mass (i.e., insulin content) also was increased when compared with control rats.[97] Streptozotocin-induced diabetes in rats was similarly inhibited by theophylline (about 9 mg/L theophylline in serum).[98]

NZW/W F-1 mice spontaneously develop an autoimmune renal disease resembling systemic lupus erythematosus in man. In these mice theophylline enhanced suppressor T-cell activity, prolonged survival, and decreased renal damage.[99] Glycerol-induced kidney damage[100] and joint inflammation in adjuvant-induced arthritis[101] could be prevented by theophylline.

Taken together, these data further demonstrate the immunomodulatory effects of theophylline in vivo and support the view that suppressor T lymphocytes (CD8+ T cells) may be involved in its anti-inflammatory actions. A protective effect in experimental allograft rejection lends support to this hypothesis.[102,103]

Anti-Inflammatory Effects in Asthma Patients

ANTIGEN-INDUCED LATE-PHASE BRONCHOCONSTRICTOR RESPONSES AND AIRWAY HYPERRESPONSIVENESS

It is generally held that the late-phase bronchoconstrictor response occurring after antigen-challenge is the consequence of an intensified inflammatory reaction in the bronchial mucosa. Eosinophils accumulate during the late-phase response and can readily be detected in tissue and lavage fluid.[104,105] Eosinophil-derived cytotoxic proteins are believed to mediate tissue damage and the subsequent increase in airways hyperresponsiveness. Theophylline almost completely inhibited this late-phase response in mild asthmatics, while having a very small, although statistically significant, effect on the immediate bronchoconstrictor response (Fig. 61-4).[25,67,106] Interestingly, Pauwels and coworkers[25] found that theophylline exerted this effect already at a plasma concentration that is considered to be at the lower end of the therapeutic range (about 10 mg/L). In their study, theophylline produced only a small bronchodilator response and the inhibition of the late-phase response could therefore not be accounted for by relaxation of airways smooth muscle.

The late asthmatic response was also inhibited in a recent study in which atopic asthmatics were treated with a "subtherapeutic" dose (the mean plasma concentration was 6.6 mg/L) of theophylline for 6 weeks.[67] An anti-inflammatory effect also was demonstrated in this later study where there were reductions in activated, EG2-positive eosinophils (Fig. 61-3), in the number of total eosinophils, and in free eosinophil cationic protein (ECP) below the basement membrane in biopsy samples.[67] There were no changes in the number of mast cells, CD25 positive cells, or lymphocyte populations in this study.[67]

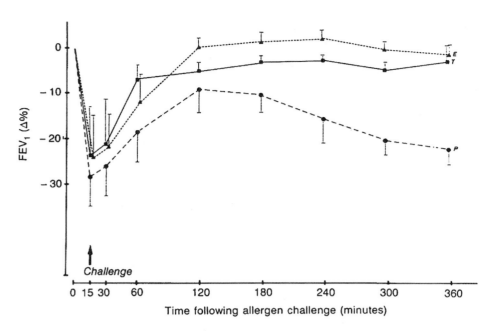

FIGURE 61-4 Relative changes in FEV_1 (mean ± SEM) following antigen-challenge in six patients who developed a late asthmatic reaction during the placebo study day (*P*). Theophylline treatment day (T), enprofylline treatment day (E). (*From Ref. 25.*)

A delayed bronchoconstrictor response, accompanied by a BAL neutrophilia and eosinophilia, also can be produced in subjects exposed to chemical sensitizers such as toluene diisocyanate (TDI). Some pathologic features of TDI asthma are similar to those of nonoccupational asthma.[107] One-week administration of theophylline significantly reduced the late asthmatic reaction.[108,109] Theophylline had no effect on the baseline airways caliber before TDI exposure, again supporting the view that it had an anti-allergic effect. TDI-challenge resulted in an increased airways hyperresponsiveness to inhaled methacholine. Unlike the late-phase response, theophylline treatment did not affect the baseline reactivity to inhaled methacholine, nor did it alter the heightened responsiveness produced by acute TDI exposure.[109]

Conflicting results have been obtained in the studies in which theophylline has been assessed on "spontaneous" airways hyperresponsiveness. Most studies would appear to indicate that this drug has only marginal[52,55] or no inhibitory effect at all[110,111] in adult asthmatics. However, in a study by Crescioli and colleagues,[106] airways hyperresponsiveness in five out of six subjects was reduced by theophylline, and, similarly, patients with allergic rhinitis showed a significant reduction in hyperresponsiveness after 30 days of treatment.[112] Theophylline has been shown to suppress the allergen-induced increase in inflammatory mediators in nasal lavage fluid,[113] which may have contributed to the reduction of airways hyperresponsiveness. Alternatively, the rhinitics had a less severe hyperresponsiveness, and were therefore more sensitive to theophylline therapy. Children treated with theophylline for one year also had a somewhat reduced airways hyperresponsiveness[36] and a suppressed ex vivo monocyte chemotactic response. Accordingly, children may be more susceptible to the long-term immunomodulatory effect of theophylline.

These data demonstrate that theophylline could prevent the occurrence of late-phase reactions produced by antigen or occupational sensitizers. Unfortunately, theophylline seems to have only a marginal effect on airways hyperresponsiveness, supporting the view that these two events are mechanistically unrelated.

EFFECTS ON INFLAMMATORY CELLS IN BLOOD AND BAL

The effects of 6-week treatment with theophylline on blood and BAL fluid composition has been examined in mild asthmatics.[114] Compared with placebo treatment, there was a significant loss of BAL CD3+ lymphocytes with the number of both CD4+ and CD8+ T cells being reduced. Furthermore, the number of CD4+ cells expressing markers of activation, such as VLA-1, HLA-DR, and CD25, was reduced.[114] Inflammatory cells in BAL fluid and the concentrations of ECP, histamine, tryptase, and PGD_2 were not significantly altered by the theophylline treatment.

In contrast to lung tissue, there was an increase in the percentage of CD4+ cells expressing HLA-DR, but not other activation markers, in peripheral blood after the 6-week theophylline therapy.[114] It was concluded that activated CD4+ lymphocytes were migrating out of lung tissue and back into the circulation and so reducing the overall sensitivity of the tissue to the allergic insult. These studies confirm earlier reports, which have shown that chronic theophylline therapy increases the number of CD8+ lymphocytes (suppressor cells) in peripheral blood.[71,74]

A reversed protocol was used by Kidney and colleagues,[43] when they studied the effect of theophylline withdrawal in asthmatic patients who had been treated chronically with the drug. Discontinuation was associated with an increase in asthma symptoms and a decrease in activated CD4+ and CD8+ lymphocytes in blood, which was mirrored by a concomitant increase in bronchial tissue.

The role of T-cell subsets in acute and provoked asthma attacks is not entirely clear, however, since antigen challenge increased CD4+ and CD8+ cells 48 h later, and this effect could be inhibited by pretreatment with theophylline.[115] An acute infusion of theophylline seems to decrease CD8+ cells in peripheral blood.[116]

These results demonstrate that theophylline can modulate the inflammatory response in the airways and that CD8+ suppressor T cells seem to be particularly sensitive to theophylline.

Conclusion

Theophylline relaxes airways smooth muscle, inhibits cell proliferation, and suppresses mediator release from inflammatory cells. Anti-inflammatory effects exerted locally in the inflamed bronchial wall are illustrated in Fig. 61-5. Interestingly, a subpopulation of CD8+ suppressor T cells seems particularly sensitive to theophylline. In animal studies, theophylline inhibits antigen-induced bronchospasm, eosinophilia, microvascular leakage of plasma proteins, the late-phase bronchoconstrictor response, and airways hyperresponsiveness. Several studies also have shown immunomodulatory effects in animal models. Theophylline is a weak cyclic nucleotide–PDE inhibitor although at present this seems to be the most likely explanation for its mode of action. However, other as yet unidentified cellular actions may contribute to the antiasthmatic effects of theophylline.

Theophylline has until now been generally regarded as a bronchodilator drug such as the β_2-adrenergic agonists. However, several clinical studies have shown that when theophylline therapy was discontinued, the degree of inflammation increased in the asthmatic airways and that in some severely ill patients even high-dose glucocorticoids could not entirely compensate for theophylline. These data demonstrate important anti-inflammatory effects in asthma patients. The observation that these beneficial effects occurred at plasma concentrations considered to be below the recommended range provides an opportunity to increase the narrow therapeutic margin and thus improve safety and acceptability of methylxanthines.

It is imperative that further clinical investigations are undertaken to confirm the findings of these experimental studies. If recognized as an anti-inflammatory agent with immunomodulatory properties, the role of theophylline would have to be reevaluated.

It is envisaged that knowledge about the precise mechanism of action of theophylline will offer new insights into the pathology of asthma and possibly unravel opportunities for the discovery of novel and more efficacious antiasthmatic agents.

References

1. Brenner M, Berkowitz R, Marshall N, Strunk RC: Need for theophylline in severe steroid requiring asthmatics. *Clin Allergy* 1988; 18:143.
2. Persson CGA: On the medical history of xanthines and other remedies for asthma: a tribute to HH Salter. *Thorax* 1985; 40:881.
3. Mitenko PA, Ogilvie RI: Rational intravenous doses of theophyllines. *N Engl J Med* 1973; 289:600.
4. Thompson JW: Cyclic nucleotide phosphodiesterases: pharmacology, biochemistry and function. *Pharmacol Ther* 1991; 51:13.
5. Beavo JA, Reifsnyder DH: Primary sequence of cyclic nucleotide phosphodiesterase isozymes and the design of selective inhibitors: *Trends Pharmacol Sci* 1990; 11:150.
6. Ichimura M, Kase H: A new cyclic nucleotide phosphodiesterase isozyme expressed in the T-lymphocyte cell lines. *Biochem Biophys Res Commun* 1993; 193:985.
7. Bergstrand H: Phosphodiesterase inhibition and theophylline: *Eur J Respir Dis* 1980; 91(suppl 109): 37.
8. Lohmann SM, Miech RP, Butcher FR: Effects of isoproterenol, theophylline and carbachol on cyclic nucleotide levels and relaxation of bovine tracheal smooth muscle. *Biophys Acta* 1977; 499:238.
9. Kolbeck RC, Speir WA, Carrier GO, Bransome ED: Apparent irrelevance of cyclic nucleotides to the relaxation of tracheal smooth muscle induced by theophylline. *Lung* 1979; 156:173.

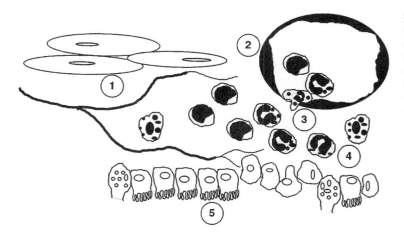

FIGURE 61-5 Anti-inflammatory effects of theophylline in the asthmatic airways are illustrated in this schematic drawing. (*1*) relaxation of airways, smooth muscle; (*2*) inhibition of microvascular leakage of plasma proteins; (*3*) inhibition of inflammatory cell migration; (*4*) inhibition of mediator release; and (*5*) protection of the integrity of the epithelial membrane and increased mucociliary clearance.

10. Nielson CP, Crowley JJ, Cusask BJ, Vestal RE: Therapeutic concentrations of theophylline and enprofylline potentiate catecholamine effects and inhibit leukocyte activation. *J Allergy Clin Immunol* 1986; 78:660.

11. Chan SC, Hanafin JM: Differential inhibitor effects on phosphodiesterase isoforms in atopic and normal leukocytes. *J Lab Clin Med* 1993; 121:44.

12. Grewe SE, Chan SC, Hanafin JM: Elevated leukocyte cyclic AMP phosphodiesterase in atopic disease: a possible mechanism for cAMP hyperresponsiveness. *J Allergy Clin Immunol* 1982; 70:452.

13. Goldberg BJ, Lad PM, Ghekiere L: Phosphodiesterase activity and superoxide production in normal and asthmatic neutrophils. *J Allergy Clin Immunol* 1994; 93:166.

14. Holden CA, Chan SC, Hanafin JM: Monocyte localization of elevated cyclic AMP phosphodiesterase activity in atopic dermatitis: *J Invest Dermatol* 1986; 87:372.

15. Chan SC, Reifsynder D, Beavo JA, Hanifin JM: Immunochemical characterization of the distinct monocyte cyclic AMP–phosphodiesterases from patients with atopic dermatitis. *J Allergy Clin Immunol* 1993; 91:1179.

16. Coulson IH, Duncan SN, Holden CA: Peripheral blood mononuclear leukocyte cyclic adenosine monophosphate specific phosphodiesterase activity in atopic dermatitis. *Br J Dermatol* 1989; 120:607.

17. Busse WW, Anderson CL: The granulocyte response to the phosphodiesterase inhibitor RO 20-1724 in asthma. *J Allergy Clin Immunol* 1981; 67:70.

18. Rott O, Cash E, Fleischer B: Phosphodiesterase inhibitor pentoxifylline, a selective suppressor of T-helper type 1- but not type 2–associated lymphokine production, prevents induction of experimental autoimmune encephalomyelitis in Lewis rats. *Eur J Immunol* 1993; 23:1745.

19. Fredholm BB: Theophylline actions on adenosine receptors. *Eur J Respir Dis* 1980; 61(suppl 109): 29.

20. Cushley MJ, Tattersfield AE, Holgate ST: Adenosine-induced bronchoconstriction in asthma: antagonism by inhaled theophylline. *Am Rev Respir Dis* 1980; 129:380.

21. Marone G, Findlay SR, Lichtenstein LM: Adenosine receptor on human basophils: modulation of histamine release. *J Immunol* 1979; 123:1473.

22. Finney MJB, Karlsson JA, Persson CGA: Effects of bronchoconstriction and bronchodilation on a novel human small airway preparation. *Br J Pharmacol* 1985; 85:29.

23. Björk T, Gustafsson LE, Dahlen S-E: Isolated bronchi from asthmatics are hyperresponsive to adenosine, which apparently acts indirectly by liberation of leukotrienes and histamine. *Am Rev Respir Dis* 1992; 145:1087.

24. Persson GCA, Erjefält I, Edholm L-E, et al.: Tracheal relaxant and cardiostimulant actions of xanthines can be differentiated from diuretic and CNS-stimulant effects. Role of adenosine antagonism? *Life Sci* 1982; 31:2673.

25. Pauwels R, van Renterghem D, van der Straeten M, et al.: The effect of theophylline and enprofylline on allergen-induced bronchoconstriction. *J Allergy Clin Immunol* 1985; 76:583.

26. Persson CGA: Development of safer xanthine drugs for the treatment of obstructive airways disease. *J Allergy Clin Immunol* 1986; 78:817.

27. Chapman KR, Bryant D, Marlin GE, et al.: A placebo controlled dose-response study of enprofylline in the maintenance therapy of asthma. *Am Rev Respir Dis* 1989; 139:688.

28. Manzini S, Meini S, Giachetti A, et al.: Pharmacodynamic profile of isbufylline, a new antibronchospastic xanthine devoid of central excitatory actions. *Arzneimittelforschung* 1990; 40:1205.

29. Persson CGA: Experimental lung actions of xanthines, in Andersson K-E, Persson CGA (eds): *Anti-asthma Xanthines and*

Adenosine. Amsterdam, The Netherlands, Excerpta Medica, 1985: 61–82.

30. Barnes PJ, Pauwels RA: Theophylline in the management of asthma: time for reappraisal? *Eur Respir J* 1994; 7:579.

31. Bowler SD, Mitchell CA, Armstrong JG: Nebulised fenoterol and i.v. aminophylline in acute severe asthma. *Eur J Respir Dis* 1987; 70:280.

32. Littenberg B: Aminophylline treatment in severe acute asthma. A meta-analysis. *J Am Med Assoc* 1988; 259:1678.

33. Siegel D, Sheppard D, Gelf A, Weinberg PF: Aminophylline increases the toxicity but not the efficacy of an inhaled β-adrenergic agonist in the treatment of acute exacerbations of asthma. *Am Rev Respir Dis* 1985; 132:283.

34. Fanta H, Rossing TH, McFadden ER: Treatment of acute asthma: is combination therapy with sympathomimetics and methylxanthines indicated? *Am J Med* 1986; 80:5.

35. Furukawa CT, Shapiro SG, Bierman CW: A double-blind study comparing the effectiveness of cromolyn sodium and sustained release theophylline in childhood asthma. *Pediatrics* 1984; 74:435.

36. Tinkelman DG, Reed CE, Nelson HS, Offord KP: Aerosol beclomethasone dipropionate compared with theophylline as primary treatment of chronic, mild to moderately severe asthma in children. *Pediatrics* 1993; 92:64.

37. Birkett DJ, Miners JO, Wing LMH, et al.: Methylxanthine metabolism in man, in Andersson K-E, Persson CGA (eds): *Anti-asthma Xanthines and Adenosine.* Amsterdam, The Netherlands, Excerpta Medica, 1985: 230–272.

38. Williamson BH, Milligan C, Griffiths K, et al.: An assessment of major and minor side effects of theophylline. *Aust N Z J Med* 1988; 19:539.

39. British Thoracic Society: Guidelines on management of asthma. *Thorax* 1993; 48(suppl):S1.

40. Sheffer AL: International consensus report on diagnosis and management of asthma. *Eur Respir J* 1992; 5:601.

41. Nassif EG, Weinberger M, Thompson R, Huntley W: The value of theophylline in steroid-dependent asthma. *N Engl J Med* 1981; 304:71.

42. Weinberger M: The pharmacology and therapeutic use of theophylline. *J Allergy Clin Immunol* 1984; 73:525.

43. Kidney JC, Dominguez M, Rose M, et al.: Immune modulation by theophylline: the effect of withdrawal of chronic treatment (abstract). *Am Rev Respir Dis* 1993; 147:A772.

44. Kidney JC, Dominguez M, Rose M, et al.: Withdrawing chronic theophylline treatment increases airway lymphocytes in asthma. 1994; 49:396.

45. Karlsson, J-A, Persson CGA: Influence of tracheal contraction on relaxant effects in vitro of theophylline and isoprenaline. *Br J Pharmacol* 1981; 74:73.

46. Goldie RG, Spina D, Henry PJ, et al.: In vitro responsiveness of human asthmatic bronchus to carbachol, histamine, beta-adrenoceptor agonists and theophylline. *Br J Clin Pharmacol* 1986; 22:669.

47. Bai TR, Mak JCW, Barnes PJ: A comparison of beta-adrenergic receptors and in vitro relaxant responses to isoproterenol in asthmatic airway smooth muscle. *Am J Respir Cell Mol Biol* 1992; 6:647.

48. Jones TR, Charette L, Garcia ML, Kaczorowski GJ: Interaction of iberiotoxin with β-adrenoceptor agonists and sodium nitroprusside on guinea-pig trachea. *J Appl Physiol* 1993; 74:1879.

49. Miura M, Belvisi MG, Stretton CD, et al.: Role of potassium channels in bronchodilator responses in human airways. *Am Rev Respir Dis* 1992; 146:132.

50. Andersson P, Brange C, Sonmark B, et al.: Anti-anaphylactic and anti-inflammatory effects of xanthines in the lung, in: Andersson KE, Persson CGA, (eds): *Anti-asthma Xanthines and*

Adenosine. Amsterdam, The Netherlands, Exerpta Medica, 1985: 187–192.

51. Cartier A, Lemaire I, L'Archevegue J, et al.: Theophylline partially inhibits bronchoconstriction caused by inhaled histamine in subjects with asthma. *J Allergy Clin Immunol* 1986; 77:570.

52. Magnussen H, Reuss G, Jörres R: Theophylline has a dose-related effect on the airway response to inhaled histamine and methacholine in asthmatics. *Am Rev Respir Dis* 1987; 136:1163.

53. Pollock J, Kiechel F, Cooper D, Weinberger M: Relationship of serum theophylline concentration to inhibition of exercise-induced bronchospasm and comparison with cromolyn. *Pediatrics* 1977; 60:840.

54. Fabbri LM, Allessandri MV, De Marzo N, et al.: Long-lasting protective effect of slow-release theophylline on asthma induced by ultasonically nebulized distilled water. *Ann Allergy* 1986; 56:171.

55. Merland N, Cartier A, L'Archeveque J, et al.: Theophylline minimally inhibits bronchoconstriction induced dry cold air inhalation in asthmatic subjects. *Am Rev Respir Dis* 1988; 137:1304.

56. Magnussen H, Reuss G, Jörres R: Methylxanthines inhibit exercise-induced bronchoconstriction at low serum theophylline concentrations and in a dose-dependent fashion. *J Allergy Clin Immunol* 1988; 81:531.

57. Orange RP, Kaliner MA, Laraia PJ, Austen KG: Immunological release of histamine and slow reacting substance of anaphylaxis from human lung. II. Influence of cellular levels of cyclic AMP. *Fed Proc* 1971; 30:1725.

58. Louis R, Bury T, Corhay JL, Radermecker M: LY 186655, a phosphodiesterase inhibitor, inhibits histamine release from human basophils, lung and skin fragments. *Immunopharmacology* 1992; 14:191.

59. Calhoun WJ, Stevens CA, Lambert SB: Modulation of superoxide production of alveolar macrophages and peripheral blood mononuclear cells by beta-agonists and theophylline. *J Lab Clin Med* 1991; 117:514.

60. Dent G, Giembycz MA, Rabe KF, et al.: Theophylline suppresses human alveolar macrophage respiratory burst through phosphodiesterase inhibition. *Am J Respir Cell Mol Biol* 1994; 10:565.

61. Endres S, Fulle HI, Sinha B, et al.: Cyclic nucleotides differentially regulate the synthesis of tumour necrosis factor-α by human mononuclear cells. *Immunology* 1991; 72:56.

62. O'Neill SJ, Sitar DS, Kilass DJ: The pulmonary dis-position of theophylline and its influences on human alveolar macrophage bactericidal function. *Am Rev Respir Dis* 1988; 134:1225.

63. Souness JE, Carter CM, Diocee BK, et al.: Characterization of guinea-pig eosinophil phosphodiesterase activity. *Biochem Pharmacol* 1991; 42:937.

64. Kita H, Abu-Ghazaleh RI, Gleich GJ, Abraham RT: Regulation of Ig-induced eosinophil degranulation by adenosine 3′,5′-cyclic monophosphate. *Immunology* 1991; 146:2712.

65. Yukawa T, Kroegel C, Chanez P, et al.: Effect of theophylline and adenosine on eosinophil function. *Am Rev Respir Dis* 1989; 140:327.

66. Venge P, Dahl R, Karlstrom R, et al.: Eosinophil and neutrophil activity in asthma in a one-year double blind trial with theophylline and two doses of inhaled budesonide. *J Allergy Clin Immunol* 1992; 89:A181.

67. Sullivan P, Bekir S, Jaffar Z, et al.: Anti-inflammatory effects of low-dose oral theophylline in atopic asthma. *Lancet* 1994; 343:1006.

68. Nielson CP, Vestal RE, Sturm RJ, Heaslip R: Effects of selective phosphodiesterase inhibitors on the polymorphonuclear leukocyte respiratory burst. *J Allergy Clin Immunol* 1990; 86:801.

69. Condino-Neto A, Vilela MM, Cambiucci EC, et al.: Theophylline therapy inhibits neutrophil and mononuclear cell

70. chemotaxis from chronic asthmatic children. *Br J Clin Pharmacol* 1991; 32:557.

70. Ghio R, Scordamaglia A, D-Elia P, et al.: Inhibition of the colony-forming capacity of human T-lymphocytes exerted by theophylline. *Int J Immunopharmacol* 1988; 10:299.

71. Scordamaglia A, Ciprandi G, Ruffoni S, et al.: Theophylline and the immune response: in vitro and in vivo effects. *Clin Immunol Immunopathol* 1988; 48:238.

72. Bruserud O, Hamann W, Patel S, Pawelec G: CD4+ TCR alpha beta+ T-cell clones derived shortly after allogeneic bone marrow transplantation: theophylline and verapamil inhibit proliferation of functionally heterogeneous T-cells. *Int J Immunopharmacol* 1992; 14:783.

73. Shohat B, Shapira Z, Joshua H, Servadio C: Lack of suppressor T cells in renal transplant recipients and activation by aminophylline. *Thymus* 1983; 5:67.

74. Fink G, Mittelman M, Shohat B, Spitzer SA: Theophylline-induced alterations in cellular immunity in asthmatic patients. *Clin Allergy* 1987; 17:316.

75. Ilfield D, Kivity S, Feierman E, et al.: Effect of in vitro colchicine and oral theophylline on suppressor cell function of asthmatic patients. *Clin Exp Immunol* 1985; 61:360.

76. Yokoyama A, Yamashita N, Mizushima Y, Yano S: Inhibition of natural killer cell activity by oral administration of theophylline. *Chest* 1990; 98:924.

77. Coskey LA, Bitting J, Roth MD: Inhibition of natural killer cell activity by therapeutic levels of theophylline. *Am J Respir Cell Mol Biol* 1993; 9:659.

78. Paliogianni F, Kincaid RL, Boumpas DT: Prostaglandin E$_2$ and other cyclic AMP elevating agents inhibit interleukin 2 gene transcription by counteracting calcineurin-dependent pathways. *J Exp Med* 1993; 178:1813.

79. Corrigan CJ, Kay AB: T cells and eosinophils in the pathogenesis of asthma. *Immunol Today* 1992; 13:501.

80. Perruchoud AP, Yerger L, Abraham W: Differential effects of aminophylline on the early and late antigen-induced bronchial obstruction in allergic sheep (abstract). *Respiration* 1984; 46:44.

81. Pretolani M, Ruffie C, Joseph D, et al.: Role of eosinophil activation in the bronchial reactivity of allergic guinea pigs. *Am J Respir Crit Care Med* 1994; 149:1167.

82. Underwood S, Foster M, Raeburn D, et al.: Time-course of antigen-induced airway inflammation in the guinea-pig and its relationship to airway hyperresponsiveness. *Eur Resp J* 1995; 8:2104.

83. Tarayre JP, Aliaga M, Barbara M, et al.: Pharmacological modulation of a model of bronchial inflammation after aerosol-induced active anaphylactic shock in conscious guinea-pigs. *Int J Immunopharmacol* 1991; 13:349.

84. Sanjar S, Aoki S, Kristersson A, et al.: Antigen challenge induces pulmonary eosinophil accumulation and airway hyperreactivity: the effect of anti-asthma drugs. *Br J Pharmacol* 1990; 99:679.

85. Tarayre JP, Aliaga M, Barbara M, et al.: Model of bronchial allergic inflammation in the Brown Norway rat. Pharmacological modulation. *Int J Immunopharmacol* 1992; 14:847.

86. Post MJ, te Biesebeek JD, Wemer J, et al.: Comparison of the anti-anaphylactic effects of milrinone, sulmazole and theophylline in the rat. *Int Arch Allergy Appl Immunol* 1989; 89:6.

87. Berti F, Rossoni G, Buschi A, et al.: Influence of theophylline on both bronchoconstriction and plasma extravasation induced by acetaldehyde in guinea-pigs. *Arzneimittelforschung* 1994; 44:323.

88. Boner A-L, Piacentini G-L, Peroni D-G, et al.: Theophylline inhibition of BCG-induced pulmonary inflammatory responses. *Ann Allergy* 1990; 64:530.

89. Pauwels RA, Kips JC, Peleman RA, Van Der Straeten ME: The

effect of endotoxin inhalation on airway responsiveness and cellular influx in rats. *Am Rev Respir Dis* 1990; 141:542.

90. Kips JC, Tavernier J, Pauwels RA: Tumor necrosis factor causes bronchial hyperresponsiveness in rats. *Am Rev Respir Dis* 1992; 145:332.

91. Pauwels RA, Kips JC, Peleman RA, Van Der Straeten ME: The effect of endotoxin inhalation on airway responsiveness and cellular influx in rats. *Am Rev Respir Dis* 1990; 141:540.

92. Harada H, Ishizaka A, Yonemaru M, et al.: The effects of aminophylline and pentoxifylline on multiple organ damage after *Escherichia coli* sepsis. *Am Rev Respir Dis* 1989; 140:974.

93. Persson CGA: Role of plasma exudation in asthmatic airways. *Lancet* 1986; ii:1126.

94. Erjefält I, Persson CGA: Pharmacologic control of plasma exudation into tracheobronchial airways. *Am Rev Respir Dis* 1991; 143:1008.

95. Boschetto P, Roberts NM, Rogers DF, Barnes PJ: The effect of anti-asthma drugs on microvascular leak in guinea-pig airways. *Am Rev Respir Dis* 1989; 139:416.

96. Raeburn D, Karlsson J-A: Effects of isoenzyme-selective inhibitors of cyclic nucleotide phosphodiesterase on microvascular leak in guinea pig airways in vivo. *J Pharmacol Exp Ther* 1993; 267:1147.

97. Rabinovitch A, Sumoski WL: Theophylline protects against diabetes in BB rats and potentiates cyclosporine protection. *Diabetologia* 1990; 33:506.

98. Ferrero E, Marni A, Ferrero ME, et al.: Effect of cyclosporine and aminophylline on streptozotocin-induced diabetes in rats. *Immunology Lett* 1985; 10:183.

99. Gelber M, Sidi Y, Ben-Bassat M, et al.: Theophylline prolongs survival and decreases renal damage in female NZB/W F-1 mice. *Thymus* 1988; 11:231.

100. Bidani AK, Churchill PC, Packer W: Theophylline-induced protection in myoglobinuric acute renal failure: further characterization. *Can J Physiol Pharmacol* 1987; 65:42.

101. Bonta IL, Parnham MJ, Van Vliet L: Combination of theophylline and protaglandin E as inhibitors of the adjuvant-induced arthritis syndrome of rats. *Ann Rheumat Dis* 1978; 37:212.

102. Ljungstrom J, Holmgren J: In vivo suppression of allograft rejection by cyclic AMP increasing agents. *Int Arch Allergy Appl Immunol* 1979; 58:99.

103. Shohat B, Volovitz B, Varsano I: Induction of suppressor T cells in asthmatic children by theophylline treatment. *Clin Allergy* 1983; 13:487.

104. De Monchy JGR, Kauffman HF: Venge P, et al.: Bronchoalveolar lavage eosinophilia during allergen induced late asthmatic reactions. *Am Rev Respir Dis* 1985; 131:373.

105. Laitinen LA, Laitinen A, Heino M, Haahtela T: Eosinophilic airway inflammation during exacerbation of asthma and its treatment with inhaled corticosteroid. *Am Rev Respir Dis* 1991; 143:423.

106. Crescioli S, Spinazzi A. Plebani M, et al.: Theophylline inhibits early and late asthmatic reactions induced by allergens in asthmatic subjects. *Ann Allergy* 1991; 66:245.

107. Fabbri LM, Maestrelli P, Saetta M, Mapp CE: Bronchial hyperreactivity: mechanisms and physiologic evaluation. *Am Rev Respir Dis* 1991; 143:S37.

108. Mapp C, Boschetto P, del Veccho L, et al.: Protective effect of anti-asthma drugs on late asthmatic reactions and increased airway responsiveness induced by toluene diisocyanate in sensitized subjects. *Am Rev Respir Dis* 1987; 136:1403.

109. Crescioli S, Marzo ND, Boschetto P, et al.: Theophylline inhibits late asthmatic reactions induced by toluene diisocyanate in sensitized subjects. *Eur J Pharmacol* 1992; 228:45.

110. Dutoit J, Salome CM, Woolcock AJ: Inhaled corticosteroids reduce the severity of bronchial hyperresponsiveness in asthma but oral theophylline does not. *Am Rev Respir Dis* 1987; 136:1174.

111. Cockcroft DW, Murdock KY, Gore BP, et al.: Theophylline does not inhibit allergen-induced increase in airway responsiveness to methacholine. *J Allergy Clin Immunol* 1989; 83:913.

112. Aubier M, Levy J, Clerici C, et al.: Protective effect of theophylline on bronchial hyperresponsiveness in patients with allergic rhinitis. *Am Rev Respir Dis* 1991; 143:346.

113. Naclerio RM, Bartenfelder D, Proud D, et al.: Theophylline reduces histamine release during pollen-induced rhinitis. *J Allergy Clin Immunol* 1986; 78:874.

114. Jaffar ZH, Sullivan P, Page C, Costello J: Low dose theophylline therapy modulates T-lymphocyte activity in subjects with atopic asthma. *Eur Respir J*, in press.

115. Ward AJM, McKenniff M, Evans JM, et al.: Theophylline—an immunomodulatory role in asthma? *Am Rev Resp Dis* 1993; 147:518.

116. Pardi R, Zocchi MR, Ferrero E, et al.: In vivo effects of a single infusion of theophylline on human peripheral blood lymphocytes. *Clin Exp Immunol* 1984; 57:722.

Chapter 62

ANTI-INFLAMMATORY EFFECTS OF PHOSPHODIESTERASE INHIBITORS

JAN-ANDERS KARLSSON

Asthma is a chronic inflammatory disease of the airways; its most characteristic symptoms are variable airflow obstruction and airway hyperresponsiveness. The eosinophil is the predominant inflammatory cell in the bronchial mucosa, and while its cytotoxic mediators can account for much of the tissue damage, T lymphocytes together with resident and migrating inflammatory cells orchestrate the inflammatory response.[1,2] The formidable network of putative mediators, cytokines, and cells contributing to the chronic inflammatory pathology indicates that anti-inflammatory and immunomodulating properties are required in novel disease-modifying treatments for asthma.

The purine cyclic nucleotides cyclic 3′,5′-adenosine monophosphate (cAMP) and cyclic 3′,5′-guanosine monophosphate (cGMP) have multiple regulatory roles in cell differentiation, proliferation, maturation, activation, and protein/mediator release. These second messengers are metabolized by cyclic nucleotide-phosphodiesterases (PDE). They were first described more than 30 years ago[3,4] as the enzymes that hydrolyze the phosphodiester bond in cAMP and cGMP to their corresponding 5′-mononucleotides (5′AMP and 5′GMP). cAMP- and cGMP-dependent protein kinases (PKA and PKG) are not activated by 5′AMP and 5′GMP; PDE activity is thus a most important inactivation pathway for these intracellular second messengers.

Multiple PDE isoenzymes have been described based on kinetic properties, substrate specificity, responsiveness to endogenous regulators, and inhibition by selective pharmacologic agents. At least seven different families of isoenzymes now have been identified.[5–7] Isolation of their cDNA has resulted in further members of this class of enzymes being identified, and it now is appreciated that each family of isoenzymes consists of several closely related subtypes. These enzymes have different cellular distributions and within the cell they can be located either in the cytosol or the membrane fraction.[8,9]

Inhibition of PDE is of particular interest in pulmonary pharmacology with the widespread use of theophylline. Although it is a weak, nonselective PDE inhibitor, theophylline possesses bronchodilator and anti-inflammatory effects in animal models and in patients with asthma[10] (see also Chap. 61). In anticipation of obtaining therapeutically more selective agents, drugs that potently and specifically inhibit one or more PDE isoenzymes have been synthesized. Together with studies describing the cellular distribution of the isoenzymes, these inhibitors have facilitated greatly experiments investigating the relative importance of PDE isoenzymes in cyclic nucleotide metabolism and cell function.

The cAMP-specific PDE (PDE IV) has been highlighted as being of particular importance in inflammatory and immunocompetent cells. Inhibitors of PDE IV consequently display anti-inflammatory effects in vitro and in animal models and several compounds are currently in preclinical or clinical development for asthma and other chronic inflammatory conditions. This chapter focuses on cyclic nucleotide–PDE isoenzymes and anti-inflammatory effects of selective inhibitors in the lung. The role of PDEs in regulation of airway smooth muscle tone is discussed in greater detail elsewhere (see Chaps. 50 and 51).

Identification of PDE Isoenzyme Families

Different PDE isoenzymes have been identified and, based on gene sequences, a uniform nomenclature has been proposed.[7] The existence of seven major families is well recognized, as shown in Table 62-1. PDE I is stimulated by μM concentrations of Ca^{2+} and calmodulin. PDE II displays a low affinity for both cAMP and cGMP and low concentrations of cGMP stimulate cAMP hydrolysis. In contrast to the PDE II, PDE III is competitively inhibited by cGMP, has a high affinity for both cAMP and cGMP, and has a Vmax that is greater for cAMP than cGMP. PDE IV has a high affinity for cAMP, is found in many inflammatory cells, and is discussed in further detail below. PDE V selectively hydrolyzes cGMP. PDE VI also is selective for cGMP, but is located exclusively in retinal rods and cones and is important in visual transduction. PDE VII has high affinity and specificity for cAMP. It differs from PDE IV by being derived from a separate gene and by not being sensitive to inhibition by rolipram (see below).

Enzymes belonging to the same isoenzyme family share 20 to 25 percent homology with isoenzymes of other families.

The parts of the enzyme with the largest homology (>60 percent amino acid identity) are the catalytic sequences consisting of about 270 amino acids and located near the carboxy terminal end.[5,6] The most recent developments include the observation that each isoenzyme family consists of two or more related subtypes, which emanate from similar but distinct genes (Table 62-2). A number of different proteins are produced from these genes by alternative mRNA splicing or by different start sites for translation of the protein.

An important contribution to the identification of the relative importance of different isoenzymes has been the development of selective pharmacologic inhibitors. In this respect, PDEs III, IV, and V have attracted the greatest attention. Inhibitors of PDE III and V have beneficial effects in various cardiovascular disorders, whereas PDE IV inhibitors have been implicated in inflammatory diseases and also may influence activity in the central nervous system (CNS). Some of the selective and most widely used inhibitors of PDE isoenzymes are shown in Table 62-1. The functional importance of different PDE isoenzymes in vitro and in vivo have been elucidated by use of these pharmacologic tools (as discussed in more detail below), but inhibitors uniquely affecting one or more of the subtypes are not yet available.

CAMP-SPECIFIC PDE (PDE IV)

The PDE IV isoenzyme consists of several different subtypes which, depending on the cell type, can be detected either in the cytosol or membrane fraction.[11–13] Four rat PDE IV subtypes have been identified as transcripts of four separate genes with highly conserved catalytic domains and variable N- and carboxy-terminal domains (see Refs. 14 and 15). Initial studies found two PDE IV subtypes in human monocyte and brain cDNA libraries, but this now has been expanded to include four subtypes, which are similar to their rat homologs[16,17] (see also Ref. 7 and Table 62-2). These enzymes seem to have a differential distribution between tissues, as shown by reverse-transcriptase–polymerase chain

TABLE 62-1   Cyclic Nucleotide-Phosphodiesterase Isoenzyme Families and Their Biochemical Properties

Isoenzyme	Modulator	Affinity, Km	Selective Antagonists
family			
PDE Iα	Ca2+/calmodulin	cAMP 2–20 μM	Vinpocetine
PDE Iβ	stimulated	cGMP 2–20 μM	
PDE II	cGMP stimulated	cAMP 30–100 μM	EHNA (MEP-1)
		cGMP 10–30 μM	
PDE III	cGMP inhibited	cAMP 0.1–0.5 μM	Milrinone
		cGMP 0.1–0.5 μM	Siguazodan
PDE IV	cAMP specific	cAMP 0.5–2 μM	Rolipram, Ro 20-1724,
		cGMP >50 μM	RP 73401
PDE V	cGMP specific	cAMP >40 μM	Zaprinast,
		cGMP 1.5 μM	SK&F 96231
PDE VI	Photoreceptor	cAMP >500 μM	Zaprinast
		cGMP 17–20 μM	
PDE VII	cAMP specific	cAMP 0.2 μM	Not sensitive to
		cGMP	rolipram

TABLE 62-2   Cyclic Nucleotide-Phosphodiesterase Isoenzyme Subtyes

Isoenzyme Family	Subtypes Identified	Cloned from Species	Splice Variants Reported
PDE I	PDE I_A	Bovine	
	PDE I_B	Bovine, rat, mouse	>9
	PDE I_C	Human, mouse	
PDE II	PDE II_A	Bovine	2
PDE III	PDE III_A	Human	
	PDE III_B	Rat	>2
PDE IV	PDE IV_A	Human, rat	
	PDE IV_B	Human, rat	
	PDE IV_C	Human, rat	>15
	PDE IV_D	Human, rat	
PDE V	PDE V_A	Bovine	2
PDE VI	PDE VI_A	Human, bovine, mouse	
	PDE VI_B	Human, bovine, mouse	>2
PDE VII	PDE VII_A	Human	1

reaction (RT-PCR).[17,18] Northern blot analysis of mRNA from different cells shows transcripts of different sizes for each of the four rat PDE IV subtypes.[13,19] Up to five different transcripts of PDE IV_A and PDE IV_C have been demonstrated in germ cells, and three PDE IV_As with different 5' ends have been found in brain cDNA libraries.[19] The PDE IV_D can also be found with different 5' ends.[20] These various forms are thought to be a result of multiple transcriptional start sites and alternative splicing of RNA.[20]

The reasons for this abundance of closely related enzymes have not been elucidated. One possibility is that intracellular localization is conferred by structural features and, for example, the PDE IV_A has a unique N-terminal domain, which seems to target the protein to the membrane.[21]

Peculiar to the PDE IV is the rolipram binding site. Despite being a relatively weak inhibitor of the catalytic activity (Ki, inhibition constant, 0.5 to 1 μM), rolipram binds with high affinity to the enzyme (Kd about 1 nM). Human recombinant PDE IV_A has high affinity (Kd, dissociation constant, 2 nM) and low affinity (Kd 40 nM) binding sites for rolipram,[22] whereas human recombinant PDE IV_B has been reported to have two noninteracting high-affinity binding sites (Kd 0.4 and 6 nM).[23] The rolipram binding site appears to be separate from the catalytic site,[22] and the (possible) interaction between the two still is unknown. The potency of rolipram at the binding and catalytic sites varies with enzyme source and in vitro treatment of the PDE IV enzyme, supporting the view that it can exist in different conformational states (see Ref. 24).

PDE IV activity can be upregulated by exposure of cells to agents that stimulate cAMP production, such as β-adrenoceptor agonists, prostaglandin E_2, and cAMP analogs.[25] The magnitude of the upregulation can be potentiated by the selective inhibitor, rolipram.[25] It is possible that not all subtypes are expressed to the same extent, since Northern blots of mRNA demonstrate that levels of PDE IV_B and PDE IV_D are specifically augmented in rat Sertoli cells by agents increasing cAMP.[13] The pattern of PDE subtype expression

conceivably could differ in other cell types. With regard to short-term (minutes) regulation, increased PDE activity can be explained by phosphorylation of the enzyme.[26] A PDE IV_D splice variant uniquely has a consensus sequence for protein kinase A (PKA) phosphorylation in its N-terminus.[26]

Histamine, lipopolysaccharide (LPS), gamma-interferon (IFN-γ and interleukin-4 (IL-4) all can increase cAMP-PDE activity in mononuclear cells.[27,28] At least in theory, this increased PDE activity could reduce intracellular concentrations of cAMP and thereby augment the proinflammatory effects of these cytokines. Mononuclear cells from subjects with atopic dermatitis have increased PDE IV activity.[29,30] Mononuclear cells from this group of patients behave somewhat differently from cells isolated from ragweed-sensitive individuals, since prolonged incubation with proliferating stimuli (ragweed antigen, tetanus toxoid, phytohemagglutinin (PHA)) did not alter PDE IV gene expression compared with control cells and cells from healthy subjects.[31] Interestingly, the PDE IV inhibitor Ro 20-1724 was equally effective in attenuating enzyme release from normal and asthmatic polymorphonuclear leukocytes.[32]

A large number of enzymes with high specificity for cAMP have been described, and it now is important to elucidate their distribution and function in health and disease. A better understanding of the significance of the rolipram binding site may unravel novel (endogenous?) control mechanisms for PDE activity.

PDE Activity in Inflammatory Cells in Vitro

PDE ISOENZYMES IN INFLAMMATORY CELLS

It now is well recognized that inflammatory cells have different profiles of PDE isoenzymes, as shown in Table 62-3. The most widely distributed family of isoenzymes is the cAMP-specific PDE, which has been shown to be present in

TABLE 62-3 Cyclic Nucleotide-Phosphodiesterase Isoenzyme Families Present in Inflammatory and Immune Cells and Effects of Selective Inhibitors

Cell Type	Species	PDE Isoenzyme	Inhibitory Response
Eosinophils	Guinea pig	IV	ROS*
	Human	IV	ROS, ECP, MBP, TXA$_2$
Monocytes	Human	IV	TNFα, ROS, phagocytosis
Macrophages	Mouse	II, III, IV	ROS, TNFα
	Guinea pig	IV	ROS
T lymphocytes	Rat	II, III, IV, (V)	
	Human	(III), IV	IL-2, cytotoxicity, proliferation
T-cell clone	Human	IV, VII	Proliferation
B lymphocytes	Human	IV	Antibody
Mast cells	Mouse	I, IV	Histamine, LTC$_4$
	Rat	V ?	Histamine
Basophils	Human	III, IV	Histamine, LTC$_4$
Neutrophils	Human	IV	ROS, enzyme
Epithelial cells	Bovine trachea	I, II, III, IV, V	
	Human airway	I, II, III, IV, V	Prostaglandin secretion
Endothelial cells	Bovine aorta	II, IV, (V)	
Platelets	Human	II, III, V	Aggregation, 5-HT, ATP

ABBREVIATIONS: ROS = reactive oxygen species; ECP = eosinophil cationic protein; MBP = major basic protein; TXA$_2$ = thromboxane A$_2$; TNFα = tumor necrosis factor α; LTC$_4$ = leukotriene C$_4$; 5-HT = 5-hydroxy tryptamine; ATP = adenosine triphosphate.

neutrophils,[33,34] monocytes,[35] basophils,[36] mast cells,[37] certain lymphocytes,[38] cosinophils,[39–41] and epithelial cells.[42,43] PDE III is found in basophils,[36] murine macrophages,[27] T lymphocytes,[38] platelets,[44,45] and epithelial cells.[42,46] PDE V, together with PDE III, is present in platelets,[45] rat mast cells,[47] and epithelial cells.[42,43] PDE I (murine mast cells,[17] epithelial cells,[42]) PDE II (murine macrophages,[27] rat mast cells,[47] platelets[44] and PDE VII (T cells[48]) have a restricted distribution.

The PDEs present in endothelial cells from the airway microvasculature, where mediator-induced plasma protein leakage occurs, are not known. However, endothelial cells from pig aorta contain PDEs II and IV.[49,50] Bovine aortic endothelial cells may also contain PDE V.[51]

EFFECTS OF SELECTIVE PDE INHIBITORS ON INFLAMMATORY CELLS IN VITRO

EOSINOPHILS

The eosinophil is thought to play a central role in asthma pathology by releasing the cytotoxic proteins eosinophil cationic protein (ECP), major basic protein (MBP), eosinophil peroxidase (EPO), and eosinophil derived neurotoxin (EDN).[1,2] These proteins slow ciliary beating, and immunoreactive ECP and MBP have been found in the asthmatic mucosa at sites of epithelial shedding and tissue damage.[2,52,53] In a detailed time-course study in antigen-challenged guinea pigs, MBP was found at sites of epithelial damage with protein deposition preceding sloughing of the epithelium, further supporting a cause-and-effect relationship.[54]

The predominant PDE in the guinea pig and human eosinophil is the PDE IV, which is tightly bound to the membrane.[39,40] There is to date no evidence for the presence of

any significant cGMP hydrolytic activity in the eosinophil. A poor correlation has been reported between the inhibitory potencies of chemically distinct compounds against bound, particulate PDE IV and whole-cell cAMP-generation or superoxide release.[39] However, when the compounds were tested against cAMP-PDE, which had been solubilized with deoxycholate and NaCl, a very close relationship was obtained, mainly due to more than a 10-fold increase in the potency of a range of rolipramlike selective PDE IV inhibitors (for example, rolipram (IC$_{50}$ decreased from 186 nM to 28 nM[55]). Incubation of freshly prepared eosinophil membranes with vanadate/glutathione complex had a similar effect.[53] These observations indicate that PDE IV can exist in at least two different conformational states and that, in the cell, it adopts a shape that is more closely akin to that of the solubilized enzyme. In contrast to rolipram, the potency of the selective PDE IV inhibitor, RP 73401 (IC$_{50}$ ≈ 1 nM), is not altered by this treatment of the isolated enzyme, indicating that RP 73401 and rolipram interact differently with the cAMP-PDE.[55,56]

Rolipram and other PDE IV inhibitors potentiate cAMP accumulation in eosinophils, whereas inhibitors of PDE III and PDE V are without effect,[39,40] as would be expected based on the isoenzyme profile. Surprisingly, the PDE IV inhibitor-mediated potentiation of β$_2$-adrenergic-agonist–induced cAMP accumulation is not accompanied by a greater inhibition of superoxide release.[24] PAF, LTB$_4$, FMLP, human recombinant C5$_a$, and opsonized zymosan–induced oxygen radical formation by guinea pig and human eosinophils is attenuated by PDE IV inhibitors.[39–41,58] Likewise, MBP release from guinea pig eosinophils and ECP release from human eosinophils are suppressed potently by RP 73401.[55,58] Chemotaxis produced in vitro by human recombinant C5$_a$, PAF and FMLP also is reduced.[59] By use of RT-PCR and immunologic methods, a range of cytokines,

TNF-α, TGF-α, TGF-β, GM-CSF, IL-3, IL-5 and IL-6, have been detected in human eosinophils (see Ref. 60), but whether compounds acting selectively on PDE IV can alter their synthesis and/or secretion has not been examined.

The survival of eosinophils is prolonged by cytokines, such as GM-CSF and IL-5, by adhesion to extracellular matrix or by cytokines released by fibroblasts.[61] Conversely, eosinophils contain TGF-α and TGF-β, which could conceivably contribute to the subepithelial fibrosis in asthmatic airways[53,62] by stimulating fibroblast proliferation and collagen production.[63]

Taken together, these data indicate that PDE IV inhibitors most effectively downregulate eosinophil function in vitro by suppressing activation, chemotaxis, and mediator release. These enzyme inhibitors are much more potent, at least in vitro, than current anti-inflammatory medications[64] and may therefore be useful in eosinophil-driven pathologies like asthma, chronic allergic inflammation, parasitic infections, and perhaps the hypereosinophilic syndrome.

MONOCYTES AND MACROPHAGES

The most important functions of monocytes and macrophages are their phagocytic activity and their capacity to act as antigen-presenting cells. When triggered by IgE (through FcϵRII receptors) or during phagocytosis, lysosomal enzymes are released into the extracellular space together with proinflammatory mediators and cytokines.

PDE IV inhibitors potently suppress TNF-α production from LPS-stimulated macrophages and human monocytes.[65–67] They act pretranscriptionally, since they reduce concentrations of TNF-α-mRNA in macrophages (Ref. 67, Maslen, Souness, Karlsson, unpublished) at concentrations also attenuating protein release. A posttranscriptional effect also has been proposed,[67] but whether this contributes to any significant degree to inhibition of protein release is uncertain. Selective PDE III inhibitors have a small effect on TNF-α release but inhibitors of PDE I and PDE V are not active.[67] In contrast to TNF-α, PDE IV inhibitors have little or no direct effect on the release of IL-1β or IL-6 from stimulated macrophages.[66,67] However, it has been demonstrated in synovial tissue in vitro that an anti-TNF-α antibody could antagonize IL-1β and IL-6 release, suggesting that PDE IV inhibitors also may exert such an effect.[68]

A study with the PDE IV inhibitor, Ro 20-1724, in human alveolar macrophages suggests that neither this compound, nor isoproterenol is able to reduce superoxide, LTB$_4$ or TXA$_2$ release.[69] These data question the existence and importance of PDE IV in human alveolar macrophages.[69] The apparent lack of effect of PDE IV inhibitors in this cell type is intriguing since their "precursor cell," the monocyte, is exquisitely sensitive to suppression by these drugs (particularly with regard to TNF-α release).

The cAMP-specific PDE has been demonstrated in mouse and guinea pig peritoneal macrophages, and PDE IV inhibitors have consequently been shown to antagonize phagocytosis,[70] arachidonic acid release,[71,72] and production of reactive oxygen species,[70,73] although being much less potent on these responses than on TNF-α production.

It would thus appear that PDE IV inhibitors, and hence cAMP, are involved in only certain intracellular processes in monocytes and macrophages. The apparent lack of effect by drugs acting on the PDE IV in human alveolar macrophages differs from the effect of blood monocytes and granulocytes and requires further study. The PDE profile in human macrophages is not known, and it is possible that other as yet unidentified PDE isoenzymes and/or subtypes are present in macrophages but not in human peripheral blood monocytes.

T LYMPHOCYTES

CD4+ T lymphocytes synthesize a range of proinflammatory cytokines, and the T-helper-2 (Th2) subtype of CD4+ lymphocytes has been proposed to initiate and direct the immune and inflammatory response in asthma (e.g., Ref. 1). This lymphocyte subtype produces a range of cytokines, which promote the growth of Th2 cells but suppresses that of Th1 cells (e.g., IL-4), regulate switching to IgE production in B lymphocytes (e.g. IL-4 and IL-13) and stimulates the differentiation and maturation of eosinophils (IL-5) (see Ref. 75). PGE$_2$ increases cAMP concentrations in both human monocytes and lymphocytes[30,75] and there is no appreciable difference in inducible cAMP concentrations between human T-cell clones producing high concentrations of IL-2 (Th0 or Th1) or high concentrations of IL-5 (Th2).[75] These effects on cAMP concentrations are, therefore, difficult to reconcile with the fact that in different T-cell clones, IL-2 and IFN-γ secretion are inhibited potently, whereas PGE$_2$ has only a small effect on IL-4 and produces a transient increase in IL-5 release.[75] Interestingly, forskolin, dibutyryl-cAMP, and IBMX have weak inhibitory effects on IL-2 and IFN-γ. This supports the view that PGE$_2$ may work through additional intracellular pathways beside cAMP.[75]

PDE IV inhibitors consistently suppress IL-2 and IFN-γ release from Th1 lymphocytes[76–78] but have little direct effect on Th2 cell proliferation or cytokine secretion. Furthermore, Mirza and coworkers[79] showed in a mouse mixed splenocyte population in vitro that inhibition of IL-2 release by rolipram and RP 73401 is the mechanism behind growth suppression and consequently reduced cytokine (IL-4, IL-5) release from Th2 cells.

Rolipram has been reported to inhibit equally well ragweed antigen (Th2)- and tetanus toxoid-(Th1)-induced proliferation of peripheral blood mononuclear cells, whereas PDE III and PDE V inhibitors are inactive.[31,80] PDE IV inhibitors suppress PHA-stimulated proliferation of human CD4+/CD8+ T lymphocytes, although maximum inhibition is greater in the presence of both a PDE III and a PDE IV inhibitor. Both isoenzymes having been identified in these cells.[31,81] Inhibition of IL-2 release from T cells[82,83] is probably not the only mechanism causing inhibition of proliferation, since concanavalin A–stimulated murine splenocyte proliferation occurred with lesser concentrations than IL-2 release from the same cells.[83]

In a preliminary study, rolipram inhibited IL-5, but not IL-4 mRNA concentrations after allergen provocation.[80] This observation contrasts with earlier data and needs confirmation.

It is not known if cytokine release from lymphocytes from asthmatic subjects also is sensitive to inhibition by selective PDE inhibitors, particularly since mononuclear cells from subjects with atopic dermatitis may have an increased PDE activity (as discussed above; Refs. 29 and 30). Ro 20-1724 reduces the spontaneous IgE synthesis by mononuclear cells from subjects with atopic dermatitis,[84] but it is possible that the drug acts on antigen-presenting monocytes rather than on the IgE-secreting B lymphocytes themselves.

Thus, presently available data suggest that PDE IV inhibitors may act on naive T cells or even Th1 cells rather than on fully differentiated Th2 cells. Suppression of growth factor release, including IL-2, from these cells could indirectly reduce the number and commitment of T-helper2 cells and therefore dampen the inflammatory response.

MAST CELLS AND BASOPHILS

Mast cells and basophils generally are believed to contribute primarily to the immediate allergic reaction by release of bronchoconstrictor mediators, such as histamine and the cysteinyl-leukotrienes. Mast cells recently have been shown to synthesize a range of cytokines, including IL-4, IL-5, IL-6 and TNF-α,[85-87] with proliferative and pro-inflammatory effects as discussed above.

It seems clear that species and tissue source (mucosal or connective tissue type, Ref. 86) influence the PDE isoenzyme profile. Antigen-induced histamine and LTC$_4$ release from murine bone marrow–derived mast cells is inhibited by rolipram,[37] whereas zaprinast (a PDE V inhibitor) inhibits mediator release from rat peritoneal mast cells.[88] The PDE isoenzymes present in human lung mast cells are not known, but rolipram has been reported to increase cAMP concentrations and suppress histamine release.[89] Somewhat surprisingly, a PDE III inhibitor more effectively inhibited histamine release than rolipram, even though the change in cAMP concentrations was minimal.[89] These data suggest that PDE III is more important than PDE IV in regulating histamine release, but whether this is true also for cytokine release is not known.

Interestingly, rolipram inhibits antigen-induced mediator release from human basophils, and this effect is potentiated by a PDE III inhibitor and by forskolin,[36] again suggesting that in humans, both the type III and IV may be important for basophil and mast cell function.

NEUTROPHILS

The neutrophil is recruited in large numbers during infection and chronic inflammatory conditions, although its precise role in asthma is unclear. Nevertheless, PDE IV inhibitors like rolipram and RP 73401 suppress superoxide anion generation and elastase release with low potency.[58] Other responses, such as chemotaxis, degranulation, and phagocytosis also can be suppressed by PDE IV inhibitors.[70,90,91] Opsonized zymosan-induced secretion of beta-glucuronidase is inhibited by Ro 20-1724, and there is no difference in the responsiveness between PMNs from normal and asthmatic subjects.[33] The PDE IV seems to be most important for neutrophil function, at least with regard to the respiratory burst activity, which has been studied in most detail (33, 34).

OTHER CELLS

Platelets as well as epithelial and endothelial cells have been proposed to contribute mediators and enzymes to inflam-

matory reactions. Increased intracellular concentrations of cAMP dampen platelet function (aggregation, mediator release). The major cAMP-hydrolyzing enzyme is the PDE III.[92] The principal PDE activity in human bronchial epithelial cells in primary culture was found to be the type IV, although PDEs I, II, III, and V were also present.[42] Almost all PDE activity was found in the cytosol. The non-selective PDE inhibitor IBMX inhibited prostaglandin secretion from these cells in culture.[42] Similarly, PDEs III and IV are the main enzymes in the human airway epithelial cell line BEAS-2B,[43] but these investigators did not explore their function or importance in functional studies. The PDE profile in endothelial cells is discussed in relation to microvascular leakage below.

Taken together, the PDE profile and activity of individual cells varies depending on genetic background, tissue microenvironment, and prior exposure to proinflammatory mediators and cytokines. The PDE IV and its various subtypes clearly are present in a wide range of cells, which are involved in the initial and chronic phases of the inflammatory reaction. Even in cells in which this is the major enzyme, it participates only in select processes exemplified in monocytes where TNF-α, but not IL-1β or IL-6, release is affected. Compared with the PDE IV, other isoenzymes have a restricted distribution in inflammatory cells and, as discussed below, selective inhibitors have limited effects in models of inflammation.

Anti-Inflammatory Effects of PDE Inhibitors in Animal Models

The anti-inflammatory and immunomodulatory effects of the non-selective PDE inhibitor theophylline have been well documented[10] (see also Chap. 61). In the lung, theophylline inhibits antigen-induced bronchospasm, and eosinophilia, and other facets of the inflammatory response. Theophylline has, however, many extrapulmonary effects that limit its clinical use, and isoenzyme-selective PDE inhibitors have been developed with the hope of obtaining more lung-specific anti-inflammatory agents. These PDE inhibitors have been studied in experimental models of inflammation.

INHIBITION OF ANTIGEN-INDUCED BRONCHOSPASM AND CELL INFILTRATION INTO THE AIRWAYS

Guinea pigs frequently are used in these types of studies, and antigen exposure of sensitized animals results in an acute bronchoconstriction, microvascular leakage of proteins, mucus secretion, and waves of inflammatory cells entering the bronchial mucosa and airway lumen. An early neutrophilia is followed by eosinophilia and sometimes also an increase in macrophages and lymphocytes.[54,93,94] The cells clearly are activated as shown by shape-change and degranulation and because increased amounts of cell-specific mediators—e.g., elastase and MBP—accumulate in tissue and bronchoalveolar lavage (BAL) fluid.[54,95] The acute inflammatory response is similar to that described in asthma patients exposed to antigen.[2,53]

Sensitized guinea pigs sometimes respond to an antigen challenge with a dual immediate and late-phase bronchoconstrictor response,[96–98] although this is often difficult to demonstrate unequivocally in animal experiments. Selective PDE inhibitors have not been studied in these models.

Nonselective PDE inhibitors such as theophylline inhibit antigen- and PAF-induced airway obstruction and eosinophilia in guinea pigs.[93,99] AH 21-132 and zardaverine, mixed PDE III/IV inhibitors, have similar effects in this species when administered repeatedly before challenge.[93,100]

Rolipram and other selective PDE IV inhibitors have potent antibronchoconstrictor and anti-inflammatory effects in models of lung inflammation (e.g., Refs. 100–103). When administered directly into the lung as a dry powder before antigen challenge, rolipram and RP 73401 completely inhibit bronchospasm in sensitized guinea pigs and rats. In addition, both the total number of inflammatory cells and the eosinophils in BAL fluid are reduced.[102] PDE III but not PDE V inhibitors reduce mediator/antigen-induced bronchospasm in different species.[101,104,105] Interestingly, neither selective PDE III (siguazodan) nor PDE V (zaprinast) inhibitors attenuate cell accumulation following antigen challenge,[64] suggesting that the effects of AH 21-132 and zardaverine are mediated through PDE IV.

The anti-inflammatory effects of rolipram also have been examined in one study in cynomolgus monkeys. Subcutaneous administration of rolipram 1 h before antigen challenge results in inhibition of BAL eosinophils and neutrophils and diminished concentrations of TNF-α and IL-8 but no change in the acute constrictor response or in IL-1β or IL-6 concentrations.[106] Repeat allergen exposure results in inflammation and airway hyperresponsiveness, which could be prevented by treatment with rolipram.[106] These effects are accompanied by an increase in BAL leukocyte cAMP concentrations, supporting PDE inhibition as its mechanism of action.

PDE IV inhibitors may act at several levels to reduce cell trafficking into the airways. They have been shown to inhibit the generation of potent eosinophil chemoattractants such as PAF and complement C_2.[107] IL-2 has recently been proposed as a particularly potent chemotactic agent for human eosinophils[108] and, as discussed above, IL-2 release from lymphocytes potently is inhibited by PDE IV inhibitors.[82]

These agents also may reduce the expression of adhesion molecules on the surface of endothelial cells or on the granulocyte itself. Agents that increase cAMP concentration decrease the number of adhesion molecules like ELAM-1 and VCAM-1 but not ICAM-1 on endothelial cells.[109] The same end effect could be achieved by inhibiting the release of cytokines like TNF-α, which potently upregulate adhesion molecules in the vasculature.[110,111] Interest-ingly, cAMP has been found to downregulate VLA-4, one of the most important integrins for association with the endothelial cells, on the surface of an eosinophil-like cell line (EoL-1; Ref. 112). Furthermore, an increase in cAMP concentrations in neutrophils is associated with a decreased adhesiveness to endothelial layers.[113]

The eosinophilia in asthma is at least partly a result of an increased production of eosinophil progenitors in the bone marrow and the numbers circulating in blood increases dramatically in both dogs and asthmatic humans after antigen provocation.[114,115] In a preliminary study, it was observed that treatment for one week with rolipram reduced bone marrow and peritoneal eosinophils in parasite (*Mesocestoides corti*)-infected mice. This results from a reduction in the number of eosinophil progenitor cells.[116] This effect is not linked to inhibition of IL-5, since neither release of this cytokine nor IL-5–mediated stimulation of eosinophil progenitors is antagonized by rolipram.[116] An effect by the PDE IV inhibitor at the level of the bone marrow could contribute to a reduced number of mature eosinophils in chronic disease.

BRONCHIAL HYPERRESPONSIVENESS

The basal responsiveness to bronchoconstrictor agents is determined by genetic, environmental, and other ill-defined factors, but it is generally increased in asthma. Inflammatory reactions in the bronchial mucosa enhance this hyperresponsiveness further. Support for this view stems from studies showing that drugs such as glucocorticoids, which stabilize inflammatory cells and suppress mediator release, also reduce airway hyperresponsiveness. In most animal models of airway hyperresponsiveness, the reactivity to standard bronchoconstrictors is increased only two- to fivefold. Even repeat antigen exposure in guinea pigs[54,94,98] and monkeys[117] rarely increase reactivity more than 10-fold.

Administration of theophylline or AH 21-132 to guinea pigs for ≤ 1 week does not reduce significantly the hyperresponsiveness caused by antigen aerosol.[93] However, the eosinophilia is markedly suppressed by this treatment, demonstrating that the compounds are absorbed. This supports the view that there is not a direct relationship between the number of circulating eosinophils but rather their activation state[55] and the degree of airway hyperresponsiveness. In contrast, LPS-challenged rats develop airway hyperresponsiveness to 5-HT, which can be reduced by the mixed PDE III/IV inhibitor zardaverine.[119] Zardaverine also inhibited the BAL neutrophilia and TNF-α production.[118]

In guinea pigs, rolipram abolishes the PAF-induced hyperreactivity to bombesin and, when administered intravenously, both rolipram and RP 73401 are exceedingly potent in reducing the PAF-induced hyperresponsiveness.[102] Together with the observations in the cynomolgus monkey,[106] it seems that potent and selective PDE IV inhibitors reduce airway hyperresponsiveness, at least in animal models.

MICROVASCULAR LEAKAGE

The endothelium of postcapillary venules usually constitutes a tight barrier to cells and macromolecules in the circulation, but a range of inflammatory mediators can cause the formation of intercellular gaps. Proteins of the complement and blood-clotting cascades have proinflammatory properties, and, together with other plasma proteins, may cause tissue injury and fluid accumulation (119). Detection of proteins in BAL fluid and sputum from asthmatic patients may be a sign of ongoing inflammation.[119] Naclerio and coworkers[120] have demonstrated that theophylline can reduce leakage of proteins into the nasal mucosa in rhinitis, and proteins in sputum are also reduced by therapeutic concentrations of this xanthine.[119] Likewise, theophylline inhibits the PAF-induced leakage of a macromolecular tracer (FITC dextran) in the guinea pig tracheobronchial tree and lavage fluid.[121,122]

Adenylyl cyclase and guanylyl cyclase activities have been found in bovine and porcine aortic endothelial cells together with PDEs types II and IV.[49,50,123] The PDE isoenzymes present in postcapillary venular endothelial cells in the tracheobronchial circulation, where active leakage occurs, is not known. Agents that increase intracellular cAMP concentration in vitro[124,125] reduce endothelial permeability. Accordingly, salbutamol and sodium nitroprusside, which increase cAMP and cGMP concentrations, respectively, as well as rolipram[122,126] and RP 73401,[64,102] inhibit plasma protein extravasation into guinea pig airways. Zaprinast administered directly into the airways also inhibits significantly leakage, whereas vinpocetine and siguazodan are without effect. These data demonstrate that PDEs IV and V but not I and III are involved in guinea pig airway microvascular leakage.[64,122] Interestingly, RP 73401 is more effective in reducing epithelial than endothelial permeability, supporting the view that epithelial and endothelial cells have separate PDE isoenzyme profiles. Rolipram and the β_2-adrenoceptor agonist, terbutaline, also have been shown to reduce directly the bradykinin-induced permeability increase in the hamster cheek pouch preparation.[127]

PDE IV inhibitors effectively reduce microvascular leakage in the tracheobronchial circulation and possibly in other vascular beds, as suggested by the effect in the hamster cheek pouch preparation. Even when study compounds are administered directly into the airways and expected to act directly on the endothelium to inhibit mediator-induced leakage, an additional effect on for example mediator release from other cells in the airway mucosa cannot be excluded.

Bronchodilator Effects of Selective PDE Inhibitors

Several recent reviews have discussed PDE inhibitors and airway smooth muscle,[37,105,128] including Chap. 50 in this volume. In human, bovine, and canine airway smooth muscle, PDEs I, II, III, IV, and V have been demonstrated.[129–132] PDE III and PDE IV inhibitors relax airway smooth muscle irrespective of the agent used to induce tone; that is, they act as functional antagonists (e.g., Refs. 102, 132–135) and are also active in vivo (e.g., Refs. 102 and 104). PDEs III and IV seem to be most effective in regulating human bronchial tone in vitro.[130,132,135] Zaprinast relaxes human isolated bronchi, but with a low potency.[132] Rolipram enhances isoproprenol- but not sodium nitroprusside-induced relaxation of human isolated bronchi.[135] The PDE V inhibitor zaprinast potentiates sodium nitroprusside-induced relaxation and cGMP

accumulation in the canine trachea, but does not cause relaxation on its own.[136]

It is interesting to note the apparent association between presence of β_2-adrenergic receptors on bronchial smooth muscle and potency of PDE IV inhibitors as brochodilators (e.g., human, guinea pig, cow) and that between β_1-adrenoceptors and PDE III inhibitors (e.g., mouse, pig).[133,135] Rolipram is thus about 100-fold more potent in human than pig bronchi, whereas the opposite is true for siguazodan. Collectively, these observations suggest that PDE IV and possibly PDE III inhibitors could dilate the airways of asthma patients.

The functions of PDE I and PDE II in control of smooth muscle are unknown, largely because of the lack of potent and selective antagonists.

These data indicate that PDE III and IV inhibitors are capable of modulating bronchial tone and organ bath studies suggest that they may be as potent as β-adrenergic agonists. It is important to remember, however, that with PDE IV inhibitors like rolipram and RP 73401 an improvement in lung function could result not only from a direct effect on the smooth muscle relaxation, but also indirectly through inhibition of mediator release from inflammatory cells.

Effects of PDE Inhibitors in Patients with Airways Disease

Despite the large amount of preclinical data, little is still known about the effects of selective PDE inhibitors in patients with asthma or other airway diseases. AH 21-132 and zardaverine relax bronchial smooth muscle in vitro and act as bronchodilators in vivo.[137,138] AH 21-132 has been shown to reverse methacholine-induced bronchospasm in healthy subjects and to induce a small, transient bronchodilation when administered intravenously.[138] The two drugs inhibit both PDE III and PDE IV and it is, therefore, impossible to deduce which of the two enzymes is most important for this effect on airway tone. On the other hand, DeBoer and coworkers[132] showed that combined PDE III/IV inhibitors cause a more marked relaxation of human bronchi in vitro than selective inhibitors alone. Whether this is the case also in human subjects remains to be demonstrated.

Of selective inhibitors, those that affect the PDE III, IV, and V have attracted the greatest interest for their potential as antiasthma drugs. PDE III inhibitors are effective bronchodilators in a number of species although they have profound cardiovascular effects at the same doses (e.g. Ref. 104). The PDE III inhibitor enoximone (MDL 17043) improves lung function in patients with chronic obstructive lung disease.[139] In a placebo-controlled, double-blind, crossover trial, zaprinast reduced exercise- but not histamine-induced bronchoconstriction in asthmatics, suggesting that it was acting indirectly, possibly on mast cells.[140]

To date, only one relatively weak PDE IV inhibitor, tibenelast (LY-186655), has been examined in subjects with asthma. At a single oral dose, a slight but nonsignificant improvement in FEV_1 was observed in asthmatics.[141] This effect may not be representative for novel, potent, and more selective PDE IV inhibitors, which may exert qualitatively different effects.

Extrapulmonary Effects of PDE Inhibitors

PDE isoenzymes have a tissue-specific distribution and are therefore of varying importance in organ functions. A prime example is PDE VI, which is uniquely found in the retinal rod and cones and is involved in vision.

PDE III is the predominant cAMP-catalysing enzyme in the cardiovasculature. Inhibitors of PDE III strengthens the contactility of the heart and relaxes vascular smooth muscle.[142] These agents also attenuate platelet aggregation[44] and stimulate lipolysis.[143] As would be expected, combined PDE III/IV inhibitors also affect the cardiovascular system, but this is almost exclusively due to the PDE III component as shown by Heaslip and coworkers in the dog.[104] PDE V is also present in platelets and vascular smooth muscle, and selective compounds have been developed with the aim of producing vasodilator and antithrombotic drugs.[37]

PDE IV is the most important cAMP-metabolizing PDE in brain and kidney, but PDEs I and II also are present in high levels in certain areas of the brain. Rolipram has effects on behavior in several animal models and was developed originally as an antidepressant but found to have inconsistent effects in patients.[144] Increased cAMP concentrations in the kidney perhaps could explain the transient decrease in plasma osmolality seen in human subjects after 24 h, but not 7 days after commencement of rolipram administration (daily dose of 3 mg).[145] PDE IV inhibitors stimulate parietal cell acid secretion, which may contribute to the general gastrointestinal irritation observed with these agents.[146] Nausea has been observed with PDE IV inhibitors in healthy subjects and patients, but whether this is caused by a local effect in the stomach/intestine or by an effect directly at the emetic center is not known.

PDE I is found in liver, brain, smooth muscle, and fat cells, but the few inhibitors that have been synthesized have been found to have insignificant effects on CNS function and smooth muscle. Some of the reported effects may be due to inhibition of the PDE V, since both isoenzymes have a high affinity for cGMP and some compounds may not be selective.

Conclusion and Future Directions

Advances in biochemistry and molecular biology have provided the foundation for the identification of at least seven different cyclic nucleotide PDE isoenzymes, each with a number of subtypes. The cellular distribution of PDEs varies greatly, and they are detected in either the cytosol or associated with membranes. Together they provide the cell with many opportunities for selective control of cyclic nucleotide levels, even between different intracellular compartments.

The cAMP-specific PDE IV is localized in granulocytes and mononuclear cells and is considered to play a key role in regulating cAMP concentrations and, consequently, cell function. Four different PDE IV subtype families (with more than 15 splice variants) have been identified. Rapid progress in PDE research is likely to identify additional members of the PDE IV subtypes and perhaps, novel isoenzymes. It should also be remembered that the most recently discovered PDE, the type VII, was found in lymphocytes and could provide an important pathway in cAMP metabolism. This could be of particular interest in allergic conditions where PDE IV inhibitors only indirectly affect release of Th2-type cytokines, such as IL-4 and IL-5. Future studies may show PDE VII to have a wider distribution and importance than what is currently appreciated. Emerging data suggest an altered PDE profile in various disease states, but this needs to be better documented.

PDE IV inhibitors, like RP 73401, represent a new generation of potent and selective drugs, which have been shown to suppress inflammatory cell function and relax airway smooth muscle in vitro and to have anti-inflammatory and anti-bronchoconstrictor properties in animal models. This type of compound thus shows potential as anti-asthma agents, and their great potency and selectivity may produce therapeutic agents with distinct advantages over theophylline. Exploratory clinical studies have pointed toward a possible use also in other allergic conditions such as rhinitis and atopic dermatitis. Whether inflammation and tissue remodeling in chronic obstructive pulmonary disease (COPD) and lung fibrosis will be sensitive to PDE IV inhibitors remains an intriguing possibility. The potent immuno-modulatory effects, including suppression of TNF-α production, suggest that these drugs may be of value in diseases with aberrant TNF-α production such as inflammatory bowel disease and rheumatoid arthritis.

Selective PDE IV or mixed PDE III/IV inhibitors are currently in preclinical and clinical development for asthma and other chronic inflammatory and/or allergic conditions. Together with rapid progress in other areas of PDE research, it is anticipated that the results from these clinical studies will further our understanding of physiologic and pathologic processes and contribute to the development of novel and more efficacious medicines.

References

1. Corrigan CJ, Kay AB: T cells and eosinophils in the pathogenesis of asthma, *Immunol Today* 1992; 13:501.
2. Djukanovic R, Roche WR, Wilson JW, et al.: Mucosal inflammation in asthma. *Am Rev Respir Dis* 1990; 142:434.
3. Sutherland EW, Rall TW: Fractionation and characterization of a cyclic adenosine nucleotide formed by tissues particles. *J Biol Chem* 1958; 232:1077.
4. Butcher RW, Sutherland EW: Adenosine 3′,5′-phosphate in biological materials. *J Biol Chem* 1962; 237:1244.
5. Beavo JA, Relfsnyder DH: Primary sequence of cyclic nucleotide phosphodiesterase isozymes and the design of selective inhibitors. *Trends Pharmacol Sci* 1990; 11:150.
6. Thompson JW: Cyclic nucleotide phosphodiesterases: Pharmacology, biochemistry and function. *Pharmacol Ther* 1991; 51:13.

7. Beavo JA, Conti M, Heaslip RJ: Multiple cyclic nucleotide phosphodiesterases. *Mol Pharmacol* 1994; 46:399.

8. Nicholson CD, Challiss RAJ, Shahid M: Differential modulation of tissue function and therapeutic potential of selective inhibitors of cyclic nucleotide phosphodiesterase isoenzymes. *Trends Pharmacol Sci* 1991; 12:19.

9. Raeburn D, Souness JE, Tomkinson A, Karlsson J-A: Isozyme-selective cyclic nucleotide phosphodiesterase inhibitors: Biochemistry, pharmacology and therapeutic potential in astham, in Jucker E (ed): *Progress in Drug Research.* Vol 40. Basel, Birkhäuser Verlag, 1993.

10. Barnes PJ, Bauwels RA: Theophylline in the management of asthma: Time for reappraisal? *Eur Respir J* 1994; 7:579.

11. Chen CN, Denome S, Davis RL: Molecular analysis of cDNA clones and the corresponding genomic coding sequences of the *Drosophila* duncc$^+$ gene, the structural gene for cyclic AMP phosphodiesterase. *Proc Natl Acad Sci USA* 1986; 83:9313.

12. Colicelli J, Birchmeier C, Michaeli T, O'Neill K, et al.: Isolation and characterisation of a mammalian gene encoding a high-affinity cyclic AMP phosphodiesterase. *Proc Natl Acad Sci USA* 1989; 86:3599.

13. Swinnen JV, Tsikalas KE, Conti M: Properties and hormonal regulation of two structurally related cyclic AMP phosphodiesterases from rat Sertoli cells. *J Biol Chem* 1991; 266:18370.

14. Conti M, Swinnen JV: Structure and function of the rolipram-sensitive, low-Km cyclic AMP phosphodiesterases: A family of highly related enzymes, in Beavo JA, Houslay MD (eds): *Molecular Pharmacology of Cell Regulation: Cyclic Nucleotide Phosphodiesterase Structures, Regulation and Drug Action.* New York, Wiley, 1990:234.

15. Souness JE, Raeburn D, Karlsson J-A: Phosphodiesterase type IV inhibitors as potential anti-asthma agent, in Pauwels R, Advenier C, O'Byrne P (eds): *Progress in Basic and Clinical Pharmacology, Antiasthmatic Drugs.* Basel, Karger, 1995, in press.

16. Bolger G, Michaeli T, Martins T, et al.: A family of human phosphodiesterase homologous to the *dunce* learning and memory gene product of *Drosophila melanogaster* are potential targets for anti-depressant drugs. *Mol Bell Biol* 1993; 13:6558.

17. Engles P, Fichtel K, Lubbert H: Expression and regulation of human and rat phosphodiesterase type IV isogenes. *FEBS Lett* 1994; 350:291.

18. Conti M, Swinnen JV, Tsikalas KE, Jin S-LC: Structure and regulation of the rat high affinity cyclic AMP phosphodiesterase. *Adv Second Messenger Protein Phosphorylation Res* 1992; 25:87.

19. Davies RL, Takaysasu H, Eberwine M, Myres J: Cloning and characterization of mammalian homologs of the *Drosophila* dunce+ gene. *Proc Natl Acad Sci USA* 1989; 86:3604.

20. Monaco L, Vicini E, Conti M: Structure of two rat genes coding for a closely related rolipram-sensitive cAMP phosphodiesterase: Multiple mRNA variants originate from alternative splicing and multiple start sites. *J Biol Chem* 1994; 269:347.

21. Shakur Y, Pryde J, Houslay MD: Engineered deletion of the unique N-terminal domain of the cyclic AMP-specific phosphodiesterase RD1 prevents plasma membrane association and the attainment of enhanced thermostability without altering it sensitivity to inhibition by rolipram. *Biochem J* 1993; 292:677.

22. Torphy TJ, Stadel JM, Burman M, et al.: Coexpression of human cyclic AMP-specific phosphodiesterase activity and high-affinity rolipram binding in yeast. *J Biol Chem* 1992; 267:1798.

23. McLaughlin MM, Cieslinski LB, Burman M, et al.: A low-Km, rolipram-sensitive, cyclic AMP-specific phosphodiesterase from human brain: Cloning and expression of cDNA, biochemical characterisation of recombinant protein, and tissue destribution of mRNA. *J Biol Chem* 1993; 268:6470.

24. Giembycz MA, Souness JE: Characteristics and properties of the cyclic AMP-specific phosphodiesterase in eosinophil leukocytes: A potential target for asthma therapy? in Postma D, Gerritsen J (eds): *Bronchitis.* Vol V. Assen, The Netherlands, Van Gorcum, 1994:319.

25. Torphy TJ, Zhou H-L, Cieslinski LB: Stimulation of *Beta*-adrenoceptors in a human monocyte cell line (U937) up-regulates cyclic AMP-specific phosphodiesterase activity. *J Pharmacol Exp Ther* 1992; 263:1195.

26. Sette C, Vicini E, Conti M: The rat PDE3/IVd phosphodiesterase gene codes for multiple proteins differentially activated by cAMP-dependent protein kinase: *J Biol Chem* 1994; 269:18271.

27. Okonogi K, Gettys TW, Uhing RJ, et al.: Inhibition of prostaglandin E$_2$-stimulated cyclic AMP accumulation by lipopolysaccharide in murine peritoneal macrophages. *J Biol Chem* 1991; 266:10305.

28. Li S-H, Chan SC, Toshitani A, et al.: Synergistic effects of interleukin 4 and interferon-gamma on monocyte phosphodiesterase activity. *J Invest Dermatol* 1992; 99:65.

29. Chan SC, Hanifin JM: Differential inhibitor effects on phosphodiesterase isoforms in atopic and normal leukocytes. *J Lab Clin Med* 1993; 121:44.

30. Chan SC, Reifsynder D, Beavo JA, Hanifin JM: Immunochemical characterization of the distinct monocyte cyclic AMP-phosphodiesterases from patients with atopic dermatitis. *J Allergy Clin Immunol* 1993; 91:1179.

31. Essayan DM, Huang S-K, Undem BJ: Antigen- and mitogen-induced proliferative responses of peripheral blood mononuclear cells by non-selective and isozyme selective cyclic nucleotide phosphodiesterase inhibitors. *J Immunol* 1994; 153:3408.

32. Busse WW, Anderson CL: The granulocyte response to the phosphodiesterase inhibitor RO 20-1724 in asthma. *J Allergy Clin Immunol* 1981; 67:70.

33. Wright CD, Kuipers PJ, Kobylarz-Singer D, et al.: Differential inhibition of neutrophil functions: Role of cyclic AMP-specific, cyclic GMP-insensitive phosphodiesterase. *Biochem Pharmacol* 1990; 40:699.

34. Nielson CP, Vestal RE, Sturm RJ, Heaslip R: Effects of selective phosphodiesterase inhibitors on the polymorphonuclear leukocyte respiratory burst. *J Allergy Clin Immunol* 1990; 86:801.

35. White JR, Torphy TJ, Christensen SB, et al.: Purification and characterization of the rolipram sensitive, low K_m phosphodiesterase from human monocytes. *FASEB J* 1990; 4:A1987.

36. Peachell PT, Undem BJ, Schleimer RP, et al.: Preliminary identification and role of phosphodiesterase isozymes in human basophils. *J Immunol* 1992; 148:2503.

37. Torphy TJ, Undem BJ: Phosphodiesterase inhibitors: New opportunities for the treatment of asthma. *Thorax* 1991; 46:512.

38. Robiscek SA, Krzanowski JJ, Szentivanyi A, Polson JB: High pressure liquid chromatography of cyclic AMP phosphodiesterase from purfied human T lymphocytes. *Biochem Biophys Res Comm* 1989; 163:554.

39. Souness JE, Carter CM, Diocee BK, et al.: Characterization of guinea-pig eosinophil phosphodiesterase activity: Assessment of its involvement in regulating superoxide generation. *Biochem Pharmacol* 1991; 42:937.

40. Dent G, Giembycz MA, Rabe KF, Barnes PJ: Inhibition of eosinophil cyclic nucleotide PDE activity and opsonised zymosan-induced respiratory burst by "type IV"-selective PDE inhibitors. *Br J Pharmacol* 1991; 103:1339.

41. Giembycz MA, Dent G, Virdee H, et al.: Cyclic nucleotide phosphodiesterases in human eosinophils: Functional and biochemical effects of isoenzyme-selective inhibitors: *Br J Pharmacol* 1994; 112:26P.

42. Rabe KF, Tenor H, Spaethe SM, et al.: Identification of the PDE isoenzymes in human bronchial epithelial cells and the effect of PDE inhibiton on PGE$_2$ secretion. *Am Rev Respir Dis* 1994; 149:A986.

43. Brennan KJ, Kelsen SG, Sheth SB, Colman RW: Phosphodiesterase in human airway epithelial cells (AEC). *Am Rev Respir Dis* 1994; 149:A988.

44. Simpson AWM, Reeves ML, Rink TJ: Effects of SK&F 94120, an inhibitor of cyclic nucleotide phosphodiesterase type III, on human platelets: *Biochem Pharmacol* 1988; 37:2315.

45. Murray KJ, England PJ, Hallam TJ, et al.: The effects of siguazodan, a selective phosphodiesterase inhibitor, on human platelet function. *Br J Pharmacol* 1990; 99:612.

46. Rousseau E, Gagnon J, Lugnier C: Soluble and particulate cyclic nucleotide phosphodiesterases characterized from airway epithelial cells. *FASEB J* 1993; 7:A146.

47. Bergstrand H, Lundqvist B, Schurmann A: Rat mast cell high affinity cyclic nucleotide phosphodiesterases: Separation of inhibitory effects of two antiallergic agents. *Mol Pharmacol* 1978; 14:848.

48. Ichimura M, Kase H: A new cyclic nucleotide phosphodiesterase isozyme expressed in the T-lymphocyte cell lines. *Biochem Biophys Res Comm* 1993; 193:985.

49. Souness JE, Diocee BK, Martin W, Moodic SA: Pig aortic endothelial cell cyclic nucleotide phosphodiesterase: Use of phosphodiesterase inhibitors to evaluate their roles in regulating cyclic nucleotide levels in intact cells. *Biochem J* 1990; 266:127.

50. Lugnier C, Schini VB: Characterization of cyclic nucleotide phosphodiesterases from cultured bovine aortic endothelial cells. *Biochem Pharmacol* 1990; 39:75.

51. Kishi Y, Ashikaya T, Numano F: Phosphodiesterases in vascular endothelial cells. *Adv Second Messenger Phosphoprotein Res* 1992; 25:201.

52. Filley WV, Holley KE, Kephart GM, Gleich GJ: Identification by immunofluorescence of eosinophil granule major basic protein in lung tissues of patients with bronchial asthma. *Lancet* 1982; 2:11.

53. Bousquet J, Chanez P, Lacoste JY, et al.: Assessment and clinical relevance of eosinophil inflammation in asthma. *N Engl J Med* 1990; 323:1086.

54. Underwood S, Foster M, Raeburn D, et al.: Time-course of antigen-induced airway inflammation in the guinea pig and its relationship to airway hyperresponsiveness. *Eur Respir J* 1995; 8:2104.

55. Souness JE, Maslen C, Webber S, et al.: Suppression of eosinophil function by RP 73401, a potent and selective inhibitor of cyclic AMP-specific phosphodiesterase: Comparison with rolipram. *Br J Pharmacol* 1995; 115:39.

56. Ashton MJ, Cook DC, Fenton G, et al.: Selective type IV phosphodiesterase inhibitors as anti-asthmatic agents: The synthesis and biological activities of 3-(cyclopentyloxy)-4-methoxybenzamides and analogues. *J Med Chem* 1994; 37:1696.

57. Barnette MS, Manning CD, Banner K, et al.: Effect of selective phosphodiesterase (PDE) IV inhibitors on responsiveness of guinea-pig eosinophils. *Am Rev Respir Dis* 1993; 147:A824.

58. Karlsson J-A, Souness JE, Webber SE, et al.: Suppression of mediator release from granulocytes by RP 73401, a novel, selective PDE IV inhibitor. *Am Rev Respir Dis* 1994; 149:A947.

59. Cohan VL, Johnson KL, Breslow R, et al.: PDE JV is the predominant PDE isozyme regulating chemotactic factor-mediated guinea-pig eosinophil functions in vitro. *J Allergy Clin Immunol* 1992; 89:663.

60. Finotto S, Ohno I, Marshall JS, et al.: TNF-α production by eosinophils in upper airways inflammation (nasal polyposis). *J Immunol* 1994; 153:2278.

61. Shock A, Rabe KF, Dent G, et al.: Eosinophils adhere to and stimulate replication of lung fibroblasts *in vitro*. *Clin Exp Immunol* 1991; 86:185.

62. Roche WR, Beasley R, Williams JH, Holgate ST: Subepithelial fibrosis in the bronchi of asthmatics. *Lancet* 1989; 1:520.

63. McAnulty RJ, Campa JS, Cambrey AD, Laurent GJ: The effect of transforming growth factor β on rates of procollagen synthesis and degradation in vitro. *Biochem Biophys Acta* 1991; 1091:231.

64. Karlsson J-A, Souness J, Raeburn D, et al.: Anti-inflammatory effects of novel selective cyclic nucleotide phospodiesterase inhibitors, in Jolles G, Karlsson J-A, Taylor J (eds): *T-Lymphocyte and Inflammatory Cell Research in Asthma*. London, Academic Press, 1993:323.

65. Semmler J, Wachtel H, Endres S: The selective type IV phosphodiesterase inhibitor rolipram suppresses tumour necrosis factor-α production by human mononuclear cells. *Int J Immunopharmacol* 1993; 15:409.

66. Molnar-Kimber K, Yonno L, Heaslip RJ, Weichman BM: Modulation of TNFα and IL-1β from endotoxin-stimulated monocytes by selective PDE isozyme inhibitors. *Agents Actions* 1993; 39:C77.

67. Probhakar U, Lipshutz D, Bartus JO, et al.: Characterization of cAMP-dependent inhibition of LPS-induced TNF alpha production by rolipram, a specific phosphodiesterase IV (PDE IV) inhibitor. *Int J Immunopharmacol* 1994; 16:805.

68. Brennan FM, Chantry D, Jackson A, et al.: Inhibitory effect of TNFα antibodies on synovial cell interleukin-1 production in rheumatoid arthritis. *Lancet* 1989; 2:244.

69. Fuller RW, O'Malley G, Baker AJ, MacDermot J: Human alveolar macrophage activation: Inhibition by forskolin but not β-adrenoceptor stimulation or phosphodiesterase inhibition. *Pulm Pharmacol* 1988; 1:101.

70. Bessler H, Gilgal R, Djaldatti M, Zahavi I: Effect of pentoxifylline on the phagocytic activity, cyclic AMP levels, and superoxide anion production by monocytes and polymorphonuclear cells. *J Leukocyte Biol* 1986; 40:747

71. Godfrey RW, Manzi RM, Gennaro DE, Hoffstein ST: Phospholipid and arachidonic acid metabolism in zymosan-stimulated human monocytes: Modulation by cyclic AMP. *J Cell Physiol* 1987; 131:384.

72. Schade FU, Schudt C: The specific type III and IV phosphodiesterase inhibitor zardaverine suppresses formation of tumour necrosis factor by macrophages. *Eur J Pharmacol* 1993; 230:9.

73. Turner NC, Wood LJ, Burns FM, et al.: The effect of cyclic AMP and cyclic GMP phosphodiesterase inhibitors on the superoxide burst of guinea-pig peritoneal macrophages. *Br J Pharmacol* 1993; 108:876.

74. Romagnani S: Human Th1 and Th2: doubt no more. *Immunol Today* 1991; 12:256.

75. Snijdewint FGM, Kalinski P, Wierenga EA, et al.: Prostaglandin E$_2$ differentially modulates cytokine secretion profiles of human T helper lymphocytes. *J Immunol* 1993; 150:5321.

76. Betz M, Fox BS: Prostaglandin E$_2$ inhibits production of Th1 lymphokines but not of Th2 lymphokines. *J Immunol* 1991; 146:108.

77. Novak TJ, Rothenberg EV: Cyclic AMP inhibits induction of interleukin 2 but not of interleukin 4 in T cells. *Proc Natl Acad Sci USA* 1990; 87:9353.

78. Munoz E, Zubiaga AM, Merrow M, et al.: Cholera toxin discriminates between T helper 1 and 2 cell receptor-mediated activation: Role of cyclic AMP in T cell proliferation. *J Exp Med* 1990; 172:95.

79. Mirza S, Withnall M, Karlsson J-A: Elevated cyclic AMP inhibits IL-4 and IL-5 release from mixed mouse splenocytes by blocking IL-2 release. *Immunology* 1994; 83(suppl 1):79.

80. Essayan DM, Kagey-Sobotka A, Lichtenstein LM, Huang S-K: Studies of phosphodiesterase (PDE) isozyme function and expression in human allergic disease. *J Allergy Clin Immunol* 1994; 93:286.

81. Robicsek SA, Blanchard DK, Djen JY, et al.: Multiple high-affinity cyclic AMP phosphodiesterases in human T lymphocytes. *Biochem Pharmacol* 1991; 42:869.

82. Averill LE, Stein RL, Kammer GML: Control of human T-lymphocyte interleukin-2 production by a cyclic AMP-dependent pathway. *Cell Immunol* 1988; 115:88.

83. Lewis GM, Caccese RG, Heaslip RL, Bansbach CC: Effects of rolipram and CI-930 on IL-2 mRNA transcription in human Jurkat cells. *Agents Actions* 1993; 39:C89.

84. Cooper KD, Kang K, Chan SC, Hanifin JM: Phosphodiesterase inhibition by Ro 20-1724 reduces hyper-IgE synthesis by atopic dermatitis cells in vitro. *J Invest Dermatol* 1985; 84:477.

85. Gordon JR, Burd PR, Galli SJ: Mast cells as a source of multifunctional cytokines. *Immunol Today* 1990; 11:458.

86. Schwartz LB: Mast cells: Function and contents: *Curr Opin Immunol* 1994; 6:91.

87. Howarth PH, Bradding P, Feather I, et al.: Mucosal cytokine expression in allergic rhinitis. *Int Arch Allergy Immunol* 1995; 107:390.

88. Frossard N, Landry Y, Pauli G, Ruckstuhl M: Effects of cyclic AMP- and cyclic GMP-phosphodiesterase inhibitors on immunological release of histamine and on lung contraction. *Br J Pharmacol* 1981; 73:933.

89. Anderson N, Peachell PT: Effect of isoenzyme-selective inhibitors of phosphodiesterase (PDE) on human lung mast cells (HLMC). *FASEB J* 1994; 8:A239.

90. Harvath L, Robbins JD, Russell AA, Seaman KB: Cyclic AMP and human neutrophil chemotaxis: Elevation of cyclic AMP differentially affects chemotactic responsiveness. *J Immunol* 1991; 146:224.

91. Fonteh AN, Winkler JD, Torphy TJ, et al.: Influence of isoproterenol and phosphodiesterase inhibitors on platelet-activating factor biosynthesis in the human neutrophil. *J Immunol* 1993; 151:339.

92. MacPhee CH, Harrison SA, Beavo JA: Immunological identification of the major low K_m cAMP phosphodiesterase: Probable target for anti-thrombotic agents. *Proc Natl Acad Sci USA* 1986; 83:6660.

93. Sanjar S, Aoki S, Kristersson A, et al.: Antigen challenge induces pulmonary eosinophil accumulation and airway hyperreactivity: The effect of anti-asthma drugs. *Br J Pharmacol* 1990; 99:679.

94. Ishida K, Kelly LJ, Thomson RJ, et al.: Repeated antigen challenge induces airway hyperresponsiveness with tissue eosinophilia in guinea pigs. *J Appl Physiol* 1989; 67:1133.

95. Pretolani M, Ruffie C, Joseph D, et al.: Role of eosinophil activation in the bronchial reactivity of allergic guinea pigs. *Am J Respir Crit Care Med* 1994; 149:1167.

96. Brattsand R, Andersson P, Wieslander E, et al.: Pathophysiological characteristics of a guinea-pig model for dual bronchial obstruction, in Hogg JC, Ellul-Micallef R, Brattsand R (eds): *Glucocorticoids, Inflammation and Bronchial Hyperreactivity*. Amsterdam, Excerpta Medica, 1985:51.

97. Iijima H, Ishii M, Yamauchi K, et al.: Bronchoalveolar lavage and histologic characterization of late asthmatic response in guinea pigs. *Am Rev Respir Dis* 1987; 136:922.

98. Karlsson J-A, Zackrisson C, Erjefält J, Forsberg K: Airway responsiveness in guinea pigs with *Ascaris suum-induced early and late bronchoconstrictor responses.* Pulm Pharmacol 1992; 5:191.

99. Andersson P, Bergstrand H: Antigen-induced bronchial anaphylaxis in actively sensitized guinea-pigs: Effect of long-term treatment with sodium cromoglycate and aminophylline. *Br J Pharmacol* 1981; 74:601.

100. Banner KH, Page CP: Acute versus chronic administration of phosphodiesterase inhibitors on allergen-induced pulmonary cell influx in sensitized guinea-pigs. *Br J Pharmacol* 1995; 114:93.

101. Howell RE, Sickles BD, Woeppel SL: Pulmonary antiallergic and bronchodilator effects of isozyme-selective phosphodiesterase inhibitors in guinea-pigs. *J Pharmacol Exp Ther* 1993; 264:609.

102. Raeburn D, Underwood SL, Lewis SA, et al.: Anti-inflammatory and bronchodilator properties of RP 73401, a novel and selective phosphodiesterase type IV inhibitor. *Br J Pharmacol* 1994; 113:1423.

103. Underwood DC, Osborn RR, Novak LB, et al.: Inhibition of antigen-induced bronchoconstriction and eosinophil infiltration in the guinea-pig by the cyclic AMP-specific phosphodiesterase inhibitor, rolipram. *J Pharmacol Exp Ther* 1993; 266:306.

104. Heaslip RJ, Buckley SK, Sickels BD, Grimes D: Bronchial vs cardiovascular activities of selective phosphodiesterase inhibitors in the anaesthetized beta-blocked dog. *J Pharmacol Exp Ther* 1991; 257:741.

105. Raeburn D, Advenier C: Isoenzyme-selective cyclic nucleotide phosphodiesterase inhibitors: Effects on airways smooth muscle. *Int J Biochem Cell Biol* 1995; 27:29.

106. Turner CR, Andresen CJ, Smith WB, Watson JW: Effects of rolipram on responses to acute and chronic antigen exposure in moneys. *Am J Respir Crit Care Med* 1994; 149:1153.

107. Lappin D, Riches DWH, Damerau B, Whaley K: Cyclic nucleotides and their relationship to complement-component-C2 synthesis by human monocytes. *Biochem J* 1984; 222:477.

108. Rand TH, Silberstein DS, Kornfeld H, Weller PF: Human eosinophils express functional interleukin 2 receptors. *J Clin Invest* 1991; 88:825.

109. Pober JS, Slowik MR, De Luca LG, Ritchie AJ: Elevated cyclic AMP inhibits endothelial cell synthesis and expression of TNF-induced endothelial leukocyte adhesion molecule-1, and vascular cell adhesion molecule-1, but not intercellular adhesion molecule-1. *J Immunol* 1993; 150:5114.

110. Wellicome SM, Thornhill MH, Pitzalis C, et al.: A monoclonal antibody that detects a novel antigen on endothelial cells that is induced by tumor necrosis factor, IL-1, or lipopolysaccharide. *J Immunol* 1990; 144:2558.

111. Thornhill MH, Haskard DO: IL-4 regulates endothelial cell activation by IL-1, tumor necrosis factor, or IFN-gamma. *J Immunol* 1990; 145:865.

112. Jung E-Y, Ohshima Y, Shintaku N, et al.: Effects of cyclic AMP on expression of LFA-1, Mac-1, and VLA-4 and eosinophilic differentiation of a human leukemic cell line, Eol-1. *Eur J Haematol* 1994; 53:156.

113. Riva CM, Morganroth ML, Marks RM, et al.: Iloprost inhibits activated human neutrophil (PMN) adherence to endothelial cells via increased cyclic AMP. *Clin Res* 1989; 37:949A.

114. Gibson PG, Manning PJ, O'Byrne PM, et al.: Allergen-induced asthmatic responses. *Am Rev Respir Dis* 1991; 143:331.

115. Woolley MJ, Wattie J, Ellis R, et al.: Effect of an inhaled corticosteroid on airway eosinophils and allergen-induced airway hyperresponsiveness in dogs. *J Appl Physiol* 1994; 77:1303.

116. DeBrito FB, Ebsworth KE, Lawrence CE: Regulation of

eosinophilia by cyclic AMP: *Proceedings International Congress on Inflammation*. Edyprint Inc. Geneva, Switzerland.

117. Gundel RH, Gerritsen ME, Wegner CD: Antigen-coated sepharose beads induce airway eosinophilia and airway hyperresponsiveness in cynomolgus monkeys. *Am Rev Respir Dis* 1989; 140:629.

118. Kips JC, Joos GF, Peleman RA, Pauwels RA: The effect of zardaverine, an inhibitor of phosphodiesterase isoenzymes III and IV, on endotoxin-induced airway changes in rats. *Clin Exp Allergy* 1993; 23:518.

119. Persson CGA: Role of plasma exudation in asthmatic airways. *Lancet* 1986; 2:1126.

120. Naclerio RM, Bartenfelder D, Proud D, et al.: Theophylline reduces histamine release during pollen-induced rhinitis. *J Allergy Clin Immunol* 1986; 78:874.

121. Erjefält I, Persson CGA: Pharmacologic control of plasma exudation into tracheobronchial airways. *Am Rev Respir Dis* 1991; 143:1008.

122. Raeburn D, Karlsson J-A: Effects of isoenzyme-selective inhibitors of cyclic nucleotide phosphodiesterase on microvascular leak in guinea pig airways *in vivo. J Pharmacol Exp Ther* 1993; 267:1147.

123. Makarski JS: Stimulation of cyclic AMP production by vasoactive agents in cultured bovine aortic and pulmonary artery endothelial cells. *In vitro* 1981; 17:450.

124. Suttorp N, Welsch T, Weber U, et al.: Activation of cAMP-dependent protein kinase blocks hydrogen peroxide-induced enhanced endothelial permeability *in vitro. Am Rev Respir Dis* 1991; 143:A572.

125. Seibert AF, Thompson WJ, Taylor A, et al.: Reversal of increased microvascular permeability associated with ischemia-reperfusion: role of cAMP. *J Appl Physiol* 1992; 72:389.

126. Ortiz JL, Cortijo J, Valles JM, et al.: Rolipram inhibits PAF-induced airway microvascular leakage in guinea-pig: A comparison with milrinone and theophylline. *Fund Clin Pharmacol* 1992; 6:247.

127. Svensjö E. Andersson KE, Bouskela E, et al.: Effects of two vasodilatory phosphodiesterase inhibitors on bradykinin-induced permeability increase in the hamster cheek pouch. *Agents Actions* 1993; 39:35.

128. Nicholson CD, Shahid M: Inhibitors of cyclic nucleotide phosphodiesterase isoenzymes—Their potential utility in the therapy of asthma. *Pulm Pharmacol* 1994; 7:1.

129. Bergstrand H: Phosphodiesterase inhibition and theophylline. *Eur J Respir Dis* 1980; 91(suppl 109):37.

130. Torphy TJ, Undem BD, Cieslinski LB, et al.: Identification, characterisation and functional role of phosphodiesterase isozymes in human airway smooth muscle. *J Pharmacol Exp Ther* 1993; 265:1213.

131. Shahid M, van Amsterdam RGM, deBoer J, et al.: The presence of five cyclic nucleotide phosphodiesterase isoenzyme activities in bovine tracheal smooth muscle and the functional effects of selective inhibitors. *Br J Pharmacol* 1991; 104:471.

132. De Boer J, Philpott AJ, van Amsterdam RGM, et al.: Human bronchial cyclic nucleotide phosphodiesterase isoenzymes: Biochemical and pharmacological analysis using selective inhibitors. *Br J Pharmacol* 1992; 106:1028.

133. Tomkinson A, Karlsson J-A, Raeburn D: Comparison of the effects of rolipram and siguazodan, selective inhibitors of phosphodiesterase type IV and type III, in airway smooth muscle preparations with differing β-adrenoceptor subtype populations. *Br J Pharmacol* 1993; 108:57.

134. Giembycz MA, Barnes PJ: Selective inhibition of a high affinity type IV cyclic AMP phosphodiesterase in bovine trachealis by AH 21-132: Relevance to the spasmolytic and anti-spasmogenic actions of AH 21-132 in the intact tissue. *Biochem Pharmacol* 1991; 42:663.

135. Qian Y, Naline E, Karlsson J-A, et al.: Effects of rolipram and siguazodan on the human isolated bronchus and their interaction with isoprenaline and sodium nitroprusside. *Br J Pharmacol* 1993; 109:774.

136. Torphy TJ, Zhou H-L, Burman M, Huang LBF: Role of cyclic nucleotide phosphodiesterase isozymes in intact canine trachealis. *Mol Pharmacol* 1991; 39:376.

137. Brunnee T, Engelstatter R, Steinijans VW, Kunkel G: Bronchodilatory effect of zardaverine, a phosphodiesterase III and IV inhibitor, in patients with asthma. *Eur Respir J* 1992; 5:982.

138. Foster RW, Rakshi K, Carpenter JR, Small RC: Trials of the bronchodilator activity of the isoenzyme selective phosphodiesterase inhibitor AH 21-132 in healthy volunteers during a methacholine challenge. *Br J Clin Pharmacol* 1992; 34:527.

139. Leeman M, Lejeune P, Melot C, Naeije R: Reduction in pulmonary hypertension and in airway resistance by enoximone (MDL 17043) in decompensated COPD. *Chest* 1987; 91:662.

140. Rudd RM, Gellert AR, Studdy PR, Geddes DM: Inhibition of exercise-induced asthma by an orally absorbed mast cell stabilizer (M&B 22948). *Br J Dis Chest* 1983; 77:78.

141. Israel E, Mathur PN, Tashkin D, Drazen JM: LY186655 prevents bronchospasm in asthma of moderate severity. *Chest* 1988; 91:71S.

142. Brunkhorst D, van der Leyen H, Meyer W, et al.: Relation of positive inotropic and chronotropic effects of pimobendan, UD-CG 212 C1, milrinone and other phosphodiesterase inhibitors to phosphodiesterase III inhibition in guinea-pig heart. *Nauny Schmiedebergs Arch Pharmacol* 1989; 339:575.

143. Elks ML, Manganiello VC: Selective effects of phosphodiesterase inhibitors on different phosphodiesterases, adenosine 3′, 5′-monophosphate metabolism, and lipolysis in 3T3-L1 adipocytes. *Endocrinology* 1984; 115:1262.

144. Bertolino A, Crippa D, Di Dio S, et al.: Roliram versus imipramine in inpatients with major, "minor," or atypical depressive disorder: A double-blind, double-dummy study aimed at testing a novel therapeutic approach. *Int Clin Psychopharmacol* 1988; 3:245.

145. Sturgess I, Searle GF: The acute toxic effect of the phosphodiesterase inhibitor rolipram on plasma osmolality. *Br J Clin Pharmacol* 1990; 29:369.

146. Puurunen J, Lucke C, Schwabe U: Effect of the phosphodiesterase inhibitor 4-(3-cyclopentyloxy-4-methoxypenyl)-2-pyrrolidone (ZK 62711) on gastric secretion and gastric mucosal cyclic AMP. *Naunyn-Schmiedeberg's Arch Pharmacol* 1978; 304:69.

METHOTREXATE

PHILIP PADRID

Introduction

For most patients with asthma, regular and aggressive treatment with inhaled corticosteroids is sufficient to control symptoms and minimize decrements in pulmonary function. In a small number of asthmatic patients, systemic corticosteroids are required to control frequent exacerbations of their disease. Within this group, an additional subset of patients may develop serious side effects related to chronic corticosteroid use, including diabetes mellitus, cataracts, obesity, osteoporosis, and psychiatric disturbances. In this clinical setting, it is important to attempt alternative therapies that will maintain the patient's level of comfort derived through corticosteroid therapy without the attendant deleterious side effects. Methotrexate (MTX) has been used for this purpose.

The notion that MTX might be valuable in the treatment of asthma has its roots in the initial observation 50 years ago that children with acute leukemia responded to folate therapy by producing more myeloblasts.[1] This led to the theory that folate antagonism might be effective in the treatment of children with leukemia. In the late 1940s, the folate antagonist aminopterin was used to induce striking, but temporary, remission in a series of leukemic patients.[2] Aminopterin was soon found to be effective also in the treatment of two small groups of patients with rheumatoid arthritis and psoriasis.[3] In 1963, Hertz[4] reported use of the next generation antifolate, MTX, in the first reported cure of a solid tumor. Recognition of the suppressive properties of folate antagonists in cell-mediated reactions led to routine use of MTX in the treatment of patients with rheumatoid arthritis and psoriasis and to clinical trials for MTX in the treatment of organ transplantation rejection, Reiter's syndrome, inflammatory bowel disease, and Wegener's granulomatosis.[5–8] In 1983, Mullarkey observed that a patient with psoriasis, arthritis, and bronchial asthma had a beneficial clinical outcome for all three diseases after taking low-dose MTX to treat the psoriasis and arthritis.[9] Mullarkey's observation led to clinical trials designed to test the hypothesis that corticosteroid-dependent asthmatic patients can benefit from low-dose MTX therapy. This chapter summarizes the pharmacologic mechanism(s) of action of MTX, outlines the theoretical basis for the use of MTX to treat bronchial asthma, and reviews and critically evaluates the results of clinical trials using MTX in patients with asthma.

Pharmacologic Mechanism of Action

Methotrexate inhibits the enzyme tetrahydrofolate reductase (THFR) in most species studied. The significance of this effect lies in the fact that THFR normally reduces folate to tetrahydrofolate (FH_4). Single carbon groups can be added enzymatically to FH_4 and then transferred in specific synthetic reactions. During these synthetic reactions, FH_4 is reduced to dihydrofolate (FH_2). To continue to function as a cofactor, FH_2 must be converted to FH_4 by THFR. Methotrexate inhibits THFR, thus limiting the conversion of FH_2 to FH_4. The resulting deficiency in FH_4 and folate coenzymes required for the single carbon fragment transfer reactions results in a deficiency in the synthesis of purines and thymidylate. This in turn leads to a deficiency in the synthesis of both DNA and RNA (Fig. 63-1). The inhibitory effects on RNA and DNA are synergistic; inhibition of RNA synthesis blocks cell division *prior to* entry into the S phase of the growth cycle, whereas inhibition of DNA synthesis blocks cells division most profoundly when the cells *have already* entered the logarithmic S phase of cell growth.

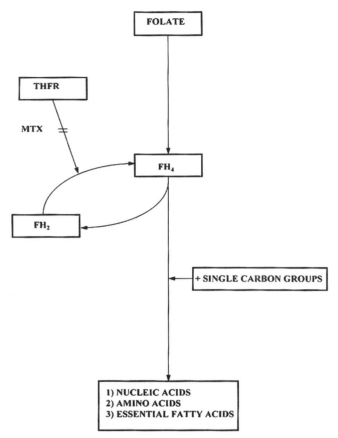

FIGURE 63-1 Folic acid cycle and mechanism of action of methotrexate.

More recently, investigators have suggested that the therapeutic effect of MTX may be linked to inhibition of folate-dependent enzymes other than THFR, including 5-aminoimidazole-4-carboxamide ribonucleotide transformylase.[10]

Pharmacokinetics and Toxicity

Methotrexate can be given orally or parenterally and is frequently administered intramuscularly. Concern regarding the potential for hepatic toxicity makes the parenteral route particularly attractive because the drug then bypasses the hepatic circulation. Sixty percent of the oral dose is absorbed, with a plasma half-life of 2 h. Fifty percent of the drug is protein bound and more than 90 percent is excreted unchanged in the urine.[11] Although MTX is frequently given in three small doses divided over 12 h, this is based on the cell cycle of psoriatic cells,[12] and it may not be an important delivery method when MTX is used to treat asthma.

Methotrexate has been studied most closely in patients with rheumatoid arthritis. The use of MTX has been associated with the development of a number of serious complications including interstitial pneumonitis and bone marrow depression. However, serious morbidity associated with low-dose MTX is the exception and most commonly occurs in the setting of occult renal disease or systemic infection. Common side effects of MTX therapy include gastrointestinal upset and headache. For patients with rheumatoid arthritis, these side effects sometimes may be relieved by supplemental folic acid. Methotrexate is also teratogenic and should be avoided in women with childbearing potential. An occasional case report describing idiosyncratic effects of MTX has been reported, including the *induction* of asthma in a patient using MTX.[13]

There have been at least eight published clinical studies involving approximately 160 adults with bronchial asthma, examining the effect of low-dose MTX (15 mg/week) as a corticosteroid-sparing agent (see below under "Clinical Trials"). Only 5 percent of the patients (8 of 160) who initially enrolled in these studies withdrew because of adverse symptoms related to use of MTX; an additional 3 patients had to withdraw because of a fourfold elevation in liver enzymes. At least 14 other patients had increases in liver enzymes that were not significant enough to warrant withdrawal from study. In one study, 15 of 26 patients had drug-related adverse reactions requiring temporary cessation of MTX for 1 week.[14] Life-threatening complications related to administration of MTX were rare, involving 3 patients. Two patients developed bacterial pneumonia.[15] One additional patient initially treated with MTX had an exacerbation of asthma requiring increased corticosteroids. This patient subsequently developed *Pneumocystis carinii* pneumonia and died.[16]

Some general guidelines have emerged from the experience using MTX in patients with rheumatoid arthritis, and these guidelines may apply to treating patients with asthma.[17,18] Specifically, the use of MTX should be avoided in patients with risk factors for hepatic toxicity including patients with a history of alcohol abuse and preexisting hepatic disease. Additional recommendations include monitoring serum alanine aminotransferase, aspartate aminotransferase, and albumin concentrations monthly, and obtaining liver biopsy in patients with persistent abnormalities in these tests.

Theoretical Basis for the Use of Methotrexate to Treat Asthma

At high doses, (50 to 150 mg/week) MTX is used commonly as a cytotoxic agent in the treatment of neoplastic diseases. In lower doses (5 to 25 mg/week) the drug has been used as an anti-inflammatory agent to treat arthritis, psoriasis, polymyositis, and Crohn's disease. As a corticosteroid-sparing agent in asthma, MTX has been used at doses ranging from 5 to 50 mg/week. As pointed out by Weinblatt,[19] even at low doses MTX has a prompt onset of action in many chronic inflammatory diseases, and symptoms reappear soon after MTX is withdrawn. This suggests that MTX has significant anti-inflammatory effects although the mechanism(s) of this general anti-inflammatory effect is unknown. It is unlikely that MTX acts as an anti-inflammatory agent through its ability to inhibit dehydrofolate reductase (DHFR). This conclusion is based on the facts that DHFR is virtually absent in inflammatory white blood cells,[20] MTX does not cause a reduction of white blood cell counts, and MTX retains anti-inflammatory properties in the setting of folinic acid supplementation.[21] It is equally true that the mechanism(s) by which methotrexate acts as a corticosteroid-sparing agent in the treatment of bronchial asthma is obscure. Methotrexate has been said to "reset the level of inflammation" in asthma[22] although this explanation seems unfulfilling. It has been suggested that the anti-inflammatory properties of MTX in asthma are related to the effect of the drug to inhibit histamine release from basophils[23] [Note: cytotoxic doses of MTX were used in this study]; the activity (not production) of interleukin-1 (IL-1) secreted from mononuclear cells[24] [Note: IL-1 may be produced from other sources including alveolar macrophages and bronchial epithelial cells], chemotactic activity of neutrophils induced by leukotriene B (LTB$_4$) and C5a,[25,26] and synthesis of lipoxygenase products.[27] There also is at least one report describing the effect of MTX in inhibiting eosinophil migration in parasitic infection in mice.[28]

Clinical Trials

In 1986, Mullarkey reported that seven of eight corticosteroid-dependent asthmatic patients were able to reduce the dose of prednisone they required to minimize their asthma symptoms after taking low-dose MTX. Since then there have been at least two studies claiming to show a corticosteroid-sparing effect of MTX in children (12 total children studied), and eight studies evaluating the potential corticosteroid-sparing effect of MTX in adult asthmatics (160 adults total). Four of the eight studies of adult asthmatics purport to show a corticosteroid-sparing effect for MTX, whereas four others concluded that low-dose MTX therapy does not have such an effect. Most of these studies used small patient populations (<25) and were completed within 12 to 24 weeks. A reduction in corticosteroid requirement was the endpoint in each clinical trial. Results of these studies are summarized in Table 63-1.

Evaluation of Results of Clinical Trials

There are not many published data on the use of MTX in children with corticosteroid-dependent asthma. In the Guss and Portnoy study,[29] seven adolescent asthmatics were enrolled. The corticosteroid dose required by these children ranged from 30 mg prednisone every other day to 60 mg daily. Four of the 7 children were able to discontinue prednisone while on MTX, over a period of time ranging from 4 to 17 months. The second evaluation of children with asthma consisted of a series of five case reports. Stempel[30] reported

that after 1 to 2 years, 3 of 5 children previously dependent on systemic prednisone to control their asthma were no longer using corticosteroids, and the remaining 2 children enjoyed a 75 to 90 percent reduction in their corticosteroid requirement. The finding that 7 of 12 children with corticosteroid-dependent asthma were able to discontinue completely corticosteroid use by introduction of low-dose MTX is, at first blush, an exciting discovery. However, serious design flaws and omissions in reporting preclude a sound scientific judgment on the efficacy of MTX in this clinical setting. For example, the Guss and Portnoy study was open and uncontrolled, and there was no attempt to optimize the corticosteroid dosage before initiating MTX therapy. It is not clear that the dose of prednisone used by these children was the dose of prednisone they required; that is, this study does not mention other doses of other drugs used, frequency of visits to their physician, compliance with the medical regimen, etc. Importantly, the natural history of childhood asthma follows a waxing and waning course over time. Without a placebo control it would be a mistake to attribute the decrease in corticosteroid requirement to the addition of MTX. In the five case reports described by Stempel, the average dose of prednisone used by four children was not reported, and in two patients the dose of MTX used also was not mentioned. Further study clearly is required before MTX can be recommended in the treatment of corticosteroid-dependent adolescent asthmatic patients.

There are four studies of adult asthmatics in which MTX had a corticosteroid-sparing effect. In the first, double-blind, crossover study, Mullarkey[31] reported that 14 patients with an average daily steroid requirement of 26 mg prednisone were able to reduce that requirement to 17 mg/week, a 36 percent reduction, compared to placebo. One of these patients was able to discontinue completely use of prednisone during the 12-week course of MTX, and 3 additional patients discontinued corticosteroids entirely while continuing to take MTX after the completion of the study. In a longer term follow-up study by the same author,[14] 25 different patients were given 15 mg MTX orally and followed for 18 to 28 months. The initial corticosteroid requirement for these patients was, on average, 26 mg prednisone per day. At the completion of the study this was reduced to an average of 6 mg prednisone daily. Importantly, 24 of 25 patients receiving MTX were able to decrease their corticosteroid dose by 50 percent or greater, and 15 of 25 patients actually discontinued regular corticosteroid use. In the largest study in this series, Shiner et al.[32] reported the results of MTX or placebo treatment for 60 asthmatic and corticosteroid-dependent patients. There was no significant difference after 12 weeks for patients in the MTX or placebo group in their ability to decrease corticosteroid use. However, in the following 12 weeks there was a reduction of 50 percent of corticosteroids in the MTX group, whereas no additional reduction in corticosteroid use was found in the group receiving placebo. Importantly, 6 of 32 patients taking MTX were able to discontinue prednisone use completely, whereas none of the 28 patients taking placebo were able to stop prednisone use entirely. Dyer[33] studied 10 corticosteroid-dependent

TABLE 63-1 Clinical Trials of Methotrexate in the Treatment of Asthma

Reference	No. of Patients Enrolled	Study Design	Length of Study	Patient Symptomatic for Steroid Toxicity?	Initial Steroid Taper Period	Minimum Daily Corticosteroid Requirement on Entry (mg)	Baseline Dose (mg/day) of Prednisone (Mean)	Prednisone Dose (mg/day) after MTX (Mean)	Poststudy Follow-up
Mullarkey (1988)[31]	14	randomized, double-blind, placebo-controlled, crossover	12 weeks MTX 12 weeks placebo	yes	no	10	26 (10–60)	17 (36% decrease compared to placebo)	1/13 patients on MTX stopped prednisone during study 3 more stopped prednisone after completion of study
Mullarkey (1990)[14]	25	open uncontrolled	18–28 months	yes	Yes, 1 month If successful patients were not included in study.	10	26.9	6.3	24/25 patients decreased steroid dose by >50% 17/25 reduced steroids by 30% within 2 months 15/25 off regular steroids use
Shiner (1990)[32]	60	randomized, double-blind, placebo-controlled	12 weeks MTX 12 weeks placebo	no	no	7.5	13.2 (MTX) 15.0 (placebo)	2 mg ↓ both groups after 12 weeks 6.6 (MTX) 12.9 (placebo) after 24 weeks	6/32 pts on MTX, 0.28 patients on placebo stopped prednisone
Dyer (1991)[33]	10	double-blind, placebo-controlled, crossover	12 weeks MTX 12 weeks placebo	no	yes, 3 weeks	7.5 daily 20 every other day	11.7	8.4 (MTX) 12.0 (placebo)	1/7 patients continuing MTX stopped prednisone
Erzurum (1991)[16]	18	randomized, double-blind, placebo-controlled	13 weeks	yes	yes	15	20	12 (MTX) 12 (placebo)	2 patients stopped steroids within 2 years of beginning MTX
Taylor (1993)[36]	9	randomized, double-blind, placebo-controlled	24 weeks MTX 24 weeks placebo	yes	yes 4–10 weeks	10	16.9 (MTX) 18.2 (placebo)	14.4 (MTX) 12.9 (placebo)	1/9 patients on MTX reduced prednisone by 7 mg daily 3/9 patients on MTX had 7 mg/day increase
Trigg (1993)[15]	12	randomized, double-blind placebo-controlled, crossover	12 weeks MTX 12 weeks placebo	no	no	10	17.5 (10–50)	10 (MTX) 13 (placebo)	
Coffey (1994)[26]	11	placebo-controlled, double-blind, crossover	12 weeks MTX 12 weeks placebo	yes	yes 4–10 weeks	10	30.8 (6.9–60)	20.1 (MTX) 24.5 (placebo)	3/11 patients on MTX, 2/11 patients on placebo decreased steroids by 33% or more

asthmatic patients who showed a reduction of more than 35 percent in steroid requirement after 12 weeks of MTX therapy.

In contrast, four later studies involving 50 patients failed to show a corticosteroid-sparing effect for MTX.[15,16,26,36] These discordant findings may be explained, in part, by the variations in patient populations and study designs used by the different authors of these clinical trials. For example, in both Mullarkey studies, patients were included *only if* their postbronchodilator forced expiratory volume in 1 s (FEV$_1$) was above 70 percent. In contrast, the *average* post bronchodilator FEV$_1$ in the study of Erzurum et al.[16] was 70 percent, with a large standard error. In the study of Dyer et al.,[33] the range of values for FEV$_1$ before using a bronchodilator was 35 to 90 percent. Clearly, different studies evaluated patients with widely varying degrees of airflow obstruction. Prednisone requirements at the initiation of each study also varied widely, from 5 to 60 mg/daily. Most importantly, while the Mullarkey studies only chose patients with symptoms of prednisone toxicity, two additional studies purporting to show a corticosteroid-sparing effect of MTX and one that failed to show a beneficial effect of MTX did not identify patients with corticosteroid toxicity for inclusion into their study.[15,32,33]

Study designs also varied in important ways. First, the long-term study by Mullarkey was open and uncontrolled. As pointed out by Coffey et al. and others,[26,34] the natural history of bronchial asthma is variable, and patient compliance with medications is often poor. In the long-term study of Dykewicz et al. of the natural history of patients on corticosteroids for asthma,[34] 25 percent discontinued corticosteroid use, and 20 percent enjoyed intervals of up to 3 years during which corticosteroids could be tapered completely. Without regard for the well-recognized placebo effect on patient compliance, and the predictably variable history of asthma symptoms when viewed over a 2-year time period, the results of the Mullarkey study must be accepted with caution. Secondly, two additional studies showing a positive effect of MTX did not include a corticosteroid taper period.[31,32] A third allowed for a 1-month period to optimize the dose of prednisone required. However, in this study,[14] the patients were allowed to adjust their dose of prednisone without direct supervision of the physician. These may be critical flaws in light of the finding of other studies[16,26] showing that patients taking MTX or placebo experienced equivalent corticosteroid reductions when their corticosteroid dose was optimized before entry into the study.

The definition of a successful outcome also varied greatly among studies. Dyer et al.[33] reported that 10 patients were able to reduce their corticosteroid requirement by greater than 30 percent after 24 weeks of low-dose (15 mg/week) MTX. This was statistically different compared to the decrease seen in the placebo group. However, the average dose of prednisone at the start of the study for both groups (after the steroid taper period) was 12 mg/day. The 30 percent decrease in corticosteroid requirement experienced by the MTX group reflects a decrease of 3.6 mg/day. Shiner[32] reported that 32 patients taking MTX for 24 weeks experienced a decrease in prednisone dosage from 13.2 mg to 6.6 mg versus 15.0 to 12.9 in the placebo group. This represents a decrease of 6.6 mg versus a decrease of 2.1 mg. Although differences between groups are *statistically* significant, it is not intuitively obvious that the decrement in corticosteroid requirement reported from these two studies represents a *biologically significant* sparing effect.

Lastly, most of the studies used relatively small patient sample sizes, and conclusions reached using these small numbers of patients have even led to debate invoking power analysis.[35]

Conclusions

For most patients with asthma, regular and aggressive treatment with inhaled corticosteroids is sufficient to control symptoms and minimize decrements in pulmonary function. A smaller population of asthmatic patients may require systemic corticosteroids to control their disease symptoms. Because of the spectrum of potentially damaging side effects related to chronic systemic corticosteroid treatment it is incumbent on the physician to maximize the nonsystemic corticosteroid regimen. This includes confirmation that the patient is compliant with the nonsteroid treatments and is using the inhalers in the prescribed manner and frequent patient examinations to determine the optimal dose of nonsteroid drugs. Only when these details are fully attended to can the corticosteroid dose for each patient be considered "optimized."

When corticosteroid-dependent asthmatic patients receive the minimum corticosteroid dose required to control their symptoms and still experience significant corticosteroid-related side effects, it becomes important to attempt to introduce alternative therapies that will maintain the patient's level of corticosteroid-derived comfort without the associated morbidity. Methotrexate has been used in this clinical setting. An equal number of studies have concluded that MTX does or does not reduce the corticosteroid requirement in asthma. It is difficult to determine the true meaning of the results of these studies because of the number of confounding variables, including spontaneous improvement in some asthmatics, initial corticosteroid overdosage before entering the MTX trial, improved medical compliance, and the well-known and well-demonstrated (in these studies) placebo effect.

Even if one suspends judgment regarding study design and focuses on the study results, it seems that for most patients, there is at best only a minor reduction in corticosteroid requirement that results from introduction of MTX. It is important to point out that a dependence on low-dose prednisone may not be associated with significant morbidity. In these cases, it may not be important to reduce the steroid dose further by adding MTX. Additionally, there is no evidence to suggest that MTX improves pulmonary function in asthma. On the other hand, even in the best designed studies, it seems clear that at least a small number of patients do benefit significantly from MTX and are able to discontinue prednisone use entirely (see Table 64-1). Unfortunately, there seems no way prospectively or retrospectively to predict which patients will have a corticosteroid-sparing effect from MTX. Additionally, it is unknown for how long to continue treatment or for how long MTX should be given before a clinical effect can be expected.

It is possible that a small subgroup of asthmatic patients may require less corticosteroid with MTX, but it is difficult to make that conclusion with the available information to date. It is likely that, for most corticosteroid-dependent asthmatics, optimization of the medical regime, including more frequent physician visits, may be the most therapeutic change in patient management.[26]

References

1. Farber S: Action of pteroylglutamic conjugates on man. *Science* 1947; 106:619.
2. Farber S: Temporary remissions in acute leukemia in children produced by folic acid antagonist 4-aminopterlyl-glutamic acid (aminopterin). *N Engl J Med* 1948; 238:787.
3. Gubner R, August S, Ginsberg V: Therapeutic suppression of tissue reactivity. II. Effect of aminopterin in rheumatoid arthritis and psoriasis. *Am J Med Sci* 1951; 221:176.
4. Hertz R: Folic acid antagonists: effects on the cell and the patient. *Ann Intern Med* 1963; 59:931.
5. Kreme J, Lee J: Long term prospective study of the use of methotrexate in rheumatoid arthritis. *Arthritis Rheum* 1988; 31:577.
6. Tugwell P, Bennett K, Gent M: Methotrexate in rheumatoid arthritis. *Ann Intern Med* 1987; 107:358.
7. Kozarek R, Patterson D, Gelfand M, et al.: Methotrexate induces clinical and histologic remission in patients with refractory inflammatory bowel disease. *Ann Intern Med* 1989; 110:353.
8. Feagen BG, Rochon J, Fedorak RN, et al.: Methotrexate for the treatment of Crohn's disease. *N Engl J Med* 1995; 332:292.
9. Mullarkey MF: Potent anti-inflammatory agents, in Weiss EB, Stein M (eds): *Bronchial Asthma*, 3d ed. Boston, Little Brown, 1993; 910–916.
10. Cronstein BN, Naime D, Ostad E: The anti-inflammatory mechanism of methotrexate: increased adenosine release at inflamed sites diminishes leukocyte accumulation in an in vivo model of inflammation. *J Clin Invest* 1993; 92:2675.
11. Yntema JL, Walker C, Aalbers R: Methotrexate in the treatment of severe asthma. *Respir Med* 1993; 87:57.
12. Weinstein GD, Frost P: Methotrexate for psoriasis. A new therapeutic schedule. *Arch Dermatol* 1971; 103:33.
13. Jones G, Mieruis E, Karsh J: Methotrexate induced asthma. *Am Rev Respir Dis* 1991; 194:179.
14. Mullarkey MF, Lammert JK, Blumenstein BA: Long term methotrexate treatment in corticosteroid dependent asthma. *Ann Intern Med* 1990; 112:577.
15. Trigg CJ, Davies RJ: Comparison of methotrexate 30 mg/week with placebo in chronic steroid-dependent asthma: a 12 week double-blind cross-over study. *Respir Med* 1993; 87:211.
16. Erzurum SC, Leff JA, Cochran JE, et al.: Lack of benefit of methotrexate in severe steroid dependent asthma. *Ann Intern Med* 1991; 114:353.
17. Kremer JM, Alarcon GS, Lightfoot RW, et al.: Methotrexate for rheumatoid arthritis: suggested guidelines for monitoring liver toxicity. *Arthritis Rheum* 1994; 37:316.
18. Whiting-O'Keefe QE, Fye KH, Sack KD: Methotrexate and histologic hepatic abnormalities: a meta-analysis. *Am J Med* 1991; 90:711.
19. Weinblatt ME: Methotrexate for chronic diseases in adults (editorial). *N Engl J Med* 1995; 332:330.
20. White A: The erythrocyte and iron metabolism: leukocyte composition and metabolism, in White A, Handler P, Smith EL (eds): *Principles of Biochemistry* New York, McGraw-Hill, 1973:876.
21. Calderon E, Coffey RG, Lockey RF: Methotrexate in bronchial asthma. *J Allergy Clin Immunol* 1991; 88:274.
22. Mullarkey MF: Methotrexate and asthma. *J Allergy Clin Immunol* 1991; 88:272.
23. Notle H, Skov PS: Inhibition of basophil histamine release by methotrexate. *Agents Actions* 1988; 23:173.
24. Segal R, Mozes E, Yaron M, Tartakovsky B: The effects of methotrexate on the production and activity of interleukin-1. *Arthritis Rheum* 1989; 32:370.
25. Cream JJ, Pole DS: The effect of methotrexate and hydroxyurea on neutrophil chemotaxis. *Br J Dermatol* 1980; 102:192.
26. Coffey MJ, Sanders G, Eschenbacher WL, et al.: The role of methotrexate in the management of steroid dependent asthma. *Chest* 1994; 105:117.
27. Kremer JM: The mechanisms of action of methotrexate in rheumatoid arthritis: the search continues. *J Rheumatol* 1994; 21:1.
28. Michael AI, Girgis RS, El-Assi LH, et al.: Effect of methotrexate on the response of eosinophils to *Schistosoma mansone* infection in mice. *East Afr Med J* 1983; 60:608.
29. Guss S, Portnoy J: Methotrexate treatment of severe asthma in children. *Pediatrics* 1992; 89:635.
30. Stempel DA, Lammert J, Mullarkey MF: Use of methotrexate in the treatment of steroid-dependent adolescent asthmatics. *Ann Allergy* 1991; 67:346.
31. Mullarkey MF, Blumenstein BA, Andrade WP, et al.: Methotrexate in the treatment of corticosteroid-dependent asthma. A double-blind cross over study. *N Engl J Med* 1988; 318:603.
32. Shiner RJ, Nunn AJ, Chung KF, Geddes DM: Randomized double blind placebo controlled trial of methotrexate in steroid dependent asthma. *Lancet* 1990; 336:137.
33. Dyer PD, Vaughan TR, Weber RW: Methotrexate in the treatment of steroid-dependent asthma. *J Allergy Clin Immunol* 1991; 88:208.
34. Dykewicz MS, Greenberger PA, Patterson R, Halwig JM: Natural history of asthma in patients requiring long term systemic corticosteroids. *Arch Intern Med* 1986; 146:2369.
35. To the editors: Methotrexate for asthma. *Ann Intern Med* 1991; 115:66.
36. Taylor DR, Flannery EM, Herbison GP: Methotrexate in the management of severe steroid dependent asthma. *N Z Med J* 1993; 106:409.

Chapter 64
CYCLOSPORINE
PHILIP PADRID

Introduction

Cyclosporine A (CsA) was discovered in 1972 by Jean F. Borel and coworkers at the Sandoz Laboratories in Basel, Switzerland.[1] The drug originally was identified by screening materials of fungal origin for antibiotic properties. The finding that CsA inhibited interleukin (IL)-2 production from activated T cells without the side effects of lymphocyte or bone marrow toxicity made an immediate and profound impact in the field of organ and tissue transplantation. In recent years, it has been established that, in addition to the effect of CsA on activated T cells, CsA also inhibits release of preformed mediators and secretion of other cytokines from non–T-cell sources such as mast cells, basophils, and epithelial cells. This has renewed interest in the possible therapeutic application of CsA in many chronic inflammatory noninfectious diseases including bullous pemphigoid, uveitis, rheumatoid arthritis, glomerulonephritis, inflammatory bowel disease, and multiple collagen vascular disorders. Additionally, the recent discovery that asthmatic airway inflammation may be mediated by products of activated T cells has generated new interest in the use of CsA to treat this chronic airway disorder. This chapter summarizes the pharmacologic mechanisms of action of CsA and reviews the results of studies using CsA in animal models of airway inflammation and hyperreactivity. A theoretical basis for the use of CsA to treat bronchial asthma is outlined, and results of clinical trials using CsA in patients with asthma are reviewed and critically evaluated.

Pharmacologic Mechanism of Action

Cyclosporine is a neutral, lipophilic, and exceedingly hydrophobic cyclic peptide produced by the fungus *Tolypocladium inflatum Gams*. It is comprised of 11 amino acids, has a 9-carbon amino acid in position 1, and no other functional groups. The biologic activity of CsA is very sensitive to alteration or modification of its stereochemical configuration or its amino acid residues, especially at positions 1, 2, 3, 10, and 11.

Cyclosporine inhibits T-cell cytokine gene transcription by a mechanism that involves binding to a specific family of proteins called cyclophilins. These proteins are found in most mammalian tissues; proteins with similar structure are found in most eukaryote organisms. Lymphoid organs are a particularly rich source of cyclophilins; thus, lymphocytes are a primary target for CsA activity. The major isoform of cyclophilin is peptidyl proline isomerase (PPI). Formation of the PPI-CsA complex inhibits PPI's rotamase activity to catalyze the cis-trans isomerization of proline imido peptide bonds, which are required for proper protein folding. Thus, CsA blocks posttranscriptional gene expression by preventing the conformational change that normally is required to confer functional status to proteins.

The best studied effect of CsA is on inhibition of T-lymphocyte production of IL-2. Antigen recognition by T cells leads to T-cell activation through coupling of the T-cell receptor to cell surface receptors, including CD_3, and results in IL-2 secretion. Cyclosporine binding to cyclophilin results in the formation of a CsA-cyclophilin complex that binds to and inhibits calcineurin, a calcium- and calmodulin-dependent serine/threonine phosphatase. The phosphatase activity of calcineurin is initiated when antigen presentation to T cells generates inositol trisphosphate (IP3), diacylglycerol, and an increase in intracellular calcium. Inhibition of calcineurin phosphatase activity inhibits or prevents DNA binding of nuclear factor in activated T cells (NF-AT) and octamer-associated protein (OAP); the importance of CsA inhibition of activator protein 3 and nuclear factor kB is controversial.[2,3] These nuclear proteins normally bind to regulatory sites on the IL-2 enhancer region and act cooperatively to initiate transcription of the IL-2 gene. Nuclear factor in activated T cells and OAP are particularly sensitive to the inhibitory effects of CsA.[3] Thus, inhibition of these nuclear regulatory proteins by CsA inhibits IL-2 production[2,4] (Fig. 64-1).

Cyclosporine also inhibits, in a dose-dependent fashion, IL-5 production from activated peripheral blood lymphocytes in vitro. Mori and colleagues[5] reported areas of strong homology between the enhancer region of the IL-5 gene and the NF-AT and AP-1 binding sites on the IL-2 enhancer. Thus, the action of CsA to inhibit IL-5 production in vitro may involve interactions with NF-AT and AP-1 during transcription of IL-5 similar to the presumed mechanisms of inhibition of IL-2 transcription.

It has also been appreciated that CsA inhibits release of preformed mediators and newly secreted cytokines from activated mast cells and basophils.[6,7] The mechanisms through which this occurs is less clear. For example, CsA binds with low affinity to calmodulin. It has been suggested that CsA interferes with calcium signaling directly through interaction with calcium-binding proteins such as calmodulin or by blocking calcium channels and thus inhibiting the increase in intracellular calcium that is required for mast cell release of stored granules.[6]

Pharmacokinetics

Cyclosporine generally is administered orally. It is absorbed poorly by the small intestine, and absorption and bioavailability are significantly variable from patient to patient. Cyclosporine blood concentrations peak 1 to 8 h after oral administration in healthy volunteers and may reach an additional second peak after food intake or possibly as a result of reabsorption following excretion into bile. Most of the CsA that is absorbed is rapidly (within minutes) taken up by blood cells; less than 40 percent of the drug is distributed in plasma where it is bound primarily to lipoproteins. Red blood cells have a particular affinity for CsA and account for approximately 50 percent of the cellular distribution of the drug. Tissue distribution of CsA is greatest where white blood cell concentrations are highest and correlates positively with increased concentrations of cy-clophilins. Cyclosporine does not cross the blood-brain barrier but is passed from the placenta into fetal blood and amniotic fluid; it is also present in breast milk.

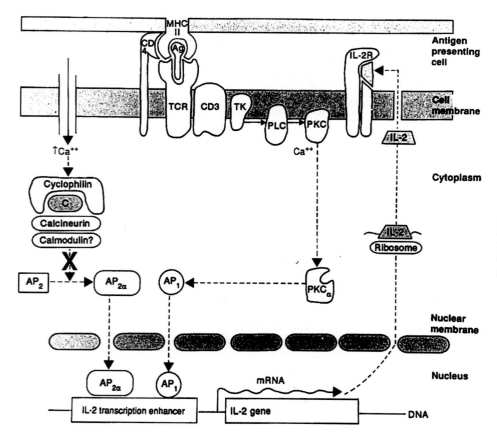

FIGURE 64-1 Schematic representation of the function of cyclosporine (C) to inhibit events associated with T-lymphocyte activation. Both AP-1 and AP-2 must bind to the interleukin (IL)-2 enhancer to initiate transcription of IL-2 messenger RNA (mRNA). Cyclosporine may inhibit T cell activation by inhibiting activation of AP-2. The cyclosporine/cyclophilin/calcineurin complex may also block nuclear translocation of AP-2. MHC II = major histocompatibility complex II; Ag = antigen; CD = cluster differentiation; TCR = T cell receptor; TK = tyrosine kinase; PLC = phospholipase; PKC = protein kinase; IL-2R = IL-2 receptor; AP = activation protein; α = activated. (*Modified from Faulds,[8] with permission.*)

Cyclosporine is primarily metabolized in the liver by the cytochrome P_{450} enzyme system and results in the creation of at least 30 metabolic by-products with little secondary immunosuppressive properties. The overwhelming majority of CsA is excreted into bile (>90 percent); the remainder is primarily lost through urine.

The elimination half-life of CsA is estimated at 19 h and is decreased in children in parallel with an increased clearance rate in this patient population. An increased dosage requirement in children would therefore be expected.

Side effects of CsA therapy are common, and the morbidity is variable. Common and relatively benign side effects include hypertrichosis and gingival hyperplasia. More significant problems associated with CsA therapy include gastrointestinal upset, hypertension, and neurologic impairment with seizure. Common laboratory abnormalities include hyperkalemia and elevated blood urea nitrogen and creatinine. In almost all cases, these side effects and laboratory abnormalities are reversible by decreasing the dose of CsA or eliminating the drug entirely. Although frank renal failure is rare, elderly patients and patients with preexisting hypertension or renal dysfunction are at risk for the development of CsA-associated renal tubular atrophy and interstitial fibrosis. For this reason, it is considered standard practice to monitor renal function at regular intervals for all patients receiving CsA.[8]

Theoretical Basis for the Use of Cyclosporine to Treat Asthma

It has been recognized for decades that the airways of patients with severe chronic asthma are strikingly abnormal. Histologic evaluation reveals profound inflammation of central airways, including hyperplasia and hypertrophy of the mucous-secreting apparatus and smooth muscle thickening. A particularly striking and commonly found feature of asthmatic airways is an eosinophil and mononuclear cell infiltration within bronchial epithelium, including the deposition of eosinophil granular products in association with epithelial denuding, erosion, and ulceration.

One of the more recent and significant advances in the understanding of the pathophysiology of bronchial asthma is the finding that airway inflammation is a feature not only of chronic severe asthma but also of mild asymptomatic asthma.[9] Even in these mild cases, eosinophil cell infiltration of bronchial epithelium is a consistent finding. Immunocytochemical staining has demonstrated CD_{25} receptor-positive activated lymphocytes within bronchial epithelium of patients with asthma. This latter finding lends itself easily to a possible relationship between activated T lymphocytes and activated eosinophils in the pathophysiology of the inflamed asthmatic airway (Fig. 64-2).

The major focus of study of T cell-eosinophil interactions has been the CD_4^+ T lymphocyte because it is the only cell that recognizes antigen after processing by antigen-presenting cells. On activation, these T cells produce cytokines, including IL-5, which have profound effects on eosinophils in vitro and in animal models of airway inflammation. These effects include eosinophilopoiesis from bone marrow stem cells, increased survival of eosinophils in vitro, enhanced adhesion of eosinophils to vascular endothelium, and degranulation of eosinophils within airways.[10–12] Thus, products of activated T cells may assist in the directed migration of eosinophils from bone marrow to airways and account for the selective accumulation of activated eosinophils in airways of asthmatics.

In addition to IL-5, the CD_4^+ T lymphocyte is capable of producing a wide range of cytokines, some of which are proinflammatory and some of which inhibit the inflammatory process. After antigen stimulation, T-lymphocyte clones

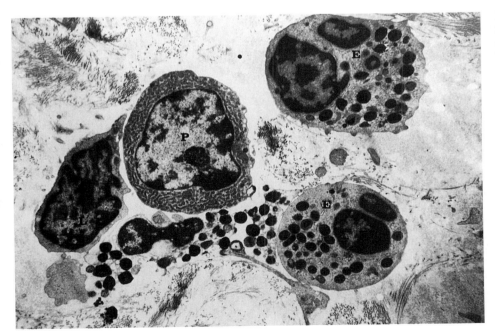

FIGURE 64-2 Transmission electron micrograph of subepithelial tissue in a bronchial biopsy from a patient with mild atopic asthma. Lymphocytes, plasma cells, and eosinophils lie in close proximity to each other. Cell-to-cell signaling may account for activation and degranulation of eosinophils within airways. L = lymphocyte; P = plasma cell; E = eosinophil. (*From Jeffrey RK: Comparative morphology of the airways in asthma and COPD. Am J Respir Crit Care Med 1994; 150:S10.*)

of mouse origin can be further subdivided on the basis of their unique pattern of cytokine secretion.[13] Thus, the Th_1 subpopulation of CD_4^+ cells secrete IL-2, interferon-γ, and tumor necrosis factor-β. The Th_2 subpopulation secretes IL-4, 5, and 6, while both subpopulations secrete IL-3 and granulocyte-macrophage colony-stimulating factor (GM-CSF). The Th_2 subpopulation has been identified as particularly important in the generation of eosinophilic inflammation in asthma by producing IL-5. However, it is not clear under what conditions the expression of the Th_1 or Th_2 phenotype occurs. In vitro, Th_0 cells can be stimulated to express the Th_2 cytokine profile by stimulation with IL-4. However, this begs the question because it is the Th_2 phenotype that produces IL-4. Recently, attention has focused on activated mast cell secretion of IL-4 as possible mechanisms by which antigen stimulation results in the generation of the Th_2 phenotype.[14,15]

GLUCOCORTICOID RESISTANCE IN VITRO

Glucocorticosteroids are the most effective therapy for chronic asthma currently available. Although most patients have a positive therapeutic response to corticosteroids, a subset of patients with asthma are resistant.[16,17] This resistance does not seem to result from decreased absorption or increased elimination. Instead, corticosteroid resistance seems to be a cellular phenomenon. Corrigan and coworkers studied a group of patients with moderate to severe asthma who failed to show a positive therapeutic response to 20 to 40 mg/day of prednisolone given over a 2-week period. Peripheral blood T cells from these patients secreted IL-2 and proliferated (assessed by uptake of tritiated thymidine at 24 to 72 h in response to stimulation with phytohemagglutinin) in vitro in an equivalent manner as T cells from corticosteroid-sensitive asthmatics. These cellular responses were attenuated or ablated when T cells from the corticosteroid-sensitive group were cocultured with dexamethasone. In contrast, T-cell proliferation and IL-2 production were unaffected by dexamethasone in the corticosteroid-insensitive group. However, T-cell proliferative responses from these same corticosteroid-insensitive patients again were attenuated or ablated if the cells were coincubated with CsA (500 ng/mL). Corrigan and colleagues extrapolated from these results that CsA may be an important therapeutic tool in the treatment of asthmatic patients whose clinical response to corticosteroids is poor.[18,19]

EFFECTS OF CsA ON MAST CELLS

In 1989, Plaut and associates and others reported that cross-linkage of IgE bound to mast cell FcεRI (high affinity Fc receptor for IgE) results in mast cell secretion of a large number of cytokines, including IL-1, 3, 4, 5, and 6, TNF-α and GM-CSF.[20,21] Production of IL-2, 3, and 4 and GM-CSF by mast cell clones was inhibited by pretreatment of CsA before mast cell stimulation.[22] Although T-cell activation occurs principally through the CD_3 membrane complex by cross-

linking the antigen-specific T-cell receptor, and mast cell activation occurs following cross-linking the FcεRI, in both cell types CsA blocks cytokine production at the level of transcription. Cyclosporine also inhibits the release of preformed mediators in a nontranscriptionally regulated fashion, such as serotonin from rat basophilic leukemia cell lines and histamine from human basophils.[23,24] Because inhibition of cytokine production is correlated positively with CsA binding affinity to cyclophilin, it has been assumed that the mechanism by which CsA inhibits mast cell cytokine production parallels the mechanism of action of CsA on T cells. Each of these events, cytokine secretion and preformed mediator release by cellular degranulation, has as a common requirement an increase in the concentration of intracellular calcium. Additionally, because CsA blocks gene expression of the same profile of cytokines in both T cells and mast cells, it seems likely that CsA works on a regulatory protein similar to both cell types.[3]

Cross-linking of mast cell IgE by antigen is fundamental to the release of mediators from activated mast cells. B-cell production of IgE requires physical interaction with T cells (or mast cells?) and involves at least three molecular contact signals. One of these cell contact signals is CD40-L ligand, which is required to induce IgE-producing cells to become plasmacytes. Mast cells express CD40-L and thus may be intimately involved in IgE production and the sensitization process. It recently has been appreciated that CsA inhibits expression of CD40–L by mast cells and so may inhibit mast cell sensitization as well as degranulation.[25]

Interestingly, although CsA can inhibit both preformed mediators and newly secreted cytokines from activated mast cells in vitro, the activity of CsA on acute mast cell degranulation in vivo is less clear. For instance, in a mouse model of cutaneous sensitivity, CsA inhibited the late phase T cell-dependent response to antigen but did not inhibit the early phase, which is dependent on release of serotonin from mast cells.[26] More recently, in an antigen-sensitized feline model of asthma, histamine release into bronchoalveolar lavage fluid (BAL) and the early phase response to acute antigen challenge was equivalent in cats pretreated with CsA or sham pretreated with saline. Airway smooth muscle of sensitized cats also contracted in vitro after exposure to antigen (Shultz-Dale response) in an equivalent manner whether or not the cats had been pretreated with CsA in vivo. Interestingly, pretreatment with CsA in vitro did abolish the Shultz-Dale response in these same tissues.[27] Thus, it remains to be seen if the effects of CsA on mast cell function in vitro parallel the effects of CsA on mast cell function in vivo.

Summary

CsA can inhibit airway inflammation in at least three ways:

1. Interleukin-2 promotes effector cell development regardless of the presence of other cytokines.[28] Perhaps the most fundamental method by which CsA inhibits airway

inflammation is by preventing T-cell secretion of IL-2 and thus prohibiting the clonal expansion of T cells in general.

2. Interleukin-4 may be important in the differentiation of Th$_0$ cells into Th$_2$.[15] It is possible that mast cell-derived IL-4 drives the Th$_2$ response. For example, human mast cells in the nose, skin, and lung contain IL-4; mast cells comprise as much as 80 percent of the cells in biopsy samples of human asthmatic airways that stain positively for IL-4. This suggests that the mast cell stores IL-4.[14] CsA can inhibit mast cell secretion of IL-4 and thus possibly inhibit the expression of the Th$_2$ phenotype of CD$_4^+$ T lymphocytes.[22]

3. Interleukin-2 is a potent chemoattractant for eosinophils.[29] Additionally, IL-2 may promote the generation of IL-5 from CD$_4^+$ T cells.[30,31] Inhibition of T-lymphocyte secretion of IL-2 may inhibit asthmatic airway inflammation by inhibiting IL-5 secretion and by downregulating the chemoattraction signal for eosinophils within airways.

It is worth emphasizing that both the Th$_1$ and Th$_2$ phenotypes probably represent activated effector T cells. Resting T cells probably secrete only IL-2 after initial stimulation with antigen.[32] Although the absolute number of T cells in airways may be low compared to other infiltrating cells, it is estimated that one T cell can make enough cytokine to have biologic effect on 10^4 effector cells. Thus, if 5 percent of airway T cells are making message for IL-5, there is probably enough secretion of IL-5, for example, to saturate all eosinophils in the airway milieu, and this makes for a very powerful response.[19]

Animal Studies

Cyclosporine has been used in a number of animal models of acute airway inflammation and hyperreactivity. Many of these studies have been designed to test the effects of CsA on the early phase response to antigen in sensitized animals. For example, following antigen challenge, ovalbumin-sensitized guinea pigs normally develop bronchoconstriction within 5 to 10 minutes, a late response within 4 to 8 h, and BAL eosinophils within 6 to 24 h. Cyclosporine A given at the time of sensitization prevented the accumulation of eosinophils into BAL fluid, which would normally have occurred in these animals.[33-35] Although CsA (25 mg/kg/day) did not inhibit the early phase response to antigen, the late phase was reduced and the predicted development of antihyaluronidase reaction (AHR) to histamine was also significantly attenuated in the sensitized guinea pigs given CsA.[35-37]

Treatment with CsA also attenuated the expected BAL eosinophilia and late-phase skin response in antigen-sensitized and challenged mice.[26,38] However, other studies of CsA-treated mice had contrasting results. Elwood et al.[39] reported that ovalbumin-sensitized and acutely challenged brown Norway rats developed BAL eosinophilia and a seven-fold increase in airway reactivity to inhaled antigen. Pretreatment with CsA (5 mg or 50 mg/day for 5 days prior

antigen challenge) attenuated the inflammatory cell influx into airways but did not affect the development of AHR. Wang and associates[39a] reported paradoxical results. They found that *Aspergillus fumigatus* sensitized C57B/6 mice treated with CsA had a 4.5 fold *increase* in eosinophils recovered in BAL fluid following antigen challenge compared to similarly challenged mice not treated with CsA. Ewart et al.[40] studied the effects of CsA on strains of mice with genetically conferred airway hyporesponsiveness (C3H/HeJ) and hyperresponsiveness (A/J). In this study, CsA pretreatment (25 to 100 mg/kg intraperitoneally for 5 to 10 days) completely attenuated, in a dose-dependent fashion, the otherwise predictable airway hyperreactivity to intravenous acetylcholine. However, in these same mice, ablation of either the CD$_4^+$ or CD$_8^+$ T-lymphocyte cell population with cell-specific monoclonal antibodies did not affect airway reactivity to acetylcholine. These authors concluded that the CD$_4^+$/CD$_8^+$ T-lymphocyte cell populations do not mediate genetically conferred AHR in this model, and speculated that CsA may have attenuated AHR by inhibiting IL-2 production by eosinophils, or may have had a direct inhibitory effect on airway smooth muscle.

Recent reports have examined the effects of acute and chronic antigen challenge in sensitized cats, a species that gets idiopathic asthma.[41] In these animals, challenge with *Ascaris suum* results in an immediate increase in lung resistance and a decrease in dynamic compliance. Twenty-four hours after antigen challenge, there is a shift to the left in the dose-response curve to acetylcholine and an influx of eosinophils into BAL fluid. Significantly, up to 40 percent of these airway eosinophils are hypodense. Chronic antigen challenge in these cats (thrice weekly for 6 weeks) resulted in a constellation of pathologic changes in airway wall structure, including an eosinophil infiltrate within epithelium, occasional foci of ulceration, hypertrophy and hyperplasia of epithelial goblet cells, hyperplasia of submucosal glands, and an increase in airway smooth muscle thickness.

To test the contribution of activated lymphocytes to changes in airway structure and function in this model, five additional cats were treated with high doses of CsA (500 to 1000 ng/mL whole blood trough levels) during the chronic antigen challenge period. Cats treated with CsA developed an equivalent early phase response compared to cats not given CsA. However, in CsA-treated cats the development of AHR and BAL eosinophilia and the structural changes in airway wall that would otherwise occur in antigen-sensitized and challenged cats were abolished or significantly attenuated.[42] Thus, immune sensitization and challenge alone resulted in changes in airway walll structure and function. These pathologic alterations were abolished in cats treated with CsA, suggesting that these changes are dependent on T-cell activation or products of activated T cells.

Although results of studies using animal models are intriguing, it should be recalled that the mechanisms resulting in AHR in animal models may be inflammatory cell dependent or independent, as well as both stimulus and species specific.[43] Experiments using animals to study asthma are most likely to be of value when they are designed to test a specific hypothesis concerning the pathogenesis of human asthma. In general then, CsA administration in most animal models of airway inflammation and airway reactivity has resulted in inhibition of late phase responses, airway eosinophilia, and the development of AHR. Results of studies using CsA-treated cats further suggest the *possibility* that future drugs might be produced that inhibit T cell activation and cytokine secretion (without the disturbing profile of side effects currently encountered), and that therefore may inhibit the pathologic histologic alterations in asthmatic airways if given early after the diagnosis is made.

Clinical Trials in Patients

A number of case reports and results of at least three studies suggest that CsA may have a beneficial role in the treatment of a subset of patients with corticosteroid-dependent asthma. Matusiewicz and coworkers[44] designed a double-blind experiment to study 30 patients with corticosteroid-dependent asthma (triamcinolone 6 to 8 mg/day for >5 years). Fifteen patients were treated with CsA (100 mg/day) for 2 years. Patients given CsA but not sham had statistically significant increases in forced vital capacity (FVC), forced expiratory volume in 1 s (FEV$_1$), and peak expiratory flowrate (PEFR) and were able to tolerate reduction in their corticosteroid dosages. Alexander and colleagues[45] also used a double-blind design to evaluate 30 corticosteroid-dependent patients with moderate to severe asthma. Patients given CsA (5 mg/kg/day) for 5 months had a mean 18 percent increase in FEV$_1$, and greater than 10 percent increase in morning PEFR and FVC compared to sham-treated patients. Additionally, patients receiving placebo had twice as many exacerbations requiring increased corticosteroid administration. In a follow-up study, these investigators showed that another group of steroid dependent asthmatic patients treated with CsA also had increased morning PEFR compared to patients receiving placebo. Additionally, improvement in PEFR was positively correlated with decreases serum concentrations of soluble interleukin-2 receptor, a marker of T-lymphocyte activation.[45a] In a similar study, Fukuda and associates reported that 6/9 steroid dependent asthmatic patients had an increase in PEFR following 12 weeks of CsA treatment. In these patients, increased PEFR was associated with a decrease in peripheral blood T-lymphocyte expression of interleukin-2 receptor, a decrease in serum concentrations of IgE, and a decrease in the number of circulated peripheral eosinophils.[45b] Finnerty[46] and Nizankowska[47] also have reported single cases in which corticosteroid-dependent asthmatics were treated with CsA. These patients had an approximately 10 percent increase in lung function associated with a decrease in their corticosteroid-dependency. Infrequent case reports also suggest a beneficial effect of CsA in patients with aspirin-induced asthma.[48]

If CsA has a therapeutic effect in patients with corticosteroid-dependent asthma, it would be important to know if these positive effects remain after the drug is discontinued. Szczeklik and associates[49,50] treated 12 corticosteroid-dependent asthmatic patients with CsA (3.5 mg/kg/day) for

9 months. Six of these patients improved enough to allow a reduction in their corticosteroid requirement from 30 to 11 mg/day. After an additional 9 months of CsA treatment, the drug was discontinued. Four of these six patients had a worsening of their symptoms and required an upward adjustment of their corticosteroid dose to the pre-CsA requirement. Although this study was not designed in a "blinded" fashion, it is the only study that addresses the question of the long-term effects of CsA treatment. Unfortunately, these results suggest that long-term CsA treatment does not result in a long-lasting improvement in lung function.

Clinical trials designed to study the efficacy of CsA therapy in patients with asthma have been limited by the side effects associated with CsA. For example, 12 patients were originally enrolled in the study of Szczeklik et al. Six patients had a positive therapeutic result. However, 3 patients had an exacerbation of preexisting hypertension, 1 patient became septic, and 1 other patient developed symptoms of peripheral polyneuropathy. Stated in another way, a positive therapeutic outcome was seen in 50 percent of patients using CsA, whereas 42 percent of patients using CsA experienced moderate to severe side effects during the course of the study.

Conclusions

The drugs that are currently used in the treatment of asthma have been available for 20 years and can be grouped into five classes (Table 64-1). Recent alterations in the way physicians treat asthmatic patients have resulted from a newer understanding of the pathophysiology of the disease. Thus, inhaled corticosteroids are now used sooner after diagnosis and β-adrenergic agonists are available with an increased duration of action. Nevertheless, new treatment approaches to asthma have revolved around different formulations and use of the five established classes of asthma drugs. Of some significance then is the realization that worldwide morbidity and mortality from asthma is rising.[51]

The recognition that inflammation is a fundamental feature of even mild asymptomatic asthma has led to new insight into the role of inflammatory mediators, cytokines, and adhesion molecules in the development and perpetuation of the asthmatic airway. This in turn has led to increased interest in the use of immunomodulating drugs to inhibit the inflammatory process. Evidence that activated T lymphocytes may play an important role in the generation of eosinophilic airway inflammation has stimulated interest in the use of CsA to treat patients with asthma. In limited clinical trials, CsA has improved lung function and acted as a corticosteroid-sparing agent for patients with moderate to

TABLE 64-1   Conventional Drugs Used to Treat Bronchial Asthma

1. Corticosteroids	4. Anticholinergics
2. Beta$_2$ agonists	5. Mast cell "stabilizing" agents
3. Methylxanthines	

severe disease. For the small subpopulation of patients with chronic severe asthma who require very large doses of corticosteroids or are steroid resistant, CsA may be a useful adjunct to therapy.[52] More widespread use of CsA to treat asthma is limited by the wide profile of significant side effects that result from CsA administration. Nevertheless, the beneficial effect of CsA in these patients further suggests a role for T lymphocytes in the pathogenesis of asthma, and therefore the need to develop additional agents that specifically target activated T cells or specific proinflammatory cytokines produced by T lymphocytes.

References

1. Borel JF, Feurer C, Gubler HHU, et al.: Biological effects of cyclosporine A: a new antilymphocytic agent. *Agents Actions* 1976; 6:468.
2. Fruman DA, Klee BC, Bierer BE, et al.: Calcineurin phosphatase activity in T lymphocytes is inhibited by FK506 and cyclosporine A. *Nat Acad Sci* 1992; 89:3686.
3. Schreiber SL, Crabtree GR: The mechanism of action of cyclosporin A and FK506. *Immunol Today* 1992; 13:136.
4. O'Keefe SJ, Tamura J, Kinkaid RL, et al.: FK506 and CsA sensitive activation of the interleukin 2 promoter by calcineurin. *Nature* 1992; 10:519.
5. Mori A, Suko M, Nishizaki Y, et al.: Regulation of interleukin-5 production by peripheral blood mononucleur cells from atopic patients with FK506, cyclosporin A and glucocorticoid. *Int Arch Allergy Immunol* 1994; 10:32.
6. Draberova L: Cyclosporin A inhibits rat mast cell activation. *Eur J Immunol* 1990; 20:1469.
7. Ezeamuzie IC, Assem ESK: Inhibition of histamine release from human lung and rat peritoneal mast cells by cyclosporin-A. *Agents Action* 1990; 30:110.
8. Faulds D, Goa KL, Benfield P: Cyclosporin. A review of its pharmacodynamic and pharmacokinetic properties and therapeutic use in immunoregulatory disorders. *Drugs* 1993; 45:953.
9. Beasley R, Roche WR, Roberts JA, et al.: Cellular events in the bronchi in mild asthma and after bronchial provocation. *Am Rev Respir Dis* 1989; 139:806.
10. Yamaguchi Y, Hayashi Y, Sugama Y, et al.: Highly purified murine interleukin 5 stimulates eosinophil function and prolongs in vitro survival. IL-5 as an eosinophil chemotactic factor. *J Exp Med* 1988; 167:1737.
11. Lopez AF, Sanderson CJ, Gamble JR, et al.: Recombinant human interleukin-5 is a selective activator of human eosinophil function. *J Exp Med* 1988; 167:219.
12. Clutterbuck EJ, Hirst EMA, Sanderson CJ: Human interleukin-5 regulates the production of eosinophils in human bone marrow cultures: comparisons and interactions with IL-1, IL-3, IL-6 and GM-CSF. *Blood* 1989; 3:1504.
13. Mosmann TR, Cherwinski H, Bond MW, et al.: Two types of murine helper T cell clones. Definition according to profiles of lymphokine activities and secreted proteins. *J Immunol* 1986; 136:2348.
14. Bradding P, Feather IH, Howarth PH, et al.: Interleukin-4 is localized to and released by human mast cells. *J Exp Med* 1992; 176:1381.
15. Cofmann RL, Chatelain R, Leal LMCC, et al.: Leishmania major infection in mice: a model of system for the study of CD_4^+ T-cell subset differentiation. *Res Immunol* 1991; 142:36.
16. Barnes PJ, Pederson S: Efficacy and safety of inhaled corticosteroids in asthma. *Am Rev Respir Dis* 1993; 148:sl.
17. Carmichael J, Paterson JC, Diaz P, et al.: Corticosteroid resistance in chronic asthma. *Br Med J* 1981; 282:1419.
18. Corrigan CJ, Brown PH, Barnes NC, et al.: Glucocorticoid resistance in chronic asthma. Peripheral blood T lymphocyte activation and comparison of the T lymphocyte inhibitory effects of glucocorticoids and cyclosporine A. *Am Rev Respir Dis* 1991; 144:1026.
19. Corrigan CJ, Kay AB: T lymphocytes in allergic asthma, in Jolles G, Karlsson JA, Taylor J (eds): *T Lymphoctye and Inflammatory Cell Research in Animals.* London, Academic Press, 1993:3-24.
20. Plaut M, Pierce JH, Watson CJ, et al.: Mast cell lines produce lymphokines in response to cross linkage of FcRI or to calcium ionophore. *Nature* 1989; 339:64.
21. Gordon JR, Burd PR, Galli SJ: Mast cells as a source of multifunctional cytokines. *Immunol Today* 1990; 11:458.
22. Hatfield SM, Roehm NW: Cyclosporine and FK506 inhibition of murine mast cell cytokine production. *J Pharmacol Exp Ther* 1992; 260:680.
23. Cirillo R, Triggiana T, Siri L, et al.: Cyclosporine A rapidly inhibits mediator release from human basophils presumably by interacting with cyclophilin. *J Immunol* 1990; 144:3891.
24. Hultsch T, Rodriguez JL, Kaliner MA, et al.: Cyclopsorine A inhibits degranulation of rat basophilic leukemia cells and human basophils. Inhibition of mediator release without affecting PI hydrolysis or $Ca_{2}+$ fluxes. *J Immunol* 1990; 144:2659.
25. Gauchet FJ, Henchoz S, Mazzei G, et al.: Induction of human IgE synthesis in B cells by mast cells and basophils. *Nature* 1993; 365:340.
26. Geba GP, Ptak W, Askenase P: Cyclosporine inhibits the late component of DTH in late phase responses without affecting early DTH or the immediate phase of IgE responses. *J Allergy Clin Immunol* 1991; 87:333.
27. Padrid PA, Ndukwu IM, Cozzi PJ, et al.: Cyclosporine treatment in vivo does not attenuate the Schultz-Dale contraction of airway smooth muscle from immune sensitized cats. *Am Rev Respir Dis* 1994; 149:A771.
28. Swain SL: Regulation of the development of distinct subsets of CD_4^+ T cells. *Res Immunol* 1991; 142:14.
29. Rand TH, Silberetein DS, Kornfeld H, et al.: Human eosinophils express functional interleukin 2 receptors. *J Clin Invest* 1991; 88:825.
30. vanHaelst PC, Kovach JS, Kita H, et al.: Administration of interleukin-2 (IL-2) results in increased plasma concentrations of IL-5 and eosinophilia in patients with cancer. *Blood* 1991; 78:1538.
31. Yamaguchi Y, Suda T, Shiozaki H, et al.: Role of IL-5 in IL-2 induced eosinophilia. *J Immunol* 1990; 145:873.
32. Mosmann TR, Moore KW: The role of IL-10 in cross regulation of the TH_1 and TH_2 responses. *Immunol Today* 1991; 12:49.
33. Norris AA, Jackson DM, Eady RP: Protective effects of cyclosphosphamide, cyclosporin A and FK506 against antigen induced lung eosinophilia in guinea pigs. *Clin Exp Immunol* 1992; 3:347.
34. Lagente V, Carre C, Boichot E, et al.: Cyclosporin A inhibits antigen aeorosol challenge induced eosinophil accumulation in lungs from sensitized guinea pigs. *Am Rev Respir Dis* 1992; 145:A697.
35. Akutsu I, Fukuda T, Makino S: Inhibition of antigen induced eosinophil infiltration, late asthmatic response and bronchial hyperresponsiveness by cyclosporin A. *Adv Asthmol* 1990; 39:427.
36. Arima A, Yukawa T, Terashi Y, et al.: Cyclosporine A inhibits allergen induced late asthmatic response and increase of airway hyperresponsiveness in guinea pigs. *Nippon Kyobe Shikkan Gakkai Zasshi* 1991; 29:1089.
37. Fukuda T, Akutsu I, Motojima S, et al.: Inhibition of antigen induced late asthmatic response and bronchial hyperrespon-

siveness by cyclosporin and FK-506. *Int Arch Allergy Appl Immunol* 1991; 94:259.

38. Nogami M, Suko M, Okudaira H, et al.: Experimental pulmonary eosinophilia in mice by *Ascaris suum* extract. *Am Rev Respir Dis* 1990; 141:1289.

39. Elwood W, Lotvall JO, Barnes PJ, et al.: Effects of dexamethasone and cyclosporin A on allergen-induced airway hyperresponsiveness and inflammatory cell responses in sensitized Brown-Norway rats. *Am Rev Respir Dis* 1992; 145:1289.

39a. Wang JM, Denis M, Fournier M, et al.: Cyclosporin a increases pulmonary eosinophilia induced by inhaled aspergillus antigen in mice. Clin Exp Immunol 1993; 93:323.

40. Ewart SL, Gavett SH, Margolick J, Wills-Karp M: Cyclosporine A attenuates genetic airway hyperresponsiveness in mice but not through inhibition of CD4 or CD8 T cells. *Am Rev Respir Cell Mol Biol* 1996.

41. Padrid PA, Snook S, Finucane T, et al.: Persistent airway hyperresponsiveness and histologic alterations after chronic antigen challenge in cats. *Am J Respir Crit Care Med* 1995; 150.

42. Padrid PA, Mitchell RW, Cozzi P, et al.: Cyclosporine treatment inhibits the development of airway hyperresponsiveness and histologic alterations after chronic antigen challenge in cats. *Am Rev Respir Dis* 1994; 149:A771.

43. Padrid PA: Animal models of asthma, in The Genetics of Asthma: Lung Biology in Health and Disease. Liggett SB, Meyers DA (eds): Marcel Dekker, 1996. (In press).

44. Matusiewicz R, Urbankowska B: Effect of cyclosporine A on the clinical state and spirometric parameters in patients with steroid-dependent bronchial asthma. *Pneumonol Alergol Pol* 1992; 60:53.

45. Alexander AG, Barnes NC, Kay AB: Trial of cyclosporine in corticosteroid dependent chronic severe asthma. *Lancet* 1992; 339:324.

45a. Alexander AG, Barnes NC, Kay AB, Corrigan CJ: Clinical response to cyclosporine in chronic severe asthma is associated with reduction in serum soluble interleukin-2 receptor concentrations. *Eur Respir J* 1995; 8:574.

45b. Fukuda T, Asakawa J, Motojima S, Makino S: Cyclosporine A reduces T-lymphocyte activity and improves airway hyperresponsiveness in corticosteroid-dependent chronic severe asthma. *Ann Allergy Asthma and Immunol* 1995; 75:65.

46. Finnerty NA, Sullivan TJ: Effect of cyclosporine on corticosteroid dependent asthma. *J Allergy Clin Immunol* 1991; 87:297a.

47. Nizankowska E, Dworski R, Szczeklik A: Cyclosporin for a severe case of aspirin-induced asthma. *Eur Respir J* 1991; 4:380.

48. Herzog CH, Walker CH, Erlich H: Cyclosporine A in aspirin-induced asthma. *J Autoimmun* 1992; 38:286a.

49. Szczeklik A, Nizankowska E, Dworski R, et al.: Cyclosporin for steroid-dependent asthma. *Allergy* 1991; 46:312.

50. Szczeklik A, Nizankowska E, Sladek K: Cyclosporin and asthma. *Lancet* 1992; 339:873.

51. US Department of Health and Human Services: International consensus report on diagnosis and treatment of asthma. Publication No. 92-3091, 1992.

52. Editorial: Cyclosporin in chronic severe asthma. *Lancet* 1992; 339.

THERAPY FOR ASTHMA DIRECTED AGAINST SPECIFIC METABOLITES

Chapter 65

LEUKOTRIENE RECEPTOR ANTAGONISTS AND SYNTHESIS INHIBITORS IN ASTHMA

MARY E. STREK

The therapeutic armamentarium available to treat asthma has not included a new class of medications since the introduction of inhaled corticosteroids. Currently, most asthmatic patients are treated with bronchodilators, usually inhaled β-adrenoreceptor agonists, and many receive anti-inflammatory therapy at an increasingly early stage with inhaled corticosteroids. Recent evidence suggests that leukotrienes cause inflammatory cell chemotaxis, bronchoconstriction, production of mucus, and increased microvascular permeability, similar to that noted in asthmatic subjects.[1,2] New pharmacologic agents have been developed that either inhibit the synthesis of leukotrienes or block their effects by (1) inhibiting the 5-lipoxygenase enzyme; (2) binding to 5-lipoxygenase–activating protein (FLAP); (3) antagonizing the leukotriene B_4 (LTB_4) receptor; or (4) binding the cysteinyl leukotriene$_1$ ($CysLT_1$) receptor for leukotriene D_4 (LTD_4) and leukotriene E_4 (LTE_4) (Fig. 65-1). The biochemistry and biologic effects of leukotrienes and their role as mediators of asthma have been discussed in Chap. 10. In this chapter, data are presented that more precisely characterize the mechanisms of action and preclinical pharmacology of leukotriene synthesis inhibitors and receptor antagonists. Clinical studies in asthmatic patients show that these compounds block the acute asthmatic response to allergen and cold, dry air challenge in most, but not all, patients. Recent studies suggest these agents are beneficial in treating pa-

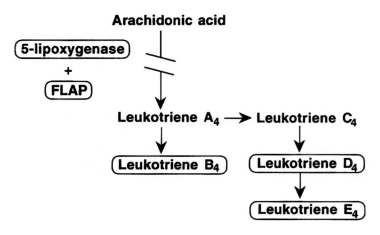

Arachidonic acid

FIGURE 65-1 Sites at which inhibition of leukotriene synthesis or receptor blockade can occur. Leukotriene synthesis can be blocked by drugs that inhibit the 5-lipoxygenase enzyme or antagonize 5-lipoxygenase–activating protein (FLAP). Distal blockade of the effects of leukotrienes occurs with compounds that selectively antagonize either leukotriene B_4 or leukotrienes D_4 and E_4 through the leukotriene B_4 or cysteinyl leukotriene$_1$ receptors, respectively.

tients with aspirin sensitivity, exercise-induced asthma, and chronic asthma, without causing significant adverse effects. In the near future, this exciting new class of medications will be available for the treatment of asthma.

5-Lipoxygenase Inhibitors

PRECLINICAL PHARMACOLOGY

MECHANISM OF ACTION
The 5-lipoxygenase enzyme catalyzes the conversion of arachidonic acid to 5-hydroperoxyeicosatetraenoic acid (5-HPETE) and then to leukotriene A_4 (LTA$_4$). Leukotriene A_4, in the presence of appropriate enzymes, is converted to LTB$_4$ or conjugated with glutathione to form leukotriene C_4 (LTC$_4$). Leukotriene B_4 is responsible for inflammatory cell chemotaxis, especially neutrophils, and to a lesser degree eosinophils.[3,4] Leukoriene C_4 is converted to LTD$_4$, which then is metabolized to LTE$_4$. Leukotrienes C_4, D_4, and E_4 are referred to as the *cysteinyl leukotrienes* and act to cause airway smooth muscle contraction. For 5-lipoxygenase to be catalytically active, 5-lipoxygenase–activating protein (FLAP) is required to translocate 5-lipoxygenase from the cytosol to the perinuclear membrane. Characterization of the precise mechanism(s) by which 5-lipoxygenase inhibition occurs is not possible since 5-lipoxygenase is regulated by complex enzyme kinetics and the need for FLAP. It is theorized that the 5-lipoxygenase reaction can be inhibited by (1) reducing agents, (2) iron chelating agents, (3) nonredox-based enzyme inhibitors, and (4) FLAP inhibitors.[5,6] Examples of representative leukotriene synthesis inhibitors are shown in Table 65-1.[7–16] A more complete list of these compounds can be found in a review by Henderson and colleagues.[17]

Phenidone and BW755C, are 5-lipoxygenase inhibitors that are thought to act as electron reducing agents.[11,13] It is postulated that these compounds reduce either iron or a radical intermediary leaving the 5-lipoxygenase enzyme in the inactive Fe^{2+} state.[5] As a group, redox inhibitors are not selective for 5-lipoxygenase as compared with cyclooxygen-

ase, and are frequently weak or inactive 5-lipoxygenase enzyme inhibitors in vivo when given orally.[5,11] These agents may interact with other biologic redox systems and form methemoglobin.[5] Problems obtaining biologic activity after oral dosing and toxicity from interaction with other oxidase systems have precluded development of this group of compounds.

It is thought that 5-lipoxygenase contains a catalytically important iron atom at its active site.[5,15] Hydroxamic acids, such as BWA4C, bind strongly to Fe^{3+} and may inhibit 5-lipoxygenase by interacting with enzyme-bound iron[5]; A-63162 and A-78773 are examples of this group of compounds.[7,9] Zileuton, formerly known as A-64077, contains a modified hydroxamic acid moiety (N-hydroxyurea) and may inhibit 5-lipoxygenase by a similar mechanism.[15] In addition, there is evidence that the 5-lipoxygenase inhibitory activity of these compounds may be mediated, at least in

TABLE 65-1   Representative Leukotriene Synthesis Inhibitors

Compound	Reference
5-Lipoxygenase inhibitors	
A-63162	7
A-69412	8
A-78773	9
BI-L-239	10
BWA4C	5
BW755C	11
Docebenone (AA-861)	12
Phenidone	13
Piripost (U-60,257)	14
Zileuton (A-64077)	15
ZD2138	16
FLAP[a] inhibitors	
BAY X 1005	21
MK-886	22
MK-0591	23
REV 5901	24
WY-50,295	25

SOURCE: Modified from Henderson.[17]
[a] FLAP = 5-lipoxygenase-activating protein.

part, by their redox properties, which are weak but may be enhanced in the presence of iron.[18] Both $R(+)$ and $S(-)$ enantiomers of zileuton are equipotent, which suggests they inhibit 5-lipoxygenase through a nonspecific interaction with the enzyme. BWA4C is approximately 20 times, while zileuton is approximately 15 times, as selective for 5-lipoxygenase as cyclooxygenase.[5,15] Zileuton and longer-acting N-hydroxyurea derivatives such as A-69412 are under active clinical investigation.[8]

Methoxyalkyl thiazoles are 5-lipoxygenase inhibitors that do not act as redox inhibitors or bind to iron. There is experimental evidence that they cause enantioselective inhibition of the 5-lipoxygenase enzyme.[19] A derivative of this group of agents, the 5-lipoxygenase inhibitor ZD2138, is an achiral compound that is highly selective for 5-lipoxygenase and does not inhibit cyclooxygenase at concentrations up to 20,000 times greater than those that inhibit 5-lipoxygenase.[16,20] ZD2138 is currently the subject of active clinical investigation.

Lastly, leukotriene biosynthesis can be inhibited by compounds that bind to FLAP, thereby preventing translocation of the 5-lipoxygenase enzyme from the cytosol to its active site on the cell membrane.[21–25] Leukotriene synthesis inhibitors that are thought to act as FLAP antagonists are listed in Table 65-1. In additon to its ability to inhibit the translocation of the 5-lipoxygenase enzyme to the cell membrane, WY-50,295 inhibits soluble, cell-free 5-lipoxygenase; thus, it may inhibit 5-lipoxygenase by more than one mechanism.[25]

POTENCY

The N-hydroxyurea 5-lipoxygenase inhibitors soon may be available for use in asthmatic patients. Zileuton is a potent 5-lipoxygenase inhibitor with an inhibitory concentration causing a 50 percent inhibition (IC_{50}) of 5-hydroxy-eicosatetraenoic acid (5-HETE) synthesis by rat basophilic leukemia cell supernatant of 0.5 μM.[15] This is four to six times as potent as phenidone (IC_{50} = 1.9 μM) and BW755C (IC_{50} = 2.0 μM) (Table 65-2).[15] Zileuton is effective when given orally; the effective dose causing a 50 percent inhibition (ED_{50}) of blood LTB_4 synthesis ex vivo in the rat is

TABLE 65-3   Comparison of Leukotriene Synthesis Inhibitors

	HUMAN BLOOD IN VITRO IC_{50} μM		RAT ED_{50} MG/KG PO AT 3 H	
	LTB_4	TXB_2	Ex Vivo Blood	Inflammatory Exudate
Zileuton	2.6	40	5	3
MK-886	1.1	NT^a	3	2
ZD2138	0.02	>500	0.9	0.3

SOURCE: Modified from Crawley.[20]
[a] NT; not tested.

2 mg/kg.[15] A-69412 has potency similar to zileuton from 0.5 to 4 h after dosing (oral ED_{50} = 5 mg/kg in the rat) but is effective twice as long as zileuton.[8] ZD2138, a newer nonredox 5-lipoxygenase inhibitor, is more potent than either zileuton or the FLAP antagonist MK-886 in human whole blood in vitro and in rat blood ex vivo (Table 65-3).[16,20] ZD2138 was approximately 10 times as potent as zileuton in inhibiting allergen-induced bronchoconstriction in sensitized guinea-pigs.[16]

ANTI-INFLAMMATORY ACTIONS

At present, there is no evidence that 5-lipoxygenase inhibition alters architectural changes of inflammation that are characteristic of asthma. In animal models, 5-lipoxygenase inhibition with zileuton or ZD2138 prevents arachidonic acid–induced edema of mouse ear[15,16] and rabbit skin.[16] In Ascaris-sensitized sheep, zileuton inhibits late-phase bronchoconstriction by 55 percent, airway hyperresponsiveness to carbachol, and bronchoalveolar lavage fluid eosinophilia after exposure to allergen.[26] In sensitized guinea-pigs, A-63162 attenuated microvascular leak and airflow obstruction caused by inhalation of ovalbumin.[7] Inhaled BI-L-239, another 5-lipoxygenase inhibitor, caused dose-related inhibition of late-phase leukocyte bronchoconstriction and neutrophil infiltration in two animal models of asthma.[10]

HUMAN CLINICAL PHARMACOLOGY

ACUTE BRONCHODILATION

Prevention of leukotriene biosynthesis by 5-lipoxygenase inhibition produces acute bronchodilation in asthmatic subjects with mild-to-moderate baseline airflow obstruction. Israel and colleagues[27] recently demonstrated that a single 600 mg dose of zileuton caused an 0.35 L, or 14.6 percent increase, in forced expiratory volume in 1 s (FEV_1) above baseline within 1 h after administration. Zileuton was previously shown to have no effect on baseline FEV_1 in patients with very mild airflow obstruction.[28,29] This suggests that continuous formation of leukotrienes may contribute to the increased bronchomotor tone observed in asthmatic patients with baseline airway obstruction. The bronchodilation observed with zileuton is less than half that generally noted after inhaled β-adrenergic agonist but nearly as great as that observed after oral or high-dose inhaled corticosteroids.[30]

TABLE 65-2   Inhibitory Effects of Zileuton and Reference Compounds on Rat Basophilic Leukemia Cell Supernatant 5-Lipoxygenase Activity (after centrifugation at 20,000 xg)

Compound	IC_{50}^a [95% CL] (μM)
Zileuton	0.5 [0.4–0.6]
Phenidone	1.9 [1.5–2.8]
BW755C	2.0 [1.8–2.3]
NDGA	0.3 [0.2–0.3]
Indomethacin	12% at 100^b

SOURCE: Reprinted with permission from Carter et al, 5-Lipoxygenase inhibitory activity of zileuton. *J Pharmacol Exp Ther* 1991; 256:929–937.[15]
[a] IC_{50} values, 95% CL shown in brackets.
[b] Percentage of inhibition of highest tested concentration.

EFFECT ON ALLERGEN-INDUCED BRONCHOCONSTRICTION

Until recently, clinical studies have not demonstrated that 5-lipoxygenase inhibitors protect against either the early- or late-phase response after allergen challenge. Hui and colleagues[29] studied the effect of a single 800 mg dose of zileuton on both early and late responses to inhaled allergen in nine atopic asthmatic subjects. Protection against antigen-induced airflow obstruction and methacholine hyperresponsiveness was assessed and correlated with urinary LTE_4 excretion and ex vivo calcium ionophore stimulated whole blood leukotriene B_4 production. After antigen challenge, zileuton did not protect against either early or late asthmatic responses as assessed by FEV_1 or against increased airway responsiveness to methacholine.[29] Ex vivo LTB_4 production was almost completely inhibited by zileuton, but urinary LTE_4 excretion was reduced by only about one-half. Zileuton caused a reduction in maximum decrease in FEV_1 during the early response which was not significantly different than placebo but was significantly correlated with the decrease in urinary LTE_4 excretion. The power of this study was limited by the small number of subjects, some of whom did not bronchoconstrict significantly to allergen challenge on either study day. In addition, the efficacy of zileuton was assessed after peak plasma concentrations had occurred. More complete inhibition of 5-lipoxygenase may be required to protect against allergen-induced bronchoconstriction. A more recent study using the FLAP antagonist MK-886 demonstrated that an oral dose of 750 mg inhibited the early asthmatic response by 58.4 percent and the late asthmatic response by 43.6 percent as assessed by the mean change from baseline of the area under the curve (AUC) for FEV_1.[22]

EFFECT ON COLD AIR–INDUCED BRONCHOCONSTRICTION

Israel and colleagues[28] demonstrated that selective inhibition of 5-lipoxygenase by zileuton protected against bronchoconstriction caused by inhalation of cold, dry air. A single 800 mg dose of zileuton given to asthmatic subjects 3 h prior to cold air hyperventilation caused a 47 percent increase in the amount of cold, dry air required to reduce the FEV_1 by 10 percent. (Fig. 65-2). Mean whole blood ex vivo synthesis of leukotriene B_4 after calcium ionophore stimulation was reduced by 74 percent while synthesis of thromboxane B_4, a cyclooxygenase product, was not affected. The authors concluded that 5-lipoxygenase inhibition can attenuate significantly bronchoconstriction from cold, dry air. In this study, 4 of the 13 subjects had little or no improvement in cold air–induced bronchoconstriction, suggesting that products of the 5-lipoxygenase pathway do not mediate cold air hyperresponsiveness in all asthmatic patients or that 5-lipoxygenase inhibition was insufficient (Fig. 65-2).

Additional studies confirm that 5-lipoxygenase inhibition reduces cold air hyperresponsiveness. ZD2138, a long-acting 5-lipoxygenase inhibitor, blocks cold air–induced bronchoconstriction for up to 24 h in subjects with mild-to-moderate asthma.[31] After a single 350 mg dose of ZD2138, significantly more cold, dry air, as assessed by mean respiratory heat exchange and minute ventilation, was required to

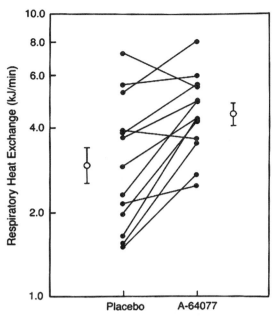

FIGURE 65-2 Effect of pretreatment with zileuton (A-64077) or placebo on airway reactivity to hyperventilation of cold, dry air. Reactivity is expressed as the respiratory heat exchange required to reduce the force expiratory volume in 1 s by 10 percent ($PD_{10}FEV_1$). The values are plotted on a log proportional scale. Open circles and attached bars indicate means ± SEM. There was a 47 percent increase in the $PD_{10}FEV_1$ 3 h after pretreatment with zileuton as compared with placebo (P < .002). (*Reprinted with permission from N Engl J Med 1990; 323:1740–4.*[28])

reduce FEV_1 by 20 percent from prechallenge baseline both 4 and 24 h after dosing.

CLINICAL EFFICACY

ASPIRIN-INDUCED BRONCHOCONSTRICTION

It is estimated that between 10 percent and 30 percent of asthmatic patients have aspirin sensitivity that is manifested by bronchospasm, rhinitis, gastrointestinal symptoms, conjunctivitis, urticaria, angioedema, and anaphylaxis occurring alone or in combination.[32] Increased synthesis of leukotrienes has been noted with increased urinary LTE_4 serving as a marker for increased LTC_4 synthesis. In addition, increased target organ sensitivity to leukotrienes may be a factor in aspirin sensitivity.[32] In a recent study by Israel and colleagues,[33] inhibition of leukotriene synthesis with zileuton in asthmatic subjects with aspirin sensitivity associated with LTE_4 hyperexcretion abolished the usual end-organ responses to aspirin ingestion. One week of zileuton 600 mg four times daily prevented both the decrease in FEV_1 and the development of nasal, gastrointestinal, and dermal symptoms after aspirin ingestion. Treatment with zileuton significantly reduced the maximum increase in urinary LTE_4 after ingestion of aspirin (3539 ± 826 pg/mg creatinine after placebo versus 1120 ± 316 pg/mg creatinine after zileuton). This substantial, but incomplete, inhibition of leukotriene synthesis completely abolished the bronchoconstriction and other end-organ symptoms associated with aspirin ingestion in patients with aspirin-sensitive asthma.

EXERCISE-INDUCED ASTHMA

There is evidence that leukotrienes are important mediators of exercise-induced bronchoconstriction (see below). However, studies evaluating the efficacy of 5-lipoxygenase inhibitors in preventing exercise-induced bronchoconstriction have not been published. In a recent study (data on file, Abbott Laboratories, Abbott Park, IL) zileuton 600 mg four times daily inhibited significantly airflow obstruction after exercise challenge in 24 patients with exercise-induced bronchoconstriction. Mean maximum decrease in FEV_1 after an exercise treadmill test performed 2 to 3 h after the morning dose on day 3 of treatment with zileuton was 0.59 L (-16.06 percent) versus 0.96 L (-28.16 percent) during treatment with placebo ($p < .001$). This is consistent with the findings of Israel and colleagues[28] that inhibition of the 5-lipoxygenase enzyme protects against cold air–induced bronchoconstriction, which is thought to be an analog of exercise-induced asthma.

CHRONIC ASTHMA

Leukotriene synthesis inhibition also is efficacious when given chronically to patients with mild-to-moderate asthma. Inhibition of the 5-lipoxygenase enzyme ameliorates asthma symptoms and improves airflow obstruction when given chronically to asthmatic subjects. Zileuton is the only 5-lipoxygenase inhibitor that has been studied in asthmatic subjects for an extended length of time. In a study of the effects of chronic 5-lipoxygenase inhibition, zileuton was given to subjects with mild-to-moderate asthma for four weeks.[27] Uri-nary LTE_4 excretion was significantly reduced in patients receiving zileuton (Fig. 65-3). Chronic therapy with zileuton resulted in improved FEV_1 (Fig. 65-4) and peak

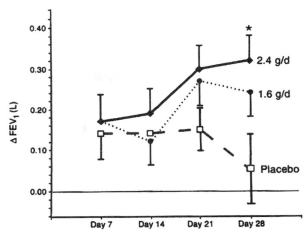

FIGURE 65-4 Change in forced expiratory volume in 1 s (ΔFEV_1) after 4 weeks of treatment with zileuton or placebo. Data are plotted as mean change ($\pm$SE) compared with values at the end of the placebo lead-in period. At 4 weeks, patients receiving 2.4 g/day of zileuton were improved compared with patients receiving placebo (*$p = .02$). (*Reprinted with permission from Ann Intern Med 1993; 119:1059–1066.*[27])

expiratory flow rate, with decreased asthma symptoms and β-adrenergic agonist use. In addition, the response to zileuton improved with time (Fig. 65-4). The improvement in FEV_1 and decreased β-adrenergic agonist use occurred by day 21 with further improvement by day 28.

Leukotriene Receptor Antagonists

PRECLINICAL PHARMACOLOGY

MECHANISM OF ACTION

An alternative to suppressing formation of LTB_4 and the cysteinyl leukotrienes (LTC_4, LTD_4, LTE_4) by 5-lipoxygenase inhibition is selective blockade of the effects of LTB_4 or the cysteinyl leukotrienes by specific receptor antagonists (Fig. 65-1). Numerous antagonists at the LTB_4 and $CysLT_1$ receptors have been developed.[34–45] A representative list of these compounds is contained in Table 65-4. A more complete list can be found in a review by Henderson and colleagues.[17]

Leukotriene B_4 receptor antagonists inhibit chemotaxis of inflammatory cells, and, most importantly in asthma treatment, eosinophils. The selective LTB_4 receptor antagonist U-75302 inhibited by 61.1 percent eosinophil influx into the bronchoalveolar lavage fluid 24 h after inhalation of antigen in ovalbumin-sensitized guinea-pigs.[36] In addition, treatment with U-75302 significantly reduced eosinophil adherence to peribronchiol capillaries with a 79 percent reduction in peribronchial eosinophil infiltration at 24 h. Neutrophil migration was not affected by treatment with U-75302. In contrast, ONO-4057, another orally active LTB_4 receptor antagonist, inhibits the binding of [³H} LTB_4 to the LTB_4 receptor on human neutrophils and inhibits LTB_4 induced aggregation, chemotaxis, and degranulation of human neu-

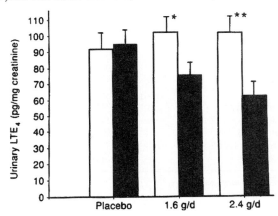

FIGURE 65-3 Mean urinary leukotriene E_4 before and after 4 weeks of treatment with zileuton. Bars represent the mean $\pm$ SE. Open: placebo lead-in urinary leukotriene E_4 (LTE_4); solid: urinary LTE_4 after 4 weeks of treatment. Patients receiving zileuton at 1.6 g/day and 2.4 g/day had decreased urinary LTE_4 concentrations of 26 percent and 39 percent, respectively, compared with placebo lead-in. (*$p < 0.05$; **$p = 0.007$). (*Reprinted with permission from Ann Intern Med 1993; 119:1059–1066.*[27])

TABLE 65-4 Representative Leukotriene Antagonists

Antagonist	Reference
Leukotriene B$_4$ antagonists	
BRL-35135	34
ONO-4057	35
U-75302	36
CysLT$_1$ receptor antagonists	
FPL-55712	37
L-648,051	38
L-649,923	39
MK-571	40
Pranlukast (ONO-1078)	41
SK&F 104353	42
Tomelukast (LY-171883)	43
Verlukast (MK-0679)	44
Zafirlukast (ICI 204,219)	45

SOURCE: Modified from Henderson.[17]

trophils.[35] BRL-35135 is an atypical β-adrenergic receptor agonist with the ability to inhibit LTB$_4$-induced guinea-pig eosinophil chemotaxis in a concentration-dependent fashion.[34]

The precise number and specificity of cysteinyl leukotriene receptors in human lung has yet to be fully elucidated. Specific LTC$_4$ receptors, while present in guinea-pig lung, have not been found in human lung tissue with receptor binding studies.[1] However, functional studies have demonstrated that LTD$_4$ receptor antagonists prevent LTC$_4$-induced smooth muscle contraction in human airways, even when bioconversion to LTD$_4$ is inhibited; thus, LTC$_4$ may interact with a common LTD$_4$ binding site.[17,42,46,47] This remains an issue of some controversy, and, at present, LTC$_4$ is thought to cause human bronchial smooth muscle contraction mainly by its bioconversion to LTD$_4$.[2,17] Both functional and receptor binding studies suggest there are specific receptors for LTD$_4$ in human airways.[1,42,46,48] Leukotriene E$_4$ binds to the LTD$_4$ receptor in guinea-pig lung and acts as a partial agonist at the LTD$_4$ receptor in human airways.[2,42,49] In early studies in human airways, blockade of the leukotriene D$_4$ receptor effectively antagonized contraction caused by all three cysteinyl leukotrienes.[42,46] This suggested that a single compound would be effective in blocking bronchoconstriction caused by LTC$_4$, LTD$_4$, and LTE$_4$, and provided the rationale for further development of leukotriene D$_4$ receptor antagonists.

Generally, CysLT$_1$ receptor antagonists, or LTD$_4$ receptor antagonists as they are more commonly known, act as competitive receptor antagonists; FPL-55712 and LY-171883 were the first such compounds developed.[46,50] However, in addition to being leukotriene receptor antagonists, these compounds inhibit cyclic nucleotide phosphodiesterase activity in canine tracheal smooth muscle.[6,42] A more selective CysLT$_1$ receptor antagonist, SK&F 104353, does not inhibit phosphodiesterase and has no effect on contractions elicited by KCl, histamine, prostaglandin D$_2$, or platelet-activating factor in guinea-pig trachea.[42] More recently developed compounds are selective CysLT$_1$ receptor antagonists.

POTENCY

The potencies of the CysLT$_1$ receptor antagonists have been well-characterized in guinea-pig and human airways in vitro. Recently developed leukotriene receptor antagonists are quite potent when assessed in functional binding assays, with pA$_2$ or pK$_B$ values of about 7.5 to 9.5 and K$_i$ values of about 0.1 to 10 nM, respectively[6] (Table 65-5). FPL-55712 is of relatively low potency in antagonizing LTD$_4$-induced contraction in human airways (pK$_B$ = 6.3) as compared with newer receptor antagonists.[46] SK&F 104353 is a more potent antagonist of LTD$_4$-induced contractions with pK$_B$ = 7.6 in human airways.[42] MK-571 competitively antagonizes contraction of human trachea elicited by LTD$_4$ (pA$_2$ = 8.5).[53] Zafirlukast, formerly known as ICI 204,219, is 1006 and 679 times as potent as LY 171883 and FPL-55712, respectively, in blocking LTD$_4$-induced contraction in guinea-pig trachea, and has a pA$_2$/pK$_B$ of 8.6 against LTD$_4$-induced contraction in human airways.[51,54] ONO-1078, or pranlukast, a relatively new CysLT$_1$ receptor antagonist, competitively antagonized LTD$_4$-induced contractions of guinea-pig trachea with a pA$_2$ of 10.71.[55]

HUMAN CLINICAL PHARMACOLOGY

POTENCY

In normal human subjects, CysLT$_1$ receptor antagonists are effective in inhibiting bronchoconstriction caused by LTD$_4$. Both LY-171883 and zafirlukast protect against airflow obstruction elicited by inhaled leukotriene D$_4$.[43,56] A single oral 40 mg dose of zafirlukast increased by 117-fold the concentration of LTD$_4$ needed to decrease specific airway conductance 35 percent 2 h after dosing, with persistent protection for 24 h after dosing.[56] A 400 mg oral dose of LY-171883 caused a mean rightward shift of the LTD$_4$ dose-response curve 4.6-fold for the provocative dose of LTD$_4$

TABLE 65-5 Relative Potency, As Expressed by pA$_2$ or Pk$_B$ Values, for Cysteinyl Leukotriene Receptor Antagonists versus Leukotriene (LT) C$_4$ and LTD$_4$.

Antagonist	COMPARATOR	
	LTC$_4$	LTD$_4$
Guinea pig trachea		
FPL-55712	6.0	6.3
Tomelukast (LY-171883)	6.2–7.1	8.1
SKF-104353	6.5	8.6
Zafirlukast (ICI-204,219)	8.5–9.5	9.7
MK-571	8.1–9.3	9.4
Human airways		
FPL-55712	6.1	6.3
SKF-104353	8.1	7.6
Zafirlukast (ICI-204,219)	8.5	8.6
MK-571	Not done	8.5

SOURCE: Modified from Chancrin.[52]
NOTE: The pA$_2$ values have been obtained from experiments in vitro measuring contraction in guinea-pig trachea or human airways. pK$_B$ values are given when pA$_2$ determination could not be performed.

TABLE 65-6   Effects of Cysteinyl Leukotriene₁ Receptor Antagonists in Asthma.

Antagonist	Route of Administration	Shift in LTD_4 Dose-Response Curve
LY-171,883	Oral	Three- to fourfold
MK-571, MK-691	Intravenous/oral	30- to 40-fold
SKF-104,353	Inhaled	Three- to fourfold
ICI-204,219	Oral/inhaled	Approximately 100-fold

SOURCE: Modified from Drazen.[2]

causing a 12 percent decrease in FEV_1.[43] More importantly, $CysLT_1$ receptor antagonists protect against LTD_4-induced bronchoconstriction in asthmatic subjects (Table 65-6). Oral LY-171883 and inhaled SK&F 104353 cause a three- to four-fold shift in the dose-response curve to LTD_4.[2] In contrast, subjects that received 100 mg of zafirlukast had a 90-fold shift in the provocative concentration of LTD_4 needed to decrease the FEV_1 by 20 percent.[57]

ACUTE BRONCHODILATION

Blockade of the $CysLT_1$ receptor causes acute bronchodilation in asthmatic subjects, suggesting that leukotrienes modulate resting bronchomotor tone in asthmatic airways. After 40 mg zafirlukast administered orally, an 8 percent improvement in FEV_1 occurred 3.5 h after dosing.[58] Intravenous administration of 500 mg MK-679 caused a mean increase in FEV_1 of 15.8 percent 15 min after the end of the bolus with a mean plasma concentration of 86.2 ± 13.9 μg/ml.[44] It is interesting to note that a nonuniform response to leukotriene receptor blockade occurred with four of nine patients bronchodilating after 125 mg and six of nine after 500 mg. Thus three patients had no response even at the highest dose. The degree of bronchodilation appeared to correlate with the degree of baseline airflow obstruction.[40]

In addition, the effect of $CysLT_1$ receptor antagonists is additive with β-adrenergic receptor agonists (Fig. 65-5).

Twenty minutes after intravenous infusion of MK-571 was begun, FEV_1 increased 22 percent above baseline. Immediately following treatment with MK-571, 180 μg of inhaled albuterol caused an additional 27 percent increase in mean FEV_1. Maximal bronchodilation was significantly greater in patients receiving MK-571 and albuterol versus those treated with placebo and albuterol.[40] That bronchodilation from combined $CysLT_1$ receptor antagonism and β-adrenergic agonist receptor stimulation was additive suggests that these compounds act to decrease airflow obstruction in asthma by different mechanisms.

EFFECT ON ALLERGEN-INDUCED BRONCHOCONSTRICTION

Blockade of the $CysLT_1$ receptor unequivocally prevents the early-phase asthmatic reaction after antigen challenge. Treatment with a 20 mg oral dose of zafirlukast caused a 2.5-fold increase in the mean provocative dose of allergen that decreased FEV_1 by 20 percent ($PD_{20}FEV_1$) when measured 2 h later,[59] while in a separate study 40 mg of zafirlukast caused a 10-fold increase in the $PD_{20}FEV_1$ after allergen exposure.[60] Inhalation of 1.6 mg of zafirlukast inhibited the early but not the late phase of allergen-induced bronchoconstriction.[61] By contrast, an oral dose of 40 mg of zafirlukast and 450 mg intravenous MK-571 inhibited both the early and late asthmatic response to allergen challenge.[62,63]

EFFECT ON BRONCHIAL HYPERREACTIVITY

It recently has been demonstrated that chronic treatment with leukotriene receptor antagonists improves underlying airway hyperreactivity. In a recent study by Taki and colleagues[41] of chronic treatment with pranlukast (ONO-1078), there was a small, but significant, improvement in the response to methacholine after both 12 and 24 weeks of treatment. This finding was confirmed in a similar study with 9 days of inhaled L-648051.[38] In this study, bronchial hyperresponsiveness to inhaled methacholine was improved by 1.5 doubling dilutions at day 9. By contrast, previous studies

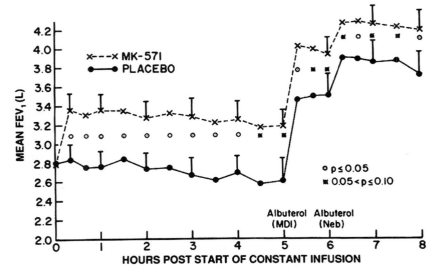

FIGURE 65-5 A comparison of the effect of intravenous MK-0571 (**x**) and placebo (closed circles) treatment and the subsequent response to inhaled and nebulized albuterol on forced expiratory volume in 1 s (FEV_1). Data are mean (±SEM) FEV_1 values (L). Alternate standard error bars have been deleted for clarity of presentation. (*Reprinted with permission from Am Rev Respir Dis 1992; 146:358–63.*[40])

using single doses of $CysLT_1$ receptor antagonists have not demonstrated improvement in airway hyperresponsiveness to histamine or methacholine.[39] This suggests that chronic leukotriene receptor blockade improves airway hyperresponsiveness by a mechanism other than simple functional antagonism of the $CysLT_1$ receptor, and concurs with recent studies of these compounds that suggest that their effects increase with time administered.[45,50]

CLINICAL EFFICACY

ASPIRIN-INDUCED BRONCHOCONSTRICTION

As with 5-lipoxygenase inhibition, blockade of the $CysLT_1$ receptor prevents aspirin-induced bronchoconstriction in sensitive subjects. Pretreatment with inhaled SK&F 104353 inhibited the response to aspirin ingestion by a mean of 47 percent.[64] An oral dose of 225 mg of the more potent leukotriene receptor blocker pranlukast increased the $PD_{20}FEV_1$ significantly in response to inhaled dipyrone.[65] In addition, analgesic-induced bronchoconstriction was completely inhibited in subjects whose plasma concentration of pranlukast was > 0.5 $\mu g/ml$. MK-0679 (750 mg orally) caused a median 4.4-fold rightward shift in the dose-response curve to inhaled lysine-aspirin for all subjects studied.[66] In a separate study, MK-0679 caused a 5 percent to 34 percent improvement in FEV_1 (average 18 percent) above pretreatment baseline in aspirin-sensitive asthmatic subjects.[67] This bronchodilator response correlated significantly with both the severity of asthma as assessed by FEV_1 and medication use and the degree of aspirin sensitivity.

EXERCISE-INDUCED ASTHMA

Several studies demonstrate that $CysLT_1$ receptor blockade protects against exercise-induced bronchoconstriction, suggesting that leukotrienes mediate this effect and that their blockade may be of benefit for patients with exercise-induced asthma.[68–70] In a study by Finnerty and colleagues,[70] 20 mg zafirlukast given orally 2 h prior to exercise challenge blocked the mean maximum percentage decrease in FEV_1 by 40 percent as compared with placebo (Fig. 65-6). Inhibition of bronchoconstriction was greatest over the latter part of the period assessed. In addition, 400 μg inhaled zafirlukast and 160 mg intravenous MK-571 blocked the mean maximal decrease in FEV_1 in response to exercise by 50 percent and 70 percent, respectively.[68,69] Makker[68] noted that protection by inhaled zafirlukast was variable in the nine subjects, with complete inhibition in three subjects, partial inhibition in three subjects and no protection in the remaining three subjects. $CysLT_1$ receptor blockade also protects against cold air–induced bronchoconstriction.[71]

CHRONIC ASTHMA

A 6-week trial of LY 171883, one of the least potent $CysLT_1$ receptor antagonists, was performed in 138 asthmatic subjects. After 6 weeks of treatment there was a 4.5 percent increase in FEV_1 versus a 2.4 percent decrease after placebo.[50] Day and nighttime wheezing and breathlessness also decreased. Greater improvement occurred in the more severely impaired patients.

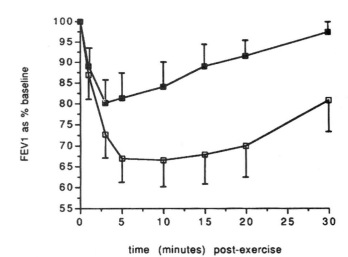

FIGURE 65-6 The mean exercise-induced bronchoconstriction (SEM) at each time point, expressed as a percentage of pre-exercise baseline forced expiratory volume in 1 s (FEV_1) over 30 min following the oral administration of placebo (open squares) and ICI 204,219 (zafirlukast) 20 mg (closed squares). (*Reprinted with permission from the Am Rev Respir Dis 1992; 145:746–749.*[70])

Spector and colleagues[45] recently reported the results of 6 weeks of therapy with oral doses of zafirlukast, a more potent $CysLT_1$ receptor antagonist, in 266 subjects with mild-to-moderate asthma. Subjects were randomized to receive zafirlukast in oral doses of 5, 10, or 20 mg twice daily or placebo. The greatest dose (40 mg per day) significantly decreased nighttime awakenings, first morning asthma symptoms, daytime asthma score, and albuterol use and increased evening peak expiratory flow rates as well as FEV_1 when compared with placebo after 4 weeks of treatment (Fig. 65-7). Compared with baseline, the 40 mg dose decreased nighttime awakenings by 46 percent, albuterol use by 30 percent, and daytime symptoms by 26 percent. Six weeks of therapy with zafirlukast increased FEV_1 by 11 percent, with most of the improvement occurring after 2 weeks of therapy. Morning peak expiratory flow rates were not significantly improved by treatment with zafirlukast. Treatment failures were significantly less in patients receiving zafirlukast (2 percent) versus placebo (10 percent).

Adverse Effects

Most studies of leukotriene synthesis inhibitors or receptor antagonists have used single doses of these compounds. More recently, studies have been published describing chronic therapy with these agents of 4 to 24 weeks duration. Overall, leukotriene synthesis inhibitors and receptor antagonists have been well-tolerated. Adverse effects from these compounds are generally mild. Headache, dyspepsia, and diarrhea are the most commonly reported side effects in clinical studies using these agents; however, headache and dyspepsia have not occurred more commonly in patients receiving study medication as compared with placebo overall.[52]

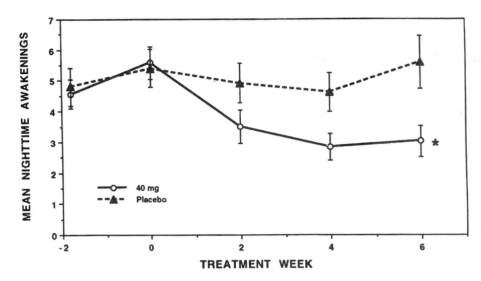

FIGURE 65-7 Mean ± SEM nighttime awakenings per week from week 2 (screening) through week 6 (endpoint) for subjects who received zafirlukast (ICI 204,219) or placebo. Treatment with 40 mg zafirlukast significantly decreased mean nighttime awakening per week as compared with placebo (*$p < .01$*). (*Reprinted with permission from the Am J Respir Crit Care Med 1994; 150:618–23.[45]*)

In the study by Israel and colleagues[27] of 4 weeks of therapy with zileuton, adverse effects were reported by equal numbers of patients in active treatment groups as in placebo groups. The most common adverse effects were headache and dyspepsia. An urticarial rash as well as increased liver function tests were noted in one patient after receiving zileuton 800 mg twice daily for 24 days. This resolved after stopping zileuton therapy. No deaths or hospitalizations were reported.

The most frequently reported side-effects in the study by Spector and colleagues[45] of 6 weeks of therapy with zafirlukast were headache, gastritis, pharyngitis, and rhinitis. None appeared to occur more frequently in patients receiving study medication versus placebo. Asymptomatic increases in SGPT levels occurred in 4 percent of subjects in both the 40 mg and placebo groups.

Specific Agents

ZILEUTON (A-64077)

Zileuton {N-(1-benzo[b]thien-2-ylethyl)-N-hydroxyurea}, formerly known as A-64077, is a potent 5-lipoxygenase inhibitor both in vitro and in vivo (Fig. 65-8; Tables 65-2 and 65-3). Zileuton has a single chiral center and is given orally as a racemic mixture with equal parts of the $R(+)$ and $S(-)$ enantiomers (data on file, Abbott Laboratories, Abbott Park, IL). As discussed in more detail above, it is thought to inhibit 5-lipoxygenase by binding to the iron atom in the 5-lipoxygenase enzyme.

PRECLINICAL PHARMACOLOGY

Preclinical studies have demonstrated that zileuton specifically and potently inhibits 5-lipoxygenase (as assessed by 5-HETE and LTB₄ synthesis) at concentrations that do not inhibit 12-lipoxygenase, 15-lipoxygenase, or cyclooxygenase.[15] As discussed above, zileuton is thought to inhibit 5-lipoxygenase by binding to iron on the active site of 5-lipoxygenase. Inhibition by zileuton was reversible, suggesting that zileuton does not covalently bind 5-LO. Zileuton inhibits 5-HETE synthesis by rat basophilic leukemia cell supernatant ($IC_{50} = 0.5$) and polymorphonuclear leukocytes ($IC_{50} = 0.3$ μM). It inhibits LTB₄ synthesis by human whole blood ($IC_{50} = 0.9$ μM). In addition, zileuton significantly decreased mouse ear edema caused by arachidonic acid ($ED_{50} = 31$ mg/kg) and reduced inflammatory leukocyte accumulation by 50 percent in the rat pleural Arthus reaction.[15]

PHARMACOKINETICS

Absorption and Bioavailability

Zileuton is well-absorbed, producing dose-dependent inhibition of LTB₄ synthesis in ex vivo blood after oral administration.[5] Leukotriene B₄ inhibition is approximately 80 percent when the zileuton plasma level is 2 μg/ml (data on file, Abbott Laboratories). Zileuton is absorbed quickly with a relatively short half-life. Zileuton manifests linear pharmacokinetics up to 2400 mg per day (600 mg four times daily). Mean pharmacokinetic parameters at steady state after oral administration of zileuton 600 mg four times daily were measured in 12 healthy adults (Table 65-7) (data on file, Abbott Laboratories). Zileuton has low aqueous solubility, which precludes intravenous administration. It will be released as film-coated tablets in 300 mg and 600 mg strengths.

It is estimated that if 100 percent of zileuton is absorbed unchanged into the portal circulation, approximately 40 percent of zileuton would be metabolized by first-pass metabolism in the liver. When 600 mg zileuton is given with food, a small but significant (27 percent) increase in mean C_{max} as compared with fasting was noted without significant changes in AUC or T_{max}. Protein binding of zileuton in human plasma varied from 92 percent to 94 percent when assessed in vitro. Zileuton was detected in the bronchoalveolar lavage fluid in both asthmatic subjects and healthy volunteers (data on file, Abbott Laboratories).

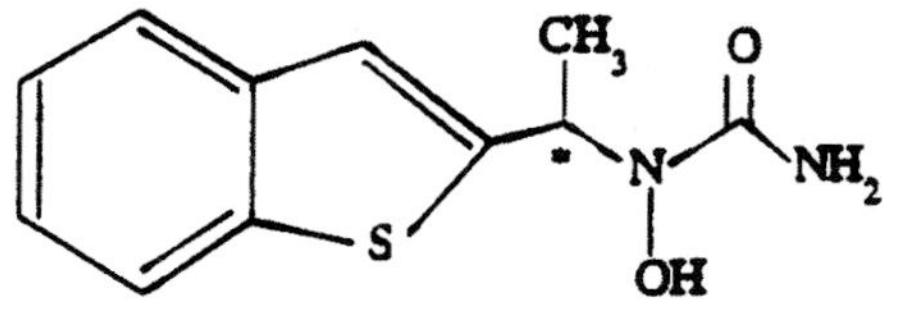

Zileuton

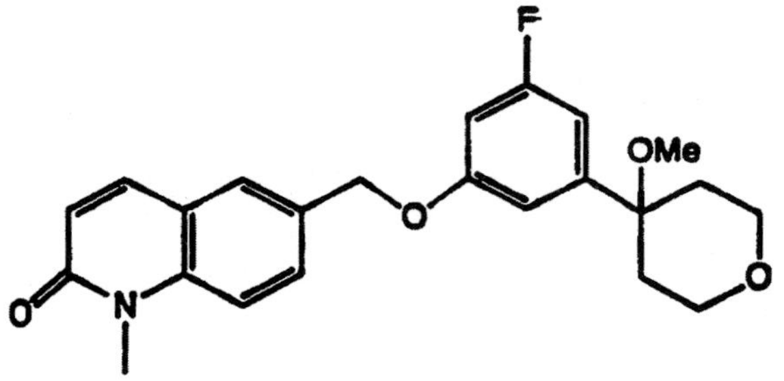

ZD2138

FIGURE 65-8 The chemical structures of the 5-lipoxygenase inhibitors zileuton (A-64077) and ZD2138. (*Reprinted with permission from Abbott Laboratories and Trends Pharmacol Sci 1992; 13:323–330.*[5])

Metabolism and Elimination

Zileuton is metabolized extensively by the liver and then excreted principally in the urine. The major metabolic pathway is O-glucuronidation to $R(+)$ and $S(-)$ zileuton glucuronides with nearly 80 percent of the dose recovered in the urine as approximately equal amounts of these $R(+)$ and $S(-)$ enantiomers. A minor metabolic pathway is N-dehydroxylation via the gut flora to A-66193, an inactive metabolite, which then is absorbed and metabolized by the liver. These metabolites and polar material account for much (8 percent) of the rest of the dose eliminated in the urine with about 2 percent being excreted in the feces (data on file, Abbott Laboratories).

TABLE 65-7   Pharmacokinetic Parameters of Zileuton at Steady State[a]

Parameter	Mean ± SD
C_{max} (μg/ml)	6.0 ± 1.0
T_{max} (h)	2.3 ± 0.6
C_{min} (μg/ml)	1.8 ± 0.6
AUC (μg•h/ml)	20.8 ± 3.4
Half-life (h)	2.5 ± 0.3
Apparent Volume of Distribution (L)	93 ± 19

SOURCE: Data on file Abbott Laboratories; $n = 12$.
[a] After administration of 600 mg four times daily in healthy human subjects.

Special Populations

Zileuton appears to be well-tolerated by both young and elderly subjects with no statistically significant difference in clearance between young (ages 20 to 40 years) and older age (ages 65 to 81 years) healthy volunteers at steady state after 600 mg zileuton every 6 h (data on file, Abbott Laboratories). Gender, race, and the presence of asthma do not seem to affect the pharmacokinetics of zileuton. Hepatic disease significantly decreases the plasma clearance of zileuton by one-half in subjects with mild or moderate liver disease (data on file, Abbott Laboratories), and zileuton thus should be administered at a reduced dose to patients with hepatic impairment. Reduction in the dose of zileuton does not appear to be necessary in patients with renal dysfunction. Zileuton pharmacokinetics are not altered by renal impairment or dialysis (data on file, Abbott Laboratories). The percentage of zileuton glucuronides recovered in the urine decreased as a function of increasing renal impairment; however, since these are thought to be pharmacologically inactive compounds, dose reduction of zileuton in renal disease is presumably not necessary.

Drug Interactions

As discussed above, zileuton is principally metabolized by glucuronidation to enantiomeric zileuton glucuronides, which suggests that zileuton can potentially interfere with drugs that share common glucuronyltransferases. In addition, there is evidence that zileuton and its metabolite A-66193 can be oxidatively metabolized by the P450 isoenzymes CYP1A2, CYP3A, and CYP2C9 and thus may interact with other drugs that are metabolized by these same isoenzymes.

Zileuton has the potential to interact with a number of commonly prescribed medications (Table 65-8). Zileuton significantly inhibits theophylline metabolism, causing mean theophylline C_{max} to increase from 12 to 21 μg/ml and mean oral theophylline clearance to decrease from 62 to 32 ml/min (data on file, Abbott Laboratories). Coadministration of zileuton and theophylline resulted in a significant increase in the number of adverse events reported in a clinical drug interaction study of these two compounds. Since zileuton reduces theophylline clearance by about one-half, the dose of theophylline must be reduced by at least 50 percent when the two drugs are given together. In addition, plasma theophylline concentrations should be followed closely.

Zileuton decreases mean clearance of oral propranolol by 42 percent (data on file, Abbott Laboratories). However, this is not likely to be encountered in asthma patients since propranolol is contraindicated. Mean clearance of R-warfarin was decreased by 15 percent in subjects also taking zileuton, resulting in a 12 percent prolongation of the prothrombin

TABLE 65-8   Drugs That May Interact with Zileuton

Theophylline
Warfarin
Terfenadine
Naproxen
Propranolol

SOURCE: Data on file, Abbott Laboratories.

time. Zileuton causes a small but statistically significant increase in plasma terfenadine concentration when these two drugs are coadministered; however, no prolongation of the QTc interval was noted on ECG. A small inhibitory effect on naproxen metabolism has been noted that is probably of no clinical significance. Drug interaction studies show that zileuton does not inhibit phenytoin, prednisone, digoxin, or sulfasalazine metabolism (data on file, Abbott Laboratories).

CLINICAL EFFICACY

Zileuton causes acute bronchodilation in subjects with pre-existing airflow obstruction. Within 1 h of oral administration of 600 mg of zileuton, 0.35 L (14.6 percent) increase in FEV_1 from baseline is observed. No effect on baseline lung function is observed in patients with very mild airflow obstruction.

Zileuton decreases cold, dry air hyperresponsiveness and thus may be beneficial for the treatment of exercise-induced asthma. A single 800 mg dose of zileuton decreases the response to cold-air bronchoprovocation by nearly 50 percent. This compares favorably with the 33 percent, 43 percent, and 32 percent improvement obtained with inhaled cromolyn sodium, terbutaline, and high-dose inhaled atropine, respectively.

Zileuton is likely to have an important role in patients with aspirin sensitivity. One week of therapy with zileuton 600 mg four times daily completely blocks aspirin-induced airflow obstruction, nasal, gastrointestinal, and dermal symptoms that occur after aspirin ingestion in sensitive patients.

Chronic therapy with zileuton is beneficial in patients with mild-to-moderate asthma. A dose- and time-related improvement in FEV_1 and decrease in β-adrenergic agonist use have been noted with chronic zileuton therapy. Chronic zileuton therapy improves FEV_1 by 13 percent at 4 weeks, and this improvement had not plateaued by the end of the study. A dose of zileuton of 600 mg four times daily or 2.4 g/day is superior to 800 mg twice daily or 1.6 g/day. In addition, chronic zileuton therapy improves morning and evening peak expiratory flow rates and daytime asthma symptoms.

At present, zileuton has undergone extensive clinical evaluation. A new drug application was recently filed with the U.S. Food and Drug Administration. It will be released as 300 mg and 600 mg tablets to be given four times daily.

ZD2138

ZD2138 (formerly ICI D2138; 6-[[3-fluoro-5-(4-methoxy-3,4,5,6-tetrahydro-2*H*-pyran-4-yl)phenoxy]methyl]-1-methylquinol-2-one) is a potent, long-acting 5-lipoxygenase inhibitor both in vitro and in vivo (Fig. 65-8; Table 65-3). ZD2138 is an achiral compound that is thought to cause enantioselective inhibition of the 5-lipoxygenase enzyme by nonredox mechanisms. Preclinical studies have demonstrated that ZD2138 selectively inhibits 5-lipoxygenase.[16] It inhibits human blood synthesis of LTB_4 in vitro with an IC_{50} of 0.02 μ*M* versus 2.6 μ*M* for zileuton (Table 65-3).[20] ZD2138 caused a dose-dependent inhibition of bronchoconstriction after antigen challenge in guinea-pigs.

At present, clinical experience with ZD2138 is rather limited. It has been given to normal volunteers and was well-tolerated at single doses up to 1 g.[72] Doses as low as 100 mg significantly inhibited LTB_4 synthesis in blood ex vivo. After single doses of 350 mg or greater, maximal inhibition of leukotriene synthesis occurred for at least 24 h. The half-life of ZD2138 in normal volunteers is about 12 h. Preliminary clinical studies in asthmatic subjects suggest that 350 mg ZD2138 blocks cold air–induced bronchoconstriction for up to 24 h.[31] ZD2138 is currently undergoing phase II clinical trials in asthma.

ZAFIRLUKAST (ICI 204,219)

Zafirlukast [4-(5-cyclopentyloxycarbonylamino-1methylindol-3-ylmethyl)-3-methoxy-*n*-*o*-tolylsulfonyl benzamide], formerly known as ICI 204,219, is a potent $CysLT_1$ receptor antagonist both in vitro and in vivo (Fig. 65-9; Tables 65-5 and 65-6). Both oral and inhaled preparations have been studied, with oral administration the most extensively studied.

PRECLINICAL PHARMACOLOGY

As discussed above, zafirlukast is a competitive antagonist of LTD_4 ($pK_B = 8.6$) and LTE_4 ($pK_B = 9.7$) induced contraction of guinea-pig lung trachea and human airways.[54] It did not antagonize LTC_4-elicited contraction when the metabolism of LTC_4 to D_4 and E_4 was inhibited. It is a competitive receptor antagonist and does not bind other receptors even at high concentrations. It is effective orally, intravenously, or

FIGURE 65-9 The chemical structure of the cysteinyl leukotriene₁ receptor antagonist zafirlukast (ICI 204,219) and pranlukast (ONO-1078). (*Reprinted with permission from Zeneca Pharmaceuticals and the Jpn J Pharmacol 1992; 60:227–237.*[55])

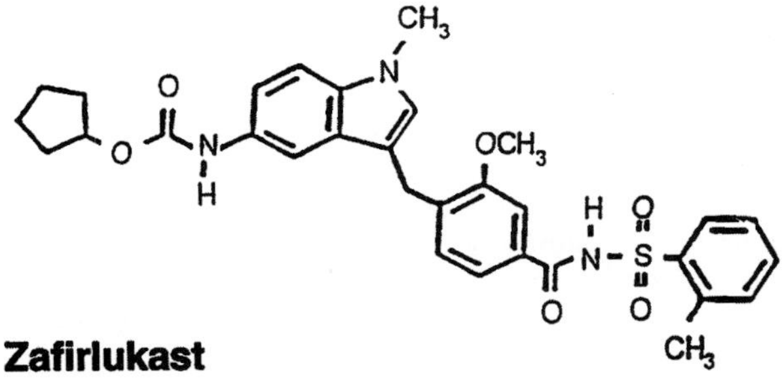

Zafirlukast

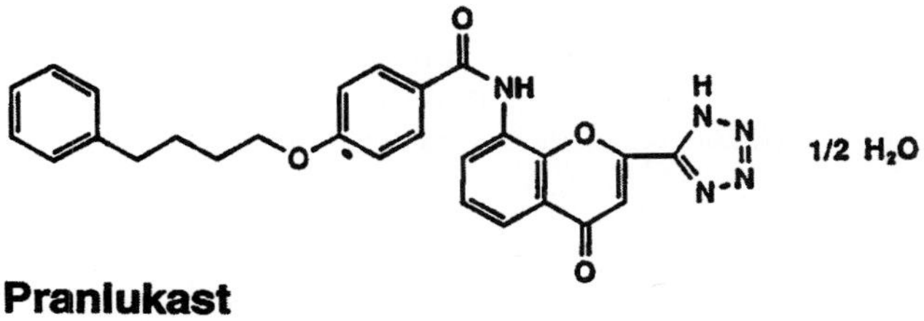

Pranlukast

by aerosol with ED_{50} values of 0.52 $\mu M/kg$, 0.046 $\mu M/kg$, and 5.1×10^{-6} M, respectively.

PHARMACOKINETICS

Absorption and Bioavailability

Peak plasma concentrations are achieved after oral administration of zafirlukast tablets in approximately 3 h (data on file, Zeneca Pharmaceuticals, Wilmington, DE). The half-life of zafirlukast is 10 h with twice-daily dosing, resulting in minimal accumulation of the drug. Steady-state plasma concentrations of zafirlukast occur after 3 days of therapy. Time- and dose-dependent changes in the pharmacokinetics of zafirlukast were not observed in 14-day trials with doses up to 80 mg twice daily of zafirlukast (data on file, Zeneca Pharmaceuticals).

Metabolism and Elimination

Zafirlukast is well-absorbed after oral administration (data on file, Zeneca Pharmaceuticals, Wilmington, DE). The administration of zafirlukast with food may reduce the absorption in some subjects. Zafirlukast undergoes extensive biotransformation, with excretion of metabolites primarily through the feces. Urinary excretion of metabolites accounts for 10 percent of the dose. Within clinically relevant ranges of plasma concentrations, the plasma protein binding of zafirlukast is 99 percent. Zafirlukast is excreted in breast milk.

Special Populations

The pharmacokinetics of zafirlukast are the same in normal volunteers and adult subjects with asthma (data on file, Zeneca Pharmaceuticals). Renal impairment does not alter the pharmacokinetics of zafirlukast. Plasma concentrations are increased by approximately twofold in the elderly, compared with healthy adult subjects receiving the same dose. Hepatic impairment may increase drug levels as measured by C_{max} and AUC when compared with matched controls.

Drug Interactions

Zafirlukast does not alter the pharmacokinetics of orally administered theophylline or oral contraceptive steroids (data on file, Zeneca Pharmaceuticals). Coadministration of zafirlukast and erythromycin decreased the absorption of zafirlukast while coadministration of zafirlukast with aspirin increased zafirlukast plasma concentrations by an unknown mechanism.

CLINICAL EFFICACY

Zafirlukast does not cause significant acute bronchodilation. Protection (> 100-fold) against LTD_4-induced bronchoconstriction in normal volunteers was obtained with a single oral 40 mg dose of zafirlukast, with doses of 10 mg, 40 mg, and 100 mg providing 10-fold protection in asthmatic subjects. In addition, 40 mg of oral zafirlukast blocks bronchoconstriction caused by platelet-activating factor in normal subjects.[73]

Zafirlukast inhibits the early response to inhaled allergen in numerous studies. Studies demonstrating protection against the late asthmatic response are less conclusive. There is considerable evidence that zafirlukast provides significant protection against exercise-induced bronchoconstriction after a single oral dose of 20 mg or 400 μg by inhalation. Protection did not occur in one-third of the subjects receiving inhaled zafirlukast, suggesting that protection is not universal.

Chronic therapy with zafirlukast is efficacious in patients with mild-to-moderate asthma. In a study of therapy with oral doses of zafirlukast of 5 mg, 10 mg, or 20 mg twice daily or placebo,[45] 6 weeks of treatment with the highest dose (40 mg per day) significantly decreased nighttime awakenings by 46 percent, daytime asthma score by 26 percent, and albuterol use by 30 percent and increased evening peak expiratory flow rates when compared with baseline. In addition, mean FEV_1 increased by 11 percent as compared with baseline.

Zafirlukast has been studied extensively, and a new drug application has been filed with the U.S. Food and Drug Administration. Its long duration of action may be of particular benefit in patients with nighttime asthma symptoms.

PRANLUKAST (ONO 1078)

Pranlukast (ONO-1078; 4-oxo-8-[4-(4-phenylbutoxy)benzoylamino]-2-(tetrazol-5-yl)-4H-1-benzopyran hemihydrate), is a relatively new potent and selective competitive $CysLT_1$ receptor antagonist (Fig. 65-9). In guinea-pig trachea and lung parenchymal strips, pranlukast competitively antagonized LTC_4- and LTD_4-induced contractions with a pA_2 range of 7.70 to 10.71.[55] When bioconversion of LTC_4 to LTD_4 was prevented, pranlukast remained a potent antagonist of LTC_4-induced contractions ($pA_2 = 7.78$). Pranlukast did not antagonize histamine, acetylcholine, 5-hydroxytryptamine, prostaglandin D_2, or U-46619, and had minimal effect on the activities of cyclooxygenase, 5-lipoxygenase, or thromboxane synthetase.

Recent studies document the clinical efficacy of pranlukast in patients with analgesic-induced asthma and for chronic therapy of patients with mild-to-moderate asthma. Taki and colleagues[41] gave eleven subjects 450 mg of pranlukast twice daily for 24 weeks. Asthma symptom score and supplemental inhaled β-adrenergic agonist use decreased significantly by 2 weeks, FEV_1 significantly improved 12 weeks after treatment, histamine responsiveness also improved, but not until the end of the study.

Conclusion

Current clinical evidence suggests that leukotriene synthesis inhibition and receptor blockade will be useful in the treatment of asthma. They are effective against acute challenge and for chronic therapy of asthma in most patients. These compounds may prove especially beneficial in patients with aspirin sensitivity. A small subset of patients are not protected against cold-air challenge, exercise-induced bronchoconstriction, and allergen challenge by these compounds. It is possible that the development of even more potent compounds will improve their efficacy. In addition, since they work by blocking a unique class of mediators, their effects may be additive when used with existing asthma medication. At present they do not appear to have significant side effects.

References

1. Lewis RA, Austen KF, Soberman RJ: Leukotrienes and other products of the 5-lipoxygenase pathway: biochemistry and relation to pathobiology in human diseases. *N Engl J Med* 1990; 323:645–655.

2. Drazen JM: Leukotrienes, in Busse W, Holgate ST (eds): *Asthma and Rhinitis*. Cambridge, Eng, Blackwell Scientific, 1995:838–850.

3. Ford-Hutchinson AW, Bray MA, Doig MV, et al.: Leukotriene B, a potent chemokinetic and aggregating substance released from polymorphonuclear leukocytes. *Nature* 1980; 286:264–265.

4. Nagy L, Lee TH, Goetzl EJ, et al.: Complement receptor enhancement and chemotaxis of human neutrophils and eosinophils by leukotrienes and other lipoxygenase products. *Clin Exp Immunol* 1982; 47:541–547.

5. McMillan RM, Walker ERH: Designing therapeutically effective 5-lipoxygenase inhibitors. *Trends Pharmacol Sci* 1992; 13:323–330.

6. Hay DWP, Griswold DE: Inhibitors of fatty acid-derived mediators, in Cunningham FM (eds): *Lipid Mediators*. San Diego, Academic Press, 1994:117–179.

7. Hui KP, Lötvall J, Chung KF, Barnes PJ: Attenuation of inhaled allergen-induced airway microvascular leakage and airflow obstruction in guinea pigs by a 5-lipoxygenase inhibitor (A-63162). *Am Rev Respir Dis* 1991; 143:1015–1019.

8. Bell RL, Bouska J, Young PR, et al.: The properties of A-69412: a small hydrophilic 5-lipoxygenase inhibitor. *Agents Actions* 1993; 38:178–187.

9. Bell RL, Brooks DW, Young PR, et al.: A-78773: a selective, potent 5-lipoxygenase inhibitor. *J Lipid Mediat* 1993; 6:259–264.

10. Wegner CD, Gundel RH, Abraham WM, et al.: The role of 5-lipoxygenase products in preclinical models of asthma. *J Allergy Clin Immunol* 1993; 91:917–929.

11. Higgs GA, Flower RJ, Vane JR: A new approach to anti-inflammatory drugs. *Biochem Pharmacol* 1979; 28:1959–1961.

12. Fujimura M, Sasaki F, Nakatsumi Y, et al.: Effects of a thromboxane synthetase inhibitor (OKY-046) and a lipoxygenase inhibitor (AA-861) on bronchial responsiveness to acetylcholine in asthmatic subjects. *Thorax* 1986; 41:955–959.

13. Batt DG, Maynard GD, Petraitis JJ, et al.: 2-Substituted-1-naphthols as potent 5-lipoxygenase inhibitors with topical antiinflammatory activity. *J Med Chem* 1990; 33:360–370.

14. Mann JS, Robinson C, Sheridan AQ, et al.: Effect of inhaled piriprost (U-60,257) a novel leukotriene inhibitor, on allergen and exercise induced bronchoconstriction in asthma. *Thorax* 1986; 41:746–752.

15. Carter GW, Young PR, Albert DH, et al.: 5-lipoxygenase inhibitory activity of zileuton. *J Pharmacol Exp Ther* 1991; 256:929–937.

16. McMillan RM, Spruce KE, Crawley GC, et al.: Pre-clinical pharmacology of ICI D2138, a potent orally-active non-redox inhibitor of 5-lipoxygenase. *Brit J Pharmacol* 1992; 107:1042–1047.

17. Henderson WR: The role of leukotrienes in inflammation. *Ann Intern Med* 1994; 121:684–697.

18. Riendeau D, Falgueyret JP, Guay J, et al.: Pseudoperoxidase activity of 5-lipoxygenase stimulated by potent benzofuranol and N-hydroxyurea inhibitors of the lipoxygenase reaction. *Biochem J* 1991; 274:287–292.

19. McMillan RM, Girodeau JM, Foster SJ: Selective chiral inhibitors of 5-lipoxygenase with anti-inflammatory activity. *Br J Pharmacol* 1990; 101:501–503.

20. Crawley GC, Dowell RI, Edwards PN, et al.: Methoxy-tetrahydropyrans. A new series of selective and orally potent 5-lipoxygenase inhibitors. *J Med Chem* 1992; 35:2600–2609.

21. Hatzelmann A, Fruchtmann R, Rohrs KH, et al.: Mode of action of the new selective leukotriene synthesis inhibitor BAY X 1005{(R)-2-[4-(quinolin-2-yl-methoxy)phenyl]-2-cyclopentyl acetic acid} and structurally related compunds. *Biochem Pharmacol* 1993; 45:101–111.

22. Friedman BS, Bel EH, Buntinx A, et al.: Oral leukotriene inhibitor (MK-886) blocks allergen-induced airway responses. *Am Rev Respir Dis* 1993; 147:839–844.

23. Prasit P, Belley M, Blouin M, et al.: A new class of leukotriene biosynthesis inhibitor: the development of MK-0591. *J Lipid Mediat* 1993; 6:239–244.

24. Anderson G, Fennessy M: Effects of REV 5901, a 5-lipoxygenase inhibitor and leukotriene antagonist, on pulmonary responses to platelet activating factor in the guinea-pig. *Br J Pharmacol* 1988; 94:1115–1122.

25. Grimes D, Sturm RJ, Marinari LR, et al.: WY-50,295 tromethamine, a novel, orally active 5-lipoxygenase inhibitor: biochemical characterization and antiallergic activity. *Eur J Pharmacol* 1993; 236:217–228.

26. Abraham WM, Ahmed A, Cortes A, et al.: The 5-lipoxygenase inhibitor zileuton blocks antigen-induced late airway responses, inflammation and airway hyperresponsiveness in allergic sheep. *Eur J Pharmacol* 1992; 217:119–126.

27. Israel E, Rubin P, Kemp JP, et al.: The effect of inhibition of 5-lipoxygenase by zileuton in mild-to-moderate asthma. *Ann Intern Med* 1993; 119:1059–1066.

28. Israel E, Dermarkarian R, Rosenberg M, et al.: The effects of a 5-lipoxygenase inhibitor on asthma induced by cold, dry air. *N Engl J Med* 1990; 323:1740–1744.

29. Hui KP, Taylor IK, Taylor GW, et al.: Effect of a 5-lipoxygenase inhibitor on leukotriene generation and airway responses after allergen challenge in asthmatic patients. *Thorax* 1991; 46:184–189.

30. Wempe JB, Postma DS, Breederveld N, et al.: Separate and combined effects of corticosteroids and bronchodilators on airflow obstruction and airway hyperresponsiveness in asthma. *J Allergy Clin Immunol* 1992; 89:679–687.

31. Strek ME, Solway J, Saller L, et al.: Effect of the 5-lipoxygenase inhibitor, ZD2138, on cold-air-induced bronchoconstriction in patients with asthma. *Am J Respir Crit Care Med* 1995; 151:A377.

32. Lee TH: Mechanism of bronchospasm in aspirin-sensitive asthma. *Am Rev Respir Dis* 1993; 148:1442–1443.

33. Israel E, Fischer AR, Rosenberg MA, et al.: The pivotal role of 5-lipoxygenase products in the reaction of aspirin-sensitive asthmatics to aspirin. *Am Rev Respir Dis* 1993; 148:1447–1451.

34. Sugasawa T, Morooka S: Effect of BRL-35135 on LTB_4-induced guinea pig eosinophil chemotaxis. *Agents Actions* 1992; 37:232–237.

35. Kishikawa K, Tateishi N, Maruyama T, et al.: ONO-4057, a novel, orally active leukotriene B_4 antagonist: effects on LTB_4-induced neutrophil functions. *Prostaglandins* 1992; 44:261–275.

36. Richards IM, Griffin RL, Oostveen JA, et al.: Effect of the selective leukotriene B_4 antagonist U-75302 on antigen-induced bronchopulmonary eosinophilia in sensitized guinea pigs. *Am Rev Respir Dis* 1989; 140:1712–1716.

37. Lee TH, Walport MJ, Wilkinson AH, et al.: Slow-reacting substance of anaphylaxis antagonist FPL 55712 in chronic asthma. *Lancet* 1981; 2ii:304–305.

38. Rasmussen JB, Eriksson LO, Tagari P, et al.: Reduced nonspecific bronchial reactivity and decreased airway response to antigen challenge in atopic asthmatic patients treated with the inhaled leukotriene D_4 antagonist, L-648,051. *Allergy* 1992; 47:604–609.

39. Barnes N, Piper PJ, Costello J: The effect of an oral leukotriene antagonist L-649,923 on histamine and leukotriene D_4-induced bronchoconstriction in normal man. *J Allergy Clin Immunol* 1987; 79:816–821.

40. Gaddy JN, Margolskee DJ, Bush RK, et al.: Bronchodilation with a potent and selective leukotriene D_4 (LTD_4) receptor antagonist (MK-571) in patients with asthma. *Am Rev Respir Dis* 1992; 146:358–363.

41. Taki F, Suzuki R, Torii K, et al.: Reduction of the severity of bronchial hyperresponsiveness by the novel leukotriene antagonist 4-oxo-8-[4-(4-phenyl-butoxy)benzoylamino]-2-(tetrazol-5-yl)-4H-1-benzopyran hemihydrate. *Drug Res* 1994; 44:330–332.

42. Hay DWP, Muccitelli RM, Tucker SS, et al.: Pharmacologic profile of SK&F 104353: a novel, potent and selective peptidoleukotriene receptor antagonist in guinea pig and human airways. *J Pharmacol Exp Ther* 1987; 243:474–481.

43. Phillips GD, Rafferty P, Robinson C, Holgate ST: Dose-related antagonism of leukotriene D_4-induced bronchoconstriction by p.o. administration of LY-171883 in nonasthmatic subjects. *J Pharmacol Exp Ther* 1988; 246:732–738.

44. Impens N, Reiss TF, Teahan JA, et al.: Acute bronchodilation with an intravenously administered leukotriene D_4 antagonist, MK-679. *Am Rev Respir Dis* 1993; 147:1442–1446.

45. Spector SL, Smith LJ, Glass M, and the Accolate™ Asthma Trialists Group: Effects of 6 weeks of therapy with oral doses of ICI 204,219, a leukotriene D_4 receptor antagonist, in subjects with bronchial asthma. *Am J Respir Crit Care Med* 1994; 150:618–623.

46. Buckner CK, Krell RD, Laravuso RB, et al.: Pharmacological evidence that human intralobar airways do not contain different receptors that mediate contractions to leukotriene C_4 and leukotriene D_4. *J Pharmacol Exp Ther* 1986; 237:558–562.

47. Buckner CK, Saban R, Castleman WL, Will JA: Analysis of leukotriene receptor antagonists on isolated human intralobar airways. *Ann N Y Acad Sci* 1988; 524:181–186.

48. Rovati GE, Giovanazzi S, Mezzetti M, Nicosia S: Heterogeneity of binding sites for ICI 198,615 in human lung parenchyma. *Biochem Pharmacol* 1992; 44:1411–1415.

49. Aharony D, Catanese CA, Falcone RC: Kinetic and pharmacologic analysis of [³H]leukotriene E_4 binding to receptors on guinea pig lung membranes: evidence for selective binding to a subset of leukotriene D_4 receptors. *J Pharmacol Exp Ther* 1989; 248:581–588.

50. Cloud ML, Enas GC, Kemp J et al.: A specific LTD_4/LTE_4-receptor antagonist improves pulmonary function in patients with mild, chronic asthma. *Am Rev Respir Dis* 1989; 140:1336–1339.

51. Aharony D, Krell RD: Pharmacology of peptide leukotriene receptor antagonists. *Ann N Y Acad Sci* 1991; 629:125–132.

52. Chanarin N, Johnston SL: Leukotrienes as a target in asthma therapy. *Drugs* 1994; 47:12–24.

53. Jones TR, Zamboni R, Belley M, et al.: Pharmacology of L-660,711 (MK-571): a novel potent and selective leukotriene D_4 receptor antagonist. *Can J Physiol Pharmacol* 1989; 67:17–28.

54. Krell RD, Aharony D, Buckner CK, et al.: The preclinical pharmacology of ICI 204,219. *Am Rev Respir Dis* 1990; 141:978–987.

55. Obata T, Okada Y, Motoishi M, et al.: In vitro antagonism of ONO-1078, a newly developed anti-asthma agent, against peptide leukotrienes in isolated guinea pig tissues. *Jpn J Pharmacol* 1992; 60:227–237.

56. Smith LJ, Geller S, Ebright L, et al.: Inhibition of leukotriene D_4-induced bronchoconstriction in normal subjects by the oral LTD_4 receptor antagonist ICI 204,219. *Am Rev Respir Dis* 1990; 141: 988–992.

57. Smith LJ, Glass M, Minkwitz MC: Inhibition of leukotriene D_4-induced bronchoconstriction in subjects with asthma: a concentration-effect study of ICI 204,219. *Clin Pharmacol Ther* 1993; 54: 430–436.

58. Hui KP, Barnes NC: Lung function improvement in asthma with a cysteinyl-leukotriene receptor antagonist. *Lancet* 1991; 337: 1062–1063.

59. Dahlén B, Zetterström O, Björck T, Dahlén SE: The leukotriene-antagonist ICI-204,219 inhibits the early airway reaction to cumulative bronchial challenge with allergen in atopic asthmatics. *Eur Respir J* 1994; 7:324–331.

60. Findlay SR, Barden JM, Easley CB, Glass M: Effect of the oral leukotriene antagonist, ICI 204,219, on antigen-induced bronchoconstriction in subjects with asthma. *J Allergy Clin Immunol* 1992; 89:1040–1045.

61. O'Shaughnessy KM, Taylor IK, O'Connor B, et al.: Potent leukotriene D_4 receptor antagonist ICI 204,219 given by the inhaled route inhibits the early but not the late phase of allergen-induced bronchoconstriction. *Am Rev Respir Dis* 1993; 147: 1431–1435.

62. Taylor IK, O'Shaughnessy KM, Fuller RW, Dollery CT: Effect of cysteinyl-leukotriene receptor antagonist ICI 204,219 on allergen-induced bronchoconstriction and airway hyperreactivity in atopic subjects. *Lancet* 1991; 337:690–694.

63. Rasmussen JB, Eriksson LO, Margolskee DJ, et al.: Leukotriene D_4 receptor blockade inhibits the immediate and late bronchoconstrictor responses to inhaled antigen in patients with asthma. *J Allergy Clin Immunol* 1992; 90:193–201.

64. Christie PE, Smith CM, Lee TH: The potent and selective sulfidopeptide leukotriene antagonist, SK&F 104353, inhibits aspirin-induced asthma. *Am Rev Respir Dis* 1991; 144:957–958.

65. Yamamoto H, Nagata M, Kuramitsu K, et al.: Inhibition of analgesic-induced asthma by leukotriene receptor antagonist ONO-1078. *Am J Respir Crit Care Med* 1994; 150:254–257.

66. Dahlén B, Kumlin M, Margolskee DJ, et al.: The leukotriene-receptor antagonist MK-0679 blocks airway obstruction induced by inhaled lysine-aspirin in aspirin-sensitive asthmatics. *Eur Respir J* 1993; 6:1018–1026.

67. Dahlén B, Margolskee DJ, Zetterström O, Dahlén SE: Effect of the leukotriene receptor antagonist MK-0679 on baseline pulmonary function in aspirin sensitive asthmatic subjects. *Thorax* 1993; 48:1205–1210.

68. Makker HK, Lau LC, Thomson HW, et al.: The protective effect of inhaled leukotriene D_4 receptor antagonist ICI 204,219 against exercise-induced asthma. *Am Rev Respir Dis* 1993; 147:1413–1418.

69. Manning PJ, Watson RM, Margolskee DJ, et al.: Inhibition of exercise-induced bronchoconstriction by MK-571, a potent leukotriene D_4-receptor antagonist. *N Engl J Med* 1990; 323: 1736–1739.

70. Finnerty JP, Wood-Baker R, Thomson H, Holgate ST: Role of leukotrienes in exercise-induced asthma. *Am Rev Respir Dis* 1992; 145:746–749.

71. Israel E, Juniper EF, Callaghan JT, et al.: Effect of a leukotriene antagonist, LY171883, on cold air-induced bronchoconstriction in asthmatics. *Am Rev Respir Dis* 1989; 140:1348–1353.

72. Yates RA, McMillan RM, Ellis SH, et al.: A new non redox 5-lipoxygenase inhibitor ICI D2138 is well tolerated and inhibits blood leukotriene synthesis in healthy volunteers. *Am Rev Respir Dis* 1992; 145:A745.

73. Kidney JC, Ridge SM, Chung KF, Barnes PJ: Inhibition of platelet-activating factor–induced bronchoconstriction by the leukotriene D_4 receptor antagonist ICI 204,219. *Am Rev Respir Dis* 1993; 147:215–217.

Chapter 66

THROMBOXANE SYNTHETASE INHIBITORS AND RECEPTOR ANTAGONISTS IN ASTHMA

MARY E. STREK

Introduction

Interest in specific pathway antagonists as a treatment for asthma has flourished in recent years. Experimental evidence suggests that prostaglandins and thromboxanes may cause airway smooth muscle contraction, airway hyperresponsiveness, and inflammatory cell chemotaxis, similar to that noted in asthmatic subjects. The biochemistry and biologic effects of prostaglandins and thromboxanes and their role as potential mediators of asthma were discussed in Chap. 12. Unfortunately, while theoretically appealing, no prostaglandin receptor antagonists are under active clinical investigation, and inhibition of cyclooxygenase results in bronchospasm in a significant percentage of asthmatic subjects (see Chap. 70). Of more clinical relevance are new pharmacologic agents that either inhibit the synthesis or block the effects of thromboxane A_2 (TXA_2). In this chapter, the preclinical pharmacology of thromboxane synthetase inhibitors and receptor antagonists is discussed. Preliminary clinical studies in asthmatic patients show that these compounds may block the acute asthmatic response to allergen and exercise challenge and improve airway hyperresponsiveness to contractile stimuli. At present, these compounds are in the early stages of development, and long-term studies have not been conducted.

Thromboxane Synthetase Inhibitors

Thromboxane synthetase catalyzes the conversion of the endoperoxide prostaglandin H_2 (PGH_2), a derivative of arachidonic acid, to TXA_2, which then is rapidly degraded to thromboxane B_2 (TXB_2) (Fig. 66-1).[1,2] Because the biologic effects of TXA_2 are short lived, the use of synthetic endoperoxides that mimic the effects of TXA_2 and measurement of its inactive and stable metabolite TXB_2 have been helpful in evaluating the role of TXA_2 in pulmonary diseases.[3] Experimental evidence suggests that TXA_2 causes airway smooth muscle contraction, hyperresponsiveness, exudation of plasma, and smooth muscle cell proliferation.[2–5] It is released from the lung tissue of atopic asthmatic subjects after allergen stimulation[3] with increased amounts of TXB_2 measured in bronchoalveolar lavage fluid[6] and urine of allergic asthmatic subjects after bronchial challenge with antigen.[7] Urinary excretion of metabolites of TXA_2 is increased significantly in patients with severe acute asthma.[8] Evidence suggests that leukotriene-mediated bronchoconstriction may occur, at least in part, through synthesis of TXA_2.[9] Unfortunately, despite preclinical studies demonstrating the effectiveness of thromboxane synthetase inhibitors, results of clinical studies have been disappointing because of the short duration of action of these compounds

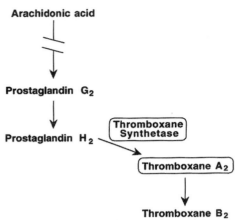

FIGURE 66-1 Schema of the sites at which inhibition of thromboxane synthesis or receptor blockade can occur. Thromboxane synthesis can be blocked by drugs that inhibit the thromboxane synthetase enzyme. Distal blockade of the effects of thromboxane occurs with compounds that antagonize the effects of thromboxane A_2 (and perhaps its precursor prostaglandin H_2) through the thromboxane A_2 receptor.

TABLE 66-1 Representative Inhibitors or Antagonists of Thromboxane A_2

Compound	Reference
Thromboxane synthetase inhibitors	
CGS 13080	10
CV 4151	11
Dazoxiben (UK-37, 248)	12
DP-1904	13
OKY-046	14
OKY-1581	15
Thromboxane receptor antagonists	
AA-2414	27
AH19437	28
AH 23848	29
BAY U 3405	30
EP092	29
GR32191	31
ICI 192605	4
ONO-3708	32
ONO NT-126	33
S-1452	33
SQ 29548	15

and the ability of the precursor endoperoxide PGH_2 to mimic the biologic activity of TXA_2 through interaction with the TXA_2 receptor.

PRECLINICAL PHARMACOLOGY

MECHANISM OF ACTION AND POTENCY

In recent years, a variety of compounds have been synthesized that prevent the formation of TXA_2 by inhibiting the thromboxane synthetase enzyme (see Fig. 66-1). A list of representative thromboxane synthetase inhibitors can be found in Table 66-1.[10–15] Many of the more recently developed compounds are imidazole derivatives; these include dazoxiben (UK-37,248), DP-1904, and OKY-046 (Fig. 66-2). Most other potent thromboxane synthetase inhibitors are substituted pyridines such as OKY-1581 and CV 4151 (see Fig. 66-2). CGS 13080 is a selective thromboxane synthetase inhibitor that contains an imidazopyridine ring.[16] The precise molecular mechanism of action of these compounds is unknown. Inhibitors of thromboxane synthetase were designed to decrease selectively the synthesis of TXA_2; however, a problem with these compounds is that they do not decrease the synthesis of PGH_2, a TXA_2 precursor that can mimic the biologic effects of TXA_2.[1]

The potency of these compounds has been studied both in vitro and in vivo. They are potent inhibitors of thromboxane synthetase with a concentration that produces 50 percent inhibition (IC_{50}) of thromboxane synthetase of 3 to 50 nM for most compounds (Table 66-2).[1,16–18] CGS 13080 selectively inhibited cell-free human platelet thromboxane synthetase with an IC_{50} of 3 nM.[16] It effectively blocked the formation of TXB_2, while prostaglandin E_2 (PGE_2) production increased, suggesting diversion of endoperoxide to PGE_2. CV 4151 has an IC_{50} of 26 nM for inhibiting horse platelet microsomal TXA_2 synthetase and little effect on cyclooxygenase.[17]

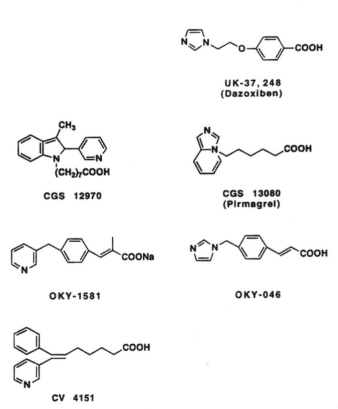

FIGURE 66-2 Names and chemical structures of representative thromboxane synthetase inhibitors. (*From Hay,*[1] *with permission.*)

TABLE 66-2   Inhibitory Effects of Thromboxane Synthetase Inhibitors on Thromboxane A_2 Production by Platelet Thromboxane Synthetase

Compound	IC_{50} (nM)
CGS 13080	3
CV 4151	26
Dazoxiben (UK-37, 248)	28

Dazoxiben was more potent than OKY-1581 in inhibiting the conversion of PGH_2 into TXA_2 by microsomes from guinea pig lung.[18]

EFFICACY IN EXPERIMENTAL MODELS

Preclinical studies show that thromboxane synthetase inhibition blocks bronchoconstriction caused by allergen, arachidonic acid, and leukotrienes in conjunction with decreased synthesis of TXB_2 in experimental models. Oral administration of OKY-046 or CV 4151 1 h before antigen challenge reduced the immediate bronchoconstrictor response to antigen challenge in sensitized guinea pigs in vivo; only OKY-046 reduced the late airway response.[11] Intravenous infusion of OKY-046 inhibited the late antigen-induced airway hyperresponsiveness to acetylcholine in ragweed-sensitized dogs.[19] There was no effect on acute antigen-induced bronchoconstriction or neutrophil influx. DP-1904 inhibited antigen-induced bronchoconstriction in sensitized guinea pigs for 12 h and bronchoconstriction caused by leukotriene D_4, arachidonic acid, platelet-activating factor, or bradykinin in nonsensitized guinea pigs.[13] Dazoxiben inhibited increased transpulmonary pressure and lung resistance caused by arachidonic acid release after calcium ionophore administration in cats in vivo.[12] Administration of OKY-1581 inhibited increased airway resistance in response to leukotrienes C_4 and D_4 in guinea pigs in vivo[20] and arachidonic acid but not PGH_2 in cats in vivo.[14] OKY-046 inhibited bronchoconstriction caused by peptidoleukotrienes in guinea pig bronchial smooth muscle strips and lung parenchyma and in vivo.[21-23]

HUMAN CLINICAL PHARMACOLOGY

EFFECT ON AIRWAY HYPERRESPONSIVENESS

Given orally or by inhalation, OKY-046 inhibited the increased responsiveness to cholinergic stimulation characteristic of asthmatic patients. In 8 asthmatic subjects, the provocative concentration of methacholine causing a 20 percent fall in forced expiratory volume in 1 s (PC_{20}-FEV_1) was measured before and after oral administration of 200 mg qid OKY-046 for 4 days and 200 mg on the morning of testing.[14] OKY-046 did not affect baseline FEV_1 or forced vital capacity; however, it caused the geometric mean value of PC_{20}-FEV_1 to increase significantly from 1.78 to 4.27 mg/mL with no change in normal subjects. In a similar fashion, aerosol administration of OKY-046 (100 mg/day) for 4 days significantly increased PC_{20}-FEV_1 in 10 asthmatic subjects.[24]

EFFECT ON ALLERGEN- AND EXERCISE-INDUCED BRONCHOCONSTRICTION

In a study of four atopic asthmatic subjects, 200 mg of OKY-046 given orally 1 h before and 1, 4, and 8 h after antigen challenge, inhibited both the early and late asthmatic response by 56 and 39 percent, respectively.[25] This was associated with a substantial decrease in TXB_2 concentrations. In a more recent study, CGS 13080 was given orally in a dose of 200 mg qid for 2 days before, the day of, and the day after allergen inhalation in 12 atopic asthmatic subjects.[10] Pretreatment with CGS 13080 inhibited increased serum TXB_2 levels before and up to 24 h after allergen challenge. There was a significant decrease in the early asthmatic response after allergen challenge, but the effect was small. Administration of CGS 13080 did not block the late asthmatic response or affect either baseline or postchallenge histamine responsiveness. Oral administration of OKY-046 in a dose of 200 mg qid for 6.5 days inhibited exercise-induced asthma in 7 of 11 asthmatic subjects.[26] In addition, there was concomitant inhibition of plasma TXB_2 concentration.

Thromboxane A_2 Receptor Antagonists

Disappointing results with thromboxane synthetase inhibitors have led to an interest in drugs that block the action of TXA_2 at its receptor. Theoretical advantages of TXA_2 receptor blockade versus synthetase inhibition include antagonism of the action of the precursor endoperoxide PGH_2, which acts at the TXA_2 receptor; shunting toward formation of detrimental eicosanoids does not occur; and it is effective when given after the formation of thromboxane.[1] As discussed above, because of the inherent instability of TXA_2, experiments often are performed with the prostaglandin endoperoxide analog, U-46619, which has biologic activity similar to TXA_2.

PRECLINICAL PHARMACOLOGY

MECHANISM OF ACTION AND POTENCY

Numerous TXA_2 receptor antagonists have been developed (see Table 66-1).[4,15,27-33] These compounds are structurally diverse (Fig. 66-3). Evidence suggests that TXA_2 and its precursor PGH_2 have a similar profile of biologic activity as discussed above and act via a common receptor; thus, blockade of the TXA_2 receptor effectively blocks the action of both mediators.[34-36] Species differences and specific tissue subtypes of TXA_2 receptors have been noted in preliminary studies.[34-36] Thromboxane A_2 receptor antagonists act both competitively and noncompetitively and have pA_2 values between 7 and 9 in human airways (Table 66-3). They are selective for the TXA_2 receptor but also block contraction caused by eicosanoids, suggesting that, in some species, eicosanoids act through the TXA_2 receptor or cause the production of eicosanoid mediators.[37]

AA-2414, a benzoquinone TXA_2 receptor antagonist, competitively inhibited contraction caused by U-46619 in guinea pig tracheal and parenchymal strips with pA_2 values of 7.69 and 8.29, respectively.[37] In addition, AA-2414 inhibited bron-

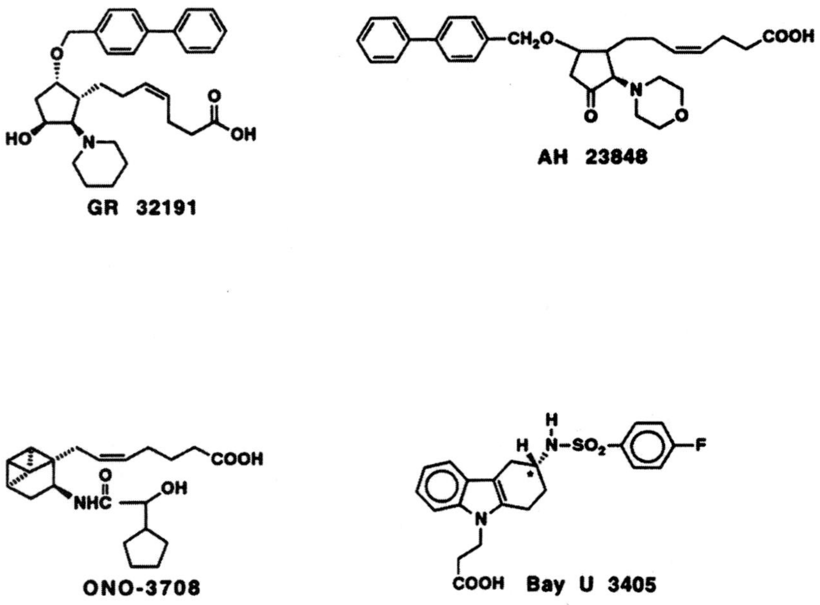

FIGURE 66-3 Names and chemical structures of representative thromboxane A_2 receptor antagonists. (*From Hay,*[1] *with permission.*)

TABLE 66-3   Relative Potency, as Expressed by pA_2 or pk_B Values for Thromboxane A_2 Receptor Antagonists versus the Thromboxane A_2 Mimetic U-46619.

Antagonist	pA_2/pk_B
Guinea pig airways	
AA-2414	7.69
AH 23848	8.5
BAY U 3405	8.7
EP092	8.7
GR32191	8.26
ONO-3708	7.78
Human airways	
AH 23848	6.9
BAY U 3405	8.8
EP092	6.8
ONO-3708	7.43

NOTE: The pA_2 values have been obtained from experiments in vitro measuring contraction in guinea pig or human airways. pK_B values are given when pA_2 determination could not be performed.

choconstriction caused by inhaled leukotriene D_4 or intravenously administered platelet-activating factor in guinea pigs in vivo. Another competitive TXA_2 receptor antagonist, AH 19437, selectively blocks all U-46619/TXA_2-sensitive receptors.[28] AH 19437 blocked the effects of U-46619 and prostaglandin F_{2a} (PGF_{2a}) on guinea pig lung strips with pA_2 values of 6.6 and 5.9, respectively. No effect on responses to acetylcholine or histamine was noted. AH 23848 appears to be a competitive TXA_2 receptor antagonist in

guinea pig and human parenchymal lung strips at low concentrations, but at greater than 10^{-8} M, antagonism did not occur.[29] By contrast, EP092 was a competitive TXA_2 receptor antagonist in guinea pig tracheal rings and lung strips and human lung strips at all concentrations tested with pA_2 values of 8.7, 8.7, and 8.9, respectively.[29] It poorly antagonized the responses to U-46619 in human bronchiolar ring with a pA_2 of 6.8. Neither compound blocked the response to noradrenaline, acetylcholine, or KCl. BAY U 3405 is a potent and selective competitive TXA_2 receptor antagonist with pA_2 values between 8.0 and 8.9 for all airway smooth muscle tested including humans.[38] BAY U 3405 is stereoselective; the R-enantiomer is the most effective in guinea pig and human airway. It competitively antagonizes human airway smooth muscle contraction caused by prostaglandin D_2 (PGD_2), PGF_{2a}, and 16, 16-dimethyl-PGE_2. At high concentrations, it had no effect on airway smooth muscle contraction caused by carbachol, histamine, 5-hydroxytryptamine, or leukotrienes C_4 or D_4. In a similar fashion, GR32191 was an equally potent competitive antagonist of the contractile responses to U-46619, PGD_2, and PGF_{2a} in guinea pig tracheal segments in vitro with pA_2 values of 8.26, 8.79, and 7.92, respectively.[39] ONO-3708 inhibited contraction of isolated guinea pig and human tracheal smooth muscle in vitro in a dose-dependent fashion (pA_2 values of 7.78 and 7.43, respectively).[32] Guinea pig tracheal smooth muscle contraction to histamine or leukotriene D_4 was not inhibited by ONO-3708. SQ 29548 blocked airway responses to PGH_2 in cats in vivo.[15]

EFFICACY IN EXPERIMENTAL MODELS

AA-2414 given orally before allergen challenge inhibited bronchoconstriction acutely[11,37,40] and during the late asthmatic response in a dose-dependent fashion in sensitized guinea pigs.[11,40] It did not inhibit either eosinophil or neutrophil accumulation in bronchoalveolar lavage fluid or airways after antigen challenge.[11] ONO-3708 prevented the increase in airway reactivity to acetylcholine caused by U-46619 in guinea pigs in vivo.[32] The thromboxane receptor antagonists, S-1452 and ONO NT-126, given intravenously to sensitized guinea pigs before antigen challenge blocked the subsequent propranolol-induced bronchoconstriction after allergen challenge.[33] Pretreatment with GR32191 inhibited neutrophil-induced bronchial hyperresponsiveness to histamine in human bronchial tissue.[41] ICI 192605 given intravenously abolished plasma exudation from trachea to distal intrapulmonary airways in response to U-46619 in guinea pigs in vivo.[4]

HUMAN CLINICAL PHARMACOLOGY

EFFECT ON AGONIST-INDUCED BRONCHOCONSTRICTION AND AIRWAY HYPERRESPONSIVENESS

Thromboxane A_2 receptor antagonists protect against bronchoconstriction caused by PGD_2 and, in some studies, methacholine but not histamine in subjects with asthma. BAY U 3405 protected against PGD_2-induced bronchoconstriction in asthmatic patients.[42] A single dose of 20 mg increased the amount of PGD_2 necessary to cause a 20 percent decrease in FEV_1 by 6-fold at 60 min and 16-fold at 90 min after drug ingestion. The 50-mg dose did not increase the efficacy at 90 min, and neither dose protected against bronchoconstriction caused by histamine. In a similar fashion, a single dose of 80 mg GR32191 caused a greater than 10-fold shift to the right in the dose-response curve to PGD_2 in asthmatic subjects.[39] There was no effect on baseline lung function or response to methacholine. The effect of AA-2414 on bronchial hyperresponsiveness to methacholine was tested at oral doses of either 20 or 40 mg/day for 4 days in 15 asthmatic subjects.[27] The PC_{20}-FEV_1 increased from 0.43 to 0.93 mg/mL after 40 mg/day of AA-2414, whereas 20 mg/day did not change the response to methacholine. Baseline lung function was not changed by either dose.

EFFECT ON ALLERGEN- AND EXERCISE-INDUCED BRONCHOCONSTRICTION

Thromboxane A_2 receptor antagonists protect against bronchoconstriction caused by allergen challenge, but they are not effective against exercise-induced bronchoconstriction in subjects with asthma. GR32191 caused a mean inhibition of 23.6 percent in the immediate bronchoconstrictor response to allergen challenge after a single oral dose of 80 mg in 7 subjects.[39] In contrast, a single 120-mg dose of GR32191 was not effective in preventing exercise-induced bronchoconstriction in 12 asthmatic subjects. The mean maximum percentage decrease in FEV_1 from baseline after exercise was 31.6 percent after GR32191 versus 30.2 percent after placebo.[43] In a similar fashion, 20 mg BAY U 3405 given 1 h before exercise challenge did not modulate exercise-induced bronchoconstriction or affect resting bronchial tone in 12 subjects with mild asthma.[30]

EFFECT OF CHRONIC THERAPY

The effect of chronic treatment with GR32191 on lung function and methacholine responsiveness was tested in 9 subjects with chronic asthma on inhaled corticosteroids.[31] Subjects were randomized to receive 40 mg qid and placebo for 3 weeks each in a double-blind, placebo-controlled, crossover fashion. Mean FEV_1 did not improve after treatment with GR32191 (2.86 L after GR32191 versus 2.94 L after placebo). In addition, airway responsiveness to methacholine was not significantly different (PC_{20}-FEV_1 38.5 μg after GR32191 versus 24.3 μg after placebo).

Conclusion

Despite theoretical reasons for using thromboxane synthetase inhibitors and receptor antagonists in asthma and preclinical data suggesting efficacy in experimental models, the results of clinical trials have been disappointing. Thromboxane synthetase inhibitors and receptor antagonists do not affect baseline airway smooth muscle tone, and the improvements in airway responsiveness to contractile agonists and allergen and exercise challenge are small and inconsistently attained. The development of more selective or potent compounds may improve their clinical efficacy; however, the results at present call into question the importance of these compounds in the overall inflammatory response of asthma.

Acknowledgments

The author wishes to thank Donna Jasutis for her assistance in typing the manuscript.

References

1. Hay DWP, Griswold DE: Inhibitors of fatty acid-derived mediators, in Cunningham FM (ed): *Lipid Mediators*. San Diego, Academic Press, 1994; 117–179.
2. Ogletree ML: Overview of physiological and pathophysiological effects of thromboxane A_2. *Fed Proc* 1987; 46:133.
3. O'Byrne PM, Fuller RW: The role of thromboxane A_2 in the pathogenesis of airway hyperresponsiveness. *Eur Respir J* 1989; 2:782.
4. Lötvall J, Elwood W, Tokuyama K, et al.: A thromboxane mimetic, U-46619, produces plasma exudation in airways of the guinea pig. *J Appl Physiol* 1992; 72:2415.
5. Noveral JP, Grunstein MM: Role and mechanism of thromboxane-induced proliferation of cultured airway smooth muscle cells. *Am J Physiol* 1992; 263:L555.
6. Lui MC, Hubbard WC, Proud D, et al.: Immediate and late inflammatory responses to ragweed antigen challenge of the peripheral airways in allergic asthmatics. *Am Rev Respir Dis* 1991; 144:51.
7. Kumlin M, Dahlen B, Björck T, et al.: Urinary excretion of leukotriene E_4 and 11-dehydro-thromboxane B_2 in response to bronchial provocations with allergen, aspirin, leukotriene D_4, and histamine in asthmatics. *Am Rev Respir Dis* 1992; 148:96.
8. Taylor IK, Ward PS, O'Shaughnessy KM, et al.: Thromboxane A_2

biosynthesis in acute asthma and after antigen challenge. *Am Rev Respir Dis* 1991; 143:119.

9. Weichman BM, Muccitelli RM, Osborn RR, et al.: In vitro and in vivo mechanisms of leukotriene-mediated bronchoconstriction in the guinea pig. *J Pharmacol Exp Ther* 1982; 222:202.

10. Manning PJ, Stevens WH, Cockcroft DW, O'Byrne PM: The role of thromboxane in allergen-induced asthmatic responses. *Eur Respir J* 1991; 4:667.

11. Matsumoto T, Ashida Y, Tsukuda R: Pharmacological modulation of immediate and late airway response and leukocyte infiltration in the guinea pig. *J Pharmacol Exp Ther* 1994; 269:1236.

12. Kriseman T, Underwood D, McNamara D, Kadowitz P: Inhibition of A23187-induced bronchoconstriction by dazoxiben, a thromboxane synthetase inhibitor. *Am J Med Sci* 1987; 293:349.

13. Takami M, Takata Y, Matsumoto K, et al.: Effect of DP-1904, a new thromboxane A_2 synthetase inhibitor, on guinea pig experimental asthma. *Ann N Y Acad Sci* 1991; 629:407.

14. Fujimura M, Sakamoto S, Matsuda T: Attenuating effect of a thromboxane synthetase inhibitor (OKY-046) on bronchial responsiveness to methacholine is specific to bronchial asthma. *Chest* 1990; 98:656.

15. Tilden SJ, Underwood DC, Cowen KH, et al.: Effects of OKY 1581 on bronchoconstrictor responses to arachidonic acid and PGH_2. *J Appl Physiol* 1987; 62:2066.

16. Ku EC, McPherson SE, Signor C, et al.: Characterization of imidazo [1, 5-a] pyridine-5-hexanoic acid (CGS 13080) as a selective thromboxane synthetase inhibitor using in vitro and in vivo biochemical models. *Biochem Biophys Res Commun* 1983; 112:899.

17. Terashita Z, Imura Y, Tanabe M, et al.: CV-4151—a potent, selective thromboxane A_2 synthetase inhibitor. *Thrombosis Res* 1986; 41:223.

18. Aiken JW: Pharmacology of thromboxane synthetase inhibitors. *Adv Prostaglandin Thromboxane Leukot Res* 1983; 11:253.

19. Chung KF, Aizawa H, Becker AB, et al.: Inhibition of antigen-induced airway hyperresponsiveness by a thromboxane synthetase inhibitor (OKY-046) in allergic dogs. *Am Rev Respir Dis* 1986; 134:258.

20. Ueno A, Tanaka K, Katori M: Possible involvement of thromboxane in bronchoconstrictive and hypertensive effects of LTC_4 and LTD_4 in guinea pigs. *Prostaglandins* 1982; 23:865.

21. Prié S, Sirois P: Mechanism of action of leukotrienes on the guinea pig bronchus. *Prostaglandins Leukot Essent Fatty Acids* 1988; 34:19.

22. Nagai H, Yakuo I, Togawa M, et al.: Effect of OKY-046, a new thromboxane A_2 synthetase inhibitor, on experimental asthma in guinea pigs. *Prostaglandins Leukot Med* 1987; 30:111.

23. Fujimura M, Ogawa H, Saito M, et al.: Inhibitory effect of inhalation of a thromboxane synthetase inhibitor on bronchoconstriction induced by aerosolized leukotriene C_4 and thromboxane A_2 analogue in anesthetized guinea pigs. *Allergy* 1991; 46:534.

24. Fujimura M, Nishioka S, Kumabashiri I, et al.: Effects of aerosol administration of a thromboxane synthetase inhibitor (OKY-046) on bronchial responsiveness to acetylcholine in asthmatic subjects. *Chest* 1990; 98:276.

25. Iwamoto I, Ra C, Sato T, et al.: Thromboxane A_2 production in allergen-induced immediate and late asthmatic responses. *J Asthma* 1988; 25:117.

26. Hoshino M, Fukushima Y: Effect of OKY-046 (thromboxane A_2 synthetase inhibitor) on exercise-induced asthma. *J Asthma* 1991; 28:19.

27. Fujimura M, Sakamoto S, Motoyasu S, et al.: Effect of a thromboxane A_2 receptor antagonist (AA-2414) on bronchial hyperresponsiveness to methacholine in subjects with asthma. *J Allergy Clin Immunol* 1991; 87:23.

28. Kennedy I, Coleman RA, Humphrey PPA, et al.: Studies on the characterization of prostanoid receptors: a proposed classification. *Prostaglandins* 1982; 24:667.

29. McKenniff M, Rodger IW, Norman P, Gardiner PJ: Characterization of receptors mediating the contractile effects of prostanoids in guinea-pig and human airways. *Eur J Pharmacol* 1988; 153:149.

30. Magnussen H, Boerger S, Templin K, Baunack AR: Effects of a thromboxane-receptor antagonist, BAY U 3405, on prostaglandin D_2- and exercise-induced bronchoconstriction. *J Allergy Clin Immunol* 1992; 89:1119.

31. Stenton SC, Young CA, Harris A, et al.: The effect of GR32191 (a thromboxane receptor antagonist) on airway responsiveness in asthma. *Pulm Pharmacol* 1992; 5:199.

32. Nagai H, Tsuji F, Inagaki N, et al.: The effect of ONO-3708, a novel TXA_2 receptor antagonist, on U-46619-induced contraction of guinea pig and human tracheal strips in vitro and on bronchoconstriction in guinea pigs in vivo. *Prostaglandins* 1991; 41:375.

33. Songur N, Fujimura M, Mizuhashi K, et al.: Involvement of thromboxane A_2 in propranolol-induced bronchoconstriction after allergic bronchoconstriction in guinea pigs. *Am J Respir Crit Care Med* 1994; 149:1488.

34. Halushka PV, Mais DE, Morinelli TA: Thromboxane and prostacyclin receptors. *Prostaglandins Clin Biol Res* 1989; 301:21.

35. Halushka PV, Mais DE, Saussy DL: Platelet and vascular smooth muscle thromboxane A_2/prostaglandin H_2 receptors. *Fed Proc* 1987; 46:149.

36. Halushka PV, Mais DE, Mayeux PR, Morinelli TA: Thromboxane, prostaglandin and leukotriene receptors. *Annu Rev Pharmacol Toxicol* 1989; 10:213.

37. Ashida Y, Matsumoto T, Kuriki H, et al.: A novel anti-asthmatic quinone derivative, AA-2414 with a potent antagonistic activity against a variety of spasmogenic prostanoids. *Prostaglandins* 1989; 38:91.

38. McKenniff MG, Norman P, Cuthbert NJ, Gardiner PJ: BAY U 3405, a potent and selective thromboxane A_2 receptor antagonist on airway smooth muscle in vitro. *Br J Clin Pharmacol* 1991; 104:585.

39. Beasley RCW, Featherstone RL, Church MK, et al.: Effect of a thromboxane receptor antagonist on PGD_2- and allergen-induced bronchoconstriction. *J Appl Physiol* 1989; 66:1685.

40. Ashida Y, Matsumoto T, Kuriki H, Saijo T: Effect of the prostaglandin endoperoxide antagonist AA-2414 on experimental allergic asthma. *Ann N Y Acad Sci* 1991; 629:394.

41. Hughes JM, McKay KO, Johnson PR, et al.: Neutrophil-induced human bronchial hyperresponsiveness in vitro- pharmacological modulation. *Clin Exp Allergy* 1992; 23:251.

42. Johnston SL, Bardin PG, Harrison J, et al.: The effects of an oral thromboxane TP receptor antagonist BAY U 3405, on prostaglandin D_2- and histamine-induced bronchoconstriction in asthma, and relationship to plasma drug concentrations. *Br J Clin Pharmacol* 1992; 34:402.

43. Finnerty JP, Twentyman OP, Harris A, et al.: Effects of GR32191, a potent thromboxane receptor antagonist, on exercise induced bronchoconstriction in asthma. *Thorax* 1991; 46:190.

STIMULANTS, ANTITUSSIVE AGENTS, AND MUCOLYTICS

Chapter 67
VENTILATORY STIMULANTS

JESSE HALL

Pharmacology of Respiratory Stimulants
    Acetazolamide
    Doxapram
    Almitrine
    Progesterones
    Naloxone and flumazenil
Clinical Use of Respiratory Stimulants
    Acute-on-chronic respiratory failure
    Sleep-disordered breathing
    Acute mountain sickness
Conclusion

A number of pharmacologic agents are available that exert stimulatory effects on ventilation by actions at the level of peripheral chemoreceptors and/or the central nervous system. The instances in which these drugs are clinically useful are extremely limited; the reason being that the vast majority of cases of chronic or acute ventilatory failure occur with normal or supranormal drive to breathe, and appropriate therapy should be directed at reducing mechanical loads on the respiratory system, enhancing neuromuscular competence or both, and not at increasing drive on an already failing system. Accordingly, this chapter will review briefly the pharmacology of respiratory stimulants, detail clinical studies proscribing their use in most patients, and comment on the limited instances in which these agents may confer benefit.

Pharmacology of Respiratory Stimulants

ACETAZOLAMIDE

Acetazolamide is a carbonic anhydrase inhibitor that causes a metabolic acidosis by diminishing renal tubular bicarbonate reclamation.[1] The effects of the drug on ventilation are secondary, as a result of attempted respiratory compensation for the metabolic disturbance. This agent has no role in the treatment of patients with or at risk for chronic or acute ventilatory failure, since the effect of combined respiratory and metabolic acidosis could be disastrous. Its use is limited to the prevention and treatment of acute mountain sickness (AMS) (see "Acute Mountain Sickness," below). Acetazolamide is available for both intravenous or oral administration but the latter route is adequate for prevention of AMS. The usual dose for this purpose is 250 mg every 8 to 12 h before and during ascent to altitude; a single daily dose of a 500 mg controlled-release tablet may be equally efficacious.

DOXAPRAM

Doxapram hydrochloride is a pyrrolidinone that can only be administered intravenously. At lesser doses (< 0.5 mg/kg intravenously), it stimulates carotid chemoreceptors and thus increases ventilatory drive. At greater doses, it likely has a direct stimulatory effect on medullary respiratory centers.[2,3] A single intravenous injection has an onset of action at 20 to 40 s, with a peak effect at 1 to 2 min. The duration of effect varies from 4 to 15 min. Because of this very short action, advocates of the drug usually recommend continuous infusion if there is an initial response to one or two "priming" doses of 2.0 mg/kg. If the drug appears to reverse incipient respiratory failure, a continuous infusion then is started, beginning at 0.5 to 1.0 mg/kg per h and gradually titrating upward against ventilatory response to a maximum dose of 4 mg/kg per h. The side effects of this agent can be substantial and include tachycardia, systemic and pulmonary hypertension, skeletal muscle hyperactivity, and seizures. Drug clearance is reduced with hepatic insufficiency, and this drug is incompatible with alkaline infusions, including aminophylline, a commonly used agent in the treatment of chronic obstructive pulmonary disease (COPD). Because of the considerable risk of side effects and the lack of proven efficacy in the vast majority of cases of acute respiratory failure, this drug is rarely, if ever, appropriate treatment (see discussion below).

ALMITRINE

Almitrine is a piperazine derivative that stimulates peripheral chemoreceptors in the presence of hypoxia with resulting increase in ventilation.[4] It also appears to potentiate hypoxic vasoconstriction and thereby improve ventilation-perfusion matching and, hence, gas exchange.[4–7] Since long-term use is complicated by a peripheral neuropathy, this agent is not currently available in the United States.[8,9]

PROGESTERONES

That hyperventilation occurs during the luteal phase of the menstrual cycle and during pregnancy has been known for many years. This normal physiologic response results from the action of progesterone. The respiratory response to this hormone appears to occur through estrogen-dependent progesterone receptor binding at hypothalamic sites and requires RNA and protein synthesis.[10] Progesterone and progesterone-analog stimulation of ventilation has been employed in the treatment of central sleep apnea and obesity-hypoventilation, although results of clinical studies have been inconsistent (see below). Recommended daily doses are 60 to 120 mg of medroxyprogesterone acetate or 50 mg of chlormadinone acetate, a synthetic progestone.

NALOXONE AND FLUMAZENIL

Naloxone and flumazenil are competitive antagonists for opioid and benzodiazepine receptors, respectively.[11,12] While there may be nonspecific stimulatory effects of these agents on ventilation, their primary use is to reverse respiratory depression arising from opiates or benzodiazepines. The depressive effects of these analgesic and sedative drugs may be particularly pronounced in elderly patients with COPD. Thus, contemplation of the use of naloxone or flumazenil in such a patient manifesting respiratory depression is perhaps more rational than use of a direct respiratory stimulant such as doxapram, certainly if the clinical context suggests recent prior use of an opioid or benzodiazepine. The usual dose of naloxone is 2 mg intravenously, which can be repeated at 2- to 4-min intervals to a total dose of 10 mg.

Reversal of opioid-induced toxicity is usually sustained for only 20 to 60 min, since the duration of most opioids exceeds the duration of action of naloxone. Thus, repeated bolus administration or continuous infusion of naloxone is often required. One potential side effect of naloxone is creation of a withdrawal state in individuals using or receiving narcotics on a chronic basis. Flumazenil may be given as an 0.6 to 1.0 mg dose intravenously. The drug should be administered slowly at a rate of approximately 0.1 mg/min. This dose can be repeated after 2 to 3 min if the suspicion of benzodiazepine overdose is high. Unfortunately, flumazenil has not consistently reversed benzodiazepine-induced respiratory depression even when it achieves an improved level of consciousness.[13,14] Thus, the clinician should be prepared to support ventilation at all times. One potential adverse effect of flumazenil is induction of seizures, perhaps by suppression of the γ-aminobutyric acid (GABA) system.

Clinical Use of Respiratory Stimulants

ACUTE-ON-CHRONIC RESPIRATORY FAILURE

Patients with COPD often present for care at the time of an acute deterioration in function, a condition termed *acute-on-chronic respiratory failure* (ACRF).[15] It is in this clinical context that some have advocated the use of respiratory stimulants, with an aim of maintaining ventilation until other therapies have taken effect, thus avoiding a need for mechanical ventilatory support.[16] This theory would be supported by a component of inadequate drive to breathe in this patient population—that in the paradigm of "won't breathe" versus "can't breathe"; some patients "won't breathe" and can be made to do so pharmacologically.[17] While there is a clinical literature claiming benefit from the use of agents such as doxapram when given to patients with ACRF, it is entirely anecdotal.[18–21] Indeed, most carefully performed prospective studies suggest that the drive to breathe in patients with ACRF is supranormal. When patients with ACRF were treated with oxygen, a further increase of baseline hypercarbia was noted but was not explained on the basis of worsened hypoventilation. A large component of the observed increase in P_{CO_2} is explained by an increase in dead space, a ventilation-perfusion alteration that could occur as a result of oxygen-mediated relaxation of airways or alteration of blood flow.[22,23] Respiratory drive measured by mouth occlusion pressure ($P_{.01}$) was three times normal despite abolition of hypoxic drive by oxygen therapy, and minute ventilation was not reduced.[24] These observations were consistent with a view that hypercarbia following oxygen therapy in ACRF does not necessarily signal worsened respiratory failure secondary to diminished drive to breathe. Indeed, attention in this disorder has increasingly turned toward respiratory muscle fatigue (resulting from the excessive mechanical load of ACRF) as an explanation for failure in these patients. When doxapram was given to patients with COPD undergoing weaning from mechanical ventilation, no change in measures of drive to breathe were seen; an increase in end-expiratory volume suggested the drug worsened gas trapping with the potential for diaphragm dysfunction.[25]

Unwarranted use of drugs to stimulate drive to breathe when it is already high is therefore likely to risk side effects without benefit. Thus administration of respiratory stimulants to patients with ACRF at the time of presentation cannot be supported. If respiratory depression is apparent clinically, it is likely to have arisen from either the effects of analgesic or sedative drugs, or because the patient has already progressed to respiratory muscle fatigue with impending respiratory arrest. Brief consideration can be given to the use of the opioid antagonist naloxone or the benzodiazepine antagonist flumazenil. Mechanical ventilatory support, if appropriate to the patient's overall condition, is the treatment of choice for advanced muscle fatigue with impending respiratory arrest.

SLEEP-DISORDERED BREATHING

The majority of patients with sleep-disordered breathing manifest obstructive sleep apnea (OSA), which can be successfully treated by elimination of precipitating factors (e.g., obesity), tracheostomy, upper airway surgery, or, most commonly, positive-pressure mask ventilation (e.g., nocturnal CPAP).[26] When central sleep apnea is present, it most commonly coexists with OSA and responds to successful treatment of OSA. Obstructive sleep apnea also may coexist with the obesity-hypoventilation syndrome; that is, patients with significant obesity, daytime hypercapnea, and nocturnal episodes of obstruction with desaturation and worsened hypercapnea.

Most clinical studies suggest that use of respiratory stimulants as adjunctive therapy for uncomplicated OSA is usually unsuccessful,[27–29] and these agents should probably be reserved for use in patients with OSA and obesity hypoventilation.[30] Medroxyprogesterone is the preferred agent and in most circumstances will be used in combination with CPAP or other therapies directed at nocturnal obstruction and desaturation.

ACUTE MOUNTAIN SICKNESS

Rapid ascent to altitudes > 3000 meters often are associated with a constellation of symptoms that include headache, anorexia, insomnia, lethargy, nausea, vomiting, dyspnea, and cough.[31] The majority of these symptoms can be ascribed to cerebral and pulmonary edema. In addition, periodic breathing with episodes of desaturation is common and perhaps universal at altitudes above 2800 meters. While the precise sequence of pathophysiologic events that may result in this clinical entity currently are debated, a number of studies have indicated that use of acetazolamide can prevent the onset of AMS as well as ameliorate symptoms once they have occurred.[32–35] How much of this beneficial effect relates to diuretic or other action as opposed to stimulation of ventilation is not clear, but this drug does tend to eliminate nocturnal desaturation.[32]

Conclusion

There are few data to support the use of respiratory stimulants in the treatment of acute respiratory failure. Indeed current understandings of the pathophysiology of this disorder suggest diminished drive to breathe is rarely a component of this disorder apart from instances of drug overdose; in this circumstance specific antidote therapy would be more rational than nonspecific respiratory stimulants. The use of respiratory stimulants in sleep-disordered breathing is presently largely limited to patients with obesity-hypoventilation and then in conjunction with other treatments directed at nocturnal events. The respiratory stimulant acetazolamide is useful in the prevention and treatment of AMS.

References

1. Heller I. Halvey J, Cohen S, et al.: Significant metabolic acidosis induced by acetazolamide. Not a rare complication. *Arch Int Med* 1985; 145:1815–1817.
2. Burki NK: Ventilatory effects of doxapram in conscious human subjects. *Chest* 1984; 85:600–04.
3. Scott RM, Whitwam JG, Chakrabarti MK: Evidence of a role for the peripheral chemoreceptors in the ventilatory response to doxapram in man. *Br J Anaesth* 1977; 49:227–31.
4. Powles ACP, Tuxen DV, Mahood CB, et al.: The effect of intravenously administered almitrine, a peripheral chemoreceptor agonist, on patients with chronic air-flow obstruction. *Am Rev Resp Dis* 1983; 127:284–289.
5. Castaing Y, Manier G, Guenard H: Improvement in ventilation perfusion relationships by almitrine in patient with chronic obstructive pulmonary disease during mechanical ventilation. *Am Rev Resp Dis* 1986; 134:910–916.
6. Connaughton JJ, Douglas NJ, Morgan AD, et al.: Almitrine improves oxygenation when both awake and asleep in patients with hypoxia and carbon dioxide retention caused by chronic bronchitis and emphysema. *Am Rev Resp Dis* 1985; 132:206–210.
7. Prost JF, Desche P, Jardin F, et al.: Comparison of the effects of intravenous almitrine and positive end-expiratory pressure on pulmonary gas exchange in adult respiratory distress syndrome. *Eur Resp J* 1991; 4:683–687.
8. Gherardi R, Louarn F, Benvenuti C, et al.: Peripheral neuropathy in patients treated with almitrine dismesilate. *Lancet* 1985; 1247–1249.
9. Gherardi R, Baudrimont M, Gray F, et al.: Almitrine neuropathy. A nerve biopsy study of 8 cases. *Acta Neuropath (Berl)* 1987; 73:20–28.
10. Baylis DA, Millhorn DE: Central neural mechanisms of progesterone action: application to the respiratory system. *J Appl Physiol* 1992; 73(2):393–404.
11. Weisman RS: Naloxone, in Goldfranks LR, et al. (eds): *Goldfrank's Toxicologic Emergencies.* Connecticut: Appleton & Lange, 1994:784–786.
12. Howland MA: Flumazenil, in Goldfranks LR, et al. (eds): *Goldfrank's Toxicologic Emergencies.* Connecticut: Appleton & Lange, 1994, 805–810.
13. Shalansky SJ, Naumann TL, Englander FA: Therapy update: effect of flumazenil on benzodiazepine-induced respiratory depression. *Clin Pharm* 1993; 12:483–487.
14. Mora CT, Torjman M, White PF: Effects of diazepam and flumazenil on sedation and hypoxic ventilatory response. *Anesth Analg* 1989; 68:473–478.
15. Geppert EF: Thoracentesis and pleural biopsy, in Hall JB, Schmidt GA, Wood DH (eds): *Principles of Critical Care,* McGraw-Hill, New York, 1992; 220–223.
16. Jeffrey AA, Warren PM, Flenley DC: Acute hypercapnic respiratory failure in patients with chronic obstructive lung disease: risk

factors and use of guidelines for management. *Thorax* 1992; 47:34–30.

17. Fahey PJ, Hyde RW: "Won't breathe" vs. can't breathe, detection of depressed ventilatory drive in patients with obstructive pulmonary disease. *Chest* 1983; 84:19–25.

18. Gilbert J, Rice WH, Johnston J: Possible doxapram reversal of ventilator dependence in a brain damaged patient. *Crit Care Med* 1985; 13:605–06.

19. Moser KM, Luchsigner PC, Adamson JS, et al.: Respiratory stimulation with intravenous doxapram in respiratory failure. *N Engl J Med* 1973; 288–427–31.

20. Haake RE, Saxon LA, Bander SJ, et al.: Depressed central respiratory drive causing weaning failure. Its reversal with doxapram. *Chest* 1989; 95:695–97.

21. McNamara RM, Euerle BD: Doxapram reversal of respiratory failure in a patient refusing assisted ventilation. *Ann Emerg Med* 1994; 24:751–754.

22. Aubier M, Murciano D, Milic-Emili J, et al.: Effects of administration of O_2 on ventilation and blood gases in patients with chronic obstructive pulmonary disease during acute respiratory failure. *Am Rev Respir Dis* 1980; 122:147–154.

23. Libby DM, Briscoe WA, King TKC: Relief of hypoxia-related bronchoconstriction by breathing 30 percent oxygen. *Am Rev Respir Dis* 1981; 123:171–175.

24. Aubier M, Murciano D, Fournier M, et al.: Central respiratory drive in acute respiratory failure of patients with chronic obstructive pulmonary disease. *Am Rev Respir Dis* 1980; 122:191–199.

25. Pourriat JL, Baud M, Lamberto C, et al.: Effects of doxapram on hypercapnic response during weaning from mechanical ventilation in COPD patients. *Chest* 1992; 101:1639–43.

26. Strohl KP, Cherniack NS, Gothe B: Physiologic basis of therapy for sleep apnea. *Am Rev Respir Dis* 1986; 134:791–802.

27. Orr WC, Imes NK, Martin RJ: Progesterone therapy in obese patients with sleep apnea. *Arch Intern Med* 1979; 139:109–111.

28. Rajagopal KR, Abbrecht PH, Jabbari B: Effects of medroxyprogesterone acetate in obstructive sleep apnea patients. *Sleep Research* 1991; 20A:446.

29. Stohol KP, Hensley MJ, Saunders NA, et al.: Progesterone administration and progressive sleep apneas. *JAMA* 1980; 245:1230–1232.

30. Kryger MJ: Management of obstructive sleep apnea, in Phillpson EA, Bradley TD (eds): *Clinics in Chest Medicine*. Philadelphia, 1992; 13(3):481–492.

31. Hsia CCW: Southwestern internal medicine conference: pulmonary complication of high-altitudes exposure. *Am J Med Sci* 1994; 307(6):448–464.

32. Burki NK, Khan SA, Hameed MA: The effects of acetazolamide on the ventilatory response to high altitude hypoxia. *Chest* 1992; 101:736–41.

33. Greene MK, Keer AM, McIntosh IB, et al.: Acetazolamide in prevention of acute mountain sickness; a double-blind controlled cross-over study. *Br Med J* 1981; 283:811–13.

34. Hackett PH, Rennie D, Levine HD: The incidence, importance, and prophylaxis of acute mountain sickness. *Lancet* 1976; ii:1149–54.

35. Larson EB, Roach RC, Schoene RB, et al.: Acute mountain sickness and acetazolamide. *JAMA* 1982; 248:328–32.

Chapter 68

PHARMACOLOGIC TREATMENT OF COUGH

ARTHUR S. BANNER

Cough is the most powerful and effective of a group of respiratory reflexes that protect the lung from injurious inhaled agents and cleanse the airways of endogenously produced debris. Although defensive in function, the response is a stereotypical one, and frequently serves no useful purpose, other than to signal the presence of abnormal conditions within the respiratory system. The proper management of cough requires an understanding of its etiology, functional significance, and deleterious consequences. Because cough may reflect important and even life-threatening conditions within the respiratory system, an explanation for the symptom always must be sought. Often the cause for cough is relatively trivial, but its identification is useful because treatment of cough is most effective when efforts are directed at the underlying condition. Cough suppressants are appropriate only when the underlying abnormality is not responsive to therapy, and a judgment is made that the deleterious consequences of cough outweigh any functionally important effects.

Physiology of the Cough Reflex

Cough is a reflex with a complicated efferent response involving both the somatic and autonomic nervous systems. Afferent information is carried to the brainstem where impulses are summed and the nature of the efferent response is determined. Higher centers are capable of further modifications and can initiate at least a portion of the efferent response without activation of the reflex arc. Cough can be triggered by a variety of mechanical and chemical stimuli, and complex interactions among stimuli occur.

AFFERENT COMPONENT

There is considerable debate concerning which receptors are responsible for cough.[1,2] A complete cough receptor never has been visualized. Nonmyelinated nerve endings have been identified within airway mucosa and within the larynx. Some of these endings are connected to rapidly adapting myelinated fibers. Evidence derived from reflex and nerve recording experiments implicate these fibers in the cough reflex.[3] Other nerve endings are connected to thin nonmyelinated fibers, known as bronchial C fibers. It is uncertain as to whether these receptors, subserve cough. Bronchial C fibers respond to some of the same stimuli that cause discharge of rapidly adapting receptors, and agents that are relatively selective for these receptors elicit cough when administered intravascularly and by inhalation.[4] However, selective stimulation of these fibers causes rapid shallow breathing rather than cough.[5] Discharge of C fibers within pulmonary parenchyma does not cause cough but actually results in cough attenuation.[6] Nerve fibers within airway smooth muscle, termed slowly adapting fibers, are inaccessible to cough stimuli and appear to subserve a proprioceptive function. However, discharge of these fibers augment the cough response elicited by other nervous receptors.[7]

Cough receptors are situated in the larynx and larger airways as well as in the ear canals and tympanic membranes. Although cough may occur when there is inflammation of the sinuses, oropharynx, pericardium, pleura, and diaphragm, it is probable that cough results from discharge of receptors located elsewhere. Afferent information is carried to the brainstem from airway receptors in the vagus nerve, from the larynx in the laryngeal nerves, and from the tympanic membranes in the glossopharyngeal nerve.

Experimentally, cough can be elicited by mechanical, chemical, and electrical stimuli. However, the precise mechanism by which the cough reflex is triggered naturally is unknown. Salem and Aviado[8] suggested that airway smooth muscle contraction was the invariable proximate cough stimulus. They based this assumption on observations that agents that produced cough also elicit bronchoconstriction and that bronchoconstriction appeared to occur concomitantly with cough. More recent evidence indicates that bronchoconstriction is not linked invariably to cough[9] and that, under certain conditions, the two responses may be conducted by different pathways.[10] It thus appears that cough is elicited by a variety of mechanical and chemical agents and that interaction between stimuli may occur. Agents such as histamine have a direct effect on receptors, but require bronchoconstriction before cough occurs.[11] Cough may also be subject to a complex interaction of sensory receptors. Thus slowly adapting fibers, although not directly responsible for cough, allow cough to occur.[7] Stimulation of irritant receptors in the airway by mechanical stimuli may lead to release of mediators, which, in turn, may trigger cough. Finally, other receptors, such as the pulmonary C fibers, may inhibit the reflex.[6]

CENTRAL MODULATION

It is uncertain if there is a separate cough center or whether cough results from excessive stimulation of expiratory neurons that are responsible for normal breathing. The fact that some antitussive agents stimulate respiration supports the existence of a separate cough center.[12] Experimental studies in cats have identified an area in the medulla that results in cough when electrically stimulated.[13] Higher centers are capable of initiating cough voluntarily, even when patients are incapable of spontaneous cough.[14] In addition, such higher centers may modulate the cough response, initiated by reflex mechanisms.

EFFERENT RESPONSE

Nerves involved in the efferent component of the cough reflex are carried within the somatic nervous system to the muscles of respiration. With most stimuli, there is also an effector response conducted by the vagus nerve, which consists of bronchoconstriction and mucosal glandular secretion. The bronchoconstrictor response may be mediated by receptors different from those that subserve cough.[9] The cough response consists of an initial inspiration, usually followed by transient glottic closure, a buildup of pressure, and finally forceful expulsion. The increased pressures result in high flows. The accompanying airway compression ensures high flow velocities, the function of which is to impart kinetic energy to airway secretions and so aid in their expulsion.

Evaluation of Cough

Uncovering the etiology of chronic cough may be an elusive goal, frustrating to both patient and physician. To provide guidelines for such an investigation, some investigators[15,16] have promoted a systematic approach based on anatomic location of cough receptors. Although this approach may seem intimidating, operationally it consists of excluding just a handful of conditions, which more often than not respond to therapy. Table 68-1 lists common causes for chronic cough and their relative frequencies based on published reports.[15,16]

TABLE 68-1   Findings in Patients Evaluated for Chronic Cough

	Irwin et al.[15] %	Poe et al.[16] %
Postnasal drip	28	27
Asthma	20	27
Asthma + postnasal drip	18	1
Asthma + chronic bronchitis	0	1
Postinfectious	0	10
Chronic bronchitis	12	4
Gastroesophageal reflux	10	5
Left ventricular failure	6	0
Metastatic cancer	2	0
Sarcoid	2	0
Psychogenic	0	1

An initial investigation consists of a history, physical examination, and a chest radiograph. Such an evaluation usually is sufficient to exclude potentially serious conditions that warrant therapy independent of the cough symptom. These conditions include airway and parenchymal lung disease, neoplasia, infection, and congestive heart failure. Specialized investigations using bronchoscopy,[17] echocardiography, and cardiac catheterization are not indicated when an initial evaluation does not point to a cardiac or pulmonary condition. An initial examination usually provides evidence for the common causes of chronic cough including asthma, postnasal drip, respiratory virus infection, and gastroesophageal reflux. When evidence for these conditions is not found, more specialized investigations are warranted. Pulmonary function studies, including measurement of flows, lung volumes, and diffusing capacity, may reveal significant lung disease not evident on physical examination and chest radiography. A diagnosis of asthma may be especially elusive because patients may complain solely of cough and pulmonary function studies may be normal.[18] Under these circumstances, bronchoprovocation may be the only evidence for asthma. Similarly, cough may be the sole presenting symptom of gastroesophageal reflux.[19] When the history does not suggest this condition, diagnosis may require prolonged measurement of esophageal pH with attempts to correlate symptoms with reflux episodes. Occasionally, these correlations are difficult to establish, and studies using acid instillation into the esophagus are necessary.[20] Ultimately a therapeutic trial of antireflux measures may be required. Once the above conditions are excluded, further investigations are usually unfruitful, and therapeutic trials with nonspecific antitussive medications are justified.

Pharmacologic Treatment of Cough

SPECIFIC TREATMENT

Therapy directed at the cause of cough has been termed specific or definitive. Treatment is termed specific when the nature of the underlying condition influences the choice of therapy. The therapy is definitive in so far that it eliminates the cough symptom. Reports of the results of specific ther-

TABLE 68-2   **Pharmacologic Treatment of Conditions Causing Cough**

Condition	Drugs
Asthma	Bronchodilators, corticosteroids, cromolyn sodium, nedocromil
Postnasal drip (sinusitis)	Antibiotics, nasal decongestants, H_1-antagonist
Postnasal drip (allergic or perennial nonallergic)	Nasal corticosteroids, H_1-antagonist, nasal decongestants
Postviral cough	Ipratropium bromide, ?corticosteroids
Gastroesophageal reflux	H_2-antagonist, omeprazole, metoclopramide
Congestive heart failure	Diuretics, digoxin, angiotensin-converting enzyme inhibitors

apy in patients with chronic cough have shown that such treatment is definitive in 80 to 98 percent of patients.[15–17,21] None of these investigations were blinded or placebo controlled, and all used patient reports rather than objective techniques for cough quantification. In addition, treatment was often prolonged, thus raising the question of spontaneous resolution of cough in some subjects. Nevertheless, the general impression of physicians is that specific therapy is highly effective in some patients and in some conditions more than others. Pharmacologic therapy of conditions resulting in cough is listed in Table 68-2.

Specific therapy is probably most effective in patients with bronchial asthma. This is especially true in patients in whom the diagnosis of asthma is made using conventional criteria of reversible airway obstruction. When the diagnosis of asthma is based solely on the finding of airway hyperreactivity as determined by bronchoprovocation, therapy directed against asthma is ineffective in 22 percent of cases.[21] When cough is the sole presenting symptom of asthma, bronchodilators alone are often ineffective, and it is necessary to use anti-inflammatory agents such as corticosteroids, disodium cromoglycate, or nedocromil.[15,16] Nedocromil sodium is especially effective in relieving asthmatic cough,[22] perhaps because of its postulated effects on airway sensory receptors.[23]

Postnasal drip commonly is associated with and may be causally related to chronic cough. It has been suggested that treatment of postnasal drip be based on the underlying cause.[24] Thus, when postnasal drip is due to sinusitis, the appropriate treatment consists of antibiotics, nasal decongestants and H_1-antagonists, whereas postnasal drip due to allergic or nonallergic perennial rhinitis is best treated with inhaled corticosteroids. Published reports indicate that such treatment is highly successful,[15,16,21] but this condition may be frustratingly resistant to treatment.

Gastroesophageal reflux has been shown to be common in patients with chronic cough.[19] Treatment of this condition with H_2-antagonists, blockers, omeprazole, and metoclopramide, as well as nonpharmacologic interventions, alleviate cough, although prolonged treatment is often necessary.[19,21] Whether, in some patients, relief of cough results from treatment or to spontaneous resolution is not clear. Preliminary findings from one controlled study suggest that treatment with ranitidine is superior to placebo.[25]

Acute upper respiratory tract infections are a frequent cause of cough. Individuals with the common cold rarely seek medical advice, but do use over-the-counter (OTC) cold formulations consisting of antitussives, nasal decongestants, and antihistamines. Some[26] but not all studies have found these medications to be effective in adults.[27,28] Cough occasionally persists for weeks to months after such infections and is usually resistant to most medications. However, one controlled, double-blind study found that treatment with inhaled ipratropium bromide was effective, to some degree, in nearly all patients studied.[29]

A variety of other conditions respond to specific measures. These include treatment of congestive heart failure with appropriate drugs, sarcoidosis and other interstitial diseases with corticosteroids, chronic bronchitis by smoking cessation, and stopping treatment with inhibitors of angiotensin-converting enzyme (ACE) in patients with cough consequent to these agents.

NONSPECIFIC TREATMENT

Nonspecific therapy consists of the use of agents that suppress the cough reflex, irrespective of the underlying condition. In general, antitussive drugs are not strikingly effective. Although patients may perceive some benefit from these agents, cough generally persists, though the intensity of the symptom may wax and wane with time.

Antitussives may act centrally within the brainstem or peripherally at the nerve receptor site. In most cases, the mechanism of action is not known with certainty. Agents are presumed to have a central action when they have other central properties or when they are capable of inhibiting cough elicited by central stimulation. However, in such cases, it is difficult to exclude a peripheral mechanism as well.

CENTRALLY ACTING DRUGS

The most effective antitussive agents are those that are thought to act at the level of the brainstem. These consist of the opiates, opiate derivatives, and nonopiates. Although there is considerable evidence that opiates act centrally,[30] recent studies suggest these agents may act peripherally as well.[31,32] Many opiates have analgesic and sedative properties and are termed narcotics. All narcotics are effective antitussive agents, but their use is limited by their abuse potential. Narcotics approved as antitussives include codeine, hydrocodone, and hydromorphone. When used as prescribed, these drugs rarely result in psychological or physical addiction. However, persons addicted to opiates occasionally will resort to cough medications when their preferred drug is unavailable. For this reason many physicians favor the opiate derivatives such as dextromethorphan or noscapine or the nonopiate centrally acting drugs caramiphan or carbetapentane. In most circumstances, there is little benefit to using nonnarcotic preparations.

PERIPHERALLY ACTING DRUGS

Peripherally acting agents are thought to inhibit cough by some direct or indirect action on peripheral nervous receptors. In many instances, these agents are combined with centrally acting agents in cough mixtures. It is unlikely that any of these agents act directly on cough receptors. Benzonatate, a drug that is related chemically to procaine and administered orally is thought to inhibit cough by inhibition of stretch receptors.[33] Local anesthetics such as benzocaine, benzyl alcohol, and phenol are frequently incorporated into throat lozenges and appear to soothe irritated throats. It is doubtful that these agents act directly on cough receptors because they do not have access to laryngeal and airway receptors. Demulcents are agents incorporated into cough mixtures that also are thought to soothe irritated throats by coating the oral mucosa. Many cough mixtures consist mostly of sugar. These mixtures may have a mild antitussive effect. It has been suggested that the sugar serves as a sialalogue, which encourages swallowing, an act that may inhibit cough.[34] The sugar may also coat receptors, protecting them from irritation or promoting discharge and thereby blocking cough through a gating effect. Although not marketed as an antitussive, inhaled lidocaine is highly effective in blocking cough provoked by bronchoscopy. Aerosol treatments with lidocaine have been used by some physicians in patients with spontaneous cough.[34] The effectiveness of this mode of treatment is not well documented and is not recommended in patients with airway hyperreactivity because lidocaine inhalation may cause bronchoconstriction.

Cough mixtures frequently contain a variety of expectorants. These agents are supposed to alter the consistency of sputum and to thereby alter the environment of the cough receptor. These agents are ineffective as antitussives.[35] These same mixtures also frequently contain sympathomimetics, which exert a drying effect on nasal mucosa. Some evidence suggests that such agents may have an antitussive effect in patients with acute upper respiratory tract infections.[26]

INDICATIONS

Antitussives are indicated when coughs are bothersome and serve no useful function or are associated with significant complications (Table 68-3). Patients with cough frequently experience adverse respiratory sensations, such as a raw feeling in the trachea, and dyspnea. In addition, patients suffer from the anxiety of being unable to predict the occurrence of the next cough paroxysm, of being unable to terminate a coughing fit, or suffering urinary or bowel incontinence. To avoid embarrassment, such patients undergo lifestyle changes, such as avoiding social events, concerts, and restau-

TABLE 68-3   Cough Complications

Psychological
  Fear of loss of control: bladder and bowel incontinence
  Sleep deprivation
  Social isolation
  Depression

Respiratory
  Adverse respiratory sensations
  Bronchoconstriction
  Barotrauma: pneumothorax, pneumomediastinum
  Laryngeal and airway trauma

Hemodynamic
  Arrhythmia
  Impaired venous return
  Transient hypotension

Musculoskeletal
  Fractured ribs and cartilage
  Ruptured rectus abdominus muscles

Cerebral
  Syncope
  Apoplexy

rants. Patients with cough are also subject to a number of complications, which are a consequence of the vigorous muscular efforts of cough, such as strained chest and abdominal muscles, hernias, vaginal prolapse, and rib fractures. The marked pleural pressure changes associated with vigorous cough may lead to circulatory changes and syncope. In the absence of such complications, patients with productive coughs rarely seek relief of cough but rather request medication to aid in cough effectiveness. In such patients expectorants such as iodinated glycerol are indicated, albeit their efficacy is not striking.[36] When patients with productive cough suffer the complications described above, antitussives may be administered with caution. Here, one must weigh the benefits of cough suppression against the hazards of retained secretions.

ANTITUSSIVE AGENTS

The relative effectiveness of one antitussive drug versus another is difficult to establish even when well-performed, controlled trials have been conducted. Antitussive drugs are evaluated using a variety of methods.[37,38] Drugs may be tested against provoked cough, using inhaled irritating substances or against spontaneously occurring cough, using patient diaries or cough recording techniques. Often, the results with one method are not confirmed when other methods are used. The lack of adequate methodologies to evaluate antitussives has resulted in the marketing of many drugs with little clinical utility, and the use of cough mixtures, with little rational basis for their ingredients. At present, only a handful of agents are approved for antitussive use. The remarkable number of cough and cold preparations available OTC and with prescriptions, actually represent nine drugs compounded with a variety of vehicles, antihistamines, expectorants, and decongestants. Prescription

TABLE 68-4   Antitussive Agents

	Number of Formulations	Antitussive Drugs		
		Site of Action	Efficacy	Availability
Codeine	50	C, ?Per		P, OTC[a]
Hydrocodone	18	C, ?Per	= Codeine	P
Hydromorphone	1	C, ?Per	= Codeine	P
Dextromethorphan	104	C	≤ Codeine	P, OTC
Noscapine	2	C	≤ Codeine	OTC
Caramiphen	2	C	≤ Codeine	P
Diphenhydramine	1	C	≤ Codeine	OTC
Carbetapentane	3	C	≤ Codeine	P, OTC
Benzonatate	1	Per, C	≤ Codeine	P

[a] In some states.

ABBREVIATIONS: C = central; Per = peripheral; P = prescription, OTC = over-the-counter.

products generally contain the opiates codeine or hydrocodone or the opiate derivative dextromethorphan. Most OTC preparations contain dextromethorphan. In some states, codeine is available OTC, as a component of antitussive mixtures. The sale of such formulations is subject to considerable regulation. Table 68-4 lists antitussive agents available as cough formulations.

CODEINE   Among the narcotic antitussives, codeine is the drug of choice, having the least abuse potential. Efficacy has been proven in a variety of animal and human studies.[30] Human studies have included provoked and spontaneously occurring cough with both subjective and objective evaluations. Many studies have been placebo controlled. No drug is superior to codeine as an antitussive. The drug is absorbed promptly by the intestinal mucosa, reaches peak antitussive effect in 2 h, and has a duration of action of 4 to 6 h. It is metabolized by the liver to morphine and norcodeine. Ninety percent is excreted in the urine within 24 h. Adverse effects are infrequent with usual doses. Respiratory depression is minimal. The most common side effects include dryness of mouth, nose, and throat; sedation; dizziness; and disturbed coordination. Less frequently noted are gastrointestinal disturbances such as nausea, vomiting, diarrhea, and urinary disturbances such as frequency and urinary retention. Abuse potential is low. Psychological dependence requires 1 to 2 months of use. Physical dependence is rare. Its antitussive effect is dose related although greater than recommended doses do not have a proportionally greater effect. Most studies have used doses between 30 and 60 mg. The usual recommended dose is 10 to 20 mg every 4 to 6 h, not to exceed 120 mg/day. Lesser doses are recommended in poor-risk patients and the elderly and in patients receiving other central nervous system (CNS) depressants. Doses in children are 1 to 1.5 mg/kg/day in six divided doses.

HYDROCODONE   Hydrocodone is a narcotic with an antitussive effect similar to that of codeine; it may be more potent than codeine. Its abuse potential is somewhat greater, and its side effect profile similar to codeine.[33] It has no therapeutic advantage over codeine. The adult dose is 5 to 10 mg every 4 to 6 h. The dose in children is 0.6 mg/kg daily in three to four divided doses.

HYDROMORPHONE   Hydromorphone is a narcotic primarily used as an analgesic, but it does have antitussive properties and is available as a cough syrup.[33] Its side effects are similar to those of codeine, but it has a greater abuse potential and gives rise to physical addiction more readily, making prolonged use inadvisable. In addition, it has a greater tendency to produce respiratory depression. Under most circumstances, it has little advantage over codeine. The usual adult dose is 1 mg every 3 to 4 h.

DEXTROMETHORPHAN   Dextromethorphan is a nonnarcotic derived from the narcotic analgesic levorphanol. It has been effective in animal studies[39,40] and in patients using both subjective evaluation[41] and objective cough counting techniques.[42] It has no analgesic effect and thus no significant abuse potential. Its antitussive effect is probably somewhat less than that of codeine. Unlike codeine, the antitussive effect is not dose-related above 20 mg. Adverse effects are few. Nausea, dizziness, and mild sedation are occasionally noted. The drug is contraindicated in patients receiving monoamine oxidase inhibitors. The adult dose and for children greater than 12 years is 10 to 20 mg every 4 h or 30 mg every 6 to 8 h, not to exceed 120 mg/day. For children 6 to 11 years, the recommended dose is 5 to 10 mg every 4 h or 15 mg every 6 to 8 h, not to exceed 60 mg/day. For children 2 to 6 years, the recommended doses are 2.5 to 5 mg every 4 h or 7.5 mg every 6 to 8 h, not to exceed 30 mg/day.

NOSCAPINE   Noscapine is a nonnarcotic opiate that may be equivalent to codeine in antitussive effect.[43] However, an insufficient number of studies have been performed to document fully its efficacy. It has no analgesic effect, no abuse potential, and no respiratory depressive effect.[33] It is available only in OTC formulations. The side effects are minimal and include mild drowsiness and mild nausea. Allergic vasomotor rhinitis and conjunctivitis have been reported. The usual dose is 15 to 30 mg every 4 to 6 h, not to exceed

120 mg/day. Children from 2 to 12 years receive 7.5 to 15 mg every 3 to 4 h, not to exceed 60 mg/day.

CARAMIPHEN AND CARBETAPENTANE Caramiphen and a related drug carbetapentane are centrally acting drugs unrelated to the opiates. Neither drug is well studied. Although some investigations have documented efficacy to be equal to that of codeine, the overall impression is that neither drug is particularly effective.[33,44] They are rarely used in cough preparations. Side effects include mild nausea and drowsiness. These drugs have weak anticholinergic properties and should be used with caution in patients with glaucoma and urinary retention. The dose of caramiphen for adults and children over 12 is 10 to 20 mg tid or qid. The dose of carbetapentane is not well established.

DIPHENHYDRAMINE Antihistamines are reported to have some antitussive actions. Chlorpheniramine, doxylamine, phenindamine, phenyltoloxamine, pheniramine maleate, and pyrilamine maleate are components of a variety of cough mixtures. Only diphenhydramine has been judged safe and effective as an antitussive by a federal panel reviewing OTC preparations.[45] Studies presented to the review panel of the Food and Drug Administration suggested that diphenhydramine was equivalent to a low dose of codeine. The side effects are occasional drowsiness, CNS excitement, and anticholinergic effects. It needs to be used with caution in patients with glaucoma and urinary retention. The adult dose is 25 mg every 4 h, not to exceed 100 mg/day. For children 6 to 12 years, the dose is 12.5 mg every 4 h, not to exceed 50 mg/day. For children 2 to 5 years, the recommended dose is 6.25 mg every 4 h, not to exceed 25 mg/day.

BENZONATATE Benzonatate is the only ingested drug that is thought to act on peripheral receptors. Intravenous administration in animals inhibits a variety of receptors including airway stretch receptors, atrial receptors, chemoreceptors, and aortic baroreceptors.[33] At least some of its effect results from central action. Benzonatate has antitussive effects in both animals and in patients with a variety of conditions. In the few controlled studies in patients, drug efficacy has been comparable to that of codeine.[46] In addition to its antitussive effect, it appears to reduce dyspnea in asthmatic subjects but does not depress respiration. Side effects are few and unusual and include sedation, headache, rash, hypersensitivity reactions, and chilly sensations. It is available in one product in the form of perles. The perle must be swallowed whole, because chewing results in oral anesthesia with choking and CNS effects such as restlessness and convulsions. The recommended dose is one perle (100 mg) tid with a maximum of 6 perles daily.

References

1. Widdicombe JG: Respiratory reflexes and defense, in Brain JD, Proctor DF, Reid CM (eds): *Respiratory Defense Mechanisms*, vol 5. New York, Marcel Dekker, 1977: 593-629.
2. Korpas J, Widdicombe JG: Aspects of the cough reflex. *Respir Med* 1991; 85(suppl A):3.
3. Widdicombe JG: Receptors in the trachea and bronchi of the cat. *J Physiol (Lond)* 1954; 123:71.
4. Coleridge JCG, Coleridge HM: Afferent vagal C-fiber innervation of the lungs and airways and its functional significance. *Rev Physiol Biochem Pharmacol* 1984; 99:1.
5. Coleridge HM, Coleridge JCG, Roberts AM: Rapid shallow breathing evoked by selective stimulation of bronchial C-fibers in dogs. *J Physiol (Lond)* 1983; 340:415.
6. Tatar M, Webber SE, Widdicombe JG: Lung C-fiber receptor activation and defensive reflexes in anesthetized cats. *J Physiol (Lond)* 1988; 402:411.
7. Hanacek J, Davies A, Widdicombe JG: Influence of lung stretch receptors on the cough reflex in rabbits. *Respiration* 1984; 45:161.
8. Salem H, Aviado DM: Antitussive drugs with special reference to a new theory for the initiation of the cough reflex and the influence of bronchodilators. *Am J Med Sci* 1964; 247:585.
9. Eschenbacher WL, Boushey HA, Sheppard D: Alteration in osmolarity of inhaled aerosols causes bronchoconstriction and cough, but absence of a permeant anion causes cough alone. *Am Rev Respir Dis* 1984; 129:211.
10. Karlsson JA, Sant'Ambrogio G, Widdicombe J: Afferent neural pathways in cough and reflex bronchoconstriction. *J Appl Physiol* 1988; 65:1007.
11. Chausow AM, Banner AS: Comparison of the tussive effects of histamine and methacholine in humans. *J Appl Physiol* 1983; 55:541.
12. Korpas J, Tomori Z: Cough and other respiratory reflexes, in Herzog H (ed): *Progress in Respiration Research*, vol 12. Basel, S Karger, 1979; 22.
13. Kase Y, Wakita Y, Kito G, et al.: Centrally induced cough in the cat. *Life Sci* 1970; 9:49.
14. Davis JN: Autonomous breathing. *Arch Neurol* 1974; 30:480.
15. Irwin RS, Carrao WM, Pratter MR: Chronic persistent cough in the adult: the spectrum and frequency of causes and successful outcome of specific therapy. *Am Rev Respir Dis* 1981; 123:413.
16. Poe RH, Harder RV, Israel RH, Kallay MC: Chronic persistent cough. Experience in diagnosis and outcome using an anatomic diagnostic protocol. *Chest* 1989; 95:723.
17. Poe RH, Israel RH, Utell MJ, Hall WJ: Chronic cough: bronchoscopy or pulmonary function testing. *Am Rev Respir Dis* 1982; 126:160.
18. Carrao WM, Braman SS, Irwin RS: Chronic cough as the sole presenting manifestation of bronchial asthma. *N Engl J Med* 1979; 300:633.
19. Irwin RS, Zawacki JK, Curley FJ, et al.: Chronic cough as the sole presenting manifestation of gastro-esophageal reflux. *Am Rev Respir Dis* 1989; 140:1294.
20. Ing AJ, Ngu MC, Breslin ABX: Pathogenesis of chronic persistent cough associated with gastroesophageal reflux. *Am Rev Respir Crit Care Med* 1994; 149:160.
21. Irwin RS, Curley FJ, French CL: Chronic cough. The spectrum and frequency of causes, key components of the diagnostic evaluation and outcome of specific therapy. *Am Rev Respir Dis* 1990; 141:640.
22. Grief J, Fink G, Smorzk Y, et al.: Nedocromil sodium and placebo in the treatment of bronchial asthma: a multivariable, double-blind parallel group comparison. *Chest* 1989; 96:583.
23. Barnes PJ: Effect of nedocromil sodium on airway sensory nerves. *J Allergy Clin Immunol* 1993; 92:182.
24. Irwin RS, Curley FJ, Bennett FM: Appropriate use of antitussives and protussives. A practical review. *Drugs* 1993; 46:80.
25. Ing AJ, Ngu MC, Breslin ABX: A randomized double blind placebo controlled crossover study of ranitidine in patients with chronic persistent cough associated with gastro-esophageal reflux. *Am Rev Respir Dis* 1992; 145:A11.
26. Smith MBH, Feldman W: Over-the-counter cold medications. A

critical review of clinical trials between 1950 and 1991. *JAMA* 1993; 269:2258.

27. Eccles R, Morris S, Jawad M: Lack of effect of codeine in the treatment of cough associated with acute upper respiratory infection. *J Clin Pharm Ther* 1992; 17:175.

28. Berkowitz RB, Connell JT, Dietz AJ, et al.: The effectiveness of nonsedating antihistamine loratadine plus pseudoephedrine in the symptomatic management of the common colds. *Ann Allergy* 1989; 63:336.

29. Holmes PW, Barter CCE, Pierce RJ: Chronic persistent cough: use of ipratropium bromide in undiagnosed cases following upper respiratory tract infection. *Respir Med* 1992; 86:425.

30. Eddy NB, Friebel H, Hahn K-J, Halbach J: Codeine and its alternatives for pain and cough relief. *Bull World Health Organ* 1969; 40:425.

31. Adcock JJ, Smith TW: Inhibitory effects of the opioid peptide BW443C on smaller diameter sensory nerve activity in the vagus. *Br J Pharmacol* 1987; 96:596P.

32. Adcock JJ, Schneider C, Smith TW: Effects of codeine, morphine and a novel pentapeptide BW443C on cough, nociception and ventilation in the unanesthetised guinea-pig. *Br J Pharmacol* 1988; 93:93.

33. Salem H, Aviado DM: *International Encyclopedia of Pharmacology and Therapeutics*, section 27, vol 111: *Antitussive Agents*. Oxford, Pergamon Press, 1970.

34. Fuller RW, Jackson DM: Physiology and treatment of cough. *Thorax* 1991; 45:425.

35. Kuhn JJ, Hendley O, Adams KF, et al.: Antitussive effect of guaifenesin in young adults with natural colds. *Chest* 1982; 82:713.

36. Petty TL: The National Mucolytic Study: results of a randomized, double-blind, placebo-controlled study of iodinated glycerol in chronic obstructive bronchitis. *Chest* 1990; 97:75.

37. Korpas J, Tomori Z: Cough and other respiratory reflexes, in Herzog H (ed): *Progress in Respiration Research*, vol 12. Basel, S Karger, 1979: 81–90.

38. Banner AS: Cough, in Simmons DH (ed): *Current Pulmonology*, vol 9. Chicago, Year Book Medical Publishers, 1988: 124–127.

39. Benson WM, Stefko PL, Randall LG: Comparative pharmacology of levorphan, racemorphan and dextromethorphan and related methyl ethers. *J Pharmacol Exp Ther* 1953; 109:189.

40. Stefko PL, Denzel J, Hickey I: Experimental investigation of nine antitussive drugs. *J Pharm Sci* 1961; 50:216.

41. Gravenstein JS, Devloo RA, Beecher HK: Effects of antitussive agents on experimental and pathologic cough in man. *J Appl Physiol* 1954; 7:119.

42. Reece CA, Cherry A, Reece AT, et al.: Tape recorder for evaluation of coughs in children. *Am J Dis Child* 1966; 112:124.

43. Barasz Z, Bonstein H, Aguet F, Favez G: Effet antitussif comparé du chlorhydrate de noscapine et du bitartrate de dihydocodeine. *Praxis* 1962; 51:317.

44. Bickerman HA: Clinical pharmacology of antitussive agents. *Clinical Pharm Ther* 1962; 3:353.

45. FDA Review Panel on over-the-counter drugs for cough and cold preparations. *Fed Reg* 1976; 41:38338.

46. Simon SW: A new non-narcotic antitussive drug. *Ann Allergy* 1957; 15:521.

Chapter 69
MUCOLYTIC THERAPIES
LUCILLE A. LESTER

A variety of common pulmonary disorders, including asthma, chronic bronchitis, and cystic fibrosis, are associated with excessive or abnormally constituted respiratory secretions. These secretions lead to variable degrees of airways obstruction and contribute to abnormalities in gas exchange and, thereby, to the morbidity associated with these diseases. There has been an improved understanding of the mechanisms by which mucous hypersecretion occurs in diseases such as asthma and chronic bronchitis, and the finding of the gene for cystic fibrosis and the understanding of the function of its product, cystic fibrosis transmembrane regulator protein (CFTR), have led to an improved understanding of the basis for the abnormally thick and viscid secretions that are the hallmark of this disease.

Normal Mucus

PRODUCTION AND SECRETION OF MUCUS

Mucus covers the surface of the conducting airways from the nasal cavity to the larger bronchioles. Mucus is the major component of the thin, watery, viscoelastic secretion that coats and protects the respiratory epithelial surface. This coat, which is generally 5 μm thick, serves a variety of functions. It acts as a barrier to infectious and irritative particles;

it is a medium for the transport and removal of trapped, inhaled particles, debris, "senescent cells," and cell products[1]; and it provides for airway humidification, waterproofing, and maintenance of an optimal environment for ciliary action.[2] Cell types responsible for airway secretions are the mucous and serous cells of the submucosal glands, which produce both mucus and serous fluid, respectively, and the goblet cells of the surface epithelium, which produce mucus (Fig. 69-1). The surface of the trachea and bronchi includes ciliated epithelial cells and goblet cells in a 5:1 ratio. Mucus production by goblet cells is stimulated by direct contact with irritants such as cigarette smoke, sulfur dioxide, ammonia, and organic vapors[3]; they also may respond to sympathomimetic agents. Submucosal glands contribute a volume of secretion that is 40 times greater than that provided by goblet cells. They are directly innervated by the parasympathetic nervous system, and therefore are affected by changes in vagal activity. Both beta- and alpha-adrenergic stimulation influence mucous secretion, and beta-adrenergic blockade decreases basal secretion. Activation of adrenergic and cholinergic receptors stimulates gland secretions with distinct properties. Many neuropeptides, such as substance P, other tachykinins, and vasoactive intestinal peptide (VIP), also have been shown to be important in regulating normal mucous secretion.[4] Animal studies suggest that the vol-

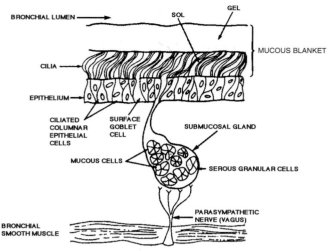

FIGURE 69-1 Cross-section schema of a bronchiole wall, illustrating the components of the mucociliary system in the lung. (From Rao.[8])

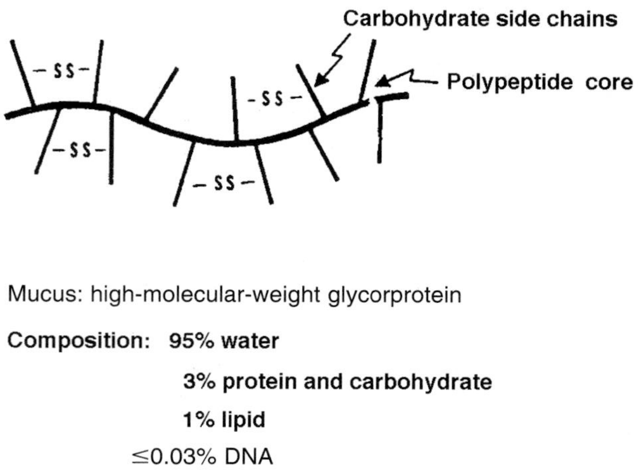

Mucus: high-molecular-weight glycorprotein

Composition: 95% water

3% protein and carbohydrate

1% lipid

≤0.03% DNA

FIGURE 69-2 Basic structure and constituents of the mucous macromolecule. (From Rao.[8])

ume of secretions produced from the lungs may approach 100 ml/day, while human studies estimate the volume under normal conditions to be as little as 10 ml/day.[5]

COMPOSITION OF MUCUS

Respiratory mucus is a mixture of a variety of proteins, glycoproteins, lipids, electrolytes, and water. Individual mucin molecules range in size between 3 and 32 million daltons, and are ≤80 percent carbohydrate.[6] The carbohydrate is in the form of oligosaccharide side chains that may be linear or branched and are linked by N-acetylglucosamine residues to threonine or serine of the mucin polypeptide backbone. Glycosylated regions, which make up 60 percent or more of the mucin monomer, are insensitive to proteolysis, while the remaining "naked" regions are sensitive to proteolysis.[7] Mucin chains are cross-linked by disulfide bonds supplied by cysteine residues, and eventually form flexible, threadlike strands 200 to 1000 mm in length. Mucous glycoprotein strands are variably cross-linked with each other by disulfide and hydrogen bonds, resulting in the formation of a gel. The gel has a high water content (approximately 95 percent), and the final gelation of mucus results from a combination of hydrogen, electrostatic, and hydrophilic bonds together with specific disulfide linkages[8] (Fig. 69-2). In the normal situation, bonding within mucus results in low viscosity but high elasticity. The hydration of mucus is controlled by transepithelial chloride secretion with some additional passive diffusion of water. The passive diffusion of water occurs as a result of the osmotic effect of other secreted materials in mucus. It is important to note that water is incorporated into mucous gel during its formation, but, once formed, mucus does not incorporate topically applied water.[9]

Mucus contains numerous other molecules that serve both to regulate the physical properties of the final secretion product and to protect the mucous membrane and contribute to host defenses. Some of these substances derive

from the blood by transudation, while others are known to be products of the serous cells of the epithelial submucous glands. Important nonmucin components include albumin, protease inhibitors, immunoglobulin, lysozyme, lactoferrin, and peroxidase.

Albumin is a major component of mucus, which enters the airway through passive transudation from local blood vessels and appears to bind and transport biologically active molecules and to act as a free-radical scavenger. Albumin also has been found to be a modulator of the viscosity of the mucous gel.[10]

Leukocytes and bacteria are the major sources of proteases in human airway secretion. Neutrophil elastase, which is released from neutrophils after they enter the airway by diapedesis through local vessels, is a serine protease that can degrade a wide range of extracellular matrix components in addition to elastin.[4] Neutrophil elastase is a powerful stimulant of both submucosal gland secretion and goblet cell hyperplasia.[11] Bacterial elastase degrades lung elastin, but other bacterial proteases also have been shown to degrade immunoglobulin, lysozymes, basement membranes, and complement components.[12] Normal airway secretions contain protease inhibitors in small amounts; in particular, α_1-antiprotease and antileukoprotease, or mucous protease inhibitor.[13] In situations of chronic airways infection, their activity may be overwhelmed, and administration of additional antiproteases, in conjunction with more specific therapeutic agents, may provide added benefit in the attempt to clear airway secretion and protect airways (see below).

Immunoglobulins, lysozyme, lactoferrin, and peroxidase are produced in serous cells of the submucosal glands, and all play specific roles in defense against infectious agents.

PHYSICAL PROPERTIES OF MUCUS

The biochemical composition of mucus determines its physical characteristics, which in turn directly affect airway mucociliary clearance. Mucins display non-Newtonian viscoelastic properties intermediate between those of a viscous fluid and an elastic gel. When ciliary force is applied to mucus, deformation occurs; when the force is released, it recovers to its original position. Thus, mucus has an elastic component in which energy can be stored. Mucus also flows when ciliary force is applied; thus, it has the viscous properties of a liquid when its energy is dissipated.[8] The resultant viscoelasticity permits the mechanical coupling of mucus with cilia. In the mucous blanket coating the airways, mucus consists of two physical phases: a *gel* that is propelled upward toward the larynx by cilia; and a thin, proteinaceous, watery *sol* layer in which cilia beat in an energy-conserving wavelike motion called *metachronism*—that is, parallel ranks of cilia beat one after another[14] (Fig. 69-3). Alterations that occur in the composition of mucus in disease states or from mucolytic agents will have a direct effect on normal mucociliary function.

MUCOCILIARY CLEARANCE

Cilia beat at frequencies of 10 to 20 Hz, and the frequency of the beat increases from the peripheral airways to the trachea. The rate of mucociliary clearance in the normal lung has been estimated at 1.5 mm/min in the periphery and 21.5 mm/min in the trachea. Clearance rates are known to be slowed by various conditions or agents; in particular, increasing age, atmospheric pollutants and cigarette smoke, hyperoxia and hypoxia, general anesthetics, parasympatholytics (atropine), narcotics,[8] and in disease situations such as chronic obstructive pulmonary disease[15] and cystic fibrosis.[16] β-Adrenergic and cholinergic drugs and methylxanthines increase mucociliary clearance to some degree. For cholinergic agents, the increase may result indirectly from an increase in the secretion of mucus.[17] The mechanism by which these various factors affect clearance rates is likely to involve a complex interaction between ciliary beat frequency, the depth of the periciliary sol phase, and the quantity and viscoelastic properties of the airway mucus and the state of hydration. Elasticity appears to be crucial for mucociliary transport, and mucolytic agents, which destroy the elasticity of mucus and reduce viscosity, may have a negative effect or impair normal physiologic mucus clearance. Rao[8] claims that facilitating the physiological clearance of mucus by optimizing viscoelasticity should be the goal of mucolytic therapy.

Disease States Associated with Altered Mucus

The normal function of respiratory tract mucus is altered in various disease entities as a result of changes in volume, changes in hydration, or changes in the composition of the secretion. Mucous hypersecretion, abnormal ion transport at the epithelial cell level, infection, and inflammation are processes that occur in pulmonary disease. The extent and nature of the mucus alteration in diseases such as chronic bronchitis, cystic fibrosis, and asthma determine to some extent the efficacy of mucolytic agents.

CHRONIC BRONCHITIS

Chronic bronchitis is a clinical diagnosis made on the basis of a history of production of sputum on most days for more than three months a year, or for two consecutive years in individuals who have no other underlying pulmonary dis-

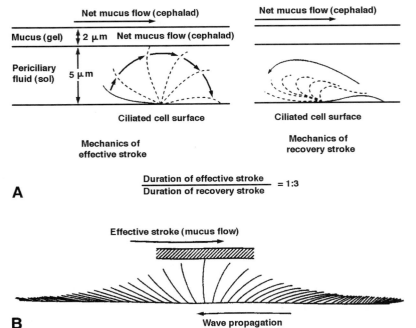

FIGURE 69-3 *A.* Schematic representation of ciliary motion and mucus flow. *B.* Wave pattern of metachronal ciliary beat. (From Witek and Schachter.[2])

ease.[18] The histology of conducting airways of individuals with this problem reflect acute and chronic inflammation with hyperplasia of the submucosal glands and goblet cells. There is an increase in the number of goblet cells as well as hypertrophy of the submucosal glands as measured by the Reid index of gland to airway wall thickness ratio.[19] In addition, airway explants and submucosal gland cells from patients with chronic bronchitis produce excessive amounts of mucous glycoprotein.[20] Tobacco smoke generally is regarded as the major predisposing factor in the mucous hypersecretion in this disease, but prior viral infection, other pollutants, or genetic predisposition also may be factors.[21] Sputum production and expectoration increases in amount and frequency as the disease progresses, and bronchial infection with mucopurulence caused by influx of neutrophils is recurrent. Slowed mucociliary clearance has been demonstrated in studies of these patients. Mucus clearance may be so impaired that cough becomes the major mechanism for removal of bronchopulmonary secretions.[22] Mucolytic agents may have limited benefit during periods of infectious exacerbation, but appear to have little impact on the underlying hypersecretory state.

ASTHMA

The pathophysiology of asthma includes bronchoconstriction, airway inflammation and edema, and mucous hypersecretion. The mucus produced by individuals with asthma ranges from copious, watery secretions to extremely viscid mucus expectorated only with difficulty. During an acute episode of asthma, 80 percent of patients report sputum production (adults > children), and a smaller percentage reportedly have bronchorrhea (>100 ml of sputum per day).[23] The sputum expectorated during an acute attack is often thick and purulent-appearing and is related to increased numbers of eosinophils. Degeneration of eosinophils gives rise to Charcot-Leyden crystals, which can be detected on microscopic examination of sputum, in addition to bronchiolar casts composed of inspissated mucus and cellular debris (Curschmann's spirals), as well as clumps of bronchial epithelial cells (Creola bodies).[2] Copius sputum production has been associated in some instances with persistent airflow obstruction, where it appears that sputum production may overwhelm normal clearance mechanisms. Mucous gland hyperplasia and increased numbers of goblet cells are usual in patients with asthma. The stimulus for hyperplasia is not known, but a large number of mediators found in bronchoalveolar lavage fluid and tissues of patients with asthma are known to be secretagogues.[24] Mucous hypersecretion is likely caused by those mediators that cause the asthma attack. Both cholinergic and adrenergic stimuli appear to contribute to hypersecretion in asthma,[25] and two enzymes, mast cell chymase[26] and neutrophil elastase,[27] recently have been shown to be potent secretagogues in airway submucosal glands. Eosinophil elastase possibly has a similar role.

The pathology of fatal cases of asthma demonstrate acute and chronic inflammatory cells in the airway, submucosal edema, bronchial smooth muscle hypertrophy, submucosal gland enlargement, increased numbers of goblet cells, and areas of focal desquamation of epithelium. In addition, extensive mucous plugging, especially in the distal airways, contributes to abnormalities of gas exchange and, in some individuals, to the development of respiratory failure.[28] Mucous plugging and obstruction of larger segmental airways leading to atelectasis is a common complication of an acute asthma episode in a young child with asthma. In general, mucolytic agents have very little role in the treatment of acute asthma, whereas treatment directed at reversing airway inflammation and effecting bronchodilatation is paramount. Certain medications, such as aerosolized corticosteroids, appear to affect sputum volume and airway clearance in asthma,[23] but are not considered mucolytic agents in the strictest sense.

CYSTIC FIBROSIS

The bronchopulmonary disease cystic fibrosis (CF) is characterized by the accumulation of viscid, thick secretions in the conducting airways, recurrent respiratory infections, and progressive deterioration in lung function leading ultimately to respiratory failure and death.[29–31] However, the lungs of newborn infants with CF appear to be histologically normal,[32,33] and neonates with CF have normal lung function.[30] The earliest microscopic changes in respiratory epithelium include dilation of acinar and ductal lumina of the submucosal glands and glandular hypertrophy thought to result from abnormal secretions and obstruction of the ductal lumen.[33] In addition to hyperplasia and hypertrophy of mucous glands, the earliest gross pathology is the plugging of bronchioles with excessive secretions.[30,34] Mucous gland hypertrophy appears to occur before inflammatory changes suggestive of infection; thus, the abnormal secretions are hypothesized to predispose to infection rather than result from it.[29]

Nearly every mucous-secreting epithelium has been found to be altered in CF. Thus, great efforts have been made to characterize the physical properties and molecular components of mucous secretions in CF to account for the pervasive mucous obstruction.[35] Subtle, but inconsistent, abnormalities in the mucous glycoprotein macromolecular structure and composition have been found, and abnormal electrolyte and water content also have been known for some time. The identification in 1989 of the gene responsible for cystic fibrosis, and the subsequent characterization of its gene product, CFTR, as a cyclic AMP–regulated chloride ion channel,[36] have greatly enhanced understanding of the basis for the abnormally viscid mucus. Sodium ion transport (specifically the rate of transepithelial sodium absorption) also is known to be increased in CF airway epithelium to values two to three times those of normal airway epithelium.[37] The combination of defective or absent chloride secretion and increased sodium absorption would be expected to generate dehydrated airway fluid. Although this is a plausible explanation for the pathogenesis of CF, little is known about how abnormal ion transport specifically translates into altered mucus and obstructed airways.

Though the respiratory tract secretions in CF are initially affected by the underlying ion transport defect, the effect of chronic airways infection and resultant inflammation leads to ineffective airway clearance and secondary mucous hypersecretion, which are of major importance as the disease progresses.[35] Chronic bacterial infection stimulates an inflammatory response including the recruitment of neutrophils, which eventually accumulate in excessive amounts in airways. Neutrophils are the predominant source of elastase, which is a potent secretagogue and causes further airway damage.[38] When neutrophils disintegrate, they release high concentrations of extracellular deoxyribonucleic acid (DNA) into airway secretions.[39] Polymerized DNA strands contribute to the increased viscoelasticity of sputum in CF. Mucous glycoproteins and extracellular DNA are responsible for the viscoelastic properties of CF sputum. However, it

is likely that the increased viscosity of infected airway secretions in CF is more attributable to extracellular DNA than to glycoproteins.[40] The mean content of DNA has been found to be 10.2 percent of the dry weight of secretions from some patients with CF,[40] and DNA from degenerating leukocytes has been found to approach concentrations averaging 6 mg/ml.[41] Solutions containing purified high-molecular-weight DNA at this concentration are highly viscous.[42]

Eventually, a cycle of airways infection, inflammation, obstruction, and destruction characterizes well-established CF lung disease (Fig. 69-4). Agents aimed at altering mucus have been sought to interrupt this cycle for treatment of CF.

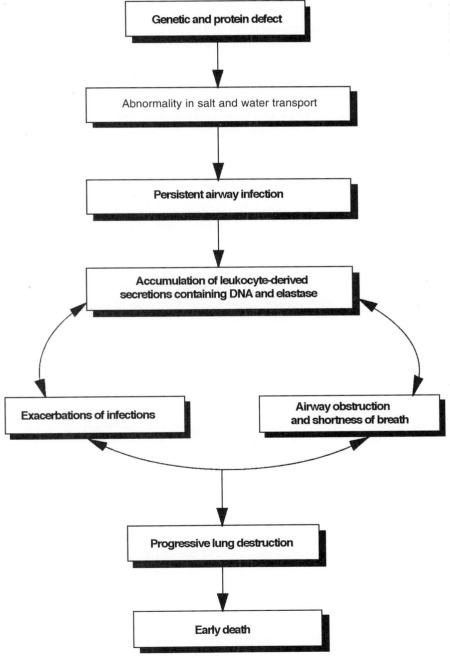

FIGURE 69-4 Pathogenesis of pulmonary involvement in cystic fibrosis. [Reproduced with permission: Pulmozyme (Dornase alfa) DNase Product Monograph. Genentech, Inc., San Francisco, CA, 1994.]

N-acetylcysteine offered the only hope for a long period of time, but its effectiveness is limited and possibly outweighed by its undesirable side effects. Newer agents such as dornase alfa (rhDNase; Pulmozyme) offer some hope for more effective alteration of airway mucus and slowing of progression of the disease (see below).

BRONCHIECTASIS

Bronchiectasis, which is defined as abnormal dilatation of bronchi or bronchioles, typically results from severe or chronic airways bacterial infection. Most often bronchiectasis results from an underlying disorder such as cystic fibrosis, B-cell immunodeficiency states, or ciliary motility defects, but it may be familial and/or idiopathic. Chronic infection, airway inflammation, and mucous hypersecretion all occur in individuals with bronchiectasis, and the same treatment considerations and possible efficacy of mucolytic agents apply here as well.

BRONCHOPULMONARY DYSPLASIA

Bronchopulmonary dysplasia is a complication of premature birth, which results in interstitial fibrosis and edema and damage to small airways. Barotrauma and hyperoxia are primary factors that act on developing premature lungs that lack surfactant and major antioxidant and antiprotease defense systems. The major clinical consequences in the fully developed syndrome are squamous metaplasia, which replaces ciliated respiratory epithelium, and ineffective clearance of airway secretions. Airways hyperreactivity is a frequent secondary problem, though hypersecretion of mucus is not documented. Facilitation of secretion clearance is important in the long-term care of these infants, and anticholinergic agents, such as glycopyrrulate, have been used to reduce airway secretions. Mucolytic agents do not appear to have a role in the management of this increasingly common pediatric disorder, but they have not been systematically evaluated.

Mucolytic Agents

METHODS OF MUCOLYSIS

Mucolytic drugs are those that alter the rheological properties of mucus by acting directly on the secretions or by modifying the metabolic activity of the cells that secrete mucus.[43] Rao[8] describes three processes by which mucous structure can be altered: *proteolysis, pH adjustment*, and *disulfide bond disruption*. All three methods of mucolysis destroy the elasticity of mucus while reducing the viscosity because the gel structure is broken down. Since elasticity appears to be critical for mucociliary transport, mucolytics may have a potentially negative effect on physiologic mucus clearance.[8] It is not desirable to liquify secretions unless a person is able to cough adequately. The goal of therapy with mucolytic agents should be to facilitate physiologic clearance by *optimizing* the viscoelasticity of mucus. Assuring adequate hydration by the oral or intravenous route is important, but water admin-

istered to the airway as a "bland aerosol" will not affect the hydration or composition of mucus, though it may aid in secretion clearance. Avoiding exposure to irritants and extremes in humidity and temperature also is important in reducing the development of mucostasis. There is some question whether any of the mucolytic agents prevent airways obstruction by tenacious secretions more effectively than hydration alone.[5] The remainder of this chapter addresses the efficacy of specific mucolytic agents currently in use and related agents that are being investigated for their ability to alter mucus and improve airway secretion clearance in specific clinical settings.

N-ACETYLCYSTEINE

CHEMISTRY

N-Acetylcysteine (Mucomyst) is the N-acetyl derivative of the amino acid L-cysteine. Single oral doses are rapidly absorbed and excreted slowly; high concentrations are still active in lung tissue up to 5 h after oral administration.[44] After aerosol administration, N-acetylcysteine–cysteine disulfide can be found in the urine, indicating the absorption of swallowed drug by this route.[45]

MECHANISM OF ACTION

N-Acetylcysteine acts as a mucolytic agent because it disrupts the structure of mucous molecules by substituting its own sulfhydryl groups for the disulfide bonds of the mucus (Fig. 69-5). The substituted sulfhydryl groups in the mucous strands do not allow for cross-linking, and, as a result, the viscosity and the elasticity of mucus is reduced. This compound is active in the presence of the cellular debris and DNA that are present in purulent secretions. Once in contact with the mucus, N-acetylcysteine begins to act immediately;

FIGURE 69-5 Mechanism of action by which N-acetylcysteine reduces the viscosity of mucus by substituting the sulfhydryl for the disulfide bonds. (From Rao.[8])

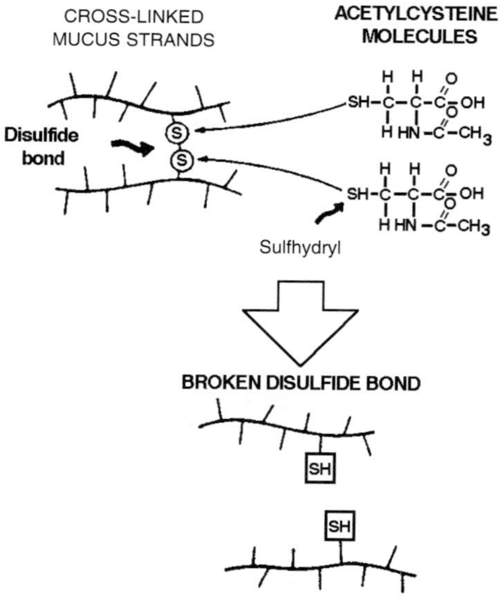

its mucolytic activity is enhanced at greater pH, and is optimal at a local pH between 7 and 9.

CLINICAL USE AND EFFICACY

N-Acetylcysteine is administered as a solution by aerosol or by direct instillation into the tracheobronchial tree. A reduction in viscosity of sputum of patients with cystic fibrosis, asthma, emphysema, or bronchitis has been demonstrated in vitro.[46] Its use during fiberoptic bronchoscopy to relieve mucous plugging in patients with asthma[47] and atelectasis[48] has been reported to be beneficial, and its usefulness when delivered directly through endotracheal tube to clear inspissated secretions has been demonstrated.[49] However, the delivery of N-acetylcysteine by metered dose inhaler did not result in clinical benefit in a group of patients with chronic bronchitis treated for a 16-week period.[50] Many clinical trials have reported efficacy based on increased sputum production after treatment with N-acetylcysteine, but few have reported beneficial effects on pulmonary function. It would appear that the efficacy of this drug in the treatment of mucostasis is highly variable from patient to patient, and the decision to continue to treat must be based on objective assessment of individual patients.

In the United States, the therapeutic use of N-acetylcysteine for respiratory care is limited to aerosol delivery; however, orally administered drug has been judged to be beneficial on the basis of objective and subjective sputum characterization, clinical improvement, and improvement in pulmonary function.[51,52] An increase in mucociliary clearance was reported in healthy subjects treated with 600 mg of N-acetylcysteine a day for 60 days[53] and in smokers with hypersecretory bronchitis on the same regimen for 10 days.[54] In an interesting unrelated study, N-acetylcysteine administered orally in the same dose of 600 mg/day resulted in increased plasma and bronchoalveolar lavage fluid glutathione levels, which appeared to enhance the antioxidant system in individuals with smoke-induced airway changes.[55] Plasma and red cell glutathione levels also were increased in association with clinical improvement when N-acetylcysteine was administered parenterally in acute respiratory diseases (ARDs).[56] Thus, the benefits of N-acetylcysteine in certain disease states may be secondary to its antioxidant properties rather than to mucolysis.

DOSAGE

N-Acetylcysteine is available in solutions of either 10% or 20% for nebulization. The 10% solution may be used undiluted; the 20% solution may be diluted with saline or water, or mixed with albuterol (0.5 ml of 0.5% solution) or isoproterenol (0.05%). The manufacturer recommends the following dosing frequencies and strengths:

- 10% solution: 3 to 5 ml three or four times daily.
- 20% solution: 6 to 10 ml three or four times daily.
- 10% solution with 0.05% isoproterenol: 3 to 5 ml four times daily.
- Direct instillation into airway: 1 to 2 ml of 10% or 20% solution.

N-Acetylcysteine is physically incompatible with ampicillin, amphotericin, erythromycin lactobionate, and tetracyclines, and should never be combined with these antibiotics for nebulization. Data are not readily available on the compatibility of N-acetylcysteine and aminoglycosides that are more likely to be used for inhalation, particularly in patients with chronic bronchial infection such as cystic fibrosis. Because it is a reducing agent, N-acetylcysteine is incompatible with rubber and some metals; it should only be administered through equipment made of glass, plastic, or aluminum.[5]

SIDE EFFECTS

N-Acetylcysteine has a disagreeable odor and taste, which may lead to nausea or vomiting; which may affect compliance for some patients. Inhalation of the drug may produce bronchospasm, particularily in those who have airways hyperresponsiveness. This has led to the recommendation for its concomitant use with an inhaled bronchodilator.[57]

DORNASE ALFA

CHEMISTRY

Recombinant human deoxyribonuclease (dornase alfa; rhDNase; Pulmozyme) is a glycoprotein containing 260 amino acids with a molecular weight of 37,000.[58] It is produced by genetically engineered Chinese hamster ovary cells containing DNA encoded for the native human protein with a primary amino acid structure of deoxyribonuclease I (DNase), which is identical to that of the native human enzyme. Native human DNase is normally present in saliva, urine, pancreatic secretions, and blood, and is responsible for the digestion of extracellular DNA.[59] In studies of pulmonary secretions in cystic fibrosis in the early 1960s, DNA was found to account for 3 percent to 4 percent of the total solids in cystic fibrosis sputum and for less than 1 percent in bronchiectasis sputum; only traces of DNA could be isolated from the "normal" mucus in laryngectomized patients in this study.[60] Bovine pancreatic DNase (dornase) was approved for human use and used with some success soon after these studies, but the preparations were found to be contaminated with proteases, the bovine proteins were antigenic, and the agent often proved to be a bronchial irritant.[61] With the advent of molecular cloning techniques and improvements in purifying recombinant proteins, renewed interest in this treatment modality arose. The gene for recombinant human deoxyribonuclease I (rhDNase) was cloned from a pancreatic cDNA library and used to express the recombinant protein in mammalian cells.[58] Human DNase I and bovine DNase I have extensive structural homology, but they have only 77 percent overall identity at the amino acid level. Almost all of the differences between the two proteins are located in potentially immunogenetic regions of the surface of the molecule, suggesting that adverse reactions to the bovine protein could be an immunologic response to foreign protein.[58]

MECHANISM OF ACTION

Catalytic amounts of rhDNase greatly reduce the viscosity of purulent cystic fibrosis sputum in vitro, rapidly transforming it from a nonflowing viscous gel to a flowing liquid. Qualitative studies of purified rhDNase, protease-free bovine DNase, heat-inactivated rhDNase, and saline showed that both rhDNase and bovine DNase, but not heat-inactivated rhDNase or saline, dramatically increased the pourability of CF sputum in a time-dependent manner. A quantitative study[58] using the Brookfield cone-plate viscometer confirmed the effect of rhDNase on viscosity. When CF sputum was incubated for 15 min at 37°C with five consecutive concentrations of rhDNase, viscosity decreased in a concentration-dependent manner (Fig. 69-6). Other enzymes similarly tested—lysosomal DNase II, RNase, trypsin, chymotrypsin, and *N*-acetylcysteine—had minimal effects on sputum viscosity.[58]

The mechanism of action of rhDNase in improving pulmonary function in patients with cystic fibrosis probably is related to selective cleavage of DNA in purulent airway secretions,[62] but the precise mechanism by which hydrolysis of extracellular DNA facilitates clearance of secretions in CF is unknown. It is speculated that biophysical properties other than viscosity are altered in cystic fibrosis secretions in vivo by treatment with rhDNase and that these alterations are responsible for the observed clinical benefits.[63]

CLINICAL USE AND EFFICACY
Phase I, II, and III clinical studies, involving from 12 to 968 patients (≥5 years of age) for 10 days to 24 weeks, were carried out in a 2-year period prior to FDA approval of the drug in January, 1994. In the initial phase I nonrandomized, repetitive, dose-escalation study of 12 patients over 10 days, pulmonary function tests and dyspnea scores improved, and a trend toward decreased sputum bacterial density was noted.[64] Two 10-day duration phase II randomized, double-blind, placebo-controlled studies of different dosing regimens indicated that inhalation of rhDNase improved pulmonary function, regardless of baseline FVC; benefit began within 3 days and was lost 18 days after cessation of therapy.[65] A long-term phase II study of intermittent dosing (2 weeks on, 2 weeks off for 24 weeks) showed that FVC and FEV$_1$ improved each time therapy was initiated, and improvement in both parameters subsided to baseline values each time therapy was interrupted. The phase III double-blind study of 968 patients continued for 24 weeks and showed a decrease, but not elimination, of the number of exacerbations of respiratory symptoms, and a significant improvement in pulmonary function (mean 5.8 ± 0.7 percent and 5.6 ± 0.7 percent increase in FEV$_1$) in those patients receiving once daily and twice daily treatment, respectively.[66] When the previously untreated (placebo) patients were given rhDNase during the subsequent 24 week open-label component of the study, they had a similar improvement from baseline in their pulmonary function (Fig. 69-7). A quantitative microbiological sputum analysis in 59 stable patients with CF treated with rhDNase showed a significant decrease in bacterial density (CFU/ml of sputum) over a 3-month period.[67] A short-term study of CF patients experiencing pulmonary exacerbations for which they required hospitalization, and a study of severely ill patients with baseline FVC less than 40 percent of predicted, showed no evidence of efficacy after 2 weeks of therapy.

Though studied extensively and currently only approved for treatment of individuals with cystic fibrosis, rhDNase is undergoing clinical trials in patients with chronic bronchitis. These patients also have increased airway secretion and chronic infection, which should increase DNA content of sputum. Phase II trials in stable outpatients and in a group experiencing acute pulmonary exacerbations showed that the drug was well-tolerated, but efficacy was not documented objectively. These were short-term studies, and more definitive phase III trials have been initiated.[68]

DOSAGE
Early phase II studies of rhDNase in cystic fibrosis showed efficacy in three different dosages (0.6, 2.5, and 10 mg); the greatest improvement in FVC and FEV$_1$ occurred in the two higher-dose groups.[65] No significant differences were found in once-a-day as compared with twice-a-day therapy with a 2.5 mg dose. Once-a-day administration of 2.5 mg/ml

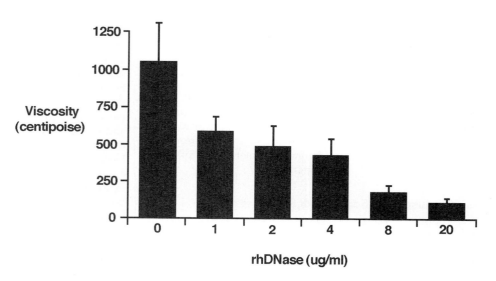

FIGURE 69-6 Effect of rhDNase on viscosity of cystic fibrosis sputum by concentration of rhDNase. [Reproduced with permission: Pulmozyme (Dornase alfa) DNase Product Monograph. Genentech, Inc., San Francisco, CA, 1994.]

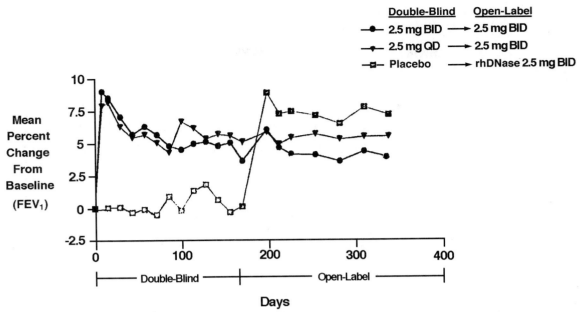

FIGURE 69-7 Mean percent change from baseline in FEV_1 of patients with cystic fibrosis ($n = 968$) treated with rhDNase by inhalation, 2.5 mg daily or twice daily. Effect of addition of drug in the open-label arm of the study to patients previously randomized to placebo. [Reproduced with permission: Pulmozyme (Dornase alfa) DNase Product Monograph. Genentech, Inc., San Francisco, CA, 1994.]

rhDNase administered through compressed-air-driven simple nebulizer is recommended for routine treatment in patients selected to receive this therapy. It is recommended that rhDNase not be mixed with other drugs in the nebulizer unit, and it must be kept refrigerated prior to use. Efficacy (or safety) has not been established in children <5 years of age, although this is a patient group in which prevention of early obstruction of small airways would be most desirable.

SIDE EFFECTS
Clinical trials as outlined above have established rhDNase to be a safe and well-tolerated drug, even for patients with cystic fibrosis with FVC < 40 percent and for individuals with acute exacerbations of chronic bronchitis. Daily administration of the drug was associated with a low, but reproducible, incidence of pharyngitis, laryngitis, or voice alteration, and rare reports of rash, chest pain, and conjunctivitis.[66] In the great majority of cases, the minor respiratory tract irritation was short-lived and disappeared in all but 2 percent of individuals reporting this problem. No sign of serious drug allergy or anaphylaxis was seen during trials or subsequent reports. Also, no evidence of clinically significant bronchoconstriction has emerged.

rhDNase is a "true" mucolytic agent in patients who have chronic airways infection and accumulation of leukocyte-derived DNA. It has been shown to be well-tolerated and efficacious in certain patients with CF, and without a doubt is a useful adjunct in a regimen of care for the CF patient.[69] It is expensive therapy; single doses cost approximately $30.

Precise guidelines for its initiation in individual patients, and its long-term efficacy, remain to be determined.

IODIDES

Iodine is a nonmetallic halide element whose ion, iodide, has several effects on the respiratory system including an improvement in ciliary activity, expectoration, and mucolytic effects.[70] Inorganic and organic iodide preparations have mucokinetic properties. In discussions of this class of drugs, the terms mucolytic, mucokinetic, and expectorant appear to be used almost interchangeably, but these terms can be considered to have distinct definitions. Table 69-1 summarizes pertinent terms from the definitive text on the subject by Ziment.[70]

INORGANIC IODIDES

Chemistry
Potassium iodide (KI) is the most commonly used inorganic iodide expectorant. It is dispensed for clinical use as a saturated solution of potassium iodide (SSKI); a clear, odorless liquid with a salty metallic taste.

Clinical Use and Efficacy
SSKI is described as a stimulant expectorant that acts like an emetic.[49] It has been shown to decrease mucus elasticity in animal studies,[71] and to have mucolytic activity in human bronchial secretions in vitro.[72] The clinical benefit of SSKI was reported in two studies in the late 1960s. In one study of

TABLE 69-1 Glossary of Terms Used to Describe Mucokinetic Drug Activity

Term	Definition
Mucolytic	Breaks up mucous glycoproteins, other proteins, DNA, and other macromolecules into smaller components. Alters the structure of mucus.
Mucokinetic	Improves the mobilization and clearance of abnormal respiratory secretions.
Mucoactive	Has a beneficial effect on respiratory secretions, without specific regard to their mechanism of action.
Expectorant	Acts reflexively on bronchial glands to increase their output of mucoid secretion.

SOURCE: Modified from Braga PC, Ziment I, Allegra L: Classification of agents that act on bronchial mucus, in Braga PC, Allegra L (eds): *Drugs in Bronchial Mucology.* New York: Raven Press, 1989; 59–67.

adults with asthma, "decreased phlegm" was reported[73]; in the other, a "favorable clinical response" was reported in children with asthma who had been treated for 12 weeks.[74] No objective data were reported in either study, and in the most recent FDA status report of nonprescription products in 1989, potassium iodide was not given efficacy approval.[49]

Dosage

A saturated solution of potassium iodide containing 1 g/ml is available in some pharmacies. The recommended adult dose is 0.3 ml (300 mg) to 0.6 ml (600 mg), diluted in water or selected flavored beverages, three to four times a day.

Side Effects

Iodides are poorly tolerated because of their metallic taste. It is of greater concern that prolonged use has been associated with hyperthyroidism.[49] The study in asthmatic children noted above reported a high incidence of thyroid enlargement during the 12 weeks of administration. In children and in pregnant women where the possibility of fetal harm, including goiter, exists, this drug has absolutely no usefulness. Potential side effects greatly outweigh likely benefit, and greatly improved therapeutic armamentarium for childhood asthma essentially precludes any usefulness of mucolytic or expectorant drugs, especially SSKI.

ORGANIC IODIDES

Chemistry

The one commonly prescribed and readily available organic iodide compound is iodinated glycerol (Organidin). It is a viscous, stable liquid that does not contain inorganic or free iodide. Its precise mechanism of action is not known; it is absorbed intact into the blood stream and then metabolized into iodide and glycerol.[75] A detailed review of the pharmacokinetics of iodides is contained in a 1989 review by Ziment,[76] but, in brief, iodide appears to be preferentially sequestered into exocrine glands, including bronchial glands, and subsequently secreted along with an augmented output of respiratory tract fluid and mucoprotein.[75] This explanation noted by Petty[75] in the National Mucolytic Study accounts for the mucokinetic or expectorant property of iodinated glycerol, but though frequent mention is made in this study and others of the mucolytic activity of this compound, the possible mechanism of mucolysis is not described.

Clinical Use and Efficacy

In 1990, Petty[75] reported the outcome of a randomized, double-blind, placebo-controlled study of iodinated glycerol administered for 8 weeks in stable outpatient adults with chronic obstructive bronchitis. All subjects had advanced disease with baseline FEV_1 of 43 percent to 45 percent predicted, and patients with asthma were excluded. Iodinated glycerol given as Organidin, 60 mg four times daily, was found to improve cough symptoms, chest discomfort, ease in expectoration, and patient well-being, as well as decrease the duration of acute exacerbations of chronic bronchitis.[75] Despite the careful attention to study design at the outset, the outcome measures were disappointingly subjective, and its final analysis has been criticized by some.[49] However, a recent report of the Task Group on Mucoactive Drugs[77] recommended guidelines for future studies of the effectiveness of mucus-altering agents that included equally subjective primary and secondary study endpoints. They noted that pulmonary function measures, though typically considered important in defining efficacy of treatment of processes producing airflow obstruction, had "a role in assessing efficacy of bronchodilators, . . . but their role for assessing efficacy of mucoactive drugs is controversial."[77]

Two more-recent studies reported the efficacy of iodinated glycerol in patients with asthma and chronic bronchitis. In one study, patients with chronic asthma symptoms had a clinically and statistically significant reduction in their cough frequency and improved expectoration of mucus.[78] In the second study, which was double-blind and placebo-controlled, improved tracheobronchial clearance was documented using a radiolabeled tracer, but this was confined to a subset of patients who produced increased sputum.[79]

Dosage

Iodinated glycerol (Organidin) is available as a solution, as tablets, and as an elixir. The recommended adult dosage of the 5% solution is 20 drops (3 mg/drop) added to juice or other liquid; the 30 mg tablet is administered as two tablets four times daily. The adult dose of the 1.2% elixir is one teaspoon four times daily; up to one-half the adult dose has been given to children based on weight.[49]

Side Effects

The side effects of organic iodides include gastrointestinal irritation with diarrhea, rash, hypersensitivity, thyroid enlargement, and acute parotitis. The chronic use of all iodides may cause iodism, with symptoms of irritation of the eyes, periorbital swelling, burning of the mouth and throat, and a metallic taste in the mouth.[5]

GUAIFENESIN

Guaifenesin (glycerol guaiacolate) is usually considered an expectorant because of evidence that it facilitates the removal of mucus from airways. However, because of its action to reduce the surface tension and the viscosity of mucus, it also may be considered a mucolytic agent.[80] It is classified by the FDA as safe and effective as an expectorant.[8] Clinical studies have suggested that it improved mucociliary clearance,[81,82] but no studies have documented improved pulmonary function from the use of this agent.

Guaifenesin is available in a variety of preparations under a variety of trade names (Naldecon, Robitussin, Humibid). It also is a very frequent additive in the hundreds of available over-the-counter cough and cold preparations; most often it is combined with an antihistamine or an antitussive agent. When administered orally as a single agent, 200 to 400 mg every 4 h is given to adults and children over 12 years; the dose for children is 100 to 200 mg every 4 h, not to exceed 1.2 g daily. In larger doses, guaifenesin may produce emesis, but gastrointestinal distress at ordinary doses is rare.[80]

Guaifenesin is included in this review in the interest of completeness, but, singly or in combination, this drug has no role in the routine management of the clinical entities described above, with the possible exception of chronic bronchitis in adults. This drug, which is readily available, should not be used in place of standard therapies for asthma, cystic fibrosis, chronic bronchitis, and bronchiectasis.

ANTICHOLINERGIC AGENTS

Though discussed elsewhere (Chaps. 52–54), brief mention of anticholinergic agents is included here, because at times, they are prescribed for the purpose of altering respiratory secretions. Mucous production and cough both result from irritation of subepithelial airway receptors in the vagal reflex arc, which leads to bronchoconstriction. Atropine, the prototypic anticholinergic drug, has been shown to depress ciliary action and overall mucociliary clearance in the airways. It also can block the production of mucous secretion caused by cholinergic agonists, but not the normal baseline secretion of airway mucus.[83] Ipratropium bromide (Atrovent)®, a quaternary ammonium derivative of atropine, is the only approved anticholinergic bronchodilator for aerosol use. It has been shown to increase mucociliary clearance[84] and to alter sputum production in chronic bronchitis.[85] Ipratropium is used primarily for its bronchodilating effects, but glycopyrrolate (Robinul)®, a related quaternary ammonium derivative of atropine, also has been used as an aerosol for its respiratory antisecretory properties. The injectable solution of glycopyrrolate was first reported for use as an aerosol in a study that documented long duration of bronchodilation that was free of the side effects of muscarinic blockade which

characterize atropine inhalation.[86] The injectable solution (0.2 mg/ml) is given in a dose of 0.1 to 0.2 mg every 4 to 8 h, diluted in saline and often in combination with a β-adrenergic bronchodilator. It is used for its antisecretory effects in infants and young children with tracheostomies, such as those with bronchopulmonary dysplasia and in those severely neurologically impaired individuals for whom secretion clearance and frequent aspiration of airway secretions may be problematic.

MUCOLYTIC AGENTS UNDER INVESTIGATION: SPECIAL SITUATIONS

AMILORIDE

Amiloride is an orally administered diuretic agent that blocks sodium reabsorption in the nephron while preventing potassium excretion. For this to occur, amiloride must be filtered in the glomerulus and act on the luminal side of the epithelium.[87] Boucher[88] and Knowles[89] have shown that amiloride applied directly to the luminal side of respiratory epithelium was able to "normalize" the increased transepithelial potential difference in patients with cystic fibrosis, and proposed it for therapy in this patient group. App and co-workers[90] reported that amiloride administered by inhalation as a single dose or as long-term therapy increased mucociliary clearance and cough clearance in patients with cystic fibrosis. They proposed that inhibition of sodium reabsorption likely altered the water content of airway secretion, allowing improved clearance. Tomikiewicz and co-workers[91] subsequently have showed that chronic (25-week) treatment with amiloride inhalation reduced mucous viscoelasticity and increased mucous clearance by mechanisms that involved electrolyte transport. The chronic therapy had resulted in increased sodium and chloride content of CF sputum, but did not measurably change sputum water content.[91] Preliminary studies of amiloride combined with the nucleotide uridine triphosphate (UTP)—which has been shown to stimulate cyclic AMP–dependent chloride ion channels that are defective (or absent) in CF—also have improved mucociliary clearance and pulmonary function in individuals with CF.[92]

Phase III multicenter clinical trials are currently under way to definitively establish long-term efficacy and safety of amiloride in cystic fibrosis; as yet, the FDA approves only the oral form of this drug as a diuretic. Inhalation of amiloride would appear to represent a very rational approach to therapy based on an understanding of the altered airway secretion in CF. Amiloride and the combination of amiloride and UTP would appear to be specific "mucolytic" therapy for a specific disease, and are unlikely to have similar beneficial effects in situations where sodium transport across airway epithelium is normal.

PROTEASE INHIBITORS

Neutrophil elastase is present in increased amounts in the sputum of patients with cystic fibrosis who are chronically infected with bacterial pathogens.[93] There is a growing body of evidence that suggests that neutrophil-derived proteases play a major role in damaging lung tissue in cystic fibrosis;

specifically, uninhibited proteases act on airway walls where proteolytic destruction of structural proteins leads to the development of bronchiectasis. Unchecked neutrophil elastase is the major cause of emphysema in patients with α_1-antiprotease deficiency.[93] α_1-Antitrypsin (α_1-protease inhibitor) purified from normal plasma is used for the treatment of this disorder, and it is safe when administered by both intravenous and aerosol routes.[94] This protein, which is produced normally by individuals with CF, is relatively deficient in the CF lung because of an excessive protease burden and inactivation.[93] A preliminary study in patients with CF demonstrated that free elastase in lung fluid could be decreased by aerosolized α_1-antitrypsin.[95] In the case of α_1-antitrypsin deficiency, aerosol delivery of this drug could be considered replacement therapy; in the case of CF, it could be considered "mucus-altering" therapy. In this sense, it may have possible usefulness in other disease states that are characterized by chronic airway infection (e.g., bronchiectasis).

Synthetic leukocyte protease inhibitor (SLPI) is a recombinant antiprotease that is entering clinical trials of patients with cystic fibrosis. This inhibitor has a lower molecular weight than α_1-antitrypsin and ionic properties that suggest improved usefulness. Also, it has the advantages of being resistant to oxidative inactivation and a more effective inhibitor of elastase already bound to elastin than is α_1-antiprotease.[96]

GELSOLIN

Sputum samples from patients with CF have been found to contain filamentous actin. Human gelsolin is a plasma protein that severs actin filaments. In an in vitro study, Vasconcellos and colleagues[97] demonstrated that gelsolin rapidly decreased the viscosity of CF sputum. Gc globulin and deoxyribonuclease I, which are known to sequester monomeric actin but do not sever actin filaments, were less efficient than gelsolin in diminishing sputum viscosity. This preliminary study concluded that gelsolin may have therapeutic potential as a mucolytic agent in CF.[97] Increased filamentous actin is likely not specific to CF, and, therefore, this agent may have a broader potential usefulness.

Summary

Mucolytic agents are those that alter the structure of mucus, with the ultimate goal of promoting clearance of secretion from airways and reversing obstructive pathophysiology. A mucolytic alone is rarely effective,[8] given the complex nature of the major clinical entities described above which are characterized by chronic infection, inflammation, and/or mucous hypersecretion. Therefore, mucolytic agents are best employed as adjuncts to more specific therapeutic interventions, such as bronchodilator, antibiotic, or anti-inflammatory agents. The understanding of the biochemistry of mucus, including the genetic aspects of its diversity, and the improved understanding of the mechanisms of mucous hypersecretion have "evolved more rapidly than our development of specific (mucolytic) therapies."[1] It will remain the purview of the clinician or the "art of medicine" to determine when and how to use the agents described herein. The future holds promise of a yet improved understanding and new and better therapies.

References

1. Lundgren JD, Shelhamer JH: Pathogenesis of airway mucus hypersecretion. *J Allergy Clin Immunol* 1990; 85:399.
2. Witek TJ, Schachter EN: Mucus and its clearance in health and disease, in Witek TJ, Schachter EN (eds): *Pharmacology and Therapeutics in Respiratory Care.* Philadelphia: WB Saunders, 1994: 87–107.
3. Nadel JD, Davis B, Phipps RG: Control of mucus secretion and ion transport in airways. *Ann Rev Physiol* 1979; 41:369.
4. Basbaum C, Welsh MJ: Mucous secretion and ion transport in airways, in Murray JF, Nadel JA (eds): *Textbook of Respiratory Medicine,* 2nd ed. Philadelphia: WB Saunders, 1994: 323–344.
5. Seligman M: Mucolytics, in Kacmarek RM, Stoller JK (eds): *Current Respiratory Care.* Toronto: BC Becker, 1988: 41–46.
6. Sheahan JK, Thornton DJ, Somerville M, Carlstedt I: The structure and heterogeneity of respiratory mucus glycoproteins. *Am Rev Respir Dis* 1991; 144(suppl):S4.
7. Lamblin G, Lhermitte M, Klein A, et al.: The carbohydrate diversity of human respiratory mucins: A protection of the underlying mucosa? *Am Rev Respir Dis* 1991; 144(suppl):S19.
8. Rao JL: Mucus-controlling agents, in Rao JL (ed): *Respiratory Care Pharmacology,* 4th ed. St. Louis: Mosby, 1994: 195–222.
9. Dulfano JJ, Adler KB: Physical properties of sputum VII. Rheologic properties and mucociliary transport. *Am Rev Respir Dis* 1975; 112:341.
10. List SJ, Findla BP, Forstner GG, Forstner JF: Enhancement of the viscosity of mucin by serum albumin. *Biochem J* 1978; 175:565.
11. Snider GL, Lucey E, Christensen TG, et al.: Emphysema and bronchial secretory cell hyperplasia induced in hamsters by human neutrophil products. *Am Rev Respir Dis* 1984; 129:155.
12. Schultz DR, Miller KD: Elastase of *Pseudomonas aeruginosa*: Inactivation of complement components and complement derived chemotactic and phagocytic factors. *Infect Immun* 1974; 10:128.
13. Fritz H: Human mucus protease inhibitor (human MPI). *Biol Chem* 1988; 369:79.
14. Sleigh MA, Blake JR, Liron N: The propulsion of mucus by cilia. *Am Rev Respir Dis* 1988; 137:726.
15. Snider GL, Faling LJ, Rennard SI: Chronic bronchitis and emphysema, in Murray JF, Nadel JA (eds): *Textbook of Respiratory Medicine,* 2nd ed. Philadelphia: WB Saunders, 1994: 1331–1398.
16. Boat TF, Cheng PW: Epithelial cell dysfunction in cystic fibrosis: Implications for airways disease. *Acta Pediatr Scand* 1989; 363(suppl):25.
17. Cammer P, Strandberg K, Phillipson K: Increased mucociliary transport by cholinergic stimulation. *Arch Environ Health* 1974; 29:220.
18. Medical Research Council Committee: The aetiology of chronic bronchitis for clinical and epidemiological purposes. *Lancet* 1965; i:286.
19. Reid L: Measurement of the bronchial mucus gland layer. *Thorax* 1960; 15:132.
20. Sturgess J, Reid L: An organ culture study of the effects of drugs on the secretory activity of human bronchial submucosal gland. *Clin Sci* 1972; 43:533.
21. Pullan CR, Hey EN: Wheezing, asthma, and pulmonary dysfunction 10 years after infection with respiratory syncytial virus in infancy. *Br Med J* 1982; 284:1665.

22. Cammer P, Mossberg B, Phillipson K: Tracheobronchial clearance and chronic obstructive lung disease. *Scan J Respir Dis* 1973; 54:272.

23. Turner-Warwick M, Openshaw P: Sputum in asthma. *Postgrad Med J* 1987; 63(suppl 1):79.

24. Nadel JA: Regulation of bronchial secretion, in Newball HH (ed): *Immunopharmacology of the Lung.* New York: Marcel Dekker, 1983; 109–139.

25. Phipps RJ, Williams IP, Richardson PS, et al.: Sympathomimetic drugs stimulate the output of secretory glycoprotein from human bronchi in vitro. *Clin Sci* 63:23, 1982.

26. Sommerhoff CP, Caughey GH, Finkbeiner WE, et al.: Mast cell chymase: A potent secretogogue for airway gland serous cells. *J Immunol* 1989; 142:2450.

27. Sommerhoff CP, Nadel JA, Basbaum CB, et al.: Neutrophil elastase and cathespin G stimulate secretion from cultured airway gland serous cells. *J Clin Invest* 1989; 85:682.

28. Kaliner M: Bronchial asthma, in Samter M (ed): *Immunologic Diseases*, 4th ed. Boston: Little, Brown, 1988: 1067.

29. Boat TF: Cystic fibrosis, in Murray JF, Nadel JA (eds): *Textbook of Respiratory Medicine.* Philadelphia: WB Saunders, 1988: 1126–1152.

30. Taussig LM, Landau LI, Marks MI: Respiratory system, in Taussig LM (ed): *Cystic Fibrosis.* New York: Thieme-Stratton, 1984: 115–174.

31. Penketh ARL, Wise A, Mearns MB, et al.: Cystic fibrosis in adolescents and adults. *Thorax* 1987; 42:526.

32. Chow CW, Landau LI, Taussig LM: Bronchial mucous glands in the newborn with cystic fibrosis. *Eur J Pediatr* 1982; 139:240.

33. Sturgess J, Imrie J: Quantitative evaluation of the development of tracheal submucosal glands in infants with cystic fibrosis and control infants. *Am J Pathol* 1982; 106:303.

34. Bedrossian CWM, Greenberg SD, Singer DB, et al.: The lung in cystic fibrosis. *Hum Pathol* 1976; 7:195.

35. Gerken TA, Gupta R: Mucus in cystic fibrosis, in Davis PB (ed): *Cystic Fibrosis. (Lung Biology in Health and Disease, vol 64.)* New York: Marcel Dekker, 1993: 53–90.

36. Frizzell RA, Cliff WH: Cystic fibrosis: back to the chloride channel. *Nature* 1991; 350:277.

37. Boucher RC, Stutts MJ, Knowles MR, et al.: Na^+ transport in cystic fibrosis respiratory epithelia: Abnormal basal rate and response to adenylate cyclase activation. *J Clin Invest* 1986; 78:1245.

38. Elborn JS, Shale DL: Lung injury in cystic fibrosis. *Thorax* 1990; 45:970.

39. Berger M: Inflammation in the lung in cystic fibrosis. *Clin Rev Allergy* 1991; 9:119.

40. Chernick WS, Barbero GJ: Composition of tracheobronchial secretions in cystic fibrosis of the pancreas and bronchiectasis. *Pediatrics* 1959; 24:739.

41. Smith AL, Redding G, Doershuk C, et al.: Sputum changes associated with therapy for endobronchial exacerbation in cystic fibrosis. *J Pediatr* 1988; 112:547.

42. Picot R, Das I, Reid L: Pus, deoxyribonucleic acid and sputum viscosity. *Thorax* 1978; 33:235.

43. Dorow P: Mucolytics: When dispensible, when necessary? *Lung* 1990; (suppl):622.

44. Rodenstein D, DeCoster A, Gazzangia A: Pharmacokinetics of oral acetylcysteine: Absorption, binding, and metabolism in patients with respiratory disorders. *Clin Pharmacokinet* 1978; 3:247.

45. Shih VE, Shulman JD: N-acetylcysteine-cysteine disulfide excretion in the urine following N-acetylcysteine administration. *J Pediatr* 1969; 74:129.

46. Sheffner AL, Medler EM, Jacobs LW, Sarett HP: The in vitro reduction in viscosity of human tracheobronchial secretions by acetylcysteine. *Am Rev Respir Dis* 1964; 90:721.

47. Millman M, Goodman AH, Goldstein IM, et al.: Treatment of a patient with chronic bronchial asthma with bronchoscopies and lavage using acetylcysteine. *J Asthma* 1985; 22:13.

48. Perruchoud A, Ehrsam R, Heitz M, et al.: Atelectasis of the lung: Bronchoscopic lavage with acetylcysteine; experience in 51 patients. *Eur J Respir Dis* 1980; 61:163.

49. Witek TJ, Schachter EN: Agents that affect mucus and cough, in Witek TJ, Schachter EN (eds): *Pharmacology and Therapeutics of Respiratory Care.* Philadelphia: WB Saunders, 1994: 239–255.

50. Dueholm M, Nielsen C, Thorshavge H, et al.: N-acetylcysteine by metered dose inhaler in the treatment of chronic bronchitis. *Respir Med* 1992; 86:89.

51. Parr GD, Huitson A: Oral N-aectylcysteine in chronic bronchitis. *Brit J Dis Chest* 1987; 81:341.

52. Strafanger G, Garne S, Howeitz P, et al.: The clinical effect and the effect on the ciliary motility of oral N-acetylcysteine in patients with cystic fibrosis and primary ciliary dyskinesia. *Eur Respir J* 1988; 1:161.

53. Todisco T, Polidori R, Rossi F, et al.: Effect of N-acetylcysteine in subjects with slow mucociliary clearance. *Eur J Respir Dis* 1985; 66:136.

54. Olivieri D, Marsico SA, Del Donno M: Improvements of mucociliary transport in smokers by mucolytics. *Eur J Respir Dis* 1985; 66:143.

55. MacNee W, Bridgeman MME, Marsden M, et al.: The effects of N-acetylcysteine and glutathione on smoke-induced changes in lung phagocytes and epithelial cells. *Am J Med* 1991; 91:3C–60S.

56. Bernard GR: N-Acetylcysteine in experimental and clinical acute lung injury. *Am J Med* 1991; 91:3C–54S.

57. Falliers CJ, Cato A: Controlled trial of bronchodilator-mucolytic aerosols, combined and separate. *Ann Allergy* 1978; 40:77.

58. Shak S, Capon DJ, Hellmiss R, et al.: Recombinant human DNase I reduces the viscosity of cystic fibrosis sputum. *Proc Natl Acad Sci USA* 1990; 87:9188.

59. Liao TH, Salnikow J, Moore S, Stein WH: Bovine pancreatic deoxynuclease A: Isolation of cyanogen bromide peptides; complete covalent structure of the polypeptide chain. *J Biol Chem* 1973; 248:1489.

60. Potter J, Matthews LW, Lemm J, Spector S: The composition of pulmonary secretions from patients with and without cystic fibrosis. *Am J Dis Child* 1960; 100:493.

61. Raskin P: Bronchospasm after inhalation of pancreatic dornase. *Am Rev Respir Dis* 1968; 98:697.

62. Hubbard RC, McElvaney NG, Birrer P, et al.: A preliminary study of aerosolized recombinant human deoxyribonuclease I in the treatment of cystic fibrosis. *N Engl J Med* 1992; 326:812.

63. Rubin BK: Aerosolized recombinant deoxyribonuclease I in the treatment of cystic fibrosis. *N Engl J Med* 1992; 327:571.

64. Aitken ML, Burke W, McDonald G, et al.: Recombinant human DNase inhalation in normal subjects and patients with cystic fibrosis. *JAMA* 1992; 267:1947.

65. Ramsey BW, Astley SJ, Aitken ML, et al.: Efficacy and safety of short-term administration of aerosolized recombinant human deoxyribonuclease in patients with cystic fibrosis. *Am J Respir Dis* 1993; 148:145.

66. Fuchs HJ, Borowitz DS, Christiansen DH, et al.: Effect of aerosolized recombinant human DNase on exacerbations of respiratory symptoms and on pulmonary function in patients with cystic fibrosis. *N Engl J Med* 1994; 331:637.

67. Shah PL, Scott S, Knight RA: Quantitative changes in sputum microbiology following treatment of stable cystic fibrosis with aerosolised recombinant human DNase I. *Pediatr Pulmonol* 1993; 9(suppl):265.

68. Genentech, Inc., San Francisco, CA, (personal communication).

69. Davis PB: Evolution of therapy for cystic fibrosis. *N Engl J Med* 1994; 331:672.

70. Ziment I: Help for an overtaxed mucociliary system: Managing abnormal mucus. *J Respir Dis* 1991; 12:21.

71. Martin R, Litt M, Marriott C: The effect of mucolytic agents on the rheologic and transport properties of canine tracheal mucus. *Am Rev Respir Dis* 1980; 121:495.

72. Marriott C, Richards JH: The effects of storage and potassium iodide, urea, N-acetylcysteine and Triton X-100 on the viscosity of bronchial mucus. *Br J Dis Chest* 1974; 68:171.

73. Bernecker C: Potassium iodide in bronchial asthma. *Br Med J* 1969; 4:183.

74. Falliers CJ, McCann WP, Chai H, et al.: Controlled study of iodotherapy for childhood asthma. *J Allergy* 1966; 38:183.

75. Petty TL: The National Mucolytic Study: Results of a randomized, double-blind, placebo controlled study of iodinated glycerol in chronic obstrucive bronchitis. *Chest* 1990; 97:75.

76. Ziment I: Inorganic and organic iodides, in Braga PC, Allegra L (eds): *Drugs in Bronchial Mucology*. New York: Raven, 1989.

77. Special Report of the Task Group on Mucoactive Drugs: Recommendations for guidelines on clinical trials of mucoactive drugs in chronic bronchitis and COPD. *Chest* 1994; 106:1532.

78. Repsher LH, Glassman JM, Soyka JP: Evaluation of iodopropylidene glycerol as adjunctive therapy in stable, chronic asthmatic patients on theophylline maintenance. *Today's Ther Trends* 1983; 1:77.

79. Pavia D, Agnew JE, Glassman JM, et al.: Effects of iodopropylidene glycerol on tracheobronchial clearance in stable, chronic bronchitis patients. *Eur J Respir Dis* 1985; 67:177.

80. Farrington E: Pharmacotherapy, in Loughlin GM, Eigen H (eds): *Respiratory Disease in Children: Diagnosis and Management*. Baltimore: Williams & Wilkins, 1994; 741–782.

81. Thomson ML, Pavia D, McNicol MW: A preliminary study of the effect of guaifenesin on mucociliary clearance from the human lung. *Thorax* 1973; 28:742.

82. Wanner A: Clinical aspects of mucociliary transport. *Am Rev Respir Dis* 1977; 116:73.

83. Wanner A: Effect of ipratropium bromide on airway mucociliary function. *Am J Med* 1986; 81(suppl 5):32.

84. Cugell DW: Clinical pharmacology and toxicology of ipratropium bromide. *Am J Med* 1986; 81(suppl 5A):27.

85. Chafouri MA, Patil KD, Kass I: Sputum changes associated with the use of ipratropium bromide. *Chest* 1984; 86:387.

86. Gal TJ, Suratt PM, Lu J: Glycopyrrolate and atropine inhalation: Comparative effects on normal airway function. *Am Rev Respir Dis* 1984; 129:871.

87. Hyams DE: Amiloride: A review. Royal Society of Medicine, International Congress and Symposium Series 1981; 44:65.

88. Boucher RC, Knowles MR, Stutts MJ, Gatzy JT: Epithelial dysfunction in cystic fibrosis lung disease. *Lung* 1983; 308:1185.

89. Knowles MR, Gatzy JT, Boucher RC: Increased bioelectric potential difference across respiratory epithelia in cystic fibrosis. *N Engl J Med* 1981; 305:1489.

90. App EM, King M, Helfesreider R, et al.: Acute and long-term amiloride inhalation in cystic fibrosis lung disease. *Am Rev Respir Dis* 1990; 141:605.

91. Tomikiewicz RP, App EM, Zayas JG, et al.: Amiloride inhalation therapy in cystic fibrosis: Influence on ion concentration, hydration, and rheology of sputum. *Am Rev Respir Dis* 1993; 148:1002.

92. Knowles MR, Clarke LL, Boucher RC: Activation by extracellular nucleotides of chloride secretion in the airway epithelia of patients with cystic fibrosis. *N Engl J Med* 1991; 325:533.

93. Konstan MW, Berger M: Infection and inflammation of the lung in cystic fibrosis, in Davis PB (ed): *Cystic Fibrosis*. New York: Marcel Dekker, 1993: 219–276.

94. Hubbard RC, Crystal RG: α_1-Antitrypsin augmentation therapy for α_1-antitrypsin deficiency. *Am J Med* 1988; 84(suppl 6A):52.

95. McElvaney NG, Hubbard RC, Birrer P, et al.: Aerosol α_1-antitrypsin treatment for cystic fibrosis. *Lancet* 1991; 337:392.

96. Vogelmeier S, Buhl R, Hoyt RF, et al.: Aerosolization of recombinant SLPI to augment antineutrophil elastase protection of pulmonary epithelium. *J Appl Physiol* 1990; 69:1843.

97. Vasconcellos CA, Allen PG, Wohl ME, Stossel TP: Reduction in viscosity of cystic fibrosis sputum in vitro by gelsolin. *Science* 1994; 263:969.

ADVERSE DRUG REACTION

Chapter 70
ASPIRIN-SENSITIVE ASTHMA

ELLIOT ISRAEL
ANDREW R. FISCHER

Introduction

Aspirin and nonsteroidal anti-inflammatory drugs (NSAIDs) produce a wide variety of adverse reactions, including gastric ulcers, gastritis, prolonged bleeding, blood dyscrasias, nephritis, and hepatitis. In addition, there exists a class of reactions to these drugs that are typically classified as "allergic" because they are caused by IgE-mediated reactions. These reactions include urticaria, rhinosinusitis, and bronchospasm. This chapter concentrates on the syndrome of bronchospasm associated with the ingestion of aspirin or other NSAIDs, such as inhibitors of cyclooxygenase. For this discussion, this syndrome is specified as ANSIA (aspirin- and nonsteroidal-induced asthma). The clinical characteristics of this syndrome, potential pathophysiologic mechanisms, and information concerning diagnosis, management, and treatment of this syndrome are reviewed.

Clinical Characteristics

The first case report of aspirin sensitivity was described by Hirschberg in 1902.[1] Vanselow and Smith described asthma occurring after indomethacin ingestion in 1967[2] followed a year later by Samter and Beers' paper describing a triad that included asthma, nasal polyps, and aspirin sensitivity.[3] Since then, asthma provoked by aspirin ingestion has been widely described and has been reported to occur in 5 to 30 percent of adult asthmatics. Its incidence appears greater among severe asthmatics, reportedly 19 percent[4] and may occur in 20 to 30 percent of asthmatics with nasal polyps and sinusitis. Although more than half of nonspecific asthma presents before the age of 20, ANSIA is rare in childhood. It presents most frequently in the third to fourth decade of life in patients without a history of prior aspirin sensitivity.

It is estimated that 80 to 90 percent of patients with true ANSIA will have some radiographic abnormality of the paranasal sinuses.[5] Sinus disease frequently precedes the onset of aspirin-induced bronchospasm by several years. Classically, patients describe a history of several years of sinusitis, frequently associated with nasal polyps, and asthmatic symptoms. Patients further report an acute asthma exacerbation associated with aspirin ingestion.

As opposed to classical anaphylactic reactions, bronchospasm associated with ingestion of aspirin or NSAIDs associated with ANSIA is slow in onset—occurring 30 min to 2 h after ingestion. Reactions occurring within several minutes of exposure are distinctly unusual. In ANSIA, the bronchospasm resulting from aspirin ingestion is associated frequently with severe rhinorrhea and occasionally accompanied by gastrointestinal pain or angioedema. These reactions are frequently profound enough to result in emergency room visits, hospitalization, or intubation.

Cross-Reactivity of Aspirin and NSAIDs and Other Agents

It appears that nearly all patients with rhinosinusitis and bronchospasm associated with aspirin ingestion experience a similar response to drugs that inhibit the enzyme cyclooxygenase. Although a small population of patients has been described to experience anaphylactoid reactions or urticaria in response to a specific NSAID, or to aspirin but not NSAIDs, these patients do not have asthma.[6]

The extent of cross-reactivity to drugs that induce reactions in ANSIA appears to be related to the ability of these agents to inhibit cyclooxygenase.[7] In fact, drugs that have minimal cyclooxygenase inhibitory effects have been documented to produce reactions when administered in sufficient doses. Thus, acetaminophen, which only weakly inhibits cyclooxygenase, caused reactions in 28 percent of aspirin-sensitive asthmatics when administered at a dose of 1000 mg but not at 500 mg.[8] In more sensitive asthmatics, reactions have been reported with doses of 600 mg as well.[9,10]

Nonacetylated salicylates with weak cyclooxygenase-inhibitory effects such as salsalate, have also been reported to cause reactions in as many as 20 percent of aspirin-sensitive asthmatics.[11] Of interest, nonacetylated salicylates, which have little or no cyclooxygenase-inhibitory effects (e.g., choline magnesium trisalicylate), block or attenuate aspirin-induced reactions.[12] These observations are consistent with the in vitro observations that these drugs can interfere with the cyclooxygenase inhibitory effect of aspirin while producing minimal to no cyclooxygenase inhibitory effects themselves.[13]

In addition to a sensitivity to drugs that inhibit cyclooxygenase, it has been suggested that ANSIA patients may be particularly sensitive to other chemicals and additives. However, systematic documentation of such reactivity is lacking. It had long been suggested that such patients are intolerant of tartrazine. However, a multicenter randomized, double-blind, placebo-controlled study of tartrazine challenge in ANSIA patients reported only a 2.6 percent incidence of tartrazine-induced asthma in those patients.[14] Similarly, there have been several reports of bronchospasm provoked by intravenous hydrocortisone sodium succinate. However, systematic study of 43 aspirin-sensitive patients did not document such a sensitivity.[15]

Pathophysiology

The reason that patients develop ANSIA is unclear; a viral precipitant has been speculated.[16] However, significant progress has been made in elucidating the underlying mechanisms of ANSIA. It was originally thought that the asthma, rhinorrhea, and skin manifestations associated with ANSIA were related to an immune hypersensitivity phenomenon. However, it has not been possible to demonstrate immune recognition of aspirin or nonsteroidals in ANSIA patients, and the various NSAIDs that also induce ANSIA have chemical structures dissimilar to aspirin. The discovery that aspirin and NSAIDs inhibit the enzyme cyclooxygenase and the correlation between the ability of a drug to inhibit cyclooxygenase in vitro and its ability to induce a reaction in sensitive asthmatics[7] clearly suggested that inhibition of cyclooxygenase is critical to the drug reaction in ANSIA.

Cyclooxygenase is an enzyme critical to the conversion of arachidonic acid to the prostanoids. Because cyclooxygenase is critical to the formation of prostaglandins, it has been postulated that ANSIA may be related to the inhibition of a bronchodilator prostanoid such as prostaglandin E_2 (PGE_2). Indeed, administration of PGE_2 has been shown to block a component of aspirin-induced bronchospasm.[17] However, this effect is incomplete, and recent evidence suggests the critical mediators in ANSIA are products of an alternative pathway of arachidonic acid metabolism—the 5-lipoxygenase pathway.

The 5-lipoxygenase pathway of arachidonic acid metabolism is outlined in Fig. 70-1. More details concerning this pathway are provided in Chapter 72. The products of this pathway mediate biologic effects associated with the pathobiology of asthma. The cysteinyl leukotrienes (LTC_4, LTD_4, and LTE_4), which are potent constrictors of the airways,[18,19] can cause edema[20] and can play a role in eosinophil recruitment.[21] Additionally, another 5-lipoxygenase pathway product, LTB_4, is a potent leukocyte chemotactic agent,[22] whereas other metabolites such as 5-hydroxyeicosatetraenoic acid (5-HETE) metabolites have been shown to be mucous secretagogues.[23]

FIGURE 70-1 The 5-lipoxygenase pathway of arachidonic acid metabolism. AA = arachidonic acid; 5-HPETE = 5-hydroperoxyeicosatetraenoic acid; 5-HETE = 5-hydroxyeicosatetraenoic acid; Gamma-GT = gamma glutamyl transpeptidase; LTA_4, B_4, C_4, D_4, E_4 = leukotriene A_4, B_4, C_4, D_4, and E_4. (Modified from Israel E: New agents in asthma treatment—inhibitors of the formation and action of products of the 5-lipoxygenase pathway of arachidonic acid; in Crommelin DJA, Midha KK, Nagai T (eds); *Topics in Pharmaceutical Sciences*. Stuttgart, Scientific Publishers, 1994:89–102.)

Conversion of Arachidonic Acid to Leukotrienes

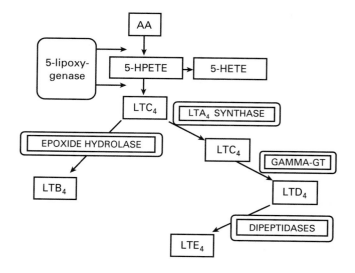

Because the effects mediated by the 5-lipoxygenase products of arachidonic acid—bronchoconstriction, inflammatory cell recruitment, airway edema, and mucous secretion—are characteristic of asthma, it had been postulated that the administration of cyclooxygenase inhibitors may produce reactions in ANSIA through elaboration of the 5-lipoxygenase products of arachidonic acid. These 5-lipoxygenase products have been detected in biologic fluids of ANSIA patients after aspirin challenge. Ferreri and colleagues first detected immunoreactive cysteinyl leukotrienes in nasal secretions after aspirin-induced reactions and noted that such levels return to normal following aspirin desensitization.[24]

Further support for leukotriene production in aspirin-induced reactions has come from quantification of LTE_4 in the urine. As can be seen in Fig. 71-1, LTC_4 is converted to LTD_4, which is subsequently converted to LTE_4. The latter product can be detected in the urine. Christie and coworkers demonstrated that LTE_4 could be detected in the urine after aspirin challenge in aspirin-sensitive asthmatics, but not in non–aspirin-sensitive patients.[25] No such elevations occurred when these patients were challenged with methacholine. Similar elevations have been reported by other investigators after aspirin challenge in ANSIA patients.[26,27] Leukotriene concentrations have also been shown to increase after provocation with inhaled lysine-aspirin in ANSIA.[28,29] In addition, these studies have noted that the basal concentration of urinary LTE_4 is increased in aspirin-sensitive asthmatics as compared to non–aspirin-sensitive asthmatics.[25,28,29]

The studies cited above have established that increased cysteinyl leukotriene production is associated with ANSIA. Recently, the availability of inhibitors of 5-lipoxygenase or antagonists of the action of the receptor for the cysteinyl leukotrienes has made it possible to establish that the action of these 5-lipoxygenase products is critical to the development of the aspirin-induced response. Christie and associates first demonstrated that an inhaled cysteinyl leukotriene antagonist inhibited the mean decrease in forced expiratory volume in 1s (FEV_1) after ingestion of aspirin in six patients by 47 percent.[30] Subsequently, an oral leukotriene antagonist has been shown to shift the pulmonary dose response curve to inhalation of lysine-aspirin in eight subjects by greater than fourfold.[31] Three subjects in this study did not experience a 20 percent decline in FEV_1 despite inhalation of the greatest dose of lysine-aspirin. In a study of eight aspirin-sensitive subjects, treatment with a 5-lipoxygenase inhibitor caused almost complete inhibition of the pulmonary response to oral aspirin.[26] In this study, the extrapulmonary responses to aspirin ingestion, including nasal, gastrointestinal, and dermal responses, also were completely inhibited.

Although these studies clearly demonstrate that 5-lipoxygenase products are critical to the development of aspirin-induced responses in ANSIA, the mechanism of the induction of these products by cyclooxygenase inhibition is as yet unclear. Such effects might occur through shunting of arachidonic acid to the 5-lipoxygenase pathway as a result of blockade of cyclooxygenase or alternatively through "disinhibition" of the 5-lipoxygenase pathway by inhibition of a cyclooxygenase product that regulates the 5-lipoxygenase

pathway. In addition to the overproduction of leukotrienes, it also appears that ANSIA patients may have selective pulmonary hyperresponsiveness to LTE_4.[32] This hyperresponsiveness appears to diminish with desensitization. The etiology of this possible selective hyperresponsiveness is also unclear.

Although it appears clear that 5-lipoxygenase products are critical to the ANSIA reaction, the cellular source of these products is not yet clear. Mast cells, eosinophils, and alveolar macrophages, among others, have the capacity to metabolize arachidonic acid via 5-lipoxygenase.[33–35] Eosinophils are present within nasal polyps and in asthmatic airways. Mast cells are present at these sites as well as in the skin and gut—additional sites that are frequently involved in the aspirin response. Currently, evidence suggests mast cells are activated in the aspirin response in ANSIA. Tryptase, an enzyme specific to mast cells, has been detected in the serum of ANSIA patients experiencing gastrointestinal reactions after aspirin ingestion.[36] Recently, nasal tryptase has been detected during these reactions in a sequence that mirrors the rise in leukotrienes.[37] In this study, inhibition of 5-lipoxygenase resulted in a decrease in nasal tryptase. This observation suggests the possibility that leukotrienes themselves may be active in an autocrine or paracrine fashion to facilitate activation of mast cells, and thus indirectly, leukotriene production.

Although eosinophils are present in nasal polyps and can synthesize LTC_4, it has been difficult to document their activation in ANSIA. One study reported a trend toward an increase in serum eosinophil cationic protein (ECP) after aspirin ingestion, but the trend was not statistically significant.[38] Paradoxically, a study of ECP concentrations in bronchoalveolar lavage fluid of ANSIA patients after lysine-ASA inhalation found a significant decrease in the levels of this mediator.[39] A consistent pattern in the change in ECP levels in the nasal lavage fluid of ANSIA patients was not found after ASA ingestion.[37] Hence, the role of the eosinophil as a major contributor to the acute increase in leukotriene production after NSAID ingestion in ANSIA patients remains unproven.

Treatment

The ANSIA asthmatic's underlying asthma should be treated with stepwise therapy along the lines outlined in generally accepted protocols.[40] However, as outlined previously, these patients tend to present with the more severe spectrum of asthma, and a larger proportion than usual of these patients will require inhaled or oral steroids.

Avoidance of NSAIDs is important in preventing exacerbations in ANSIA patients. Patients must avoid preparations that contain aspirin or NSAIDs. Avoiding chronic use of compounds that contain salicylates may be advisable as well. Acetaminophen generally can be used with safety, although, as noted earlier, high doses may precipitate reactions in very sensitive patients. If severe sensitivity is suspected, it may be advisable to have patients slowly titrate acetaminophen doses up to routine doses. Dextropropoxyphene and other narcotic analgesics that do not have cyclooxygenase inhibitory activity can be used without fear of initiating aspirin-induced responses.

Aggressive treatment of the nasal and sinus disease commonly associated with ANSIA is important in improving asthma control in these patients. Polyp growth can be retarded and, in some cases, regression of nasal polyps can be promoted with the aggressive use of nasal steroids. Decongestants to promote drainage and prolonged (4 to 6 weeks) courses of antibiotics are advisable for treatment of sinus infections. Although polypectomy promotes drainage, the rapid regrowth of nasal polyps generally provides only short-term relief. On a case by case basis, sinus surgery may need to be contemplated to improve sinus drainage.

Aspirin desensitization clearly decreases the sensitivity of ANSIA patients to inhibitors of cyclooxygenase and, in some cases, appears to decrease the underlying severity of their asthma.[41–43] Desensitization may be desirable in clinical situations where chronic aspirin ingestion is required, such as chronic rheumatologic conditions or coronary artery disease prophylaxis. This procedure involves administering increasing doses of aspirin over several days until the chronic dose to be administered is achieved without precipitating exacerbations. Patients must continue to take daily aspirin after desensitization, because discontinuation of chronic aspirin results in recovery of sensitivity within several days. Desensitization requires an appropriate inpatient facility with experienced physicians and available emergency care.

The recent elucidation of the critical role of the 5-lipoxygenase products in mediating aspirin-induced reactions has provided an avenue for pharmacotherapeutic interventions. The 5-lipoxygenase inhibitor, zileuton, eliminated all manifestations of the aspirin-induced response in a group of treated aspirin-sensitive asthmatics.[26] Other inhibitors of leukotriene synthesis have blunted the response to aspirin challenge, as have leukotriene receptor antagonists.[30,31,44] These antileukotriene drugs have been shown to be of benefit in the treatment of asthma in asthmatics who are not necessarily aspirin sensitive and the benefits of long-term treatment with antileukotriene drugs in ANSIA patients is currently being investigated.

Summary

Asthmatics with nasal polyps or sinusitis who wheeze in response to ingestion of inhibitors of cyclooxygenase form a biochemically distinct subgroup of asthmatics. These patients appear to have an alteration in the control of the 5-lipoxygenase arachidonic acid pathway characterized by overproduction of the 5-lipoxygenase products of arachidonic acid in response to inhibition of cyclooxygenase. Although the etiology of this abnormality is unclear, its expression is frequently delayed in onset, usually occurring after age 20. Antagonizing the effects of leukotrienes has been shown to inhibit the pulmonary response in this reaction and inhibition of 5-lipoxygenase has been shown to inhibit all the manifestations of the aspirin induced response. Mast cells are activated in ANSIA and may be a major source of the mediators of this reaction. Aspirin desensitization and antileukotriene drugs prevent the reaction to

aspirin and NSAIDs in these patients. The long-term effects of antileukotriene drugs on the underlying asthma of these patients is being explored.

References

1. Hirschberg: Mittheilung uber einen Fall von Nebenwirkung des Aspirin. *Dtsch Med Wochenschr* 1902; 28:416.
2. Vanselow NA, Smith JR: Bronchial asthma induced by indomethacin. *Ann Intern Med* 1967; 66:568.
3. Samter M, Beers RF: Intolerance to aspirin: clinical studies and consideration of its pathogenesis. *Ann Intern Med* 1968; 68:975.
4. McDonald JR, Mathison DA, Stevenson DD: Aspirin intolerance in asthma, detection by oral challenge. *J Allergy Clin Immunol* 1972; 50:198.
5. Stevenson DD, Mathison DA, Tan EM, Vaughan JH: Provoking factors in bronchial asthma. *Arch Intern Med* 1975; 135:777.
6. Settipane RA, Constantine HP, Settipane GA: Aspirin intolerance and recurrent urticaria in normal adults and children. Epidemiology and review. *Allergy* 1980; 35:149.
7. Szczeklik A, Gryglewski RJ, Czerniawska-Mysik G: Relationship of inhibition of prostaglandin biosynthesis by analgesics to asthma attacks in aspirin-sensitive patients. *BMJ* 1975; 1:67.
8. Delaney JC: The diagnosis of aspirin idiosyncrasy by analgesic challenge. *Clin Allergy* 1976; 6:177.
9. Szczeklik A, Gryglewski RJ, Czerniawska-Mysik G: Clinical patterns of hypersensitivity to nonsteroidal anti-inflammatory drugs and their pathogenesis. *J Allergy Clin Immunol* 1977; 60:276.
10. Spector SL, Wangaard CH, Farr RS: Aspirin and concommitant idiosyncracies in adult asthmatic patients. *J Allergy Clin Immunol* 1979; 64:500.
11. Stevenson DD, Hougham AJ, Schrank PJ, et al.: Salsalate cross-sensitivity in aspirin-sensitive patients with asthma. *J Allergy Clin Immunol* 1990; 86:749.
12. Nizankowska E, Dworski R, Soja J, Szczeklik A: Salicylate pretreatment attenuates intensity of bronchial and nasal symptoms precipitated by aspirin in aspirin-intolerant patients. *Clin Exp Allergy* 1990; 20:647.
13. Vargaftig BB: The inhibition of cyclo-oxygenase of rabbit platelets by aspirin is prevented by salicylic acid and by phenanthrolines. *Eur J Pharmacol* 1978; 50:231.
14. Virchow C, Szczezklik A, Bianco S, et al.: Intolerance to tartrazine in aspirin-induced asthma: results of a multicenter study. *Respiration* 1988; 53:20.
15. Stevenson DD, Simon RA: Sensitivity to aspirin and nonsteroidal antiinflammatory drugs, in Middleton E, Reed CE, Ellis EF, et al. (eds): *Allergy Principles and Practice*, 4th ed. St. Louis, CV Mosby, 1993; 1747–1765.
16. Szczeklik A: Aspirin-induced asthma as a viral disease. *Clin Allergy* 1988; 18:15.
17. Pasargiklian M, Bianco S, Allegra L, et al.: Aspects of bronchial reactivity to prostaglandins and aspirin in asthmatic patients. *Respiration* 1977; 34:78.
18. Weiss JW, Drazen JM, McFadden ER Jr, et al.: Airway constriction in normal humans produced by inhalation of leukotriene D. Potency, time course, and effect of aspirin therapy. *JAMA* 1983; 249:2814.
19. Davidson AB, Lee TH, Scanlon PD, et al.: Bronchoconstrictor effects of leukotriene E_4 in normal and asthmatic subjects. *Am Rev Respir Dis* 1987; 135:333.
20. Shore SA, Austen KF, Drazen JM: Eicosanoids and the lung, in L'Enfant C (ed): *Lung Biology in Health and Disease: Lung Cell Biology*. New York, Marcel Dekker, 1989:1011.
21. Laitinen LA, Laitinen A, Haahtela T, et al.: Leukotriene E_4 and

granulocytic infiltration into asthmatic airways. *Lancet* 1993; 341:989.

22. Palmblad J, Malmsten C, Uden A, et al.: Leukotriene B_4 is a potent and stereospecific stimulator of neutrophil chemotaxis and adherence. *Blood* 1981; 58:658.

23. Marom Z, Shelhamer J, Sun F, Kaliner M: Human airway mono-hydroxyeicosatetraenoic acid generation and mucus release. *J Clin Invest* 1983; 72:122.

24. Ferreri NR, Howland WC, Stevenson DD, Spiegelberg HL: Release of leukotrienes, prostaglandins, and histamine into nasal secretions of aspirin-sensitive asthmatics during reaction to aspirin. *Am Rev Respir Dis* 1988; 137:847.

25. Christie PE, Tagari P, Fordhutchinson AW, et al.: Urinary leukotriene-E_4 concentrations increase after aspirin challenge in aspirin-sensitive asthmatic subjects. *Am Rev Respir Dis* 1991; 143:1025.

26. Israel E, Fischer AR, Rosenberg MA, et al.: The pivotal role of 5-lipoxygenase products in the reaction of aspirin-sensitive asthmatics to aspirin. *Am Rev Respir Dis* 1993; 148:1447.

27. Knapp HR, Sladek K, FitzGerald GA: Increased excretion of leukotriene E_4 during aspirin induced asthma. *J Lab Clin Invest* 1992; 119:48.

28. Christie PE, Tagari P, Ford-Hutchinson AW, et al.: Urinary leukotriene E_4 after lysine-aspirin inhalation in asthmatic subjects. *Am Rev Respir Dis* 1992; 146:1531.

29. Kumlin M, Dahlen B, Bjorck T, et al.: Urinary excretion of leukotriene E_4 and 11-dehydro-thromboxane B_2 in response to bronchial provocations with allergen, aspirin, leukotriene D_4 and histamine in asthmatics. *Am Rev Respir Dis* 1992; 146:96.

30. Christie PE, Smith CM, Lee TH: The potent and selective sulfidopeptide leukotriene antagonist, SK&F 104353, inhibits aspirin-induced asthma. *Am Rev Respir Dis* 1991; 144:957.

31. Dahlen B, Kumlin M, Margolskee DJ, et al.: The leukotriene-receptor antagonist MK-0679 blocks airway obstruction induced by bronchial provocation with lysine-aspirin in aspirin-sensitive asthmatics. *Eur Respir J* 1993; 6:1018.

32. Arm JP, O'Hickey SP, Spur BW, Lee TH: Airway responsiveness to histamine and leukotriene E_4 in subjects with aspirin-induced asthma. *Am Rev Respir Dis* 1989; 140:148.

33. Owen WF Jr, Soberman RJ, Yoshimoto T, et al.: Synthesis and release of leukotriene C_4 by human eosinophils. *J Immunol* 1987; 138:532.

34. MacGlashan DW Jr, Schleimer RP, Peters SP, et al.: Generation of leukotrienes by purified human lung mast cells. *J Clin Invest* 1982; 70:747.

35. Rankin JA, Schrader CE, Smith SM, Lewis RA: Recombinant interferon-gamma primes alveolar macrophages cultured in vitro for the release of leukotriene B_4 in response to IgG stimulation. *J Clin Invest* 1989; 83:1691.

36. Bosso JV, Schwartz LB, Stevenson DD: Tryptase and histamine release during aspirin-induced respiratory reactions. *J Allergy Clin Immunol* 1991; 88:830.

37. Fischer AR, Rosenberg MA, Lilly CM, et al.: Direct evidence for a role of the mast cell in the nasal response to aspirin in aspirin-sensitive asthma. *J Allergy Clin Immunol* 1994; 94:1046.

38. Sladek K, Szczeklik A: Cysteinyl leukotrienes overproduction and mast cell activation in aspirin-provoked bronchospasm in asthma. *Eur Respir J* 1993; 6:391.

39. Sladek K, Dworski R, Soja J, et al.: Eicosanoids in bronchoalveolar lavage fluid of aspirin-intolerant patients with asthma after aspirin challenge. *Am J Respir Crit Care Med* 1994; 149:940.

40. National Heart, Lung, and Blood Institute. National Asthma Education Program. Expert Panel Report: Guidelines for the diagnosis and management of asthma. *J Allergy Clin Immunol* 1991; 88:425.

41. Pleskow WW, Stevenson DD, Mathison DA, et al.: Aspirin desensitization in aspirin-sensitive asthmatic patients: clinical manifestations and characterization of the refractory period. *J Allergy Clin Immunol* 1982; 69:11.

42. Chiu JT: Improvement in aspirin-sensitive asthmatic subjects after rapid aspirin desensitization and aspirin maintenance (ADAM) treatment. *J Allergy Clin Immunol* 1983; 71:560.

43. Stevenson DD: Aspirin desensitization. *N Engl Reg Allergy Proc* 1986; 7:101.

44. Nasser SM, Bell GS, Foster S, et al.: Effect of the 5-lipoxygenase inhibitor ZD2138 on aspirin-induced asthma. *Thorax* 1994; 49:749.

Chapter 71

SEDATIVE HYPNOTIC AGENTS IN PULMONARY AND CRITICAL CARE MEDICINE

MICHAEL F. O'CONNOR AND THEODORE LEWIS, JR.

Opiates

Benzodiazepines

Haloperidol

Propofol

Barbiturates

Complications of ICU Sedation
   Hypotension
   Respiratory depression
   Inability to examine the patient

Sedatives and hypnotic agents are used for a wide range of purposes in pulmonary medicine, from the light sedation used to facilitate bronchoscopy to the deep sedation used in the treatment of tetanus. Consequently, pulmonary and critical care physicians must be knowledgeable about the use of sedative drugs. Newer agents, such as fentanyl, midazolam, and propofol recently have come into general use. The wide range of agents available for use as sedatives today makes it much easier to choose a drug that is suited to both the patient and the procedure being undertaken.

Increased sensitivity to the complications of oversedation frequently has resulted in institutional guidelines regarding the use and monitoring of patients undergoing sedation for procedures. Many institutions now require that an individual not actually performing the procedure monitor the patient during the procedure and that patients be monitored in a supervised setting until they demonstrate adequate recovery from the effects of sedation. Many also mandate or encourage strongly the use of routine ECG and pulse oximetry monitoring during sedation for procedures.

Opiates

Opiates are used widely for their analgesic properties as well as for their ability to suppress the subjective sensation of dyspnea and reduce cough. Opiates provide dose-dependent analgesia, no amnesia, and dose-dependent depression of consciousness. They act through a variety of receptors (mu 1 and 2, delta, kappa, and sigma) in both the central nervous system (CNS) and the peripheral nervous system (PNS).[2] The primary site of action for most commercially available opiates appears to be mu receptors in the CNS. Mu receptors mediate analgesia, hypoventilation, bradycardia, euphoria, ileus, and physical dependence. The role of the delta-receptors appears to be to modulate the activity of the mu receptors. Kappa-receptors mediate analgesia, sedation, hypoventilation, and miosis. Agonist-antagonist agents, such as butorphanol, act at the kappa-receptor.[2] Unfortunately, there is a high incidence of excitation reactions and a very low therapeutic effect from kappa-agonists. Activation of the sigma-receptor results in dysphoria, hypertonia, tachycardia, and tachypnea. Hence, although discussion of opiate receptors is interesting, clinicians at present must choose among agents that act primarily at mu receptors in the CNS.

Almost all critically ill patients have pain, so a case can be made to include opiates in the sedation regimen of all critically ill patients. However, in addition to their analgesic properties, opiates have the unique ability to suppress the subjective sensation of dyspnea. It is this characteristic that makes opiates so attractive for use in the intensive care setting. The physiologic mechanisms by which opiates relieve the sensation of dyspnea are poorly understood. Hypoxia, hypercarbia, and decreased lung compliance may all play a role in the sensation of dyspnea. Opiates are well known to diminish the respiratory response to both hypoxia and hypercarbia in humans. Other factors, not yet described, may also play important roles in the sensation of dyspnea.

There are a number of opiates from which to choose for sedation in the intensive care unit (ICU). Morphine may be given by either bolus or continuous infusion. The infusion should be initiated at 0.05 mg/kg/h and titrated to effect. Most patients will require morphine infusion rates of between 0.05 and 0.2 mg/kg/h. Loading doses in the form of boluses of 0.05 to 0.1 mg/kg are appropriate to provide analgesia prior to the initiation of the infusion. Bolus doses of morphine in this range are suitable for sedation for patients undergoing procedures such as bronchoscopy. Levorphanol and hydromorphone are also suitable as agents for bolus dosing of patients requiring sedation. Fentanyl is best given as a loading bolus and continuous infusion. A bolus of 0.5 μg/kg to 2 μg/kg followed by an infusion rate of 0.5 μg/kg/h is a reasonable strategy for using fentanyl. The rapid occurrence of tolerance may require titration to relatively large doses of fentanyl. Boluses of 50 to 100 μg are adequate for sedation for procedures. Higher doses of fentanyl should be avoided in outpatients as they may be associated with excessive respiratory depression and nausea and vomiting, which may delay or preclude discharge following the procedure.[6] Methadone may be the ideal opiate for sedation in the ICU. Bolus administration of 0.5 mg/kg per day in divided doses (q 6 to 12 h) will provide adequate analgesia for most patients. Doses of methadone of up to 2 mg/kg per day are well tolerated by most patients. Opiate-tolerant patients may require very high rates of infusion of any of the opiates and may be best served by starting with and sticking to methadone.

Strong consideration should be given to prescribing laxatives to maintain gut motility in all patients being treated with opiates in the ICU. A wide variety of agents are available for this purpose, and one should be chosen which is consistent with the patient's coexisting medical conditions and treatment plan.

In general, opiates have little direct effect on cardiac or vascular function. These agents have achieved enormous popularity and success in the perioperative care of patients with limited cardiovascular reserve. All opiates, with the exception of meperidine, are associated with bradycardia.[2,7] Meperidine, because of its atropine-like structure, is associated with tachycardia.[2] Both morphine and fentanyl can be given in large doses with little or no myocardial depression.[8,9] Meperidine is the only opiate that has been demonstrated to depress myocardial contractility in clinically relevant doses.[10,11] Morphine may cause mild decreases in systemic vascular resistance and increases in venous capacitance.[12] It has been associated with histamine release, but only when relatively large doses of the drug are given over a relatively short period of time.[13] The hemodynamic consequences of histamine release associated with high dose morphine administration can be prevented or attenuated by pretreatment with H_1- and H_2-receptor antagonists.[14] Other commonly used opiates, including fentanyl, sufentanil, hydromorphone, and levorphanol have no significant hemodynamic side effects.[15] Potent opiates (fentanyl, alfentanil),

when used in conjunction with benzodiazepines in the operating room, have been associated with a decrease in afterload and blood pressure.[16,17] The frequency and severity of this syndrome have not been ascertained in the critical care setting.

Routine reversal of opiate analgesia with naloxone should be avoided. Although naloxone is inexpensive and readily available, reversal of opiate-induced sedation may cause significant risk. Many patients treated with naloxone demonstrate hypertension and tachycardia and may develop pulmonary edema.[18–21] The use of naloxone to establish the diagnosis of opiate overdose in relatively young patients in the emergency department is warranted and relatively safe.

Benzodiazepines

Benzodiazepines are the principal anxiolytic agents used in clinical practice. Benzodiazepines bind to the alpha-subunit of the gamma-aminobutyric acid (GABA) receptor, increasing the affinity of the receptor for GABA.[22] This results in increased action of GABA, an inhibitory neurotransmitter, which in turn results in decreased CNS function. Benzodiazepine receptors are found on neurons throughout the CNS but are not present in large quantities elsewhere in the body. This is probably the explanation for why benzodiazepines have potent effects on CNS function but little effect on other organs.

Because of their lack of effect on the circulation and overall very high therapeutic index, benzodiazepines have achieved enormous popularity as sedative agents in the ICU. Nevertheless, understanding their pharmacology can enhance the safety and efficacy of their use. Most benzodiazepines are heavily protein bound, and hence only a very small percentage of the drug that is injected into a patient is bioavailable for activity at cellular receptors.[23] Hypoproteinemic patients consequently will demonstrate an exaggerated response to the injection of benzodiazepines, which will last until the drug is redistributed into the fatty tissues. Surprisingly, the duration of effect of benzodiazepines is also shorter in hypoproteinemic patients, because the drug also is more available for clearance by the liver. Almost all benzodiazepines are hepatically metabolized. Only oxazepam does not require hepatic clearance.

Lorazepam, midazolam, and diazepam are all used commonly to produce a combination of sedation, anxiolysis, and amnesia. Other benzodiazepines, such as oxazepam, chlordiazepoxide, and clonazepam, are used less commonly for sedation in the ICU. Benzodiazepines in high doses may reduce requirement for analgesic medicines by up to 15 percent. Benzodiazepines have no known effect upon the sensation of dyspnea. They provide dose-dependent depression of consciousness, anxiolysis, and variable amnesia. Greater doses of the more potent benzodiazepines (midazolam, lorazepam) cause amnesia. Benzodiazepines do not cause direct cardiovascular effects when used in sedating doses.[24,25] When given in doses sufficient to induce general anesthesia, midazolam causes a 10 to 15 percent decrease in blood pressure and cardiac output.[26,27] As mentioned above, benzodiazepines, when used in conjunction with potent opiates, have been associated with a decrease in afterload and blood pressure.[16,17] The mechanism of this interesting drug-drug interaction has not been elucidated (it is not mediated by either histamines or catecholamines). Benzodiazepines depress the drive to breathe. The response to hypoxia is depressed severely (frequently obliterated), and the response to hypercarbia is reduced in a dose-dependent fashion.

Lorazepam and midazolam are the two most commonly used benzodiazepines in the ICU. Lorazepam can be given either by bolus or continuous infusion. Most patients obtain satisfactory sedation with boluses of 0.5 to 4 mg every 1 to 4 h. Patients who are to be sedated with a continuous infusion should be loaded with the appropriate bolus doses, followed by an infusion of 0.5 to 4 mg/h. Most patients will require infusion rates of about 4 mg/h to obtain satisfactory sedation. When used to sedate critically ill patients, midazolam should be given as a constant infusion, as it is too short acting to be used in repeated boluses. This is quite the opposite of patients undergoing awake procedures, where prolonged sedation is not a desired effect. Infusions should be initiated with a loading dose of 0.05 to 0.2 mg/kg of midazolam, given in increments of 0.05 mg/kg over a brief period (30 min). An infusion can then be started and titrated to patient comfort. Most patients are comfortable at rates of approximately 0.1 mg/kg/h. Tolerance tends to occur rapidly to continuous infusions of midazolam, and rates of 0.2 to 0.3 mg/kg/h are typical after 3 days. The requirement for benzodiazepines can be reduced by increasing the amount of opiate used to sedate a patient.

Tolerance to both lorazepam and midazolam occurs rather quickly after the initiation of continuous infusion for sedation. The mechanism of this tolerance remains unclear but is probably a combination of both downregulation of receptors at the cell membrane and increased hepatic clearance. Recovery from these agents is not straightforward. Lorazepam, which has a very long duration of action compared to midazolam when given as a single bolus dose (8 h versus 1 h), has a substantially shorter recovery (4 h) than midazolam (30 h) in ICU patients sedated to the same levels by continuous infusion.[28] The reason for this is also unclear. Possible explanations include greater storage of midazolam in body fat, resulting in an increased washout time, or the accumulation of a long-acting active metabolite, resulting in prolonged sedation. All other benzodiazepines presently available have known active metabolites, which create similar problems when used for prolonged sedation in the ICU.

Withdrawal syndromes frequently have been associated with prolonged sedation with benzodiazepines in the ICU. These syndromes are characterized by agitation, tachycardia, hypertension, and tachypnea. In patients who have been sedated with benzodiazepines for one to several days, a slow taper is the best way to avoid this.

The routine reversal of benzodiazepines with flumazenil is ill advised. Nausea and vomiting frequently accompany reversal of benzodiazepines, as may an acute and severe withdrawal syndrome.[29–34] Seizures have been reported in patients treated with flumazenil in the presence of cyclic antidepressants, and the use of flumazenil is discouraged in these patients.[32,33,34] Flumazenil, like naloxone, does not last as long as any of the commercially available benzodiazepines. Hence, it may have a role as diagnostic tool for oversedation with benzodiazepines, rather than for the therapeutic reversal of benzodiazepine sedation. Repeated doses or a continuous infusion are required to maintain therapeutic reversal of a benzodiazepine overdose.

Haloperidol

Haloperidol is a major tranquilizing drug that has achieved popularity as a sedative agent in the ICU. Haloperidol is a butyrophenone, chemically related to droperidol. Its major clinical use is as an antipsychotic medication. Haloperidol antagonizes dopamine binding at dopamine-2-receptors in the CNS.[35] Dopamine-2-receptors are postsynaptic dopamine receptors and appear to be the major dopamine receptors in the CNS. Haloperidol appears to have little activity at dopamine-1-receptors, which are the major postsynaptic receptors for dopamine outside the CNS.

Haloperidol is sedative and anxiolytic but is not analgesic or amnestic. Consequently, patients experiencing pain should be sedated with an analgesic in addition to haloperidol. Droperidol, a closely related drug, potentiates the analgesic properties of opiates and has antiemetic effects as well. Unfortunately, droperidol is associated with a high percentage of dysphoric reactions, and its popularity has waned as a consequence.[36]

Haloperidol is an excellent sedative for critically ill patients for a number of reasons. There is little or no tolerance to the drug. It depresses only minimally the CO_2 drive to breathe. There is evidence to suggest that butyrophenones, such as haloperidol actually may increase the ventilatory response to hypoxia.[37] Haloperidol is mildly vasodilating in a dose-dependent manner but is occasionally associated with substantial decrease in blood pressure. Rapid injection will result in high peak concentrations of the drug and concomitant sedation. As the drug is redistributed to the tissues of the body, the level of sedation will decline. The elimination half-life of haloperidol is long, and it may take a patient days to eliminate large doses of the drug. Large doses of antipsychotic medications such as haloperidol precipitate a number of well-described side effects. A small percentage of patients will experience extrapyramidal side effects, which can be prevented or treated with benzodiazepines.[38] Tolerance to haloperidol has not been described, and there is no known withdrawal syndrome associated with the drug.

Haloperidol customarily is given by intermittent bolus. Individual patients may require very high daily doses to maintain adequate sedation. Elderly, hypovolemic, and debilitated patients may respond to very small doses and may demonstrate hypotension or prolonged sedation in response to even small doses. Small boluses should be used at first (1.25 to 2.5 mg). Rapid escalation of dose, (bolus doses of up to 10 mg) is permissible if the patient demonstrates hemodynamic stability and need for more sedation. Patients may benefit from treatment with benzodiazepines to prevent extrapyramidal symptoms with large daily doses of haloperidol.

Propofol

Propofol is a sedative-hypnotic agent that has achieved widespread use as a sedative agent for critically ill patients. Its site of action remains unknown, but it is thought to have effects on the CNS similar to benzodiazepines and barbiturates. Onset of action following intravenous injection of propofol is very rapid, approximating one circulation time. Termination of activity, even after very long infusions, is by redistribution of drug into the fatty tissues of the body and slow elimination.[39] Patients typically wake up within an hour of termination of infusion, even if the infusion has lasted for weeks. Propofol is profoundly anxiolytic, sedative in a dose-dependent fashion, and has no analgesic properties. Titrated to large doses, it can be the mainstay of an intravenous general anesthetic. As it is not analgesic, all patients sedated with propofol will require treatment with an analgesic for whatever pain they may have. Propofol produces amnesia reliably only when it is titrated to relatively high doses.

Propofol is both a vasodilator and a myocardial depressant.[40–44] Bolus doses of propofol can cause precipitous decreases in blood pressure in healthy, euvolemic patients. Bolus doses in the ICU are frequently associated with hypotension. Consequently, propofol is best administered as a continuous infusion. Because propofol is dissolved in a lipid emulsion, patients may become hyperlipidemic during continuous infusion of large doses. This problem can be either ignored or treated by decreasing the dose of propofol and using another agent in its place. Propofol is also a potent respiratory depressant and should only be used in settings where respiration is carefully monitored.[40,46] As greater rates of infusion of propofol can induce general anesthesia and loss of airway reflexes, patients who are at risk for aspiration should be intubated while undergoing deep sedation with propofol. Its use is restricted to intubated, mechanically ventilated patients in the ICU.

Propofol is best used by continuous infusion only. The infusion should be started at 5 μg/kg/min, and titrated up until satisfactory sedation is achieved or until unacceptable decreases in blood pressure occur. Patients who have received large doses of opiates, such as postsurgical patients, will tend to require lesser infusion rates of propofol (around 10 to 20 μg/kg/min). Patients who have not received large doses of opiates will require greater infusion rates, typically in the range of 30 to 50 μg/kg/min. Infusion rates of higher than 70 to 80 μg/kg/min rarely are necessary.

Barbiturates

Barbiturates have lost favor as sedating agents in the ICU for many reasons. Profound negative inotropic effects, antianalgesic effects, and tachyphylaxis all have contributed to the decline in popularity of these agents in the ICU.

Nevertheless, they remain effective agents. Barbiturates act principally by binding to GABA receptors in the reticular activating system and preventing the disassociation of GABA from its receptor. This increased activity of GABA, an inhibitory neurotransmitter, results in decreased reticular activating system activity, which in turn results in decreased consciousness.

Barbiturates directly depress the myocardium; as a consequence, their use for sedation frequently is associated with hemodynamic deterioration in adults. The longer-acting barbiturates, such as phenobarbital, are less likely to cause this than shorter acting agents, such as thiopental. Barbiturates have an antianalgesic effect, actually heightening the sensation of pain in patients; this phenomenon is well described but poorly understood. Tachyphylaxis, or tolerance, also is a well-described phenomenon associated with sedation with barbiturates in the ICU.

Why might one choose to use barbiturates in the ICU? Barbiturates have several desirable properties; they increase the seizure threshold (methohexital is an exception to this), reduce intracranial pressure (ICP), and can be used to induce coma. The utility of barbiturates for lowering the ICP long has been recognized as a major asset of this class of drug. Barbiturates cause a decrease in the cerebral metabolic rate, are cerebral arterial vasoconstrictors, and cause a decrease in cerebral blood flow. All of these physiologic changes are particularly desirable in patients with increased ICP. Because the cerebral metabolic rate is depressed far more than the blood flow, it is accepted widely (but not proven) that the decrease in blood flow takes place in a situation that results in a favorable change in the balance of cerebral oxygen delivery and uptake. Barbiturates probably will continue to play an important role in the management of CNS-injured patients for the foreseeable future.

Complications of ICU Sedation

In addition to side effects that are attributable to the individual agents, there are side effects of sedation in the ICU that are common to all agents and that merit discussion separately. These side effects include hypotension, respiratory depression, and inability to examine the patient.

HYPOTENSION

Although opiates and benzodiazepines are not myocardial depressants or vasodilators, hypotension frequently is observed in critically ill patients shortly after boluses of these medications are administered. Understanding the physiology of this hypotension helps to treat it in a manner that is consistent with the goals for the management of that patient.

Sedative agents depress CNS function nonspecifically. A consequence of this is that all of them depress CNS outflow to the sympathetic nervous system. This in turn results in a decrease in sympathetic outflow to the periphery, including the heart and circulation. Decreased venous return, decreased myocardial contractility, and decreased arterial tone all may accompany a decrease in sympathetic nervous system activity. Patients who do not require their sympathetic nervous system to maintain their venous return, myocardial contractility, or arterial tone typically do not demonstrate hemodynamic response even to general anesthetic doses of opiates and benzodiazepines. Patients who are hypovolemic or have severely impaired myocardial function may have significant changes in blood pressure and cardiac output when treated with these agents. In these latter patients, negative inotropic agents, such as propofol or thiopental, may produce disastrous decreases in cardiac output and blood pressure. Vasodilating agents, such as haloperidol, also can cause decreases in blood pressure when given in large doses.

Rapid infusion of volume and treatment with either inotropic or vasoactive agents are among the appropriate responses to decreases in blood pressure associated with boluses of sedative agents. Individual caretakers should choose which of these interventions to use, based upon their suspicion of what the primary cause of the hypotension is in a particular patient. Administration of lesser doses more frequently also may result in less hypotension but a greater workload for nursing staff. Constant infusion may result in a continuous depression of hemodynamics, which is more tolerable to the patient than any regimen of bolus infusions.

RESPIRATORY DEPRESSION

Almost all sedatives and anesthetics obliterate the hypoxic drive to breathe and depress the CO_2 drive to breathe. Different agents depress respiration in different patterns. Opiates tend to slow respiration, while having minimal effect on tidal volume. Greater doses of benzodiazepines are associated with rapid shallow breathing, as are barbiturates.[48] Patients receiving bolus doses of barbiturates may take several large tidal volumes immediately prior to becoming apneic. Sedation with propofol is associated with rapid shallow breathing.

Sedated patients will not respond to hypoxia. This is why patients require monitoring with pulse oximeters in the operating room, procedure suite, and recovery room. Monitoring respiration by observing the frequency and strength of respiration, along with pulse oximetry, should be considered as the standard for monitoring patients undergoing sedation. ECG and blood pressure monitoring should be used when deep levels of sedation are anticipated. Monitoring of respiration should continue until the patient recovers from sedation, the effects of which may last much longer than the procedure for which the patient was sedated.

INABILITY TO EXAMINE THE PATIENT

Perhaps the most important side effect of both sedation and paralysis is the impaired ability to examine the patient. It may be difficult or impossible to perform a neurologic or abdominal examination on a deeply sedated patient. Moderate or deep levels of paralysis preclude these kinds of examination altogether. Critically ill patients who are deeply sedated or paralyzed frequently undergo imaging studies because neurologic and abdominal examinations cannot be reliably performed at the bedside. Neurologic or abdominal catastrophes can go unrecognized for long periods of time in these patients, with the attendant increase in morbidity and mortality.

References

1. Council on Scientific Affairs, AMA: The use of pulse oximetry during conscious sedation. *JAMA* 1993; 270(12):1463.
2. Stoelting RK: Opioid agonists and antagonists, in *Pharmacology and Physiology in Anesthetic Practice,* 2d ed. Philadelphia, Lippincott, 1991.
3. Weil et al.: Diminished ventilatory response to hypoxia and hypercapnea after morphine in normal man. *N Engl J Med* 1975; 292:1103.
4. Eckenhoff JE, Oech SR: The effects of narcotics and antagonists upon respiration and circulation in man. *Clin Pharmacol Ther* 1960; 1:483.
5. Arunasalam et al.: Ventilatory response to morphine in old and young subjects. *Anesthesia* 1983; 38:529.
6. Rising et al.: Isoflurane vs fentanyl for outpatient laparoscopy. *Acta Anaesthesiol Scand* 1985; 29:251.
7. Liu WS et al.: Cardiovascular dynamics after large doses of fentanyl and fentanyl plus N_2O in the dog. *Anesth Analg* 1976; 55:168.
8. Strauer B: Contractile responses to morphine, piritramine, meperidine, and fentanyl. *Anesthesiology* 1972; 37:304.
9. Bovill JG, Sebel PS: Pharmacokinetics of high-dose fentanyl: A study in patients undergoing cardiac surgery. *Br J Anaesth* 1980; 52:795.
10. Stanley TH, Liu WS: Cardiovascular effects of nitrous oxide-meperidine anesthesia before and after pancuronium. *Anesth Analg* 1977; 56:669.
11. Freye E: Cardiovascular effects of high doses of fentanyl, meperidine, and naloxone in dogs. *Anesth Analg* 1974; 53:40.
12. Hsu et al.: Morphine decreases peripheral vascular resistance and increases capacitance in man. *Anesthesiology* 1979; 59:98.
13. Rosow CE et al.: Histamine release during morphine and fentanyl anesthesia. *Anesthesiology* 1982; 56:93.
14. Philbin DM et al.: The use of H1 and H2 histamine antagonists with morphine anesthesia: A double blind study. *Anesthesiology* 1982; 55:292.
15. Rosow et al.: Hemodynamics and histamine release during induction with sufentanil or fentanyl. *Anesthesiology* 1984; 60:489.
16. Tomicheck et al.: Diazepam-fentanyl interaction: Hemodynamic and hormonal effects in coronary artery surgery. *Anesth Analg* 1983; 62:881.
17. Rosow et al.: The effect of diazepam on induction of anesthesia with alfentanil. *Anesth Analg* 1986; 65:71.
18. Andree RA: Sudden death following naloxone administration. *Anesth Analg* 1980; 59:782.
19. Flacke et al.: Acute pulmonary edema following naloxone reversal of high-dose morphine anesthesia. *Anesthesiology* 1977; 47:376.
20. Tanaka GY: Hypertensive response to naloxone. *JAMA* 1974; 288:25.
21. Michaelis LL et al.: Ventricular irritability associated with the use of naloxone. *Ann Thorac Surg* 1974; 18:608.
22. Levine RL: Pharmacology of intravenous sedatives and opioids in critically ill patients. *Crit Care Clin* 1994; 10:4,709.
23. Stoelting RK: Benzodiazepines, in *Pharmacology and Physiology in Anesthetic Practice*, 2d ed. Philadelphia, Lippincott, 1991.
24. Dundee JW, Keeilty SR: Diazepam. *Int Anesthesiol Clin* 1969; 7:91.

25. Dalen JE et al.: The hemodynamic and respiratory effects of diazepam. *Anesthesiology* 1969; 30:259.

26. Liebowitz et al.: Comparative cardiovascular effects of midazolam and thiopental on healthy patients. *Anesth Analg* 1983; 61:771.

27. Marty J et al.: Effects of midazolam on the coronary circulation in patients with coronary artery disease. *Anesthesiology* 1986; 64:206.

28. Pohlman AS et al.: Continuous infusions of lorazepam vs midazolam for sedation during mechanical ventilatory support: A prospective, randomized study. *Crit Care Med* 1994; 22:1241.

29. Amrein R et al.: Flumazenil in benzodiazepine antagonism. *Med Toxicol* 1987; 2:411.

30. Bodenham A et al.: Reversal of sedation by prolonged infusion of flumazenil. *Anaesthesia* 1988; 43:376.

31. Griffiths RR et al.: Intravenous flumazenil following acute and repeated exposure to lorazepam in healthy volunteers: Antagonism and precipitated withdrawal. *J Pharmacol Exp Ther* 1993; 265:1163.

32. Spivey WH et al.: A clinical trial of escalating doses of flumazenil for reversal of suspected benzodiazepine overdose in the emergency department. *Ann Emerg Med* 1993; 22:1813.

33. Mordel et al.: Seizures after flumazenil administration in a case of combined benzodiazepine and tricyclic antidepressant overdose. *Crit Care Med* 1992; 20:1733.

34. The Flumazenil in Benzodiazepine Intoxication Multicenter Study Group: Treatment of benzodiazepine overdose with flumazenil. *Clin Ther* 1992; 14:978.

35. Ellenbroek BA et al.: The involvement of dopamine D1 and D2 receptors in the effects of the classical neuroleptic haloperidol and the atypical neuroleptic clozapine. *Eur J Pharmacol* 1991; 196:103.

36. Lee CM, Yeakel AE: Patients refusal of surgery following innovar premedication. *Anesth Analg* 1975; 54:224.

37. Ward DS: Stimulation of the hypoxic respiratory drive by droperidol. *Anesth Analg* 1984; 63:106.

38. Tonda ME, Guthrie SK: Treatment of acute neuroleptic-induced movement disorders. *Pharmacotherapy* 1994; 14:543.

39. Gepts E et al.: Disposition of propofol administered as a constant rate infusions in humans. *Anesth Analg* 1987; 66:1256.

40. Fong SY et al.: Comparison of propofol and thiopental as induction agents. *Semin Anesth (suppl 1)* 1988; 7:52.

41. Boer F et al.: Effects of propofol on peripheral vascular resistance during cardiopulmonary bypass. *Br J Anaesth* 1990; 65:184.

42. Mulier JP et al.: Cardiodynamic effects of propofol in comparison with thiopental: Assessment with transesophageal echocardiographic approach. *Anesth Analg* 1991; 72:28.

43. Coetzee A et al.: Effect of various propofol plasma concentrations on regional myocardial and left ventricular afterload. *Anesth Analg* 1989; 69:473.

44. Patel PS, Warltier DC: Negative inotropic effects of propofol as evaluated by the regional preload recruitable stroke work relationship in chronically instrumented dogs. *Anesthesiology* 1993; 78:100.

45. Eddleston JM, Shelly MP: The effect on serum lipid concentrations of a prolonged infusion of propofol—hypertriglyceridemia associated with propofol administration. *Intens Care Med* 1991; 17:424.

46. Dundee JW et al.: Sensitivity to propofol in the elderly. *Anaesthesia* 1986; 41:482.

DRUG-INDUCED PULMONARY DISEASES

CHERYL L. RENZ

Drug reactions constitute a significant health hazard. Drug-induced illness accounts for nearly 5 percent of all hospital admissions and complicates the course of as many as 15 percent of hospitalized patients.[1]

While only 2 percent of patients experiencing drug reactions report respiratory symptoms,[2] drug-induced pulmonary diseases are associated with life-threatening events in > 10 percent of these cases.[3] This is not surprising; the lungs are the only organ system exposed to the entire circulation,[4,5] and the lungs also are capable of various metabolic functions, such as N-alkylation, N-dialkylation, N-oxidation, reduction of N-oxide, and C-hydroxylation,[6] which can generate toxic products from initially innocuous substances.

The recognition of drug-induced pulmonary diseases requires a high index of suspicion. The affected patients often have complex disorders with multiple reasons for pulmonary complications. The clinical and pathologic features are often nonspecific, as are the interpretations of diagnostic tests, particularly chest radiographs. The drug-induced pulmonary diseases discussed in this chapter are classified into four categories relative to their mechanism of lung injury: (1) oxidant-induced injury, (2) hypersensitivity injury, (3) phospholipidosis, and (4) noncardiogenic pulmonary edema. Other drug-induced thoracic disorders, pertaining to the pleura, mediastinum, neuromuscular control of breathing,

airflow obstruction, and cough, are discussed elsewhere in this text.

Oxidant-Induced Lung Disease

Drugs causing oxidant-induced lung injury are listed in Table 72-1. Chemotherapeutic agents, the most frequent offenders, have been investigated in detail.[7–11]

Risk factors for oxidant-induced lung injury include increased age, preexisting pulmonary disease, tobacco exposure, remote or concurrent radiotherapy, oxygen therapy (especially at high concentrations, including during general anesthesia), and previous or simultaneous use of other cytotoxic drugs. Although the precise incidence of many of the drugs listed in Table 72-1 has not been established, dose-response relationships have been documented for busulfan, bleomycin, carmustine (BCNU) and mitomycin-C.

Busulfan, used extensively in the treatment of chronic myelogenous leukemia, was the first chemotherapeutic agent reported to cause lung disease.[12] Toxicity occurs in approximately 4 percent of patients receiving the drug, usually after a total dose of 500 mg.[9] The onset of disease is latent and occurs from 1 month to 12 years after therapy commences, with a mean of 3.5 years, and a median of 3 years.

TABLE 72-1 **Drugs that Cause Oxidant-Induced Lung Disease**

I. Chemotherapeutic agents
   A. Alkylating agents
      Busulfan
      Chlorambucil
      Cyclophosphamide
      Melphalan
      Uracil mustard
      Nitrosoureas
        a. Carmustine (BCNU)
        b. Lomostine (CCNU)
        c. Semustine (methyl-CCNU)
   B. Cytotoxic antibiotics
      Bleomycin
      Mitomycin
      Pepleomycin
      Neocarzinostatin
   C. Antimetabolites
      Azathioprine
      Cytosine arabinoside
      Methotrexate
   D. Miscellaneous
      Vinblastine
      Vindesine
      Teniposide (VM-26)
II. Noncytotoxic agents
   A. Ganglionic blockers
      Hexamethonium
      Mecamylamine
      Pentolinium
   B. Dilantin
   C. Nitrofurantoin

There is considerable information on the pulmonary toxicity of bleomycin because of its widespread use in various malignancies such as lymphomas and squamous cell and testicular carcinomas. In addition, it is administered to previously healthy young males with germ-cell tumors, and it can produce animal models of oxidant-induced lung injury. The incidence of toxicity ranges from 3 percent to 5 percent; the risk increases dramatically after a total cumulative dose of 450 mg.[8,9] Symptoms can occur when the drug first is administered,[13] or within weeks to 6 months following completion of therapy.[14,15] In the absence of bone marrow suppression, the amount of bleomycin that can be given is limited by its pulmonary toxicity.

Carmustine (BCNU) has the highest incidence of lung toxicity at 20 percent to 30 percent[16]; the incidence approaches 50 percent with cumulative doses of 1.5 gm/m[2] or more.[17] A history of cigarette smoking is associated with increased risk.[17] Latent periods range from 1 month after therapy initiation to 17 years after therapy cessation.[16,18]

On rarer occasions, other chemotherapeutic agents elicit oxidant-induced lung injury. The dose-response relationship for mitomycin-C occurs after a cumulative dose of 30 mg/m[2].[19,20,21] For cyclophosphamide no specific dose nor relationship to duration of therapy has been noted. Reported latent periods range from only 2 weeks to 13 years after cessation of therapy.[16,18,22] Toxicity produced by L-phenylala-

nine mustard and chlorambucil is not dose related. The latent period for chlorambucil ranges from 2 months to nearly 5 years after treatment initiation[23,24]; for L-phenylalanine mustard the latent period ranges from 2 to 16 months.[25–29]

MECHANISM OF INJURY

The prototype that best describes the mechanism of injury caused by the listed drugs is oxygen-induced lung damage. The drug forms a complex with O_2 and iron to produce oxygen free radicals [superoxide anion (O_2^-), hydrogen peroxide (H_2O_2), hydroxyl radical ($\cdot OH$), and singlet oxygen ($^1O_2$)].[16,30–32] These short-lived molecules generate singlet electron transfers that damage DNA, destroy lipid membranes, and inactivate crucial intracellular enzymes. The result is both inflammation, acute then chronic, and cell death, manifested as a capillary endothelial leak, loss of type I pneumocytes, and abnormal stimulation of type 2 pneumocytes and fibroblasts.

In addition, BCNU and cyclophosphamide impede cellular detoxification defenses by inhibiting the antioxidant enzymes superoxide dismutase, catalase, and glutathione peroxidase.[33,34] Studies in experimental animals demonstrate that pretreatment with superoxide dismutase and catalase reduces toxicity.[16]

Oxygen free radicals also are associated with the lung damage caused by radiation therapy and/or the administration of oxygen at high concentrations, which justifies their synergistic toxicities with drug-induced injury. For example, the incidence and severity of pulmonary fibrosis is increased in animals[35,36] and patients[37–40] exposed to bleomycin with previous or concurrent lung irradiation and/or use of high inspired oxygen concentrations.[7,8,29,37,41]

HISTOPATHOLOGY

The histopathology of oxidant-induced injury is characterized by diffuse alveolar damage[42–46] (Fig. 72-1). The alveolar septa are thickened secondary to edema, collagen deposition, and infiltration by mononuclear cells, which, at later stages, progresses to interstitial and intraalveolar fibrosis with variable degrees of organization or honeycomb change.[46,47] The type II pneumocytes are enlarged and dysplastic, with pleomorphic nuclei and prominent nucleoli. These pathologic changes have been observed in the absence of overt clinical disease as well as with normal radiologic findings.[48] For example, approximately 50 percent of patients treated with busulfan had subclinical damage apparent at autopsy.[17] Therefore, the anticipated cytologic atypia is not diagnostic of, but supportive of, oxidant-induced lung injury.

CLINICAL SPECTRUM

The presenting symptoms of patients with oxidant-induced lung injury are insidious and include malaise, dyspnea, and nonproductive cough. Occasionally, the patient is febrile, but without complaints of rigors or diaphoresis. Physical exami-

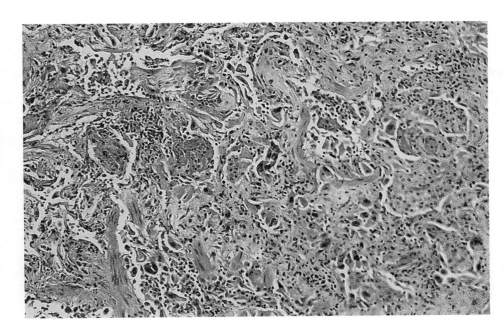

FIGURE 72-1 Diffuse alveolar damage from bleomycin toxicity characterized by alveolar septal thickening and dysplastic type II pneumocytes.

nation reveals end-inspiratory crackles. The chest radiographs may demonstrate a bibasilar or diffuse reticular or reticulonodular pattern,[49] and gallium scanning may show increased uptake by involved areas in the lungs.[16,50] Computer tomographic scanning may identify abnormalities that are not present on the routine chest film.[51] A more sensitive indicator of toxicity is a reduction in carbon monoxide diffusing capacity (DLCO).[16] A decrease of ≥ 20 percent in the DLCO is an accepted indication for discontinuing therapy.[16] However, the DLCO may be decreased in patients who never progress to overt pulmonary disease.[49] Thus, the presence of an isolated reduction in DLCO does not predict subsequent pulmonary injury. Finally, given the complexity of the clinical picture in patients prescribed cytotoxic drugs, pulmonary complications such as congestive heart failure, opportunistic infections, or relapse of underlying malignancy must be excluded.

MANAGEMENT

Once a diagnosis of oxidant-induced lung injury is established, the subsequent course is variable; discontinuation of the offending drug may result in resolution, stabilization or even progression of disease. Whenever possible, high concentrations of supplemental oxygen must be avoided. Multiple prospective series and case reports have documented response to corticosteroid therapy in doses equivalent to 60 to 100 mg/day of prednisone.[13,15,52–55] Tapering may lead to recurrence. Some patients die of fulminant injury, despite steroid therapy.[13,56–58] No known factors distinguish steroid responders from nonresponders. The impact of oxidant-induced lung injury is staggering; of all patients receiving bleomycin, nearly 2 percent die of pulmonary toxicity.[13,15,55] Novel approaches with antioxidants and iron chelating agents currently are under investigation.

Hypersensitivity-Induced Lung Disease

Hypersensitivity-induced lung disease involves stimulation of the host's own immune regulatory system and includes two categories: acute hypersensitivity with eosinophilia, and drug-induced systemic lupus erythematosus.

HYPERSENSITIVITY WITH EOSINOPHILIA LUNG DISEASE

The drugs associated with hypersensitivity with eosinophilia (HSE) lung disease are listed in Table 72-2. Reaction to these agents is idiosyncratic and there are no known risk factors. Severity and reversibility of lung injury are unrelated to cumulative dose or duration of therapy.[59]

MECHANISM OF INJURY
The offending drug apparently stimulates the host's immune system and induces a hypersensitivity reaction to an antigenic site on the drug or drug-hapten complex. The resultant sensitized T cells release lymphokines (interleukin-2, interleukin-5) that attract inflammatory cells, particularly eosinophils.

HISTOPATHOLOGY
The histopathologic features are interstitial, alveolar, and perivascular inflammation with infiltration by a mixed group of inflammatory cells, eosinophils are prominent.[60–63] There is little, if any, fibrosis.[64] Tissue from patients receiving methotrexate[65] and nitrofurantoin[66] occasionally reveals granuloma formation.

CLINICAL SPECTRUM
The presenting symptoms of HSE include fever, nonproductive cough, sensation of chest constriction, and dyspnea.

TABLE 72-2 Drugs that Cause Hypersensitivity with Eosinophilia Lung Disease

I. Cytotoxic drugs
  Bleomycin
  Methotrexate
  Procarbazine
II. Noncytotoxic drugs
  Ampicillin
  Aspirin
  Azathioprine
  Captopril
  Carbamazepine
  Chlorpromazine
  Chlorpropamide
  Cromolyn
  Dantrolene
  Diclofenac
  Diphenylhydantoin
  Febarbamate
  Fenbufen
  Gold
  Hydralazine
  Imipramine
  Isoniazid
  Mecamylamine
  Mephenesin carbamate
  Mercaptopurine
  Methylphenidate
  Minocycline
  Naproxen
  Niridazole
  Nitrofurantoin
  para-Aminosalicylic acid
  Penicillin
  Penicillamine
  Propranolol
  Salazopyrin
  Sodium dicromoglycate
  Streptomycin
  Sulfasalazine
  Tetracycline
  Tolazamide
  Tolbutamide

These symptoms may be accompanied by a pruritic skin rash that is macular and generalized in a pattern resembling erythema multiform. Arthralgias also may be present. The symptoms may occur acutely, over several hours, or develop over a period of days. Physical examination reveals auscultatory crackles and, on occasion, signs of a pleural effusion. The chest radiographs display a nonspecific pattern, suggesting diffuse alveolar or interstitial infiltrates; these may be symmetric or at other times peripheral—similar to eosinophilic pneumonia. Pleural effusions, when present, are generally unilateral; they may be an isolated finding or accompany parenchymal changes.[66] Pulmonary function tests reveal restrictive defects and a mild reduction in DLCO.[41,67] The striking laboratory finding is the presence of eosinophilia that may reach 10 percent to 20 percent of the total white blood cell count.[68] Overall, the clinical course is uncomplicated and the prognosis is favorable. The symp-toms remit rapidly and radiographic changes resolve over several days after withdrawal of the offending drug.[41]

MANAGEMENT

There are anecdotal reports that corticosteroids hasten recovery. However, the rapid improvement that follows discontinuation of the drug is so striking that corticosteroid use is not recommended. Rechallenging the patient with the offending drug may result in an exacerbation after a shortened latent period.[66,68] Still, there are case reports in which a drug was not suspected and the disease progressed to the irreversible stage of pulmonary fibrosis.

DRUG-INDUCED SYSTEMIC LUPUS ERYTHEMATOSUS

The drugs associated with a syndrome similar to systemic lupus erythematosus (SLE) are listed in Table 72-3.[69,70] Drug-induced lupus (DIL) accounts for approximately 5 percent to 10 percent of all patients with SLE.[71,72] Such patients are usually older than those with idiopathic lupus; a female predominance and HLA correlate are lacking.[73] Although the list of drugs in Table 72-3 is large, most offending agents have been documented in a limited number of case reports; the majority of cases involve procainamide and hydralazine.

Procainamide is the most frequent cause of DIL. The syndrome may occur one year or more after chronic use in approximately 30 percent of patients prescribed the drug[71,74,75]; 50 percent of whom develop pulmonary complications.[59] The syndrome may occur 1 month or as late as 12 years after initiation of treatment.[75–77] Hydralazine-induced lupus occurs in approximately 7 percent of patients using the drug[79–81]; the risk increasing when dose schedules exceed 200 mg/day and the cumulative dose is ≤ 110 gms.[81,82] Isoniazid induces a positive antinuclear antibody test in as many as 25 percent of patients, however, less than 1 percent of patients develop the clinical features of the disorder.[84]

MECHANISM OF INJURY

The offending drugs apparently manipulate the immune response by inducing the production of autoantibodies to histone components. Patients with the slow-acetylation phenotype are homozygous for a recessive gene that controls activity of hepatic acetyltransferase, an enzyme involved in the metabolism of certain drugs such as hydralazine, procainamide, and isoniazid.[84] Slow acetylators tend to develop antinuclear antibodies and DIL after shorter duration of therapy and at lower cumulative doses of offending drug.[75,85–87] T cell–directed DNA methylation is inhibited by the suspect drugs, resulting in altered gene expression[88] and upregulation of T-cell activity. The autoregulated T cells produce interleukin-4 (IL-4) and interleukin-6 (IL-6), which promote B-cell differentiation into antibody secreting plasma cells.[89] Intriguingly, T cell DNA methylation is impaired in patients with idiopathic lupus.[90,91] In addition, drug-DNA complex formation may enhance histone antigenicity[93]; conformational change of the nucleoprotein may produce new antigenic determinants or expose hidden moieties.[93]

TABLE 72-3   Drugs Implicated in Drug-Induced Lupus

Acebutolol	Nalidixic acid
Aminoglutethimide	Nitrofurantoin
Amoproxan	Nomifensine
Anthiomaline	
Atenolol	Oxyphenisatin
	para-Aminosalicylic acid
Benoxaprofen	Penicillamine
Canavanine (L-)	Penicillin
Captopril	Perazine
Carbamazepine	Pephenazine
Chlorpromazine	Phenelzine
Chlorprothixene	Phenopyrazone
Cinnarazine	Phenylbutazone
Clonidine	Phenylethyacetylurea
	Practolol
Danazol	Prazosin
Diclofenac	Primidone
Digitalis	Prinolol
1-2-dimethyl-3-hydroxypyride-4-1	Procainamide
Diphenylhydantoin	Promethazine
Disopyramide	Propylthiouracil
	Psoralen
Ethosuximide	Pyrathiazine
	Pyrithoxine
Gold salts	
Griseofulvin	Quinidine
Guanoxan	
	Reserpine
Hydralazine	
Hydrazine	Spironolactone
	Streptomycin
Ibuprofen	Sulindac
Interferon (alpha, gamma)	Sulfadimethoxine
Isoniazid	Sulfamethoxypyridazine
	Sulfasalazine
Labetalol	Sulfonamides
Leuprolide acetate	
Levo-dopa	Tetracycline
Levomeprazone	Tetrazine
Lithium carbonate	Thiazides
Lovastatin	Thionamide
	Thioridazide
Mephenytoin	Timolol (eye drops)
Methimazole	Tolazamide
Methyldopa	Tolmetin
Methylsergide	Trimethadione
Methylthiouracil	
Metrizamide	
Minoxidil	

HISTOPATHOLOGY

There is a paucity of histologic data from patients with DIL, since lung biopsies are rarely performed in these patients. Presumably, the lung lesions reflect a capillaritis, mediated by immune mechanisms,[94] the vascular equivalent of small vessel disease manifest in the skin.

CLINICAL SPECTRUM

Pulmonary involvement is a common feature of DIL. The patients may complain of dyspnea, chest discomfort, and, rarely, hemoptysis. The pulmonary manifestations include pleuritis, pleural effusions, and pneumonitis that may progress to a fibrotic stage.[95,96] Patients also complain of fever, (as high as 41 °C)[97] weight loss, myalgias, (diffuse, proximal, and distal), joint symptoms, (either arthralgias or

arthritis, nondeforming, multiple symmetric joints, sometimes migratory),[76,97,99] skin rashes, (discoid lupus or malar rash,)[97] and chest pain (pericarditis.)[98] Renal involvement is rare[76,98]; mild hematuria or proteinuria without compromised renal function is not uncommon and resolves after discontinuation of the drug.[78,97,99] Neurologic impairment and vasculitis also are rare. As expected, chest radiographs may display diffuse pulmonary infiltrates and/or pleural effusions. The most common serologic abnormality is a positive antinuclear antibody titer (homogenous pattern) due to antihistone antibodies.[100] However, many patients treated with the drugs known to cause DIL develop antihistone antibodies but never manifest overt clinical disease.[101,102] The specificity of antibodies against the different histone proteins varies from drug to drug and between symptomatic and asymptomatic patients.[103] Anti-Sm and double-stranded DNA antibodies are rare and, if detected, suggest the possibility that idiopathic SLE is present. Detection of LE cells[104–106] or antinuclear antibodies[107] in pleural fluid aids in establishing a diagnosis.

MANAGEMENT

Drug-induced lupus usually is self-limiting, and remits once the offending drug is discontinued. However, it may take >1 year for the symptoms and/or the serologic abnormalities to resolve completely.[71] On occasion, corticosteroid therapy may be necessary to produce more rapid resolution of disabling symptoms. Nonsteroidal anti-inflammatory drugs are an effective treatment for pleuritis. If the offending drug cannot be withdrawn for clinical reasons, the lowest dose should be used in conjunction with corticosteroids.[108]

Phospholipidosis-Induced Lung Disease

Drugs that produce in the lung histologic and ultrastructural changes termed *phospholipidosis* are listed in Table 72-4. Amiodarone, the prototype, is the most clinically significant. Five percent to 7 percent of the patients prescribed amiodarone develop pulmonary complications[110]; of these patients, 5 percent to 10 percent die from pulmonary disease.[111]

Nonpulmonary complications of amiodarone include blue-gray skin discoloration and photodermatitis, thyroid dysfunction, both hypo- and hyperthyroidism, corneal microdeposits, gastrointestinal symptoms, neurotoxicity (manifest by muscle weakness), peripheral neuropathy, extrapyramidal symptoms, hepatic dysfunction, myelosuppression, and bradycardia.[41,112,113] The most serious side effect, which limits clinical utility, is pulmonary toxicity.

Risk factors for amiodarone-induced lung injury include advanced age,[114] preexisting lung disease,[114–122] and maintenance dose greater than 400 mg/day.[116,120,121,123–126] There are, however, reports of toxicity with doses as small as 200 mg/day. Disease onset occurs a month and up to several years after initiation of therapy.[41,109,110,113] Neither the total cumulative dose, duration of therapy, or serum drug level correlate with the risk of lung toxicity.

Amiodarone-treated patients are at increased risk of developing acute respiratory distress syndrome (ARDS),

TABLE 72-4   Drugs that Cause Phospholipidosis-Induced Lung Disease

Amiodarone	Haloperidol
Amitriptyline	Homochlorcyclizine
Boxidine	Hydroxyzine
Chlorcyclizine	Imipramine
Chloroquine	Iprindole
Chlorphentermine	Meclizine
Chlorpromazine	Norchlorcyclizine
Cloforex	Nortriptyline
Clomipramine	Noxiptiline
Cyclizine	Perhexiline
4,4'-Diethylaminoethoxyhexestrol	Phentermine
Erythromycin	Quinacrine
Ethyl fluclozepate	Thioridazine
Fenfluramine	Triparanol
Fluoxetine	Zimelidine

beginning 18 to 72 h after pulmonary angiography, cardiothoracic surgery, and other surgical procedures requiring general anesthesia.[126–131] It has been postulated that the high fraction of inspired oxygen given perioperatively contributes to this complication.

MECHANISM OF INJURY

The drugs listed in Table 72-4 are amphiphilic and accumulate in organs and tissues with high lipid content, such as fat, the liver, and the lungs.[132,133] For example, the concentration of amiodarone in the lungs can increase to 4 to 7 times the concentration in other organs.[121] The hydrophobic regions of the drug intercalate into membranes, specifically of lysosomes, binding to phospholipids in the lysosomes. In the lungs, the metabolism of phospholipids occurs primarily in macrophages and type II pneumocytes, which produce phospholipid-rich surfactant. In these cells, the drug-phospholipid complex inhibits lysosomal enzyme phospholipase A.[134–143] Phospholipid-drug complex accumulates in the lysosomes, termed *phospholipidosis*. The accumulation of this phospholipid-rich material interferes with cellular metabolic functions,[144–146] compresses organelles, and can rupture the cell, similar to lysosomal storage diseases. Ultimately, the phospholipidosis incites inflammation and fibrosis in the lungs.[120] Additionally, the impaired macrophages can decrease systemic resistance to bacterial and fungal infections.[147]

HISTOPATHOLOGY

The histologic features of phospholipidosis include interstitial pneumonitis and, occasionally, diffuse alveolar damage with fibrosis.[148] Also present are characteristic "foamy" alveolar macrophages and type II pneumocytes (Fig. 72-2). By electron microscopy, these cells contain lamellar inclusions[149] that consists of a surfactant-like material with a repeat 5- to 10-nm apart (Fig. 72-3).[109,117,119,120,149,150] Similar inclusions have been identified within alveolar epithelial cells, interstitial inflammatory cells, and endothelial cells,[151] sometimes at extrapulmonary sites such as lymph nodes, the spleen, and thymus.[152,153] The presence of these foamy or phospholipid-laden cells is not necessarily diagnostic of drug-induced injury. Similar foamy changes have been detected in patients without evidence of clinical or radiographic toxicity.[117–119,148]

CLINICAL SPECTRUM

The presenting symptoms of phospholipidosis include the insidious onset of exertional dyspnea and nonproductive

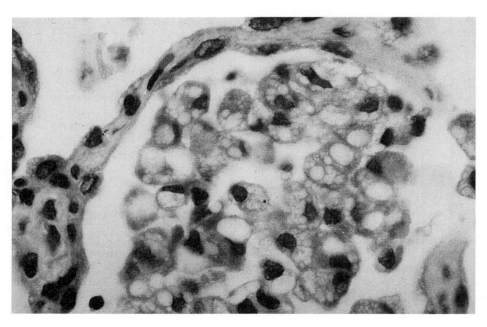

FIGURE 72-2 Phospholipidosis from amiodarone toxicity characterized by the accumulation of foamy macrophages in this alveolus. Note cytoplasmic vacuoles of varying sizes. *Reproduced with permission from* Atlas of Pulmonary Surgical Pathology, *1991: Figure 1-92.*

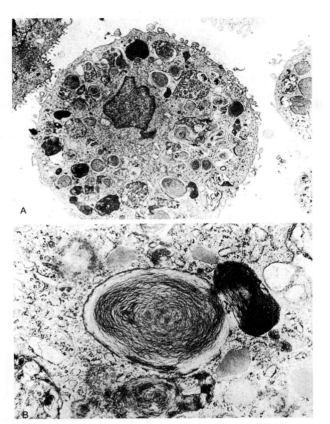

FIGURE 72-3 *Ultrastructural findings in the lung associated with amiodarone exposure.* **(A)** Electron micrograph showing a vacuolated alveolar macrophage. The cytoplasm is filled with membrane-bound lamellar bodies as well as lysosomes. (Uranyl acetate-lead citrate stain; original magnification ×6600.) **(B)** Higher-magnification electron micrograph detailing the membrane-bound lamellar bodies from (*A*). The lamellae are concentrically arranged and are focally obscured by areas of increased electron density. (Uranyl acetate-lead citrate stain; original magnification ×33,000.) *Reproduced with permission from Clinics in Chest Medicine, March 1990, JI Kennedy,* Clinical Aspects of Amiodarone Pulmonary Toxicity, *figure 3.*

cough, sometimes accompanied by fever, malaise, weight loss, and pleuritic chest pain.[109,115,120,154] Physical examination reveals tachypnea, end-inspiratory crackles (either focal or diffuse) and, occasionally, pleural rubs. Usually, there is no evidence of congestive heart failure.[40,109,120] The chest radiographs demonstrate diffuse infiltrates, sometimes asymmetric, other times with upper lobe predominance. Pleural effusions are uncommon.[112,119,155] Gallium scanning often confirms lung involvement.[156] Computer tomographic scans also demonstrate the parenchymal abnormalities as well as increased density from accumulation of the iodinated amiodarone. Pulmonary function tests may demonstrate a pattern of restrictive lung disease[116,122] and a reduction in the DLCO.[116,117] Bronchoalveolar lavage fluid may contain the characteristic foamy alveolar macrophages.[112,157] An elevated sedimentation rate is present in more than 50 percent of patients; although not pathognomonic, it is

not expected in congestive heart failure or pulmonary embolism.[109,121,158–160]

MANAGEMENT

A baseline chest radiograph and pulmonary function tests with DLCO measurement should be obtained on all patients prior to the initiation of amiodarone therapy. Subsequently, history, chest radiographs, and repeat PFTs with DLCO should be obtained approximately every three months for surveillance of potential toxicity.

Once toxicity is suspected, withdrawal of the drug has an unpredictable outcome. Some patients have complete or partial resolution. In general, the more insidious the onset of disease, the slower the resolution. The long half-life of amiodarone, estimated at 45 to 60 days,[161–164] as well as the tendency to concentrate in the lungs, contributes to the slow resolution. Some patients die of progressive disease despite discontinuation of the drug. The value of corticosteroid therapy is uncertain and substantiated only by anecdotal reports.[109,117,120,124,126,160,165] Corticosteroids are recommended for patients with severe toxicity, in doses equivalent to prednisone 40 to 60 mg daily tapered over a two- to six-month period. Withdrawal of corticosteroids too quickly can induce a recurrence.[160]

Once amiodarone is discontinued, the arrhythmia control also dissipates and may necessitate alternative therapy. Some patients have been successfully treated with the lowest dose of amiodarone to control the dysrhythmia and concurrent lower-dose corticosteroids (for example, prednisone 10 mg every other day) to stabilize the pulmonary toxicity.[166]

Drug-Induced Noncardiogenic Pulmonary Edema

The drugs listed in Table 72-5 may precipitate noncardiogenic pulmonary edema (NCPE). The highest incidence of NCPE is associated with narcotic analgesics. Narcotic-induced pulmonary edema most commonly results from intravenous heroin injection but also occurs after use of morphine, methadone, meperidine, and propoxyphene.[41,59,167] Symptoms may develop after the first administration of these drugs. Onset may occur within minutes of intravenous heroin and hours following methadone.[41] There also are case reports of NCPE from administration of the opiate agonist naloxone.[41,168]

Pulmonary edema occurs with salicylate use; sometimes after intentional overdose, other times (in approximately one-third of the cases) from chronic use of large doses for musculoskeletal complaints.[169–171] Risk factors include increasing age and a history of smoking. Patients may exhibit effects of salicylate intoxication, such as tinnitus, respiratory alkalosis followed by metabolic acidosis, pyrexia, and disorientation.[41] The serum salicylate concentration often is > 45 mg/dL, although cases have been associated with concentrations in the therapeutic range.[41]

Hydrochlorothiazide-induced NCPE results from intermittent dosing, presumably for episodic fluid retention

TABLE 72-5   Drugs that Cause Noncardiogenic Pulmonary Edema

Amitriptyline	Lidocaine
Ampicillin	Magnesium sulfate
Bleomycin	Metaraminol
Bromocarbamide	Methadone
Chlordiazepoxide	Methotrexate (intrathecal)
Chlorpromazine	Mitomycin-C
Codeine	Morphine
Colchicine	Nalbuphine
Cyclophosphamide	Naloxone
Cyclosporine	Nitrofurantoin
Cytosine arabinoside	Nitrogen mustard
Dextran-40	Nitroprusside
Epinephrine	Paraldehyde
Erythromycin	Penicillin
Ethchlorvynol	Perphenazine
Febarbamate	Propoxyphene
Fluorescein	Protamine
Flurazepam	
Haloperidol	Ritodrine
Heroin	Salbutamol
Hydrochlorothiazide	Salicylate
	Streptokinase
Ifosfamide	
Iodide	Terbutaline
Imipramine	Trimethoprim-sulfamethoxazole
Interleukin-2	
Isoxsuprine	

rather than daily dosing for hypertension.[172–178] The onset may be acute, occurring within an hour of the first dose, or anytime during the course of therapy. Rechallenges result in more severe reactions.[179]

Various chemotherapeutic agents induce NCPE. High-dose cytosine arabinoside has the highest incidence of approximately 20 percent. Onset occurs either during therapy or within four weeks of completion of therapy.[180,181] Noncardiogenic pulmonary edema also has been documented to follow the administration of bleomycin,[182] cyclophosphamide,[183,184] ifosfamide,[183] intrathecal methotrexate[185–188] and cyclosporine.[189–191]

Lidocaine-induced NCPE may occur after oropharyngeal application and subcutaneous administration for local anesthesia.[192] Cocaine-induced pulmonary edema may occur after either freebase inhalation,[193] intravenous injection,[193] or "body packing."[194]

MECHANISMS OF INJURY

The proposed mechanism(s) of injury include neurogenic pulmonary edema from CNS-mediated increased pulmonary capillary permeability,[170,195–198] direct injury to the alveolar capillary membrane,[41,199] and complement activation with subsequent alveolar capillary damage.[200,201] Analysis of pulmonary edema fluid from heroin overdose, salicylate intoxication, and hydroclorothiazide-induced NCPE confirms high protein content and chemistries similar to plasma, while pulmonary capillary wedge pressure measurements were normal.[170,202–204]

TOCOLYTIC-INDUCED PULMONARY EDEMA

Noncardiogenic pulmonary edema has been documented with various tocolytic agents, including albuterol, terbutaline, ritodrine, isoxsuprine, salbutamol, and magnesium sulfate.[41,200,205–218] The incidence varies from 0.5 percent to 5 percent.[210] Risk factors include multiparous state, fluid overload, anemia, twin gestation, and use of corticosteroids to accelerate fetal lung maturation.[208,210] These drugs produce peripheral vasodilation resulting in increased intravascular fluid volume. Upon discontinuation of the drug, the vasomotor tone returns to normal, and the excess fluid is exuded into the tissue beds, especially the lungs.

MANAGEMENT

Drug-induced NCPE usually responds quickly and completely to discontinuation of the offending drug and supportive therapy, such as supplemental oxygen, positive pressure or mechanical ventilation, and forced diuresis. Additional therapies include forced alkaline diuresis for salicylate intoxication and naloxone for opiate overdose. Symptoms dissipate within the first 24 to 48 h[219] although complete resolution may take several weeks.[220] Fatalities have been reported.

Drug-Induced Bronchiolitis Obliterans with Organizing Pneumonia

The drugs listed in Table 72-6 can induce bronchiolitis obliterans with organizing pneumonia (BOOP).[221–225] The morphologic changes are indistinguishable from idiopathic BOOP. Most patients recover with discontinuation of the offending drug; corticosteroid therapy may hasten resolution of the disease.

Conclusion

The diagnosis of drug-induced pulmonary diseases does not rely on the skilled histopathologist; rather, on the judgment and suspicion of the experienced clinician. The diagnosis of drug-induced pulmonary diseases is a diagnosis of exclusion. A small yet significant number of patients exposed to

TABLE 72-6   Drugs that Cause Bronchiolitis Obliterans with Organizing Pneumonia

Acebutolol	Mecamylamine
Amiodarone	Methotrexate
Amphotericin B	Mitomycin-C
Bleomycin	Nitrofurantoin
Chlorozotocin	Penicillamine
Cocaine	Phenytoin
Cromolyn	Sulindac
Cyclophosphamide	Sulfasalazine
Deferoxamine	Sulfametopyrazine
Gold salts	Tocainide
Hexamethonium	

the listed drugs develop the injury, in part, due to host susceptibility. The genetic or environmental factors that contribute to host susceptibility need further elucidation. The additive or synergistic effects of polypharmacy, which may independently induce lung injury, are poorly understood and difficult to study. Continued study of patients and animal models of drug-induced pulmonary diseases may enhance the understanding of and treatment of lung diseases at large.

References

1. Classen DC, Pestotnik SL, Evan RS, et al.: Computerized surveillance of adverse drug events in hospital patients. *JAMA* 1991; 266:2847.

2. Martys CR: Adverse reactions to drugs in general practice. *Br Med J* 1979; 2:1194.

3. Levy M, Kewitz H, Altwein W, et al.: Hospital admissions due to adverse drug reactions: a comparative study from Jerusalem and Berlin. *Eur J Clin Pharmacol* 1980; 17:25.

4. Heinemann HO: Alcohol and the lung: a brief review. *Am J Med* 1977; 63:81.

5. Hyman AL, Spannhake EW, Kadowitz PJ: Prostaglandins and the lung. *Am Rev Resp Dis* 1978; 117:111.

6. Kelly HW: Drug-induced pulmonary diseases, in DiPiro JT, Talbert RL, Hayes PE, et al.: (eds): *Pharmacotherapy: A Pathophysiologic Approach*, 2nd ed. Connecticut, Appelton & Lange, 1993: 482–493.

7. Batist G, Andrews Jr J: Pulmonary toxicity of antineoplastic drugs. *JAMA* 1981; 246:1449.

8. Cooper Jr J, White D, Matthay R: Drug-induced pulmonary disease, part 1: cytotoxic drugs. *Am Rev Respir Dis* 1986; 133:321.

9. Ginsberg S, Comis R: The pulmonary toxicity of antineoplastic agents. *Semin Oncol* 1982; 9:34.

10. Sostman H, Putman C, Gamsu G: Diagnosis of chemotherapy lung. *Am J Roentgenol* 1981; 136:33.

11. Weiss R, Muggia F: Cytotoxic drug-induced pulmonary disease: update 1980. *Am J Med* 1980; 68:259.

12. Oliner H, Schwartz R, Rubio F, Dameshek W: Interstitial pulmonary fibrosis following busulfan therapy. *Am J Med* 1961; 31:134.

13. Bauer KA, Skarin AT, Balikian JP, et al.: Pulmonary complications associated with combination chemotherapy programs containing bleomycin. *Am J Med* 1983; 74:557.

14. DeLena M, Guzzon A, Monfardini S, et al.: Clinical radiologic and histopathologic studies on pulmonary toxicity induced by treatment with bleomycin (NSC-125066). *Cancer Chemother Rep* 1972; 56:343.

15. White DA, Stover DE: Severe bleomycin-induced pneumonitis. Clinical features and response to corticosteroids. *Chest* 1984; 86:723.

16. Spector J, Zimbler H, Ross J: Early-onset cyclophosphamide-induced interstitial pneumonitis. *JAMA* 1979; 242:2852.

17. Aronin P, Mahaley M, Rudnick S, et al.: Prediction of BCNU pulmonary toxicity in patients with malignant gliomas. An assessment of risk factors. *N Engl J Med* 1980; 303:183.

18. Topilow A, Rothenberg S, Cottrell T: Interstitial pneumonia after prolonged treatment with cyclophosphamide. *Am Rev Respir Dis* 1973; 108:114.

19. Niell H, Griffin J, West W, Neely C: Combination chemotherapy with mitomycin C, methotrexate, cisplatin, and vinblastine in the treatment of non-small cell lung cancer. *Cancer* 1984; 54:1260.

20. Verweij J, Van Zanten T, Souren T, et al.: Prospective study on the dose relationship of mitomycin C–induced interstitial pneumonitis. *Cancer* 1987; 60:756.

21. Bedrossian C: Pathology of drug-induced lung diseases. *Semin Respir Med* 1982; 4:98.

22. Burke D, Stoddart J, Ward M, Simpson C: Fatal pulmonary fibrosis occurring during treatment with cyclophosphamide. *Br Med J* 1982; 285:696.

23. Cole S, Myers T, Klatsky A: Pulmonary disease with chlorambucil therapy. *Cancer* 1978; 41:455.

24. Godard P, Marty J, Michel F: Interstitial pneumonia and chlorambucil. *Chest* 1979; 76:471.

25. Codling B, Chakera T: Pulmonary fibrosis following therapy with melphalan for multiple myeloma. *J Clin Pathol* 1972; 25:668.

26. Goucher G, Rowland V, Hawkins J: Melphalan-induced pulmonary interstitial fibrosis. *Chest* 1980; 77:805.

27. Schallier D, Impens N, Warson F, et al.: Additive pulmonary toxicity with melphalan and busulfan. *Chest* 1983; 84:492.

28. Taetle R, Dickman P, Feldman P: Pulmonary histopathologic changes associated with melphalan therapy. *Cancer* 1978; 42:1239.

29. Westerfield B, Michalski J, McCombs C, Light R: Reversible melphalan-induced lung damage. *Am J Med* 1980; 68:767.

30. Freeman BA, Crapo JD: Biology of disease: free radicals and tissue injury. *Lab Invest* 1982; 47:412.

31. Fantone JC, Ward PA: Role of oxygen-derived free radicals and metabolites in leukocyte-dependent inflammatory reactions. *Am J Pathol* 1982; 107:397.

32. Lewis RA, Austen KF: The biologically active leukotrienes: biosynthesis, metabolism, receptors, functions and pharmacology. *J Clin Invest* 1984; 73:889.

33. Arrick BA, Nathan CF: Glutathione metabolism as a determinant of therapeutic efficacy: a review. *Cancer Res* 1984; 44:4224.

34. Nathan CF, Arrick BA, Murray HW, DeSantos NM, Cohn ZA: Tumor cell anti-oxidant defenses: inhibition of the glutathione redox cycle enhances macrophage-mediated cytolysis. *J Exp Med* 1981; 53:766.

35. Berend N: Protective effect of hypoxia on bleomycin lung toxicity in the rat. *Am Rev Respir Dis* 1984; 130:307.

36. Tryka AF, Skornick WA, Godleski JJ, et al.: Potentiation of bleomycin-induced lung injury by exposure to 70% oxygen. *Am Rev Respir Dis* 1982; 126:1074.

37. Goldiner PL, Carlon GC, Cvitkov E, et al.: Factors influencing postoperative morbidity and mortality in patients treated with bleomycin. *Br Med J* 1978; 1:1664.

38. Hakkinen PJ, Whitely JW, Witschi HR: Hyperoxia, but not thoracic x-irradiation, potentiates bleomycin and cyclophosphamide-induced lung damage in mice. *Am Rev Respir Dis* 1982; 126:281.

39. Rinaldo J, Goldstein RH, Snider GL: Modification of oxygen toxicity after lung injury by bleomycin in hamsters. *Am Rev Respir Dis* 1982; 126:1030.

40. Tryka AF, Godleski JJ, Brain JD: Differences in effects of immediate and delayed hyperoxia exposure on bleomycin-induced pulmonary injury. *Cancer Treat Rep* 1984; 68:759.

41. Cooper Jr J, White D, Matthay R: Drug-induced pulmonary disease. Part 2: noncytotoxic drugs. *Am Rev Respir Dis* 1986; 133:488.

42. Gyorkey F, Gyorkey P, Sinkovics J: Origin and significance of intranuclear tubular inclusions in type II pulmonary alveolar epithelial cells of patients with bleomycin and busulfan toxicity. *Ultrastruc Pathol* 1980; 1:211.

43. Bedrossian C, Luna M, MacKay B, Lichtiger B: Ultrastructure of pulmonary bleomycin toxicity. *Cancer* 1973; 32:44.

44. Daskal Y, Gyorkey F, Gyorkey P, Busch H: Ultrastructural study of pulmonary bleomycin toxicity. *Cancer Res* 1976; 36:1267.

45. Iacovino J, Leitner J, Abbas A, et al.: Fatal pulmonary reaction from low doses of bleomycin. An idiosyncratic tissue response. *JAMA* 1976; 235:1253.

46. Luna M, Bedrossian C, Lichtiger B, Salem P: Interstitial pneumonitis associated with bleomycin therapy. *Am J Clin Pathol* 1972; 58:501.

47. Lehne G, Lote K: Pulmonary toxicity cytotoxic and immunosuppressive agents. *Acta Oncologica* 1990; 29(2):113.

48. Heard B, Cooke R: Busulphan lung. *Thorax* 1968; 23:187.

49. Pascual RS, Mosher MB, Sikand RS, et al.: Effects of bleomycin on pulmonary function in man. *Am Rev Respir Dis* 1975; 108:211.

50. Richman SD, Levenson SM, Bunn PA, et al.: ^{67}Ga accumulation in pulmonary lesions associated with bleomycin therapy. *Cancer* 1975; 6:1966.

51. Bellamy EA, Husband JE, Blaquiere RW, Law MR: Bleomycin related lung damage: CT evidence. *Radiology* 1985; 156:155.

52. Brown WG, Hasan FM, Barbee R: Reversibility of severe bleomycin-induced pneumonitis. *JAMA* 1978; 239:2012.

53. Gilson AJ, Sahn SA: Reactivation of bleomycin lung toxicity following oxygen administration. *Chest* 1985; 88:304.

54. O'Neill TJ, Kardinal CG, Tierney LM: Reversible interstitial pneumonitis associated with low dose bleomycin. *Chest* 1975; 68:265.

55. Yagoda A, Mukherji B, Young C et al.: Bleomycin, an antitumor antibiotic: clinical experience in 274 patients. *Ann Intern Med* 1972; 77:861.

56. Bennett WM, Pastore L, Houghton DC: Fatal pulmonary bleomycin toxicity in cisplatin-induced acute renal failure. *Cancer Treat Rep* 1980; 64:921.

57. McLeod BF, Lawrence HJ, Smith DW, et al.: Fatal bleomycin toxicity from a low cumulative dose in a patient with renal insufficiency. *Cancer* 1987; 60:2617.

58. Van Barneveld PWC, Sleijfer DTH, van Der Mark THW, et al.: Natural course of bleomycin-induced pneumonitis. A follow-up study. *Am Rev Respir Dis* 1987; 135:48.

59. Brewis RAL: Respiratory disorders, in Davies DM (ed): *Textbook of Adverse Drug Reactions*, 2nd ed. New York, Oxford University Press, 1981:154–178.

60. Geddes D, Brostoff J: Pulmonary fibrosis associated with hypersensitivity to gold salts. *Br Med J* 1976; 1:1444.

61. Camus P, Degat OR, Justrabo E, Jeannin L: D-Penicillamine–induced severe pneumonitis. *Chest* 1982; 81:376.

62. Donlan CJ, Scutero JV: Transient eosinophilic pneumonia secondary to use of a vaginal cream. *Chest* 1975; 67:232.

63. Holoye PY, Luma MA, Mackay B, Bedrossian CWM: Bleomycin hypersensitivity pneumonitis. *Ann Intern Med* 1978; 88:47.

64. Smith GJ: The histopathology of pulmonary reactions to drugs. *Clin Chest Med* 1990; 11:95.

65. Sostman HD, Matthay RA, Putnam CE: Methotrexate-induced pneumonitis. *Medicine* 1976; 55:371.

66. Hailey FJ, Glascock HW, Hewitt WF: Pleuropneumonic reactions to nitrofurantoin. *N Engl J Med* 1969; 281:1087.

67. Cooper JA, Matthay RA: Drug-induced pulmonary disease. *Dis Mon* 1987; 33:61.

68. Holmberg L, Bowman G: Pulmonary reactions to nitrofurantoin. 447 cases reported to the Swedish Adverse Drug Reaction Committee 1966–1976. *Eur J Respir Dis* 1981; 62:180.

69. Weinstein A: Drug-induced systemic lupus erythematosus. *Prog Clin Immunol* 1980; 4:1.

70. Yung RL, Chb MB, Richardson BC: Drug-induced lupus. *Rheum Dis Clin North Am* 1994; 20:61.

71. Henningsen NC, Cederberg A, Hanson A, et al.: Effects of long-term treatment with procainamide. A prospective study with special regard to ANF and SLE in fast and slow acetylators. *Acta Med Scand* 1975; 198:475.

72. Lee SL, Rivero I, Siegel M: Activation of systemic lupus erythematosis by drugs. *Arch Intern Med* 1966; 117:620.

73. Brand C, Davidson A, Littlejohn G, et al.: Hydralazine-induced lupus: no association with HLA-DR4. *Lancet* 1984; i:462.

74. Sonnhag C, Karlsson E, Hed J: Procainamide-induced lupus erythematosus–like syndrome in relation to acetylator phenotype and plasma levels of procainamide. *Acta Med Scand* 1979; 206:245.

75. Woosley RL, Drayer DE, Reidenberg MM, et al.: Effect of acetylator phenotype on the rate at which procainamide induces antinuclear antibodies and the lupus syndrome. *N Engl J Med* 1978; 298:1157.

76. Blomgren SE, Condemi JJ, Vaughn JH: Procainamide-induced lupus erythematosus. Clinical and laboratory observations. *Am J Med* 1972; 52:338.

77. Harle JR, Weiller C, Durand JM, et al.: Systemic lupus erythematosus diagnosed after 12 years' treatment with procainamide (letter). *Ann Med Interne (Paris)* 1976; 137:599.

78. Dustan HP, Taylor RD, Corcoran AC, et al.: Rheumatic and febrile syndromes during prolonged hydralazine therapy. *JAMA* 1954; 154:23.

79. Morrow JD, Schroeder HA, Perry Jr HM: Studies on the control of hypertension by Hyphex: II. Toxic reactions and side effects. *Circulation* 1953; 8:829.

80. Perry HM, Schroeder HA: Syndrome simulating collagen disease caused by hydralazine (Apresoline). *JAMA* 1954; 154:670.

81. Cameron HA, Ramsay LE: The lupus syndrome induced by hydralazine: a common complication with low dose treatment. *BMJ* 1984; 289:410.

82. Roden DM, Reele SB, Higgins SB, et al.: Antiarrhythmic efficacy, pharmacokinetics and safety of N-acetylprocainamide in human subjects: comparison with procainamide. *Am J Cardiol* 1980; 46:463.

83. Rothfield NF, Bierer WF, Garfield JW: Isoniazid induction of antinuclear antibodies. A prospective study. *Ann Intern Med* 1978; 88:650.

84. Weber WW: Acetylation of drugs, in *The Acetylator Genes and Drug Response*. New York, Oxford University Press, 1987:50–84.

85. Litwin A, Adams LE, Zimmer H, et al.: Immunologic effects of hydralazine in hypertensive patients. *Arthritis Rheum* 1981; 24:1074.

86. Mansilla-Tinoco R, Harland SJ, Ryan PJ, et al.: Hydralazine, antinuclear antibodies, and the lupus syndrome. *BMJ* 1982; 284:936.

87. Reidenberg MM: Aromatic amines and the pathogenesis of lupus erythematosus. *Am J Med* 1983; 75:1037.

88. Cornacchia E, Golbus J, Maybaum J, et al.: Hydralazine and procainamide inhibit T cell DNA methylation and induce autoreactivity. *J Immunol* 1988; 140:2197.

89. Richardson BC, Liebling MR, Hudson JL: CD4+ cells treated with DNA methylation inhibitors induce autologous B cell differentiation. *Clin Immunol Immunopathol* 1990; 55:368.

90. Corvetta A, Della Bitta R, Luchetti MM, et al.: 5-Methylcytosine content of DNA in blood, synovial mononuclear cells and synovial tissue from patients affected by autoimmune rheumatic diseases. *J Chromatogr* 1991; 566:481.

91. Crisp AJ, Hoffbrand BI: Sulphasalazine-induced systemic lupus erythematosus in a patient with Sjogren's syndrome. *J R Soc Med* 1980; 73:60.

92. Tan EM: Drug-induced autoimmune disease. *Fed Proc* 1974; 33:1894.

93. Wheeler JF, Adams LE, Heineman WR, et al.: Interactions of N-oxidized procainamide metabolites with mouse and human hemoglobin and histone subfractions (abstract) *FASEB J* 1990; 4:A2108.

94. Fauci AS, Haynes BF, Katz P: The spectrum of vasculitis: clinical, pathologic, immunologic, and therapeutic considerations. *Ann Intern Med* 1978; 89:660.

95. Asherson RA, Benbow AG, Speirs CJ, et al.: Pulmonary hypertension in hydralazine induced systemic lupus erythematosus: association with C4 null allele. *Ann Rheum Dis* 1986; 45:771.

96. Cush JJ, Goldings EA: Drug-induced lupus: clinical spectrum and pathogenesis. *Am J Med Sci* 1985; 290:36.

97. Alarcon-Segovia D, Wakin KG, Worthington JW, et al.: Clinical and experimental studies on the hydralazine syndrome and its relationship to systemic lupus erythematosus. *Medicine (Baltimore)* 1967; 46:1.

98. Dubois EL: Procainamide induction of a systemic lupus erythematosus–like syndrome. Presentation of six cases, review of the literature, and analysis and followup of reported cases. *Medicine (Baltimore)* 1969; 48:217.

99. Perry HM Jr: Late toxicity to hydralazine resembling systemic lupus erythematosus or rheumatoid arthritis. *Am J Med* 1973; 54:58.

100. Fritzler MJ, Tan EM: Antibodies to histones in drug-induced and idiopathic erythematosus. *J Clin Invest* 1978; 62:560.

101. Epstein A, Barland P: The diagnostic value of antihistone antibodies in drug-induced lupus erythematosus. *Arthritis Rheum* 1985; 28:158.

102. Mongey AB, Donovan-Brand R, Thomas TJ, et al.: Serologic evaluation of patients receiving procainamide. *Arthritis Rheum* 1992; 35:219.

103. Burlingame RW, Rubin RL: Drug-induced anti-histone autoantibodies display two patterns of reactivity with substructures of chromatin. *J Clin Invest* 1991; 88:680.

104. Carel RS, Shapiro MS, Shoham D, et al.: Lupus erythematosus cells in pleural effusion: the initial manifestation of procainamide-induced lupus erythematosus. *Chest* 1977; 72:670.

105. Kaplan AI, Zakher F, Sabin S: Drug-induced lupus erythematosus with in vivo lupus erythematosus cells in pleural fluid. *Chest* 1978; 73:875.

106. Weinstein J: Hypocomplementemia in hydralazine-associated systemic lupus erythematosus. *Am J Med* 1978; 65:553.

107. Leechawengwong M, Berger HW, Sukumaran M: Diagnostic significance of antinuclear antibodies in pleural effusion. *Mt Sinai J Med* 1979; 46:137.

108. Ginsberg WW: Drug-induced systemic lupus erythematosus. *Semin Respir Med* 1980; 2:51.

109. Marchlinski FE, Gansler TS, Waxman HL, et al.: Amiodarone pulmonary toxicity. *Ann Intern Med* 1992; 97:839.

110. Raeder EA, Podrid PJ, Lown B: Side effects and complications of amiodarone therapy. *Am Heart J* 1985; 109(5 pt 1):975.

111. Colgan T, Simon CT, Kay JM, et al.: Amiodarone pulmonary toxicity. *Ultrastruct Pathol* 1984; 6:199.

112. Martin WJ and Rosenow EC. Amiodarone pulmonary toxicity recognition and pathogenesis (part 1). *Chest* 1988; 93(5):1067.

113. Pesola A, Consentino G, Vercillo C, et al.: Lung disease associated with amiodarone treatment. *C Ital Cardiol* 1985; 15:552.

114. Mason JW: Drug therapy: amiodarone. *N Engl J Med* 1987; 316:455.

115. Dean PJ, Groshart KD, Porterfield JG, et al.: Amiodarone-associated pulmonary toxicity: a clinical and pathologic study of eleven cases. *Am J Clin Pathol* 1987; 87:7.

116. Kudenchuk PJ, Pierson DJ, Green HL, et al.: Prospective evaluation of amiodarone pulmonary toxicity. *Chest* 1984; 86:541.

117. Adams PC, Gibson GJ, Morley AR, et al.: Amiodarone pulmonary toxicity: clinical and subclinical features. *QJ Med* 1986; 59:449.

118. Liu FL, Cohen RD, Downer E, et al.: Amiodarone pulmonary

toxicity: functional and ultrastructural evaluation. *Thorax* 1986; 41:100.

119. Kennedy JI, Myers JL, Plumb VJ, Fulmer JD: Amiodarone pulmonary toxicity: clinical, radiologic, and pathologic correlations. *Arch Intern Med* 1987; 147:50.

120. Rakita L, Sobol SM, Mostow N, Vrobel T: Amiodarone pulmonary toxicity. *Am Heart J* 1983; 106:906.

121. Darmanata JI, van Zandwijk N, Düren DR, et al.: Amiodarone pneumonitis: three further cases with review of published reports. *Thorax* 1984; 39:56.

122. Veltri EP, Reid PR: Amiodarone pulmonary toxicity: early changes in pulmonary function tests during amiodarone rechallenge. *J Am Coll Cardiol* 1985; 6:802.

123. Rotmensch HH, Belhassen B, Swanson BN, et al.: Steady-state serum amiodarone concentrations: relationships with antiarrhythmic efficacy and toxicity. *Ann Intern Med* 1984; 101:462.

124. Olson LK, Forrest JV, Friedman PJ, et al.: Pneumonitis after amiodarone therapy. *Radiology* 1984; 150:327.

125. Dan M, Greif J: Amiodarone and pneumonitis (letter to editor). *Ann Intern Med* 1983; 99:732.

126. Marton II WJ, Osborn MJ: Amiodarone pulmonary toxicity: clinical presentation and possible mechanisms. *Clin Prog Electrophysiol Pac* 1986; 4:371.

127. Rosenow E, Myers J, Swensen S, and Pisani R: Drug-induced pulmonary disease. An update. *Chest* 1992; 102:239.

128. Greenspon A, Kidwell G, Hurley W, Mannion J: Amiodarone-related postoperative adult respiratory distress syndrome. *Circulation* 1991; 84(suppl III):407.

129. Kupferschmid J, Rosengart T, McIntosh C, et al.: Amiodarone-induced complications after cardiac operation for obstructive hypertrophic cardiomyopathy. *Ann Thorac Surg* 1989; 48:359.

130. Wilson B, Clarkson C, Lippman M: Amiodarone-induced pulmonary inflammation. Correlation with drug dose and lung levels of drug, metabolite, and phospholipid. *Am Rev Respir Dis* 1991; 143:1110.

131. Wood D, Osborn M, Rooke J, Holmes D Jr: Amiodarone pulmonary toxicity: Report of two cases associated with rapidly progressive fatal adult respiratory distress syndrome after pulmonary angiography. *Mayo Clin Proc* 1985; 60:601.

132. Adams PC, Holt DW, Storey GCA, et al.: Amiodarone and its desethyl metabolite: tissue distribution and morphologic changes during long-term therapy. *Circulation* 1985; 72:1064.

133. Maggioni AP, Maggi A, Volpi A, et al.: Amiodarone distribution in human tissues after sudden death during Holter recording. *Am J Cardiol* 1983; 52:217.

134. Kehrer JP, Kacew S: Systematically applied chemicals that damage lung tissue. *Toxicology* 1985; 35:251.

135. Lüllman-Rauch R: Drug-induced lysosomal storage disorders, in Dingle JT, Jacques PJ, Shaw IH (eds.): *Lysomomes in Biology and Pathology*, vol 6. North-Holland, New York, 1979:49–130.

136. Seiler KU, Thiel JH, Wasserman O: Die chloroquinkeratopathie als biespiel einer arzneimittelinduzierten phospholipidosis. *Klin Monatsbl Augenheilkd* 1977; 170:64.

137. Allan D, Michell RH: Enhanced synthesis de novo of phosphatidylinositol in lymphocytes treated with cationic amphi–philic drugs. *Biochem J* 1975; 148:471.

138. Michell RH, Allan D, Bowley M, Brindley DN: A possible metabolic explanation for drug-induced phospholipidosos. *J Pharm Pharmacol* 1976; 28:331.

139. Ohkuma S, Poole B: Fluorescence probe measurement of the intralysosomal pH in living cells and the perturbation of pH by various agents. *Proc Natl Acad Sci USA* 1978; 75:3327.

140. Heath MF, Costa-Jussa FR, Jacobs JM, et al.: The induction of pulmonary phospholipidosis and the inhibition of lysosomal phospholipidoses by amiodarone. *Br J Exp Pathol* 1985; 66:391.

141. Hostetler KY, Reasor MJ, Walter ER, et al.: Role of phospholipase A inhibition in amiodarone pulmonary toxicity in rats. *Biochim Biophys Acta* 1986; 875:400.

142. Martin WJ II, Kachel DL, Vilen T, et al.: Amiodarone pulmonary toxicity: mechanism of phospholipidosis in cultured pulmonary endothelial cells. *Clin Res* 1987; 35:535.

143. Reasor MJ: Drug-induced lipidosis and the alveolar macrophage. *Toxicology* 1981; 20:1.

144. Brindley DN, Allan D, Michell RH: The redirection of glyceride and phospholipid synthesis by drugs including chlorapromazine, fenfluramine, imipramine, mepyramine and local anesthetics. *J Pharm Pharmacol* 1975; 27:462.

145. Lüllman H, Plösch H, Ziegler A: Ca replacement by cationic amphiphilic drugs from lipid monolayers. *Biochem Pharmacol* 1980; 29:2969.

146. Schwarting H, Seiler KU, Wasserman O: On the mechanism of drug-induced phospholipidosis. *Naunyn Schmiedebergs Arch Pharmacol* 1976; 293(suppl):R57.

147. Hruban Z, Swift H, Slesers A: Effect of triparanol and diethanolamine on the fine structure of hepatocytes and pancreatic acinar cells. *Lab Invest* 1965; 14:1652.

148. Myers JL, Kennedy JI, Plumb VJ: Amiodarone lung: pathologic findings in clinically toxic patients. *Hum Pathol* 1987; 18:349.

149. Hruban Z, Slesers A, Hopkins E: Drug-induced and naturally occurring myeloid bodies. *Lab Invest* 1972; 27:62.

150. Myers JL, Kennedy JI, Plumb VJ: Amiodarone lung: pathologic findings in clinically toxic patients. *Hum Pathol* 1987; 18:349.

151. Myers JL: Diagnosis of drug reactions in the lung, in Churg A, Katzenstein AL (eds): *The Lung: Current Concepts.* Maryland, Williams & Wilkens, 1993:32–54.

152. Karabelnik D, Zbinden G, Baumgartner E: Drug-induced foam cell reactions in rats. I. Histopathologic and cytochemical observations after treatment with chlorphentermine, RMI 10.393, and RO 4:4318. *Toxicol Appl Pharmacol* 1974; 27:395.

153. Gray JE, Weaver RN, Stern KF, Phillips WA: Foam cell response in the lung and lymphatic tissues during long-term high-level treatment with erythromycin. *Toxicol Appl Pharmacol* 1978; 45:701.

154. Gefter WB, Epstein DM, Pietra GG, et al.: Lung disease caused by amiodarone, a new antiarrhythmia agent. *Radiology* 1983; 147:339.

155. Gonzalez-Rothi R, Hannan S, Hood I, Franzini D: Amiodarone pulmonary toxicity presenting as bilateral exudative pleural effusions. *Chest* 1987; 92:179.

156. Zhu YY, Botvinick E, Dae M, et al.: Gallium lung scintigraphy in amiodarone pulmonary toxicity. *Chest* 1988; 93:1126.

157. Kennedy JI: Clinical aspects of amiodarone pulmonary toxicity. *Clin Chest Med* 1990; 11:119.

158. Suarez LD, Poderosos JJ, Elsner B, et al.: Subacute pneumopathy during amiodarone therapy. *Chest* 1983; 83:566.

159. Dake MD, Madison JM, Montgomery CK, et al.: Electron microscopic demonstration of lysosomal inclusion bodies in lung, liver, lymph nodes, and blood leukocytes of patients with amiodarone pulmonary toxicity. *Am J Med* 1985; 78:506.

160. Joelson J, Kluger J, Cole S, Conway M: Possible recurrence of amiodarone pulmonary toxicity following corticosteroid therapy. *Chest* 1984; 85:284.

161. Andreasen P, Agerback H, Bjerregard P, et al.: Pharmacokinetics of amiodarone after intravenous and oral administration. *Eur J Clin Pharmacol* 1981; 19:293.

162. Canada AT, Lesko LJ, Haffajee CI, et al.: Amiodarone for tachyarrhythmias: pharmacology, kinetics, and efficacy. *Drug Intell Clin Pharm* 1983; 17:100.

163. Holt DW, Tucker GT, Jackson PR, et al.: Amiodarone pharmacokinetics. *Am Heart J* 1983; 206:840.

164. Kannan R, Nademanee K, Hendrickson JA, et al.: Amiodarone kinetics after oral doses. *Clin Pharmacol Ther* 1982; 31:445.

165. Gefter WB, Epstein DM, Pietra GG, Miller WT: Lung disease caused by amiodarone, a new antiarrhythmic agent. *Radiology* 1983; 147:339.

166. Zaher C, Harner A, Peter T, et al.: Low-dose steroid therapy for prophylaxis of aiodaxone-induced pulmonary infiltrates (letter). *N Engl J Med* 1983; 308:779.

167. Kilburn KH: Pulmonary disease induced by drugs, in Fishman AP (ed): *Pulmonary Diseases and Disorders.* New York, McGraw-Hill, 1980; 707–724.

168. Flacke JW, Flacke WE, Williams GD: Acute pulmonary edema following naloxone reversal of high-dose morphine anethesia. *Anesthesiology* 1977; 47:376.

169. Heffner JE, Sahn SA: Salicylate-induced pulmonary edema: clinical features and prognosis. *Ann Intern Med* 1981; 95:405.

170. McGuigan MA: A two-year review of salicylate deaths in Ontario. *Arch Intern Med* 1987; 147:510.

171. Thisted B, Krantz T, Strom J et al.: Acute salicylate self-poisoning in 177 consecutive patients treated in ICU. *Acta Anesthesiol Scand* 1987; 31:312.

172. Kavaru MS, Ahmed M, Amirthalingam KN: Hydrochlorothiazide-induced acute pulmonary edema. *Cleve Clin J Med* 1990; 57:181.

173. Kinnunen E, Viljanen A: Pleuropulmonary involvement during bromocriptine treatment. *Chest* 1988; 94:1034.

174. Bell RT, Lippmann RM: Hydrochlorothiazide-induced pulmonary edema. *Arch Intern Med* 1979; 139:817.

175. Beaudry C, Laplante L: Severe allergic pneumonitis from hydrochlorothiazide. *Ann Intern Med* 1973; 78:251.

176. Weddington WW, Mulroy MF, Sandri SR: Pneumonitis and hydrochlorothiazide. *Ann Intern Med* 1973; 79:283.

177. Dorn MR, Walker BK: Noncardiogenic pulmonary edema associated with hydrochlorothiazide therapy. *Chest* 1981; 79:482.

178. Farrell Jr TC, Schillaci RF: Hydrochlorothiazide-induced pulmonary edema mimicking metastic carcinoma of the breast. *Cardiopulmonary Med* 1976; 15:16.

179. Biron PB, Dessureault J, Napke E: Acute allergic interstitial pneumonitis induced by hydrochlorothiazide. *Can Med Assoc J* 1991; 145(1)28.

180. John J, Göldel N, Rienmuller R, et al.: Noncardiogenic pulmonary edema complicating intermediate and high-dose Ara C treatment for relapsed acute leukemia. *Med Oncol Tumor Pharmacother* 1988; 5:41.

181. Andersson BS, Luna MA, Yee C, et al.: Fatal pulmonary failure complicating high-dose cytosine arabinoside therapy in acute leukemia. *Cancer* 1990; 65:1079.

182. Agre KA: Overview of clinical evaluation in the United States, in Soper WT, Glott AB (eds.): *New Drug Seminar on Bleomycin.* Bethesda, MD, National Institutes of Health, 1974:66–82.

183. Kehl A, Bergholz M, von Heyden HW, Nagel GA: Toxischallergisches lungenödem nach cyclophosphamide- und iphosphamide-therapie. *Onkologie* 1983; 6:84.

184. Maxwell I: Reversible pulmonary edema following cyclophosphamide treatment. *JAMA* 1974; 229:137.

185. Bernstein ML, Sobel DB, Wimmer RS: Noncardiogenic pulmonary edema following injection of methotrexate into cerebrospinal fluid. *Cancer* 1982; 50:866.

186. Lascari AD, Strano AJ, Johnson WW, Collins JGP: Methotrexate-induced sudden fatal pulmonary reaction. *Cancer* 1977; 40:1393.

187. Hamous JE, Guffy MM, Aschenbrener CA: Fatal acute respiratory failure following intrathecal methotrexate administration. *Cancer Treat Rep* 1983; 67:1025.

188. Gutin PH, Green MR, Bleyer WA, et al.: Methotrexate pneu-

monitis induced by intrathecal methotrexate therapy. *Cancer* 1976; 38:1529.

189. Powell-Jackson PR, Carmichael FJL, Calne RY, Williams R: Adult respiratory distress syndrome and convulsions associated with administration of cyclosporine in liver transplant recipients. *Transplantation* 1984; 38:341.

190. Blaauw AAM, Leunissen KML, Cheriex EC, et al.: Disappearance of pulmonary capillary leak syndrome when intravenous cyclosporine is replaced by oral cyclosporine. *Transplantation* 1987; 43:758.

191. Cabone L, Appel GB, Benvenisty AI, et al.: Adult respiratory distress syndrome associated with oral cyclosporine. *Transplantation* 1987; 43:767.

192. Howard JJ, Mohsenifar Z, Simons SM: Adult respiratory distress syndrome following administration of lidocaine. *Chest* 1982; 81:644.

193. Alfred RJ, Ewer S: Fatal pulmonary edema following intravenous "freebase" cocaine use. *Ann Emerg Med* 1981; 10:441.

194. Wetli V, Mittleman RE: The 'body packer syndrome'—Toxicity following ingestion of illicit drugs packaged for transportation. *J Forensic Sci* 1981; 26:492.

195. Felman AH: Neurogenic pulmonary edema. *AJR* 1971; 112:393.

196. Stern WZ, Spear PW, Jacobson HG: The roentgen findings in acute heroin intoxication. *AJR* 1968; 103:522.

197. Steinberg AD, Karliner JS: The clinical spectrum of heroin pulmonary edema. *Arch Intern Med* 1968; 122:122.

198. Mahutte CK, Nakasato SK, Light RW: Haloperidol and sudden death due to pulmonary edema. *Arch Intern Med* 1982; 142:1951.

199. Fisher HK: Drug-induced asthma syndromes, in Weiss EB, Segan MS, Stein M (eds.): *Bronchial Asthma: Mechanisms and Therapeutics*, 2nd ed. Boston, Little, Brown, 1985; 938–949.

200. Bowen RE, Dedhia HV, Beatty J, et al.: ARDS associated with the use of sympathomimetics and glucocorticoids for the treatment of premature labor. *Crit Care Med* 1983; 11:671.

201. Smith WR, Wells ID, Glauser FL, Novey HS: Immunologic abnormalities in heroin lung. *Chest* 1975; 68:651.

202. Hrnicek G, Skelton J, Miller WC: Pulmonary edema and salicylate intoxication. *JAMA* 1974; 230:866.

203. Hormaechea E, Carlson RW, Rogove H, et al.: Hypovolemia, pulmonary edema and protein changes in severe salicylate poisoning. *Am J Med* 1979; 66:1046.

204. Katz S, Aberman A, Frand UI, et al.: Heroin pulmonary edema. Evidence for increased pulmonary capillary permeability. *Am Rev Respir Dis* 1972; 106:472.

205. Elliott J, O'Keeffe D, Greenberg P, Freeman R: Pulmonary edema associated with magnesium sulfate and betamethasone administration. *Am J Obstet Gynecol* 1979; 134:717.

206. Guernsey B, Villarreal Y, Snyder M, Gabert H: Pulmonary edema associated with the use of betamimetic agents in preterm labor. *Am J Hosp Pharmacol* 1981; 38:1942.

207. Gupta R, Foster S, Romano P, Thomas III H: Acute pulmonary edema associated with the use of oral ritodrine for premature labor. *Chest* 1989; 95:479.

208. Jacobs M, Knight A, Arias F: Maternal pulmonary edema resulting from betamimetic and glucocorticoid therapy. *Obstet Gynecol* 1980; 56:56.

209. Mabie W, Pernoll M, Witty J, Biswas M: Pulmonary edema induced by betamimetic drugs. *South Med J* 1983; 76:1354.

210. Pisani R, Rosenow III E: Pulmonary edema associated with tocolytic therapy. *Am Intern Med* 1989; 110:714.

211. Whitehead M, Mander A, Hertogs K, et al.: Acute congestive cardiac failure in a hypertensive woman receiving salbutamol for premature labour. *Br Med J* 1980; 2:1221.

212. Anderson H: Adult respiratory distress syndrome in obstetrics and gynecology. *Obstet Gynecol* 1980; 55:291.

213. Stubblefield P: Pulmonary edema occurring after therapy with dexamethasone and terbutaline for premature labor. *Am J Obstet Gynecol* 1978; 132:341.

214. Tinga DJ, Aarnoudse JG: Post-partum pulmonary oedema associated with preventive therapy for premature labour. *Lancet* 1979; i:1026.

215. Elliott HR, Abdulla U, Hayes PJ: Pulmonary oedema associated with ritrodine infusion and betamethasone administration in premature labour. *Br Med J* 1978; 2:799.

216. Brodey PA, Fisch AE, Huffacker J: Acute pulmonary edema resulting from treatment for premature labor. *Radiology* 1981; 140:631.

217. Benedetti TJ, Hargrove JC, Rosene KA: Maternal pulmonary edema during premature labor inhibition. *Obstet Gynecol* 1982; 59(suppl):33.

218. Gleicher N, Bazile F, Elrad H: Pulmonary edema after ritrodine therapy in a patient with preeclampsia. *N Engl J Med* 1982; 306:174.

219. Light RW, Dunham TR: Severe slowly resolving heroin-induced pulmonary edema. *Chest* 1975; 67:61.

220. Louria DB, Hensle T, Rose J: The major medical complications of heroin addiction. *Ann Intern Med* 1967; 67:1.

221. Myers JL: Pathology of drug-induced lung disease, in Katzenstein AL, Askin F (eds.): *Surgical Pathology of Non-Neoplastic Lung Disease*. Philadelphia, WB Saunders, 1990.

222. Cohen MB, Austin JH, Smith-Vaniz A, et al.: Nodular bleomycin toxicity. *Am J Clin Pathol* 1989; 92:101.

223. Santrach PJ, Askin FB, Wells RJ, et al.: Nodular form of bleomycin-related pulmonary injury in patients with osteogenic sarcoma. *Cancer* 1989; 15:806.

224. Patel RC, Dutta D, Schonfeld SA: Free-base cocaine use associated with bronchiolitis obliterans organizing pneumonia. *Ann Intern Med* 1987; 107:186.

225. Kaufman J, Komorowski R: Bronchiolitis obliterans: a new clinical-pathologic complication of irradiation pneumonitis. *Chest* 1990; 97:1243.

PART 3

TREATMENT OF OBSTRUCTIVE LUNG DISEASES

ASTHMA: THERAPEUTIC PRINCIPLES

Definition

Diagnosis

Physiologic Evaluation

Diagnostic Algorithm

Differential Diagnosis

Definition

The word *asthma* is an English corruption of the Greek αρσμα, a generic expression that can be loosely translated as "panting" or "difficult breathing." Since its first recorded use in the writings of Hippocrates until the early part of this century, asthma has been a synonym for noisy respirations associated with tachypnea. To distinguish the cause of a given patient's problem, physicians began adding adjectives such as "cardiac," "foreign body," "Baker's," and so forth to the term. This approach did little to clarify the nature of asthma; rather, it helped solidify the notion that asthma was only a descriptive word for a collection of illnesses instead of a specific disease. With the advent of practical means of examining the pathogenesis and pathophysiology of the obstructive pulmonary syndromes, the meaning of asthma began to be narrowed to encompass a distinct medical entity, and the spate of recent studies in airway histology and cell and molecular biology have further refined its focus.

Presently, asthma is defined as a chronic disease of the tracheobronchial tree that causes widespread narrowing of the air passages. Asthma is characterized by acute symptomatic episodes of varying degrees of severity that can resolve spontaneously or with treatment. These exacerbations can fluctuate in intensity over time and in unusual circumstances can cause death. In autopsies of patients dying from asthma, hypertrophy of the bronchial smooth muscle, mucosal edema, denudation of the surface epithelium, thickening of the basement membrane, eosinophilic infiltration of the mucosa and submucosa, and widespread mucous plugging of the airways are seen. Some believe that asthma

should be viewed in terms of the factors thought to be important in its etiology or pathogenesis and the concepts of airway inflammation and bronchial hyperresponsiveness have been included in the definition. Although these elements are clearly present in many patients, they are not seen in all. Further, they are also found in other forms of airway disease, such as cystic fibrosis and chronic bronchitis, as well as in patients with atopic rhinitis without lower respiratory problems. Consequently, the additional information gained by defining asthma with these modifiers is uncertain. The evolution of the definition of asthma to its current state as a specific illness in which acute exacerbations are superimposed on a background of chronic disease has important diagnostic and therapeutic implications. Asthma can be detected in many of its more subtle presentations long before the patient's discomfort has reached a point demanding immediate intervention, and therapy has moved beyond symptomatic relief toward controlling the disease by modifying any cellular and biochemical abnormalities that may be present.

Diagnosis

Asthma is diagnosed solely by clinical criteria. No immunologic, physiologic, or biochemical tests are specific for this illness. Rather, asthma is suspected when a characteristic pattern of signs, symptoms, and physiologic abnormalities develop. The usual history is that of episodic paroxysms of dyspnea, cough, and wheezing that are interspersed with symptom-free periods. Patients may also complain of a sense of chest constriction and an inability to inspire fully. It is rare for asthma to have an explosive onset. Typically the initial symptoms are intermittent and short lived, lasting from minutes to hours. With time, however, they might become more frequent and severe. Complaints may last for a considerable period, but invariably the symptoms wax and wane.

Ordinarily, the symptoms of asthma coexist, but it is possible for one or more of them to dominate the picture. Wheezing is the usual manifestation, but patients also may experience cough, dyspnea, or chest discomfort as isolated entities. When dealing with cough, typically, it is paroxysmal in nature, dry or productive of scant amounts of mucoid sputum, and nocturnal. The paroxysms tend to terminate in acute breathlessness or wheezing. They can be of sufficient intensity to produce vomiting, stress incontinence, and syncope. Fractured ribs and trauma to the muscles of the thorax also may occur.

The dyspnea variant is more subtle. The patient complains of episodic inappropriate breathlessness with exertion that fluctuates in intensity. On close questioning, the patient invariably admits to wheezing. In the chest discomfort variant, patients experience a sense of heaviness or pressure over the sternum associated with an inability to take a deep breath. Dyspnea, but not necessarily tachypnea, is a frequent accompaniment. Wheezing can be present but is not a prominent symptom. Because of the predominance of the substernal distress, this constellation of complaints in middle-aged patients is often mistaken for cardiac disease. Frequently, it is only after stress tests, echocardiograms, and even cardiac catheterization have proven unrewarding that the true nature of the problem is appreciated.

When the disease is active, patients awaken at night or early in the morning with one or more of the above complaints. In fact, nocturnal symptoms are such a common feature of this illness, that their absence is cause to consider other diagnoses. Another cardinal feature of asthma is the history of acute exacerbation after exposure to various environmental stimuli (Table 73-1). Upper respiratory tract infections, exercise, frigid air, irritant vapors, emotional stress, aeroallergens, air pollutants, occupational factors, and pharmacologic stimuli can all induce symptoms in susceptible individuals. The first six tend to be the most common in the general asthmatic population.

In a survey of 430 consecutive patients with asthma referred to the clinics of the University Hospitals of Cleveland, 97 percent indicated that infections were a major cause of acute decompensation. Well-controlled investigations have demonstrated that respiratory viruses and not bacteria are the major factors in this situation. In young children the most important agents are respiratory syncytial viruses and para influenza viruses. In older children and adults, rhino viruses and influenza predominate. Infection with these pathogens increases airway reactivity in both normal and asthmatic individuals for periods of up to 2 to 8 weeks. During this time of increased risk, asthma will often destabilize.

In 94 percent of patients, exercise was also a major precipitant. This stimulus is most frequently operational in children and young adults because of their spontaneous high levels of physical activity; however, it can be seen in asth-

TABLE 73-1   Naturally Occurring Stimuli Eliciting Acute Episodes of Asthma

- Upper respiratory tract infection
- Exercise
- Frigid environmental temperature
- Irritant vapors
- Emotional stress
- Aeroallergens
- Air pollutants
- Occupational factors
- Pharmacologic stimuli

matics of all ages when they exert themselves. The patient's sensitivity to exercise and the intensity of the subsequent obstruction are related to the state of the underlying airway hyperresponsiveness, the ventilation required to complete the task, and the temperature and water content of the inspired air. For any given degree of airway reactivity, the more strenuous the physical effort, and the lower the temperature, the more severe is the resultant asthma attack.

Exposure to cold air also will induce airway obstruction in asthmatics. Eighty-two percent of participants surveyed in the clinics of the University Hospitals of Cleveland found this to be a particularly troubling trigger, and activities such as going outdoors on a cold winter day or even entering an air-conditioned room could produce acute bronchospasm. If exercise is added (e.g., shoveling snow, hurrying to catch a bus in low ambient temperatures etc.), the asthma attack can be quite disabling. Asthmatics are also sensitive to environmental vapors and smells; 62 percent of the patients relayed that contact with colognes, cooking odors, scents from laundry detergents and soaps, perfumes, and fine particulates would induce immediate response. Psychological factors are known to interact with the asthmatic diathesis to enhance or diminish the disease process, and 51 percent of the subjects related that their asthma worsened during times of emotional stress.

Although it is commonly written that asthma is an allergic disease, only 35 percent of patients surveyed by the University Hospitals of Cleveland related a positive history of acute exacerbations of their illness on contact with aeroallergens. Although many more suspected that this association existed, they were unable to recall specific instances of cause and effect. When antigens are involved, the history is frequently one of seasonal fluctuations in disease activity, which is most often observed in children and young adults after exposure to spring and fall pollens. A nonseasonal or perennial form of asthma may result from allergy to feathers, pets, dust mites, molds, and other allergens present continuously in the environment. Exposure to antigens produces an immediate response in which airway obstruction develops in minutes and then resolves. In 30 to 50 percent of patients, a second wave of bronchoconstriction, the so-called late reaction, develops 6 to 10 hours later. In a minority, only a late reaction occurs. Immunologic triggers, like upper respiratory tract infections, increase airway reactivity. Thus, a single exposure to this type of stimulus can produce recurrent episodes of asthma that can last a week or more.

The environmental air pollutants of concern are ozone, sulfur dioxide (and related compounds), and the oxides of nitrogen (see Chap. 37). Not many patients complain of these factors as a primary cause of their symptoms. They will, however, develop symptoms if the pollutants reach high enough local concentrations. The specific effects of these chemicals—and those of the various occupational factors known to adversely influence asthma—are considered elsewhere in this book.

No history of potential asthma precipitants is complete without an in-depth exploration of medication use. β-adrenoceptor antagonists delivered as eyedrops and nonsteroidal anti-inflammatory drugs can produce acute airway obstruction in susceptible individuals, as can preservatives such as sulfites and some industrial dyes. In sensitive subjects, ingestion of even small quantifies of the first two classes of agents can have severe consequences.

Physiologic Evaluations

There are no specific laboratory tests for asthma. If the patient is asymptomatic, chest radiographs are usually normal or may show nonspecific hyperinflation. The levels of immunoglobulin E (IgE) and eosinophils in the blood of asthmatics may be increased, but these are nonspecific events that may be seen in patients with atopic illnesses such as rhinitis. Sputum eosinophilia also is observed in asthmatics as compared to normal, but this, too, is nondiagnostic and has been reported in chronic bronchitis. Analysis of mediators of inflammation in sputum and blood have shown quantitative differences in asthmatics versus normal individuals, but here as well, there is considerable overlap with other nonasthmatic illnesses with allergic backgrounds. Skin tests demonstrate sensitivity to specific antigens but do not offer any insights into diagnosis or pathogenesis.

Some have advocated the use of bronchial biopsies or bronchoalveolar lavage as a means of establishing the diagnosis of asthma. Although this approach is appealing intuitively, the current data do not permit firm conclusions to be drawn. The histology of the airways of asthmatics and normals can be similar, and all of the biochemical, immunohistochemical, and molecular biologic defects thus far described in asthmatics have been observed in atopic rhinitis without any evidence of lower airway disease.

To confirm the presence of asthma, the clinical impression must be verified objectively by demonstrating reversible airflow limitation. Many patients with this illness will have functional defects even when asymptomatic. The subtlest manifestation is an isolated reduction in flows in the mid vital capacity range during a forced exhalation, with or without a concomitant increase in residual volume (RV). In such individuals, evaluation of gas exchange shows ventilation-perfusion mismatching with hypoxemia and an increase in the alveolar-arterial oxygen gradient. When the obstruction is more pronounced, asthmatics have reduced forced expiratory volumes and flow rates, with maximal expiratory flow volume curves that are concave to the volume axis. Bronchial narrowing typically is associated with gas trapping as manifested by increase in RV and functional residual capacity. Total lung capacity is normal. When the patient is symptomatic, the alternations in pulmonary mechanics can be quite dramatic and values for RV of 400 percent of expected and forced expiratory volume in 1 s (FEV_1) of 25 percent of predicted or less are common.

Airway obstruction is considered to be reversible if the FEV_1 increased by $\geq$ 15 percent after a standard dose (2 puffs) of a β-adrenergic agonist. This criterion has been determined arbitrarily, but long use has established its validity. From time to time, changes in other measures of pulmonary mechanics such as flows in the mid vital capacity or specific resistance have been proposed as being more sensitive or selective. It is important to appreciate that normal subjects also respond to a bronchodilator with an increase in airway diameter, thereby, causing large changes in those parameters. The FEV_1, however, will only improve a few percent in these circumstances.

If the presenting spirometric data are normal, the criterion for reversibility may not be fulfilled. Improvement of the FEV_1 from its expected range to a supernormal value after administration of sympathomimetic agonists cannot be relied upon as evidence of increased airway tone. When lung function is normal, the diagnosis of asthma can be established by demonstrating the increased airway responsiveness so characteristic of this illness. The provocative stimuli that currently are used are listed in Table 73-2. It is important to appreciate that no one test detects all the patients at risk. Histamine and methacoline traditionally have been used most frequently, are well validated, and have a high degree of concordance. They are easily performed, do not require special equipment, and have few contraindications. With large doses, histamine may produce glottic edema, which can confound interpretation of the results. This agent can also induce tachyphylaxis if repetitive challenges are performed over short periods.

The next most commonly used challenge is exercise. Its chief limitation is the need for the subject to perform exhausting work, and so it may not be suitable for patients who are physically disadvantaged, those with cardiac disease, or the elderly. Moreover, it is difficult to obtain stimulus-response curves. To overcome these disadvantages, isocapnic hyperventilation with frigid or dry air has been used as a surrogate. Although there has been some controversy, hyperventilation is now known to share the same mechanism of action as exercise. Because exercise and hyperventilation can be encountered in the daily lives of patients,

TABLE 73-2   Clinical Techniques Used to Measure Bronchial Responsiveness

Tests in Frequent Use
■ Histamine
■ Methacholine
■ Distilled water
■ Hypertonic saline
■ Allergen
■ Exercise
■ Hyperventilation of cold or dry air
■ Occupational sensitizers
■ Propranolol

they are highly relevant clinically. Hyperventilation can be performed by almost anyone, and stimulus-response curves are readily generated. The response to exercise and hyperventilation correlates with histamine and methacholine. Like histamine, repetitive exercise challenges induce tachyphylaxis when they are performed within 40 minutes of each other.

Some laboratories use nonisotonic aerosols as provocative agents. Solutions of distilled water or 2.7%, 3.6% or 4.5% saline are aerosolized from ultrasonic nebulizers and inhaled for different periods of time to generate dose-response curves. Nonisotonic aerosols correlate with exercise, as well as the pharmacologic stimuli, but they are selective for the more reactive asthmatics; thus, they are poor survey tools. The nonisotonic aerosols may produce nonspecific osmotic damage to the epithelium even in normal individuals, so that false-positive results may occur. Bronchial provocation tests with antigen also can be undertaken but their routine use is not recommended. They may, however, have a place in specific industrial exposures that require documentation for medical-legal purposes.

The changes in pulmonary mechanics induced by the stimuli listed in Table 73-2 usually are expressed as a percentage decrease in FEV_1, using the baseline or postdiluent value as the reference. There is little advantage to be gained from other indices derived from a spirogram or maximal expiratory flow volume curve, such as the $FEV_{25-75\%}$. Sensitivity of detection can be enhanced somewhat by using either specific conductance or specific resistance as endpoints because these variables will reflect reductions in airway geometry before the FEV_1 begins to change. Unfortunately, this approach does not enhance the basic selectivity of the challenge. The three variables most often examined in quantitating the magnitude of the response are the concentration of agonist that induces a fixed fall in lung function (i.e., a 20 percent reduction in FEV_1), the slope of the dose-response curve, and the dose at which a plateau can be produced. The first is traditional, whereas the others remain research tools at present. Typically, the response is expressed as either a provocative dose (PD_{20}) or provocative concentration (PC_{20}). PD_{20} represents the cumulative dose delivered, and PC_{20} represents the concentration administered from a nebulizer adjusted to a standard output. Both measure the same phenomenon. Values of PC_{20} of 8 mg/mL or less or PD_{20} of 7.8 μmol or less of either histamine or methacholine are generally considered to indicate the increased bronchial reactivity. It is important to appreciate that these are arbitrary values and not precise endpoints.

It generally is believed that changes in airway reactivity have direct clinical correlates in asthma. As bronchial hyperresponsiveness increases, symptoms worsen, the need for medication increases, and diurnal fluctuation in airway function becomes larger. As with other aspects of asthma, such phenomena do not always occur. It now is recognized that symptoms can develop in asthmatics who have normal values for PC_{20}, and the clinical course of any given patient can worsen or improve without a concomitant reflection in measured airway sensitivity. Further, increased airway responsiveness can be found in many people who do not have asthma including atopic rhinitis, and first-degree rela-

tives of asthmatics. Some patients with obstructive lung disease such as chronic bronchitis, bronchiectasis, and cystic fibrosis also show this effect. Thus, the interpretation of increased airway reactivity must be put into the overall clinical context, and it cannot be used as the sole marker to diagnose or exclude asthma.

Diagnostic Algorithm

At initial presentation, the health-care provider should obtain a detailed history of the patient's complaints. Essential points to record include the exact symptoms that develop, the type of stimuli that induce them, the conditions that modify them, and their onset relative to exposure to the provocational event. The patients should be queried specifically about nocturnal awakening and whether the intensity, duration, and frequency of their symptoms change with time. It is important to judge how disabling the disease is because this information will frequently be a clue to the intensity of the initial therapy needed to control the symptoms. Important ancillary information includes a personal or family history of allergic disease such as rhinitis, eczema, or urticaria.

It is helpful to assess the relative contributions to all of the triggers listed above. Here too, specific questioning about each is essential. General inquiries are often unrewarding or provide misleading information because patients have not made appropriate associations or have focused on erroneous ones. A history of bizarre triggers that exacerbate acute airway obstruction is cause for skepticism for the diagnosis of asthma, as is the absence of nocturnal complaints. Symptom patterns other than those described are also useful information. For example, cough and sputum production is associated with the resolution of acute airway obstruction in uncomplicated asthmatics and is not a daily occurrence as in chronic bronchitis. Likewise, persistent unremitting symptoms are less likely to be asthmatic in origin.

In patients with appropriate histories, the next step is to conduct pulmonary function tests. Spirometry alone is not sufficient, and measurement of lung volumes is required. Dyspnea and wheezing are nonspecific complaints that can be seen in any form of primary or secondary airway disease. If airflow obstruction is found, the patient should be given a bronchodilator to determine reversibility. If the standard criteria are not met, it has been suggested that the patient be treated aggressively with bronchodilators and anti-inflammatory agents for several weeks and then be reevaluated. This approach has a very low yield. If a patient does not respond in the laboratory acutely, it is unlikely that asthma is the cause of the problem unless he or she is extremely ill. Even then, some improvement can be expected. Even patients with status asthmaticus will show an increase in lung function with inhaled β-agonist drugs. Consequently when faced with a poor therapeutic response, one considers other causes for airflow obstruction.

In individuals without airflow obstruction who have a history compatible with asthma, it has been recommended that they be followed with measurements of peak flow at home. If there are fluctuating readings, this may be evidence of reversibility, and no further testing is undertaken. However, this approach may be problematic. Such patterns of changing peak flow recordings are commonly seen in patients with psychogenic airway narrowing and can even occur with intrinsic and extrinsic tracheal compression. When confronted with the combination of apparent history and normal lung function, bronchoprovocation should be performed during which clinical and physiologic responses of the patient are monitored. If these two entities do not match (i.e., appropriate symptoms for appropriate airway obstruction, a diagnosis other than asthma should be considered.

Differential Diagnosis

The diagnosis of asthma is usually not difficult to make, particularly if the patient is seen during an acute episode. The constellation of physical findings and symptoms listed above, compiled with the episodic history are characteristic in adults. The major differential diagnosis is the other forms of chronic obstructive lung disease (COPD), such as chronic bronchitis and emphysema (Table 73-3). Chronic bronchitis is a disease of airways and to some extent lung parenchyma that is associated with excessive sputum production that is sufficient to cause cough with expectoration for most days for at least 3 months of the year for 2 consecutive years. Physiologically, such individuals develop slowly progressive irreversible airway obstruction that is associated with minimal increases in airway reactivity. In this illness, the symptoms of airway obstruction are progressive, and any acute episode of dyspnea and wheezing that the patient develops is superimposed on a background of persistent respiratory complaints. In chronic bronchitis the symptoms are not rhythmic or nocturnal, nor are they associated with acute traumatic changes in pulmonary function. Emphysema is a disease of the parenchyma associated with distension of airspaces distal to the terminal bronchi, with obstruction of the alveolar septa. Patients with this illness are frequently asymptomatic until they develop airway dysfunction at which time they complain of progressive dyspnea. Wheezing is uncommon and cough and sputum production are much less frequent than with chronic bronchitis. Airway

TABLE 73-3   Differential Diagnosis

- Chronic bronchitis
- Bronchiectasis
- Common variable hypogammaglobulinemia
- Emphysema
- Laryngeal obstruction
- Endobronchial space-occupying lesion
- Glottic dysfunction
- Occult cardiac disease
- Multiple pulmonary emboli
- Eosinophilic pneumonia syndromes
- Systemic vasculitis
- Gastroesophageal reflux
- Cough secondary to drugs
- Carcinoid

reactivity in COPD tends to be normal and nocturnal awakenings are uncommon unless heart failure supervenes.

Bronchiectasis and all its variants are characterized by cough and copious sputum production. When this occurs, the patient may wheeze and have dyspnea. This illness can frequently mimic asthma particularly when associated with recurrent sinusitis. Differentiation rests on the unremitting nature of the symptoms and the poor response to bronchodilators.

Upper airway construction by tumor or laryngeal edema occasionally can be confused with asthma (See Chap. 82). Typically, such patients present with stridor and harsh respiratory sounds can be localized to the area of the trachea; however, they can radiate widely. Diffuse wheezes throughout both lung fields are usually absent. As with bronchiectasis, response to bronchodilators is poor, and maximum inspiratory and expiratory flow volume curves will show evidence of variable or fixed extrapulmonic obstruction. Computer assisted tomography or endoscopy may be required to establish the diagnosis. Persistent wheezing localized to one area of the chest in association with paroxysms of cough indicates endobronchial disease such as foreign body aspiration, neoplasia, or bronchial stenosis. Asthma-like symptoms have been described in patients with vocal cord dysfunction. These individuals narrow their glottis during inspiration in response to psychic stress and produce episodic attacks of severe airway obstruction. On occasion the obstruction can be sufficiently severe to cause carbon dioxide retention. Unlike asthma, however, the arterial oxygen tension decreases in proportion to the increase in CO_2, and the alveolar-arterial gradient of oxygen narrows or remains normal. In this condition, the patient's symptoms often are incited by bizarre triggers.

The signs and symptoms of acute left ventricular decompensation can occasionally mimic asthma, particularly if cough is the only complaint. The findings of moist basilar rales, gallop rhythms, and other signs of heart failure allow the appropriate diagnosis to be reached. Recurrent small pulmonary emboli can be difficult to differentiate from asthma if the patient is pain free. Most often, affected individuals will present with episodic dyspnea, particularly on exertion, which will eventually become chronic, but sometimes they will wheeze. Unlike asthma, the dyspnea is disproportionate to the changes found in pulmonary mechanics.

Eosinophilic pneumonia and systemic vasculitis can be associated with asthmatic symptoms, particularly dyspnea and wheezing. The systemic complaints and parenchymal manifestations are a means of distinguishing them from bronchial asthma.

Gastroesophageal reflux occasionally can result in episodic nocturnal coughing. Associated coexisting symptoms of hoarseness eructations or esophagitis lead to the correct diagnosis. Episodic or even paroxysmal cough can be seen in patients without heightened airway reactivity who take angiotensin-converting enzyme inhibitors and cessation of the medication eliminates the symptoms. Bronchial carcinoids can secrete histamine and produce high enough regional levels to cause airway narrowing and wheezing. Cough can also occur. The diagnosis can be made with endoscopy. This is not a usual part of the carcinoid syndrome induced by serotonin-secreting gastrointestinal tumors.

References

1. Christopher KL, Wood RP II, Eckert RC, et al.: Vocal-cord dysfunction presenting as asthma. *N Engl J Med* 1983; 308:1566.

2. Burrows B, Martinez FD, Halonen M, et al.: Association of asthma with serum IgE levels and skin-test reactivity to allergens. *N Engl J Med* 1989; 320:271.

3. McFadden ER, Jr, Gilbert IA: Exercise induced asthma. *N Engl J Med* 1994; 330:1362.

4. O'Byrne PM, Dolovich J, Hargreave FE: Late asthmatic responses. *Am Rev Respir Dis* 1987; 136:740.

5. Wardlaw AJ: The role of air pollution in asthma. *Clin Exp Allergy* 1993; 23:81.

6. McFadden: Clinical and physiologic correlates in asthma. *J Allergy Clin Immunol* 1986; 77:1–5.

7. Busse WW. Respiratory infection: their role in airway responsiveness and the pathogenesis of asthma. *J Allergy Clin Immunol* 1990; 85:671.

8. McFadden ER, Jr.: Exertional dyspnea and cough as preludes to acute attacks of bronchial asthma *N Engl J Med* 1975; 292:555.

9. Stevenson DD, Simon RA, Mathison DA: Aspirin sensitive asthma: tolerance to aspirin after positive oral aspirin challenges. *J Allergy Clin Immunol* 1980; 66:82.

Chapter 74 _____
GENETICS OF ASTHMA*
MALCOLM N. BLUMENTHAL

Asthma was described in ancient times.[1,2] The term *asthma* appeared very early in medical literature but referred to dyspnea in general. The first valid description of asthma in terms of difficult breathing was by Aretaeus. This was followed by other descriptions of asthma by Hippocrates, Galen, and Celsus. Asthma, like many diseases, was not understood initially. It was thought to be caused by mysterious and magical forces; people with asthma were seen as possessed. Hippocrates noted that asthma had a spasmodic nature and stated: "The occurrence of asthma was so sudden as to induce the vulgar and uninformed spectators to believe it was sent by the gods for some particular purpose." He believed that asthma was related to the four humors: the blood, the phlegm, and the black and yellow bile. Its relationship to the nervous system was initially suggested by Thomas Willis in the seventeenth century. The connection between asthma and the immune system was suggested by the work of Blackley, who reported skin reactivity to grass pollen in 1873.[3–5] In 1910, Samuel Maltzer demonstrated the relationship of reaginic antibodies with asthma in his description of "Bronchial Asthma as a Phenomenon of Anaphylaxis."[6] In 1966, Ishizaka and Ishizaka described the immunoglobulin group IgE and demonstrated that it was the globulin that was called reaginic antibody.[7,8] Further characterization of the immune system and its relationship to asthma resulted in a model to study its pathogenesis. This included the definition of cytokines and T and B cells as well as of the role inflammation has in the production of asthma.

Through the years, it has become evident that asthma has a familial, if not a genetic, basis. Its familial nature was suggested as early as the fifth century, at which time Hippocrates noted that asthma occurred more frequently in certain families. The familial factor in asthma was further stressed by Floyer in 1698. The first systematic study of the genetics of asthma and allergy was reported by Cooke and Vander Veer in 1916.[9]

Environmental factors also were noted to be associated with the development of asthma. Cardan, in 1545, reported that asthma was triggered by feathers. In the seventeenth century, Van Helmont described attacks of asthma caused by house dust and by eating fish fried in oil.

It is now well established that asthma is a complex disease involving an interaction of environmental and genetic factors. It is evident at the present time that more information is needed regarding its biology.

Understanding the Genetics of Asthma

Several major areas of investigation are needed to understand the genetics of asthma. The first should be directed to defining the mode of inheritance of allergic diseases. Is there a genetic determinant of asthma? If there is, then what is the mode of inheritance? In addition, is a major gene involved and, if so, is it dominant, recessive, or codominant? The second major area of investigation concerns the characteristics of the gene involved. This involves knowing everything about the gene: its chromosomal location, its DNA sequence, how its expression is controlled, and what its product does.

Despite early anecdotal evidence and the more recent, systematic studies of Cooke and others indicating a familial, if not a genetic, basis of asthma, investigations in these areas were hampered by many problems, such as inadequate knowledge of the biology of asthma and lack of a definition

* Supported by NIH Grant 5401-HL49609

of the phenotype of asthma. The parameters to be measured, study design, selection of subjects, and methods of statistical analysis also needed to be improved. Advances in several fields are now making it possible to understand the genetics of asthma and allergies.[10] A better understanding of the pathogenesis of atopic conditions is allowing researchers to characterize the phenotype of asthma and allergies. This understanding has consisted of the characterizations of IgE, T cells, and cytokines. Other advances have been those made in molecular genetics, such as the identification of recombinant DNA, cloning of DNA fragments, the discovery that DNA fragments can be separated by electrophoresis, and development of the polymerase chain reaction, which allows the rapid amplification of short regions of DNA. Statistical methods have improved as well, permitting the analysis of the genetics of complex diseases such as allergies. Methods to define the genetics of asthma can be performed using associations and disequilibrium studies, determinations of heritability and risk to relatives, segregation analysis, and linkage analysis and mapping.

HERITABILITY

Heritability for a given phenotype is useful in determining the importance of genetic factors. These can be performed in population, twin, and family populations.[11]

Segregational analysis is helpful to determine whether a genetic model is consistent with the family data.[12] This involves answering the question of whether the qualitative or quantitative trait being measured segregates as a Mendelian dominant, recessive, or codominant trait. These analyses are performed using data from families. Single locus, mixed, oligogenic, and regressive models have been used. Some of these models are inappropriate for complex inheritance, such as that seen in asthma, in which no locus may be sufficient for the affliction and different genotypes may exist in different families. Another problem is that segregation analysis of a quantitative trait is sensitive to distributional assumptions.

CHARACTERIZATION OF THE GENE(S)

The characterization of the genes involved in asthma can be examined using a variety of methods. A common way to map genes to specific chromosomal locations is linkage analysis. This application is based upon the fact that loci that are physically close together on a segment of a chromosome tend to be inherited together, or linked.

There are several routes to understanding the molecular basis of inherited diseases. The main methods used are those of forward and positional (reverse) genetics and the candidate gene approach.

FORWARD GENETICS
Forward genetics has been one of the initial methods for studying the genetics of human disease. Examples of forward genetics include the study of the hemoglobinopathies and inborn errors of metabolism in which the defective item is identified and characterized. For asthma, studies of the transcriptional control of airway inflammation may provide the necessary information to study its forward genetics. The cell adhesion molecule gene(s) and, in turn, the gene products that control them are candidates for abnormal expression in inflammation. If the defective factor is known, forward genetics can be performed by first identifying the DNA, next the gene sequence, and ultimately its location.

POSITIONAL GENETICS
Positional genetics is a method used for many diseases, such as asthma and allergies, where the underlying defect is not known. Identification of any single gene of unknown function is a complex problem. The human genome comprises 3×10^9 base pairs; thus, any specific gene represents only a very small fraction of the total DNA. The first step in this process is to identify the gene location. Researchers therefore are mapping the chromosomal location of the gene and cloning the gene knowing nothing about it except for its location. Once this is done, researchers can then determine the gene sequence, its DNA structure, and ultimately the gene product that results in the production of the disease. This process has been called *positional* or *reverse genetics*.

CANDIDATE GENE APPROACH
Another approach is the candidate gene approach. Using this method, researchers identify a gene or group of genes that appears to be important in the development of the phenotype under study. An example would be the phenotype for IgE, which appears to be influenced by several genes already identified, such as those for the interleukins IL-4, IL-5, and IL-9. Studies are then set up to evaluate the relationships between these candidate genes, which are located on chromosome 5, and measures of IgE.

Of these methods, positional genetics and the candidate gene approach are being used for the study of the complex disease of asthma, which is multifactorial and appears to be genetically heterogeneous. In other words, it involves several genes along with an array of environmental factors that influence its expression. All these advances are allowing researchers to define the molecular basis of diseases such as asthma and allergies. As a result, we will be able to have not only the information that will give us the "blueprint" of the causes of asthma but also the substances that will allow us to treat the symptoms and the disease as well as to correct the DNA that causes the disease. With these new methodologies, there have been many genetic studies undertaken, making many claims and counterclaims but few triumphs.[10]

Model of Asthma

Based upon the accumulated data, we know that multiple cell types and numerous cellular control mechanisms influence the development of asthma and its response to treatment. According to our current understanding, the following model is being used for the investigation of the genetics of atopic asthma.[13–15]

SENSITIZATION

Exposure to the allergen (antigen) occurs, following which it is taken up by an antigen-presenting cell (APC) such as a dendritic or B cell. Afterwards the allergen (antigen) will, through intracellular processing, be broken down into a specific peptide that becomes associated with a class II major histocompatibility complex (MHC) molecule selected from an MHC library. The allergen (antigen) peptide-MHC complex then moves to the surface of the APC complex where it can interact with a subset of T cells, designated CD4+ cells, which have T-cell receptors (TCR) specific for the class II peptide complex chosen from a TCR library. These CD4+ cells may differentiate either into cells called T_H1, which produce the cytokine IL-4 and a set of associated molecules, or to cells called T_H2, which produce largely interferon γ (IFN-γ) as the main cytokine. IL-4 appears to be necessary for IgE production and is important in all forms of antibody production. IFN-γ is a principal regulator of cellular immunity and associated with a decrease in IgE production. There appears to be in atopic individuals the preferential development of a disproportionate number of T_H2 as opposed to T_H1 cells; the T_H2 cells interact with the allergen (antigen)-binding B-cell clones through the production of cytokines and directly through their action on B cells. This interaction results in signals for the B cells to differentiate and produce antigen-specific antibodies, whose immunoglobulin has been chosen from a V(h) library for its ability to bind the allergen (antigen). This step may result in two major effects: (1) B cells mature to plasma cells; in the allergen-specific response, isotope switching occurs, followed by the production of allergen-specific IgE; (2) stimulation of new B and T cells to further diversify the immune response. After the specific IgE is formed, it will interact with a cell containing an IgE receptor.

REEXPOSURE

Upon reexposure, the allergen (antigen) will interact with allergen-specific IgE on the surfaces of cells, which will initiate the release of inflammatory mediators. It appears that intracellular adhesion molecules 1 (ICAM-1), vascular cell adhesion molecules 1 (VCAM-1), and endothelial cell adhesion molecules 1 (ELAM-1) are involved in airway inflammation. The end-organ response to these and other mediators will result in the clinical picture of asthma and allergy.

Clearly, each of these activities must be coordinated to produce asthma. It is equally clear that there are a multitude of steps where the process can be enhanced or attenuated. Many of these steps are under genetic control and many involve environmental interactions. While the specificity of each step may be relatively low, the overall specificity is much greater as a result of sequential gating of independent points of recognition. By studying this proposed mechanism, researchers should be able to define the biology of asthma and allergies further and develop an understanding of the genetics involved. With this blueprint of the development of asthma identified we then should be able to answer the three questions about asthma posed by British biostatistician Bradford Hill[16]: (1) What is wrong? (2) What's going to happen? and (3) What can be done about it?

Genetic Studies of Asthma

Early studies presented evidence of a hereditary factor in asthma.[1,2] Defining the phenotype to be studied has been difficult. Researchers have attempted to define phenotypes clinically, biochemically, and genetically. In view of the problem of pleiotropism (multiple effects of a single mutant gene) and genetic heterogeneity, there has been a tendency among investigators studying the genetics of asthma to fall into one of two groups: "lumpers" and "splitters." Initially the lumpers were more common. They used complex phenotypes to study the genetics of asthma. One of the major problems in studying asthma in this manner is defining the phenotype to be used. Most phenotypes of asthma have consisted of symptoms of coughing, wheezing, and shortness of breath as well as evidence of bronchial hyperreactivity demonstrated by reversibility and/or a bronchial challenge with an agent such as histamine or methacholine. Others have suggested using IgE responsiveness as a parameter. Morton[17] defines asthma as a disorder characterized by wheezing and bronchial hyperresponsiveness, for which atopy is the major cause. Atopy is defined as a condition characterized by a persistent and a heritable IgE response to protein allergens. Using these definitions, the two traits are correlated and multivariate, including total and specific IgE titer, skin prick tests, medical history, and tests of bronchial reactivity.[17] Studies by Burrows et al.[18] and Sears et al.[19] have stressed the relationship between IgE concentrations and asthma, whether the latter is defined as atopic or idiopathic (intrinsic). They have presented evidence that there may be a major gene for asthma that is different than the gene for IgE. We have found that IgE concentrations are increased in patients with asthma along with an increased specific *Amb a* V IgE response. Further studies have indicated, when subjects were selected with regard to their HLA DR2 haplotypes, that ragweed-sensitive specific *Amb a* V responders have greater IgE concentrations than ragweed-sensitive *Amb a* V–negative individuals and a normal control population.[20]

Early studies used the complex phenotype of asthma to study its genetics. Although they identified that asthma had heritability, its mode of inheritance and characterization of the gene(s) involved were not possible with the knowledge and methods available at that time. Because of the complexity of the phenotype of asthma and lack of agreement regarding its definition, many investigators became so-called splitters and used the less complex, or intermediate, phenotypes to study asthma, such as the specific immune response, IgE regulation, mediator release, and end-organ responses.

INTERMEDIATE PHENOTYPES

SPECIFIC IMMUNE RESPONSE

The specific immune response has been studied and its overall mechanism defined. Studies of the specific immune response should involve using an allergen that is well defined with regard to size, structures, sequence, epitopes, and binding capacity to T- and B-cell sites. The smaller and fewer the epitopes, the better the allergen is for study. Ragweed has been used as one of the models to study the immune response in atopic conditions. It contains at least 55 allergens, of which approximately 22 have been reported to be important clinically and bind to IgE.[21,22] One of the major purified allergens of short ragweed is *Amb a* I, with a molecular weight of 35,000.[23] *Amb a* V, the smallest ragweed allergen identified, has been used to characterize the specific immune response. It has a molecular weight of 4500 and has been sequenced and shown to have 45 amino acids. Its structure is known. At least three epitopes that bind to immunoglobulins have been identified. The binding capacity for *Amb a* V IgE antibodies ranges from 0.9×10^{-10} to 26×10^{-10}, compared to 1×10^{-7} for *Amb a* V IgG. It also has been demonstrated that in the same individual, different epitopes can bind to different immunoglobulin groups, that is, the epitope for binding IgE may be different from that for IgG in the same individual. Using the ragweed system, early studies by Levine et al. demonstrated that *Amb a* I was associated with the HLA system.[24] Blumenthal et al. also showed that *Amb a* I was linked with the HLA system.[25] Because of its large size and multiple epitopes, *Amb a* V then was studied. It has been noted to be associated strongly with HLA DR2 *1500.[26] The β chain appears to be the chain needed for presentation.[27] In addition, it also has been shown that *Amb a* V from short, giant, and false ragweed was associated with HLA DR2, although the three types of *Amb a* V are immunologically different.[23] Atopic *Amb a* V–sensitive and nonsensitive DR2-positive individuals do not differ with regard to their sequence, suggesting that *Amb a* V responders have no unique sequences with regard to the HLA DR2 loci.[28] Therefore, it appears that the immune response to *Amb a* V requires involvement of the HLA DR system but that other factors are also involved.

Other purified allergens have been found to be associated with HLA class II allergens, including those of olive (*Ole* I), giant ragweed (*Amb t* V), and rye grass (*Lol p* I).[23] There is growing evidence that the specific immune response is associated with the HLA system, specifically the DR region. The presence of a particular DR-associated class II molecule appears to provide a necessary, but not the only, condition for responsiveness to that particular epitope.

The next step in the immune response involves the interaction of the HLA class II allergen complex from the APC interacting with the T-cell receptors. The arrangement of TCR elements on the α and β chains also appears to determine the antigen specificity of the T cell. Renz et al. demonstrated in mice that specific V β-expressing T-cell subpopulations are involved in the stimulation of IgE/IgG1 production and increased airway responsiveness.[29] Recently, Moffatt et al. suggested genetic linkage of TCR α/δ complex to the specific IgE responses.[30] These studies suggest that chromosome 14 may be important in the specific atopic response.

IgE REGULATION

The phenotype of IgE regulation has been investigated genetically. Current understanding of the immune system suggests that the upregulation of IgE synthesis in atopy is due to the induction of IgE isotope utilization at the DNA level in B cells. IgE synthesis appears to involve signals following direct T cell–B cell interaction. One is delivered by an IgE isotype-specific signal, provided by the activated CD4 T cell or T$_H$2 cell–derived IL-4. Others are the CD40 ligand (CD40-L) and FcεRII B-cell activation signal, which requires the engagement of the TCR with antigenic fragments (peptides) that are recognized with the MHC class II molecules on APC. IFN-γ appears to downregulate IgE synthesis.[14]

Serum IgE level heritability has been demonstrated in twins, families, and population studies. A major gene appears to be involved. The mode of inheritance and location of the gene has not been well delineated.[11]

Studies by Marsh et al.[31] and Meyers et al.[32] presented evidence suggesting that one of the genes involved in the synthesis of IgE regulation is located on 5q 31.1. Subsequent work performed elsewhere did not confirm these findings.[33] No HLA associations with serum IgE concentrations have been adequately demonstrated.

IgE RECEPTORS

The IgE receptors recently have been studied regarding their genetics. High-affinity receptors on basophils and mast cells and low-affinity receptors on eosinophils and lymphocytes have been identified and characterized. Sandford[34] and Shirakawa[35] from the same group reported that the gene regulating the β chain of the high-affinity receptor for IgE (FcεRII-β) is on chromosome 11q. This finding has not been confirmed. Other candidate genes for study include those for the low-affinity IgE receptor (FcεRII-β) and its ligand CD40.

ALLERGEN/IgE RECEPTOR INTERACTION AND MEDIATOR RELEASE

The mechanisms of the interactions of IgE with IgE receptors and allergens and the regulation of the release of mediators and cytokines are just being characterized. The genetics of the regulation of the release of mediators or cytokines involving the interaction of IgE with cells and their ability to release mediating substances also have not been extensively investigated. A variety of mast cell mediators have been investigated, including secretory granule preformed mediators (e.g., histamine, heparin, tryptase), cytokines (i.e., IL-4, IL-5, IL-6), and lipid mediators (e.g., leukotriene B4, leukotriene C4, prostaglandin D_2). In a twin study by Marone et al.[36] and a nuclear family study by Roitman-Johnson and Blumethal,[37] the phenotype of histamine release following the anti-IgE challenge of peripheral blood basophils has been noted to have heritability.

END-ORGAN RESPONSE

The pathogenesis of the end-organ response also has not been well defined. The genetic polymorphism of the β_2-adrenergic receptors was investigated and showed no evidence of a genetic defect in asthma.[38] Bronchial hyperreactivity (BHR), one of the main end-organ responses studied in asthma, is poorly defined genetically. Bronchial reactivity may be a result of different steps ranging from the stimulus; receptors; state of the smooth muscle; and airway characteristics including its circumference, external diameters, wall thickness, and secretion. Familial factors have been reported to be involved in the development of bronchial hyperresponsiveness, defined principally as the bronchial response to methacholine and histamine inhalation challenge. Many studies have provided evidence of heritability of bronchial hyperreactivity, but there is distinct heterogeneity.[39,40] The chromosomal region 5q 31-33 has been suggested to be important in the regulation of BHR in allergy and asthma.[40]

INFLAMMATION

The mechanisms involved in the inflammatory response in asthma and its genetics are just being studied. New factors influencing inflammation, such as chemical mediators (i.e., cytokines) and cell adhesion molecules, as well as other mediators of the inflammatory response (i.e., heat shock proteins) have been identified, characterized, and localized to specific chromosomal regions. The activation of transcription factors as well as the roles of transforming growth factor β (TGF-β), epidermal growth factor (EGF), ICAM, CD-23, HLA DR, tumor necrosis factor γ (TNF-γ), IL-10, IL-4, and IL-5 are a few of the many areas being studied that may be involved in the development of asthma.[41]

SUMMARY

There are many steps hypothesized for the development of asthma. It is evident that the specific immune response to certain aeroallergens is genetically influenced by a gene(s) located on chromosome 6 at the DR locus. The T-cell receptors may play a role in the specific IgE response. Regulation of IgE is heritable and due to a major gene. Its mode of inheritance and the characterization of the gene or genes involved are under intense study, especially on chromosome 5q, but at the present time the location is unknown. The IgERI receptor for IgE has been suggested[34,35] to be under genetic control on chromosome 11q and related to the development of atopy. Histamine release and BHR appear to have heritability, but their mode of inheritance and whether there is a major gene involved and where it is located are not known at the present time. A recent study suggests chromosome 5 may be involved.[40] Phenotypes of the inflammatory processes in asthma are being studied.

COMPLEX PHENOTYPES

It has been recognized for many years that the general expression of the complex phenotype of asthma and allergic diseases is familial. The first serious modern study of the heritability of asthma and hayfever was undertaken by Cook and Vander Veer in 1916.[9] These and other early investigators emphasized the familial nature of asthma and atopic diseases and provided evidence of a genetic predisposition. Depending upon the study, as many as 40 to 80 percent of patients with allergic rhinitis or bronchial asthma have been noted to have a positive family history of allergy, as opposed to 20 percent or fewer of nonallergic individuals with a positive family history. There is no question that there is heritability of asthma. The problem of definition of phenotypes in these early studies is apparent. Recently, investigators have been attempting to study the complex phenotypes of diseases such as atopy and asthma using updated parameters and more sophisticated molecular genetic and statistical approaches to their analyses.[10]

ATOPY

Atopy may be defined using a variety of parameters including those of IgE responses. It has been estimated that 10 to 30 percent of the general population has some form of atopic disease. Cookson et al. investigated families by looking not only at total serum IgE concentrations but also at the specific IgE response to allergens as determined by skin testing and a radioallergosorbent test (RAST) in patients with asthma and allergic rhinitis.[42] They defined atopy as an increased serum IgE concentration and/or an increased specific IgE as measured by RAST or skin test. They suggested that atopy, as defined by the ability to produce IgE response using several parameters, is inherited as an autosomal dominant trait and is linked to chromosome 11q. Similar linkage was suggested by Collee et al.,[43] Shirakawa et al.,[44] and Hizawa et al.[45] Rich et al. investigated the same complex phenotypes of atopy with respect to their genetics and environmental determinants.[46] Using several phenotypes including that of Cookson et al.,[42] no evidence for linkage was found in three large pedigrees using the dominant mode of inheritance. In separate studies, Lympany et al.,[47,48] Hizawa et al.,[45] Brereton et al.,[49] and Amelung et al.[50] also could not confirm the observations of Cookson et al.[42] More recently, Cookson et al. suggested that the 11q13-linked atopy gene is inherited preferentially from the maternal side, possibly due to either paternal genetic imprinting or maternal modification of the infants' IgE responses through the placenta or breast milk.[51] These studies have not been confirmed by other groups.

ASTHMA

It has been estimated that between 5 and 15 percent of the general population has asthma.[52] The incidence varies with definition and geographic location. The complex phenotype of asthma has been investigated with regard to its genetics and relationship to known genetic markers. One of the major problems of studying asthma is the definition of the phenotype that should be used. As already discussed, most phenotypes of asthma have consisted of symptoms as well as evidence of bronchial hyperreactivity, while others have suggested using IgE levels as a parameter. Evidence has been presented that there may be a major gene for asthma that is different than the gene for IgE.[40]

Investigation of markers on chromosome 6 has yielded conflicting results regarding the location of the gene regulating asthma.[10,15,53] Thorsby,[54] Morris,[55] and Turner[56] all noted an increase in HLA B8 associated with asthma. On the other hand, Rachelefsky et al.[57] found an increase in HLA A2 but a decrease in HLA B8 in patients with bronchial asthma. Geerts and Bruce[58] found no changes in the B8 frequencies in asthma. These studies stress the importance of having a well-defined phenotype. In view of the problems of defining asthma, investigators directed their attention to phenotypes involving known triggers of asthma.

The phenotype of mite-sensitive allergic asthma has been investigated in relationship with HLA antigens. Caraballo and Hernandez studied HLA haplotype segregation in families with mite-sensitive allergic asthma.[59] They studied 20 families with allergic asthma and *Dermatophagoides fariniae* sensitivity and 8 families with intrinsic or nonallergic asthma. Genetic analysis was performed using the means of affected sib pair method. Their results suggest the existence of an HLA-linked recessive gene controlling the IgE immune responsiveness to mite allergens and conferring susceptibility to allergic asthma. Associations of other specific triggers, such as aspirin-induced asthma, have been reported with antigens of the HLA system.[60,61]

The general expression of certain diseases has been associated with the presence of the extended HLA haplotypes. It is suggested that different extended haplotypes contain a different pattern of chromosomal deletions and insertions, some of which may influence the level of gene expression. As a result, certain combinations of alleles, especially of the D/DR and complement loci, are seen to be highly associated with a disease. We have studied the association of ragweed allergic rhinitis and bronchial asthma with the extended HLA haplotype.[11] Total serum IgE concentrations and titers of IgE specific anti-*Amb a* V were measured in 144 patients with ragweed pollen allergy. MHC haplotypes were determined for 50 of these patients and 28 nonatopic controls.

Total IgE concentrations were unimodally distributed in all study groups and were greater in the atopic patients in general compared with nonatopic individuals. Although anti-*Amb a* V IgE concentrations were all low in the nonatopic patient population, a group within the atopic group had high concentrations of IgE *Amb a* V. It was noted that those with asthma had distinctly higher concentrations than those with rhinitis only and the nonatopic population. When the HLA loci were analyzed, it was noted that the frequencies of HLA-DR2 and the extended MHC haplotype B7, SC31, DR2 were significantly increased among the patients with asthma and high titers of IgE anti-*Amb a* V. Conversely, this group had decreased frequencies of HLA-DR3 and the extended haplotype HLA B8, SC01, DR3 compared with patients with only rhinitis; the latter group had an increased number of individuals with the extended haplotype HLA B8, SC01, DR3 and low levels of IgE *Amb a* V. These findings are consistent with a dominant MHC-linked gene or genes on

HLA B7, SC31, DR2 controlling the IgE immune response to *Amb a* V and predisposing to asthma. Other chromosomal regions which have been suggested to be involved in the development of the complex disease of asthma include TNF-α on chromosome 6,[62] cystic fibrosis regulator factor on chromosome 7,[63] and allotype[64] and gene variants for α-antitrypsin on chromosome 14.[65]

Benefits of Understanding the Genetics of Asthma

With a better understanding of the genetics of asthma we can start to answer the three questions raised by the British biostatistician Bradford Hill.[16]

1. What is wrong? As a result of genetic studies, researchers will be better able to understand the underlying biology of asthma and redefine asthma in terms of its genetic basis. The diagnostic armamentarium will increase greatly. Accurate diagnosis is important and will be enhanced by chromosomal and biochemical methods. Asthma most likely is a disease of many different phenotypes based on different genetic mechanisms and pathways.
2. What's going to happen? Risk estimates can be obtained regarding the occurrence of asthma as well as its severity based on the proper characterization of the disease. Potentially, researchers will be able to predict whether—and how severely—a person may suffer from asthma before he or she develops it. Even though there is agreement that these findings would be very helpful, much controversy has developed over the benefits of genetic studies. Many do not agree that human beings are constructed from "blueprints" that we can learn to read. It has been stated that we can never make predictions because we will never know enough. This is because development is dialectical and not linear. What happens to a person all along the way, and what that person makes happen, may continuously affect her or his biologic, psychological, and social growth as well as the development of conditions such as asthma. In addition, other individuals point out that having this information, although it can provide a benefit, is not without a cost. The question of a threat to one's civil liberties is being discussed. Can this information be used against an affected individual? Will it prevent a person from acquiring insurance? It has been stated that "Genetic privacy will be the major constitutional issue of the next generation."[66]
3. What are we going to do about it? This will involve asthma management ranging from programs of prevention, such as gene manipulation, to those involving the interference with pathways activated by this environmental-genetic interaction. This type of treatment has generated a great deal of discussion. Although most individuals favor this variety of treatment, others feel that altering the human gene and its actions is against the will of God. Many ethical questions will arise. It has been suggested that the equating of genetic prediction with prevention at this time may not be valid.[66]

Despite arguments against genetic studies, this knowledge is giving us needed information to understand asthma and allergies and to manage individuals in a rational way using methods of prevention and active treatment. Prevention may involve genetic counseling, gene therapy, and interference with disease-producing pathways, as well as avoidance of known high-risk environmental factors for individuals who are themselves at high risk. Once the gene(s), gene product(s), and the pathways involved are identified, we should be able to prevent or reverse the progress of the disease. The affected individuals, once in possession of all the available information, can then decide how they wish to proceed.

References

1. Silverstein A: *The History of Immunology*. San Diego, Academic Press, 1989.
2. Unger L: *The History of Bronchial Asthma*. Springfield, IL, Charles C. Thomas, 1945.
3. Major R: *A History of Medicine*, vol 2. Springfield, IL, Charles C. Thomas, 1954.
4. Blackley CH: Experimental researches on the causes and nature of *catarrhus aestivus* (hay fever or hay asthma). London, Baillière, Tindall and Cox, 1873.
5. Blackley CH: Hayfever: Its causes, treatment and effective prevention, in Blackley CH (ed): *Experimental Research*, 2d ed. London; Baillière, Tindall and Cox, 1880.
6. Maltzer SJ: Bronchial asthma as a phenomenon of anaphylaxis. *JAMA* 1910; 55:102.
7. Ishizaka K, Ishizaka T: Physiochemical properties of reaginic antibody: I. Association of reaginic activity with an immunoglobulin other than γA- or γG-globulin. *J Allergy* 1966; 37:169.
8. Ishizaka K, Ishizaka T: Physiochemical properties of reaginic antibody: III. Further studies on the reaginic antibody in γA-globulin preparation. *J Allergy* 1966; 38:108.
9. Cooke RA, Vander Veer A: Human sensitization. *J Immunol* 1916; 1:201.
10. Blumenthal MN, Björkstén B (eds): *Genetics of Allergy and Asthma: Methods for Investigative Studies*. New York, Marcel Dekker. In press, 1996.
11. Blumenthal MN, Bonini S: Immunogenetics of specific immune responses to allergens in twins and families, in Marsh DG, Blumenthal MN (eds): *Genetic and Environmental Factors in Clinical Allergy*. Minneapolis, University of Minnesota Press, 1990; 132.
12. Rich S: Human genetics, in Blumenthal MN, Björkstén B (eds): *Genetics of Allergy and Asthma: Methods for Investigative Studies*. New York; Marcel Dekker. In press, 1996.
13. Abbas AK, Lichtman AH, Pober JS: *Cellular and Molecular Immunology*. Philadelphia, Saunders, 1991.
14. Sutton BJ, Gould HJ: The human IgE network. *Nature* 1993; 66:421.
15. Blumenthal MN: Family, twin and population studies of allergic responsiveness, in Marsh DG, Lockhart A, Holgate S (eds): *The Genetics of Asthma*. Oxford, Blackwell Scientific, 1993; 133.
16. McKusick VA, Claiborne R: Introduction in, *Medical Genetics*. New York, HP Publishing, 1973.
17. Morton N: Statistical methods, in Blumenthal MN, Björkstén B (eds): *Genetics of Allergy and Asthma: Methods for Investigative Studies*. New York, Marcel Dekker. In press, 1996.
18. Burrows B, Martinez F, et al.: Association of asthma with serum IgE level and skin test reactivity to allergens. *N Engl J Med* 1989; 320:271.
19. Sears M, Burrows B, Flannery G, et al.: Relationship between airway responsiveness and serum IgE in children with asthma and in apparently normal children. *N Engl J Med* 1991; 325:1067.
20. Blumenthal MN, Marcus-Bagley D, Adweh Z, et al.: Extended major: HLA-DR2 [HLA B-7, SC31, DR3] haplotypes distinguish subjects with asthma from those with only rhinitis in ragweed pollen allergy. *J Immunol* 1992; 411.
21. Lowenstein H, Marsh DG: Antigens of *Ambrosia elatior* (short ragweed) pollen: I. Cross immunoelectrophoretic analysis. *J Immunol* 1981; 126:943.
22. Lowenstein H, Marsh DG: Antigens of *Ambrosia elatior* (short ragweed) pollen: III. Cross radioimmunoelectrophoresis of ragweed and allergic patients' sera with special attention to quantifications of IgE response. *J Immunol* 1983; 130:727.
23. Marsh DG: Immunogenetic and immunochemical factors determining immune responsiveness to allergens: Studies in unrelated subjects, in Marsh DG, Blumenthal MN (eds): *Genetic and Environmental Factors in Clinical Allergy*. Minneapolis, University of Minnesota Press, 1990; 97.
24. Levine B, Stember R, Fontino M: Ragweed hayfever: Genetic control and linkage to HLA haplotypes. *Science*. 198:1201.
25. Blumenthal MN, Amos DB, Noreen H, et al.: Genetic mapping of Ir locus in man: Linkage to second locus of HLA. *Science* 1974; 184:1301.
26. Marsh DG, Blumenthal MN, Ishikawa T, et al.: HLA and specific immune responsiveness to allergens, in Tsuji K, Aizawa M, Sasazuki T (eds): *HLA 1991: Proceedings of the 11th International Histocompatibility Workshop*. New York, Oxford University Press, 1992; 765.
27. Huang S, Zwollo P, Marsh DG: Class II major histocompatibility complex restriction of human T cell responses to short ragweed allergen *Amb a* V. *Eur J Immunol* 1991; 21:1469.
28. Zwollo P, Ehrlich Kautzky E, Scharf S, et al.: Sequences of HLA D in responders and nonresponders to short ragweed *Amb a* V. *Immunogenetics* 1991; 33:141.
29. Renz H, Saloga J, Bradley KL, et al: Specific V β T cell subsets mediate the immediate hypersensitivity response to ragweed allergy. *J Immunol* 1993; 151:1907.
30. Moffatt M, Mill M, Cornelis F, et al.: Genetic linkage of T cell receptors and α-δ complex to specific IgE response. *Lancet* 1994; 343:1597.
31. Marsh DG, Needly J, Breazeale D, et al.: Linkage analysis of IL4 and other chromosomes Sq31, 1 markers and total serum immunoglobulin E concentration. *Science* 1994; 264:1152.
32. Meyers DA, Postma DS, Panhuysen CIM, et al.: Evidence for a locus regulating total serum IgE levels mapping to chromosome 5. *Genomics* 1994; 23:464.
33. Blumenthal MN, Wang Z, Weber J, Rich S. Absence of linkage between 5q markers and serum IgE levels in four large atopic families. *Clin Exp Allergy* 1996; 26: In press.
34. Sandford AO, Shirakawa TS, Moffatt M: Localization of atopy and the β sub-unit of the high-affinity IgE receptor (FcϵR1) on chromosome 11q. *Lancet* 1993; 341:332.
35. Shirakawa T, Airong L, Dubowitz M, et al: Association between atopy and variants of the β sub unit of the high-affinity immunoglobulin E receptor. *Nat Genet* 1984; 7:125.
36. Marone G, Poto S, Celestino D, Bonino S: Human basophil releasability: III. Genetic controls of the human basophil releasability. *J Immunol* 1986; 137:3588.
37. Roitman-Johnson B, Blumenthal MN: Family analysis of histamine release (abstract). *J Allergy Clin Immunol* 1988; 81: 232.
38. Reishaus E, Innis M, MacIntyre N, Liggett S: Mutation in the

gene encoding for the β 2 adrenergic receptor in normal and asthma subjects. *Am J Respir Cell Mol Biol* 1993; 8:334.

39. Hopp RJ, Nair NM, Bewtra AK, Townley RG: Genetic aspects of bronchial hyperreactivity, in Marsh DG, Blumenthal MN (eds): *Genetic and Environmental Factors in Clinical Allergy*. Minneapolis, University of Minnesota Press, 1990; 143.

40. Bleecker EW: Bronchial hyperreactivity, in Blumenthal MN, Björkstén B (eds): *Genetics of Allergy and Asthma: Methods for Investigative Studies*. New York, Marcel Dekker. In press 1996.

41. Lympany P, Lee TH: Inflammation, in Blumenthal MN, Björkstén B (eds): *Genetics of Allergy and Asthma: Methods for Investigative Studies*. New York, Marcel Dekker. In press 1996.

42. Cookson WOCM, Sharp PA, Faux JA, Hoplin JM: Linkage between immunoglobulin E responses underlying asthma and rhinitis and chromosome 11q. *Lancet* 1989; 1:1292.

43. Collee JM, ten Kate LP, de Vries, et al.: Allele sharing on chromosome 11q in sibs with asthma and atopy. *Lancet* 1993; 342:936.

44. Shirakawa T, Hashimoto T, Furuyama J, Morimoto K: Linkage between severe atopy and chromosome 11q13 in Japanese families. *Clin Genet* 1994; 46:228.

45. Hizawa N, Yamaguchi E, Ohe M, et al.: Lack of linkage between atopy and locus 11q13. *Clin Exp Allergy* 1992; 22:1065.

46. Rich SS, Roitman-Johnson B, Greenberg B, et al.: Genetic analysis of atopy in three large kindreds: No evidence of linkage to D11S97. *Clin Exp Allergy* 1992; 22:1070.

47. Lympany P, Welsh K, MacCochrane G, et al.: Genetic analysis using DNA polymorphism of the linkage between chromosome 11q13 and atopy and bronchial hyperresponsiveness to methacholine. *J Allergy Clin Immunol* 1992; 89:619.

48. Lympany P, Welsh KI, Cochrane GM, et al.: Genetic analysis of the linkage between chromosome 11q and atopy. *Clin Exp Allergy* 1992; 22:1085.

49. Brereton HM, Ruffin RW, Thompson PJ, Turner DR: Familial atopy in Australian pedigrees: Adventitious linkage to chromosome 8 is not confirmed nor is there evidence of linkage to high-affinity IgE receptor. *Clin Exp Allergy* 1994; 24:868.

50. Amelung PJ, Panhuysen CIM, Postma DS, et al.: Atopy and bronchial hyperresponsiveness: Exclusion of linkage to markers on chromosomes 11q and 6q. *Clin Exp Allergy* 1992; 22:1077.

51. Cookson WOCM, Young RP, Sandford AJ, et al.: Maternal inheritance of atopic responsiveness on chromosome 11q. *Lancet* 1992; 340:381.

52. Friedhoff LR: Epidemiology of atopic allergy, in Marsh DG, Blumenthal MN (eds): *Genetic and Environmental Factors in Clinical Allergy*. Minneapolis, University of Minnesota Press, 1990; 53.

53. DeWeck AL, Blumenthal MN, Yunis E, Jeannet M: HLA and allergy, in Dausset J (ed): *HLA and Disease*. Copenhagen, Munksgaard, 1977; 196.

54. Thorsby E, Lie SO: Relationship between the HLA system and susceptibility to disease. *Transplant Proc* 1971; 1305.

55. Morris MJ, Vaughan H, Lane DJ, Morris PJ: HLA in asthma, in deWeck AL, Blumenthal MN (eds): *HLA and Allergy: Monographs in Allergy II*. Basel, New York, Karger, 1977; 30.

56. Turner MN, Brostoff J, Wells SR, Soothill JF: Histocompatibility antigens in atopy with special reference to eczema and hayfever, in deWeck AL, Blumenthal MN (eds): *HLA and Allergy: Monographs in Allergy II*. Basel, New York, Karger, 1977; 19.

57. Rachelefsky GS, Teraski PI, Katz RM, Siegel SC: β-lymphocyte and histocompatibility antigens in extrinsic asthma, in deWeck AL, Blumenthal MN (eds): *HLA and Allergy: Monographs in Allergy II*. Basel, New York, Karger, 1977; 35.

58. Geerts SJ, Pöttgens H, Limburg M, van Rood JJ: Predisposition for atopy or allergy linked to HLA. *Lancet* 1975; 1:461.

59. Caraballo LR, Hernandez M: HLA haplotype segregation in families with allergic asthma. *Tissue Antigens* 1990; 35:182.

60. Krishnamoorthy R: HLA class II haplotypes in aspirin-induced asthma, in Marsh DG, Lockhart A, Holgate ST (eds): *The Genetics of Asthma*. Oxford, Blackwell Scientific Publications, 1993; 223.

61. Lympany P, Welsh KI, Christie PE, et al.: An analysis with sequence-specific oligonucleotide probes of the association between aspirin-induced asthma and antigens of the HLA system. *J Allergy Clin Immunol* 1993; 92:114.

62. Morrison J: Class III MHC polymorphisms and asthma in, *Genetics of Asthma*. Worcestershire, 1995.

63. Schroeder SA, Gaughan DM, Swift M: Protection against bronchial asthma by CFTR-δ 508 mutation: A heterozygote advantage in cystic fibrosis. *Nature Med* 1995; 1:703.

64. Colp CR, Lieberman J: Asthma and alpha-1 antitrypsin, in Weiss EB, Stein M (eds): *Bronchial Asthma: Mechanisms and Therapeutics*, 3rd ed. Boston; Little, Brown, 1993:1185.

65. Max EE: Immunoglobulins: Molecular genetics, in Paul WE (ed): *Fundamental Immunology*, 2nd ed. New York; Raven Press, 1989: 235.

66. Elmer-Dewitt P: The genetic revolution. *Time Magazine* 1994; 143:46.

Chapter 75 _____

THE EPIDEMIOLOGY OF ASTHMA

EUGENE F. GEPPERT

Introduction

The epidemiology of asthma is the field of study concerned with the factors that influence the frequency and distribution of asthma in the population. The epidemiologist follows trends in health statistics and tries to identify specific risk factors that play a role in causing asthma or in making it more prevalent or severe. Epidemiology also concerns itself with the economic costs of asthma to society. Most recently, epidemiology has extended its concern to discover the impact of asthma on the quality of life of patients with the disease. In the near future, it will be the responsibility of epidemiologic studies to determine whether the United States is reaching its set goals for reducing asthma morbidity and mortality by the year 2000.[1]

Epidemiologic studies are most successful when the disease being studied is easily defined and it has a unique biologic marker. Unfortunately, asthma has so far resisted easy definition, and it has no unique biologic marker. For this reason, the literature on the epidemiology of asthma suffers from nonuniformity and sometimes vagueness that makes comparisons between statistics from different geographic regions impossible. However, despite the limits imposed by an imprecise definition, epidemiologic studies from the last several decades have detected trends that are useful in guiding health policy.

Because there is no universal definition of asthma, individual epidemiologic investigators have defined asthma separately for different purposes, the so-called operational definition. In the previous decade, there was hope that bronchial hyperresponsiveness might turn out to be a biologic marker for asthma. Bronchial hyperresponsiveness is an increase above normal in both the ease and magnitude of airway narrowing on exposure to a number of nonsensitizing bronchoconstrictive stimuli, such as histamine, methacholine, or cold, dry air.[2] Epidemiologic studies that have used field tests of bronchial hyperresponsiveness have now shown conclusively that many people with bronchial hyperresponsiveness do not have asthmalike symptoms. The converse is also found in population studies: many children and adults with asthmalike symptoms do not have bronchial hyperresponsiveness. Yet another factor that must be considered in the definition of asthma is the possibility that a patient might be in remission during the time of an epidemiologic study. Current asthma must be distinguished from asthma that is not currently active. Recently, Toelle and associates[3] proposed a melding of these characteristics for an operational definition of asthma that would be useful in epidemiology: current asthma is the presence of symptomatic bronchial hyperresponsiveness. Among the symptoms most common in the patients with asthma defined in this way are wheezing and nocturnal cough.

This chapter reviews the literature on the epidemiology of asthma and discusses the factors that may incite and influence the course of asthma.

Terminology in the Epidemiology of Asthma

The most important event in the natural history of asthma is the event that converts the patients from nonasthmatic to asthmatic. Almost nothing currently is known about this event, sometimes called "sensitization" or "inception." Because one of the aims of epidemiology in asthma is to provide data that allow hypotheses to be formed about inception, much attention is exerted on events that happen to a patient at the time of inception, which for most patients is early childhood.

Other terms that are useful to define in this discussion include incidence, prevalence, morbidity, mortality, and some of the unique ratios that provide the basic units of measurement in epidemiology.

The *incidence of asthma* is the number of new cases beginning during a specified interval of time. For example, Butcher and associates[4] prospectively studied a group of workers exposed to the chemical toluene diisocyante and found an incidence of 0.8 cases per 100 workers per year. Studies of the incidence of asthma are few in number.

The *prevalence of asthma* is the number of cases that exist in a population at a given point in time. The *cumulative prevalence* of asthma refers to the number of people in a population who have ever had asthma and includes patients with current wheeze and patients who are in remission. Studies of the prevalence of asthma are abundant, but most have suffered from the limitations imposed by the methods of data collection and lack of a uniform definition. For example, studies of cumulative prevalence may turn out to be inaccu-

rate due to the difficulty of persons with a remote history of asthma to recall their illness. Because human memory is limited, a practical solution has been to ask about asthma prevalence during the previous year.[5] There are other types of prevalence besides cumulative prevalence. *Point prevalence* is the number of cases existing in a population at a point in time. *Period prevalence* is the number of cases existing during a specified interval of time. In asthma epidemiology, it is common to use a standard questionnaire to measure the cumulative presence of asthma and the period prevalence of symptoms (typically, wheeze during the previous year). If the questionnaire asks a question such as, "Has a doctor ever diagnosed you to have asthma?", the goal is to gather data on cumulative prevalence, because the patient is asked to consider a lifetime. If the epidemiologic investigation involves a visit to the site of a population with measurement of bronchial challenge testing or spirometry, these measurements happen on a single day of the patient's life, and therefore only provide insight into the point prevalence of asthma. It should not be surprising that the results of cumulative prevalence of asthma, period prevalence of symptoms, and point prevalence of bronchial hyperresponsiveness often do not coincide.

The morbidity of asthma in the epidemiologic sense of the word refers to all of the nonfatal consequences of the disease on the patient and on society. The morbidity of asthma includes the economic costs of time lost from school and work, hospitalizations, and other usage of health-care resources. The new epidemiologic field that examines quality of life is related to morbidity. This field measures the impact of the disease on the patient's life or on the family.

The mortality of asthma refers to deaths in which asthma was listed as a major cause of death. A major concern of epidemiologists who study mortality is the accuracy of the diagnosis listed on death certificates.

In epidemiologic studies, the results usually are expressed as statistics. A major purpose of epidemiology is to make associations between diseases and possible risk factors. The strength of such an association is based on odds ratios. For example, some epidemiologic studies of asthma have examined the usefulness of a test of bronchial hyperresponsiveness, such as a methacholine inhalation test, for detecting cases of asthma in a population. Tests such as this are examined by epidemiologists for their sensitivity, specificity, positive predictive value, negative predictive value, and accuracy. These terms are defined in Table 75-1.

In general, too little is known about asthma to allow categorization into subtypes. However, occupational asthma is

TABLE 75-1 Definitions of Terms Used to Assess Diagnostic Tests in Epidemiology

Sensitivity = true positives/(true positives + false negatives)
Specificity = true negatives/(true negatives + false positives)
Positive predictive value = true positives/all positives
Negative predictive value = true negatives/all negatives
Accuracy = (true positives + true negatives/all tested

often given a separate definition. Occupational asthma, as defined by Smith,[6] has six criteria:

1. The asthma is characterized by variable airway obstruction; there should be symptoms which may include shortness of breath, wheezing, chest tightness, and cough. The asthma needs to be persistent and not related to an isolated chemical spill, viral illness, heart failure, or other causes.
2. A known occupational asthma provoking agent must be present in the workplace.
3. There must be exposure to this agent for a sufficient time for hyperreactivity to develop.
4. Pulmonary function tests must show airway obstruction after exposure to a specific agent in the actual or recreated environment, either at work or by provocation challenge.
5. The asthmatic condition usually develops when inhaling low concentrations of the specific agent (far below the threshold limit value set for the irritant effect of that agent).
6. Symptomatic improvement occurs in many cases when the patient is away form the workplace and there is a return of symptoms during the workday or workweek.

Methods Used in Studying the Epidemiology of Asthma

Methods used in asthma epidemiology have focused mainly on three variables: symptoms, variable airway obstruction, and airway hyperresponsiveness; these all can occur independently of each other. Another domain of asthma epidemiology includes ongoing studies of incidence, prevalence, health-care utilization, morbidity, and mortality. Finally, methods used to study risk factors in asthma may reveal valuable epidemiologic clues; these include studies of atopy, the indoor environment, the outdoor environment, and the workplace.

QUESTIONNAIRES IN POPULATION STUDIES

No questionnaire has been written that is capable of identifying accurately patients with asthma. Instead, the best that a questionnaire can hope to achieve is to identify the group of persons in the study population who have either asthma or asthmalike symptoms. Questionnaires for detecting asthma and asthmalike symptoms in adults have been reviewed recently.[7] In evaluating the results of a questionnaire during its field testing, it must be compared to some other measure, such as a test of bronchial hyperresponsiveness or a clinical diagnosis of asthma. The best method for identifying subjects with asthma when a questionnaire is undergoing validation is to use a combination of a clinical physiologic investigation, such as a methacholine inhalation test, and a clinical judgment of the symptoms. It seems clear that the questionnaires that are currently available are too limited because one of the best potential uses of a questionnaire in epidemiologic studies is to study the incidence of asthma, and special questions relating to the timing of onset of the disease are currently lacking. Questions relating to the

quality of the patient's life or to acculturation for patients from minority groups might also be useful in the future. Nevertheless, when questionnaires are used together with tests of bronchial hyperresponsiveness and clinical judgment, excellent epidemiologic investigations can result.[8]

SPIROMETRY AND PEAK FLOW RATE MEASUREMENTS IN POPULATION STUDIES

Spirometry has been used to detect variable airway obstruction in epidemiologic studies,[9–13] and it also has been used to follow prospectively the natural history of the disease.[11] In addition to detecting airway obstruction in subjects with active asthma, the performance of spirometry before and after inhalation of bronchodilator can detect variability of airflow obstruction, and the finding of 15 percent improvement in flows after bronchodilator is widely accepted as an insensitive but valuable finding.[14] Spirometry provides useful data on the severity of asthma, but it is insufficiently sensitive to be used by itself as a screening test in population studies; typically, spirometry has been used as an adjunct to questionnaire surveys. Spirometry is expensive and time consuming. Measuring the forced expiratory volume in 1 s (FEV_1) before and after a work shift has been found to be an unreliable method in investigating occupational asthma.[15]

Peak flow rate measurements are more dependent on patient effort than spirometry but are much less expensive and time consuming to perform. Comparative studies of asthmatic patients who are not suffering an acute attack have shown that variability of the peak expiratory flow correlates somewhat with the results of bronchial challenge testing,[16–18] although these tests measure different things and the correlation is not strong.[17] Peak flow rate measurements have been helpful in epidemiologic investigations of occupational asthma because the apparatus is portable and can be used in the workplace to detect acute changes and in the patient's home for detecting late reactions to allergens inhaled in the workplace.[9,15,19] The epidemiologic variables of interest in peak flow measurement testing are any acute decreases that occur after an exposure and the diurnal variability that is seen in chronic asthmatics who are not currently suffering an acute exacerbation.

BRONCHIAL CHALLENGE TESTING IN POPULATION STUDIES

Bronchial challenge testing is a test in which the subject inhales an agent that is capable of provoking bronchoconstriction in susceptible subjects. Positive challenges result in ≥ 20 percent decrease in FEV_1, and the results are usually expressed as the provocative concentration necessary to cause this decrease. Typical agents used include methacholine, histamine, and cold, dry air. Bronchial challenge testing is used both in clinical practice and in epidemiologic investigations, with very different purposes in the two areas. In clinical practice, bronchial challenge testing is used for excluding or confirming a diagnosis of asthma, investigating possible occupational asthma, and assessing the severity of asthma and monitoring asthma treatment.[2] There is widespread acceptance of the value of bronchial challenge testing in clinical practice. In epidemiology, bronchial challenge testing has very different purposes. By itself, bronchial challenge testing is not a strong enough tool to distinguish cases of asthma in population studies.[10,20] Because there is no unique biologic marker for defining asthma, the current level of understanding necessitates that an operational definition of asthma should include both bronchial challenge testing and clinical criteria.[3] The methodologic problems that detract from the value of bronchial challenge testing in epidemiologic studies are these. In population studies that have used bronchial challenge testing, up to one half of the subjects discovered to have a positive test are without clinical symptoms of asthma.[20,21] Conversely, about half of those subjects with asthmalike symptoms do not have a positive bronchial challenge test. Another problem is that bronchial hyperresponsiveness is not fixed; it varies with time and with exposures. For this reason, a truly asthmatic subject who is tested during a period of wellness may lack bronchial hyperresponsiveness. Finally, when bronchial challenge testing is used in population studies of adults that contain many smokers, this method cannot separate subjects with asthma from subjects with chronic bronchitis.[10] Despite its limitations, it is clear that even if bronchial hyperresponsiveness is not unique to asthma, it is strongly related to asthma, and this method will continue to be used in future studies together with other methods for combined-method epidemiologic studies.

SURVEILLANCE OF ASTHMA STATISTICS IN LARGE MOBILE POPULATIONS

A number of methods are available to epidemiologists to study asthma in large populations, such as whole countries or their subdivisions. Weiss and colleagues have recently reviewed these methods.[22] In the United States overall there are no ongoing national studies of the incidence of asthma. The prevalence, however, is tracked by means of two population-based surveys, the National Health Interview Survey (NHIS) and the National Health and Nutrition Examination Survey (NHANES). A related survey, the Hispanic Health and Nutrition Examination Survey (HHANES), conducted from 1982 to 1984, was designed to collect prevalence data on asthma and other diseases for Mexican-Americans in the Southwest, Cubans in Miami, and Puerto Ricans in the New York City area.[23] Health-care utilization at the national level is measured by the National Ambulatory Medical Care Survey and the National Hospital Discharge Survey. Important information on health-care utilization can be derived from the National Ambulatory Medical Care Survey, which was conducted in 1985 and 1986 and which contains data on visits by asthmatic patients to physicians.[24] Data on outpatient prescribing of anti-asthma drugs can be obtained from the National Prescription Audit[25] and from private companies such as the Computerized On-line Medicaid Pharmaceutical Analysis and Surveillance System (Health Information Designs, Inc., Arlington, VA).[26] Information on trends in asthma morbidity and mortality is traced using national health information systems kept at the National Center for Health Statistics. Data from death certificates is available from the health departments of individual states.

Previous experience in judging mortality rates in patients with asthma has shown that the identification of asthma as the correct cause of death is most accurate in the group from 5 to 34 years old.[27,28] This is probably because death from asthma in the very young is easily confused with bronchiolitis, and death in older patients is easily confused with chronic bronchitis and emphysema.

In large study populations, one of the problems that makes it hard to obtain accurate data is the investigator's inability to estimate the size of a changing population. Not only is the overall size of the stable population unknown, the size of the pool of people at risk is unknown, that is, the population of potential asthmatics (for incidence studies) and the population of asthmatics (for morbidity and mortality studies).

Surveillance of death from asthma in minority groups in the United States has been possible in cases where ethnicity is reported in public records. Better data are available for African-Americans than for Hispanic-Americans, because Hispanic-Americans have been listed as "white" in the past without further identification of ethnicity. When recent Hispanic immigrants are part of the study population, there is even more uncertainty about the size of the population that is being studied in collecting mortality information from death certificates because the immigrant population is mobile and may not be counted in census data.

SURVEILLANCE OF ASTHMA STATISTICS IN SMALL STABLE POPULATIONS

Valuable studies of the epidemiology of asthma have come from data collection in small subsets of the population who can be studied using accurate record systems. One approach has been to identify a small political grouping such as a city or county and to perform a thorough epidemiologic study on a large percentage of the entire population.[11,29–35] Another source of epidemiologic data in small groups is the expanding networks of health maintenance organizations, which are now a potential means to obtain information on asthma incidence, prevalence, utilization of health-care resources,[36] morbidity, and mortality.

SURVEILLANCE OF ASTHMA STATISTICS IN OCCUPATIONAL HEALTH

In the United States, the National Institute for Occupational Safety and Health (NIOSH) has experimented in two states, Michigan and Massachusetts, with a surveillance program called SENSOR (Sentinel Event Notification System for Occupational Risks).[37] Nevertheless, a national surveillance system is not currently in operation, and most cases are reported in the medical literature as case reports or investigations of small groupings of workers. In Britain, a national surveillance system called SWORD, Surveillance of Work-related and Occupational Respiratory Disease, has been in place for 5 years.[38,39] This system uses a sampling strategy to report new cases of occupational lung disease based on data from pulmonologists and occupational physicians.

EPIDEMIOLOGIC METHODS FOR EXAMINING RISK FACTORS: ATOPY

Atopy is characterized by the production of abnormally large amounts of immunoglobulin E (IgE) in response to allergens. Epidemiologists can study the role of atopy by creating first an operational definition of atopy for the study and then taking measurements in the form of IgE in the blood or by performing cutaneous tests such as scratch tests. Recent studies by Burrows[40] and Sears[41] have affirmed the potential role for this type of examination in epidemiologic studies of asthma in patients of all age groups. Many studies have also collected blood for total eosinophil counts because this variable is related to atopy and asthma.

EPIDEMIOLOGIC METHODS FOR EXAMINING RISK FACTORS: STUDIES OF THE OUTDOOR ENVIRONMENT

Outdoor air can be analyzed by a number of techniques that provide useful collateral data for epidemiologic studies. Pollen is collected from the air with fiberglass filters and identified after elution by means of immunologic techniques.[42] Sulfates and nitrates in the air can be measured by ionic chromatography and higher oxides of nitrogen by chemoluminescence.[43] Municipal departments of public health in the United States also often measure ozone, carbon monoxide, and particulate matter (particles < 10 μm in diameter).[44]

EPIDEMIOLOGIC METHODS FOR EXAMINING RISK FACTORS: STUDIES OF THE INDOOR ENVIRONMENT

Possible risk factors for the inception of asthma or its exacerbation are recognized in the indoor environment.[45] Cutaneous scratch tests or radioallergosorbent tests (RAST) can be used in epidemiologic investigations to determine what environmental antigens are causing an IgE response in the study subjects. Analysis of indoor allergens now uses sensitive methods, such as the double-antibody inhibition radioimmunoassay, to detect the potent antigen of the house dust mite, *Dermatophagoides pteronyssinus*, called *Der p* I. Sensitive two-site monoclonal antibody assays also are available for other allergens and can be used in epidemiologic studies. Questionnaires should also survey data on the indoor environment, especially the presence of smokers in the household.

For epidemiologic investigations of the workplace, the scope of each investigation is unique and depends on the array of possible allergens or irritants present. Some epidemiologic studies in occupational asthma have been conducted at the workplace itself[8,9] using spirometry and bronchial challenge testing to document the worker's sensitivity to the work environment. Others have been conducted in specialized laboratories using "specific" inhalation challenge testing in which the patient is exposed to the probable provoking agent under controlled conditions in a specially equipped laboratory.

Incidence of Asthma

There are only a small number of studies on the incidence of asthma in the United States, but there is remarkable concurrence among them.[12,30,34,46] The incidence rate of asthma varies with age, with the higher rates in the very young and a striking stability of rates in adults. The overall incidence varies from about 2.38 to 4 new cases per 1000 residents per year.[12,30,34,46] The rate in children less than 5 years old in the Tucson, Arizona and Tecumseh, Michigan studies is: boys, 8.1 to 14/1000/year; girls, 4.5 to 9/1000/year. In the Olmstead County, Minnesota study, the high incidence rates of infancy were even more strikingly documented, with the rate in boys less than 1 year of age approaching 40/1000/year (see Fig. 76-4, Chapter 76). In the latter study, the median age of onset was 3 years for boys and 8 years for girls; an increase in incidence rates was documented for the years 1964 to 1983, but only in children and in adolescents. It is important to point out that these data come from a community-based study in a population that is more than 96 percent white and likely do not represent the situation among communities with high percentages of minority residents. No similar data exist on the incidence rate of asthma for minority groups.

Although the NHANES did not carefully examine the incidence of asthma, Gergen and coworkers[47] commented that most asthmatics had their first episode before their third birthday.

Data on the incidence of occupational asthma are rare. Butcher and colleagues[4] carried out a prospective longitudinal study of occupational asthma in an isocyanate manufacturing plant during 5.5 years. They were able to define the incidence of asthma in that industry as 8 cases per 1000 workers per year. Although few other data are available on the incidence of occupational asthma, it seems likely from the extremely wide variance among prevalence data that the incidence would be expected to vary widely among different occupational settings. Prospective incidence studies would be especially informative in industries where large numbers of newly hired workers leave their jobs in response to symptoms of occupational asthma.

Prevalence

In general, data on the prevalence of asthma differ more widely than do the available data on incidence. This is due to very different methods of case finding and differing definitions of asthma. The major usefulness of prevalence data in given population groups is to identify very low or very high prevalence and to relate these unusual situations to living conditions so that hypotheses can be formed about why the prevalence of asthma is different from the expected. A persistent problem in all population studies of asthma is the presence of asthmalike symptoms in a substantial percentage of the population who do not fit the operational definition of asthma. This is sometimes called "persistent wheeze" or just "wheeze." Although some authorities have the strong impression that patients with only asthmalike symptoms and no response to bronchial challenge testing have a very mild condition, little is known of the natural history of patients with asthmalike symptoms and it will be important to study this group more in the future.

PREVALENCE OF ASTHMA IN THE UNITED STATES OVERALL

Data for the overall point prevalence of asthma in the United States for different age groups are shown in Fig. 76-2 in Chap. 76. These data from the NHIS show that the 1992 overall prevalence is 49.2/1000 residents, increased from 34.8 cases of asthma per 1000 residents in 1982. The same survey shows that the prevalence of asthma decreases as family income increases. This inverse relationship between the prevalence of asthma and affluence within the United States contrasts with the conclusion that Gregg[48] drew on the basis of his review of asthma worldwide. Gregg believed that asthma was distinctly less prevalent in less affluent countries. Nevertheless, the results of the NHANES summarized by Mcwhorter[46] confirm that in the United States, lower income was strongly related to asthma in both whites and African-Americans. The latter study reported an overall prevalence of asthma of 26/1000 residents. These overall prevalence rates for the United States are comparable to published rates in Western countries that vary from 10 to 60 cases of asthma per 1000 residents.[48,49]

Overall prevalence data show only trivial difference between the sexes, but among children there is a higher prevalence in boys.[47]

Using the above numbers, the current total number of persons with asthma in the United States is over 12 million.

PREVALENCE OF ASTHMA IN SUBSETS OF THE U.S. POPULATION

Data for the period prevalence of asthma in the Michigan Medicaid population[26] are shown in Fig. 76-3, Chap. 76. In this study, no questionnaire was used; instead, cases were collected by using the billing codes of health-care providers. These data are probably less sensitive and more specific than questionnaire data, and for this reason the prevalence rate is lower than the rate from the NHIS above. These data are most interesting for what they tell us of the age distribution of medication-requiring asthma in the Medicaid population, and they also document a slightly rising prevalence in recent years. These data also confirm the findings of Dodge and Burrows[33] in their Tucson study that asthma is more common in young children, least in adolescence, and increased again in early adult life.

When children are singled out in prevalence studies, it becomes obvious that asthma is much more prevalent among children than adults. In 1989, the NHIS showed that the prevalence of asthma was 6.1 percent for Americans ≤ 18 years old compared with 4.8 percent among all other age groups (see Fig. 76-1, Chap. 76). Gergen and associates[47] reported that asthma was present in 6.7 percent of youths between ages 3 and 17, and there was higher prevalence in boys than girls (9.4 percent in boys versus 6.2 percent in girls).

African-Americans are a minority group that have been shown to have a higher prevalence of asthma in several studies.[46,47,50] Overall, the percent of African-Americans with asthma is 5.3 percent as opposed to 4.7 percent in whites.[51] A number of studies have measured the comparative prevalence of asthma in American children with separate attention to African-Americans. In the national surveys reviewed by Gergen,[47] asthma prevalence was reported as 9.4 percent in African-American youths and 6.2 percent in white youths. Schwartz and associates[52] analyzed the prevalence data of the Second National Health and Nutrition Survey and concluded that the relative odds of asthma for African-American children as opposed to white children were 2.5.

Prevalence data for Hispanic-Americans are few and it will take future studies to present the epidemiologic profile of this important minority group in more detail. In 1982, Samet and associates[32] reported their questionnaire survey of 633 Hispanics and 1038 Anglos in Bernalillo County, New Mexico. They found asthma to be significantly less common among Hispanics. The overall prevalence of current, physician-confirmed asthma were 9/1000 for Hispanic males and 23/1000 for Hispanic females. The prevalence for Anglos was 33/1000 for males and 48/1000 for females. Dodge[12] collected data on Mexican-American children in three small Arizona communities and found a point prevalence of 19/1000 among Mexican-American children but 65/1000 among Anglo children from the same communities. In contrast to these studies that seem to show a lower prevalence of asthma among Mexican-Americans, the data collected on Puerto Ricans living in the United States show a larger problem with asthma. Karetzky[53] studied an adult emergency room population in Bronx, New York and found that although Puerto Ricans made up approximately 25 percent of the population served by the emergency room, they made up 59 percent of the patients entered into the asthma registry. Carter-Pokras and Gergen[54] analyzed the data collected from 1982 to 1984 from the Hispanic Health and Nutrition Examination Survey (NHANES) II. The study population was Hispanic-American children from ages 6 months to 11 years and it included Puerto Rican, Mexican-American, and Cuban children. These investigators found large differences in prevalence among groups from different countries of origin. The highest prevalence of active asthma was in the Puerto Rican children (11.2 percent) compared with 3.3 percent for non-Hispanic whites, 5.9 percent for non-Hispanic African-Americans, 5.2 percent for Cubans, and only 2.7 percent for Mexican-Americans.

PREVALENCE OF OCCUPATIONAL ASTHMA

The prevalence of occupational asthma varies remarkably depending on the industrial process, the concentration of exposure, and the working conditions.[55] Prevalence data are important in epidemiologic investigations of occupational asthma because a comparison of "before and after" prevalence is necessary to know whether efforts at prevention are successful.[39] Approximately 5 percent of workers exposed to volatile isocyanates develop asthma[56]; the prevalence in many other workplaces is much higher.

Risk Factors for Asthma

ATOPY

Atopy has long been suspected of being a risk factor for asthma. The relationship of atopy to asthma has been studied by applying skin tests to asthmatics and nonasthmatics and by measuring IgE antibodies. A number of studies have documented a high percentage of atopic patients among populations with asthma.[40,41] In addition to these measurements, which are useful in defining the population of atopic people, studies of potential aeroallergens in the environment have strengthened the case for possible cause-effect relationships between atopy and asthma. O'Hollaren and associates studied the relationship between exposure to the aeroallergen *Alternaria alternata* and respiratory arrest in children and young adults.[42] They were able to document a temporal clustering between asthma deaths and the *Alternaria* season. Sunyer and associates studied epidemics of asthma caused by soybean dust released during unloading of soybeans into a silo. They found increased serum IgE antibody specific for soybean antigen in 74 percent of epidemic patients. Interestingly, the data showed that epidemic asthma provoked by aeroallergens had its strongest effect in older adults, and children were largely unaffected by exposure to soybean dust.[57]

Studies that have focused on the role of atopy in childhood asthma have shown a striking correlation between asthma and IgE antibodies specific for dust mites. In a recent review of the association between allergy and asthma, Platts-Mills noted that the association between sensitization to indoor allergens and asthma is very strong, with odds ratios varying from 6 to more than 20.[45] This association has been observed in many different countries and is specific for asthma in the sense that immediate hypersensitivity to common allergens has not been related to any other lung disease. Many studies have shown a dose-response relationship between exposure to dust-mite allergens and the prevalence of sensitization to mite allergens.[58] Provocation of the lungs with nebulized dust mite is capable of provoking bronchospasm and bronchial hyperresponsiveness. As a final point, a series of studies have shown that avoidance of specific allergens can both reduce asthma symptoms and decrease bronchial hyperresponsiveness.[45]

In addition to sensitization to dust mites, other allergens, including cockroach, cat, and pollens have been reported to be important in the atopic aspect of asthma.[59–62]

Burrows and associates[40] studied the relationship of atopy to asthma in a population of children and adults. The definition of asthma used in this study was rather subjective,[63] but they found that the prevalence of asthma was closely associated with the serum IgE concentration standardized for age and sex and this was true for all age groups.

OTHER POSSIBLE RISK FACTORS

A number of risk factors have been proposed, but the evidence for their connection with asthma is not fully worked out.

The evidence for a genetic basis for asthma has not been strong, but ongoing studies should contribute a great deal to our understanding of the genetics of asthma in the future.

Except for the stronger predilection for boys than girls in childhood asthma, gender is not a risk factor of note. As mentioned earlier, studies show a higher prevalence and mortality among African-Americans, but in many studies the role of race seems to represent an effect of poverty with decreased access to health care.

Although one study[64] discusses air pollution as a possible risk factor in asthma, a recent study by Lang[44] showed that a progressive increase in the air quality of Philadelphia had no beneficial relationship with asthma mortality. Changes of rates of breast-feeding have not played any role in the changing picture of asthma epidemiology.[22] Any possible relationship between the increasing number of babies who survive low birthweights and asthma awaits further investigation. Tobacco smoke in the indoor environment of children has been studied. It has been implicated in an earlier onset of asthma,[65] with development of asthma before 12 years of age,[66] and in increases in the overall severity of asthma[65,67] but not in the primary causation of asthma.

RISK FACTORS FOR OCCUPATIONAL ASTHMA

Potential risk factors that have been studied in occupational asthma include atopy, cigarette smoking, and bronchial hyperresponsiveness before starting work.

A role for atopy as a risk factor has been found in some, but not all, forms of the disease. In general, workplace exposures that result in the sensitization of some workers as indicated by specific IgE have shown that atopy is a risk factor in an exposed worker. Other forms of occupational asthma, such as asthma caused by Western Red Cedar dust, have not been associated with atopy.[68] Atopy has an inconsistent role in asthma caused by isocyanates.[55]

The role of cigarette smoking as a risk factor in occupational asthma has been mainly as a risk factor that interacts with atopy.[39] In a survey of workers with occupational asthma caused by tetrachlorophthalic anhydride, more smokers were found in the group who had specific IgE antibodies to the chemical compared to the group without specific antibody. In contrast, workers with occupational asthma caused by Western Red Cedar, who do not form specific IgE antibodies, were not found to have an increased risk associated with cigarette smoking.[68]

Although it seems counterintuitive, bronchial hyperresponsiveness before beginning workplace exposure has not been shown to be a risk factor for the development of occupational asthma.[4,55]

Social Costs and Morbidity of Asthma

One goal of many epidemiologic studies is to measure the impact of asthma on the patient and on society. Morbidity includes all the undesirable effects of asthma except death, which is considered separately. Thus, morbidity includes such measures as numbers of scheduled and unscheduled visits to health-care providers, admission to hospital, loss of time from school or work, decrease in functional status, decrease in quality of life, and the impact of the illness on the family.

Weiss and coworkers[24] performed an economic evaluation of asthma in the United States in 1992. They estimated the cost of this illness to society to be $6.2 billion in 1990. Of the different direct expenditures, the most expensive was inpatient hospital care.

There are a number of studies on health-care utilization in asthma. Vollmer and associates[36] studied the utilization of hospital-based resources of a large health maintenance organization for treatment of asthma during a 20-year period. They created the concept of "episode of acute asthma care" that was defined as "a collection of one or more emergency room visits or hospitalizations that cluster in time with no two adjoining visits separated by more than two days." Using this concept, they found a statistically significant increase in asthma episodes among boys younger than 5 years of age that continued unabated from 1967 to 1987. They suggested that this novel concept might be a more useful one in the context of managed health-care systems than studies of hospital admission for the study of changes in the epidemiology of asthma in the future. This would be especially true if alternatives to hospitalization become more common in coming years. Their finding of an increasing rate of asthma admission for boys under age 5 was also seen in data collected by the National Hospital Discharge Survey.[22]

Data from the National Center for Health Statistics have shown a steady increase in the number of hospital discharges for asthma in children for 1982 to 1992 (see Fig. 76-5 in Chap. 76). Gergen and Weiss[69] analyzed data from the National Hospital Discharge Survey for 1979 to 1987 and found that asthma hospitalizations for children aged 0 to 17 years increased 4.5 percent per year. They were also able to analyze racial differences and reported that African-Americans had approximately 1.8 times the increase of whites. Wissow and associates[35] analyzed data from the Maryland hospital discharges to determine a similar racial difference in hospitalization rates for children. They found an annual discharge rate for African-American children aged 0 to 19 years of 3.75/1000; the rate for white children was 1.25/1000. Interestingly, most of this racial difference disappeared when asthma discharge rates were adjusted for poverty. They concluded that African-American children are at increased risk for hospitalization for asthma but that some of the increase is related to poverty rather than race. Wood and associates[13] studied the morbidity of asthma in Hispanic children. They studied a highly selected population of Hispanic children with moderate asthma without non-Hispanic controls. They documented a relatively low rate of hospitalization of 1.3 days per child per year but a rather high rate of impact of the disease on the children's daily lives in the form of school absenteeism, days with impairment, exercise limitation, and the need for acute care visits. Through use of a scale that measures the impact of disease on the family they discovered that the impact was higher if there was a smoker in the household. The impact on the family was lower when knowledge about asthma was high. This epidemiologic study thus uncovered factors that contributed to morbidity of asthma in this population.

In the near future, instruments that have been developed for measuring the quality of life in asthma[70–72] likely will reveal much new data on the morbidity of asthma.

The morbidity of occupational asthma could be measured in all the ways already mentioned plus one more: potential removal from the workplace of the victim with loss of livelihood. In a British study, Venables[73] found the following outcomes in workers with occupational asthma who were followed for an average of 6 years: 90 percent were improved, 72 percent still took medications, 40 percent reported limitation in their activities, 33 percent were unemployed, and 10 percent required hospital admission.

Mortality

Data on mortality from asthma for all age groups are shown in Fig. 76-8 in Chap. 76. The mortality rate for the whole of the United States is very low. Although the rate has been and continues to be low, there has been an increasing tendency in mortality rates collected from different sources.[44,74–77] This increase in mortality is problematic when one considers that it has been recorded during a period of advances in the therapy of asthma and progress in the battle against air pollution.[44] It is also regrettable in the sense that many assume death from asthma to be a preventable form of death. One source of possible optimism in this picture is that it remains possible that despite the slight increase in the U.S. asthma death rate, mortality as a percentage of prevalence may have actually decreased.[22] Also, a recent study of the long-term survival of a cohort of community residents in Olmstead County, Minnesota showed that among this sample of patients, which is not representative of the U.S. population as a whole, the survival among patients with asthma but no other lung disease was not significantly different from the expected survival.[31]

One of the most important recent epidemiologic discoveries has been the uncovering of geographic pockets of high asthma mortality within impoverished urban areas of the United States.[24,44,77–82] Many studies also have found a greater asthma mortality rate in African-Americans[44,74,76,79–81] and in Puerto Ricans[44,78] but not in other Hispanic groups.[32,74] Currently the asthma death rate is almost three times greater among African-Americans than whites in the United States as a whole. Within the poor neighborhoods of cities such as New York, Chicago, and Philadelphia, the asthma death rate has been recorded to be much higher than elsewhere in the country. The majority of analyses link the greater asthma death rate in African-Americans to poverty. In Philadelphia, for example, Lang found that African-American race was only associated with an increased rate of death from asthma in census tracts with higher poverty rates.[44] In Chicago, Targonski presented evidence that the high asthma mortality rate among African-Americans is linked to lack of access to health care.[82] Targonski noted that between 1979 and 1991, outpatient and emergency department deaths due to asthma increased significantly, whereas the proportion of dead-on-arrival cases remained stable. This shift to non-inpatient death suggested that lack of access to health care may play a role in increasing asthma mortality.

Data on asthma mortality among Hispanic-Americans are not yet as substantial as among other population groups. Nevertheless, many studies suggest a high asthma death rate among impoverished Puerto Ricans.[44,78] The asthma death rate appears to be low among Mexican-Americans.[32,74]

Mortality appears to be a rare event in occupational asthma, although at least one death has been documented in a worker with toluene diisocyante-induced asthma.[83]

Epidemics of Asthma

The prevalence and mortality of asthma in the United States has been nearly stable overall with a small rising trend in the last decade. Epidemiology has been used to track these trends in the effects of asthma in the United States and in many other nations.

Abrupt short-term epidemics of asthma have also been investigated and the data show interesting and often unexplained trends in asthma morbidity and mortality. Asthma epidemics have occurred in New Orleans,[84] New York,[85] and Birmingham, England,[86] but the causes of these epidemics were never found. Castor bean dust was responsible for several epidemics in past decades.[87–89] More recently, an acute epidemic of asthma morbidity was investigated in Barcelona, Spain, and epidemiologic investigations succeeded in identifying the causative agent as soybean dust that was being dispersed into the outdoor air during unloading into a silo at the harbor.[43,90–92] The investigation of the Barcelona epidemic was a triumph of modern epidemiology. Before the epidemiologic investigation succeeded there were 26 epidemics of asthma that overloaded the emergency departments and intensive care units of Barcelona. Twenty-six people died of asthma during these epidemics. After the cause was determined and soybean dust was prevented from being dumped into the air, the epidemics ceased.

Several epidemics of increased asthma mortality of more prolonged duration have been described in recent years.[93] The first of these epidemics happened in the United Kingdom, Australia, and New Zealand[94] and the second was limited to New Zealand.[93] Despite a great deal of thought and study, the causes of these epidemics, each of which lasted for years, have not been elucidated. These two epidemics have been limited to asthma deaths with no concomitant rise seen in other respiratory diseases. For the more recent epidemic in New Zealand, speculation on causes centers on the fact that asthma medications were available free of charge during the epidemic but the costs of primary care visits were increasing. This might have led to inappropriate self-medication.[95] Another possible cause may have been delays in receipt of potentially lifesaving care in emergencies.[96]

Conclusions

The epidemiology of asthma is a field of knowledge that has made progress against great odds, most significantly, the roadblock posed by a lack of a definition of its object of study. Nevertheless, epidemiology has contributed greatly to the formation of current hypotheses about the causes of asthma and the populations who will require special attention if the disease is to be brought under better control.

References

1. *Healthy People 2000*. National health promotion and disease prevention objectives. Washington: GPO, DHHS publication no. (PHS)91-50213:105.
2. Cockcroft DW, Hargreave FE: Airway hyperresponsiveness: relevance of random population data to clinical usefulness. *Am Rev Respir Dis* 1990; 142:497.
3. Toelle BG, Peat JK, Salome CM, et al.: Toward a definition of asthma for epidemiology. *Am Rev Respir Dis* 1992; 146:633.
4. Butcher BT, Jones RN, O'Neil CE, et al.: Longitudinal study of workers employed in the manufacture of toluene diisocyanate. *Am Rev Respir Dis*, 1977; 116: 411–421.
5. Anderson HR: Is the prevalence of asthma changing? *Arch Dis Child* 1989; 64:172.
6. Smith DD: Medical-legal definition of occupational asthma. *Chest* 1990; 98:1007.
7. Torén K, Brisman J, Järvholm B: Asthma and asthma-like symptoms in adults assessed by questionnaires: a literature review. *Chest* 1993; 104:600.
8. Malo JL, Carier A, L'Archeveque J, et al.: Prevalence of occupational asthma among workers exposed to Eastern White Cedar. *Am J Respir Crit Care Med* 1994; 150:1697.
9. Desjardins A, Bergeron JP, Ghezzo H, et al.: Aluminum potroom asthma confirmed by monitoring of forced expiratory volume in one second. *Am J Respir Crit Care Med* 1994; 150:1714.
10. Enarson DA, Vedal S, Schulzer M, et al.: Asthma, asthma-like symptoms, chronic bronchitis, and the degree of bronchial hyperresponsiveness in epidemiologic surveys. *Am Rev Respir Dis* 1987; 136:613.
11. Schachter EN, Doyle CA, Beck GJ: A prospective study of asthma in a rural community. *Chest* 1984; 85:623.
12. Dodge R: A comparison of the respiratory health of Mexican-American and non-Mexican-American white children. *Chest* 1983; 84:587.
13. Wood PR, Hidalgo HA, Prihoda TJ, Kromer ME: Hispanic children with asthma: morbidity. *Pediatrics* 1993; 91:62.
14. Burney PGJ: The classification and epidemiology of asthma, in Holgate ST, Church MK (eds): *Allergy*. London, Gower Medical Publishing, 1993: 12.1–12.10.
15. Burge PS: Single and serial measurements of lung function in the diagnosis of occupational asthma. *Eur J Resp Dis* 1982; 63:47.
16. Ryan G, Latimer KM, Dolovich J, Hargreave FE: Airway responsiveness to histamine: relationship to diurnal variation of peak flow rate, improvement after bronchodilator, and airway calibre. *Thorax* 1982; 37:423.
17. Higgins B: Unpublished data shown in Burney PGJ: The classification and epidemiology of asthma, in Holgate ST, Church MK (eds): *Allergy*. London, Gower Medical Publishing, 1993: 12.1–12.10.
18. Woolcock AJ, Yan K, Salome CM: Effect of therapy on bronchial hyperresponsiveness in the long-term management of asthma. *Clin Allergy* 1988; 18:165.
19. Kongerud J, Soyseth V, Burge S: Serial measurements of peak expiratory flow and responsiveness to methacholine in the diagnosis of aluminum potroom asthma. *Thorax* 1992; 27:292.
20. Pattemore PK, Asher MI, Harrison AC, et al.: The interrelationship among bronchial hyperresponsiveness, the diagnosis of asthma, and asthma symptoms. *Am Rev Respir Dis* 1990; 142:549.
21. Cockcroft DW, Berscheid BA, Murdock KY, Gore BP: Sensitivity and specificity of histamine PC_{20} measurements in a random population. *J Allergy Clin Immunol* 1985; 75:142(A).

22. Weiss KB, Gergen PJ, Wagener DK: Breathing better or wheezing worse? The changing epidemiology of asthma morbidity and mortality. *Annu Rev Public Health* 1993; 14:491.

23. Maurer KR (ed): *Plan and Operation of the Second National Health and Nutrition Examination Survey, 1982–84.* Vital Health Stat [1] 19, 1985. DHHS publication PHS 90-1232.

24. Weiss KB, Gergen PJ, Hodgson TA: An economic evaluation of asthma in the United States. *N Engl J Med* 1992; 326:862.

25. Bosco LA, Knapp DE, Gerstman B, Graham CF: Asthma drug therapy trends in the United States, 1972 to 1985. *J Allergy Clin Immunol* 1987; 80:398.

26. Gerstman BB, Bosco LA, Tomita DK, et al.: Prevalence and treatment of asthma in the Michigan Medicaid patient population younger than 45 years, 1980–1986. *J Allergy Clin Immunol* 1989; 83:1032.

27. Sears MR, Rea HH, de Boer G, et al.: Accuracy of certification of deaths due to asthma: a national study. *Am J Epidemiol* 1986; 124:1004.

28. Subcommittee of the BTA research committee. Accuracy of death certificates in bronchial asthma: accuracy of certification procedures during the confidential inquiry by the British Thoracic Association. *Thorax* 1984; 39:505.

29. Hunt LW Jr, Silverstein MD, Reed CE, et al.: Accuracy of the death certificate in a population-based study of asthmatic patients. *JAMA* 1993; 269:1947.

30. Yuninger JW, Reed CE, O'Connell EJ, et al.: A community-based study of the epidemiology of asthma: incidence rates, 1964–1983. *Am Rev Respir Dis* 1992; 146:888.

31. Silverstein MD, Reed CE, O'Connel EJ, et al.: Long-term survival of a cohort of community residents with asthma. *N Engl J Med* 1994; 331:1537.

32. Samet JM, Schrag SD, Howard CA, et al.: Respiratory disease in a New Mexico population sample of Hispanic and non-Hispanic whites. *Am Rev Respir Dis* 1982; 125:152.

33. Dodge RR, Burrows B: The prevalence and incidence of asthma and asthma-like symptoms in a general population sample. *Am Rev Respir Dis* 1980; 122:567.

34. Broder I, Higgins MW, Mathews KP, Keller JB: Epidemiology of asthma and allergic rhinitis in a total community, Tecumseh, Michigan: III. Second survey of the community. *J Allergy Clin Immunol* 1974; 53:127.

35. Wissow LS, Gittelsohn AM, Szklo M, et al.: Poverty, race, and hospitalization for childhood asthma. *Am J Public Health* 1988; 78:777.

36. Vollmer WM, Osborne M, Buist AS: Temporal trends in hospital-based episodes of asthma care in a health maintenance organization. *Am Rev Respir Dis* 1993; 147:347.

37. Matte TD, Hoffman RE, Rosenman KE, Stanbury M: Surveillance of occupational asthma under the SENSOR model. *Chest* 1990; 98:173S.

38. McDonald JC, Meredith SK: Would a SWORD-like surveillance scheme be useful and feasible in the USA (abstract). *Am Rev Respir Dis* 1993; 147:A903.

39. Beckett WS: The epidemiology of occupational asthma. *Eur Respir J* 1994; 7:161.

40. Burrows B, Liebowitz MD, Bargee RA: Respiratory disorders and allergy skin test reactions. *Ann Intern Med* 1976; 84:134.

41. Sears MR, Burrows B, Flannery EM, et al.: Relation between airway responsiveness and serum IgE in children with asthma and in apparently normal children. *N Engl J Med* 1991; 325:1067.

42. O'Hollaren MT, Yuninger JW, Offord KP, et al.: Exposure to aeroallergen as a possible precipitating factor in respiratory arrest in young patients with asthma. *N Engl J Med* 1991; 324:359.

43. Antó MJ, Sunyer J, and the Asthma Collaborative Group of Barcelona: A point-source asthma outbreak. *Lancet* 1986; 1:900.

44. Lang DM, Polansky M: Patterns of asthma mortality in Philadelphia from 1969 to 1991. *N Engl J Med* 1994; 331:1542.

45. Platts-Mills TAE: Allergen-specific treatment for asthma: III. *Am Rev Respir Dis* 1993; 148:553.

46. Mcwhorter WP, Polis MA, Kaslow RA: Occurrence, predictors, and consequences of adult asthma in NHANESI and follow-up survey. *Am Rev Respir Dis* 1989; 139:721.

47. Gergen PJ, Mullally DI, Evans R III: National survey of prevalence of asthma among children in the United States, 1976 to 1980. *Pediatrics* 1988; 81:1.

48. Gregg I: Epidemiological aspects, in Clark TJH, Godfrey S (eds): *Asthma*, 2nd ed. London, Chapman and Hall, 1983; 242–284.

49. Division of Lung Diseases, National Heart, Lung and Blood Institute: Report of Task Force on Epidemiology of Respiratory Diseases. Bethesda, MD: National Institutes of Health, 1980; NIH publication No. 81-2019.

50. Turkeltaub PC, Gergen PJ: Prevalence of upper and lower respiratory conditions in the US population by social and environmental factors: data from the second National Health and Nutrition Examination Survey, 1976–1980 (NHANES II). *Ann Allergy* 1991; 67:147.

51. National Heart, Lung, and Blood Institute: *Data Fact Sheet: Asthma Statistics.* Publication of the U.S. Department of Health and Human Services, May, 1992.

52. Schwartz J, Gold D, Dockery DW, et al.: Predictors of asthma and persistent wheeze in a national sample of children in the United States: association with social class, perinatal events, and race. *Am Rev Respir Dis* 1990; 142:555.

53. Karetzky MS: Asthma in the South Bronx: clinical and epidemiologic characteristics. *J Allergy Clin Immunol* 1977; 60:383.

54. Carter-Pokras OD, Gergen PJ: Reported asthma among Puerto Rican, Mexican-American, and Cuban children, 1982 through 1984. *Am J Public Health* 1993; 83:580.

55. Chan-Yeung M, Lam S: Occupational asthma. *Am Rev Respir Dis* 1986; 133:686.

56. *NIOSH Criteria for a Recommended Standard. Occupational Exposure to Diisocyanate.* Washington, DC: U.S. Department of Health, Education and Welfare, September 1978 (NIOSH Publication No. 78-215).

57. Sunyer J, Antó JM, Rodrigo MJ, Morell F: Case-control study of serum immunoglobulin-E antibodies reactive with soybean in epidemic asthma. *Lancet* 1989; 1:179.

58. Sporik R, Holgate ST: Platts-Mills TAE, Cogswell JJ: Exposure to house-dust mite allergen (*Der p* I) and the development of asthma in childhood: a prospective study. *N Engl J Med* 1990; 323:502.

59. Sears MR, Herbison GP, Holdaway ME, et al.: The relative risks of sensitivity to grass pollen, house dust mite and cat dander in the development of childhood asthma. *Clin Exp Allergy* 1989; 19:419.

60. Kang B, Chang JL: Allergenic impact of inhaled arthropod material. *Clin Rev Allergy* 1985; 3:363.

61. Van Metre TE, Marsh DG, Adkinson NFJ, et al.: Dose of cat (*Felis domesticus*) allergen I (Fel d I) that induces asthma. *J Allergy Clin Immunol* 1986; 78:62.

62. Pollart SM, Chapman ME, Fiocco GP, et al.: Epidemiology of acute asthma: IgE antibodies to common inhalant allergens as a risk factor for emergency room visits. *J Allergy Clin Immunol* 1989; 83:875.

63. McFadden ER Jr, Gilbert IA: Asthma. *N Engl J Med* 1992; 327:1928.

64. Goren AI, Hellmann S: Prevalence of respiratory symptoms and diseases in school children living in a polluted and in a low polluted area in Israel. *Environ Res* 1988; 45:28.

65. Weitzman M, Gortmaker S, Walker DK, Sobol A: Maternal smoking and childhood asthma. *Pediatrics* 1990; 85:505.

66. Martinez FD, Cline M, Gurrows B: Increased incidence of asthma in children of smoking mothers. *Pediatrics* 1992; 89:21.

67. Murray AB, Ferguson AC, Morrison BJ: Passive smoking and the seasonal difference of severity of asthma in children. *Chest* 1988; 94:701.

68. Chan-Yeung M: Immunologic and non-immunologic mechanisms due to Western Red Cedar (*Thuja plicata*). *J Allergy Clin Immunol* 1982; 70:32.

69. Gergen PJ, Weiss KB: Changing patterns of asthma hospitalization among children: 1979 to 1987. *JAMA* 1990; 264:1688.

70. Hyland ME, Finnis S, Irvine SH: A scale for assessing quality of life in adult asthma sufferers. *J Psychosom Res* 1991; 35:99.

71. Marks G, Dunn S, Woolcock A: A scale for the measurement of quality of life in adults with asthma. *J Clin Epidemiol* 1992; 45:461.

72. Bousquet J, Knani J, Dhivert H, et al.: Quality of life in asthma: I. Internal consistency and validity of the SF-36 questionnaire. *Am J Respir Crit Care Med* 1994; 149:371.

73. Venables KM, Davidson AG, Newman Taylor AJ: Consequences of occupational asthma. *Respir Med* 1989; 83:437.

74. Schenker MB, Gold EB, Lopez RL, Beaumont JJ: Asthma mortality in California, 1960–1989. *Am Rev Respir Dis* 1993; 147:1454.

75. Asthma—United States, 1980–1987. *MMWR* 1990; 39:493.

76. Evans R III, Mullally DI, Wilson RW, et al.: National trends in the morbidity and mortality of asthma in the US: prevalence, hospitalization and death from asthma over two decades: 1965–1984. *Chest* 1987; 91:65S.

77. Weiss KB, Wagener DK: Changing patterns of asthma mortality: identifying target populations at high risk. *JAMA* 1990; 264:1683.

78. Carr W, Zeitel L, Weiss K: Variations in asthma hospitalizations and deaths in New York City. *Am J Public Health* 1992; 82:59.

79. Marder D, Targonski P, Orris P, et al.: Effect of racial and socio-economic factors on asthma mortality in Chicago. *Chest* 1992; 101(suppl 6):426S.

80. Evans R: Asthma among minority children: a growing problem. *Chest* 1992; 101(suppl):368S.

81. Kaplan KM: Epidemiology of deaths from asthma in Pennsylvania, 1978–87. *Public Health Rep* 1993; 108:66.

82. Targonski PV, Persky VW, Orris P, Addington WA: Trends in asthma mortality among African Americans and whites in Chicago, 1968 through 1991. *Am J Public Health* 1994; 84:1830.

83. Fabbri LM, Danieli D, Crescioli S, et al.: Fatal asthma in a toluene diisocyanate-sensitized subject. *Am Rev Respir Dis* 1988; 137:1494.

84. Weill H, Ziskind MM, Dicerson RC, Derbes VJ: Epidemic asthma in New Orleans. *JAMA* 1964; 190:811.

85. Greenburg L, Field F, Reed JI, Erhard CL: Asthma and temperature change. *Arch Environ Health* 1964; 8:642.

86. Packe GE, Ayres JG: Asthma outbreak during a thunderstorm. *Lancet* 1985; 2:199.

87. Figley KD, Elrod RH: Endemic asthma due to castor bean dust. *JAMA* 1928; 90:79.

88. Ordman D: An outbreak of bronchial asthma in South Africa, affecting more than 200 persons, caused by castor bean dust from an oil-processing factory. *Int Arch Allergy Appl Immunol* 1955; 7:10.

89. Mendes E, Ulhôa CA: Collective asthma, simulating an epidemic, provoked by castor-bean dust. *J Allergy* 1954; 25:253.

90. Sunyer J, Antó J, Sabrià J, et al.: Risk factors of soybean epidemic asthma: the role of smoking and atopy. *Am Rev Respir Dis* 1992; 145:1098.

91. Antó J, Sunyer J, Rodriguez-Roisin R, et al. and the Toxicoepidemiological Committee: Community outbreaks of asthma associated with inhalation of soybean dust. *N Engl J Med* 1989; 320:1097.

92. Antó JM, Sunyer J, Reed CE, et al.: Preventing asthma epidemics due to soybeans by dust-control measures. *N Engl J Med* 1993; 329:1760.

93. Jackson R, Beaglehole R, Rea HH, Sutherland DC: Mortality from asthma: a new epidemic in New Zealand. *BMJ* 1982; 285:771.

94. Stolley PD, Schinnar R: Association between asthma mortality and isoproterenol aerosols: a review. *Prev Med* 1978; 7:319.

95. Jackson R, Sears MR, Beaglehole R, Rea HH: International trends in asthma mortality: 1970 to 1985. *Chest* 1988; 94:914.

96. Rea HH, Sears MR, Beaglehole R, et al.: Lessons from the National Asthma Mortality Study: circumstances surrounding death. *N Z Med J* 1985; 100:10.

Asthma is a common disease. It affects 4 to 5 percent of the population in the United States[1] and is responsible for substantial morbidity. Asthma was defined classically as a disease of reversible airflow obstruction.[2,3] It is best described as a syndrome consisting of episodic, reversible airflow obstruction, airway inflammation, and airway hyperreactivity. As outlined below, the syndrome of asthma may, in fact, represent more than one disease. Epidemiologic studies have added greatly to our understanding of the natural history of asthma. This chapter will describe the natural history of asthma, and the next chapter will discuss the epidemiologic and etiologic factors that may incite asthma and influence its course.

Methodologic Problems in Describing the Natural History of Asthma

There are some substantial difficulties in studying the natural history of asthma. One of the most vexing is that of defining the disorder. Several potential asthma syndromes exist, each overlapping others. Early childhood-onset asthma differs substantially from adult-onset asthma in presentation, presence of atopy, potential inciting factors, and prognosis. Exercise-induced asthma differs substantially from asthma associated with atopy. The syndrome of asthmatic bronchitis, in which asthma symptoms and airways hyperresponsiveness are found in older adults with a smoking history, differs from asthma in children and young adults. Asthma, therefore, is several syndromes with some common clinical findings. The delineation of these asthma variants on epidemiologic grounds is quite incomplete, so that any large population study is bound to include all types

of asthma. Such mixing of populations renders difficult any interpretation of incidence, prevalence, and remission.

Population studies that examine the clinical findings that are ordinarily but not exclusively associated with asthma (e.g., the presence of atopy or the presence of airways hyperreactivity) may include subjects who ought not to be classified as asthmatic. For example, a history of wheezing in a young child is characteristic not only of asthma but of bronchitis and bronchiolitis, or it may not indicate any special clinical diagnosis at all.[4] A study that includes all children with a history of wheezing may incorporate a substantial number who do not and will not have asthma. The problem will be compounded if the claim then is made that these children are "in remission." The use of airways responsiveness as a surrogate for asthma in population studies may be inappropriate, as several studies have demonstrated that normal, nonatopic, nonsmoking subjects without the clinical signs of asthma nevertheless may show a response to an inhaled provocative agent that is "greater than normal"[5,6] (Fig. 76-1). The predictive power of airways responsiveness may be poor because of the overlap in responsiveness between symptomatic and asymptomatic individuals, the low prevalence of symptoms in the general population, and the high prevalence of asymptomatic hyperresponsiveness.

Defining asthma simply on the basis of a history of the disease also introduces bias into a study. Studying only children known to have "asthma" may underestimate vastly the magnitude of reactive airways diseases in children by focusing on the most severe and "characteristic" children in the population. In the Tecumseh study of asthma, in which the population of a single community, Tecumseh, MI, was studied in the 1960s, characteristic diagnostic findings in children reporting a history of asthma were absent in many of the children studied.[7] As shown in Table 76-1, even among the

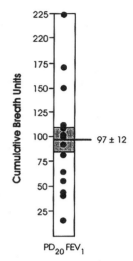

FIGURE 76-1 Range of provocative dose of methacholine needed to cause a 20 percent decrease in forced expiratory volume in 1 second (PD$_{20}$FEV$_1$) for the 14 normal subjects, of 50 tested, who were found to be responsive to methacholine. Each subject had a positive methacholine challenge test, defined as a PD$_{20}$FEV$_1 \leq$ 225 cumulative breath units. Shaded area represents mean ± SE. The remaining 36 normal subjects had a PD$_{20}$FEV$_1 >$ 225 cumulative breath units. None of the 50 subjects had clinical evidence of pulmonary disease. The wide variation in PD$_{20}$FEV$_1$ values obtained in otherwise normal subjects is demonstrated. (*From Casale et al.,*[5] *with permission.*)

subjects thought probably to have asthma, attacks of shortness of breath were found in 80 percent, and only two-thirds were thought to have asthma by an examiner. The variable histories of symptoms and the mislabeling of symptomatology by previous examiners make the tracking of subjects in a longitudinal study difficult.

Another problem in studying the natural history of asthma is the inherent variability of the syndrome, both among subjects and in a given subject over time. As discussed below, the mortality of asthma is low, the prevalence is high in industrialized countries, and the spectrum of the disease is broad. Standard epidemiologic approaches, such as the use of questionnaires and surveys, suffer from a sub-

stantial recall bias in subjects with mild asthma or asthma in remission. Use of clinical series is problematic, because the spectrum of disease found in a university or research-oriented clinic is different than that in the general population. Studies that examine subjects at the time of presentation to a physician for an acute exacerbation are biased against subjects with milder disease. Studies that examine incidence and prevalence over a relatively short period underestimate the remission potential, particularly in children and adolescents.

One of the cardinal features of asthma is its responsiveness to bronchodilator therapy. The influence of adequate treatment on the long-term natural history of asthma may be difficult, if not impossible, to determine, as the goal is not to have a control (untreated) group of ill asthmatics. One then is reduced to describing the natural course of the disease in subjects receiving ordinary medical care.

In examining the natural history in the many studies done across several continents, one thus must be careful to consider the bias of the definition of asthma. Perhaps the best definition for general population studies is the simplest: patients have asthma if they, or their physician, report a history of asthma. While this definition is neither precise nor physiologic, it is more inclusive. Active asthma then can be defined as asthma requiring the use of medication or consultation with a physician, whereas quiescent asthma is marked by the absence of treatment.

Inception and Course of Asthma

Asthma may begin in early life and is common throughout adult life. The overall prevalence of asthma in the United States has been defined in several national studies. The United States Public Health Service conducted a survey in 1970 on the basis of household interviews done by trained census bureau personnel.[8] The survey did not include clinical examinations or a review of clinical symptoms; instead, subjects simply were asked if anyone in the household had asthma. This survey, which included about 116,000 people, estimated a 12-month prevalence of 3 percent and a 12-month incidence of about 0.22 percent. The prevalence was higher in the southern and western regions of the United States. If one considers that chronic diseases generally are

TABLE 76-1 Components of Diagnostic Criteria for Asthma in Persons Reporting Asthma or Wheezing, by Diagnosis, Tecumseh, 1962 through 1965[a]

Diagnostic Component	PROBABLE ASTHMA		SUSPECTED ASTHMA		OTHER CONDITIONS	
	Male	Female	Male	Female	Male	Female
Number of subjects	322	286	291	268	714	676
Attacks of shortness of breath	80.7	79.4	49.5	54.5	13.0	9.8
Trouble breathing out	74.5	77.3	48.1	53.4	11.8	17.3
Chest tightness	78.9	78.3	56.4	66.4	46.1	43.8
Cough	75.8	75.5	71.8	71.6	76.1	73.5
Phelgm	63.4	61.9	57.0	57.1	64.1	57.0
Asthma by diagnosis	64.3	69.6	16.2	10.8	0.0	0.0

[a]Values represent percent of total in that group.
SOURCE: From Broder et al.,[7] with permission.

underreported in such surveys, the adjusted prevalence is about 4.3 percent.[9] In an ongoing series of later studies beginning in 1982, the Public Health Service estimated the prevalence of asthma and other obstructive airways diseases as part of the National Health Interview Survey.[10] Approximately 40,000 households are surveyed each year, for a total of about 115,000 civilian, noninstitutionalized respondents, with a response rate of >95 percent. Whether a subject had asthma was determined by responses to a questionnaire. As shown in Fig. 76-2, the prevalence of asthma has increased from 34.8 per 1000 in 1982 to 49.2 per 1000 in 1992.[10] Much of the increased prevalence of asthma in the study population can be explained by an increased prevalence in subjects younger than 18 (Fig. 76-2). The western region of the United States has a slightly higher prevalence, and the prevalence of asthma decreases as family income increases. Using 1990 census data and the most recent prevalence value for asthma, the total number of individuals with asthma in the United States is >12 million. Asthma thus is one of the more common chronic medical conditions in the United States.

It is useful to consider the natural history of asthma by the major age groups afflicted with the syndrome: children, young adults, and older adults. Each has a characteristic presentation and natural history.

ASTHMA IN CHILDHOOD

Asthma is one of the most common chronic and disabling diseases in childhood.[11] Estimates of the prevalence and incidence of asthma differ greatly in published studies, owing to the varying criteria used to make the diagnosis. Two large community studies used a physician diagnosis of asthma as the criterion. Both studies, one the Tecumseh, MI study of the 1960s and the second from Tucson, AZ, in the 1970s, found a similar incidence and prevalence of asthma[7,12] (Tables 76-2 and 76-3). In both studies, the incidence peaks in children under age 5 and declines slowly to a stable baseline incidence of 0.2 to 0.6 percent by age 15. The point prevalence (the incidence rate minus the rate of remission) also is highest in young children, with a decline to the early twenties and a gradual increase thereafter to old age. The inci-

TABLE 76-2   Prevalence and Cumulative Prevalence of Probable and Suspected Asthma, by Sex and Age, Tecumseh, 1962 through 1965[a]

Sex and Age	PREVALENCE		CUMULATIVE PREVALENCE	
	Probable	Suspected	Probable	Suspected
Males				
0–4	4.6	7.2	5.3	8.4
5–9	5.3	3.6	8.9	6.4
10–15	6.0	1.9	10.7	4.4
16–24	3.4	3.2	7.0	6.8
25–34	3.6	2.1	5.6	4.3
35–44	3.0	3.8	6.3	6.7
45–54	3.6	4.7	6.9	6.9
55–64	3.1	4.7	5.4	8.1
65–74	3.1	8.4	5.3	10.7
75+	3.6	7.1	5.4	8.9
All ages	4.2	4.0	7.2	6.5
Females				
0–4	2.7	6.4	3.0	7.6
5–9	3.0	2.2	4.4	4.3
10–15	3.7	1.1	7.6	3.6
16–24	2.5	2.4	4.6	4.1
25–34	5.2	4.6	7.4	6.8
35–44	3.7	4.0	6.6	6.9
45–54	3.9	3.4	8.0	6.6
55–64	2.9	3.9	6.4	7.5
65–74	3.5	3.5	9.9	5.2
75+	3.2	0.0	3.2	1.1
All ages	3.5	3.4	6.0	5.7

[a]Values presented represent percent of total.
SOURCE: From Broder et al.,[7] with permission.

dence of asthma was higher in boys to the adolescent years, and thereafter higher in women.

These findings are confirmed in a large study of patients receiving public assistance from the Medicaid program in Michigan.[13] Over 52,000 cases of asthma were identified in the total population on the basis of a Medicaid billing database used for postmarketing drug surveillance. The prevalence of asthma was greatest in the age group from 0 to 4 years and lowest in the age group from 15 to 29 years, with

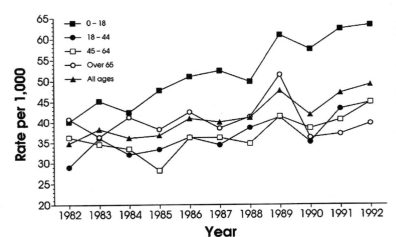

FIGURE 76-2 Prevalence of asthma in the United States. The prevalence rate for asthma is shown for the years 1982 through 1992 as estimated by the National Health Interview Survey each year. The rate represents the number of subjects with asthma, as ascertained by questionnaire, per 1000 study subjects. While the prevalence rate generally is increased in all age groups, it has increased by over 50 percent in the age group from 0 to 18 years from 1982 to 1992. For details of the survey, see text. (*Data from the National Health Interview Survey for the years 1982 through 1992, National Center for Health Statistics, Public Health Service.*)

TABLE 76-3   Prospective Incidence of Asthma by Age and Sex[a]

Age at Entry	Males	Females
0–4	1.4	0.9
5–9	1.0	0.7
10–14	0.2	0.3
15–19	0.0	0.0
20–29	0.2	0.4
30–39	0.0	0.4
40–49	0.0	0.4
50–59	0.0	0.5
60–69	0.3	0.8
70+	0.2	0.6

[a]Values represent incidence per year at risk.
SOURCE: From Dodge and Burrows,[12] with permission.

a gradual increase thereafter to age 45 (Fig. 76-3). As in the Tucson study,[12] males had a higher prevalence to age 20; thereafter women had a higher prevalence. African-American children and young adults had a higher prevalence than white persons or persons of other races, which may reflect a socioeconomic bias in the data collection. Urban children and adults had a higher prevalence than rural individuals: the prevalence was 3.8 per 100 Medicaid recipients for urban children and 2.1 per 100 recipients for rural children in the age group from 0 to 4 years, and 1.8 per 100 urban Medicaid recipients and 0.7 per 100 rural recipients in the age group from 20 to 29 years. This difference may reflect a bias in data collection or population distribution, differences in access to health care, or true differences in the urban and rural environments.

There is thus some evidence that the prevalence of asthma has been increasing in the past two decades. In the 7 years of the Michigan Medicaid study, the prevalence of asthma in the study population increased, from 2.0 per 100 recipients in 1980 to 2.8 per 100 recipients in 1986. This increase was due almost completely to an increased prevalence in younger children.[13] Yunginger and associates conducted an extensive community-based study of asthma in Rochester,

MN from 1964 through 1983.[14] In this study, subjects with asthma were identified through a review of medical records in the community. As medical care in this city was virtually self-contained, all details of the medical care provided to the study population were available for review. The annual age- and sex-adjusted incidence of asthma (defined as definite plus probable asthma) increased from 183 per 100,000 in 1964 to 284 per 100,000 in 1983. This increase was entirely accounted for by increased incidence rates in children 1 to 14 years old (Fig. 76-4).[14] These data are supported by prevalence data obtained from the National Health Interview Survey. The increased prevalence of asthma from 1982 to 1992, as shown in Fig. 76-2, is explained almost entirely by the increased prevalence in persons younger than 18.[10]

Further evidence for the increasing prevalence of asthma in children compared to adults comes from the National Hospital Discharge Survey of the Public Health Service. This survey covers discharges from noninstitutional, non-Federal, acute-care hospitals, and in 1992 reported almost 31 million discharges from a sample of 495 hospitals across the United States.[15] While the rate of discharges has decreased in every age group over the past 10 years, reflecting better utilization of hospital resources and the trend towards outpatient management of many medical problems, the rate of discharges for asthma has decreased only slightly from 1982 to 1992. Asthma discharges for all age groups over age 15 have been stable or declined slightly in this time, whereas asthma discharges for the age group from 0 to 15 years have increased significantly, even while the overall discharge rate for this age group has decreased (Fig. 76-5). The rate of asthma discharges increased even as the length of stay for this age group decreased, from an average of 3.6 days in 1982 to 2.9 days in 1992.[15] This survey is limited in that it does not distinguish new admissions from readmissions and, therefore, cannot distinguish an increased prevalence (more hospitalized children) from an increased severity of illness (children hospitalized more often).

Most of the data, then, suggest that the increasing prevalence of asthma in the United States is due to an increased prevalence in children. One point that is not clear from these

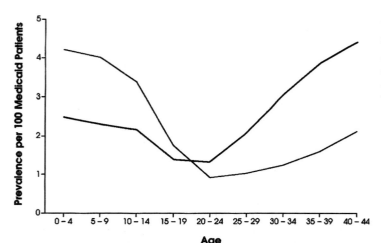

FIGURE 76-3 Average annual prevalence of asthma in subjects aged 0 to 44 years in the Michigan Medicaid population, by age and sex for 1980 through 1986. The solid line represents males; the dotted line represents females. Asthma is more common in males to about age 19, and in women thereafter. For details of the study, see text. (*From Gerstman et al.,*[13] *with permission.*)

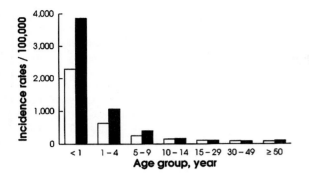

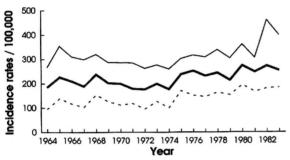

FIGURE 76-4 Incidence of asthma among residents of Rochester, Minnesota, 1964 through 1983. (*Top*) Annual incidence rates of definite and probable asthma per 100,000 person-years by sex and age. Open bars represent females, solid bars represent males. As in the Michigan Medicaid study (Fig. 76-3), asthma is more common in boys through adolescence, and thereafter in women. (*Bottom*) Overall annual incidence rates per 100,000 person-years for definite cases of asthma (dashed line), definite plus probable cases of asthma (heavy solid line), and total cases of definite asthma, probable asthma, and single wheezing episodes (light solid line) among residents. Rates shown are age- and sex-adjusted to the 1970 U.S. white population. The incidence of asthma increased slowly over the study period. For details of the study, see text. (*From Yunginger et al.,*[14] *with permission.*)

studies is whether the prevalence of childhood asthma truly is increasing, or whether physicians are more willing to give the diagnosis. The perception among pediatricians may be changing so that asthma may be diagnosed instead of bronchitis or bronchiolitis, and complaints of episodic wheezing may be considered more seriously now than in the past. Practitioners also may be more willing to treat asthma, as studies have shown that treatment can be effective in children younger than 2 years.[16,17]

Studies done over the past 40 years suggest that about half of all childhood asthmatics become symptom-free as adults.[18–20] The prognosis of asthma in childhood depends on several factors, the most prominent being the age of onset of symptoms. About half of all children who begin wheezing before age 7 will be symptom-free in early adulthood.[20–22] Childhood asthma is more persistent in women,[20] in those with more severe asthma,[22] and in those with onset before the age of 3 years.[23] Derrick demonstrated that patients with onset between birth and 9 years had a worse prognosis than patients with later onset.[24] In one large study, Anderson and colleagues studied 8806 children born in 1958 as part of the National Child Development Study in the United Kingdom.[21] Interviews were done at ages 7, 11, and 16 to track symptoms of asthma and wheezing; of the children who entered the study at birth, 87 percent were available for interview at age 16. Over 75 percent of the children had no history of asthma or wheezing over the course of the study. The prevalence of current asthma was greatest at age 7 (8.3 percent of all children) and least at age 16 (3.5 percent of all children). The prognosis was related to both the presence and the severity of asthma at age 7.[21] These figures are in substantial agreement with those of McNicol and Williams, who performed a population-based survey of children in Melbourne, Australia, and demonstrated that, of children with wheezing at age 7, only 30 percent had symptoms at age 10 and only 25 percent at age 14.[25] It should be noted, however, that questionnaire-based surveys may underesti-

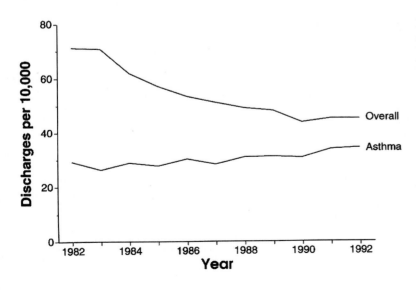

FIGURE 76-5 Hospital discharges of children for asthma in the United States. The rate of discharges per 10,000 population is shown for children aged 0 to 15 years from 1982 to 1992 for the principal diagnosis of asthma (ICD-9 code 493), versus the total number of discharges for the same age group per 10,000. While the overall discharge rate for children has decreased substantially since 1982, the discharge rate for asthma has increased slightly, suggesting a greater prevalence of asthma in hospitalized children compared to overall discharges. (*Data from the National Hospital Discharge Survey for the years 1982 through 1992, National Center for Health Statistics, Public Health Service.*)

mate the severity of asthma. Subjects who are symptom-free for prolonged periods nevertheless may have persistent airways hyperreactivity.[26] In a study of childhood asthmatics who were symptom-free as young adults, Martin and colleagues, demonstrated that 60 percent had persistent airways hyperreactivity; 31 percent of these subjects had recurrent wheezing by age 28.[27] In a later study, Gerritsen and colleagues demonstrated that the outcome of childhood asthma is predicted primarily by the initial degree of bronchial obstruction and responsiveness to histamine.[28] In their study, 101 adults who were asthmatic as children were evaluated for symptoms and airways responsiveness. The mean age of the adults was 26 years, and at least 16 years had elapsed between the childhood and adult evaluations. Of these subjects, 43 percent had symptoms as adults, and all demonstrated airways hyperreactivity to histamine. Of the 58 subjects who no longer had symptoms, only 4 demonstrated sensitivity to histamine. The symptomatic and asymptomatic adults had had similar rates of respiratory symptoms as children, although the asymptomatic adults had been less responsive to histamine as children.[28] These data suggest that both asthma symptoms and airways hyperresponsiveness can be "outgrown," but that this is not necessarily the most likely course.

One important point concerning the prognosis of childhood-onset asthma is that the prognosis will appear progressively worse the longer the interval over which the subjects are studied. A retrospective study by the Royal Army Medical Corps examined a cohort of military recruits discharged from service for asthma.[29] Of 108 discharged soldiers with a history of childhood asthma, 64 percent had a remission between ages 10 and 14. Relapse was most common between 17 and 21 years of age (76 percent of subjects). Of interest, 58 of the total 201 soldiers discharged for asthma had a new onset of asthma after entering service, with symptoms appearing for the first time between ages 17 and 20. Earlier studies, which predicted that many childhood-onset asthmatics would enter remission as young adults, generally studied their subjects for <5 years. More recent studies that have followed children into the third and fourth decades of life have demonstrated relapse, even if the subjects had a period of remission.[18,19] Therefore, a history of childhood asthma or wheezing in an adult with new symptoms compatible with asthma suggests strongly that the original childhood disease has relapsed.

ASTHMA IN YOUNG ADULTS

Asthma is a disease of both adults and children. While the incidence of asthma is less in young adults than in children, new-onset adult asthma (adult asthma without a history of childhood asthma, wheezing, or respiratory complaints) has an incidence of up to 2 percent.[30] Combining both persistent and relapsing childhood-onset asthma cases with new adult-onset asthma yields a total prevalence of asthma in the United States as great as 5 percent.[7,30] Several potential etiologies are cited for adult-onset asthma: respiratory infection causing persistent wheezing; occupational exposure; exposure to environmental pollutants; and occurrence in association with nonallergic rhinitis.[31] Asthmatics with an initial

presentation after the age of 40 may have a history of respiratory complaints and of "chronic bronchitis," to which the diagnosis of "asthma" is added.[12] While asthmatic subjects diagnosed at a young age generally have a history of atopy, that is not necessarily true in older asthmatics.[32]

Remission rates for asthma decline dramatically in adults. In the study of Bronnimann and Burrows, remission rates were 60 percent in adolescents between ages 10 and 19, 30 percent in adults aged 20 to 29, and < 20 percent in adults aged 30 to 39.[33] Coincident with the decline in remission rates was an increase in the relapse rate, which was about 25 percent in the age group 10 to 19 years and almost 50 percent in adults 40 to 49 years old.[33] Lower remission rates for asthma in adults than in children have been confirmed in other studies.[24] Overall, relapse in quiescent asthmatics is a likely event, particularly if there are even mild respiratory symptoms persisting from childhood. Asthma presenting in or persisting into adult years is not likely to remit and carries a prognosis of continued activity and exacerbations throughout adult life.

In children, most studies find more boys than girls with asthma. Among young adults asthma is more common in young adult women than men.[7,34] Estimates from the 1992 National Health Interview Survey show that slightly more women than men under the age of 45 years have asthma: 53.5 per 1000 women versus 50.7 per 1000 men.[10] Similar data are not presented for younger age groups, unfortunately, so that it is not clear when the shift in prevalence from men to women occurs in this survey. In the Michigan Medicaid study, asthma was more prevalent in males to about age 19, and thereafter more prevalent in women (Fig. 76-3).[13]

ASTHMA IN OLDER ADULTS

Asthma in older adults often is confused with chronic bronchitis and emphysema. As originally stated in the Ciba symposium of 1959 and by the American Thoracic Society in 1962, reversible airflow obstruction was defined as asthma, whereas patients with fixed or irreversible airflow obstruction were defined as having either emphysema or chronic bronchitis, even though it was recognized that their condition may respond somewhat to bronchodilators.[2,3] However, the use of variability or hyperreactivity of airflow obstruction as a means of separating asthmatic subjects from those with chronic airflow obstruction (CAO), such as emphysema, chronic bronchitis, and the combined chronic obstructive pulmonary disease, (COPD), has an obvious difficulty—how much reversibility or hyperreactivity is required to merit the diagnosis of asthma? Even apart from the considerable technical difficulties of expressing the difference, deciding what tests to perform in either a clinical or an epidemiologic setting, and deciding just how much of a change is significant, one problem is insurmountable: there are many older patients, particularly those with smoking histories, who have both fixed and relatively fixed airflow obstruction.[35,36] Labeling such patients with both diagnoses (asthma and COPD) seems contrived at best.[37] Further, as described below, many older patients in whom a diagnosis of asthma is firmly established by history, demonstration of atopy, eosinophilia, airways hyperresponsiveness, and clinical response, also may have both fixed and reversible airflow obstruction. Over time, the fixed component may become more pronounced and the reversible component less pronounced, so that the individual appears to have both diseases.[38] The use of bronchodilator responses to separate the two groups of patients has been demonstrated to be unworkable.[39] Once again, the best definition for the natural history of asthma in older adults is the same as for children and young adults: simply a history of asthma reported by either the patient or the physician.

The incidence of new asthma in older adults may be appreciable. Dodge and colleagues have estimated the incidence of asthma in adults aged 40 to 49 years to be about 0.4 new cases per 100 person-years, compared to 1.6 new cases per 100 person-years in children under the age of 5.[38] The incidence of new asthma did not appreciably decline with advancing age to 70 years. Other studies suggest that up to 15 percent of all asthmatic subjects may experience their first symptoms after the age of 40,[40] although only 3 percent develop their first symptoms after age 60.[41] While many elderly asthmatic subjects have smoked and thereby have compounded the difficulty of distinguishing them from subjects with CAO, a study of nonsmoking elderly asthmatics demonstrated that these individuals had the usual sensitivity to histamine provocation, negative skin test responses to common allergens, and normal serum immunoglobulin E concentrations and eosinophil counts.[42]

The prevalence of asthma in older adults also is appreciable. Dodge and Burrows report that 7.1 percent of people over age 70 report symptoms of asthma.[12] A population survey from New South Wales, Australia, showed that about 3 percent of subjects over age 70 had symptomatic asthma, and an additional 3.6 percent had mild asthma with intermittent attacks.[43] Both of these studies included smokers and thus may have overestimated the true prevalence of the disease. Estimates from the 1992 National Health Interview Survey show that in subjects 65 years old and older, the prevalence of asthma is approximately one-third that of chronic bronchitis and emphysema combined.[10] Again, there is no estimate of the number of asthmatic subjects with a smoking history, nor of subjects with chronic airflow obstruction who have significant airways hyperreactivity, so that an appreciable number of subjects may be misclassified. Even allowing for this, the prevalence of asthma in the elderly is significant.

Asthma in older subjects is much less likely to remit over time. In a 9-year study of active asthmatics, the remission rate for subjects over age 50 was 20 to 30 percent, compared to over 60 percent for subjects between the ages of 10 and 19[33] (Fig. 76-6). Lower remission rates for older adults with asthma have been confirmed in other studies.[24,44]

Consequences of Asthma

A potential end point of any chronic, untreated illness is either incapacity or death. With asthma, incapacity may take the form of more severe, more labile reversible airflow obstruction, or the development of new, irreversible airflow

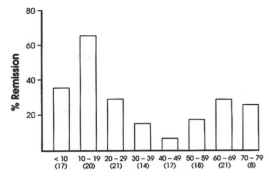

FIGURE 76-6 The rate of remission of asthma by decade of age in a cohort of 136 asthmatic subjects followed over 10 years. The younger asthmatic subjects tend to have a remission, although it may be temporary. The older subjects have a much lower remission rate. Numbers in parentheses indicate the number of subjects in each decade of age. For details of the study, see text. (*From Bronnimann and Burrows,*[33] *with permission.*)

obstruction. The latter consequence, and the potential mortality of asthma, are considered below.

IRREVERSIBLE AIRFLOW OBSTRUCTION

Asthma is defined as a disease of reversible airflow obstruction.[2,3] However, it is clear that at least in some patients, this airflow obstruction is not completely reversible. Finucane and colleagues examined the reversibility of asthma in a cohort of patients treated aggressively with both bronchodilators and oral prednisone to normalize pulmonary function. Even with aggressive therapy, some patients had an element of obstruction that was fixed and not reversible.[45] This irreversible component correlated with both the duration and the severity of their asthma but not with smoking. The predominant mechanism of airflow obstruction was diffuse narrowing of the airways, as opposed to peripheral destruction of small airways as in emphysema. Elderly asthmatic subjects with new-onset asthma often do not respond completely to inhaled bronchodilators and retain an element of fixed airflow obstruction.[42]

Irreversible airflow obstruction and a decrease in lung function may develop over time in asthmatic patients. What is not clear is whether control of asthma symptoms with appropriate therapy prevents the development of irreversible airflow obstruction. In a population study in West Australia, Peat and colleagues demonstrated a decrease in lung function in subjects with asthma over an 18-year period; this decrease was due in nearly equal measures to worsening bronchial hyperresponsiveness and to the development of irreversible airflow limitation.[46] However, their study population was too small to allow them to examine the effect of smoking on this decline. Burrows and colleagues examined the decline in lung function and mortality in 117 patients with "asthmatic bronchitis," chronic bronchitis, and emphysema over a 10-year period. Those with asthmatic bronchitis had a small decline in lung function, with a slope of decline that was substantially less than that for the group classified as having emphysema.[47] Mortality also was less

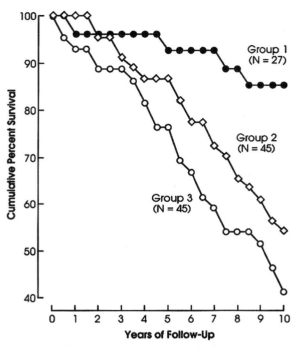

FIGURE 76-7 Comparison of 10-year survival rates in three groups of subjects with chronic airways obstruction. Group 1 included subjects with a diagnosis of asthma who were also atopic, nonsmokers, or both. Group 3 included subjects who were nonatopic smokers without asthma. Group 2 included the remaining subjects. Patients in groups 1 (with asthma) had a mortality that was much less than patients in group 3 who had emphysema. For details of the study, see text. (*From Burrows et al.,*[47] *with permission.*)

in the asthmatic group (15 percent) than in the group with emphysema (60 percent) (Fig. 76-7).[47] It is not clear whether the patients with asthma had been aggressively and adequately treated, so it is not known whether their smaller decline in lung function represents the natural history of asthma as compared to emphysema or was simply the result of effective treatment.

There has been a concern that the presence of asthma, even in a subclinical form, is a risk factor for the development of CAO in later life. A predisposition to airways hyperreactivity, combined with smoking, has been suggested as an etiology of CAO in adults to explain the fact that smoking alone does not cause CAO in all adults.[48] This so-called Dutch hypothesis suggests that the CAO is caused by the combination of airway hyperreactivity and smoking. Asthma in childhood has been associated with reduced pulmonary function in some cross-sectional studies, as has a history of childhood respiratory infection.[49] However, the preferential recall of such histories by those with significant disease introduces a substantial selection bias. Clinical signs seen in asthmatic patients, such as increased concentrations of serum IgE[50,51] and eosinophilia,[52,53] also have been associated with chronic airflow limitation in older adults. A reanalysis of these data by Burrows and colleagues suggests that these factors appear to be important only in subjects with "chronic asthmatic bronchitis" and not in those with

predominant emphysema.[54] Airway hyperreactivity plus smoking is associated with an accelerated rate of decrease in FEV_1 in a cohort of middle-aged, nonasthmatic adult working men studied prospectively over up to 6 years.[55] Hyperreactivity was not associated with an accelerated rate of decrease in pulmonary function in nonsmokers and exsmokers. It is not clear that these subjects had airways hyperreactivity prior to the onset of smoking, and one could argue that such reactivity is an epiphenomenon rather than being causal.

It is clear that some but not all subjects with asthma will develop irreversible airflow obstruction over time, and that this problem will worsen with advancing age. It is not clear that asthma per se is a risk factor for the development of CAO or that it somehow worsens the risk for CAO in subjects who smoke. Further long-term longitudinal studies are required to determine if the natural history of asthma, entwined with deleterious effects of smoking, becomes the natural history of chronic obstructive pulmonary disease.

MORTALITY

At the beginning of this century, Sir William Osler wrote that asthmatic patients don't die, they just pant into old age.[56] Only as this century has progressed has it been appreciated that asthma can be fatal. Asthma mortality has been recorded separately and distinguished reliably from mortality for other obstructive airways diseases in the records of the United States Vital Statistics since 1968. As shown in Fig. 76-8, mortality has increased from 1.3 per 100,000 in 1968 to 2.0 per 100,000 (provisional) in 1993.[57] The sharp increase in mortality in 1979 is explained best by changes in diagnosis coding as a result of the transition from the eighth to the ninth revision of the *International Classification of Diseases*. Following this change, asthma was coded more frequently as such and not as bronchitis.[58,59] The trend downward from 1969 to 1978 may be a result of coding in favor of the more general diagnosis of chronic obstructive lung disease.[59] There has been a trend upward since 1981 that has been seen in all age groups, although it is most pronounced in the elderly asthmatic population. Children and adolescents, in particular, have a low mortality rate from asthma compared to older adults (Fig. 76-8).

What is notable is that, while asthma is a common disease, mortality from asthma is very low compared to that for COPD and other common illnesses. Deaths caused by chronic bronchitis, emphysema, and COPD combined outnumber asthma deaths for all ages $\geq$ 45 years, and the disparity widens rapidly with advancing age. For example, in 1991, the prevalence of chronic bronchitis plus emphysema in individuals aged 65 to 74 years in the United States in the National Health Interview Survey is about 2.4 times greater than that of asthma (88.9 per 1000 persons for chronic bronchitis plus emphysema versus 38.0 per 1000 persons for asthma).[60] However, the mortality from chronic bronchitis, emphysema, and COPD in the same year for subjects aged 65 to 74 years is almost 24 times greater than that for asthma (149.9 per 100,000 for the three combined diseases of CAO versus 6.3 per 100,000 for asthma).[61] While there has been an increasing focus on asthma mortality in the industrialized

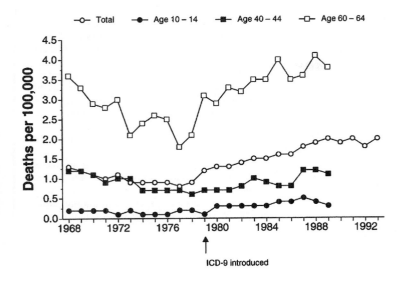

FIGURE 76-8 The mortality rate for asthma in the United States, 1968 through 1993. Asthma mortality (ICD-8 code 493 through 1978; ICD-9 code 493.0 thereafter) is shown for the population overall (through 1993) and for selected 5-year age groups (through 1989). The sharp increase from 1978 to 1979 in both overall mortality and mortality in the age group from 60 through 64 represents the change in coding from ICD-8 to ICD-9. These data suggest that the upward trend in asthma mortality since 1980 may be the result of worsening mortality in elderly asthmatic subjects, as opposed to young or middle-aged subjects. (*) provisional values. (*Data from the Vital and Health Statistics for the years 1968 through 1993, National Center for Health Statistics, Public Health Service.*)

countries, reflecting the prevailing notion that most, if not all, asthma mortality is preventable, the proper context for the following discussion is that asthma mortality is low relative to the prevalence of the disease and is increasing slowly.

What are the factors that have increased asthma mortality, and are these factors part of the natural history of the disorder? Trends in asthma mortality since 1970 in the industrialized Western countries demonstrate a wide variation in asthma mortality rates in young adults, though little change in asthma mortality in children.[62] A gradual increase has been noted in most countries since the mid-1970s. Several factors may account for this. As with prevalence data, the increase in asthma mortality may be due to an increased willingness on the part of practitioners to list asthma instead of a more general diagnosis. Asthma may be diagnosed correctly in more cases now that it is recognized as a disease of reversible airflow obstruction and now that tests to distinguish asthma from other diseases of airflow obstruction are more available. The prevalence of asthma may be increasing, as noted above. There has been increased recognition of the disease and of the need for early intervention. Treatment requires not only knowledge and appropriate therapy, but also access to that therapy. Lack of access and deteriorating socioeconomic status may worsen mortality by preventing appropriate treatment. It is interesting to note that in the United States, asthma deaths are concentrated in four regions: New York, NY, Cook County, IL (including Chicago), Fresno County, CA, and Maricopa County, AZ.[1] Cook County (Chicago) and the city of New York alone account for 21.1 percent of all asthma deaths in the United States aged 5 to 34 years, although they contain only 6.8 percent of the population.[1] Small-area analyses of the cities of Chicago and New York demonstrate that disproportionate numbers of deaths occur in a few inner-city neighborhoods.[63,64] Social factors, language and cultural barriers, poverty, and city pollution, combined with poor access to health care, may constitute as great a barrier to the control of asthma as they did for the control of tuberculosis. These data suggest that whatever the effects of specific drug therapies

may be (see below), the natural history of asthma surely is modified by effective medical intervention.

Does corticosteroid treatment modify the natural history of asthma? Certainly, effective treatment lessens the risk of death, which is a potential outcome of untreated asthma. But, as demonstrated above, death is not the usual outcome in all but the most severe cases of asthma. Regular use of inhaled corticosteroids is associated with a lessening of airways inflammation,[65] but, again, there is no conclusive demonstration that this effect prevents the progression of asthma or the development of irreversible airflow obstruction. Clearly, however, these agents control asthma symptoms and reduce the risk of death.

Recent evidence suggests that some therapies may, paradoxically, worsen the natural history of asthma. Treatment with potent β-adrenergic agonists, a traditional mainstay of first-line therapy, recently has been reported to increase asthma mortality.[66–71] The mechanisms proposed to explain how β-adrenergic agonists worsen mortality and morbidity include development of hypokalemia, induction of cardiac ventricular irritability, and worsening of airway reactivity by development of tolerance or tachyphylaxis. These data are interesting but not yet compelling. Several of the major claims are subject to methodologic problems.[1] A major case-control study suggests that regular use of β-adrenergic agonists is associated with an increased risk of death.[66] However, this study has some problems concerning the adjustments for the severity of illness, the difficulty of measuring exactly how much β-adrenergic agonist the subjects actually were taking, and the selection of proper controls.[1,67] Further, the estimated risk of death associated with the use of albuterol (salbutamol), a major β agonist used in the United States, was 2.4 times the risk when the agent was not used. This is a small increment in risk even if true, since the risk of death from asthma is small compared to its overall prevalence, as noted above. Finally, it is curious that albuterol, a selective $β_2$-adrenergic agonist, is associated with death in this study from Canada, whereas there has been no sudden increase in asthma mortality in other coun-

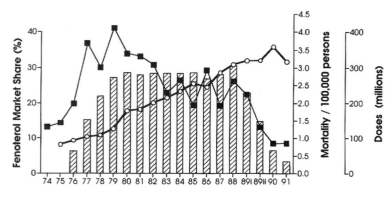

FIGURE 76-9 The potential relation of the use of the potent, nonspecific β-adrenergic agonist, fenoterol, to asthma mortality in New Zealand. Total sales of β-adrenergic agonists (*open circles*, in millions of doses), fenoterol market share (*bars*, as a percentage of total sales) and asthma mortality (*closed squares*, in mortality per 100,000 persons) are shown. While the sales of β-adrenergic agonists continued to increase, the decrease in asthma mortality from 1988 to 1991 was associated with warnings about the use of fenoterol in severe asthmatics (first half of 1989) and the subsequent decline in fenoterol use (second half of 1989). This association suggests that the use (or overuse) of potent β-adrenergic agonists may be related to asthma mortality, but it does not implicate the use of other β-adrenergic agonists, such as albuterol (salbutamol) and terbutaline. (*From Ernst et al.,*[65] *with permission.*)

tries in which this agent has been used, such as the United States. In fact, only the non-subtype-specific β-adrenergic agonists such as isoproterenol and fenoterol have been associated with broad, though small, changes in mortality[68–71]; these agents may have greater cardiac side effects than equivalent doses of the more selective β2-adrenergic agonists. Health care costs, in-patient days for patients hospitalized for asthma, and sick leave all declined in Sweden after the introduction of the specific β2-adrenergic agonists albuterol and terbutaline.[72]

A series of case-control studies from New Zealand examined mortality allegedly caused by fenoterol.[68,70,71] These studies suggested strongly that fenoterol, but not other β-adrenergic agonists, was associated with a severalfold increase in death in asthmatic patients. However, the control group also had an increased risk of death associated with the use of theophylline and oral corticosteroids, as in the Saskatchewan studies.[66,70] These data suggest that the control subjects were poorly matched and had a severity of illness different from those using β agonists on a regular basis. However, it is clear that the high-potency formulation of fenoterol used, combined with its lack of specificity for β-adrenergic receptor subtypes, was associated with increased mortality. Withdrawal of this agent from the New Zealand market was associated with reduction in mortality, though the total use of β-adrenergic agonists did not change[67] (Fig. 76-9).

Another study has suggested that the regular use of fenoterol in high concentrations can result in deteriorating control of asthma, compared to as-needed use of the same drug.[73] However, there are no estimates of variability in these observations, and therefore no way to validate the conclusions.[1] The issue of compliance with a regular-use regimen was not addressed adequately in this study, nor was the issue of the proper use of as-needed regimens for symptom relief, which may be likened to "titration to suffering." Finally, another study has demonstrated that the regular use of salmeterol, a β-adrenergic agonist with a longer duration of action than albuterol, results in better control of asthma symptoms without changing intrinsic airways reactivity.[74]

Taken together, these data suggest, but do not demonstrate with certainty, that the excessive use of β-adrenergic agonists or the use of nonspecific β-adrenergic agonists may cause worsening of asthma symptoms and thereby alter control of the illness. It is not clear that this alters the natural history, though it is claimed that small changes in airways reactivity due to overuse of β-adrenergic agonists would shift the population distribution towards more patients with worsened disease.[75] This remains to be demonstrated conclusively.

The worst consequence of the natural history of asthma—mortality—has been increasing slowly in the United States over the past two decades. It is difficult to prove in epidemiologic studies that treatment lessens mortality, though it is clear that aggressive therapy in the most severe asthmatic patients prevents complications, hospitalizations, and, one hopes, death from asthma.

Conclusions

Asthma is a common disease in both children and adults. The incidence of asthma is greatest in childhood, but the disease can appear at any age. Remission rates are substantial in adolescents and young adults, but remission is uncommon in older adults. Individuals in remission should be considered to have a substantial risk of relapse, and perhaps should be considered as having "asthma in remission." With prolonged and severe asthma, irreversible airflow obstruction may develop, even in lifelong nonsmokers. Asthma mortality is increasing in the industrialized world despite advances in therapy, though it is clear that aggressive medical therapy can prevent complications and death. Perhaps the best hope in preventing the progression of the natural history of asthma will come through better access to health care, as opposed to specific improvements in pharmacologic therapy.

Acknowledgments

Data from specific years of the National Health Interview Survey, National Hospital Discharge Survey, and Vital and Health Statistics are cited in the references. Space limitations do not permit citing each year of each of these surveys separately. Therefore, I thank the many people at the National Center for Health Statistics, Public

Health Service, for their compilation of the surveys used in this chapter.

This work is supported in part by grants HL 48696 and HL 02484 from the National Heart, Lung and Blood Institute, and by a grant from the American Lung Association.

References

1. McFadden ER, Gilbert IA: Asthma. *N Engl J Med* 1992; 327:1928.
2. Ciba Guest Symposium: Terminology, definitions and classifications of chronic pulmonary emphysema and related conditions. *Thorax* 1959; 14:286.
3. American Thoracic Society: Chronic bronchitis, asthma, and pulmonary emphysema. A statement by the committee on diagnostic standards for nontuberculous respiratory diseases. *Am Rev Respir Dis* 1962; 85:762.
4. Burrows B, Lebowitz MD, Barbee BA: Respiratory disorders and allergy skin-test reactions. *Ann Intern Med* 1976; 84:134.
5. Casale TB, Rhodes BJ, Donnelly AL, Weiler JM: Airway reactivity to methacholine in nonatopic asymptomatic adults. *J Appl Physiol* 1988; 64:2558.
6. Rijcken B, Schouten JP, Weiss ST, et al.: The distribution of bronchial responsiveness to histamine in symptomatic and in asymptomatic subjects. A population-based analysis of various indices of responsiveness. *Am Rev Respir Dis* 1989; 140:615.
7. Broker I, Higgins MW, Mathews KP, Keller JB: Epidemiology of asthma and allergic rhinitis in a total community, Tecumseh, Michigan. III. Second survey of the community. *J Allergy Clin Immunol* 1974; 53:127.
8. Wilder CS: Prevalence of selected chronic respiratory conditions. *Vital Health Stat* 1973; 10:1.
9. Schachter J: Measurement of the prevalence of respiratory allergies by interview questionnaire. *J Allergy Clin Immunol* 1975; 55:249.
10. Benson V, Marano MA: Current estimates from the National Health Interview Survey, 1992. *Vital Health Stat* 1994; 10:189.
11. Siegel SC, Rachelefsky GS: Asthma in infants and children: part I. *J Allergy Clin Immunol* 1985; 76:1.
12. Dodge RR, Burrows B: The prevalence and incidence of asthma and asthma-like symptoms in a general population sample. *Am Rev Respir Dis* 1980; 122:567.
13. Gerstman BB, Bosco LA, Tomita TK, et al.: Prevalence and treatment of asthma in the Michigan Medicaid patient population younger than 45 years, 1980–1986. *J Allergy Clin Immunol* 1989; 83:1032.
14. Yunginger JW, Reed CE, O'Connell EJ, et al.: A community-based study of the epidemiology of asthma. Incidence rates, 1964–1983. *Am Rev Respir Dis* 1992; 146:888.
15. Graves EJ: *1992 Summary: National Hospital Discharge Survey. Advance Data from Vital and Health Statistics*, no 249. Hyattsville, MD; National Center for Health Statistics, 1994.
16. Tal A, Bavilski C, Yohai D, et al.: Dexamethasone and salbutamol in the treatment of acute wheezing in infants. *Pediatrics* 1983; 71:13.
17. Lenney W, Milner AD: At what age do bronchodilators work? *Arch Dis Child* 1978; 53:532.
18. Ryssing E: Continued follow-up investigation concerning the fate of 298 asthmatic children. *Acta Pediatr* 1959; 48:255.
19. Blair H: Natural history of childhood asthma. *Arch Dis Child* 1977; 52:613.
20. Martin AJ, McLennan LA, Landau LI, Phelan PD: The natural history of childhood asthma to adult life. *Br Med J* 1980; 280:1397.
21. Anderson HR, Bland JM, Patel S, Peckham C: The natural history of asthma in childhood. *J Epidemiol Commun Health* 1986; 40;121.
22. Jönsson JA, Boe J, Berlin E: The long-term prognosis of childhood asthma in a predominantly rural Swedish county. *Acta Paediatr Scand* 1987; 76:950.
23. Martin AJ, Landau LI, Phelan PD: Natural history of allergy in asthmatic children followed to adult life. *Med J Aust* 1981; 2:470.
24. Derrick EH: The significance of the age of onset of asthma. *Med J Aust* 1971; 1:1317.
25. McNicol KN, Williams HE, Allan J, McAndrew I: Spectrum of asthma in children. III, Psychological and social components. *Br J Med* 1973; 4:16.
26. Blackhall M: Ventilating function in subjects with childhood asthma who have become symptom free. *Arch Dis Child* 1970; 45:363.
27. Martin AJ, Landau LI, Phelan PD: Lung function in young adults who had asthma in childhood. *Am Rev Respir Dis* 1980; 122:609.
28. Gerritsen J, Koëter GH, Postma DS, et al.: Prognosis of asthma from childhood to adulthood. *Am Rev Respir Dis* 1989; 140:1325.
29. Dickenson JG: Asthma in the army: a retrospective study and review of the natural history of asthma and its implications for recruitment. *J R Army Med Corps* 1988; 134:65.
30. Broder I, Higgins MW, Mathews KP, Keller JB: Epidemiology of asthma and allergic rhinitis in a total community, Tecumseh, Michigan. IV. Natural history. *J Allergy Clin Immunol* 1974; 54:100.
31. Nelson HS: The natural history of asthma. *Ann Allergy* 1991; 66:196.
32. Burrows B: The natural history of asthma. *J Allergy Clin Immunol* 1987; 80:373.
33. Bronnimann S, Burrows B: A prospective study of the natural history of asthma remission and relapse rates. *Chest* 1986; 90:480.
34. Wormald PJ: Age-sex incidence in symptomatic allergies an excess of females in the childbearing years. *J Hyg* 1977; 79:39.
35. Anthonisen NR, Wright EC: IPPB Trial Group: Bronchodilator response in chronic obstructive pulmonary disease. *Am Rev Respir Dis* 1986; 133:814.
36. Nisar M, Walshaw M, Earis JE, Pearson MG: Calverley PMA: Assessment of reversibility of airway obstruction in patients with chronic obstructive airways disease. *Thorax* 1991; 45:190.
37. Gross NJ: COPD: a disease of reversible air-flow obstruction. *Am Rev Respir Dis* 1986; 133:725.
38. Dodge R, Cline MG, Burrows B: Comparisons of asthma, emphysema, and chronic bronchitis diagnoses in a general population sample. *Am Rev Respir Dis* 1986; 133:981.
39. Eliasson O, DeGraff AC: The use of criteria for reversibility and obstruction to define patient groups for bronchodilator trials. Influence of clinical diagnosis, spirometric, and anthropometric variables. *Am Rev Respir Dis* 1985; 132:858.
40. Broder I, Barlow PPO, Horton RJM: The epidemiology of asthma and hay fever in a total community, Tecumseh, Michigan. *J Allergy* 1962; 33:513.
41. Ford RM: Aetiology of asthma: a review of 11,551 cases. *Med J Aust* 1969; 1:628.
42. Braman SS, Kaemmerlen JT, Davis SM: Asthma in the elderly: a comparison between patients with recently acquired and long-standing disease. *Am Rev Respir Dis* 1991; 143:336.
43. Burr ML, Charles TJ, Roy K, Seaton A: Asthma in the elderly: an epidemiological survey. *Br Med J* 1979; 1:1041.
44. Ogilvie AG: Asthma: a study in prognosis of 1000 patients. *Thorax* 1962; 17:183.
45. Finucane KE, Grevill HW, Brown PJE: Irreversible airflow obstruction: evolution in asthma. *Med J Aust* 1985; 142:602.
46. Peat JK, Woolcock AJ, Cullen K: Rate of decline of lung function in subjects with asthma. *Eur J Respir Dis* 1987; 70:171.
47. Burrows B, Bloom JW, Traver GA, Cline MG: The course and

prognosis of different forms of chronic airways obstruction in a sample from the general population. *N Engl J Med* 1987; 317:1309.

48. Oire NGM, Slutier HJ, DeVries K, et al.: The host factor in bronchitis, in Orie NGM, Slutier HJ, (eds): *Bronchitis.* Assen, Royal Vangorcum, 1969:43–59.

49. Burrows B, Knudson RJ, Lebowitz MD: The relationship of childhood respiratory illness to adult obstructive airway disease. *Am Rev Respir Dis* 1977; 115:751.

50. Burrows B, Halonen M, Lebowitz MD, et al.: The relationship of serum immunoglobulin E, allergy skin tests, and smoking to respiratory disorders. *J Allergy Clin Immunol* 1982; 70:199.

51. Dow L, Coggon D, Campbell MJ, et al.: The interaction between immunoglobulin E and smoking in airflow obstruction in the elderly. *Am Rev Respir Dis* 1992; 146:402.

52. Burrows B, Hasan FM, Barbee RA, et al.: Epidemiologic observations on eosinophilia and its relation to respiratory disorders. *Am Rev Respir Dis* 1980; 122:709.

53. Mensinga TT, Schouten JP, Weiss ST, Van der Lenge R: Relationship of skin test reactivity and eosinophilia to level of pulmonary function in a community-based population study. *Am Rev Respir Dis* 1992; 146:638.

54. Burrows B, Knudson RJ, Cline MG, Lebowitz MD: A reexamination of risk factors for ventilatory impairment. *Am Rev Respir Dis* 1988; 138:829.

55. Frew AJ, Kennedy SM, Chan-Yeung M: Methacholine responsiveness, smoking and atopy as risk factors for accelerated FEV_1 decline in male working populations. *Am Rev Respir Dis* 1992; 146:878.

56. Osler W: *The Principles and Practice of Medicine,* 4th ed. Edinburgh, Pentland, 1901.

57. National Center for Health Statistics: Annual summary of births, marriages, divorces and deaths: United States, 1993. *Month Vital Stat Report* 1994; 42(13).

58. Evans R, Mullally DI, Wilson RW, et al.: National trends in the morbidity and mortality of asthma in the US. Prevalence, hospitalization and death from asthma over two decades: 1965–1984. *Chest* 1987; 91:65S.

59. Gergen PJ, Weiss KB: Changing patterns of asthma hospitalization among children: 1979 to 1987. *JAMA* 1990; 264:1688.

60. Benson V, Marano MA: Current estimates from the National Health Interview Survey, 1991. *Vital Health Stat* 1993; 10(184).

61. National Center for Health Statistics: Advance report of final mortality statistics, 1991. *Month Vital Stat Rep* 1993; 42(2).

62. Jackson R, Sears MR, Beaglehole R, Rea HH: International trends in asthma mortality: 1970 to 1985. *Chest* 1988; 94:914.

63. Carr W, Zeitel L, Weiss KB: Asthma hospitalization and mortality in New York City. *Am J Public Health* 1992; 82:59.

64. Marder D, Targonsky P, Orris P, et al.: Effect of racial and socioeconomic factors on asthma mortality in Chicago. *Chest* 1992; 101:427S.

65. Ernst P, Spitzer WO, Suissa S, et al.: Risk of fatal and near-fatal asthma in relation to inhaled corticosteroid use. *JAMA* 1992; 268:3462.

66. Spitzer WO, Suissa S, Ernst P, et al.: The use of β-agonists and the risk of death and near death from asthma. *N Engl J Med* 1992; 326:501.

67. Pearce NE, Beasely R, Crane J, Burgess C: Epidemiology of asthma mortality, in Busse WW, Holgate ST (eds): *Asthma and Rhinitis.* Boston, Blackwell Scientific 1994: 58.

68. Beaglehole R, Jackson R, Sears M, Rea H: Asthma mortality in New Zealand: a review with some policy implications. *NZ Med J* 1987; 100:231.

69. Beasley R, Pearce N, Crane J, et al.: Asthma mortality and inhaled beta agonist therapy. *Aust NZ J Med* 1991; 21:753.

70. Grainger J, Woodman K, Pearce NE, et al.: Prescribed fenoterol and death from asthma in New Zealand 1981–7: a further case-control study. *Thorax* 1991; 46:105.

71. Pearce NE, Grainger J, Atkinson M, et al.: Case-control study of prescribed fenoterol and death from asthma in New Zealand, 1977–1981. *Thorax* 1991; 45:170.

72. Lofdahl CG, Svemyr N: Beta-agonists—friends or foes? *Eur Respir J* 1991; 4:1161.

73. Sears MR, Taylor DR, Print CG, et al.: Regular inhaled beta-agonist treatment in bronchial asthma. *Lancet* 1990; 336:1391.

74. Cheung D, Timmers MC, Zinderman AH, et al.: Long-term effects of a long-acting $β_2$-adrenoceptor agonist, salmeterol, on airway hyperresponsiveness in patients with mild asthma. *N Engl J Med* 1992; 327:1198.

75. Mitchell EA: Is current treatment increasing asthma mortality and morbidity? [Editorial] *Thorax* 1989; 44:81.

Chapter 77 _____

SELECTING A
TREATMENT REGIMEN
FOR ASTHMA

ALAN R. LEFF

Asthma will be encountered in the treatment of patients as a coincident process by physicians of all specialties, as there currently are 12 million to 15 million persons with asthma in the United States. An assessment of the severity and requisite treatment of asthma is essential even for patients whose asthma is under good control if they are facing situations of potential physiologic risk or stress (e.g., surgical anesthesia with intubation). As asthma is inherently an unstable process, contingency plans may be essential for many asthma patients who contemplate travel to either distant locations where medical therapy may not be readily available, or to high altitudes or physiologically stressful environments that may provoke otherwise quiescent asthma.

It is important to recognize that asthma is not a disease, but rather a syndrome of reversible bronchospasm characterized by a variable degree of inflammation.[1,2] Accordingly, different therapies are required for different patients. This has become obvious particularly with the development of selective "designer" therapies, which appear to have selective efficacy among asthma patients.[3] There is yet no established paradigm for assessing which patients with asthma may benefit from specific therapies, and with the few exceptions cited below, the implementation of polypharmacy for the treatment of asthma largely is based on the severity of ill-ness as assessed clinically and physiologically. While treatments directed toward etiology (i.e., allergy, inflammation) are esthetically appealing, bronchodilation, physical comfort, and prevention of tragic, premature death are the guiding principles of asthma therapy. Selection of a treatment regimen must account the therapeutic benefit against the therapeutic risk, and herein lies the common ground on which optimal therapy is based.

Treatment of Asthma in the Ambulatory Setting

ASSESSMENT OF SEVERITY

For all but the most severe asthma patients, treatment resides solely in the outpatient setting. Accordingly, evaluation and formulation of a therapeutic regimen is a customized formulation for each patient. Nearly all patients with inadequately controlled asthma experience nocturnal awakenings.[4,5] In a survey conducted by Turner-Warwick,[4] > 93 percent of all patients with asthma experienced one nocturnal awakening per month, and approximately two-thirds of all patients were awakened > 3 nights per week

TABLE 77-1   Frequency of Nocturnal Awakenings in Untreated Asthma

Once per month	94%
Once per week	74%
≥ 3 times per week	64%
Every night	39%

SOURCE: Adapted from Turner-Warwick.[4]

with dyspnea related to asthma (Table 77-1). The frequency of nocturnal awakenings also corresponded to the severity of airflow obstruction observed in the subsequent physiologic assessment of these patients. In the initial assessment of the adequacy of the need for therapy or of an existing treatment regimen, inquiry into the sleep patterns of asthma patients serves as a simple index of the adequacy of control of the patient's asthma. Airway caliber follows a circadian rhythm. In the late afternoon (around 4:00 P.M.), airflow obstruction is least severe; in the early morning hours (around 4:00 A.M.), airflow obstruction is maximal. This pattern, which is observed among normal individuals, is accentuated among asthmatics. Hence, physical examination of historical information about a patient's symptoms during "office hours" may belie what is actually a more serious situation.

Physical examination of the asthma patient is most useful when remarkable findings are overt. An obviously tachypneic individual who is using accessory respiratory muscles requires prompt attention (see below). However, even patients with episodic severe asthma may not demonstrate wheezing on tidal respiration. Auscultation during forced expiration may reveal wheezing that is not obvious during tidal inspiration; forced inspiratory or expiratory maneuvers also may cause reflex cough (i.e., cough irritability).[6] This reflex causing cough in patients having bronchoconstriction is poorly understood and may relate to simultaneous irritability of cough receptors in the upper airways[7]; however, the reason for improvement in cough threshold with bronchodilation remains unclear.[8] It is possible that patients experiencing episodic severe symptoms will demonstrate no diagnostic physiologic findings during examination. For these patients, further evaluation includes lung function testing. At a minimum, this should include a spirometric assessment of airflow obstruction and, if obstruction is demonstrated, attempted reversal of airflow obstruction with inhaled bronchodilator. For patients with a history of cigarette smoking, industrial exposure, or other potential causes of chronic obstructive pulmonary disease, a full battery of pulmonary function tests that includes plethysmographic measurement of lung volume, airway resistance, and diffusing capacity is useful. In some young patients with no significant spirometric evidence of airflow obstruction, a mild degree of hypoxemia may reveal an underlying ventilation-perfusion mismatch that results from subtle airflow obstruction. For patients with nondiagnostic findings from these tests of lung function, but with convincing history of symptoms, bronchial challenge testing may reveal airway hyperreactivity[9,10] (see also Chap. 73). While airway hyper-

responsiveness sometimes is found in patients who do not have asthma, a positive bronchial challenge test (defined as a decrease in FEV_1 of > 20 percent at a concentration of methacholine < 8 to 10 mg/mL) is considered diagnostic of "latent" asthma. In patients with cough-variant asthma,[11] this may be the only positive finding.

The collated results of history, physical findings, and physiologic evaluation are the basis upon which the need for and extent of therapy is made. In the simplest terms, the requirement for therapy falls into one of two categories: symptomatic treatment and mandatory therapy. For patients with rare nocturnal awakenings, minimal symptoms, and a sedentary lifestyle, little or no therapy may be required, and treatment under these circumstances certainly can be administered on an episodic (as needed) basis. For patients with history of frequent hospitalization, severe airflow obstruction, and prior history of emergency treatment or hospitalization for asthma, continuous maintenance therapy is essential.

Marquette and colleagues[12] followed 145 asthmatics previously hospitalized for status asthmaticus of severity sufficient to require mechanical ventilation. Approximately 20 percent of these patients died of their asthma within the next 6 years.[12] For patients < 40 years of age, asthma death over the next 5 years was rare. However, > 40 percent of all patients > 40 years of age died within 5 to 6 years after requiring mechanical ventilation for treatment of their asthma (Fig. 77-1). This study demonstrates the need for continued vigilance among a subset of patients who can be identified by selected risk factors to be at increased risk for asthma death (Table 77-2). In recent years, such patients have been classified as having "fatal asthma syndrome" or "sudden onset fatal asthma."[13–15] This complex identifies patients who require oral corticosteroid for treatment of their disease and who have a prior history of hospitalization, especially those who have required mechanical ventilation for their asthma and who thus are at greater risk for asthma death. This is a particular concern for patients who have a high threshold for dyspnea caused by increased work of breathing. Such patients may be unaware of development of severe airflow obstruction, which further may delay lifesaving therapy. A separate concern exists as to whether certain therapies independently increase the risk of asthma death. Beta-adrenergic agonists, oral corticosteroids, and theophylline all have been correlated to increased death rates among asthmatics.[15,16] Yet, there has been no report relating the physiologic severity of airflow obstruction to the patients taking these drugs. As these are the drugs used most frequently by patients with severe airflow obstruction, a reasonable concern remains as to whether there is a causal, rather than merely correlative, relationship in these retrospective observations.[17] It is difficult to conceive of how three different drugs, all having very different toxicities, could each be associated with increased asthma death, except as markers of disease severity. It is even more difficult to conceive how one would manage severe asthma without substantial use of these drugs, particularly given the high mortality rate associated with the most severe forms of airflow obstruction.[12]

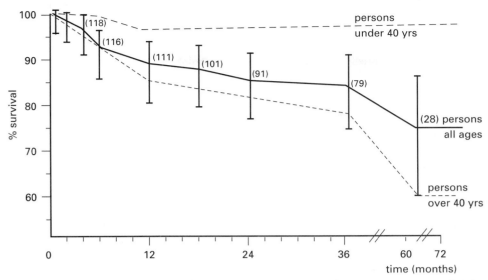

FIGURE 77-1 Mechanical ventilation required for treatment of asthma in patients over and under 40 years of age.

TABLE 77-2   Risk Factors in Asthma Deaths

1. History of frequent emergency visits/hospitalizations.
2. Prior necessity of mechanical ventilation for treatment, especially if > 40 years old.
3. Frequent or constant use of oral corticosteroid medications.
4. High threshold for perception of dyspnea with increased work of breathing.
5. Associations: Frequent use of β-adrenoceptor drugs, cortico-steroids, or theophylline.

BETA-ADRENERGIC AGONISTS

Beta-adrenergic agonists cover the gamut of the severity of asthma. For patients with minimal asthma induced only after exercise, those who have very infrequent nocturnal awakenings, or those having no symptoms except those induced by specific infrequent or avoidable environmental conditions, a relatively short-acting β-adrenoceptor agonist (e.g., albuterol) administered as needed is the only required therapy. It also should be noted, however, that β-adrenoceptor agonists are roughly twice as effective as all other therapies (except oral corticosteroids) in causing bronchodilation (see below). Hence, their inclusion in treatment regimens of patients with severe asthma is universal. There is, however, substantial debate about how these agents should be used in the treatment of severe asthma. Virtually all investigators agree that when β-adrenergic agonists are used routinely in asthma, they should be administered with corticosteroids (inhaled or orally administered). The concern is whether β-adrenoceptor agonists induce tolerance after sustained use or whether they actually cause asthma deaths that would not otherwise occur.[18] However, there have been no prospective studies that have implicated causally β-adrenoceptor agonists in increased asthma deaths, and prior retrospective studies have been decidedly deficient in separating causality from correlation (i.e., severity of illness from frequency of therapy)[19] (see also above). The β-adrenergic agonist, fenoterol was correlated to increased asthma deaths after its introduction in New Zealand, and this increase in asthma deaths diminished after the drug was withdrawn from use by the government.[20] Withdrawal, however, also corresponded to increased access to health care among the indigenous population of that country, and a causal relationship between fenoterol and asthma death thus cannot be established with certainty. There are some reasons to consider that certain β-adrenergic agonists could theoretically cause potentially fatal cardiotoxic arrhythmias (see Chap. 47), and thus, as for other medication, monitoring, vigilance, and *prospective* study are warranted.

A recent evaluation of the long-acting β-adrenergic agonist salmeterol against albuterol, conducted by Glaxo Pharmaceutical Corporation in the United Kingdom, examined prospectively the risk of death between these two agents in ~ 25,000 subjects. A statistically significant difference in asthma deaths between the groups was not found. However, the period of study was short (16 weeks), and no comparisons were made to subjects not receiving any β-adrenergic agonist. A recent investigation of quality of life indicated that patients treated with regularly administered salbutamol demonstrated better control of asthma than those receiving "as needed" treatment.[21] Presumably, the use of new, long-acting β-adrenoceptor agonists affords the opportunity for steady-state bronchodilation and improved therapeutic compliance. The burden of evidence suggests that for any patient with persistent symptoms, regular use of

TABLE 77-3 Potency, Specificity, and Intrinsic Activity of β-Adrenoceptor Agonists

	RELATIVE POTENCY		
Compound	β_1-adrenoceptor/atrium	β_2-adrenoceptor/bronchus	Selectivity β_2:β_1
Isoproterenol	1.0	1.0	1.0
Albuterol	0.0004	0.55	1375
Fenoterol	0.005	0.6	120
Formoterol	0.05	20.0	400
Salmeterol	0.0001	8.5	85,000

SOURCE: Adapted with permission from Johnson et al.[51]

β-adrenoceptor agonists, including long-acting agents such as salmeterol or formoterol, are both safe and desirable. Formoterol is not yet available in the United States. These drugs have both high potency and selectivity for the β_2-adrenoceptor (Table 77-3). In theory, this offers the optimal therapeutic approach to the use of β-adrenergic agonist for patients with persistent symptoms who otherwise frequently require daily use of β-adrenoceptor agonists (e.g., albuterol). A recent report[22] has suggested that continued use of β-adrenoceptor agonists causes increased airway responsiveness (e.g., as assessed by methacholine challenge); however, there is no demonstration of lack of efficacy from continued use, and many studies conducted over many years indicate that true tachyphylaxis from use of β-adrenoceptor agonists is not a concern (see Chap. 48). This seems especially true for patients who simultaneously are taking inhaled corticosteroids. Although not mandated in the United States, in many European countries inhaled corticosteroids are required by law to be administered concomitantly with salmeterol. This seems wise; patients who require sustained bronchodilation with β-adrenergic agonists likely also require a second medication to optimize bronchodilation, and a drug with a different mode of action (e.g., an anti-inflammatory agent) having nonadditive toxicity is an optimal choice.

INHALED CORTICOSTEROIDS

Inhaled corticosteroids have been demonstrated unequivocally to cause improvement in spirometric measurements of airflow obstruction,[23] presumably through their anti-inflammatory effects. These drugs are delivered topically through metered-dose inhalers, and are most frequently used in combination with inhaled β-adrenergic agonists. For patients with persistent asthma symptoms of a mild to moderate nature, a combination of these two medications may suffice. As noted, longer-acting β-adrenoceptor agonists need to be administered only twice daily, and thus are considered preferable to shorter-acting agents in improving therapeutic compliance. In the United States, beclomethasone dipropionate (84 to 168 μg twice daily to four times daily) and triamcinolone acetate (200 to 400 μg twice daily to four times daily) are the two most frequently used compounds. These drugs are administered through metered-dose inhalers. Flunisolide is an inhaled corticosteroid designed for twice-daily use. It is not clear that this compound is significantly more effective than larger doses of either beclomethasone or triamcinalone administered twice daily, and many patients complain of its taste. Regardless of the compound selected, regular use of inhaled corticosteroids is essential. The onset of improvement also is slow and may not be maximal for several weeks after initiation of therapy. Hence, patients may be unaware of the incremental benefit of inhaled corticosteroids. Likewise, without the knowledge that these are slow-acting anti-inflammatory agents, patients may be tempted to use these agents on an "as needed" basis.

In regimens where both long-acting β-adrenergic agonists and corticosteroids are used optimally, "breakthrough" symptoms still may persist. One current recommendation is for the use of supplemental short-acting β_2-adrenergic agonists (not more frequently than 4 h apart) for patients who are receiving treatment with salmeterol and inhaled corticosteroids. If frequent use is required (more than twice daily), the patient should seek advice from the prescribing physician. It is important that patients avoid self-treatment of acute asthma symptoms with long-acting agents. These are slow in onset, and anticipation that improvement would occur with the use of salmeterol in this circumstance, as for albuterol, is speculated as a potential (but unsubstantiated) cause of as many as 20 asthma deaths in the United States over an 18-month period. The necessity of supplementing inhaled long-acting β-adrenoceptor agonists with further doses of short-acting analogs may depend in large part on the efficacy of the inhaled corticosteroid preparation that is used. Fluticasone[24] and budesonide[25] are significantly more potent than the inhaled corticosteroids that are licensed for use in the United States, and their ability to abrogate use of supplemental treatment with short-acting β-adrenergic agonists has not been assessed here.

Some have advocated the use of these compounds as the exclusive first-line agents in mild asthma. This reasoning is based largely on the anti-inflammatory mechanism of the action of the compounds. The practicality of this is another matter. For patients who require only intermittent treatment on a symptomatic basis, the continuous use of compounds that must be administered more than once daily is a questionable therapeutic strategy.

THEOPHYLLINE

Theophylline is a compound that has been in use for many decades, and in its different forms it has had many lives. It has been delivered by intravenous administration, suppository, orally in elixir form, as tablet and time-released tablet preparations, and even by smoking. It is ineffective when delivered as an aerosol (e.g., by metered-dose inhaler). The reason for this remains unclear. Thirty years ago, it was thought that theophylline could not be absorbed through the upper gastrointestinal tract, and it was thus administered as a suppository. Subsequently, it was demonstrated that aminophylline could be delivered as an alcoholic elixir, and, shortly thereafter, in tablet form as a salt of aminophylline. Dozens, perhaps hundreds, of preparations have been concocted from various salts of theophylline, each claiming particular advantages related to the undesirable side effects of the drug. None of these claims are, in fact, justified. Toxicity is directly related to plasma concentration (see below). While doses of various theophylline-based preparations are based on the total molecular weight of the compound, the side effects are related to that proportion of the salt that is the active ingredient. Hence 200 mg of a salt that is 64 percent aminophylline may appear to be less toxic than one that is 85 percent aminophylline, but the same 200-mg dose will be less efficacious.

Theophylline has a narrow toxic/therapeutic ratio. As a bronchodilator, it is largely ineffective at blood concentrations < 10 mg/L. At concentrations exceeding 20 mg/L nausea, gastrointestinal hypermotility, and, occasionally, vomiting ensue. Patient tolerance at even this level is entirely variable, and some patients experience these undesirable side effects even at "therapeutic" concentrations. Cardiac arrhythmias are common at concentrations exceeding 40 mg/L, and at plasma concentrations > 60 mg/L seizures may occur. Theophylline has often been called the "digitalis of pulmonary medicine." While theophylline has unquestionable bronchodilator effects[26] that are addictive to β-adrenergic agonists,[27] it can cause serious toxicity. As for digitalis, some individuals pass through all "preliminary" planes of toxicity and progress directly to seizures. The mortality rate for seizures[28] from theophylline is high—as great as 50 percent. Yet, the various compounds of theophylline are widely used, largely because of their efficacy and because of their availability as sustained-release compounds, which make them important in suppression of nocturnal symptoms of asthma.

The role of theophylline in the treatment of asthma continues to be debated. With the advent of inhaled long-acting β-adrenoceptor agonists, theophylline cannot be considered as other than a "second-line" drug. For patients receiving both β-adrenergic agonists and inhaled corticosteroids and who still require frequent supplemental use of inhaled short-acting β-adrenergic agonists, oral theophylline administration may help control breakthrough symptoms. Compliance is not a problem with theophylline, since it can be given once or twice daily as a sustained-action preparation. Administration of theophylline, even as an oral agent, is nonetheless complicated. A number of factors affect theophylline metabolism, including liver disease and concomitant administration of other compounds. Other interactions are somewhat more inexplicable; for example, history of cigarette smoking or degree of airflow obstruction.[29] Treatment with theophylline also entails a commitment to monitor plasma concentration on a regular basis and a knowledge of the multiple interactions of theophylline with other drugs

(see Chap. 49). It cannot be assumed that steady-state plasma concentrations demonstrated on one or two occasions will persist, and for patients having achieved steady-state concentration, monitoring on an average of every 6 months is advisable. Because of these concerns for monitoring theophylline concentrations, many physicians have advocated abandonment of this drug from the therapeutic armamentarium for asthma. While it is likely that theophylline will be replaced in the future either by a specific phosphodiesterase isozyme inhibitor (see Chap. 62) or by an alternative oral preparation of a different class, it remains a widely used and potentially beneficial compound for the treatment of more severe asthma.

Recently, it has been suggested that theophylline may have anti-inflammatory properties at plasma concentrations below those currently regarded as therapeutic.[30–32] This view is a projection of still-limited in vitro investigations to the clinical situation, and it seemingly disregards the observation that theophylline is ineffective as a bronchodilator at plasma concentrations less than currently recommended. Whether theophylline has a supplemental anti-inflammatory effect to that currently conferred by corticosteroids remains to be investigated, but this does not justify its prescription as an anti-inflammatory agent per se.

ORAL β-ADRENERGIC AGONISTS

The use of these compounds as supplements to short-acting inhaled β-adrenergic agents was controversial even before the advent of long-acting β-adrenoceptor agonists (e.g., salmeterol and formoterol). Orally administered albuterol and terbutaline have a longer duration than their inhaled counterparts, despite substantial first-pass clearance by the liver. In the circulation, these drugs have a therapeutic duration of 6 to 8 h and as long as 12 h in the sustained-release forms, whereas mucociliary clearance limits the duration of therapeutic doses of the same compounds to 3 to 6 h when administered by aerosol. These have never been first-line drugs for use in the treatment of asthma, and their use was largely confined to improvement of patient compliance and control of nocturnal symptoms. For patients receiving long-acting β-adrenoceptor agonists, the simultaneous administration of a second long-acting β-adrenergic agent could pose a significant concern. The advisability of using these drugs in deference to a sustained-release compound of theophylline also is questionable as a strategy of polypharmacy. Accordingly, the use of these compounds is viewed in most cases as being largely obsolete now that long-acting inhaled β-adrenergic agonists are available.

PATHWAY INHIBITORS AND ANTAGONISTS OF 5-LIPOXYGENASE PRODUCTS

These drugs represent a new concept in the treatment of asthma. In contrast to all of the compounds cited above, they are inhibitors of receptor antagonists, rather than agonists. They do not stimulate relaxation; they block contraction caused by released products of the 5-lipoxygenase pathway, either by blocking directly the 5-lipoxygenase enzyme or the leukotriene receptor on airway smooth muscle per se. The development and design of these compounds represents a direct application of a knowledge of the pathogenesis of asthma into the development of therapeutic agents.[33] (The mechanism and development of these novel compounds is discussed extensively in Chap. 65.) While these drugs inhibit the activity of inflammatory cells, these are presumed to be cells that already have transmigrated into airways. This is particularly true for leukotriene-receptor antagonists. Thus, their actions are not equivalent to oral corticosteroids, and their efficacy is correspondingly substantially less. Their positioning in the therapeutic armamentarium for asthma treatment remains to be defined.

Several aspects of these agents are appealing. The best characterized of the 5-lipoxygenase inhibiting agents is zileuton, which is being tested for imminent release at the time of this writing (see Chap. 65). A potential limitation to the use of this drug is the need to administer zileuton four times daily to maintain bronchodilation[34] and the question of hepatotoxicity, which, although infrequent, remains to be resolved.[35] Zileuton causes 12 percent to 15 percent bronchodilation within 1 h of administration, and this bronchodilation may be superimposable upon that elicited by albuterol. Hence, the bronchodilator effects of β-adrenoceptor agonists and zileuton may be both "acute" and truly additive. In contrast to inhaled corticosteroids, patients perceive this bronchodilator effect as incremental, and, particularly for patients receiving inhaled corticosteroids four times daily, this property of zileuton could lead to improved compliance. Zileuton is available in tablet form, obviating both the concern of using a fluorohydrocarbon propellant and the reluctance of many patients to use metered-dose inhalers in public. A sustained-release version of this compound is under development. Data for other compounds still are somewhat preliminary.

Several compounds have been tested that block directly the leukotriene receptor (see Chap. 65). As currently reported, they have a therapeutic profile that parallels that for zileuton[34,36]; however, zafirlukast, a leukotriene D$_4$ antagonist, may be administered twice daily. It has no significant toxicity at a dose of 40 mg and currently is being tested at greater doses to determine if greater efficacy will be obtained. Pranlukast, another LTD$_4$-receptor antagonist, has been evaluated extensively in Japan and is undergoing testing in the United States. These are the drugs of the near future. There is no doubt that sustained-release preparations of 5-lipoxygenase inhibitor also will be developed, and hence there is no specific rationale at present to limit the use of any of these compounds other than their potential toxicity.

Zileuton has been shown to cause inhibition of a limited aspirin challenge in aspirin-sensitive asthmatics[3] and is more effective in patients with moderate to severe bronchoconstriction than for mild bronchoconstriction. There appears to be a subset of patients nonetheless in which it is ineffective. Whether this is a unique property of zileuton, or a unique concern in the analysis and testing of this compound, remains to be defined. Other than the parameters cited above, one cannot predict the efficacy of this drug for a particular patient except by empirical trial. A reasonable

question is whether compounds that inhibit leukotriene synthesis or its action more distally at the receptor are a reasonable substitute for inhaled corticosteroids as first-line drugs, assuming they prove to have low toxicity and can be administered with equal or lesser frequency than inhaled corticosteroids. About 30 percent of patients taking inhaled corticosteroids develop some degree of dysphonia, which can be a significant occupational impediment,[37] and concerns persist about systemic absorption in children.[38–40] A counterargument for the substitution of these compounds in place of inhaled corticosteroids is that the anti-inflammatory effects of corticosteroids could prevent airway remodeling changes, which some have postulated to lead to chronic, intractable asthma.[41] It should be noted that there is yet little foundation for this concern, since the mechanism by which some patients develop intractable asthma is not defined, nor has the use of corticosteroids, either oral or inhaled, been shown to be preventative. It is not known whether inhaled corticosteroids and zileuton are additive in their therapeutic effects as are these same compounds with inhaled β-adrenergic agonists. Finally, it is worth noting that these are the first of what promises to be a generation of new drugs, and there is potential for the development of related, innovative therapies that will obviate or replace existing regimens.

MAST CELL STABILIZING COMPOUNDS

A review of disodium cromoglycate and nedocromil sodium is included in Chaps. 58 and 59. These compounds are effective in both exercise-induced bronchoconstriction and in allergic asthma in children. Exercise-induced bronchoconstriction, however, is easily aborted by the preemptive use of β-adrenergic agonists, and maintenance therapy thus is not essential if symptoms are limited to this condition. Pure allergic asthma is rare in adults, and inhaled corticosteroids have accordingly become the first line of treatment accompanying inhaled β-adrenergic agonists in adult asthma in the United States and in many places in Europe and Asia. There is no convincing evidence that the addition of these compounds to inhaled corticosteroids confers an incremental therapeutic benefit, and they add to the cost of treatment. In the United States, disodium cromoglycate and nedocromil sodium often are used as first-line therapy in children as an alternative to inhaled corticosteroids. Where adequate control of symptoms is achieved, this is a reasonable strategy. Children often have atopic asthma and have unquestionable requirements for vigorous exercise.

ORAL CORTICOSTEROIDS

All but the most resistant asthmatics demonstrate dramatic improvement with these compounds, which are truly anti-inflammatory, very inexpensive, and, unfortunately, laden with numerous and potentially disastrous side effects (see Chaps. 55 and 56). These are probably the most underused drugs in the therapeutic arsenal for the treatment of asthma. The medical (and legal) literature is filled with incidents of asthma death that are unquestionably attributed to the failure to prescribe oral corticosteroids in sufficient doses for severe asthmatics. The reluctance to prescribe these drugs in sustained and substantial doses is understandable, but this must be balanced against the clear recognition that some patients do indeed have corticosteroid-dependent asthma. This is defined for the purposes of this presentation as asthma not adequately controlled by any or all of the drugs enumerated above given in combination.

Oral corticosteroids also are extremely useful for treatment of acute exacerbations of asthma; for example, during a viral infection or for patients with mild to moderate asthma to achieve symptomatic relief, even if it is obvious that hospitalization is not imminent. Patients with a history of multiple emergency visits, prior hospitalizations for asthma, or, especially, with a history of intubation and mechanical ventilation for asthma, often have a substantial requirement for oral corticosteroid therapy. While every attempt should be made to wean patients from oral corticosteroids, some patients demonstrate rapid recurrence of symptoms and objective demonstration of worsening airflow obstruction shortly after—or even during—weaning, even when a new exacerbating cause is not evident. Demonstration on several occasions that patients cannot sustain adequate control of severe symptoms of asthma diagnoses corticosteroid-dependent asthma. The next step is to determine the dose of oral corticosteroid that ameliorates symptoms successfully. The use of corticosteroids should always be superimposed on an aggressive regimen of other agents, including long-acting inhaled β-adrenoceptor agonists, supplemental short-acting inhaled β-adrenergic agonists, inhaled corticosteroids, and theophylline. While these drugs may not always be tolerable by all patients in therapeutic doses and in combination, it should be recognized that oral prednisone is not a substitute for routine therapy, including the use of inhaled corticosteroids, which may be sparing of greater doses of oral corticosteroid medications. Other inhaled compounds that are more potent than preparations available in the United States ameliorate or—in some cases—abolish the need for use of oral corticosteroids. However, even these more efficacious agents (see above) do not obviate the need for use of oral corticosteroids for some patients.

Patients receiving oral corticosteroids require frequent monitoring in the outpatient clinic. This includes measurement of spirometry on clinic visits and a diary of peak flow measurement at home.[39] There is no particular reason for use of corticosteroid medications other than prednisone in most patients. Methylprednisolone may cause slightly less sodium retention in some patients and is possibly somewhat more potassium sparing.[40] It also is substantially more expensive than prednisone. This is important to patients who already are bearing the cost of multiple clinic visits and polypharmacy with other agents for the treatment of their asthma. Determination of the optimal dose of oral corticosteroid is empirical and is based on reports of symptoms, peak flow measurements at home, and assessment through customized interactions with patients in the ambulatory clinic. Routine schedules or "kits" for tapering corticosteroids by a universal formula for all patients cannot be encouraged. The tapering and final adjustment of cortico-

steroid dose should be based on the response of each patient to preceding decrement in dose. Telephone consultation between visits is a useful adjunct in this regard.

IMMUNOTHERAPY

Immunotherapy has largely been supplanted by the development of inhaled corticosteroid-containing regimens and a new generation of other compounds for the treatment of asthma in adults, where asthma is largely perennial and frequently not related to atopy (see Chap. 35). Its use is strictly adjunctive and should be based on careful consideration of a unique circumstance that cannot be otherwise addressed. Immunotherapy is relatively expensive, highly inconvenient, and not without risk of anaphylaxis. It should be administered only by skilled specialists with specific training in administration of this mode of therapy.

IMMUNOSUPPRESSIVE THERAPIES

Immunosuppressive therapies are those that employ systemic suppression of the immune system for treatment of otherwise intractable asthma. Current therapies have been directed against the T cell (cyclosporine)[41] and the granulocyte.[42–44] It is recognized that treatment with oral corticosteroids causes systemic immunosuppression. Nonetheless, these alternative therapies are toxic and currently cannot be recommended even in the most severe asthma. Cyclosporine has been shown to cause improvement in severe asthma,[41] but its expense (including monitoring for toxicity) and the dangers of nephrotoxicity preclude its use, even in severe asthma. Previous investigations have suggested that methotrexate could be used to decrease the dose of oral corticosteroid used in the treatment of corticosteroid-dependent asthma, but only for the patients requiring lesser doses of corticosteroid to begin; treatment also was not free of toxicity.[42–44] Unfortunately, these data have been occasionally misinterpreted and applied as supplemental or alternative therapy for patients with very severe asthma, where there has been no claim of efficacy. Methotrexate is potentially hepatotoxic, and its questionable efficacy also suggests that it has limited (if any) indication in the treatment of asthma.

ASTHMA IN PREGNANCY

The treatment of asthma in pregnancy represents a special situation that fortunately is reasonably uncomplicated. The goal of all treatment in pregnancy is to minimize risk to both fetus and mother and to avoid therapies that will cause congenital malformations. Good control of the mother's asthma is essential in this circumstance, for a severe asthma attack is a substantial risk to fetal survival. Fortunately, virtually all drugs used to treat asthma are known to be safe for use in pregnancy. These include β-adrenoceptor agonists, oral and inhaled corticosteroids, and theophylline.[45] Only beclomethasone dipropionate has been shown specifically to be *unassociated* with fetal malformation, and so it is usually the drug of choice during pregnancy.[46] Given the absence of risk in treating pregnant women, asthma can and should be treated optimally without withholding medications during pregnancy, and failure to do so has been regarded by some as inadequate medical practice.[45]

Treatment of Status Asthmaticus

ASSESSMENT OF SEVERITY AND INITIAL TREATMENT

Status asthmaticus is a severe exacerbation of asthma that is refractory to emergent supplemental therapy. Failure of severe, acute asthma to improve may lead to failure of the respiratory muscles and sudden respiratory arrest. This is the mechanism of death in asthma, and presentation of acute asthma that is refractory to treatment is worrisome. (The supportive treatment of those patients who are intubated and receiving mechanical ventilation is considered in Chap. 78.) This section considers the phase that precedes the decision to intubate.

The typical presentation in status asthmaticus is that of a diaphoretic, dyspneic patient using the accessory muscles of inspiration. Labored breathing is obvious, and often accompanied by loud wheezing both on inspiration and expiration. A somewhat later presentation may obscure these signs. If respiratory muscle fatigue or severe mucus plugging has occurred, airflow is reduced greatly, wheezing subsides, and labored breathing may not be obvious, as respiratory muscle fatigue ensues. In this circumstance, death is imminent without proper intervention. Assessment often can be made quickly, solely on the basis of clinical observation, and there is no immediate further need for diagnostic assessment until therapy is begun. If time permits, peak flow measurements should be attempted.

Therapy should begin at once with inhaled, relatively short-acting β-adrenoceptor agents (e.g., albuterol or isoproterenol administered by nebulization through a mask). Use of a metered-dose inhaler (MDI) is not possible because patients cannot hold their breath after inspiration for a sufficient period of time. Other methods of administration requiring patient cooperation likewise should be discouraged. The use of longer-acting β-adrenoceptor agonists (e.g., salmeterol) should be avoided; the onset of action is too slow for emergent situations, and "overshoot" is more difficult to correct. Although albuterol is more β_2-specific than isoproterenol (which has equivalent β_1-adrenergic intrinsic activity) and has a longer duration of action, it also has a slightly longer onset of action. On balance, neither drug is preferable to the other; rapid initiation of therapy is the only consideration. Where nebulized β-adrenergic agonists are not immediately available, subcutaneous administration can be substituted with almost equivalent efficacy. Either subcutaneous epinephrine (non-β–specific) or subcutaneous terbutaline can be used. Onset of bronchodilation may be rapid, but may be of short duration (< 30 min). This affords, nonetheless, time to assess the potential reversibility of the

patient's asthma with longer-acting preparations and the simultaneous institution of other therapies in the emergency setting.

The response to β-adrenoceptor agonists is to a large degree predictive of the severity of the status asthmaticus and the subsequent need for hospitalization.[47] For this reason, continuous nebulization, when possible, seems preferable to bolus administration of β-adrenergic agonist by subcutaneous injection. Patients not responding to this and other therapies within the first hour will not respond satisfactorily during the next 24 h.[47] They should be admitted to an intensive care unit or another unit permitted extremely close observation, even if intubation is not imminent.

Immediately after establishing therapy with β-adrenoceptor agents, arterial blood gases should be obtained, and supplemental oxygen (2 to 4 L/min by nasal cannula) administered. The arterial blood gas measurement will indicate the extent of lactic acidosis and CO_2 retention. Both are ominous signs.[48–49] Acute airflow obstruction is a powerful ventilatory stimulus; Pa_{CO_2} in the face of an acute increase in respiratory flow should be substantially < 40 mmHg. A patient demonstrating anaerobic metabolism (metabolic acidosis) and a P_{O_2} between 35 and 40 mmHg is likely on the verge of imminent respiratory arrest. When the P_{CO_2} exceeds 40 mmHg and is not rapidly decreased by bronchodilator therapy, intubation almost certainly is indicated (see Chap. 78). A decrease in Pa_{O_2} rarely is the problem in asthma; supplemental oxygen therapy is designed to delay the onset of lactic acidosis in more marginal patients; however, death occurs from hypoventilation and respiratory arrest, which are marked by Pa_{CO_2}. High-flow oxygen also may be irritating to already inflamed airways.

Patients treated by mechanical ventilation for asthma should be transferred immediately to a critical care unit. If therapy with intravenous corticosteroids has not already begun, this is now most certainly indicated (see Chap. 78). Theophylline, which is not particularly useful acutely in the treatment of status asthmaticus, should not be administered until plasma theophylline concentration is first determined.[49] Dozens of preparations contain theophylline, and it is difficult to conduct a sufficient interview with patients who are acutely dyspneic. Administration of a loading dose of theophylline may supplement an adequate or overly aggressive home regimen and induce severe, even life-threatening toxicity.

In recent years, the recommended dose of theophylline used for loading patients having no significant existing plasma concentration has been reduced. A dose of 5 to 6 mg/kg intravenously over 20 min is then followed by a continuous infusion of 0.5 mg/kg per h.[29] The loading dose is constant, but the dose for continuous infusion is affected by many variables, and it must be adjusted accordingly. Frequently monitoring (at least twice daily) is desirable while patients with unstable asthma remain on intravenous theophylline therapy. Intravenous corticosteroids can be tapered to orally administered doses, and intravenous theophylline can be changed to orally administered medication once stability has been established. The details of management of the patient while receiving mechanical ventilation once again are referred to Chap. 78.

HOSPITAL DISCHARGE REGIMEN: RETURN TO THE HOME ENVIRONMENT

Once the patient has recovered, it is necessary to establish a regimen for the home environment. This may include oral theophylline and should always include oral corticosteroid. There is little rationale for tapering patients from oral corticosteroids while in hospital. This delays discharge and exposes the patient to the initial environment from which they were admitted with a relatively lesser degree of pharmacologic protection. Most patients can tolerate a dose of 60 mg of prednisone or the equivalent at home. Tapering then can be accomplished in the outpatient clinic. Discharge regimens should include β-adrenoceptor agents. In these patients, there is a strong rationale for sustained-acting preparations that afford steady-state β-adrenergic activity. As for less severe asthma, other therapies are adjunctive, and the patient moves now to the clinical arena in which most asthma is treated—the outpatient setting.

PROGNOSIS

Status asthmaticus is a marker of severe, potentially life-threatening asthma. Even a single episode of asthma requiring hospital admission (and, especially, if accompanied by intubation) indicates a high-risk patient with an overall mortality of as great as 40 percent over the next 5 years. Among these patients, death rates are substantially greater for patients having prior hospital admissions versus those admitted for the first time.[12] Such patients are reasonable candidates for follow-up in a subspecialty clinic with ready accessibility to the care of nurse and physician subspecialists in asthma. These patients are rarely, if ever, truly well, and routine clinic visits to monitor the clinical status of these patients, insure administration of vaccinations against influenza and pneumonia, and anticipate difficulties arising from routine respiratory infections, may be invaluable in minimizing exacerbations and preventing asthma deaths. The ability to communicate rapidly with a knowledgeable physician or nurse, preferably one who knows the patient well, is essential. The increase in asthma deaths in the United States is alarming, but not especially difficult to understand. In the last 12 years, the number of asthma deaths has doubled from about 2,500 per year to 5,000 per year.[50] At the same time, the prevalence of asthma also has increased, largely in the pediatric population. This may be the result of increased recognition of asthma in the younger pediatric population. It is noteworthy that asthma deaths have *not* increased among white Americans and that the increase in asthma death can be accounted largely by the increase in deaths among African-Americans. In 1979, asthma deaths were 2.0-fold greater among black Americans than whites; in 1989, asthma deaths were 3.5-fold greater. At the same time, there has been a substantial withdrawal of health care from inner-city populations. Among some inner-city populations,

deaths from tuberculosis among children increased approximately 8-fold, and once were almost nonexistent. It is clear that access to medical care may be the single most important factor in preventing mortality, especially among patients now recognized to be at special risk (i.e., those having experienced prior episodes of status asthmaticus).

Risk Management: Managed Care Paradigms

At present, there is little insight into the effect of managed care on the treatment of asthma. Motivation to minimize treatment costs has no predictable effect on either physician utilization or allocation of treatment regimens. In one paradigm, primary care physicians serve largely as gatekeepers, and asthma is managed as a component of other common disorders handled by general internists. This is, of course, largely how asthma is managed today, and there is no particular necessity for mild- or low-risk asthma to be managed by a subspecialist. Here the role of education of the physician community is particularly important, especially as new products and treatment regimens are introduced. As indicated in other chapters in this book, this is likely to be substantial over the next 5 years, and there is a promise for even more innovative and complex therapies for the more distant future.

It is not clear that the "gatekeeping" approach to asthma treatment will necessarily dominate asthma management for higher-risk patients (i.e., those requiring emergency treatment or episodic emergency room visits and/or hospital admission). Some patients and physicians fear that large managed-care facilities seek only the lowest bid in patient care management and are as indifferent as is legally feasible to outcome. These fears have not been ameliorated by recent attempts of the U.S. Congress and many state legislatures to limit legal liability in medical litigation. Nonetheless, outcome analysis is a vital component of asthma management when the goal precisely is to conserve financial resources. Use of innovative therapies and optimal outpatient management may generate incremental costs at the outset, but if emergency room visits and hospitalizations are reduced even in a relatively small fraction of patients, these costs are more than offset. It remains to be determined if managed care is likely to cause a "chilling" effect on product development, as industry weighs the economic cost of new product development against attempts of the health-care industry to minimize treatment costs. Based on experiences in European and Asian countries, the prospects for innovative treatment regimens and further product developments are good.

References

1. Leff AR: State of the art review: endogenous regulation of bronchomotor tone. *Am Rev Respir Dis* 1988; 137:1198–1216.
2. Leff AR, Hamann K, Wegner C: Inflammatory and cell-cell inter-

actions in airway hyperresponsiveness. *Am J Physiol: Lung Cell Mol Physiol* 1991; 260:L189–L206.

3. Israel E, Fisher AR, Rosenbergy MA, et al.: The pivotal role of 5-lipoxygenase products in the reaction of aspirin-sensitive asthmatics to aspirin. *Am Rev Respir Dis* 1993; 148:1447–1451.

4. Turner-Warwick M: Epidemiology of nocturnal asthma. *Am J Med* 1988; 88:6–8.

5. Ballard RD, Saathof MC, Patel DK, et al.: Effect of sleep on nocturnal bronchoconstriction and ventilatory patterns I asthmatics. *J Appl Physiol* 1989; 67:243–249.

6. Simonsson BG, F Jacobs, Nadel JA: Role of the autonomic nervous system and the cough reflex in the increased responsiveness in patients with obstructive lung disease. *J Clin Invest* 1967; 46:1812–1818.

7. Stone RA, Fuller RW: Mechanism of cough, in Busse WW, Holgate ST (eds): *Asthma and Allergic Rhinitis.* Blackwell Scientific, 1995: 1075–1081.

8. Banner AS: Pharmacologic treatment of cough, in Leff AR (ed): *Pulmonary Pharmacology and Therapeutics.* New York, McGraw-Hill, 1996: 673–679.

9. Murphy TM, Leff AR: Airway reactivity and respiratory smooth muscle tone, in Chernick V, Mellins RB (eds): *Basic Mechanisms of Pediatric Respiratory Disease: Cellular and Integrative.* Philadelphia, BC Becker, 1991: 221–236.

10. James AL, Pare PD, Hogg JC: The mechanics of airway narrowing in asthma. *Am Rev Respir Dis* 1989; 139:242–246.

11. McFadden ER: Exertional dyspnea and cough as preludes to acute attacks of bronchial asthma. *N Engl J Med* 1975; 292:555–559.

12. Marquette CH, Saulnier F, Leroy O, et al.: Long-term prognosis of near fatal asthma: a 6-year followup study of 145 asthmatic patients who underwent mechanical ventilation for a near fatal attack of asthma. *Am Rev Respir Dis* 1992; 146:76–81.

13. Crane J, Pearce NE, Burgess C, et al.: Markers of risk of asthma death or readmission in the 12 months following a hospital admission for asthma. *Int J Epidemiol* 1992; 21:737–744.

14. Strunck RC, Mrazek DA, Wolfson-Furhman GS, LaBrecque JF: Physiologic and psychological characteristics associated with deaths due to asthma in childhood. *JAMA* 1985; 254:1193–1198.

15. Spitzer WO, Suissa S, Ernst P, et al.: The use of beta-agonists and the risk of death and near death from asthma. *N Engl J Med* 1992; 326:501–506.

16. Pearce NE, Grainger J, Atkinson M, et al.: Case-control study of prescribed fenoterol and death from asthma in New Zealand, 1977–1981. *Thorax* 1991; 46:105–111.

17. Burrows B, Lebowityz MD: The beta-agonist dilemma (editorial). *N Engl J Med* 1992; 326:560–561.

18. Harden TK: Agonist-induced desensitization of the β-adrenergic receptor-linked adenylate cyclase. *Pharmacol Rev* 1983; 37:5–32.

19. Barrett TE, Strom BL: Inhaled beta-adrenergic receptor agonists in asthma: more harm than good? *Am Rev Respir Dis* 1995; 151:574–577.

20. Pearce N, Crane J, Burgess C, et al.: Beta-agonists and asthma mortality: deja vu. *Clin Exp Allergy* 1991; 21:401–410.

21. Chapman K, Kesten S, Szalai J: Regular vs. as needed inhaled salbutamol in asthma control. *Lancet* 1994; 343:1379–1382.

22. Sears MR, Taylor DR, Print CG, et al.: Regular inhaled beta agonist treatment in bronchial asthma. *Lancet* 1990; 336:1391–1396.

23. Ryan G, Latimer KM, Juniper EF, et al.: Effect of beclomethasone diproprionate on bronchial responsiveness to histamine in controlled nonsteroid-dependent asthma. *J Allergy Clin Immunol* 1985; 75:25–30.

24. Svedsen UG: Fluticasone proprionate (a new inhaled steroid): clinical developments in mild to moderate adult asthmatics (abstract). *Eur Respir J* 3:(suppl 10)250S.

25. Barnes P: Inhaled glucocorticoids for asthma. *N Engl J Med* 1995; 332:868–875.

26. Weinburger M: The pharmacology and therapeutic use of theophylline. *J Allergy Clin Immunol* 1984; 73:525–540.

27. Handslip PDJ, Dart AM, Davies BTI: Intravenous salbutamol and aminophylline in asthma: a search for synergy. *Thorax* 1981; 36:741–744.

28. Eason J, Makowe HLJ: Aminophylline toxicity—how many hospital asthma deaths does it cause? *Respir Med* 1989; 83:219–226.

29. Piafsky KM, Ogilvie RI: Dosage of theophylline in bronchial asthma. *N Engl J Med* 1975; 292:1218–1222.

30. Erjefält I, Persson CGA: Pharmacologic control of plasma exudation into tracheobronchial airways. *Am Rev Respir Dis* 1991; 143:1008–1104.

31. Naclerio RM, Bartenfelder D, Proud D, et al.: Theophylline reduces histamine release during pollen-induced rhinitis. *J Allergy Clin Immunol* 1986; 78:874–876.

32. Pauwels R, van Renterghem D, van der Sataeten M, et al.: The effect of theophylline and enprophylline on allergen-induced bronchoconstriction. *J Allergy Clin Immunol* 1985; 76:583–590.

33. Lewis RA, Drazen JM, Austen KF, et al.: Contractile activities of structural analogs of leukotrienes C and D: role of the polar substituents. *Proc Natl Acad Sci U S A* 1981; 78:4579–4583.

34. Strek ME: Leukotriene receptor blockers and synthesis inhibitors in asthma, in Leff AR (ed): *Pulmonary Pharmacology and Therapeutics.* New York, Mc-Graw-Hill, 1996.

35. Data on file, Abbott Laboratories.

36. Kidney JC, Ridge SM, Chung KF, Barnes PJ: Inhibition of platelet-activating factor-induced bronchoconstriction by the leukotriene D_4 receptor antagonist ICI 204,219. *Am Rev Respir Dis* 1993; 147:215–217.

37. Toogood JH, Jennings B, Greenway KRW, Chuang L: Candidiasis and dysphonia complications of beclomethasone treatment of asthma. *J Allergy Clin Immunol* 1980; 65:145–153.

38. Koenig P: Inhaled corticosteroids—their present and future role in the management of asthma. *J Allergy Clin Immunol* 1988; 60:231–238.

39. National Institutes of Health, Expert Panel Report: *Guides for the Diagnosis and Management of Asthma.* Publication No. 91-3042, Bethesda, MD, National Institutes of Health, 1991.

40. Hayes RC Jr, Murad F: Adrenocorticotropic hormone; adrenocortical steroids and their synthetic analogs: inhibitors of adrenocortical steroid biosynthesis, in Gilman AG, Goodman LS, Rall TW, Murad F (eds): *The Pharmacological Basis of Therapeutics.* New York, MacMillan, 1985:1459–1489.

41. Alexander AG, Barnes NC, Kay AB: Trial of cyclosporine in corticosteroid dependent chronic severe asthma. *Lancet* 1992; 339:324–328.

42. Mullarkey MF, Blumenstein BA, Andrade WP, et al.: Methotrexate in the treatment of corticosteroid-dependent asthma. A double-blind cross over study. *N Engl J Med* 1988; 318:603.

43. Mullarkey MF, Lammert JK, Blumenstein BA: Long term methotrexate treatment in corticosteroid-dependent asthma.

44. Mullarkey MF: Methotrexate and asthma. *J Allergy Clin Immunol* 1991; 88:272–274.

45. Barron WM, Leff AR: Asthma in pregnancy. *Am Rev Respir Dis* 1993; 147:510–511.

46. National Heart, Lung, and Blood Institute, Report of the Work

Group on Asthma and Pregnancy, Executive Summary. *Management of Asthma during Pregnancy*. Publication No. 93-3279A.

47. Beasley R, Burgess C, Crane J, D'Souza W: Management of exacerbations of asthma in adults, in Busse WW, Holgate ST (eds): *Asthma and Rhinitis*. Blackwell Scientific, 1995:1349–1364.

48. Appel D, Rubenstein R, Schrager K, et al.: Lactic acidosis in severe asthma. *Am J Med* 1983; 75:580.

49. Hall JB, Wood LDH: Status asthmaticus, in Hall JB, Schmidt GA, Wood LDH (eds): *Principles of Critical Care*. New York, McGraw-Hill, 1992:1670–1679.

50. USPHS, National Institutes of Health, Division of Lung Diseases. Estimates from personal communication.

51. Johnson M, Butchers PR, Coleman RA, et al.: The pharmacology of salmeterol. *Life Sci* 1993; 52:2131–2143.

Chapter 78 _____

PHARMACOTHERAPY OF STATUS ASTHMATICUS

THOMAS CORBRIDGE AND JESSE HALL

Standard Pharmacologic Management of Status Asthmaticus
Oxygen therapy
β-adrenergic agonists
Corticosteroids
Anticholinergics
Theophylline

Innovative Therapies
Magnesium sulfate
Heliox

Pharmacologic Adjuncts to Intubation and Mechanical Ventilation in Status Asthmaticus
Sedatives
Paralytics
Inhalational anesthetics

Many asthma patients are at risk to develop airflow obstruction that is so severe that ventilatory failure results, with risk of death. This condition is termed *status asthmaticus*.[1,2] The mechanisms for rapidly progressive, or *sudden asphyxic asthma*, may be different than for more slowly progressive forms of airflow obstruction.[3] Regardless of potential mechanisms and pace of illness, status asthmaticus is treated aggressively with combinations of anti-inflammatory and bronchodilator drugs.

While the mainstay of therapy for status asthmaticus involves the same drugs that are utilized in the treatment of asthma in the ambulatory setting (see Chap. 77), the tempo and endpoints of treatment are quite different. In outpatient treatment of asthma, the goal of therapy is control of disease with as few side effects as possible. In patients with status asthmaticus, drug therapy should be titrated rapidly and individually to the maximum tolerated doses, with the goal of interrupting progression of airflow obstruction to ventilatory failure. Standard doses may need to be repeated to the limits of tolerance. This chapter will describe these modified goals of pharmacology applied to the treatment of status asthmaticus. Some therapeutic agents that have little or no role in ambulatory patients—oxygen, magnesium, and heliox—will be discussed as well. Finally, specific agents used for intubation, sedation, muscle relaxation, and anesthesia in the critically ill patient will be discussed. It is beyond the scope of this chapter to discuss the important issues of clinical assessment, mechanical ventilation, and

prevention of recurrent episodes in patients with status asthmaticus. For these important topics, the reader is referred to several excellent reviews.[1,2,4]

Standard Pharmacologic Management of Status Asthmaticus

OXYGEN THERAPY

Obstruction of peripheral airways by bronchoconstriction, airway inflammation and edema, and by mucus causes ventilation-perfusion mismatch and hypoxemia in patients with status asthmaticus (SA). True shunt in acute asthma averages only 1.5 percent,[5] and so low-flow oxygen concentration typically reverses arterial hypoxemia. While few patients with mild-to-moderate asthma exhibit significant hypoxemia,[6] routine use in patients with SA is recommended since it is safe, will be lifesaving in the small fraction of patients with significant hypoxemia, and confers the potential benefits of improved oxygen delivery to peripheral tissues, reversal of hypoxic vasoconstriction, and airway bronchodilation.[2] Oxygen also is useful to avoid the modest decrease in Pa_{O_2} that is typically encountered after administration of β-adrenergic agonists.[7] Failure of low-flow oxygen to correct hypoxemia should prompt a search for causes of true intrapulmonary shunt (e.g., lobar collapse, acute lobar pneumonia).

TABLE 78-1   Drugs Used in the Treatment of Status Asthmaticus

STANDARD THERAPIES

Albuterol	0.5 mL of 0.5% solution (2.5 mg) in 2.5 mL normal saline by nebulization or 4 puffs by MDI with spacer every 20 min × 3; for intubated patients, titrate to physiologic effect and side effects (see text).
Epinephrine	0.3 mL of a 1:1000 solution subcutaneously every 20 min × 3. Terbutaline is favored in pregnant patients when parenteral therapy is indicated. Use with caution in patients over age 40 and in patients with coronary artery disease.
Corticosteroids	Methylprednisolone 60 to 125 mg IV every 6 h or prednisone 30 to 40 mg PO every 6 h.
Oxygen	1 to 3 L/min by nasal cannula; titrate using pulse oximeter.
Anticholinergics	Ipratropium bromide 0.5 mg by nebulization hourly or 4 to 10 puffs by MDI with spacer every 20 min. Or: glycopyrrolate 2 mg by nebulization every 2 h × 3.
Theophylline	5 mg/kg IV over 30 min loading dose in patients not on theophylline followed by 0.4 mg/kg per h IV maintenance dose. Check serum concentration within 6 h of loading dose. Watch for drug interactions and disease states that alter clearance rates (see text).

UNPROVEN ALTERNATIVE THERAPIES

Magnesium sulfate	1 g IV over 20 min, repeat in 20 min (total dose 2 g). If hypomagnesemic, dose adequately to normalize serum levels.
Heliox	80:20, 70:30, or 60:40 helium:oxygen mix by tight fitting, non-rebreathing face mask. Higher helium concentrations are needed for maximal effect.

β-ADRENERGIC AGONISTS

Inhaled β-adrenergic agonists are the drugs of choice to treat bronchoconstriction in SA (see Chap. 77 and Table 78-1). While various epidemiologic studies have raised concern that long-term use of these drugs may be associated with asthma deaths [8–10] (see Chaps. 47 and 48), there is little dispute that these drugs are essential to the management of SA. When misused in the setting of SA, it is most often the case that patients are undertreated.

Long-acting congeners such as salmeterol are not indicated in SA because of their slow onset of action. Among the agents with rapid onset, many clinicians prefer albuterol because it has a slightly longer duration of action and more β2-selectivity than other drugs, such as metaproterenol.[11]

Large doses of β-adrenergic agonists typically are required in the treatment of SA. This relates in part to the adverse effects of extreme bronchoconstriction on the dose-response and duration of action of these agents, as well as to diminished delivery by inhalation related to airway narrowing, altered breathing patterns, and poor patient cooperation. Initial treatment in the adult should be 2.5 or 5.0 mg of albuterol (0.5 or 1.0 mL of an 0.5% solution with saline dilution to a total of 3 mL) by nebulization every 20 min for three doses. Dosing can be reduced in patients who exhibit a dramatic response. Alternatively, inhaled treatments can be given continuously to severely obstructed patients until a clinical response is seen or adverse effects (e.g., excessive tachycardia, arrhythmias, tremor) limit further drug administration.

In most circumstances β-adrenergic agonists should be administered by inhalation alone, although there are circumstances in which alternative routes of administration are warranted. Intravenous administration of these drugs has been evaluated in patients with severe asthma and in most studies is not superior to administration by inhalation.[12–15] Bloomfield and co-workers[15] compared salbutamol given as a 0.5-mg intravenous (IV) infusion over 3 min with a 0.5% solution of salbutamol given by inhalation over 3 min. Peak expiratory flow rate (PEFR) improvements were similar in both groups, but the resolution of pulsus paradoxus was greater and tachycardia less in patients treated by inhalation. Salmeron and colleagues[13] compared the efficacy of albuterol given by nebulization versus IV infusion. The mean increase in PEFR at 1 h was greater in the patients treated by inhalation as was the decrease in Pa_{CO_2}; in addition, there was less hypokalemia in the patients treated with nebulized drug. In one clinical study,[14] salbutamol given by continuous IV infusion (0.72 mg/h) over 4 h caused a greater increase in PEFR than did 5 mg salbutamol nebulized at 30 and 120 min. The difference between groups was modest, however (25 percent increase in the IV group versus 14 percent in the inhaled group), and IV drug administration was associated with more tachycardia. It also is notable that the doses given by inhalation in this study were rather low, and the groups may have achieved equivalency if inhalation doses more comparable to current clinical practice had been utilized.

There is no advantage to subcutaneous β-adrenergic agonist administration over inhaled drug unless patients are unable to cooperate with therapy,[16,17] such as patients with impaired sensorium or those in cardiopulmonary arrest. Subcutaneous therapy also should be considered in patients not responding to inhalation therapy.[18] Epinephrine and terbutaline are the agents typically used, largely for historical reasons. There is little advantage of one drug over the other except in the special circumstance of pregnancy. Since epinephrine can reduce placental blood flow and has been associated with congenital malformations, terbutaline is the preferred agent in this circumstance.[19] Typical doses for subcutaneous epinephrine or terbutaline are given in Table 78-1.

While most data support exclusive use of an inhalational route for administration of β-adrenergic agonists in SA, some controversies exist concerning optimal methods of inhalation. It is clear, however, that prior use of inhaled drugs prior to arrival in the emergency department or clinic should not preclude continued use unless clear-cut toxic side effects are identified. Many patients demonstrate a beneficial response despite recent self-administration of drug at home.[20] For nonintubated patients, metered-dose inhalers (MDIs) combined with a spacing device may be equivalent in effect to nebulizers.[21,22] In addition, they are generally quicker and cheaper to use. Nonetheless, many clinicians prefer first treatments for patients with SA to be administered by handheld nebulizers since fewer instructions are required and less coordination is necessary from the severely dyspneic patient.

If ventilatory failure has supervened and endotracheal intubation and mechanical ventilation have been instituted, β-adrenergic agonist administration should continue. Many questions remain unanswered regarding optimal drug administration under these conditions, since aspects of the ventilator circuit, ventilator settings, connectors, and circuitry for nebulizers or MDIs, endotracheal tube, and intrinsic properties of the patient's airways likely influence drug delivery and efficacy.[23] Whether nebulizers or MDIs are used, there is consensus that higher drug doses are required to achieve physiologic effect than in nonintubated patients. In studies using radioactively labeled drug delivered by either MDI or nebulizer in intubated patients or lung models, only small fractions of drug can be demonstrated to be delivered to distal airways[23-31]; in one such study of nebulized drug, the fraction deposited in lungs of mechanically ventilated patients was less than 3 percent.[24] Various routes of administration may be totally ineffective during mechanical ventilation. Manthous and colleagues[31] compared administration of nebulized albuterol to drug delivered by MDI through a simple inspiratory adapter to patients having airflow obstruction on mechanical ventilatory support. Using the peak-to-pause pressure gradient at constant inspiratory flow as a measure of airway resistance (see Fig. 78-1), they found no effect and no side effects of up to 100 puffs (9.0 mg) of albuterol delivered by MDI. Albuterol delivered by nebulizer to a total dose of 2.5 mg reduced the flow-resistive pressure by 18 percent. Increasing the nebulized dose to a total of 7.5 mg caused further reduction in the pressure gradient in 8 of 10 patients but also caused toxic side effects in 4 of the 8. In an accompanying editorial,[32] Newhouse and Fuller commented that "the major importance of this study is its potential for raising the awareness of physicians to the need to study aerosol delivery systems as thoroughly as they study the pharmacologic agents themselves, since both are equally important determinants of the therapeutic response."

If MDIs are used to deliver β-adrenergic agonists to mechanically ventilated patients, use of a spacer device on the inspiratory limb of the ventilator may improve drug delivery significantly.[33] Whether drug is delivered by nebulizer or MDI, dosage should be titrated to a physiologic end-

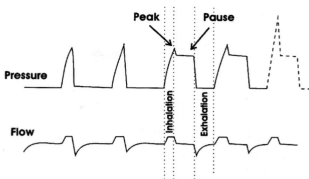

FIGURE 78-1 Simultaneous plots of airflow and airway pressure in a mechanically ventilated patient. The airway peak-to-plateau gradient is determined by temporarily occluding inspiratory flow (usually with an inspiratory pause). Under conditions of constant inspiratory flow and absence of patient effort, this gradient is a useful parameter to gauge airway resistance and bronchodilator efficacy. With increases in airflow obstruction, the peak-to-plateau gradient will widen (as in the dotted line breath).

point such as peak-to-pause airway pressure gradient (see Fig. 78-1). In the majority of patients with SA who are receiving mechanical ventilation, continuous nebulization of albuterol should be prescribed until an improvement in the airway peak-to-pause gradient is observed, or toxic side effects limit further use. When a response is obtained, drug administration can be decreased to 2.5 mg of albuterol every h, and then every 2 h as airway pressures continue to decrease. Exacerbation of airflow obstruction requires increased doses of β-adrenergic agonists. In all patients it is important to exclude other causes of elevated airway pressure, such as gas trapping, with intrinsic end-expiratory pressure or endotracheal tube kinking or plugging.

CORTICOSTEROIDS

Corticosteroids treat airways inflammation, decrease mucous production, potentiate the effect of β-adrenergic agonists, and decrease β-agonist tachyphylaxis[34,35] (see Chaps. 56, 77). These drugs offer the best opportunity to interrupt the spiral of worsening airflow obstruction. When patients present to the emergency room with SA, they almost invariably have received inadequate doses of corticosteroids.

The benefits of corticosteroid therapy in the emergency setting were recently summarized in a meta-analysis of prior randomized, controlled studies of severe asthma.[36] It was concluded that emergency department use of corticosteroids significantly reduced the rates of admission and the number of future relapses in the subsequent 7 to 10 days. Large differences between oral, parenteral, and intravenous routes were not seen as long as a minimum of 30 mg of prednisone or its equivalent was given every 6 h in the first day of management. In a review of guidelines for corticosteroid dosing in SA, McFadden recommended 150 to 225 mg/day of prednisone be given to reach maximum benefit; a typical regimen achieving equivalence would be 40 mg of methylprednisolone IV every 6 h.[37] Haskell and coworkers[38] showed that patients receiving 125 mg of methylprednisolone every 6 h improved more rapidly than patients receiving 40 mg every 6 h, although there was no difference in ultimate improvement in airflow obstruction.

While more studies would be helpful to define further the benefit of higher doses of corticosteroids in the more severely ill patients, current data support use of 60 to 125 mg IV methylprednisolone every 6 h during the initial 24 to 36 h of treatment. Regardless of the dose of corticosteroids used at home, an initial supplemented dose should be administered in the emergency department since benefits are not seen clinically for hours.[34] As patients improve, corticosteroid dose may be reduced to 60 to 80 mg of prednisone daily, which is then continued until peak flow determinations have returned to baseline. Oral corticosteroids are generally continued for a minimum of 14 days and should not be tapered until pulmonary function has returned to baseline. Most patients with a prior episode of SA should be committed to long-term asthma therapy (see Chap. 77). Aggressive use of inhaled corticosteroids should be pursued without fail and may be an effective means of limiting or eliminating systemic corticosteroids.

In all patients so treated, steroid-induced side effects should be expected and appropriate monitoring conducted. Typical problems encountered (albeit in a minority of patients) include hyperglycemia, ketoacidosis, hypertension, hypokalemia, and major mood alterations. When patients are managed concurrently with corticosteroids and muscle relaxants during mechanical ventilatory support, the incidence of myopathy may be increased (see below).

ANTICHOLINERGICS

Three drugs in this class are currently available in the United States: atropine sulfate, ipratropium bromide, and glycopyrrolate (see Chaps. 52–54). Since atropine is well absorbed from the airways and causes undesirable systemic effects, it should not be used in asthma. The quartenary amine structures of ipratropium and glycopyrrolate limit their absorption, and they may be beneficial in acute asthma. Ipratropium has been shown to augment the bronchodilating effect of β-adrenergic agonists.[39] Some authors[39,40] have suggested that a subset of patients with asthma may exhibit a paradoxical bronchoconstrictive response to ipratropium; the incidence has been estimated to be 4 percent to 20 percent. While the true incidence of this possible adverse effect is likely to be low, clinicians opting to employ anticholinergics in the management of SA should be aware of this possibility and should be prepared to discontinue drug use if this phenomenon is encountered.

The optimal dose of ipratropium or glycopyrrolate is not known. Most studies utilizing ipratropium have evaluated doses of 0.25 to 0.50 mg by nebulization in nonintubated patients, which would be equivalent to more than 10 puffs by MDI (0.018 mg/puff). Ipratropium currently is available in the United States as a premixed unit-dose inhalation solution for nebulization (0.5 mg diluted in saline). Ipratropium solution can be mixed directly with a number of β-adrenergic agonists for conebulization,[41] but the efficacy of combined therapy requires further study. A reasonable approach is to utilize ipratropium or glycopyrrolate as second-line agents in patients with SA not responding to therapy with corticosteroids and β-adrenergic agonists. Recommended initial doses for anticholinergics in SA are given in Table 78-1.

THEOPHYLLINE

Despite a history of use that predates the development of β-adrenergic agonists, the precise role of theophylline and its congeners in the management of asthma in general and SA in particular continues to be debated (see Chaps. 51 and 77). Several studies have demonstrated that as monotherapy, theophylline is inferior to β-adrenergic agonists as a bronchodilator and increases the incidence of undesirable side effects.[42–44] In addition, when theophylline is added to other standard medications in severe asthma, there is little additional improvement in measures of airflow obstruction such as PEFR.[44] Nonetheless, some studies suggest that improvement over the first 48 h of management occurs in patients treated with theophylline in addition to β-adrenergic agonists and corticosteroids[45,46] and that some of this benefit may derive from effects of methylxanthines unrelated to bronchodilation.[47,48]

While debate concerning methylxanthine use in SA will likely continue until further studies are performed,[49,50] it is still reasonable to administer IV theophylline to patients not responding to β-adrenergic agonists and corticosteroid therapy or to those patients who are so severely ill as to require mechanical ventilatory support. Loading and maintenance doses of theophylline are given in Table 78-1 (see Chaps. 51 and 61). Several studies have established the safety of theophylline use in severe asthma if appropriate monitoring of serum concentrations is conducted.[51] In patients arriving to the health-care facility with prior use of theophylline, serum concentrations should be checked *before* additional drug is given. In patients loaded with theophylline IV, serum concentrations should be checked within 6 h to avoid toxicity and to guide subsequent dosing. Factors influencing methylxanthine metabolism and drugs interacting with methylxanthine metabolism are discussed elsewhere in this text (see Chaps. 51 and 61).

Innovative Therapies

MAGNESIUM SULFATE

There are several effects of magnesium that suggest it could have direct or synergistic bronchodilating effects in SA. Magnesium inhibits calcium channels of airway smooth muscle and thus could inhibit calcium-mediated contraction.[52] Magnesium has been shown to reduce histamine- and methacholine-induced bronchoconstriction in asthmatics.[53,54] Magnesium also decreases acetylcholine release and thus could reduce bronchoconstriction associated with parasympathetic stimulation.

While a number of anecdotal reports have suggested a dramatic effect from magnesium administration in SA,[55–60] the two largest prospective studies did not demonstrate a benefit from magnesium administration to ambulatory patients with severe SA treated with β-adrenergic agonists and corticosteroids.[61,62] Nonetheless, these observations may not be sufficient to completely preclude magnesium use in critically ill patients requiring mechanical ventilatory support, in whom even small benefits in reduction of airflow obstruction could be useful. We recommend use of magnesium in patients undergoing mechanical ventilatory support who have failed standard therapies. It should be noted that this is fortunately a very small patient pool. Such patients should receive 1 g magnesium sulfate IV over 20 min and repeat 20 min later; if the patient is hypomagnesemic, we normalize serum levels with additional doses. All patients receiving magnesium should have serum levels monitored and maintained at < 6 mg/dL. Neuromuscular weakness is a potential side effect but is not usually encountered with the doses recommended and is without consequence during mechanical ventilatory support, which typically requires sedation if not muscle relaxation (see below).

HELIOX

Heliox is a blend of helium and oxygen that has a density less than that of air. It can be administered to patients with SA through a rebreather mask or can be administered through the gas blender of most ventilators. Because of its low density, heliox decreases airway resistance in bronchi with turbulent flow regimes. This may decrease work of breathing in the spontaneously breathing patient and forestall ventilatory failure until bronchodilators and anti-inflammatories take effect; in the mechanically ventilated patient, heliox may be useful to diminish hyperinflation and risk of barotrauma. Since the decreased density effect of heliox is only significant at high helium concentrations, it is advisable to use as close to an 80:20 helium:oxygen mix as possible. This can usually be accomplished in SA because supplemental oxygen requirements are minimal (see above).

Manthous and colleagues[63] observed a significant increase in PEFR and a significant decrease in pulsus paradoxus in patients with acute asthma breathing heliox for 15 min as compared with controls. To the extent that these observations indicate a reduction in both inspiratory and expiratory airway resistance, heliox may diminish muscle fatigue and lung hyperinflation in SA and serve as a bridge to effective bronchodilator/anti-inflammatory therapy. Similarly, Gluck and coworkers[64] administered heliox to intubated patients with SA and observed a decrease in peak airway pressure and Pa_{CO_2} in all patients within minutes.

Although these results are promising, further studies are required to define better the use of heliox in patients with SA. If heliox is used during mechanical ventilatory support, it is important to recognize that recalibration of gas blenders and flow meters is required. This is not easily undertaken in the midst of managing the critically ill, mechanically ventilated patient with SA and is a procedure that should be performed in advance, with careful training of respiratory therapy staff before attempting routine clinical application.

Pharmacologic Adjuncts to Intubation and Mechanical Ventilation in Status Asthmaticus

If clinical deterioration occurs in the face of aggressive pharmacologic therapy in SA, intubation and mechanical ventilation should be performed electively, well in advance of respiratory arrest.[1] Patients with SA represent some of the most challenging clinical scenarios in critical care management. During mechanical ventilatory support, many patients have extraordinary increases in proximal airway pressure (often so extreme as to impair delivery of set tidal volume) in association with severe gas trapping, as reflected by the measurement of static airway pressure, intrinsic positive end-expiratory pressure (PEEP$_i$)[1] (see Fig. 78-2), or the volume of gas at end-inspiration above FRC (V_{EI}).[65] The risk of barotrauma is substantial under these conditions. General approaches to this challenging derangement of pulmonary mechanics are to (1) tolerate high peak airway pressures, since much of this pressure dissipates across the resistance of the robust central airways and does not necessarily reflect increased alveolar volume; (2) seek minimal gas trapping by reducing inspiratory times and minute ventilation; and (3) accept a degree of hypoventilation (e.g., permissive hypercapnea) if necessary to reduce static airway pressure

FIGURE 78-2 Measurement of intrinsic PEEP (PEEP$_i$). Under normal conditions, alveolar pressure (P_{alv}) closely tracks the pressure at the airway opening (P_{ao}), which is reported on the ventilator manometer. At end-expiration, P_{alv} falls to atmospheric pressure (0 cmH$_2$O) and is accurately reflected by P_{ao}. In severe airflow obstruction, P_{alv} may increase because of gas trapping, and at end-expiration P_{alv} has not fallen to atmospheric pressure and does not equal P_{ao}. If an expiratory hold maneuver is performed, P_{ao} will increase, reflecting the degree of gas trapping. (*From Corbridge T, Hall JB: Status asthmaticus in the adult: assessment, drug therapy, mechanical ventilation.* Choices Respir Mgmt 1991; 21(5):199; with permission).

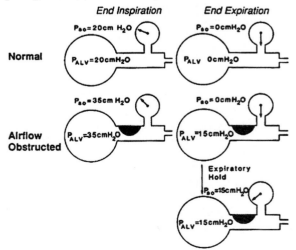

TABLE 78-2   Sedatives Used in Status Asthmaticus

Agent	Dose	Cautions
	PERI-INTUBATION PERIOD	
Midazolam	1 mg IV slow infusion. Repeat every 2 to 3 min as needed.	Hypotension Respiratory depression
Ketamine	1 to 2 mg/kg IV at a rate of 0.5 mg/kg per min.	Sympathomimetic effects Respiratory depression Mood changes Delerium-type reactions
Propofol	60 to 80 mg/min IV initial infusion up to 2.0 mg/kg, followed by an infusion of 5 to 10 mg/kg per h as needed.	Respiratory depression
	SEDATION FOR PROTRACTED MECHANICAL VENTILATION	
Lorazepam	1 to 5 mg/h IV continuous infusion or IV bolus as needed.	Drug accumulation
Morphine sulfate	1 to 5 mg/h IV continuous infusion; avoid bolus.	Ileus
Ketamine	0.1 to 0.5 mg/min IV.	Sympathomimetic effects Delerium-type reactions
Propofol	1 to 4.5 mg/kg per h IV.	Seizures Hypertriglyceridemia

< 30 cmH$_2$O, PEEP$_i$ < 15 cmH$_2$O, and V$_{EI}$ < 20 mL/kg. The specifics of implementing these goals have been detailed elsewhere, and the reader is referred to several extensive reviews.[1–3] To manage these patients during mechanical ventilatory support, sedation is invariably required and muscle relaxation often is required. The details of these pharmacologic interventions are offered below (see Tables 78-2 and 78-3).

SEDATIVES

Drugs typically used to sedate the patient in preparation for mechanical ventilation are listed in Table 78-2. Midazolam is given in doses of 1 mg IV every 2 to 3 min until the patient allows positioning and inspection of the airway. Morphine sulfate is usually avoided in this setting because of the propensity to cause hypotension (particularly in the face of elevated intrathoracic pressures secondary to gas trapping), histamine release, and opioid-induced vomiting. Ketamine,

an intravenous general anesthetic with analgesic, anesthetic, and bronchodilating properties also is useful during airway management of patients with SA.[66,67] A dose of 1 to 2 mg/kg IV given at a rate of 0.5 mg/kg per min usually provides 10 to 15 min of general anesthesia, often without profound respiratory depression.[68] While bronchospasm may improve acutely after IV administration of ketamine, the effect usually dissipates over 20 to 30 min.[69] This agent does have sympathomimetic effects and is relatively contraindicated in patients with vascular disease, hypertension, increased intracranial pressure (e.g., postcardiac arrest), and preeclampsia. Ketamine also can decrease seizure threshold and provoke delirium.

Propofol is a lipid-soluble anesthetic available for intravenous use. In a recent study comparing propofol to a benzodiazepine in sedation for asthmatics undergoing fiberoptic bronchoscopy, propofol appeared more titratable, with a more rapid onset and resolution of sedation.[70] Initial IV infusions of 60 to 80 mg/min to ≤ 2.0 mg/kg will usually

TABLE 78-3   Paralytics Used in the Management of Status Asthmaticus

Agent	Initial Paralyzing Dose (mg/kg)	Duration of Action of Bolus (min)	Initial Drip Rate (mg/kg per h)
Vecuronium (Norcuron)	0.08	30–45	0.07
Atracurium (Tracrium)	0.5	30–45	0.7
Pancuronium (Pavulon)	0.08	60–80	0.025

achieve adequate sedation, which can then be maintained with an infusion beginning at 5 to 10 mg/kg per h, titrated as necessary. Some data suggest that generalized seizures may complicate long-term propofol infusion.[71,72]

Once an airway is secured and the patient is stabilized on the mechanical ventilator, ongoing sedation over the first hours to days of management is usually required. Either of the short-acting benzodiazepines, lorazepam or midazolam, are useful for this purpose (see Table 78-2). Unfortunately, even these agents may accumulate significantly in critically ill patients when used on a continuous basis and may cause protracted periods of recovery after drug discontinuation.[73] Use of small doses of morphine may allow significant reductions in benzodiazepine dosing. Since safety data are still lacking, neither propofol nor ketamine can be recommended for long-term sedation in SA.

PARALYTICS

Paralysis can augment the beneficial effects of sedation to reduce oxygen consumption and hence carbon dioxide production (thus reducing minute ventilation requirement), lactic acid production, and patient dysynchrony with the ventilator. *Paralytics never should be used until attempts at sedation have been exhausted, and paralyzed patients should always be reassessed for the adequacy of sedation.*

Vecuronium and atracurium are the preferred paralytic agents in SA. These nondepolarizing agents are largely free of cardiovascular side effects. Vecuronium is metabolized and excreted via hepatic and renal routes and thus may accumulate in patients with failure of either organ system. These drugs may be administered by intermittent bolus injection or continuous IV infusion. In either case, drug should be withheld every 4 to 6 h to avoid drug accumulation and assess the need for ongoing paralysis. Dosing guidelines are given in Table 78-3.

Many difficulties arise in the course of maintaining the patient undergoing therapeutic paralysis. Mental status and other aspects of the physical examination are difficult or impossible to assess, making it difficult for the clinician to identify new complications of critical illness. It is likely these agents increase the risk of deep venous thrombosis and disuse muscle atrophy. Importantly, these drugs also appear to play a causative role in the development of myopathy in severe acute asthma. In one recent study,[74] more than 75 percent of patients undergoing mechanical ventilation and muscle relaxation for SA demonstrated a significant increase in serum creatine kinase (CK), and 36 percent of patients had clinically detectable myopathy. Other studies[75,76] have suggested a somewhat lower incidence of this complication and have implicated the coadministration of corticosteroids and paralytics in the development of significant neuromuscular weakness.

In view of these data, efforts to limit paralytic use are important. As better regimens for sedation are established, use of paralytics will be curtailed and doses reduced. When paralytics are used, dosing in accord with peripheral nerve stimulation is helpful to define least required doses.[1] Paralytics should be stopped periodically to assess on-going need, serum CK levels should be followed serially, and confounding electrolyte disorders that may contribute to muscle weakness should be aggressively sought and corrected.

INHALATIONAL ANESTHETICS

The pharmacologic and ventilator strategies delineated above will be effective in the majority of patients. On occasion, patients will fail all of these measures during their acute management, and consideration can be given to general anesthesia. Both enflurane and halothane have bronchodilating properties, but this effect is almost invariably lost soon after the drug is discontinued.[77,78] If inhalational anesthesia is employed, staff familiar with the expected side effects of myocardial depression, arterial vasodilation, and arrhythmias should be involved in management. This usually requires the consultation of a skilled anesthesiologist in management and in some institutions can only be accomplished in the operating room.

References

1. Corbridge T, Hall JB: Assessment and Management of the adult with status asthmaticus: A state-of-the-art. *Am J Respir Crit Care Med* 1995; 151:1296.
2. Hall JB, Wood LDH: Management of the critically ill asthmatic patient, in Dosman JA, Cockcroft DW, (eds): *Obstructive Lung Disease. Med Clin N Amer* 1990; 74(3):1–18.
3. Wasserfallen JB, Schaller MD, Feihl F, Perret Ch: Sudden asphyxic asthma: a distinct entity? *Am Rev Respir Dis* 1990; 142:108–11.
4. Leatherman J: Life-threatening asthma. *Clin Chest Med* 1994; 15:453–479.
5. Rodriquez-Roisin R, Ballester E, Roca J, et al.: Mechanisms of hypoxemia in patients with status asthmaticus requiring mechanical ventilation. *Am Rev Rspir Dis* 1989; 139:732–39.
6. McFadden ER Jr, Lyons HA: Arterial-blood gas tension in asthma. *N Engl J Med* 1968; 278:1027–32.
7. Ballester E, Reyes A, Roca J, et al.: Ventilation-perfusion mismatching in acute severe asthma: effects of salbutamol and 100% oxygen. *Thorax* 1989; 44:258–67.
8. Sears MR, Taylor DR, Print CG, et al.: Regular inhaled beta-agonist treatment in bronchial asthma. *Lancet* 1990; 336:1391–96.
9. Spitzer WO, Suissa S, Ernst P, et al.: The use of beta-agonists and the risk of death and near death from asthma. *N Engl J Med* 1992; 326:501–06.
10. Suissa S, Ernst P, Boivin JF: A cohort analysis of excess mortality in asthma and the use of inhaled beta-agonists. *Am J Respir Crit Care Med* 1994; 149:604–10.
11. Gern JE, Lemanske RF: Beta-adrenergic agonist therapy. *Immunol Allergy Clin N Am* 1993; 13(4):839–860.
12. Williams SJ, Winner SH, Clark TJH: Comparison of inhaled and intravenous terbutaline in acute severe asthma. *Thorax* 1981; 36:629–631.
13. Salmeron S, Brochard L, Mal H, et al.: Nebulized versus intravenous albuterol in hypercapnic acute asthma: a multicenter, double-blind, randomized study. *Am J Respir Crit Care Med* 1994; 149:1466–70.
14. Cheong B, Reynolds SR, Rajan G, et al.: Intravenous beta-agonist in severe acute asthma. *Br Med J* 1988; 297:448–450.
15. Bloomfield P, Carmichael J, Petrie GR, et al.: Comparison of salbutamol given intravenously and by intermittent positive-

pressure breathing in life-threatening asthma. *Br Med J* 1979; 1:848–850.

16. Uden DL, Goetz DR, Kohen DP, et al.: Comparison of nebulized terbutaline and subcutaneous epinephrine in the treatment of acute asthma. *Ann Emerg Med* 1985; 14:229–232.

17. Becker AB, Nelson NA, Simons FER: Inhaled salbutamol (albuterol) vs injected epinephrine in the treatment of acute asthma in children. *J Pediatr* 1983; 102:465–469.

18. Appel D, Kapel JP, Sherman M: Epinephrine improves expiratory airflow rates in patients with asthma who do not respond to inhaled metaproterenol sulfate. *J Allergy Clin Immunol* 1989; 84:90–98.

19. Schmidt G, Hall JB: Pulmonary disease, in Barron WM, Lindheimer MD (eds): *Medical Disorders during Pregnancy.* St. Louis, Mosby Year Book, 1994; 197–231.

20. Rossing TH, Fanta CH, McFadden ER: Effect of outpatient treatment of asthma with beta agonists on the response to sympathomimetics in an emergency room. *Am J Med* 1983; 75:781–84.

21. Idris AH, McDermott MF, Raucci JC, et al.: Emergency department treatment of severe asthma: metered-dose inhaler plus holding chamber is equivalent in effectiveness to nebulizer. *Chest* 1993; 103:665–72.

22. Newhouse MT: Emergency department management of life-threatening asthma: are nebulizers obsolete? *Chest* 1993; 103:661–63.

23. Manthous CA, Hall JB: Administration of therapeutic aerosols to mechanically ventilated patients. *Chest* 1994; 106:560–71.

24. MacIntyre NR, Silver RM, Miller CW, et al.: Aerosol delivery in intubated, mechanically ventilated patients. *Crit Care Med* 1985; 13(2):81–4.

25. O'Doherty MJ, Thomas SHL, Page CG, et al.: Delivery of a nebulized aerosol to a lung model during mechanical ventilation. *Am Rev Respir Dis* 1992; 146:383–88.

26. O'Riordan TG, Greco MJ, Perry RJ, et al.: Nebulizer function during mechanical ventilation. *Am Rev Respir Dis* 1992; 145:1117–22.

27. Fuller HD, Dolovich MB, Posmituck G, et al.: Pressurized aerosol versus jet aerosol delivery to mechanically ventilated patients. *Am Rev Respir Dis* 1990; 141:440–44.

28. Bishop MJ, Larson RP, Buschman DL: Metered dose inhaler aerosol characteristics are affected by the endotracheal tube actuator/adaptor used. *Anesthesiology* 1990; 73:1263–65.

29. Taylor RH, Lerman J, Chambers C, et al.: Dosing efficiency and particle size characteristics of pressurized metered-dose inhalers in narrow catheters. *Chest* 1993; 103:920–24.

30. Niven RW, Kacmarek RM, Brain JD, et al.: Small bore nozzle extensions to improve the delivery efficiency of drugs from metered dose inhalers: laboratory evaluation. *Am Rev Respir Dis* 1993; 147:1590–94.

31. Manthous CA, Hall JB, Schmidt GA, et al.: Metered-dose inhaler versus nebulized albuterol in mechanically ventilated patients. *Am Rev Respir Dis* 1993; 148:1567–70.

32. Newhouse MT, Fuller HD: Rose is a rose is a rose? Aerosol therapy in ventilated patients: nebulizers versus metered-dose-inhalers—a continuing controversy. *Am Rev Respir Dis* 1993; 148:1444–46.

33. Chatila W, Hall JB, Manthous CA: Treatment of bronchospasm by metered-dose-inhaler albuterol via spacer in mechanically ventilated patients. *Am J Respir Crit Care Med* 1994; 149:A190.

34. Barnes NC: Effects of corticosteroids in acute severe asthma. *Thorax* 1992;47:582–583.

35. Townley RG, Reeb R, Fitzgibbons T, et al.: The effects of corticosteroids on the beta-adrenergic receptors in bronchial smooth muscle. *J Allergy* 1970; 45:118.

36. Rowe BH, Keller JL, Oxman AD: Effectiveness of steroid therapy in acute exacerbations of asthma: a meta-analysis. *Am J Emerg Med* 1992; 10(4):301–10.

37. McFadden ER Jr: Clinical commentary: dosages of corticosteroids in asthma. *Am Rev Respir Dis* 1993; 147:1306–10.

38. Haskell RJ, Wong BM, Hansen JE: A double-blind, randomized clinical trial of methylprednisolone in status asthmaticus. *Arch Intern Med* 1983; 143L1324–27.

39. Bryant DH, Rogers P: Effects of ipratropium bromide nebulizer solution with and without preservatives in the treatment of acute and stable asthma. *Chest* 1992; 102:742–47.

40. Rafferty P, Beasley R, Howarth PH: Bronchoconstriction induced by ipratropium bromide in asthma: relation to bromide ion. *Br Med J* 1986; 293:1538–39.

41. Fitzgerald JM: A study of the efficacy and safety of nebulization therapy combining ipratropium bromide 0.5 mg with salbutamol sulphate 3.0 mg versus salbutamol sulphate 3.0 mg alone in acute asthma. *Am J Respir Crit Car Med* 1994; 149:A190.

42. Rossing TH, Fanta CH, Goldstein DH, et al.: Emergency therapy of asthma: comparison of the acute effects of parenteral and inhaled sympathomimetics and infused aminophylline. *Am Rev Respir Dis* 1980; 122:365–371.

43. Siefel D, Sheppard D, Gelb A, et al.: Aminophylline increases the toxicity but not the efficacy of an inhaled beta-adrenergic agonist in the treatment of acute exacerbations of asthma. *Am Rev Respir Dis* 1985; 132:283–86.

44. Murphy DG, McDermott MF, Rydman RF, et al.: Aminophylline in the treatment of acute asthma when beta two adrenergics and steroids are provided. *Arch Intern Med* 1993; 153:1784–88.

45. Huang D, O'Brien RG, Harman E, et al.: Does aminophylline benefit adults admitted to the hospital for an acute exacerbation of asthma? *Ann Intern Med* 1993; 119:1155–60.

46. Wrenn K, Slovis CM, Murphy F, et al.: Aminophylline therapy for acute bronchospastic disease in the emergency room. *Ann Intern Med* 1991; 115:241–47.

47. Milgrom H, Bender B: Current issues in the use of theophylline. *Am Rev Respir Dis* 1993; 147:S33–S39.

48. Milgrom H: Theophylline. *Immunol Allergy Clin N Am* 1993; 13(4):819–38.

49. Newhouse MT: Is theophylline obsolete? *Chest* 1990; 98:1–2.

50. McFadden ER: Methylxanthines in the treatment of asthma: the rise, the fall, and the possible rise again. *Ann Intern Med* 1991; 115:323–24.

51. George RB: Preventing arrhythmias in acute asthma. *J Respir Dis* 1991; 12(6):545–61.

52. Spivey WH, Skobeloff EM, Levin RM: Effect of magnesium chloride on rabbit bronchial smooth muscle. *Ann Emerg Med* 1990; 19:1107–12.

53. Rolla G, Bucca C, Bugiani M, et al.: Reduction of histamine-induced bronchoconstriction by magnesium in asthmatic subjects. *Allergy* 1987; 42:186–88.

54. Rolla G, Bucca C, Arossa W, et al.: Magnesium attenuates methacholine-induced bronchoconstriction in asthmatics. *Magnesium* 1987; 6:201–04.

55. Skobeloff EM, Spivey WH, McNamara RM, et al.: Intravenous magnesium sulfate for the treatment of acute asthma in the emergency department. *JAMA* 1989; 262:1210–3.

56. Noppen M, Vanmaele L, Impens N, et al.: Bronchodilating effect of intravenous magnesium sulfate in acute severe asthma. *Chest* 1990; 97:373–76.

57. Okayama H, Okayama M, Aikawa T, et al.: Treatment of status asthmaticus with intravenous magnesium sulfate. *J Asthma* 1991; 28:11–17.

58. Okayama H, Aikawa T, Okayama M, et al.: Bronchodilating effect of intravenous magnesium sulfate in bronchial asthma. *JAMA* 1987; 257:1076–78.

59. McNamara RM, Spivey WH, Skobeloff EM, et al.: Intravenous magnesium sulfate in the management of acute respiratory failure complicating asthma. *Ann Emerg Med* 1989; 2:197–99.

60. Sydow M, Crozier TA, Zielmann S, et al.: High-dose intravenous magnesium sulfate in the management of life-threatening status asthmaticus. *Inten Care Med* 1993; 19:467–471.

61. Green SM, Rothrock SG: Intravenous magnesium for acute asthma: failure to decrease emergency treatment duration or need for hospitalization. *Ann Emerg Med* 1992; 21:260–65.

62. Tiffany BR, Berk W, Todd IK, et al.: Magnesium bolus or infusion fails to improve expiratory flow in acute asthma exacerbations. *Chest* 1993; 104:831–34.

63. Manthous CA, Hall JB, Caputo ME, et al.: The effect of heliox on pulsus paradoxus and peak flow in non-intubated patients with severe asthma. *Chest* 1993; 104:29S.

64. Gluck EH, Onorato DJ, Castriotta R: Helium-oxygen mixtures in intubated patients with status asthmaticus and respiratory acidosis. *Chest* 1990; 98:693–98.

65. Williams TJ, Tuxen DV, Scheinkestel CD, et al.: Risk factors for morbidity in mechanically ventilated patients with acute severe asthma. *Am Rev Respir Dis* 1992; 146:607–15.

66. Corseen G, Gutierrez J, Reves JG, et al.: Ketamine in the anaesthetic management of asthmatic patients. *Anesth Analg* 1972; 51(4):588–96.

67. L'Hommedieu CS, Arens JJ: The use of ketamine for the emergency intubation of patients with status asthmaticus. *Ann Emerg Med* 1987; 16(5):568–71.

68. Roy TM, Pruitt VL, Garner PA, et al.: The potential role for anesthesia in status asthmaticus. *J Asthma* 1992; 29(2):73–77.

69. Sarma VJ: Use of ketamine in acute severe asthma. *Acta Anaesthesiol Scand* 1992; 36:106–7.

70. Clarkson K, Power CK, O'Connell F, et al.: A comparative evaluation of propofol and midazolam as sedative agents in fiberoptic bronchoscopy. *Chest* 1993; 104:1029–31.

71. Valente JF, Anderson GL, Branson RD, et al.: Disadvantages of prolonged propofol sedation in the critical care unit. *Crit Care Med* 1994; 22:710–12.

72. McManus KF: Convulsions after propofol. *Anaesth Intensive Care* 1992; 20:396–97.

73. Pohlman A, Simpson K, Hall J: Continuous intravenous infusions of lorazepam vs. midazolam for sedation during mechanical ventilatory support: a prospective, randomized study. *Crit Care Med* 1994; 22:1241–1248.

74. Douglass JA, Tuxen D, Horne M, et al.: Myopathy in severe asthma. *Am Rev Respir Dis* 1992; 146:517–19.

75. Fluegel W, Iber C, Davies S, et al.: Risk factors for acute myopathy in patients with severe asthma who require mechanical ventilation. *Am J Respir Crit Care Med* 1994; 149:A432.

76. Griffin D, Fairman N, Coursin D, et al.: Acute myopathy during treatment of status asthmaticus with corticosteroids and steroidal muscle relaxants. *Chest* 1992; 102:510–14.

77. Saulnier FF, Durocher AV, Deturck RA, et al.: Respiratory and hemodynamic effects of halothane in status asthmaticus. *Inten Car Med* 1990; 16:104.

78. Echeverria M, Gelb AW, Wexler HR, et al.: Enflurane and halothane in status asthmaticus. *Chest* 1986; 89:153.

INNOVATIVE ASTHMA THERAPIES AND SPECIAL PROBLEMS

Chapter 79

CYTOKINE THERAPY OF ASTHMA

GARY P. ANDERSON
VOLKER BRINKMANN

Aberrant T Cell Mucosal Immunity and Airways Inflammation in Asthma

Current therapies for asthma are neither preventative nor curative. In this section, we outline recent advances in the understanding of T lymphocyte (T cell) mediated mucosal immunity are outlined, which suggest the possibility of improved disease control and, perhaps, prophylaxis of asthma. It currently is believed (but not proven) that T cells acting by the release of cytokines are central regulators of human airways inflammation and, in turn, that the abnormalities in lung physiology in asthma (such as wide spontaneous fluctuation in airway caliber, bronchial hyperreactivity, and airflow obstruction) are the direct consequence of inflammation of the bronchial mucosa.[1,2] T-cell derived interleukin-5 (IL-5) is crucial for the induction of eosinophilia,[3] and interleukin-4 (IL-4) promotes production of IgE antibodies[4–6]: both cytokines are produced mainly by a specialized subset of helper T cells termed the T$_H$2 cell.[7] The distinct subsets of T cells implicated in asthma and atopy are themselves regulated by cytokines, and these cross-regulatory processes[8,9] may provide the basis of new therapeutic approaches with much greater specificity than currently available (nonspecific) immunosuppressors such as glucocorticosteroids, cyclosporin, FK506, and rapamycin. However, formidable problems associated with cytokine treatment remain to be overcome, most notably questions of safety, administration, antibody formation, and the determination of whether cytokine-based therapy will be more useful in preventing rather than reversing established pathologies.

The majority of mature T cells in the periphery display the surface phenotype markers CD4 or CD8. These markers define fundamental functional differences. CD4+ T cells recognize processed foreign antigen in the context of MHC class II on the surface of specialized antigen presenting cells, such as airways dendritic cells, and help B-cell antibody production. CD8+ cells, in contrast, recognize somatic (self) antigens or intracellular pathogen antigens (notably viral antigens) presented in the context of MHC class I molecules, and mediate direct cytolysis of target cells.[10–12] Studies on mouse CD4+ T-cell clones have identified two further phenotypes, currently indistinguishable by their surface markers, but recognized by their production of a restricted panel of cytokines, which contribute to highly specialized functions (Fig. 79-1). The T_H2 cell subset produces IL-4, IL-5, IL-10, and IL-13. T helper-1 (T_H1) cells, in contrast, produce IFN-γ, TNF-β, and IL-2. Both subsets produce IL-2 and GM-CSF.[7,8] [See also Chap. 31]

There is good evidence that T-cell subsets analogous to those identified from mouse T-cell clones exist in human allergic disease. The majority of allergen-specific T-cell clones derived from the peripheral blood of atopic individuals produce increased amounts of IL-4 and IL-5 but lower levels of IFN-γ.[13,14] Furthermore, immunohistochemistry and in situ hybridization studies have shown IL-4/IL-5 cytokine protein or mRNA in biopsies from the airways of asthmatics,[15,16] and these T_H2 cytokines also are increased in bronchioalveolar lavage fluid after antigen challenge.[17] The production of T_H2 cytokines in allergic disease has prompted the search for therapeutic methods to control the delicate balance between T_H1 (IFN-γ) and T_H2 (IL-4, IL-5, IL-13) mucosal immune responses.

Interleukin-5 may be one of the critical mediators of atopic inflammation in asthma. Eosinophilia is both IL-5– and T cell–dependent.[18–20] Eosinophils directly damage the airway epithelium by degranulation of highly cationic proteins,[20–22] release cysteinyl-leukotrienes causing bronchospasm,[23] and, possibly, over the longer term, fibrinogenic growth factors such as transforming growth factors α and β (TGF α and TGF β),[24–26] thus contributing to intractable airways obstruction.

IL-4 and IL-13 induce B cells expressing surface IgM and IgD (IgM+D+ B cells) to rearrange genomic DNA coding for immunoglobulins, leading to the production of IgE by a process termed *isotype switching*.[4,6,27–29] Immunoglobulin E bound to high- (FceIR) and low-affinity (FceIIR) cellular receptors mediates activation and degranulation of metachromatic and other cells, leading to direct airways obstruction and recruitment of inflammatory cells. During this process, released inflammatory mediators (e.g., histamine and eicosanoids) may also feed back on B and T lymphocytes.[30] Furthermore, IL-4 (but not IL-13) may serve as an

Important cytokine producing cellular phenotypes in asthma

CD4+ (TH1 and TH2), CD8+

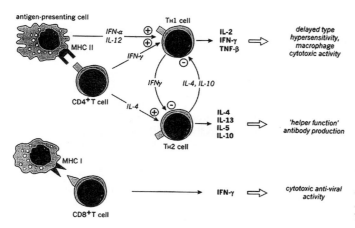

FIGURE 79-1 *Important cytokine-producing cellular phenotypes in asthma.* The upper panel shows cytokines produced by T cells bearing the surface markers CD4+ (T_H1 and T_H2 cells) and CD8+ (cytotoxic T cells). Processed antigenic epitopes of an inhaled allergen are shown presented by an antigen-presenting cell to a naïve CD4+ T cell, which recognizes the processed antigen bound to the MHC class II molecules. These naïve CD4+ T cells can commit to either a T_H1 or T_H2 phenotype, which are defined by the panel of cytokines they produce. Commitment to the T_H1 phenotype is favored (+) by IFN-α, IL-12, or IFN-γ, whereas IL-4 favors commitment to the T_H2 phenotype. Mature committed T_H1 cells inhibit (-) T_H2 cells via secretion of IFN-γ, whereas T helper-2 (T_H2) cells suppress the activity of T_H1 cells via secretion of IL-4 and IL-10. T helper-1 (T_H1) cells mediate delayed hypersensitivity reactions and induce cytotoxicity in macrophages by secretion of IL-2, IFN-γ, and TNF-β. Conversely, T_H2 cells promote B-cell antibody production via cytokine secretion. Interleukin-4 promotes further T_H2 commitment and, together with IL-13, B-cell IgE switch. Interleukin-5 promotes eosinophilia of mucosal tissues. CD8+ T cells recognize either self-antigen (which normally elicits no response) or the antigenic determinant of intracellular pathogens such as virus expressed on the cell surface by MHC class I. In this case CD8+ cells are activated, secrete IFN-γ, and mount a cytotoxic defense against the infected cell. Metachromatic cells (mast cells, basophils, and non-B, non-T cells (NBNT cells) can be triggered by cross-linking of surface-bound allergen-specific IgE to release a range of preformed and newly synthesized anaphylatic mediators, but also the cytokines IL-4, IL-5, IL-3, and GM-CSF. Note that the schema is somewhat generalized for clarity; there are, for example, established examples of non-MHC I restricted antigen presentation to CD8+ cells. The models are based predominantly on studies in rodents but strong evidence favoring analogous phenotypes in humans has been obtained.

autocrine growth and differentiation factor for the commitment of naïve T_H0 cells to a functional T_H2 phenotype.[31,32]

The factors controlling the development of T_H1 versus T_H2 cells in vivo are increasingly better understood. During antigen stimulation, T_H1 and T_H2 cells develop from a common, nonspecialized precursor (T_H0) with an unrestricted cytokine production profile. During this process, termed *commitment*, selective cytokine gene induction and suppression occurs.[7,8] The commitment to differential phenotypes may be regulated by the nature of the antigenic stimulation, the duration of T-cell stimulation, and, particularly, by the nature of soluble signals uncommitted CD4+ T_H0 cells encounter during the commitment process.[8,9,13] Studies in mice suggest that only a small subset of CD4 T-cells (bearing the NK1.1 surface marker) secretes IL-4 upon primary T-cell receptor stimulation in the absence of preformed IL-4,[33] and that repletion of IL-4–deficient mice with lymphoid but not myeloid lineages restores the capability of mounting a T_H2 response. The secreted IL-4 may then favor T_H2 commitment of neighboring T cells (*by-stander effect*), either of the same specificity or of distinct antigen specificities.

T helper-1 and T_H2 cells reciprocally inhibit each other through secretion of cytokines.[8,34] Known regulatory pathways between T_H1 and T_H2 cells are shown diagrammatically in Fig. 79-1, and are discussed in detail below. These cross-regulatory pathways, provide a rational basis for the use of cytokine manipulations to treat asthma. In addition, several cytokines produced by established T_H2 cells are excellent therapeutic targets for pharmacologic inhibition.

Alternative Sources of T_H2 Cytokines

T helper-2 cells are not the unique source of IL-4 and IL-5 in human disease (Fig. 79-2). Metachromatic cells [basophils and mast cells, and so-called non-B non-T cells (NBNT cells)], eosinophils, and CD8+ T cells or CD4-8– T cells also can produce a "T_H2-like" cytokine profile.[35–43] Mast cell metaplasia is a pathologic feature of the inflamed mucosa and these cells are sources of IL-4 and IL-5 in asthma.[35–37,40] Human eosinophils, especially in disease, produce IL-5, IL-3, IL-8, IL-1, and granulocyte/macrophage colony-stimulating factor (GM-CSF) mRNA or protein,[39,44,45] which may serve as autocrine or paracrine survival and activation factors reducing the dependency of this lineage on T_H2 lymphocyte cytokine secretion. IL-4/IL-5 production from mast cells and eosinophils may be important, since IL-4 would drive T_H2 cell development independent of the nature of the antigen/allergen stimulus and induce IgE switching of B cells, and IL-5 would maintain eosinophilic infiltration to the airways mucosa.

CD8+ cells, which normally produce IFN-γ, can be induced to produce IL-4 and IL-5 in vitro.[37,41–43,46] CD8+ cells also can convert "double negative" (i.e., lose surface expression of CD4+ and CD8+ markers), and help B cell IgE isotype switch, but lose their potential to kill their normal targets.[38,43] The existence of these subsets in asthma is not established but it represents a potential source of IL-4 and IL-5 in MHC class I restricted immune responses; for example, CD8+ mediated defense of virus-infected respiratory epithelial cells.

Therapeutic Effects of Cytokines in Airways Disease

Interrupting cytokine-mediated T_H2 commitment or the use of cytokines to suppress T_H2 cell function would be expected to prevent B cell–IgE switch, leading to reductions in allergen-specific and total IgE, and to prevent eosinophilic inflammation of the airways mucosa (Table 79-1). In addi-

Other potential cytokine producing cellular phenotypes in asthma

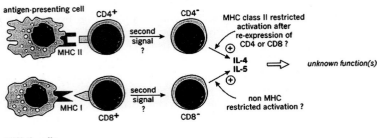

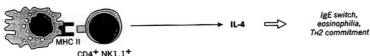

FIGURE 79-2 *Other potential cytokine-producing cellular phenotypes in asthma.* **Several other potentially important cytokine-producing cellular phenotypes have been identified in animal studies but to date have not been unequivocally demonstrated in human asthma. In the upper panel of the diagram, CD4+ and CD8+ T cells are shown receiving a primary activation signal from an antigen-presenting cell. Under the influence of a number of second signals, both surface markers can be completely downregulated, producing so-called *T_H2-like double negative* T cells that lack surface CD4 or CD8. In the case of CD8 cells, a concomitant conversion from IFN-γ to IL-4 and IL-5 production occurs. The in vivo reactivation path of these cells is currently uncertain but may involve both MHC restricted and non-MHC restricted mechanisms. NK1.1 cells are a rare subpopulation of CD4+ cells in the periphery, expressing the surface markers CD4+ and NK1.1+ and distinguished by their production of IL-4 on primary stimulation (i.e., in the absence of a prior IL-4–mediated commitment process). These cells may represent an early source of IL-4 to drive the T_H2 commitment process, but the in vivo significance of the phenotype is yet to be established.**

TABLE 79-1   Potential Cytokine-Based Therapies for the Treatment of Asthma

Cytokine Treatment	Action
IFN-γ	Inhibits T_H2 commitment and B-cell IgE switch
IFN-α	Induces IFN-γ, inhibits T_H2 commitment and function, inhibits B-cell IgE switch
IL-12	Inhibits T_H2 commitment and function

Inhibition of Cytokine Action	Effect of Inhibitor
anti–IL-4	Prevents B-cell IgE switch, reduces T_H2 commitment
anti–IL-13	Prevents B-cell IgE switch
anti–IL-5	Prevents eosinophilia
anti–IL-1	Reduces eosinophilic inflammation
anti–IL-10	Inhibits T_H2 commitment

NOTE: The table is based on in vitro and in vivo animal studies. The term "anti-" denotes any effective inhibition of production or action of the specified interleukin (IL); for example, neutralizing antibodies, soluble cytokine decoy receptors, synthesis inhibitors, signal transduction inhibitors, and so on.

tion, although it is not proven for T_H2 cells, CD4+ T cells release the smooth muscle growth factor basic fibroblast growth factor (bFGF),[47] and directly stimulate airways smooth muscle mitosis in vitro, suggesting a possible role in longer-term alterations to airways architecture.[48] Although cytokines are pleiotrophic, exerting a wide range of biologic activities, this complexity of action is reduced during more extreme responses (e.g., allergic reactions due to polarization of cytokine patterns). The clinical outcome of cytokine manipulations is theoretically less unpredictable in these polarized conditions. However, to date, no blinded, placebo-controlled studies of cytokine therapy in asthma have been reported.

The presence of IL-4 in the early stages of T-cell activation leads to strong polarization of the T cells toward the T_H2 phenotype.[31,32,49] However, T_H1 differentiation to the same stimuli can be induced by IFN-α,[49,50] IFN-γ,[49] or IL-12.[51,52] This suggests that the soluble cytokine signal present at the time of T_H0 commitment is possibly more important than the type of inhaled allergen as a determinant of the nature of the airways mucosal immune response (Fig. 79-1). Animal studies have demonstrated the possibility of directing the outcome of T_H0 commitment by neutralizing cross-regulatory cytokine[8,32,53–56] or using cytokines at the time of immunization to bias the commitment process away from T_H2 immunity.[57] As discussed below, IFN-α, IFN-γ, and IL-12 represent potential therapeutic paradigms for redirecting T_H2 commitment and suppressing T_H2 function. By contrast, neutralization of IL-4, IL-13, IL-10, or IL-5 are approaches that would suppress the effects of established T_H2 cells in human asthma.

Effect of Interferon-α, Interferon-γ, and IL-12 on T_H2 Immune Responses

Interferon-α (IFN-α) has a wide range of antiviral, antitumor, and immunomodulatory activities.[58–61] The monocyte/macrophage product IFN-α inhibits IL-4/T cell–dependent IgE-responses in vitro[6] and in vivo[32,62] by interfering with the initial T-cell activation process.[28] Interferon-α directly increases IFN-γ production by human CD4 (but not CD8) T cells on the mRNA level[50] and suppresses production of IL-4 and IL-5[49] (Brinkman and colleagues, unpublished). It is reasonable to assume that IFN-α also may counteract already established T_H2 immune responses, since it antagonizes the suppressive effect of IL-4 on IFN-γ production.[50] These data also may explain why IFN-α suppresses the generation of allergen-specific T_H2 clones in vitro from PBMC of patients sensitive to the major house dust mite allergen Der p I.[43] The in vitro effects of IFN-α strongly correlate to its activities in vivo. In ovalbumin-sensitized mice, IFN-α produced a dose-dependent inhibition of inhaled allergen-induced eosinophilia.[63] In human disease, IFN-α reduces IL-4–dependent IgE production in the hyper-IgE syndrome[62] and reduces IL-5–dependent eosinophil levels in hyper-eosinophilia syndromes.[64] Taken together, the effects of IFN-α observed in vivo most likely relate to its potential to (1) suppress IL-4 and IL-5 production by T cells,[49] (2) to increase IFN-γ production by T cells,[50] and (3) to antagonize the suppressive effect of high concentrations of IL-4 on IFN-γ production.[50]

Interferon-γ (IFN-γ), a major T_H1 cytokine product, inhibits proliferation of T_H2 cells,[65] prevents T_H2 commitment,[49] and suppresses IL-4/IL-5 production from mature T_H2 cells.[8,34] Interferon-γ antagonizes several IL-4–mediated effects on B cells such as induction of MHC class II antigens,[66] CD23 expression,[67] and isotype switching to IgE.[32,68,69] The importance of IFN-γ as an in vivo regulator of T_H0 commitment is strongly suggested by the observation that neutralization of IFN-γ in *Leishmania major* resistant mice (genetically predisposed to T_H1 responses) favors the development of IL-4–producing T_H2 cells and abolishes resistance to progressive disease.[70] Exogenous IFN-γ produced a dose-dependent suppression of eosinophilia and CD4+ T-cell infiltration into the airways mucosa of ovalbumin-sensitized and aerosol-challenged mice.[71] In humans, defective production and IFN-γ by T cells has been observed in atopic dermatitis[72] and in hyper-IgE syndrome,[73] where it may account for the massive IgE concentrations accumulating in sera of such individuals. Systemic treatment of patients with atopic dermatitis with IFN-γ reduces serum IgE levels and spontaneous IgE production in vitro, resulting in clinical improvements in pruritis and erythema.[72,74] Single case reports also suggest improvement in hypereosinophilia syndrome.[64,73] However, patients with seasonal allergic rhinitis did not show any changes in symptom scores or in serum IgE concentrations.[75] Clinical studies in asthma are in progress.

Interleukin-12 (IL-12) is produced by macrophages and B cells.[76] Interleukin-12 promotes the growth of activated T cells and NK cells,[77] stimulates these cells to secrete IFN-γ, and synergizes with other IFN-γ inducers in this effect.[77] In murine and human systems, IL-12 has been shown to act directly on CD4+ T cells to enhance priming for IFN-γ production.[51,52,78] In vivo in mice, IL-12 induces protective T_H1 immune responses and counteracts T_H2 development in several parasite infections.[55,79–81] In mice infected with the T_H2-inducing helminth *Nippostrongylus brasiliensis*, IL-12 stimulates IFN-γ and inhibits IL-3, IL-4, and IL-5 expression, and, as a consequence, blocks IgE, mucosal mast cell, and blood and tissue eosinophil responses.[55] Taken together, the balance of IL-12 (and IFN-α, IFN-γ) versus IL-4 (and IL-10, see below) during a primary immune response may be crucial for the development of a T_H1 or T_H2 response, respectively. As discussed below, IL-12 has recently been used successfully as an adjuvant to induce a specific T_H1 response to *Leishmania* antigens in vivo in mice.[57]

Effects of Blocking T_H2 Cytokines in Airways Disease Models

A number of highly original strategies have been developed to manipulate the synthesis and actions of cytokines. Recombinant technologies have permitted the development of "humanized" or reshaped monoclonal antibodies used to neutralize cytokine; to produce human recombinant soluble cytokine receptors that serve as decoys; to produce pure recombinant cytokines; natural cytokine receptor antagonists; or, to produce mutant antagonistic cytokine proteins lacking intrinsic activity. Classical pharmacologic antagonists, synthesis inhibitors, inducers of selected cytokines, or signal transduction inhibitors have already been described for other high-molecular-weight signaling proteins, and T_H2-selective drugs are actively sought as potential antiasthmatics. In addition, it seems likely that cytokines will be combined with antigens in the near future to bias the outcome of vaccination and desensitization.

SUPPRESSION OF IL-4 AND IL-13: MANIPULATION OF T_H2 COMMITMENT AND LONG-TERM IgE MEMORY

The genes for IL-4 and IL-13 are related closely and linked closely on human chromosome 5q31, possibly reflecting similar biology and signal transduction pathways.[29,82] The T_H2 cytokine IL-4 directs mouse and human B cells to produce, respectively, IgG1 and IgE or IgG4 and IgE.[4,5,6,83] In animal models, eosinophilic inflammation and the development of T_H2 mucosal immunity assessed by ex vivo restimulation of lung T cells was suppressed markedly after antigen challenge in mice lacking the IL-4 gene or after pretreatment with polyclonal or monoclonal anti–IL-4 antibodies.[84,85] The timing of anti–IL-4 administration is critical: neutralizing monoclonal antibodies administered in doses preventing B-cell IgE switch were without benefit in the allergen-challenged mouse when administered immediately prior to allergen challenge,[85] suggesting that IL-4 is not as important for eosinophil recruitment as in vitro experiments suggest.[86] However, pronounced inhibition of pulmonary eosinophil influx was observed when monoclonal antibodies were administered prior to secondary immunization, suggesting an important role for IL-4 in expanding or maintaining the T_H2 population induced on primary allergen exposure.[85]

Interleukin-13 induces IgE production by human but not murine B cells.[30,87] Whereas IL-4 serves as an autocrine factor to drive T_H2 development,[8,13,31,34] IL-13 has not been shown to display effects directly on T cells. However, both IL-4 and IL-13 inhibit transcription of IFN-α and IL-12 by macrophages,[29] and may thereby directly suppress the development of T_H1 cells during presentation of antigen by macrophages to T cells. Interleukin-13 mRNA can be found in CD4+ T-cell clones of T_H0, T_H1, and T_H2 phenotypes, as well as in CD8+ clones.[29] Human CD4+ T cells can coexpress large amounts of IL-13, IL-5, and IFN-γ without expressing IL-4, and such cells help efficient IgE production by B cells via IL-13 exclusively (Brinkmann and colleagues, unpublished). In vivo, cells of this phenotype would be extremely efficient in exacerbating atopic inflammation, since they would drive IL-13–dependent IgE production, IL-5–dependent eosinophilia, and IFN-γ dependent macrophage activation but would not suppress IFN-γ production by other T cells via IL-4. Indeed, IgE production in atopic patients may be only partly IL-4 dependent, since lymphocytes from nonatopic subjects activated in vitro showed a good correlation between IL-4 and IgE production, whereas atopic patients did not.[88] Furthermore, T cells from atopic but not from nonatopic individuals produced an IgE-inducing activity that could not be blocked by anti–IL-4 in vitro.[89] Together the data suggest a critical role for a second IgE switch factor, most likely IL-13, in atopy and asthma.

The data seem at variance with the finding that IL-4–deficient mice have no detectable circulating IgE following helminth infections.[90,91] However, it is possible that primary murine B cells may require repetitive stimulation or additional signals to express IL-13 receptors and to respond to IL-13. Although the relative roles of IL-4 and IL-13 in human IgE responses remain to be established, the present observations imply that the use of antagonists specific for IL-4 will not be sufficient to prevent IgE-mediated allergic disease. Since the receptors for IL-4 and IL-13 share a common subunit,[29,92] an agent such as the recently described IL-4 mutant protein, which acts on both IL-4 and IL-13 receptor systems,[93,94] may provide the most efficient way to block both IL-4 and IL-13 action in vivo.

SUPPRESSION OF IL-5: LINEAGE-SPECIFIC INHIBITION OF EOSINOPHIL DIFFERENTIATION AND ACTION

Interleukin-5 supports the terminal differentiation of lineage committed progenitors into mature eosinophils in vitro and to date is the only cytokine known to exert this effect.[19] Although there currently is controversy surrounding the role of IL-5 in basal, very-low-level eosinophil production in healthy animals, it is clear from numerous experiments that IL-5 is critical for the manifestation of eosinophilia and that eosinophilia is CD4+ T cell–dependent.[18] In humans, IL-5 has been located by immunohistochemistry and identified in lung lavages and blood, suggesting IL-5 is a major determinant of eosinophilic inflammation consequent to allergen challenge in asthmatics.[95,96] Pharmacologic inhibitors of IL-5 production or action have not yet been discovered, but animal experiments with neutralizing antibodies suggest such drugs would be useful in asthma. In presensitized mice or guinea-pig, allergenic challenge leads to an eosinophilic inflammation of the airways which is profoundly suppressed by neutralizing antibodies against IL-5.[97] Similarly, soluble recombinant IL-5 receptors reduce eosinophilia. However, as predicted by in vitro studies, anti–IL-5 has no effect on IgE production.

SUPPRESSION OF IL-10: COMMITMENT TO THE T_H1 PHENOTYPE

Interleukin-10 (IL-10) plays a major role in suppressing immune and inflammatory responses. Interleukin-10 is produced by various cell types, including CD4+ and CD8+ T cells, B cells, and macrophages/monocytes.[98] The inhibitory effect of IL-10 on the secretion of proinflammatory cytokines, and the enhancing effect on production of IL-1 receptor antagonist (IL-1RA), which itself is an antiinflammatory agent, may suggest a role of IL-10 as a natural dampener of immune proliferative and inflammatory responses.[98] In the context of allergic asthma, it is important that IL-10 inhibits production of IFN-γ by T cells through an effect on the antigen-presenting cells, thereby favoring T_H2 responses.[9] Like IL-4, IL-10 inhibits several T_H1 effector functions, notably the induction by IFN-γ of cytokine production (IL-1, TNF-α, IL-6),[98,99] and inhibits production of reactive nitrogen oxides by macrophages and monocytes.[100] The inhibitory effects of IL-4 and IL-10 seem to be complementary, since both cytokines synergize with TGF-β to inhibit macrophage cytotoxicity, and a combination of IL-4 and IL-10 inhibits DTH (delayed hypersensitivity) responses more efficiently than either cytokine alone.[9]

INHIBITION OF IL-1: REDUCTION OF REACTIVATION OF ANTIGEN-EXPERIENCED T CELLS IN CHRONIC DISEASE?

Interleukin-1α and IL-1β are produced rapidly by mononuclear/macrophage lineages in response to insult but also are very widely expressed in other cell types reflecting an extremely diverse biology. The proliferation of T_H2, but not T_H1 cells (which do not express the functionally coupled type 1 IL-1 receptor), is promoted by IL-1.[101,102] A subset of antigen-experienced or "memory" (recently activated?) CD4+ cells is particularly sensitive to IL-1–induced proliferation. Indeed there is evidence that T_H2 cells produce IL-1 as an autocrine growth factor[103] and that IL-1 favors the in vitro development of T_H2 cells[78] acting through IL-4 upregulated type 1 receptors.[104] Furthermore, IL-1 promotes adhesion of eosinophils to cultured endothelial cells through VCAM-1[105] and may act synergistically with IL-4 to induce VCAM-1,[106] but unlike IL-4 does not appear to mediate transmigration through cultured endothelial cell monolayers.[86] Recombinant human IL-1 receptor antagonist (rhIL-1RA) was found to reduce substantially the intensity of inhaled allergen-provoked eosinophilic airways inflammation and hyperreactivity in guinea-pigs.[107] rhIL-1RA has been administered to humans, but no studies in asthma have been reported. In view of the selective action of IL-1 on postcommitted T_H2 cells, drugs targeted at IL-1 may be used preferentially in established rather than early disease. The situation in allergic asthma may, however, be somewhat more complex than predicted by animal models, since IL-4 has recently been discovered to upregulate the synthesis and release of the soluble IL-1 type II receptor that serves as a decoy for IL-1, reducing its biologic effects.[111]

Role of Long-Term "Memory" versus "Primary" T_H Cells in Allergy: Differential Cytokine Production and Sensitivity to Immunomodulators

A still-unresolved question is the involvement of long-term "memory" versus "primary" T_H cells in the maintenance of allergy and asthma. We found that the potential of human CD4+ T_H cells to secrete IL-4 and IL-5 drastically increased upon repetitive T-cell receptor stimulation in vitro and coincided with expression of the memory surface marker CD45RO+. In contrast, the potential to secrete IL-10 declined, and the potential to secrete IFN-γ remained unchanged (Brinkmann and colleagues, unpublished). Compared with "primary" CD4+ T cells, CD4+45RO+ memory cells were 10,000-fold less sensitive to glucocorticosteroids. Interestingly, glucocorticosteroids specifically suppressed production of the T_H2 cytokines IL-4 and IL-5, but not of the T_H1 cytokine IFN-γ (Brinkmann and colleagues, unpublished). The finding that topical treatment of atopic asthmatics with corticosteroids recently has been reported to reduce mRNA expression for IL-4 and IL-5 and to increase mRNA expression for IFN-γ in bronchioalveolar lavage T cells[109] may indicate the presence of highly activated memory T_H cells of low glucocorticoid sensitivity in asthma. The differential effects of immunomodulators suggest that animal models of IgE production and eosinophilia after primary immunization should be interpreted very cautiously since they may not reflect adequately memory T_H2 cell–driven pathologic immune responses occurring in human disease. It is important to realize that the use of cytokines or cytokine antagonists in the treatment of atopic diseases may depend critically on their effects on memory rather than primary T cell populations. In practical terms of disease therapy, a successful manipulation to suppress development of T_H2 immunity in recently diagnosed mild disease may be without benefit in long-standing disease.

Special Patient Subpopulations: Glucocorticosteroid-Insensitive Asthma, Intrinsic and Isocyanate-Induced Asthma

On the basis of current knowledge the patients most likely to benefit from manipulation of the T_H1/T_H2 balance are those with extrinsic asthma associated with identifiable allergens and elevated IgE titers. It is less clear whether patients with corticosteroid-insensitive asthma, intrinsic asthma (defined as asthma in the absence of identifiable IgE response to relevant allergens), or patients with occupational asthma induced by isocyanates would benefit from T_H2 cytokine inhibitors. A small subgroup of asthmatics are insensitive to glucocorticosteroids. One major mechanism of corticosteroid insensitivity that has been very recently discovered is IL-4–induced reversible decreases in glucocorticosteroid receptor affinity both in vitro and in clinical asthma.[100,110] This suggests that treatment to suppress IL-4 may restore corticosteroid responsiveness in this patient subpopulation. It is less clear whether manipulation of the T_H2 system would benefit those suffering from intrinsic and isocyanate-induced asthma. Intrinsic asthmatics have increased IL-5 concentrations and eosinophilia, but seldom abnormal IgE titers, and show a different pattern of cytokine-like activity as compared with atopic asthmatics.[95] Isocyanate-induced asthma appears histopathologically similar to extrinsic or allergic asthma,[114] has clear involvement of IL-5, but may represent a form of chemically induced T-cell activation not readily amenable to cytokine manipulation. It is probable that patients with isocyanate and intrinsic asthma would benefit from inhibitors of IL-5, but cytokine treatment to alter the T_H1/T_H2 balance seems less relevant to these patients. It also should be noted that there may be distinct "immunotypes" even within atopic asthma: immunogenetic studies have already identified possible linkages to the β subunit of the high affinity IgE receptor found on human chromosome 11q, and to chromosome 5q31 (which contains multiple candidate genes such as IL-3, IL-4/IL-13, IL-5, GM-CSF, the β_2-adrenoceptor, and glucocorticosteroid receptor), but *not* linkage between these putative disease-relevant chromosome regions.[112,113]

Use of Cytokines to Bias Immune Responses during Desensitization and the Prospects of Vaccination Against Atopy

A major challenge for successful immunotherapy directed at T_H cell subsets is to convert an already established, but inappropriate, T_H response into one that is beneficial, or at least not pathologic. To do this requires a clear understanding of how growth and cytokine production by T_H1 and T_H2 cells are regulated (Fig. 79-1). Vaccination/desensitization strategies against allergy/asthma aim to selectively induce T_H1 (IFN-γ) but not T_H2 (IL-4/IL-5) immune responses. Currently, "desensitization" is less successful in atopic patients with asthma than with hayfever and carries a certain risk of anaphylaxis. This could result in part from the fact that repetitive inoculation of allergic patients with allergens may lead to a selective clonal expansion of already existing allergen-specific T_H2-like cells, which further increase rather than suppress the allergic immune response.

A more efficient immunotherapy may be vaccination with allergens in combination with cytokines/anticytokines that favor T_H1 immune responses. As discussed above, the presence of selected cytokines during the activation of T cells critically determines their cytokine secretion pattern (Fig. 79-1). In vivo studies showed that neutralization of IFN-γ in *Leishmania major*–resistant mice favored an inappropriate T_H2 response.[79] Conversely, neutralization of IL-4 in susceptible mice favored generation of IFN-γ–producing T_H1 cells and allowed mice to heal. Most interestingly, vaccination of susceptible mice with a cocktail of *Leishmania* antigens alone induced a T_H2 response and no protection, whereas vaccination with the same antigens plus IL-12 favored induction of T_H1 cells and protection.[57] The data clearly show that the induction of either T_H1- or T_H2-like cells is linked genetically, but also demonstrate that the genetic predisposition to mount a T_H2 response can be overcome by supplying cytokines that favor T_H1 responses. It may prove possible to exploit these observations to develop effective immunotherapy methods in atopic asthma and, perhaps, prophylactic vaccinations against major allergen immunogenic epitopes.

T Helper-1 Immunity, Interferons, and Virally Induced Asthma

Viral infections of the upper respiratory tract are frequent in asthma and atopy, and positive serology for recent viral illness is associated strongly with hospitalization for acute severe asthma.[114] Viruses, like other intracellular pathogens, normally stimulate macrophage production of IFN-α[60] and promote IFN-γ production from infected cells.[10] In viral infection of the airways T_H cells normally may be presented simultaneously with processed antigen and IFN-α, which induces them to differentiate toward a T_H1-like phenotype.[28] However, asthmatics and atopics, for unknown reasons, are more susceptible to viral respiratory tract infections. Possible explanations include upregulation on epithelial cells by inflammatory mediators of an integrin, ICAM-1, known to act as a receptor for rhinovirus, a major precipitant of human asthma.[115] T helper-2 immune responses are poorly suited to antiviral defense. Anderson and Coyle[116] have proposed an alternative hypothesis that genetic predisposition to T_H2 immunity may compromise IFN-mediated antiviral host defense reaction, leading to an increased rate of infections and/or a more protracted and severe illness due to impaired viral clearance. This concept is supported indirectly by studies in mice where intense T_H2 immune responses induced by helminth infection decreased viral clearance as well as CD8+ cytotoxicity and T_H1 cytokine responses,[117] and would contribute to understanding the susceptibility of asthmatic airways to infection by virus *not* binding to upregulated adhesion molecules. Similarly, indirect support for the concept that a T_H2 mucosal immune response would both predispose asthmatics to viral infections and augment the severity of viral infection comes from studies in mice where the gene for IFN-γ has been deleted. In such mice, influenza virus infection of the lung leads to an increased production of virus specific IgG1, and the cytokines IL-4 and IL-5.[118] Numerous clinical studies have attested to the usefulness of IFN in viral infection,[75] although studies are lacking in airways disease. Therapeutic administration of IFN might realign the T_H1/T_H2 balance in humans and provide an adjunct therapy to reduce the risk of severe or recurrent virally mediated exacerbations.

Conclusion

Studies on T_H1 and T_H2 biology and mucosal immunity have suggested potential strategies to selectively downregulate T_H2 immune responses and thereby reduce IgE and eosinophilic inflammation. However, much remains to be understood. One of the most crucial issues, still only poorly understood in humans, is the susceptibility of T cells to cross-regulation by cytokines in different severity grades of the disease. Treatments intended to block or reduce T_H2 immunity (induction of IFN-α/IFN-γ, inhibition of IL-4/IL-5/IL-13) might be very much more effective in newly diagnosed disease early in life. In long-established disease, targets such as IL-5 may prove the more useful approaches to treat asthma. The pleotrophic nature of the cytokines of potential therapeutic interest in asthma could lead to numerous, potentially severe side effects, thus limiting their usefulness. In addition, the high molecular weight of these molecules means that they are not systemically available unless administered topically or parenterally, a severe limitation in chronic disease. The use of parenterally administered native cytokines in minute quantities, probably combined with allergens or recombinant allergen epitopes, may circumvent these problems and could prove of greatest benefit when used as adjuncts in immunotherapy/vaccination protocols. However, the risk of an immune response against recombinant cytokines leading to neutralizing antibodies cannot be excluded. Research into cytokine biology will almost certainly deliver drugs affecting T_H2 cytokines— either cytokine mimetics; direct cytokine inhibitors or selective cytokine inducers; inhibitors of cytokine signal transduction or receptor-complex antagonists—in the near future. These awaited discoveries may fundamentally change current views on the treatment and prevention of asthma.

References

1. Busse WW, Reed CE: Asthma: definition and pathogenesis, in *Allergy, Principles and Practice*, 3rd ed. Middleton E Jr, Reed CE, Ellis EF, Adkinson NF Jr, and Yunginger JW, ed: CV Mosby, St. Louis. 969–998.
2. McFadden ER Jr, Gilbert IA: Asthma. *N Engl J Med* 1992; 327:1928.
3. Lopez AL, Sanderson CJ, Gamble JR, et al.: Recombinant human interleukin 5 is a selective activator of human eosinophil function. *J Exp Med* 1988; 167:219.
4. Coffman RL, Ohara J, Bond MW, et al.: B cell stimulatory factor-1 enhances the IgE response of lipopolysaccharide-activated B cells. *J Immunol* 1986; 151:5053.
5. Snapper CM, Paul WE: Interferon gamma and B cell stimulatory factor-1 reciprocally regulate Ig isotype production. *Science* 1987; 251:949.
6. Pene J, Rousset F, Briere F, et al.: IgE production by normal human lymphocytes is induced by interleukin 4 and suppressed by interferons gamma and alpha and by prostaglandin E2. *Proc Natl Acad Sci U S A* 1988; 85:6880.
7. Mosmann TR, Coffman RL: TH1 and TH2 cells: different patterns of lymphokine secretion lead to different functional properties. *Ann Rev Immunol* 1989; 7:150.
8. Mosmann TR: Cytokine secretion patterns and cross-regulation of T cell subsets. *Immunol Res* 1991; 10:183.
9. Powrie F, Coffman RS: Cytokine regulation of T-cell function: potential for therapeutic intervention. *Immunol Today* 1993; 14:270.
10. Zingernagel RM, Doherty PC: Major transplantation antigens, viruses and specificity of surveillance T cells. *Contemp Top Immunol* 1977; 7:179.
11. Lukacher AE, Braciale VL, Braciale TJ: In vivo effector function of influenza-virus specific cytotoxic T lymphocyte clones is highly specific. *J Exp Med* 1984; 160:814.
12. Morrison LA, Lukacher AE, Braciale VL, et al.: Differences in antigen presentation to MHC class I and class II restricted influenza virus specific CTL clones. *J Exp Med* 1986; 163:903.
13. Romagnani S: Induction of TH1 and TH2 responses: a key role for natural immune response? *Immunol Today* 1992; 13:529.
14. Yssel H, Johnson KE, Schneider PV, et al.: T cell activation-inducing epitopes of the house dust mite allergen Der p I. Proliferation and lymphokine production patterns of Der p I–specific CD4+ T cell clones. *J Immunol* 1992; 148:738.
15. Hamid Q, Azzawi M, Ying S, et al.: Expression of mRNA for interleukin-5 in mucosal bronchial biopsies from asthma. *J Clin Invest* 1991; 87:1541.
16. Kay AM, Ying S, Varney V, et al.: Messenger RNA expression of the cytokine gene cluster, interleukin (IL)-3, IL-4, IL-5 and GM-CSF in allergen-induced late phase reactions in atopic subjects. *J Exp Med* 1991; 173:775.
17. Robinson DS, Hamid W, Ying S, et al.: Predominant T_H2-like bronchoalveolar T-lymphocyte population in atopic asthma. *N Engl J Med* 1992; 326:298.
18. Baston A, Beeson PB: Mechanism of eosinophilia. II. Role of the lymphocyte. *J Exp Med* 1970; 131:1288.
19. Sanderson CJ, O'Garra A, Warren DJ, Klaus GGB: Eosinophil differentiation factor also has B cell growth factor activity. Proposed name interleukin-4. *Proc Nat Acad Sci U S A* 1986; 83:437.
20. Frigas E, Loegering DA, Gleich GJ: Cytotoxic effects of guinea-pig major basic protein on tracheal epithelium. *Lab Invest* 1980; 42:35.
21. Spry CKF, Tai PC, Barkans J: Tissue localization of human eosinophilic cationic proteins in allergic disease. *Int Arch Allergy Appl Immunol* 1985; 77:252.
22. Filley WV, Kephart GM, Holly KE, et al.: Identification by immunofluorescences of eosinophil granule major basic protein

in lung tissues of patients with bronchial asthma. *Lancet* 1982; ii:11–15.

23. Owen WF, Soberman RJ, Yoshimoto T, et al.: Synthesis and release of leukotriene C4 by human eosinophils. *J Immunol* 1987; 138:532.

24. Wong DTW, Weller PF, Galli SJ, et al.: Human eosinophils express transforming growth factor α. *J Exp Med* 1990; 172:673.

25. Wong DTW, Elovic A, Matossian K, et al.: Eosinophils from patients with blood eosinophilia express transforming growth factor β1. *Blood* 1991; 78:2702.

26. Ohno I, Lea RG, Flanders KC, et al.: Eosinophils in chronically inflammed human airway tissues express transforming growth factor beta 1 gene (TGF beta 1). *J Clin Invest* 1992; 89:1662.

27. Brinkmann V, Heusser C: T cell dependent differentiation of human B cells into IgM, IgG, IgA, or IgE plasma cells: high rate of antibody production by IgE plasma cells, but limited clonal expansion of IgE precursors. *Cell Immunol* 1993; 152:323.

28. Brinkmann V, Heusser C, Baer J, et al.: Interferon alpha suppresses the capacity of T cells to help antibody production by human B cells. *J Interferon Res* 1992; 12:267.

29. Zurawski G, De Vries JE: Interleukin 13, an interleukin 4–like cytokine that acts on monocytes and B cells, but not on T cells. *Immunol Today* 1994; 15:19.

30. Bray MA, Brinkmann V, Heusser CH: Cytokines and inflammatory mediators in the regulation of IgE formation, in Bray MA, Anderson WH (eds): *Mediators of Pulmonary Inflammation*, Marcel Dekker, New York, 1991; 81–143.

31. Le Gros G, Ben Sasson SZ, Seder R, et al.: Generation of IL-4–producing cells in vivo and in vitro: IL-2 and IL-4 are required for the in vitro generation of IL-4 producing cells. *J Exp Med* 1990; 172:921.

32. Finkelman FD, Holmes J, Katona IM, et al.: Lymphokine control of in vivo immunoglobulin isotype selection. *Annu Rev Immunol* 1990; 8:303.

33. Yoshimoto T, Paul WE: CD4^pos, NK1.1^pos T cells promptly produce interleukin 4 in response to in vivo challenge with anti-CD3. *J Exp Med* 1994; 179:1285.

34. Mossmann TR: Cytokines: is there biological meaning? *Curr Opin Immunol* 1991; 3:511.

35. Seder RA, Plaut M, Barbieri S, et al.: Purified Fc epsilon R⁺ bone marrow and splenic non-B, non-T cells are highly enriched in the capacity to produce IL-4 in response to immobilized IgE, IgG2a, or ionomycin. *J Immunol* 1991; 147:903.

36. Heusser C, Brinkmann V, LeGros G, et al.: New aspects of IgE regulation, in Wüthrich B (ed): *Highlights in Allergy and Clinical Immunology*. Hogrefe & Huber, Seattle, 1992; 30–34.

37. Piccini M-P, Macchia D, Parronchi P, et al.: Human bone marrow Non-B, Non-T cells produce interleukin-4 response to cross-linkage of Fcepsilon and Fcgamma. *Proc Nat Acad Sci U S A* 1991; 88:8656.

38. Erard F, Wild MT, Garcia-Sanz JA, LeGros G: Switch of CD8 T cells to noncytolytic CD8⁻CD4⁻ cells that make Th2 cytokines and help B cells. *Science* 1993; 260:1802.

39. Desreumaux P, Janin A, Colombel JF, et al.: Interleukin 5 messenger RNA expression by eosinophils in the intestinal mucosa of patients with coeliac disease. *J Exp Med* 1992; 175:293.

40. Seder RA, Paul WE, Bensasson SZ, et al.: Production of interleukin-4 and other cytokines following stimulation of mast cell lines and in vivo mast cells/basophils. *Int Arch Allergy Appl Immunol* 1991; 94:137.

41. Salgame P, Abrams JS, Clayberger C, et al.: Differing lymphokine profiles of functional subsets of CD4+ and CD8+ T cell clones. *Science* 1991; 254:279.

42. Seder RA, Boulay J-L, Finkelman F, et al.: CD8+ T cells can be primed in vitro to produce IL-4. *J Immunol* 1992; 148:1652.

43. Maggi E, Giudizi MG, Biagiotti R, et al.: Th2-like CD8+ T cells showing B cell helper function and reduced cytolytic activity in human immunodeficiency virus type 1 infection. *J Exp Med* 1994; 180:489.

44. Kita H, Ohnishi T, Okubo Y, et al.: Granulocyte/macrophage colony stimulating factor and interleukin 3 release from human peripheral blood eosinophils and neutrophils. *J Exp Med* 1991; 174:745.

45. Mobqel R, Hamid Q, Ying S, et al.: Expression of mRNA and immunoreactivity for the granulocyte/macrophage colony stimulating factor in activated human eosinophils. *J Exp Med* 1991; 174:749.

46. Kemeny DM, Noble A, Holmes BJ, Diaz-Sanchez D: Immune regulation: a new role for the CD8+ T cell. *Immunol Today* 1994; 15:107.

47. Blotnick S, Peoples GE, Freeman MR, et al.: T lymphocytes synthesize and export heparin-binding epidermal growth factor-like growth factor and basic fibroblast growth factor, mitogens for vascular cells and fibroblasts: differential production and release by CD4+ and CD8+ T cells. *Proc Natl Acad Sci U S A* 1994; 91:2890.

48. Lazaar A, Albelda SM, Pilewski JM, et al.: T lymphocytes adhere to airway smooth muscle cells via integrins and CD44 and induce smooth muscle cell DNA synthesis. *J Exp Med* 1994; 180:807.

49. Demeure CE, Wu CY, Shu U, et al.: In vitro maturation of human neonatal CD4 T lymphocytes. II Cytokines present at priming modulate the development of lymphokine production. *J Immunol* 1994; 152:4775.

50. Brinkmann V, Geiger T, Alkan S, Heusser C: IFNα increases the frequency of IFNg-producing human CD4-positive T cells. *J Exp Med* 1993; 178:1655.

51. Hsieh CS, Macatonia SE, Tripp CS, et al.: Development of TH1 CD4+ T cells through IL-12 produced by Listeria-induced macrophages. *Science* 1993; 260:547.

52. Seder RA, Gazzinelli R, Sher A, Paul WE: IL-12 acts directly on CD4+ T cells to enhance priming for IFNγ production and diminishes IL-4 inhibition of such priming. *Proc Natl Acad Sci U S A* (in press).

53. Sadick MD, Heinzel FP, Holaday BJ, et al.: Cure of murine leishmaniasis with anti–IL-4 monoclonal antibody. *J Exp Med* 1989; 169:115.

54. Finkelman FD, Svetic A, Gresser I, et al.: Regulation by interferon alpha of immunoglobulin isotype selection and lymphokine production in mice. *J Exp Med* 1991; 174:1179.

55. Finkelman FD, Madden KB, Cheever AW, et al.: Effects of interleukin 12 on immune responses and host protection in mice infected with intestinal nematode parasites. *J Exp Med* 1994; 179:1563.

56. Pearce EJ, Caspar P, Grzych JM, et al.: Down regulation of T_H1 cytokine production accompanies induction of Th2 responses by a parasitic helminth. *J Exp Med* 1991; 173:159.

57. Afonso LC, Scharton TM, Vieira LQ, et al.: The adjuvant effect of interleukin 12 in a vaccine against *Leishmania major*. *Science* 1994; 263:235.

58. DeMaeyer E, DeMaeyer-Guignard J (eds): *Interferons and Other Regulatory Cytokines*. New York, John Wiley & Sons, 1988.

59. DeMaeyer E, DeMaeyer-Guignard J: The anti-viral effects of interferons, in DeMaeyer E, DeMaeyer-Guignard J (eds): *Interferons and Other Regulatory Cytokines*. John Wiley & Sons, New York, 1988: 114–153.

60. DeMaeyer E, J. DeMaeyer-Guignard: The effects of interferons on tumor cells, in DeMaeyer E, DeMaeyer-Guignard J (eds):

Interferons and Other Regulatory Cytokines. John Wiley & Sons, New York, 1988: 534–513.

61. DeMaeyer E, DeMaeyer-Guignard J: Macrophages as interferon producers and interferons as modulators of macrophage activity, in DeMaeyer E, Demaeyer-Guignard J, (eds): *Interferons and Other Regulatory Cytokines*. John Wiley & Sons, New York, 1988; 194–220.

62. Souillet G, Rousset F, DeVries JE: Alpha interferon treatment of a patient with hyper IgE syndrome. *Lancet* 1989; 1:1534.

63. Nakajima H, Nakao A, Watanabe Y, et al.: IFNα inhibits antigen-induced eosinophil and CD4+ T cell recruitment into tissue. *J Immunol* 1994; 153:1264.

64. Zielinski RM, Lawrence WD: IFNγ for the treatment of hyper-eosinophilic syndrome. *Ann Int Med* 1990; 113:716.

65. Gajewski TF, Fitch F: Anti-proliferative effect of IFNγ in immune regulation. I. IFNγ inhibits the proliferation of TH2 but not TH1 murine helper T lymphocyte clones. *J Immunol* 1988; 150:5250.

66. Mond JJ, Carman J, Sharma C, et al.: Interferon-gamma suppresses B cell stimulatory factor (BSF-1) induction of class II MHC determinants on B cells. *J Immunol* 1986; 137:3534.

67. Rousett F, de Waal-Malefijt R, Slierendregt B: Regulation of FC receptor for IgE (CD23) and class II MHC antigen expression on Burkitts lymphoma cell lines by human IL-4 and IFNg. *J Immunol* 1988; 140:2625.

68. Coffman RL, Seymour BWP, Lebman DA, et al.: The role of helper T cell products in mouse B cell differentiation and isotype regulation. *Immunol* 1988; 102:5.

69. Romagnani S: Regulation and deregulation of human IgE synthesis. *Immunol Today* 1990; 11:516.

70. Heinzel FP, Sadick MD, Mutha SS, Locksley RM: Production of interferon g, interleukin 2, interleukin 4, and interleukin 10 by CD4+ lymphocytes in vivo during healing and progressive murine leishmaniasis. *Proc Natl Acad Sci U S A* 1991; 88:7011.

71. Iwamoto I, Nakajima H, Endo H, Yoshida S: Interferon γ regulates antigen induced eosinophil recruitment into the mouse airways by inhibiting the infiltration of CD4+ T cells. *J Exp Med* 1993; 177:573.

72. Reinhold U, Wehrmann W, Kukel S, Kreisel HW: Evidence that defective interferon-γ production in atopic dermatitis patients is due to intrinsic abnormalities. *Clin Exp Immunol* 1990; 79:524.

73. Del Prete G, Tiri A, Maggi E, et al.: Defective in vitro production of gamma interferon and tumor necrosis factor alpha by circulating T cells from patients with the hyper IgE syndrome. *J Clin Invest* 1989; 84:1830.

74. Boguniewicz M, Jaffe HS, Izu A, et al.: Recombinant gamma interferon in treatment of patients with atopic dermatitis and elevated IgE levels. *Am J Med* 1991; 88:365.

75. Volz MA, Kirkpatrick CH: Interferons 1992. How much of the promise has been realised? *Drugs* 1992; 43:285.

76. Trinchieri G, Wysocka M, DÀndrea A, et al.: Natural killer cell stimulatory factor (NKSF) or interleukin 12 is a key regulator of immune response and inflammation. *Prog Growth Factor Res* 1992; 4:355.

77. Chan SH, Perussia B, Gupta JW, et al.: Induction of IFNγ production by natural killer cell stimulatory factor: characterization of the responder cells and synergy with other inducers. *J Exp Med* 1991; 173:869.

78. Manetti R, Parronchi P, Giudizi MG, et al.: Natural killer cell stimulatory factor (interleukin 12) induces T helper type 1 (TH1)-specific immune responses and inhibits the development of IL-4-producing Th cells. *J Exp Med* 1993; 177:1199.

79. Heinzel FP, Schoenhaut DS, Rerko RM, et al.: Recombinant IL-12 cures mice infected with *Leishmania major*. *J Exp Med* 1993; 177:1505.

80. Sypek JP, Chiung CL, Mayor JM, et al.: Resolution of cutaneous leishmaniasis: interleukin 12 initiates a protective T helper type 1 immune response. *J Exp Med* 1993; 177:1797.

81. Morris SC, Madden KB, Adamovicz JJ, et al.: Effects of IL-12 on in vivo cytokine gene expression and Ig isotype selection. *J Immunol* 1994; 152:1047.

82. Boulay J-L, Paul WE: Haematopoietin sub-family classification based on size, gene organisation and sequence homology. *Curr Opin Immunol* 1993; 3:573–581.

83. Gascan H, Gauchat JF, Roncarolo MG, et al.: Human B cell clones can be induced to proliferate and to switch to IgE and IgG4 synthesis by interleukin 4 and a signal provided by activated CD4+ T cell clones. *J Exp Med* 1991; 173:747.

84. Lukacs NW, Strieter RM, Chensue SW, Kunkel SL: Interleukin-4–dependent pulmonary eosinophil infiltration in a murine model. *Am J Respir Cell Mol Biol* 1994; 10:526–532.

85. Coyle AJ, Le Gros G, Bertrand C, et al.: IL-4 is required for the induction of lung Th2 mucosal immunity. *Am J Respir Cell Mol Biol* in press.

86. Moser R, Fehr J, Bruijnzeel PL: IL-4 controls the selective endothelium driven transmigration of eosinophils from allergic individuals. *J Immunol* 1992; 149:1432.

87. Punnonen J, Aversa G, Cocks BG, et al.: Interleukin 13 induces interleukin 4-independent IgG4 and IgE synthesis and CD23 expression by human B cells. *Proc Natl Acad Sci U S A* 1993; 90:3730.

88. Van der Pouw Kraan CTM, Aalbersee RC, Aarden LA: IgE production in atopic patients is not related to IL-4 production. *Clin Exp Immunol* 1994; 97:254.

89. Zhang X, Polla B, Hauser C, Zubler RH: T cells from atopic individuals produce an IgE-inducing activity incompletely blocked by anti–interleukin-4 antibody. *Eur J Immunol* 1992; 22:829.

90. Kühn R, Rajewski K, Müller W: Generation and analysis of interleukin-4 deficient mice. *Science* 1991; 254:707.

91. Kopf M, Le Gros G, Bachmann M, et al.: Disruption of the murine IL-4 gene blocks Th2 cytokine responses. *Nature* 1993; 362:245.

92. Zurawski SM, Vega F, Huyghe B, Zurawski G: Receptors for interleukin 13 and interleukin 4 are complex and share a novel component that functions in signal transduction. *EMBO J* 1993; 12:2663–2670.

93. Kruse N, Tony HP, Sebald W: Conversion of human interleukin 4 into a high affinity antagonist by a single amino acid replacement. *EMBO J* 1992; 11:3237–3244.

94. Aversa G, Punnonen J, Cocks BG, et al.: An interleukin 4 (IL-4) mutant protein inhibits both IL-4 or IL-13–induced human immunoglobulin G4 (IgG4) and IgE synthesis and B cell proliferation: support for a common component shared by IL-4 and IL-13 receptors. *J Exp Med* 1993; 178:2213.

95. Walker C, Virchow JC, Bruijnzeel PLB, Blaser K: T cell subsets and their soluble products regulate eosinophilia in allergic and nonallergic asthma. *J Immunol* 1991; 146:1829.

96. Ohishi T, Kita K, Weiller D, et al.: IL-5 is the predominate eosinophil-active cytokine in the allergen-induced pulmonary late phase reaction. *Am Rev Respir Dis* 1993; 147:901.

97. Chand N, Harrison JE, Rooney S, et al.: Anti–IL-5 monoclonal antibody inhibits allergic late phase bronchial eosinophilia in guinea-pigs: a therapeutic approach. *Eur J Pharmacol* 1992; 211:121–123.

98. DeWaal Malefyt R, Yssel H, Roncarolo MG, et al.: Interleukin-10. *Curr Opin Immunol* 1992; 4:314.

99. Fiorentino DF, Zlotnik A, Mosmann TR, et al.: IL-10 inhibits cytokine production by activated macrophages. *J Immunol* 1991; 147:3815.

100. Sher ER, Leueng DYM, Surs W, et al.: Steroid resistant asthma. Cellular mechanisms contributing to inadequate response to glucocorticoid therapy. *J Clin Invest* 1994; 93:33.

101. Weaver CT, Hawrylowicz CM, Unanue ER: T helper cell subsets requires the expression of distinct costimulatory signals by antigen presenting cells. *Proc Natl Acad Sci U S A* 1988; 85: 8181–8185.

102. Solari R, Smithers N, Page K, et al.: Interleukin 1 responsiveness and receptor expression by murine Th1 and Th2 clones. *Cytokines* 1990; 2:129–141.

103. Zubiaga AM, Munoz E, Huber BT: Production of IL-1α by activated Th type 2 cells. Its role as an autocrine growth factor. *J Immunol* 1991; 146:3849–3856.

104. Koch KC, Ye K, Clark BD, Dinarello CA: Interleukin (IL) 4 upregulates gene and surface IL1 receptor type 1 in murine T helper type 2 cells. *Europ J Immunol* 1992; 22:153–157.

105. Bochner BS, Luscinskas FW, Gimbrone MAJ, et al.: Adhesion of human basophils, eosinophils, and neutrophils to IL-1 activated vascular endothelial cell adhesion molecules. *J Exp Med* 1991; 173:1553–1557.

106. Masinovsky B, Urdal D, Gallatin WM: IL-4 acts synergistically with IL-1β to promote lymphocyte adhesion to microvascular endothelium by induction of vascular cell adhesion molecule-1, dependent and independent mechanisms. *J Immunol* 1991; 145:2886.

107. Watson ML, Smith D, Bourne AD, et al.: Cytokines contribute to airway dysfunction in antigen challenged guinea-pigs: inhibition of airway hyperreactivity, pulmonary eosinophil accumulation, and tumor necrosis factor generation by pretreatment with an interleukin-1 receptor antagonist. *Am J Respir Cell Mol Biol* 1993; 8:365.

108. Colotta F, Muzio FRM, Bertini R, et al.: Interleukin-1 type II receptor: a decoy target for IL-1 that is regulated by IL-4. *Science* 1993; 261:472–475.

109. Robinson D, Hamid Q, Ying S, et al.: Prednisolone treatment in asthma is associated with modulation of bronchoalveolar lavage cell interleukin-4, interleukin-5, and interferon gamma gene expression. *Am Rev Respir Dis* 1993; 148:401.

110. Kam JC, Szefler SJ, Surs W, et al.: Combination of IL-2 and IL-4 reduces glucocorticoid receptor binding affinity and T cell response to glucocorticoids. *J Immunol* 1993; 151:3460–3466.

111. Bentley AM, Maestrelli P, Saetta M, et al.: Activated T lymphocytes and eosinophils in the bronchial mucosa in isocyanate-induced asthma. *J Allergy Clin Immunol* 1992; 89:821–828.

112. Marsh DG, Neely JD, Breazeale DR, et al.: Linkage analysis of IL-4 and other chromosome 5q31.1 markers and total serum immunoglobulin E concentrations. *Science* 1994; 264:1152.

113. Shirakawa T, Li A, Dubowitz M, et al.: Association between atopy and variants of the β subunit of the high-affinity immunoglobulin E receptor. *Nature Genetics* 1994; 7:125.

114. McIntosh K, Ellis EF, Hoffman LS, et al.: The association of viral and bacterial respiratory infections with exacerbations of wheezing in young asthmatic children. *J Pediatr* 1973; 83:578–590.

115. Greve JM, Davis G, Meyer AM: The major human rhinovirus reeptor is ICAM-1. *Cell* 1989; 56:839–847.

116. Anderson GP, Coyle AJ: TH-2 and TH2-like cells in allergy and asthma: pharmacological perspectives. *Trend Pharmacol Sci* 1994; 15:324–332.

117. Actor JK, Shirai M, Kullberg MC, et al.: Helminth infection results in decreased virus specific CD8+ cytotoxic T cell and Th1 cytokine responses as well as delayed virus clearance. *Proc Nat Acad Sci U S A* 1993; 90:948–952.

118. Graham MB, Dalton DK, Giltinan D, et al.: Response to influenza infection in mice with a targeted disruption in the interferon γ gene. *J Exp Med* 1993; 178:1725–1732.

Chapter 80

IMMUNOSUPPRESSIVE AGENTS
ANDREW G. ALEXANDER

NEIL C. BARNES

There is a wide clinical spectrum in asthma, ranging from infrequent episodes of mild symptoms requiring only occasional bronchodilators to severe intractable corticosteroid-dependent asthma with considerable disruption of lifestyle and life-threatening acute exacerbations. Corticosteroids, administered by inhalation[1] or, where necessary, systemically, are the mainstay of treatment for asthma. Although their mechanism of action is still unclear, corticosteroids appear to act in various ways, including inhibition of mediator and cytokine release, reduction of microvascular leakage, inhibitory effects on inflammatory cell function (particularly lymphocytes and monocytes), and prevention and reversal of the down-regulation of pulmonary β-adrenergic receptors.[2]

For most patients, asthma can be controlled by regularly inhaled corticosteroids, in high doses where necessary, together with other effective antiasthma drugs, as discussed in the National Asthma Education Program guidelines.[3] The term *corticosteroid-dependent* commonly is given to the difficult minority of patients whose asthma requires the additional oral corticosteroids for adequate control. Although these patients probably comprise < 2 percent of all asthmatics, they account for a high proportion of attendances at respiratory out-patient clinics and hospital admissions for asthma. Some patients with chronic severe asthma are refractory to the effects of corticosteroids, despite showing reversibility of airflow obstruction after β$_2$-adrenergic agonist.[4] The mechanism of corticosteroid resistance is unclear but there is evidence that it may be associated with defects in lymphocyte and monocyte function and in the skin vasoconstrictor response. Patients whose asthma remains poorly controlled despite treatment with oral corticosteroids may be at risk of progressive irreversible airflow obstruction.

Long-Term Maintenance Oral Corticosteroid Therapy

Where asthma control remains difficult despite inhaled corticosteroids and bronchodilators, potential contributing factors should be considered and remedied where possible. These include smoking, drugs such as β-adrenoceptor antagonist, and aspirin, rhinitis and sinusutis, allergens at work or at home (e.g., pets) and psychological factors. Poor compliance and poor inhaler technique are common and should be addressed. These usually can be improved with appropriate explanation and alternative inhaler devices where necessary. A large volume spacer is recommended for doses of inhaled corticosteroids above 800 μg daily. It is essential that the dosage and delivery of all other drugs should be optimized before the addition of long-term oral corticosteroid therapy is considered, usually in conjunction with a hospital-based asthma clinic. However, where control remains poor despite all these measures, regularly administered oral prednisolone may improve both symptoms and lung function and reduce the frequency of disease exacerbations. In patients already using oral prednisolone, optimization of other therapies, particularly by inhaled corticosteroids in high doses (up to 2 mg daily), may permit a reduction in maintenance dose, and those taking small doses of prednisolone may be weaned from oral corticosteroids altogether. Open, uncontrolled studies suggests that high-dose nebulized corticosteroid may also spare use of cortico-steroids.

The long-term side effects of chronic oral corticosteroid usage are of considerable concern. In adult patients, the commonest effects that cause problems are osteoporosis,[5] skin thinning and easy bruising, hypertension, induction or worsening of diabetes mellitus, obesity, muscle weakness, and cataract formation. In children, growth retardation is a concern. Such adverse effects are common with a daily prednisolone dose >10 mg and are reduced when a single morning-dose is used. Where control permits, alternate-day dosing may reduce unwanted effects in patients on small doses. Intramuscular triamcinolone has been shown to be more effective than low-dose prednisolone in one group of patients, but adverse effects were more severe.[6] Measures to prevent osteoporosis should be considered particularly in peri- and postmenopausal women. These may include calcium, bisphosphonates, hormone replacement therapy, and referral to an osteoporosis clinic. The need for continued oral corticosteroid therapy should be kept under close review with regular attempts to determine the current minimum adequate maintenance dose, and, where possible, to wean completely.

Immunosuppressive Agents

Many chronic severe asthmatics remain controlled inadequately despite oral corticosteroid therapy. These individuals must contend with the morbidity both of their asthma and the unwanted effects of their therapy. Because of these concerns, there has been interest in the use of immunosuppressive agents in asthma in an attempt to decrease or eliminate the requirement for oral corticosteroids and improve asthma control. Since the 1950s, attempts to find a corticosteroid-sparing agent have led to the use of many immunosuppressive drugs including nitrogen mustard, chlorambucil, 6-mercaptopurine, thioguanosine, and azathioprine for treatment of refractory asthma.[7] Interest in this approach has been heightened by controlled trials of various immunosuppressants in a number of other inflammatory diseases (particularly rheumatoid arthritis), which have shown clinical benefit, as well as by the increasing evidence that the activated T lymphocyte plays a role in the pathogenesis of asthma.[8]

A number of well-controlled clinical trials of immunosuppressants now have been performed and show beneficial effects in asthma. However, the longest of these was only for 36 weeks and, on cessation of the various drugs studied, improvements in lung function and corticosteroid requirement returned to the pretreatment baseline. Thus, there is a lack of data from controlled studies on long-term treatment with these drugs. Furthermore, all of the agents used have been compared with placebo, and there has been no comparison of the relative efficacy of different immunosuppressants.

The decision to treat an asthmatic patient with long-term oral corticosteroids should be made only when disease control remains poor despite optimizing all other asthma treatment and after addressing any possible contributing factors. Similarly, the addition of an immunosuppressive agent should only be considered when disease control remains poor despite long-term oral corticosteroid therapy or when there are troublesome side effects from corticosteroids. All other means of decreasing oral corticosteroid requirement should be attempted. In addition to the factors previously addressed, there is some limited evidence that oral theophyllines may decrease requirement for oral corticosteroids, and a trial of oral theophyllines should be performed. If, despite these measures, patients still require long-term oral corticosteroids in dosage sufficient to cause concern, then the physician may wish to consider a trial of immunosuppressants.

METHOTREXATE

Worldwide the most commonly employed immunosuppressant in asthma is the dihydrofolate reductase inhibitor methotrexate (see also Chap. 81). This is partly due to its established role as a corticosteroid-sparing agent in rheumatoid arthritis and as an effective therapy for psoriasis; and partly to the observation in 1986 that an asthmatic patient given methotrexate for psoriasis noted an improvement in her asthma and was able to decrease her corticosteroid requirement. Following this observation there have been a number of controlled trials of methotrexate in oral corticosteroid-dependent asthmatics. These studies have produced conflicting results with some studies showing marked benefit,[9] others showing modest benefit, and some showing no evidence of any difference between methotrexate and placebo.[10]

The largest and best-controlled trial was performed by Shiner and colleagues in >60 patients with oral corticosteroid-dependent asthma.[11] They showed a 50 percent reduction in oral corticosteroid requirement in the group treated with low-dose oral methotrexate (15 mg/week) compared with a 14 percent improvement in the placebo-treated group (Fig. 80-1). In addition, there was a decrease in exacerbations of asthma but no improvement in pulmonary function. Several other features of this study are of interest. First, there was a substantial lag in benefical effect with the methotrexate and placebo groups not diverging until after 12 weeks of therapy. Second, the methotrexate-treated group was still improving at the end of the 24-week study period. Third, the oral corticosteroid requirement returned to baseline within 10 weeks of stopping methotrexate. Five patients had to stop because of nausea or liver function test abnormalities. Controversy exists about the need for liver biopsies on long-term methotrexate treatment, but baseline liver function tests need to be performed with regular monitoring thereafter.

The place of methotrexate in the treatment of chronic severe asthma has yet to be elucidated. Methotrexate has effects on all dividing cells, and therefore its mechanism of

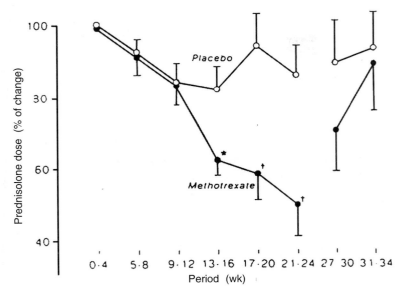

FIGURE 80-1 Effect of methotrexate or placebo on mean (SEM) daily dose of prednisolone. (*$p < .05$; †$p < .05$) (*Reprinted with permission.*[11])

action in asthma is not clear. It has been shown to decrease neutrophil chemotaxis and to reduce the wheal and flare reaction of skin testing, which raises the possibility that at low doses methotrexate exerts an anti-inflammatory action rather than acting as an immunosuppressant. Increasing use of the drug has raised questions about both long-term efficacy and adverse effects. It is recognized in rheumatoid arthritis that the efficacy of methotrexate may not be sustained, and there are now anecdotal reports of this occurring in asthma. An increasing number of adverse effects now are recognized with low-dose methotrexate, including methotrexate-induced asthma, methotrexate-induced pneumonitis, and *Pneumocystis carinii* pneumonia occurring both in patients with rheumatoid arthritis and, more recently, asthma. Nevertheless, methotrexate is the most-used immunosuppressive agent in asthma and is worthy of consideration in corticosteroid-dependent patients who remain poorly controlled or who are suffering unwanted effects.

CYCLOSPORIN A

Cyclosporin A, an inhibitor of T-lymphocyte activation, has revolutionized organ transplantation and also has been used extensively in low dosage for the treatment of autoimmune diseases in which activated T lymphocytes are believed to play a role, such as psoriasis, atopic dermatitis, Crohn's disease, and rheumatoid arthritis.[12] The rationale for its use in asthma is based on the accumulating evidence that activated T lymphocytes also play a role in asthma pathogenesis. Cyclosporin A now has been the subject of three controlled clinical trials, and there have been a number of reports of uncontrolled experience with cyclosporin A. In the first randomized, double-blind, placebo-controlled cross-over trial, oral cyclosporin therapy (5 mg/kg per day) resulted in a mean increase above placebo of 12.0 percent in morning PEF_R and 17.6 percent in FEV_1 in a group of patients with

corticosteroid-dependent asthma.[13] The improvement in PEF_R with cyclosporin was in addition to, rather than in place of, the component sensitive to β_2-adrenergic agonist and appeared to be continuing at the end of the 12-week treatment period (Fig. 80-2). Diurnal variation in PEF_R decreased by a mean of 27.6 percent, and there was a 48 percent decrease in the frequency of disease exacerbations requiring rescue prednisolone. No attempt was made in this study to decrease the dosage of oral corticosteroids.

In two further studies attempting to decrease the requirement for oral corticosteroids, cyclosporin A allowed a significantly greater reduction in oral corticosteroid dosage than placebo, with a reduction in exacerbations of asthma in one study. Again, an increase in pulmonary function was seen, despite a decrease in oral corticosteroid dosage. Experience from these controlled trials and from the open use of cyclosporin has shown the effects of cyclosporin A to be variable, with approximately one-half of patients showing little or no response and a wide range of improvement in those who do respond. In psoriasis, a dose-response relationship has been established, but this has not been explored in asthma. On cessation of therapy, treatment requirement and asthma severity return to baseline over a variable period of one week to several months, but there is no evidence of rebound exacerbation below baseline.

Like other immunosuppressive drugs, cyclosporin A has many unwanted effects.[12] Those observed in the trials in asthma are similar to those seen in studies of low-dose cyclosporin A in autoimmune diseases.[14] The main concerns are nephrotoxicity[15] and hypertension, but many other adverse effects also have been reported, including hypertrichosis, gingival hyperplasia, nausea, hepatotoxicity, tremor, paresthesia, headache, and cramps. Small reversible decreases in renal function were observed and, although irreversible renal damage appears to be largely dose-related, it remains to be seen whether this will occur with long-term

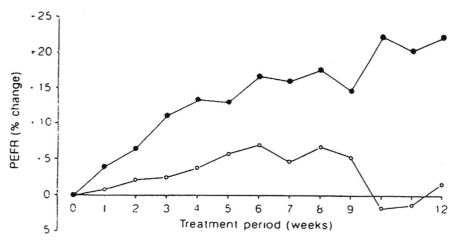

FIGURE 80-2 Percentage change from baseline in mean weekly morning PEF_R (before bronchodilator) plotted by week for cyclosporin A (closed circles) or placebo (open circles). (*Reprinted with permission.*[11])

use even of low doses of cyclosporin with careful monitoring of blood concentrations and renal function. A number of patients have had to start (or increase) antihypertensive therapy during cyclosporin A treatment but were able to stop (or return to pretrial therapy) on cessation of cyclosporin A. The long-term efficacy and safety of cyclosporin in asthma therefore remain to be established, and, at present, its use outside clinical trials is limited.

The mechanism of action of cyclosporin A in asthma is unknown. It is believed to act principally through inhibition of T-lymphocyte activation, and in one study clinical improvement was associated with a reduction in serum concentrations of soluble interleukin-2 receptor, a marker of T-lymphocyte activation. However, cyclosporin A also exerts inhibitory effects on antigen-presenting cells and on mediator and cytokine release from human basophils, mast cells, and eosinophils, which may be relevant in asthma.

ORAL GOLD

Parenteral gold salts (chrysotherapy) have been used in Japan for the treatment of asthma for <20 years, but there is

a high incidence of proteinuria and other adverse effects that necessitate withdrawal of therapy. There have been open uncontrolled studies suggesting benefit from oral gold (auranofin), and recently a controlled clinical trial of auranofin (3 mg twice daily) in patients with corticosteroid-dependent asthma showed a small, but statistically significant, reduction in oral corticosteroid requirement with a small increase in lung function and a decrease in asthma exacerbation rate[17] (Fig. 80-3). Side effects were less severe than with parenteral gold and included exacerbation of atopic dermatitis, nausea, and diarrhea. Auranofin has also been shown in a placebo-controlled study to reduce bronchial hyperresponsiveness in patients with mild asthma. The mechanism of action of gold salts in asthma remains obscure. Oral gold salt preparations have been shown to inhibit anti-IgE–induced release of histamine and leukotriene C_4 from human lung mast cells and to inhibit histamine-induced contraction of guinea-pig tracheal smooth muscle rings. In addition, oral gold salts inhibit mitogen-induced T-lymphocyte proliferation in vitro. Whether or not these actions of gold salts are relevant to a corticosteroid-sparing effect in asthma is not known, but it is

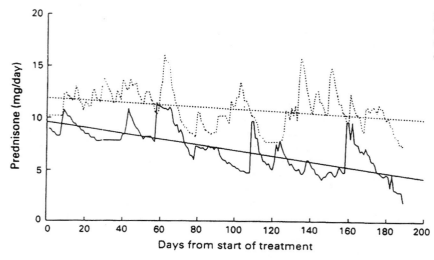

FIGURE 80-3 Mean daily dose of oral corticosteroids during the study in the placebo group (dotted lines) and in the auranofin group (continuous lines). (*Reprinted with permission.*[11])

thought that in rheumatoid arthritis, gold salts exert at least part of their action by interfering with T-lymphocyte function.

AZATHIOPRINE

In 1971, two short studies of the use of azathioprine in small numbers of patients found no benefit,[18] but subsequent experience with other drugs suggest that the duration of these trials was probably insufficient. It is possible that, if studied in sufficient numbers of patients for an adequate period of time, azathioprine would be effective, but in the absence of controlled trials, it is difficult to advocate its use. Purine antagonists have relatively little effect on delayed-type hypersensitivity reactions in man or on T-lymphocyte proliferative responses in vitro. Their main mode of action appears to be directed at killer cell activity and antibody production.

CYCLOPHOSPHAMIDE

There are anecdotal reports of the use of cyclophosphamide in asthma but no controlled clinical trials.

INTRAVENOUS IMMUNOGLOBULIN

There have been small uncontrolled trials of the use of intravenous immunoglobulin in corticosteroid-dependent asthma. The results of some of these studies have been quite dramatic,[19] but in the absence of controlled trials, it is difficult to advocate its use.

TROLEANDOMYCIN

Troleandomycin is a macrolide antibiotic with the odd property of blocking the metabolism of methylprednisolone but not prednisolone. Thus, when troleandomycin is given with methylprednisolone, the clinical effect of methylprednisolone is enhanced, and the dosage of methylprednisolone can be decreased while its therapeutic effect and side effects remain unchanged. In addition, it has been claimed that troleandomycin has vaguely defined immunosuppressant properties. A number of uncontrolled trials of troleandomycin have been performed, but the best-performed studies have shown no evidence of beneficial effects.[70] It has significant liver toxicity, and it is thus difficult to justify its use.

HYDROXYCHLOROQUINE

Hydroxychloroquine has been shown to be corticosteroid-sparing in rheumatoid arthritis. A small, open study in corticosteroid-dependent asthma showed impressive improvements in symptoms and lung function with virtually no adverse effects,[21] but, obviously double-blind placebo-controlled studies are awaited. Hydroxychloroquine inhibits both leukotriene and histamine release from human lung and antagonizes directly the effects of histamine and acetylcholine on guinea-pig tracheal rings. It also exerts anti-inflammatory effects by stabilizing lysosomes and

inhibiting superoxide release. Of interest in this study was a significant decrease in mean serum IgE concentrations while reducing oral corticosteroid dosage, in contrast to the increase usually seen on reducing corticosteroid dosage.

Clinical Use of Immunosuppressive Agents

In the absence of controlled clinical trials of other agents, the choice of immunosuppressants lies between methotrexate, cyclosporin A, and oral gold. Before embarking on the use of any such strategy, the dose of oral corticosteroid needs to be minimized by other methods, and the physician will need to weigh the relative risks and benefits to the individual patient. In poorly controlled asthma, greater doses of oral corticosteroids are required, and more severe adverse effects occur. In these instances, there is greater justification for a trial of an immunosuppressant. Before embarking on the use of immunosuppressants, safety checks need to be performed. In particular, hepatitis B status needs to be ascertained and patients need to be questioned about risk factors for HIV infection. Previous malignancy is a contraindication to cyclosporin A. Patients should be made fully aware of the possible risks and benefits. Most patients who respond to cyclosporin A do so within 3 months, but the response to methotrexate may be slower. A 4- to 6-month trial of immunosuppressant therefore should be given with careful monitoring of unwanted effects, and an attempt to decrease the dose of oral corticosteroids should be made. If, after 4 to 6 months, no benefit has been found and there are no extenuating reasons for this, the therapy should be discontinued. If a decrease in corticosteroid dosage and/or improvement in asthma control has been achieved, it may be appropriate to continue treatment. A few patients, however, despite a lack of improvement in lung function or reduction in maintenance prednisolone dosage, nevertheless note an overall improvement in asthma control with fewer exacerbations requiring temporary increases in prednisolone and/or hospitalization, and these patients also may benefit from an extended trial of treatment. It is worth noting that in the trials of methotrexate, cyclosporin, and oral gold, there was no evidence of plateauing of the beneficial effect at the end of the study, and it is possible that greater effects would have been seen had treatment been continued for longer (Figs. 80-1–3). When the dose of oral corticosteroids has been reduced to a minimum, it may be worth trying to decrease the dose of immunosuppressant. Anecdotal experience suggests this can be done with cyclosporin A. Alternatively, the physician may wish to make a judgment as to the optimal balance between the dose of immunosuppressant and dose of corticosteroid, electing for a small dose of each, rather than elimination of oral corticosteroids with use of a greater dosage of immunosuppressant. The possibility of opportunistic infections is a constant concern. These have been reported with low-dose methotrexate but not low-dose cyclosporin A, although this may reflect the longer experience with methotrexate and should be considered in any asthmatic patient who becomes more breathless.

The Future

There is, at present, no effective alternative to oral corticosteroids for patients with chronic severe asthma. The potential risks and benefits of any immunosuppressive agent must be balanced against those of poorly controlled asthma and the unwanted effects of its therapy with corticosteroids and other corticosteroid-sparing agents. While the toxicity of these oral immunosuppressants means that, currently, they only may be appropriate for a minority of severe corticosteroid-dependent asthmatics, it is likely in the future that more effective or safer immunosuppressants will be developed.[22] Possibilities include the macrolide immunosuppressants tacrolimus and rapamycin, specific cytokine antagonists such as antiinterleukin-5, and humanized or chimeric monoclonal antibodies directed at T cells,[23] such as anti-CD4, or at adhesion molecules, such as anti-ICAM-1. Clinical trials of tacrolimus and anti-CD4 in autoimmune disease are already in progress. It also may be possible to develop a lung-specific immunosuppressant.

Another approach may be to inhale immunosuppressants. Cyclosporin A has been shown to be effective by the inhaled route in antigen-challenge models in animals, and limited short-term experience shows that it can be given in humans by the inhaled route. If these and future drugs could be delivered effectively by the inhaled route, this form of therapy might be of benefit not only in chronic severe asthmatics but also in the much larger numbers of patients with milder disease.

References

1. Barnes PJ: Inhaled glucocorticoids for asthma. *N Engl J Med* 1995; 332:868–875.
2. Schleimer RP: Effects of glucocorticosteroids on inflammatory cells relevant to their therapeutic applications in asthma. *Am Rev Respir Dis* 1990; 141:S59–S69.
3. National Asthma Education Program Expert Panel Report: *Guidelines for the Diagnosis and Management of Asthma.* Washington, DC, US Department of Health and Human Services, August 1991.
4. Carmichael J, Patterson IC, Diaz P, et al: Corticosteroid-resistance in chronic asthma. *Br Med J* 1981; 282:1419–1422.
5. Adinoff AD, Hollister JR: Steroid-induced fractures and bone loss in patients with asthma. *N Engl J Med* 1983; 309:265–8.
6. Ogirala RG, Aldrich TK, Prezant DJ, et al: High-dose intramuscular triamcinolone in severe, chronic, life-threatening asthma. *N Engl J Med* 1991; 324:585–9.
7. Asmundsson T, Kilburn KH, Lazzlo J, Krock CJ: Immunosuppressive therapy of asthma. *J Allergy* 1971; 47:136–147.
8. Kay AB: Asthma and inflammation. *J Allergy Clin Immunol* 1991; 87:893–910.
9. Mullarkey MF, Blumenstein BA, Andrade WP, et al: Methotrexate in the treatment of corticosteroid-dependent asthma. A double-blind crossover study. *N Engl J Med* 1988; 318:603–607.
10. Erzurum SC, Leff JA, Cochran JE, et al: Lack of benefit of methotrexate in severe, steroid-dependent asthma. A double-blind placebo-controlled study. *Ann Intern Med* 1991; 114:353–360.
11. Shiner RJ, Nunn AJ, Chung KF, Geddes DM: Randomised, double-blind, placebo-controlled trial of methotrexate in steroid-dependent asthma. *Lancet* 1990; 336:137–140.
12. Kahan BD: Cyclosporine. *N Engl J Med* 1989; 321:1725–1738.
13. Alexander AG, Barnes NC, Kay AB: Trial of cyclosporin A in corticosteroid-dependent chronic severe asthma. *Lancet* 1992; 339:324–328.
14. von Graffenried B, Friend D, Shand N, et al: Cyclosporin A (Sandimmun®) in autoimmune disorders, in Thomson AW (ed): *Cyclosporin. Mode of Action and Clinical Applications.* London, Eng, Kluwer, 1989:213–50.
15. Feutren G, Mihatsch MJ: Risk factors for cyclosporine-induced nephropathy in patients with autoimmune diseases. *N Engl J Med* 1992; 326:1654–60.
16. Sigal NH, Dumont FJ: Cyclosporine A, FK-506, and rapamycin: pharmacological probes of lymphocyte signal transduction. *Annu Rev Immunol* 1992; 10:519–60.
17. Nierop G, Gijzel WP, Bel EH, et al: Auranofin in the treatment of steroid-dependent asthma: a double blind study. *Thorax* 1992; 47:349–354.
18. Hodges NG, Brewis RAL, Howell JBL: An evaluation of azathioprine in severe chronic asthma. *Thorax* 1971; 26:734–739.
19. Mazer BD, Gelfand EW: An open-label study of high-dose intravenous immunoglobulin in severe childhood asthma. *J Allergy Clin Immunol* 1991; 87:976–83.
20. Nelson HS, Hamilos DL, Corsello PR, et al: A double-blind study of troleandomycin and methylprednisolone in asthmatic subjects who require daily corticosteroids. *Am Rev Respir Dis* 1993; 147:398–404.
21. Charous BL: Open study of hydroxychloroquine in the treatment of severe symptomatic or corticosteroid-dependent asthma. *Ann Allergy* 1990; 65:53–58.
22. Kahan BD. New immunosuppressive drugs—pharmacologic approaches to alter immunoregulation. *Therapeutic Immunol* 1994; 1:33–44.
23. Waldmann H: Manipulation of T-cell responses with monoclonal antibodies. *Annu Rev Immunol* 1989; 7:407–44.

Chapter 81
NOVEL ANTI-INFLAMMATORY DRUGS IN ASTHMA

ALLAN GARLAND AND JULIAN SOLWAY

Modulation of the Leukotriene Mediator System

Modulation of the Prostanoid Mediator System

Selective Histamine-Receptor Antagonists

Bradykinin

Neuropeptides

Platelet-Activating Factor

Miscellaneous Anti-Inflammatory Agents

Over the past 20 years, a large body of evidence has accumulated implicating numerous elements of the inflammatory cascade in the pathogenesis of asthma and/or nonspecific bronchial hyperresponsiveness (BHR). Both inflammatory cells and soluble mediators appear to be important. Attempts to synthesize this mass of information into a unified picture of clinical asthma have as yet been unrewarding. Complex interactions have been discovered among the various elements of inflammation present in the airways. Different studies, carefully performed, have sometimes rendered apparently contradictory results. Undoubtedly, a large part of this difficulty derives from the wide variety of clinical and experimental settings that have been utilized to generate these data. Both in vivo and in vitro methods have been used to study spontaneous bronchoconstriction, bronchoconstriction in response to provocative challenge, or bronchial hyperresponsiveness in asthmatic and nonasthmatic humans as well as in other species.

Endogenous inflammatory mediators implicated in the pathophysiology of asthma include histamine; lipid mediators such as prostanoids, leukotrienes, and platelet activating factor; peptide mediators including bradykinin and the tachykinins; other inflammatory substances including cytokines; and oxygen radicals. Other components of inflammation are undoubtedly also involved, including immune cells and intercellular adhesion molecules. Until recently, evaluation of the roles of individual mediators among the complex mix probably present in asthmatic airways has been thwarted by the inadequate specificities or activities of pharmacologic tools available. However, aggressive and innovative research efforts have recently resulted in the synthesis of new anti-inflammatory agents. Novel drugs include those that act with high specificity to either block synthesis or

receptor binding of endogenous bioactive substances; their use has or will soon permit investigators to more clearly identify the contribution of many important mediators to the pathogenesis of asthma. This chapter reviews the results of studies that have used these new specific anti-inflammatory agents and also discusses possible future directions. As regards human drug studies, except as noted, this chapter is confined to experiments of blinded, randomized, placebo-controlled trials.

Modulation of the Leukotriene Mediator System

Leukotrienes comprise a class of lipid-based substances that are synthesized upon demand rather than stored within cells and whose production begins with the action of various intracellular lipoxygenase enzymes on cell membrane phospholipids liberated by the action of phospholipase A_2. The predominant family of leukotrienes—LTA_4, B_4, C_4, D_4, and E_4—originate from the effect of 5-lipoxygenase (5-LO) on arachadonic acid. LTB_4 is chemotactic for leukocytes, and the sulfidopeptide leukotrienes LTC_4, D_4, and E_4 (the combination previously known collectively as "slow-reacting substance of anaphylaxis") are potent bronchoconstrictor substances that also induce secretion of airway mucus[1,2] and increase the permeability of the airway microvasculature.[3]

A significant role for leukotrienes in the pathogenesis of asthma has been suggested by indirect evidence. Asthmatic patients demonstrate hyperresponsiveness to inhaled LTC_4 or LTD_4.[4] Production of leukotrienes is augmented by airway challenge with either antigen[5] or isocapnic hyperpnea.[6]

Additionally, Sasagawa and coworkers observed that the serum concentrations of LTB_4, C_4, D_4, and E_4 were dramatically higher in patients having acute spontaneous asthma exacerbations than in normal patients; in that study, all six of the asthmatics who had blood tested both during an exacerbation and while in remission had higher leukotriene levels during the attack.[7]

New investigational drugs have been developed that block the synthesis of leukotrienes by specific inhibition of 5-LO activity either by direct action on the enzyme (e.g., A-64077, subsequently named zileuton) or indirectly by binding to the 5-lipoxygenase activating protein FLAP (e.g., MK-886). Another class of novel drugs blocks the action of leukotrienes by competing at the cell surface receptor to which LTC_4, D_4, and E_4 bind to initiate their biologic actions (e.g., MK-571, MK-679, SKF-104353, and ICI-204219, now called Accolate). Studies using these agents have demonstrated significant effects upon both spontaneous asthma and asthmatic bronchoconstriction elicited by aspirin, thermal challenges, or antigen.

Thermal challenges performed either with exercise or voluntary hyperventilation with dry and/or cold gas result in bronchoconstriction in asthmatics through cooling and/or drying of the airways.[8] Both 5-LO inhibition and leukotriene receptor blockade inhibit the bronchoconstriction that results from these challenges. In three crossover trials of stable patients with exercise-induced asthma, single doses of the leukotriene-receptor antagonists MK-571 (160 mg IV[9]), ICI-204219 (20 mg PO[10]), and SKF-104353 (0.8 mg inhaled[11]) were tested. In each case, the mean exercise-induced decline in FEV_1 after placebo was >25 percent; but for the same amount of exercise, the active agents attenuated this decline by 63, 40, and 38 percent, respectively. The salutary prophylactic effect of SKF-104353 was comparable to that of disodium cromoglycate.[11] In the two studies in which it was evaluated, the leukotriene-receptor antagonists caused a more rapid recovery to preexercise baseline FEV_1.[9,11] Using the related stimulus of isocapnic ventilation of frigid air, Israel et al. observed that pretreatment with a single 800 mg oral dose of the 5-LO inhibitor zileuton increased by 38 percent the minute volume of cold, dry air that subjects needed to breathe to elicit a 15 percent decrease in FEV_1.[12] In that study, 5-LO was inhibited 74 percent as measured by the reduction in calcium ionophore-stimulated production of LTB_4 by leukocytes ex vivo.

Sensitivity to peripheral cyclooxygenase (CO)-inhibiting drugs, such as aspirin, is not rare among asthmatics. Since CO and 5-LO compete for arachadonic acid as their substrate, it has long been hypothesized that blockade by CO inhibitors of one arm of the eicosanoid pathway might contribute to aspirin-induced asthma through "shunting" of arachadonic acid toward production of excess amounts of bronchoconstrictive leukotrienes. Indirect evidence that leukotrienes play an important role in this reaction[13] has recently been supplemented by the following direct evidence. Israel et al. found that pretreatment of aspirin-sensitive asthmatics with oral zileuton (600 mg qid) for 6 to 8 days caused *ablated* the decrease in FEV_1 induced by aspirin challenge.[14] This clinical response was accompanied by a reduc-

tion in the associated nasal, gastrointestinal, and dermal symptoms, though by only a 69 percent reduction in the urinary excretion of LTE_4, the excreted metabolic product of the sulfidopeptide leukotrienes. Using pretreatment with a single 750 mg oral dose of the leukotriene-receptor antagonist MK-679, Dahlen et al.[15] found similar results—a mean 4.4-fold leftward shift in the lysine-aspirin dose-response curve, with 3 of the 8 patients failing to sustain a >20 percent fall in FEV_1 even at the highest dose of lysine-aspirin. These investigations strongly imply that leukotrienes are the major mediators in asthmatic bronchoconstriction triggered by CO inhibitors.

The evidence for a clinically important effect of leukotriene-modulating drugs on antigen-induced bronchoconstriction in atopic asthmatics is less impressive than that for either exercise, cold/dry air, or aspirin-induced bronchospasm. Two well-designed studies have observed only modest effects. Friedman et al.[16] found that 750 mg of the orally active FLAP antagonist MK-886 resulted in statistically significant attenuations of 29 percent in the early asthmatic FEV_1 response and 19 percent in the late asthmatic response, accompanied by approximately 50 percent declines in ex vivo LTB_4 production and urinary LTE_4 excretion. Findlay et al.[17] measured a 0.65 log shift in the dose-response curve to inhaled cat allergen after pretreatment with 40 mg of the oral leukotriene-receptor antagonist ICI-204219. On the other hand, a similarly well-done study performed by Hui et al.,[18] using an 800 mg oral dose of zileuton, did not demonstrate a significant effect either upon the early or late asthmatic responses, despite a 93 percent inhibition of ex vivo LTB_4 production and 50 percent decrease in urinary LTE_4 excretion.

The effects of inhibition of leukotriene production or receptor binding on symptoms and measures of spontaneous asthmatic bronchoconstriction have also been modest. The finding of statistically significant 8 to 22 percent increases in resting FEV_1 soon after the first dose of either 5-LO inhibitor (600 mg po zileuton[19]) or leukotriene-receptor blockers (334 mg IV MK-571[20] or 40 mg PO ICI-204219[21]) suggests that in patients with mild to moderate stable asthma, there is an element of baseline airway tone attributable to leukotrienes. However, other studies have not shown an immediate bronchodilator effect of these classes of agents.[9–12,16,17]

Studies of the effects over longer time periods have been somewhat more encouraging. After 4 weeks of oral therapy, Israel et al. found that patients with stable mild to moderate asthma who received zileuton (600 mg qid) experienced a 0.32-L (13.4 percent) increase in FEV_1, while the increase in the placebo group was only 0.06 L.[19] This change was accompanied by a 37 percent decrease in the asthma symptom score (versus a 17 percent decrease for placebo), a 24 percent decline in as-needed use of inhaled β_2-agonists (versus a 7 percent decline for placebo), and a 39 percent decline in the urinary recovery of LTE_4. A similarly conducted 6-week study of ICI-204219 showed that 20 mg bid of this leukotriene-receptor antagonist, a 0.23-L (11 percent) rise in FEV_1 (versus 1 percent for placebo), a 27 percent decrease in symptom score (versus a 13 percent decrease for placebo), and a 31 percent decrease in use of inhaled β_2-adrenergic agonists (versus a 15 percent decrease for placebo). In both of these studies, the bronchodilator effect of inhaled β_2-adrenergic agonists was additive to that of the leukotriene modulating agents.

Taken together, these results show that leukotrienes play a variable role in asthma. They appear to play a predominant role in aspirin-induced asthma, to be of moderate importance in exercise- or hyperpnea-induced asthma, and seem to be one class of mediators among many which conspire to produce antigen-induced bronchoconstriction in atopic asthmatics. Overall, the 5-LO inhibiting agents and leukotriene-receptor antagonists now in trials appear to have equivalent clinical efficacy. The actual role of these agents in the management of asthma is yet to be defined, but it seems likely that some patients will find them quite helpful.

Modulation of the Prostanoid Mediator System

Prostanoids comprise a large group of mediators whose synthesis begins with the action of cyclooxygenase (CO) on arachadonic acid liberated from cell membranes by the action of phospholipase A_2. They have numerous biologic actions, including effects upon airway smooth muscle. Included among the prostanoid family are prostaglandins and thromboxanes, among which there are bronchoconstrictors, such as thromboxane A_2 (TXA_2), PGD_2, and $PGF_{2\alpha}$, and also bronchodilators such as PGI_2 and PGE_2.[1] Evidence that suggests a role for prostanoids in the pathogenesis of asthma includes findings of increased concentrations of prostaglandins and TXA_2, or their degradation products, in the urine and bronchoalveolar lavage (BAL) fluid of asthma patients either after antigen challenge or during an acute asthma exacerbation.[5,22,23] Numerous and complex interactions with other mediators—including PAF, histamine, bradykinin, and tachykinins—have been observed[24–29] and may have clinical relevance.

In light of (1) the opposing effects of different prostanoids, (2) the existence of aspirin-induced asthma, and (3) the potential that CO inhibitors might shunt arachadonic acid toward production of proinflammatory and bronchoconstrictive leukotrienes, it is not surprising that nonspecific CO inhibitors have proven ineffective against asthmatic bronchoconstriction. Thus, pretreatment for 2 days with indomethacin has no effect upon either the early or late antigen response.[5,30] When tested against exercise-induced bronchoconstriction, oral CO inhibitors were similarly of little or no benefit.[31,32]

Although nonspecific inhibition of prostanoid synthesis has not proven useful in asthma, it remains possible that individual members of this class of mediators may be important in its pathogenesis. Thus, new drugs have been developed that modulate the effects of the powerful bronchoconstrictor TXA_2 either through inhibition of its synthesis or by competitive antagonism at the common TXA_2 and PGD_2 receptor.

The best-studied and most consistent property that these newer agents demonstrate against asthma is a rather slight diminution in airway hyperresponsiveness to cholinergic agonists, observed after pretreatment with thromboxane synthase inhibitors[33,34] and some[35] but not all[36] receptor antagonists. When it was tested against exercise-induced bronchoconstriction, Magnussen et al. found no effect of pretreatment with the thromboxane-receptor antagonist BAY-u-3405 at a dose that elicited a >10-fold shift in the dose-bronchoconstriction response to inhaled PGD_2.[37] In a group of atopic, mildly asthmatic patients, Beasley et al. observed that a single 80 mg oral dose of the receptor antagonist GR-32191 led to modest 24 percent mean attenuation in the antigen-induced decrease in FEV_1.[36] In that study, as in many investigations of drugs that influence only one or a few of the mediators postulated to be involved in the pathogenesis of asthma, it was noted that a minority of patients had a rather significant response, while in most there was no effect.

Selective Histamine-Receptor Antagonists

Histamine is a potent bioactive substance in the airways, inducing bronchoconstriction, mucus production, and bronchovascular hyperpermeability. These effects are mediated mainly through interaction with the H_1 subtype of histamine receptor on airway target cells. Histamine is produced and stored primarily by mast cells, with secretion initiated by interaction of specific antigen with bound idiotype-specific IgE. Patients with asthma almost universally demonstrate bronchial hyperresponsiveness to histamine, and increased amounts are found both in the BAL fluid and the blood after antigen challenge or spontaneous exacerbations in atopic asthmatics.[38] Despite such indirect evidence of the importance of histamine in allergic asthma, use of antihistaminic agents in the therapy of asthma has historically been so disappointing that they have no established role. However, the more recent synthesis of potent and somewhat more specific H_1-receptor antagonists such as ketotifen, azelastine, cetirizine, terfenadine, and clemastine has led to a new series of clinical studies, the interpretation of which is clouded by the fact that some of these agents have other potentially significant biologic actions.

A beneficial effect of these drugs upon inhaled antigen-induced bronchoconstriction has been inconsistently demonstrated. In one of the most dramatically positive published trials, Rafferty et al.[39] found that a single 180 mg oral dose of terfenadine administered 3 h prior to challenge led to a 50 percent attenuation in the antigen-induced decrease in FEV_1 (from 36 to 19 percent); a similar result was obtained with three daily oral doses (30 mg) of the structurally unrelated drug astemizole. Prior to that, Phillips et al.[40] found that pretreatment with 0.5 mg of inhaled clemastine or ketotifen led to only minor increases in the inhaled antigen PD_{20}; FEV_1 of 2.1- and 1.6-fold, respectively. However, other well-designed studies using azelastine[41] or cetirizine[42,43] found no benefit of these drugs in the early-phase response to antigen. The effects upon the late asthmatic response to antigen are similarly inconsistent; Twentyman et al.[41] found no effect of 4 days of oral azelastine, while Wasserfallen et al.[43] measured a 17 percent reduction in the late decrease in FEV_1 after cetirizine, compared to a 1 percent rise after placebo.

When tested against exercise-induced bronchoconstriction, benefits of the newer H_1-receptor antagonists are equivocal as well. While Patel observed that pretreatment with a single 120 mg dose of terfenadine resulted in a small but significant reduction in exercise-induced decline in FEV_1 from 33 to 23 percent,[44] Gong et al. found no benefit from a 20 mg dose of cetirizine.[42] Only a small number of blinded, placebo-controlled studies have been published using the new generation of H_1-receptor antagonists in spontaneous clinical asthma. As identified in the excellent review by Bousquet et al.,[38] the beneficial effects of these agents in both seasonal and perennial asthma have been quite mild, and a number of other studies, which found no effect, were never published.

Bradykinin

Bradykinin (BK) is a nonpeptide generated from the action of kallikrein upon circulating high-molecular-weight kininogen. In asthmatics but not in normal subjects, it causes bronchoconstriction through mechanisms that involve binding to the BK_2 subtype of bradykinin receptor.[45,46] Most or all of this effect is mediated indirectly; BK is only a weak bronchoconstrictor in vitro,[47] and evidence exists to implicate release of tachykinins, thromboxane, acetylcholine, and possibly also histamine in the mechanism of BK-induced bronchoconstriction in humans.[28,47–49]

Currently, evidence for a significant role of BK in the pathogenesis of asthma is indirect. Symptomatic but not asymptomatic atopic asthmatics have increased amounts of BK in their BAL fluid.[50] Antigen challenge also elicits further increases of kininogen, kallikrein, and BK in BAL fluid.[22,50,51] In an allergic sheep model, Abraham et al. showed that the BK_2-receptor antagonist NPC-567 ablated metabisulfite-induced bronchoconstriction[52] and attenuated subsequent cholinergic bronchial hyperresponsiveness after inhaled antigen challenge.[53] Direct investigation of the role of BK in asthma will have to await human trials of the highly potent and specific BK_2-receptor antagonists, which have been developed and are continuing to undergo study in animals.

Neuropeptides

Nociceptive nerve endings of the C-fiber type contain the tachykinins substance P (SP) and neurokinin A (NKA) and also calcitonin gene-related peptide (CGRP). These mediators are released upon local nerve stimulation or by the axon reflex. C-fiber nerve endings are present throughout the airways, innervating airway smooth muscle, mucous glands, microvessels, and airway epithelium. By interaction with the NK-1 and NK-2 subtype of neurokinin receptors, tachykinin release leads to "neurogenic inflammation" in the airways,

consisting of bronchoconstriction, mucus production, and bronchovascular hyperpermeability.[1,54,55] The role of tachykinins may be complex; there is evidence that their release may be elicited or potentiated by bradykinin, histamine, and leukotrienes.[29,48,57,58] Additionally, tachykinins stimulate release of histamine.[59]

The importance of tachykinins in various animal models of asthma has been demonstrated clearly. In guinea pigs, they are the key mediators in dry-gas hyperpnea-induced bronchospasm and bronchovascular hyperpermeability[60] and are important as well in antigen-induced bronchoconstriction.[57,61]

Currently, the evidence for potential involvement of tachykinin in asthma is indirect and equivocal. Inhaled SP or NKA causes bronchoconstriction in asthmatics, primarily through activation of the NK-2 receptor, but not in normal subjects.[55,62] Ollerenshaw reported that immunohistopathologic evaluation of airway tissues from asthmatics demonstrated more and longer substance P immunoreactive nerve fibers than did those of nonasthmatics,[54] but Lilly et al. found smaller quantities of immunoreactive SP in tracheas obtained from asthmatic subjects compared with those of normals.[63] It is also possible that some of the antiasthma effect of cromolyn sodium and nedocromil sodium derives from their ability to inhibit release of neuropeptides from airway C-fiber neurons.[62,64]

Within the next several years, studies using neuropeptide-receptor antagonists should elucidate the role of tachykinins in asthma. To date, the only published trial of such drugs administered to asthmatics utilized the combined NK-1- and NK-2-receptor antagonist FK-224 to attenuate bronchoconstriction induced by inhaled bradykinin.[48] It seems likely that these agents will be found to have a significant effect in selected subsets of patients (e.g., those for whom exercise or cold air inhalation is their predominant asthma trigger) but might, as the experience has been with many other modulators of individual bronchoactive mediators, be unimpressive if tested in an unselected crosssection of asthmatics.

Platelet-Activating Factor

Platelet-activating factor (PAF) is a lipid-derived mediator synthesized by a variety of cell types, including eosinophils. It elicits a number of responses; in airways these include bronchoconstriction, mucus secretion, and diverse inflammatory effects which include very potent eosinophil chemotaxis and stimulation.[65] It appears that some of these effects, especially a portion of the bronchoconstriction, results from PAF-induced production and release of leukotrienes.[66,67] The similarity of these functions with abnormalities present in asthma suggests a possible pathophysiologic role.

Indirect evidence suggesting such a role includes observations that (1) plasma PAF concentrations are increased two- to eightfold during acute asthma exacerbations, (2) atopic asthmatic children who respond well to immunotherapy have lower plasma PAF concentrations than do nonresponders, and (3) antigen challenge in atopic asthmatics results in augmented PAF secretion into the systemic circulation.[68–70] In addition, there are conflicting data on whether inhalation of PAF increases nonspecific bronchial responsiveness.[71,72]

Attempts to use new PAF antagonists to modulate asthmatic responses have been unproductive until very recently. While Hsieh found a minor beneficial shift in the allergen dose-response curve after acute inhalational pretreatment with BN-52021,[73] other studies using pretreatment with either UK-74505 acutely or WEB-2086 for 1 week did not find any effect either upon the early or late asthmatic responses to antigen, despite using doses demonstrated to antagonize PAF-induced effects.[74,75] Similarly, there was no significant effect of acute pretreatment with BN-52063 upon exercise- or cold air-induced bronchoconstriction,[76] and Spence et al. found that compared to placebo, 12 weeks of therapy with WEB-2086 had no beneficial effects upon a cohort of atopic asthmatics.[77] However, Hozawa et al.[78] showed that 2 week treatment with a new PAF-receptor antagonist, Y-24180, reduced slightly airway responsiveness to methacholine slightly in asthmatics.

Miscellaneous Anti-Inflammatory Agents

In addition to those humoral mediators already discussed, other mediators, as well as a variety of other elements of the inflammatory response, almost certainly are involved in the pathogenesis of asthma and thus could supply potential targets for antiasthma drug development. A variety of agents that influence inflammation, some new and some well established in other settings, have been or will soon be tested against the symptoms and signs of asthma.

Activated helper T lymphocytes (i.e., CD25-positive CD4 cells) are increased in the airways of asthmatics, with greater increases during acute asthma symptoms[79]; this may have some pathophysiologic significance. Cyclosporine is an immunosuppressive agent that is believed to act largely, though probably not exclusively, by inhibiting activation of T lymphocytes. In a well-designed crossover trial, Alexander et al. demonstrated in 33 corticosteroid-dependent patients that 12 weeks of low-dose cyclosporine resulted in a 17.6 percent improvement in FEV_1 and a 48 percent reduction in the frequency of clinical exacerbations, though there were no differences in asthma symptom score, corticosteroid use, or bronchodilator usage.[80] Despite this encouraging result, one recalls that while early studies of the use of methotrexate were likewise encouraging, further studies failed to demonstrate a convincing benefit of that immunosuppressive agent.[81]

The anticoagulant, heparin, has anti-inflammatory effects that may be mediated by its ability to block receptors to the ubiquitous intracellular second messenger inositol triphosphate.[82] Heparin has been observed to attenuate mast cell histamine release in vitro,[83] and in separate trials in asthmatics, pretreatment with aerosolized heparin attenuated bronchoconstriction after exercise by 74 percent, and it had a small beneficial effect upon antigen-induced constriction.[82,84]

Another possible target for development of antiasthma drugs are the "adhesion molecules," which mediate cell-cell adherence. Given the somewhat unclear but unquestioned role of inflammatory cells in asthma, it seems certain that such proteins must be of importance. Adhesion molecules on eosinophils, mast cells, vascular endothelial cells, lymphocytes, and other cells are upregulated by many of the putative mediators involved in asthma, including histamine, PAF, leukotrienes, substance P, and cytokines.[85] For example, PAF stimulates expression of proteins that result in increased adherence of eosinophils to endothelium. Thus, agents that interfere with the adherence of inflammatory cells to endothelial or epithelial surfaces may be useful antiasthma drugs. In a primate model of allergen-induced bronchial hyperresponsiveness, treatment with a monoclonal antibody against the adhesion molecule ICAM-1 resulted in attenuation of airway eosinophilia and a 10-fold decrease in bronchial responsiveness to inhaled antigen.[86] While no such specific agents have yet been tested on humans, it is possible that some of the demonstrated antiasthma behavior of cyclosporine, cromolyn sodium, glucocorticoids, and other drugs may be mediated partly by their effects upon adhesion molecules.[85]

The vital and varied roles of cytokines in inflammation make it appear likely that, at least in some patients, this class of molecules might play a significant part in the pathogenesis of asthma. Indirect support for this hypothesis comes from observations that various cytokines—including GM-CSF, IL-5, IL-6, IL-1β—are expressed in increased amounts by airway cells of asthmatics, and that concentrations increase both after antigen challenge and during acute asthma attacks.[87–89] It is possible that some of the antiasthma effect of corticosteroids derives from their ability to influence cytokine production,[89] and in the future, novel pharmacologic agents that modulate production, receptor binding, or action of cytokines should be tested for possible beneficial clinical effect in asthma.

Oxygen radicals, produced as part of the inflammatory cascade, could be involved in the pathogenesis of asthma. Production of such reactive molecules by ozone inhalation or other methods generates bronchoconstriction and/or bronchial hyperresponsiveness in animals[90,91] and humans.[92] The finding of increased plasma concentrations of free-radical lipid peroxidation products in stable asthmatics, with an additional increase during acute attacks,[93] also is suggestive. Observations such as that of Lansing et al. that pretreatment of allergic sheep with aerosolized catalase (to reduce oxygen radical generation) attenuates antigen-induced bronchial responsiveness,[94] suggest that antioxidant strategies could possibly be of utility in asthma.

The nonselective phosphodiesterase (PDE) inhibitor theophylline has a long and successful history in the therapy of asthma. Since the major PDE isoform present in human airways is PDE IV, selective inhibitors of that isoform have been recently tested in animal models of asthma. Recent studies in animals using specific PDE IV inhibitors (e.g., rolipram), have demonstrated that these agents possess anti-inflammatory activities,[95,96] the ability to dilate airways in vitro and in vivo,[97] to attenuate leukotriene-induced bronchoconstriction, and to inhibit antigen-induced bronchial hyperresponsiveness.[98] It would not be surprising if the mechanism of the antiasthma effect of both selective and nonselective PDE inhibitors were related at least in part to their anti-inflammatory activities.

Last, some of the other currently available effective antiasthma drugs have varied anti-inflammatory activities that may contribute to their efficacy. Thus, in addition to the inhibitory effect upon C-fiber neuropeptide release mentioned above for cromolyn sodium and nedocromil sodium, some of the newer β-adrenergic agonist drugs (e.g., salmeterol), appear to possess anti-inflammatory influences upon neutrophils, eosinophils, and endothelium, some of which are β-adrenergically mediated, while others are not.[99,100]

References

1. Shore SA, Austen KF, Drazen JM: Eicosanoids and the lung, in Massaro D (ed): *Lung Cell Biology*, vol 41. New York: Marcel Dekker, 1989: 1011–1089.
2. Henderson WR Jr: Role of leukotrienes in asthma. *Ann Allergy* 1994; 72:272.
3. Persson CGA, Erjefalt I, Andersson P: Leakage of macromolecules from guinea pig tracheobronchial microvasculature: Effects of allergen, leukotrienes, tachykinins, and anti-asthma drugs. *Acta Physiol Scand* 1986; 127:95.
4. Henderson WR Jr: Eicosanoids and lung inflammation. *Am Rev Respir Dis* 1987; 135:1176.
5. Sladek K, Dworski R, Fitzgerald GA, et al.: Allergen-stimulated release of thromboxane A_2 and leukotriene E_4 in humans. *Am Rev Respir Dis* 1990; 141:1441.
6. Pliss LB, Ingenito EP, Ingram RH, Pichurko B: Assessment of bronchoalveolar cell and mediator response to isocapnic hyperpnea in asthma. *Am Rev Respir Dis* 1990; 142:73.
7. Sasagawa M, Satoh TL, Takemoto A, et al.: Blood levels of leukotrienes in asthmatic patients during attack and remission. *Jpn J Allergol* 1994; 43:28.
8. McFadden ER, Gilbert IA: Exercise-induced asthma. *N Engl J Med* 1994; 330:1362.
9. Manning PJ, Watson RM, Margolskee DJ, et al.: Inibition of exercise-induced bronchoconstriction by MK-571, a potent leukotriene D_4-receptor antagonist. *N Engl J Med* 1990; 323:1739.
10. Finnerty JP, Wood-Baker R, Thomson H, Holgate ST: Role of leukotrienes in exercise-induced asthma. *Am Rev Respir Dis* 1992; 145:746.
11. Robuschi M, Riva E, Fuccella LM, et al.: Prevention of exercise-induced bronchoconstriction by a new leukotriene antagonist (SK&F) 104353. *Am Rev Respir Dis* 1992; 145:1285.
12. Israel E, Dermarkarian R, Rosenberg M, et al.: The effects of a 5-lipoxygenase inhibitor on asthma induced by cold, dry air. *N Engl J Med* 1990; 323:1740.
13. Lee TH: Mechanism of bronchospasm in aspirin-sensitive asthma. *Am Rev Respir Dis* 1993; 148:1442.
14. Israel E, Fischer AR, Rosenberg MA, et al.: The pivotal role of 5-lipoxygenase products in the reaction of aspirin-sensitive asthmatics to aspirin. *Am Rev Respir Dis* 1993; 148:1447.
15. Dahlen B, Kumlin M, Margolskee DJ, et al.: The leukotriene-receptor antagonist MK-0679 blocks airway obstruction induced by inhaled lysine-aspirin in aspirin-sensitive asthmatics. *Eur Respir J* 1993; 6:1018.
16. Friedman BS, Bel EH, Buntinx A, et al.: Oral leukotriene inhibitor (MK-886) blocks allergen-induced airway responses. *Am Rev Respir Dis* 1993; 147:839.
17. Findlay SR, Barden JM, Easley CB, Glass M: Effect of the oral leukotriene antagonist, ICI 204,219, on antigen-induced bronchoconstriction in subjects with asthma. *J Allergy Clin Immunol* 1992; 89:1040.
18. Hui KP, Taylor IK, Taylor GW, et al.: Effect of a 5-lipoxygenase inhibitor on leukotriene generation and airway responses after allergen challenge in asthmatic patients. *Thorax* 1991; 46:184.
19. Israel E, Rubin P, Kemp JP, et al.: The effect of inhibition of 5-lipoxygenase by zileuton in mild-to-moderate asthma. *Ann Intern Med* 1993; 119:1059.
20. Gaddy JN, Margolskee DJ, Bush RK, et al.: Bronchodilation with a potent and selective leukotriene D_4 receptor antagonist (MK-571) in patients with asthma. *Am Rev Respir Dis* 1992; 146:358.
21. Hui KP, Barnes NC: Lung function improvement in asthma with a cysteinyl-leukotriene receptor antagonist. *Lancet* 1991; 337:1063.
22. Liu MC, Hubbard WC, Proud D, et al.: Immediate and late inflammatory responses to ragweed antigen challenge of the peripheral airways in allergic asthmatics. *Am Rev Respir Dis* 1991; 144:51.
23. Taylor IK, Ward PS, O'Shaughnessy KM, et al.: Thromboxane A_2 biosynthesis in acute asthma and after antigen challenge. *Am Rev Respir Dis* 1991; 143:119.
24. O'Connor BV, Uden S, Carty TJ, et al.: Inhibitory effect of UK-74505, a potent and specific oral platelet activating factor receptor antagonist on airway and systemic responses to inhaled PAF in humans. *Am J Respir Crit Care Med* 1994; 150:35.
25. Ward PS, Taylor IK, Fuller RW: TxA_2 formation in vivo following inhaled PAF in human asthma. *Thorax* 1990; 45:790.
26. Platshon LF, Kaliner M: The effects of the immunologic release of histamine upon human lung cyclic nucleotide levels and prostaglandin generation. *J Clin Invest* 1978; 62:1113.
27. Curzen N, Rafferty P, Holgate ST: Effects of a cyclo-oxygenase inhibitor, flurbiprofen, and an H_1 histamine receptor antagonist, terfenadine, alone and in combination on allergen induced immediate bronchoconstriction in man. *Thorax* 1987; 42:946.
28. Hulsmann AR, Raatgeep HR, Saxena KF, et al.: Bradykinin-induced contraction of human peripheral airways mediated by both bradykinin β_2 and thromboxane prostanoid receptors. *Am J Respir Crit Care Med* 1994; 150:1012.
29. Garland A, Jordan JE, Ray DW, et al.: Role of eicosanoids in hyperpnea-induced airway responses in guinea pigs. *J Appl Physiol* 1993; 75:2792.
30. Kirby JG, Hargreave FE, Cockcroft DW, O'Byrne PM: Effect of indomethacin on allergen-induced asthmatic responses. *J Appl Physiol* 1989; 66:578.
31. Finnerty JP, Holgate ST: Evidence for the roles of histamine and prostaglandins as mediators in exercise-induced asthma: The inhibitory effect of terfenadine and flurbiprofen alone and in combination. *Eur Respir J* 1990; 3:540.
32. O'Byrne PM, Jones GL: The effect of indomethacin on exercise-induced bronchoconstriction and refractoriness after exercise. *Am Rev Respir Dis* 1986; 134:69.
33. Fujimura M, Sasaki F, Nakatsumi Y, et al.: Effects of a thromboxane synthetase inhibitor and a lipoxygenase inhibitor on bronchial responsiveness to acetylcholine in asthmatic subjects. *Thorax* 1986; 41:955.
34. Fujimura M, Sakamoto S, Matsuda T: Attenuating effect of a thromboxane synthetase inhibitor on bronchial responsiveness to methacholine is specific to bronchial asthma. *Chest* 1990; 98:656.
35. Fujimura M, Sakamoto S, Saito M, et al.: Effect of a thromboxane A_2 receptor antagonist on bronchial hyperresponsiveness to

methacholine in subjects with asthma. *J Allergy Clin Immunol* 1991; 87:23.

36. Beasley RCW, Feathersone RL, et al.: Effect of a thromboxane receptor antagonist on PGD$_2$- and allergen-induced bronchoconstriction. *J Appl Physiol* 1989; 66:1685.

37. Magnussen H, Boerger S, Templin K, Baunack AR: Effects of a thromboxane-receptor antagonist, BAY u 3405, on prostaglandin D$_2$- and exercise-induced bronchoconstriction. *J Allergy Clin Immunol* 1992; 89:1119.

38. Bousquet J, Bodard P, Michel FB: Antihistamines in the treatment of asthma. *Eur Respir J* 1992; 5:1137.

39. Rafferty P, Beasley R, Holgate ST: The contribution of histamine to immediate bronchoconstriction provoked by inhaled allergen and adensoine 5' monophosphate in atopic asthma. *Am Rev Respir Dis* 1987; 136:369.

40. Phillips MJ, Ollier S, Gould C, Davies RJ: Effect of antihistamines and antiallergic drugs on responses to allergen and histamine provocation tests in asthma. *Thorax* 1984; 39:345.

41. Twentyman OP, Ollier S, Holgate ST: The effect of H$_1$-receptor blockade on the development of early- and late-phase bronchoconstriction and increased bronchial responsiveness in allergen-induced asthma. *J Allergy Clin Immunol* 1993; 93:1169.

42. Gong H Jr, Tashkin DP, Dauphinee B, et al.: Effects of oral cetirizine, a selective H$_1$ antagonist, on allergen- and exercise-induced bronchoconstriction in subjects with asthma. *J Allergy Clin Immunol* 1990; 85:632.

43. Wasserfallen J, Leuenberger P, Pecoud A: Effects of cetirizine, a new H$_1$ antihistamine, on the early and late allergic reactions in a bronchial provocation test with allergen. *J Allergy Clin Immunol* 1993; 91:1189.

44. Patel KR: Terfenadine in exercise induced asthma. *Br Med J* 1984; 288:1496.

45. Polosa R, Holgate ST: Comparative airway response to inhaled bradykinin, kallidin, and [des-Arg^9] bradykinin in normal and asthmatic subjects. *Am Rev Respir Dis* 1990; 142:1367.

46. Barnes PJ: Bradykinin and asthma. *Thorax* 1992; 47:979.

47. Fuller RW, Dixon CMS, Cuss FMC, Barnes PJ: Bradykinin-induced bronchoconstriction in humans. *Am Rev Respir Dis* 1987; 135:176.

48. Ichinose M, Nakajima N, Takahashi T, et al.: Protection against bradykinin-induced bronchoconstriction in asthmatic patients by neurokinin receptor antagonist. *Lancet* 1992; 340:1248.

49. Polosa R, Phillips GD, Lai CKW, Holgate ST: Contribution of histamine and prostanoids to bronchoconstriction provoked by inhaled bradykinin in atopic asthma. *Allergy* 1990; 45:174.

50. Baumgarten CR, Lehmkuhl B, Henning R, et al.: Bradykinin and other inflammatory mediators in BAL-fluid from patients with active pulmonary inflammation. *Agents Actions Suppl* 1992; 38:475.

51. Christiansen SC, Proud D, Sarnoff RB, et al.: Elevation of tissue kallikrein and kinin in the airways of asthmatic subjects after endobronchial allergen challenge. *Am Rev Respir Dis* 1992; 145:900.

52. Mansour E, Ahmed A, Cortes A, et al.: Mechanisms of metabisulfite-induced bronchoconstriction: evidence for bradykinin B$_2$-receptor stimulation. *J Appl Physiol* 1992; 72:1831.

53. Soler M, Sielczak M, Abraham WM: A bradykinin-antagonist blocks antigen-induced airway hyperresponsiveness and inflammation in sheep. *Pulm Pharmacol* 1990; 3:9.

54. Ollerenshaw SL, Jarvis D, Sullivan CE, Woolcock AJ: Substance P immunoreactive nerves in airways from asthmatics and nonasthmatics. *Eur Respir J* 1991; 4:673.

55. Solway J, Leff AR: Sensory neuropeptides and airway function. *J Appl Physiol* 1991; 71:2077.

56. Martling C: Sensory nerves containing tachykinins and CGRP in the lower airways. *Acta Physiol Scand Suppl* 1987; 563:1.

57. Lundberg JM, Alving K, Karlsson JA, et al.: Sensory neuropeptide involvement in animal models of airway irritation and of allergen-evoked asthma. *Am Rev Respir Dis* 1991; 143:1429.

58. Saria A, Martling CR, Yan Z, et al.: Release of multiple tachykinins from capsaicin-sensitive sensory nerves in the lung by bradykinin, histamine, dimethylphenyl piperazinium, and vagal nerve stimulation. *Am Rev Respir Dis* 1988; 137:1330.

59. Johnson AR, Erdos EG: Release of histamine from mast cells by vasoactive peptides. *Proc Soc Exp Biol Med* 1973; 142:1252.

60. Solway J, Kao BM, Jordan JE, et al.: Tachykinin receptor antagonists inhibit hyperpnea-induced bronchoconstriction in guinea pigs. *J Clin Invest* 1993; 92:315.

61. Kawano O, Kohrogi H, Yamaguchi T, et al.: Neutral endopeptidase inhibitor potentiates allergic bronchoconstriction in guinea pigs in vivo. *J Appl Physiol* 1993; 75:185.

62. Joos GF, Pauwels RA, Van Der Streten ME: The effect of nedocromil sodium on the bronchoconstrictor effect of neurokinin A in subjects with asthma. *J Allergy Clin Immunol* 1989; 83:663.

63. Lilly CM, Bai TR, Shore SA, et al.: Neuropeptide content of lungs from asthmatic and non-asthmatic patients. *Am J Respir Crit Care Med* 1995; 151:548.

64. Barnes PJ: Effect of nedocromil sodium on airway sensory nerves. *J Allergy Clin Immunol* 1993; 92:182.

65. Henson PM, Barnes PJ, Banks-Schlegel SP: Platelet-activating factor: Role in pulmonary injury and dysfunction and blood abnormalities. *Am Rev Respir Dis* 1992; 145:726.

66. Taylor IK, Ward PS, Taylor GW, et al.: Inhaled PAF stimulates leukotriene and thromboxane A$_2$ production in humans. *J Appl Physiol* 1991; 71:1396.

67. Kidney JC, Ridge SM, Chung KF, Barnes PJ: Inhibition of platelet-activating factor-induced bronchoconstriction by the leukotriene D$_4$ receptor antagonist ICI 204,219. *Am Rev Respir Dis* 1993; 147:215.

68. Hsieh K, Ng C: Increased plasma platelet-activating factor in children with acute asthmatic attacks and decreased in vivo and in vitro production of platelet-activating factor after immunotherapy. *J Allergy Clin Immunol* 1993; 91:650.

69. Kurosawa M, Yamashita T, Kurimoto F: Increased levels of blood platelet-activating factor in bronchial asthma patients with active symptoms. *Allergy* 1994; 49:60.

70. Burgers JA, Bruynzeel PLB, Mengelers HJ, et al.: Occupancy of platelet receptors for platelet-activating factor in asthmatic patients during an allergen-induced bronchoconstrictive reaction. *J Lipid Med* 1993; 7:135.

71. Cuss FM, Dixon CMS, Barnes PJ: Effects of inhaled platelet-activating factor on pulmonary function and bronchial responsiveness in man. *Lancet* 1986; 2:189.

72. Lai CKW, Jenkins JR, Polosa R, Holgate ST: Inhaled PAF fails to induce airway responsiveness to methacholine in normal human subjects. *J Appl Physiol* 1990; 68:919.

73. Hsieh K: Effects of PAF antagonist, BN52021, on the PAF- and methacholine-, and allergen-induced bronchoconstriction in asthmatic children. *Chest* 1991; 99:877.

74. Kuitert LM, Hui KP, Uthayarkumar S, et al.: Effect of the platelet-activating factor antagonist UK-74505 on the early and late response to allergen. *Am Rev Respir Dis* 1993; 147:82.

75. Freitag A, Watson RM, Matsos G, et al.: Effect of a platelet activating factor antagonist, WEB 2086, on allergen induced asthmatic responses. *Thorax* 1993; 48:594.

76. Wilkens JH, Wilkens H, Uffmann J, et al.: Effects of a PAF antagonist on bronchoconstriction and platelet activation during exercise asthma. *Br J Pharmacol* 1990; 29:85.

77. Spence DP, Johnston SL, Calverley PM, et al.: The effect of the

orally active platelet-activating factor antagonist WEB 2086 in the treatment of asthma. *Am J Respir Crit Care Med* 1994; 149:1142.

78. Hozawa S, Haruta Y, Ishioka S, Yamakido M: Effects of a platelet-activating factor antagonist, Y-24180, on bronchial hyperresponsiveness in patients with asthma. *Am J Respir Crit Care Med* 1995; 152:1198.

79. Robinson DS, Bentley AM, Hartnell A, et al.: Activated memory T helper cells in bronchoalveolar lavage fluid from patients with atopic asthma: Relation to asthma symptoms, lung function, and bronchial responsiveness. *Thorax* 1993; 48:26.

80. Alexander AG, Barnes NC, Kay AB: Trial of cyclosporin in corticosteroid-dependent chronic severe asthma. *Lancet* 1992; 339:324.

81. Coffey MJ, Sanders G, Eschenbacher WL, et al.: The role of methotrexate in the management of steroid-dependent asthma. *Chest* 1994; 105:117.

82. Ahmed T, Garrigo J, Danta I: Preventing bronchoconstriction in exercise-induced asthma with inhaled heparin. *N Engl J Med* 1993; 329:90.

83. Ahmed T, Syriste T, Lucio J, et al.: Inhibition of antigen-induced airway and cutaneous responses by heparin: A pharmacologic study. *J Appl Physiol* 1993; 74:1492.

84. Bowler SD, Smith SM, Lavercombe PS: Heparin inhibits the immediate response to antigen in the skin and lungs of allergic subjects. *Am Rev Respir Dis* 1993; 147:160.

85. Calderon E, Lockey RF: A possible role for adhesion molecules in asthma. *J Allergy Clin Immunol* 1992; 90:852.

86. Wegner CD, Gundell RH, Reilly P, et al.: Intercellular adhesion molecules-1 (ICAM-1) in the pathogenesis of asthma. *Science* 1990; 247:456.

87. Broide DH, Lotz M, Coumo AJ, et al.: Cytokines in symptomatic asthma airways. *J Allergy Clin Immunol* 1992; 89:958.

88. Robinson DH, Ying S, Bentley AM, et al.: Relationships among numbers of bronchoalveolar lavage cells expressing messenger ribonucleic acid for cytokines, asthma symptoms, and airway methacholine responsiveness in atopic asthma. *J Allergy Clin Immunol* 1993; 929:397.

89. Robinson DH, Durham SR, Kay AB: Cytokines in asthma. *Thorax* 1993; 48:845.

90. Lansing MW, Mansour E, Ahmed A, et al.: Lipid mediators contribute to oxygen-radical-induced airway responses in sheep. *Am Rev Respir Dis* 1991; 144:1291.

91. Matsui S, Jones GL, Woolley MJ, et al.: The effect of antioxidants on ozone-induced airway hyperresponsiveness in dogs. *Am Rev Respir Dis* 1991; 144:1287.

92. Linn WS, Shamoo DA, Anderson KR, et al.: Effects of prolonged, repeated exposure to ozone, sulfuric acid, and their combination in healthy and asthmatic volunteers. *Am J Resp Crit Care Med* 1994; 150:431.

93. Owen S, Pearson D, Suarez-Mendez V, et al.: Evidence of free-radical activity in asthma. *N Engl J Med* 1991; 325:586.

94. Lansing MW, Ahmed A, Cortes A, et al.: Oxygen radicals contribute to antigen-induced airway hyperresponsiveness in conscious sheep. *Am Rev Respir Dis* 1993; 147:321.

95. Griswold DE, Webb EF, Breton J, et al.: Effect of selective phosphodiesterase type IV inhibitor, rolipram, on fluid and cellular phases of inflammatory response. *Inflammation* 1993; 17:333.

96. Newsholme SJ, Schwartz L: cAMP-specific phosphodiesterase inhibitor, rolipram, reduces eosinophil infiltration evoked by leukotrienes or by histamine in guinea pig conjunctiva. *Inflammation* 1993; 17:25.

97. Cortijo J, Bou J, Beleta J, et al.: Investigation into the role of phosphodiesterase IV in bronchorelaxation, including studies with human bronchus. *Br J Pharmacol* 1993; 108:562.

98. Howell RE, Sickels BD, Woeppel SL: Pulmonary antiallergic and bronchodilator effects of isozyme-selective phosphodiesterase inhibitors in guinea pigs. *J Pharmacol Exp Ther* 1993; 264:609.

99. Whelan CJ, Johnson M, Vardey CJ: Comparison of anti-inflammatory properties of formoterol, salbutamol and salmeterol in guinea pig skin and lung. *Br J Pharmacol* 1993; 110:613.

100. Whelan CJ, Johnson M: Inhibition by salmeterol of increased vascular permeability and granulocyte accumulation in guinea pig lung and skin. *Br J Pharmacol* 1992; 105:831.

Chapter 82
VOCAL CORD DYSFUNCTION MIMICKING ASTHMA
BERNARD MARSH AND ROBERT NACLERIO

Case Report

Discussion

Diagnosis

Management

Summary

Intermittent wheezing and dyspnea, while characteristic of asthma, may result from a poorly understood form of vocal cord dysfunction. This condition, characterized by upper airway obstruction with varying degrees of stridor and wheezing, typically is misidentified as bronchial asthma. Furthermore, the symptoms, which can be quite severe, fail to respond to bronchodilators or steroids, sometimes leading to emergency airway intervention. This condition represents a psychiatric disorder in which a correct diagnosis not only leads to symptom relief but spares the patient from inappropriate therapy. The episodic and variable wheezing of this disorder helps to differentiate it from tracheal tumors, stenosis, and other anatomic airway obstructions. This disorder differs from others discussed in this text in that a correct diagnosis leads to decreased pharmacotherapy.

Case Report

A 15-year-old boy with a history of asthma was hospitalized for a severe acute attack.[1] He had a history of episodic wheezing and had required hospitalization once or twice per year for several years. The current episode could not be controlled by his usual medications or aggressive emergency room management. He was admitted to the hospital and given intravenous aminophylline and hydrocortisone in addition to nebulized β-adrenergic drugs. The wheezing improved some initially, but then reached a plateau. Because of the refractory nature of his wheezing, evaluation for other causes of wheezing was undertaken. At no time during his hospitalization did he develop hypercarbia or significant hypoxemia. The results of pulmonary function studies indicated combined expiratory obstruction and an extrathoracic upper airway obstruction (Fig. 82-1). The chest radiograph showed minimal bibasilar peribronchial thickening. Physical examination demonstrated expiratory wheezing associated

with mild inspiratory stridor both were reduced dramatically when the patient was asleep but recurred immediately on awakening. The wheezing was localized to the extrathoracic trachea. Fiberoptic laryngoscopy performed under local anesthesia showed adduction of the vocal cords during expiration and minimal abduction with inspiration. When the patient took a breath while being distracted his vocal cords momentarily functioned normally with relief from wheezing. Psychiatric consultation discovered a history of psychological dysfunction and recent distress about the departure of his older brother to the army. Concurrent with the successful treatment of his depression with a tricyclic antidepressant and psychotherapy, the patient's pulmonary status improved substantially. In the 10 years since this episode, he has required no further hospitalization for respiratory distress but continues to require bronchodilator therapy for asthma.

Discussion

During the past 20 years, considerable attention has been focused on obstructive airways disorders that have no apparent organic basis. Terms applied to such disorders include *episodic laryngeal dyskinesia, variable vocal cord dysfunction, paradoxical vocal cord dysfunction, psychogenic laryngeal dyskinesia, factitious asthma, emotional laryngeal wheezing, Munchausen's stridor,* and *vocal cord dysfunction presenting as asthma.* Some patients present with a history of chronic asthma, while others do not. Most reports of episodic airways distress describe patients with multiple hospital admissions and unsatisfactory response to maximal bronchodilator therapy. Symptoms vary from purely inspiratory stridor to expiratory wheezing or some combination of both. The typical patient is a young woman. Male patients and patients ranging in age from childhood to middle age have

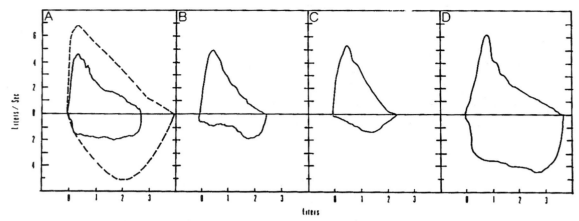

FIGURE 82-1 Flow-volume curves obtained during patient's hospital course. (*A–C*) Examples of variable extrathoracic airway obstruction. The dashed curve in *A* depicts a normal inspiratory (below baseline) and expiratory (above baseline) flow-volume curve. (*D*) Improvement of extrathoracic obstruction but persistence of a small airway obstruction after intensive therapy.

been described, however. Other characteristics include above average intelligence and a connection with the medical profession. There is often a history of psychiatric care or stress factors and interpersonal difficulties. Symptoms result from inappropriate vocal cord activity during any phase of the respiratory cycle. Vocal cord function is under both voluntary motor and respiratory control, but a patient with this disorder seems unaware of his or her role in producing the obstruction.

Normally, the glottis opens during inspiration and narrows slightly on expiration (Figs. 82-2, 82-3). In asthmatics, some have observed that glottal width appears to adjust in parallel with changes in caliber of the intrapulmonary airways. The greater the reduction in FEV_1, the more the glottis narrows during expiration. Some data suggest that there also may be an inspiratory obstruction, perhaps providing airflow regulation in and out of the lungs in the patient with asthma. Nevertheless, such "regulatory changes" should rarely be so marked as to obscure the diagnosis of a psychogenic disorder.

Diagnosis

The diagnosis of vocal cord dysfunction should be suspected when a patient who is presumed to have asthma does not respond to standard therapy and when the symptoms are dramatically *reduced* during sleep. Auscultation demonstrates wheezing/stridor localized to the neck and poorly audible in the lower lung fields. Ultrasonography has been used as a noninvasive screening tool, especially in children, but the diagnosis must be established by fiberoptic laryngoscopy during an attack. The findings from this examination will be normal between attacks. Typical findings include adducted vocal cords that appear similar to those in bilateral vocal cord paralysis (Fig. 82-4). A considerable period of observation may be required in some individuals before the diagnosis can be confirmed. The vocal cords may seem to adduct paradoxically during inspiration while separating only slightly during expiration. The false cords function normally. Often the severity of the dyspnea accompanying an episode causes a sense of urgency to intervene. Some

FIGURE 82-2 Glottis open during inspiration.

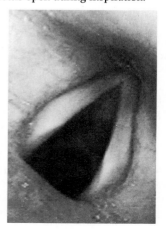

FIGURE 82-3 Glottis slightly closed during expiration.

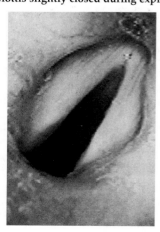

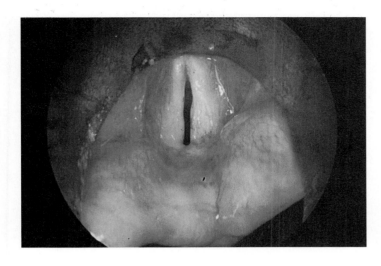

FIGURE 82-4 Endoscopic view of the glottis during inspiration in a patient with posterior glottic fibrosis. This condition simulates bilateral vocal cord paralysis, arytenoid fixation, and some cases of psychogenic dysfunction.

patients have been intubated, and others have undergone a tracheotomy before the diagnosis was established. Curiously, the patient often seems less concerned about the condition than his medical attendants. The voice varies from strained and high-pitched to relatively normal. A laryngologist must differentiate this condition from both vocal cord paralysis and fixation, which it simulates and which require very different interventions. The larynx should be visualized without sedation or anesthesia to determine whether it functions normally during any part of the respiratory cycle. Often the laryngologist must resort to distraction techniques to achieve a correct diagnosis. The patient can be asked to take a deep breath and then count from 100 backwards by threes as far as possible before taking another breath. A momentary inspiratory vocal cord abduction may be seen as the patient inspires to continue the task. Such an abduction may not be a completely normal excursion, but it is sufficient to rule out arytenoid fixation and to establish that there is an intact neuromotor system. It is also helpful to observe the response of the larynx to cough and to panting. A video recording of this examination proves helpful in communicating the findings to colleagues, the patient, and the family.

Electromyogram of the larynx can determine the functional state of nervous innervation. Flow-volume loops are abnormal, with evidence of a variable extrathoracic airway obstruction that is manifested as a flat inspiratory loop with variable expiratory airflow limitation. Chest radiographs are normal, lacking the classic hyperinflation typical of asthmatic patients. Arterial blood gases are frequently normal, but hypoxia sometimes is seen.

Management

The acute management of these patients may be difficult. Some patients appear so dyspneic that airway intervention precedes a firm diagnosis. In most cases, a brief period of investigation should suffice to confirm the diagnosis. The dysfunction sometimes can be interrupted by anesthetizing the pharynx with lidocaine. How this intervention functions is unknown. Other techniques include the use of sedation (midazolam or a small dose of intravenous propofol), breathing a gas mixture of 70 percent helium and 30 percent oxygen, and autosuggestion. Psychiatric consultation should be obtained early. Psychiatric conditions associated with this disorder include conversion disorders, depression, personality disorders, and post-traumatic stress disorder. There also appears to be an increased incidence of childhood sexual abuse. Speech therapists have been helpful in the management of some cases.

Summary

Psychogenic upper airway obstruction is a poorly recognized cause of dyspnea and wheezing that mimics asthma or an upper airway obstruction. It represents a spectrum of diseases, which some prefer to designate "functional upper airway obstruction," although it may occur in patients with asthma. When wheezing is refractory to bronchodilator therapy, especially in an adolescent, the possibility of laryngeal dysfunction should be entertained. The diagnosis may be difficult, but it can usually be confirmed by typical physical findings and laboratory results. A thorough understanding of laryngeal function assists in correctly interpreting the multiple manifestations of this disorder. Prompt psychiatric care is the cornerstone of therapy.

References

1. Barnes SD, Grob CS, et al.: Psychogenic upper airway obstruction presenting as refractory wheezing. *J Pediatr* 1986; 109;1067.
2. Christopher KL, Wood RP, Echert RC, et al.: Vocal cord dysfunction presenting as asthma. *N Engl J Med* 1983; 308:1566.
3. Selner JC, Staudenmayer H, Koephe JW, et al.: Vocal cord dysfunction: the importance of psychologic factors and provocation challenge testing. *J Allergy Clin Immunol* 1987; 79:726.
4. Tomares SM, Flotte TR, Tunkel DE, et al.: Real time laryngoscopy with olfactory challenge for diagnosis of psychogenic stridor. *Ped Pulm* 1993; 16:259.

TREATMENT OF CHRONIC OBSTRUCTIVE PULMONARY DISEASE AND BRONCHIECTASIS

Chapter 83

DIAGNOSIS OF CHRONIC OBSTRUCTIVE PULMONARY DISEASE

NEIL S. CHERNIACK AND M. D. ALTOSE

Chronic obstructive pulmonary disease (COPD; also called *chronic obstructive lung disease* and *chronic airway obstruction*) is a disease spectrum that results in a progressive reduction in expiratory flow rates.[1-4] Ultimately, the pathologic processes that underlie the disease impair lung function and blood oxygenation. Unlike asthma, which produces episodes of airway obstruction that resolve without causing permanent damage, a significant portion of the obstruction in COPD cannot be reversed even by intensive treatment. Although there is no cure, the progress of COPD can be slowed if the patient stops smoking, and the symptoms of the condition can be relieved by a wide variety of measures, including the use of bronchodilators or anti-inflammatory agents, and, when necessary, inhalation of increased concentrations of oxygen.[4-6]

At one end of the spectrum of COPD are patients in whom the disease primarily affects the airways, causing chronic bronchitis with increased cough and sputum production. Although not all patients with bronchitis develop obstruction, it occurs when secretions fill the airways so as to hinder the egress of air or when the inflammatory process produces actual narrowing of the airways.[7] At the other end of the spectrum are patients with emphysema, in which the disease leads to destruction of the alveolar walls and dilation of the airway spaces beyond the terminal bronchioles.[5] This loss of lung tissues diminishes the elastic pull of the tissues on the airway, allowing the airways to collapse during expiration. In most patients with COPD, the disease affects both the airways and the lung parenchyma in varying degrees.

Cigarette smoking is the chief cause of COPD, but other injurious agents in the inhaled air can contribute to the disease and maintain a persisting inflammation in which leukocyte and macrophage release of oxidants and proteases damage respiratory tissues.[8–14] Abnormalities in the mechanisms that protect the lung and airways against injury (the immune system, the mucociliary escalator, and antiproteases) all increase susceptibility to COPD.[15–21] COPD is also more common in individuals who had severe lung diseases in childhood, and it can occur in families.[9,22,23] Most patients with COPD are > 40 years old, reflecting the time required for the inflammatory process to produce tissue damage.[24] COPD is more common in men, but it is common in women as well.[24]

Pathophysiologic Basis for the Diagnosis of COPD

A diagnosis of COPD depends on the objective demonstration of airway obstruction by physiologic measurement.[4,25–27] A number of different techniques can be used to determine whether the resistance to airflow is increased. Most often, spirometry is employed; in COPD, a reduction of the FEV_1 (forced expiratory volume in 1 s) occurs with little reduction in the forced vital capacity (FVC).[28] In normal individuals, the FEV_1 is $\geq$ 80 percent of the FVC. In those with COPD, it is less. In a sense, the diagnosis of COPD is similar to the diagnosis of hypertension in requiring the demonstration of a specific physiologic abnormality. Like high blood pressure, airflow reduction indicates the presence of a process that can lead to disabling and even life-threatening changes in function.

Another essential criterion for the diagnosis of COPD is that the airflow reduction be permanent.[5,25,29] Hence, the diagnosis is made most confidently when repeated physiologic measurements demonstrate the airflow abnormality even after the best treatment efforts.

Airway obstruction frequently leads to overinflation of the lungs.[24,30] Hyperinflation shortens the resting length of the inspiratory muscles, decreasing the force they can generate when they contract.[12] In addition, hyperinflation flattens the diaphragm and changes the direction of the force vectors produced by diaphragm contraction, reducing the ability of the diaphragm to lift the chest wall.[12,31–34] As a result, the accessory respiratory muscles are brought into play and are used even during quiet breathing. Both the greater airway resistance and the diminished capacity of the inspiratory muscles increase the work of breathing and its O_2 cost.[35–38] Dyspnea, often an incapacitating symptom of COPD, arises from the increasing inability of the respiratory muscles to satisfy breathing demands despite increased efforts.

Neither bronchitis nor emphysema affects all parts of the respiratory system uniformly. As COPD becomes more severe, the mechanisms that help maintain the balanced distribution of ventilation to perfusion in the lung fail.[12,39,40] A greater fraction of the inspired air is wasted, not reaching the gas-exchanging surfaces in the alveoli and filling the dead space instead. More of the pulmonary arterial blood traverses the lung without being exposed to the fresh inspired air, so the proportion of deoxygenated blood rises. As a consequence, hypoxia and hypercapnia develop and worsen. Ultimately, pressures in the pulmonary circulation rise, leading to right-sided heart failure.[41] The eventual consequence is malfunction in multiple organ systems.

Because of the many factors that can worsen airway obstruction, and because patients present in different stages of the natural history of the disease, the history and physical examination of the patient and selected additional tests can provide useful information concerning potentially helpful therapeutic measures. Therefore, the evaluation of patients with COPD should be directed to the following objectives:

1. Assessing the severity of the disease and hence the prognosis and the need for treatment
2. Identifying factors that exacerbate airflow obstruction and that could be reversible, such as allergic or infectious factors, as well as factors that decrease the ability of the respiratory system to compensate for the obstructions, such as respiratory muscle weakness, muscle fatigue, or decreased sensitivity to changes in P_{O_2} or PC_{O_2} in the arterial blood
3. Uncovering systemic complications caused by hypoxia and/or hypercapnia that may be treatable

Methods of Assessing Patients with COPD

HISTORY

The value of the history of COPD is difficult to overestimate. It frequently provides the only clues to potentially remediable conditions or to complications that should be evaluated and treated further. Almost every patient with COPD has smoked cigarettes, and if there is no history of cigarette smoking, conditions other than COPD should be sought.[8–10,17] Passive inhalation of cigarette smoke rarely if ever causes COPD. The greater the pack-years of smoking, the greater the risk of COPD, but accurate histories of cigarette smoking are difficult to obtain. Patients often stop smoking because they have developed respiratory symptoms, and it is useful to ask the reasons for quitting smoking.

Dyspnea is the most common symptom in patients with COPD, correlating roughly with the degree of obstruction.[42–44] However, shortness of breath is common with other diseases as well. COPD-associated dyspnea may occur only during exertion; unlike the dyspnea associated with exercise-induced asthma, it will improve rather than worsen in the postexercise period. COPD-associated dyspnea rarely wakens the patient from sleep, as does the dyspnea caused by obstruction in sleep apnea or the breathlessness occasioned by nocturnal asthma. It is not improved by sitting up, thus differing from the shortness of breath of congestive heart failure. However, the patient with COPD may adopt certain characteristic positions to relieve breathing, such as leaning forward with arms supported, a posture that improves the force the accessory respiratory muscles of the neck can produce.[45]

The severity of the disease and the need for treatment can be gauged by determining the activities of daily living that bring on dyspnea. An accurate determination of the level of dyspnea before treatment is started is useful in evaluating the effects of medications.[44] Dyspnea may limit the ability of the patient to maintain good nutrition and may lead to other complications such as muscle weakness and atrophy because it limits activity.[37,46] Weight loss is not uncommon in COPD.

Cough is another common symptom in COPD and is often productive. Purulent-appearing sputum can be due to infections or allergies (eosinophilia), which can be treated.[47,48] Exertion can trigger coughing in COPD, or increased coughing may be related to meals, suggesting that gastroesophageal reflux is the problem. In persons with COPD, colds frequently settle into the chest and cause prolonged periods of productive cough.

Chest pain is uncommon in COPD except after coughing. Some patients describe a burning substernal sensation, which can be caused by gastroesophageal reflux and occasionally by severe bronchitis.[49–51] Wheezing or noisy breathing may be present in COPD patients and may be particularly prominent during exposure to cold air.

Some patients with COPD have breathing disturbances during sleep and obstructive apneas, which significantly worsen arterial blood O_2 saturation.[52–54]

It is most important to obtain a good history of the progression of the disease. Are symptoms about the same or have they worsened over the years? What medications have been taken? Have there been hospitalizations for respiratory conditions? Severe and repeated respiratory infections may indicate the presence of chronic sinusitis, bronchiectasis, or some problem in the immune system. Securing previous chest radiographs or results of previous pulmonary function tests is important. Valuable information can be obtained by questions about potential allergens in the home and exposure to sick friends, and by a history of travel experiences.

Family histories can be important in detecting the rare cases of familial COPD and in distinguishing COPD from cystic fibrosis, which can cause symptoms resembling those of COPD.[22,55,56]

PHYSICAL EXAMINATION

Physical evidence of airway obstruction, hyperinflation, ineffectual respiratory muscle function, and right-sided heart failure all can be present in patients with COPD. Even when the COPD patient breathes quietly, expiration may be prolonged (more than twice the length of respiration), and wheezing may be detected.[57] However, breath sounds during quiet breathing may be difficult to hear because of lung hyperinflation.[58] More often, wheezing can be produced by having the patient perform maximal inspirations and expirations or simulate a maximal voluntary ventilation test (by breathing as rapidly and as deeply as possible for 10 to 15 s).[28] When expiratory obstruction is severe, active contraction of the abdominal and/or accessory muscles is observed.[38] Stridor and other signs of inspiratory obstruction are not part of COPD; they may indicate the presence of complicating diseases, or they may be sequelae of previous tracheal intubations for respiratory failure.

Pursed-lips breathing is also a sign of severe airway obstruction.[59] Its physiologic effects are not well understood. It slows the usual tachypneic breathing of COPD, and it may help keep the airways open during expiration by producing a back-pressure to counter the increased pleural pressure, thereby evening out the distribution of ventilation.

Because of hyperinflation, the diaphragm may move less than the usual 5 to 6 cm during maximal inspiration and expiration. In addition, because the flattened diaphragm is less able to expand the rib cage, the lower ribs may move inward rather than outward during inspiration (Hoover's sign).[50] Hyperinflation also can cause tracheal tug and decreases the distance between the cricoid cartilage and the sternal notch to less than three finger-breadths.

The greater negative pleural pressure required to further expand the overinflated lungs in patients with COPD is transmitted to the left ventricle, decreasing the difference between left ventricular pressure and the pressure in extrathoracic arteries. Hence, pulsus paradoxus, a decrease in systolic pressure by 10 mmHg or more during inspiration, may be present in COPD.

When the thoracic wall is overexpanded, the inspiratory muscles are shortened and cannot generate as much force as usual, which changes the pattern of chest wall movement during breathing. Such changes may arise from ineffectual diaphragm contractions. For example, the abdomen may move toward rather than away from the spine during inspiration, indicating greater use of the intercostal muscles.[38] Because the weakened inspiratory muscles are more likely to fatigue, the muscles of respiration in the neck tend to become prominent, particularly when the FEV_1 decreases to < 1 liter.[31,35]

Oxygenation eventually becomes subnormal in COPD, leading to cyanosis. Right-sided heart failure (cor pulmonale) is likely to occur when the arterial O_2 saturation decreases to < 60 percent.[41] With right-sided heart failure, the jugular venous pulse may be visible more than 3 cm above the sternal notch when the head and thorax are 45 degrees from the horizontal. Peripheral edema may be obvious. The second pulmonic heart sound becomes prominent, and there may be a right ventricular gallop.[60] Murmurs of tricuspid or pulmonary insufficiency can be discerned. Physical examination may not detect evidence of cardiac enlargement because lung hyperinflation decreases the area of dullness to percussion, and the point of maximal cardiac impulse (PMI) may be obscured. Sometimes the PMI is most prominent in the subxiphoid area even in the absence of right-sided heart failure, and the heart sounds are best heard in this area.

It is important to search for physical signs of diseases that may complicate COPD, such as signs of thromboembolic disease or clubbing or other evidence of pulmonary osteoarthropathy. Inguinal hernias are common in COPD patients. All the adverse complications of smoking can be present.

PULMONARY FUNCTION TESTS

In COPD, an increase in airway resistance always can be demonstrated by appropriate tests of pulmonary function. If measurements show that this increase is not present, then some other condition accounts for the patient's symptoms. Airway resistance is the ratio of the change in airway pressure to the change in airflow. The resistance of the airways is related inversely to their cross-sectional area, and this quantity in turn depends on lung volume.[28,61,62] At total inspiratory capacity, the airways are dilated maximally by the stretched elastic tissue of the lung parenchyma; airway caliber decreases as lung volume diminishes.

It is difficult to use the usual measurement of airway resistance in a body plethysmograph to separate the resistance to flow offered by the airways from that caused by the viscosity of lung or chest wall tissues.[61,62] Complicated tests are required, and normal values are based on a relatively small number of subjects and show a wide scatter. In most instances, therefore, measurements of airway resistance are not used to diagnose COPD.[28,63] More reliable, reproducible results can be obtained by indirectly evaluating resistance during maximal expiratory efforts. The measurement most frequently used is the FEV_1, the volume of air that can be expired in 1 s with maximal effort.[4] This test, which can be simply and quickly performed, is supported by a very large number of normal values, which show a relatively small variation around the mean (coefficient of variation $\pm$ 20 percent). Patients with COPD will have an FEV_1 less than 80 percent of predicted normal values and will require a long time to expire fully during a maximal inhalation (more than 6 s). The FEV_1 is used frequently to grade the severity of the obstruction. An $FEV_1 < 35$ percent of the predicted normal value indicates severe obstructive disease.[25]

Unlike patients with asthma, COPD patients will not respond to treatment with an appreciable improvement in FEV_1. If the spirogram is recorded after the administration of bronchodilators, the increase in FEV_1 will be < 15 percent. Better information about the severity of airway obstruction and its reversibility can be obtained by making several serial FEV_1 measurements as obstruction is treated.

A number of factors besides airway resistance influence the FEV_1. For example, as it is essential that maximal effort be exerted, the test depends on patient cooperation. The first 20 to 30 percent of the volume expired in 1 s is effort-dependent.[39,40] As lung volume decreases during exhalation, the airways are compressed, and flow rates become independent of effort. Thus, it is useful to examine the entire spirogram. If volume on the vertical axis is plotted against time on the horizontal, the expiratory portion of the spirogram characteristically will show a downward convexity in patients with COPD. Measurement of FEV_1 will not detect patients whose vital capacity is at the upper limits of normal and those with very mild disease. Because of the lack of effort-dependence, the flow at low lung volumes may offer a more sensitive way to measure airway obstruction from the FEV_1, but normal values are less well established.

If airflow is directly measured during a forced vital capacity maneuver, both inspiratory and expiratory flow can be plotted against volume (flow-volume curve), and upper airway obstruction can be detected by decreases in inspiratory flow.[64,65] Usually the airflow midway through a forced expiration is less than airflow midway through inspiration. A reversal of this ratio suggests obstruction in the upper airways.

Respiratory muscle weakness will diminish the vital capacity as well as flow rates. Any pulmonary disease that decreases the vital capacity also will decrease the FEV_1, but in COPD, the FEV_1 will be < 80 percent of the vital capacity.[66]

Other tests help in confirming the diagnosis of COPD and grading the severity of the disease, but they do not substitute for the spirogram. Characteristically, patients with COPD have an increased residual volume and an enlarged functional residual capacity, and total lung capacity is greater than normal. Lung compliance is normal, and diffusing capacity is either normal or mildly reduced.[67,68] Arterial blood gas measurements show hypoxemia and a widened alveolar-arterial O_2 gradient, and with severe disease there may be hypercapnia.[69,70]

Measurements of respiratory muscle strength are useful in patients with COPD, because hyperinflation and malnutrition may reduce the maximal force that can be generated. Low potassium or phosphate levels are possible causes of muscle weakness in COPD.[34,71–73]

Patients with decreased sensitivity to changes in O_2 and CO_2 levels may not be able to compensate well for the increased load on the respiratory muscles caused by airway obstruction.[29,69,70,74,76,78] In some cases, poor chemosensitivity is familial; in other cases, it is caused by a metabolic alkalosis produced by treatment with diuretics or by the sleep apnea syndrome. Ventilation is a poor index of respiration output in COPD because respiratory mechanics are impaired. Thus, tests of chemosensitivity in COPD patients frequently use occlusion pressure or even the electrical activity of the respiratory muscles as a measure of the response to changes in respiratory gases.[29,69,77]

Finally, in some patients, exercise testing can be useful in the design of rehabilitation programs, which can reduce both the lactic acidosis and the ventilation levels produced by exertion.[80,81] Arterial O_2 saturation may decrease during exercise in COPD patients, unlike normal individuals, and pulmonary artery pressures may increase inordinately as cardiac output increases with exertion.[80,81]

IMAGING

Imaging of the chest is extremely valuable in detecting most lung diseases (usually more so than the physical examination), but it is much less important in the diagnosis of COPD.[82]

Typically the chest radiograph in COPD patients shows some or all of the following signs: a low, flattened diaphragm, an increased retrosternal airspace (greater than 4.5 cm), and a vertical heart.[83,84] In panlobular emphysema, bullae may be present and vascular markings are decreased, but in centrilobular emphysema, vascular markings may be more prominent than normal. When there is significant bronchitis, bronchial markings may be enhanced. At times, some degree of fibrosis complicates COPD, causing cystic changes on radiographs; this finding also can occur with bronchiectasis. As pulmonary vascular pressure increases, blood vessels become prominent in the hila and may need to be distinguished from tumor masses. Computed tomography (CT) or magnetic resonance imaging (MRI) may be useful in this regard.[85–87] CT also is useful in delineating bullae.[88,89] In emphysema, the usual density gradient observable in CT scans may disappear. Thin-section CT scans can help in the detection of bronchiectasis.

Radioisotope scans may be helpful not just in localizing pulmonary abnormalities but in the evaluation of lung function as well.[90] Inhalation of radioactive gases or particles and injection of the same materials can be useful in assessing the unevenness of ventilation and perfusion. The time required to expel radioactive foreign gases and particles also can serve as an index of the evenness and efficiency of ventilation. On the other hand, because uneven ventilation and perfusion are so common in COPD, they can make the detection of important complications of COPD such as pulmonary embolism more difficult and necessitate angiography.

OTHER DIAGNOSTIC PROCEDURES

Clues to the presence of remediable components of COPD or to complications can be obtained from a wide range of noninvasive and invasive diagnostic procedures, which are briefly summarized here.

Erythrocytosis can be a result of hypoxemia and occasionally requires treatment. Leukocytosis suggests infection, and eosinophilia the presence of allergies. Elastic fibers in the sputum suggest an infection with tissue destruction. Research studies have shown increases in the concentrations of lysozymes, meyeloperoxidase, and lactoferrin in the sputum of patients with pulmonary infection.[48,91,92]

Microscopic examination and culture of the sputum is useful.[48,91] The most frequently encountered bacterial organisms in COPD are *Hemophilus*, *Streptococcus pneumoniae*, *Klebsiella*, *Staphylococcus*, and *Moraxella*, but many infections in COPD are viral. Bronchoscopy using the protected brush technique or bronchoalveolar lavage may be necessary in some patients with pneumonic processes recalcitrant to treatment to determine the cause of the infection. Eosinophils as well as neutrophils may give the sputum a purulent appearance. The presence of Charcot-Leyden crystals or Curschmann's spirals supports the diagnosis of asthma. Many patients with COPD show exaggerated airway responses when challenged with histamine aerosols, but autonomic control of the airways is normal in COPD, unlike asthma.[92] In patients with recurrent infections, an otorhinolaryngologic examination is useful, as well as sinus radiographs. Measurements of serum immunoglobulins should also be made. Defects in IgG subgroups and in IgA have been implicated in lung infections. Recent studies suggest that H_2O_2 or NO are detectable in the expired air in patients with infected lungs, but this is still an experimental procedure.[93,94]

Determination of serum α_1-antitrypsin concentrations or of chloride concentrations in the sweat can assist in the diagnosis and treatment of nonsmoking patients who develop COPD. Low concentrations of prealbumin may confirm the presence of malnutrition.[15,95–98]

The electrocardiogram in COPD typically shows exaggerated P waves in leads II, III, and aV_F; prominent T_a waves in the same leads; and a vertical heart with counterclockwise rotation.[99–101] Increased pulmonary vascular pressures may cause electrocardiographic signs of right ventricular hypertrophy and necessitate a more extensive evaluation with catheterization of the heart to evaluate the pulmonary circulation. The right ventricular ejection fraction is often decreased in patients with COPD because of the increased pulmonary afterload. This change may become obvious only during exercise that causes the ejection fraction to increase at least 5 percent.

Finally, in some patients, it may be useful to quantify dyspnea objectively at rest and at different levels of exercise to better evaluate the effects of new therapeutic options. This can be done using Borg or visual analog scales.[44]

Clinical Patterns of COPD

Attempts have been made to subdivide patients with COPD according to clinical patterns of presentation.[102] Two distinctive types of patients with COPD have been described—the "blue bloater" (type B) and the "pink puffer" (type A).[103] The blue bloater is cyanotic and develops peripheral edema (bloating from right-sided heart failure). These patients were believed to have depressed chemosensitivity and were said to rarely complain of shortness of breath. Bronchitis or centrilobular emphysema was regarded as the underlying pathology. On the other hand, the pink puffer has labored breathing and complains of severe dyspnea (puffing). Panacinar emphysema was believed to be the underlying pathology in the pink puffer. It was believed that ventilation and perfusion remained well matched in these patients, allowing them to preserve normal levels of arterial O_2 saturation (and thus remain "pink"). While occasional patients exhibit the features of one of these two types, they are exceedingly rare as pure forms of the disease.

Early Diagnosis and Differential Diagnosis of COPD

Since the damage caused by COPD is irreversable largely, repeated attempts have been made to detect patients with minimal COPD and to identify patients who are at high risk for severe complications if COPD develops.[104] Efforts to achieve early detection have centered on identifying disease in the small airways. Because the cross-sectional area of the airways is much greater at the level of the terminal bronchioles than at the central bronchi, considerable inflammation may be present in the small airways before there is a noticeable change in either airway resistance or the FEV_1.[105] Several ingenious tests to diagnose small airway disease have been developed under the assumption that the physiologic abnormalities occurring in smokers are early manifestations of COPD.[106] These tests, which aim at detecting subtle abnormalities in the distribution of the inspired air, include the closing volume and measurements of the frequency dependence of dynamic compliance. Other tests attempt to detect early narrowing of the terminal airways, using, for example, the effect of gases of different density on the flow-volume curve (e.g., volume at isoflow).[107,108]

Although these tests have expanded substantially our understanding of lung physiology, they have not proved useful clinically. Almost all smokers show abnormal findings with these tests, yet most do not develop frank COPD.[109]

Some individuals seem unusually susceptible to the complications of COPD, developing hypercapnia with only relatively mild abnormalities in lung function. It has been suggested that these individuals have decreased sensitivity to hypoxia and/or hypercapnia and fail to increase their ventilation normally.[69,74–77] Most patients with COPD seem to breathe at greater than normal levels though a smaller group does not.[69] Members of the latter subgroup often have reduced respiratory responses to CO_2 and low arterial blood levels of oxygen.[44,69] In addition, some patients with COPD seem to have a diminished perception of added respiratory loads.[44] It has been suggested that chemosensitivity and load perception be examined in patients who show abnormalities in gas exchange that are disproportionate to the decreases in FEV_1. In most patients with COPD, hypercapnia, for example, does not occur until the FEV_1 is less than 1 L.

DIFFERENTIAL DIAGNOSIS

None of the symptoms of COPD are unique to the disease. It is often quite difficult to separate patients with asthma from those with COPD, because infection often complicates asthma, and asthmatics may smoke. Similarly, some patients with COPD have an allergic component that complicates their disease.

Since COPD is relatively common, many patients with mild COPD have other serious illnesses. Hypoxemia should not be attributed to COPD when the changes in FEV_1 are only moderate; other possible causes of hypoxemia, such as intracardiac or intrapulmonary shunts, should be sought. Neurologic disease of the central nervous system, peripheral neuropathies, and primary muscle disease can produce hypoxia and hypercapnia. Finally, COPD that produces blood gas abnormalities may present as a neurologic or psychiatric disease. Peptic ulcer is common in patients with COPD.[51] The burning substernal pain of bronchitis can be confused with cardiac angina.

Summary

The diagnosis of COPD depends on physical measurements that demonstrate increased airway resistance that cannot be reversed completely by treatment. The history, the physical examination, and chest imaging may suggest COPD, but the diagnosis is not established without physiologic measurements. The evaluation of the COPD patient should be directed to finding factors that can be treated. While smoking cessation is the most important measure to be taken, treatment of allergies, infections, and poor nutrition, as well as regimens to improve muscle strength and endurance can substantially improve the life of COPD patients.

References

1. Ciba Guest Symposium: Terminology, definitions and classifications of chronic pulmonary emphysema and related conditions. *Thorax* 1959; 14:286.
2. Fletcher C, Pride N: Definitions of emphysema, chronic bronchitis, asthma, and airflow obstruction; 25 years from the CIBA Symposium. *Thorax* 1984; 89:81.
3. Cherniack NS, Altose MD: Mechanisms of dyspnea. *Clin Chest Med* 1987; 8:297.
4. American Thoracic Society: Standards for the diagnosis and care of patients with chronic obstructive pulmonary disease (COPD) and asthma. *Am Rev Respir Dis* 1987; 136:225.
5. Thurlbeck W: Aspects of chronic airflow obstruction. *Chest* 1977; 72:341.
6. Brown CA, Crombie IK, Smith WCS, Tunstil-Pedoe H: The impact of quitting smoking on symptoms of chronic bronchitis: results of the Scottish Heart Health Study. *Thorax* 1991; 46:112.
7. Vermeire P: Chronic bronchitis: definition (or redefinition). *Respiration* 1991; 58(Suppl 1):6.
8. Burrows B, Knudson RJ, Chine MG, Lebowitz MD: Quantitative relationships between cigarette smoking and ventilatory function. *Am Rev Respir Dis* 1977; 115:195.
9. Huchon G: Risk factors for chronic bronchitis and obstructive lung disease. *Respiration* 1991; 58(Suppl 1):10.
10. Kauffman F, Drovet D, Lelouch J, Brille D: Twelve years of spirometric changes among Paris area smokers. *Int J Epidemiol* 1979; 8:201.
11. Schenker MB, Samet JM, Speizer FE: Effect of cigarette tar content and smoking habits on respiratory symptoms in women. *Am Rev Respir Dis* 1982; 125:684.
12. Thurlbeck WM: Pathophysiology of chronic obstructive pulmonary disease. *Clin Chest Med* 1990; 11:389.
13. Burrows B: Airways obstructive diseases: pathogenetic mechanisms and natural histories of the disorders. *Med Clin North Am* 1990; 74:547.
14. Becklake MR: Occupational exposures: evidence for a causal association with chronic obstructive pulmonary disease. *Am Rev Respir Dis* 1989; 140(Suppl):S85.
15. Hutchinson DC: Natural history of alpha-1-protease inhibitor deficiency. *Am J Med* 1988; 84:3.
16. Holland WW: Chronic obstructive lung disease prevention. *Br J Dis Chest* 1988; 82:32.
17. American Thoracic Society: Cigarette smoking and health. *Am Rev Respir Dis* 1985; 131:1133.
18. Riley DJ, Kerr JS: Oxidant injury to the extracellular matrix: Potential role in the pathogenesis of pulmonary emphysema. *Lung* 1985; 163:1.
19. Agnew JE, Little F, Pavia D, Clarke SW: Mucus clearance from the airways in chronic bronchitis—smokers and ex-smokers. *Bull Eur Physiopathol Respir* 1982; 18:473.
20. Eiason R, Mossberg B, Cammer P, Afzelius BA: The immotile cilia syndrome: a congenital ciliary abnormality as an etiological factor in chronic airways infections and male sterility. *N Engl J Med* 1977; 97:1.
21. Mossberg B, Afzelius BA, Cammer P: Mucociliary clearance in obstructive lung diseases. Correlations to the immotile cilia syndrome. *Eur J Respir Dis* 1985; 69(Supple 146):295.
22. Kauffman F: Genetics of chronic obstructive pulmonary diseases. Searching for their heterogeneity. *Bull Eur Physiolpathol Respir* 1984; 20:163.
23. Burrows B, Knudson RJ, Lebowitz MD: The relationship of childhood respiratory illness to adult obstructive airway disease. *Am Rev Respir Dis* 1977; 115:751.
24. Fletcher CM, Peto R, Tinker CM, Speizer FS: *The Natural History*

of Chronic Bronchitis and Emphysema. Oxford, Oxford University Press, 1986.

25. American Thoracic Society: Definitions and classifications of chronic bronchitis, asthma, and pulmonary emphysema. *Am Rev Respir Dis* 1962; 85:762.

26. Medical Research Council: Definition and classification of chronic bronchitis for clinical and epidemiologic purposes. *Lancet* 1965; 1:775.

27. Pride N, Vermeire P, Allegra L: Diagnostic labels in chronic airflow obstruction: responses to a questionnaire with model case histories in North America and Western European countries. *Eur Respir J* 1986; 2:702.

28. Pride NB: The assessment of airflow obstruction: role of measurement of airway resistance and tests of forced expiration. *Br J Dis Chest* 1971; 65:135.

29. Weil J, Zwillich CW: Assessment of ventilatory response to hypoxia: methods and interpretation. *Chest* 1976; 70(Suppl): 124.

30. O'Donnell DE, Sanij R, Anthonisen NR, Younes M: Effect of dynamic airway compression on breathing pattern and respiratory sensation in severe chronic obstructive pulmonary disease. *Am Rev Respir Dis* 1987; 135:912.

31. Efthimiou J, Fleming J, Spiro SG: Sternomastoid muscle function and fatigue in breathless patients with severe respiratory disease. *Am Rev Respir Dis* 1987; 136:1099.

32. Killian KJ, Jones NL: Respiratory muscles and dyspnea. *Clin Chest Med* 1988; 91:237.

33. Gilmartin JJ, Gibson GJ: Mechanisms of paradoxical rib cage motion in patients with chronic obstructive pulmonary disease. *Am Rev Respir Dis* 1986; 1134:683.

34. Koulourio N, Mulvey DA, LaRoche C: The measurement of inspiratory muscle strength by sniff, eosphageal and mouth pressure. *Am Rev Respir Dis* 1989; 139:641.

35. Bellemare F, Grassino A: Force reserve of the diaphragm in patients with chronic obstructive pulmonary disease. *J Appl Physiol* 1983; 55:8.

36. Roussos CS, Macklem PT: Diaphragmatic fatigue in man. *J Appl Physiol* 1977; 43:189.

37. Arora NS, Rochester DP: Respiratory muscle strength and maximal voluntary ventilation in undernourished patients. *Am Rev Respir Dis* 1982; 126:5.

38. Ashutosh K, Gilbert R, Auchincloss JH, Peppi D: Asynchronous breathing movement in patients with chronic obstructive pulmonary disease. *Chest* 1975; 67:553.

39. Mead J, Turner JM, Macklem PT, Little JB: Significance of the relationship between lung recoil and maximum expiratory flow. *J Appl Physiol* 1967; 22:95.

40. Marthan R, Castaing I, Manier G, Guenard H: Gas exchange alterations in patients with chronic obstructive lung disease. *Chest* 1985; 87:470.

41. Fishman AP: Hypoxia and its effect on the pulmonary circulation. *Circ Res* 1976; 38:221.

42. Altose MD, Cherniack NS, Fishman AP: Respiratory sensations and dyspnea. *J Appl Physiol* 1985; 58:1051.

43. Campbell EJM, Howell JBL: The sensation of breathlessness. *Br Med Bull.*

44. Altose MD: Assessment and management of breathlessness. *Chest* 1985; 85:77.

45. Sharp JT, Druz WS, Moisan T, et al.: Postural relief of dyspnea in severe chronic obstructive pulmonary disease. *Am Rev Respir Dis* 1980; 122:201.

46. Hunter AMB, Carey MA, Larsh HW: Nutritional stakes of patients with chronic obstructive pulmonary disease. *Am Rev Respir Dis* 1981; 129:376.

47. Brand PLP, Postma DS, Kerstjens HAN, et al.: Relationship of airway hyper-responsiveness to respiratory symptoms and diurnal peak flow variation in patients with obstructive lung disease. *Am Rev Respir Dis* 1991; 143:916.

48. Chodosh S: Examination of sputum cells. *N Engl J Med* 1970; 282:854.

49. David P, Denis P, Nouvet G, et al.: Lung function and gastroesophageal reflux during chronic bronchitis. *Bull Eur Physiopathol Respir* 1985; 18:81.

50. Hoover CF: Diagnostic significance of inspiratory movements of costal margin. *Am J Med Sci* 1920; 159:663.

51. Zasly L, Baum GL, Rumball JM: The incidence of peptic ulceration in chronic obstructive pulmonary emphysema: a statistical study. *Dis Chest* 1960; 37:400.

52. Flenly DC: Sleep in chronic obstructive lung disease. *Clin Chest Med* 1985; 6:652.

53. Arand DL, McGinty DJ, Littner MR: Respiratory patterns associated with hemoglobin desaturation during sleep in chronic obstructive pulmonary disease. *Chest* 1981; 80:183.

54. Strohl KP, Cherniack NS, Gothe B: Physiological basis of therapy for sleep apnea. *Am Rev Respir Dis* 1986; 134:791.

55. Umetsu DT, Ambrosino DM, Quinti I, et al.: Recurrent sinopulmonary infection and impaired antibody response to bacterial capsular polysaccharide antigen in children with selective IgG-subclass deficiency. *N Engl J Med* 1985; 313:1247.

56. Gibson LE, Cooke RE: A test for concentration of electrolytes in sweat and cystic fibrosis of the pancreas utilizing pilocarpine by iontophoresis. *Pediatrics* 1959; 23:549.

57. Lai S, Ferguson AD, Campbell EJM: Forced time: a simple test for airways obstruction. *Br Med J* 1969; 1:814.

58. Bohadan AB, Peslin R, Uffholtz H: Breath sounds in the clinical assessment of airflow obstruction. *Thorax* 1978; 33:345.

59. Ingram RH, Schilder DP: Effect of pursed lips expiration on the pulmonary pressure flow relationship in obstructive lung disease. *Am Rev Respir Dis* 1967; 96:381.

60. Matthay RA, Berger JH: Cardiovascular function in cor pulmonale. *Clin Chest Med* 1983; 4:269.

61. DuBois AB, Botellio SY, Comroe JH Jr: A new method for measuring airway resistance in man using a body plethysmograph: values in normal subjects and in patients with respiratory disease. *J Clin Invest* 1956; 35:327.

62. Ferris BG Jr, Mead J, Opie LH: Partitioning of respiratory flow-resistance in man. *J Appl Physiol* 1964; 19:653.

63. Burrows B: Differential diagnosis of chronic obstructive pulmonary disease. *Chest* 1990; 97(Suppl 2):16.

64. Knudson RJ, Satin RC, Lebowitz MD, Burrows B: The maximal expiratory flow-volume curve. Normal standards, variability and effects of age. *Am Rev Respir Dis* 1976; 1113:587.

65. Hyatt RE, Black LF: The flow-volume curve: a current perspective. *Am Rev Respir Dis* 1973; 107:191.

66. Hutcheon M, Griffen P, Levison H, Samel N: Volume isoflow: a new test in detection of mild abnormalities of lung mechanics. *Am Rev Respir Dis* 1974; 110:458.

67. Woolcock AJ, Vincent NJ, Macklem PT: Frequency dependence of compliance as a test for obstruction in the small airways. *J Clin Invest* 1969; 48:1097.

68. Bryan AC, Bentivoglio LG, Beerel F, et al.: Factors affecting regional distribution of ventilation and perfusion in the lung. *J Appl Physiol* 1964; 19:395.

69. Sorli J, Grassino A, Lorarje G, Milic-Emil J: Control of breathing in patients with chronic obstructive lung disease. *Clin Sci Mol Med* 1978; 54:295.

70. Flenly DC, Franklin DH, Millar JS: The hypoxic drive to breathing in chronic bronchitis and emphysema. *Clin Sci* 1970; 38:503.

71. Dhingra S, Solven F, Wilson A, McCarthy DS: Hypomagnesemia and respiratory muscle power. *Am Rev Respir Dis* 1984; 129:497.

72. Newman JH, Neff TA, Ziporin P: Acute respiratory failure

associated with hypophosphatema. *N Engl J Med* 1977; 296: 1101.

73. Edelman NH, Rucker RB, Peary HH: NIH workshop summary. Nutrition and the respiratory system. Chronic obstructive pulmonary disease (COPD). *Am Rev Respir Dis* 1986; 134:347.

74. Zakon H, Despas I, Anthonisen NR: Occlusion pressure responses in asthma and chronic obstructive pulmonary disease. *Am Rev Respir Dis* 1976; 114:917.

75. Altose MD, McCauley WC, Kelson SG, Cherniack NS: Effect of hypercapnia and inspiratory flow-resistance on respiratory activity in chronic airways obstruction. *J Clin Invest* 1977; 59:500.

76. Burki NK: Breathlessness and mouth occlusion pressure in patients with chronic obstruction of the airways. *Chest* 1979; 76:527.

77. Lourenco RV, Miranda JM: Drive and performance of the ventilatory apparatus in chronic obstructive lung disease. *N Engl J Med* 1968; 18:43.

78. Abraham AS, Hedworth-Whitty RB, Bishop JM: Effects of acute hypoxia and hypervolemia singly and together upon the pulmonary circulation in patients with chronic bronchitis. *Clin Sci* 1967; 33:371.

79. Oliven A, Cherniack NS, Deal EC, Kelsen SG: The effects of acute bronchoconstriction on respiratory activity in patients with chronic obstructive pulmonary disease. *Am Rev Respir Dis* 1985; 131:236.

80. Dantzger DR, D'Alonzo GE: The effect of exercise on pulmonary gas exchange in patients with severe chronic obstructive pulmonary disease. *Am Rev Respir Dis* 1986; 134:1325.

81. Jones NL, Jones G, Edwards RHT: Exercise tolerance in chronic airways obstruction. *Am Rev Respir Dis* 1971; 103:477.

82. Nicklaus TM, Stowell DW, Chrisiansen WR, Renzetti ADJ: The accuracy of the roentgenologic diagnosis of chronic pulmonary emphysema. *Am Rev Respir Dis* 1966; 93:889.

83. Pratt CP: Role of conventional chest radiography in diagnosis and exclusion of emphysema. *Am J Med* 1987; 82:998.

84. Sutinen S, Christofondis AJ, Clogh GA, Pratt PC: Roentgenologic criteria for the recognition of nonsymptomatic pulmonary emphysema: correlation between roentgenographic findings and pulmonary pathology. *Am Rev Respir Dis* 1965; 91:69.

85. Gould GA, MacNee W, McClean A, et al.: CT measurements of lung density in life can quantitate distal air enlargement: an essential defining feature of human emphysema. *Am Rev Respir Dis* 1988; 137:380.

86. Robinson PJ, Keel L: Pulmonary tissue attenuation with computed tomography: comparison of inspiration and expiration scan. *J Comput Assist Tomogr* 1979; 3:740.

87. Borgin CJ, Muller NL, Miller RR: CT in the qualitative assessment of emphysema. *J Thoracic Imaging* 1986; 1:94.

88. Simon G: *Principles of Chest X-Ray Diagnosis*, 4th ed. London, Butterworth, 1978.

89. Hayhorst MD, MacNee W, Flenely DC, et al.: The diagnosis of emphysema. A computer tomographic-pathologic correlation. *Am Rev Respir Dis* 1986; 133:541.

90. Potchen EJ, Evens RG: The physiologic factors affecting regional ventilation and perfusion. *Semin Nucl Med* 1980; 10:218.

91. Epsten RL: Constituents of sputum. A simple method. *Am Intern Med* 1972; 77:259.

92. DeJonste JC, Jongejan RC, Kerrebun KF: Control of airway caliber by autonomic nerves in asthma and chronic obstructive pulmonary disease. *Am Rev Respir Dis* 1991; 143:1421.

93. Alving K, Weitzberg E, Lundberg JM: Increased amount of nitric oxide in exhaled air of asthmatics. *Eur Respir J* 1993; 6:1368.

94. Dohlman SW, Black HR, Royall JA: Expired breath hydrogen peroxide is a marker of acute airway inflammation in pediatric patients with asthma. *Am Rev Respir Dis* 1993; 148:955.

95. Larsson C: Natural history and life expectancy in severe alpha$_1$-antitrypsin deficiency. *Acta Med Scand* 1978; 204:345.

96. Janoff A: Elastases and emphysema. Current assessment of protease-antiprotease hypothesis. *Am Rev Respir Dis* 1985; 132:417.

97. Campbell EJ, Senior RM, Welgus HG: Extracellular matrix injury during lung inflammation. *Chest* 1987; 92:161.

98. Hubbard RC, Crystal RG: Antiproteases and antioxidants: strategies for the pharmacological prevention of lung destruction. *Respiration* 1986; 50:56.

99. Millard FTC: The electrocardiogram in chronic lung disease. *Br Heart J* 1967; 29:43.

100. Philips RW: The electrocardiogram in cor pulmonale secondary to pulmonary emphysema: a study of 18 cases proved by autopsy. *Am Heart J* 1958; 56:352.

101. Wasserborger RH, Kelly JR, Rasmussen HK, Juhl JH: The electrocardiographic pentology of pulmonary emphysema. *Circulation* 1959: 20:831.

102. Burrows B, Fletcher CM, Heard BE, et al.: The emphysematous and bronchial types of chronic airways obstruction: a clinicopathological study in London and Chicago. *Lancet* 1966; 1:830.

103. Dornhorst AC: Respiratory insufficiency. *Lancet* 1955; 1:1185.

104. Thurbeck WM: Small airways disease. *Hum Pathol* 1973; 4:150.

105. Macklem PT, Mead J: Resistance of central and peripheral airways measured by a retrograde catheter. *J Appl Physiol* 1967; 22:395.

106. McCarthy DS, Spencer R, Green R, Milic-Emili J: Measurement of closing volume as a simple and sensitive test for early detection of small airway disease. *Am J Med* 1972; 52:747.

107. Boist AS, Vollmer WM, Johnson LR, McCamant LE: Does the single breathe N$_2$ test identify the smoker who will develop chronic airflow limitation? *Am Rev Respir Dis* 1988; 137:293.

108. Hutcheon M, Griffen P, Levison H, Zamel N: Volume of isoflow: a new test in detection of mild abnormalities of lung mechanics. *Am Rev Respir Dis* 1974; 110:458.

109. Stanescu DC, Robenstein DO, Hoeven C, Robert A: "Sensitive tests" are poor predictors of the decline in forced expiratory volume in one second in middle-aged smokers. *Am Rev Respir Dis* 1987; 135:585.

Chapter 84 _____

EPIDEMIOLOGY AND NATURAL HISTORY OF COPD

GORDON L. SNIDER

Explication of COPD

Pulmonary Pathology
  Airways
  Emphysema
  The cause of airflow obstruction in COPD

Epidemiology
  Morbidity
  Mortality
  Trends over time

Risk Factors for COPD
  Gender, race, socioeconomic status, and genetic influences
  Tobacco smoking
  Asthma and atopy
  Nonspecific airways hyperresponsiveness
  Occupational and environmental air pollution

Natural History

Prognosis

To discuss the epidemiology and natural history of chronic obstructive pulmonary disease (COPD), this chapter begins with a definition and review of the pathology of COPD and the disorders that it encompasses. The definition was developed by a committee of the American Thoracic Society:[1a]

Chronic obstructive pulmonary disease is defined as a disease state characterized by the presence of chronic bronchitis or emphysema associated with airflow obstruction; the airflow obstruction may be accompanied by airways hyperreactivity and may be partially reversible (Fig. 84-1).

The two disease entities included in COPD have widely accepted definitions.

Chronic bronchitis is defined as the presence of chronic productive cough for at least 3 months in each of two successive years in a patient in whom other causes of chronic cough, such as infection with *Mycobacterium tuberculosis*, carcinoma of the lung, or chronic congestive heart failure, have been excluded.[1]

Emphysema, one of three forms of permanent respiratory airspace enlargement, is defined in morphologic terms.[2]

Simple airspace enlargement is defined as enlargement of the respiratory airspaces without destruction. It may be congen-

ital, as in Down's syndrome, or acquired, as in the overdistension of the contralateral lung that follows pneumonectomy.

Emphysema is defined as a condition of the lung characterized by abnormal permanent enlargement of the airspaces distal to the terminal bronchioles accompanied by destruction of their walls and without obvious fibrosis. Destruction is defined as nonuniformity in the pattern of respiratory airspace enlargement; the orderly appearance of the acinus and its components is disturbed and may be lost.

Airspace enlargement with fibrosis, occurs *with* obvious fibrosis, associated with infectious granulomatous disease such as tuberculosis, noninfectious granulomatous disease such as sarcoidosis, or fibrosis of undetermined etiology. The scarring is readily evident in the chest radiograph or is apparent to the naked eye in the inflation-fixed lung specimen. This form of airspace enlargement with fibrosis was formerly termed irregular or paracitatricia.

Some patients with asthma also may be included under the rubric COPD.

Asthma is defined[1] as a disease characterized by an increased responsiveness of the trachea and bronchi to various stimuli and manifested by a widespread narrowing of the airways that changes in severity either spontaneously or as a result of therapy.

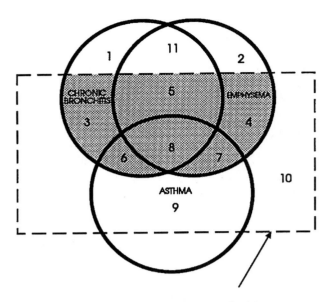

AIRFLOW OBSTRUCTION

FIGURE 84-1 Schema of chronic obstructive pulmonary disease. A nonproportional Venn diagram shows subsets of patients with chronic bronchitis, emphysema, and asthma in three overlapping circles; the subsets comprising COPD are shaded. The areas of the subsets are not proportional to the size of the subset. Some patients have only chronic bronchitis (subset 3), others have only emphysema (subset 4). Most patients with severe disease have features of both chronic bronchitis and emphysema and fall into subset 5; some patients have features of asthma as well and fall into subset 8. Patients with features of asthma and chronic bronchitis (asthmatic bronchitis or the asthmatic form of COPD) fall into subset 6. Patients with asthma whose airflow obstruction is completely reversible (subset 9) and patients with chronic bronchitis or emphysema without airflow obstruction (subsets 1, 2 and 11) are not classed as COPD.

Explication of COPD

In the American Thoracic Society definition, patients who have features of chronic bronchitis or emphysema without airflow obstruction are not considered to have COPD (see Fig. 84-1). Most patients with COPD have features of both chronic bronchitis and emphysema. Patients who have completely reversible airways obstruction without features of chronic bronchitis or emphysema are classified as having asthma and are not included within COPD. As a practical matter, patients whose asthma is characterized by incomplete remission of airways obstruction are included as a subset of COPD because it often is not possible to differentiate these individuals from persons with chronic bronchitis and emphysema who have reversible airways obstruction (see Chap. 83) It is important to point out that some physicians include all asthma under the rubric of COPD.

Pulmonary Pathology

AIRWAYS

The bronchial glands are enlarged and goblet cell frequency is increased. Polymorphonuclear neutrophils and lymphocytes sparsely infiltrate the mucous membrane. Airway smooth muscle is increased. The bronchioles, which are membranous airways less than 2 mm in diameter, show varying degrees of plugging with mucus, goblet cell metaplasia, inflammation, increased smooth muscle, and distortion due to fibrosis and loss of alveolar attachments. This small airways disease is a consistent and persistent feature of COPD.[3]

EMPHYSEMA

Two main types of emphysema, centrilobular and panacinar, are seen in COPD (Table 84-1). Centriacinar emphysema begins in the respiratory bronchioles. Scarring and focal dilation of the bronchioles and of the adjacent alveoli result in the development of an enlarged airspace or microbulla in the center of the secondary lung lobule. Airspace enlargement spreads peripherally from the centriacinar region. Centrilobular emphysema (CLE), which begins in the respiratory bronchioles, is the form of emphysema most frequently associated with prolonged cigarette smoking. This lesion involves the upper and posterior portions of the lungs more than the lower portions. Panacinar emphysema results from dilation of all of the respiratory airspaces of the secondary lung lobule and may be either focal or diffuse. The diffuse form occurs in α_1-protease inhibitor API deficiency. Focal panacinar emphysema commonly occurs in the lung bases of smokers with normal serum proteins in association with CLE in the lung apices.[3]

THE CAUSE OF AIRFLOW OBSTRUCTION IN COPD

Bronchial gland enlargement is not related to airflow obstruction, presumably because the process gives rise to only slight thickening of the mucosa. Bronchiolitis or disease of the small airways is an important cause of airflow obstruction in COPD. Emphysema also causes airflow obstruction as a result of loss of elastic recoil of the lung and rupture of alveolar attachments to small airways, which results in their distortion and premature collapse as lung volume diminishes in expiration. In mild COPD, bronchiolar inflammation and accompanying pathologic changes play the major role in causing airflow obstruction. As the airflow obstruction accompanying COPD worsens, emphysema becomes progressively more severe and becomes the predominant cause of airflow obstruction.[4]

Epidemiology

MORBIDITY

It is estimated from the National Health Survey that in 1991, about 12 million men and women in the United States had

TABLE 84-1   Classification of Respiratory Airspace Enlargement

			Remarks
Simple Airspace Enlargement	Congenital	Lobar inflation	Seen in infancy
		Down's syndrome	
	Acquired	Secondary to loss of lung volume	Accompanying atelectasis or lung resection
Emphysema	Proximal Acinar Emphysema	Focal emphysema	Widespread, in coal worker's pneumoconiosis
		Centrilobular emphysema	The main type in smokers, predominant in upper lung fields
	Panacinar Emphysema	Focal	Occurs at the lung bases; may accompany CLE in smokers
		Widespread	Begins and is more severe at the lung bases; occurs in API deficiency
	Distal Acinar (Paraseptal) Emphysema	Apical bullae	Focal; airflow obstruction absent; the cause of spontaneous pneumothorax
		Giant bullous disease	May be severe, compressing normal lung; amenable to surgical resection
Airspace Enlargement with Fibrosis			Occurs with fibrosing disease such as sarcoidosis and tuberculosis

ABBREVIATIONS: API = α_1-protease inhibitor; CLE = centrilobular emphysema.

chronic bronchitis and about 2 million had emphysema. The overall prevalence of COPD cannot be precisely estimated from these data because the number of persons reporting more than one condition is not given.[5]

MORTALITY

In 1991, there were 85,544 deaths certified as due to COPD and allied conditions, a death rate of 18.6/100,000; this category ranked as the fourth leading cause of death in the United States.[5] In 1985, COPD was the underlying cause for 3.6 percent of all deaths in the United States and was a contributory factor in an additional 4.3 percent of deaths. COPD takes its toll primarily at the older ages; more than 95 percent

of all deaths from COPD in 1985 occurred in persons over the age of 55. Men and women have similar mortality rates for COPD before age 55 years, but men have appreciably higher rates thereafter. Thus, mortality for men is more than double that for women at age 70 and is more than 3.5 times that for women at age 85 years and over.[6]

TRENDS OVER TIME

The age-adjusted death rate for COPD increased 71 percent between 1966 and 1986, during which time the death rate from all causes declined by 22 percent and the rates for heart disease and cerebral vascular disease declined by 45 and 58 percent, respectively.[7] Age-adjusted prevalence rates for men rose only slightly over the period 1979 to 1985, with a prevalence of 110/1000 in 1985. However, among women, prevalence rates increased by more than one third between 1979 and 1985, with a prevalence of 119/1000 in 1985. The mortality attributed to COPD increased nearly 32.9 percent between 1979 and 1991.

Much of the trend of increasing morbidity and mortality from COPD appears to be due to past temporal trends in cigarette smoking. The current data are explainable from the effects of cigarette smoking on members of birth cohorts now reaching an advanced age. In contrast to cardiovascular mortality rates, COPD mortality rates are relatively insensitive to intermittent or short-term smoking cessation. Part of the continued rise in morbidity and mortality may be due to the increasing numbers of people living to an advanced age; the increases are particularly striking in those who continue to smoke. Because smoking frequency has decreased sharply in the United States over the past three decades, there should be an appreciable decrease in COPD mortality in the decades to come.[8]

Risk Factors for COPD

GENDER, RACE, SOCIOECONOMIC STATUS, AND GENETIC INFLUENCES

Most population studies have reported a greater prevalence of respiratory symptoms in men than in women, even when the data are controlled for smoking. About 20 percent of COPD patients have a family history of the disease. Mortality rates for COPD are greater in whites than in nonwhites, but the difference is becoming less among males. Morbidity and mortality rates are related inversely to socioeconomic status as measured by level of education and income and, generally, are greater in blue collar workers than in white collar workers.[7,9,11]

Homozygous API deficiency is the single, fully established genetic disorder that gives rise to severe premature emphysema; however, the disorder accounts for less than 1 percent of COPD in large clinics (see Chap. 85). α_1-Antichymotrypsin deficiency is a rare genetic disorder, inherited in autosomal dominant fashion, which is associated with lung disease.[12] A point mutation occurring in a 3' flanking, region of the API gene is associated with chronic lung disease.[13] There is an increased frequency of the $\Delta F508$ and some rarer forms of the cystic fibrosis (CFTR) gene in patients with mucous hypersecretion, bronchiectasis, and normal sweat electrolyte levels[14,15]; these patients are better classified as having a variant form of cystic fibrosis rather than COPD because there is a known (genetic) etiology for their respiratory symptoms.

TOBACCO SMOKING

Cigarette smoking is established firmly as the most important risk factor for COPD. Tobacco smoking accounts for most of the risk of developing COPD in the United States. It has been calculated that the smoking-attributable fraction of COPD mortality in the United States during the 1980s was

0.850 for men and 0.694 for women.[16] Data from longitudinal, cross-sectional, and case control studies show that in comparison with nonsmokers, cigarette smokers have greater death rates for chronic bronchitis and emphysema. They have higher prevalence and incidence for chronic bronchitis, emphysema, and obstructive airways disease, and a greater frequency of respiratory symptoms and lung function abnormalities (Figs. 84-2 and 84-3). Cigarette smokers also have a greater average annual rate of decline in forced expiratory volume in 1 s (FEV_1). Differences between cigarette smokers and nonsmokers increase as cigarette consumption increases. Pipe and cigar smokers have higher morbidity and mortality rates for COPD than nonsmokers, although their rates are lower than for cigarette smokers. Only a minority, or about 15 percent of smokers, develop clinically significant COPD.[11] Cigarette smoking is a continuous-effect variable. Despite controlling for individual variability of FEV_1 in never-smokers and for variability in measurements of cigarette smoke dose, there is a large interindividual variability in the rate of decline of the FEV_1. With the same smoke exposure, persons at the 97.5th percentile of the distribution suffer 18 times as large an effect of FEV_1 as persons at the 2.5th percentile.[17] The reason for the increased susceptibility of a small subset of smokers is not known.[7,9–11,18–22]

Passive or involuntary smoking is the exposure of nonsmokers to cigarette smoke in the indoor environment. Cigarette smoke in the air can irritate the eyes. The children of smoking parents have higher prevalence of respiratory symptoms and respiratory disease and appear to have a small but measurable difference in tests of pulmonary function when compared with children of nonsmoking parents. The significance of these findings in relation to the future development of lung disease is unknown.[11]

ASTHMA AND ATOPY

In 1960, Orie and colleagues from the Netherlands[23] proposed that an "asthmatic constitution," consisting of a predisposition to atopic disease, airway hyperresponsiveness, and sometimes eosinophilia, underlies the development of chronic airflow obstruction. Smoking was only one extrinsic factor that could lead to chronic airflow obstruction. This formulation has come to be known as the Dutch hypothesis.[24]

Many studies have since focused on this hypothesis. Skin test reactivity to allergens, elevated serum IgE concentration, and eosinophilia, while all markers of atopy, are apparently not interchangeable and have different relations to clinical manifestations such as asthma and hay fever. In contrast to asthma, neither the diagnoses of chronic bronchitis or emphysema nor the presence of ventilatory impairment in the absence of asthma are related to age-sex standardized serum IgE concentrations. Smokers tend to be less atopic than nonsmokers but have higher concentrations of serum IgE.[11,25] As has been noted (see Fig. 84-1), even in the absence of smoking, asthma can progress to severe, nonremitting chronic airflow obstruction so that the disease is inseparable from COPD. Asthma also may be made worse by smoking, with development of chronic sputum production and the

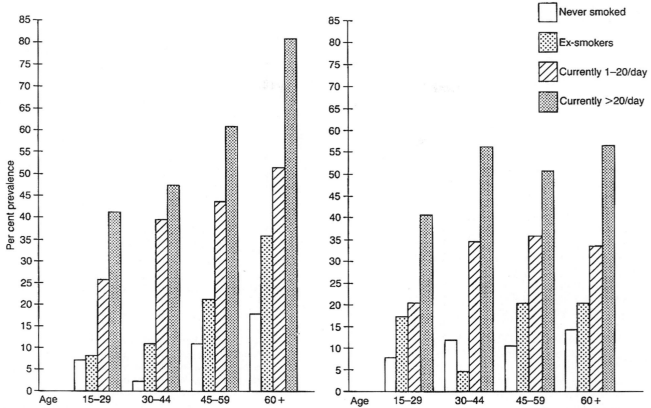

FIGURE 84-2 Prevalence of chronic cough with or without sputum production among samples of men and women in Tucson, Arizona, depicted by age and smoking history. The prevalence of symptoms increases with age even in nonsmokers, but the increase is greater in ex- and current smokers. The prevalence is greater in 20+/day than in 1 to 20 cigarette per day smokers. (*From Liebowitz,*[20] *with permission.*)

FIGURE 84-3 Mean difference (residual) of height adjusted FEV$_1$ (L) from expected values for healthy smokers versus lifetime pack-years in 8842 adults from six U.S. cities. Note the linear relation between mean residual and pack-years of smoking, suggesting a cumulative and irreversible effect of cigarette smoking that was directly related to the number of cigarettes smoked. (*From Dockery DW, Speizer FE, Ferris BG Jr, et al.: Cumulative and reversible effect of lifetime smoking on simple tests of lung function in adults. Am Rev Respir Dis 1988; 137:286.*)

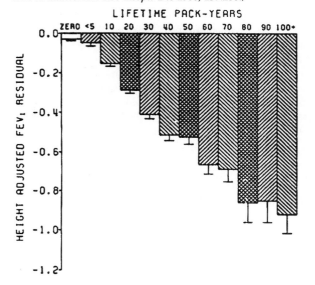

overlap condition often referred to as "asthmatic bronchitis." A group of patients with chronic airflow obstruction and features of asthma have been identified who have a better prognosis than patients with usual COPD.[26] Although they consider that an atopic constitution *may* be associated with COPD, American investigators generally do not consider asthma and atopy as *necessary* risk factors for COPD.[27]

NONSPECIFIC AIRWAYS HYPERRESPONSIVENESS

The possibility that nonspecific airways hyperresponsiveness (NAH) in response to histamine or methacholine challenge might be a risk factor for COPD was first raised as a part of the Dutch hypothesis. The presence of NAH is inversely related to the FEV$_1$. For example, in the Lung Health study, NAH was noted in a significantly greater percentage of women (85.1 percent) than men (58.9 percent). Moreover, nearly twice as many women as men responded to ≤5 mg/mL methacholine (46.6 and 23.9 percent, respectively), and in both genders, baseline degree of airflow obstruction was highly correlated with NAH but age was not.[28] In a subsequent analysis,[28a] the authors concluded that the higher prevalence of NAH in women was due to their having a smaller airway caliber than their male counterparts. Although evidence is steadily accumulating that NAH is predictive of an accelerated rate of decline of lung function in smokers, it is not yet clear whether NAH is a risk factor that predisposes to the development of COPD in smokers or whether it is a result of the airway inflammation that regularly accompanies the development of smoking-related chronic airflow obstruction.[29–31]

OCCUPATIONAL AND ENVIRONMENTAL AIR POLLUTION

Having an occupation in which the atmosphere is polluted with chemical fumes or nonhazardous dust gives rise to increased prevalence of chronic airflow obstruction, increased rates of decline of FEV_1, and greater mortality from COPD. Interaction between cigarette smoking and exposure to hazardous dust such as cotton dust and crystalline silica results in higher rates of COPD. Smoking effects generally are much greater than the occupational effects.[32]

High levels of urban air pollution are harmful to persons with heart or lung disease, but the role of environmental air pollution in producing COPD in the United States is small compared with that of cigarette smoking. In developing countries, the use of various solid fuels for cooking and heating without adequate ventilation may result in very high levels of indoor air pollution and the development of COPD.[11]

Natural History

The natural history of airflow obstruction is still described only partial. Longitudinal studies show that ventilatory function as measured by the FEV_1 in nonsmokers without respiratory disease declines by 25 to 30 mL/year beginning at about age 25 to 30 (Fig. 84-4). The rate of decline of FEV_1 with age is steeper for smokers than for nonsmokers. It also is steeper for heavy smokers than for light smokers. The decline in function occurs along a slowly accelerating curvilinear path. In most persons the loss occurs uniformly, but in some it develops in stages with relatively steep declines. There is a direct relation between the level of the initial FEV_1 and the slope of FEV_1 decline. Age, which cannot be separated from the number of years of cigarette smoking, is clearly a risk factor for more rapid decline of lung function; so are lifetime smoking history and the number of cigarettes currently smoked.[19,27,33]

Individuals with COPD have more frequent acute chest illnesses than those without COPD. Transient decreases of lung function, which occur with most episodes, usually are restored after about 90 days.[19] Mucous hypersecretion in smokers plays little or no role in the rate of decline of lung function or the mortality from COPD.[34–36] The most powerful predictor of the development of disability and death from the disease is the presence of airflow obstruction, best measured as the postbronchodilator FEV_1 or the ratio of FEV_1 and forced vital capacity (FVC). Tests reflecting emphysema (diffusing capacity of the lung for carbon monoxide, functional residual capacity, total lung capacity) predict survival in a relatively minor way.[37]

After the cessation of smoking, lung function lost as a result of smoking is regained minimally; the rate of decline of lung function with increasing age in former smokers slows by about the fifth ex-smoking year to that seen in non-

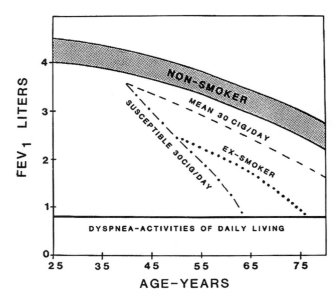

FIGURE 84-4 Schema shows relationships among FEV_1, age, and smoking. Nonsmokers lose FEV_1 at an accelerating rate with age; the average loss is about 30 mL/year. Smokers of 30 cigarettes per day average a slightly greater rate of decline and have FEV_1 values slightly below average when first studied at age 40 years. A small proportion of susceptible smokers (about 15 percent) lose function much more rapidly, 150 mL/year, and have an FEV_1 of 0.8 L at age 65, a level that is so low that they experience dyspnea during activities of daily living. A susceptible smoker who stops smoking at age 50 does not regain any lost function but subsequently loses function at the rate for nonsmokers. Dyspnea on activities of daily living will develop at age 76, 11 years later than if he had continued to smoke. *(From Snider GL, Faling LJ, Rennard SI: Chronic bronchitis and emphysema, in Murray JF, Nadel JA (eds): Textbook of Respiratory Medicine. Philadelphia, WB Saunders, 1994:1342.)*

smokers of the same age[9,19,38] (see Fig. 84-4). Data from several studies strongly suggest that the susceptible subgroup of smokers having more rapid decline of lung function in the mid-years of life can be defined by their greater loss of FEV_1 or FEV_1/FVC ratio. For example, it has been suggested that a smoker of 20 to 30 cigarettes per day for 20 years with an FEV_1 that is more than 1L below the predicted value for age and height[19,22] or an FEV_1/FVC ratio less than 70 percent[38] is in the susceptible group. The goal of smoking cessation is to delay the rate of decline of ventilatory function and, therefore, the onset of dyspnea and disability; persons shown by spirometry to be at risk of developing COPD should be especially targeted for efforts at smoking cessation.

Prognosis

The prognosis of patients with COPD who have mild airflow obstruction is favorable; survival in a group with initial postbronchodilator FEV_1 of ≥50 percent of predicted is only slightly worse than in a group smokers without airflow obstruction. The prognosis worsens as the FEV_1 decreases, especially if there is accompanying hypercapnia. In patients presenting with values of FEV_1 <0.75 L, the approximate mortality rate at 1 year is 30 percent and at 10 years 95 percent.[39] Death generally occurs as a result of some medical complication, such as acute respiratory failure, an overwhelming infection, retained secretions with atelectasis and pneumonia, pneumothorax, cardiac arrhythmia, or pulmonary embolism. The correction of severe persistent hypoxemia by long-term oxygen therapy improves survival.[40,41] Patients surviving a bout of heart failure due to cor pulmonale or an episode of acute respiratory failure may live for many years. Some patients with severe obstructive airways disease may survive for as long as 15 years. Assiduous management and ready access to medical care during an exacerbation are important in maximally prolonging life.

References

1. American Thoracic Society: Chronic bronchitis, asthma and pulmonary emphysema. A statement by the Committee on Diagnostic Standards for Nontuberculous Respiratory Diseases. *Am Rev Respir Dis* 1962; 85:762.

1a. American Thoracic Society. Standards for the diagnosis and care of patients with chronic obstructive pulmonary disease. *Am J Respir Crit Care Med* 1995; 152:S78–S121.

2. Snider GL, Kleinerman J, Thurlbeck WM, Bengali ZH: The definition of emphysema. Report of a National Heart, Lung, and Blood Institute, Division of Lung Diseases Workshop. *Am Rev Respir Dis* 1985; 132:182.

3. Thurlbeck WM: Pathology of chronic obstructive pulmonary disease. *Clin Chest Med* 1990; 11:389.

4. Snider GL: Chronic obstructive pulmonary disease: a definition and implications of structural determinants of airflow obstruction for epidemiology. *Am Rev Respir Dis* 1989; 140:S3.

5. Schultz D: Lung disease data 1994. New York, American Lung Association, 1994.

6. Feinlieb M, Rosenburg HM, Collins JG, et al.: Trends in COPD morbidity and mortality in the United States. *Am Rev Respir Dis* 1989; 140:S9.

7. Higgins MW, Thom T: Incidence, prevalence, and mortality: intra- and intercountry differences, in Hensley MJ, Saunders NA (eds): *Clinical Epidemiology of Chronic Obstructive Pulmonary Disease.* New York, Marcel Dekker, 1990:23–43.

8. Speizer FE: The rise in chronic obstructive pulmonary disease mortality; overview and summary. *Am Rev Respir Dis* 1989; 140:S106.

9. U.S. Surgeon General. *The Health Consequences of Smoking: Chronic Obstructive Lung Disease.* Washington DC: U.S. Department of Human Services, 1984. USDHHS publication 84-50205.

10. Sherrill DL, Lebowitz MD, Burrows B: Epidemiology of chronic obstructive pulmonary disease. *Clin Chest Med* 1990; 11:375.

11. Buist SA: Smoking and other risk factors, in Murray JF, Nadel JA (eds): *Textbook of Respiratory Medicine,* 2nd ed. Philadelphia, WB Saunders, 1994: 1259–1287.

12. Poller W, Faber J-P, Scholtz S, et al.: Mis-sense mutation of α_1-antichymotrypsin gene associated with chronic lung disease. Lancet 1992; 339:1538.

13. Kalsheker N, Morgan J: The alpha$_1$-antitrypsin gene and chronic lung disease. *Thorax* 1990; 45:759.

14. Gervais, Lafite J-J, Dumur V, et al.: Sweat chloride and F508 mutation in chronic bronchitis or bronchiectasis. *Lancet* 1993; 342:997.

15. Highsmith WE, Burch LH, Zhou Z, et al.: A novel mutation in the cystic fibrosis gene in patients with pulmonary disease but normal sweat chloride concentrations. *N Engl J Med* 1994; 331:974.

16. Davis RM, Novotny TE: The epidemiology of cigarette smoking and its impact on chronic obstructive pulmonary disease. *Am Rev Respir Dis* 1989; 140:S82.

17. Silver K, Hatis D: *Human Interindividual Variability in Susceptibility to FEV_1 Decline from Smoking.* CTPID 90-8. Cambridge MA, M.I.T. Center for Technology Policy and Industrial Development, 1990.

18. Auerbach O, Hammond EC, Garfinkel L, Benante C: Relation of smoking and age to emphysema: whole lung section study. *N Engl J Med* 1972; 286:853.

19. Fletcher CM, Peto R, Tinker C, Speizer FE: *The Natural History of Chronic Obstructive Lung Disease in Working Men in London.* New York, Oxford University Press, 1976.

20. Lebowitz MD, Burrows B: Quantitative relationships between cigarette smoking and chronic productive cough. *Int J Epidemiol* 1977; 6:107.

21. Burrows B, Knudson RJ, Cline MG, Lebowitz MD: Quantitative relationships between cigarette smoking and ventilatory function. *Am Rev Respir Dis* 1977; 115:195.

22. Higgins MW, Keller JB, Becker M, et al.: An index of risk for obstructive airways disease. *Am Rev Respir Dis* 1982; 125:144.

23. Orie NG, Sluiter HJ, DeVries K, et al.: The host factor in bronchitis, in Orie NGM, Sluiter HJ (eds): *Bronchitis.* Assen Royal Vangorcum, 1961:43–59.

24. Burrows B, Bloom JW, Traver GA, Cline MG: The course and prognosis of different forms of chronic airways obstruction in a sample from the general population. *N Engl J Med* 1987; 317:1309.

25. Burrows B, Martinez FD, Halonen M, et al.: Association of asthma with serum IgE levels and skin-test reactivity to allergens. *N Engl J Med* 1989; 320:271.

26. Burnett D, Chamba A, Hill SL, Stockley RA: Neutrophils from subjects with chronic obstructive lung disease show enhanced chemotaxis and extracellular proteolysis. *Lancet* 1987; 2(8567): 1043.

27. Burrows B: Airways obstructive diseases: pathogenetic mechanisms and natural histories of the disorders. *Med Clin North Am* 1990; 74:547.

28. Tashkin DP, Altose MD, Bleeker ER, et al, and the Lung Health Study Research Group: The Lung Health Study: airway responsiveness to inhaled methacholine in smokers with mild to moderate airflow limitation. *Am Rev Respir Dis* 1992; 145:301.

28a. Kanner RE, Conett JE, Altose MD, Buist AS, Lee WW, Tashkin DP, Wise RA: Gender difference in airway hyperresponsiveness in smokers with mild COPD; the lung health study. *Am J Respir Crit Care Med* 1994; 150:956–61.

29. Redline S, Tager IB: The relationship of airway reactivity to the occurrence of chronic obstructive pulmonary disease: an epidemiologic assessment, in Hensley MJ, Saunders NA (eds): *Clinical Epidemiology of Chronic Obstructive Pulmonary Disease.* New York, Marcel Dekker, 1989:169–199.

30. O'Connor GT, Sparrow D, Weiss ST: The role of allergy and nonspecific airway hyperresponsiveness in the pathogenesis of chronic obstructive pulmonary disease. *Am Rev Respir Dis* 1989; 140:225.

31. Burrows B: Epidemiologic evidence for different types of chronic airflow obstruction. *Am Rev Respir Dis* 1991; 143:1452.

32. Becklake MR: Occupational exposures: evidence for a causal association with chronic obstructive pulmonary disease. *Am Rev Respir Dis* 1989; 140:S85.

33. Burrows B, Knudson RJ, Camilli AE, et al.: The "horse-racing effect" and predicting decline in forced expiratory volume in

one second from screening spirometry. *Am Rev Respir Dis* 1987; 135:788.

34. Peto R, Spiezer FE, Cochrane AL, et al.: The relevance in adults of air-flow obstruction, but not of mucus hypersecretion, to mortality from chronic lung disease: results from 20 years of prospective observation. *Am Rev Respir Dis* 1983; 126:491.

35. Ebi-Kryston KL: Respiratory symptoms and pulmonary function as predictors of 10 year mortality from respiratory disease, cardiovascular disease, and all causes in the Whitehall study. *J Clin Epidemiol* 1988; 41:251.

36. Lange P, Nyboe J, Appleyard M, et al.: Relation of ventilatory impairment and of chronic mucus hypersecretion to mortality from obstructive lung disease and from all causes. *Thorax* 1990; 45:579.

37. Anthonisen NR: Prognosis in chronic obstructive pulmonary disease: results from multicenter clinical trials. *Am Rev Respir Dis* 1989; 133:S95.

38. Camilli AE, Burrows B, Knudson RJ, et al.: Longitudinal changes in forced expiratory volume in one second in adults; effects of smoking and smoking cessation. *Am Rev Respir Dis* 1987; 135:794.

39. Hodgkin JE: Prognosis in chronic obstructive pulmonary disease. *Clin Chest Med* 1990; 11:555.

40. Nocturnal Oxygen Therapy Trial Group: Continuous or nocturnal oxygen therapy in hypoxemic chronic obstructive lung disease. *Ann Intern Med* 1980; 93:391.

41. Medical Research Council Working Party: Long-term domiciliary oxygen therapy in chronic hypoxic cor pulmonale complicating chronic bronchitis and emphysema. *Lancet* 1981; 1:681.

α₁-PROTEASE INHIBITOR DEFICIENCY AND THE PREVENTIVE THERAPY OF EMPHYSEMA

GORDON L. SNIDER

Severe α₁-protease inhibitor (API) deficiency is the one genetic defect that is unequivocally and importantly linked to the development of emphysema. In this chapter, the genetics of API deficiency, the lung disease caused by the deficiency, and its treatment by augmentation therapy with human API are reviewed. The number of people who smoke in the United States population has decreased from 41 percent in 1964 to approximately 26 percent in 1994. This represents about 50 million U.S. residents. A great many of these persons, some with chronic obstructive pulmonary disease (COPD), are unable to stop smoking despite the best efforts of specialists in smoking cessation. Because emphysema is a slowly progressive disease, it is rational to attempt to develop drugs for the preventive therapy of emphysema. The hope is that drug therapy will slow the rate of decline of lung function, thereby delaying the onset of disability and prolonging life. In the second portion of this chapter, theories of the pathogenesis of emphysema are summarized to provide a foundation for a discussion of the potential development of antiproteases as a treatment to prevent emphysema in API-replete persons who cannot stop smoking.

α₁-Protease Inhibitor Deficiency

The serum protein API is an inhibitor of serine proteases. Its main substrate in vivo is neutrophil elastase (NE).[1] Severe API deficiency is associated with the development of pulmonary emphysema in early or mid life. The emphysema is panacinar and is usually more severe in the lung bases. In about 50 percent of cases, the onset of emphysema is accompanied by chronic bronchitis. The mucous hypersecretion may be due to bronchial secretory cell metaplasia induced by proteases.[2] Liver disease occurs in about 10 percent of API-deficient infants[3] but usually subsides by age 6 months. In adult men, there is an increased risk of cirrhosis, often with hepatoma.[4]

GENETICS

α₁-Protease inhibitor is a 54-kD glycoprotein composed of 394 amino acids, which is coded for by a single gene on chromosome 14. The API serum phenotype (the protease inhibitor or Pi phenotype) is determined by the independent expression of the two parental alleles. The API gene is highly pleomorphic, with some 75 alleles known. They have been classified into normal, associated with normal serum concentrations of normally functioning API; deficient, associated with API having altered electrophoretic properties and lesser-than-normal serum concentrations of API; null, associated with undetectable API in the serum; and dysfunctional, in which API is present in normal amount but does not function normally.[5]

The variants of API occur because of point mutations that result in a single amino acid substitution. The normal M alleles (the alleles are assigned a letter code) occur in about 90 percent of persons of European descent with normal serum API levels; their phenotype is designated Pi MM. Normal values of serum API are 150 to 350 mg/dL (commercial standard) or 20 to 48 μM (true laboratory standard). More than 95 percent of persons in the severely deficient category will be homozygous for the Z allele, designated Pi ZZ, and will have serum API levels of 2.5 to 7 μM (mean, 16 percent normal). Almost all of these persons are Caucasians of northern European descent because the Z allele is rare in Orientals and African Americans. Rarely observed phenotypes that are associated with these low concentrations of serum API include Pi SZ and persons with nonexpressing alleles: Pi-null, occurring in homozygous form (Pi null-null) or, in heterozygous form with a deficient allele, Pi Znull. Persons with phenotype Pi SS have API values ranging from 15 to 33 μM (mean, 52 percent of normal). The threshold protective level of 11 μM or 80 mg/dL (35 percent of normal) is based on the knowledge that Pi SZ heterozygotes, with serum API values of 8 to 19 μM (mean, 37 percent of normal), rarely develop emphysema. Pi MZ heterozygotes have serum API levels that are intermediate between Pi MM normals and Pi ZZ homozygotes (12 to 35 μM; mean, 57 percent of normal) and are not at increased risk for emphysema.

Estimates of the frequency of the Pi ZZ phenotype in North America and Europe range from about 1/1600 to 1/4000,[6] a prevalence approximating that of cystic fibrosis, and suggesting that severe API deficiency is among the most common potentially serious genetic conditions. Nevertheless, in large studies in both Sweden[7] and Great Britain,[6] rigorous attempts to collect all available cases have garnered 10 percent of estimated cases at most. This suggests that either most subjects who are type Pi Z are asymptomatic or they are masquerading under other diagnoses such as asthma.

NATURAL HISTORY OF API DEFICIENCY

Knowledge of the natural history of lung disease in API deficiency is derived mostly from a few large case series.[5,7-10] Most patients in these series have been diagnosed as type Pi Z because they have had pulmonary symptoms, and they are called index cases; nonindex cases have been discovered through studies of blood donors or family members of subjects who are type Pi Z. Symptoms or signs of pulmonary disease rarely develop before age 25 years. A recent report of a follow-up of 22 subjects, ages 12 to 18 years with API deficiency discovered through neonatal screening, showed that all had normal spirometric values after bronchodilator

aerosol inhalation as well as normal lung volume and carbon monoxide diffusing capacity values.[10]

Tobacco smoking is strongly associated with the development of pulmonary disease. Dyspnea begins at an earlier age in smokers than in nonsmokers; smokers who are type Pi Z have a significantly lower life expectancy than nonsmokers who are type Pi Z, although nonsmokers also have a reduced life expectancy.[7-9] Annual decline of forced expiratory volume in 1 s (FEV_1) is greater than normal in nonsmokers who are type Pi Z, but is much greater in smokers who are type Pi Z than in nonsmokers.[9]

Severity of lung disease varies markedly; lung function is well preserved in some smokers who are type Pi Z and severely impaired in some nonsmokers.[5,7-9] Nonindex cases tend to have better lung function, whether they smoke or not, than index cases.[8] The annual decline in FEV_1 of nonindex cases tends to be only moderately greater than normal[11]; however, even nonindex cases usually develop obstructive airways disease late in life[7,9,12]; such persons may live into their eighth[12] or ninth[9] decade. Obstructive airways disease occurs more frequently in men than in women. More than half of Pi Z subjects die from pulmonary disease; cirrhosis, often with hepatoma, is the next most common cause of death.[4,7,8] In addition to cigarette smoking, asthma, recurrent respiratory infections, and unidentified familial factors have been identified as possible risk factors for chronic airflow obstruction.[10] It is surprising that increased frequency of respiratory infections as a risk factor for chronic airways obstruction has been clearly noted in only two studies.[7,10]

AUGMENTATION THERAPY FOR API DEFICIENCY

Augmentation therapy with purified human API for patients with severe API deficiency is based on the concept that a deficient protein is being restored to protective levels.[13] It is presumed, but not proved, that augmentation therapy will halt the progression of emphysema; because emphysema produces a permanent structural change, augmentation therapy cannot improve lung structure or function. Because of inherent difficulties,[13,14] a controlled trial of efficacy has not been carried out. The cost of the drug for 1 year of augmentation therapy in a 70-kg patient is about $25,000.

The American Thoracic Society[15] recommends that augmentation therapy should be reserved for patients whose serum concentration of API is less than 11 μM; it is not indicated for patients with cigarette smoking-related emphysema who have normal or heterozygous phenotypes. It is also not indicated in patients who have the liver disease associated with API deficiency, unless they also have lung disease. Persons with normal lung function should be followed but not treated; augmentation therapy should be considered when lung function is abnormal and especially if serial studies show deterioration. The American Thoracic Society makes the point that it is inappropriate to define a lower limit of lung function or an upper limit of age for administration of augmentation therapy because it is unethical to withhold treatment that may have benefit even in very severe end-stage disease.

However, it seems reasonable to weigh carefully the advantages and disadvantages of augmentation therapy and to jointly reach a decision with elderly persons or those with severe lung function impairment (FEV_1 values under 0.8 L). The addition of the Food and Drug Administration-approved, weekly, intravenous infusions to an already onerous treatment regimen, despite little expectation of real benefit may be unacceptable. (Bi-weekly or monthly augmentation therapy now is used widely.[16]) The effects of an expensive therapy on the patient's and the long-term health insurance benefits must be weighed. For the severely impaired person under 50 years of age, lung transplantation is a reasonable consideration.[17]

Pathogenesis of Emphysema

The elastase-antielastase hypothesis of emphysema, which posits that emphysema results from elastic fiber degradation that occurs because of an imbalance between elastases and antielastases in the lungs,[18] is shown schematically in Fig. 85-1.

SOURCES OF ELASTASE

Neutrophils are rich in a protease of broad specificity, which because of its ability to solubilize elastin, is known as neutrophil elastase (NE). Cathepsin G is plentiful in neutrophils and with protease 3 can also solubilize human lung elastin.

Macrophages comprise 90 percent of the lavageable cells in the lungs. Together, human macrophage metalloproteases (collagenase, stromelysins 1 and 2, and gelatinase) are capable of degrading matrix collagens, proteoglycans, elastin, fibronectin, laminin, and gelatin. Degradation of elastin by macrophages requires contact between the cell and matrix. The elastin degradation is inhibited by the tissue inhibitor of metalloproteases. Both neutrophils and macrophages are increased by four- to fivefold in smokers and it seems likely that both of these cell types are involved in the tissue damage and repair that leads to emphysema in smokers.[19]

THE ANTIELASTASE SHIELD

The main defense against damage from NE is API, which is normally present in the lungs. Oxidants derived from neutrophils and macrophages or from cigarette smoke may inactivate API inhibitor and may interfere with lung matrix repair. Endogenous antioxidants such as superoxide dismutase, glutathione, and catalase protect the lung against oxidant injury. α_2-Macroglobulin enters the lungs only if capillary permeability is increased. Secretory leukocyte protease inhibitor (SLPI) is secreted by bronchial glands and goblet cells; its main role is to protect the airway epithelium from proteolytic injury, but it may also play a role in preventing alveolar elastic fiber injury. Other antielastases, present in small amount, such as elafin, also play a role.[20]

EVIDENCE FOR VALIDITY OF THE ELASTASE-ANTIELASTASE HYPOTHESIS

Experimentally, only elastolytic enzymes can induce emphysema when they are instilled into the lungs; proteolytic but nonelastolytic enzymes do not do so. In young animals made copper deficient or fed lathyrogens and in several genetic models of emphysema (beige, tight-skin and blotchy mice), airspace enlargement appears to result from impaired elastin cross-linking.[18,21,22]

One study using immunoultrastructure has reported that NE is bound to elastic fibers in the lungs of smokers and that the amount of elastase is proportional to the amount of emphysema that is present.[23] Another group reports inability to reproduce these findings.[24]

More direct evidence for elastin degradation in the body can be obtained by measuring plasma and urine elastin peptide levels using an enzyme-linked immunosorbent assay[25,26] or by measuring the cross-link amino acids desmosine and isodesmosine in the urine.[27] Such studies have

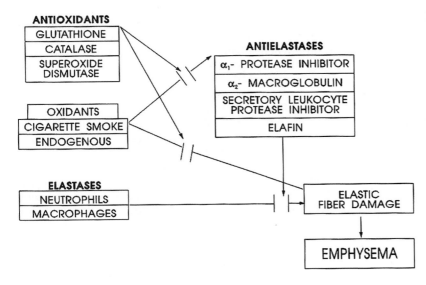

FIGURE 85-1 Schema of elastase-antielastase hypothesis of emphysema. The lung is protected from elastolytic damage by the antielastases, α_1-protease inhibitor (API), secretory leukocyte protease inhibitor and elafin, which are normally present in the lungs; α_2-macroglobulin enters the lungs only with increased capillary permeability. Elastolytic enzymes are derived from neutrophils and macrophages. Oxidants derived from neutrophils and macrophages or from cigarette smoke may inactivate API and may interfere with matrix repair. Endogenous antioxidants such as superoxide dismutase, glutathione, and catalase protect the lung from oxidant injury.

shown evidence of increased elastin degradation in patients with COPD compared with never-smokers; smokers without airflow obstruction have intermediate values.[28]

NONELASTOLYTIC MECHANISMS CAUSING EMPHYSEMA

Experimentally, neonatally formed lung elastin was not destroyed in cadmium chloride-induced airspace enlargement in hamsters.[29] There was no measurable alteration of lung elastin in the emphysema of oxygen-exposed rats and preventing synthesis of cross-linked collagen prevented the airspace enlargement.[30]

The different types of emphysema are variably distributed in the secondary lung lobule and in the lung (see previous chapter) and they have other differentiating features. The microbullae of centrilobular emphysema (CLE) contain fibrous tissue and are less compliant than the lungs that contain them and than normal lungs.[31,32] Lung tissue contains increased collagen in CLE but not in panacinar emphysema (PAE); elastin is decreased in all grades of PAE but only in severe CLE.[33] The ratio of FEV_1 to the forced vital capacity (FEV_1/FVC), an index of airflow obstruction, is significantly related to small airways disease score in CLE (r = 0.69) but not in PAE (r = 0.29). Conversely, FEV_1/FVC is related to elasticity of the lung (the exponential constant of the volume-pressure curve, k) in PAE (r = 0.72) but not in CLE (r = 0.08).[34]

In summary, although the elastase/antielastase hypothesis has dominated the literature, evidence is accumulating that airspace enlargement need not always be accompanied by elastin degradation. Airspace enlargement may result from a number of different lung injuries followed by repair processes that are unable to preserve the normal alveolated structure of the lungs (see Table 84-1). Antielastase drugs that are specific for NE would not be expected to affect elastolysis and emphysema caused by enzymes other than NE. Neither would such drugs affect emphysema caused by nonelastolytic mechanisms such as fibrosis.

PREVENTIVE STRATEGIES

A number of different strategies, all based on the elastase-antielastase hypothesis, might be pursued in developing drugs for emphysema prevention. Antioxidants might be expected to prevent oxidation of antiproteases, but little work has been done with these agents. An attempt to decrease the elastase burden of the lungs with colchicine, which prevents degranulation of neutrophils by preventing microtubule assembly, was not successful in smokers.[35] The third approach is to supplement the naturally occurring antiproteases in the lungs by treatment with a naturally occurring or synthetic antiprotease.

ANTIPROTEASES AS POTENTIAL DRUGS

FUNCTIONAL CLASSIFICATION OF ANTIPROTEASES

Elastase inhibitors include small molecular weight synthetic compounds and larger molecules such as API and SLPI of natural or recombinant DNA origin. These may be classified on the basis of the relations between their in vitro properties, their rate of clearance from the lungs, and their ability to prevent emphysema in hamsters when administered intratracheally prior to intratracheal NE.[36]

- *Category 1: Sparingly Soluble Agents*
  Sparingly water-soluble agents (approximately 1 mM or less) generally are ineffective in preventing emphysema, possibly because, relative to inhibitory potency, adequate amounts of the inhibitor are not in solution in the lungs or because lipophilic compounds clear rapidly from the lungs.
- *Category 2: Irreversible Inhibitors*
  High molecular weight, slowly clearing, irreversible inhibitors such as API, are effective in ameliorating emphysema for many hours in a dose-dependent fashion.
- *Category 3: Tight-binding Slowly Clearing Inhibitors*
  Tight-binding, high molecular weight inhibitors, such as SLPI, that clear slowly from the lungs, prevent emphysema in a dose-dependent fashion for many hours.
- *Category 4: Reversible Rapidly Clearing Inhibitors*
  Reversible, rapidly clearing inhibitors have the potential for worsening emphysema.

INHIBITORS THAT WORSEN EMPHYSEMA

Methoxy succinyl-L-alanyl-L-alanyl-L-prolyl-ambo-boro-val pinacol (BOROVAL), a small molecular weight agent, is a reversible, highly effective in vitro inhibitor of NE. Treatment of hamsters with as much as 1 mg BOROVAL 1 h before NE, a molar ratio of NE to BOROVAL of 1:600, prevented lung hemorrhage but did not ameliorate emphysema (Fig. 85-2). Intratracheal administration of 250 μg human NE (HNE), premixed with and inactivated by 200 μg BOROVAL (1:40 molar ratio) resulted in production of emphysema comparable in severity to that produced by 250 μg of NE alone (see Fig. 85-2). The administration of 500 μg NE premixed with a 1:40 molar ratio of BOROVAL resulted in emphysema of a severity not previously seen with NE—the mean linear intercept was almost double the negative control instead of the approximately 20 percent increase usually achieved with 250 to 300 μg HNE (Fig. 85-3). Doses of NE greater than 300 μg, which are not complexed with inhibitor, have consistently caused massive fatal pulmonary hemorrhage within 2 h of instillation. In contrast, 500 μg of NE premixed with a 40-fold molar excess of BOROVAL produced neither pulmonary hemorrhage nor death.[37]

It is hypothesized that the transient inactivation of NE by BOROVAL prevented the destructive effects of NE on the alveolar epithelium and capillary walls. Alveolar hemorrhage and the associated heavy influx of antiproteases, which partially inactivate the NE, does not occur. At the same time, the NE-BOROVAL complex is transported across the alveolar epithelium into the interstitium of the alveolar wall. Once in the interstitium, the complex dissociates and the BOROVAL clears; the NE digests the elastin, thus giving rise to emphysema. In effect, the BOROVAL provides safe passage for the NE into the alveolar wall.

A recent study of a novel peptidyl carbamate inhibitor, methoxysuccinyl-L-alanyl-L-alanyl-L-propyl-CH$_2$N

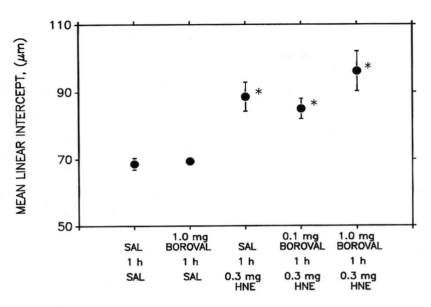

FIGURE 85-2 Mean linear intercept (MLI) values (mean ± SE) for lungs of hamsters given doses of saline (SAL) or BOROVAL intratracheally followed in 1 h by an intratracheal dose of SAL or human neutrophil elastase (HNE). The asterisks denote that the values for hamsters treated with HNE, whether preceded by BOROVAL or SAL, are significantly greater than the values for the SAL-1h-SAL and 1 mg BOROVAL-1h-SAL negative control groups.[37] (*From Stone,[37] with permission.*)

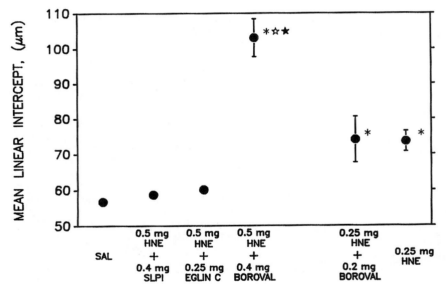

FIGURE 85-3 Mean linear intercept (MLI) values (mean ± SE) for lungs of hamsters given a single intratracheal dose of human neutrophil elastase (HNE) or a mixture of HNE and secretory leukocyte protease inhibitor (SLPI), eglin C, or BOROVAL. There was no significant increase in MLI values of hamsters receiving HNE + SLPI or HNE + eglin C, compared with the negative saline control group (SAL). The groups receiving 0.25 mg HNE, 0.25 mg HNE + 0.2 mg BOROVAL or 0.5 mg HNE + 0.4 mg BOROVAL had MLI values significantly greater than those of the negative control group (*asterisk*). The group receiving 0.5 mg HNE + 0.4 mg BOROVAL also has MLI values significantly greater than those of the positive control group (0.25 mg HNE) and the group receiving 0.25 mg HNE + 0.2 mg BOROVAL (*open star*).[37] (*From Stone,[37] with permission.*)

(i-Pr)CO₂-p-nitrophenol (PCI) studied both alone and covalently bound to a water-soluble polymer, N(2-hydroxyethyl)-D,L-aspartamide, (PPCI) provides evidence in support of this theory. The molecular mass of the PCI is 591, that of PPCI is 22,000. The in vitro molar ratio for 50 percent inhibition of NE was 4.5 for PCI and 0.5 for PPCI. The half-time of lung clearance is 4 min for PCI and 7 h for PPCI. Significant amelioration of emphysema did not occur when 300 μg NE was mixed with a gross excess (503-fold) of PCI prior to intratracheal administration to hamsters (Fig. 85-4). Emphysema was virtually eliminated in all groups by intratracheal administration to hamsters of PPCI for 8 hours before intratracheal administration of 300 μg NE (Fig. 85-5). Thus, unless PCI is bound to a polymer, with a resultant marked increase in molecular weight and lung clearance

time, the reversible inhibitor PCI fails to ameliorate emphysema, even when present in gross excess as compared with HNE.[38]

The interaction among three factors likely determines the behavior of a soluble elastase inhibitor in preventing NE-induced emphysema: the rate of dissociation of the NE-inhibitor complex, the rate of clearance of the inhibitor from the lungs, and the rate of transport of the NE-inhibitor complex across the alveolar epithelium.

The theory of potentiation of emphysema by small molecular weight reversible elastase inhibitors, a potential pitfall in the development of antiprotease drugs, is not proven. Even if true, it is not known whether the theory might apply to NE already in the lungs of a human smoker under treatment with a reversible inhibitor. What is clear from experi-

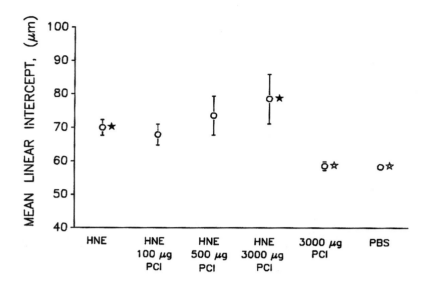

FIGURE 85-4 Dose-response study of ability of peptidyl carbamate inhibitor (PCI) mixed with human neutrophil elastase (HNE) to prevent induction of emphysema. Mean linear intercept values are shown 56 days following intratracheal instillation of a mixture of 100, 500, or 3000 μg PCI mixed with 300 μg HNE. The positive control group received 300 μg HNE and the negative control groups received 3000 μg PCI or phosphate buffered saline alone (PBS). Groups that are significantly different from the negative control groups are shown by a solid star. Groups that are significantly different from the positive control groups are shown by an open star. The mixture of PCI+HNE does not protect against emphysema at any dose.[38] (*From Stone,[38] with permission.*)

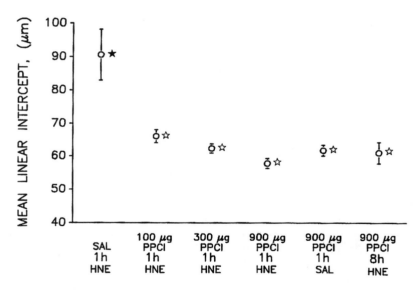

FIGURE 85-5 Dose-response study of ability of a water-soluble polymer of peptydil carbamate inhibitor (PPCI) given 1 or 8 h before human neutrophil elastase (HNE) to prevent induction of emphysema. Mean linear intercept values are shown 56 days following intratracheal instillation of a mixture of 100, 300, or 900 μg PPCI followed in 1 h by 300 μg HNE intratracheally, both in 0.5 mL saline. One group was given 900 μg PPCI intratracheally, followed in 8 h by 300 μg HNE. The positive control group received 0.5 mL saline (SAL) followed in 1 h by 300 μg of HNE; the negative control group received 900 μg of PPCI followed in 1 h by SAL. Groups that are significantly different from the negative control groups are shown by a solid star. Groups that are significantly different from the positive control groups are shown by an open star. Note that in contrast to the results with PCI in Fig. 85-4, all groups receiving PPCI were protected against HNE-induced emphysema.[38] (*From Stone,[38] with permission.*)

ence with BOROVAL and PCI/PPCI is that the protection by an inhibitor against NE-induced pulmonary hemorrhage in an animal must not be equated with protection against NE-induced emphysema. In vivo experiments of the protective effects of elastase inhibitors on NE-induced emphysema should be part of the preclinical process of developing NE inhibitors for use as drugs for the preventive treatment of emphysema.

Testing of Antiprotease Drugs in Humans

Testing the preventive effect of antiprotease drugs raises the questions of the route of administration of the drug, what population is to be studied, and how the population should be studied.

ROUTE OF ADMINISTRATION OF ANTIPROTEASES

The intravenous route is obviously not suitable for the widespread preventive therapy of emphysema in COPD because of expense, discomfort, and inconvenience. Aerosol administration has the drawback that even with particles of the appropriate aerodynamic diameter, only about 10 percent of an orally inhaled aerosol is deposited in the lungs. Thus, it might require long periods of inhalation each day to administer sufficient drug to alter the elastolytic burden of the lungs. The ideal drug would be bioavailable after oral administration, would appear in adequate concentration in the lungs when given orally, and would not interfere with the function of proteases elsewhere in the body.

STUDY OF THE PROCESS OF EMPHYSEMA DEVELOPMENT

There are two main approaches to study of the process believed to lead to emphysema: evaluation of the elastolytic burden of the lungs from measurements of elastolytic potency and neutrophil numbers in sputum or bronchoalveolar lavage fluid[35] and detection of degradation of elastin as indicated by an increase in the level of metabolites of elastin in blood or urine.[25-27] From the ability of drug treatment to affect these parameters, it should be possible to do a dose-ranging study and to estimate the economic feasibility and patient acceptance of a drug regimen. Recent studies have shown a decrease in desmosine excretion in 2 Pi ZZ patients after augmentation therapy with human API was begun. A pilot study on as few as 10 smokers with airflow limitation, studied in the control state and while the subjects were receiving an antiprotease, should indicate whether elastolytic potency of lung fluids and the level of elastin degradation products in urine could be diminished by drug treatment. If there were only a trend in the right direction, the information could be used to carry out a power analysis to determine the number of subjects needed to do a study that would answer the question.

STUDY OF OUTCOME

The efficacy of antielastase treatment in preventing the progression of emphysema in susceptible smokers can be determined by a surrogate for emphysema such as a decrease in the rate of loss of FEV_1 with age. A study of outcome will be difficult and expensive, requiring the study of several hundred subjects over several years. Certainly, such an expensive and difficult study will never be done with an antielastase agent until there is some evidence in humans of its possible efficacy from a process study.

References

1. Travis J: Alpha₁-proteinase inhibitor deficiency, in Massaro M (ed): *Lung Cell Biology.* New York, Marcell Dekker, 1989:1227–1246.
2. Snider GL: Pulmonary disease in alpha-1-antitrypsin deficiency. *Ann Intern Med* 1989; 111:957.
3. Sveger T: Liver disease in alpha₁-antitrypsin deficiency detected by screening of 200,000 infants. *N Engl J Med* 1976; 294:155.
4. Eriksson S, Carlson J, Velez R: Risk of cirrhosis and primary liver cancer in alpha₁-antitrypsin deficiency. *N Engl J Med* 1986; 314:736.
5. Brantly M, Nukiwa T, Crystal RG: Molecular basis of alpha-1-antitrypsin deficiency. *Am J Med* 1988; 84:13.
6. Hutchison DC: Natural history of alpha-1-protease inhibitor deficiency. *Am J Med* 1988; 84:3.
7. Larsson C: Natural history and life expectancy in severe alpha₁-antitrypsin deficiency, Pi Z. *Acta Med Scand* 1978; 204:345.
8. Tobin MJ, Cook PJ, Hutchison DC: Alpha₁-antitrypsin deficiency: the clinical and physiological features of pulmonary emphysema in subjects homozygous for Pi type Z. A survey by the British Thoracic Association. *Br J Dis Chest* 1983; 77:14.
9. Janus ED, Phillips NT, Carrell RW: Smoking lung function, and alpha₁-antitrypsin deficiency. *Lancet* 1985; 1:152.
10. Silverman EF, Pierce JA, Province MA, et al.: Variability of pulmonary function in alpha-1-antitrypsin deficiency: clinical correlates. *Ann Intern Med* 1989; 111:982.
11. Buist AS, Burrows B, Eriksson S, et al.: The natural history of airflow obstruction in PiZ emphysema. *Am Rev Respir Dis* 1983; 127:S43.
12. Black LF, Kueppers F: Alpha₁-antitrypsin deficiency in nonsmokers. *Am Rev Respir Dis* 1978; 117:421.
13. Wewers MD, Casolaro A, Sellers SE, et al.: Replacement therapy of alpha₁-antitrypsin deficiency associated with emphysema. *N Engl J Med* 1987; 316:1055.
14. Burrows B: A clinical trial of efficacy of antiproteolytic therapy: can it be done? *Am Rev Respir Dis* 1983; 127:S42.
15. Buist AS, Burrows B, Cohen A, et al.: Guidelines for the approach to the patient with severe hereditary alpha-1-antitrypsin deficiency. *Am Rev Respir Dis* 1989; 140:1494.
16. Hubbard RC, Brantly ML, Sellers SE, et al.: Anti-neutrophil-elastase defenses of the lower respiratory tract in alpha-1-antitrypsin deficiency directly augmented with an aerosol of alpha-1-antitrypsin. *Ann Intern Med* 1988; 111:206.
17. Levine SM, Anzueto A, Gibbons WJ, et al.: Graft position and pulmonary function after single lung transplantation for chronic obstructive lung disease. *Chest* 1993; 103:444.
18. Snider GL: Experimental studies on emphysema and chronic bronchial injury. *Eur J Respir Dis* 1986; 69s:17.
19. Snider GL, Lucey EC, Stone PJ: Pitfalls in antiprotease therapy of emphysema. *Am J Respir Crit Care Med* 1994; 150:S131.
20. Snider GL, Stone PJ, Lucey EL: Development and evaluation of antiproteases as drugs for preventing emphysema, in Grassi C, Travis J, Caseli L, Luisetti M (eds): *Current Topics in Rehabilitation.* London, Springer Verlag, 1992:143–158.
21. Starcher B, James H: Evidence that genetic emphysema in tight-skin mice is not caused by neutrophil elastase. *Am Rev Respir Dis* 1991; 143:1365.
22. Starcher B, Williams I: The beige mouse: role of neutrophil elastase in the development of pulmonary emphysema. *Exp Lung Res* 1989; 15:785.
23. Damiano VV, Tsang A, Kucich U, et al.: Immunolocalization of elastase in human emphysematous lungs. *J Clin Invest* 1986; 78:482.
24. Fox B, Bull TB, Guz A, et al.: Is neutrophil elastase associated with elastic tissue in emphysema? *J Clin Pathol* 1988; 41:435.
25. Akers S, Kucich U, Swartz M, et al.: Specificity and sensitivity of the assay for elastin-derived peptides in chronic obstructive pulmonary disease. *Am Rev Respir Dis* 1992; 145:1077.
26. Schriver EE, Davidson JM, Sutcliffe MC, et al.: Comparison of elastin peptide concentrations in body fluids from healthy volunteers, smokers and patients with chronic obstructive pulmonary disease. *Am Rev Respir Dis* 1992; 145:762.
27. Stone PJ, Bryan-Rhadfi J, Lucey EC, et al.: Measurement of urinary desmosine by isotope dilution and high performance liquid chromatography: correlation between elastase-induced airspace enlargement in the hamster and elevation of urinary desmosine. *Am Rev Respir Dis* 1991; 144:284.
28. Stone PJ, Gottlieb DJ, O'Connor GT, et al.: Elastin and collagen degradation products in urine of smokers with and without COPD. *Am J Respir Crit Care Med* 1995; 151:952.
29. Snider GL, Lucey EC, Faris B, et al.: Cadmium chloride-induced

airspace enlargement with interstitial pulmonary fibrosis is not associated with destruction of lung elastin. Implications for the pathogenesis of human emphysema. *Am Rev Respir Dis* 1988; 137:918.

30. Riley DJ, Kramer MJ, Kerr JS, et al.: Damage and repair of lung connective tissue in rats exposed to toxic levels of oxygen. *Am Rev Respir Dis* 1987; 135:441.

31. Leopold JG, Gough J: The centrilobular form of hypertrophic emphysema and its relation to chronic bronchitis. *Thorax* 1957; 12:219.

32. Hogg JC, Nepszy SJ, Macklem PT, Thurlbeck WM: Elastic properties of the centrilobular emphysematous space. *J Clin Invest* 1969; 48:1306.

33. Cardoso WV, Sekhon HS, Hyde DM, Thurlbeck WM: Collagen and elastin in human pulmonary emphysema. *Am Rev Respir Dis* 1993; 147:975.

34. Kim WD, Eidelman DH, Izquierdo JL, et al.: Centrilobular and panlobular emphysema in smokers; two distinct morphologic and functional entities. *Am Rev Respir Dis* 1991; 144:1385.

35. Cohen AB, Girard W, McLarty J, et al.: A controlled trial of colchicine to reduce the elastase load in the lungs of cigarette smokers with chronic obstructive pulmonary disease. *Am Rev Respir Dis* 1990; 142:63.

36. Snider GL: Emphysema: the first two centuries—and beyond; a historical overview, with suggestions for future research: part 2. *Am Rev Respir Dis* 1992; 146:1615.

37. Stone PJ, Lucey EC, Snider GL: Induction and exacerbation of emphysema in hamsters with human neutrophil elastase inactivated reversibly by a peptide boronic acid. *Am Rev Respir Dis* 1990; 141:47.

38. Stone PJ, Lucey EC, Noskova D, et al.: Covalently linking a peptidyl carbamate elastase inhibitor to a hydrophilic polymer increases its effectiveness in preventing emphysema and secretory cell metaplasia in the hamster. *Am Rev Respir Dis* 1992; 146:457.

Chapter 86

THERAPEUTIC REGIMENS IN CHRONIC OBSTRUCTIVE PULMONARY DISEASE

ALEJANDRO C. ARROLIGA AND RICHARD A. MATTHAY

Prevention
   Smoking cessation
   Pneumococcal vaccine
   Influenza vaccine and chemoprophylaxis

Pharmacologic Therapy
   Anticholinergic agents
   β-Adrenergic agonists
   Theophylline
   Corticosteroids
   Mucolytic agents
   Almitrine
   Vasodilators
   Nitric Oxide

α_1**-Antiprotease Deficiency Therapy**

The management of patients with chronic obstructive pulmonary disease (COPD) includes primary and secondary prevention, adequate nutrition, surgery, rehabilitation, and pharmacologic treatment. This chapter provides an overview of the most commonly used preventive and pharmacologic measures. Nutritional management as well as surgical therapy (bullectomy, lung volume reduction, and lung transplantation) are beyond the scope of this chapter. Rehabilitation and oxygen and antibiotic therapy in patients with COPD are covered in other chapters in this book.

Prevention

SMOKING CESSATION

Cigarette smoking is the most important preventable cause of morbidity and mortality in the United States.[1] Smoking significantly accelerates the rate of decline of lung function associated with aging; therefore smokers with COPD should be vigorously encouraged to discontinue smoking.[2] Nicotine addiction is treated with nonpharmacologic as well as pharmacologic modalities.[3] Nicotine replacement therapy, which alleviates the symptoms of nicotine withdrawal, is beneficial in the first 3 weeks after smoking cessation when clinical manifestations of nicotine withdrawal are most intense.[4] When combined with behavior modification, nicotine

replacement is more effective than placebo in helping the smoker to quit.[3,4] Nicotine replacement therapy has been beneficial in highly nicotine-dependent subjects, as indicated by their strong desire to smoke within 30 min after waking up, smoking 20 cigarettes or more per day, and strong craving for cigarettes during previous attempts to quit.[4]

Nicotine replacement therapy is available as nicotine polacrilex (chewing gum), as a nasal solution, and as a patch for transdermal delivery. Side effects of nicotine replacement therapy are minimal.[4-6] Recommended exclusion criteria for nicotine replacement are listed in Table 86-1.

Other pharmacologic agents that have been used but are of unproven efficacy in smoking cessation include clonidine, propranolol, naloxon, and tricyclic antidepressants.

PNEUMOCOCCAL VACCINE

The currently used 23-valent pneumococcal vaccine was initially licensed in 1984, and its composition has been determined by the relative distribution of 83 pneumococcal serotypes that cause invasive infections.[7] The 23-valent vaccine has capsular polysaccharide representing 85 to 90 percent of the pneumococci responsible for invasive infection.[7,8]

Healthy young adults have an excellent antibody response to the vaccine; 80 percent or more show at least a twofold increase in antibody concentrations.[9] Most healthy elderly persons have a similar response, although antibody concen-

TABLE 86-1 Exclusion Criteria for Nicotine Replacement Therapy

Postmyocardial infarction
Severe peripheral vascular disease
Serious cardiac arrhythmia
Systemic hypertension
Vasospastic disease
Active peptic ulcer disease
Active esophagitis
Pheochromocytoma
Hyperthyroidism
Insulin-dependent diabetes mellitus
Pregnancy
Breast-feeding

SOURCE: Modified from Lee and D'Alonzo,[4] with permission.

trations after vaccination are lower and tend to decrease over time; revaccination in the elderly is usually followed by a new increase in antibody concentrations.[9] Compared with age-matched controls, patients with COPD attain a lower concentration of antibody and respond to fewer antigens. However, the overall vaccination efficacy in patients with COPD is 60 to 70 percent.[9]

Patients with COPD are at increased risk for serious pneumococcal infection, and the current recommendation is that such patients receive the pneumococcal vaccine,[7,8,10] which can be administered intramuscularly or subcutaneously.[10] Minor self-limited local reactions—such as erythema, induration, and pain—occur in as many as half of recipients.[7,8,10] Severe reactions are rare.[8]

Patients at high risk who received the previously available 14-valent vaccine should be revaccinated with the 23-valent vaccine.[10] Revaccination after 6 years is recommended for patients who received the 23-valent vaccine and are considered to be at risk for fatal pneumococcal infection—for example, asplenic and transplant patients.[10] Patients with COPD probably require revaccination because they are at risk for rapid decline in the antibody concentrations.

INFLUENZA VACCINE AND CHEMOPROPHYLAXIS

Influenza is associated with significant morbidity and mortality and a high economic cost. Influenza viruses cause as many as 40,000 excess deaths in the United States during epidemic years, and the annual cost associated with epidemics exceeds $12 billion.[11,12] Influenza is preventable, but unfortunately influenza vaccine is underutilized. As many as 60 percent of the elderly population at risk have never received the vaccine.[11]

The vaccine is a combination of two strains of influenza A virus and one strain of influenza B virus. The current-year vaccine is based on antigenic analysis of isolates of the previous year. The viruses contained in the vaccine are inactivated and grown on eggs.[10] The vaccine is administered in mid-October and November; thus the period of maximum antibody titer coincides with the period of most likely exposure to the influenza virus (December to March).[10,11] The vaccine has been proven to be associated with less frequent hospitalization for pneumonia and influenza, congestive heart failure, and acute and chronic respiratory problems.[11] Furthermore, influenza vaccine decreases mortality and is associated with direct savings in health care costs; therefore the vaccine is indicated in patients with COPD.[11,12]

The vaccine is given intramuscularly, and one-third of vaccinated patients have minor side effects such as local soreness, swelling, and erythema.[10] Because the vaccine contains inactivated virus, it does not cause a viruslike illness and is not associated with an increased incidence of Guillian-Barré syndrome.[10] The antibody response after vaccination is not affected by concominant corticosteroid therapy in patients with COPD.[13]

Antiviral prophylaxis with amantadine or rimantadine is effective for high-risk patients during outbreaks of influenza A. Chemoprophylaxis is not useful against influenza B virus. Chemoprophylaxis may be particularly useful during outbreaks of a strain of influenza A that is not contained in the vaccine used in that particular season. Amantadine prevents influenza A in 70 to 90 percent of cases and may reduce the duration of constitutional symptoms if given within 48 h of the onset of influenza A. Amantadine and rimantadine may also be useful as an adjunct to late immunization, as supplemental protection in patients expected to have a weak immunologic response, or when influenza vaccine is contraindicated—for example, in patients who are allergic to eggs. Amantadine is also useful to control nosocomial outbreaks of influenza A.[10]

The recommended dosage of amantadine for normal adults below 65 years of age is 200 mg per day in one or two doses for at least 10 days after exposure; in patients 65 years of age and older, the dosage is reduced to 100 mg per day. Amantadine is excreted by the kidneys, and the dosage must be adjusted in patients with impaired renal function. The side effects of therapy include light-headedness, insomnia, nervousness, and dyspepsia. Rimantadine is as effective as amantadine in the prevention of influenza A infection. The recommended dosage is 100 mg twice a day, but in the elderly and in patients with liver and renal dysfunction, this must be reduced to 100 mg per day. The duration of therapy should be at least 10 days after exposure. Rimantadine is well tolerated. The influenza virus may become resistant to the drug during treatment.[10]

Pharmacologic Therapy

ANTICHOLINERGIC AGENTS

Herbal medications containing anticholinergic drugs have been used in India and the Americas for centuries.[14,15] Anticholinergic agents have become more widely used in patients with COPD, primarily because of the availability of the new quaternary anticholinergic drugs (for example, ipratropium bromide), which are significantly less toxic than their tertiary ammonium precursors, such as atropine sulfate.[14,15]

The activity of the vagus nerve causes an increase in the bronchomotor tone and is responsible for the reflex bronchoconstriction that occurs in response to noxious stimuli. Anticholinergic agents antagonize the vagal innervation of central airways, thereby producing bronchodilatation.[15] None of the anticholinergic agents have anti-inflammatory effects, but they alleviate dyspnea, increase exercise tolerance, and improve gas exchange in patients with COPD.[14,15] In acute exacerbations of COPD, ipratropium bromide produces at least the same degree of bronchodilatation as maximal doses of β-adrenergic agonists.[14,16] Ipratropium bromide has been shown to reduce the volume of sputum without altering its viscosity.[16]

The anticholinergic agents consist of two classes: tertiary and quaternary ammonium compounds.[14,15] The most important tertiary ammonium compound is atropine sulfate. Generally, atropine sulfate is used in nebulized form in a dosage of 0.5 to 2.5 mg every 4 to 6 h. The tertiary ammonium compounds are lipid-soluble and easily absorbed, and they can cause significant toxic effects, including dry mouth, flushing of the skin, blurred vision, mood changes, and psychosis. Tachycardia is common.[14,15] The quaternary ammonium compounds, however, are water-soluble and poorly absorbed and therefore cause fewer side effects when administered directly to the airways. The most commonly used quaternary ammonium compounds are ipratropium bromide, oxitropium bromide, atropine methylnitrate, and glycopyrrolate. Ipratropium bromide and glycopyrrolate are frequently used in clinical practice, but only ipratropium bromide is approved in the United States for treatment of patients with COPD[14,15] (see Table 86-2).

Ipratropium bromide is available in a metered-dose inhaler (MDI) and as an 0.02 percent solution for nebulized administration. Each puff of the MDI provides 18 μg of drug. The recommended dose of MDI preparation is two puffs four times a day, but most patients require four to eight puffs four times a day.[14,16] These high doses unfortunately double or triple the cost of treatment and contribute significantly to the poor compliance of patients with COPD.[15,17]

Ipratropium bromide has been shown in short- and long-term studies to be superior to therapy with β-adrenergic agonists; these findings and the lack of side effects make ipratropium bromide MDI the preferred bronchodilator in outpatients with COPD.[14-16] Although the use of a combination of an anticholinergic agent and β-adrenergic agonist in the stable patient with COPD is controversial, an additive effect may be expected.[14,15,18] Anticholinergic agents cause bronchodilation predominantly in the major airways and β-adrenergic agonist agents exert their major effect in the smaller airways. In patients with COPD, the combination of ipratropium bromide and the β-agonist albuterol elicits a greater bronchodilator response than that caused by either agent used alone.[18,19] During acute exacerbations of COPD, ipratropium bromide and β-adrenergic agonists appear to have at least similar and probably additive effects.[20]

β-ADRENERGIC AGONISTS

β-Adrenergic agents have been used since ancient times. The modern use of these agents dates from the 1930s, when epinephrine became available in a nebulized form.[14,15]

There are two classes of β-adrenergic bronchodilators: catecholamines (e.g., epinephrine) and the more commonly used noncatecholamines, which are less biodegradable and therefore have a more persistent effect.[14] The β-adrenergic agents activate adenylate cyclase. A cyclic adenosine monophosphate–dependent protein kinase phosphorylates a myosin kinase, reducing its affinity for calmodulin (a calcium-binding protein) and thus changing the actin-myosin interaction and producing bronchodilation.[15,21,22]

Besides producing bronchodilation, β-adrenergic agonists improve mucociliary clearance and may reduce airway inflammation in patients with inflammatory airways disease.[15] Despite their long-time use, optimal dosing for patients with COPD has not been well evaluated, and in general, commonly used doses may result in submaximal bronchodilatation.[16] However, doses of more than four puffs of albuterol by MDI do not cause further increment in FEV_1.[23]

In patients with COPD, a small component of the airways obstruction is frequently reversible. The acute response to inhaled bronchodilators is not a reproducible guide to reversibility of airflow obstruction, and testing for the reversibility of airways obstruction is imperfect in patients with COPD.[23,24] The response is heterogeneous with different drugs. But even in the absence of reversible airways obstruction, β-adrenergic agents alone or in combination

TABLE 86-2   Inhaled Anticholinergic Medication

Drug	Dose, μg	Peak Effect, min	Dose Interval, h
Ipratropium bromide[a]			
MDI[b]	36–144	60–120	6
Nebulization	500	60–120	6
Atropine sulfate (1%)			
Nebulization	500–2500	30–170	6
Glycopyrrolate			
Nebulization	200–1000	120–180	6–12
Atropine methylnitrate			
Nebulization	1500	60–180	6–10
Oxitropium bromide			
MDI	200–500	40–120	6–12

[a] Approved by the U.S. Food and Drug Administration.
[b] MDI = metered-dose inhaler.
SOURCE: Modified from Ziment[14] and Skorodin,[15] with permission.

TABLE 86-3 Inhaled β-Adrenergic Agonists

Drugs	MDI Dose, mg/puffs	Three-Puff Dose, mg approx.	Nebulization Dose, 4–6 h	β RECEPTOR ACTIVITY		EFFECT, min		
				β₁	β₂	Onset	Peak	Duration
Albuterol	0.09	0.3	1.5 mg	+	+ + + +	5–15	60–90	240–360
Metaproterenol	0.65	2.0	15 mg	+	+ + +	5–15	10–60	60–180
Bitolterol	0.37	1.0		+	+ + + +	5–10	60–90	300–480
Terbutaline	0.20	0.6	0.3 mg	+	+ + + +	5–30	60–120	180–360
Pirbuterol	0.20	0.6		+	+ + +	5–10	30–60	180–240
Isoproterenol	0.08	0.2	0.7–3 mg	+ + +	+ + +	3–5	5–10	60–90
Isoetharine	0.34	1.0		+ +	+ +	3–5	5–20	60–150

a MDI = Metered-Dose inhaler.
SOURCE: Modified from Skorodin[15] and Feguson and Cherniack,[16] with permission.

with theophylline and anticholinergic agents, may decrease dyspnea and improve functional activity and gas exchange.[14,15]

Several β-adrenergic agents are available. They differ in their activity at the different β-adrenoceptors and in the onset and duration of action (Table 86-3). The preferred agents are albuterol, metaproterenol, bitolterol, pirbuterol, and terbutaline, which are associated with a low incidence of cardiovascular side effects because they predominantly stimulate the $β_2$-adrenoceptor.[14,15]

These drugs may be administered by oral, parenteral subcutaneous and intravenous, and inhalational routes. Inhalation (MDI and nebulizer) provides adequate bronchodilation without significant toxic effects and therefore is the preferred route.[14,15]

Oral β-adrenergic agonists may be as effective as theophylline for chronic airways obstruction, but because of the high incidence of side effects, oral β-adrenergic agonists are used only if the patient cannot use inhaled agents.[16] Nebulized preparations may be useful in acute exacerbations.[14,15] Doses delivered by a nebulizer are greater than the doses delivered by MDI; however, even in hospitalized patients, an MDI with a spacer device is less expensive and may be as effective as a jet nebulizer. Parenteral administration of β-adrenergic agonists sometimes is used in the emergency setting. Administration of the drug by subcutaneous or intravenous routes is possible, but these routes do not offer any advantage over delivery by MDI with a spacer or by nebulizer. Furthermore, parenteral administration may be hazardous because of the high incidence of cardiovascular side effects (for example, cardiac arrhythmia).[14,15]

The patient must be taught the correct technique for using the MDI, and the patient's technique must be reviewed frequently. After a gentle exhalation to residual volume, the MDI is activated by the patient simultaneously with a slow, deep inhalation to total lung capacity.[25] The breath should be held for 8 to 10 s to maximize the deposition of the drug in the tracheobronchial tree. The use of a spacer has been advocated to increase delivery of the drug to the bronchial tree and to decrease its deposition in the oropharynx; this decreases the systemic absorption of the drug and reduces side effects of therapy.[15]

The most common side effects of β-adrenergic agonists are tremors, nervousness, and palpitations. The β-adrenergic

agents have positive inotropic and chronotropic effects and cause a minor increase in the blood pressure; tachycardia and simple arrhythmias may also occur. These cardiovascular effects are dose-dependent and are minimal when the agent is administered by MDI, but they increase progressively when the medication is given by nebulizer, oral, and parenteral administration. Excessive doses may produce fatal arrhythmias and myocardial ischemia.[14,15]

The β-adrenergic agonists may cause electrolyte abnormalities. Serum concentration of potassium may decrease because of a shift of potassium into the intracellular compartment. The decrease may be accentuated in patients taking theophylline and diuretics. Similar decreases may occur in serum phosphate, calcium, and magnesium, whereas serum glucose, insulin, and fatty acids may increase.[14–16]

β-adrenergic agonists also may temporarily worsen arterial hypoxemia because they produce pulmonary vasodilatation and a transient worsening of the ventilation-perfusion relationship. Careful administration of supplemental oxygen may overcome this problem. Tolerance of β-adrenergic agonists and rebound bronchoconstriction may occur; deterioration of pulmonary function in patients with COPD and asthma has been reported with prolonged administration of bronchodilators, although the mechanism of this effect is unknown.[14,15]

THEOPHYLLINE

Theophylline, a xanthine derivative, has been used to treat obstructive airways disease since the beginning of the century, and despite controversy about its current role in COPD, theophylline continues to be used in patients with airways disease.[14,15]

Theophylline may be beneficial in patients with COPD. However, with the increased use of other pharmacologic agents, the place of theophylline in the treatment of patients with COPD must be redefined. Theophylline is a bronchodilator and probably has anti-inflammatory properties.[14–16] It can increase the FEV_1 by 10 to 15 percent and improve forced vital capacity and maximal voluntary ventilation. Even in the absence of spirometric changes, dyspnea may be alleviated and gas exchange improved. Besides the improvement in ventilatory indices, significant improvement in exercise performance after 1 month of therapy with theophylline has been documented.[26–28]

The mechanism of action of theophylline is unknown, but some of the proposed modes of action responsible for the smooth muscle relaxation and the inhibition of inflammatory cell function are inhibition of leukotriene and oxygen radicals production by neutrophils, inhibition of neuropeptide release, antagonism of adenosine receptors, inhibition of phosphodiesterase isozymes and calcium ion sequestration and stimulation of calcium efflux in airway muscle. Other therapeutic actions of theophylline that probably have clinical implication include improvement of mucociliary clearance in vitro and in vivo, augmentation of diaphragmatic strength and delay in the onset of fatigue of the diaphragm, improvement in the cardiovascular performance of the right and, in some studies, of the left ventricle, and enhancement of the neurorespiratory drive of the central nervous system.[14–16,29]

The reasons for the controversy about the use of theophylline in COPD include uncertainty about the mechanism of action of the drug, confusion about its absorption and clearance, complexities in dosing, and toxic effects of the medication. Moreover, studies documenting the efficacy of theophylline have been contradictory, and there has been a lack of standardization, with variation in the populations studied, treatment duration, and follow-up evaluation.[29]

Theophylline is available in many oral preparations and for intravenous use as aminophylline, which consists of approximately 80 percent anhydrous theophylline. Multiplying the oral dose of theophylline by 1.2 equals the dose of aminophylline, and multiplying the dose of aminophylline by 0.8 approximates the dose of oral anhydrous theophylline. Theophylline therapy should be started if the patient has not responded adequately to less toxic agents such as ipratropium bromide and β-adrenergic agonists or when the patient has cor pulmonale. Therapy is begun at a low dosage of 200 mg once or twice daily and gradually increased over the next 2 weeks by 100 to 200 mg per day every second or third day. The final dosage is determined by the presence of side effects, intercurrent infection, cardiac and liver dysfunction, or hypoxemia, which tend to increase the blood theophylline concentration.[14–16]

Theophylline metabolism is affected by various drugs and intercurrent disease. Theophylline clearance is enhanced by therapy with phenytoin, phenobarbital, rifampin, carbamazapine, and furosemide as well as the smoking of tobacco and cannabis. The effect of tobacco on theophylline metabolism decreases within 1 week of abstinence and is not affected by pharmacologic nicotine. Medical conditions that enhance clearance include hyperthyroidism and cystic fibrosis. Theophylline clearance is slowed by quinolone and macrolide antibiotics, isoniazid, propranolol, calcium channel blockers, cimetidine, oral caffeine, and influenza vaccine. When these drugs are used, theophylline concentration must be measured and the dose adjusted.[14,15]

Intravenous theophylline therapy is valuable in patients with an acute exacerbation of COPD.[14] In such patients who have no detectable serum theophylline, an initial bolus of 6 mg/kg is given, followed by a drip of 0.4 to 0.6 mg/kg/h. This dose should be adjusted to achieve a serum concentra-

tion between 8 and 10 μg/mL. The dose in the elderly usually is lower than that in a younger patient. In the patient receiving theophylline before admission to the hospital, each 1-mg/kg bolus of aminophylline increases the serum concentration by approximately 2 μg/mL.

Toxic effects are common in patients taking theophylline, and symptoms of toxicity tend to appear at a lower serum concentration in elderly patients and patients with a low albumin level. In general, symptoms are mild, but they may be life-threatening. The most common side effects are gastrointestinal distress, including epigastric pain, nausea, dyspepsia, and occasionally gastrointestinal bleeding. Anxiety, nervousness, irritability, and tremor are common. Alteration in sleep habits and insomnia have been reported, even in patients with therapeutic levels of theophylline. Serious toxic effects include cardiac arrhythmias and even cardiac arrest with rapid intravenous injection (administration of the initial bolus over 30 min avoids this problem). Seizures and death occur with acute and chronic overdosage. The diagnosis of theophylline toxicity requires a high clinical suspicion. Patients with severe toxicity require hemoperfusion or hemodialysis; in patients with recent oral ingestion, nasogastric lavage and administration of activated charcoal and a cathartic are helpful.[15,30]

CORTICOSTEROIDS

Although the role of corticosteroid therapy in stable disease and acute exacerbations of COPD is controversial, few patients may benefit.[14,15] A recent meta-analysis concluded that patients receiving oral corticosteroids had more frequent increases in FEV_1 than patients receiving placebo.[31] A closely monitored corticosteroid trial may be appropriate in patients with stable COPD receiving maximal inhaled bronchodilator therapy who remain symptomatic, functionally impaired, or show a progressive decrease in the FEV_1.[16,31–33] The patient with variability in flow rate is more likely to respond. The most commonly used corticosteroid preparations are prednisone and methylprednisolone. Prednisone 40 mg (or its equivalent in methylprednisolone) is given in the morning for 2 weeks. An improvement ≥ 20 percent in baseline FEV_1 is considered a positive trial. Besides improvement in the FEV_1, dyspnea and functional status must be measured during the trial. Occasionally, dyspnea may be alleviated and functional capacity improved without improvement in spirometry. If the patient responds to the corticosteroid trial, the dose should be slowly tapered over 3 to 4 weeks. The goal is to achieve the lowest dosage that provides an objective response and minimal side effects. Usually this goal is achieved at 5 to 15 mg per day or 10 to 25 mg on alternate days.[14–16]

Corticosteroids also are used during an acute exacerbation of COPD, in which their role is equally controversial. In spite of this uncertainty, therapy with high-dose intravenous methylprednisolone (60 to 120 mg every 6 h) frequently is used in acute exacerbations.

Corticosteroids also may be delivered by inhalation. Although inhaled corticosteroids are beneficial in patients with bronchial asthma, the effect is less conclusive in patients with COPD.[34] The subgroup of patients with chronic bronchitis have evidence of inflammation in the airways, although less severe than in patients with asthma, and therapy with inhaled corticosteroids may reduce the airways obstruction and decrease inflammation of the bronchial tree in such patients.[35,36] However, most reports have involved heterogeneous populations, including patients with reversible and nonreversible airways disease.[34] Patients with some degree of reversibility in the airways obstruction are most likely to respond. Patients with COPD and rapidly declining lung function also may benefit from inhaled corticosteroid therapy.[33] Other anti-inflammatory agents, such as cromolyn sodium and nedocromil, are not beneficial in the vast majority of patients with COPD.[15]

The side effects of systemic corticosteroid therapy are significant. The most common such side effects include weight gain, thinning of the skin, and cataracts. Other common and severe side effects include osteoporosis, hyperglycemia, and gastrointestinal bleeding. In addition, systemic and respiratory muscle dysfunction may occur with prolonged therapy.[37] Finally, corticosteroid therapy may facilitate opportunistic infection, including gram-negative rods and fungi (for example, aspergillosis). Inhaled corticosteroid therapy is associated with fewer systemic complications than oral or parenteral therapy. Irritation of the oropharynx and hoarseness are common side effects of inhalation; mouthwash and gargling after use of inhaled corticosteroids may decrease local complications and the likelihood of systemic absorption.[14,15]

MUCOLYTIC AGENTS

Mucolytic therapy plays a minor role in the therapy for COPD. The agents most commonly used are water, iodide, guaifenesin, and acetylcysteine. Antibiotic therapy decreases mucus production associated with infection. Ipratropium bromide may reduce the volume of sputum but does not change its viscosity, and the β-adrenergic agonists increase mucociliary function and thus may facilitate the kinesis of the mucus.[14]

Even though water administration loosens secretions, its therapeutic value has not been demonstrated. However, patients with COPD should be well hydrated, especially during acute exacerbations. Aerosolized water may increase bronchospasm. Isotonic aerosols and humidifiers may have demulcent action, although there is no proof that this benefits patients with COPD.[14]

The iodide preparations used as mucolytic agents include saturated solution of potassium iodide (SSKI) and iodinated glycerol. The dosage of SSKI is 10 to 20 drops three or four times a day. Side effects range from a cutaneous reaction and a bad taste in the mouth to hypothyroidism. Iodinated glycerol (Organidin) was the only mucolytic agent that was studied in a randomized, double-blind, placebo-controlled trial.[38] Iodinated glycerol was recently discontinued from the market.

Expectorants, such as guaifenesin 200 to 400 mg orally every 4 to 6 h, have not been shown to be of value in patients with COPD. Acetylcysteine, a mucolytic agent, is available in the United States for nebulization, whereas an oral formulation is available in Europe and has been associated with some benefit in patients with COPD. When acetylcysteine is given by nebulizer, bronchospasm may be induced; therefore, prior administration of a β-adrenergic agent is indicated.[14]

Recombinant human DNase, a genetically engineered ribonuclease recently approved for treatment of cystic fibrosis, may be useful in patients with COPD. Clinical trials with this agent are being conducted, but because of its high cost and probably marginal effect, it will be unlikely to play a significant role in the management of patients with COPD.

ALMITRINE

Almitrine has been available outside of the United States for the last decade. Its role in the therapy of patients with COPD is uncertain. Almitrine increases the Pa_{O_2} by 5 to 10 mmHg and decreases the Pa_{CO_2} by about 4 mmHg in hypoxemic patients with COPD. Although its mode of action is unclear, it has been thought to stimulate the carotid and aortic bodies. Moreover, almitrine improves the ventilation-perfusion relationship. Unfortunately, therapy with almitrine has been associated with worsening of dyspnea. Furthermore, a significant increase in the mean pulmonary arterial pressure has been documented, with enhancement of the vasopressor response in the presence of hypoxia. Neuropathy has also been reported in patients with almitrine, although this important side effect may be avoided by using low doses of the drug.[39,40]

VASODILATORS

Approximately 50 percent of patients with COPD 50 years of age or older develop pulmonary hypertension.[41] The increase of mean pulmonary arterial pressure is usually mild to moderate, and the mean pressure generally does not exceed 40 mmHg. The best available vasodilator is oxygen, which attenuates and sometimes even reverses the progression of pulmonary hypertension in COPD.[41,42] Oxygen administration is discussed in Chapter 87.

Other conventional pulmonary vasodilators include β-adrenergic agonists, α-adrenergic antagonists, calcium channel blockers, angiotensin-converting enzyme inhibitors, nitrates, and such direct vasodilators as diazide and hydralazine.[41,42] The calcium channel blockers nifedipine, diltiazem, and felodipine exert an acute vasodilating effect, although long-term studies have failed to demonstrate sustained improvement in pulmonary hemodynamics at rest and during exercise.[41–44] Therapy with calcium channel blockers may be associated with systemic hypotension and decreased cardiac output due to a negative inotropic effect. At present, there is no indication for long-term use of oral vasodilators in patients with pulmonary hypertension and COPD.[41,42]

NITRIC OXIDE

Nitric oxide, which has been associated with selective pulmonary vasodilation, may have therapeutic potential in view of its lack of systemic effects.[45,46] Long-term studies are necessary, however, before nitric oxide can be recommended for use in patients with COPD.

Therapy for α_1-Antiprotease Deficiency

Deficiency of α_1-antiprotease, a codominant autosomal recessive disease, is present in 2 to 5 percent of patients with emphysema; α_1-antiprotease is an enzyme that protects against the effect of neutrophil elastase. Patients who have deficiency of α_1-antiprotease are at increased risk for lung damage and development of emphysema. The current strategies for treatment of the enzyme deficiency include pharmacologic stimulation with tamoxifen and danazol, augmentation therapy with human pooled α_1-antiprotease, and lung transplantation. Genetic therapy, including retrovirus and adenovirus-mediated transfer, will probably be available in the future.[47]

The clinical efficacy of augmentation therapy is unproven, although it is assumed that increasing the serum concentration of the enzyme decreases the rate of decline of airflow. Currently, the preferred treatment is administration of human pooled α_1-antiprotease by intravenous infusion, which can be given weekly, biweekly, or monthly. The recommended weekly dose is 60 mg/kg and the recommended monthly dose is 250 mg/kg. Both dose schedules increase antineutrophil elastase activity above levels considered pose a risk for emphysema. The U.S. Food and Drug Administration has approved weekly infusion, although monthly infusion probably has equal efficacy. The biweekly dose is 120 mg/kg, but because biweekly dosing offers less consistent serum levels above the protective threshold, it is not recommended. The following criteria have been suggested to select candidates for α_1-antiprotease replacement: (1) a high-risk phenotype, (2) an α_1-antiprotease concentration less than 11 μmol/L, (3) airflow obstruction on spirometry, (4) compliance with the treatment protocol, (5) age above 18 years, and (6) being a nonsmoker.[47]

References

1. Bartecchi CE, MacKenzie TD, Schrier RW: The human costs of tobacco use: Parts 1 and 2. *N Engl J Med* 1994; 330:907, 975.
2. Anthonisen NR, Connett JE, Kiley JP, et al.: Effects of smoking intervention and the use of an inhaled anticholinergic bronchodilator on the rate of decline of FEV$_1$: The Lung Health Study. *JAMA* 1994; 272:1497.
3. Fisher EB Jr, Lichtenstein E, Haire-Joshu D, et al.: Methods, successes, and failures of smoking cessation programs. *Annu Rev Med* 1993; 44:481.
4. Lee EW, D'Alonzo GE: Cigarette smoking, nicotine addiction, and its pharmacological treatment. *Arch Intern Med* 1993; 153:34.
5. Silagy C, Mant D, Fowler G, Lodge M: Meta-Analysis on efficacy of nicotine replacement therapies in smoking cessation. *Lancet* 1994; 343:139.
6. Imperial Cancer Research Fund General Practice Research Group: Randomized trial of nicotine patches in general practice: Results at one year. *Br Med J* 1994; 308:1476.
7. Butler JC, Breiman RF, Campbell JF, et al.: Pneumococcal polysaccharide vaccine efficacy: An evaluation of clinical recommendations. *JAMA* 1993; 270:1826.
8. Fine MJ, Smith MA, Carson CA, et al.: Efficacy of pneumococcal vaccination in adults: A meta-analysis of randomized controlled trials. *Arch Intern Med* 1994; 154:2666.
9. Fedson DS, Musher DM: Pneumococcal vaccine, in Plotkin SA, Mortimer EA Jr, (eds): *Vaccines* 2d ed. Philadelphia: Saunders, 1994: 517–564.
10. Clinical issues regarding specific vaccines, in *Guide for Adult Immunization*, 3d ed. Philadelphia: American College of Physicians, 1994: 79–149.
11. Nichol KL, Margolis KL, Wuorenma J, Von Sternberg T: The efficacy and cost effectiveness of vaccination against influenza among elderly persons living in the community. *N Engl J Med* 1994; 331:778.
12. Mullooly JP, Bennett MD, Hornbrook MC, et al.: Influenza vaccination programs for elderly persons: Cost-effectiveness in a Health Maintenance Organization. *Ann Intern Med* 1994; 121:947.
13. Kubiet MA, Gonzalez-Rothi RJ, Bender B, Cottey R: Antibody response to influenza vaccine in pulmonary patients receiving corticosteroids (abstr). *Chest* 1994; 106:163S.
14. Ziment I: Pharmacologic therapy of obstructive airway disease. *Clin Chest Med* 1990; 11:461.
15. Skorodin MS: Pharmacotherapy for asthma and chronic obstructive pulmonary disease. *Arch Intern Med* 1993; 153:814.
16. Ferguson GT, Cherniack RM: Management of chronic obstructive pulmonary disease. *N Engl J Med* 1993; 328:1017.
17. Rogol PR: Bronchodilator therapy with or without inhaled corticosteroid therapy for obstructive airways disease (letter). *N Engl J Med* 1993; 328:1044.
18. Newnham DM, Dhillon DP, Winter JH, et al.: Bronchodilator reversibility to low and high dose of terbutaline and ipratropium bromide in patients with chronic obstructive pulmonary disease. *Thorax* 1993; 48:1151.
19. Combivent Inhalation Aerosol Study Group: In chronic obstructive pulmonary disease, a combination of ipratropium and albuterol is more effective than either agent alone: An 85 day multicenter trial. *Chest* 1994; 105:1411.
20. Rebuck AS, Chapman KR, Abboud R, et al.: Nebulized anticholinergic and sympathomimetic treatment of asthma and chronic obstructive airways disease in the emergency room. *Am J Med* 1987; 82:59.
21. Adelstein RS, Sellers JR, Conti MA, et al.: Regulation of smooth muscle contractile proteins by calmodulin and cyclic AMP. *Fed Pro* 1982; 41:2873.
22. Lefkowitz RJ, Stadel JM, Caron M: Adenylate cyclase-coupled beta-adrenergic receptors: Structure and mechanisms of activation and desensitization. *Annu Rev Biochem* 1983; 52:159.
23. Jaeschke R, Guyatt GH, Cook D, et al.: The effect of increasing doses of β-agonists on airflow in patients with chronic airflow limitation. *Respir Med* 1993; 87:433.
24. Nisar M, Earis JE, Pearson MG, Calverly PMA: Acute bronchodilator trials in chronic obstructing pulmonary disease. *Am Rev Respir Dis* 1992; 146:555.
25. Hindle M, Newton DAG, Chrystin H: Investigations of an optimal inhaler technique with the use of urinary salbutamol excretion as a measure of relative bioavailability to the lung. *Thorax* 1993; 48:607.
26. McKay SE, Howie CA, Thomson AH, et al.: Value of theophylline treatment in patients handicapped by chronic obstructive lung disease. *Thorax* 1993; 48:227.
27. Mulloy E, McNicholas WT: Theophylline improves gas exchange during rest, exercise and sleeping in severe chronic obstructive pulmonary disease. *Am Rev Respir Dis* 1993; 148:1030.

28. Fink G, Kaye C, Sulkes J, et al.: Effect of theophylline on exercise performance in patients with severe chronic obstructive pulmonary disease. *Thorax* 1994; 49:332.

29. Vaz Fragoso CA, Miller MA: Review of the clinical efficacy of theophylline in the treatment of chronic obstructive pulmonary disease. *Am Rev Respir Dis* 1993; 147:S40.

30. Shannon M: Predictors of major toxicity after theophylline overdose. *Ann Intern Med* 1993; 119:1161.

31. Callahan CM, Dittus RS, Katz BP: Oral corticosteroid therapy for patients with stable chronic obstructive pulmonary disease. *Ann Intern Med* 1991; 114:216.

32. Stoller JK: Systemic corticosteroids in stable chronic obstructive pulmonary disease: Do they work (editorial). *Chest* 1987; 91:155.

33. Dompeling E, van Schayck CP, van Grunsven PM, et al.: Slowing the deterioration of asthma and chronic obstructive pulmonary disease observed during bronchodilator therapy by adding inhaled corticosteroids. *Ann Intern Med* 1993; 118:770.

34. Wedzicha JA: Inhaled corticosteroids in COPD: Awaiting controlled trials. (editorial). *Thorax* 1993; 48:305.

35. Linden M, Rasmussen JB, Piitulainen E, et al.: Airway inflammation in smokers with nonobstructive and obstructive chronic bronchitis. *Am Rev Respir Dis* 1993; 148:1226.

36. Thompson AB, Mueller MB, Heires AJ, et al.: Aerosolized beclomethasone in chronic bronchitis: Improved pulmonary function and diminished airway inflammations. *Am Rev Respir Dis* 1992; 146:389.

37. DeCramer M, Lacquet LM, Fagard R, Rogiers P: Corticosteroids contribute to muscle weakness in chronic airflow obstruction. *Am J Respir Crit Care Med* 1994; 150:11.

38. Petty TL: The national mucolytic study: Results of a randomized, double-blind, placebo-controlled study of iodinated glycerol in chronic obstructive bronchitis. *Chest* 1990; 97:75.

39. Winkelmann BR, Kullmer TH, Kneissl DG, et al.: Low-dose almitrine bismesylate in the treatment of hypoxemia due to chronic obstructive pulmonary disease. *Chest* 1994; 105:1383.

40. Saadjian AY, Philip-Joet FF, Barret A, et al.: Effect of almitrine bismesylate on pulmonary vaso-reactivity to hypoxia in chronic obstructive pulmonary disease. *Eur Respir J* 1994; 7:862.

41. Salvaterra CG, Rubin LJ: Investigation and management of pulmonary hypertension in chronic obstructive pulmonary disease. *Am Rev Respir Dis* 1993; 148:1414.

42. Weitzenblum E, Kessler R, Oswald M, Fraisse PH: Medical treatment of pulmonary hypertension in chronic lung disease. *Eur Respir J* 1994; 7:148.

43. Sajkov D, McEvoy RD, Cowie RJ, et al.: Felodipine improves pulmonary hemodynamics in chronic obstructive pulmonary disease. *Chest* 1993; 103:1354.

44. Mols P, Huynh CH, Dechamps, P, et al.: Acute effects of nifedipine on systolic and diastolic ventricular function in patients with chronic obstructive pulmonary disease. *Chest* 1993; 103:1381.

45. Adnot S, Kouyoumdjian C, De-Fouilloy C, et al.: Hemodynamic and gas exchange responses to infusion of acethylcholine and inhalation of nitric oxide in patients with chronic obstructive lung disease and pulmonary hypertension. *Am Rev Respir Dis* 1993; 148:310.

46. Moinard J, Manier G, Pillot O, Castaing Y: Effect of inhaled nitric oxide on hemodynamics and V/Q inequalities in patients with chronic obstructive pulmonary disease. *Am J Respir Crit Care Med* 1994; 149:1482.

47. Rovner MS, Stoller JK: Therapy for alpha 1-antitrypsin deficiency: Rationale and strategic approach. *Clin Pulm Med* 1994; 1:135.

Chapter 87

OXYGEN THERAPY IN CHRONIC OBSTRUCTIVE PULMONARY DISEASE

JESSE HALL AND LAWRENCE D. H. WOOD

Gas Exchange Impairment and Its Consequences in COPD

Patients with chronic obstructive pulmonary disease (COPD) exhibit various degrees of chronic hypoventilation and ventilation-perfusion (VA/Q) mismatch because of the large numbers of air spaces that are poorly ventilated in relation to their perfusion. Under these conditions, air inspired with a Pi_{O_2} of about 140 mmHg into alveoli with low VA/Q has sufficient oxygen removed to approach the mixed venous P_{O_2} of 40 mmHg, whereas less CO_2 is added to the alveolar gas as it approaches mixed venous P_{CO_2} of 50 mmHg. This degree of alveolar hypoxia stimulates hypoxic pulmonary vasoconstriction, which in turn causes pulmonary hypertension, right-heart dysfunction, and reduced cardiac output (Q_t). This same degree of alveolar hypoxia also causes incomplete saturation of arterial hemoglobin (Sa_{O_2}). Arterial hemoglobin desaturation reduces arterial oxygen content. This decreases oxygen delivery (the product of arterial oxygen content and cardiac output) to peripheral tissues, thus causing tissue hypoxia.

Hypoxic pulmonary vasoconstriction is only one of the causes of pulmonary hypertension and consequent cor pulmonale in patients with COPD.[1] Other potential contributors include other metabolic disturbances (e.g., hypercapnia, acidosis), pulmonary capillary loss related to emphysema, pulmonary arterial and arteriolar anatomic changes, neurohumoral changes, and lung mechanical effects. Nonetheless, treatment of hypoxic vasoconstriction may represent the most successful therapy currently available to the clinician to reverse cardiovascular dysfunction in patients with COPD. Even modest enrichment of the inspired oxygen concentration may reverse alveolar hypoxia (thus eliminating the component of hypoxic vasoconstriction contributing to pulmonary hypertension and right-heart failure) and arterial desaturation, thus eliminating the potential for tissue hypoxia. For example, increasing Fi_{O_2} from 0.2 to 0.4 raises Pi_{O_2} to 280 mmHg and virtually eliminates alveolar hypoxia and desaturation in all but the very low VA/Q units. Thus, the goals for oxygen therapy in those chronic lung diseases, which produce these gas exchange and circulatory disturbances, are to provide sufficient oxygen enrichment at home or in the hospital to ensure that Sa_{O_2} is > 90 percent, usually at a Pa_{O_2} of 65 to 70 mmHg, in a cost-efficient, convenient manner.[2]

Studies Evaluating Benefit and Risk of Oxygen Therapy in COPD

LONG-TERM OXYGEN THERAPY IN CHRONIC LUNG DISEASE

Early anecdotal experience in treatment of chronic lung disease with supplemental oxygen suggested that this intervention could correct secondary erythrocytosis, diminish pulmonary artery pressures, improve central nervous system, and decrease hospital admissions for disease exacerbations characterized by cor pulmonale. The effect of oxygen therapy on pulmonary artery pressure was felt to be particularly significant, since pulmonary hypertension with cor pulmonale long had been recognized as a poor prognostic sign in COPD, with a mortality > 65 percent over 4 years.[3] These and other clinical observations suggesting improved function and survival resulted in frequent use of LTOT, despite the expense of this therapy and the frequency of COPD. To their credit, early clinical investigators of pulmonary disease submitted LTOT to rigorous evaluation in prospective, randomized, placebo-controlled trials that could serve as models for future clinical studies.[4,5]

In a British study supported by the Medical Research Council of the United Kingdom,[4] 87 patients were enrolled and randomized between no oxygen therapy and 2 L/min for at least 15 h/day, including the sleeping hours. Patients were followed for 5 years. In an American study supported by the National Institutes of Health,[5] 203 patients at six centers were enrolled and randomized to receive oxygen either nightly for 12 h or continuously for at least 19 h/day. The dose of oxygen used was the amount necessary to increase the arterial P_{O_2} to 65 mmHg, with 1 L/min additional oxygen flow at night. Both studies showed a clear difference in survival between the groups (Fig. 87-1); together, these studies strongly supported the notion that LTOT improved survival in COPD and that continuous therapy was preferable. The American study included detailed evaluation of neurologic, psychologic, and social function. Both patient groups showed improvement in these parameters after 6 months of treatment, but these differences were not significantly different between the oxygen and room-air placebo groups.

Data from these trials regarding the effects of LTOT on pulmonary hypertension and cardiovascular function were not entirely consistent. In analysis of the British trial, no difference in pulmonary artery pressure or pulmonary vascular resistance was noted between the two groups.[4] In the North American series, neither group normalized baseline elevations of pulmonary artery pressure and resistance while on supplemental oxygen, but the group receiving continuous therapy did exhibit a decrease in resting pulmonary artery pressure of about 3 mmHg with a 20 percent decrease in pul-

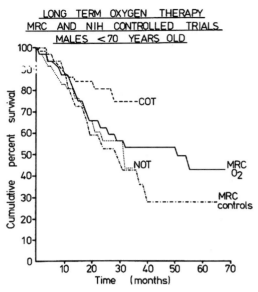

Figure 87-1 Survival data for the Medical Research Council (MRC) and North American (NOT, COT) long-term oxygen therapy trials. Note that in the MRC study, patients receiving nocturnal oxygen therapy had improved survival over controls receiving none. In the North American trial, patients receiving continuous oxygen therapy (COT) had improved survival over patients receiving only nocturnal oxygen therapy (NOT).

monary vascular resistance. This was associated with an increase in stroke volume index; hemodynamics were slightly more improved during exercise.[6] For both groups, the early change in pulmonary artery pressure was associated with subsequent survival. Of note, oxygen therapy was most effective in reducing mortality in patients with an initial low pulmonary artery pressure and resistance, suggesting that early therapy to prevent more severe pulmonary vascular disease may be a desirable goal.

It has been suggested in other studies that the hemodynamic response to 24 h of oxygen therapy might be useful as a means for predicting long-term benefit from LTOT. In 28 patients with COPD and cor pulmonale, responders, defined as those with > 5-mmHg decrease in mean pulmonary artery pressure, had an 85 percent survival over 2 years compared with only 22 percent in nonresponders.[7] The progressive increase in pulmonary arterial pressure and resistance in these patients can be halted and partially reversed by LTOT (Fig. 87-2), although normalization of these values rarely is observed.[8] Removing oxygen from patients receiving LTOT also has been demonstrated to increase pulmonary vascular resistance at rest and during exercise, with an associated decrease in stroke volume.[9]

Although these findings are consistent with a view that resolution of hypoxia-mediated pulmonary hypertension explains survival benefit in LTOT, other studies suggest that improved oxygen delivery to peripheral tissues may be an alternative and independent mechanism to explain this finding.[10-12] These studies do not clarify if benefit from LTOT is

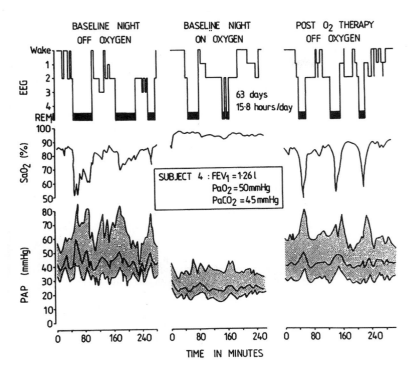

Figure 87-2 Response of pulmonary artery pressure to nocturnal oxygen therapy in patients with COPD. Several representative tracings of continuously monitored pulmonary artery pressure are shown.

conferred by prevention of progression of pulmonary vascular disease or by augmentation of oxygen delivery to key tissues, or by both. Nonetheless, it is well demonstrated that LTOT in hypoxemic patients with COPD will improve survival. Analysis of data combined from prospective studies indicates that nocturnal oxygen therapy is preferable to no therapy, and that continuous therapy (> 19 h/day) is better still for patient survival.[4,5] Incremental benefit to be derived from 24 h/day use of oxygen has not been determined.

OXYGEN THERAPY FOR NOCTURNAL DESATURATION

It appears that many patients with COPD with normal oxygenation while awake may exhibit nocturnal oxyhemoglobin desaturation during sleep.[13-15] Some studies have estimated that as many as 25 percent of the nonhypoxemic COPD patient population may exhibit this gas exchange abnormality.[13] Nocturnal desaturation is typically accompanied by increases in pulmonary artery pressure, which can be prevented by supplemental oxygen.[14,15] Some investigators have suggested that nocturnal oxygen desaturation results in transient pulmonary hypertension, which is a precursor to fixed pulmonary hypertension in patients with COPD.[16,17] Nocturnal desaturation in patients with COPD has been shown to correlate with prognosis.[18] Some data suggest that low-flow oxygen therapy in patients with nocturnal desaturation may delay deterioration of cardiovascular function in patients with COPD, but there has been no confirmation of improved survival or quality of life by treatment of this patient group with nocturnal oxygen.[19] Further evaluation of this issue is required.

OXYGEN FOR ACUTE-ON-CHRONIC RESPIRATORY FAILURE

Patients with COPD often experience acute deteriorations characterized by worsened hypoxemia and hypoventilation, a phenomenon termed *acute-on-chronic respiratory failure* (ACRF).[20] As in chronic stable lung disease, this hypoxemia is caused by mismatching of ventilation and perfusion and is corrected with modest oxygen enrichment of inspired air.[21] Despite the obvious potential benefit to correcting hypoxemia during these episodes of ACRF, some clinicians have advocated a constrained use of oxygen therapy because of concerns that excessive oxygen administration in ACRF could precipitate a need for mechanical ventilatory support, since patients with COPD might rely on a hypoxic drive to breathe.[22] This notion has been well studied, and these concerns are not supported by currently available information.[23,24] When patients with COPD are treated with oxygen, a further increase of baseline hypercarbia is encountered almost invariably, but this increment in Pa_{CO_2} is not explained on the basis of worsened hypoventilation. A large component of the observed increase in P_{CO_2} is explained by an increase in dead space, a ventilation-perfusion alteration that could occur as a result of oxygen-mediated relaxation of airways or alteration of blood flow.[25,26] Respiratory drive measured by mouth occlusion pressure ($P_{.01}$) is three times normal despite abolition of hypoxic drive by oxygen therapy, and minute ventilation is not reduced.[23] These observations are consistent with a view that hypercarbia following oxygen therapy in ACRF does not necessarily signal worsened respiratory failure secondary to diminished drive to breathe. Indeed, attention in this disorder has increasingly turned toward respiratory muscle fatigue (resulting from the excessive mechanical load of ACRF) as an explanation for failure in these patients.[20] Unwarranted reluctance to provide oxygen might actually contribute to ventilatory failure by adverse effects on muscle function or through hypoxic impairment of the patient's compliance with other therapies.

The precise mechanism(s) of benefit from acute administration of oxygen in ACRF are not entirely clear.[27-29] Some investigators have demonstrated that acute administration of oxygen in ACRF causes a fall in pulmonary artery pressure,[27] while others have shown that pulmonary artery pressure remains the same or may actually increase.[28,29] Acute benefits from oxygen therapy (e.g., reduction in pulmonary artery pressure) may be blunted by increases in Pa_{CO_2} with an associated acidosis. Effects of oxygen therapy over the days of recovery from ACRF have not been well studied.

Recommendations for LTOT in COPD

In the United States, recommendations for prescription of oxygen therapy for patients with COPD are formulated in light of the frequently required Certificate of Medical Necessity (HCFA Form 484), which regulates government reimbursement for this therapy.[30-32] Current recommendations for home oxygen therapy in patients with COPD are that LTOT be prescribed when $P_{O_2} < 55$ mmHg at rest in a patient with COPD who is stable and receiving optimal therapy, or when $P_{O_2} = 56$ to 59 mmHg and cor pulmonale, erythrocytosis, or peripheral edema is present. Ideally, the dose of oxygen prescribed should be determined for exercise, sleep, and the awake resting state separately, as determined by some measure of continuous saturation such as pulse oximetry. The utility of beginning LTOT at an earlier point in the course of COPD, as well as the usefulness of oxygen during exercise in patients who desaturate only during activity, remains to be defined. These guidelines for LTOT in COPD generally have been used for patients with chronic lung disease of all types, despite the lack of large reported series of other patient groups. Current HCFA guidelines allow reimbursement for supplemental oxygen during sleep in COPD patients with nocturnal oxygen desaturation who otherwise do not qualify for continuous home oxygen therapy, although long-term benefit has not been demonstrated in this patient group (see above).

For patients with ACRF, a reasonable approach is to use sufficient amounts of supplemental oxygen to achieve 90 percent arterial saturation, titrated by applying nasal prongs and increasing flow while saturation is measured by pulse oximetry.[20] If bedside measures of airflow obstruction and respiratory muscle function (respiratory rate, use of accessory muscles, pulsus paradoxus, chest auscultation) indicate improvement with oxygen and other therapies, measurement of blood gases is not necessary, because hypercapnia is not likely to signal a deteriorating course. This titrated therapy should be conducted in a closely monitored setting, since progression of ventilatory failure may occur despite correction of hypoxemia.

Techniques of Oxygen Administration and Monitoring

OXYGEN DELIVERY SYSTEMS

The ubiquitous need for oxygen in health-care facilities requires these locations to have bulk storage of oxygen with gas piped to all patient-care areas. Long-term oxygen therapy in the outpatient setting as prescribed by the physician involves use of compressed gas, liquid oxygen, or oxygen concentrators.

Tanks of compressed gas are widely used but require frequent refilling and are minimally transportable for extended periods of time. Table 87-1 lists characteristics of these storage devices. These compressed gas tanks do not meet the requirements of a lightweight source for prolonged use between fillings.

Liquid oxygen may be stored at home in insulated reservoirs at -300 °C for direct use by the nonambulatory patient. Transfilling of portable devices by the patient allows up to 8 h of continuous oxygen delivery at a rate of 2 L/min, thus facilitating out-of-home activities. Liquid delivery systems may increase cost in some care settings.[33] These systems may have an incidence of inaccurate oxygen delivery higher than compressed gas systems, creating a potential for inadequate treatment of hypoxemia.[34]

Oxygen concentrators extract oxygen from atmospheric gas, employing either a molecular sieve or membrane concentration design.[33] Molecular sieve devices are capable of generating low flows at high oxygen concentration (> 90 percent). Membrane concentration devices are only capable of doubling ambient oxygen concentration and thus greater flows are required for correction of any given degree of hypoxemia; these high flows may compromise patient compliance. Concentrators are relatively cheap and eliminate the need for transport of oxygen to the patient's home, but they require a constant electric source, consume considerable power, and presently are not portable.

OXYGEN CONSERVATION DEVICES

The cost of home oxygen therapy is difficult to estimate. There are wide regional differences in charges and distinctions between rental and purchase of equipment. An estimate based on Congressional Budget Office data in 1988 indicated that 500,000 to 800,000 individuals used home oxygen in the United States at an annual cost of $2 billion to $3 billion, 60 percent of which was paid by the federal government through Medicare reimbursement.[35] Cost considerations such as these have resulted in governmental overview of indications for oxygen therapy as well as the creation of guidelines to promote the use of devices to conserve oxygen and reduce cost. Currently available devices may be classified as reservoirs, demand or pulse systems, and transtracheal catheters.

Reservoir devices collect oxygen during noninspiratory portions of the respiratory cycle, thus enhancing Pi_{O_2}. Typical devices that provide 20 mL of stored oxygen permit a

TABLE 87-1 Characteristics of Oxygen Storage Cylinders

Cylinder Type	Size (inches)	Weight (pounds)	Hours of use (1 L/min)
H	9 × 56	135	115
G	8 × 55	100	88
M	7 × 47	66	50
E	4 × 29	15	10
D	4 × 20	10	6
B	3 × 16	5	2.3
A	3 × 10	2	1

40 percent to 75 percent reduction in flow rates.[36] Reservoirs are particularly useful in preventing arterial desaturation during exercise, a time during which oxygen flow requirements would otherwise increase.[37] For this particular application the pendant-type reservoir may be preferable, since some authors have reported arterial desaturation during exercise occurring with reservoir devices that are attached directly to the nasal cannula at the nares. Unfortunately the magnitude of oxygen conservation is extremely variable and difficult to predict for a given patient, and patient acceptance of these devices is not high.[38]

Demand systems provide oxygen delivery, which is synchronized to inspiration, thus avoiding loss of gas during the expiratory phase.[36] A variety of techniques have been utilized to provide this synchronization, including actuation by measurement of chest wall impedance, nasal temperature fluctuation, or airway pressure excursion. Despite theoretical benefits, these devices have not gained wide acceptance because of the considerable initial cost and maintenance difficulties.

Continuous delivery of oxygen by a transtracheal route is the most widely employed method of oxygen conservation during long-term therapy.[39-41] Significant cost reduction, reasonable patient acceptance, and a reasonable incidence of complications have been observed in several studies. Transtracheal delivery of oxygen may be particularly useful in the relatively rare patient who cannot achieve adequate arterial hemoglobin saturation with high flows through nasal cannula. Transtracheal oxygen delivery also may relieve dyspnea and increase exercise tolerance in patients with chronic lung disease by mechanisms distinct from resolution of arterial hypoxemia.[41,42] In patients with COPD and restrictive lung disease, transtracheal gas flow of 6 L/min was associated with a decrease in inspired minute ventilation of 50 percent. This reduction in ventilation and associated improvement in dyspnea appeared to be unrelated to changes in oxygen delivery or arterial hemoglobin saturation, since transtracheal air administration resulted in similar effects. One possible explanation for these findings is that transtracheal oxygen delivery decreases inspiratory work in these patients. Treatment of chronic lung disease patients with oxygen thus may confer benefit by mechanisms apart from correction of hypoxemia.

Fi_{O_2} IN THE NONINTUBATED PATIENT

The use of a low-flow oxygen system necessarily results in mixing of ambient air to meet inspiratory flow demand. A largely unwarranted concern is the notion that patients with COPD depend on components of hypoxic drive to breathe during exacerbations, and that excessive oxygen therapy could readily precipitate frank respiratory failure. This point has been discussed above. It should be noted that the various Venturi and high-flow mask delivery systems utilized to administer this "controlled" oxygen therapy have been validated largely on simulators and that there is a striking deviation from predicted Fi_{O_2} when tracheal oxygen concentrations are measured in volunteers with hyperventilatory breathing patterns.[43] However, under clinical conditions in nonintubated patients with respiratory distress, the following statements apply: (1) Fi_{O_2} cannot be determined accurately and lung gas-exchange efficiency cannot be assessed unless the patient is breathing room air; (2) it is not necessary to know Fi_{O_2} for prevention of depressed drive to breathe; and (3) even with high-flow systems with rebreathing reservoirs, Fi_{O_2} will often be considerably less than 0.5 and vary widely in different clinical settings, so monitoring Sa_{O_2} is important.

MONITORING OXYGEN THERAPY

To the extent that the endpoint of oxygen therapy is resolution of hypoxemia, direct measurement of P_{O_2} or hemoglobin saturation would provide the most reasonable monitors of efficacy. Arterial blood gas analysis has become routine and is useful in the setting of critical illness in view of the information regarding ventilatory and acid-base status that it additionally provides. This therapy is far from ideal, however, given the cost, invasive nature, and, most importantly, the difficulties with providing continuous information. This last point is crucial in settings such as sleep or during exercise in stable ambulatory patients, or during an acute exacerbation of COPD, since arterial oxygenation is a very dynamic property. The development of pulse oximetry in the past decade has improved the ability to assess saturation on an ongoing basis.[44] By analyzing the pulsatile component of the absorbance of hemoglobin in red and infrared light, these devices eliminate much of the difficulty in calibration and operation of the older generation oximeters. These measurements compare favorably with direct arterial oximetry. Errors in measurement of saturation will occur in the presence of increased bilirubin concentrations, carboxyhemoglobinemia, or methemoglobinemia. In typical clinical practice, light and motion artifacts are even more commonly encountered problems. These devices are now the standard of care for monitoring patients in the clinic and hospital setting, and are finding increasing application in home monitoring as well.

References

1. Macnee W: Pathophysiology of cor pulmonale in chronic obstructive pulmonary disease, state-of-the-art: Parts one and two. *Am J Respir Crit Care Med* 1994; 150:833–852; 1158–1168.

2. Hall JB, Wood LDH: Oxygen therapy in, Crystal RG, West JB, (eds): *The Lung: Scientific Foundations.* New York, Raven Press, 1995.

3. Renzetti AD, McClement JH, Litt BD: The Veterans Administration cooperative study of pulmonary function: III. Mortality in relation to respiratory function in chronic obstructive pulmonary disease. *Am J Med* 1966; 41:115–129.

4. Stuart-Harris C, Bishop JM, Clark TJH, et al.: Long term domiciliary oxygen therapy in chronic hypoxic cor pulmonale complicating chronic bronchitis and emphysema. *Lancet* 1981; 181–685.

5. Kvale PA, Anthonisen NR, Cugell W, et al.: Continuous or nocturnal oxygen therapy in hypoxemic chronic obstructive lung disease. *Ann Intern Med* 1980; 93:391–398.

6. Timms RM, Khaja FU, Williams GW: The Nocturnal Oxygen Therapy Trial Group: Hemodynamic response to oxygen therapy in chronic obstructive pulmonary disease. *Ann Intern Med* 1985; 102:29–36.

7. Ashutosh K, Mead G, Dunsky M: Early effects of oxygen administration and prognosis in chronic obstructive pulmonary disease and cor pulmonale. *Am Rev Respir Dis* 1983; 127:399–404.

8. Weitzenblum E, Sautegeau A, Ehrhart M, et al.: Long-term oxygen therapy can reverse the progression of pulmonary hypertension in patients with chronic obstructive pulmonary disease. *Am Rev Respir Dis* 1985; 131:493–498.

9. Selinger SR, Kennedy TP, Buescher P: Effects of removing oxygen from patients with chronic obstructive pulmonary disease. *Am Rev Respir Dis* 1987; 136:85–91.

10. Kawakami Y, Kishi F, Yamamoto H, Miyamoto K: Relation of oxygen delivery, mixed venous oxygenation, and pulmonary hemodynamics to prognosis in chronic obstructive pulmonary disease. *N Engl J Med* 1983; 308(18):1046–1049.

11. Douglass A, Morrison RH, Goldman S: Preliminary study of the effects of low flow oxygen on oxygen delivery and right ventricular function in chronic lung disease. *Am Rev Respir Dis* 1986; 133:390–395.

12. Macnee W, Wathen CG, Flenley DC, Muir AD: The effects of controlled oxygen therapy on ventricular function in patients with stable and decompensated cor pulmonale. *Am Rev Respir Dis* 1988; 137:1289–1295.

13. Fletcher EC, Miller J, Divine GW, et al.: Nocturnal oxyhemoglobin desaturation in COPD patients with arterial oxygen tensions above 60 torr. *Chest* 1987; 92:604–8.

14. Boysen PG, Block AJ, Wynne JW, et al.: Nocturnal pulmonary hypertension in patients with chronic obstructive pulmonary disease. *Chest* 1979; 76:536–42.

15. Fletcher EC, Levin DC: Cardiopulmonary hemodynamics during sleep in subjects with chronic obstructive pulmonary disease: The effect of short- and long-term oxygen. *Chest* 1984; 85:6–14.

16. Flenley DC: Clinical hypoxia: Causes, consequences, and correction. *Lancet* 1978; i:542–6.

17. Block AJ, Boyson PG, Wynne JW: The origins of cor pulmonale: A hypothesis. *Chest* 1979; 75:109.

18. Fletcher EC, Donner CF, Midgren B, et al.: Survival in COPD patients with a daytime $Pa_{O_2} > 60$ torr with and without nocturnal oxyghemoglobin desaturation (NOD) *Chest* 1992; 101:649–55.

19. Fletcher EC, Luckett RA, Goodnight-White S, et al.: A double-blind trial of nocturnal supplemental oxygen for sleep desaturation in patients with chronic obstructive pulmonary disease and a daytime Pa_{O_2} above 60 torr. *Am Rev Respir Dis* 1992; 145(2):1070–6.

20. Schmidt GA, Hall JB: Acute chronic respiratory failure. Assessment and management of patients with COPD in the emergent setting. *JAMA* 1989; 261:3444–3453.

21. Wagner P, Dantzker D, Dueck D, et al.: Ventilation-perfusion inequality in chronic obstructive pulmonary disease. *J Clin Invest* 1977; 59:203–216.

22. Campbell EJM: The J Burns Amberson Lecture: The management of acute respiratory failure in chronic bronchitis and emphysema. *Am Rev Respir Dis* 1967; 96:626–639.

23. Aubier M, Murciano D, Fournier M, et al.: Central respiratory drive in acute respiratory failure of patients with chronic obstructive pulmonary disease. *Am Rev Respir Dis* 1980; 122:191–199.

24. Aubier M, Murciano D, Milic-Emili J, et al.: Effects of administration of O_2 on ventilation and blood gases in patients with chronic obstructive pulmonary disease during acute respiratory failure. *Am Rev Respir Dis* 1980; 122:147–154.

25. Libby DM, Briscoe WA, King TKC: Relief of hypoxia-related bronchoconstriction by breathing 30 percent oxygen. *Am Rev Respir Dis* 1981; 123:171–175.

26. Lee J, Read J: Effect of oxygen breathing on distribution of pulmonary blood flow in chronic obstructive lung disease. *Am Rev Respir Dis* 1967; 96:1173–1180.

27. Abraham AS, Cole RB, Greene ID, et al.: Factors contributing to the reversible pulmonary hypertension in patients with acute respiratory failure studied by serial observations during recovery. *Circ Res* 1969; 26:51–60.

28. Degaute D, Dominghetti G, Naeije R, et al.: Oxygen delivery in acute exacerbation of chronic obstructive pulmonary disease: Effects of controlled oxygen therapy. *Am Rev Respir Dis* 1981; 124:26–30.

29. Lejeune P, Mois P, Naeije R, et al.: Acute hemodynamic effects of controlled oxygen therapy in decompensated chronic obstructive pulmonary disease. *Crit Care Med* 1984; 12:1032–5.

30. Petty TL, O'Donohue WJ Jr: Further recommendations for prescribing, reimbursement, technology development, and research in long-term oxygen therapy. *Am J Respir Crit Care Med* 1994; 150:875–877.

31. Summary of the Third Consensus Conference held in Washington, DC, March 15–16, 1990. New problems in supply, reimbursement, and certification of medical necessity for long-term oxygen therapy. *Am Rev Respir Dis* 1990; 142:721–724.

32. Levin DC, Neff TA, O'Donohue WJ, et al.: Conference report: further recommendations for prescribing and supplying long-term oxygen therapy. *Am Rev Respir Dis* 1988; 138:745–747.

33. Flenley DC: Long-term home oxygen therapy. *Chest* 1985; 87(1):99–103.

34. Massey LW, Hussey JD, Albert RK: Inaccurate oxygen delivery in some portable liquid oxygen devices. *Am Rev Respir Dis* 1988; 137:204–205.

35. O'Donohue WJ Jr: The future of home oxygen therapy. *Respir Care* 1988; 33(12):1125–1130.

36. Tiep BL, Lewis MI: Oxygen conservation and oxygen-conserving devices in chronic lung disease. *Chest* 1987; 92(2):263–272.

37. Arlati S, Rolo J, Micaleff E, et al.: A reservoir nasal cannula improves protection given by oxygen during muscular exercise in COPD. *Chest* 1988; 93(6):1165–1169.

38. Claiborne RA, Paynter DE, Dutt AK, et al.: Evaluation of the use of an oxygen conservation device in long-term oxygen therapy. *Am Rev Respir Dis* 1987; 136:1095–1098.

39. Heimlich JH, Carr GC: Transtracheal catheter technique for pulmonary rehabilitation. *Ann Otol Rhinol Laryngol* 1985; 94:502–504.

40. Christopher KL, Spofford BT, Brannin PK, et al.: Transtracheal oxygen therapy for refractory hypoxemia. *JAMA* 1986; 256:494–497.

41. McCarty DC, Goodman JR, Petty TL: A program for transtracheal oxygen delivery: assessment of safety and efficacy. *Ann Intern Med* 1987; 107:802–808.

42. Couser JI Jr, Make BJ: Transtracheal oxygen decreases inspired minute ventilation. *Am Rev Respir Dis* 1989; 139:627–631.

43. Gibson RL, Comer PB, Beckham RW, et al.: Actual tracheal oxygen concentrations with commonly used oxygen equipment. *Anesthesiology* 1976; 44(1):71–73.

44. Tremper KK: Pulse oximetry. *Chest* 1989; 95(4):713–715.

Chapter 88

PHYSIOTHERAPY AND REHABILITATION FOR PATIENTS WITH CHRONIC OBSTRUCTIVE PULMONARY DISEASE

MICHAEL H. RIES

Exercise Training

Exercise Training for the Upper Extremities

Ventilatory Muscle Training

Respiratory Muscle Rest Therapy

Controlled Breathing Techniques

Conclusion

Comprehensive pulmonary rehabilitation programs have demonstrated benefits in (1) improvement in exercise tolerance, which frequently translates into improved functional capacity and activities of daily living (ADLs); (2) improved sense of the patient's well-being with reduction in the symptoms of dyspnea, anxiety, and depression; (3) reduction in number of hospital days and number of hospitalizations; and (4) moderate success in retaining or resuming gainful employment.[1] Patients with chronic obstructive pulmonary disease (COPD) are frequently limited by symptoms of dyspnea and fatigue; these generally are secondary to limitation in performance of exercise to inappropriately low work rates. The reduction in exercise capacity is the result of a reduction in maximum oxygen consumption. The reduced maximum oxygen consumption is an end result of both an increased ventilatory requirement from the patient's underlying abnormal gas exchange and a reduced ventilatory capacity that is secondary to the patient's abnormal ventilatory mechanics (see Fig. 88-1). As the patient with chronic obstructive pulmonary disease is limited in his exercise capacity, his physical activity diminishes, resulting in further inactivity and deconditioning. This causes a vicious cycle of further dyspnea resulting in further deconditioning, and so on. As a result, the patient experiences depression, anxiety, frustration, and anger.

Exercise training is one of the more important aspects of pulmonary rehabilitation.[2,3] With time, it has been realized that the exercise prescription of patients with COPD differs markedly from that of normal individuals or patients with other disease processes. This difference is because the abnormal responses to exercise in obstructive lung disease are unique to this patient population (see Table 88-1). The purpose of this chapter is to present an overview of the present-day standards of exercise training, which are aimed at reducing these symptoms and restoring as great a functional capacity as possible to patients with COPD. These strategies include leg exercises, arm exercises, ventilatory muscle training, controlled breathing and postural techniques, and noninvasive intermittent ventilatory support.

Exercise Training

The benefits of exercise training in patients with COPD are both physiologic[4–9] and psychological.[10–12] Exercise prescription needs to be individualized not only to the patient's physical capabilities but also to the patient's motivation, goals, interests, and environmental situation. The actual physical training prescription needs to be individualized since the functional abnormalities among patients with COPD in pulmonary rehabilitation programs varies considerably.[9,10]

Normal patients are limited primarily in their maximal exercise tolerance by cardiovascular and muscle function. Recommendations for exercise prescription by the American College of Sports Medicine are relatively standard. They rec-

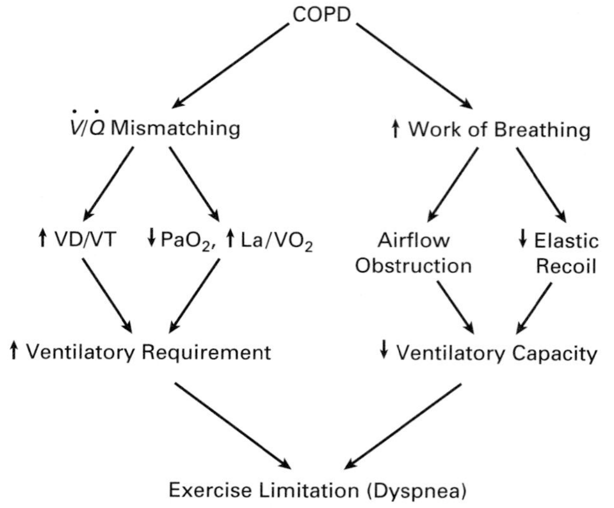

COPD

$\dot{V}/\dot{Q}$ Mismatching   ↑ Work of Breathing

↑ VD/VT   ↓ PaO₂, ↑ La/V̇O₂   Airflow   ↓ Elastic
                                   Obstruction   Recoil

↑ Ventilatory Requirement   ↓ Ventilatory Capacity

Exercise Limitation (Dyspnea)

FIGURE 88-1 Factors that play a role in the onset of exercise limitation and dyspnea in patients with COPD. Chronic obstructive pulmonary disease patients have both an increase in ventilatory requirement to perform exercise and a reduction in ventilatory capacity. (See text for a detailed discussion of each of the factors shown.) (V/Q: ventilation-perfusion ratio; VDS/VT: dead space-tidal volume ratio; La/$\dot{V}_{O_2}$: ratio of lactate to oxygen consumption.) (Modified from Wasserman K, Hansen JE, Sue KY, Whipp BJ: *Principles of Exercise Testing and Interpretation.* **Philadelphia: Lea & Febiger, 1987:52.)**

erature up to 1991. He noted that improved endurance was judged either by an ability to tolerate a greater level of exercise or by the ability to exercise at a given level for a longer period of time. In 31 of the 32 studies that looked at exercise tolerance, tolerance was found to increase after such a program. Without specific physiologic testing, however, it was not obvious from these studies whether or not improvement in exercise was based on improved motivation or improved maximum oxygen uptake.

It was felt for a long time that because of exercise limitations patients with severe COPD could not train above an anaerobic threshold. Many of these patients would achieve a rapid heart rate and significant oxygen uptake at low levels of work because of their abnormal ventilatory function and/or pulmonary gas exchange. Since patients with severe COPD could not attain the usual physiologic levels of training (an increase in maximum oxygen uptake and a higher work level before the onset of anaerobic metabolism), they were exercised either by using subjective measures (such as increasing exercise as tolerated) or criteria used for normal individuals (such as heart rate or oxygen uptake). In 1987, Ries and Archibald[6] described an exercise program for patients with COPD whereby patients trained at near-maximal exercise tolerance. They made the point that the usual training intensities based on heart rate or oxygen uptake criteria that were adequate for healthy subjects would be inappropriately low for patients with COPD. It also was shown that contrary to common belief a significant number of patients with severe COPD could reach work rates above the anaerobic threshold and reach levels of oxygen uptake resulting in lactate production.[8]

The work of Punzal and colleagues,[5] Ries and Archibald,[6] Carter and Nicotra,[15] Casaburi and colleagues,[8] and Smerts and colleagues,[7] suggests that a "critical training intensity" exists and that a relatively high intensity training is warranted in patients with severe COPD. Their studies revealed an increase in maximum oxygen uptake, less lactate production with higher work rates, and a reduced sense of dyspnea with near-maximal exercise training. Their exercise protocols used near-maximal ventilation. Their data support the assumption that patients with severe COPD differ from normal individuals in that they can sustain levels of exercise at

ommend achieving 60 percent to 90 percent of maximum heart rate reserve or 50 percent to 85 percent of maximum oxygen uptake.[13] In addition to the exercise intensity, the characteristics of an effective training program also must include session duration, session frequency, duration of exercise (before increasing the intensity of the exercise), the mode of exercise, and subsequent maintenance of fitness.

There are favorable responses to exercise training in patients with COPD. A recent review by Casaburi,[14] however, revealed a significant variation in the duration, training frequency, and type of exercise that has been reported in the literature. In his review, he summarized 37 reports of exercise training that included 933 patients presented in the lit-

TABLE 88-1   Typical Responses to Exercise Testing in Patients with Chronic Obstructive Pulmonary Disease[a]

At Maximal Exercise	At Submaximal Exercise
Low peak $\dot{V}_{O_2}$ and peak work rate	Normal or near normal $\dot{V}_{O_2}$
Low $\dot{V}_E$	High $\dot{V}_E$
High $\dot{V}_E$/maximal voluntary ventilation	High respiratory frequency, low VT
Low VT	High arterial P_{CO_2}, low arterial P_{O_2}
Normal or slightly reduced VT/vital capacity ratio	Normal cardiac output (usually)
Low heart rate (usually)	High heart rate, low stroke volume
Low oxygen pulse	Increased metabolic acidosis (at least in some patients)
Reduced metabolic acidosis (usually)	

[a] Data are shown in comparison to normal subjects of the same sex, age, and body size. See text for details.
SOURCE: *From Gallagher CG: Exercise limitation and clinical exercise testing in chronic obstructive pulmonary disease, in Weisman IM, Zeballos RJ (eds): Clinics in Chest Medicine 1994, 15:308.*

greater percentages of maximum and even patients with severe disease can train at these levels with safety. All five of these protocols relied on some of the training methods used in normal individuals whereby patients were exercised for 20 to 30 min a day (in one to two sessions per day) and five days a week. In Casaburi's study[8] patients were exercised both at maximal and submaximal levels of work, and even the lesser intensity exercises resulted in a training effect.

There are patients with severe COPD who cannot reach an anaerobic threshold and do not develop a significant lactic acidosis during maximal exercise testing. Punzal and colleagues[5] have shown that these patients can be exercised at 95 percent of their baseline maximum treadmill work load with an improvement in maximum oxygen uptake, endurance exercise time, an increase in maximum treadmill work load, and a reduction in perceived symptoms. Based on these studies there appears to be a training intensity threshold for patients with COPD beyond which a physiologically documented change will occur. Whereas most of the recent studies have shown an exercise training effect at these high-intensity work loads, there is a paucity of data regarding any beneficial effect of physiologic improvement with lower-intensity exercise programs. There also is a paucity of data regarding the duration, frequency, or length of training. Even the five studies cited above relied on the duration, frequency, and length of exercise based on healthy individuals.

Exercise training is relatively specific to the muscles and activities involved. Therefore, the type of activity chosen must be tailored to the needs of the individual patient. For this reason, walking (6-min or 12-min walks), treadmill, or cycle ergometer are the most common exercises prescribed. The type of exercise testing and mode also depends on the availability of equipment in the pulmonary rehabilitation program. The bicycle ergometer is very efficacious when the physiologic responses to exercise are studied and allows one to quantitate the amount of work more precisely. The treadmill or walking exercises result in a higher metabolic cost and are less precise in quantitating amount of work; but are more available than a bicycle ergometer. If a full exercise study that includes oxygen uptake and CO_2 production can be obtained, then patients are given a program whereby they exercise at a work load around 90 percent of the anaerobic threshold. If patients do not reach an anaerobic threshold, their exercise intensity is a workload of 90 percent of their maximum achieved workload.[3,5,7,8] Their maximum work load is obtained by determining the maximum speed at which the patient's dyspnea or fatigue limit exercise.

If the patient's exercise evaluation is performed on a treadmill, the same principles are involved. No incline is used to test the patient. If the patient is tested on a cycle ergometer, his treadmill/walking speed can be predicted and his exercise prescription obtained.[16] If the program does not have a treadmill or a cycle ergometer or if the patient either is too debilitated or intimidated by a treadmill or ergometer, he can be tested with a 6- or 12-min walk (distance patient is able to walk in either 6 or 12 min). Since there is a "learning effect," the patient should be exercised one or two times prior to actual exercise efficiency testing. The threshold exercise is determined by the distance covered and the patient's subjective sense of dyspnea. The target intensity is then 80 percent to 90 percent of the work achieved.

Exercise prescription does not require sophisticated equipment. If oxygen uptake and CO_2 production cannot be measured, then a simple exercise study can be performed and maximum work load can be determined by quantification of mechanical work and the patient's sensation of dyspnea on whatever mode of exercise is available. Although less precise, the patient merely is asked to exercise at maximum exercise tolerance based on limitation of sense of dyspnea and a general assessment of mechanical work at that threshold. All that is required is an electrocardiogram and an ear oximeter for a very simple, but effective, assessment of exercise tolerance.

To help the patient gain confidence and experience success with the exercise program, exercise training is initiated with 5 min at approximately 60 percent of the target intensity. As the patient feels comfortable, the time gradually is increased to 20 min and then the intensity is increased to 90 percent of the threshold. Initially, the patient is able to rest and then is instructed to resume exercise so that a total time of 20 min is achieved. With time, the patient is able to exercise for 20 min continuously without a rest period. The duration is subsequently increased to 30 min, and once 30 min of continuous exercise at the target intensity work load is achieved, the intensity of the exercise can be increased further. The patient is instructed to exercise for 20 to 30 min per day and four to five times per week. After six to eight weeks, a repeat exercise study is performed to determine any need for upgrading further his endurance program.

Maintaining fitness is very important. Substantial loss of improvement can occur within two weeks of not exercising. A return to pretraining status can occur in as little as 10 weeks.[14] The most problematic aspect of a maintenance program is the exacerbations frequently encountered by patients with COPD. Therefore, as soon as the patient's exacerbation has resolved, they are asked to return to the pulmonary rehabilitation program for a reassessment of their exercise program.

Pulmonary patients, unlike normal individuals and patients with other diseases, can develop oxygen desaturation with exercise. Therefore, if either the pulse oximeter or the indwelling arterial cannula reveals any significant desaturation below 90 percent at rest or with exercise, the patient has an oxygen prescription study performed. The patient exercises on the treadmill, bicycle ergometer, or takes a 6-min walk. If the P_{O_2} decreases to < 55 mmHg or oxygen saturation is less than 90 percent at rest, the patient is placed on supplemental oxygen in incremental flows. Arterial blood gases are drawn with each change of the supplemental oxygen to determine the flow of oxygen required to maintain the P_{O_2} > 55 mmHg and the oxygen saturation at greater than 90 percent. The patient then is exercised at that determined oxygen flow. If further desaturation is noted with exercise, greater increments of oxygen flow are provided until acceptable levels are obtained. Once the oxygen prescription study is performed, final recommendations as to the dose of oxygen either at rest or with exercise are made.[1]

Currently, there are no data available describing the long-term benefits of supplemental oxygen during exercise. Supplemental oxygen during exercise reduces respiratory rate, exercise ventilation, and the ventilatory equivalents for oxygen.[17,18] The greater availability of oxygen to the tissues also may shift the anaerobic threshold to a higher work load, reducing the necessity of hyperventilation to compensate for the metabolic acidosis that develops at the anaerobic threshold. Another mechanism for which supplemental oxygen may reduce the ventilatory requirement is by removing the hypoxemic drive on the carotid bodies.

Exercise Training for the Upper Extremities

Exercise programs for patients with COPD have traditionally focused on prescribing lower extremity training. Patients with COPD, however, frequently report dyspnea with activities of daily living (ADLs) such as eating, lifting, grooming, dressing, and so on. The same muscles that are used for ADLs also serve frequently as accessory muscles of respiration.

The external intercostals, the parasternal part of the internal intercostal, and the scalene are essential muscles of respiration because they are active during quiet breathing. The accessory inspiratory muscles are inactive during quiet breathing in normal individuals; however, they can be inspiratory in action when the patient's ventilatory capacity is stressed.[19] Activities involving the arms can produce dyspnea and dyscoordination of the respiratory muscles in patients with COPD.[20] Thus, upper extremity exercises may prove to be advantageous in a pulmonary rehabilitation program.[21] Unfortunately the data in this area of exercise are scant, and additional research is necessary. It has been shown that lower extremity training does not improve upper extremity muscle function. Therefore, the training of upper extremities is specific.[22]

Many of the data in upper extremity exercise prescription are related to supported arm exercise such as ergometers or cranking. It has been shown that an exercise program involving arm cranking increases upper extremity performance; however, the training is quite specific and results in no reduction in symptoms with activities of daily living.[23] Most activities of daily living are carried out by unsupported arm activity. It has been shown that unsupported arm activity (UAE) results in dyssynchronous thoracoabdominal excursion and dyspnea at a lower oxygen uptake than more metabolically active leg exercises.[20] The conclusions from the studies in the literature indicate that the recruitment of the respiratory muscles is complex and when the upper arm muscles are recruited for performance of nonventilatory work, their participation in ventilation is reduced.[24] Thus, respiratory muscle recruitment results in increased diaphragmatic dysfunction during inspiration.[25]

There are few studies on the effect of unsupported arm training in patients with COPD. Table 88-2 summarizes three of these studies. Interestingly, maximum inspiratory pressure increases significantly in one of the studies and ventilatory muscle endurance increased in all three studies. Upper extremity training should focus principally on the use of repetitive, endurance-type, task-specific exercises. The muscles of the arm and shoulder girdle should be trained specifically. There are presently no available results on strength training in COPD patients and the possibility that it may result in respiratory muscle recruitment.

An occupational therapist would be expected to have the most expertise among members of the rehabilitation team in developing and initiating an upper extremity exercise program. In general, high repetition, low resistance exercises, which mimic activities commonly performed by patients during ADLs, usually are recommended. Such exercises could include the use of a pegboard with pegs separated 10 cm vertically and the patient shifting the rings with extended arms at the shoulder level, intermittent vertical and oblique lifting of a dowel[19] or lifting small objects at shoulder height and passing a beanbag over the head. The frequency of the exercises should equal the respiratory rate, should be repeated in three to five sets per session, and may include the use of light weights (one-quarter to five pounds). Since dyspnea with activities of daily living is a common complaint of patients with moderate to severe obstructive lung disease, this is an area where more research is necessary.

Ventilatory Muscle Training

One of the major pathophysiologic abnormalities in patients with COPD is an increase in ventilatory requirements with a reduction in ventilatory capacity. A common finding in patients with COPD is hyperinflation, which can be augmented by either exercise or tachypnea. Hyperinflation results in further increase in functional residual capacity, resulting in reduction in diaphragmatic strength. The effect is one of shortening the diaphragmatic fibers, thus placing the diaphragm at a more inefficient point on its length-tension curve. This results in a reduction in diaphragmatic strength and possibly diaphragmatic muscle fatigue. In an attempt to improve ventilatory muscle endurance, and reduce the potential development of diaphragmatic fatigue with exercise, ventilatory muscle training (VMT) has been introduced. There have been three methods of VMT: voluntary isocapneic hyperpnea, inspiratory resistive loading, and inspiratory threshold loading.

In voluntary isocapneic hyperpnea, the patient exercises repeatedly against a submaximal work load over a 15- to 30-min period. The patient hyperventilates by breathing rapidly and deeply into a device that prevents hypocapnia. This exercise provides a low tension and a high level of repetitive activity for the diaphragm and other inspiratory muscles. An expression of ventilatory muscle endurance is known as the maximum sustained ventilatory capacity (MSVC), which is defined as the maximal level of ventilation that can be sustained under isocapneic conditions for 15 min.[26,27] Belman and Mittman[28] and Ries[29] have demonstrated an improvement in the MSVC and oxygen uptake as well as improvements in submaximal arm and leg exercise endurance with

TABLE 88-2   Controlled Studies of Arm Exercise in Patients with Chronic Obstructive Lung Disease

Authors	Number of Patients	Duration	Course	Type	Results
Keens[a]	7 arms	1.5 h daily	4 week	Swimming	↑ VME (56%)
					Canoeing
	4 VMT	15 min daily	4 week	VMT	↑ VME (52%)
	4 control	—	—	VMT	↑ VME (22%)
Ries et al.[b]	8 gravity resistance arms	15 min daily	6 week	Low resistance/ high repetition	↑ Arm endurance Dyspnea
	9 neuromuscular facilitation arms	15 min daily	6 week	Weight lifts	↑ Arm endurance Dyspnea
	11 controls	—	6 week	Walk	No change
Epstein et al.[c]	13 arm	30 min daily	8 week	UAE	$\dot{V}_{O_2}$ and $\dot{V}_E$ for arm elevation ↑ PI$_{max}$
	10 VMT	30 min daily	8 week	VMT	↑ PI$_{max}$ and VME

NOTE: VMT = Ventilatory muscle training; VME = ventilatory muscle endurance; PFT = pulmonary function tests; PI$_{max}$ = maximal inspiratory pressure; UAE = unsupported arm exercise.
SOURCE: *From Celli BR: The clinical use of upper extremity exercise, in Weisman IM, Zeballs RJ (eds): Clin Chest Med 1994; 15:345.*
[a] Reprinted with permission.
[b] Reprinted with permission.[1]
[c] Reprinted with permission.[43]

isocapneic hyperpnea training. Thus voluntary isocapneic hyperpnea can improve ventilatory muscle endurance; however, the complexity of the equipment required has resulted in relatively few studies and difficulty in most pulmonary rehabilitation programs acquiring the necessary equipment.

Inspiratory resistive loading exercises result both in an increase in respiratory muscle strength as well as respiratory muscle endurance.[30] For endurance training, the work load is set at 30 percent of PI$_{max}$ and training involves breathing with a maximum inspiratory effort for 15 to 30 min continuously per day with a frequency of four to five days per week minimum.[31] The studies in the literature are conflicting in that some show both improvement in ventilatory muscle endurance as well as reduction in dyspnea and improved exercise tolerance.[27] Other studies fail to show any significant improvement. Since the work load imposed by the inspiratory resistive trainer is accomplished by breathing through smaller orifices, the pattern of breathing has a direct effect on the actual work load.[32] Inspiring slowly through the orifice creates little resistance whereas aggressive inspiratory effort imposes disproportionately greater resistances and consequently higher work loads. Without information on the breathing strategy, therefore, it is difficult to know whether the ability to breath through a smaller orifice represents a true training response or just a more favorable breathing strategy.[33] One study revealed that a change from a regular breathing pattern to one involving long, slow breaths resulted in immediate improvement in endurance. When prescribing the inspiratory resistive devices, therefore, the control of breathing strategy during training is essential to ensure any possible benefits in ventilatory muscle or exercise endurance.

In an attempt to avoid the problem with breathing pattern, another inspiratory resistive device has been developed whereby resistance was provided by a threshold loading device that permitted inspiration only after a certain threshold mouth pressure was reached.[35,36] This device allows for the development of an inspiratory pressure that is independent of the inspiratory flow rate so that the breathing pattern does not affect the training effect of the inspiratory loading exercise.

Thus, it would seem appropriate to recommend a resistive device for VMT in patients with COPD undergoing a pulmonary rehabilitation program. Future studies are required to confirm the benefits of the resistive devices, including studies that assess whether these devices can prevent respiratory failure during exacerbations of COPD or even result in faster weaning from the ventilator should intubation be required. This would require studying strength training methods (breathe maximally for 2- to 3-min periods) in addition to the endurance methods explained above.

Respiratory Muscle Rest Therapy

Increased airways resistance and reduction in lung elastic recoil results in hyperinflation. Hyperinflation results in shortening of the ventilatory muscles and subsequent decreased ability of the inspiratory muscles to generate adequate ventilatory pressures. Superimposed on this inspiratory muscle fatigue, one sees malnutrition in patients with severe COPD and subsequent muscle weakness. As with any overused muscle, it has been proposed that resting the respiratory muscles (using intermittent ventilation) might improve ventilatory muscle function. Although several early studies indicated that external negative-pressure ventilation resulted in improvement in blood gas parameters, exercise capacity, MSVC, and hypercarbia,[37] subsequent larger studies have failed to confirm this. In addition, many patients found the equipment cumbersome and inconvenient to use.

A major problem with external negative-pressure ventilation is upper airway obstruction at night.[38] These difficulties resulted in the use of nasal positive-pressure ventilation via continuous positive airway pressure masks and bilevel positive airway pressure (BIPAP).[47] Preliminary studies have shown some promise for this modality.[39,40] Electrophysiologic studies have shown reduction in diaphragm electromyographic activity and other studies have revealed reduction in transdiaphragmatic pressure with nasal positive-pressure ventilation.[41] Although most of the experience with nasal positive-pressure ventilation is in patients with chest wall or neuromuscular diseases, this area of respiratory muscle rest therapy needs further study.

Controlled Breathing Techniques

Controlled breathing techniques such as pursed-lip breathing (PLB), the bending forward posture, and diaphragmatic breathing exercises have been utilized for years in pulmonary rehabilitation programs. Few studies exist that analyze the true benefits of these breathing techniques. The theoretical purpose of these breathing techniques is to restore the diaphragm to a more normal position (allowing for more efficient and stronger contractions), decrease the respiratory rate by increasing tidal volume, reducing the work of breathing, and reduce dyspnea by reducing patient anxiety.

Studies have shown that PLB can reduce P_{CO_2}, increase P_{O_2}, increase alveolar ventilation, increase tidal volume[42] with a reduction in respiratory rate and minute ventilation,[43] and decrease functional residual capacity by increasing bronchial diameter and delaying airways collapse (by increasing expiratory airways pressure). Despite these improvements, however, PLB actually results in an increased work of breathing because of the added expiratory resistance and also increased inspiratory work of breathing. Pursed-lip breathing is performed by inhaling through the nose for several seconds with the mouth closed. The patient then exhales slowly for 4 to 6 s through pursed lips held in a whistling or kissing position. The patient is instructed to use PLB during any exercise or any period of tachypnea or increased dyspnea.

The bending forward position has been shown to improve the mechanical efficiency of the diaphragm and thereby relieve dyspnea.[44] The position is attained by the patient bending forward 20° to 45° from the vertical axis. This position can be assumed while the patient is seated or walking and explains why so many patients with severe COPD find it easier to walk leaning on a shopping cart. Although this position can be achieved by using a walker or two canes, this defeats the purpose of exercise training and should be discouraged (unless the patient is extremely debilitated). Physiologic improvement from the forward posture has been confirmed by electromyographic recordings of respiratory muscle activity as well as transdiaphragmatic pressure monitoring.[45] A study by Delgado[46] revealed that the bending forward posture resulted in a reduction in dyspnea and an improvement in exercise tolerance during walking.

Nevertheless, more studies are needed to confirm these findings.

Diaphragmatic breathing exercises have been a standard in pulmonary rehabilitation programs for years. Physiologic studies, however, have been inconclusive as to its effectiveness. Until further studies are available, the technique should only be used when it results in reduced dyspnea that may merely represent a reduction in patient anxiety.

Conclusion

Pulmonary rehabilitation programs have been available since the 1970s. Exercise has been shown to play a critical role in both the physiologic and psychological benefits of these programs. Only recently, however, has there been an understanding of the physiologic basis by which to develop an exercise prescription. In addition to routine lower extremity exercise programs for patients with severe chronic obstructive disease, the role of upper extremity exercises, ventilatory muscle training, respiratory muscle rest therapy, and controlled breathing techniques have been recognized. It is these latter modalities that require further study to confirm and maximize their contribution to the care of the patient with chronic obstructive pulmonary disease.

References

1. Ries M: Rehabilitation of the patient with chronic obstructive pulmonary disease, in Kaplan PE (ed): *The Practice of Physical Medicine*. Springfield, Illinois, Charles C. Thomas, 1984.
2. Casaburi R, Petty TL (eds): *Principles and Practice of Pulmonary Rehabilitation*. Philadelphia, WB Saunders, 1993.
3. Ries AL: The importance of exercise in pulmonary rehabilitation, in Weisman IM, Zeballos RJ (eds): *Clinics in Chest Medicine*. Philadelpha, WB Saunders. 1994; 15(2):327.
4. Carter R, Coast JR, Idell S: Exercise training in patients with chronic obstructive pulmonary disease. *Medicine and Science in Sports and Exercise* 1992; 24:281.
5. Punzal PA, Ries AL, Kaplan RM, Prewitt, LM: Maximum intensity exercise training in patients with chronic obstructive pulmonary disease. *Chest* 1991; 100:618.
6. Ries AL, Archibald CJ: Endurance training in maximal targets in patients with chronic obstructive pulmonary disease. *J Cardiopulmonary Rehabil* 1987; 7:594.
7. Swerts PMJ, Kretzers LMJ, Terpstra-Lindeman E, et al.: Exercise training as a mediator of increased exercise performance in patients with chronic obstructive pulmonary disease. *J Cardiopulmonary Rehabil* 1992; 12:188.
8. Casaburi R, Patessio A, Ioli F, et al.: Reductions in exercise lactic acidosis and ventilation as a result of exercise training in patients with obstructive lung disease. *Am Rev Respir Dis* 1991; 143:9.
9. Corriveau ML, Harris CM, Chun DS, et al.: Relationship between multiple physiologic variables and change in exercise capacity after a pulmonary rehabilitation program. *J Cardiopulmonlary Rehabil* 1988; 8:303.
10. Niederman MS, Clemente PH, Rein AM, et al.: Benefits of a multidisciplinary pulmonary rehabilitation program. *Chest* 1991; 99:798.
11. Mahler DA: The measurement of dyspnea during exercise in patients with lung disease. *Chest* 1992; 101:2425.

12. Haas F, Salazar-Schicchi J, Axen K: Desensitization to dyspnea in chronic obstructive pulmonary disease, in Casaburi R, Petty TL (eds): *Principles and Practice of Pulmonary Rehabilitation.* Philadelphia, WB Saunders, 1993.

13. Faryniarz K, Mahler, DA: Writing an exercise prescription for patients with COPD. *Journal of Respiratory Diseases* 1990; 11:638.

14. Casaburi R: Exercise training in chronic obstructive lung disease, in Casaburi R, Petty TL (eds): *Principles and Practice of Pulmonary Rehabilitation.* Philadelphia, WB Saunders, 1993.

15. Carter R, Nicotra B: Exercise conditioning in the rehabilitation of patients with chronic obstructive pulmonary disease. *Arch Phys Med Rehabil* 1988; 69:118.

16. Ries AL, Moser KM: Predicting treadmill/walking speed from cycle ergometry exercise in chronic obstructive pulmonary disease. *Am Rev Respir Dis* 1982; 126:924.

17. Bye PTP, Esau SA, Walley KR, et al.: Ventilatory muscles during exercise in air and oxygen in normal men. *J Appl Physiol: Respir Environ Exercise Physiol* 1984; 56:464.

18. Zack MB, Palange AV: Oxygen supplemented exercise of ventilatory and nonventilatory muscles in pulmonary rehabilitation. *Chest* 1985; 88:669.

19. Celli, BR: The clinical use of upper extremity exercise in Weisman IM, Zaballos RJ (eds): *Clinics in Chest Medicine.* Philadelphia, WB Saunders, 1994; 15(2):339.

20. Celli BR, Rassulo J, Make BJ: Dyssynchronous breathing during arm but not leg exercise in patients with chronic airflow obstruction. *N Engl J Med* 1986; 314:1485.

21. Martinez FJ, Vogel PD, Dupont DN, et al.: Supported arm exercise vs unsupported arm exercise in the rehabilitation of patients with severe chronic airflow obstruction. *Chest* 1993; 103:1397.

22. Lake FR, Henderson K, Briffa T, et al.: Upper-limb and lower-limb exercise training in patients with chronic airflow obstruction. *Chest* 1990; 97:1077.

23. Ries AL, Ellis B, Hawkins RW: Upper extremity exercise training in chronic obstructive pulmonary disease. *Chest* 1988; 93:688.

24. Couser, JI, Martinez FJ, Celli BR: Pulmonary rehabilitation that includes arm exercise reduces metabolic and ventilatory requirements for simple arm elevation. *Chest* 1993; 103:37.

25. Martinez FJ, Couser JI, Celli BR: Respiratory response to arm elevation in patients with chronic airflow obstruction. *Am Rev Respir Dis* 1991; 143:476.

26. Tiep BL: Biofeedback and respiratory muscle training, in Hodgkin JE, Connors GL, Bell CW (eds): *Pulmonary Rehabilitation: Guidelines to Success.* Philadelphia, JB Lippincott, 1993.

27. Carter R, Coast JR: Respiratory muscle training in patients with chronic obstructive pulmonary disease. *J Cardiopulmonary Rehabil* 1993; 13:117.

28. Belman MJ, Mittman C: Ventilatory muscle training improves exercise capacity in chronic obstructive pulmonary disease patients. *Am Rev Respir Dis* 1980; 121:273.

29. Ries AL, Moser KM: Comparison of isocapneic hyperventilation and walking exercise training at home pulmonary rehabilitation. *Chest* 1986; 90:285.

30. Belman MJ: Ventilatory muscle training and unloading, in Casaburi R, Petty TL (eds): *Principles and Practice of Pulmonary Rehabilitation.* Philadelphia, WB Saunders, 1993.

31. Mahler DA: Therapeutic strategies, in Mahler DA (ed): *Dyspnea.* New York, Futura Publishing, 1990; 231–263.

32. Belman MJ, Thomas SG, Lewis MI: Resistive breathing training in patients with chronic obstructive lung disease. *Chest* 1986; 90:662.

33. Smith K, Cook D, Guyatt GH, Madhavan J, Oxman AD: Respiratory muscle training in chronic airflow limitation: a meta-analysis. *Am Rev Respir Dis* 1992; 145:533.

34. Harver A, Mahler DA, Daubenspeck JA: Targeted inspiratory muscle training improves respiratory muscle function and reduces dyspnea, in *Patients with Chronic Obstructive Pulmonary Disease. Ann Intern Med* 1989; 111:117.

35. Larson JL, Kim MJ, Sharp JT, et al.: Inspiratory muscle training with a pressure threshold breathing device, in *Patients with Chronic Obstructive Pulmonary Disease. Am Rev Respir Dis* 1988; 138:689.

36. Flynn MG, Barter CE, Nosworthy, JC, et al.: Threshold pressure training, breathing pattern and exercise performance in chronic airflow obstruction. *Chest* 1989; 95:535.

37. Cropp A. DiMarco AF: Effects of intermittent negative pressure ventilation on respiratory muscle function in patients with severe chronic obstructive pulmonary disease. *Am Rev Respir Dis* 1987; 135:1056.

38. Levine S, Hensen D, Levy S: Respiratory muscle rest therapy, in Belman MJ (ed): *Clinics in Chest Medicine,* Philadelphia, WB Saunders 1988; 9:297.

39. Marin JC, Levy RD: Respiratory muscle rest. *Prob Resp Care* 1990; 3:534.

40. Carrey Z, Gottfied SB, Levy RD: Ventilatory muscle support in respiratory failure with nasal positive pressure ventilation. *Chest* 1990; 97:150.

41. Belman MJ, Soohoo G, Kuei J, et al.: Efficacy of positive vs negative pressure ventilation in unloading the respiratory muscles. *Chest* 1990; 98:850.

42. Mueller RE, Petty TL, Filley GF: Ventilation and arterial blood gas changes induced by pursed lips breathing. *J Appl Physiol* 1970; 28:784.

43. Roa J, Epstein S, Preslin E, et al.: Work of breathing and ventilatory muscle recruitment during pursed lips breathing in patients with chronic airway obstruction. *Am Rev Respir Dis* 1991; 143:77.

44. Sharp JT, Drutz WS, Moisan T, et al.: Postural relief of dyspnea in severe chronic obstructive pulmonary disease. *Am Rev Respir Dis* 1980; 122:201.

45. Druz WS, Sharp JT: Electrical and mechanical activity of the diaphragm accompanying body position in severe chronic obstructive pulmonary disease. *Am Rev Respir Dis* 1982; 125:275.

46. Delgado HR, Braun SR, Skatrud JB, et al.: Chest wall and abdominal motion during exercise in patients with chronic obstructive pulmonary disease. *Am Rev Respir Dis* 1982; 126:200.

Chapter 89 _____

ANTIBIOTICS FOR RESPIRATORY TRACT INFECTIONS

MICHAEL S. NIEDERMAN

Pharmacologic Principles of Antibiotic Therapy for Respiratory Infections
    Mechanisms of antimicrobial activity
    Pharmacodynamics in the treatment of lung infections
    Profiles of common antibiotics

An Antibiotic Approach to Common Respiratory Tract Infections
    Bronchitic exacerbations of chronic obstructive pulmonary disease
    Community-acquired pneumonia
    Nosocomial pneumonia

Summary

Antibiotics remain the cornerstone of therapy for common respiratory tract infections, including bronchitic exacerbations of chronic obstructive pulmonary disease (COPD) as well as pneumonia. There are convincing data to show that the use of antibiotics is associated with an improved outcome in these illnesses. Patients with COPD who are given antibiotics at the time of an exacerbation are more likely to have resolution of symptoms than are patients who do not receive antibiotics, and the symptoms also resolve more quickly.[1] Similarly, patients with community-acquired pneumonia (CAP) have a better chance of survival if given antibiotics, particularly if the antibiotics are administered early, before the onset of severe septic complications.[2,3] Even among seriously ill patients with hospital-acquired pneumonia (HAP), appropriate therapy gives a better outcome than inappropriate therapy.[4]

The therapy for respiratory tract infections often must be selected empirically, because the pathogen is not identified reliably at the time of diagnosis. Sputum Gram stain long has been used to guide antibiotic selection, but a recent consensus statement about the therapy of CAP has questioned the accuracy of this approach.[2] Therefore, it is important to use a number of clinical and epidemiologic features to define a list of likely pathogens and to select empirical therapy from available antimicrobials. In recent years, this approach has required some modification because of the emergence of antibiotic-resistant bacteria. In some areas, penicillin-resistant pneumococcus makes up ≥10 percent of all bacterial respiratory isolates, while methicillin-resistant *Staphylococcus aureus* is an emerging nosocomial pathogen.[5,6] *Pseudomonas aeruginosa* is a tenacious enteric gram-negative bacillus that can cause airway infection in patients with bronchiectasis

and cystic fibrosis, as well as nosocomial pneumonia in mechanically ventilated patients, and this organism commonly develops resistance during therapy if only a single antimicrobial agent is used.[7]

This chapter considers the principles of antibiotic therapy of common respiratory tract infections. The mechanisms of antimicrobial action, the relevant pharmacokinetic principles, and the empirical approach to therapy for bronchitis and pneumonia are presented.

Pharmacologic Principles of Antibiotic Therapy for Respiratory Infections

MECHANISMS OF ANTIMICROBIAL ACTIVITY

Antibiotics eliminate bacteria by interfering with the integrity of their cell wall or by interfering with basic protein synthesis or common metabolic pathways. Agents are classified often as *bactericidal* or *bacteriostatic*. Bactericidal agents act either by interfering with cell wall synthesis or by interrupting the protein synthesis or metabolic function of the organism. These agents include the penicillins, the cephalosporins, the aminoglycosides, the fluoroquinolones, vancomycin, rifampin, and metronidazole.[8] Bacteriostatic agents do not interfere with cell wall synthesis and include the macrolides, the tetracyclines, the sulfa drugs, chloramphenicol, and clindamycin. These terms only define broad categories, and some agents are bactericidal against some organisms but bacteriostatic against others. Both categories include agents that are effective against lung infections, and the distinction between the two types of effect may be most

859

relevant in the treatment of neutropenic patients or those with endocarditis, meningitis, or osteomyelitis.

The antimicrobial activity of an antibiotic often is expressed by the concentration required to eliminate an organism. The *minimal inhibitory concentration* (MIC) is the minimum concentration of antibiotic needed to inhibit the growth of 90 percent of a standard-sized bacterial inoculum (resulting in no visible growth in a broth culture), while the *minimal bactericidal concentration* (MBC) is the minimum concentration required to eradicate 99.9 percent of the bacterial growth (a reduction by three orders of magnitude). In general, the MBC for a given organism exceeds the MIC, and a ratio of the two concentrations can be used as a measure of the likelihood that an antibiotic can eradicate a serious infection. Antimicrobial susceptibility patterns are defined by MIC values measured in a laboratory against a given clinical isolate of bacteria. "Sensitivity" to a given antibiotic implies that the measured MIC is low enough that an appropriate concentration of antibiotic will reach the infecting organism under normal dosing conditions. The laboratory report does not take into account the site of infection, however. Clearly, an agent that achieves the MIC for an organism in serum but not at the site of infection may not eradicate the infection. Therefore, it is important to consider the penetration of a proposed antibiotic to respiratory sites.

PHARMACODYNAMICS IN THE TREATMENT OF LUNG INFECTIONS

The dosage and method of delivery used for a chosen antibiotic should reflect the mechanism of action of the drug. For example, some bactericidal antibiotics kill in a time-dependent fashion (that is, dependent on the length of time the local concentration remains above the MIC), while others kill in a concentration-dependent fashion (Table 89-1). Agents such as the aminoglycosides and the fluoroquinolones act in a concentration-dependent fashion, killing bacteria more

rapidly the greater the concentration at the site of infection.[9] To optimize efficacy, these agents should be given to produce high peak concentrations; dosing intervals may be less critical. On the other hand, agents such as the beta-lactam antibiotics and vancomycin act in a time-dependent fashion—the rate of bacterial killing is concentration-dependent at relatively low concentrations, but it becomes saturated once the concentration exceeds approximately four times the MIC.[10] These agents must be administered often, and it is important not to let trough concentrations fall below the MIC of the target organism for too long.

Another property of many antibiotics is the *post-antibiotic effect* (PAE), defined as the ability of the drug to suppress bacterial growth after concentrations decrease to < the MIC of the organism. Most antibiotics exhibit a post-antibiotic effect against susceptible gram-positive cocci. For gram-negative bacilli, antibiotics that inhibit protein and nucleic acid synthesis have a prolonged PAE; these include the aminoglycosides, the quinolones, the tetracyclines, the macrolides, and rifampin. In general, bactericidal agents that kill by a concentration-dependent mechanism also have a prolonged PAE. This has led to the suggestion that aminoglycosides that fit this profile can be given once daily.[11,12] Such a dosing regimen can achieve high peak concentrations, thereby maximizing antimicrobial killing, and low trough concentrations, which minimizes toxicity; the prolonged PAE continues to suppress bacterial growth while concentrations are < the MIC. Agents that kill in a time-dependent fashion generally have little or no PAE against gram-negative bacteria. These agents include the beta-lactam antibiotics. One exception among the beta-lactam antibiotics are the penem agents (such as imipenem), which have a modest PAE against *Pseudomonas aeruginosa*.[9] A similar effect, *post-antibiotic leukocyte enhancement* (PALE), tends to parallel the PAE. PALE is an enhanced susceptibility of an organism to the antibacterial effect of functioning white cells while the organism is in the post-antibiotic phase of growth. Thus, in the presence of functioning white cells, the PAE of some agents is extended by the existence of PALE.[9]

The penetration of a drug to a given site depends on the permeability of the capillary bed at the site, the degree of protein binding of the drug, and the presence or absence of an active transport pump at the target organ.[8,13] In the case of lung infections, there are several sites where the concentration of antibiotics may be relevant. For bronchitic infections, the relevant site is the sputum.[13] For parenchymal lung infections, such as pneumonia, the concentration achieved in the bronchial mucosa or epithelial lining fluid, as well as in macrophages and neutrophils, may be more important.[13,14] If the infection involves an intracellular pathogen, such as *Legionella pneumophila* or *Chlamydia pneumoniae*, then concentration in macrophages may be particularly relevant. Finally, even if an antibiotic gets to a site of infection, it may be inactivated by local conditions. For example, in patients with pneumonia, the lung parenchyma commonly has an acidic pH, and agents such as aminoglycosides have reduced activity under these conditions. In some infections, the etiologic organism produces enzymes such as beta lactamases, which can inactivate a number of common beta-lactam antibiotics.

TABLE 89-1   Pharmacodynamic Properties of Common Antimicrobials Used for Respiratory Tract Infections

Bactericidal in a concentration-dependent fashion
   Aminoglycosides
   Quinolones
Bactericidal in a time-dependent fashion
   Beta-lactams
   Vancomycin
Prolonged PAE against gram-negative bacteria
   Aminoglycosides
   Quinolones
   Macrolides
   Tetracyclines
   Rifampin
Little or no PAE against gram-negative bacteria
   Beta-lactams (except for penem agents)
      Penicillins
      Cephalosporins
      Monobactams

As mentioned, the penetration of a drug into lung tissue depends partly on the local capillary permeability and on the protein binding of the drug. The bronchial circulation is fenestrated, whereas that of the pulmonary endothelium is not. Thus, antibiotics can reach lung tissue (through the bronchial circulation) in proportion to their molecular size and protein binding. Small molecules with low protein binding readily pass into lung tissue through fenestrated capillaries, and this mechanism of drug delivery is enhanced in the presence of inflammation, which can increase capillary permeability. Antibiotics reach the epithelial lining fluid through the nonfenestrated capillaries of the pulmonary endothelium, and thus drugs that are lipophilic are most likely to enter by this mechanism. In general, lipophilic drugs enter the epithelial lining fluid well and independently of inflammation, whereas drugs that are less lipophilic tend to depend on inflammation for entry into the lung. Inflammation-independent (lipid-soluble) antibiotics include chloramphenicol, the macrolides, clindamycin, the tetracyclines, the quinolones, and trimethoprim/sulfamethoxazole. Inflammation-dependent (poorly lipid soluble) antibiotics include the penicillins, cephalosporins, aminoglycosides, carbapenems, and monobactams[14] (Table 89-2).

Active transport may enhance the concentration of certain antibiotics in the lung. Agents such as the macrolides, clindamycin, and the fluoroquinolones may be concentrated in phagocytes and macrophages by this mechanism,[8,13] thereby raising their measured concentration in lung tissue. On the other hand, beta-lactam antibiotics achieve only 40 percent of their serum concentration in lung tissue, because they are not concentrated in cells and remain primarily in the extracellular space, which constitutes about 40 percent of the weight of bronchial tissue.[13]

When all these factors affecting drug concentrations in the lung are taken into account, some general categories of antibiotic penetration can be distinguished. Drugs that generally penetrate well into sputum or bronchial secretions include the quinolones, the newer macrolides (azithromycin and clarithromycin), the tetracyclines, clindamycin, and trimethoprim/sulfamethoxazole. Drugs that penetrate poorly into these sites include the aminoglycosides and, to some extent, the beta-lactam agents.[14]

TABLE 89-2   Penetration of Antibiotics into Sputum and Bronchial Secretions

Good penetration[a]
  Quinolones
  New macrolides: clarithromycin, azithromycin
  Tetracyclines
  Clindamycin
  Trimethoprim/sulfamethoxizole
Poor penetration[b]
  Aminogycosides
  Beta lactams

[a] These drugs are lipid soluble and show inflammation-independent penetration into lung sites.
[b] These drugs have poor lipid solubility and show inflammation-dependent penetration into lung sites.

PROFILES OF COMMON ANTIBIOTICS

BETA-LACTAM ANTIBIOTICS

The beta-lactam antibiotics include a number of agents that have in common the presence of a beta lactam ring. In the case of penicillins, this beta-lactam nucleus is bound to a five-membered thiazolidine ring, while in the case of cephalosporins, it is bound to a six-membered dihydrothiazine ring.[8,15] Modifications in the thiazolidine ring produce the penem antibiotics (such as imipenem), while the absence of a second ring structure bound to the beta-lactam core defines the monobactams (such as aztreonam). All beta-lactam antibiotics (penicillins, cephalosporins, carbapenems, monobactams, and beta-lactam/beta-lactamase inhibitor combinations) act to interfere with the synthesis of bacterial cell wall peptidoglycan by binding to bacterial penicillin-binding proteins. They are bactericidal.

Among the penicillins that are used for respiratory tract infections are the natural penicillins (penicillins G and V), the aminopenicillins (ampicillin and amoxicillin), the antistaphylococcal penicillins, the extended-spectrum antipseudomonal penicillins, and the combinations of a beta-lactam with a beta-lactamase inhibitor. Among the antipseudomonal penicillins are the older carboxypenicillins (ticarcillin) and the ureidopenicillins (piperacillin, azlocillin, and mezlocillin), with piperacillin and azlocillin being the most active against *Pseudomonas aeruginosa*. The available beta-lactam/beta-lactamase inhibitor combinations include clavulanic acid with either amoxicillin or ticarcillin, sulbactam with ampicillin, and tazobactam with piperacillin. The addition of the beta-lactamase inhibitor extends the spectrum of the antibiotic to cover more organisms, particularly those that produce beta-lactamase enzymes.

The cephalosporins include first-, second-, and third-generation drugs. In general, as one moves from the first to the third generation, the activity against gram-positive organisms declines, whereas specialized activity against certain anaerobes and gram-negative bacteria increases. The only third-generation agents active against *Pseudomonas aeruginosa* are ceftazidime and cefoperazone. Some of the second-generation agents (such as cefuroxime) and the third-generation agents are active against beta-lactamase–producing *Hemophilus influenzae*, while the first-generation agents generally are not.

Imipenem is the broadest-spectrum antibiotic currently available, but when it is used as the sole agent for *P. aeruginosa* respiratory tract infections, resistance emerges in as many as 50 percent of all cases.[7] Aztreonam is a monobactam with only gram-negative activity; it is so antigenically different from other beta-lactams that it can be used in penicillin-allergic patients.

MACROLIDES

The macrolides consist of erythromycin and its derivative drugs. These agents are important for the treatment of community-acquired bronchitis and pneumonia. Erythromycin is active against pneumococcus and atypical pathogens (*Mycoplasma pneumoniae* and *Chlamydia pneumoniae*). Like all macrolides, it acts by binding to the 50S ribosomal subunit of the target bacteria and inhibiting RNA-dependent protein synthesis.[8] The newer macrolides, clarithromycin, and azithromycin (the latter often referred to as an azalide), have additional antimicrobial activity against *Hemophilus influenzae*, including beta-lactamase–producing strains. Erythromycin also has activity against *Moraxella catarrhalis*, but the newer macrolides have enhanced antimicrobial effects against this organism. Among the macrolides, azithromycin is the most active agent against *Hemophilus influenzae*, *Moraxella catarrhalis*, and *Mycoplasma pneumoniae*, while clarithromycin (in combination with its active 14-OH metabolite) is the most active agent against *Streptococcus pneumoniae*, *Legionella*, and *Chlamydia pneumoniae*.[8,14] The newer macrolides also are active against the *Mycobacterium avium-intracellulare* complex, and this represents an expanding indication for their use.[16] Both of the newer macrolides are more easily tolerated by the gastrointestinal tract than is erythromycin, and they penetrate well into sputum, lung tissue, and phagocytes. Azithromycin has an exceedingly long tissue half-life and can be given once daily for a total of 5 days when treating pneumonia and bronchitis. By virtue of its sustained tissue levels, azithromycin may be bactericidal, while the other macrolides are usually bacteriostatic.[14]

QUINOLONES

Three fluoroquinolones are currently available for the therapy of respiratory tract infections: ciprofloxacin, ofloxacin, and lomefloxacin. These agents are bactericidal and act by interfering with bacterial DNA gyrase, leading to impaired DNA synthesis and cell lysis.[8] These agents are active against aerobic gram-negative bacilli, but only ciprofloxacin is active enough against *Pseudomonas aeruginosa* to be used against this organism in the respiratory tract. Because they have marginal MICs against pneumococcus, there is some concern (in spite of generally good clinical experience) about using these agents as monotherapy for CAP, although they may be effective as a single agent in the therapy of severe HAP and in the treatment of bronchitic exacerbations of COPD, especially in older and debilitated patients.[7,17] They are active against *Hemophilus influenzae*, including beta-lactamase–producing strains, and they penetrate well into the respiratory tract, achieving high concentrations in bronchial mucosa, sputum, and lung phagocytes. Serum and tissue concentrations are similar for oral and intravenous administration.

AMINOGLYCOSIDES

The aminoglycosides, which are derived from bacteria, act as bactericidal agents; they act as antimicrobials by binding to the 30S ribosomal subunit and interfering with bacterial protein synthesis, along with other less-well-defined effects. These drugs are used primarily to treat infections with aerobic gram-negative bacilli, including *Pseudomonas aeruginosa*. When combined with antipseudomonal beta-lactam antibiotics, these agents demonstrate antibacterial synergy. Tobramycin is more active against *P. aeruginosa* than gentamicin, while amikacin is less susceptible to enzymatic inactivation than the other agents in this class. Because these agents penetrate poorly into lung tissue, some investigators have supplemented systemic therapy with endotracheal instillation, but this approach has not led to any clear bene-

fit in the treatment of serious respiratory tract infections.[8,18] Given the penetration issues and the potential nephrotoxicity of these drugs, there often is some reluctance to use them for severely ill patients with pneumonia.[19]

TETRACYCLINES

The tetracyclines are bacteriostatic agents that act by binding to the 30S ribosomal subunit, interfering with bacterial protein synthesis. Although tetracyclines generally are active against *Hemophilus influenzae* and atypical pathogens, there are reports of increasing resistance by pneumococcus.[8] Photosensitivity reactions limit the safety of these agents in sun-exposed individuals.

CLINDAMYCIN AND METRONIDAZOLE

Clindamycin and metronidazole are used primarily to treat anaerobic lung infections, although clindamycin has good gram-positive antibacterial effects and can be used to treat complex pneumonias in penicillin-allergic patients if it is combined with an agent active against aerobic gram-negative bacilli. Clindamycin acts by binding to the 50S ribosomal subunit, while metronidazole interacts with cellular DNA. Metronidazole should not be used alone to treat lung infections.

TRIMETHOPRIM/SULFAMETHOXAZOLE

Trimethoprim and sulfamethoxazole are used together in a fixed 1:5 ratio. The two drugs act on sequential sites of folate metabolism to inhibit bacterial purine and DNA synthesis. Because of a broad spectrum of activity against gram-positive and gram-negative pathogens, as well as *Legionella* and *Pneumocystis carinii*, trimethoprim/sulfamethoxazole has applications in the therapy of both pneumonia and bronchitis. It is not active against *Pseudomonas aeruginosa*, however.

An Antibiotic Approach to Common Respiratory Tract Infections

BRONCHITIC EXACERBATIONS OF CHRONIC OBSTRUCTIVE LUNG DISEASE

RATIONALE FOR USING ANTIBIOTICS FOR COPD EXACERBATIONS

Not all clinicians believe that antibiotics are useful for patients with COPD who have acute exacerbations, many of which are due to bronchitis. The arguments against the routine use of antimicrobials include the observation that no more than half of all bronchitic exacerbations are bacterial in origin; that the exacerbations are self-limited and can improve without specific antibiotic therapy; and that widespread use of antibiotics in these patients will contribute to the problem of drug-resistant organisms. In spite of these arguments, it is common practice to use antimicrobials in this clinical situation, often with good justification.

The main argument in favor of the routine use of antibiotics for exacerbations of COPD is that a prospective, randomized, controlled trial has shown this approach to be beneficial.[1] COPD exacerbations can be classified by how many of the following three "cardinal" symptoms are present: increased sputum volume, increased sputum purulence, and increased dyspnea.[1] An exacerbation that has all three of these symptoms is classified as type I; one with two of the symptoms is of type II; and one with only one of the symptoms is of type III.[1] In a study of 362 exacerbations in 173 patients, approximately 80 percent of all the episodes were of type I or II. For these more severe bronchitis events, antibiotic therapy was superior to placebo therapy, although the benefits did not extend to patients with more mild, type III exacerbations. Patients treated with antibiotics had a greater likelihood of symptom resolution, more rapid resolution, and a more rapid return of peak flow rates than patients who had been given placebo.[1] These results firmly established the usefulness of antibiotics for COPD exacerbations but suggested that they be limited to type I or II exacerbations. The findings were not antibiotic-specific, and a variety of agents were employed in the study.

In addition to the unequivocal benefits of antibiotics discussed above, there are several theoretical reasons for widespread use of these agents for exacerbations of COPD. There is evidence from quantitative bronchoscopy sampling that some exacerbations (up to half) are associated with as many bacteria in the lung as are seen in patients with pneumonia.[20] If antibiotics were used, they could reduce this bacterial burden, possibly preventing some patients from progressing from bronchitis to pneumonia. If one accepts that antibiotics should be used for bacterial exacerbations, then it would seem unnecessary to use them for viral and other nonbacterial episodes. However, on clinical grounds, it is virtually impossible to distinguish bacterial from non-bacterial exacerbations, since in severely ill patients both have the same degree of fever, leukocytosis, hypoxemia, and symptoms.[20] Thus, it may be necessary to use antibiotics even for these non-bacterial exacerbations. In addition, there are some data to show that even viral exacerbations can be complicated by secondary bacterial infection, and possibly the use of antibiotics might prevent some of these episodes, even in the setting of a viral bronchitis.[21] Finally, there is evidence in patients with bronchiectasis that the degree of airways obstruction may increase as a result of bronchial infection and its associated inflammatory response. This "vicious circle hypothesis" states that infection may lead to airways injury and recurrent infection; possibly antibiotic therapy could break this cycle.[22] All of these theoretical benefits of antibiotic therapy, along with the data showing clearcut clinical benefit, justify the use of these agents for patients with exacerbations of COPD.

CHOOSING AN ANTIBIOTIC FOR COPD EXACERBATIONS

In cases of COPD exacerbation, one would like to use an agent that has the following characteristics: (1) Ease of administration, few side effects, and infrequent dosing; (2) activity against the three most common pathogens (nontypable *Hemophilus influenzae*, pneumococcus, and *Moraxella catarrhalis*); activity against atypical pathogens would also be desirable; (3) resistance to bacterial beta-lactamases, since up to 40 percent of *H. influenzae* and 75 percent of *M. catarrhalis* isolates produce such enzymes; (4) good penetration into

respiratory secretions, achieving high concentrations in the sputum and bronchial mucosa; (5) minimal potential for drug interactions, particularly with theophyllines; (6) proven efficacy and superiority to other agents; and (7) low expense.

Unfortunately, no such antibiotic exists, and, thus, choosing the antibiotic treatment that will best serve the patient involves making some compromises. For many patients, cost is a major consideration, and therefore an older and less expensive agent is often chosen, even if doing so means compromising on antimicrobial spectrum or ease of administration. For example, amoxicillin must be given three times a day and is not active against beta-lactamase–producing organisms or atypical pathogens. Erythromycin must be given three or four times daily and has no activity against *H. influenzae*, while first-generation cephalosporins are not active against beta-lactamase–producing organisms or atypical pathogens. Tetracyclines are commonly used for exacerbations of COPD but are not as reliable against pneumococcus as are other agents. If an agent with a limited antimicrobial spectrum is chosen, then the patient should be followed carefully; if there is no clinical improvement after 3 to 5 days, the antibiotic should be changed to one that fills in the gaps in the antimicrobial spectrum of the original agent.

For some patients, it is necessary to choose a newer and often more expensive antibiotic that has a more complete antimicrobial spectrum. If, for example, the patient used antibiotics recently and showed no response, or if the patient is at risk for enteric gram-negative bronchitis, then a specific agent may be needed. Quinolones may be a good choice for bronchitic exacerbations of COPD in certain patients because they are active against beta-lactamase and non-beta-lactamase producing *Hemophilus influenzae* and *Moraxella catarrhalis* strains, as well as against enteric gram-negative organisms. Because of their excellent bronchial penetration, these agents are likely to be adequate for pneumococcal bronchitis as well, in spite of concerns about their efficacy in pneumococcal pneumonia. The new macrolides also represent good choices for bronchitic exacerbations of COPD, having activity against the three most common pathogens, as well as atypical ones, and achieving high levels in sputum, lung tissue, and phagocytes. The newer macrolides may also offer better patient compliance, because they can be given either once daily (azithromycin) or twice daily (clarithromycin). A theophylline interaction has been shown for clarithromycin but not for azithromycin, and the theophylline dosage should be reduced and levels monitored when this drug is used with clarithromycin.

If compliance is a major concern, then drugs that can be administered once or twice daily should be considered. Agents that are available for this type of schedule are listed in Table 89-3.

COMMUNITY-ACQUIRED PNEUMONIA

CHOOSING AN ANTIBIOTIC ON THE BASIS OF THE MOST LIKELY PATHOGEN(S)

The American Thoracic Society has published guidelines for the initial therapy of CAP. This approach involves making an empirical choice of the initial therapy on the basis of a pre-

TABLE 89-3 Antimicrobials for Exacerbations of COPD that Can Be Given Once or Twice Daily

Once daily
    Beta lactams: cefixime
    Macrolides: azithromycin
    Quinolones: lomefloxacin
Twice Daily
    Beta lactams: cefprozil, cefuroxime, loracarbef
    Macrolides: clarithromycin
    Quinolones: ciprofloxacin, ofloxacin
    Others: doxycycline, trimethoprim/sulfamethoxazole

diction of the likely etiologic pathogens for a given patient. Patients fall into one of four categories, each with its own list of likely pathogens and appropriate therapy.[2] Neither the sputum Gram stain, clinical presentation (typical or atypical syndromes), nor extensive diagnostic testing is used in categorizing patients. Instead, the following three clinical and epidemiologic assessments are made. (1) How ill is the patient when initially seen—is the pneumonia mild, moderate, or severe? (2) Will the patient be treated in the hospital or at home? (3) Does the patient have comorbid illness or an age >60 years? On the basis of these assessments, patients fall into the following four categories: (1) patients who are mildly to moderately ill, who are treated outside the hospital, and who neither are elderly nor have comorbid disease; (2) patients who are mildly to moderately ill, who are treated outside the hospital, and who are elderly and/or have comorbid disease; (3) patients whose illness is moderately severe, who are treated in the hospital but not in an intensive care unit, and who may be elderly and/or have comorbid disease; and (4) patients who are severely ill, who are treated in an intensive care unit, and who may be elderly and/or have comorbid disease.

Outpatients fall in the first two categories and are treated with oral agents. Patients in the first category are likely to be infected with pneumococcus, atypical pathogens, respiratory viruses, or *Hemophilus influenzae*. A macrolide or tetracycline is recommended. The newer macrolides, clarithromycin and azithromycin, can be used if *H. influenzae* is likely (as in a cigarette smoker) or if erythromycin intolerance is present. For patients in the second category, the presence of advanced age and/or comorbid illness alters the list of likely pathogens, which includes pneumococcus, *H. influenzae*, enteric gram-negative bacteria, and respiratory viruses. Since atypical pathogens are less likely in this category, recommended therapy is with an oral second-generation cephalosporin (such as cefuroxime), trimethoprim/sulfamethoxazole, or a beta-lactam/beta-lactamase inhibitor combination (amoxicillin/clavulanate). A macrolide can be added as a second agent if atypical pathogens seem likely.

For the third and fourth categories, patients are treated intravenously to begin because they are admitted to the hospital. Patients in the third category are likely to be infected with pneumococcus, *H. influenzae*, enteric gram-negative bacteria (but not *Pseudomonas aeruginosa*), anaerobes, and possibly *Legionella* spp. or *Staphylococcus aureus*. This list dictates that initial therapy be with a second-generation

cephalosporin, a non-antipseudomonal third-generation cephalosporin, or a beta-lactam/beta-lactamase inhibitor combination (such as ampicillin/sulbactam). If *Legionella* infection is likely, then a macrolide should be added as a second agent. For patients in the fourth category—those with severe CAP—multiple drugs are needed to cover the likely pathogens, which include pneumococcus, *Legionella* spp., enteric gram-negative bacteria (including *Pseudomonas aeruginosa*), *Mycoplasma pneumoniae*, and respiratory viruses.[23] These patients should receive a macrolide (plus rifampin if *Legionella* is documented), along with a combination of two antipseudomonal agents.

Antipseudomonal antibiotics (Table 89-4) include the aminoglycosides, the third-generation cephalosporins ceftazidime and cefoperazone, ciprofloxacin, the antipseudomonal penicillins (piperacillin, azlocillin, and mezlocillin), aztreonam, imipenem, and the beta-lactam/beta-lactamase inhibitor combinations (ticarcillin/clavulanate). When it is necessary to combine agents from this list, acceptable combinations include an aminoglycoside with a beta-lactam, an aminoglycoside with a quinolone, and a quinolone with a beta-lactam.[19] Only the aminoglycoside/beta-lactam combination will achieve antipseudomonal synergy, but a quinolone/beta-lactam combination may be effective because of the excellent penetration of the quinolone into respiratory sites of infection. A combination of two beta-lactams generally is not a good idea because of the possibility of inducing a bacterial beta-lactamase enzyme that could inactivate both agents simultaneously.

If the patient is not responding to one of these empirical regimens, then several alternative diagnoses and complications should be considered, and extensive diagnostic testing may be necessary.[2] One possibility is that the initial pathogen is antibiotic-resistant, an increasing concern with pneumococcal infections.[5,6] Penicillin resistance can be at an intermediate or high level. Highly resistant organisms should be treated with cefotaxime, ceftriaxone, or vancomycin, while high intravenous doses of cefo may be effective for moderately resistant organisms.

TABLE 89-4 Antipseudomonal Antibiotics

Aminoglycosides
    Gentamicin
    Tobramycin
    Amikacin
Beta-lactams
    Third-generation cephalosporins[a]: ceftazidime, cefoperazone
    Monobactams: aztreonam
    Carbapenems[b]: imipenem
    Penicillins: piperacillin, azlocillin, mezlocillin, ticarcillin
    Beta-lactam/beta-lactamase inhibitor combinations:
        ticarcillin/clavulanate, piperacillin/tazobactam
    Fluoroquinolones[c]: ciprofloxacin

[a] A new-generation cephalosporin, cefipime, may soon be available for this indication.
[b] A new carbapenem, meropenem, may soon be available for this indication.
[c] Several new fluoroquinolones with antipseudomonal activity are being developed.

CHANGING FROM INTRAVENOUS TO ORAL THERAPY
When a hospitalized patient begins to improve, oral therapy may appropriately replace intravenous therapy. In clinical practice, this process can involve one of three approaches: (1) *streamlining*, which means focusing therapy on a narrower bacteriologic spectrum on the basis of initial culture results or other data; (2) *sequential* or *switch therapy*, which involves changing to an oral regimen that is equivalent in potency to the intravenous regimen (as could be accomplished with a quinolone)[17]; and (3) *stepdown therapy*, which means changing to an oral regimen less potent than the intravenous regimen.

The clinical indications for each of these scenarios still are being defined. However, as a patient improves, and provided signs of life-threatening illness are absent, step-down therapy is appropriate. One recent study found that one-third of 503 CAP patients could have been switched to oral therapy by day 3 because they were defined as "low-risk." This designation was given if the patient was not severely ill, did not have a "high-risk" pathogen, and did not have any other life-threatening complications.[24] The authors estimated that early switching, using similar criteria, could have reduced the length of the hospital stay by several days for low-risk patients.

NOSOCOMIAL PNEUMONIA

DEFINING AN EMPIRICAL APPROACH

The clinical definition of nosocomial pneumonia may be inaccurate in some patients because of its high sensitivity and poor specificity. The presence of a new lung infiltrate in a patient with fever, leukocytosis, and purulent sputum who has been in the hospital for at least 48 h is not pathognomonic for respiratory infection. This realization has led to the proliferation of invasive diagnostic methods for nosocomial pneumonia that involve the collection of respiratory secretions that can be cultured quantitatively to define whether pneumonia actually is present.[25] Controversy abounds about the accuracy of these methods, and some clinicians will not start antibiotics unless the clinical diagnosis of HAP is confirmed microbiologically, while others will initiate empirical therapy if the clinical picture is compatible with HAP.[25,26]

In selecting initial empirical therapy, the likely pathogens can be predicted by defining the severity of illness and the presence of specific risk factors for certain pathogens, although local patterns of bacteriology and antimicrobial resistance always should be considered. If a patient has mild to moderate illness, and no unusual risk factors, then he is at risk for a "core" group of bacteria that include pneumococcus, *Hemophilus influenzae, Staphylococcus aurus, Klebsiella pneumoniae, Enterobacter* spp., *Escherichia coli, Proteus* spp., and *Serratia marcescens*.[19,27] These organisms can be treated with a second-generation cephalosporin, a non-antipseudomonal third-generation cephalosporin, a beta-lactam/beta-lactamase inhibitor combination, or a fluoroquinolone.

If specific risk factors are present, then, in addition to the core organisms, the patient is at risk for other bacteria, the identity of which depends on the risk factor.[19,27] Anaerobes are a concern in the presence of witnessed aspiration, but many such patients are infected with a mixed flora of gram-positive and gram-negative organisms.[28] *S. aureus* infection is a concern in patients with diabetes, coma, head injury, or renal failure and is also common in patients who develop pneumonia within the first 4 days of hospitalization.[19,29,30] *Legionella* is a concern if the patient is receiving high-dose corticosteroids; and highly resistant gram-negative bacteria are a concern if the patient has had prolonged hospitalization or has received multiple antibiotics.[31] Appropriate therapy involves the same antibiotics as are used against the core organisms, with additional agents directed against the organisms that are of special concern.

Patients with severe HAP are usually being ventilated mechanically and are at risk for the core organisms plus *Pseudomonas aeruginosa* and other highly resistant gram-negative bacteria. Therapy should include two antipseudomonal agents (listed above), which can be combined in the ways that have been discussed. If methicillin-resistant *S. aureus* is common in the ICU, then consideration should be given to adding vancomycin empirically in patients who have received prior antibiotics.

CONTROVERSIES IN THE ANTIBIOTIC THERAPY OF HAP

When a patient is severely ill and develops nosocomial pneumonia, combination therapy is commonly used, but in many such patients monotherapy may be adequate. Only a few situations absolutely necessitate combination therapy. Dual antipseudomonal coverage is needed if *P. aeruginosa* pneumonia is complicated by bacteremia or neutropenia.[19,32] Combination therapy also may be needed if the list of likely pathogens is so long that a single agent cannot provide adequate antimicrobial coverage. Combination regimens also may prevent the emergence of antimicrobial resistance during therapy (as can occur with *P. aeruginosa*). Certain regimens, such as an aminoglycoside/beta-lactam combination, can provide anti-bacterial synergy against organisms such as *P. aeruginosa*.

Patients with HAP who lack these specific indications but are treated with a combination regimen may be exposed to more antibiotics than are necessary. Some studies have shown that monotherapy is as effective as combination therapy for mild and moderate forms of nosocomial pneumonia.[19,33] However, the role of monotherapy in severely ill patients is unclear. One recent study has shown that monotherapy of severe nosocomial pneumonia, using either ciprofloxacin or imipenem, is effective provided that *P. aeruginosa* is not the etiologic agent.[7] This organism was absent in 70 percent of the patients studied, but in the 30 percent who had *P. aeruginosa*, monotherapy was associated with a poor rate of bacterial eradication and a high rate of resistance emerging during therapy.[7] In practical terms, these findings suggest that patients with severe HAP should be started on a combination therapy regimen that includes two antipseudomonal agents, but if this organism is not isolated, switching to a single agent (such as ciprofloxacin or imipenem) will provide effective therapy.

Another therapeutic controversy relevant to patients with HAP is whether the capacity of an antibiotic to induce an adverse host inflammatory response should be considered in deciding whether to use the agent. When certain antibiotics kill bacteria, they produce cell wall lysis products that can interact with the patient's cytokine-producing cells and lead to an excessive release of inflammatory mediators, such as tumor necrosis factor (TNF). Clinically, this response could cause a sepsis syndrome to develop after the initiation of antibiotic therapy. In-vitro systems have been developed to measure the potential of antibiotic lysis products to induce cytokine production by inflammatory cells, but the relevance of these observations to clinical events is not established. In these systems, high concentrations of TNF can be produced by mononuclear cells in response to the bacterial lysis products produced when *E. coli* is incubated with ceftazidime or aztreonam, but lower concentrations result from incubation with amikacin, ciproflaxacin, or imipenem.[34] Investigators have speculated that antibiotics that kill rapidly lead to less cytokine release than antibiotics that kill slowly and that act by binding to penicillin-binding protein 3, leading to the production of an abnormal, filamentous cell wall.[34-36] Again, the clinical relevance of these in-vitro observations is not known.

One last therapeutic question is whether topical antibiotic therapy can supplement systemic therapy in patients with HAP. In one double-blind, randomized study, endotracheal tobramycin was added to systemic therapy in patients with gram-negative pneumonia. Although topical therapy did not lead to an improved clinical outcome, it did result in greater rates of bacterial eradication.[18] These findings have led to the suggestion that topical therapy may be useful for some patients with highly resistant pathogens, as an adjunct to systemic therapy.

Summary

A large number of antimicrobial agents are available for the treatment of respiratory infections, and selection among them should be based on a number of factors in addition to their antimicrobial spectra of activity. Pharmacodynamic factors such as the mechanism of killing, the presence or absence of a postantibiotic effect, the frequency of administration, and the ability to penetrate to the site of infection must all be considered. These principles can be applied to develop guidelines for empirical therapy of bronchitic exacerbations of COPD, community-acquired pneumonia, and nosocomial pneumonia. Many of the recommended regimens have not yet been proved to work better than other regimens, and they often are based on the theoretical pharmacologic and bacteriologic advantages of certain antimicrobial agents. Many therapeutic issues remain unresolved, and this complicates the selection of therapy, particularly for patients with nosocomial pneumonia.

References

1. Anthonisen NR, Manfreda J, Warren CPW, et al.: Antibiotic therapy in exacerbations of chronic obstructive pulmonary disease. *Ann Intern Med* 1987; 106:196.
2. Niederman MS, Bass JB, Campbell GD, et al.: Guidelines for the initial management of adults with community-acquired pneumonia: diagnosis, assessment of severity, and initial antimicrobial therapy. *Am Rev Respir Dis* 1993; 148:1418.
3. Fang GD, Fine M, Orloff J, et al.: New and emerging etiologies for community-acquired pneumonia with implication for therapy. A prospective multicenter study of 359 cases. *Medicine* 1990; 69:307.
4. Celis R, Torres A, Gatell J, et al.: Nosocomial pneumonia: a multivariate analysis of risk and prognosis. *Chest* 1988; 93:318.
5. Breiman RF, Butler JC, Tenover FC, et al.: Emergence of drug-resistant pneumococcal infections in the United States. *JAMA* 1994; 271:1831.
6. Friedland IR, McCracken GH: Management of infections caused by antibiotic-resistant *Streptococcus pneumoniae*. *NEJM* 1994; 331:377.
7. Fink MP, Snydman DR, Niederman MS, et al.: Treatment of severe pneumonia in hospitalized patients: results of a multicenter, randomized, double-blind trial comparing intravenous ciprofloxacin with imipenem-cilastatin. *Antimicrob Agents Chemother* 1994; 38:547.
8. Mandell LA: Antibiotics for pneumonia therapy. *Med Clin North Am* 1994; 778:997.
9. Craig W: Pharmacodynamics of antimicrobial agents as a basis for determining dosage regimens. *Eur J Clin Microbiol Infect Dis* 1993; 12:6.
10. Redington J, Craig WA: Pharmacology of antimicrobials in the elderly, in Niederman MS (ed): *Respiratory Infections in the Elderly.* New York, Raven Press, 1991:239.
11. Prins JM, Buller HR, Kuijper EJ, et al.: Once versus thrice daily gentamicin in patients with serious infections. *Lancet* 1993; 341:335.
12. Miyagawa CI: Aminoglycosides in the intensive care unit: an old drug in a dynamic environment. *New Horizons* 1993; 1:172.
13. Honeybourne D: Antibiotic penetration into lung tissues. *Thorax* 1994; 49:104.
14. Sonnesyn SW, Gerding DN: Antimicrobials for the treatment of respiratory infection, in Niederman MS, Sarosa GA, Glassroth J (eds): *Respiratory Infections: A Scientific Basis for Management.* Philadelphia, W. B. Saunders, 1994:511.
15. Nolan PE, Bass JB: New drugs for treating lung infection. *Chest* 1988; 94:1076.
16. Wallace RJ, Brown BA, Griffith DE, et al.: Initial clarithromycin monotherapy for *Mycobacterium avium-intracellulare* complex lung disease. *Am J Respir Crit Care Med* 1994; 149:1335.
17. Khan FA, Basir R: Sequential intravenous–oral administration of ciproflaxacin vs. ceftazidime in serious bacterial respiratory tract infections. *Chest* 1989; 96:528.
18. Brown RB, Kruse JA, Counts GW, et al.: Double blind study of endotracheal tobramycin in the treatment of gram-negative bacterial pneumonia. *Antimicrob Agents Chemother* 1990; 34:269.
19. Niederman MS: An approach to empiric therapy of nosocomial pneumonia. *Med Clin North Am* 1994; 78:1123.
20. Fagon JY, Chastre J, Trouillet JL, et al.: Characterization of distal bronchial microflora during acute exacerbation of chronic bronchitis: use of the protected specimen brush technique in 54 mechanically ventilated patients. *Am Rev Respir Dis* 1990; 142:1004.
21. Smith CB, Golden C, Klauber MR, et al.: Interaction between viruses and bacteria in patients with chronic bronchitis. *J Infect Dis* 1976; 134:552.
22. Murphy TF, Sethi S: Bacterial infection in chronic obstructive pulmonary disease. *Am Rev Respir Dis* 1992; 146:1067.
23. Torres A, Serra-Batlles J, Ferrer A, et al.: Severe community-acquired pneumonia. Epidemiology and prognostic factors. *Am Rev Respir Dis* 1991; 144:312.
24. Weingarten SR, Riedinger MS, Varis G, et al.: *Chest* 19XX; 105:1109.

25. Chastre J, Fagon JY: Invasive diagnostic testing should be routinely used to manage ventilated patients with suspected pneumonia. *Am J Respir Crit Care Med* 1994; 150:570.

26. Niederman MS, Torres A, Summer W: Invasive diagnostic testing is not needed routinely to manage suspected ventilator-associated pneumonia. *Am J Respir Crit Care Med* 1994; 150:565.

27. Mandell LA, Marrie TJ, Niederman MS: Initial antimicrobial treatment of hospital acquired pneumonia in adults: a conference report. *Can J Infect Dis* 1993; 4:317.

28. Mier L, Dreyfuss D, Darchy B, et al.: Is penicillin G an adequate initial treatment for aspiration pneumonia? A prospective evaluation using a protected specimen brush and quantitative cultures. *Intensive Care Med* 1993; 19:279.

29. Rello J, Quintana E, Ausina V, et al.: Risk factors for *Staphylococcus aureus* nosocomial pneumonia in critically ill patients. *Am Rev Respir Dis* 1990; 142:1320.

30. Prod'hom G, Leuenberger P, Koerfer J, et al.: Nosocomial pneumonia in mechanically ventilated patients receiving antiacid, ranitidine, or sucralfate as prophylaxis for stress ulcer: a randomized controlled trial. *Ann Intern Med* 1994; 120:653.

31. Rello J, Ausina V, Ricart M, et al.: Impact of previous antimicrobial therapy on the etiology and outcome of ventilator-associated pneumonia. *Chest* 1993; 104:1230.

32. Hilf M, Yu VL, Sharp J, et al.: Antibiotic therapy for *Pseudomonas aeruginosa* bacteremia: outcome correlations in a prospective study of 200 patients. *Am J Med* 1989; 87:540.

33. Mangi RJ, Greco T, Ryan J, et al.: Cefoperazone versus combination antibiotic therapy of hospital-acquired pneumonia. *Am J Med* 1988; 84:68.

34. Simon DM, Koenig G, Trenholme GM: Differences in release of tumor necrosis factor from THP-1 cells stimulated by filtrates of antibiotic-killed *Escherichia coli*. *J Infect Dis* 1991; 164:800.

35. Arditi M, Kabat W, Yogev R: Antibiotic-induced bacterial killing stimulates tumor necrosis factor-∂ release in whole blood. *J Infect Dis* 1993; 167:240.

36. Prins JM, Van Deventer S, Kuijper EJ, Speelman P: clinical relevance of antibiotic-induced endotoxin release. *Antimicrob Agents Chemother* 1994; 38:1211.

BRONCHIECTASIS
EUGENE F. GEPPERT

Pathogenesis and Etiologies

Diagnosis

Treatment

Bronchiectasis is a pathologic condition in the lung that is characterized anatomically by the presence of single or multiple lung segments whose middle-sized bronchi have become permanently dilated as a result of a previous or ongoing injury to the structural elements of the airway walls. Bronchiectasis has many different etiologies, and the proper treatment depends upon the cause and degree of severity of the disease process in the patient. Bronchiectasis can be an asymptomatic condition that is diagnosed incidentally from computed tomography (CT) of the thorax that is done for another purpose, or it can be a symptomatic condition with a variety of possible complications.

Pathogenesis and Etiologies

Bronchiectasis is not a single disease but rather an anatomic abnormality with many different possible causes. Some of these are listed in Table 90-1. Since bronchiectasis is very rarely congenital,[1] the different etiologies usually depend on the appearance of a process of injury that causes severe damage to the middle-sized bronchi.

The pathogenesis of bronchiectasis usually starts with a structurally normal lung in which a sequence of injury and attempted repair leads to the chronic disease. Most investigators who have studied the pathogenesis of bronchiectasis agree that some inherent weakness of the bronchial wall is likely to be present,[2] although the precise nature of this defect is unknown in the majority of cases of idiopathic bronchiectasis. In cases of bronchiectasis associated with a systemic disease, it more often is possible to speculate on the nature of the compromised defense mechanisms that makes the patient vulnerable to excessive bronchial injury. For example, the patient with primary ciliary dysfunction lacks a normal mucociliary clearance mechanism, for removing bacteria and other harmful agents from the surface of the bronchus, making it more susceptible to injury.

Illustrative of the pathogenesis of one type of bronchiectasis, the postinfectious type, is the transformation from healthy to diseased lung (Fig. 90-1). An example is the child who develops bronchiectasis from lobar pneumonia caused by *Staphylococcus aureus*. Prior to development of the pneumonia, the child's lung and bronchial tree are normal,

although an underlying cellular or molecular abnormality of the bronchial mucosa may be present ("unknown mucosal vulnerability factor"). During the acute pneumonia, prior to any treatment, the lower lobe of the right lung is infiltrated with neutrophils and organisms. Since these organisms induce a necrotizing response, the pus-filled middle-sized bronchi, which initially had a cartilaginous skeleton, are damaged in such a manner that their cartilage and smooth muscle layers disappear, and only the lumen and a floppy membranous wall remain. The daughter branches of these middle-sized bronchi, the smallest bronchi and bronchioles, are damaged in such a way that they either become stenosed or their lumens disappear completely, leaving fibrous remnants behind. Many air spaces are destroyed as well, and because of this loss of air spaces, the middle-sized bronchi

TABLE 90-1   Conditions Associated with Bronchiectasis

Idiopathic
Process that promotes damage to bronchial wall is known
  Postinfectious (after a necrotizing pneumonia)
  Primary ciliary dyskinesia
  Cystic fibrosis
  Hypogammaglobulinemia
  Deficiency of immunoglobulin A and IgG subclasses
  Congenital absence of cartilages of segmental bronchi
    (Williams-Campbell syndrome)
  Chronic bronchial obstruction (e.g., from bronchial carcinoid
    tumor)
  Allergic bronchopulmonary aspergillosis
  Inflammatory bowel disease
  Rheumatoid arthritis
  Infection with human immunodeficiency virus (HIV)
  Inhalation of ammonia fumes
  Sarcoidosis
 Process that promotes damage to bronchial wall is unknown
  Young's syndrome (azoospermia without an abnormal
    sweat test)
  Alpha$_1$-antiprotease deficiency
  Tracheobronchomegaly
  Yellow nail syndrome
  Ehlers-Danlos syndrome
  Marfan's syndrome
  Heroin addiction

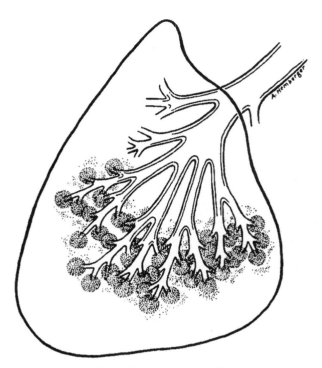

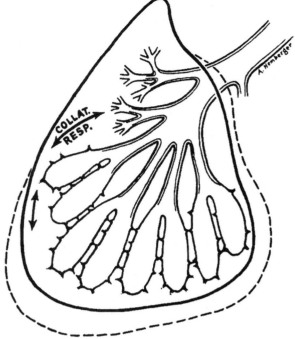

FIGURE 90-1 Diagram illustrating two stages in the pathogenesis of postinfectious bronchiectasis. The drawing on the left shows finely dotted zones that indicate areas of alveolar pus in a necrotizing pneumonia caused by *Staphylococcus aureus*. The middle-sized bronchi near the pus-filled air spaces are damaged by proteolytic enzymes released by the bacteria and inflammatory cells. The drawing on the right shows the end result of this type of pneumonia in a patient whose bronchial mucosa is susceptible to this type of damage. The middle-sized bronchi that were formerly involved by the pneumonia are rendered floppy by destruction of their rigid tissues, such as cartilage. During the healing process, scars form in the periphery of these bronchi; as the scars contract, the bronchi are pulled open and assume a clubbed shape. These bronchi end blindly and the air spaces distal to them can receive air only through collateral respiration by way of the pores of Kohn and canals of Lambert. (*From Mark and Baldwin,*[33] *with permission.*)

move closer together in the shrunken lobe. The lobar bronchus proximal to the infected region is not destroyed but it is injured slightly and, as a result, is more readily compressed during forced exhalation. This leads to exaggerated dynamic compression and airflow limitation during maximal exhalation.[3] After the injury has progressed to this point, the child is treated for the pneumonia. Although the child survives, the residual damage to the bronchi remains for the rest of life as lobar bronchiectasis. Thus, the acute bacterial pneumonia resolves, but the anatomic deformity that it leaves behind is a group of dilated middle-sized bronchi, tethered open by the contracting radial scars that hold the floppy bronchial walls to the adjoining lung tissue. These bronchiectatic bronchi terminate in stenotic or obliterated terminals. They are blind pouches, and no stream of exhaled air flows through them to propel bronchial mucus toward the larynx during forceful exhalation. If the entire lobe is affected by bronchiectasis, the lobe may collapse partially or totally. If less than a lobe is involved, its air spaces may remain inflated as a result of collateral airflow channels.

Bronchiectasis of any etiology can be complicated by hypersecretion of mucus, diffuse airway obstruction, cachexia, bleeding, recurrent pneumonia, and pulmonary hypertension. The pathogenesis of mucous hypersecretion is as follows. In some patients, the dilated bronchi fill with clear mucus from nearby bronchial glands and from goblet cells. This static mucus can become chronically infected with bacteria such as *Streptococcus pneumoniae, Haemophilus influenzae,* or *Pseudomonas aeruginosa.* Neutrophils migrate into the infected mucus and contribute to an inflammatory state. Elastase released from these neutrophils is capable of stimulating the secretion of even more mucus.[4] The end result of this process of infection of the bronchi and hypersecretion is exaggerated production of mucus, which can continue indefinitely. Whenever the excessive mucus is propelled into the large central bronchi by a change of body position (gravitational mucus flow) or through the effects of exercise, the patient is stimulated to cough, and the cough propels a large quantity of purulent sputum into the large central bronchi. From these the purulent mucus can spread to other regions of the lungs. If the patient's disease is extensive and bilateral, enough tiny bronchioles will be plugged with inspissated mucus to result in airway obstruction. This airflow limitation leads to mismatching of ventilation and pulmonary blood flow, hypoxemia, and consequently dyspnea on exertion. The systemic effects of chronic bronchial infection include weight loss and even cachexia in some patients as well as chronic fatigue. In the minority of the patients who also have bronchial hyperactivity, as shown by methacholine or histamine challenge testing, wheezing is present.[5] Hemoptysis results indirectly from the process by which the infected bronchi heal.[6] The infected bronchial mucosa is transformed by the growth of new capillaries from the bronchial arteries in the form of granulation tissue. The capillaries are infected easily with the nearby bacteria, and this infected granulation tissue bleeds easily. As the chronic infection proceeds, new granulation tissue replaces the old and the bronchial arteries undergo progressive hypertrophy. Thus, an artery with systemic pressure supplies blood to a fragile, chronically infected capillary bed; the results can be hemoptysis that is occasionally massive. The last complication is recurrent pneumonia, which is a problem only in a minority of patients with bronchiectasis (Fig. 90-2). It is thought to result from the proximity of chronically infected bronchiectatic bronchi to regions of intact lung. The bacteria spill over into neighboring regions and cause an acute pneumonia. The most severe cases of bronchiectasis are complicated by pulmonary hypertension. Pulmonary hypertension complicates bronchiectasis when the patient suffers from chronic hypoxemia with the resultant hypoxic vasoconstriction of the pulmonary arteries. Over many years, chronic pulmonary hypertension leads to right ventricular hypertrophy and failure. Destruction of more than two-thirds of the pulmonary capillary bed can also result in pulmonary hypertension and chronic cor pulmonale.

The degree of bronchial dilatation that results from this pathogenetic process is variable. Three types are described.[7] The mildest form of bronchiectasis is cylindrical bronchiectasis (Fig. 90-3). In this form, the middle-sized bronchi are dilated in the shape of cylinders and the small bronchi and bronchioles distal to the dilated bronchi are present but often obstructed by mucus or stenosis. In the form known as varicose bronchiectasis, the middle-sized bronchi are distorted into the irregular shape of varicose veins (Fig. 90-4), and many of the distal bronchioles are destroyed. The most severe anatomic form of bronchiectasis is saccular bronchiectasis (Fig. 90-5), in which the middle-sized bronchi are pulled open into the form of sacks; most of the distal bronchi and bronchioles are destroyed. All three of these different anatomic forms of bronchiectasis can be recognized on high-resolution CT (HRCT) of the lungs.

The preceding discussion of the pathogenesis of bronchiectasis is based on the type of injury to the middle-sized bronchi that takes place in some patients with necrotizing pneumonia. The reason why only a subset of patients with necrotizing pneumonia develop bronchiectasis and others are spared is unknown. In other types of bronchiectasis, such as that associated with inflammatory bowel disease, the pathogenesis is probably different in detail[8,9] but similar in the end result. Once the transformation of the bronchi into

FIGURE 90-2 Posteroanterior chest roentgenograms taken about 1 month apart in a 40-year-old woman with severe cystic bronchiectasis of the left lower lobe. The film on the left (*A*) shows volume loss in the left lower lobe together with some loss of definition of the diaphragm. The film on the right (*B*) shows that the infiltrate seen in the previous film now extends upward into the left midlung field. The first film was taken at a time when the patient's bronchiectasis was stable. The second film was taken when the patient had signs and symptoms of bacterial pneumonia together with an elevated leukocyte count. Blood cultures were positive for *Streptococcus pneumoniae.*

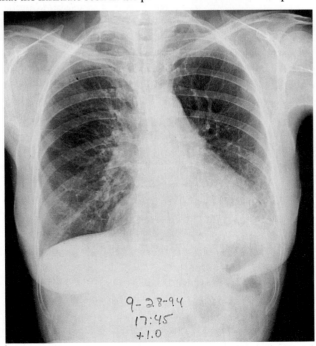

A

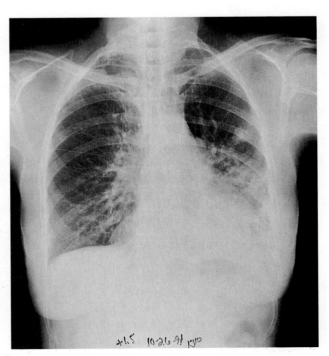

B

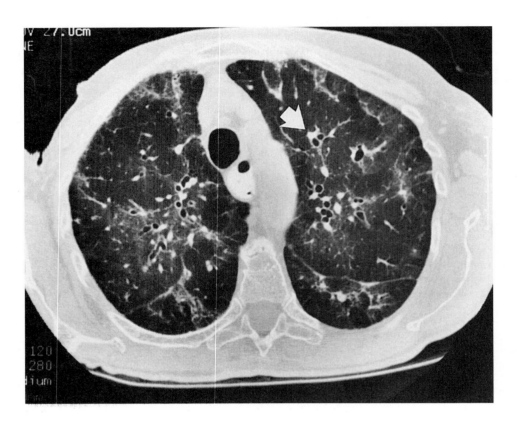

FIGURE 90-3 High-resolution computed tomography of the midlung area showing cylindrical bronchiectasis. Note that the vertically oriented bronchi appear as white rings with black centers and the accompanying branches of the pulmonary arteries are white dots. The "signet-ring" sign is shown at the arrow, where a bronchus is dilated to a diameter larger than that of the accompanying artery.

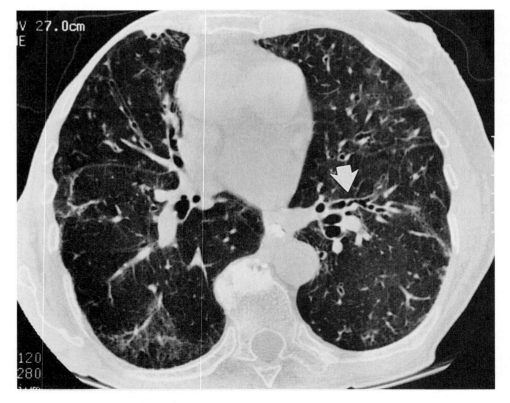

FIGURE 90-4 High-resolution computed tomography of the midlung area showing varicose bronchiectasis. Horizontally oriented bronchi are dilated in the shape of varicose veins and extend abnormally far out toward the lung periphery. Several of these bronchi show parallel lines, or "tram lines," that represent thickening of the walls. The walls of these bronchi show occasional beading, the "string of pearls" sign.

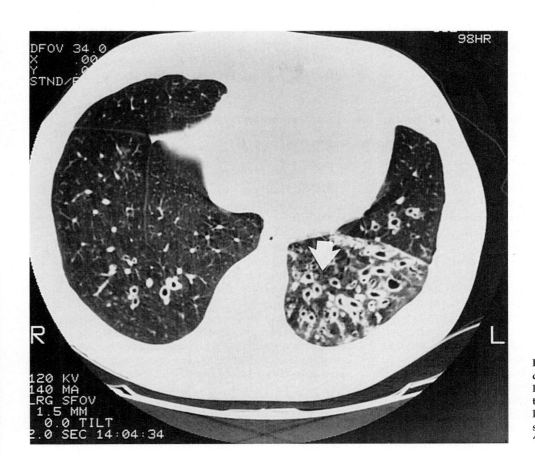

FIGURE 90-5 High-resolution computed tomography of the lower lobes showing bilateral cystic bronchiectasis. In the left lower lobe, many dilated ring shadows are close together, the "cluster of grapes" sign.

dilated tubes has taken place, the anatomic pathology can remain totally stable for many years. In some systemic diseases, however, a second form of lung disease may complicate simple bronchiectasis. For example, in patients with cystic fibrosis, progressive bronchiolitis obliterans caused by heavy infection with *P. aeruginosa* does progressive damage to lung tissue.[10] Patients with allergic bronchopulmonary aspergillosis have a distinctive form of exudative bronchiolitis that can eventually result in extensive lung destruction that is separate from the patient's central bronchiectasis.[11]

It is useful to divide the etiologies of bronchiectasis into three categories: idiopathic bronchiectasis, bronchiectasis associated with systemic etiologies where the nature of the process that damages the bronchial wall is known, and bronchiectasis associated with systemic etiologies where the pathogenetic factor is completely unknown (Table 90-1).

Idiopathic bronchiectasis is defined as disease in which the known causes and risk factors have been excluded by a careful history, physical examination, and a standard laboratory workup that includes (1) a serum protein electrophoresis for α_1-antitrypsin deficiency; (2) immunoglobulin levels including IgG subclasses; (3) a sweat test; (4) determination of immunoglobulins and *Aspergillus* precipitins for allergic bronchopulmonary aspergillosis, and (5) an electron microscopic examination of sperm or respiratory epithelium for primary ciliary dyskinesia.[2] The history is most useful in documenting past episodes of pneumonia that left the

patient with chronic sputum production thereafter. Although they are rare, cases of bronchiectasis following the inhalation of toxic fumes such as ammonia[12] would be diagnosed only from a history of serious exposure with the appearance of chronic symptoms from that point on. A positive family history of bronchiectasis or cystic fibrosis is useful in suggesting one of the familial forms of bronchiectasis, such as cystic fibrosis or primary ciliary dyskinesia. A positive history of heroin-induced pulmonary edema,[13] inflammatory bowel disease,[9] rheumatoid arthritis,[14] Elhers-Danlos syndrome,[15] or Marfan's syndrome[16] can provide a possible etiology for bronchiectasis. Physical examination can suggest a possible cause of bronchiectasis. In the latter three diseases with their distinctive physical findings and, in addition, in the yellow nail syndrome,[17] where examination of the patient's fingernails may provide an immediate diagnosis.

In bronchiectasis associated with systemic diseases where the nature of the process that damages the bronchial wall is known, the process that makes the bronchi vulnerable to permanent damage is at least partially understood. In postinfectious bronchiectasis, the injurious agent is the microbe that causes the necrotizing pneumonia, leaving the bronchi permanently dilated, such as adenovirus type 7, *S. aureus,* and many others. In primary ciliary dyskinesias, the patient has a congenital defect in the structure of the ciliary apparatus throughout the body, including the cilia of the respiratory epithelia cells.[18] The abnormal action of the cilia of the bronchial mucosa makes the airways prone to infection because of poor clearance of inhaled or aspirated microbes. In cystic fibrosis, the bronchial mucosa is compromised by abnormal surface water content that impairs mucociliary clearance. In congenital or acquired deficiencies of immunoglobulin,[19–22] the patient is more prone to bronchial infections that may result in damage and deformation. In bronchiectasis secondary to bronchial obstruction, as is seen in aspiration of foreign bodies, impedance of clearance of airway mucus beyond the obstruction leads secondarily to infection behind the obstruction. In the Williams-Campbell syndrome, it is thought that the patients are born with a deficiency of the cartilages of the segmental bronchi, which makes the bronchi floppy, and that this promotes the formation of bronchiectasis in the daughter bronchial branches. Chronic obstruction of large bronchi is also the major problem in lung tumors that cause bronchiectasis, as seen in chronic endobronchial carcinoid tumors. More is known about allergic bronchopulmonary aspergillosis, where the bronchus appears to be damaged as an "innocent bystander" in the "battle" between *Aspergillus* organisms in the bronchial lumen and the patient's activated immune system.[11,23] In patients with inflammatory bowel disease, pathologic studies have shown that the bronchi are damaged by cellular inflammation in the bronchial walls, somewhat reminiscent of the process that occurs in the wall of the bowel.[9] In rheumatoid arthritis, less is known about the tissue histopathology of the process, but bronchiectasis is considered to be one of the extraarticular manifestations of the disease.[14] In the newly described form of bronchiectasis associated with human immunodeficiency virus (HIV) infection, the cause of the injury is hypothesized to be a chronic bacterial bronchitis.[24] Bronchiectasis in HIV infection is associated with bronchial infection with *H. influenzae, S. pneumoniae*, and *P. aeruginosa*. A toxic inhalant that is capable of injuring the bronchi and causing bronchiectasis is ammonia.[12] Finally, in some cases of sarcoidosis, the chronic lung disease is complicated by bronchiectasis,[25] and the injurious process is most likely the granulomatous inflammation that localizes itself predominantly in the bronchial lymphatics.

The final category of etiologies of bronchiectasis comprises situations in which nothing is known about the fundamental pathophysiology of the systemic disease. Young's syndrome has some similarities to cystic fibrosis, but the bronchiectasis and azoospermia are not coupled with a positive sweat test. In α_1-antiprotease deficiency, it seems clear from the association between the disease and bronchiectasis that the absence of this enzyme deprives the bronchial mucosa of an important defense mechanism, but the identity of the mechanism is still unknown.[26] Tracheobronchomegaly (Mounier-Kuhn disease) is probably characterized by an abnormality of the structural elements of the tracheobronchial walls, but its identity is not known. Little is known about the biochemical abnormalities in yellow nail syndrome, Ehlers-Danlos syndrome, or the Marfan's syndrome, but extensive experience shows that in many cases these patients develop bronchiectasis. Although an association has been documented between heroin-induced pulmonary edema and subsequent bronchiectasis, the pathogenesis is not understood.[13]

In summary, the factors that come together to cause bronchiectasis are an inherent weakness or defect of the bronchial mucosa together with some form of bronchial inflammation. Once the bronchi have been dilated by this event, they remain permanently dilated and obstructed; in many cases, this results in a chronic respiratory disease with intermittent exacerbations characterized by dyspnea on exertion, fatigue, chronic productive cough, and sometimes hemoptysis or chronic hypoxemia.

Diagnosis

A diagnostic evaluation for bronchiectasis should be done in patients who have an unexplained cough productive of more than 30 mL of sputum per day. The daily sputum volume is best quantitated by giving the patient a clear plastic volumetric jar with a tight-fitting lid and asking him or her to save all sputum expectorated during a 24-h period. It is also reasonable to look for bronchiectasis in patients with unexplained nonproductive cough or unexplained hemoptysis. This is true because bronchiectasis of the upper lobes is sometimes not associated with sputum production but may be a cause of cough or bleeding. Patients with bronchiectasis often have a variety of other less specific symptoms: dyspnea, wheezing, chest pain, fatigue, and anorexia. Some patients with mild bronchiectasis are completely asymptomatic. Physical exam often yields information increasing the likelihood that the patient has bronchiectasis. The most classical physical finding in patients with moderate to severe bronchiectasis is the auscultation of early inspiratory crackles, sometimes both early and late inspiratory crackles together. Patients with severe bronchiectasis may also have wheezing, clubbing, and cachexia. Patients with advanced, end-stage bronchiectasis have physical findings of cor pulmonale: edema, jugular venous distension while in the upright position, and a right ventricular heave in the subxiphoid area.

The most reliable and sensitive way to diagnose bronchiectasis is with (HRCT) of the thorax. Figures 90-3 through 90-5 show examples of diagnostic images taken with HRCT. The diagnosis of bronchiectasis can be made by first looking for vertically and horizontally oriented bronchi.[27] The finding on vertically oriented bronchi indicating bronchiectasis is the "signet-ring" sign—i.e., the shadow composed of a bronchus together with its accompanying pulmonary artery; the dilated bronchus is the "ring" and the pulmonary artery is the "jewel in the ring." The findings on horizontally oriented bronchi are "tram tracks" and the "string of pearls." Tram tracks are the parallel thickened walls of bronchi, which are much more prominent than in normal lungs. Strings of pearls are beaded images along the wall of a bronchus in varicose bronchiectasis. In other situations, the "cluster of grapes" sign may be seen, indicating severe cystic bronchiectasis. Finally, when mucoid impaction fills a bronchiectatic bronchus, it shows as a high-attenuation (white) tubular structure that does not taper as a branch of the pulmonary artery tapers.

Other laboratory findings may help to refine the diagnosis or to define the patient's current clinical status. The typical microscopic findings in the sputum of patients with bronchiectasis are large numbers of neutrophils mixed with the debris of lysed neutrophils, whose overall color is yellow or green or mixed with blood. If the patient's associated illness is allergic bronchopulmonary aspergillosis, fungal hyphae are seen together with eosinophils and sometimes Charcot-Leyden crystals. Sputum culture should be performed about once per year in patients with bronchiectasis to look for mucoid *P. aeruginosa*. It is worthwhile to alert the microbiology laboratory that this organism is being sought, so that it can be identified specifically. Most patients who have cystic fibrosis and some patients who have other diseases associated with bronchiectasis have chronic bronchial infection with mucoid *P. aeruginosa*. It is not yet known whether patients infected with this organism who do not have cystic fibrosis are at special risk of suffering complications.

The diagnosis of bronchiectasis often can be made from a plain chest roentgenogram. As in the high-resolution CT, chest films show tram tracking, which is a representation of thickened bronchial walls seen longitudinally, or ring shadows that have the appearance of a cluster of grapes (these latter correspond to shadows of lesions of saccular or cystic bronchiectasis)(Fig. 90-2).

When the diagnosis of bronchiectasis is made initially, it is important to extend the diagnostic evaluation to look for known etiologies and to assess the extent of impairment that can be attributed to the disease. A sweat test or gene test should be done to look for cystic fibrosis. Blood should be assayed for quantitative immunoglobulins, and the subclasses of immunoglobulin G should be assayed. A serum α_1-antiprotease inhibitor assay should be obtained. To perform screening for allergic bronchopulmonary aspergillosis, a scratch test with fungal antigens should be performed on the skin of the patient's forearm. If a wheal and flare reaction results within 20 min, serum should be sent for immunoglobulin G and E concentrations and for immunoglobulins specific for *Aspergillus fumigatus*. When a primary disorder of ciliary motility is suspected, electron microscopy should be performed on a sample of cilia taken from the patient. In male patients, sperm tails provide a convenient source of diagnostic material; in female patients, a sample of respiratory mucosa can be obtained by bronchoscopy and endobronchial biopsy. The extent of bronchiectasis can be determined by both HRCT and pulmonary function testing. The HRCT scan should include sections from all bronchopulmonary segments to determine whether disease is bilateral and to determine how many segments are involved. This is important, since a patient with only one unilateral focus of disease may be a candidate for lobectomy with the goal of enhancing the patient's quality of life by removing a single focus of disease. Pulmonary function testing together with a measurement of oxyhemoglobin saturation determines the amount of functional impairment caused by the disease. Many different patterns are seen in the pulmonary function tests of patients with bronchiectasis. It is not rare for patients to have completely normal pulmonary function, even when the disease appears widespread on HRCT. In patients who suffer functional impairment, both restrictive and obstructive patterns can be seen, and sometimes both

are present in the same patient. The restrictive pattern is seen when enough bronchopulmonary segments have been destroyed fully to decrease the patient's total lung capacity. In patients with airway obstruction, patients who have coincident bronchial hyperreactivity will have an obstructive pattern on the flow-volume loop and some degree of improvement after inhalation of bronchodilators. Patients who do not have bronchial hyperreactivity but have widespread plugging of structurally normal airways show an obstructive pattern with no acute improvement after inhalation of bronchodilators. Most patients with extensive bilateral bronchiectasis have obstructive airways pattern with no substantial change after inhalation of bronchodilating drugs (Fig. 90-6).

In summary, bronchiectasis can be readily diagnosed with HRCT of the lungs. A search should be made for a specific etiology, as outlined above. In the majority of cases, no specific etiology will be found and the patient will carry the diagnosis of idiopathic bronchiectasis.

Treatment

The goal of medical treatment in patients with bronchiectasis is to reduce the severity of symptoms and prevent the disease from extending into uninvolved segments. The therapies available for patients with bronchiectasis include preventive and secondary therapies, since no specific therapy is available for the condition. Preventive therapy includes annual inoculation for influenza, and the patient should receive other vaccines against respiratory pathogens, such as the polyvalent pneumococcal vaccine. Secondary therapies include nutritional support, physical therapy, antimicrobial therapy, mucolytic therapy, and bronchodilator therapy. Patients who are cachectic should receive nutritional supplements to counteract inanition. Physical therapy should include measures that promote the expectoration of sputum from bronchiectatic segments of the lungs. Simple exercise, such as walking, is beneficial in promoting bronchial toilet. In the technique of percussion and postural drainage, the patient with bronchiectasis is trained to lie in a position that allows a bronchiectatic segment to drain by gravity into the large central bronchi, and the patient then expels the mobilized sputum by coughing. External percussion of the chest by a physical therapist or other caretaker can aid in this process. In addition, mechanical vibrating vests are now available for use by patients without the assistance of others. A new hand-held "flutter" device (Scandipharm, Inc., Birmingham, AL) creates small vibrations that move retrograde through the bronchial tree, loosen secretions adherent to the bronchial walls, and promote expectoration of sputum.

Pharmacologic therapy of patients with bronchiectasis includes agents to reduce the burden of bronchial bacterial infection, agents that liquify the sputum, and drugs that dilate constricted bronchi.

The use of antimicrobial drugs[18,28,29] in most patients with bronchiectasis is empiric—i.e., it is not always based on the results of sputum culture and the documented sensitivities of the organisms to specific antimicrobials. This practice is in

Lung volumes, L	Actual	% Pred	Predicted			
Total lung capacity	3.9 L	88	4.4 L			
Functional residual cap	2.5 L	105	2.4 L			
Residual volume	2.3 L	155	1.5 L			

	PREDRUG			POSTDRUG		Change, %
Spirometry	Actual	% Pred	Predicted	Actual	% Pred	
FEV_1 (L)	1.08 L	49	2.22 L	1.07 L	48	−1%
FVC (L)	1.64 L	56	2.94	1.70 L	58	+4%
FEV_1 %	66		76		63	
Inspiratory capacity	1.4 L	69	2.03			

Airway resistance Raw (cmH_2O/L/s)	3.82	(normal <2.0)	
Diffusing capacity DL_{CO} (mL/min/mmHg)	100%		
pH	7.46		
P_{CO_2} (mmHg)	43		
P_{O_2} (mmHg)	80		

FIGURE 90-6 Pulmonary function tests of a 51-year-old woman with severe bilateral postinfectious bronchiectasis resulting from a severe necrotizing pneumonia experienced at age 16. She had a daily cough productive of up to a cup of purulent sputum, occasional hemoptysis, and dyspnea on walking two blocks. Chest roentgenogram showed bilateral cystic bronchiectasis. In these tests, the flow-volume loop has a concave shape (not shown), indicative of airway obstruction. The obstructive pattern is also shown by the elevated airway resistance and decreased FEV_1, FVC, and FEV_1%. Note that there is no substantial change in the spirometric values after inhalation of albuterol ("drug"). DL_{CO} and arterial blood gases are normal.

contrast to the treatment of patients with cystic fibrosis, where the goal is to identify whether mucoid *Pseudomonas* is present and if so, to specify the drugs that should be used against it through sensitivity testing. Nevertheless, a minority of patients with bronchiectasis who do not have cystic fibrosis also have bronchial infection with mucoid *Pseudomonas*.[30,31] In this group of patients, antipseudomonal drugs such as oral ciprofloxacin should be used for 2 weeks.

The goal of antimicrobial therapy in patients with bronchiectasis is to reduce the extent of bronchial infection and thereby reduce the daily sputum volume and promote the patient's well-being through reduction of cough frequency and severity and amelioration of systemic symptoms. For patients with bronchiectasis who do not have cystic fibrosis, antimicrobial drugs are typically chosen from a list such as that shown in Table 90-2. In patients with severe bronchiectasis who have *P. aeruginosa* in their sputum, intermittent therapy (as often as every 4 months) with intravenous antimicrobials active against *P. aeruginosa* can be used to reduce the degree of bronchial infection. These drugs can be given to outpatients through the use of peripheral intravenous central catheters (PICC lines) under the supervision of home-care nursing agencies.

There are two methods of administering antimicrobial drugs to patients with bronchiectasis: intermittent and nearly continuous. Intermittent therapy is a 2-week course of daily oral antimicrobials administered to outpatients with mild or moderate symptoms in exacerbation. After therapy has reduced the patient's symptoms, it is reasonable to stop the drugs and resume them only at the onset of the next exacerbation.

Nearly continuous antimicrobial therapy is used for patients with severe bronchiectasis who are almost never free of symptoms. In these patients, therapy should be given in 2-week cycles in which the antimicrobial drugs are alternated among those that have been found through previous experience to be beneficial to the patient (usually chosen from thé list in Table 90-2). Many patients will identify no more than three or four drugs that are effective at reducing

TABLE 90-2   Oral Antimicrobials Used in Empirical Treatment of Bronchiectasis

Tetracycline	250–500 mg qid
Ampicillin	250–500 mg qid
Amoxicillin	250–500 mg tid
Amoxicillin-clavulanate	250–500 mg tid
Trimethoprim/sulfamethoxazole	160 gm/800 mg bid
Erythromycin	250–500 mg qid
Clarithromycin	500 mg bid
Azithromycin	250 mg qd (500 mg day 1)
Ciprofloxacin	500–750 mg bid
Ofloxacin	400 mg bid
Cefaclor	250 mg tid
Cefuroxime axetil	250–500 mg bid
Doxycycline	100–200 mg qd

symptoms, and these should be prescribed for rotating use in future cycles of therapy. At the end of a cycle of three or four drugs, each given daily for 2 weeks, the patient is given a 2-week "drug holiday." Usually the patient's symptoms will worsen during the period of abstinence from antimicrobials, and the rotating cycle can be reinitiated by the patient. A typical rotating cycle for an adult with bronchiectasis is tetracycline 250 mg tid for 2 weeks, then amoxicillin 250 to 500 mg tid or qid for 2 weeks, then trimethoprim/sulfamethoxazole double strength bid for 2 weeks, then cefaclor 250 mg tid for 2 weeks, then no antimicrobial for 2 weeks.

Only one mucolytic agent can be recommended currently. DNase (Pulmonzyme) is a recombinant human enzyme that has been shown to be of benefit in the treatment of selected patients with cystic fibrosis when inhaled with a nebulizer[32] (see Chap. 69). The first studies showed that use of DNase was associated with improved pulmonary function, improved sensation of dyspnea, and a better sense of well-being. Although no studies have been published on its effectiveness in bronchiectasis that is not associated with cystic fibrosis, the main action of this drug is to cleave DNA molecules in neutrophil-laden sputum and purulent sputum, which is a symptom in many patients with bronchiectasis. In the absence of specific data, it still is reasonable to use DNase in selected patients with *severe* bronchiectasis for whom thick, purulent sputum is a major symptom.

Bronchodilators are useful in patients with bronchiectasis if an empirical trial shows an improvement in the patient's pulmonary function or if the patient reports that the use of the drugs enhances the effectiveness of physical therapy in promoting bronchial toilet. Some patients with bronchiectasis have an improvement in their values for FEV_1 and/or FVC on spirometry immediately after inhaling bronchodilator drugs, and such patients should receive one of these drugs on a regular basis. The first drug to be prescribed in most patients is either salmeterol 2 puffs (42 µg) every 12 h or albuterol 2 puffs (180 µg) every 6 h. In some patients, a trial of oral theophylline is worthwhile if the patient notes improved dyspnea and exercise tolerance on this drug. Since no data are available on the most desirable serum theophylline level for these patients, we recommend achieving a stable serum concentration between 5 and 12 mg/L, since this level has been useful for patients with asthma.

In rare instances, surgery may have a role in the treatment of bronchiectasis. When a patient with troublesome symptoms has been shown by high-resolution CT to have bronchiectasis localized to a single lobe or segment, lobectomy can remove the entire focus of disease. In most patients, the disease is too widespread for surgical excision to be considered.

In summary, the medical treatment of patients with bronchiectasis is graduated and should match the severity of the disease. Very mild cases with few or no symptoms require only preventive therapy with vaccines. Mild to moderate bronchiectasis should be treated with intermittent courses of rotating antimicrobials, supplemented with bronchodilators as needed to control symptoms and physical therapy with a "flutter" device. Patients with severe bronchiectasis should be treated with nearly continuous 2-week courses of oral antimicrobials; if they are infected with

P. aeruginosa, antimicrobial therapy should be given in the form of a 2-week intravenous course of drugs approximately every 4 to 6 months. The exact drug should be dictated by sputum culture with drug sensitivities. Severely ill patients will also benefit from bronchodilators and an agent to help liquify sputum, such as DNase. Physical therapy with a flutter device or other mechanism should be performed daily on patients with severe disease. Hypoxemic patients should be treated with supplemental oxygen at a flow that increases the peripheral oxygen saturation to at least 89%.

References

1. Mitchell RE, Bury RG: Congenital bronchiectasis due to deficiency of bronchial cartilage (Williams-Campbell syndrome). *Am Rev Respir Dis* 1976; 114:15.
2. Luce JM: Bronchiectasis, in Murray JF, Nadel JA (eds): *Textbook of Respiratory Medicine*, 2d ed. Philadelphia: Saunders, 1994:1398.
3. Fraser RG, Macklem PT, Brown WG: Airway dynamics in bronchiectasis: A combined cinefluorographic-manometric study. *Am J Roentgenol* 1965; 93:821.
4. Fahy JV, Schuster A, Ueki I, et al.: Mucus hypersecretion in bronchiectasis: The role of neutrophil proteases. *Am Rev Respir Dis* 1992; 146:1430.
5. Pang J, Chan HS, et al.: Prevalence of asthma, atopy, and bronchial hyperreactivity in bronchiectasis: A controlled study. *Thorax* 1989; 44:948.
6. Liebow AA, Hales MR, Lindskog GE: Enlargement of the bronchial arteries and their anastomoses with the pulmonary arteries in bronchiectasis. *Am J Pathol* 1949; 25:211.
7. Reid LM: Reduction in bronchial subdivisions in bronchiectasis. *Thorax* 1950; 5:233.
8. Kraft SC, Earle RH, Roesler M, Esterly JR: Unexplained bronchopulmonary disease with inflammatory bowel disease. *Arch Intern Med* 1976; 136:454.
9. Camus P, Piard F, Ashcroft T, et al.: The lung in inflammatory bowel disease. *Medicine* 1993; 72:151.
10. Baltimore RS, Christie CDC, Smith GJW: Immunohistopathologic localization of *Pseudomonas aeruginosa* in lungs from patients with cystic fibrosis: Implications for the pathogenesis of progressive lung deterioration. *Am Rev Respir Dis* 1989; 140:1650.
11. Bosken CH, Myers JL, Greenberger PA, Katzenstein AL: Pathologic features of allergic bronchopulmonary aspergillosis. *Am J Surg Pathol* 1988; 12:216.
12. Kass I, Zamel N, Dobry CA, Holzer M: Bronchiectasis following ammonia burns of the respiratory tract: A review of two cases. *Chest* 1972; 62:282.
13. Banner AS, Rodriguez J, Sunderrajan EV, et al.: Bronchiectasis: A cause of pulmonary symptoms in heroin addicts. *Respiration* 1979; 37:232.
14. Shadick NA, Fanta CH, Weiblatt ME, et al.: Bronchiectasis: A late feature of severe rheumatoid arthritis. *Medicine* 1994; 73:161.
15. Robitaille G: Ehler-Danlos syndrome and recurrent hemoptysis. *Ann Intern Med* 1964; 61:710.
16. Foster ME, Foster DR: Bronchiectasis and Marfan's syndrome. *Postgrad Med J* 1980; 56:718.
17. Hiller E, Rosenow EC, Olsen AM: Pulmonary manifestations of the yellow nail syndrome. *Chest* 1972; 61:452.
18. Murray JF: New presentations of bronchiectasis. *Hosp Pract* March 30, 1991.
19. Marcy TW, Reynolds HY: Pulmonary consequences of congenital and acquired primary immunodeficiency states. *Clin Chest Med* 1989; 10:503.

20. Knowles GK, Stanhope R, Green M: Bronchiectasis complicating chronic lymphatic leukaemia with hypogammaglobulinaemia. *Thorax* 1980; 35:217.

21. Beck CS, Heiner DC: Selective immunoglobulin G4 deficiency and recurrent infections of the respiratory tract. *Am Rev Respir Dis* 1981; 124:94.

22. Umetsu DT, Ambrosino DM, Quinti I, et al.: Recurrent sinopulmonary infection and impaired antibody response to bacterial capsular polysaccharide antigen in children with selective IgG subclass deficiency. *N Engl J Med* 1985; 131:1247.

23. Panchal N, Pant C, Bhagat R, Shah A: Central bronchiectasis in allergic bronchopulmonary aspergillosis: Comparative evaluation of computed tomography of the thorax with bronchography. *Eur Respir J* 1994; 7:1290.

24. Verghese A, Al-Samman M, Nabhan D, et al.: Bacterial bronchitis and bronchiectasis in human immunodeficiency virus infection. *Arch Intern Med* 1994; 154:2086.

25. Hamper UM, Fishman EK, Khouri NF, et al.: Typical and atypical CT manifestations of pulmonary sarcoidosis. *J Compu Assist Tomogr* 1986; 10:928.

26. Shin MS, Ho KJ: Bronchiectasis in patients with α_1-antitrypsin deficiency: A rare occurrence? *Chest* 1993; 104:1384.

27. Webb WR, Muller NL, Naidich DP: *High-Resolution CT of the Lung*, 1st ed. New York: Raven Press, 1992:123–129.

28. Tsang KWT, Roberts P, Read RC, et al.: The concentrations of clarithromycin and its 14-hydroxy metabolite in sputum of patients with bronchiectasis following single dose oral administration. *J Antimicrob Chemother* 1994; 33:289.

29. British Medical Research Council: Prolonged antibiotic treatment of severe bronchiectasis. *B Med J* 1957; 255.

30. Rivera M, Nicotra MB: *Pseudomonas aeruginosa* mucoid strain: Its significance in adult chest diseases. *Am Rev Respir Dis* 1982; 126:833.

31. Pang JA, Cheng A, Chan HS, et al.: The bacteriology of bronchiectasis in Hong Kong investigated by protected catheter brush and bronchoalveolar lavage. *Am Rev Respir Dis* 1989; 139:14.

32. Ramsey BW and associates: Efficacy and safety of short-term administration of aerosolized recombinant human deoxyribonuclease in patients with cystic fibrosis. *Am Rev Respir Dis* 1993; 148:145.

33. Mark JBD, Baldwin JC: Pneumonia, lung abscess, and bronchiectasis, in Glenn WL (ed): *Glenn's Thoracic and Cardiovascular Surgery*, 5th ed. Norwalk, CT: Appleton and Lange, 1991.

TREATMENT OF CYSTIC FIBROSIS

Chapter 91

INTRODUCTION, PATHOPHYSIOLOGY, GENETICS

THOMAS M. MURPHY, CHRIS RUDD,
AND WAYNE SAMUELSON

Overview

Cystic fibrosis (CF) is an autosomal recessive disorder of exocrine and sweat glands that causes premature death from progressive respiratory failure in >95 percent of affected individuals. It is the most common fatal genetic disorder of the Caucasian population. With a carrier rate of about 5 percent, it affects one out of 2500 live births. It is less common in African Americans (1/17,000 live births)[1] and rare in individuals of Asian ancestry (<1/100,000). While CF probably has affected individuals for thousands of years, it was clinically described only 50 years ago.

Fanconi first described a celiac syndrome with pancreatic changes that differed from the classic disease. In the first English-language description of cystic fibrosis in 1936, Andersen described meconium ileus and recommended treatment.[2] Changes induced by CF were noted earlier than this.

"*Das Kind stirbt bald wieder, dessen Stirne beim Küssen salzig schmeckt*" ("The child will die soon, whose forehead tastes salty when kissed"). This phrase, taken from German children's songs from Switzerland, suggests that earlier folk recognized that the defect that led to an early death was associated with an abnormal salt content of sweat. It is likely that many "bewitched" children or even adults died of CF while their deaths were attributed to other causes. Frederic Chopin died of respiratory failure at the age of 39. He suffered from steatorrhea, was underweight (45 kg), was apparently sterile, and his postmortem did not reveal the characteristic features of tuberculosis, the presumed cause of his death. Accordingly, there is suspicion that he died of CF.

While the early descriptions of CF emphasized malabsorption and growth retardation,[3] lung involvement has come to be the central feature of CF illness.[4–6] Progressive lung disease develops as a result of thick, viscid secretions, not cleared from lung airways, which compromise normal breathing and pulmonary function. The problem is further compounded by impaired clearance of mucus. The airways are congested and become colonized by bacteria as a result of repeated respiratory infections. Eventually bronchiectasis results from the chronic infectious processes. Patients develop chronic airway obstruction, with eventual respiratory failure and death.

Other organs are affected by CF. Pancreatic insufficiency and malabsorption require continuous treatment.[7] Nutrition is a major challenge because of malabsorption, poor appetite, a catabolic state arising from chronic infection, and increased energy needs related to coughing and to increased work of breathing. Evidence is accumulating that aggressive approaches to chronic nutritional management result in prolonged survival.[8]

Thirty years ago, death from CF was almost universal within the first decade of life. Improvements in diagnosis and treatment have dramatically altered this statistic. Current survival statistics demonstrate a median life expectancy of approximately 30 years[9] (Fig. 91-1). Many patients now marry and pursue graduate education and professional careers.[10] Survival into the fourth and fifth decades of life is now common.[9]

A key insight into the cellular nature of CF was provided during the hot New York summer of 1949, when di Sant'Agnese demonstrated that heat prostration in children with CF was caused by serum NaCl depletion. This condition results from excessive perspiration containing elevated sodium and chloride and is found in virtually every CF patient. This discovery led Gibson and Cooke, in 1959,[11] to develop pilocarpine iontophoresis as a tool in the diagnosis of CF by sweat testing. This remains the cardinal laboratory confirmation of a diagnosis of CF.

Identification of patients with CF led to a more complete description of the clinical manifestations of the disease. The treatment of CF improved greatly in the 1960s with the creation of the national Cystic Fibrosis Foundation and the establishment of multidisciplinary care centers that promulgated models of empiric therapy,[12] but the mechanisms of the disease remained a mystery. However, the 1980s brought

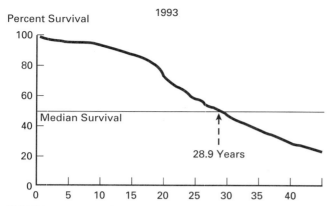

FIGURE 91-1 Survival curve for all cystic fibrosis patients. (*From Fitzsimmons,*[9] *with permission.*)

remarkable progress in defining the cellular pathophysiology of CF. Quinton showed that the epithelia of sweat ducts in CF patients are impermeable to chloride transport.[13] Knowles and colleagues demonstrated abnormal ion transport at the cellular level by careful measurements of transmembrane potential.[14–16] Further studies in CF airway epithelium revealed decreased secretion of chloride ion from the apical membrane to the airway lumen and excessive sodium reabsorption from lumenal fluid.

This work led to the clarification of the pathway by which chloride secretion is normally initiated by a β-adrenergic epithelial stimulus that is defective in CF.[17] Following β-adrenoceptor binding, G proteins are activated, with stimulation of adenylate cyclase to produce cyclic 5′-3′ adenosine monophosphate (cAMP), followed by cAMP-mediated activation of protein kinase A (PKA). This causes the apical membrane to increase its permeability to chloride. The defect in CF cells appears at the point of PKA activation, where, unlike the normal case, CF membranes do not become permeable to chloride ions. This suggested that the core defect in CF is related to epithelial chloride channel dysfunction.

In 1989, following the localization of the gene to the long arm of chromosome 7, region q21-q22, in 1987,[18] the gene responsible for CF was isolated and cloned.[19–21] The protein derived from this gene was named cystic fibrosis transmembrane conductance regulator, or CFTR, which normally appears to function as a channel-modulating transporter of the chloride ion. As demonstrated in Fig. 91-2, the presumed structure derived from the cDNA sequence is anchored in the epithelial membrane by two hydrophobic membrane-spanning domains (MSD_1 and MSD_2) that each are attached to a hydrophilic nucleotide-binding domain (NBD_1 and NBD_2); the latter are thought to interact with adenosine triphosphate (ATP).[22] An additional regulatory (R) domain is a highly charged polypeptide that has multiple potential sites for phosphorylation by cyclic adenosine monophosphate (cAMP)–dependent PKA and by protein kinase C (PKC). This structure is thought to provide a key role in the cAMP-dependent gating of chloride by way of the apical cell membrane through the CFTR, which establishes an electrochemical and osmotic gradient to attract sodium and water from the cell to the epithelial lining fluid in order to hydrate the mucus lining the epithelial duct. This is postulated to be the molecular basis for the defect governing the disease. Innovative strategies for treating the manifestations of the disease have been and are being developed based on improved understanding of the fundamental nature of the disease process.[6] (See also Table 91-1.)

Diagnosis

The diagnosis of CF was simplified by the introduction of the sweat test.[11] However, several other conditions cause increases in sweat chloride concentration[23,24] (see Table 91-2). While the sweat test is useful and relatively easily applied, it requires an experienced operator who adheres rigorously to the proposed NCCLS laboratory guidelines. Results can vary substantially if the test is performed in laboratories that are not experienced or the test is done infrequently.[23,24] The diagnosis of CF is usually made by

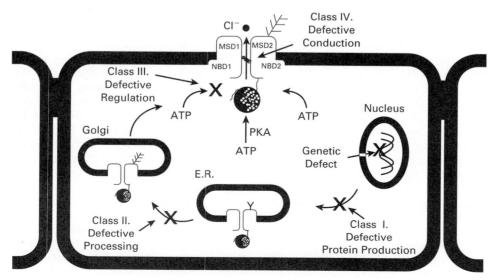

FIGURE 91-2 Biosynthesis and cellular circulation of CFTR in an epithelial cell. MSD = membrane-spanning domain; NBD = nucleotide-binding domain; R = regulatory domain. (*From Welsh and Smith,*[22] *with permission.*)

TABLE 91-1   Mechanism-Specific Therapies in Cystic Fibrosis

Defect	Conventional	New
Abnormal gene		Gene replacement
⇓		
Abnormal or absent CFTR		Replace protein ?Phosphatase inhibitors
⇓		
Desiccated secretions Impacted mucus ? Abnormal mucus	Cough/chest percussion	Block Na⁺ uptake Amiloride Stimulate Cl-secretion UTP/ATP
⇓		
Bacterial colonization and Infection	Acute antibiotics (oral, IV)	Aerosolized antibiotics
⇓		
Chronic infection	Intermittent and chronic Antibiotics (oral, IV)	Aerosolized antibiotics
⇓ ⇑		
↑ Mucopurulent secretions	Cough/chest percussion	rhDNase/gelsolin Colfosceril palmitate
⇓ ⇑		
↑ Airways obstruction Hyperresponsiveness	Chest percussion/antibiotics bronchodilators/corticosteroids	
⇓ ⇑		
Chronic inflammation		
Bacterial exoproducts	Antibiotics	Bacterial vaccine
↑ PMN recruitment		?ICAM-1, CD-18
Blockade		
PMN degradation		
Proteases		Antiproteases
DNA		rhDNase
Actin		Gelsolin
Hyperimmune response		Ibuprofen/corticosteroids
⇓		
Bronchiectasis	Resectional surgery	
⇓		
End-stage lung disease	Oxygen, diuretics	Lung transplantation

SOURCE: Adapted from Turpin and Knowles[6] and from Fiel,[36] with permission.

TABLE 91-2   Causes of Increased Sweat Chloride

Technical

    Inadequate sweat collection
    Evaporative water loss
    Laboratory error

Disease

    Cystic fibrosis
    Malnutrition
    Adrenal insufficiency
    Pseudohypoaldosteronism
    Panhypopituitarism
    Hypothyroidism
    Ectodermal dysplasia
    Nephrogenic diabetes insipidus
    Glycogen storage disease type 1
    Fucosidosis
    Mucopolysaccharidosis

increased sweat chloride concentration (i.e., > 60 mEq/L) in the appropriate clinical context (Table 91-3). Atypical cases may present with a "normal" sweat chloride. In these unusual cases the chloride concentration is usually > 40 mEq/L.

Presenting symptoms of CF vary. Approximately 12 percent of pediatric patients present with meconium ileus at birth. Other common pediatric presentations include failure to thrive, cough, recurrent bronchitis or pneumonia, and asthma. Patients who are diagnosed in adulthood have often had minor symptoms for many years. Adults may present with symptoms of asthma, bronchitis, sinusitis, or infertility. Malabsorption or pancreatitis may also be manifestations of CF; 85 percent of children and adults with CF have evidence of malabsorption.[4,5]

Genetics

Cystic fibrosis is transmitted by the homozygous inheritance of an autosomal recessive gene. Beginning with the identification of the genetic locus on the long arm of chromosome 7

TABLE 91-3   Clinical Presentations of Cystic Fibrosis

Infancy	Childhood	Adolescence/Adulthood
Meconium ileus	Recurrent bronchitis	Bronchitis/bronchiectasis
Failure to thrive	Recurrent pneumonia	Clubbing
Steatorrhea	Asthma	Glucose intolerance
Bronchiolitis	Nasal polyposis	Diabetes mellitus
Bronchitis	Intestinal obstruction	Intestinal obstruction
Pneumonia	Malabsorption	Delayed puberty
Heat prostration	Growth failure	Recurrent pancreatitis
Hyponatremia	Clubbing	Biliary cirrhosis
Obstructive jaundice	Intussusception	Portal hypertension
Hypoprothrombinemia		Gallstones
Rectal prolapse		Aspermia/infertility

in 1987,[18] a vigorous collaborative effort to identify and clone the gene succeeded in September 1989.[19–21] The most common mutation (ΔF508) consists of a deletion (Δ) of three nucleotides in exon 10, which leads to the absence of a phenylalanine residue (F) at position 508 on the CFTR protein. This mutation accounts for about 70 percent of CF alleles worldwide. More than 450 additional mutations have been identified since the discovery and cloning of the ΔF508 mutation.

According to Welsh and Smith, four classes of mutations disrupt normal CFTR function.[22] **Class I mutations**, exemplified by the G542X nonsense mutation, cause premature termination signals and *defective production* before the CFTR arrives at the endoplasmic reticulum for processing (Fig. 91-2). **Class II mutations**, exemplified by the ΔF508/ΔF508 mutation, are characterized by a posttranslational *defective trafficking* of the protein to its correct cellular location. It is hypothesized that these CFTR mutants are recognized by the cell as abnormally folded and are degraded. This implies that the most common genotype, ΔF508/ΔF508, in CF is characterized by a CFTR that usually does not attain its final destination in the apical cell membrane. **Class III mutations** involve *defective regulation* of CFTR, causing decreased chloride channel activity. Since all of these mutations occur in the nucleotide binding domains (as with the G551D mutation), the mechanism probably occurs through decreased function of ATP in stimulating chloride channel opening. **Class IV mutations** involve *defective conduction* through the channel. Regulatory mechanisms involving cAMP-dependent phosphorylation and ATP appear unaffected. All class IV mutations involve the membrane-spanning domain. An example is the R117H mutation. In general, class I and II mutations are associated with malabsorption, class III mutations are mixed, and class IV mutations are free of malabsorption.[22]

The disease tends to follow the migration of Europeans throughout the world. It is rare among African blacks and is also extremely uncommon among Orientals. Until relatively recently, the majority of CF patients died before childbearing age. Even now, almost all males with CF are sterile, and fertility among females is lower than usual. Despite this, the disease continues to be a factor in the health of the world's Caucasian population.

Approximately 1 in 25 Caucasians are carriers of the gene. Why the gene for CF occurs so frequently is a question that continues to mystify investigators. Of the variety of possible explanations that have been advanced, the possibility that the CF gene may have afforded higher resistance to chloride-secreting diarrheas such as cholera (leading to increased survival of heterozygous infants) has the most support. The frequency of the ΔF508 allele differs across Europe, suggesting that migration of CF genes occurred in chronologically distinct expansions. In northern Europe and North America, the frequency of ΔF508 reaches 70 to 90 percent. However, it is much less frequent in the Mediterranean region, where fewer than 50 percent of the CF chromosomes carry the mutation. Nonetheless, the ΔF508 deletion accounts for 70 percent of the world's CF chromosomes. Since the discovery of the CFTR gene, more than 450 additional mutations have been detected.

Cystic fibrosis is a homozygous disease, which implies that the presence of one normal allele eliminates the expression of the disease. This presents opportunities for treatment at the gene level, without the need for a complete overhaul of the genome.

There are approximately 60,000 patients with documented CF worldwide. About 33,000 of them reside in North America, with another 20,000 in Europe. It has been estimated that there are potentially as many as 10,000 asymptomatic (and undiagnosed) additional patients in the United States alone. Roughly 1 in 2500 Caucasian children and 1 in 17,000 African American children are born with CF. An average four to five children with CF are born daily in the United States. Approximately 1300 new cases are diagnosed each year. The majority of these are identified within the first 3 years of life.

The discovery of numerous mutations of the CF gene and the recognition of differing frequencies of the ΔF508 mutation in various populations has stirred interest in the relationship between genotype and phenotype in CF. The expression of the disease, or phenotype, is influenced by both genetic and environmental factors. However, some relationships may be identifiable. Patients with pancreatic insufficiency tend to have more severe disease.[25] Current data suggest a correlation between ΔF508/ΔF508 gene expression and pancreatic insufficiency. Most patients carrying the R117H mutation are pancreatic-sufficient. No clear associations between any specific mutation and the severity of respiratory illness have been identified.[25]

Pathophysiology

Respiratory disease is responsible for >95 percent of mortality and much of the morbidity resulting from CF.[4–6] The pulmonary pathophysiologic effects of CF occur after birth. The lungs of affected neonates appear morphologically normal,[26] but excessive secretion of mucus from airway epithelial glands begins as soon as the cycle of mucus impaction of small airways and the establishment of recurrent airways infections begins, so that airway changes occur early.[27] Bronchiolectasis and bronchitis are common autopsy findings in patients above 1 month of age. Bronchiectasis associated with lung infection is an almost universal finding in patients 2 years of age or older.[28]

The natural role of mucus and the mucociliary transport system is subverted in CF. In normal airways, the mucus serves as a trap for foreign particles such as bacteria. Beneath the naturally occurring layer of mucus, the airway is lined with hairlike cilia whose rhythmic and continuous beating moves the mucus toward the oropharynx, where it can be swallowed or expectorated. Patients with CF produce mucus that is dehydrated and more viscous than normal. This tenacious mucus accumulates on airway surfaces and is difficult to clear. A consequence of mucus impaction is that the airways are easily colonized by bacteria. Once respiratory infections take root, a relentless cycle of airway obstruction and infection, accompanied by inflammation and immune response, begins. This cycle has its onset early in childhood. By adolescence, most CF patients have cough and sputum production.[29] Microbial colonization and susceptibility to specific pathogens are usually age-related and tend to follow a sequence.[30] In the early stages of CF, *Staphylococcus aureus* and *Haemophilus influenza* are the most common pathogens. Partly due to the common use of effective antistaphylococcal and other broad-spectrum antibiotics[31] and partly as a result of a specific predilection for the airways of patients with CF,[32] *Pseudomonas aeruginosa* has emerged as the major bacterial pathogen in chronic respiratory infections in CF. Once established, *P. aeruginosa* never is fully eradicated from the CF lung.[31,33]

Pseudomonas aeruginosa is a toxigenic and immunoevasive bacterial parasite.[32] Elastase, alkaline protease, and exotoxin A released by the organism are major promoters of tissue damage as well as efficient immunomodulators. In the CF lung, factors such as altered mucus and possibly an increased number of receptors for *P. aeruginosa* on the surface of epithelial cells may delay the elimination of infectious bacteria. Other factors native to *Pseudomonas* contribute to adherence and colonization during the early phase of infection. Numerous virulence factors (elastase, alkaline protease, exotoxin A, leukocidin PMN inhibitor, phospholipase C, pyocyanine pigments, and mucoid exopolysaccharide) not only initiate and amplify a nectrotizing inflammatory response but also suppress normal immune defenses, thus aiding the invasion of bacteria and the establishment of chronic infection. The proteases and toxins released by the microorganisms also promote tissue destruction. Damage occurs when chronic inflammation results from the constant local formation of immune complexes with the antigens of a

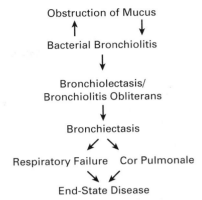

FIGURE 91-3 Progression of pulmonary pathophysiology in CF.

microorganism that cannot be eradicated from the respiratory tract.[34]

The accumulation of mucus and the cycle of infection/inflammation cause bronchial obstruction, areas of atelectasis, and uneven ventilation (Fig. 91-3). This becomes more marked with time, leading to airway necrosis, the loss of airway elasticity, and the creation of areas of emphysema within the lung, as well as airways hyperresponsiveness. This process may not be manifest clinically until later in life. Patients may function normally for some time, becoming symptomatic only when the reserve capacity of the lung is depleted. Eventually, this process leads to a degree of ventilation-perfusion imbalance, which exceeds the capacity of the patient to compensate, and hypoxemia ensues.

Airway obstruction correlates with the deterioration in pulmonary function in CF. Progression of disease leads to ventilation-perfusion mismatching, with subsequent impairment of gas exchange. Increased anatomic dead space also develops, with resultant increase in the resting arterial P_{CO_2}. Late-stage disease is characterized by severe hypoxemia and CO_2 retention. Pulmonary hypertension and cor pulmonale eventually develop (Fig. 91-3).

Other pulmonary complications are associated with late-stage disease. Hemoptysis is a common occurrence in patients with significant disease. The degree of severity correlates with the age of the patient and the severity of bronchiectasis. Persistent infection causes neovascularization, and the frequency of hemoptysis increases with more frequent infectious exacerbations. Massive hemoptysis (>300 mL in 24 h) occurs in less than 1 percent of CF patients.[9,35] It usually responds to appropriate antibiotic therapy.[31] Life-threatening hemoptysis occurs less frequently.[9] Intubation for airway protection and embolization of the bronchial artery may be necessary to control the bleeding.[35,36] Lobar resection rarely is required for control of bleeding.[37]

Cor pulmonale develops in severely ill CF patients.[37] Hypoxemia resulting from alterations of the ventilation-perfusion relationship in the lung causes pulmonary hypertension, associated with right ventricular hypertrophy and enlargement. Fulminant right heart failure may develop and usually heralds the terminal stage of the illness.

The progression of pulmonary changes is accompanied by other constitutional changes. Nutrition, consistently impaired by pancreatic insufficiency and malabsorption, is further challenged by the increased energy costs of breathing with diseased lungs and the catabolic state associated with chronic pulmonary infection.[7] Hepatobiliary disease— which, like lung involvement, may remain asymptomatic until well advanced—often complicates management of end-stage disease. Most of the small proportion of the mortality from CF not attributable to lung disease is accounted for by liver failure.[38]

General Principles of Treatment

The fundamentals of CF therapy have changed little since the 1960s.[12] Antibiotics and pulmonary toilet remain the mainstays of treatment. Aerosolization of medications including antibiotics has become an important part of the standard regimen.[39] An appreciation of the nutritional needs of CF patients has resulted in better dietary counseling, enzyme replacement, and caloric supplementation.[7,8]

References

1. Kulczycki LL, Schauf V: CF in blacks in Washington, DC: Incidence and characteristics. *Am J Dis Child* 1974; 127:64.
2. Andersen DH: Cystic fibrosis of the pancreas and its relation to celiac disease: A clinical and pathological study. *Am J Dis Child* 1938; 56:344.
3. Schwachman H, Kulczycki LL: Long-term study of 105 patients with cystic fibrosis. *Am J Dis Child* 1958; 96:6.
4. Wood RE, Boat TF, Doershuk CF: Cystic fibrosis. *Am Rev Respir Dis* 1976; 113:841.
5. Maclusky I, Levison H: Cystic fibrosis, in Chernick V (ed): *Disorders of the Respiratory Tract in Children,* 5th ed. Philadelphia, Saunders, 1990: 692–730.
6. Turpin SV, Knowles MR: Treatment of pulmonary disease in patients with cystic fibrosis, in Davis PB (ed): *Cystic Fibrosis.* New York; Marcel Dekker, 1993; 277–344.
7. Ramsey B, Farrell PM, Pencharz P, et al.: Nutritional assessment and management in cystic fibrosis: A consensus report. *Am J Clin Nutr* 1992; 55:108.
8. Corey M, McLaughlin FJ, Williams M, Levison H: A comparison of survival, growth, and pulmonary function in patients with cystic fibrosis in Boston and Toronto. *J Clin Epidemiol* 1988; 41:483.
9. Fitzsimmons SC: *Cystic Fibrosis Foundation Patient Registry: 1993 Annual Data Report.* Bethesda, MD: CFF, September 1994.
10. di Sant'Agnese PA, Davis PB: Cystic fibrosis in adults. *Am J Med* 1979; 66:121.
11. Gibson LF, Cooke RE: A test for concentration of electrolytes in sweat in cystic fibrosis of the pancreas utilizing pilocarpine iontophoresis. *Pediatrics* 1959; 23:545.
12. Doershuk CF, Matthews LW, Tucker AS, et al.: A 5-year clinical evaluation of a therapeutic program for patients with cystic fibrosis. *J Pediatr* 1964; 65:677.
13. Mastella G, Quinton PM (eds): *Cellular and Molecular Traits of Cystic Fibrosis.* San Francisco: San Francisco Press, 1988.
14. Knowles M, Gatzy J, Boucher R: Modulation of nasal epithelium ion permeability in normal and cystic fibrosis subjects *in vivo* (abstr). *Clin Res* 31:858A.
15. Knowles M, Gatzy J, Boucher R: Relative ion permeability of nor-

16. mal and cystic fibrosis nasal epithelium. *J Clin Invest* 1983; 71:1410.
16. Knowles MR, Stutts MJ, Yankaskas JR, et al.: Abnormal respiratory epithelial ion transport in cystic fibrosis. *Clin Chest Med* 1986; 7:285.
17. Dubinsky WP: Resolution and reconstitution of the factors controlling chloride permeability in the trachea. *Prog Clin Biol Res* 1987; 254:167.
18. Lathrop GM, Farrall M, O'Connell P, et al.: Refined linkage map of chromosome 7 in the region of the cystic fibrosis gene. *Am J Hum Genet* 1988; 42:38.
19. Rommeus JM, Iannuzzi MC, Kerem BS, et al.: Identification of the cystic fibrosis gene: Chromosome walking and jumping. *Science* 1989; 245:1059.
20. Riordan JR, Rommeus JM, Kerem BS, et al.: Identification of the cystic fibrosis gene: Cloning and characterization of the complementary DNA. *Science* 1989; 245:1066.
21. Kerem BS, Rommeus JM, Buchanan JA, et al.: Identification of the cystic fibrosis gene: Genetic analysis. *Science* 1989; 245:1073.
22. Welsh MJ, Smith AE: Molecular mechanisms of CFTR chloride channel dysfunction in cystic fibrosis. *Cell* 1993; 73:1251.
23. Littlewood JR: The sweat test. *Arch Dis Child* 1986; 61:1041.
24. LeGrys VA, Wood RE: Incidence and implications of false-negative sweat test reports in patients with cystic fibrosis. *Pediatr Pulmonol* 1988; 4:169.
25. Kerem E, Corey M, Kerem B, et al.: The relationship between genotype and phenotype in cystic fibrosis: Analysis of the most common mutation (ΔF508). *N Engl J Med* 1990; 323:1517.
26. Chow CW, Landau LI, Taussig LM: Bronchial mucous glands in the newborn with cystic fibrosis. *Eur J Pediatr* 1982; 139:240.
27. Girod S, Galabert, Lecuire A, et al.: Phospholipid composition and surface active properties of tracheobronchial secretions from patients with cystic fibrosis and chronic obstructive pulmonary diseases. *Pediatr Pulmonol* 1992; 13:22.
28. Oppenheimer EH, Esterley JR: Pathology of cystic fibrosis: Review of the literature and comparison of 146 autopsied cases. *Perspect Pediatr Pathol* 1975; 2:241.
29. Hodson ME, Warner JO: Respiratory problems and their treatment. *Br Med Bull* 1992; 48:931.
30. Friend PA: Pulmonary infection in cystic fibrosis. *J Infect* 1986; 13:55.
31. Kulczycki LL, Murphy TM, Bellanti JA: *Pseudomonas* colonization in cystic fibrosis: A study of 160 patients. *JAMA* 1978; 240:30.
32. Buret A, Cripps AW: State of the art: The immunoevasive activities of *Pseudomonas aeruginosa*—Relevance for cystic fibrosis. *Am Rev Respir Dis* 1993; 148:793.
33. Hoiby N: Epidemiological investigations of the respiratory tract bacteriology in patients with cystic fibrosis. *Acta Pathol Microbiol Scand* 1974; 82:541.
34. Moss RB, Hsu Y, Lewiston NJ, et al.: Association of systemic immune complexes, complement activation, and antibodies in *Pseudomonas aeruginosa* lipopolysaccharide and exotoxin A with mortality in cystic fibrosis. *Am Rev Respir Dis* 1986; 133:648.
35. Stern RC, Wood RE, Boat TF, et al.: Treatment and prognosis of massive hemoptysis in cystic fibrosis. *Am Rev Respir Dis* 1978; 117:825.
36. Fiel SB: Clinical management of pulmonary disease in cystic fibrosis. *Lancet* 1993; 341:1070.
37. Stern RC: Pulmonary complications, in David PB (ed): *Cystic Fibrosis.* New York, Marcel Dekker, 1993:345–380.
38. Cotton CU, Davis PB: The pancreas in cystic fibrosis, in Davis PB (ed): *Cystic Fibrosis.* New York: Marcel Dekker, 1993: 161–192.
39. Ramsey BW, Dorkin HL, Eisenberg JD, et al.: Efficacy of aerosolized tobramycin in patients with cystic fibrosis. *N Engl J Med* 1993; 328:1740.

Chapter 92

THERAPIES OTHER THAN ANTIBIOSIS

THOMAS M. MURPHY, CHRIS RUDD,
AND WAYNE SAMUELSON

Nonpharmacologic Pulmonary Therapy

CLEARANCE OF AIRWAY MUCUS

Chest physiotherapy (CPT) has assumed an important role in the care of CF patients.[1,2] While there is little documentation of immediate functional improvement in response to regularly administered therapy, a 3-week period without chest physiotherapy results in functional deterioration.[3] Traditionally, CPT has been administered by parents or family members. This is both time-consuming and labor-intensive. Modified techniques, such as autogenic drainage and active cycle breathing, are also useful and may be more acceptable to patients. The need for independence makes regular CPT a difficult goal for patients to reach. Associated conditions, such as gastroesophageal reflux, may complicate the administration of CPT.[4] New devices offer options to patients that may improve their access to effective CPT. These include the high-frequency chest-compression vest, the intrapulmonary percussive ventilator, the positive expiratory pressure (PEP) mask, and the flutter device.[5]

NUTRITION

Pancreatic enzyme (pancreatin) replacement therapy and nutritional supplementation appear to be important not only to prevent malabsorption and malnutrition, but also to maintain the long-term health of the lungs.[6,7] Bovine and porcine pancreatin is available as powder, tablets, enteric-coated tablets, or enteric-coated microspheres packaged in capsules. The microspheres appear to be the most effective approach to bypassing stomach acid intact (a pH < 4 inactivates lipase) and allowing dissolution in the intestine, where a higher pH permits greater lipase activity.[8] However, in patients with cystic fibrosis, small-intestinal pH is less than normal because of inadequate pancreatic alkalinization.[9] This helps to explain why pancreatin replacement therapy is seldom fully corrective in cystic fibrosis. Nonetheless, enzyme therapy, sometimes aided by therapy to suppress gastric acid secretion, usually succeeds in controlling symptoms of malabsorption and promoting better nutritional balance.[6] Short-term trials of pancreatin in association with gastric histamine H_2-receptor blockade by cimetidine or ranitidine have demonstrated improved weight gain and reduced stool fat and nitrogen over pancreatin alone.[10–12] Pancreatin administered as microspheres appears to be free of side effects—such as oral and anal mucositis and hyperuricemia—that were associated with prior formulations.[8] Recommended doses of pancreatin products are listed in Table 92-1. Doses that are significantly larger than recommended may be associated with colonic stricture formation, particularly in younger children.[13]

A second strategy to minimize malnourishment is to increase caloric intake. In infants with CF, this is accomplished by feeding predigested formulas that are often concentrated to a higher caloric density and supplemented with polymerized glucose. In all age groups, oral, enteral, or intravenous nutritional supplements are administered when weight gain, weight maintenance, or growth are deemed inadequate.[6] Oral supplementation is limited by the inherent anorexia that accompanies chronic illness and the reality that oral supplements diminish appetite for regular meals.[8] The fundamental approach that works in most CF patients is to provide a high-calorie, high-fat diet targeted to achieve about 200 percent of age-related caloric needs. The prior concern that high-fat diets worsen symptoms of malabsorption has given way to the realization that intake of dietary fat is the most efficient way to provide increased calories, and that symptoms of malabsorption usually can be controlled by adjusting doses of pancreatin with or without antacid. Water-soluble vitamins are given as standard multivitamin preparations. Fat-soluble vitamins A, D, E, and K require age-appropriate supplementation and are usually given in water-soluble preparations.[6]

Approaches to Drug Therapy in Cystic Fibrosis

Several organ-specific and metabolic factors differ in the CF population and modify the approach to drug therapy. This is targeted to the airways, the site of mucous desiccation, abnormal clearance, and chronic infection. Medications administered intravenously and orally are delivered to the airways primarily through the bronchial arterial circulation, which accounts for only about 1 percent of the cardiac output. Therefore, only 1 percent of these drugs are presumed to

TABLE 92-1   Suggested Lipase-Based Doses of Pancreatin Replacement

Infants
1000 to 2000 IU lipase per 4 oz formula
(Upper range: 8000 IU per 4 oz formula)[a]
    OR
200 IU/kg/feeding
(Upper range: 1000 IU/kg/feeding)[a]

Older children and adults
1000 to 2000 IU lipase/kg/meal
(Upper range: 6000 IU/kg/meal)[a]

[a]Once upper dose range is reached, consider the addition of an H_2 blocker or look for another cause of malabsorption.

achieve delivery to their target. For this and a variety of other reasons, including decreased bioavailability at the site and increased plasma and renal clearance, drug doses are often substantially increased to generate adequate tissue levels. In order to increase the therapeutic index (the ratio of benefit to toxicity), the aerosol route of delivery is increasingly employed.[14]

Drug metabolism in patients with CF is substantially altered. Because CF patients are typically small for age, a greater percentage of body weight is lean body mass.[15] This relatively low body-fat composition results in a higher apparent volume of distribution for hydrophilic agents (e.g., aminoglycosides) compared to a lower apparent volume of distribution for lipophilic agents (e.g., phenobarbital). This increased apparent volume of distribution has been described for penicillins, cephalosporins, aminoglycosides, theophylline, and cimetidine.[16] In addition, renal and blood clearance of several medications, especially antibiotics, is increased substantially in CF.[17] The renal clearance of penicillin and aminoglycoside antibiotics is increased 20 to 30 percent (Fig. 92-1), while plasma clearance of the same drugs is increased 20 to 80 percent. For these reasons, dosing

FIGURE 92-1 Percent increase in plasma clearance (mL/min/ 1.73 m2) in cystic fibrosis patients. (*Adapted from Kavanaugh et al.,*[17] *with permission.*)

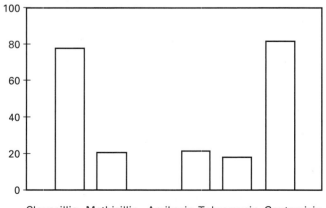

schedules for aminoglycoside antibiotics are approximately double those for non-CF patients (Tables 92-2, 92-3, and 92-4).

Pulmonary Pharmacology (Other than Antibiotics)

BLAND AEROSOLS AND BRONCHODILATORS

Bland aerosols of saline with or without a bronchodilating drug such as albuterol are administered commonly prior to sessions of chest percussion or other forms of chest physiotherapy. While there is no objective evidence that this aids the processes of cough and clearance of secretions, many patients report less dyspnea. Inhalation of a bronchodilating drug may help to alleviate the bronchoconstriction that frequently attends coughing and the mobilization of secretions. Inhalation of distilled water should be avoided because of its capacity to induce bronchoconstriction.

There is no evidence that bland aerosols hydrate CF secretions. For approximately two decades, infants and younger children were treated with several hours a day of mist-tent therapy.[18] In 1972, a controlled study demonstrated no clinical improvement,[19] and biophysical interventions did not reduce sputum viscosity,[20] so that the practice largely was abandoned.[21]

A variety of bronchodilators have been utilized in treating CF. Bronchial hyperresponsiveness to methacholine inhalation challenge has been demonstrated in CF patients[22] and correlated with disease severity,[23] but long-term studies to document a beneficial effect of bronchodilator therapy applicable to most CF patients have not been performed. A bronchodilatory effect of methylxanthines has been demonstrated,[24] but this appears to be less than that demonstrated by β-adrenergic drugs, and the side effects (nausea, dyspepsia, vomiting, tremulousness, palpitations) occur frequently (particularly in younger children) and can interfere with nutritional therapy. In addition, methylxanthine kinetics in CF may be difficult to determine and to translate into consistent therapy.[25] Nonetheless, symptoms of airways hyperreactivity may be well controlled by methylxanthine therapy in individual patients. As with asthmatic patients, doses of theophylline should be adjusted to achieve therapeutic serum concentrations, usually 10 to 20 μg/mL. Other indications for theophylline therapy include failure of response to β-adrenergic therapy, nocturnal asthma, and exercise limitation attributable to respiratory muscle dysfunction.[5]

The popularity of β-adrenergic drugs in the treatment of a variety of obstructive airway disorders has translated into extensive utilization in CF. Both oral and inhaled preparations are used, but since the oral form is associated with a greater incidence of side effects (tremulousness, tachycardia, insomnia) and is no more effective,[26] the inhaled preparation enjoys greater usage. In the CF population, doses of inhaled medications, in contrast to oral and intravenous forms, tend to be similar to those in non-CF patients.[27] Evidence for putative benefits of treatment in CF extends beyond relief of

TABLE 92-2   Dosing Schedules for Commonly Used Parenteral Antibiotics in CF

Parenteral Antibiotic	Dose, mg/kg/24h	Number of Doses/Day	Max Daily Dose, g	Pathogen(s)
Aminoglycosides				
Tobramycin gentamicin, and Netilmicin	6–15	2–3	Peak 8–12 μg/mL Trough <2 μg/mL	*P. aeruginosa, S. aureus H. influenzae*
Amikacin	5–10	2–3	Peak 25–30 μg/mL Trough < 5 μg/mL	*P. aeruginosa, S. aureus, H. influenzae*
Penicillins				
Ureidopenicillins azlocillin, mezlocillin, and piperacillin	500	4–6	20.0	*P. aeruginosa, H. influenzae*
Carboxypenicillins Ticarcillin carbenicillin, and timentin	750	4–6	30.0	*P. aeruginosa, S. aureus*—timentin only
Ampicillin-Sulbactam	100–150	4	8.0	*S. aureus, H. influenzae*
Nafcillin	200	4	8.0	*S. aureus*
Cephalosporins				
Ceftazidime	150–200	3	12.0	*P. aeruginosa, P. cepacia, H. influenzae*
Cefsulodin	200	3–4	12.0	*P. aeruginosa, H. influenzae*
Cefuroxime	100–150	3	5.0	*S. aureus, H. influenzae*
Others				
Imipenem/cilastin	50–100	4	12.0	*P. aeruginosa, S. aureus H. influenzae*
Ciprofloxacin	8–16	4	0.8	*P. aeruginosa, S. aureus H. influenzae*
Aztreonam	150	4	8.0	*P. aeruginosa, H. influenzae*
Chloramphenicol	40–60	4	4.0	*P. cepacia, H. influenzae*
Trimethoprim/sulfamethoxazole	12–20[a]	3–4	1.5	*S. aureus, H. influenzae P. cepacia*
Vancomycin	30–40	2	2.0	*S. aureus*
Clindamycin	40–80	3–4	4.0	*S. aureus*

[a]Dose of trimethoprim. Doses frequently require modification in the setting of hepatic or renal impairment.[86]
SOURCE: Adapted from Turpin et al.,[5] with permission.

airways obstruction by relaxation of airway smooth muscle and reduction of airway hyperreponsiveness[28,29] to enhancement of mucociliary clearance[30] and modification of mucous secretions.[31] Nonetheless, several concerns should be weighed in selecting this therapy on an individual basis. Since the natural evolution of CF in the (distal) airways results in the progressive loss of elastance, it is reasonable to query whether in individual cases administration of smooth-muscle-relaxant therapy might *increase* chronic airway obstruction. Indeed, in one study, a decrease was detected in half of the CF patients whose airflows changed when given an inhaled β-adrenergic agonist.[32] Another possible concern[5] is that stimulation of airway β-adrenoceptors might increase the already excessive reabsorption of sodium by the apical

epithelium.[33] However, there is no evidence that this effect alters sputum biorheology or clinical outcomes. Taken together, these concerns suggest that β-adrenergic agonists not be administered to patients who demonstrate paradoxical bronchoconstriction and that the clinical and pulmonary function response to treatment be periodically assessed.

AMILORIDE AND NUCLEOTIDE TRIPHOSPHATE AEROSOL

In response to the observation that CF epithelium demonstrated excessive reabsorption of sodium ion,[33,34] Boucher and Knowles suggested that this problem of ion traffic combined with the failure of cAMP-mediated chloride secretion

TABLE 92-3 Dosing Schedules for Commonly Used Oral Antibiotics in CF

Oral Antibiotic	Dose, mg/kg/24h	Number of Doses/Day	Max Daily Dose, g	Pathogen(s)
Quinolones				
Ciprofloxacin	10–20	2–3	2.0	*P. aeruginosa, S. aureus H. influenzae*
Ofloxacin	5–10	2–3	0.8	*P. aeruginosa, S. aureus H. influenzae*
Penicillins				
Amoxicillin	25–50	3	1.5	*S. aureus, H. influenzae*
Augmentin	25–50	3	1.5	*S. aureus, H. influenzae*
Dicloxacillin	25–50	4	2.0	*S. aureus*
Cephalosporins				
Cefuroxime	25–50	2	2.0	*S. aureus, H. influenzae*
Cefaclor	25–50	3	1.5	*S. aureus, H. influenzae*
Cephalexin	50–100	4	4.0	*S. aureus*
Others				
Trimethoprim/ sulfamethoxazole	12–20[a]	2	0.64	*S. aureus, H. influenzae P. cepacia*
Clindamycin	20–30	4	2.0	*S. aureus*
Erythromycin	25–50	4	2.0	*S. aureus*
Tetracycline	25–50	4	2.0	*H. influenzae*
Doxycycline	2–5	4	2.0	*H. influenzae*

[a]Dose of trimethoprim. Doses frequently require modification in the setting of hepatic or renal impairment.[86]
SOURCE: Adapted from Turpin et al.,[5] with permission.

TABLE 92-4 Guidelines for Oxygen Therapy in Cystic Fibrosis

Daytime room air:	$Pa_{O_2} < 55$ torr or $Pa_{O_2} < 59$ torr, plus one of the following: Edema Hematocrit $> 55\%$ P-pulmonale wave pattern on ECG
Nocturnal:	Oxygen saturations $< 88–90\%$ for 10% of total sleep time
Exercise:	Oxygen saturations $< 88–90\%$

SOURCE: Adapted from Schidlow et al.,[83] with permission.

into the airway lumen would result in less sodium and chloride, and, subsequently, less water in airway lining fluid and in airway mucus. They postulated that inhibition of active sodium reabsorption with amiloride would relieve this fundamental problem and bring long-term clinical benefit. A pilot study of the effect of aerosolized amiloride on the progression of lung disease in CF suggested improvement in sputum viscosity, retardation in the rate of deterioration of pulmonary function, and an increase in mucociliary clearance.[35] A potential limitation of this therapy is the apparent need for four-times-daily treatment for effective results. Results of these preliminary studies are currently being confirmed in a large clinical trial. More recent work[36,37] indicated that aerosols of triphosphate nucleotides—adenosine triphosphate (ATP) and uridine triphosphate (UTP)—stimulate chloride secretion through non-CFTR channels from the apical surface of airway epithelial cells by calcium-dependent stimulation of extracellular 5'-nucleotide receptors in a dose-dependent fashion. Because ATP aerosol treatment has been associated with airway hyperresponsiveness, UTP is preferred. When therapy with UTP was combined with amiloride aerosols, results were enhanced.[38]

MUCOLYTIC THERAPY

N-ACETYLCYSTEINE
The search for effective mucolytic agents began in the 1970s with the introduction of *N*-acetylcysteine (NAC), which demonstrated effective mucolysis in vitro but was less beneficial in the clinical setting.[39,40] Its utility was further limited by its irritant effect on oral and nasal mucous membranes and its propensity to cause airway hyperresponsiveness.[41] The vigorous and sometimes violent cough induced by NAC was probably related to the clinical perception of enhanced airway clearance. Further progress in mucolytic therapy awaited the realization that much of the adverse rheology of CF sputum was related to degradation products of polymorphonuclear leukocytes, such as deoxyribonuclease (DNase) and filamentous action.

HUMAN RECOMBINANT DNASE (RHDNASE; DORNASE ALPHA) [SEE ALSO CHAP. 69]
Extracellular DNA is released from leukocytes and accumulates in the airway secretions. At concentrations commonly found in CF sputum, DNA forms a highly viscous solution.[42] Deoxyribonuclease I is a human enzyme—normally present in saliva, urine, pancreatic secretions and blood—that is responsible for the digestion of extracellular DNA.

Recombinant human DNase (rhDNase) reduces the viscosity of CF sputum in vitro[43] by mechanisms that include both lysis of DNA and binding of monomeric actin and depolymerization of filamentous actin.[44] When administered in aerosolized form to patients with CF as a mucolytic agent, it generally has been well tolerated and has been shown to reduce exacerbations of respiratory symptoms and to improve pulmonary function moderately.[45] In short-term follow-up, the rate of decline of pulmonary function appears to be reduced. The usual dose is 2.5 mg administered once daily.

GELSOLIN

Approximately 10 percent of leukocyte protein is actin filaments, which are long, protease-resistant, and viscoelastic.[44] As infection progresses in CF, the proportion of actin filaments in sputum from lysed neutrophils appears to change.[46] Gelsolin, a plasma protein that severs actin filaments, rapidly and substantially reduced the viscosity of CF sputum in vitro when given alone and synergistically in combination with rhDNase.[44,46] Human studies are being initiated.

COLFOSCERIL PALMITATE

Several research groups believe that CF sputum viscoelasticity, by standard biophysical measurements, is similar to that of sputum from subjects with asthma and chronic bronchitis. What is more consistently problematic (in comparison with chronic bronchitis) is the "clearability" of CF mucus, measured either directly as tracheal cough clearance[47] or cough clearability of expectorated mucus in a simulated cough machine.[48,49] Since altering the viscoelasticity of CF sputum may not be required if the clearance is facilitated, an aerosolized surfactant, colfosceril palmitate (Exosurf), is proposed to reduce surface adhesion of CF sputum and to enhance clearance, and clinical trials in CF patients have begun. In a study of neonates with respiratory distress syndrome given colfosceril palmitate, mucociliary clearance of mucous secretions was significantly increased.[50]

ANTI-INFLAMMATORY THERAPY

The inefficient clearance of chronic bacterial infection in CF airways is associated with tissue expression of high titers of antibodies to multiple antigens of *Pseudomonas aeruginosa*[51] and other bacteria, immune complex formation,[52,53] activation of complement,[54] and the consequent vigorous infiltration by polymorphonuclear leukocytes,[55] which undergo autolysis with the release of a number of lytic enzymes, including elastases. These have been detected on bacterial and neutrophil immunoreceptors.[56,57] Taken together, this results in a hyperimmune response that is thought to cause tissue destruction.[5] Several therapies are directed to interrupt this inflammatory cascade.

IBUPROFEN

As a prototypical nonsteroidal anti-inflammatory drug, ibuprofen (IBP) inhibits cyclooxygenase in tissues throughout the body. At serum concentrations > 25 μg/mL (which are safely feasible), IBP *also* inhibits products of the 5-lipoxygenase pathway, decreasing the production of the chemoattractant leukotriene B_4.[58] Thus, administration of higher-dose IBP would be expected to reduce the influx of neutrophils into the lungs. In a rat model of CF chronic *Pseudomonas* infection, IBP-treated animals demonstrated a 30 percent reduction in the area of infection.[58] A preliminary study in CF patients of higher-dose IBF treatment individualized with plasma concentrations demonstrated minimal side effects.[59] A 4-year phase III study of 85 patients with mild lung disease who were given twice-daily therapy with IBP in a dose (20 to 30 mg/kg, mean 25 mg/kg) sufficient to generate plasma concentrations always above 35 μg/mL and above 50 μg/mL demonstrated an about 40 percent decrease in the annualized decline of FEV_1 and appeared to reduce hospitalizations.[60] Because of substantial intrasubject dose variability, sequential plasma levels were required. Gastrointestinal side effects were not increased above those seen in the placebo group. Adverse renal effects were also not noted in the IBP-treated group. The importance of pharmacokinetic studies is underscored by the observation in the rat model that lower-dose therapy with IBP appears to *increase* pulmonary inflammation.

CORTICOSTEROIDS

Glucocorticoid preparations have been used for several years to treat exacerbations of reactive airways in the context of cystic fibrosis. Observations that lower concentrations of serum immunoglobulins in CF patients were associated with a better prognosis[61] suggested that anti-inflammatory immunosuppressive therapy might be more universally beneficial, particularly in younger, less affected patients. Accordingly, a controlled study of alternate-day therapy with prednisone in children with CF demonstrated better pulmonary function and growth and stable concentrations of immunoglobulins in the treated group.[62] A 4-year multicenter placebo-controlled, double-blinded study of 285 CF patients who were given treatment regimens of either 1 mg/kg or 2 mg/kg every other day confirmed some benefits (stabilization of pulmonary function in the treated group), but it demonstrated significant side effects. After 6 months of therapy, both regimens were associated with growth retardation, and the higher-dose treatment group demonstrated an increase in glucose intolerance. Because of these side effects, the study was terminated prior to completion, and chronic corticosteroid therapy is not recommended for prophylactic treatment of CF patients with mild pulmonary involvement.[63]

ANTIPROTEASES (α_1-ANTITRYPSIN, SLPI, PENTOXYPHYLLINE, ICI 200,880)

Therapeutic strategies in recent years have focused on the inflammatory and lung-damaging effects of neutrophil proteases. Concern regarding the burden of bacterial and neutrophil proteases and the potential inactivation of antiproteases in CF sputum has resulted in the clinical testing of several protease inhibitors. Therapy for α_1-antiprotease deficiency has been achieved safely by administering intravenous and aerosolized α_1-antiprotease inhibitor (α_1-PI) purified from normal plasma.[64,65] Accordingly, it has been hypothesized that the relative excess of neutrophil proteases in CF airways might be countered by the administration of large doses of α_1-PI. A pilot study of α_1-PI administered by aerosol to CF adults demonstrated that free lung-fluid elastase could be decreased.[66] Clinical efficacy has not been confirmed.

Secretory leukocyte protease inhibitor (SLPI) is a low-molecular-weight inhibitor that is resistant to oxidation[67] and is more effective than α_1-PI in inhibiting elastin-bound elastase.[68] Clinical trials with human recombinant SLPI have been initiated. A multicenter study of pharmacologic leukocyte protease inhibition with pentoxyphylline also has begun. An additional protease inhibitor, the tripeptide ketone ICI 200,880, is being developed.[69]

OTHER ANTI-INFLAMMATORY THERAPIES

Studies of other anti-inflammatory therapies, such as the immunosuppressive antimetabolite azathioprine[70] and the cyclooxygenase inhibitor piroxicam,[71] have been initiated. Therapies directed at interrupting the influx of neutrophils into the airway parenchyma by blocking tissue and leukocyte adhesion molecules, such as ICAM-1 and CD-18, have been studied in animals.

OXYGEN, DIGOXIN

Terminal care of cor pulmonale with digoxin and diuretics has given way to earlier, more prospective, and more aggressive therapy with supplemental oxygen designed to retard or diminish the impact of this complication. With progression of bronchiectasis with age in CF, several factors in addition to hypoxemia contribute to the development of pulmonary artery hypertension and subsequent cor pulmonale. These include increased arterial P_{CO_2}, mediators of vasoconstriction elaborated by inflammatory cells; loss of the pulmonary vascular bed through fibrosis; atelectasis or disordered autoregulation; and alteration of the capability of the endothelial bed to metabolize vasoconstrictor mediators or to elaborate relaxant factors.[72,73] However, these factors are usually minor in comparison with the overall importance of local pulmonary tissue hypoxia.[74,75] Since this mechanism is driven in individual arteriolar beds scattered throughout the more diseased areas of the lungs, it is possible to develop pulmonary hypertension prior to the onset of systemic arterial hypoxemia. Indeed, in one study, 24 percent of CF patients with overt right heart failure complicating cor pulmonale demonstrated a normal arterial P_{CO_2}.[76] As expected, patients with more severe lung disease ($FEV_1 < 50$ percent of predicted) are more likely to develop exercise-[77] or sleep-[78] induced desaturation. Supplemental oxygen has been demonstrated to delay the progression of hypoxemia and to improve exercise tolerance in chronic obstructive lung disease (COPD) of diverse etiologies.[79,80] Two major clinical trials, the Nocturnal Oxygen Therapy Trial Group and the Medical Research Council Working Party, also demonstrated improved survival in severely affected COPD patients.[81,82] Consensus guidelines for oxygen therapy in cystic fibrosis are listed in Table 92-3. If daytime therapy is required, then oxygen is administered best on a continuous basis. When oxygen therapy is instituted in this fashion, there is usually no indication for chronic digoxin therapy for cor pulmonale.[83]

PHARMACOLOGY OF LUNG TRANSPLANTATION

For advanced lung disease, bilateral lung transplantation is a therapeutic option. Because of their youth and cardiovascular fitness, CF patients are well suited for this procedure. The first CF pulmonary transplant occurred in 1984, when a CF patient received a heart-lung combination.[84] Since then, numerous technical innovations have improved survival. Better means of controlling organ rejection and dealing with postoperative complications have also improved the outlook for CF patients. The pulmonary abnormalities of CF do not recur in the transplanted lung.[85]

Drugs commonly employed to suppress immune rejection of the heterologous lung and heart-lung transplants are listed in Table 92-4 along with representative dosages. In addition to these drugs, anti-thymocyte globulin is used in several centers.

TABLE 92-5 Drugs Used for Immunosuppression in CF Heart/Lung Transplantation

	Drug	Dosage	Route	Notes
Preoperative				
	Azathioprine	2 mg/kg	PO, IV	
	Cyclosporine	5 mg/kg	PO	
		1 mg/kg	IV	2 h
Intraoperative				
	Methylprednisolone	10 mg/kg	IV	
Postoperative				
	Cyclosporine	5 mg/kg or	PO	q12h Blood levels
		1.5 mg/kg/24h	IV, continuous infusion	
	Azathioprine	2 mg/kg/24h	IV,PO	WBC >4000
	Methylprednisolone then	10 mg/kg q8h; 2 mg/kg	IV X3 IV q24h X3	

References

1. Reisman JJ, Rivington-Law B, Corey M, et al.: Role of conventional physiotherapy in cystic fibrosis. *J Pediatr* 1988; 113:636.

2. Rossman CM, Waldes R, Sampson D, Newhouse MT: Effect of chest physiotherapy on the removal of mucus in patients with cystic fibrosis. *Am Rev Respir Dis* 1982; 126:131.

3. Desmond KJ, Schwenk WF, Thomas E, et al.: Immediate and long-term effects of chest physiotherapy in patients with cystic fibrosis. *J Pediatr* 1983; 103:538.

4. Vandenplas, Diercix A, Blecker U, et al.: Esophageal pH monitoring data during chest physiotherapy. *J Pediatr Gastroenterol Nutr* 1991; 13:23.

5. Turpin SV, Knowles MR: Treatment of pulmonary disease in patients with cystic fibrosis, in Davis PB (ed): *Cystic Fibrosis.* New York: Marcel Dekker, 1993:277–344.

6. Ramsey B, Farrell PM, Pencharz P, et al.: Nutritional assessment and management in cystic fibrosis: A consensus report. *Am J Clin Nutr* 1992; 55:108.

7. Corey M, McLaughlin FJ, Williams M, Levison H: A comparison of survival, growth, and pulmonary function in patients with cystic fibrosis in Boston and Toronto. *J Clin Epidemiol* 1988; 41:483.

8. Cotton CU, Davis PB: The pancreas in cystic fibrosis, in Davis PB (ed): *Cystic Fibrosis.* New York: Marcel Dekker, 1993: 161–192.

9. Youngberg CA, Berardi RR, Howatt WF, et al.: Comparison of gastrointestinal pH in cystic fibrosis and healthy subjects. *Digest Dis Sci* 1987; 32:472.

10. Hubbard VS, Dunn GF, Lester LA: Effectiveness of cimetidine as an adjunct to supplemental pancreatic enzymes in patients with cystic fibrosis. *Am J Clin Nutr* 1980; 33:2281.

11. Zentler-Munro PL, Fine DR, Batten JC, Northfield TC: Effect of cimetidine on enzyme inactivation, bile acid precipitation, and lipid solubilisation in pancreatic steatorrhoea due to cystic fibrosis. *Gut* 1985; 26:892.

12. Heijerman HGM, Lamers CB, Dijkman JH, Bakker W: Ranitidine compared with dimethylprostaglandin E₂ analogue enprostil as adjunct to pancreatic enzyme replacement in adults cystic fibrosis. *Scand J Gastroenterol* 1990; 25(suppl 178):26.

13. Smyth RL, van Velzen D, Smyth AR, et al.: Strictures of the ascending colon in cystic fibrosis and high strength pancreatic enzymes. *Lancet* 1994; 343:85.

14. Ramsey BW, Dorkin HL, Eisenberg JD, et al.: Efficacy of aerosolized tobramycin in patients with cystic fibrosis. *N Engl J Med* 1993; 328:1740.

15. Morgan DJ, Bray KM: Lean body mass as a predictor of drug dosage: Implications for drug therapy. *Clin Pharmacokinet* 1994; 26:292.

16. Groot de R, Smith AL: Antibiotic pharmacokinetics in cystic fibrosis: Differences and clinical significance. *Clin Pharmacokinet* 1987; 13:228.

17. Kavanaugh RE, Unadkat JD, Smith AL: Drug disposition in cystic fibrosis, in Davis PB (ed): *Cystic Fibrosis.* New York, Marcel Dekker, 1993: 91–136.

18. Matthews LW, Doershuk CF, Spector S: Mist tent therapy of the obstructive pulmonary lesion of cystic fibrosis. *Pediatrics* 1967; 39:176.

19. Waring WW, Seleny FL: Mist tent effects on ventilatory mechanics and other factors in cystic fibrosis (abstr). *Pediatr Res* 1972; 6:431.

20. Rosenbluth M, Pagtakhan RD, Chernick V: Influence of mist tent therapy on sputum viscosity in cystic fibrosis. *Clin Res* 1971; 19:805.

21. Taussig LM: Mist and aerosols: New studies, new thought. *J Pediatr* 1974; 84:619.

22. Holzer FJ, Olinsky A, Phelan PD: Variability of airways hyperreactivity and allergy in cystic fibrosis. *Arch Dis Child* 1981; 56:455.

23. Eggleston PA, Rosenstein BJ, Stackhouse CM, Alexander MF: Airway hyperreactivity in cystic fibrosis: Clinical correlates and possible effects on the disease. *Chest* 1988; 94:360.

24. Larsen GL, Barron RJ, Cotton EK, Brooks JG: Intravenous aminophylline in patients with cystic fibrosis. *Am J Dis Child* 1980; 134:1143.

25. Isles A, Spino M, Tabachnik E, et al.: Theophylline disposition in cystic fibrosis. *Am Rev Respir Dis* 1983; 127:417.

26. Barnes PJ: Airway pharmacology, in Murray JF, Nadel JA (eds): *Textbook of Respiratory Medicine.* Philadelphia: Saunders, 1988: 249–268.

27. National Asthma Education Program Expert Panel: *Guidelines for the Diagnosis and Treatment of Asthma.* Washington, DC: U.S. Department of Health and Human Services Public Health Service Publication No. 91-3042, August 1991.

28. Hordvik NL, Koenig P, Morris D, et al.: A longitudinal study of bronchodilator responsiveness in cystic fibrosis. *Am Rev Respir Dis* 1985; 131:889.

29. Pattishall EN: Longitudinal response of pulmonary function to bronchodilators in cystic fibrosis. *Pediatr Pulmonol* 1990; 9:80.

30. Wood RE, Boat TF, Doershuk CF: Cystic fibrosis. *Am Rev Respir Dis* 1976; 113:841.

31. Sutton PP, Gemmell HG, Innes N, et al.: Use of nebulised saline and nebulised terbutaline as an adjunct to chest physiotherapy. *Thorax* 1988; 43:57.

32. Landau LI, Phelan PD: The variable effect of a bronchodilating agent on pulmonary function in cystic fibrosis. *Pediatr Pharmacol Ther* 1981; 82:863.

33. Boucher RC, Stutts MJ, Knowles MR, et al.: Na⁺ transport in cystic fibrosis respiratory epithelia: Abnormal basal rate and response to adenylate cyclase activation. *J Clin Invest* 1986; 78:1245.

34. Waltner WE, Boucher RC, Gatzy JT, Knowles MR: Pharmacotherapy of airway disease in cystic fibrosis. *Trends Pharmacol Sci* 1987; 8:316.

35. Knowles MR, Church NL, Waltner WE, et al.: A pilot study of aerosolized amiloride for the treatment of lung disease in cystic fibrosis. *N Engl J Med* 1990; 322:1189.

36. Mason SJ, Paradiso AM, Boucher RC: Regulation of transepithelial ion transport and intracellular calcium by extracellular adenosine triphosphate in human normal and cystic fibrosis airway epithelium. *Br J Pharmacol* 1991; 103:1649.

37. Knowles MR, Clarke LL, Boucher RC: Activation by extracellular nucleotides of chloride secretion in the airway epithelia of patients with cystic fibrosis. *N Engl J Med* 1991; 325:533.

38. Knowles MR, Olivier KN, Bennett W, et al.: Aerosolized uridine triphosphate (UTP) ± amiloride: Safety and effect on mucociliary clearance in normal subjects and CF patients (abstr). *Pediatr Pulmonol Suppl* 1994; 10:99.

39. Waring WW: Current management of cystic fibrosis. *Adv Pediatr* 1976; 23:401.

40. Kuhn RJ, Nahata MC: Therapeutic management of cystic fibrosis. *Clin Pharm* 1985; 4:555.

41. Rao S, Wilson DB, Brooks RC, Sproule ABJ: Acute effects of nebulization of N-acetylcysteine on pulmonary mechanics and gas exchange. *Am Rev Respir Dis* 1970; 102:17.

42. White JC, Elmes PC: The rheological problem in chronic bronchitis. *Rheol Acta* 1958; 1(2–3):96.

43. Shak S, Capon DJ, Hellniss R, et al.: Recombinant human DNase I reduces the viscosity of cystic fibrosis sputum. *Proc Natl Acad Sci U S A* 1990; 87:9188.

44. Vasconcellos CA, Allen PG, Wohl ME, Drazen JM, et al.: Reduction in viscosity of cystic fibrosis sputum in vitro by gelsolin. *Science* 1994; 263:969.

45. Fuchs HJ, Borowitz DS, Christiansen DJ, et al.: Effect of aerosolized recombinant human DNase on exacerbations of respiratory symptoms and on pulmonary function in patients with cystic fibrosis. *N Engl J Med* 1994; 331:637.

46. Stossel TP, Allen PG, Janmey PA, et al.: Actin, DNA, and mucolysis of CF sputum in vitro (abstr). *Pediatr Pulmonol Suppl* 1994; 10:102.

47. App EM, King M, Helfesrieder R, et al.: Acute and long-term amiloride inhalation in cystic fibrosis lung disease. *Am Rev Respir Dis* 1990; 141:605.

48. Rubin BK, Ramirez O, Gourishankar S, et al.: Cough clearability of human respiratory mucus (abstr). *Am Rev Respir Dis* 1991; 143:A707.

49. Rubin BK, Ramirez O, Zayas JG, King M: Is cystic fibrosis sputum abnormal? *Chest* 1990; 98:81S.

50. Rubin BK, Ramirez O, King M: Mucus rheology and transport in neonatal respiratory distress syndrome and the effect of surfactant therapy. *Chest* 1992; 101:1080.

51. Eichler I, Joris L, Hus Y-P, et al.: Nonopsonic antibodies in cystic fibrosis. *J Clin Invest* 1989; 84:1794.

52. Moss RB, Hsu Y, Lewiston NJ, et al.: Association of systemic immune complexes, complement activation, and antibodies in *Pseudomonas aeruginosa* lipopolysaccharide and exotoxin A with mortality in cystic fibrosis. *Am Rev Respir Dis* 1986; 133:648.

53. van Bever HP, Gigase PL, de Clerck, et al.: Immune complexes and *Pseudomonas aeruginosa* antibodies in cystic fibrosis. *Arch Dis Child* 1988; 63:1222.

54. Berger M, Sorensen RU, Tosi MF, et al.: Complement receptor expression on neutrophils at an inflammatory site, the *Pseudomonas*-infected lung in cystic fibrosis. *J Clin Invest* 1989; 84:1302.

55. Banda MJ, Rice AF, Griffin GL, Senior RM: 1-Proteinase inhibitor is a neutrophil chemoattractant after proteolytic inactivation by macrophage elastase. *J Biol Chem* 1988; 263:4481.

56. Döring G, Goldstein W, Botzenhart K et al.: Elastase from polymorphonuclear leukocytes: A regulatory enzyme in immune complex disease. *Clin Exp Immunol* 1986; 64:597.

57. Tosi MF, Zakem H, Berger M: Neutrophil elastase cleaves C3bi on opsonized pseudomonas as well as CR1 on neutrophils to create a functionally important opsonin-receptor mismatch. *J Clin Invest* 1990; 86:300.

58. Konstan MW, Vargo KM, Davis PB: Ibuprofen attenuates the inflammatory response to *Pseudomonas aeruginosa* in a rat model of chronic pulmonary infection: Implications for anti-inflammatory therapy in cystic fibrosis. *Am Rev Respir Dis* 1990; 141:186.

59. Konstan MW, Hoppel CL, Chae B-L, Berger M: Ibuprofen in children with cystic fibrosis: Pharmacokinetics and adverse effects. *J Pediatr* 1991; 118:956.

60. Konstan MW, Davis PB, Byard PJ, Hoppel CL: Results of a four-year, randomized, placebo-controlled, double-blind trial of high-dose ibuprofen in CF patients with mild lung disease (abstr). *Pediatr Pulmonol Suppl* 1994; 10:103.

61. Matthews WJ Jr, Williams M, Oliphint B, et al.: Hypogamma-globulinemia in patients with cystic fibrosis. *N Engl J Med* 1980; 302:245.

62. Auerbach HS, Williams M, Kirkpatrick JA, Colten HR: Alternate-day prednisone reduces morbidity and improves pulmonary function in cystic fibrosis. *Lancet* 1985; 2:686.

63. Rosenstein BJ, Eigen H: Risks of alternate-day prednisone in patients with cystic fibrosis. *Pediatrics* 1991; 87:245.

64. Hubbard RC, Crystal RG: α₁-Antitrypsin augmentation therapy for α₁-antitrypsin deficiency. *Am J Med* 1988; 84(suppl 6A):52.

65. Hubbard RC, Brantly ML, Sellers SE, et al.: Anti-neutrophil-elastase defenses of the lower respiratory tract in α₁-antitrypsin deficiency directly augmented with an aerosol of α₁-antitrypsin. *Ann Intern Med* 1989; 111:206.

66. McElvaney NG, Hubbard RC, Birrer P, et al.: Aerosol α₁-antitrypsin treatment for cystic fibrosis. *Lancet* 1991; 337:392.

67. Vogelmeier C, Buhl R, Hoyt RF, et al.: Aerosolization of recombinant SLPI to augment antineutrophil elastase protection of pulmonary epithelium. *J Appl Physiol* 1990; 69:1843.

68. Bruch M, Bieth JG: Influence of elastin on the inhibition of leukocyte elastase by α₁ proteinase inhibitor and bronchial inhibitor. *Biochem J* 1986; 238:269.

69. Williams JC, Falcone RC, Knee C, et al.: Biologic characterization of ICI 200,880 and ICI 200,355, novel inhibitors of human neutrophil elastase. *Am Rev Resp Dis* 1991; 144:875.

70. Raeburn J: Studies of azathioprine in cystic fibrosis (CF), in *XIXth International Congress of Pediatrics, Paris, Abstract Book*, 1989:63.

71. Sordelli DO, Macri CN, Maillie AJ: A study on the effect of piroxicam (PIR) treatment to prevent lung damage in CF patients with *Pseudomonas aeruginosa* (Psa) pneumonia (abstr). *Pediatr Pulmonol Suppl* 1990; 5:247.

72. Stern RC: Cystic fibrosis and the gastrointestinal tract, in Davis PB (ed): *Cystic Fibrosis*. New York, Marcel Dekker, 1993: 401–434.

73. Gotz MH, Burghuber OC, Salzer-Muhar, et al.: Cor pulmonale in cystic fibrosis. *J R Soc Med* 1989; 82(suppl 16):26.

74. Goldring RM, Fishman AP, Turino GM, et al.: Pulmonary hypertension and cor pulmonale in cystic fibrosis of the pancreas. *J Pediatr* 1964; 65:601.

75. Bowden DH, Fischer VW, Wyatt JP: Cor pulmonale in cystic fibrosis. *Am J Med* 1965; 38:226.

76. Stern RC, Borkat G, Hirschfeld SS, et al.: Heart failure in cystic fibrosis: Treatment and prognosis of cor pulmonale with failure of the right side of the heart. *Am J Dis Child* 1980; 134:267.

77. Nixon PA, Orenstein DM, Curtis SE, Ross EA: Oxygen supplementation during exercise in cystic fibrosis. *Am Rev Respir Dis* 1990; 59:807.

78. Tepper RS, Skatrud JB, Dempsey JA: Ventilation and oxygenation changes during sleep in cystic fibrosis. *Chest* 1983; 84:388.

79. Woodcock AA, Gross ER, Geddes DM: Oxygen relieves breathlessness in "pink puffers." *Lancet* 1981; 1:907.

80. McKeon JL, Hensley MJ, Saunders NA: Efficacy of current therapy for patients with chronic obstructive lung disease, Hensley MJ, Saunders NA (eds): in *Clinical Epidemiology of Chronic Obstructive Pulmonary Disease*: vol. 43 *Lung Biology in Health and Disease*. New York: Marcel Dekker, 1989:305–354.

81. Nocturnal Oxygen Therapy Trial Group: Continuous or nocturnal oxygen therapy in hypoxemic chronic obstructive lung disease: A clinical trial. *Ann Intern Med* 1980; 93:391.

82. Medical Research Council Working Party: Long term domiciliary oxygen therapy in chronic hypoxic cor pulmonale complicating chronic bronchitis and emphysema. *Lancet* 1981; 1:681.

83. Schidlow DV, Taussig LM, Knowles MR: Cystic Fibrosis Foundation consensus conference report on pulmonary complications of cystic fibrosis. *Pediatr Pulmonol* 1993; 15:187.

84. Yacoub MH, Banner NR, Khaghani A, et al.: Heart-lung transplantation for cystic fibrosis and subsequent domino heart transplantation. *J Heart Transplant* 1990; 9:459.

85. Wood, Alison, Higenbottam T, et al.: Airway mucosal bioelectric potential difference in cystic fibrosis after lung transplantation. *Am Rev Respir Dis* 1989; 140:1645.

86. Mouton JW, Kerribijn KF: Antibacterial therapy in cystic fibrosis. *Med Clin North Am* 1990; 74:837.

ANTIBIOTIC THERAPY

THOMAS M. MURPHY, CHRIS RUDD,
AND WAYNE SAMUELSON

General Principles
  What is being treated?
  Doses and routes of delivery
  Dosing interval

Antibiotic Treatment of *Staphylococcus aureus* **and** *Haemophilus*
influenzae

Antipseudomonal Antibiotics

Aerosolized Antibiotics

General Principles

WHAT IS BEING TREATED?

Chronic bacterial infection of the airways in CF is at the heart of the pathophysiology of progressive pulmonary failure.[1] The spectrum of bacterial flora involved in this process is illustrated in Fig. 93-1.[2] During the first several years of life, the dominant bacteria are *Staphylococcus aureus*, *Haemophilus influenzae*, and a variety of gram-negative bacteria. Inevitably *Pseudomonas* species—most often *Pseudomonas aeruginosa*—dominate the respiratory flora; once established, they are seldom eradicated.[3] The age-specific frequency of bacterial flora is illustrated in Fig. 93-2.[2] In addition to those bacteria that are cultured routinely, anaerobic species may be important.[4,5] The goal of antimicrobial therapy is to reduce as much as possible the burden of bacterial growth, the elaboration of toxic exoproducts, the chemoattractant stimulus for vigorous infiltration with neutrophils, and the secondary stimulus for a chronic hyperimmune inflammatory response. A secondary benefit is to reduce an important stimulus for chronic hypersecretion of desiccated mucopurulent secretions (Table 91-1). Clinical indications for antibiotic administration are listed in Table 93-1.[6–8]

DOSES AND ROUTES OF DELIVERY

Antibiotics have been administered to CF patients orally and intravenously and increasingly by the aerosolized route. Doses of commonly used antibiotics and their targeted microorganisms are listed in Tables 92-2 and 92-3. Because of an increased volume of distribution and increased plasma and renal clearance, antibiotic doses in patients with CF are typically significantly greater than in unaffected patients. Oral antibiotics are used primarily in the outpatient setting and are most effective against *S. aureus*, *H. influenzae*, sensitive strains of gram-negative bacteria, and anaerobes.

However, clinical benefit sometimes appears to result from this group of antibiotics even if sputum culture results suggest resistance. Putative reasons are as follows.

1. The commensal and anaerobic oropharyngeal flora that are cultured from sputum and are assumed to represent contamination may represent pathogenic microbes[5,9] that are often sensitive to commonly used oral antibiotics.
2. Major pathogens such as *S. aureus* may be difficult to grow in culture, particularly when patients are concomitantly treated with antibiotics.[10]
3. Noncidal concentrations of antibiotics may inhibit bacterial multiplication or production of toxic exoproducts, or they may exert anti-inflammatory effect.[11–13]
4. The standard laboratory tool to assess bacterial susceptibility to antimicrobial therapy is the minimal inhibitory concentration (MIC), which does not always correlate with bacterial killing (see "Antipseudomonal Antibiotics," below).

FIGURE 93-1. Percent prevalence of microorganisms in cystic fibrosis patients. (*From Konstan and Berger,[2] with permission.*)

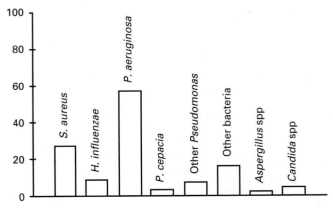

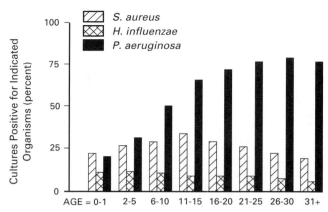

FIGURE 93-2. Age-related prevalence of CF pathogens. (*From Konstan and Berger,*[2] *with permission.*)

Despite these considerations, the results of treatment using standard oral antibiotics in patients whose dominant sputum pathogen is *P. aeruginosa* are often disappointing. A significant recent addition to the oral antibiotic regimen are the fluoroquinolones,[14] which are currently the only oral antibiotics with significant activity against *Pseudomonas* species. Use of fluoroquinolone antibiotics is usually limited to relatively short-term administration because of potential problems with headache, nausea, and depression.[15] A major concern regarding toxicity are reports in animals of cartilage erosion in weight-bearing joints.[16] To date, such reports in humans are rare. Nonetheless caution is recommended when ciprofloxacin or ofloxacin are used either in children below 14 years of age or in pregnant mothers.[6] A collaborative study has been initiated to assess the safety and efficacy of ciprofloxacin in school-aged children with CF. Standard doses are listed in Tables 92-2 and 92-3.

Infectious exacerbations of *Pseudomonas* bronchiectasis that do not respond to treatment with oral antibiotics are still treated primarily by the intravenous administration of specific antipseudomonal antibiotics. While intravenous therapy can be administered in part in the patient's home (assuming all the rest of the necessary therapy—such as chest physiotherapy and nutritional support—is in place), this usually is initiated in the hospital. The aerosol route of treatment is utilized increasingly because of the greater therapeutic index associated with it (i.e., greater organ-specific dose relative to toxicity). A recent study demonstrated that treatment with high-dose aerosolized tobramycin (600 mg bid) generated sputum concentrations more than 10 times the MIC of the *Pseudomonas*, produced no significant toxicity,[17] and yielded clinically significant clinical improvement.[18]

DOSING INTERVAL

The tactical goal in choosing a dosing interval is to maximize the effect of an antibiotic while minimizing toxicity. A secondary concern of the interval is one of logistics, i.e., the interval must not be so frequent as to conflict unrealistically with school or job responsibilities. Drugs rarely are administered continuously in CF. Therefore, orally and intravenously administered drugs generate blood concentrations that peak to a maximum within 20 to 30 min (IV) to a few hours after administration (PO) and then decay exponentially to a trough concentration determined just prior to the next dose. Because of the difficulties in achieving adequate bronchial tissue and sputum concentrations of antibiotics in CF with less than maximal tolerated doses,[19,20] peak concentrations are targeted at a maximal concentration limited by the potential toxicity of the drug. Because these peak concentrations demonstrate a rapid exponential decay, average blood concentration tends to be less than that of unaffected individuals. It would appear likely that only the blood concentrations in the neighborhood of the peak concentration contribute to tissue concentrations of drug. Since the incidence of bacteremia in CF patients is very low, there appears to be little point in maintaining high trough concentrations. The end result of these considerations is that peak antibiotic concentrations are targeted to be therapeutic, while trough concentrations are targeted to be sufficiently low to minimize the likelihood of toxicity. Since antibiotic agents in CF are cleared at an increased rate, the dosing interval can often be shortened. However, the shortening of this interval often is associated with an unacceptable increase in trough blood concentrations (See "Anti-pseudomonal Antibiotics," below).

Antibiotic Treatment of Staphylococcus aureus and Haemophilus influenzae

Staphylococcus aureus has been recognized as an important pathogen in CF lung disease since the initial description of the disorder by Dorothy Andersen in 1938.[21] For the next three decades antimicrobial strategies were designed to control the virulence of this organism.[22] Perhaps because of the development and increased use of β-lactamase–resistant penicillins, the prevalence of *S. aureus* declined beginning in

---

TABLE 93-1 Indications for Additions or Changes in Antimicrobial Therapy

Symptoms
Increase in productive cough
Increased dyspnea
Decreased appetite
Fatigue or reduced exercise tolerance
Signs
Increased respiratory rate, chest retractions
Fever
Weight loss or failure to gain weight
Change in volume, appearance, or color of sputum
New chest auscultative findings
Laboratory
Deterioration in pulmonary function tests and/or oxygen saturation
New radiologic chest infiltrates
Newly isolated bacterial pathogen
Increased white blood count or erythrocyte sedimentation rate

SOURCES: Adapted from Rubio et al.[7] and Smith et al.,[8] with permission.

the 1960s.[23] Despite the emergence of *Pseudomonas* species as the current dominant organism in CF respiratory infections, *S. aureus* remains a clinically important pathogen capable of causing rapidly progressive bronchiectasis. Microbiologic identification is sometimes difficult because of the tendency of the upper respiratory tract to be colonized with this organism.[2] In one study comparing culture results from throat culture and bronchoalveolar lavage (BAL) in CF, *S. aureus* was present in throat cultures more than 50 percent of the time when it was absent from BAL fluid.[24] Throat cultures may also be negative in non-sputum-producing patients who harbor the organism in their lower respiratory tracts.[25] Treatment strategies vary among clinical centers, but all seem to agree on the need to treat symptomatic pulmonary exacerbations in respiratory colonized CF patients with specific antistaphylococcal drugs (Tables 92-2 and 92-3). Because of the more severe complications related to this organism that can affect infants with CF, many clinicians treat *S. aureus* prospectively ("prophylactically") with daily antimicrobial therapy in this age group. However, the benefits of this approach are not yet well established. To evaluate this approach, a 6-year, multicenter, double-blind, placebo-controlled trial of daily treatment with cephalexin in CF patients < 2 years of age is under way.

The role of *H. influenzae* as an agent of progressive CF bronchiectasis is less certain. While its overall prevalence is relatively low (< 10 percent), its presence is likely to be intermittent; therefore it may play a role similar to that of *H. influenzae* in other forms of chronic lung disease, as chronic bronchitis.[24] Multiple antibodies to antigens of *H. influenzae* are detectable in the serum of most patients with CF.[26] The phenotype in CF sputum is nonencapsulated, and biotype I ("nontypable *H. influenzae*"), which is generally sensitive to β-lactamase–resistant penicillins and a variety of cephalosporins, predominates.[26–28] Its recovery is increased during respiratory exacerbations, and specific antimicrobial therapy appears to be associated with clinical improvement.[28] However, in another 5-year study, sputum recovery of *H. influenzae* among 226 CF patients was associated with a worsened prognosis.[29] Some have speculated that the role of *S. aureus* and *H. influenzae* is to cause early airway damage, setting the stage for chronic colonization and infection with species of *Pseudomonas* that are usually not virulent in patients without CF.[6,24]

Antipseudomonal Antibiotics

With the emergence in the 1960s and 1970s of *Pseudomonas* species as the dominant pathogen in CF (displacing the more sensitive *S. aureus*), a de facto therapeutic barrier manifested itself as greater resistance to vigorous antibiotic therapy. In the next two decades, several new agents were introduced to treat the most common pathogen, *P. aeruginosa*. Popular examples of these new agents include the extended penicillins piperacillin and azlocillin as well as ceftazidime, ciprofloxacin, aztreonam, and imipenem/cilastatin. While each of these antibiotics is useful in managing the acute infectious exacerbations, none can eradicate established *Pseudomonas* airway infections.[30]

Aminoglycosides have been shown to demonstrate increased activity in vitro when used in combination with one of the newer antibiotics. Although there is no evidence from controlled clinical studies that combination therapy is superior to monotherapy, aminoglycosides used in combination with an extended penicillin, cephalosporin, or fluoroquinolone is an accepted therapeutic regimen for treating serious pulmonary exacerbations due to *P. aeruginosa*.[31,32] Gentamicin, tobramycin, and amikacin are commonly prescribed aminoglycosides for patients with susceptible *P. aeruginosa*. Netilmicin, the newest addition to this class, also has activity against *Pseudomonas* species, but it is not widely used, because of MICs that are greater than those of the more commonly used agents.

Susceptibility of strains of *P. aeruginosa* to various antibiotics are evaluated in vitro using the MIC. For the treatment of serious infections, the MIC of an antibiotic should be less than the concentration of the antibiotic at the site of infection. It is suggested that plasma and/or tissues concentrations of the antibiotic should be four to eight times the MIC to treat infections in compromised patients effectively.[33–35] An alternative in vitro test is the minimum bactericidal concentration (MBC), which does not always correlate well with the reported MIC for a cultured infectious pathogen. Ansorg and coworkers found a poor correlation between the inhibitory and bactericidal activity of antipseudomonal antibiotics against *P. aeruginosa* strains isolated from patients with CF.[36] When MIC values were evaluated, imipenem, ciprofloxacin, tobramycin, amikacin, ceftazidime, cefsulodin, piperacillin, and azlocillin were effective against cultured strains of *P. aeruginosa*. In contrast, MBC values for the same strains only supported the use of ciprofloxacin, tobramycin, amikacin, and imipenem in the same patients. Microbiology laboratories routinely report MIC data for a given sputum culture, and clinical decisions are made without the availability of MBC data for the same cultures. The discrepancy between these reported values may be responsible for the sometimes poor correlation between in vitro predictions and the clinical success of antipseudomonal chemotherapy in patients with CF.

As with all chronic infections, the underlying disease process determines the relative effectiveness of an inhibitory or cidal antibiotic regimen. In CF, *P. aeruginosa* colonizes the respiratory tract early and causes chronic infection.[23] Tobramycin, gentamicin, and amikacin are bactericidal agents that have proven efficacy in the treatment of pulmonary infections; however, toxicity limits the effectiveness of these agents. Penetration into the lungs and achievement of therapeutic concentrations at the site of infection is directly related to the serum concentration of an antimicrobial agent.[37] Unfortunately, serum concentrations are limited by nephrotoxicity and ototoxicity occurring in a dose-related fashion.

Several physiologic factors influence drug penetration to the site of infection and the resultant therapeutic activity. Inflammation and sputum production may decrease the amount of aminoglycoside reaching the site of infection. Furthermore, the mucoid anion matrix in the lung of a CF patient decreases drug penetration and efficacy of the aminoglycoside and thus protects the *Pseudomonas*.[38] This mucoid anion matrix serves to protect *P. aeruginosa* from the aminoglycoside agent. Compared to amikacin and gentamicin, tobramycin has the highest penetration in bronchial secretions and the lowest MIC for *P. aeruginosa*.[39]

A recommended dosing strategy is to achieve sufficiently increased peak serum concentrations (8 to 12 μg/mL for tobramycin and gentamicin, 20 to 30 μg/mL for amikacin) 30 min after infusion to achieve bronchial tissue and secretion penetration while maintaining sufficiently low trough concentrations (≤ 2 μg/mL mg/L for tobramycin and gentamicin, ≤ 5 to 10 μg/mL mg/L for amikacin) to minimize the risk of nephrotoxicity and ototoxicity.[40] The pharmacokinetic disposition profile for aminoglycoside agents in CF is unique. Total body clearance is increased both from an increase in the apparent volume of distribution and from enhanced renal elimination; the composite results in a reduced elimination half-life and increased plasma clearance.[41]

Because of this increased clearance, patients with CF commonly require approximately twice the daily recommended dose of aminoglycosides—compared to the general pediatric and adult patient populations—to achieve and maintain therapeutic plasma concentrations of aminoglycosides.[42] Thus, it is not surprising that nephrotoxicity associated with aminoglycoside therapy is rarely observed in patients with cystic fibrosis. The lower potential for renal toxicity in these patients allows aggressive dosing to control infectious exacerbations; however, long-term high-dose therapy has occasionally resulted in irreversible ototoxicity.[43]

As noted, CF patients are typically small for age and have a greater percentage of body weight that is lean body mass.[44] This relatively low body fat composition results in a higher apparent volume of distribution for hydrophilic agents (e.g., aminoglycosides) compared to a lower apparent volume of distribution for lipophilic agents (e.g., phenobarbital). This increased apparent volume of distribution has been well described for penicillins, cephalosporins, aminoglycosides, theophylline, and cimetidine.[41]

Several published studies have quantified the increased clearance of aminoglycosides in CF.[41,42,45–48] Enhanced elimination has been reported for all aminoglycosides studied in patients with cystic fibrosis. The volume of distribution in this patient population ranges from 0.31 to 0.35 L/kg compared to 0.24 L/kg in the general population.[45,48] The increased volume of distribution reflects the relative decrease in adipose tissue. The half-life for aminoglycosides in CF patients (in comparison with unaffected children and adults) is reported at the low-normal range of 1.8 to 2.5 h. In addition to an increased apparent volume of distribution and decreased elimination half-life, several physiologic factors result in enhanced renal clearance. These include (1) increased kidney size (as well as glomeruli); (2) increased plasma volume; and (3) increased elimination through sputum and biliary tract.

Whether the glomerular filtration rate (GFR) is increased in CF is a matter of controversy. Several studies show a 20 percent increase in creatinine clearance in CF, while others indicate little difference relative to control populations.[49–51] At autopsy CF kidneys are 1.5 to 2.0 times normal size with evident glomerulomegaly.[52,53] Patients with CF have decreased free-water clearance, which is proposed to result from increased reabsorption of sodium in the proximal renal tubules with decreased sodium delivery in the distal segments of the nephron.[54,55] Increases in GFR may be explained by increased filtration pressure. Patients with CF have a 25 to 40 percent greater mean venous plasma volume, which causes an increase in filtration pressure.[56] Increased filtration pressure with an increase in kidney size and glomerulomegaly results in a higher filtration coefficient for drugs as well as endogenous creatinine.[57] Thus, increased filter pressure, decreased free-water clearance, and kidney size all contribute to increased renal clearance of aminoglycosides and other agents commonly prescribed in this patient population.

Another potential site of drug elimination is through the copious bronchial secretions, which may increase as sputum production escalates.[45] The clearance of aminoglycosides appears to increase as the severity of the pulmonary disease progresses.[58] This clearance change is associated with an increased apparent volume of distribution as well as an increase in sputum production.[47]

A reasonable goal for gentamicin/tobramycin dosing in CF patients is to target peak serum concentrations of 8 to 12 μg/mL 30 min postinfusion while maintaining a trough serum concentration ≤ 2 μg/mL. Consistent achievement of these target concentrations can be difficult. Several dosing guidelines and strategies have been evaluated over the years; however, no single recommendation is applicable to all patients with CF.[42,48,59–62] Generally, dosing is initiated at 10 mg/kg/day divided in 6 to 8 h intervals. If the target plasma concentrations are not achieved with 10 mg/kg/day, then the daily dose should be adjusted based on a linear one-compartment open model.[63]

Studies have suggested that a shorter dosing interval (6 h) results in better pulmonary function as measured by sustained improvement of FEV_1 at follow-up and a significantly longer time before the next hospitalization.[59] However, a routine 6-h dosing interval may be complicated by enhanced drug accumulation, which can result in a sustained trough serum concentration ≥ 2 mg/L, with the attendant risks of nephrotoxicity and ototoxicity. Guidelines for selecting dosing intervals can be based on the half-life of the drug. Six-hour intervals may be used if the individual half-life is < 1.5 h and an 8-h interval may be used if the half-life is 1.5 to 2.5 h. For greater half-lives, the dosing interval will have to be further extended.

Because of the shorter half-life and an increase in the apparent volume of distribution in younger children with CF, many pediatric patients may require tobramycin doses in the range of 10 to 20 mg/kg/day to achieve the desired peak and trough serum concentrations. An individualized pharmacokinetic profile should be kept on file for prompt retrieval to initiate therapy on future admissions. This will shorten the time required to achieve targeted serum levels to within 24 to 48 h of admission. Attaining appropriately high peak serum concentrations in patients with CF is necessary to achieve adequate sputum aminoglycoside concentrations.[40]

Aminoglycoside dosing in adults can be similarly difficult. Alterations in both plasma clearance and volume of distribution have been suggested as explanations for the higher dose requirements often seen.[63–65] The disposition of aminoglycoside may also be influenced by the severity of illness in CF.[66] Serum concentration of drug also can be influenced by the method used to infuse the drug.[67] Hendeles and colleagues studied gentamicin dosing in 15 children and 7 adults with CF in whom dose and dosing intervals were adjusted empirically on the basis of a pair of peak and trough serum measurements.[68] Mean half-life and incremental increase in serum concentration from previous trough to subsequent peak (which indirectly reflects volume of distribution) were not significantly different between children or adults with cystic fibrosis and pediatric control subjects. The investigators concluded that the high dose requirements in CF were related more to high target serum concentrations than to altered pharmacokinetics in CF patients. They recommended an initial dosing regimen of 3 mg/kg every 8 h for adults, with later adjustments to be made on the basis of subsequent paired peak and trough measurements obtained after steady state has been reached. These recommendations are widely followed.

Several recent studies have supported the use of "once daily" aminoglycoside dosing.[69,70] The goal of this therapy is to administer the entire daily dose in one infusion to achieve a peak gentamicin or tobramycin level of 20 to 30 µg/mL. This scheme still permits the trough serum concentration to remain ≤ 2 µg/mL for several hours daily. With this regimen, there is evidence of a "postantibiotic effect," that is, continued bacterial growth suppression in the presence of subtherapeutic concentrations of the drug at the site of infection.[71] To date, limited studies of adults have documented efficacy equivalent to that of the traditional regimens and no increased nephrotoxicity or ototoxicity. Studies in pediatric CF patients are needed. If further studies confirm the safety and efficacy of this approach, this might simplify hospital and home antibiotic regimens for CF patients.

Aerosolized Antibiotics

The administration of antibiotics by nebulization offers a rational approach to the challenge of delivering a high concentration of antipseudomonal antibiotic directly to the airways while minimizing the potential for toxicity. Only recently has evidence of the efficacy of this approach appeared. Several indications have been promoted.[72]

1. *Maintenance of suppression of chronic Pseudomonas infection.* Hodson and coworkers demonstrated that twice-daily administration of 80 mg of gentamicin and 1 g of carbenicillin appeared to retard the decline in pulmonary function and decreased hospitalization in adults with CF.[73] Similar results were obtained with inhaled ceftazidime[74] and with nebulized colistin given between courses of intravenous antibiotics.[75]

2. *Supplementation of intravenous therapy.* The addition of inhaled amikacin to a regimen of intravenous amikacin and ceftazidime appeared acutely to reduce further the quantity of *Pseudomonas* in the sputum but failed to produce longer-term benefits.[76]

3. *Treatment of acute respiratory exacerbations.* In uncontrolled studies, 80 mg tobramycin and 1 g carbenicillin administered twice daily[77] and 80 mg tobramycin administered twice to three times daily[78] appeared to give results comparable to those of intravenous therapy.

4. *Delay of early colonization with Pseudomonas species.* A preliminary study demonstrated a reduction in cultures positive for *Pseudomonas* when colistin aerosols were initiated soon after the discovery of respiratory colonization.[79]

There has been little toxicity using this approach, including the use of high-dose (600 mg bid) tobramycin given for 28 days.[18] The major concerns that previously limited this approach have been (1) the quantity of drug delivered (usually < 10 percent of the total nebulized) to the airways might be less than required; (2) the more rapid emergence of bacterial resistance to antimicrobial treatment; (3) selection of organisms with high virulence, such as *Pseudomonas cepacia (Burkholderia cepacia)*; and (4) elicitation of bronchial hyperresponsiveness. In addition to refuting these concerns in a short-term study, the high-dose tobramycin study demonstrated two key endpoints: (1) a consistent increase in FEV_1 of 10 percent in the treated group and (2) sputum concentrations of antibiotic that were at least 10 times the MIC of the underlying microorganism.[18,80] Currently, a more moderate dose of tobramycin (300 mg) in a preservative-free vehicle is being studied in a similar multicenter trial after a preliminary study demonstrated improvement in clinical status and pulmonary function.[81] A major advantage of this preparation will be reduced cost. Doses of commonly used nebulized antibiotics are listed in Table 93-2.

The optimal method of aerosol delivery is still a matter of concern and debate.[72] The nebulizer must be able to produce

TABLE 93-2   Doses of Aerosolized Antibiotics for CF Respiratory Exacerbations

Antibiotic	Low Dose	High Dose	Doses/Day	Pathogens
Tobramycin	40–80 mg	200–600	2–4	*P. aeruginosa, S. aureus, H. influenzae*
Gentamicin	40–80 mg	200–600	2–4	*P. aeruginosa, S. aureus, H. influenzae*
Colistin	50–75 mg	75–150	2–3	*P. aeruginosa, S. aureus, H. influenzae*
Ceftazidime	1000 mg		1–2	*P. aeruginosa, P. cepacia, H. influenzae*
Ticarcillin	1000 mg		1–2	*P. aeruginosa, H. influenzae*
Carbenicillin	1000 mg		1–2	*P. aeruginosa, H. influenzae*

SOURCES: Adapted from Turpin and Knowles,[6] Ramsey et al.,[18] and Eisenberg,[81] with permission.

aerosol droplets of diameter 0.5 to 5.0 μm to be respirable.[82] The mass median diameter should be in the range of 3 to 5 μm.[83,84] To do this, the nebulizer usually will require a flow > 10 L/min.[84,85] Since the efficiency of generating respirable medication is increased with volume, a total nebulizer volume of 4 mL is recommended by some as a compromise between efficiency and time.[72,83,86] Because ultrasonic nebulizers heat their solutions and the impact of heat on antibiotics is unknown, jet nebulizers generally are preferred. Several new delivery systems are under investigation.

References

1. Govan WJRW, Harris GS: *Pseudomonas aeruginosa* and cystic fibrosis: Unusual bacterial adaptation and pathogenesis. *Microbiol Sci* 1986; 3:302.

2. Konstan MW, Berger M: Infection and inflammation of the lung in cystic fibrosis, in Davis PB (ed): *Cystic Fibrosis*. New York, Marcel Dekker, 1993; 219–276.

3. Kulczycki LL, Murphy TM, Bellanti JA: *Pseudomonas* colonization in cystic fibrosis: A study of 160 patients. *JAMA* 1978; 240:30.

4. Lester LA, Egge A, Hubbard VS, di Sant'Agnese P: Aspiration and lung abscess in cystic fibrosis. *Am Rev Respir Dis* 1983; 127:786.

5. Jewes LA, Spencer RC: The incidence of anaerobes in the sputum of patients with cystic fibrosis. *J Med Microbiol* 1990; 3:271.

6. Turpin SV, Knowles MR: Treatment of pulmonary disease in patients with cystic fibrosis, in Davis PB (ed): *Cystic Fibrosis*. New York: Marcel Dekker, 1993; 277–344.

7. Rubio TT: Infection in patients with cystic fibrosis. *Am J Med* 1986; 81(suppl A):73.

8. Smith AL, Redding G, Doershuk C, et al.: Sputum changes associated with therapy for endobronchial exacerbation in cystic fibrosis. *J Pediatr* 1988; 112:547.

9. Myers MG, Koontz FP, Weinberger M: Lower respiratory infections in patients with cystic fibrosis, in Lloyd-Still JD (ed): *Textbook of Cystic Fibrosis*. Boston: John Wright, 1983; 91–107.

10. Williams RF: Persistence of thymine-dependent Staphylococci in CF sputum: A pitfall for the unwary, in Sturgess JM (ed): *Perspectives in Cystic Fibrosis*. Toronto: Canadian Cystic Fibrosis Foundation, 1980; 352–358.

11. Govan JRW: In vivo significance of bacteriocins and bacteriocin receptors. *Scand J Infect Dis Suppl* 1986; 49:31.

12. Morris G, Brown MRW: Novel modes of action of aminoglycoside antibiotics against *Pseudomonas aeruginosa*. *Lancet* 1988; 2:1359.

13. Goswami SK, Kivity S, Marom Z: Erythromycin inhibits respiratory glycoconjugate secretion from human airways *in vitro*. *Am Rev Respir Dis* 1990; 141:72.

14. Rubio TT: Ciprofloxacin: Comparative data in cystic fibrosis. *Am J Med* 1987; 82(suppl 4A):185.

15. Fass RJ: Efficacy and safety of oral ciprofloxacin in the treatment of serious respiratory infections. *Am J Med* 1987; 82(suppl 4A):202.

16. Schlueter G: Ciprofloxacin: Review of potential toxicologic effects. *Am J Med* 1987; 82(suppl 4A):91.

17. Smith AL, Ramsey BW, Hedges DL, et al.: Safety of aerosol tobramycin administration for 3 months to patients with cystic fibrosis. *Pediatr Pulmonol* 1989; 7:265.

18. Ramsey BW, Dorkin HL, Eisenberg JD, et al.: Efficacy of aerosolized tobramycin in patients with cystic fibrosis. *N Engl J Med* 1993; 328:1740.

19. Medelman PM, Smith AL, Levy J, et al.: Aminoglycoside penetration, inactivation, and efficacy in cystic fibrosis sputum. *Am Rev Respir Dis* 1985; 132:761.

20. Smith BR, Le Frock JL: Bronchial tree penetration of antibiotics. *Chest* 1983; 83:904.

21. Andersen DH: Cystic fibrosis of the pancreas and its relation to celiac disease: A clinical and pathological study. *Am J Dis Child* 1938; 56:344.

22. di Sant'Agnese PA: The pulmonary manifestations of fibrocystic disease of the pancreas. *Dis Chest* 1955; 27:654.

23. Mearns MB, Hunt GH, Rushworth R: Bacterial flora of respiratory tract in patients with cystic fibrosis. *Arch Dis Child* 1972; 47:902.

24. Konstan MW, Hilliard KA: Comparison of throat with bronchoalveolar lavage cultures in determining lower airway bacterial colonization in cystic fibrosis. *Pediatr Pulmonol Suppl* 1991; 6:281.

25. Ramsey BW, Wentz KR, Smith AL, et al.: Predictive value of oropharyngeal cultures for identifying lower airway bacteria in cystic fibrosis patients. *Am Rev Respir Dis* 1991; 144:331.

26. May JR, Herrick NC, Thompson D: Bacterial infection in cystic fibrosis. *Arch Dis Child* 1972; 47:908.

27. Hoiby N, Killian M: *Haemophilus* from the lower respiratory tract of patients with cystic fibrosis. *Scand J Respir Dis* 1976; 57:103.

28. Rayner RJ, Hiller EJ, Ispahani P, Baker M: *Haemophilus* infection in cystic fibrosis. *Arch Dis Child* 1990; 65:255.

29. Knoke JD, Stern RC, Doershuk CF, et al.: Cystic fibrosis: The prognosis for five-year survival. *Pediatr Res* 1978; 12:676.

30. Hoiby N: Clinical uses of nalidixic acid analogues: the fluoroquinolones. *Eur J Clin Microbiol* 1986; 5:138.

31. Nelson JD: Management of acute pulmonary exacerbations in cystic fibrosis: A critical appraisal. *J Pediatr* 1985; 106:1030.

32. Watkins J, Francis J, Kuzemko JA: Does monotherapy of pulmonary infections in cystic fibrosis lead to early development of resistant strains of *Pseudomonas aeruginosa*? *Scand J Gastroenterol* 1988; 23(suppl 143):81.

33. BSAC Working Party: Breakpoints in in-vitro antibiotic sensitivity testing. *J Antimicrob Chemother* 1988; 21:701.

34. Scribner RK, Marks MJ, Weber AH, et al.: Activities of various β-lactams and aminoglycosides, alone and in combination, against isolates of *Pseudomonas aeruginosa* from patients with cystic fibrosis. *Antimicrob Agents Chemother* 1982; 21:939.

35. Washington II JA: Susceptibility tests: agar dilution; in Lennette EH, Balows A, Hausler WJ, Shadomy HJ (eds): *Manual of Clinical Microbiology* 4th ed. Washington, DC: American Society of Microbiology 1985; 967–971.

36. Ansorg R, Muller KD, Wiora J: Comparison of inhibitory and bactericidal activity of antipseudomonal antibiotics against *Pseudomonas aeruginosa* isolates from cystic fibrosis patients. *Chemother* 1990; 36:22.

37. Levy J, Baran D, Klastersky, J: Comparative study of the antibacterial activity of amikacin and tobramycin during *Pseudomonas* pulmonary infection in patients with cystic fibrosis. *J Antimicrob Agents Chemother* 1982; 10:227.

38. Lam J, Chan R, Lam K, et al.: Production of mucoid microcolonies by *Pseudomonas aeruginosa* within infected lungs in cystic fibrosis. *Infect Immunol* 1980; 28:546.

39. Mandelman PM, Smith AL, Levy J, et al.: Aminoglycoside penetration, inactivation, and efficacy in cystic fibrosis. *Am Rev Respir Dis* 1985; 132:761.

40. McCrae WM, Raeburn JA, Hanson EJ: Tobramycin therapy of infections due to *Pseudomonas aeruginosa* in patients with cystic fibrosis: Effect of dosage and concentration of antibiotic in sputum. *J Infect Dis* 1976; 134(suppl):S191.

41. Groot de R, Smith AL: Antibiotic pharmacokinetics in cystic

fibrosis: Differences and clinical significance. *Clin Pharmacokinet* 1987; 13:228.

42. Horrevorts AM, Driessen OMJ, Michel MF, Kerrebijn KF: Pharmacokinetics of antimicrobial drugs in cystic fibrosis: Aminoglycoside antibiotics. *Chest* 1988; 94:S120.

43. McRorie TI, Bosso J, Randolph L: Aminoglycoside ototoxicity in cystic fibrosis: Evaluation by high-frequency audiometry. *Am J Dis Child* 1989; 143:1328.

44. Morgan DJ, Bray KM: Lean body mass as a predictor of drug dosage. Implications for drug therapy. *Clin Pharmacokinet* 1994; 26:292.

45. Levy J, Smith AL, Loup JR, et al.: Disposition of tobramycin in patients with cystic fibrosis: A prospective controlled study. *J Pediatr* 1984; 105:117.

46. Kildoo CW, Harralson AF, Folli HL, et al.: Direct determination of tobramycin clearance in patients with mild-to-moderate cystic fibrosis. *DICP* 1987; 21:639.

47. Prandota J: Drug disposition in cystic fibrosis: Progress in understanding pathophysiology and pharmacokinetics. *Pediatr Infect Dis* 1987; 6:1111.

48. Kearns GL, Hilman BC, Wilson JT: Dosing implications of altered gentamicin disposition in patients with cystic fibrosis. *J Pediatr* 1982; 100:312.

49. Jusko WJ, Mosovich LL, Gerbract LM, et al.: Enhanced renal excretion of dicloxacillin in patients with cystic fibrosis. *Pediatrics* 1975; 56:1038.

50. Spino M, Chai RP, Isles AF, et al.: Assessment of glomerular filtration rate and effective renal plasma flow in cystic fibrosis. *J Pediatr* 1985; 107:64.

51. Aladjem M, Lotan, Boichis H, et al.: Renal function in patients with cystic fibrosis. *Nephron* 1983; 34:84.

52. Vawter GF, Shwachman H: Cystic fibrosis in adults: An autopsy study. *Pathol Annu* 1979; 14:357.

53. Abramowsky CF, Swinehart GL: The nephropathy of cystic fibrosis: A human model of chronic nephrotoxicity. *Human Pathol* 1982; 13:934.

54. Robson AM, Tateishi S, Inglefinger JR, et al.: Renal function in patients with cystic fibrosis. *J Pediatr* 1971; 79:42.

55. Berg V, Kusoffsky E, Strandvik B: Renal function in cystic fibrosis with special reference to the renal sodium handling. *Acta Paediatr Scan* 1982; 71:833.

56. Rosenthal A, Button LN, Khaw KT: Blood volume changes in patients with cystic fibrosis. *Pediatrics* 1977; 59:588.

57. Brenner BM, Baylis C, Deen WM: Transport of molecules across renal glomerular capillaries. *Physiol Rev* 1976; 56:502.

58. MacDonald NE, Anas NG, Peterson RG, et al.: Renal clearance of gentamicin in cystic fibrosis. *J Pediatr* 1983; 103:985.

59. Winnie GB, Cooper JA, Witson J, et al.: Comparison of 6 and 8 hourly tobramycin dosing intervals in treatment of pulmonary exacerbations in cystic fibrosis patients. *Pediatr Infect Dis J* 1991; 10:381.

60. Touw DJ, Vinks ATMM, Heijerman HGM, et al.: Suggestions for the optimization of the initial tobramycin dose in adolescent and adult patients with cystic fibrosis. *Ther Drug Monit* 1994; 16:125.

61. Hsu MC, Aguila HA, Schmidt VL, et al.: Individualization of tobramycin dosage in patients with cystic fibrosis. *Pediatr Infect Dis* 1984; 3:526.

62. Touw DJ, Vinks AA, Heijerman HG, et al.: Validation of tobramycin monitoring in adolescent and adult patients with cystic fibrosis. *Ther Drug Monit* 1993; 15:52.

63. Kelly HB, Menendez R, Fan L, Murphy S: Pharmacokinetics of tobramycin in cystic fibrosis. *J Pediatr* 1982; 100:318.

64. Kearns G, Hilman BC, Wilson JT: Dosing implications of altered gentamicin disposition in patients with cystic fibrosis. *J Pediatr* 1982; 100:312.

65. Levy J, Smith AL, Koup JR, et al.: Disposition of tobramycin in patients with cystic fibrosis. *J Pediatr* 1984; 105:117.

66. Pleasants R, Williams D, Waltner W, et al.: Comparative disposition of tobramycin in adult cystic fibrosis patients and normal adults (abstr). *Clin Pharmacol Ther* 1989; 45:150.

67. Pleasants RA, Williams DM, Waltner WE, Knowles MR: Influence of infusion method on serum concentrations in adults with cystic fibrosis. *Clin Pharm* 1990; 9:541.

68. Hendeles L, Iafrate RP, Stilwell PC, Mangos JA: Individualizing gentamicin dosage in patients with cystic fibrosis: Limitations to pharmacokinetic approach. *J Pediatr* 1987; 110:303.

69. Bates RD, Nahata MC: Once-daily administration of aminoglycosides. *Ann Pharmacother* 1994; 28:757.

70. Barclay ML, Begg EJ, Hickling KG: What is the evidence for once-daily aminoglycoside therapy? *Clin Pharmacokinet* 1994; 27:32.

71. Vogelman BS, Craig WA: Postantibiotic effects. *J Antimicrob Chemother* 1985; 15:37.

72. Littlewood JM, Smye SW, Cunliffe H: Aerosol antibiotic treatment in cystic fibrosis. *Arch Dis Child* 1993; 68(6):788.

73. Hodson ME, Penketh ARL, Batten JC: Aerosol carbenicillin and gentamicin treatment of *Pseudomonas aeruginosa* infection in patients with cystic fibrosis. *Lancet* 1981; 2:1137.

74. Stead RJ, Hodson ME, Batten JC: Inhaled ceftazidime compared with gentamicin and carbenicillin in older patients with cystic fibrosis infected with *Pseudomonas aeruginosa*. *Br J Dis Chest* 1987; 81:272.

75. Jensen T, Pedersen SS, Garne S, et al.: Colistin inhalation therapy in cystic fibrosis patients with chronic *Pseudomonas aeruginosa* lung infection *J Antimicrob Chemother* 1987; 19:831.

76. Schaad UB, Wedgwood-Krucko J, Suter S, Kraemer R: Efficacy of inhaled amikacin as adjunct to intravenous combination therapy (ceftazidime and amikacin) in cystic fibrosis. *J Pediatr* 1987; 111:599.

77. Cooper DM, Harris M, Mitchell I: Comparison of intravenous and inhalation antibiotic therapy in acute pulmonary deterioration in cystic fibrosis. *Am Rev Respir Dis* 1985; 131:A242.

78. Semsarian C: Efficacy of inhaled tobramycin in cystic fibrosis. *J Paediatr Child Health* 1990; 26:110.

79. Littlewood JM, Miller MG, Ghonheim AT, Ramsden CH: Nebulised colomycin for early *Pseudomonas* colonisation in cystic fibrosis. *Lancet* 1985; 1:865.

80. Levy J, Smith AL, Kenny MA, et al.: Bioactivity of gentamicin in purulent sputum from patients with cystic fibrosis or bronchiectasis: Comparison with activity in serum. *J Infect Dis* 1983; 148:1069.

81. Eisenberg J: Safety, efficacy and pharmacokinetics of tobramycin (Tobra) administered by three different nebulizer delivery systems: Late-breaking science abstracts. Eighth Annual North American Cystic Fibrosis Conference, Session S5.6, 1994.

82. Newman SP, Agnew JE, Pavia D, Clarke SW: Inhaled aerosols: Lung deposition and clinical applications. *Clin Phys Physiol Meas* 1987; 3:1.

83. Newman SP, Clarke SW: Nebulisers: Uses and abuses. *Arch Dis Child* 1986; 61:424.

84. Clay MM, Pavia D, Newman SP: Factors influencing the size distribution of aerosols from jet nebulisers. *Thorax* 1983; 38:755.

85. Clay MM, Pavia D, Newman SP, et al.: Assessment of jet nebulisers for lung aerosol therapy. *Lancet* 1983; 2:592.

86. Newman SP, Pellow PGD, Clay MM, Clark SW: Evaluation of jet nebulisers for use with gentamicin solution. *Thorax* 1985; 40:671.

Chapter 94

ALLERGIC BRONCHOPULMONARY ASPERGILLOSIS AND PREGNANCY IN CYSTIC FIBROSIS

THOMAS M. MURPHY, CHRIS RUDD, AND WAYNE SAMUELSON

Allergic Bronchopulmonary Aspergillosis

Pregnancy

Allergic Bronchopulmonary Aspergillosis

The progressive airway disease in cystic fibrosis (CF) predisposes patients to colonization by *Aspergillus* species. However, this seldom results in parenchymal destruction. Instead, *Aspergillus fumigatus* is capable of inducing an intense hypersensitivity reaction in the airways known as allergic bronchopulmonary aspergillosis (ABPA). This process presents clinically as mucoid impaction of proximal bronchi, segmental or lobar collapse, and bronchiectasis. It first was described in CF patients more than 25 years ago.[1] The incidence in CF patients is estimated variously at rates of 0.5 to 11 percent, depending on the criteria used and the location.[2–4]

Major and minor diagnostic criteria have been established for the diagnosis of ABPA in CF (Table 94-1). The diagnosis is made in the presence of five major criteria or four major and two minor criteria. Making a firm diagnosis is frequently difficult because the typical CF exacerbation is associated with many of the signs and symptoms of ABPA. Many CF patients have evidence of immunologic response to *Aspergillus*. Thirty percent of apparently unaffected CF patients may have positive immediate skin tests and precipitating antibodies to *Aspergillus*.[5–7] *Aspergillus* is recovered incidentally from up to 70 percent of sputum cultures of CF patients. The severity of lung disease in CF does not appear to correlate with the development of ABPA.[8]

The treatment for ABPA is corticosteroid therapy in doses of 0.5 to 1 mg/kg/day of prednisone. There are no clear recommendations for duration of therapy. Prednisone is generally administered at the higher dose range for 2 to 3 weeks, followed by a taper over 2 to 6 months. Symptoms, serum IgE concentrations, and radiographs can be used to monitor the efficacy of therapy.[9,10]

Pregnancy

There has long been concern about the effects of pregnancy on women with CF. In a 1976 survey of CF clinics in North America comprising 129 pregnancies in 100 women, 97 (75.2 percent) pregnancies went to term.[11] Twenty-six deliveries (26.8 percent) were preterm and 6 (4.7 percent) were spontaneous abortions. An association was noted between preterm delivery, perinatal death, and a weight gain of less than 4.5 kg during the course of the pregnancy. Corkey and colleagues described a worse outcome in patients who had pancreatic insufficiency, noting that two patients who required enzyme replacement therapy had a greater deterioration in lung function than five who did not require replacement.[12] A more optimistic view was offered by Canny and associates,[13] half of whose patients required pancreatic enzyme replacement. In 38 pregnancies in 25 patients, no difference in outcome was seen on the basis of pancreatic function. The investigators also disputed Larson's earlier conclusions[14] that a prepregnancy forced vital capacity (FVC) of < 50 per-

TABLE 94-1 Diagnostic Criteria of Allergic Bronchopulmonary Aspergillosis (ABPA) in CF[a]

Major criteria
1. Pulmonary infiltrate (often segmental or lobar atelectasis)
2. Bronchodilator-responsive bronchoconstriction
   or
   Clinical airway hyperresponsiveness
   or
   Positive methacholine challenge
3. Positive immediate skin test to extract of *A. fumigatus*
4. Elevated serum IgE (> 300 IU/mL)
5. Precipitating IgG antibodies to *A. fumigatus*

Minor criteria
1. Positive sputum culture for *A. fumigatus*
2. Bronchiectasis of central airways
3. Blood eosinophilia (> 1000/mm³)
4. Russet mucus plugs in sputum

[a] A diagnosis of ABPA is made on the basis of five major criteria or four major criteria plus two minor criteria.
SOURCES: Adapted from Kolls and Beckerman,[8] Rosenberg et al.,[9] and Turpin and Knowles,[15] with permission.

cent of that predicted or the presence of cor pulmonale constituted grounds for termination of pregnancy. Two patients in Canny's series with FVC < 50 percent of predicted completed their pregnancies. The pulmonary status of both patients prior to pregnancy had been stable.

In the Canny series, all patients continued their usual regimens during pregnancy. These consisted of enzymes, vitamins, antibiotics (aminoglycosides, semisynthetic penicillins, cephalosporins), and aerosolized bronchodilators along with chest physiotherapy and nutritional support. Of the 38 pregnancies, 34 were completed. Two infants were preterm, but birthweights were appropriate for gestational age. One term infant delivered by cesarean section to a mother with a pregravid FVC of 49 percent of predicted was small for gestational age. One infant delivered at 31 weeks' gestation died of sepsis after birth. No other neonatal deaths occurred. No congenital abnormalities were noted. The maternal mortality rate within 6 weeks of delivery was zero. However, because maternal pulmonary health may deteriorate during pregnancy, it is recommended that vigorous pulmonary therapy be continued throughout while avoiding certain medications, such as ciprofloxacin, for which there are specific concerns regarding fetal effects.

References

1. Mearns M, Young W, Batten J: Transient pulmonary infiltrations in cystic fibrosis due to allergic aspergillosis. *Thorax* 1965; 20:385.
2. Brueton MJ, Ormerod LP, Shah KJ, Anderson CM: Allergic bronchopulmonary aspergillosis complicating cystic fibrosis in childhood. *Arch Dis Child* 1980; 55:348.
3. Maguire S, Moriarty P, Tempany E, Fitzgerald M: Unusual clustering of allergic bronchopulmonary aspergillosis in children with cystic fibrosis. *Pediatrics* 1988; 82:835.
4. Zeaske R, Bruns WT, Fink JN, et al.: Immune responses to *Aspergillus* in cystic fibrosis. *J Allergy Clin Immunol* 1988; 82:73.
5. Mearns M, Longbottom J, Batten J: Precipitating antibodies to *Aspergillus fumigatus* in cystic fibrosis. *Lancet* 1967; ii:538.
6. Warner JO, Taylor BW, Norman AP, Soothill JF: Association of cystic fibrosis with allergy. *Arch Dis Child* 1976; 51:507.
7. Silverman L, Hobbs FDR, Gordon IRS, Carswell F: Cystic fibrosis, atopy, and airways lability. *Arch Dis Child* 1978; 53:873.
8. Kolls JK, Beckerman RC: Will ABPA occur in your patient with cystic fibrosis? *J Respir Dis* 1991; 12:137.
9. Rosenberg M, Patterson R, Mintzer R, et al.: Clinical and immunologic criteria for the diagnosis of allergic bronchopulmonary aspergillosis. *Ann Intern Med* 1977; 86:405.
10. Hiller JC: Pathogenesis and management of aspergillosis in cystic fibrosis. *Arch Dis Child* 1990; 65:397.
11. Cohen LF, di Sant'Agnese PA, Friedlander J: Cystic fibrosis and pregnancy: A national survey. *Lancet* 1980; ii:842.
12. Corkey CWB, Newth CJL, Corey M, Levison H: Pregnancy in cystic fibrosis: A better prognosis in patients with pancreatic function? *Am J Obstet Gynecol* 1981; 140:737.
13. Canny GJ, Corey M, Livingstone RA, et al.: Pregnancy and cystic fibrosis. *Obstet Gynecol* 1991; 77:850.
14. Larson JW: Cystic fibrosis and pregnancy. *Obstet Gynecol* 1972; 39:880.
15. Turpin SV, Knowles MR: Treatment of pulmonary disease in patients with cystic fibrosis, in Davis PB (ed): *Cystic Fibrosis*. New York: Marcel Dekker, 1993:277–344.

Chapter 95

GENE THERAPY
FOR CYSTIC FIBROSIS

THOMAS M. MURPHY, CHRIS RUDD,
AND WAYNE SAMUELSON

General Considerations

The most exciting development in the pulmonary pharmacology of CF is gene therapy. With identification of the CFTR gene in 1989,[1–3] attention rapidly shifted to the potential for treating the disease by altering genetic structure.[4–7] Evidence for the feasibility of transfer of human CFTR to lung epithelial cells rapidly accumulated.[8–10]

A therapeutic issue that required early clarification was to determine the percentage of cells within the airway that must undergo physiologic correction to achieve clinical benefit. Johnson et al. mixed populations of a CF airway cell line expressing either the normal CFTR cDNA (corrected cells) or a reporter gene in defined percentages.[11] Sheets of cells containing as few as 6 to 10 percent corrected cells within an demonstrated chloride ion transport properties similar to those in sheets made up of 100% corrected cells. This implies an intercellular connection and suggests that in vivo correction of all CF airway cells is probably not necessary to achieve a therapeutic benefit.

It is widely believed that the target for gene therapy most likely to prolong the life of the patient is the airway epithelium.[8] However, because of uncertainty regarding the relative importance of CFTR function in epithelial cell subtypes, it is not known which epithelial cell—ciliated, basal, or mucus-secreting—should be targeted. Hepatobiliary disease also may be amenable to gene therapy.[12] The complex structure of the airways and concomitant infection, inflammation, and mucus hypersecretion pose significant challenges to gene therapy. The bronchial epithelial cells rarely divide, so that there is little opportunity for a transformed cell to propagate. Ex vivo therapy is not an option, as the bronchial epithelium cannot be removed, treated, and reimplanted.

There are several potential methods for delivering gene therapy to the lung. These include (1) receptor-mediated delivery approaches; (2) instilled or aerosolized liposomes; (3) retrovirus-based vectors; (4) adeno-associated virus-based vectors; and (5) virus-mediated plasmid delivery. Each presents its own advantages and disadvantages.

A key principle that permits gene therapy for the recessive genetic disorder of CF is the fact that heterozygotes express a normal phenotype. The normal gene is expressed without interference from the mutant allele. In this sort of "gene augmentation" therapy, the gene is inserted at a site distant from the original locus. Therefore the transcription promoter and other desired regulatory elements must be provided with it.[6] The principal viral vectors felt to be useful for gene transfer are *retroviruses, adenoviruses,* and *adeno-associated viruses.*

Retroviral Vectors

Retroviruses have a single-stranded RNA genome that is converted to DNA by reverse transcriptase carried in the virus particles. Once the retrovirus gains entry into the cell, its genetic information is efficiently inserted into the genome of the host cell.[13] The DNA provirus is integrated randomly into the host-cell genome if the infected cell is dividing rapidly. Viral genes are expressed and new RNA copies are transcribed, with resultant formation of new particles. These virions bud from the producer cell membrane and infect other cells, perpetuating the cycle.[6] A retrovirus vector was used to demonstrate the first successful complementation of the CF defect in vitro.[114] Functional CFTR cDNA was transduced into a pancreatic adenocarcinoma cell line derived from a patient with CF. The cells subsequently demonstrated restoration of cAMP-regulated chloride conductance, consistent with normal CFTR function.

Gene transfer by retrovirus vectors seems to occur only in cells that are dividing rapidly.[15] As noted above, only a small percentage of bronchial epithelial cells are actively dividing at any given time. This limits the effectiveness of the vector.[16] The low titer and the worrisome possibility of insertional mutagenesis are additional disadvantages of the retroviral vector.[17]

Adenoviral Vectors

Adenoviruses (Ad) commonly infect the respiratory and intestinal tracts of humans and thus provide a natural tropism for important target tissues in CF patients. In some initial studies, the tropism of Ad for ciliated epithelial cells proved to be significantly less than that for basal or undifferentiated cells.[18] Unlike the retrovirus, the Ad does not insert into the genome but functions extrachromosomally. While this avoids the theoretical problem of insertional mutagenesis, the genetic program cannot be passed on to target-cell progeny. Thus, it is likely that gene therapy will have to be administered repetitively. Vectors of Ad can be used to transfer genes to nonproliferating cells. Because of extensive experience with certain serotypes of Ad vaccine in the United States military, types 2 and 5 have been utilized. Successful gene transfer was identified in rhesus monkey bronchial epithelium 6 days after exposure to an adenovirus vector.[19] Zabner et al. demonstrated a decrease in the basal transepithelial voltage and restoration of normal response to cAMP after administration of an Ad vector to a defined area of nasal airway epithelium.[20] The same Ad was applied repeatedly to intrapulmonary epithelia in cotton rats and nasal airway epithelia in rhesus monkeys.[21] The vector did not replicate and was cleared rapidly. There was no evidence of a local or systemic inflammatory response. Despite the appearance of an antibody response, the expression of the gene appeared intact, leading the authors to conclude that repeat administration of the Ad vector was both safe and efficacious. Further modification of the Ad was associated with longer recombinant gene expression and less inflammatory response.[22]

Crystal and colleagues administered an Ad vector to the nasal and bronchial epithelium of four individuals with cystic fibrosis.[23] No adverse effects were noted in response to nasal administration. One individual developed transient leukocytosis, fever, and pulmonary infiltrates following bronchial administration of the vector. Another had a more severe response characterized by headache, fatigue, fever, tachycardia, hypotension, and dyspnea. Changes in pulmonary function and radiographic changes also were observed. Despite this, all four individuals have had similar safety parameters throughout a 1-year follow-up.

Adeno-Associated Viral Vectors

The adeno-associated virus (AAV) is a small, single-stranded DNA virus of the parvovirus family. It normally replicates productively only in the presence of a coinfecting adenovirus or herpesvirus. In the absence of helper virus, the AAV undergoes high-frequency stable DNA integration. Because of its integrating capability, the AAV offers potential long-term correction of defective CFTR function. AAV-CFTR vectors have been demonstrated to be effective in complementing the chloride transport defect in CF bronchial epithelial cells.[24] Selective bronchoscopic delivery of AAV-CFTR vectors to the right lower lobe of New Zealand white rabbits resulted in detection of the presence and expression of the vector genome from the airway surface for periods as long as 6 months after infection.[25] The degree of efficiency of expression from the AAV vector suggests that active division of the epithelial cells is not necessary for gene expression. The principal theoretical advantage of AAV over retroviral vectors is relative site-specificity, with less risk of insertional mutagenesis. Adverse immunologic reactions are possible with AAV, and coincident adenovirus infection could lead to unexpected consequences.[6]

Liposome-DNA Complexes

Hyde et al. used liposomes to deliver a CFTR expression plasmid to airway epithelia and to alveoli deep in the lungs

of transgenic mice.[26] Human CFTR expression was seen in the airways of 3 out of 4 animals; in 1 animal, CFTR sequences were detected in all five lobes of the lung. In other studies, variable levels of transgene expression were found both within a single animal (trachea, peripheral lung, rectum) as well as between animals.[27] Although liposomes are less immunogenic than viral vectors, it is still uncertain whether the lower efficiency of this system will prove sufficient to achieve clinical benefit.

Receptor-Mediated Endocytosis

Receptor-mediated endocytosis has also been exploited as a means of delivering genetic material. Molecular conjugates linked to DNA-binding agents have produced transfection in cell-culture studies.[28] The utility of this and all other gene delivery schemes will be best evaluated when the ability to define and evaluate important clinical endpoints improves.[29]

References

1. Rommeus JM, Iannuzzi MC, Kerem BS, et al.: Identification of the cystic fibrosis gene: Chromosome walking and jumping. *Science* 1989; 245:1059.
2. Riordan JR, Rommeus JM, Kerem BS, et al.: Identification of the cystic fibrosis gene: Cloning and characterization of the complementary DNA. *Science* 1989; 245:1066.
3. Kerem BS, Rommeus JM, Buchanan JA, et al.: Identification of the cystic fibrosis gene: Genetic analysis. *Science* 1989; 245:1073.
4. Coutelle C, Caplen N, Hart S, et al.: Gene therapy for cystic fibrosis. *Arch Dis Child* 1993; 68:437.
5. Crystal RG: Gene therapy strategies for pulmonary disease. *Am J Med* 1992; 92(6A):44S.
6. Flotte TR: Prospects for virus-based gene therapy for cystic fibrosis. *J Bioenerg Biomembr* 1993; 25(1):37.
7. Tizzano EF, Buchwald M: Cystic fibrosis: Beyond the gene to therapy. *J Pediatr* 1992; 120:337.
8. Rich DP, Couture LA, Cardoza LM, et al.: Development and analysis of recombinant adenoviruses for gene therapy of cystic fibrosis. *Hum Gene Ther* 1993; 4:461.
9. Rosenfeld MA, Yoshimura K, Trapnell BC, et al.: In vivo transfer of the human cystic fibrosis transmembrane conductance regulator gene to the airway epithelium. *Cell* 1992; 68:143.
10. Whitsett JA, Dey CR, Stripp BR, et al.: Human cystic fibrosis transmembrane conductance regulator directed to respiratory epithelial cells of transgenic mice. *Nature Genet* 1992; 2:13.
11. Johnson LG, Olsen JC, Sarkadi B, et al.: Efficiency of gene transfer for restoration of normal airway epithelial function in cystic fibrosis. *Nature Genet* 1992; 2:21–25.
12. Yang Y, Raper SE, Cohn JA, et al.: An approach for treating the hepatobiliary disease of cystic fibrosis by somatic gene transfer. *Proc Natl Acad Sci USA* 1993; 90:4601.
13. Miller AD: Progress toward human gene therapy. *Blood* 1990; 76:271.
14. Drumm ML, Pope HA, Cliff WH, et al.: Correction of the cystic fibrosis defect in vitro by retrovirus-mediated gene transfer. *Cell* 1990; 62:1227.
15. Miller DG, Adam MA, Miller D: Gene transfer by retrovirus vectors occurs only in cells that are actively replicating at the time of infection. *Mol Cell Biol* 1990; 10:4239.

16. Wilke M, Bout B, Verbeek E, et al.: Amphotropic retroviruses with a hybrid long terminal repeat as a tool for gene therapy of cystic fibrosis. *Biochem Biophys Res Commun* 1992; 187:187.

17. Nusse R, Varmus HE: Many tumors induced by the mouse mammary tumor virus contain a provirus integrated in the same region of the host genome. *Cell* 1982; 32:99.

18. Pickles RJ, Grubb BR, Johnson LG, et al.: Inefficiency of adenoviral gene transfer to airway epithelia in vivo: Cell phenotype dependent transduction. Late-breaking science abstracts. Gene Therapy Session S5a.5, Eighth North American Cystic Fibrosis Conference, 1994.

19. Bout A, Perricaudet M, Gaskin G, et al.: Lung gene therapy: *In Vivo* adenovirus-mediated gene transfer to rhesus monkey airway epithelium. *Hum Gene Ther* 1994; 5:3.

20. Zabner J, Couture LA, Gregory RJ, et al.: Adenovirus-mediated gene transfer transiently corrects the chloride transport defect in nasal epithelia of patients with cystic fibrosis. *Cell* 1993; 75:207.

21. Zabner J, Peterson DM, Puga AP, et al.: Safety and efficacy of repetitive adenovirus-mediated transfer of CFTR cDNA to airway epithelia of primates and cotton rats. *Nature Genetics* 1994; 6:75.

22. Yang Y, Nunes FA, Berencsi K, et al.: Inactivation of E2a in recombinant adenoviruses improves the prospect for gene therapy in cystic fibrosis. *Nature Genetics* 1994; 7:362.

23. Crystal RG, McElvaney NG, Rosenfeld MA, et al.: Administration of an adenovirus containing the human CFTR cDNA to the respiratory tract of individuals with cystic fibrosis. *Nature Genetics* 1994; 8:42.

24. Flotte TR, Solow RA, Owens RA, et al.: Gene expression from adeno-associated virus vectors in airway epithelial cells. *Am J Respir Cell Mol Biol* 1992; 7:349.

25. Flotte TR, Afione SA, Conrad C, et al.: Stable in vivo expression of the cystic fibrosis transmembrane conductance regulator with an adeno-associated virus vector. *Proc Natl Acad Sci USA* 1993; 90:10613.

26. Hyde SC, Gill DR, Higgins CF, et al.: Correction of the ion transport defect in cystic fibrosis transgenic mice by gene therapy. *Nature* 1993; 362:250.

27. Alton EWFW, Middleton PG, Caplen NJ, et al.: Non-invasive liposome-mediated gene delivery can correct the ion transport defect in cystic fibrosis mutant mice. *Nature Genetics* 1993; 5:135.

28. Curiel DT, Agarwal S, Romer MU, et al.: Gene transfer to respiratory epithelial cells via the receptor-mediated endocytosis pathway. *Am J Respir Cell Mol Biol* 1992; 6:247.

29. Alton E, Geddes D: A mixed message for cystic fibrosis gene therapy. *Nature Genetics* 1994; 8:8.

PART 4

PHARMACOLOGY OF PULMONARY EMBOLIC DISEASE

TREATMENT OF PULMONARY EMBOLISM

Chapter 96

NATURAL HISTORY OF PULMONARY EMBOLISM

GREGORY A. SCHMIDT

Incidence of Pulmonary Embolism

In spite of great strides in the understanding of venous thromboembolism, pulmonary embolism (PE) continues to cause substantial morbidity and mortality. Accurate estimates for its incidence and lethality are notoriously difficult to calculate, for reasons largely related to difficulties in diagnosis and data collection.[1,2] In 1975, Dalen and Alpert generated estimates for the numbers of PE deaths in acute hospitals, nursing homes, and the community, using reasonable approximations or extrapolating from known data.[3] They concluded that there were approximately 630,000 cases of pulmonary embolism in the United States each year, of which about 200,000 were lethal. The incidence of PE over the past two decades may be decreasing,[4] but this is controversial.[1] Mortality varies substantially across the United States with highest rates in the South Atlantic and Central States.[5] Men are at increased risk compared with women, as are nonwhites compared to whites, at least during middle age.[4,5]

It has been estimated further that of the roughly 630,000 cases of PE per year, 67,000 die within 1 h, leaving no real chance for diagnosis and medical intervention.[3] Of the remaining 560,000 patients who survive for more than 1 h, the diagnosis is never made in about 400,000. While some of this failure to diagnose is surely a part of appropriate management in patients who are hopelessly or terminally ill, often such failure results from misunderstanding of the presenting manifestations of PE and of the limitations of tests commonly used to diagnose PE.[6] There are two important points to draw from this: (1) since about one-third of patients who will ultimately die of PE die within the first hour after embolism, prophylaxis against PE is vitally important and the only effective way to reduce these 67,000 deaths (see Chap. 99); (2) physicians need to understand better the clinical presentation of PE and its diagnosis (see Chap. 97).

Risk Factors

In the majority of patients with proven thromboembolism, a risk factor for thrombosis can be discerned. This point is most useful in the patient lacking in risk factors, who is very unlikely to have PE. For such patients, an alternative expla-

TABLE 96-1 Risk Factors for Venous Thromboembolism.

Malignancy, especially metastatic, mucinous adenocarcinoma
Trauma, including surgery, and fractures
Pregnancy, but more importantly postpartum and postcesarean section
Estrogen therapy
Heart failure and myocardial infarction
Chronic obstructive lung disease and pulmonary hypertension
Stroke and spinal cord injury
Prior venous thromboembolism
Hypercoagulable states
    Deficiencies of proteins C, S, and antithrombin III
    Excessive plasiminogen activator inhibitor
    Antiphospholipid antibody syndromes
    Paroxysmal nocturnal hemoglobinuria
    Polycythemia
Advanced age
Obesity
Immobility
Central venous catheters

nation for symptoms prompting consideration of the diagnosis of PE should be sought. In patients who appear to have idiopathic venous thrombosis, a significant minority have occult malignancy. For example, when patients with no apparent predisposing risk factor were followed for 2 years after venous thromboembolism (VTE), 7.6 percent were found to have a malignancy, compared with only 1.9 percent of a group of patients with VTE caused by a recognized risk factor.[7]

Established risk factors for venous thromboembolism include malignancy, heart failure, obstructive airway disease, fractures, trauma, recent surgery, myocardial infarction, obesity, stroke, advanced age, pregnancy and the puerperium, spinal cord injury, prior thromboembolism, hypercoagulable states such as protein C deficiency, and the presence of intravascular catheters[8-21] (Table 96-1). The magnitude of risk resulting from these predisposing factors is known rarely except for postoperative VTE[22] and deep venous thrombosis (DVT) related to spinal cord injury.[23] Studies revealing the incidence of VTE in patients with acute myocardial infarction predate the era of thrombolytic therapy and frequent use of anticoagulation, and probably cannot be applied usefully to the modern era. Similarly, the reduced dose of estrogen used now in oral contraceptives and for postmenopausal replacement may not significantly increase the risk of VTE.[24] Moreover, some factors, such as age, clearly increase the risk of VTE—but without a clear threshold that separates those at risk from those who are not—and these are therefore not very helpful in estimating clinical probability of VTE in an individual patient.

Pathophysiology of Venous Thromboembolism

Although the two clinical syndromes, DVT and PE often are discussed separately, there are reasons to consider them as part of a spectrum of illness called venous thromboembolism.[6] This seems especially useful given the high incidence of DVT found in patients with proven PE (43 to 57 percent[25,26]) and the high likelihood of PE in patients with proximal DVT, even in those lacking symptoms (40 to 50 percent[27]). In most patients, venous thrombosis begins with the formation of microthrombi at a site of venous stasis or injury, typically in the vicinity of a venous valve in the calf. Thrombosis impedes flow and generates further vascular injury, favoring progressive clot formation. The thrombus activates the clotting cascade and also the endogenous fibrinolytic system. If thrombosis outpaces fibrinolysis, clot becomes substantial and propagates. Alternatively, the thrombus may resolve or organize, potentially damaging the venous valve, leading to venous incompetence.

In the postoperative setting, about 20 percent of distal thrombi enlarge to involve proximal veins,[28] where they have a far greater potential to embolize to the pulmonary circulation than a distal thrombus. In a comparison of patients with proximal versus distal DVT, 8 of 15 with proximal thrombosis had PE, whereas none of 21 with calf-only thrombosis had PE.[29] From the proximal leg veins, thrombus occasionally extends to the iliac veins or the vena cava. In a large group of patients diagnosed with DVT, 42 of 364 had thrombus confined to the tibial veins, while 30 patients had clot extending just to the popliteal vein. More proximal extension to the femoral vein was seen in 166 patients, to the iliac vein in 69, and into the inferior vena cava in 57.[27] Thus, 72 of 364 (20 percent) had distal thrombosis and 80 percent had proximal DVT. Occasionally, thrombus appears to originate in a proximal vein, such as the iliac vein, but this is uncommon. For example, in one study, only 2 of 49 limbs examined with impedance plethysmography (IPG) and duplex ultrasound had isolated iliac thrombus.[30] However, there are important exceptions to the general rule that popliteal and femoral thrombosis precedes pelvic thrombosis. In pregnancy, there appears to be an unusually high incidence of isolated iliac vein or iliofemoral thrombosis. In one study, 5 of 17 gravidas had isolated pelvic thrombosis.[31] This difference in incidence of pelvic thrombosis implies a different pathophysiology of DVT in pregnancy, often ascribed to compression of the iliac veins by the enlarged uterus. Other patients may have an alternative anatomic basis for an atypical, isolated iliac thrombus, such as pelvic malignancy, femoral vein catheterization, or iliac artery aneurysm. Occasionally emboli originate in the upper limbs,[32] the pelvic or renal veins, or the right heart.

More than 90 percent of clinically relevant pulmonary emboli originate from proximal venous thrombi in the lower extremities.[6,25] Pulmonary embolism occurs when thrombi detach and are carried through the great veins to the pulmonary circulation, an event estimated to complicate 50 percent of proximal DVTs.[27,33] The number of patients in whom embolization is asymptomatic is striking. In several large studies of patients with DVT, asymptomatic PEs were found in nearly 50 percent.[27,33,34] Most often, however, pulmonary vascular occlusion has important physiologic consequences, which lead to manifestations of illness as well as to clues to diagnosis. Pulmonary embolization affects most notably gas exchange and the circulation.

GAS EXCHANGE

Physical obstruction to pulmonary artery flow creates dead space in the segments served by the affected arteries. This creation of dead space tends to raise P_{CO_2}, but this is offset in most patients by an increment in minute ventilation. Thus, most patients with PE have a decreased P_{CO_2} unless they are unable to augment minute ventilation (e.g., severe lung disease or mechanical ventilation). A widened alveolar-to-arterial gradient for oxygen is present in the majority of patients with PE. However, since hyperventilation is the rule, the arterial P_{O_2} may not be decreased. In fact, only two-thirds of patients with proven PE demonstrate a $P_{O_2} < 70$ mmHg.[35,36] Neither a normal P_{O_2} nor a normal alveolar-arterial gradient excludes a diagnosis of PE.[35,37]

The mechanisms of hypoxemia have been elucidated by applying the multiple inert gas elimination technique (MIGET) to patients with PE.[38,39] Shunt is found in only a few patients. In some, this may be due to opening of a probe-patent foramen ovale when right atrial pressure increases following PE, which causes intracardiac right-to-left shunt. Since shunt is more commonly found when patients are studied after some delay, atelectasis caused by impaired surfactant production may contribute. In most patients, however, the most important pulmonary derangement is mismatching of ventilation and perfusion. In addition, the decrease in cardiac output that accompanies most pulmonary emboli leads to a decrease in mixed venous saturation.[39,40] This lowered venous saturation magnifies any hypoxemia caused by shunt or ventilation-perfusion mismatch.

While impaired oxygenation is important and often provides a clue to the diagnosis of PE, it is typically responsive to modest oxygen enrichment of inspired gas. Similarly, most patients are able to double or triple minute ventilation if necessary so that ventilatory failure is uncommon following PE. In fact, the greatest impact of pulmonary embolization is on the circulation, not on gas exchange. While there are exceptions (e.g., some patients with severe chronic obstructive pulmonary disease), morbidity and mortality from PE relate to cardiovascular compromise—not respiratory failure.

CIRCULATION

Pulmonary embolization obstructs the pulmonary vascular bed mechanically as well as through presumed humoral and other mechanisms. This increases right ventricular (RV) afterload which, compounded by tachycardia, increases right ventricular oxygen consumption. The right ventricle dilates and thins, its wall tension rises, and coronary perfusion is impeded. At the same time, pulmonary vascular obstruction hinders cardiac output and additionally causes hypoxemia. Therefore, just at the time when the right ventricle needs increased oxygen delivery, the left ventricle may not be able to supply it. The superposition of increased right heart oxygen demand on decreased oxygen supply puts the right ventricle at risk for ischemia, which can cause failure of the right heart (acute cor pulmonale). Studies in dogs with acute experimental PE support the hypothesis that ischemia underlies acute cor pulmonale.[41] Similarly, in patients with PE, the MB isoenzyme fraction of creatinine kinase occasionally suggests the presence of right ventricular infarction.[42]

If acute pulmonary vascular obstruction is sufficiently massive to cause mean pulmonary artery pressure to exceed approximately 40 mmHg to maintain cardiac output, the right heart will fail abruptly. This likely is the cause of sudden death in patients with large pulmonary emboli. On the other hand, small pulmonary emboli are unlikely to compromise the circulation (or lead to death), but instead manifest as dyspnea, hypoxemia, or chest pain (or remain undetected).

Following massive, but sublethal, PE the right ventricle dilates to a larger end-diastolic volume. This is associated with increased right atrial and ventricular pressures and abnormally low cardiac output. Echocardiographic evidence of RV hypokinesis also predicts patients at greater than usual risk of recurrence.[43] One consequence of increased right atrial pressure is the potential for right-to-left shunting across a probe-patent foramen ovale. This could allow paradoxical embolization to the systemic circulation as well as contribute to hypoxemia. The increase in right ventricular pressure and volume also affects the left heart. A change in shape of the right ventricle and corresponding shift of the interventricular septum from right to left alters the diastolic pressure-volume characteristics of the left ventricle. The consequent reduction in left ventricular compliance impairs diastolic filling, thereby reducing left ventricular preload and creating yet another obstacle to cardiac output.

The Pace of Recovery Following Pulmonary Embolism

The typical recovery of the pulmonary circulation following PE is known from studies in which patients underwent repeat right heart catheterization, echocardiography, or serial perfusion lung scanning. The rate of restoration of pulmonary flow as demonstrated by these studies is slower than is generally believed by clinicians. For example, when patients were treated with heparin or caval ligation (or both), there was only minimal angiographic and hemodynamic resolution at 7 days.[44] By 10 to 21 days, right-sided heart pressures had returned nearly to normal, but the earliest complete resolution of any patient's angiogram was at 14 days. The earliest reported complete resolution of an embolus is at 7 days following the acute embolism.[45] In 1967, Tow and Wagner reported on serial lung scans in patients with PE, most of whom had received standard anticoagulant therapy.[46] Of those with minimal embolic involvement (1 to 15 percent of the pulmonary circulation affected on the initial scan), only 25 percent of patients showed complete recovery of perfusion at 2 weeks, while of those with intermediate involvement (16 to 30 percent), 15 percent had normal scans after that interval. In the latter group, the earliest evidence of significant improvement of perfusion was on the sixth day and the earliest complete resolution was on the eighth day. In patients with severe involvement (31 to 50 percent), the earliest recovery was seen on the 60th day.[46] In

1968, Murphy and Bulloch studied 31 episodes of pulmonary embolism and found that 4 of 12 scans had normalized 1 week following embolization, 3 of 13 at 2 weeks, and 3 of 9 at 4 weeks.[47]

Even when thrombolytic therapy is given, perfusion scans and angiograms can remain abnormal for several days to months. In the report of the Urokinase Pulmonary Embolism Trial (UPET),[48] patients receiving urokinase plus heparin demonstrated greater angiographic resolution at 24 h compared with patients given only heparin, but in both groups the improvement was slight (8 versus 22 percent). Nevertheless, this degree of improvement may be hemodynamically (and potentially clinically) significant, even within the first few hours, as demonstrated by echocardiography (RV end-diastolic diameter from 3.9 to 2.0 cm at 9 h) and pulmonary artery pressures (PA systolic pressure from 42 to 26 mmHg).[49] Perfusion lung scanning following either a 0.6 mg/kg bolus of rt-PA or 100 mg over 2 h showed only a 10 to 13 percent improvement in pulmonary perfusion at 24 h.[50,51] Pulmonary perfusion assessed by lung scanning improved 50 percent only after 14 days in the UPET trial.[48] In a more recent study with rt-PA, a similar degree of resolution was noted (percent vascular obstruction as determined by perfusion scintigraphy from 74 percent at baseline to 43 percent at day 10).[52] The relevance of these findings is that diagnostic studies for PE need not be performed on an urgent basis out of concern for detecting a "fleeting" abnormality. Often it may be appropriate to begin heparin anticoagulation, planning for diagnostic evaluation when the patient is stabilized and high-quality studies can be assured.

RECURRENCE DESPITE ANTICOAGULATION

Recurrent embolism is uncommon in patients who are adequately anticoagulated.[53] In a study that compared subcutaneous versus intravenous heparin, only 1.6 percent of patients experienced recurrence when adequately anticoagulated by 24 h.[54] In contrast, those who were not adequately heparinized had a much higher rate of recurrence (24.5 percent). In another survey of anticoagulated patients with both PE and proximal DVT, the rate of recurrence was only 4 percent.[55] These investigators also concluded that new perfusion defects in therapy were not a specific indicator of recurrence, since three of four such patients had no new findings on repeat angiography. At 1-year follow-up, 21 of 160 patients (13 percent) had recurrences in the Prospective Investigation of Pulmonary Embolism Diagnosis (PIOPED) trial, 4 of them fatal.[24]

PROGRESSION TO CHRONIC PULMONARY HYPERTENSION

Despite the persistence of perfusion defects for many days to months, it appears that very few patients progress to pulmonary hypertension following a single episode of acute embolization. In a group of patients who had angiography at the time of initial diagnosis, then again several years (average 4.8 years) later, none of 12 patients with a single acute PE subsequently developed pulmonary hypertension.[56]

This contrasted with patients who initially had subacute embolism or occult embolism or were being treated for recurrent embolism. These patients often died of cor pulmonale during follow-up or had persistent severe pulmonary hypertension at reevaluation. In another follow-up study of 60 patients who had PE, perfusion defects had completely resolved in 65 percent (mean time to reevaluation, 29 months), were partially resolved in 23 percent, and were unresolved in only 12 percent.[57] Chronic cor pulmonale was present in only one patient.

Further evidence supporting the generally good outcome of adequately treated PE comes from a large series of patients operated on for chronic thromboembolic pulmonary hypertension.[58] Of 42 such patients at the University of California, San Diego, < 20 percent ever had their acute embolus diagnosed and treated. Combined with the rarity of chronic thromboembolic pulmonary hypertension, the small fraction who had a diagnosis of acute PE suggests that chronic sequelae of PE are quite uncommon. Otherwise, there should be large numbers of patients with chronic thromboembolic pulmonary hypertension resulting from prior PE, and they should dominate series of thromboembolectomy. Thus, improvements in the long-term outcome of patients with PE probably will be based not on better thrombolytic regimens or more aggressive surgical embolectomy, but instead on more accurate early diagnosis and institution of effective anticoagulation.

References

1. Alpert JS, Dalen JE: Epidemiology and natural history of venous thromboembolism. *Prog Cardiovasc Dis* 1994; 36:417.
2. Carter CJ: The natural history and epidemiology of venous thrombosis. *Prog Cardiovasc Dis* 1994; 36:423.
3. Dalen JE, Alpert JS: Natural history of pulmonary embolism. *Prog Cardiovasc Dis* 1975; 17:259.
4. Lilienfeld DE, Chan E, Ehland J, et al.: Mortality from pulmonary embolism in the United States: 1962 to 1984. *Chest* 1990; 98:1067.
5. Lilienfeld DE, Godbold JH: Geographic distribution of pulmonary embolism mortality rates in the United States, 1980 to 1984. *Am Heart J* 1992; 124:1068.
6. Moser KM: Venous thromboembolism. *Am Rev Respir Dis* 1990; 141:235.
7. Prandoni P, Lensing AWA, Büller HR, et al.: Deep-vein thrombosis and the incidence of subsequent symptomatic cancer. *N Engl J Med* 1992; 327:1128.
8. Anderson FA, Wheeler HB, Goldberg RJ, et al.: A population-based perspective of the hospital incidence and case-fatality rates of deep venous thrombosis and pulmonary embolism. *Arch Intern Med* 1991; 151:933.
9. Laissue JA, Gebbers JO, Musy JP: Embolie pulmonaire: Epidemiologie et pathologie. *Schwiez Med Wschr* 1984; 114:1711.
10. Treffers PE, Huidekoper BI, Weenink GH, et al.: Epidemiological observations of thromboembolic disease during pregnancy and in the puerperium in 56,022 women. *Int J. Gynaecol Obstet* 1983; 21:327.
11. Bonnar J: Venous thromboembolism and pregnancy. *Clin Obstet Gynaecol* 1981; 8:456.
12. Rutherford SE, Phelan JP: Thromboembolic disease in pregnancy. *Clin Perinatol* 1986; 13:719.
13. Aaro LA, Juergens JL: Thrombophlebitis associated with pregnancy. *Am J Obstet Gynecol* 1971; 109:1129.

14. Sachs BP, Brown DAJ, Driscoll SG: Maternal mortality in Massachusetts: Trends and prevention. *N Engl J Med* 1987; 316:667.

15. Chastre J, Cornud F, Bouchama A, et al.: Thrombosis as a complication of pulmonary-artery catheterization via the internal jugular vein. *N Engl J Med* 1982; 306:278.

16. Goldhaber SZ, Savage DD, Garrison RJ, et al.: Risk factors for pulmonary embolism: The Framingham study. *Am J Med* 1983; 74:1023.

17. Winter JH, Buckler PW, Bautista AP, et al.: Frequency of venous thrombosis in patients with an exacerbation of chronic obstructive lung disease. *Thorax* 1983; 38:605.

18. Ginsberg KS, Liang MH, Newcomer L, et al.: Anticardiolipin antibodies and the risk for ischemic stroke and venous thrombosis. *Ann Intern Med* 1992; 117:997.

19. Bolan CD, Krishnamurti C, Tang DB, et al.: Association of protein S deficiency with thrombosis in a kindred with increased levels of plasminogen activator inhibitor-1. *Ann Intern Med* 1993; 119:779.

20. Demers C, Ginsberg JS, Hirsh J, et al.: Thrombosis in antithrombin-III-deficient persons: Report of a large kindred and literature review. *Ann Intern Med* 1992; 116:754.

21. Broekmans AW, Veltkamp JJ, Bertina RM: Congenital protein C deficiency and venous thromboembolism: A study of three Dutch families. *N Engl J Med* 1983; 309:340.

22. Clagett GP, Anderson FA, Levine MN, et al.: Prevention of venous thromboembolism. *Chest* 1992; 102(suppl):391S.

23. Weingarden SI: Deep venous thrombosis in spinal cord injury: Overview of the problem. *Chest* 1992; 102(suppl):636S.

24. Quinn DA, Thompson BT, Terrin ML, et al.: A prospective investigation of pulmonary embolism in men and women. *JAMA* 1992; 268:1689.

25. Hull RD, Hirsh J, Carter CJ, et al.: Pulmonary angiography, ventilation lung scanning, and venography for clinically suspected pulmonary embolism with abnormal perfusion lung scan. *Ann Intern Med* 1983; 98:891.

26. Hull RD, Hirsh J, Carter CJ, et al.: Diagnostic value of ventilation-perfusion lung scanning in patients with suspected pulmonary embolism. *Chest* 1985; 88:819.

27. Monreal M, Ruíz J, Olazabel A, et al.: Deep venous thrombosis and the risk of pulmonary embolism: A systemic study. *Chest* 1992; 102:677.

28. Kakkar VV, Howe CT, Flanc C, et al.: Natural history of postoperative deep vein thrombosis. *Lancet* 1969; ii:230.

29. Moser KM, LeMoine JR: Is embolic risk conditioned by location of deep venous thrombosis? *Ann Intern Med* 1981; 94:12.

30. Mantoni M: Deep venous thrombosis: Longitudinal study with duplex US. *Radiology* 1991; 179:271.

31. Bergqvist A, Bergqvist D, Hallbook T: Deep vein thrombosis during pregnancy: A prospective study. *Acta Obstet Gynecol Scand* 1983; 62:443.

32. Monreal M, Lafoz E, Ruiz J, et al.: Upper-extremity deep venous thrombosis and pulmonary embolism: A prospective study. *Chest* 1991; 99:280.

33. Huisman MV, Büller HR, ten Cate JW, et al.: Unexpected high prevalence of silent pulmonary embolism in patients with deep venous thrombosis. *Chest* 1989; 95:498.

34. Moser KM, Fedullo PF, LittleJohn JK, et al.: Frequent asymptomatic pulmonary embolism in patients with deep venous thrombosis. *JAMA* 1994; 271:223.

35. D'Alonzo GE, Dantzker, DR: Gas exchange alterations following pulmonary thromboembolism. *Clin Chest Med* 1984; 5:411.

36. Stein PD, Terrin ML, Hales CA, et al.: Clinical, laboratory, roentgenographic, and electrocardiographic findings in patients with acute pulmonary embolism and no pre-existing cardiac or pulmonary disease. *Chest* 1991; 100:598.

37. Stein PD, Goldhaber SZ, Henry JW: Alveolar-arterial oxygen gradient in the assessment of acute pulmonary embolism. *Chest* 1995; 107:139.

38. Huet Y, Lemaire F, Brun-Buisson C, et al.: Hypoxemia in acute pulmonary embolism. *Chest* 1985; 88:829.

39. Manier G, Castaing Y, Guenard H: Determinants of hypoxemia during the acute phase of pulmonary embolism in humans. *Am Rev Respir Dis* 1985; 132:332.

40. Manier G, Castaing Y: Influence of cardiac output on oxygen exchange in acute pulmonary embolism. *Am Rev Respir Dis* 1992; 145:130.

41. Vlahakes GJ, Turley K, Hoffman JIE: The pathophysiology of failure in acute right ventricular hypertension: Hemodynamic and biochemical correlates. *Circulation* 1981; 63:87.

42. Adams JE, Siegel BA, Goldstein JA, et al.: Elevations of CK-MB following pulmonary embolism: A manifestation of occult right ventricular infarction. *Chest* 1992; 101:1203.

43. Wolfe MW, Lee RT, Feldstein ML, et al.: Prognostic significance of right ventricular hypokinesis and perfusion lung scan defects in pulmonary embolism. *Am Heart J* 1994; 127:1371.

44. Dalen JE, Banas JS, Brooks HL, et al.: Resolution rate of acute pulmonary embolism in man. *N Engl J Med* 1969; 280:1194.

45. Fred HL, Axelrod MA, Lewis JM, et al.: Rapid resolution of pulmonary thromboemboli in man. *JAMA* 1966; 196:1137.

46. Tow DE, Wagner HN: Recovery of pulmonary arterial blood flow in patients with pulmonary embolism. *New Eng J Med* 1967; 276:1053.

47. Murphy ML, Bulloch RT: Factors influencing the restoration of blood flow following pulmonary embolization as determined by angiography and scanning. *Circulation* 1968; 37:1116.

48. Urokinase Pulmonary Embolism Trial (Phase 1 Results): *JAMA* 1970; 214:2163.

49. Come PC, Kim D, Parker JA, et al.: Early reversal of right ventricular dysfunction in patients with acute pulmonary embolism after treatment with intravenous tissue plasminogen activator. *J Am Coll Cardiol* 1987; 10:971.

50. Sors H, Pacouret G, Azarian R, et al.: Hemodynamic effects of bolus vs 2-h infusion of alteplase in acute massive pulmonary embolism: A randomized controlled multicenter trial. *Chest* 1994; 106:712.

51. Goldhaber SZ, Agnelli G, Levine MN, et al.: Reduced dose bolus alteplase vs conventional alteplase infusion for pulmonary embolism thrombolysis: An international multicenter randomized trial. *Chest* 1994; 106:718.

52. Diehl JL, Meyer G, Igual J, et al.: *Am J Cardiol* 1992; 70:1477.

53. Pineo GF, Hull RD: Classical anticoagulant therapy for venous thromboembolism. *Prog Cardiovasc Dis* 1994; 37:59.

54. Hull RD, Raskob GE, Hirsh J, et al.: Continuous intravenous heparin compared with intermittent subcutaneous heparin in the initial treatment of proximal-vein thrombosis. *N Engl J Med* 1986; 315:1109.

55. Girard P, Mathieu, M Simonneau G, et al.: Recurrence of pulmonary embolism during anticoagulant treatment: A prospective study. *Thorax* 1987; 42:481.

56. Riedel M, Stanek V, Widimsky J, et al.: Longterm follow-up of patients with pulmonary thromboembolism: Late prognosis and evolution of hemodynamic and respiratory data. *Chest* 1982; 81:151.

57. Paraskos JA, Adelstein SJ, Smith RE, et al.: Late prognosis of acute pulmonary embolism. *N Engl J Med* 1973; 289:55.

58. Moser KM, Daily PO, Peterson K, et al.: Thromboendarterectomy for chronic, major-vessel thromboembolic pulmonary hypertension. *Ann Intern Med* 1987; 107:560.

Chapter 97

DIAGNOSIS OF PULMONARY EMBOLISM

GREGORY A. SCHMIDT

The diagnosis of pulmonary embolism (PE) is one of the most challenging in medicine. Often the symptoms and signs are nonspecific and they may resolve spontaneously without diagnosis or treatment. Readily available clinical tests for PE are commonly abnormal, but often in a nonspecific way. Moreover, the diagnostic stratagems are sometimes complex and often must be tailored to the peculiarities of a particular patient. Arriving at the diagnosis may depend on navigating a complicated path of subtle hints, vague abnormalities, indeterminate tests, and an extensive literature. Thus, physicians often fail to diagnose PE, despite potentially serious consequences.[1] For example, it has been estimated that fewer than one-third of PEs are diagnosed antemortem.[2] To do better, clinicians should (1) consider the diagnosis, (2) make the greatest diagnostic efforts in patients with risk factors (see Chap. 96), and (3) know the limitations of their diagnostic tests.

Occasionally, an empirical diagnosis of pulmonary embolism seems clear cut. There may be no alternative diagnoses that seem plausible, or further diagnostic steps (e.g., pulmonary angiography) seem too much trouble. While this approach may at times seem attractive, it often is incorrect. First, the clinical diagnoses of both venous thrombosis and PE are too unreliable, even for the most experienced clini-

cian. Second, one always can expand the differential diagnosis beyond PE. Finally, the doubt that lingers after an empirical diagnosis too frequently haunts subsequent management. Progression of symptoms or signs despite therapy raises questions about failure of treatment or the need for alternative treatments. Complications of treatment (usually hemorrhage due to heparin, occasionally thrombocytopenia) create uncertainty about the necessity of the toxic therapy or precipitate more diagnostic interventions in a newly unstable state. For these reasons, empiricism is rarely appropriate. Recommendations for diagnostic management are discussed below and summarized in Fig. 97-1.

Symptoms and Signs

Most patients with PE will complain of dyspnea, pleuritic chest pain, and apprehension.[3–5] Less common symptoms are cough, wheezing, central chest pain, diaphoresis, and hemoptysis. Syncope can be seen in up to 13 percent.[6] (See Table 97-1) Of course, these symptoms are nonspecific and merely serve to raise the suspicion of PE. Since the symptoms, signs, and laboratory findings of PE are usually nonspecific, to wait for a patient with classic, unmistakable clues

TABLE 97-1   Symptoms of Pulmonary Embolism[a]

Symptom	Frequency,%
Dyspnea	73
Pleuritic pain	66
Cough	37
Leg swelling	28
Leg pain	26
Hemoptysis	13
Wheezing	9
Angina	4

[a]Data taken from Ref. 5.

before pursuing a diagnosis risks missing the majority of patients with this potentially lethal disease. However, since nonspecific indicators of potential pulmonary embolism are ubiquitous, indiscriminate pursuit of the diagnosis is prohibitively costly and dangerous. Most patients with PE have identifiable risk factors as described in Chap. 96. Absence of such risk factors should lead to seeking of alternative explanations other than thromboembolism for the patient's findings. On the other hand, when numerous risk factors are present, or when there is no alternative explanation for the clinical presentation, the diagnosis of PE should be considered more seriously.

The majority of patients will demonstrate tachypnea and crackles but most will not have a heart rate > 100 beats per minute (see Tables 97-1 and 97-2). Fever is more common than is generally appreciated and seen in as many as half of patients,[3] but only rarely is the temperature higher than 38.5°C. It is notable that most patients will not have symptoms or signs of venous thrombosis. Patients with large emboli may have the typical findings of any patient with low output shock such as hypotension, narrow pulse pressure, and poor peripheral perfusion.

Ancillary Clinical Tests

CHEST RADIOGRAPHY

A chest radiograph (CXR) usually is obtained early in the evaluation of a patient with chest complaints, but is rarely diagnostic of PE. More often, the CXR serves to exclude alternative diagnoses such as pneumonia or rib fracture. In patients with proven PE, the CXR is usually abnormal,

TABLE 97-2   Signs of Pulmonary Embolism[a]

Sign	Frequency, %
Tachypnea	70
Rales	51
Tachycardia	30
Increased P2	23
T > 38.5° C	7
Wheezes	5
Homan's sign	4
Pleural rub	3

[a]Data taken from Ref. 5.

revealing atelectasis or infiltrate (68 percent), pleural effusion (48 percent), a pleural-based opacity (35 percent), or decreased pulmonary vascularity (Westermark's sign, 21 percent), but may be normal (16 percent).[5] The typical (albeit nonspecific) findings of basilar atelectasis, elevation of the diaphragm, and pleural effusion should always suggest pulmonary embolization when there is no alternative explanation for the abnormal radiograph.

ELECTROCARDIOGRAPHY

The electrocardiogram (ECG) is normal in only 30 percent of patients, but reveals findings highly suggestive of PE (acute right heart strain) in < 6 percent. The most common finding is nonspecific ST segment and T-wave abnormalities (48 percent). Atrial arrhythmias were seen in < 10 percent of patients in the Prospective Investigation of Pulmonary Embolism Diagnosis (PIOPED) trial.[5]

ARTERIAL BLOOD-GAS ANALYSIS

Arterial hypoxemia, as revealed by arterial blood-gas analysis, is a hallmark of PE. Nevertheless, as many as one patient in four has a P_{O_2} > 80 mmHg while breathing room air, and about 10 percent have a P_{O_2} > 90 mmHg.[5,7] Even when the P_{CO_2} is taken into account, 11 to 14 percent of patients will have a normal alveolar-to-arterial (A/a) gradient for oxygen.[8] Further, neither the P_{O_2} nor the A/a gradient allows one to distinguish patients suspected of having PE in whom the diagnosis will be excluded from those in whom it will be proved.[5,9] On the other hand, a change in arterial oxygenation, coupled with additional measures of lung function, may provide a clue to the diagnosis of PE. For example, in a large group of mechanically ventilated trauma patients, a decrease in arterial oxygen saturation (Sa_{O_2}) of > 10 percent with no corresponding decrement in respiratory system static compliance or new radiographic infiltrate, was highly predictive of PE (positive predictive value, 95 percent[10]).

D-DIMER ASSAYS

A simple blood test which could reliably exclude PE would be a welcome addition to the clinical armamentarium. D-dimer is a specific product of the endogenous fibrinolysis of a cross-linked fibrin clot. It is released into the circulation and can be detected following PE or deep venous thrombosis (DVT). In one study of an enzyme-linked immunosorbent assay (ELISA) kit for the determination of plasma D-dimer, only 3 of 35 patients with a concentration < 500 ng/mL had angiographically proven PE.[11] In a larger trial, a value < 300 ng/mL was found to exclude the diagnosis of PE, but was seen in such a small proportion of patients as to have little clinical value.[12] These same investigators studied a latex agglutination assay for D-dimer, finding a sensitivity of 90 percent in patients with nonhigh probability ventilation-perfusion (VQ) lung scans, but the 95 percent confidence interval was wide. It is possible that with further validation D-dimer assays may find a role in some patients suspected of PE.

Neural Networks

In the complex setting of suspected PE, the clinician may find it difficult to sort through the many nonspecific symptoms and signs to request appropriate diagnostic procedures or begin anticoagulation. Standardized questionnaires have the potential to facilitate the collection of large amounts of information and process it objectively. A further benefit of such studies may be the discovery of clinical clues, which have greater than generally appreciated discriminate power. For example, in one study neck vein distention, syncope, and recent surgery were particularly valuable in separating those with PE from those without.[13] A neural network is an artificial intelligence paradigm, which integrates multiple input variables to generate an output probability. The network "learns" from a training set of data, then attempts to apply its rules to a validation set. This technique compares favorably with clinicians experienced in the diagnosis of PE, proving to be equally accurate.[14] Although this sophisticated technique has not been shown to be superior to an experienced clinician, it might assist physicians less experienced than those involved in clinical studies of PE diagnosis. More refined neural networks might yet be able to outperform even experienced clinicians with more complex network design or more extensive data input, and this approach bears further study.

Ventilation-Perfusion Lung Scan

The ventilation-perfusion (VQ) lung scan is one of the more important tools available to the diagnostician. At the same time, however, its interpretation is complex and its limitations remain greatly underappreciated. It is well established that when the perfusion scan is normal, PE is excluded with a high degree of certainty, and it is safe to withhold anticoagulation, even when PE had been clinically suspected.[15] There has also long been unanimity regarding the utility of high-probability scans, since approximately 85 percent of such patients will have PE. Such a high likelihood of PE makes anticoagulation of all such patients preferable to performing pulmonary angiography to detect the 15 percent who have not had PE. The areas of greatest interest are VQ scan results that are not normal and not high probability. The role of low-probability scans has changed significantly since the introduction of this category, due in large part to the results of two large, prospective trials performed in the 1980s. The Canadian study enrolled 305 consecutive patients with suspected PE and abnormal perfusion scans and subjected essentially all of them to pulmonary angiography.[16] In the PIOPED trial, 755 patients underwent VQ scanning and angiography.[17] These studies showed that the probability of PE in patients with low-probability scans ranged from 16 to 40 percent (depending on the specific low-probability subgroup), results which most clinicians would not regard as low probability. Indeed, most experienced clinicians now interpret VQ scan findings to be either normal (excluding PE), high probability (leading to treatment, typically anticoagulation), or clinically indeterminate and requiring further investigation (see Fig. 97-1). An exception to this is the group

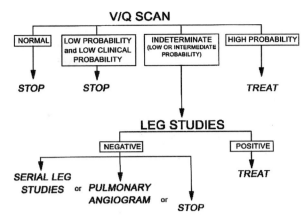

FIGURE 97-1 An algorithm for the diagnosis of pulmonary embolism. Stop means to shift the diagnostic efforts from pulmonary embolism to one of the alternative diagnoses. Treat typically means to begin (or continue) heparin, but additional therapeutic choices are discussed in Chap. 98.

of patients with low-probability scan findings in whom the pretest clinical estimate of PE likelihood is also low (0 to 19 percent clinical probability). Only 4 percent of such patients will have positive angiograms, a rate low enough to be considered truly low probability.[17]

Since low-probability scans can no longer be used to reliably exclude PE, the majority of VQ scans will not be sufficient, in and of themselves, to conclude the investigation for PE when that diagnosis is suspected. For example, of 931 scans performed in the PIOPED trial, 131 were normal (or near normal), 124 were high probability, 90 were low probability associated with a low clinical estimate, leaving 586 patients with clinically indeterminate scans.[17] Yet most of these patients need not be subjected to pulmonary angiography. For example, it may be possible to refine the definition of high-probability scans, especially in patients without prior cardiopulmonary disease, to include many scans which are currently rated as intermediate. When the PIOPED scans of patients without prior cardiopulmonary disease were grouped according to the number of mismatched segmental equivalent perfusion defects, fewer defects were found necessary to reliably predict PE than the initial PIOPED criteria required.[18] Whereas the PIOPED definition of high probability required two or more such defects, it was subsequently shown that only one or more defects was indicative of PE in 86 percent of patients. It is possible that additional refinements of VQ scan interpretation or combination with clinical or radiographic findings will further reduce the number of indeterminate scans. An even greater number of patients can be spared angiography by shifting the focus of diagnosis from the lungs to the legs.

Studies for Deep Venous Thrombosis

NONINVASIVE LEG STUDIES

Noninvasive leg studies include impedance plethysmography (IPG), phleborrheography, venous Doppler examination, and B-mode ultrasound scanning of leg veins. The technical details of these procedures and differences between them are beyond the scope of this chapter, but which particular test to choose is largely a function of local expertise. IPG has been extensively validated and found to have a sensitivity of about 92 percent and a specificity of 95 percent,[19] but attention to proper technique is extremely important.[20,21] Several studies have now shown the safety of withholding anticoagulation in patients with repeated (for example, on days 1, 3, 7, and 14) negative IPG findings, providing a potentially useful way to avoid performing pulmonary angiography in some patients with nonhigh probability ventilation-perfusion lung scans (see Fig. 97-1).[22–26] IPG is less useful for detecting calf vein thrombi and has a poor sensitivity in asymptomatic, postoperative patients.[12] This test can be falsely normal if thrombi are nonocclusive or if there are well established collaterals. Falsely abnormal results can be seen with nonthrombotic compression of the vein, increased central venous pressure, and chronic obstructive pulmonary disease.[27] B-mode ultrasound scanning has become increasingly utilized since it yields direct anatomic detail rather than indirect waveforms, it occasionally facilitates diagnosis of a nonthrombotic cause of leg pain (e.g., Baker's cyst), and is easily portable. This technique has been reported to be highly accurate, with a sensitivity of 95 percent and specificity of 99 percent.[28] However, isolated iliac and calf vein thrombi cannot be reliably seen, the experience with this technique is more limited than with impedance plethysmography, and its true utility unknown.[29] In a direct, randomized comparison of the safety of IPG and B-mode ultrasound used to withhold anticoagulation in patients with a negative study, the incidence of thromboembolism after 6 months of follow-up (2.5 percent and 1.5 percent, respectively) did not statistically differ between these techniques.[22] However, ultrasonography had a superior positive predictive value (94 percent versus 83 percent), allowing fewer patients to be unnecessarily anticoagulated.

Noninvasive leg studies cannot make or exclude the diagnosis of PE. Nevertheless, the wide availability of accurate noninvasive leg studies provides a simple method for managing many patients who have nondiagnostic VQ scans. Demonstration of venous thrombosis provides grounds for treatment (usually anticoagulation), so the question of PE may cease to be important. In patients with angiographically proven PE, 43 to 57 percent will have detectable DVT.[16,30] Using the PIOPED database it has been estimated that of 640 patients with indeterminate scans, 108 would have had detectable proximal DVT.[31] A remaining challenge involves those patients with nondiagnostic VQ scans and negative leg studies. The probability of PE in such patients varies with the prevalence of the disease, the VQ scan reading, and the clinical estimate of PE, but ranges from as low as 4 percent to as high as 66 percent.[31] Such patients should generally undergo serial noninvasive determinations while withholding anticoagulation (as described above) or have further studies (usually pulmonary angiography) to exclude thromboembolism. This combined approach of using clinical estimate, VQ scanning, and noninvasive leg studies is summarized in Fig. 97-1.

Cardiac Echocardiography

Echocardiography is increasingly used to assess cardiac function, volume status, pericardial disease, and hypoperfusion states. Occasionally, a study requested for evaluation of dyspnea or hypotension may unexpectedly reveal findings strongly suggestive of pulmonary embolization. These include a dilated, thin-walled, poorly contracting right ventricle, and bowing of the interventricular septum to the left at both end-diastole and end-systole.[32,33] Tricuspid insufficiency indicates the pressure overload typical of acute PE and, when present, may allow quantitation of the right ventricular peak systolic (and therefore, pulmonary artery systolic) pressure. The left ventricle is usually small with normal fractional shortening. Rarely, echocardiography may demonstrate a thrombus in the right atrium, right ventricle, inferior vena cava, or main pulmonary artery.[34,35]

The role of echocardiography in the evaluation of suspected PE has not been delineated. Its attractions include portability, especially for the evaluation of critically ill patients, noninvasiveness, potential to elucidate competing diagnoses (such as myocardial infarction or pericardial disease), and rapid availability. Furthermore, in one series of hemodynamically stable patients, recurrent embolism was associated strongly with baseline echocardiographic abnormalities in right ventricular wall motion, suggesting that this finding might be useful in identifying a subgroup who might benefit from thrombolytic therapy or vena caval interruption.[36] However, the sensitivity of echocardiography remains to be determined. Moreover, the classic findings of PE are nonspecific, being common to a number of causes of acute right ventricular pressure overload such as the adult respiratory distress syndrome or status asthmaticus.

Pulmonary Angiography

Pulmonary angiography is widely considered the "gold standard" for the diagnosis of PE. Experienced radiologists agree on 98 percent of studies showing lobar embolism.[37] However, agreement decreases to 90 percent with segmental embolism, and only 66 percent in those with subsegmental clots. Thus, even this test has limitations. Its sensitivity is sufficiently high to occasionally detect embolism even weeks to months after the acute episode. The earliest documented resolution of an angiogram to normal following a pulmonary embolus is one week, although faster resolution has been seen in animal studies.[38] Thus, this test can exclude reliably embolism if a negative study is obtained even a week following the onset of symptoms.[39] Since it is invasive, costly, somewhat riskier than VQ scanning, and requires the presence of an interventional radiologist (rather than a nuclear medicine technician), it is usually reserved for the patients in whom the diagnosis cannot be made or excluded by less invasive means. However, pulmonary angiography is safer than generally appreciated. Mortality is around 0.2 percent as shown in several large series.[40–42] Several patients who have died had severe pulmonary hypertension and cor pulmonale at the time of the procedure, leading some to conclude that pulmonary hypertension is a contraindication to pulmonary angiography. The degree of risk in such patients was directly addressed in one review of pulmonary angiography.[41] Increased pulmonary systolic pressure (> 70 mmHg) and elevated right ventricular diastolic pressure (> 20 mmHg) were identified as risk factors. Even in these sickest patients, however, the mortality was only 2 percent. In patients with severe chronic pulmonary hypertension who are being considered for surgical endarterectomy (admittedly a different population) angiography has been performed quite safely.[43] Nonionic, low osmolality contrast agents may be able to reduce risk even further, although this remains to be shown, but do improve image quality.[44]

Failure to diagnose PE presents substantial risks to patients. Therefore, when noninvasive evaluation has failed to establish or exclude the diagnosis, pulmonary angiography may be useful. It is most applicable to patients with low- or intermediate-probability lung scans, those in whom VQ scanning is predicted to be unhelpful (COPD, asthma, very abnormal chest radiograph), or those too ill to cooperate with VQ scanning (critically ill).

Special Situations

SIGNS FROM INVASIVE MONITORING

Valuable signs of PE may come from many of the devices used to monitor critically ill patients. Clues may be derived from the ventilator, the expired gas analysis, or the pulmonary artery catheter. The sensitivity and specificity of these monitors for the diagnosis of PE are not known. Nevertheless, it is wise to attempt to incorporate all available data into the synthesis of the patient's problem.

THE VENTILATOR

To maintain P_{CO_2}, the patient with PE must increase minute ventilation (V_E). Therefore, any unexplained increase in V_E should prompt consideration of PE. Of course, any cause of increased dead space (airflow obstruction, hypovolemia, PEEP), decreasing arterial pH, or increased CO_2 production (anxiety, pain, fever, sepsis, etc.) also will increase V_E. However, when none of these is apparent, especially when other clues to venous thromboembolism are evident, PE becomes more likely.

EXPIRED CARBON DIOXIDE

The increment in dead space after pulmonary embolization causes a detectable decrease in end-tidal CO_2 (ET-CO_2). With technological improvements in these devices, noninvasive assessment of expired CO_2 is becoming increasingly practical in the ICU. In one series of mechanically ventilated COPD patients, a group in which it is particularly difficult to diagnose PE, capnography was used successfully to distinguish embolism from COPD exacerbation.[45] A corollary of the decrease in ET-CO_2 with PE is that if V_E does not increase (e.g., muscle relaxed or deeply sedated patient), the total excretion of CO_2 (expired CO_2 concentration × V_E) must

transiently decrease. Therefore, arterial P_{CO_2} will increase progressively until a new steady state is achieved at a greater P_{CO_2}. Again, in the muscle-relaxed patient there are many explanations for an increasing CO_2, but if no explanation is forthcoming, a diagnosis of pulmonary embolism should be considered.

PULMONARY ARTERY CATHETER

The most obvious clues from the pulmonary artery (PA) catheter are the increases in right atrial, right ventricular, and PA pressures and the decrease in cardiac output that occur with PE. Along with the reduced cardiac output, there will be widening of the arterial (A) to venous (V) oxygen content difference (Fick principle) and a decrement in the mixed venous oxygen saturation. Recognition of this may be facilitated with an oximetric catheter. A final clue from the PA catheter may lie in the difference between the PA diastolic pressure and the wedge pressure (P_{PW}). Normally flow through the pulmonary circulation is pulsatile, so that by the end of diastole, there is no more flow from PA to left atrium (LA). Without flow, there can be no pressure gradient from PA to LA. Thus the end-diastolic PA pressure and the P_{PW} are nearly equal. When there is obstruction of the pulmonary vascular bed, however, flow is not completed by the end of diastole and there remains a pressure gradient. A discrepancy between the PA diastolic pressure and P_{PW} may provide a clue to PA obstruction.

Unfortunately each of these is certainly nonspecific (and probably not sensitive), so that only rarely do such changes indicate PE. For example, cardiac dysfunction (systolic or diastolic) causes an increase in right heart pressures and a fall in cardiac output; any cause of low cardiac output causes a widened AV oxygen content difference; and any cause of tachycardia or increased cardiac output may increase the PA diastolic to wedge pressure gradient.

UPPER EXTREMITY SOURCE FOR PE

It generally is accepted that the great majority of emboli arise in the veins of the lower extremities.[46] Yet over the past several years, venous thrombosis in the upper extremities has been increasingly recognized, especially in patients with indwelling central venous catheters used for chemotherapy, parenteral nutrition, and hemodynamic monitoring. In contrast to primary upper extremity thrombosis, which appears to have a very low propensity to embolize, catheter-related thrombosis is more frequently associated with PE. For example, in a survey of 30 consecutive patients with upper extremity thrombosis, 9 of 10 with primary thrombosis had normal lung scans, whereas only 13 of 20 with catheter-related thrombosis had normal scans and 4 of 20 had high-probability scans.[47]

ISOLATED PELVIC THROMBOSIS AS A SOURCE FOR PE

A weakness of the increasingly utilized duplex ultrasonography for the diagnosis of deep venous thrombosis is its inability to reliably detect isolated pelvic vein thrombus.

Owing to the natural history of deep venous thrombosis, in which most clots begin in small, muscular sinuses of the calf, then extend proximally, most thrombi in the pelvic veins are associated with extensive thrombus in the thigh, which is readily detected by all noninvasive techniques. For example, in one study, only 2 of 49 limbs examined with IPG and duplex ultrasound had isolated iliac thrombus[48] and one of these was adequately detected with the duplex study. However, there are important exceptions to the general rule that popliteal and femoral thrombosis precedes pelvic thrombosis. In pregnancy, there appears to be an unusually high incidence of isolated iliac vein or iliofemoral thrombosis. In one study, 5 of 17 pregnant women with DVT had isolated pelvic thrombosis.[49] This difference in incidence of pelvic thrombosis implies a different pathophysiology of DVT in pregnancy, often ascribed to compression of the iliac veins by the enlarged uterus. Other patients may have an alternative anatomic basis for an atypical, isolated iliac thrombus, such as pelvic malignancy, femoral vein catheterization, or iliac artery aneurysm. In addition, there are additional veins within the pelvis that are susceptible to thrombosis, but which are not interrogated by conventional venous studies, such as the uterine, ovarian, or prostatic veins. Disease in these veins is typically related to malignancy, gynecologic surgery, pelvic inflammatory disease, endometritis, septic abortion, or systemic chemotherapy. In such patients, a negative noninvasive leg study may not adequately exclude venous thrombosis.

Computed tomographic scanning (CT) and magnetic resonance imaging (MRI) are often useful in patients with isolated pelvic thrombus and can establish the diagnosis in those with ovarian vein thrombus.[50,51] These tests have the added advantage of potentially demonstrating ancillary anatomic abnormalities. Alternative diagnostic methods include IPG, which when performed serially has been validated in pregnant patients with suspected DVT,[26] and contrast venography.

An Algorithm for the Diagnosis of PE

Figure 97-1 describes an approach to the diagnosis of pulmonary embolism, emphasizing the roles of the VQ scan and noninvasive leg studies. A high-probability scan should lead to treatment for pulmonary embolism (see Chap. 98). A normal scan or a low-probability scan associated with a low prior clinical suspicion of pulmonary embolism should conclude the evaluation for PE and direct the clinician to alternative explanations for the symptoms which prompted the VQ scan. All other scan results should lead to noninvasive leg studies (impedance plethysmography or duplex ultrasound), which if positive, serve as a basis for treatment.

Patients with nondiagnostic scans and negative leg studies present a challenge. In some settings, for example a patient with a high clinical suspicion, an intermediate-probability scan, and negative duplex scanning, the overall probability of PE is quite high, and pulmonary angiography is probably the best approach. In contrast, a patient with a low-probability scan, an intermediate clinical suspicion, and negative leg studies has a probability of PE of < 10 percent,

and no further evaluation is necessary. When serial noninvasive leg studies are practical, they provide a cost-effective and safe alternative to pulmonary angiography, since very few patients so managed will suffer PE.

There are several situations in which the algorithm provided in Fig. 97-1 may not be the best approach. For example, there are some patients whose chest radiograph (diffuse severe disease) or clinical presentation (status asthmaticus or severe chronic obstructive pulmonary disease) predicts a VQ scan result which cannot be normal and will likely be indeterminate. In such patients, leg studies should precede VQ scanning, since a positive result will be clinically useful. In other patients, for example, a mechanically ventilated patient with shock after a syncopal episode, echocardiography, because of its portability and ability to diagnose competing conditions, should be performed first.

References

1. Dalen JE, Alpert JS: Natural history of pulmonary embolism. *Prog Cardiovasc Dis* 1975; 17:259.
2. Goldhaber SZ, Hennekens CH, Evans DA, et al.: Factors associated with correct antemortem diagnosis of major pulmonary embolism. *Am J Med* 1982; 73:822.
3. Stein PD, Willis PW, DeMets DL: History and physical examination in acute pulmonary embolism in patients without preexisting cardiac or pulmonary disease. *Am J Cardiol* 1981; 47:218.
4. Quinn DA, Thompson BT, Terrin ML, et al.: A prospective investigation of pulmonary embolism in women and men. *JAMA* 1992; 268:1689.
5. Stein PD, Terrin ML, Hales CA, et al.: Clinical, laboratory, roentgenographic, and electrocardiographic findings in patients with acute pulmonary embolism and no pre-existing cardiac or pulmonary disease. *Chest* 1991; 100:598.
6. Fulkerson WJ, Coleman RE, Ravin CE, et al.: Diagnosis of pulmonary embolism. *Arch Intern Med* 1986; 146:961.
7. Dantzker DR, Bower JS: Alterations in gas exchange following pulmonary thromboembolism. *Chest* 1982; 81:495.
8. Stein PD, Goldhaber SZ, Henry JW: Alveolar-arterial oxygen gradient in the assessment of acute pulmonary embolism. *Chest* 1995; 107:139.
9. Robin ED, McCauley RF: The diagnosis of pulmonary embolism: When will we ever learn (editorial). *Chest* 1995; 107:3.
10. Braithwaite CEM, O'Malley KF, Ross SE, et al.: Continuous pulse oximetry and the diagnosis of pulmonary embolism in critically ill trauma patients. *J Trauma* 1992; 33:528.
11. Goldhaber SZ, Simons GR, Elliot G, et al.: Quantitative plasma D-dimer levels among patients undergoing pulmonary angiography for suspected pulmonary embolism. *JAMA* 1993; 270:2819.
12. Ginsberg JS, Caco CC, Brill-Edwards P, et al.: Venous thrombosis in patients who have undergone major hip or knee surgery: Detection with compression ultrasound and impedance plethysmography. *Radiology* 1991; 181:651.
13. Celi A, Palla A, Petruzzelli S, et al.: Prospective study of a standardized questionnaire to improve clinical estimate of pulmonary embolism. *Chest* 1989; 95:332.
14. Patel S, Henry JW, Rubenfire M, et al.: Neural network in the clinical diagnosis of acute pulmonary embolism. *Chest* 1993; 104:1685.
15. Kipper MS, Moser KM, Kortman KE, et al.: Longterm follow-up of patients with suspected pulmonary embolism and a normal lung scan. *Chest* 1982; 82:411.
16. Hull RD, Hirsh J, Carter CJ, et al.: Diagnostic value of ventila-

tion-perfusion lung scanning in patients with suspected pulmonary embolism. *Chest* 1985; 88:819.

17. The PIOPED Investigators: Value of the ventilation/perfusion scan in acute pulmonary embolism: Results of the prospective investigation of pulmonary embolism diagnosis (PIOPED). *JAMA* 1990; 263:2753.

18. Stein PD, Gottschalk A, Henry JW, et al.: Stratification of patients according to prior cardiopulmonary disease and probability assessment based on the number of mismatched segmental equivalent perfusion defects: Approaches to strengthen the diagnostic value of ventilation/perfusion lung scans in acute pulmonary embolism. *Chest* 1993; 104:1461.

19. Koopman MMW, van Beek EJR, ten Cate JW: Diagnosis of deep vein thrombosis. *Prog Cardiovasc Dis* 1994; 37:1.

20. Prandoni P, Lensing AWA, Büller HR, et al.: Failure of computerized impedance plethysmography in the diagnostic management of patients with clinically suspected deep-vein thrombosis. *Thromb Haemostas* 1991; 65:233.

21. Grant BJB: Noninvasive tests for acute venous thromboembolism. *Am J Respir Crit Car Med* 1994; 149:1044.

22. Heijboer H, Büller HR, Lensing AWA, et al.: A randomized comparison of the clinical utility of real-time compression ultrasonography versus impedance plethysmography in the diagnosis of deep vein thrombosis in symptomatic outpatients. *N Engl J Med* 1993; 329:1365.

23. Huisman MV, Büller HR, ten Cate JW, et al.: Management of clinically suspected acute venous thrombosis in outpatients with serial impedance plethysmography in a community hospital setting. *Arch Intern Med* 1989; 149:511.

24. Huisman MV, Büller HR, ten Cate JW, et al.: Serial impedance plethysmography for suspected deep venous thrombosis in outpatients: The Amsterdam general practitioner study. *N Engl J Med* 1986; 314:823.

25. Hull RD, Hirsh J, Carter CJ, et al.: Diagnostic efficacy of impedance plethysmography for clinically suspected deep-vein thrombosis: A randomized trial. *Ann Intern Med* 1985; 102:21.

26. Hull RD, Raskob GE, Carter CJ: Serial impedance plethysmography in pregnant patients with clinically suspected deep-vein thrombosis: Clinical validity of negative findings. *Ann Intern Med* 1990; 112:663.

27. Prescott SM, Richards KL, Tikoff G, et al.: Venous thromboembolism in decompensated chronic obstructive disease. *Am Rev Respir Dis* 1981; 123:32.

28. White RH, McGahan JP, Daschbach MM, et al.: Diagnosis of deep-vein thrombosis using duplex ultrasound. *Ann Intern Med* 1989; 111:297.

29. Lensing AWA, Prandoni P, Brandjes D, et al.: Detection of deep-vein thrombosis by real-time B-mode ultrasonography. *N Engl J Med* 1989; 320:342.

30. Hull RD, Hirsh J, Carter CJ, et al.: Pulmonary angiography, ventilation lung scanning, and venography for clinically suspected pulmonary embolism with abnormal perfusion lung scan. *Ann Intern Med* 1983; 98:891.

31. Stein PD, Hull RD, Saltzman HA, et al.: Strategy for diagnosis of patients with suspected acute pulmonary embolism. *Chest* 1993; 103:1553.

32. Jardin F, Dubourg O, Guéret P, et al.: Quantitative two-dimensional echocardiography in massive pulmonary embolism: Emphasis on ventricular interdependence and leftward septal displacement. *J Am Coll Cardiol* 1987; 10:1201.

33. Come PC: Echocardiographic recognition of pulmonary arterial disease and determination of its cause. *Am J Med* 1988; 84:384.

34. Mancuso L, Marchi S, Mizio G, et al.: Echocardiographic detection of right-sided cardiac thrombi in pulmonary embolism. *Chest* 1987; 92:23.

35. Cheriex EC, Sreeram N, Eussen YFJM, et al.: Cross sectional Doppler echocardiography as the initial technique for the diagnosis of acute pulmonary embolism. *Br Heart J* 1994; 72:52.

36. Wolfe MW, Lee RT, Feldstein ML, et al.: Prognostic significance of right ventricular hypokinesis and perfusion lung scan defects in pulmonary embolism. *Am Heart J* 1994; 127:1371.

37. Stein PD, Athanasoulis C, Alavi A, et al.: Complications and validity of pulmonary angiography in acute pulmonary embolism. *Circulation* 1992; 85:462.

38. Fred HL, Axelrad MA, Lewis JM, et al.: Rapid resolution of pulmonary thromboemboli in man. *JAMA* 1966; 196:1137.

39. Dalen JE, Banas JS, Brooks HL, et al.: Resolution rate of acute pulmonary embolism in man. *N Engl J Med* 1969; 280:1194.

40. Mills SR, Jackson DC, Older RA, et al.: The incidence, etiologies, and avoidance of complications of pulmonary angiography in a large series. *Radiology* 1980; 136:295.

41. Perlmutt LM, Braun SD, Newman GE, et al.: Pulmonary angiography in the high-risk patient. *Radiology* 1987; 162:187.

42. Goodman PC: Pulmonary angiography. *Clin Chest Med* 1984; 5:465.

43. Nicod P, Peterson K, Levine M, et al.: Pulmonary angiography in severe chronic pulmonary hypertension. *Ann Intern Med* 1987; 107:565.

44. Saeed M, Braun SD, Cohan RH, et al.: Pulmonary angiography with iopamidol: Patient comfort, image quality, and hemodynamics. *Radiology* 1987; 165:345.

45. Chopin C, Fesard P, Mangalaboyi J, et al.: Use of capnography in diagnosis of pulmonary embolism during acute respiratory failure of chronic obstructive pulmonary disease. *Crit Care Med* 1990; 18:353.

46. Moser KM: Venous thromboembolism. *Am Rev Respir Dis* 1990; 141:235.

47. Monreal M, Lafoz E, Ruiz J, et al.: Upper-extremity deep venous thrombosis and pulmonary embolism: A prospective study. *Chest* 1991; 99:280.

48. Mantoni M: Deep venous thrombosis: Longitudinal study with duplex US. *Radiology* 1991; 179:271.

49. Bergqvist A, Bergqvist D, Hallbook T: Deep vein thrombosis during pregnancy: A prospective study. *Acta Obstet Gynecol Scand* 1983; 62:443.

50. Savader SJ, Otero RR, Savader BL: Puerperal ovarian vein thrombosis: Evaluation with CT, US, and MR imaging. *Radiology* 1988; 167:637.

51. Erdman WA, Jayson HT, Redman HC, et al.: Deep venous thrombosis of extremities: Role of MR imaging in the diagnosis. *Radiology* 1990; 174:425.

TREATMENT OF THROMBOEMBOLISM

GREGORY A. SCHMIDT

The goals of treatment for acute pulmonary thromboembolism (PE) are both to counter the detrimental effects of the embolus and to prevent recurrence. The impact of already embolized clot can be reduced through supportive strategies (such as oxygen, appropriate fluids, or vasoactive drugs), thrombolytic therapy, or embolectomy. Recurrent embolism typically is prevented with bed rest and anticoagulation, but at times vena caval interruption (VCI) is useful.

Supportive Therapy

Since most patients with PE are mildly to moderately hypoxemic, it is appropriate to administer oxygen. Not only does oxygen increase the Pa_{O_2}, but it also allows adequate systemic oxygen transport at lower cardiac output,[1] a benefit in those patients with impairment of right heart function. In occasional patients whose circulatory function is compromised sufficiently, mechanical ventilation can reduce further the demand for oxygen transport by decreasing breathing,[2]

thus potentially redirecting blood flow to critical organs. Two areas of controversy relate to appropriate fluid and vasoactive drug therapy in PE patients with shock.

FLUID THERAPY

In many patients with shock, large volumes of crystalloid or colloid form the keystone of resuscitation. However, patients with acute massive PE often have increased right heart filling pressures signaled by elevated neck veins or increased central venous pressure. Based on the pathophysiology of shock as outlined in Chap. 96, in which a dilated, poorly contracting right ventricle reduces left ventricular filling, one might predict that volume loading could be detrimental. Such therapy might distend further the right ventricle, shift the interventricular septum even more to the left, and progressively impair left heart function.[3,4] In patients with right ventricular infarction, especially when right atrial pressure is increased, volume loading often fails to increase cardiac output and may be detrimental.[5,6] Similar findings have been seen in a canine model of pulmonary embolism, in which animals were ventilated mechanically and monitored with sonomicrometry.[7] The effects of volume loading were determined before autologous clot embolism, after one episode of embolization, and after repeated emboli. With volume loading, the calculated left ventricular (LV) volume (preload) increased before embolization, was unchanged after initial embolization, but decreased significantly following multiple emboli. This decreased LV volume was associated with an increase in the septum to right ventricular (RV) free wall diameter, consistent with leftward shift of the septum. Further, when fluid was given following multiple emboli, the transseptal pressure gradient (which can be estimated clinically from pulmonary artery wedge pressure minus right atrial pressure) decreased, indicating that the added volume preferentially distended the right ventricle rather than the LV. The authors suggested that this finding might be useful in patients with a pulmonary artery catheter in place as a means to predict when a fluid bolus might cause hemodynamic deterioration, although this has not been tested.

It is not possible to give a simple recommendation to guide fluid administration that is appropriate for all patients with PE. When the circulation is compromised, fluid loading should not be assumed to be beneficial. Rather, a fluid bolus should be given while measuring the hemodynamic effects. If cardiac output or blood pressure increase with a bolus, additional fluid administration might be beneficial. On the other hand, if a fluid challenge causes hemodynamic deterioration or no clear improvement, fluid should be withheld. Greater caution is appropriate in those with echocardiographic evidence of leftward septal displacement or those in whom fluid challenge reduces the transseptal pressure gradient.

VASOACTIVE DRUG THERAPY

Many different vasoactive drugs have been used in acute PE, including isoproterenol,[8] epinephrine,[9] norepinephrine,[8,10,11] dobutamine,[12] dopamine,[13] amrinone,[14] and hydralazine.[15] In a comparative trial in a canine model of PE, norepinephrine was shown to be hemodynamically superior to fluid loading and isoproterenol.[8] The investigators speculated that the beneficial effect of norepinephrine might be due to its vasoconstrictor effect in the systemic circulation, increasing the right ventricular perfusion pressure, and thus relieving RV ischemia. However, a subsequent study compared norepinephrine (which has inotropic activity in addition to its vasoconstrictor properties) and phenylephrine (which is a pure vasoconstrictor) in an animal model of massive PE.[10] Although both drugs increased mean arterial pressure to a similar degree, only norepinephrine augmented cardiac output. This suggests that systemic vasoconstriction does not explain fully the benefit of norepinephrine and that its inotropism may be more important. In human PE there is more published experience with dobutamine than most other drugs. In nine patients with shock caused by PE who were given an average dobutamine infusion of 8 μg/kg/min, cardiac index increased from 1.7 to 2.3 L/min/m² and mean arterial pressure from 81 to 86 mmHg, while heart rate and wedge, right atrial, and pul-

monary artery pressures decreased.[12] These results are superior to the hemodynamic effects of dopamine infusion, during which cardiac output and blood pressure also increase, but at the cost of increased heart rate and pulmonary artery pressure.[13] Vasodilator drugs should be given with extreme caution, if ever, because they typically have little effect on pulmonary vascular resistance and thus fail to increase cardiac output. At the same time, they decrease systemic resistance, which causes a decrease in blood pressure that potentially threatens right ventricular perfusion.

A reasonable approach to vasoactive drug therapy in shock caused by PE is to begin with infusion of dobutamine (starting at 5 μg/kg/min) and to add or substitute norepinephrine if there is insufficient response. In one published case, epinephrine was beneficial when dobutamine and norepinephrine had failed.[9] Hemodynamic benefit should be judged not just by an increase in blood pressure, but also by improved renal function and mentation, and raised cardiac output, oxygen transport, or mixed venous oxyhemoglobin saturation when these indices are available.

Thrombolytic Therapy

The thrombolytic armamentarium for the treatment of PE consists of three drugs: streptokinase (SK), urokinase (UK), and recombinant tissue type plasminogen activator (rt-PA). These drugs all convert plasminogen to plasmin, thereby stimulating fibrinolysis. They differ in their mechanism of plasminogen activation, their fibrin specificity, and their pharmacokinetics. The advantage of thrombolytic agents is their ability to lyse clots that already have formed; this same quality also accounts for their hemorrhagic tendency. The role of these drugs in the management of PE has not been clearly delineated, but it is likely that, when used judiciously, they can reduce morbidity and mortality.

ACTIONS AND ADMINISTRATION

The mechanisms of action of this class of drugs can best be understood by reviewing the normal process of intrinsic clot lysis (fibrinolysis). (See Fig. 98-1.) The coagulation cascade, which forms and propagates thrombus, is opposed by fibrinolysis, which dissolves thrombus and limits its propagation. Initiation of clotting simultaneously activates fibrinolysis through depression of inhibitors of tissue type plasminogen activator (t-PA) and possibly through a direct action of factor XIIa on plasminogen. Thrombolytic agents exploit this intrinsic system by converting plasminogen to the active plasmin, thereby spurring fibrinolysis.

Some of the differences in thrombolytic agents relate to their fibrin specificity. Plasmin produced in the bloodstream is rapidly inactivated by α_2-antiplasmin. However, the unleashing of fibrinolysis results in the consumption of available α_2-antiplasmin. Subsequent excess plasmin is not specific for fibrin, but rather nonspecifically proteolyzes fibrinogen, factor V, factor VIII, and von Willebrand factor as well. This results in a generalized breakdown of hemostasis. Since fibrinogen repletion requires greater than 24 h once these drugs are stopped, the hemorrhagic diathesis is pro-

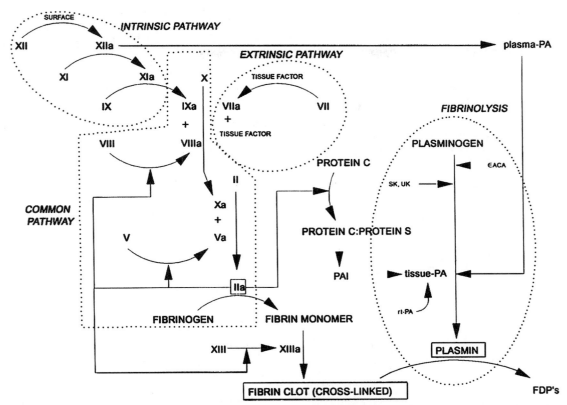

FIGURE 98-1 The coagulation and fibrinolytic pathways. The endpoint of both the intrinsic and extrinsic pathways is to activate factor X. The key step of the common pathway is the generation of thrombin (IIa), which has important actions on clotting and fibrinolysis. Thrombin causes the formation of fibrin monomer. At the same time, it feeds back positively to facilitate the common pathway by activating factors VIII and V. It also activates factor XIII, thereby leading to a cross-linked clot. Thrombin initiates fibrinolysis as well, by leading to the formation of the active protein C:protein S complex, which in turn inhibits plasminogen activator inhibitor (PAI). This leaves the action of tissue-plasminogen activator (t-PA) unchecked, and plasmin is formed. Plasmin is the final step leading to clot lysis. The sites of action of SK, UK, and rt-PA are noted: all lead to plasmin generation. Epsilon aminocaproic acid (ϵACA), an antifibrinolytic agent, inhibits the conversion of plasminogen to plasmin. Solid lines indicate stimulation, dotted lines indicate inhibition. Plasma-PA is plasma plasminogen activator. FDPs are fibrin degradation products.

tracted. The advantage of newer thrombolytic agents is that plasmin activation is dependent on fibrin, and is therefore relatively more localized to the area of clot. Nevertheless, even these fibrin-specific drugs generate a systemic lytic state.

STREPTOKINASE

Streptokinase binds to circulating plasminogen, creating a complex, which is then a potent plasminogen activator. This lack of clot specificity accounts for the relative inefficiency of clot lysis and the systemic nature of the lytic state. SK is a highly purified 47-kDa protein derived from group C streptococci and is associated with a significant incidence of febrile reactions. For this reason, pretreatment with acetaminophen, diphenhydramine, and hydrocortisone is advised. Antigenicity precludes retreatment with SK for at least 6 months. Treatment usually is initiated with a bolus of 250,000 units, followed by a continuous infusion of 100,000 units per hour for 24 h. (See Table 98-1).

UROKINASE

Urokinase is a 37-kDa serine protease derived from cultured fetal kidney cells which directly cleaves plasminogen to plasmin. This specificity for plasminogen is beneficial since fibrinogen is not consumed. UK is not antigenic and can therefore be given repeatedly. The optimal regimen for UK infusion has not been determined, and several methods are in use. One approach is to infuse 1 million units as a bolus, followed by 2 million units over 110 min.[16] Alternatives are to give a bolus of 4400 units per kilogram followed by 4400 units per kilogram per hour for 12 to 24 h,[17] or simply 15,000 units per kilogram as a 10 min bolus.[18]

RT-PA

Endothelial cells release an endogenous mediator of thrombolysis, the 56-kDa protein, called t-PA. A commercial product, produced through recombinant DNA technology, is called recombinant t-PA, rt-PA, or alteplase. This drug binds

TABLE 98-1   Selected Thrombolytic Regimens

Urokinase,[a] 4400 units per kilogram bolus, followed by 4400 units per kilogram per hour for 24 h[17]
Urokinase, 1,000,000 units bolus over 10 min, followed by 2,000,000 units over 110 min[19]
Urokinase, 15,000 units per kilogram bolus over 10 min[18]
rt-PA, 0.6 mg/kg bolus over 2 min[21]
rt-PA, 1 mg/kg over 10 min[30]
rt-PA,[a] 100 mg over 2 to 3 h
Streptokinase,[a] 250,000 units over 30 min, followed by 100,000 units per hour for 24 h

[a] Approved by the U.S. Food and Drug Administration.
NOTE: Heparin is infused at 1300 units per hour when the aPTT decreases below twice normal.

to plasminogen on the surface of clot, thereby producing plasmin locally. This fibrin specificity partly explains the efficacy of rt-PA. A systemic fibrinolytic state is generated, but it is of lesser magnitude than that created by the other thrombolytic drugs as assayed in vitro. However, bleeding seems no less common with rt-PA than with SK and UK. Several therapeutic regimens have been employed, including 100 mg over 2 or 3 h[19,20] and 0.6 mg/kg as a single bolus.[21]

THE POTENTIAL FOR THROMBOLYTIC THERAPY

Potential advantages to thrombolytic therapy over anticoagulation include reduction in the postphlebitic syndrome, removal of the thrombotic source, more rapid restoration of a normal circulation, prevention of chronic pulmonary thromboembolism and pulmonary hypertension, and improved survival. Regarding the first of these, there is conflicting evidence regarding the value of thrombolytic therapy for the treatment of proximal deep venous thrombosis (DVT) or the prevention of the postphlebitic syndrome. Although the National Institutes of Health has published a consensus statement supporting the use of thrombolytic therapy for DVT treatment,[22] two subsequent thorough reviews of the topic reached contradictory conclusions regarding therapeutic benefit.[23,24] When patients were surveyed regarding their preferences, taking into account the best estimates of complications and benefits of thrombolysis (and ignoring the higher immediate monetary cost of this therapy), they unanimously chose heparin alone.[25] Since the available evidence does not clearly support the use of thrombolytic therapy for the treatment of DVT, it seems that the burden of proof rests with those who choose to use it outside clinical trials. Perhaps certain subgroups of patients could be identified who might be more likely to have a favorable therapeutic response.

As regards the treatment of PE, more rapid clot lysis and more prompt reduction of right heart pressures have been unequivocally demonstrated.[17,26,27] A long-term beneficial effect on pulmonary diffusing capacity has also been shown.[28] Unfortunately, no impact has been demonstrated on more relevant endpoints such as mortality or clinical morbidity. Although increasing experience with thrombolytic therapy has made it progressively safer, it is clearly more risky than standard anticoagulation. It is for these reasons that thrombolysis is not as widely accepted for the treatment of PE as for acute myocardial infarction. A recent survey of pulmonary physicians showed that only 11 percent would seriously consider giving thrombolytic therapy to a patient with a large PE but lacking shock or severe hypoxemia.[29]

There are some patients who may derive benefit from the proven ability of thrombolytic therapy to improve right heart pressures rapidly. For example, death in the patient with massive embolism and shock is from acute cor pulmonale. Thus, rapid reduction in right heart pressures might allow survival.[27] Indeed, in an open trial of rt-PA (1 mg/kg over 10 min) in 54 patients with massive PE, 11 of 15 patients in shock demonstrated clinical improvement within 2 h.[30] In addition, patients in shock are critically sensitive to even minor recurrent embolism. Removal of the embolic source might therefore confer additional survival benefit. For example, in a trial of heparin versus rt-PA (100 mg over 2 h), there were five probable recurrences (two fatal) in 55 patients treated with heparin compared with none in 46 patients randomized to rt-PA.[31] Because these arguments are attractive and since such patients are so likely to die, thrombolytic therapy should be given in the setting of proven massive embolism and shock.[32] However, clear benefit in randomized trials has yet to be demonstrated in such patients. Therefore, any contraindications always should be reviewed (Table 98-2).

TABLE 98-2   Contraindications to Thrombolytic Therapy

Absolute
   Recent puncture in a noncompressible site
   Active or recent internal bleeding
   Hemorrhagic diathesis
   Recent CNS surgery or active intracranial lesion
   Uncontrolled hypertension (BP >180/110)
   Known hypersensitivity, or for SK, use of SK within 6 months
   Diabetic hemorrhagic retinopathy
   Acute pericarditis
   Recent obstetrical delivery
   History of stroke

Relative
   Trauma (including CPR) or major surgery within 10 days
   Pregnancy
   High likelihood of left heart thrombus
   Advanced age
   Liver disease

The optimal regimen for thrombolytic therapy has not been established. In a canine model of PE, rt-PA was shown to be superior to urokinase in hastening clot lysis, judged both by hemodynamic improvement and by gamma counting over radiolabeled emboli.[33] However, these two drugs gave similar results in a human comparison when given by a comparable method.[34] Nevertheless, most human trials have subsequently focused on this rt-PA. Animal experiments have also suggested that bolus administration of rt-PA causes less bleeding than the 2-h infusion. In several human trials comparing rt-PA 100 mg over 2 h (the FDA-approved regimen) and 0.6 mg/kg (maximum 50 mg) over 15 min, these regimens appear similar in terms of bleeding, scintigraphic improvement, and hemodynamic resolution.[35–37] Probably the most common clinical approach is to give rt-PA, 100 mg intravenously over 2 h, followed by heparin when the aPTT falls to twice control.[19] Alternative thrombolytic strategies are outlined in Table 98-1.[18,19,21] There is no advantage to infusing the thrombolytic agent directly into the pulmonary artery.[38]

MONITORING AND HEPARINIZATION

Currently, there are no useful guidelines for monitoring the degree of lysis. In general, both arterial and venous punctures should be avoided during the use of thrombolytic drugs. Various measures of the lytic state correlate poorly with both efficacy and incidence of bleeding, so that outside clinical research protocols, routine monitoring is not indicated. When SK is given, the manufacturer recommends that the thrombin time be assayed at 4 h to ensure that a lytic state is achieved. This is based on the concern that if plasminogen is fully consumed, none will remain to complex with SK and form the active plasminogen activator. With no residual plasminogen or plasminogen activator present, a paradoxical hypercoagulable state is possible. An adequate lytic state can be assumed if the thrombin time is prolonged above the normal limits of the laboratory, or if the fibrinogen level is reduced.

Clinical monitoring should include serial neurologic examinations to detect central nervous system hemorrhage and frequent vital signs to detect gastrointestinal or retroperitoneal hemorrhage. Patients who have undergone catheterization should have the groin puncture examined and preferably have repeated measurements of thigh girth. Huge volumes of blood can be lost into the thigh and groin, especially in obese patients, with little external evidence of bleeding. In patients with pulmonary embolism, the adequacy of oxygenation should be assessed using oximetry, rather than arterial blood gases to reduce punctures.

After the thrombolytic agent is discontinued, heparin typically is begun (without a bolus) when the thrombin time or the aPTT decrease to 2 times control. Heparin is begun as an intravenous infusion at 1300 units per hour and titrated to aPTT of 1.5 to 2 times control. Comcomitant infusion of low-molecular-weight heparin (LMWH) was not beneficial when added to rt-PA in a comparative trial of canine experimental embolism.[39]

COMPLICATIONS

The greatest limitation of the thrombolytic drugs and the factor that has limited their acceptance for the treatment of venous thromboembolism, is the consequential incidence of bleeding. In the initial Urokinase Pulmonary Embolism Trial, 45 percent of patients given urokinase suffered serious bleeding, compared with 27 percent of those who received heparin.[17] In contrast, in recent, noninvasive trials using streptokinase in patients with acute myocardial infarction, the incidence of severe bleeding has been only 0.6 to 5.9 percent.[40,41] The risk of bleeding has been reduced through the accumulated experience with these drugs, in particular by avoiding vascular punctures. The importance of maintaining vascular integrity is demonstrated by reviewing recent trials in which coronary arteriography was part of the protocol; the incidence of severe bleeding has been about 15 percent.[42] In patients treated for pulmonary embolism, in whom pulmonary angiography is commonly performed, the risk of major hemorrhage is around 15 percent.[30] In a decision analysis based on data from trials of rt-PA in acute myocardial infarction, the risk of major hemorrhage in PE patients in whom angiography was performed was estimated to be 14 percent, compared with those without angiography in whom the risk was calculated at only 4.2 percent.[43] The authors recommended that in patients who are prospective candidates for thrombolytic therapy, nonangiographic diagnosis was likely to be safer.

One of the hopes for the second-generation, fibrin-specific thrombolytic agents has been that the risk of serious bleeding would be reduced. While fibrin specificity probably accounts for the improved efficacy of these agents, the risk of hemorrhage is no less than with streptokinase. In the trials of rt-PA in myocardial infarction, most of which have necessitated coronary arteriography, the incidence of major hemorrhage has been about 12 percent.[42] While there is some evidence that hemorrhage is related to the degree of systemic lysis, the relationship is weak. The most important predictors of risk seem to be the number of vascular punctures, the duration of lytic therapy, and the coadministration of antiplatelet drugs or heparin. It is extremely important when anticipating the use of a lytic drug to limit invasive procedures as much as possible.[43] For example, a patient with massive pulmonary embolism might be managed with pulse oximetry and serial examinations rather than arterial blood gases or an arterial catheter. When vascular punctures are necessary, prolonged local compression is mandatory.

When serious bleeding occurs, the lytic agent should be immediately discontinued, and reliable, multiple, large-bore catheters secured. Direct compression of bleeding vessels may stop or slow ongoing blood loss. If heparin has been given, it should be stopped and consideration given to reversing heparinization with protamine. Most patients will be managed adequately without the transfusion of clotting factors. If it becomes necessary to reverse the lytic state, cryoprecipitate, which contains fibrinogen and factor VIII (both of which are consumed by plasmin) is the preferred blood product.[44] The initial dose is 10 units, after which the fibrinogen level should be assayed. Fresh frozen plasma (as a source of factors V and VIII), platelets, and antifibrinolytic drugs (e.g., epsilon aminocaproic acid 5 g over 30 min) all may play a role in the critically bleeding patient.[44]

ALLERGIC EFFECTS

Allergic reactions, including skin rashes, fever, and hypotension are rare except with SK. Mild reactions can be treated with antihistamines and acetaminophen. More severe reactions should prompt the addition of hydrocortisone. Hypotension usually responds to volume administration.

Embolectomy

Surgical embolectomy is a major procedure that rarely is employed. In part, this is related to the availability of other, more benign, therapies such as heparin and thrombolysis. Additionally, it takes time to organize a surgical team, operating room, cardiopulmonary bypass and so on, by which time the patient often is improved hemodynamically or moribund. Yet embolectomy has its advocates, who maintain that thrombolytic therapy is often contraindicated in patients who could benefit from it, the operative mortality for embolectomy is now acceptable, and chronic cor pulmonale can be averted.

In one review of 87 patients with PE, 34 were treated with heparin, 28 with streptokinase, and 25 with embolectomy.[45] Pretreatment embolic scores were most severe in the embolectomy group.[45] Hospital mortality in the heparin, streptokinase, and surgery groups was 6, 21, and 20 percent, respectively. However, cumulative survival at 5 years was 68, 64, and 80 percent, a trend favoring embolectomy. However, most late deaths were due to malignancy, not recurrent PE or chronic pulmonary hypertension. Although the authors recommended surgical embolectomy for all patients with emboli in the main pulmonary arteries based on their results, regardless of hemodynamic consequences, this study was not randomized, and the possibility seems great that the long-term benefit for embolectomy was related to selection of patients.

Mortality caused by surgical embolectomy is in the range of 30 to 40 percent,[46,47] but may be as low as 11 percent in those who have not sustained cardiac arrest preoperatively.[47] Even if this lower number reflects improvements in anesthetic or operative technique, this mortality is still comparable to that of patients with massive embolism treated less invasively.[48] The argument that embolectomy might reduce the long-term consequences of chronic pulmonary hypertension lacks force since this complication seems quite rare. (See Chap. 96.) Thus, it never has been demonstrated in a well performed trial that embolectomy confers any advantage over thrombolytic therapy or heparin alone. Patients who could benefit would be those with hemodynamically significant embolism in whom thrombolytic therapy is contraindicated and who are in a center with a rapidly responding cardiopulmonary bypass team having a surgeon experienced in the technique of embolectomy. In all such cases, it is prudent to confirm the diagnosis by pulmonary angiography given the false-positive rate of high-probability ventila-tion-perfusion lung scans (15 percent) and the limited accuracy of clinical diagnosis.

Several new devices have been tested that aim to remove pulmonary emboli less invasively than the direct surgical approach. For example, a 10F suction catheter, inserted through a jugular or femoral venotomy and advanced into the pulmonary artery, has been used to extract clot,[49] and 11 of 18 patients improved immediately. Suction embolectomy was more likely to be successful in patients treated promptly after hemodynamic deterioration. Alternative methods to reestablish pulmonary artery patency use rotational catheter devices[50] and endovascular stents,[51] but experience with all these techniques is limited.

Short-Term Anticoagulation

It generally is accepted that patients with PE benefit from immediate anticoagulation, the purpose of which is to prevent recurrence and not to treat the embolus which led to clinical symptoms or diagnosis. This approach relies on the natural fibrolytic system to clear the pulmonary circulation of clot and restore hemodynamic stability. Endogenous clot lysis seems effective in reducing the hemodynamic burden of embolism, although at a slower pace than can be achieved with thrombolytic therapy.[52] When patients in the Urokinase Pulmonary Embolism Trial (UPET) were reevaluated with perfusion lung scans 5 days following initial therapy, there was no difference between those who had received urokinase and those given only heparin.[52] Yet the preferred clinical dosing of heparin, the route of administration (intravenous versus subcutaneous), and type of heparin (unfractionated versus low-molecular-weight) are areas of active investigation.

HEPARIN ANTICOAGULATION

The standard treatment for most patients with PE is intravenous infusion of heparin, a naturally occurring glycosaminoglycan. The anticoagulant effect of heparin depends on a pentasaccharide sequence which binds to antithrombin III (AT-III), inhibiting the actions of thrombin and activated factor X. By a separate pathway, heparin inactivates thrombin through binding to heparin cofactor II, another endogenous plasma cofactor.[53] Heparin also binds to platelets, endothelial cells, and other sites, possibly explaining its tendency to cause hemorrhage and accounting for its variable interpatient anticoagulant effect. The anticoagulant effect of heparin begins immediately following intravenous administration, decreases rapidly in the first 15 min, then decreases linearly and more slowly.[54] The half-life of heparin is approximately 90 min, but is faster when lesser doses are given and in patients with larger thrombotic burdens.[55] By the subcutaneous route, heparin concentrations peak at 4 to 6 h and the anticoagulant effect lasts approximately 12 h.[56]

By inhibiting the coagulation pathway, heparin is highly effective in preventing propagation of thrombus when given in sufficient dose.[56,57] For example, in a study comparing continuous intravenous heparin with intermittent subcutaneous heparin in the treatment of proximal deep vein thrombosis, only 1 of 61 patients who achieved an activated partial thromboplastin time (aPTT) >1.5 times control suffered recurrent venous thromboembolism (VTE). In contrast, 13 of 53 patients whose aPTT was <1.5 for 24 h had recurrence, independent of the method of administration of heparin (relative risk 15:1[56]). Further support for the efficacy of heparin comes from a trial in which initial oral anticoagulation (without concomitant heparin) was compared with the conventional approach of heparin followed by oral agents.[57] Recurrent VTE was seen in 12 to 60 patients in whom heparin was withheld, compared with only 4 of 60 patients who were immediately anticoagulated with heparin. These studies provide convincing support for a cornerstone of heparin anticoagulation; that is, it is crucial to give sufficient heparin to increase the aPTT to >1.5 times control (or alternatively to achieve a heparin level of 0.2 to 0.4 units per milliliter by the protamine sulfate titration assay[58] or 0.35 to 0.67 units per milliliter by antifactor Xa assay[59]) as soon as possible.

The importance of prompt anticoagulation has somewhat dampened the enthusiasm for administering unfractionated heparin by the subcutaneous route. Subcutaneous administration has advantages of ease of use and reduced cost, it has been shown to effectively prevent thrombus extension,[56,60,61] and in a metaanalysis was demonstrated to be as safe and effective as intravenous heparin.[62] Its disadvantage when compared with intravenous heparin is that effective anticoagulation takes longer,[56] and the accumulated evidence is not sufficiently reassuring to conclude that this will not lead to a higher rate of recurrent VTE. Nevertheless, if the aPTT is increased to therapeutic levels, subcutaneous therapy appears as effective as the intravenous route.

While the evidence supporting a lower therapeutic limit for heparin of 1.5 times control as judged by the aPTT is quite strong, the conventional upper limit (2.5 times control) is arbitrary. For years, it had been assumed that the risk of hemorrhage was significantly related to the level of the aPTT, but a recent trial has cast doubt on this assumption.[63]

In this study, hemorrhagic complications were related to underlying predisposing factors (e.g., recent surgery, ulcer disease, or cancer) rather than to supratherapeutic levels of the aPTT. Patients were treated initially with heparin plus warfarin or with heparin alone. Of 99 patients in the combined treatment group, 69 (69 percent) had aPTT levels >2.5 times control for more than 24 h. By contrast, in the heparin-only group, 24 of 100 patients (24 percent) had supratherapeutic aPTT levels. Bleeding complications were similar in the two groups (combined therapy, 9.1 percent; heparin alone, 12.0 percent). In addition, bleeding complications were seen in only 8 of 93 patients with supratherapeutic aPTT regardless of therapeutic arm, compared with 13 of 106 patients without such elevation. These findings refute an association between modestly increased aPTT and hemorrhage and, combined with the importance of prompt, adequate anticoagulation, suggest the value of an approach that aims to assure enough heparin in the first hours of treatment, rather than to avoid too much.

Series of patients treated with heparin show that physicians do a poor job of attaining therapeutic levels of heparin.[64,65] For example, in one review at university-associated hospitals, 60 percent of patients had subtherapeutic levels of heparin after 24 h of treatment.[65] A more recent audit showed somewhat better, but still inadequate, results, with only 77 percent of patients adequately treated after 24 h.[66] Better results can be obtained by abandoning the conventional recommendation to give a 5000-unit bolus followed by 1000 units per hour by continuous infusion. For example, when patients were given a bolus of 5000 units followed by 1680 units per hour (or 1240 units per hour if risk factors for bleeding were present), with subsequent dose adjustments guided by a nomogram, 99 percent achieved therapeutic aPTT levels by 24 h.[63] This approach is summarized in Table 98-3.[67] Similarly, a weight-based nomogram (80 units per kilogram bolus, 18 units per kilogram per hour infusion) had a success rate of 97 percent.[66] These studies show that an infusion of 1000 units per hour is inadequate initial heparin therapy for many patients.

TABLE 98-3   Guidelines for Heparin in Patients with VTE[a]

Heparin bolus, 5000 units intravenously
Continuous intravenous heparin infusion at 1680 units per hour except in the following patients who should receive only 1240 units per hour (surgery in the past 2 weeks; prior history of peptic ulcer disease, gastrointestinal bleeding, or genitourinary bleeding; thrombotic stroke in past 2 weeks; platelet count less than 150,000 per cubic millimeter; other bleeding risk)
Perform aPTT 4 h following the bolus, then adjust the dose as follows:

aPTTs	Dose Change, Units per Hour	Additional Action
<45	+240	Repeat aPTT in 4–6 h
46–54	+120	Repeat aPTT in 4–6 h
55–85	None	Repeat aPTT in 4–6 h the first day, thereafter only once daily unless subtherapeutic
86–110	−120	Stop heparin for 1 h; repeat aPTT 4–6 h after restarting heparin
>110	−240	Stop heparin for 1 h; repeat aPTT 4–6 h after restarting heparin

a Adapted from Ref.[67]

COMPLICATIONS OF HEPARIN

Complications of heparin, in addition to hemorrhage, include heparin-associated thrombocytopenia (HAT), osteoporosis, hypersensitivity, and (rarely) hyperkalemia. The most important complication of heparin is bleeding. In a pooled analysis of its use in deep venous thrombosis, major bleeding (bleeding greater than 1 L, bleeding requiring blood transfusion, intracerebral bleeding) was reported in 2 of 59 patients (3 percent).[68] In a group of 121 patients given heparin for all indications, 8 percent developed major hemorrhage (fatal, life-threatening, potentially life-threatening, leading to reoperation, or requiring at least three units of blood).[69] When heparin dosing is guided by nomogram as described above, the risk of hemorrhage was 9 to 12 percent.[63] Hemorrhage typically occurs from the gastrointestinal or urinary tract, or from surgical incisions. Less common sites of serious bleeding include the retroperitoneum, adrenal glands, soft tissues, nose, and pleural space. Intracranial hemorrhage is uncommon in patients anticoagulated with heparin.

The approach to treatment of the patient who bleeds on heparin depends on the severity of bleeding. When bleeding is minor, simply stopping the heparin may be sufficient. Bleeding related to needle punctures may respond to sustained direct pressure. When hemorrhage endangers life or organ function, a more aggressive approach is mandatory. Transfusion of fresh frozen plasma usually is ineffective, since circulating heparin inhibits the function of transfused factors. Protamine sulfate is an antidote to heparin. The dose of protamine depends on heparin concentrations and is therefore related to dose, route of administration, and time since the last dose. When hemorrhage immediately follows a bolus of heparin, sufficient protamine to neutralize completely the heparin (l mg protamine per 100 units of heparin) should be administered. In the more usual situation where heparin therapy is ongoing, the dose of protamine should be based on the approximate half-life of heparin (90 min). Since protamine, too, is an anticoagulant, the dose should be calculated to only half-correct the estimated circulating heparin. Protamine has been known to cause hypotension, shock, dyspnea, and pulmonary hypertension upon intravenous injection. The incidence is reduced by giving the drug very slowly (no more than 50 mg in 10 min). When protamine is administered, a physician should be present in case of an anaphylactoid reaction. Alternatives for the treatment of underlying conditions should be considered once heparin is stopped. For example, the patient with pulmonary embolization should have vena caval interruption with a percutaneous filter (vide infra).

Thrombocytopenia is a relatively common complication of heparin administration, typically occurring after several days of therapy. It is more common in patients given bovine lung heparin (10 percent) than in those treated with porcine heparin (<5 percent)[70] and may be related to the heparin lot. The mechanism of thrombocytopenia in most patients is thought to be related to specific IgG directed against heparin. Heparin binds normally to platelets, and in individuals who develop antiplatelet IgG, an IgG:platelet—antigen immune complex forms on the platelet surface. Through the platelet Fc receptor, the immune complex may result in activation and aggregation of platelets.[71] Thrombocytopenia is not seen with highly purified low-molecular-weight heparins, suggesting that higher-molecular-weight components may be responsible. It is also rare in patients given prophylactic, minidose heparin, occurring in only 1 of 348 patients.[71] This suggests that heparin-associated thrombocytopenia also is dose-related. The onset of thrombocytopenia usually is on the 3d to 15th day (mean = day 10), but can occur after several hours in patients previously sensitized. The severity of thrombocytopenia is variable (commonly to 50,000 cells per cubic centimeter), but can be severe (<5000 per cubic centimeter). Most patients remain asymptomatic, but some suffer major arterial or venous thrombosis, or life-threatening hemorrhage. Rarely, this syndrome is associated with skin bullae, which progress to necrosis (heparin necrosis). These may occur at sites of injection or at distant sites. Any time heparin is given, it is prudent to measure platelet counts on a daily basis. An otherwise unexplained decrease in platelet count of 30 percent has been suggested as the threshold and should prompt discontinuation of heparin,[71] although there is little on which to base this. Heparin-dependent IgG should be sought in the patient serum, since a positive result may simplify management decisions. None of the available assays are fully sensitive, so that a negative test is no guarantee against recurrent thrombocytopenia or thrombosis if the patient is rechallenged with heparin.

LOW-MOLECULAR-WEIGHT HEPARIN

The promise of LMWHs is a simple, once daily, outpatient therapy for venous thromboembolism which does not require monitoring of anticoagulant effect. This potential is based on several characteristics of LMWHs, more fully discussed in Chap. 99, but include excellent bioavailability when given subcutaneously (about 90 percent of that achieved with an equal intravenous dose),[57] long half-life (2 to 4.4 h[72,73]), high correlation between anticoagulant response and body weight,[74] and equal or better antithrombotic effect than unfractionated heparin.[75] There now have been more than 10 trials, involving more than 2000 patients, comparing LMWHs (subcutaneously or intravenously) with unfractionated heparin.[72,75,76] Pooling these results shows that LMWHs are superior with regard to venographic score improvement, recurrence rate of VTE, and hemorrhage. There is also a trend toward an all-cause mortality benefit for LMWHs.[76] However, these trials vary substantially in their details, such as the specific LMWH given, the dosing schedule, the route of administration, and the duration of treatment prior to warfarin. The prospect is good that one of the LMWHs will eventually replace unfractionated heparin for the treatment of VTE, at least in some patients, but there are yet insufficient data to discard the standard, clearly effective therapy.

ALTERNATIVES TO HEPARIN

If heparin must be discontinued in a patient who remains at high risk of recurrent embolism, a vena caval filter should generally be inserted. Alternative antithrombotic agents include the heparinoid Org 10172, which only rarely cross-reacts with the immunoglobulin responsible for heparin-associated thrombocytopenia, and ancrod (1 unit per kilogram IV over 6 to 12 h, not currently available in the United States, except on a compassionate basis from Knoll Pharma, Inc.). There is little published experience with these agents. Dextran is not effective in established thrombosis and should not be used.

Long-Term Anticoagulation

Following initial anticoagulation, long-term treatment is necessary to prevent recurrence.[77,78] For example, in patients with proximal vein thrombosis, long-term treatment with warfarin reduces the incidence of recurrence from 47 to 2 percent.[77] New information from well-designed clinical trials has dramatically changed the clinical application of warfarin. Most significant is the recognition that less intense anticoagulation than was traditionally used can be prescribed, leading to reduced complications with no loss of efficacy. In addition, the need to monitor anticoagulation with the international normalized ratio (INR), rather than the prothrombin time (PT), has been established (vide infra). There are occasional patients (e.g., during pregnancy or when outpatient monitoring is burdensome or impossible) in whom outpatient anticoagulation with subcutaneous heparin (adjusted to maintain the 6 h postinjection aPTT > 1.5 times control) is preferred to oral anticoagulation.[79] The initial subcutaneous dose should be one-third of the total prior daily intravenous dose, administered every 12 h (typically 10,000 units twice daily). However, the potential for osteoporosis is real, and long-term heparin is only appropriate when oral anticoagulants cannot be given.

ACTION OF WARFARIN SODIUM

Factors II, VII, IX, and X, as well as proteins C and S, require the hydroquinone form of vitamin K_1 to attain biologic activity. These factors are synthesized as inactive zymogens and require carboxylation of glutamic acid residues for activity. The reduced form of vitamin K_1 is oxidized during these carboxylation reactions, and must then be reduced to the active form (the vitamin K cycle). This reduction is accomplished by vitamin K_1 epoxide reductase, an enzyme which is competitively antagonized by warfarin. By preventing the post-ribosomal modification of the procoagulant factors to their active forms, warfarin acts as an anticoagulant.[80] At the same time, however, it inhibits the functions of the naturally occurring anticoagulant substances, proteins C and S. Protein C is a circulating proenzyme, which is converted by the thrombin-thrombomodulin complex to its active form. Activated protein C directly inhibits activated factor VIII and, combined with protein S, also inhibits factor V.[81] Thus warfarin has a dual-edge effect, acting both as an anticoagulant and as a procoagulant. Once all the coagulation factor levels fall, which takes several days, the anticoagulant effect dominates. However, for the first few days of oral anticoagulation it is essential to continue heparin therapy to ensure adequate anticoagulation.

CONVERSION FROM HEPARIN TO WARFARIN

Warfarin can be initiated on the first day of treatment, typically in a dose of 10 mg per day for the first 2 days. Subsequent doses should be based on the anticoagulant response, since there is great patient-to-patient variability in the response to warfarin.[82] Greater initial loading doses (e.g., 40 mg) do not cause quicker equilibration of factor levels and should not be given.[83] Warfarin is absorbed rapidly and completely from the gastrointestinal tract, then circulates almost exclusively bound to albumin. Peak plasma concentrations are seen in about 90 min,[58] although the peak effect does not occur until 36 to 72 h later, depending on the half-lives of previously synthesized clotting factors. The half-life of warfarin itself is about 35 h. Drugs that displace warfarin from albumin have the potential to potentiate its anticoagulant effects. Many classes of drugs can enhance or inhibit its actions, through various mechanisms[84] (Table 98-4). In addition, dietary changes, intercurrent illness, and malabsorptive syndromes all can have an impact on the anticoagulant effect.

Following administration of warfarin, factor VII concentrations decrease most rapidly, prolonging the PT, although the full antithrombotic effect (which depends on reduced levels of the other vitamin K-dependent coagulation factors) is not seen for 72 to 96 h.[85] This provides the rationale for overlapping heparin and warfarin therapies for at least 4

TABLE 98-4   Drugs which Interact with Warfarin

Increased Effect	Decreased Effect
Allopurinol	Antacids
Amiodarone	Antihistamines
Anabolic steroids	Barbiturates
Anesthetics, inhalation	Carbamazepine
Cefamandol	Cholestyramine
Clofibrate	Corticosteroids
Chloramphenicol	Diuretics[a]
Chlordiazepoxide	Estrogens
Chlorpromazine	Griseofulvin
Cimetidine	Haloperidol
Cotrimoxazole	Methylxanthines
Diazepam	Paraldehyde
Diuretics[a]	Phenytoin
Methyldopa	Ranitidine[a]
Metronidazole	Rifampin
Moxalactam	Tetracycline
Neomycin	Vitamin K
Nortriptyline	
Phenylbutazone	
Phenytoin	
Quinidine	
Ranitidine[a]	
Salicylate	
Sulfonamides	

[a] Both increased and decreased effects are seen.

days, even though the PT will increase sooner. The optimal duration of concomitant warfarin and heparin therapy has not been established clearly. On the one hand, there are several studies showing the adequacy of 7 to 10 days of initial heparin therapy followed by warfarin. However, if heparin anticoagulation can be decreased to 4 or 5 days the cost of treatment can be reduced substantially. In one trial, warfarin was begun after 7 days of heparin or within 3 days (typically on day 1), while the patients were followed with symptoms, perfusion lung scans, ^{125}I fibrinogen leg scanning, and ultimate outpatient outcome.[86] There was no significant difference in recurrence of VTE, proximal extension of thrombus, asymptomatic pulmonary embolism, outpatient recurrence of VTE, or bleeding complications. Hospital stay was decreased by an average of 3.9 days, a tremendous cost saving. In another study of patients with proximal venous thrombosis, heparin was given for 5 days (warfarin given on day 1) versus 10 days (warfarin begun on day 5).[87] There was no difference in the rate of objectively documented recurrence of VTE. This approach of shorter duration heparin treatment has the potential to save $500 million yearly in the United States.[88]

MONITORING WARFARIN ANTICOAGULATION

The adequacy of warfarin anticoagulation generally has been assessed by measuring the PT. It has been difficult to compare the degree of anticoagulation between different centers, however, because they employ several different thromboplastins of varying sensitivities. For example, a rabbit brain thromboplastin often used in the United States is relatively unresponsive to the effect of warfarin. On the other hand, the thromboplastins used in the United Kingdom are much more responsive, whereas those used in Europe are of intermediate sensitivity. Even in North America there is substantial variation in the responsiveness of different thromboplastins.[89,90] Studies in which the particular thromboplastin used is not stated, which was the rule until the last few years, cannot be used to provide a basis for therapeutic recommendations when anticoagulant intensity is monitored with a different thromboplastin. To do so is potentially dangerous, since patients may be overtreated, as was formerly common in the United States, or undertreated.[91] To facilitate comparison of anticoagulation, it is now appropriate to express the anticoagulant effect referenced to an internationally accepted standard thromboplastin. This expression, the INR, reports the result that would have been obtained had the internationally accepted standard thromboplastin been used.[92] The relationship between the PT and the INR is

$$INR = \left(\frac{control\ PT}{patient\ PT} \right)^{ISI}$$

where ISI (international sensitivity index) is a measure of the sensitivity of the thromboplastin, available from the provider of the reagent.[84] The desired anticoagulant effect is an INR of 2.0 to 3.0 (this corresponds to a PT of about 1.3 to 1.5 when a relatively insensitive rabbit brain thromboplastin is used). This less intensive regimen (as compared with the prior recommendation to raise the PT to 1.5 to 2.5 times control) is as effective for the treatment of deep vein thrombosis with far fewer bleeding complications (4.3 versus 22.4 percent).[93] Warfarin should be continued for 3 months for a first episode of VTE. If there is an ongoing risk factor, or the patient has had prior VTE, anticoagulation should be continued indefinitely, or until the risk factor resolves. Guidelines for oral anticoagulation are summarized in Table 98-5.

COMPLICATIONS OF WARFARIN

As with heparin, the most important side effect of warfarin use is hemorrhage, occurring in 2.4 to 22.4 percent of patients chronically anticoagulated.[93,94] In contrast to bleeding due to heparin, the risk is strongly related to the prolongation of the INR. Spontaneous hemorrhage during oral anticoagulant therapy should prompt consideration of an underlying structural lesion. The sites of hemorrhage parallel those of patients who bleed while on heparin. The hemorrhagic diathesis can be reversed immediately by transfusing fresh frozen plasma (2 to 4 units). The use of more concentrated factor products, such as prothrombin complex concentrates, should be reserved for urgent situations unresponsive to fresh frozen plasma. Vitamin K_1 (phytonadione, not vitamin K_3, menadione, or vitamin K_4 menadiol, which are ineffective) can be given to antagonize the effects of warfarin, but its action is delayed for 3 to 6 h, requiring synthesis of new clotting factors by the liver. For this reason, and because it makes reinstitution of warfarin therapy complicated, vitamin K_1 is only occasionally indicated. A limited study showed that very low doses of vitamin K (0.5 to 1.0 mg IV)

TABLE 98-5 Guidelines for Oral Anticoagulation

Begin warfarin sodium, 10 mg orally, for the first 2 days.
Adjust subsequent daily doses based on the INR (goal 2.0–3.0).
Discontinue heparin on day 5, as long as INR is therapeutic.
Monitor INR daily until the warfarin dose is stable, then weekly thereafter.
Continue warfarin for 3 months for a first episode of VTE. If there is an ongoing
  risk factor, or the patient has had prior VTE, anticoagulation should be continued
  indefinitely, or until the risk factor resolves. For patients anticoagulated
  indefinitely, it may be appropriate to monitor the INR monthly.
Remain aware of the potential for drug-drug and diet-drug interactions to change the
  patient's response to warfarin, increasing the frequency of monitoring as needed.

NOTE: Warfarin is contraindicated in pregnancy.

decreased INR concentrations from 10–20 to 3–7.5 by 8 h, then further to 1.5 to 5.0 by 24 h, without interfering with continued warfarin treatment.[95]

As noted above, one of the early effects of warfarin is to impair the function of protein C in addition to its effects on procoagulant factors. Since the half-life of protein C is very short (similar to that of factor VII), warfarin may cause a paradoxical hypercoagulable state.[96] This can result in thrombosis in the skin, causing necrosis and occasionally requiring amputation. Patients with congenital deficiencies of protein C may be at particular risk for this rare condition. Warfarin necrosis occurs usually in the first week of therapy and typically manifests in areas with abundant subcutaneous tissue such as abdomen, breast, and buttocks, or in the periphery (tip of the nose, penis).

Warfarin given during pregnancy can be teratogenic. Its use during the 6th to 12th weeks of gestation may result in a typical embryopathy consisting of a variety of skeletal abnormalities. Given later in pregnancy, it may cause central nervous system abnormalities and optic atrophy. For these reasons, heparin is the anticoagulant of choice during pregnancy, even for long-term anticoagulation.

Role of Vena Caval Interruption

Since most thromboemboli originate in the legs, pelvis, or inferior vena cava (IVC),[97] inferior vena caval interruption (VCI) is effective therapy for PE. While it does nothing for the embolized clot, VCI is highly effective in preventing reembolization and death. Although data from systematically evaluated patients has not been published, the recurrence rate of PE following VCI placement is on the order of 2 percent.[98] Fatal embolism is quite rare, but reported.[99] Several methods have been devised for VCI, including surgical ligation or plication, balloon occlusion, and percuta-neous placement of filters. Placement of filters by interventional radiologists and vascular surgeons has replaced all the earlier methods since the new devices are easily placed and maintain caval patency in most instances.[100] Conventional indications for the use of VCI in patients with venous thromboembolism include contraindications to anticoagulation, hemorrhage following anticoagulation, failure of anticoagulation to prevent recurrent embolization, and postpulmonary embolectomy.

As VCI devices have evolved, they have become smaller and more easily placed. As physicians have become more experienced with them, these devices have become safer as well, although complete safety information is not available. In addition, new devices are being tested which are retrievable from the vena cava and could reduce concerns about the long-term consequences of having an intravascular foreign body. It is not surprising then that indications for VCI use are expanding. Additional potential indications include extensive free-floating vena caval thrombus (since the efficacy of heparin in this setting is controversial),[101] prepulmonary embolectomy, as primary treatment in patients with malignancy (since anticoagulants seem less effective and less safe in this setting), prophylactically in patients with minimal cardiopulmonary reserve and pulmonary hypertension, prophylactically in high risk patients (e.g., those with a history of VTE undergoing major surgery), patients with COPD and DVT, and others.[102]

Complications include filter fracture (occasionally with embolization of fragments), improper placement of the filter, venous thrombosis at the insertion site (seen in 8 to 25 percent),[102] caval occlusion (which is now far less common than when the Mobin-Uddin "umbrella" filters were in use), and erosion or perforation of the caval wall and other viscera. A final point about VCI is that while it prevents most recurrent emboli, it does not treat the (presumed) leg source. Therefore, when these devices are used, concomitant antico-

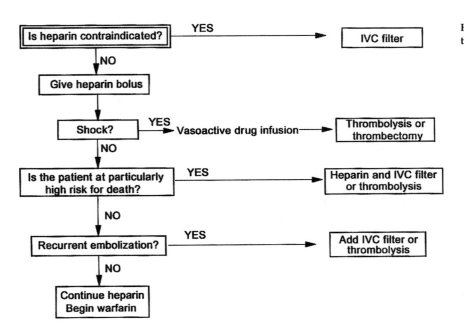

FIGURE 98-2 An integrated approach to therapy of PE.

agulation is necessary (unless the indication for VCI is contraindicated to anticoagulation).

Treatment of Pulmonary Embolism: An Integrated Approach

In most patients with objectively documented PE, pharmacologic treatment will consist of the following: (1) heparin, 5000 units IV immediately, followed by a continuous intravenous infusion of 1680 units per hour to be adjusted based on the aPTT (goal = 1.5 to 2.5 times control); (2) warfarin, 10 mg orally on each of the first 2 days following diagnosis, with subsequent doses adjusted based on the INR (goal = 2.0 to 3.0); (3) discontinuation of heparin after 5 days, if the INR is therapeutic; (4) continued warfarin to maintain the INR between 2.0 and 3.0 for ≥3 months. However, at many steps along this "ideal" treatment course, many alternative or additional strategies, such as thrombolytic therapy or vasoactive drug infusion should be considered. An approach to managing such patients is presented in Fig. 98-2.

References

1. Manier G, Castaing Y: Influence of cardiac output on oxygen exchange in acute pulmonary embolism. *Am Rev Respir Dis* 1992; 145:130.
2. Manthous CA, Hall JB, Kushner R, et al.: The effect of mechanical ventilation on oxygen consumption in critically ill patients. *Am J Respir Crit Care Med* 1995; 151:210.
3. Ozier Y, Dubourg O, Farcot JC, et al.: Circulatory failure in acute pulmonary embolism. *Intens Care Med* 1984; 10:91.
4. Jardin F, Dubourg O, Gueret P, et al.: Quantitative two-dimensional echocardiography in massive pulmonary embolism: Emphasis on ventricular interdependence and leftward septal displacement. *J Am Coll Cardiol* 1987; 10:1201.
5. Dell'Italia LJ, Starling MR, Blumhardt R, et al.: Comparative effects of volume loading, dobutamine, and nitroprusside in patients with predominant right ventricular infarction. *Circulation* 1985; 72:1327.
6. Chatterjee K: Pathogenesis of low output in right ventricular myocardial infarction. *Chest* 1992; 102:590S.
7. Belenkie I, Dani R, Smith ER, et al.: Effects of volume loading during experimental acute pulmonary embolism. *Circulation* 1989; 80:178.
8. Molloy WD, Lee KY, Girling L, et al.: Treatment of shock in a canine model of pulmonary embolism. *Am Rev Respir Dis* 1984; 130:870.
9. Boulain T, Lanotte R, Legras A, et al.: Efficacy of epinephrine therapy in shock complicating pulmonary embolism. *Chest* 1993; 104:300.
10. Hirsch LJ, Rooney MW, Wat SS, et al.: Norepinephrine and phenylephrine effects on right ventricular function in experimental canine pulmonary embolism. *Chest* 1991; 100:796.
11. Angle MR, Molloy DW, Penner B, et al.: The cardiopulmonary and renal hemodynamic effects of noreprinephrine in canine pulmonary embolism. *Chest* 1989; 95:1333.
12. Jardin F, Genevray B, Brun-Ney D, et al.: Dobutamine: A hemodynamic evaluation in pulmonary embolism shock. *Crit Care Med* 1985; 13:1009.
13. Bourdarias JP, Dubourg O, Gueret P, et al.: Inotropic agents in the treatment of cardiogenic shock. *Pharmacol Ther* 1983; 22:53.
14. Wolfe MW, Saad RM, Spence TH: Hemodynamic effects of amrinone in a canine model of massive pulmonary embolism. *Chest* 1992; 102:274.
15. Bates ER, Crevey BJ, Sprague FR, et al.: Oral hydralazine therapy for acute pulmonary embolism and low output state. *Arch Intern Med* 1981; 141:1537.
16. Goldhaber SZ: Thrombolysis in venous thromboembolism: An international perspective. *Chest* 1990; 97(suppl):176S.
17. UPET Study Group: Urokinase pulmonary embolism trial: Phase 1 results. *JAMA* 1970; 214:2163.
18. Petitpretz P, Simmoneau G, Cerrina J, et al.: Effects of a single bolus of urokinase in patients with life-threatening pulmonary emboli: A descriptive trial. *Circulation* 1984; 70:861.
19. Goldhaber SZ, Kessler CM, Heit J, et al.: A randomized controlled trial of recombinant tissue plasminogen activator versus urokinase in the treatment of acute pulmonary embolism. *Lancet* 1988; ii:293.
20. Wilcox RG: Thrombolysis with tissue plasminogen activator in suspected acute myocardial infarction: The ASSET study. *Chest* 1989; 95(suppl):270S.
21. Levine MN, Weitz J, Turpie AGG, et al.: A new short infusion dosage regimen of recombinant tissue plasminogen activator in patients with venous thromboembolic disease. *Chest* 1990; 97(suppl):168S.
22. Thrombolytic therapy in thrombosis: A National Institutes of Health Consensus Development conference. *Ann Intern Med* 1980; 93:141.
23. Rogers LQ, Lutcher CL: Streptokinase therapy for deep vein thrombosis: A comprehensive review of the English literature. *Am J Med* 1990; 88:389.
24. Goldhaber SZ, Buring JE, Lipnick RJ, et al.: Pooled analyses of randomized trials of streptokinase and heparin in phlebographically documented acute deep vein thrombosis. *Am J Med* 1984; 76:393.
25. O'Meara JJ, McNutt RA, Evans AT, et al.: A decision analysis of streptokinase plus heparin as compared with heparin alone for deep-vein thrombosis. *N Engl J Med* 1994; 330:1864.
26. PAIMS 2: Alteplase combined with heparin vs heparin in the treatment of acute pulmonary embolism. Plasminogen activator Italian multicenter study 2. *J Am Coll Cardiol* 1992; 20:520.
27. Come PC, Kim D, Parker JA, et al.: Early reversal of right ventricular dysfunction in patients with acute pulmonary embolism after treatment with intravenous tissue plasminogen activator. *J Am Coll Cardiol* 1987; 10:971.
28. Sharma GVRK, Burleson VA, Sasahara AA: Effect of thrombolytic therapy on pulmonary-capillary blood volume in patients with pulmonary embolism. *N Engl J Med* 1980; 303:842.
29. Witty LA, Krichman A, Tapson VF: Thrombolytic therapy for venous thromboembolism. *Arch Intern Med* 1994; 154:1601.
30. Diehl J-L, Meyer G, Igual J, et al.: Effectiveness and safety of bolus administration of alteplase in massive pulmonary embolism. *Am J Cardiol* 1992; 70:1477.
31. Goldhaber SZ, Haire WD, Feldstein ML, et al.: Alteplase versus heparin in acute pulmonary embolism: Randomised trial assessing right-ventricular function and pulmonary perfusion. *Lancet* 1993; 341:507.
32. Hirsh J, Hull RD: Treatment of venous thromboembolism. *Chest* 1986; 89(suppl):426S.
33. Prewitt RM, Hoy C, Kong A, et al.: Thrombolytic therapy in canine pulmonary embolism: Comparative effects of urokinase and recombinant tissue plasminogen activator. *Am Rev Respir Dis* 1990; 141:290.
34. Goldhaber SZ, Kessler CM, Heit JA, et al.: Recombinant tissue-

type plasminogen activator versus a novel dosing regimen of urokinase in acute pulmonary embolism: A randomized controlled multicenter trial. *J Am Coll Cardiol* 1992; 20:24.

35. Goldhaber SZ, Feldstein ML, Sors H: Two trials of reduced bolus alteplase in the treatment of pulmonary embolism: An overview. *Chest* 1994; 106:725.

36. Goldhaber SZ, Agnelli G, Levine MN, et al.: Reduced dose bolus alteplase vs conventional alteplase infusion for pulmonary embolism thrombolysis: An international multicenter randomized trial. *Chest* 1994; 106:718.

37. Sors H, Pacouret G, Azarian R, et al.: Hemodynamic effects of bolus vs 2-h infusion of alteplase in acute massive pulmonary embolism: A randomized controlled multicenter trial. *Chest* 1994: 106:712.

38. Verstraete M, Miller GAH, Bounameaux H, et al.: Intravenous and intrapulmonary recombinant tissue-type plasminogen activator in the treatment of acute massive pulmonary embolism. *Circulation* 1988; 77:353.

39. Werier J, Ducas J, Gu S, et al.: Effect of low-molecular-weight heparin on recombinant tissue plasminogen activator-induced thrombolysis in canine pulmonary embolism. *Chest* 1991; 100:464.

40. The ISAM Study Group: A prospective trial of intravenous streptokinase in acute myocardial infarction (I.S.A.M.). *N Engl J Med* 1986; 314:1465.

41. ISIS-2: Randomized trial of intravenous streptokinase, oral aspirin, both, or neither among 17,187 cases of suspected acute myocardial infarction. *Lancet* 1988; ii:349.

42. Fennerty AG, Levine MN, Hirsh J: Hemorrhagic complications of thrombolytic therapy in the treatment of myocardial infarction and venous thromboembolism. *Chest* 1989; 95(suppl):88S.

43. Stein PD, Hull RD, Raskob G: Risks for major bleeding from thrombolytic therapy in patients with acute pulmonary embolism. *Ann Intern Med* 1994; 121:313.

44. Sane DC, Califf RM, Topol EJ, et al. Bleeding during thrombolytic therapy for acute myocardial infarction: Mechanisms and management. *Ann Intern Med* 1989; 111:1010.

45. Lund O, Nielsen TT, Schifter S, et al.: Treatment of pulmonary embolism with full-dose heparin, streptokinase, or embolectomy—results and indications. *Thorac Cardiovasc Surgeon* 1986; 34:240.

46. DelCampo C: Pulmonary embolectomy: A review. *Can J Surg* 1985; 28:111.

47. Gray HH, Miller GAH, Paneth M: Pulmonary embolectomy: Its place in the management of pulmonary embolism. *Lancet* 1988; i:1441.

48. Alpert JS, Smith RE, Ockene IS, et al.: Treatment of massive pulmonary embolism: The role of pulmonary embolectomy. *Am Heart J* 1975; 89:413.

49. Timsit J-F, Reynaud P, Meyer G, et al.: Pulmonary embolectomy by catheter device in massive pulmonary embolism. *Chest* 1991; 100:655.

50. Schmitz-Rode T, Gunther RW: Percutaneous mechanical thrombolysis: A comparative study of various rotational catheter systems. *Invest Radiol* 1991; 26:557.

51. Haskal ZJ, Soulen MC, Huettl EA, et al.: Life-threatening pulmonary emboli and cor pulmonale: Treatment with percutaneous pulmonary artery stent placement. *Radiology* 1994; 191:473.

52. Urokinase Pulmonary Embolism Trial Study Group: Urokinase pulmonary embolism trial: Phase 1 results. *JAMA* 1970; 214:2163.

53. Tollefsen DM, Majerus DW, Blank MK: Heparin cofactor II: Purification and properties of thrombin in human plasma. *J Biol Chem* 1982; 257:2162.

54. de Swart CAM, Nijmeyer B, Roelofs JMM, et al.: Kinetics of intravenously administered heparin in normal humans. *Blood* 1982; 60:1251.

55. Simon TL, Hyers TM, Gaston JP, et al.: Heparin pharmacokinetics: Increased requirements in pulmonary embolism. *Br J Haematol* 1978; 39:111.

56. Hull R, Raskob G, Hirsh J, et al.: Continuous intravenous heparin compared with intermittent subcutaneous heparin in the initial treatment of proximal-vein thrombosis. *N Engl J Med* 1986; 315:1109.

57. Brandjes DPM, Heijboer H, Büller HR, et al.: Acenocoumarol and heparin compared with acenocoumarol alone in the initial treatment of proximal-vein thrombosis. *N Engl J Med* 1992; 327:1485.

58. Brill-Edwards P, Ginsberg S, Johnston M, et al.: Establishing a therapeutic range for heparin therapy. *Ann Intern Med* 1993; 119:104.

59. Levine MN, Hirsh J, Gent M, et al.: A randomized trial comparing activated thromboplastin time with heparin assay in patients with acute venous thromboembolism requiring large daily doses of heparin. *Arch Intern Med* 1994; 154:49.

60. Andersson G, Fagrell B, Holmgren K, et al.: Subcutaneous administration of heparin: A randomized comparison with intravenous administration of heparin to patients with deep-vein thrombosis. *Thromb Res* 1982; 27:631.

61. Bentley PG, Kakkar VV, Scully MF, et al.: An objective study of alternative methods of heparin administration. *Thromb Res* 1980; 18:177.

62. Hommes DW, Bura A, Mazzolai L, et al.: Subcutaneous heparin compared with continuous intravenous heparin administration in the initial treatment of deep vein thrombosis. A meta-analysis. *Ann Intern Med* 1992; 116:279.

63. Hull RD, Raskob GE, Rosenbloom DR, et al.: Optimal therapeutic levels of heparin therapy in patients with venous thrombosis. *Arch Intern Med* 1992; 152:1589.

64. Fennerty A, Thomas P, Backhouse G, et al.: Audit of control of heparin treatment. *Br Med J* 1985; 290:27.

65. Wheeler AP, Jaquiss RD, Newman JH: Physician practices in the treatment of pulmonary embolism and deep-venous thrombosis. *Arch Intern Med* 1988; 148:1321.

66. Raschke RA, Reilly BM, Guidry JR, et al.: The weight-based heparin dosing nomogram compared with a "standard care" nomogram: A randomized controlled trial. *Ann Intern Med* 1993; 119:874.

67. Pineo GF, Hull RD: Classical anticoagulant therapy for venous thromboembolism. *Prog Cardiovasc Dis* 1994; 37:59.

68. Goldhaber SZ, Buring JE, Lipnick RJ, et al.: Pooled analyses of randomized trials of streptokinase and heparin in phlebographically documented acute deep venous thrombosis. *Am J Med* 1984; 76:393.

69. Landefeld CS, Cook EF, Flatley M, et al.: Indentification and preliminary validation of predictors of major bleeding in hospitalized patients starting anticoagulant therapy. *Am J Med* 1987; 82:703.

70. Green D, Martin GJ, Shoichet SH, et al.: Thrombocytopenia in a prospective randomized double-blind trial of bovine and porcine heparin. *Am J Med Sci* 1984; 288:60.

71. Warkentin TE, Kelton JG: Heparin and platelets. *Hematol/Oncol Clin North Am* 1990; 4:243.

72. Green D, Hirsh J, Heit J, et al.: Low molecular weight heparin: A critical analysis of clinical trials. *Pharmacol Rev* 1994; 46:89.

73. Spiro TE, Johnson GJ, Christie MJ, et al.: Efficacy and safety of enoxaparin to prevent deep venous thrombosis after hip replacement surgery. *Ann Intern Med* 1994; 121:81.

74. Matzsch T, Bergqvist D, Hedner U, et al.: Effects of an enzymat-

ically depolymerized heparin as compared with conventional heparin in healthy volunteers. *Thromb Haemost* 1987; 57:97.

75. Hull RD, Pineo GF: Low molecular weight heparin treatment of venous thromboembolism. *Prog Cardiovasc Dis* 1994; 37:71.

76. Leizorovicz A, Simonneau G, Decousus H, et al.: Comparison of efficacy and safety of low molecular weight heparins and unfractionated heparin in initial treatment of deep venous thrombosis: A meta-analysis. *Br Med J* 1994; 309:299.

77. Hull R, Delmore T, Genton E, et al.: Warfarin sodium versus low-dose heparin in the long-term treatment of venous thrombosis. *N Engl J Med* 1979; 301:855.

78. Lagerstedt CI, Olsson C-G, Fagher BO, et al.: Need for long-term anticoagulant treatment in symptomatic calf-vein thrombosis. *Lancet* 1985; ii:515.

79. Hull R, Delmore T, Carter C, et al.: Adjusted subcutaneous heparin versus warfarin sodium in the long-term treatment of venous thrombosis. *N Engl J Med* 1982; 306:189.

80. Freedman MD: Oral anticoagulants: Pharmacodynamics, clinical indications, and adverse effects. *J Clin Pharmacol* 1992; 32:196.

81. Clouse LH, Comp PC; The regulation of haemostasis: the protein C system. *N Engl J Med* 1986; 314:1298.

82. O'Reilly RA, Aggeler PM: Determinants of the response to oral anticoagulant drug in man. *Pharmacol Rev* 1970; 22:35.

83. O'Reilly RA, Aggeler PM: Studies on coumarin anticoagulant drugs: Initiation of warfarin therapy without an initial loading dose. *Circulation* 1968; 38:169.

84. Hirsh J, Dalen JE, Deykin D, et al.: Oral anticoagulants: Mechanism of action, clinical effectiveness, and optimal therapeutic range. *Chest* 1992; 102(suppl):312S.

85. Hellemans J, Vorlat M, Verstraete M: Survival time of prothrombin and factors VII, IX, and X after complete synthesis blocking doses of coumarin derivatives. *Br J Haematol* 1963; 9:506.

86. Gallus A, Jackaman J, Tillett J, et al.: Safety and efficacy of warfarin started early after submassive venous thrombosis or pulmonary embolism. *Lancet* 1986; ii:1293.

87. Hull RD, Raskob GE, Rosenbloom D, et al.: Heparin for 5 days as compared with 10 days in the initial treatment of proximal venous thrombosis. *N Engl J Med* 1990; 322:1260.

88. Rooke TW, Osmundson PJ: Heparin and the in-hospital management of deep-venous thrombosis: Cost considerations. *Mayo Clin Proc* 1986; 61:198.

89. Bussey HI, Force RW, Bianco TM, et al.: Reliance on prothrombin time ratios causes significant errors in anticoagulation therapy. *Arch Intern Med* 1992; 152:278.

90. Eckman MH, Levine HJ, Pauker SG: Effect of laboratory variation in the prothrombin-time ratio on the results of oral anticoagulant therapy. *N Engl J Med* 1993; 329:696.

91. Hirsh J: Substandard monitoring of warfarin in North America: Time for change [editorial]. *Arch Intern Med* 1992; 152:257.

92. Hirsh J, Poller L, Deykin D, et al.: Optimal therapeutic range for oral anticoagulants. *Chest* 1989; 95(suppl):5S.

93. Hull R, Hirsh J, Jay R, et al.: Different intensities of oral anticoagulant therapy in the treatment of proximal-vein thrombosis. *N Engl J Med* 1982; 307:1676.

94. Levine MN, Raskob G, Hirsh J: Hemorrhagic complications of long-term anticoagulant therapy. *Chest* 1989; 95(suppl):26S.

95. Shetty HG, Backhouse G, Bentley DP, et al.: Effective reversal of warfarin-induced excessive anticoagulation with low dose vitamin K1. *Thromb Haemost* 1992; 67:13.

96. Vigano S, Mannucci PM, Solinas S, et al.: Decrease in protein C antigen and formation of an abnormal protein soon after starting oral anticoagulant therapy. *Br J Haematol* 1984; 57:213.

97. Moser KM: Venous thromboembolism. *Am Rev Respir Dis* 1990; 141:235.

98. Becker DM, Philbrick JT, Selby JB: Inferior vena caval filters: Indications, safety, and effectiveness. *Arch Intern Med* 1992; 152:1985.

99. Millward SF, Marsh JI, Peterson RA, et al.: LGM (Vena Tech) vena cava filter: clinical experience in 64 patients. *J Vasc Intervent Radiol* 1991; 2:439.

100. Jones TK, Barnes RW, Greenfield LJ: Greenfield vena caval filter: Rationale and current indications. *Ann Thorac Surg* 1986; 42(suppl):S48.

101. Cohen JR, Grella L, Citron M: Greenfield filter instead of heparin as primary treatment for deep-venous thrombosis or pulmonary embolism in patients with cancer. *Cancer* 1992; 70:1993.

102. Bergqvist D: The role of vena caval interruption in patients with venous thromboembolism. *Prog Cardiovasc Dis* 1994; 37:25.

Chapter 99

PROPHYLAXIS AGAINST VENOUS THROMBOEMBOLISM

GREGORY A. SCHMIDT

Overview

Methods of Thromboprophylaxis

Evidence for Efficacy in Specific Risk Groups

Specific Recommendations in Various Risk Groups

Overview

Venous thromboembolism (VTE) is a major health problem, accounting for substantial morbidity and mortality. Twenty years ago it was estimated that more than 600,000 cases of pulmonary embolism (PE) occurred in the United States each year.[1] Although some investigators have described a decreasing incidence of PE since then,[2,3] other data show little significant change over time.[4,5] Some of these events complicate the terminal stages of advanced malignancy or debilitating illness, but many occur in patients who would otherwise return to independent function. It is this segment of the population at risk for VTE in whom prophylaxis is particularly attractive. Several features of the natural history of VTE make it an appropriate target for prophylactic measures. These include the fact that most of the patients who will die from PE will do so within 30 min of the onset of symptoms—too soon for clinical diagnosis and institution of therapy[6]; the clinically silent nature of venous thrombosis and pulmonary embolism, with fatal PE unsuspected antemortem in about 75 percent of cases discovered at autopsy[7,8]; and the difficulty of establishing a diagnosis because of the lack of accurate, noninvasive diagnostic tests. Thus, prevention may do more to reduce deaths than any evaluation or treatment stratagem. The routine use of perioperative prophylaxis in patients undergoing elective general surgery could save as many as 8000 lives per year in the United States.[9]

Over the last 20 years, a large volume of information regarding the risks and benefits of numerous prophylactic strategies has been collected. The greatest accumulated experience is with low-dose heparin, typically 5000 units administered subcutaneously either bid or tid in both surgical and medical patients. Other methods of thromboprophylaxis also are available and may have a role in special subsets of patients, patients in whom heparin is ineffective or contraindicated or those who are at unusually high (or low) risk of VTE. These alternatives include low-molecular-weight heparins (LMWH), adjusted-dose heparin, heparin combined with dihydroergotamine (DHE), aspirin, warfarin, dextrans, antiembolism stockings, intermittent pneumatic (or sequential) compression cuffs, and vena caval interruption. Despite clear evidence of efficacy, practice surveys continue to show that many clinicians fail to use thromboprophylaxis.[10] Reasons include a lack of knowledge about available prophylactic measures, a poor appreciation of the magnitude of the problem of VTE, or an exaggerated fear of the complications of prophylaxis.[11] In many settings, the optimal approach has not yet been clarified. Nevertheless, for most patients at risk of VTE, some method that is both safe and effective is available. By identifying patients at risk of VTE (see Chap. 96) and employing currently available therapy, clinicians have an opportunity to reduce dramatically the morbidity and mortality of VTE.

Methods of Thromboprophylaxis

LOW-DOSE HEPARIN

Unfractionated heparin (UFH) consists of a heterogenous collection of glycosaminoglycans, typically derived from porcine or bovine lung and intestine, ranging in molecular weight from 1800 to 30,000 (mean, 15,000). Its anticoagulant activity is found in a pentasaccharide sequence with a high binding affinity for antithrombin III (AT-III). Heparin induces a conformational change in AT-III, greatly enhancing its ability to inactivate the coagulation factors thrombin, factor Xa, and factor IXa. The heparin/AT-III complex interacts differently with thrombin (heparin acting as a template for the binding of both AT-III and thrombin in a ternary complex) when compared to its role in inhibiting factor Xa (no ternary complex needed). Only heparin molecules of 18 saccharides or greater are capable of binding simultaneously AT-III and thrombin. Thus, low-molecular-weight heparins (LMWH), which consist largely of heparins with fewer than

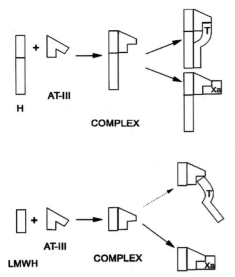

FIGURE 99-1 Both unfractionated heparin (H) and low-molecular-weight heparins (LMWH) bind to antithrombin III (AT-III), inducing a comformational change in AT-III. This structural change enhances the ability of AT-III to inactivate factors Xa and IXa. The unfractionated heparin/AT-III complex can bind further with thrombin (T), forming a ternary complex and inactivating thrombin. In contrast, the LMWH/AT-III complex is incapable of inactivating thrombin because most LMWH are < 18 saccharides in length and therefore incapable of forming the required ternary complex.

18 saccharides (see below), cannot speed the inactivation of thrombin as well as UFH yet remain able to catalyze the inhibition of factor Xa (see Fig. 99-1). Part of UFH's anticoagulant effect is mediated through heparin cofactor II, which does not bind the pentasaccharide sequence but requires a chain length of at least 24 saccharide units. With the exception of the heparinoid lomoparin, LMWH cannot use this pathway of thrombin inactivation. Differences in chain length influence not only the anticoagulant properties of unfractionated heparin but also its clearance from the body. Higher-molecular-weight components are more readily cleared, leading to a relative accumulation of the low-molecular-weight molecules, which retain their anti–factor Xa effect but have little effect on the partial thromboplastin time.

Following administration, heparin binds to several plasma proteins, such as histidine-rich glycoprotein, von Willebrand factor (VWF), and platelet factor IV, which reduces its bioavailability, especially at the low doses given for thromboprophylaxis. In addition, binding of heparin to VWF inhibits platelet function, potentially contributing to hemorrhagic complications. Following subcutaneous administration, heparin binds to macrophages and endothelial cells, where it is internalized and catabolized. This further contributes to its unpredictable effect in low doses. Some of these features are not true of LMWH, leading to a more predictable pharmacokinetic profile and making them attractive alternatives to UFH for thromboprophylaxis in some settings.

The efficacy of low-dose heparin for the prevention of deep venous thrombosis (DVT) in the perioperative setting was clearly established by the early 1970s. The important International Multicenter Trial, published in 1975, extended these findings to the ability of low doses of heparin to reduce fatal postoperative pulmonary embolism.[12] In this trial of more than 4000 patients over the age of 40 undergoing major elective surgery, half of whom served as controls, heparin was administered subcutaneously in a dose of 5000 units, beginning 2 h preoperatively and continued postoperatively every 8 h for 7 days. If patients were not ambulatory at 1 week, low-dose heparin was continued. Heparin was shown to reduce effectively the incidence of DVT and PE as well as the number of fatal PEs. Nine patients died of hemorrhage, five in the control arm and four among those who were heparin treated. There was no difference in the operative or postoperative transfusion requirement or in the decline in postoperative hemoglobin concentration. There was a statistically significant increase in wound hematomas in the treated patients. A subsequent metaanalysis of all available randomized trials in general, orthopedic, and urologic surgery[13] as well as two further metaanalyses in general surgical patients[14,15] showed that DVT could be reduced by about 65 percent, PE by about 50 percent, and fatal PE by more than 60 percent with low-dose heparin. These overviews also revealed a one-half to two-thirds increase in the risk of bleeding, but the overall magnitude of such bleeding was small. Although there is debate about whether more aggressive preventive measures are beneficial in certain very high risk patients, it is clear that heparin is effective in these settings. Twice-daily administration of 5000 units has not been compared directly with a three times per day regimen, but one metaanalysis showed that the higher-dose regimen was more effective.[14] There is also evidence for the efficacy of low-dose heparin in some groups of general medical patients (see below).

In addition to a small but significant increase in wound hematomas of surgical patients, complications of low-dose heparin prophylaxis include bleeding, heparin-associated thrombocytopenia (HAT), osteoporosis, and, very rarely, anaphylaxis, skin necrosis, local urticaria, or hypoaldosteronism. While the risk of wound hematomas is real, it is small and generally outweighed by the benefits. Exceptions include surgery of the central nervous system and eye, where heparin is contraindicated, and possibly operations in which foreign material is being implanted. In medical patients selected to be at low risk of bleeding, this complication is very uncommon (below 1 percent).[16] Thrombocytopenia is a well-established complication of heparin therapy but is relatively rare in patients receiving low-dose heparin (less than 1 percent of patients[17]). The platelet count typically returns to normal within a few days of stopping heparin, but severe or protracted thrombocytopenia and thrombotic complications are possible.[18] This complication is discussed more fully in Chap. 98. Osteoporosis is an uncommon adverse effect of heparin but is particularly worrisome in subsets of patients who receive it for long periods of time. The mechanism of osteoporosis is unknown, but its severity may be related to dose and duration of therapy. Most cases of symptomatic spinal fracture have been described in patients given more than 15,000 units per day for at least several months.[19] Yet there are exceptions, as during the thromboprophylaxis of pregnant women with a history of VTE, who are often treated with > 10,000 units per day of heparin. In a study of 184 women treated prophylactically during pregnancy and the puerperium, 4 developed osteoporotic spinal fractures.[20] Although three of these women were treated with rather high doses (25,000, 30,000, and 28,000 IU/24 h for 27, 9, and 25 weeks respectively), one was given only 15,000 IU/24 h for 7 weeks. Another single case has been described in which one woman suffered spinal fracture after treatment with only 10,000 IU/day.[21] Two recent studies have failed to show any relationship between heparin dose and osteoporosis during pregnancy.[22,23] In a group of women treated with a mean dose of 17,300 IU/day for a mean of 28 weeks during pregnancy, there was a 5 percent reduction in trabecular bone mass.[24] In the 6 weeks postpartum, a small degree of reversibility was noted, but the long-term consequences of this bone loss are not known.

LOW-MOLECULAR-WEIGHT HEPARINS

Low-molecular-weight heparins (LMWH) are derived from unfractionated heparin (UFH) through chemical or enzymatic depolymerization. The resulting products, which include Fraxiparin (also called Seleparin), Enoxaparin (also called Clexane, Lovenox), Fragmin, RD heparin, Parnaparin, Tinzaparin, Fluxum, Ardeparin (also called Normiflo), Embolex NM, Clivarin (also called Reviparin), Bioparin, Miniparin, and Logiparin (also called Innohep), have molecular weights between 4000 and 6500 kDa. A similar agent is Lomoparin, which is actually a mixture of heparan sulfate, dermatan sulfate, and chondroitin sulfates. Lomoparin is not a true heparin, although it has a molecular weight of 6500 kDa; its half-life is unusually long (1100 min), and its action is mediated wholly through heparin cofactor II rather than antithrombin III. There are potentially significant differences between the various LMWH, related to differences in average molecular weight, ratio of anti-factor IIa to anti-factor Xa, or pharmacokinetics. When more information is available, clear advantages of one agent over the others, or certain agents in particular subsets of patients may become appar-

ent. There have been no direct comparisons between these drugs. Since these agents resemble each other in many regards and tend to share features that distinguish them from UFH, they are considered together.

Several differences between LMWH and UFH have led to the increasing clinical interest in LMWH both for thromboprophylaxis and therapy of established thrombosis (see Table 99-1). These LMWH retain their ability to inhibit factor Xa by binding to AT-III but have a substantially reduced ability to catalyze the inactivation of thrombin, because only larger oligosaccharides (at least 18 monosaccharides in length) are capable of forming the ternary complex between heparin, AT-III, and thrombin required for inhibition.[25] The available LMWH have ratios of anti-factor Xa to antithrombin ranging between 2:1 and 4:1. LMWH do not bind to most heparin-binding proteins or to endothelial cells. This accounts in part for their very high bioavailability at low doses and for their predictable anticoagulant effect when given in fixed doses.[26,27] Their lack of binding to VWF may contribute to the reduced incidence of bleeding seen in some animal and clinical trials of LMWH.[28,29] This potential advantage has not been borne out in clinical trials at prophylactic doses[30] but is evident when LMWH are used in full anticoagulant doses.[29,31]

The half-lives of LMWH range from roughly 2 to 4.4 h, compared to about 35 min for heparin, and their clearance is dose-independent.[25,32] This characteristic makes once-daily dosing of LMWH possible, and they are known to be effective on such a schedule. One of the remaining questions about LMWH is whether efficacy is sacrificed with a once-daily regimen compared to twice-daily administration. In one trial of VTE prophylaxis in total hip replacement (THR), two regimens of Fragmin were used, 2500 U bid and 5000 U qd.[33] The incidence of venographic DVT was not different between these regimens (5.3 and 7.7 percent respectively) and was low in both. On the other hand, in two other studies, a twice-daily regimen of LMWH appeared more effective than a once-daily dose, although the total dose was not precisely equal in the two groups.[34,35] Further trials will be necessary to determine whether the more convenient once-daily use of LMWH is as effective as twice-daily dosing. The FDA has approved only the twice-daily regimen for prophylaxis in patients undergoing THR. LMWH are cleared

TABLE 99-1   Advantages and Disadvantages of LMWH

Advantages of LMWH over UFH	Disadvantages of LMWH
Greater prophylactic effect in certain subsets, e.g., THR	Greater cost
More predictable dose response; monitoring generally unnecessary	Little effect on PTT; monitoring difficult
Longer half-life; less frequent dosing needed	Longer half-life disadvantageous if patient bleeds
Possibly less bleeding for equivalent antithrombotic effect	Less neutralizable by protamine
Reduced incidence of HAT	
Possibly lower risk of osteoporosis	

ABBREVIATIONS: LMWH = low-molecular-weight heparins; UFH = unfractionated heparin; THR = total hip replacement; HAT = heparin-associated thrombocytopenia; PTT = partial thromboplastin time.

by the renal route, and their half-life is increased in renal failure.[25]

There is now evidence that LMWH are less likely to cause heparin-associated thrombocytopenia (HAT) than UFH.[36] This might be predicted from their lesser tendency to interact with platelets. The LMWH may also cause less osteoporosis, a feature which, if supported in further studies, would be especially important for thromboprophylaxis in pregnancy. LMWH have been shown to demineralize bone to a similar degree as UFH in experimental animals,[37] but in a small series of pregnant women followed with dual-photon absorptiometry, no loss of bone mass was seen.[38] Whether these agents have any advantage in bone mass sparing for thromboprophylaxis in pregnant women remains speculative.

ADJUSTED-DOSE HEPARIN

Although low-dose heparin is effective in moderate-risk patients, in those at highest risk of VTE, the rate of DVT remains unacceptable despite its use. A more intensive alternative approach uses greater doses of heparin, typically an amount sufficient to increase the partial thromboplastin time (PTT) to 31 to 36 s, determined 6 h following subcutaneous injection. This regimen is more effective than low-dose heparin in reducing DVT and proximal thrombosis in high-risk patients.[39,40] The number of units of blood transfused, the incidence of wound hematoma, and the postoperative drop in hemoglobin are not increased with this regimen compared to low-dose heparin. However, 2 preoperative days have been used to determine the amount of heparin needed to raise the PTT, and the cumbersomeness of this regimen lessens its attraction, despite its efficacy and safety.

HEPARIN COMBINED WITH DIHYDROERGOTAMINE

Dihydroergotamine mesylate (DHE) is a vasoconstrictor drug, which is combined with heparin in a fixed dose of 0.5 mg and 5000 IU. DHE preferentially increases venous smooth muscle tone compared to arterial tone, significantly increasing venous blood flow velocity and reducing venous diameter intraoperatively.[41] The rationale for this approach is to reduce venous stasis and, possibly, to reduce endothelial injury, in addition to providing anticoagulation.

Heparin/DHE is effective in reducing DVT in general and orthopedic surgery. The relative risk reduction is similar in magnitude to that of heparin or IPC (risk reduction, 0.64[42]); but in comparative trials of heparin versus heparin/DHE, the combined approach was found to be superior. A complication of heparin/DHE is severe vasospasm; therefore its use is contraindicated in patients with hypotension, sepsis, trauma, and ischemia. Although there is potential for this agent in very high risk patients, concern over vasospastic complications apparently has led the manufacturer to stop marketing the drug in the United States.

ASPIRIN

Aspirin generally has been considered to be ineffective in surgical patients, although it may have some efficacy in pre-

venting proximal vein thrombosis in patients having total hip replacement.[42] However, a recent overview of all antiplatelet trials (including, in addition to aspirin, dipyridamole, hydroxychloroquine, and ticlopidine) showed that aspirin has some effect in general surgery, orthopedic surgery, and high-risk medical patients.[43] The risk reduction for DVT was similar in these three groups (0.37, 0.49, and 0.42, respectively), and an effect was also shown for prevention of PE. Yet several questions remain, since specific drugs and doses that are effective cannot be ascertained from this metaanalysis. Moreover, the reduction in risk attributed to antiplatelet drugs was much less than that seen with better agents, and, at least for the time being, aspirin will continue to have no significant role in thromboprophylaxis as a single agent.

WARFARIN

Warfarin sodium, in doses less than those required for full anticoagulation, has been tested in patients at very high risk of perioperative VTE in whom low-dose heparin does not provide adequate prophylaxis. Various approaches include giving a fixed dose of 2 mg preoperatively; giving sufficient warfarin to prolong the prothrombin time (PT) by 1.5 to 3 s beginning 10 days before surgery (then boosting the dose postoperatively to a PT of 1.5 times control[44]); or beginning warfarin postoperatively to an international normalized ratio (INR) of 2 to 2.5 (or 3 for total hip replacement). Warfarin has been found to be one of the most effective of all prophylactic regimens,[40,45] but its use is limited by concern for bleeding, the need to begin treatment 1 week or more preoperatively (for most regimens), and the difficulty of adjusting the dose to the recommended degree of anticoagulation (which requires intensive testing). Despite the concern for bleeding, studies have shown warfarin to be safe, and the risk of bleeding is similar to or slightly less than that caused by LMWH or low-dose heparin.[46] The added burden of monitoring this effect of this drug is justifiable in patients at high risk of VTE, although alternative measures (such as LMWH) may be preferred.

DEXTRANS

Dextran has effects on platelets, endothelium, fibrinolysis, and blood flow, which combine to make this drug moderately effective.[40,46] Since it must be given intravenously and its use is occasionally complicated by fluid overload or anaphylaxis and since more effective drugs are now available (LMWH, warfarin), dextran will probably not continue to be used for thromboprophylaxis.

GRADUATED COMPRESSION STOCKINGS

One of the simplest methods for prophylaxis against DVT is the application of graduated compression stockings (GCS). Typically these stockings provide 18 mmHg compression at the ankle, which gradually decreases to 6 to 8 mmHg at the upper thigh. There is no risk of bleeding, but the use of GCS is not entirely without risk. Several patients have suffered serious ischemic complications, and GCS should not be used in the setting of significant peripheral vascular disease or diabetic neuropathy. Although thigh-high and knee-high stockings have occasionally been compared and found to be equivalent, too few patients wearing knee-high stockings have been studied to enable confident prediction of efficacy. A recent metaanalysis of GCS in general surgery (nearly all patients had thigh-high stockings) showed them to be remarkably effective in the prevention of DVT (risk reduction, 0.68[47]). There is only one study with acceptable methods in patients undergoing THR, and GCS appeared to be effective in that setting as well (risk reduction 0.65[48]). It is not known if GCS is effective in reducing the incidence of PE, but it may be reasonable to conclude this, based on the usual progression of DVT to PE.

INTERMITTENT PNEUMATIC COMPRESSION

Intermittent pneumatic compression (IPC) devices compress the lower extremity rhythmically, inflating for roughly 10 s/min with a pressure of about 35 mmHg, then slowly deflating. These devices should be used intraoperatively and continued until the patient is ambulatory. Short periods with the cuffs off are typically allowed to facilitate nursing care, limited ambulation, and patient comfort. The IPC device limits venous stasis, thereby reducing the propensity to clot formation. In addition, there appears to be an enhancement of systemic fibrinolysis, since application of cuffs to the arms reduces the risk of DVT in the legs.[49] This modality is of established efficacy in urologic surgery,[50] neurologic surgery, general surgery,[51] and orthopedic surgery of the lower extremities.[52] One of its greatest limitations is poor compliance, especially in alert patients.

VENA CAVAL INTERRUPTION

Several devices on the market make percutaneous vena caval interruption (VCI) relatively safe and easy. These devices effectively prevent embolization through the inferior vena cava while allowing the flow of blood to pass unobstructed. While VCI is useful in preventing PE, it does nothing to reduce the risk of DVT. Thus, it is generally not an appropriate prophylactic approach for most patients. It may be useful, however, in patients who are at extremely high risk of death if they were to suffer PE (e.g., severe pulmonary hypertension or cor pulmonale) or in those with established DVT who need perioperative protection against PE, or who suffer a complication of anticoagulation, and in patients for whom other methods of prophylaxis are contraindicated or ineffective (e.g., patients with combined brain and spinal cord injury).

THE ROLE OF EPIDURAL ANESTHESIA

The risk of DVT in patients who undergo major orthopedic surgery of the lower extremities or prostate surgery can be reduced by epidural or spinal anesthesia.[53–55] A reduction of risk of about 50 percent has generally been seen.[55] This is attributed to sympathetic blockade with vasodilation and increased blood flow to the extremities. Benefit from

hypotensive anesthesia in terms of thrombosis risk has also been reported.[56] These effects have typically been seen in patients who have not been given standard thromboprophylaxis; whether the type of anesthesia has any influence when other methods of prophylaxis are used is unknown.

In early recommendations for the use of anticoagulant thromboprophylaxis, spinal or epidural anesthesia was thought to be contraindicated because of the potential for spinal hematoma and neurologic injury. Although this complication has been reported, it appears to be extremely rare. There is now published experience with more than 10,000 patients who have undergone concomitant spinal/epidural anesthesia and prophylaxis with LMWH or low-dose heparin. With this experience, there is increasing sentiment that the combination is safe.[57] Nevertheless, any patient given the combination should have careful serial assessment of neurologic function should this potentially catastrophic complication develop.

Evidence for Efficacy in Specific Risk Groups

TOTAL HIP REPLACEMENT

The efficacy of VTE prophylaxis has been most extensively studied following total hip replacement (THR). The incidence of DVT without prophylaxis is 40 to 60 percent; of proximal extension, about 20 percent; pulmonary embolism, 10 percent or more; and fatal PE as high as 7 percent[58] but more typically about 4 percent.[25] Aspirin, heparin (low-dose, adjusted-dose, LMWH, and combined with dihydroergotamine), warfarin, dextrans, graded compression stockings (GCS), and intermittent pneumatic compression (IPC) have all been employed (see Table 99-2).

Intermittent pneumatic compression can lower significantly the overall incidence of DVT[59] but provides relatively less protection against the more clinically relevant proximal vein thrombi.[60] Although some trials have shown aspirin to be effective and one large overview of antiplatelet prophylaxis also showed this,[43] aspirin appears substantially less efficacious than other methods and probably should be abandoned for this indication. Low-dose heparin is less effective and no safer than LMWH in these patients.[61] Of the agents studied, LMWH and warfarin stand out for established efficacy and safety. In a direct comparison of these two agents, LMWH was found to reduce the DVT rate more than warfarin, but at a cost of more frequent hemorrhage.[45] Although LMWH is easier to administer than warfarin and requires no monitoring, it is more costly, even taking into account the need to monitor warfarin's effect. Enoxaparin, Fragmin, Fraxiparin, Logiparin, RD heparin, Tinzaparin, and Lomoparin all appear to be useful,[25,45] and there have as yet been no direct comparisons between these LMWH. The FDA has now approved LMWH for thromboprophylaxis in THR.

TOTAL KNEE ARTHROPLASTY

The incidence of DVT may be even greater following total knee arthroplasty (TKA) than following THR (as high as 84 percent).[25] Proximal extension is less common, however, and

TABLE 99-2   Thromboprophylaxis in Patients Undergoing Total Hip Replacement

Drug	Dose	Risk of DVT Compared to Control (IM1,MO1)	Risk of Clinically Important Bleeding (%) (MO1)
Aspirin	150–650 mg q 12 h	0.80	0.4
Heparin, low-dose	10,000–15,000 IU divided bid or tid	0.50	2.6
Heparin, adjusted-dose	PTT 31.5–36s	0.35	
LMWH	Enoxaparin 30 mg (2400 anti-factor Xa U) q 12 h	0.30	1.8
Heparin + DHE	5000 IU/0.5 mg	0.60	-
Warfarin	INR 2–2.7	0.45	1.3
Dextran	various	0.60	0.8
GCS	NA	0.80	0
IPC	NA	0.45	0

ABBREVIATIONS: LMWH = low-molecular-weight heparins; DHE = dihydroergotamine; GCS = graded compression stockings; IPC = intermittent pneumatic compression device; DVT = deep venous thrombosis; PTT = partial thromboplastin time; INR = international normalized ratio; NA = not applicable.

pulmonary embolism may complicate only a few percent of cases (2 to 7 percent[25]). The use of LMWH is much more effective than placebo, leading to a 71 percent reduced incidence of DVT.[62] In contrast to THR, warfarin is not as effective as LMWH[45,63] for DVT prevention following TKA.

GENERAL SURGERY

Many investigators have studied the effect of thromboprophylaxis in general surgical patients over the age of 40. These studies have included a diverse population of subjects, typically having gastrointestinal surgery. However, some studies have also included patients undergoing thoracic, breast, vascular, or pelvic surgery. For procedures involving general anesthesia lasting more than 30 min, it is generally agreed that the risk of DVT is moderately high. The incidence of DVT is 19 to 25 percent (depending on the detection method used); of proximal DVT, 7 percent; of clinically recognized PE, 1.6 percent; and of fatal PE, 0.8 percent.[42] Patients under the age of 40 without additional risk factors for VTE and those having brief procedures (less than 30 min) are at low risk; the impact of thromboprophylaxis in them has not been studied. In these low-risk patients, early mobilization is probably sufficient prophylaxis.

In moderate-risk surgical patients, low-dose heparin is effective in reducing the risk of DVT from 25 to 8 percent when begun 2 h preoperatively and continued every 8 or 12 h for 1 week or until full ambulation is achieved. Several studies have also shown that heparin reduces fatal PE by 50 percent.[12–14] It is likely that the higher-dose regimen (every 8 h) is more effective, as demonstrated in a metaanalysis of trials comparing these two approaches.[14] Heparin slightly increases the risk of wound hematomas, but not of serious bleeding, life-threatening hemorrhage, or transfusion requirement.[13,14]

The use of LMWH has been compared with that of low-dose heparin in more than 10,000 general surgery patients. In a metaanalysis, LMWH were shown to be as safe and more effective than standard heparin, reducing the risk of DVT (relative risk 0.79; 95 percent confidence limits, 0.65 to 0.95) and of PE (relative risk 0.44; 95 percent confidence limits, 0.21 to 0.95), with no increase in the risk of bleeding.[64] When analysis was limited to the studies with strongest methodology, however, the advantage for LMWH was small (DVT relative risk, 0.91; PE relative risk, 0.62), and there was a suggestion of increased bleeding (relative risk, 1.32).[64] In a subsequent large trial comparing low-dose heparin and LMWH begun preoperatively, rates of DVT were very low and similar in both groups (0.7 percent), while wound hematomas and severe bleeding were less frequent in the LMWH group.[65] Since the risk of VTE is less in general surgery than in orthopedic surgery, the incremental benefit of LMWH is less significant. Many more general surgery patients than THR patients would have to be treated to provide benefit, and this would be at a substantial cost. For this reason, most authorities do not believe LMWH should replace standard heparin as the prophylactic method of choice for most moderate-risk general surgery patients.

Intermittent pneumatic compression (IPC) devices have also been shown in a metaanalysis to be effective in reducing the incidence of DVT in general surgical patients.[14] Although it is reasonable to presume that this will be translated into a reduction in PE and deaths, such reductions have not been shown, and IPC cannot be used with as much confidence as better-tested methods (i.e., heparin). Other disadvantages include the limited availability of the apparatus and poor compliance rate with IPC, which, in the best circumstances, is only about 65 percent. On the other hand, IPC does not increase the risk of bleeding and may be appropriate in patients at high risk of hemorrhage, those in whom heparin is contraindicated, and those in whom foreign material is being implanted (since hematoma around a foreign body may increase the risk of serious infection). Further, IPC may prove useful when combined with heparin or LMWH in patients at very high risk of VTE.

HIGH-RISK GENERAL SURGERY

Some patients having general surgical procedures are at exceptionally high risk of VTE, such as those who have had prior DVT or PE, those with extensive malignant disease undergoing large operations, or those with multiple risk factors for VTE. The risk of DVT in this subset may be similar to that in patients having major orthopedic surgery (40 to 80 percent), with a correspondingly increased risk of PE.[66] Such patients would probably benefit from more aggressive prophylaxis than is appropriate in moderate-risk general surgery patients, such as LMWH, adjusted-dose heparin, low-dose heparin plus IPC or GCS, or warfarin.[42,66] There are insufficient data in this subset from which to draw firm conclusions about which methods may be useful.

NEUROSURGERY

The risk of DVT in a general neurosurgical population ranges from 20 to 50 percent.[67] At particularly high risk are patients with spinal cord injury or stroke (discussed below) and those with brain tumors. Intermittent pneumatic compression or GCS is preferred in neurosurgical patients because these mechanical methods do not increase the risk of hemorrhage. The highest-risk patients may benefit from more intensive prophylaxis, such as the addition of an anticoagulant postoperatively or LMWH.[67]

SPINAL CORD INJURY

Patients with acute spinal cord injury are at great risk of DVT, especially in the first weeks following injury, such that as many as 80 percent will have detectable thrombosis and roughly 3 percent will die of PE.[68] Heparin has been shown to be ineffective in low doses when given alone. Intermittent pneumatic compression should be initiated in virtually all patients and supplemented with anticoagulant drugs 72 h following injury, typically LMWH,[69] warfarin (INR 2 to 3), adjusted-dose heparin, or low-dose heparin plus continuous electrical stimulation of the calf muscles.[70] An alternative approach is to place a VCI device, especially if coincident brain injury makes anticoagulation risky. Prophylaxis is usually continued for 3 months in those who do not regain motor function. The subsequent incidence of thrombosis is about 6 percent when prophylaxis is discontinued 8 weeks following injury.

GENERAL MEDICAL CONDITIONS

Studies of the preventive effect of low-dose heparin in medical patients are fewer than those in many surgical patient groups. Nevertheless, heparin is effective for the prevention of DVT in patients with acute myocardial infarction,[71] in whom the risk of DVT is about 25 percent; in patients with ischemic stroke and leg paralysis,[72] almost half of whom would otherwise develop DVT; in those with congestive heart failure or pulmonary infection;[73] and probably in general medical inpatients over the age of 40.[74] One of these studies was sufficiently large to detect a reduction in all-cause mortality attributed to prophylaxis, from 10.9 to 7.8 percent,[74] a proportional reduction in deaths approximately equal to that achieved with perioperative prophylaxis (4.2 to 3.4 percent[13]).

In the subset of patients with acute stroke and limb paralysis, in whom the risk of DVT is high, LMWH have a potential role. It is essential to rule out intracranial hemorrhage or metastatic disease with computed tomography before utilizing anticoagulant thromboprophylaxis. In clinical trials, Lomoparin has been shown to be more effective than placebo and more effective than low-dose heparin in reducing the incidence of DVT.[75,76] Hemorrhagic transformation of the stroke was seen in 9 percent of those given Lomoparin versus 6 percent given heparin, which compares with about 7 percent of placebo-treated patients in the earlier trial. The role of Lomoparin is being investigated in a larger trial.

PREGNANCY

Women with a history of prior venous thromboembolism are at substantial risk of a recurrence during subsequent pregnancy and the postpartum period. This risk ranges from 4 to 20 percent[77–79] and may be highest in those women whose prior VTE occurred under an estrogenic stimulus.[77] Many questions remain, however, regarding the true magnitude of the risk of recurrence, which women are at highest risk of recurrence, and the optimal management of these patients. Many prophylactic strategies utilizing heparin have been advocated, but it remains unclear whether such prophylaxis is effective or completely safe. A constant dose of heparin, 5000 IU bid, throughout pregnancy appears to confer no protection compared to no prophylaxis,[77] so most authorities recommend dose escalation in the third trimester, when most recurrences are seen. One approach is to give an empiric dose of 5000 units subcutaneously every 12 h until the middle of the third trimester and then to increase the dose to prolong the midinterval (6 h postinjection) PTT to 1.5 times control.[80] Alternatively, one can more simply increase the dose to 7500 or 10,000 units every 12 h in the third trimester.[81] There are insufficient data to evaluate the effectiveness of these regimens, however. Such uncertainty regarding effectiveness could argue against the use of heparin, given the risk of osteoporosis. In one study designed to assess the risks of prophylactic heparin (10,000 units given twice daily throughout pregnancy and labor), 1 of 20 women developed severe, debilitating osteoporosis.[78] In addition, the investigators thought that the withholding of epidural analgesia in the women given heparin might have contributed to maternal and fetal morbidity, although the numbers were too small for certainty.

There is reason to be optimistic that the recent use of heparin assays, rather than the much less sensitive PTT, may lead to safe and effective prophylactic therapies. When 26 pregnant women with prior thromboembolism were given prophylactic heparin in a dose to maintain heparin levels between 0.08 to 0.15 IU/mL (measured 3 h after injection), no thromboembolic complications occurred, bleeding during delivery was not increased, and no spinal fractures were found.[82] The LMWH have also been used in pregnancy, and they appear not to cross the placenta.[83] Very preliminary evi-

TABLE 99-3   Recommended Prophylactic Regimens

Condition	Preferred Prophylaxis	Alternate
Total hip replacement	LMWH	Warfarin; INR 2-2.7
Knee arthroplasty	LMWH	IPC
General surgery; age over 40	Heparin 5000 IU SQ q 12	IPC; LMWH
General surgery; very high risk	LMWH	IPC + heparin; warfarin
Neurosurgery	IPC	
Spinal cord injury	IPC + LMWH or warfarin	VCI
General medical inpatient; age over 40	Heparin 5000 IU SQ bid	
Pregnancy with prior VTE	Heparin; for dose, see text	

ABBREVIATIONS: VTE = venous thromboembolism; LMWH = low-molecular-weight heparins, (e.g., Enoxaparin 30 mg q 12 h); INR = international normalized ratio; IPC = intermittent pneumatic compression; GCS = graded compression stockings; VCI = vena caval interruption. For specifics regarding these regimens, see their respective sections above.

dence suggests that they may not cause as much osteoporosis as UFH,[38] but this, as well as the general safety of LMWH in pregnancy, must be confirmed in further trials.

Specific Recommendations in Various Risk Groups

The preferred methods of prophylaxis for several subsets of medical and surgical patients are summarized in Table 99-3. It is important to assess each patient for potential contraindications before prescribing a particular method. For example, active bleeding or planned surgery in a critical site (eye, central nervous system) should lead to choosing a physical method rather than an anticoagulant. Also, prior heparin-associated thrombocytopenia or allergy should lead to selection of a non-heparin-based method of prophylaxis (LMWH may be acceptable). While there is still some controversy regarding the best or safest form of prophylaxis for some of these subsets, there now is unanimity that some method is preferable to no method.

References

1. Dalen JE, Alpert JS: Natural history of pulmonary embolism. *Prog Cardiovasc Dis* 1975; 17:259.

2. Goldhaber SZ, Hennekens CH: Time trends in hospital mortality and diagnosis of pulmonary embolism. *Am Heart J* 1982; 104:305–306.

3. Lilienfeld DE, Chan E, Ehland J, et al.: Mortality from pulmonary embolism in the United States: 1962 to 1984. *Chest* 1990; 98:1067–1072.

4. Lilienfeld DE, Godbold JH: Geographic distribution of pulmonary embolism mortality rates in the United States, 1980 to 1984. *Am Heart J* 1992; 124:1068–1072.

5. Anderson FA, Wheeler HB, Goldberg RJ, et al.: A population-based perspective of the hospital incidence and case-fatality rates of deep venous thrombosis and pulmonary embolism. *Arch Intern Med* 1991; 151:933–938.

6. Donaldson GA, Williams C, Scannell JG, et al.: A reappraisal of the application of the Trendelenburg operation to massive fatal embolism: Report of a successful pulmonary-artery thrombectomy using a cardiopulmonary bypass. *N Engl J Med* 1963; 268:171–174.

7. Goldhaber SZ, Hennekens CH, Evans DA, et al.: Factors associated with correct antemortem diagnosis of major pulmonary embolism. *Am J Med* 1982; 73:822–826.

8. Rubenstein I, Murray D, Hoffstein V: Fatal pulmonary emboli in hospitalized patients. *Arch Intern Med* 1988; 148:1425–1426.

9. Fratanoni J, Wessler S: *Prophylactic Therapy of Deep-Vein Thrombosis and Pulmonary Embolism.* Washington DC: United States Government Printing Office, DHEW publication no. (NIH) 76-866, 1975.

10. Anderson FA, Wheeler HB, Goldberg RJ, et al.: Physician practices in the prevention of venous thromboembolism. *Ann Intern Med* 1991; 115:591–595.

11. Laverick MD, Croal SA, Mollan RAB: Orthopedic surgeons and thromboprophylaxis. *Br Med J* 1991; 303:549–550.

12. Kakkar VV, Corrigan TP, Fossard DP, et al.: Prevention of fatal postoperative pulmonary embolism by low doses of heparin: An international multicenter trial. *Lancet* 1975; ii:45–51.

13. Collins R, Scrimgeour A, Yusuf S, et al.: Reduction in fatal pulmonary embolism and venous thrombosis by perioperative administration of subcutaneous heparin. *N Engl J Med* 1988; 318:1162–1173.

14. Clagett GP, Reisch JS: Prevention of venous thromboembolism in general surgical patients: Results of meta-analysis. *Ann Surg* 1988; 208:227–240.

15. Colditz GA, Tuden RL, Oster G: Rates of venous thrombosis after general surgery: Combined results of randomised clinical trials. *Lancet* 1986; i:143–146.

16. Freedman MD: Pharmacodynamics, clinical indications, and adverse effects of heparin. *J Clin Pharmacol* 1992; 32:584–596.

17. Phillips YY, Copley JB, Stor RA: Thrombocytopenia and low-dose heparin. *South Med J* 1983; 76:526–528.

18. Kelton JG: Heparin induced thrombocytopenia. *Haemostasis* 1986; 16:173–186.

19. Hirsh J, Dalen JE, Deykin D, et al.: Heparin: Mechanism of action, pharmacokinetics, dosing considerations, monitoring, efficacy, and safety. *Chest* 1992; 102 (suppl):337S–351S.

20. Dahlmann TC: Osteoporotic fractures and the recurrence of thromboembolism during pregnancy and the puerperium in 184 women undergoing thromboprophylaxis with heparin. *Am J Obstet Gynecol* 1993; 168:1265–1270.

21. Griffith HT, Liu DTY: Severe heparin osteoporosis in pregnancy. *Postgrad Med J* 1984; 60:424–425.

22. Dahlmann T, Lindvall N, Hellgren M: Osteopenia in pregnancy during long-term heparin treatment. *Br J Obstet Gynaecol* 1990; 97:221–228.

23. Ginsberg JS, Kowalchuk G, Hirsh J, et al.: Heparin effect on bone density. *Thromb Haemost* 1990; 64:286–289.

24. Dahlmann TC, Sjöberg HE, Ringertz H: Bone mineral density

during long-term prophylaxis with heparin in pregnancy. *Am J Obstet Gynecol* 1994; 170:1315–1320.

25. Green D, Hirsh J, Heit J, et al.: Low molecular weight heparin: A critical analysis of clinical trials. *Pharmacol Rev* 1994; 46:89–109.

26. Bara L, Billaud E, Gramond G, et al.: Comparative pharmaco-kinetics of low molecular weight heparin (PK 10169) and un-fractionated heparin after intravenous and subcutaneous administration. *Thromb Res* 1985; 39:631–635.

27. Handeland GF, Abidgaard GF, Holm U, et al.: Dose adjusted heparin treatment of deep venous thrombosis: A comparison of unfractionated and low molecular weight heparin. *Eur J Clin Pharmacol* 1990; 39:107–112.

28. Berqvist D, Nilsson B, Hedner U, et al.: The effects of heparin fragments of different molecular weight in experimental thrombosis and haemostasis. *Thromb Res* 1985; 38:589.

29. Prandoni P, Lensing AWA, Büller HR, et al.: Comparison of low-molecular-weight heparin with intravenous standard heparin in proximal deep-vein thrombosis. *Lancet* 1992; 339:441–445.

30. German Hip Arthroplasty Trial Group: Prevention of deep venous thrombosis with low-molecular-weight heparin in patients undergoing total hip replacement: A randomized trial. *Arch Orthop Trauma Surg* 1992; 111:110–120.

31. Hull R, Raskob GE, Pineo G, et al.: Subcutaneous low-molecular-weight heparin compared with continuous intravenous heparin in the treatment of proximal-vein thrombosis. *N Engl J Med* 1992; 326:975–982.

32. Spiro TE, Johnson GJ, Christie MJ, et al.: Efficacy and safety of enoxaparin to prevent deep venous thrombosis after hip replacement surgery. *Ann Intern Med* 1994; 121:81–89.

33. Dechavanne M, Ville D, Berruyer M, et al.: Randomized trial of a low molecular weight heparin (Kabi 2165) versus adjusted-dose subcutaneous standard heparin in the prophylaxis of deep-vein thrombosis after elective hip surgery. *Haemostasis* 1989; 1:5–12.

34. Hirsh J: Low-molecular-weight heparin vs warfarin for prophylaxis against deep-vein thrombosis (letter). *N Engl J Med* 1994; 330:862–863.

35. Hull RD, Pineo GF: Low-molecular-weight heparin vs warfarin for prophylaxis against deep-vein thrombosis (letter). *N Engl J Med* 1994; 330:863.

36. Warkentin TE, Levine MN, Hirsh J, et al.: Heparin-induced thrombocytopenia in patients treated with low-molecular-weight heparin or unfractionated heparin. *N Engl J Med* 1995; 332:1330–5.

37. Mätzsch T, Bergqvist D, Hedner U, et al.: Effects of low molecular weight heparin and unfragmented heparin on induction of osteoporosis in rats. *Thromb Haemost* 1990; 63:505–509.

38. Melissari E, Parker CJ, Wilson NV, et al.: Use of low molecular weight heparin in pregnancy. *Thromb Haemost* 1992; 68:652–656.

39. Leyvraz PF, Richard J, Bachmann F, et al.: Adjusted versus fixed-dose subcutaneous heparin in the prevention of deep-vein thrombosis after total hip replacement. *N Engl J Med* 1983; 309:954–958.

40. Mohr DN, Silverstein MD, Murtaugh PA, et al.: Prophylactic agents for venous thrombosis in elective hip surgery. *Arch Intern Med* 1993; 153:2221–2228.

41. Comerota AJ, White JV: The use of dihydroergotamine and heparin in the prophylaxis of deep venous thrombosis. *Chest* 1986; 89:389S–395S.

42. Clagett GP, Anderson FA, Levine MN, et al.: Prevention of venous thromboembolism. *Chest* 1992; 102(suppl):391S–407S.

43. Antiplatelet Trialist's Collaboration: Collaborative overview of randomized trials of antiplatelet therapy: III. Reduction in venous thrombosis and pulmonary embolism by antiplatelet prophylaxis among surgical and medical patients. *Br Med J* 1994; 308:235–246.

44. Francis CW, Marder VJ, Evarts M, et al.: Two-step warfarin therapy: Prevention of postoperative venous thrombosis without excessive bleeding. *JAMA* 1983; 249:374–378.

45. Hull R, Raskob G, Pineo G, et al.: A comparison of subcutaneous low-molecular-weight heparin with warfarin sodium for prophylaxis against deep-vein thrombosis after hip or knee implantation. *N Engl J Med* 1993; 329:1370–1376.

46. Imperiale TF, Speroff T: A meta-analysis of methods to prevent venous thromboembolism following total hip replacement. *JAMA* 1994; 271:1780–1785.

47. Wells PS, Lensing AWA, Hirsh J: Graduated compression stockings in the prevention of postoperative venous thromboembolism. *Arch Intern Med* 1994; 154:67–72.

48. Fredin H, Bergqvist D, Cederholm C, et al.: Thromboprophylaxis in hip arthroplasty: Dextran with graded compression or preoperative dextran compared in 150 patients. *Acta Orthop Scand* 1989; 60:678–681.

49. Knight MTN, Dawson R: Effect of intermittent compression of the arms on deep venous thrombosis in the legs. *Lancet* 1976; 2:1265–1268.

50. Coe NP, Collins REC, Klein LA, et al.: Prevention of deep vein thrombosis in urological patients: A controlled, randomized trial of low-dose heparin and external pneumatic compression. *Surgery* 1978; 83:230–234.

51. Oster B, Tuden RL, Colditz GA: Prevention of venous thromboembolism after general surgery: Cost-effectiveness analysis of alternative approaches to prophylaxis. *Am J Med* 1987; 82:889–899.

52. Hull RD, Raskob GE, Gent M, et al.: Effectiveness of intermittent pneumatic leg compression for preventing deep vein thrombosis after total hip replacement. *JAMA* 1990; 263:2313–2317.

53. Davis FM, Laurenson VG, Gillespie WJ, et al.: Deep vein thrombosis after total hip replacement: A comparison between spinal and general anesthesia. *J Bone Joint Surg* 1989; 71B:181–185.

54. Nielsen PT, Jorgensen LN, Albrecht-Beste E, et al.: Lower thrombosis risk with epidural blockade in knee arthroplasty. *Acta Orthop Scand* 1990; 61:29–31.

55. Prins M, Hirsh J: A comparison of general anesthesia and regional anesthesia as a risk factor for deep vein thrombosis following hip surgery: A critical review. *Thromb Haemost* 1990; 64:497–500.

56. Sharrock NE, Ranawat CS, Urquhart B, et al.: Factors influencing deep vein thrombosis following total hip arthroplasty under epidural anesthesia. *Anesth Analg* 1993; 76:765–777.

57. Bergqvist D, Lindblad B, Mätzsch T: Risk of combining low molecular weight heparin for thromboprophylaxis and epidural or spinal anesthesia. *Semin Thromb Hemost* 1993; 19:147–151.

58. Haake DA, Berkman SA: Venous thromboembolic disease after hip surgery: Risk factors, prophylaxis, and diagnosis. *Clin Orthop* 1989; 242:212–231.

59. Lieberman JR, Geerts WH: Prevention of venous thromboembolism after total hip and knee arthroplasty. *J Bone Joint Surg* 1994; 76A:1239–1250.

60. Francis CW, Pellegrini VD, Marder VJ, et al.: Comparison of warfarin and external pneumatic compression in prevention of venous thrombosis after total hip replacement. *JAMA* 1992; 267:2911–2915.

61. Anderson DR, O'Brien BJ, Levine MN, et al.: Efficacy and cost of low-molecular-weight heparin compared with standard heparin for the prevention of deep vein thrombosis after total hip arthroplasty. *Ann Intern Med* 1993; 119:1105–1112.

62. LeClerc JR, Geerts WH, Desjardins L, et al.: Prevention of deep vein thrombosis after major knee surgery: A randomized, double-blind trial comparing a low-molecular-weight heparin fragment (enoxaparin) to placebo. *Thromb Haemost* 1992; 67:417–423.

63. RD Heparin Arthroplasty Group: RD Heparin compared with

warfarin for prevention of venous thromboembolic disease following total hip or knee arthroplasty. *J Bone Joint Surg* 1994; 76A:1174–1185.

64. Nurmohamed MT, Rosendaal FR, Büller HR, et al.: Low-molecular-weight heparin versus standard heparin in general and orthopaedic surgery: A meta-analysis. *Lancet* 1992; 340:152–156.

65. Kakkar VV, Cohen AT, Edmonson RA, et al.: Low molecular weight versus standard heparin for prevention of venous thromboembolism after major abdominal surgery. *Lancet* 1993; 341:259–265.

66. Hull RD, Raskob GE, Hirsh J: Prophylaxis of venous thromboembolism: An overview. *Chest* 1986; 89(suppl):374S–383S.

67. Hamilton MG, Hull RD, Pineo GF: Venous thromboembolism in neurosurgery and neurology patients: A review. *Neurosurgery* 1994; 34:280–296.

68. Weingarten SI: Deep venous thrombosis in spinal cord injury: Overview of the problem. *Chest* 1992; 102(suppl):636S–639S.

69. Green D, Twardowski P, Wei R, et al.: Fatal pulmonary embolism in spinal cord injury. *Chest* 1994; 105:853–855.

70. Green D: Prophylaxis of thromboembolism in spinal cord-injured patients. *Chest* 1992; 102(suppl):649S–651S.

71. Emerson PA, Marks P: Preventing thromboembolism after myocardial infarction: effect of low-dose heparin or smoking. *Br Med J* 1977; 1:18–20.

72. McCarthy ST, Turner JJ, Robertson D, et al.: Low dose heparin as a prophylaxis against deep venous thrombosis after acute stroke. *Lancet* 1977; ii:800–801.

73. Belch JJ, Lowe GDO, Ward AG, et al.: Prevention of deep venous thrombosis in medical patients by low dose heparin. *Scot Med J* 1981; 26:115–117.

74. Halkin H, Goldberg J, Modan Michaela, et al.: Reduction of mortality in general medical in-patients by low-dose heparin prophylaxis. *Ann Intern Med* 1982; 96:561–565.

75. Turpie AGG, Hirsh J, Levine MN, et al.: Double-blind, randomised trial of ORG 10172 low-molecular weight heparinoid in prevention of deep-vein thrombosis in thrombotic stroke. *Lancet* 1987; i:523–526.

76. Turpie AGG, Gent M, Cote R, et al.: A low-molecular-weight heparinoid compared with unfractionated heparin in the prevention of deep vein thrombosis in patients with acute ischemic stroke. *Ann Intern Med* 1992; 117:353–357.

77. Tengborn L, Bergqvist D, Mätzsch T, et al.: Recurrent thromboembolism in pregnancy and puerperium: Is there a need for thromboprophylaxis? *Am J Obstet Gynecol* 1989; 160:90–94.

78. Howell R, Fidler J, Letsky E, et al.: The risks of antenatal subcutaneous heparin prophylaxis: A controlled trial. *Br J Obstet Gynaecol* 1983; 90:1124–1128.

79. Lao TT, DeSwiet M, Letsky E, et al.: Prophylaxis of thromboembolism in pregnancy: An alternative. *Br J Obstet Gynaecol* 1985; 92:202–206.

80. Ginsberg JS, Hirsh J: Use of anticoagulants during pregnancy. *Chest* 1989; 95(suppl):156S–160S.

81. Bonnar J: Venous thromboembolism and pregnancy. *Clin Obstet Gynecol* 1981; 8:456.

82. Dahlman TC, Hellgren SE, Blomback M: Thrombosis prophylaxis in pregnancy with use of subcutaneous heparin adjusted by monitoring heparin concentration in plasma. *Am J Obstet Gynecol* 1989; 161:420–425.

83. Sturridge F, deSwiet M, Letsky E: The use of low molecular weight heparin for thromboprophylaxis in pregnancy. *Br J Obstet Gynecol* 1994; 101:69–71.

PART 5

TREATMENT OF SYSTEMIC CRITICAL ILLNESS AND DISORDERED BREATHING

PHARMACOLOGY OF ACUTE LUNG INJURY: ADULT RESPIRATORY DISTRESS SYNDROME

Chapter 100

DEFINITION AND ETIOLOGIES

JESSE HALL

GREGORY A. SCHMIDT

Definition of Acute Respiratory Distress Syndrome

The Time Course of Acute Lung Injury

Etiologies of ARDS

There is no "standard" pharmacologic regimen for the treatment of acute respiratory distress syndrome (ARDS) at present. This chapter reviews clinical studies which have rigorously evaluated various agents, highlighting areas that hold promise for the future. Since current "state-of-the-art" treatment of patients with ARDS is supportive and physiologically based, the discussion concludes with a description of the methods of mechanical ventilatory and circulatory support.

Definition of Acute Respiratory Distress Syndrome

It is important to emphasize that acute respiratory distress syndrome (ARDS) is defined by a series of bedside parameters common to patients with diffuse acute lung injury resulting in pulmonary capillary leak, quite apart from the underlying mechanism(s) resulting in such injury (see Table 100-1). A recent international consensus conference proposed that acute lung injury be defined as a condition or conditions resulting in impaired gas exchange with a ratio of arterial partial pressure of oxygen to fraction of inspired

oxygen (Pa_{O_2}/Fi_{O_2}) < 300, apart from the level of positive end-expiratory pressure (PEEP); bilateral lung infiltrates on the chest radiograph; and a pulmonary capillary wedge pressure (Pcwp) < 18 mmHg or, if not directly measured, the clinical absence of an elevated left atrial pressure.[1] Acute respiratory distress syndrome is defined by these same criteria, with Pa_{O_2}/Fi_{O_2} < 200.

These definitions of acute lung injury and ARDS are intentionally broad to encompass the range of lung injury encountered in both medical and surgical settings. In the performance of clinical studies and to appraise critically the medical literature, it is useful to be familiar with various scoring systems that are used to quantitate the severity of lung injury[2,3] (see Table 100-2).

The Time Course of Acute Lung Injury

In considering both pathogenesis and treatment, it is useful to distinguish between the early and late phases of acute lung injury[3,4] (see Fig. 100-1). The early phases of ARDS are characterized by noncardiogenic pulmonary edema. Pathologically, flooding of the lung interstitium and alveoli with proteinaceous fluid is prominent. By light microscopy evi-

TABLE 100-1   Criteria for Diagnosis of ARDS

Clinical presentation
  Tachypnea and dyspnea
  Crackles on auscultation

Clinical setting
  Direct lung insult (e.g., aspiration) or systemic process with potential for lung injury (e.g., sepsis)

Radiologic appearance
  Three or four quadrant alveolar flooding

Lung mechanics
  Diminished compliance (< 40 mL/cmH$_2$O)

Gas exchange
  Severe hypoxemia refractory to oxygen therapy ($Pa_{O_2}/Fi_{O_2} < 200$)

Normal pulmonary vascular pressures
  Pulmonary capillary wedge pressure < 18 mmHg

TABLE 100-2   Scoring System for ARDS

Chest roentgenogram score	
No alveolar consolidation	0
1 quadrant consolidation	1
2 quadrant consolidation	2
3 quadrant consolidation	3
4 quadrant consolidation	4
Hypoxemia score	
$Pa_{O_2}/Fi_{O_2} \geq 300$	0
Pa_{O_2}/Fi_{O_2} 225–299	1
Pa_{O_2}/Fi_{O_2} 175–224	2
Pa_{O_2}/Fi_{O_2} 100–174	3
$Pa_{O_2}/Fi_{O_2} \leq 100$	4
Compliance (when ventilated) mL/cmH$_2$O	
≥ 80	0
60–79	1
40–59	2
20–39	3
≤ 19	4
PEEP required (when ventilated) (cmH$_2$O)	
≤ 5	0
6–8	1
9–11	2
12–14	3
≥ 15	4

Final value is obtained by dividing the aggregate sum by the number of components used

Score:	
No injury	0
Mild to moderate injury	0.1–2.5
Severe injury (ARDS)	> 2.5

SOURCE: Modified and reproduced with permission from Murray et al.[2]

dence of cellular injury is minimal. By electron microscopy, changes of endothelial cell swelling, widening of intercellular junctions, increased numbers of pinocytotic vesicles, and disruption and denudation of the basement membrane are prominent. This early phase of diffuse alveolar damage (DAD) has been termed *exudative*, since pulmonary edema and its consequences are the most prominent morphologic and physiologic aberrations.

Over the ensuing days hyaline membrane formation in the alveolar spaces is prominent, attributed to precipitation of serum proteins. Inflammatory cells become more numerous within the lung interstitium. Necrosis of type I alveolar epithelial cells may occur. This latter phase of DAD is dominated by disordered healing and has been termed the *proliferative* phase of DAD. It can occur as early as 7 to 10 days into the course of lung injury and involves abnormal collagen deposition. Alveolar flooding may be much diminished at this point, and the clinical picture is often dominated by large dead space fraction and high minute ventilation requirements, progressive pulmonary hypertension, slightly improved intrapulmonary shunt (which is less responsive to PEEP), further reduction in lung compliance, and a tendency toward creation of zone I lung conditions if the patient develops hypovolemia.[5,6] It is important for the clinician to distinguish between these phases of ARDS, since treatment approaches and goals will differ.

Etiologies of ARDS

The clinical conditions that predispose to ARDS include both those resulting in direct lung injury (e.g., aspiration or other inhalational injury) and those characterized by a systemic inflammatory process with multiple organ injury including the lung (e.g., pancreatitis, sepsis syndrome).[6] In many series

the triad of blood product resuscitation following trauma, acid aspiration, and sepsis account for the vast majority of instances of ARDS. With some of these predisposing entities, the risk of subsequent ARDS is high (e.g., 30 percent to 40 percent in cases of bacterial sepsis or acid aspiration) and with multiple risk factors, the incidence of acute lung injury increases.[7,8] Identification of risk factors has facilitated the evaluation of therapies both for prevention of ARDS as well as for treatment of early phases of the syndrome.

The predisposing cause of acute lung injury is an important determinant of mortality and outcome. Mortality is high (typically reported as > 50 percent) in patients with sepsis and/or multiorgan failure.[7,8] Tocolytic-associated pulmonary edema,[9] postictal pulmonary edema,[10] and pulmonary edema associated with air emboli typically have a benign course and often can be treated with supplemental oxygen and diuresis alone. When mechanical ventilation is required, it is usually for a brief period of time, and many of the monitoring and circulatory manipulations (see Chaps. 101 and 102) are not indicated.

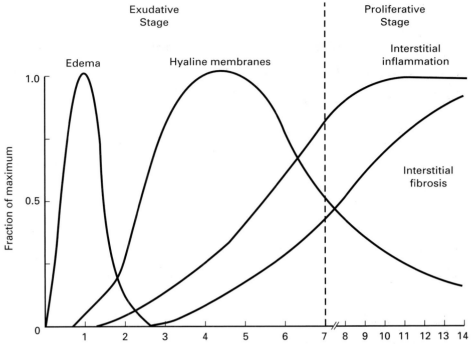

FIGURE 100-1 A schematic representation of the time course of evolution of the acute respiratory distress syndrome (ARDS). During the early or exudative phase the lesion is characterized by a pulmonary capillary leak with edema and then shortly thereafter hyaline membrane formation. Within as short a period of time as 7 to 10 days, a proliferative phase may appear, with marked interstitial inflammation, fibrosis, and disordered healing. (*Reproduced with permission from Katzenstein AA, Askin FB:* **Surgical Pathology of Non-Neoplastic Lung Disease.** *Philadelphia, WB Saunders, 1982.*)

References

1. Bernard GR, Artigas A, Brigham KL, et al.: The American-European Consensus Conference of ARDS: definitions, mechanisms, relevant outcomes, and clinical trial coordination. *Am J Respir Crit Care Med* 1994; 149:818.

2. Murray JF, Matthay MM, Luce J, et al.: An expanded definition of the adult respiratory distress syndrome. *Am Rev Resp Dis* 1988; 138:720.

3. Hall JB, Wood LD: Acute hypoxemic respiratory failure, in Hall JB, Schmidt GA, Wood LDH (eds): *Principles of Critical Care.* New York, McGraw-Hill, 1992: 1634–1658.

4. Katzenstein A, Askin FB: *Surgical Pathology of Non-Neoplastic Lung Disease,* 2nd ed. Philadelphia, WB Saunders, 1990: 9–36.

5. Meduri GU, Belenchia JM, Estes RJ, et al.: Fibroproliferative phase of ARDS: clinical findings and effects of corticosteroids. *Chest* 1991; 100(4):943.

6. Hall JB, Schmidt GA, Wood LDH. Acute hypoxemic respiratory failure, in Murray, Nadel (eds): *Textbook of Respiratory Medicine.* 1994: 2589.

7. Fowler A, Hamman R, Good J, et al.: Adult respiratory distress syndrome: risk with common predispositions. *Ann Intern Med* 1983; 98:593.

8. Kollef MH, Schuster DP: The acute respiratory distress syndrome. *N Engl J Med* 1995; 332:27.

9. Pisani RJ, Rosenow EC: Pulmonary edema associated with tocolytic therapy. *Ann Intern Med* 1989; 110(9):714.

10. Teplinsky K, Hall JB: Postictal pulmonary edema: report of a case. *Arch Intern Med* 1986; 146:801.

CHAPTER 101

PHARMACOTHERAPIES FOR ARDS

JESSE HALL
GREGORY A. SCHMIDT

SEPSIS AND RISK OF ARDS

For the purposes of this and subsequent discussions, *sepsis* is defined as an identifiable active infection with systemic manifestations including tachycardia, tachypnea, and abnormal thermoregulation[1] (see Chap. 102). The *sepsis syndrome* is defined as sepsis with signs of hypoperfusion or end-organ injury, specifically lactic acidosis, oliguria, impaired mental status, or hypoxemic respiratory failure. *Septic shock* is the sepsis syndrome plus volume-refractory hypotension, often treated with vasoactive drugs. These details are semantic, and are useful merely as a rough grading system for severity.

Of the predisposing conditions for acute respiratory distress syndrome (ARDS), sepsis is used best to define a population for the study of prevention of ARDS. This is because (1) the stages of the sepsis are reasonably well-identified clinically; (2) the incidence of ARDS following in the wake of sepsis syndrome and septic shock is high; (3) in most clinical settings, sepsis is the most, or one of the most, frequent predisposing conditions to ARDS; and (4) despite the wide variety of infecting organisms and sites, the specific patterns of inflammation may share many of the same pathways and mediators.[1,2]

Thus, sepsis and its relation to ARDS provides a research paradigm both for the study of mechanisms of lung injury as well as for evaluation of prophylactic and early treatments of injury. Accordingly, some of the recent studies in this area are reviewed below.

MICROBIAL ANTIGENS AND CYTOKINE ACTIVATION

The interaction of infecting agent antigen(s) and host effector cells, such as the macrophage, is likely a central component in the initiation of inflammatory pathways that ultimately may result in host cellular injury and dysfunction.[2–4] The gram-negative bacterial endotoxins are one such group of initiators or antigenic triggers to this process, although other bacterial, viral, fungal, and parasitic products are important in specific settings.

Endotoxin initiates host responses by binding to a receptor with subsequent activation of various intracellular processes. A soluble *lipopolysaccharide binding protein* (LBP) has been reported as a trace constituent of plasma (< 500 ng/ml) in many species, and its presence reduces the dose of *Escherichia coli* endotoxin required for macrophage production of tumor necrosis factor (TNF) by two orders of magnitude.[5] It seems likely that LBP provides a central initial detection mechanism for the presence of endotoxin.[2] The soluble endotoxin-LBP complex binds to CD14 receptors on leukocytes,[6] thereby triggering synthesis and release of TNF, one of several cytokines which play an important role in the genesis of a septic response.[7] Other cytokines detectable in increased amounts during the human septic response include interleukins-1 and 6 (IL-1, IL-6); the plasma concentrations of these mediators have been shown to correlate with survival in humans[8] (see Chap. 102).

CORTICOSTEROID TRIALS IN SEPSIS AND ARDS

A number of clinical trials have attempted to ameliorate the consequences of sepsis by reducing cytokine release, binding circulating cytokines, or blocking their receptors. Corticosteroids long have been known to attenuate mortality in endotoxin-treated animals.[9,10] Corticosteroids prevent TNF release by macrophages and blunt the endotoxin-induced increase in TNF concentrations in vivo. Extended exposure to corticosteroids is necessary to exert these effects, and corticosteroid administration limits TNF synthesis at a translational level.[11]

Thus, it is not surprising that corticosteroids were among the earliest agents proposed to treat sepsis and ARDS. However, when evaluated prospectively in patients with sepsis syndrome as their predisposition to lung injury, high-dose methylprednisolone did not prevent the development of ARDS or reduce the mortality compared with a placebo-treated control group.[12,13] In another prospective randomized trial of corticosteroid administration begun after ARDS was well-established, no beneficial effect on gas exchange or lung mechanics could be demonstrated, nor was outcome improved.[14] In this latter study a number of conditions predisposing to ARDS were present, including sepsis, aspiration, and pancreatitis.

Based on these well-conducted clinical trials, the use of corticosteroids cannot be supported for sepsis syndrome or established ARDS in the exudative phase. An exception to this generalization is the patient with acute lung injury characterized by significant lung (as detected by bronchoalveolar lavage) eosinophilia.[15] This acute eosinophilic pneumonia syndrome, while rare, does appear to respond promptly to corticosteroid therapy and may represent an acute allergic alveolitis. Rather than support the general use of corticosteroids, this exception to the rule simply makes the point that the successful outcome from ARDS entails identification and treatment of underlying disease(s).

A separate question remains concerning the benefit of corticosteroids in the treatment of the disordered healing and fibrosis of the proliferative phase of ARDS. A number of anecdotal reports and brief series have suggested that high-dose corticosteroid therapy may be helpful in reversing the pulmonary fibrosis encountered in "late" (> 10 to 14 days) ARDS.[16–18] Since gram-negative nosocomial pneumonia is such a common cause of late superinfection in patients with ARDS, immunosuppressive therapy likely carries significant risks that may outweigh benefits derived from effects on disordered healing and lung scarring. Many authors who advocate the use of corticosteroids for proliferative-phase ARDS recommend that weekly or more frequent surveillance quantitative lung cultures be obtained by sterile brush or bronchoalveolar lavage (BAL) technique and that this therapy be discontinued at the earliest evidence of superinfection. Until adequate prospective, randomized trials have clarified efficacy of corticosteroids in this setting, routine use cannot be recommended.

BIOLOGICS

Since the cascade described above appears initiated by an interaction of microbial antigen and host cell and then involves release of a large number of cytokines, strategies involving specific mediator blockade with monoclonal antibodies have been studied. While some preliminary results suggested potential benefit from monoclonal antibody therapy directed against endotoxin in the treatment of sepsis syndrome, recently published prospective trials failed to demonstrate improvement in survival.[19,20]

Similar strategies have been explored to block the action of tumor necrosis factor (anti-TNF monoclonal antibody) or interleukin-1 (interleukin-1 receptor antagonist). In two prospective trials recently completed, no improvement in survival was noted.[21,22] Currently, further multicenter trials are in progress, attempting to evaluate other antiendotoxin and anti-TNF antibodies, and to define further patient subgroups (e.g., septic shock as opposed to sepsis syndrome) that may benefit from therapy. Until such evaluations have been performed, the safety and efficacy of these agents remain undetermined, and they must be considered experimental. This is a particular concern; theoretically, diminishing circulating cytokine concentrations could have deleterious effects.[23,24]

Cytokines may promote cell-mediated tissue injury, in part by upregulating adhesion molecules, which increase and prolong contact between the circulating neutrophil and the endothelium.[25,26] Use of monoclonal antibodies to block this interaction is a promising therapy to limit lung and other tissue injury. A number of animal and human investigations suggest this strategy will be beneficial in a variety of inflammatory, immune, and ischemia-reperfusion injuries.[27–37]

POTENTIAL FOR ANTIOXIDANT PREVENTION OF ARDS

Cytokines, by direct activation or initiation of coagulation and complement cascades, increase toxic oxygen metabolite production and trigger degranulation by neutrophils.[38] While generation and release of oxidants is a primary mechanism of neutrophil-mediated injury,[39] direct participation by superoxide ion or hydroxyl radical is difficult to demonstrate in sepsis or ARDS; these species have extremely short half-lifes. Nonetheless, indirect information supports the role of oxidants in acute lung injury, including (1) analysis of more stable reactive oxygen species such as hydrogen peroxide (H_2O_2) in the expired breath or urine of patients with ARDS[40–42]; (2) observation of increased oxidant activity in the BAL fluid of patients with ARDS[43]; and (3) demonstration that pretreatment with free-radical scavengers attenuates lung injury in animal models.[44–46]

These findings support a hypothesis that lung injury under diverse conditions and inflammatory states, such as sepsis, results in part from generation of oxidants that overwhelm the usual protective mechanisms. The circulating neutrophil (PMN) may play a central role in oxidant-mediated lung injury. It has been shown that there is a transpulmonary gradient of H_2O_2 production by zymosan-activated PMNs in septic and lung-injured patients compared with controls.[47] The gradients observed (higher mixed venous H_2O_2 production in sepsis, higher arterial H_2O_2 production in lung injury) were consistent with a hypothesis that in septic patients PMNs are primed in the periphery and downregulated or sequestered in the lung, and in lung injury, PMNs are primed in the lung and sequestered in the periphery. These may be mechanisms by which sufficient oxidant generation occurs to overwhelm the normal mechanisms of protection: (1) low-molecular-weight free-radical scavengers (e.g., vitamins C and E); (2) sulfhydryl group donors (e.g., glutathione); (3) sulfhydryl-containing proteins; and (4) enzymatic conversion (e.g., superoxide dismutase, catalase). The sulfhydryl group donor glutathione may be particularly relevant to lung injury in view of the following observations: (1) under normal conditions, the lung is a net importer of glutathione[48]; (2) glutathione levels in BAL fluid from patients with ARDS are reduced[49]; and (3) the antioxidant *N*-acetylcysteine (NAC) that restores glutathione ameliorates lung injury in animal[50–54] and human studies.[55,56]

In a small pilot study by Bernard and colleagues,[55] 30 patients were randomized prospectively to receive NAC or placebo therapy; these patients had preconditions known to predispose to ARDS and already had evidence of lung injury, with both radiologic and gas exchange abnormalities. *N*-acetylcysteine was administered as a loading dose followed by 16 maintenance doses repeated every 4 h. Total thoracic compliance and chest radiograph score at 48 h were significantly improved in the NAC-treated patients. Radiographic scores continued to improve in the NAC-treated group, with further improvement over controls by 120 h. The improvement in lung mechanics was transient, and compliance returned to pretreatment levels after discontinuation of NAC. While there was a trend toward a greater early improvement in gas exchange in the NAC group, this was not significant. Suter and colleagues[56] also have reported on patients treated with NAC with intent to prevent progression to acute respiratory failure. These investigators administered NAC or placebo to 61 patients at risk for development of ARDS; only a small number of these patients had sepsis as their primary risk factor (11/61 = 18 percent). Treatment with NAC for 72 h improved systemic oxygenation and reduced the need for ventilatory support in patients presenting with mild-to-moderate lung injury. The incidence of ARDS was not affected by treatment. While there was a "trend" toward improved survival in the NAC-treated patients, the observed difference was not significant.

N-acetylcysteine has been administered in other studies. Sawyer and colleagues[57] randomized ARDS patients (entry criteria not defined) to receive placebo or multimodality antioxidant therapy, including NAC, vitamins E, and C, and selenium. In this small series of 32 patients, a significant difference in survival at 4 weeks was reported. This study exists only in abstract form, included a large number (14/32) of postcardiac surgery patients, did not report plasma glutathione or cysteine concentrations, and does not supply adequate information to assess equivalence of study groups or status of patients upon study entry. Jepsen and colleagues[58] randomized 66 patients in a medical/surgical ICU to receive NAC or placebo over a 6-day period after the onset of ARDS. They did not observe a difference in gas exchange, chest radiographic infiltrates, or survival between the groups. Lung compliance tended to be greater in the NAC-treated group throughout the treatment period, but this difference did not reach statistical significance.

In summary, both the studies by Suter and colleagues[56] and Bernard and colleagues[55] suggest potential physiologic benefits of NAC therapy for patients at risk of developing ARDS; the diverse patients treated in these studies raise a question concerning whether restriction of entry criteria to risk groups with more clearly delineated elements of inflammation (e.g., sepsis syndrome and septic shock) might not enhance response to therapy. Arguably, the major differences between these studies and that of Jepsen and colleagues[58] were the severity and stage of ARDS; the more advanced disease in the latter study may explain the failure of significant response to treatment with NAC.

While these preliminary studies are of interest, there is at present insufficient information to support the use of NAC or other antioxidants as routine therapy for ARDS.

POTENTIAL FOR ANTILIPID PREVENTION OF ARDS

Activation of neutrophils by the pathways described also results in generation of lipid-derived mediators. Phospholipases are stimulated, and cleave arachidonic acid from membrane phospholipids. Arachidonic acid, in turn, may be converted by 5-lipoxygenase to leukotrienes, and through cyclooxygenase (CO) to prostaglandins (including prostacyclins) and thence [by action of thromboxane synthetase (TS)] to thromboxane (see Fig. 101-1). Both animal and human studies suggest leukotriene generation may contribute to the pathogenesis of sepsis and ARDS.[59–63] Urinary levels of the cysteinyl leukotriene, LTE_4, a metabolite reflecting net in vivo leukotriene production, is increased 40-fold in patients with ARDS as compared with normal controls.[59] In animal models, inhibition of 5-lipoxygenase (5-LO) attenuates lung injury associated with sepsis.[60,61] As safety profiles in critically ill patients are established for a number of 5-LO inhibitors now available from industry, and as pilot studies help to determine effects in acute lung injury, it is likely that such agents will enter trials for the treatment of ARDS.

Alternatively, arachidonic acid metabolism may be blocked at the level of CO or TS. Michie and colleagues[64]

FIGURE 101-1 Pathways for lipid-derived mediators of acute lung injury.

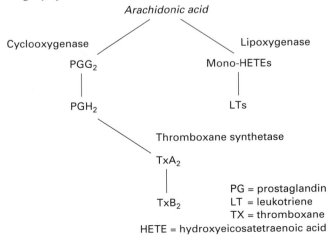

studied 13 volunteers pretreated with ibuprofen before endotoxin administration. Ibuprofen prevented the typical hyperthermia and tachycardia, but did not attenuate the leukocytosis or increased TNF levels in these subjects. In a controlled pilot study in patients with sepsis syndrome, treatment with the CO inhibitor ibuprofen resulted in decreases in heart rate, body temperature, minute ventilation, and peak pressure on the ventilator.[65] There was a positive correlation between the thromboxane metabolites measured in the urine and peak airway and pulmonary arterial pressures and an inverse correlation between urinary prostacyclin metabolite and systemic blood pressure. These findings were consistent with the known constrictor and dilator effects of thromboxane A_2 and prostacyclin on blood vessel and airway smooth muscle. Extension of these data in continued clinical trials is ongoing.

Human data concerning the use of TS inhibitors also are available.[66–70] Ketoconazole is an imidazole antibiotic that has a significant inhibitory effect on TS. It has been routinely used in the treatment of fungal disease, and, hence, its safety profile has been established in diverse clinical conditions. In view of its safety in humans and its potential to inhibit thromboxane-mediated injury in sepsis and subsequent ARDS, trials of ketoconazole in humans have been undertaken.

Slotman and colleagues[68] randomized patients at high risk for development of ARDS to receive ketoconazole, 200 mg orally once a day, or placebo. The incidence of ARDS was significantly reduced by therapy (6 percent in treated patients, versus 31 percent in controls). Data were not reported reflecting serum drug, thromboxane, or prostaglandin concentrations. Methods for controlling disease severity and comorbid conditions also were not reported. In a more recent investigation, 54 consecutive patients admitted to a surgical ICU with sepsis were randomized to receive either 400 mg ketoconazole per nasogastric tube (or orally) daily or placebo for 21 days or until discharge.[70] Study design was double-blind and characterization of study populations with Acute Physiology and Chronic Health Evaluation (APACHE) II and Therapeutic Intervention Scoring System (TISS) scores revealed no significant differences between the groups. A significant reduction in ARDS was noted with therapy (15 percent versus 64 percent in controls), and, in addition, mortality was reduced significantly from 39 percent in the placebo group to 15 percent in the treatment group. Adverse consequences ascribable to drug administration were not noted. While these results are encouraging, they are preliminary and larger studies are required to properly identify the role of ketoconazole in the treatment of ARDS.

PROSTAGLANDIN ADMINISTRATION

Strategies for treatment of ARDS have included not only antilipid inhibition of prostaglandin pathways, but administration of prostaglandins as well. Since prostaglandin E_1 (PGE_1) inhibits platelet aggregation and neutrophil chemotaxis and is a pulmonary arterial vasodilator, it has been hypothesized to have salutary effects in patients with acute lung injury. When PGE_1 was administered to surgical patients with acute respiratory failure, an improvement in gas exchange was noted as well as a trend toward improvement in long-term survival.[71] These promising results were not supported by a more recent investigation of PGE_1 infusion for treatment of ARDS associated with both medical and surgical predispositions.[72] In this study, the trend toward increased survival was present in the placebo-treated group, and many complications were noted in the treatment group, including hypotension, diarrhea, and fever. In addition, follow-up studies have failed to confirm any significant improvement in gas exchange following PGE_1 administration.[73] At the present time PGE_1 infusion cannot be considered either routine or proven therapy for ARDS.

EXOGENOUS SURFACTANT

In both animal models of acute lung injury and in bronchoalveolar lavage (BAL) from patients with ARDS, decreased concentrations or abnormal ratios of components of surfactant have been described.[74,75] The BAL from patients with ARDS also has diminished surface tension–reducing properties, which is consistent with low levels of surfactant or presence of inhibitor(s) of its action. Accordingly, surfactant replacement has been considered a potential therapy for this disorder.

Clinical data supporting the use of surfactant are most compelling in studies involving patients with the neonatal respiratory distress syndrome, a condition characterized by known surfactant deficiency.[76,77] Use of surfactant replacement in premature infants is almost invariably associated with decreased requirement for PEEP, less barotrauma, improved gas exchange, and improved respiratory system compliance.[76–78] Some, but not all, studies have demonstrated a reduced incidence of bronchopulmonary dysplasia and improved survival.[79] Clinical trials are more limited in adults, and benefits may be less.[80] One recent large trial of surfactant replacement was terminated because of absence of benefit noted at mid-study analysis.[81] Until more completely investigated in adults, this therapy should still be considered experimental.

INHALED NITRIC OXIDE

Nitric oxide is an endogenous nitrovasodilator that produces relaxation of vascular smooth muscle by stimulation of synthesis of cyclic guanosine monophosphate.[2] When inhaled at 5 to 80 ppm, nitric oxide acts as a selective pulmonary vasodilator, since rapid binding to hemoglobin prevents systemic effects.[82] Rossaint and coworkers[83] evaluated nitric oxide administered by inhalation to 10 patients with severe ARDS. They observed a significant decrease in intrapulmonary shunt and pulmonary artery pressures without changes in mean systemic arterial pressure or cardiac output. This suggested that nitric oxide acted as a selective pulmonary vasodilator in these patients, causing preferential increases in blood flow to ventilated units with improved gas exchange. These acute improvements in physiologic function also were observed over an extended period of time when administration of nitric oxide was continued. The potential survival benefit of this therapy requires further study.

References

1. Bone RC, Balk RA, Cerra FB, et al.: Definitions for sepsis and organ failure and guidelines for the use of innovative therapies in sepsis. *Chest* 1992; 101:1644–55.
2. Manthous CA, Hal JB, Samsel RW: Endotoxin in human disease: Part 1. Biochemistry, assay and possible role in diverse disease states. *Chest* 1993; 104:1572–1581.
3. Miyamoto K, Schultz E, Heath T, et al.: Pulmonary intravascular macrophages and hemodynamic effects of liposomes in sheep. *Physiology* 1986; 29:117–20.
4. Staub NC: Pulmonary intravascular macrophages. *Chest* 1988; 93:84S–85S.
5. Tesh VI, Vukajlovich SW, Morrison DC: Endotoxin interactions with serum proteins and relationships to biological activity. *Prog Clin Biol Res* 1988; 272:47–61.
6. Wright SD, Ramos RA, Tobias PS, et al.: CD14, a receptor for complexes of lipopolysaccharide (LPS) and LPS binding protein. *Science* 1990; 249:1431–33.
7. Fong Y, Lowry SF: Tumor necrosis factor in the pathophysiology of infection and sepsis. *Clin Immunol Immunopathol* 1990; 55:157–70.
8. Casey LC, Balk RA, Bone RC: Plasma cytokine and endotoxin levels correlate with survival in patients with the sepsis syndrome. *Ann Intern Med* 1993; 119:771–778.
9. Thomas CS, Brockman SK: The role of adrenal corticosteroid therapy in *Escherichia coli* endotoxin shock. *Surg Gynecol Obstet* 1968; 126:61–9.
10. White GI, Archer LJ, Beller BK, et al.: Increased survival with methylprednisolone treatment in canine endotoxin shock. *J Surg Res* 1978; 25:357–64.
11. Beutler B, Milsark I, Cerami A: Cachectin/tumor necrosis factor: production, distribution and metabolic fate in vivo. *J Immunol* 1986; 135:3972–77.
12. Luce JM, Montgomery B, Marks JD, et al.: Ineffectiveness of high-dose methylprednisolone in preventing parenchymal lung injury and improving mortality in patients with septic shock. *Am Rev Respir Dis* 1988; 138:62–68.
13. Bone RC, Fisher, CJ Jr, Clemmer TP, et al.: Early methylprednisolone treatment for septic syndrome and the adult respiratory distress syndrome. *Chest* 1987; 92(6):1032–6.
14. Bernard GR, Luce JM, Sprung CL, et al.: High-dose corticosteroids in patients with adult respiratory distress syndrome. *N Engl J Med* 1987; 317:1565–1570.
15. Allen JN, Pacht ER, Gadek JE, et al.: Acute eosinophilic pneumonia as a reversible cause of noninfectious respiratory failure. *N Engl J Med* 1989; 321:569–74.
16. Ashbaugh DG, Maier RV: Idiopathic pulmonary fibrosis in adult respiratory distress syndrome: diagnosis and treatment. *Arch Surg* 1985; 120:530–5.
17. Hooper RG, Kearl RA: Established ARDS treated with a sustained course of adrenocortical steroids. *Chest* 1990; 97:138–43.
18. Meduri GU, Belenchia JM, Estes RJ, et al.: Fibroproliferative phase of ARDS: clinical findings and effects of corticosteroids. *Chest* 1991; 100:943–52.
19. Ziegler EJ, Fisher CJ Jr, Sprung CL, et al.: Treatment of gram-negative bacteremia and septic shock with HA-1A human monoclonal antibody against endotoxin: a randomized, double-blind, placebo-controlled trial. *N Engl J Med* 1991; 324:429–36.
20. Wenzel R, Bone R, Fein A, et al.: A controlled clinical trial of E5 murine monoclonal IgM antibody to endotoxin in the treatment of gram-negative sepsis. *JAMA* 1991; 266:1097–102.
21. Fisher CJ, Dhainaut JA, Opal SM, et al.: Recombinant human interleukin 1 receptor antagonist in the treatment of patients with sepsis syndrome. *JAMA* 1994; 271:1836–1843.
22. Wherry J, Wenzel R, Wunderink R, et al.: Monoclonal antibody to human tumor necrosis factor (TNF Mab): multicenter efficacy and safety study in patients with the sepsis syndrome. Presented at the 33rd Interscience Conference on Antimicrobial Agents and Chemotherapy. American Society for Microbiology, New Orleans, Louisiana, October 17–20, 1993, Abstract No. 696:246.
23. Luger A, Graf H, Schwarz HP, et al.: Decreased serum interleukin 1 activity and monocyte interleukin 1 production in patients with fatal sepsis. *Crit Care Med* 1986; 14:458–61.
24. Munoz C, Misset B, Fitting C, et al.: Dissociation between plasma and monocyte-associated cytokines during sepsis. *Eur J Immunol* 1991; 21:2177–84.
25. Wortel CH: *Immunotherapy of Gram-Negative Sepsis with Monoclonal Anti-Endotoxin Antibodies.* Thesis, University of Amsterdam. Thesis Publishers, Amsterdam, The Netherlands, 1993.
26. Shealy D, Siegel S, Nakada M, et al.: Functional neutralization of human TNF by cA2, a mouse/human chimeric anti-TNF monoclonal antibody (abstract). *European Cytokine Network* 1992; 2:219.
27. Jasin HE, Lightoot E, Davis LS, et al.: Amelioration of antigen-induced arthritis in rabbits treated with monoclonal antibodies to leukocyte adhesion molecules. *Arthritis Rheum* 1992; 35:541–549.
28. Tuomanen EA, Saukkonen K, Sande S, et al.: Reduction of inflammation, tissue damage, and mortality in bacterial meningitis in rabbits treated with monoclonal antibodies against adhesion promoting receptors of leukocytes. *J Exp Med* 1989; 170:95–969.
29. Flavin T, Ivens K, Rothlein R, et al.: Monoclonal antibodies against intercellular adhesion molecule 1 prolong cardiac allograft survival in cynomolgus monkeys. *Transplant Proc* 1991; 23:533–534.
30. Wegner CD, Gundel RH, Reilly P, et al.: Intercellular adhesion molecule-1 (ICAM-1) in the pathogenesis of asthma. *Science* 1990; 247:456–459.
31. Mulligan MS, Varani J, Dame MK, et al.: Role of endothelial-leukocyte adhesion molecule-1 (ELAM-1) in neutrophil mediated lung injury in rats. *J Clin Invest* 1991; 88:1396–1404.
32. Arfors KE, Lundberg D, Lindbom L, et al.: A monoclonal antibody to the membrane glycoprotein complex CD18 inhibits polymorphonuclear leukocyte accumulation and plasma leakage in vivo. *Blood* 1987; 69:338–340.
33. Lindbom L, Lundberg D, Prieto J, et al.: Rabbit leukocyte adhesion molecules CD11/CD18 and their participation in acute and delayed inflammatory responses and leukocyte distribution in vivo. *Clin Immunol Immunopathol* 1990; 57:105–119.
34. Simpson PJ, Todd RF, Mickelson JK, et al.: Sustained limitation of myocardial reperfusion injury by a monoclonal antibody that alters leukocyte function. *Circulation* 1990; 81:226–237.
35. Horgan MJ, Wright SD, Malik AB: Antibody against leukocyte integrin (CD18) prevents reperfusion induced lung vascular injury. *Am J Physiol* 1990; 259:L315–L319.
36. Vedder NB, Winn RK, Rice CL, et al.: A monoclonal antibody to the adherence-promoting leukocyte glycoprotein, CD18, reduces organ injury and improves survival from hemorrhagic and resuscitation in rabbits. *J Clin Invest* 1988; 81:939–994.
37. Mileski WJ, Winn RK, Vedder NB, et al.: Inhibition of CD18-dependent neutrophil adherence reduces injury after hemorrhagic shock in primates. *Surgery* 108:206–212.
38. Ferrante A, Nandoskar AM, Waltz D, et al.: Effects of tumor necrosis factor alpha and interleukin-1 alpha and beta on human

neutrophil migration, respiratory burst, and degranulation. *Int Arch Allergy Appl Immunol* 1988; 86:82–91.

39. Weiss SJ: Tissue destruction by neutrophils. *N Engl J Med* 1989; 320:365–376.

40. Baldwin SR, Simon RH, Grum CM: Oxidant activity in expired breath of patients with adult respiratory distress syndrome. *Lancet* 1986; i:11–14.

41. Sznajder JI, Fraiman A, Hall JB, et al.: Increased hydrogen peroxide in the expired breath of patients with acute hypoxemic respiratory failure. *Chest* 1989; 96:606–12.

42. Mathru M, Rooney MW, Dried DJ, et al.: Urine hydrogen peroxide during adult respiratory distress syndrome in patients with and without sepsis. *Chest* 1994; 150:232–36.

43. Cochrane CG, Spragg R, Revak SD: Pathogenesis of the adult respiratory distress syndrome: evidence of oxidant activity in bronchoalveolar lavage. *J Clin Invest* 1983; 71:754–61.

44. Toth KM, Clifford DP, Berger EM, et al.: Intact human erythrocytes prevent hydrogen peroxide–mediated damage to isolated perfused rat lungs and cultured bovine pulmonary artery endothelial cells. *J Clin Invest* 1984; 74:292–95.

45. Fox RB: Prevention of granulocyte-mediated oxidant lung injury in rats by a hydroxyl radical scavenger, dimethylthiourea. *J Clin Invest* 1984; 74:1456–64.

46. Turrens JF, Crapo JD, Freeman BA: Protection against oxygen toxicity by intravenous injection of liposome entrapped–catalase and superoxide dismustase. *J Clin Invest* 1984; 73:879–85.

47. Martensson J, Jain A, Frayer W, et al.: Glutathione metabolism in the lung: inhibition of its synthesis leads to lamellar body and mitochondrial defects. *Proc Natl Acad Sci USA* 1989; 86:5286–5300.

48. Pacht ER, Timerman AP, Lykens MG, et al.: Deficiency of alveolar fluid glutathione in patients with sepsis and the adult respiratory syndrome. *Chest* 1991; 100:1397–1403.

49. Heffner JE, Repine JE: Pulmonary strategies of antioxidant defence. *Am Rev Respir Dis* 1989; 140:531–554.

50. Moldeus P, Cotgreave IA, Berggren M, et al.: Lung protection by thiol-containing antioxidant: *N*-acetylcysteine. *Respiration* 1986; 50(suppl 1):31–42.

51. Lucht BD, English DK, Bernard GR, et al.: Prevention of release of granulocyte aggrents into sheep lung lymph following endotoemia by *N*-acetylcysteine. *Am J Med Sci* 1987; 249: 161–167.

52. Bernard GR, Lucht WD, Niedermeyer ME, et al.: Effect of *N*-acetylcysteine on the pulmonary responses to endotoxin in the awake sheep and upon granulocyte function. *J Clin Invest* 1984; 73:1772–1784.

53. Wegener T, Sandhagen B, Saldeen T: Effect of *N*-acetylcysteine on pulmonary damage due to microembolism in the rat. *Eur J Respir Dis* 1987; 70:205–212.

54. Groeneveld ABJ, Hollander W, Straub J, et al.: Effects of *N*-acetylcysteine and terbutaline treatment on hemodynamics and regional albumin extravasation in porcine septic shock. *Circ Shock* 1990; 30:185–205.

55. Bernard GR: *N*-acetylcysteine in experimental and clinical acute lung injury. *Am J Med* 1991; 91(suppl 3C):54–59.

56. Suter PM, Domenighetti G, Schaller MD, et al.: *N*-acetylcysteine enhances recovery from acute lung injury in man—A randomized, double-blind, placebo-controlled clinical study. *Chest* 1994; 105:190–94.

57. Sawyer MAJ, Mike JJ, Chavin K, et al.: Antioxidant therapy and survival in ARDS (abstract). *Crit Care Med* 1989; 17:S153.

58. Jepsen S, Herlevsen P, Knudsen P, et al.: Antioxidant treatment with *N*-acetylcysteine during adult respiratory distress syndrome: a prospective, randomized, placebo-controlled study. *Crit Care Med* 1992; 20(7):918–923.

59. Bernard GR, Korley V, Chee P, et al.: Persistent generation of peptido leukotrienes in patients with the adult respiratory distress syndrome. *Am Rev Respir Dis* 1991; 144:263–267.

60. Coggeshall JW, Christman BW, Lefferts PL, et al.: Effect of inhibition of 5-lipoxygenase metabolism of arachidonic acid on response to endotoxemia in sheep. *J Appl Physiol* 1988; 65:1351–1359.

61. Gross D, Dahan JB, Landau EH, et al.: Effect of leukotriene inhibitor LY-171883 on the pulmonary response to *Escherichia coli* endotoxemia. *Crit Care Med* 1990; 18:190–197.

62. Davis JM, Yurt RW, Barie PS, et al.: Leukotriene B generation in patients with established pulmonary failure. *Arch Surg* 1989; 124:1451–1455.

63. Davis JM, Meyer JD, Barbie PS, et al.: Elevated production of neutrophil leukotriene B4 precedes pulmonary failure in critically ill surgical patients. *Surg Gynecol Obstet* 1990; 170:495–500.

64. Michie HR, Manogue KR, Spriggs DR, et al.: Detection of circulating tumor necrosis factor after endotoxin administration. *N Engl J Med* 1988; 310:1461–66.

65. Bernard GR, Reines HD, Halushka PV, et al.: Prostaglandin and thromboxane A2 formation is increased in human sepsis syndrome: effects of cyclooxygenase inhibition. *Am Rev Respir Dis* 1991; 144:1095–1101.

66. Lelcuk S, Huval WV, Valeri CR, et al.: Inhibition of ischemia-induced thromboxane synthesis in man. *J Trauma* 1984; 24:393–396.

67. Krausz MM, Utsunomiya T, Dunham B, et al.: Inhibition of permeability edema with imidazole. *Surgery* 1982; 92:299–308.

68. Slotman GJ, Burchard KW, D'Arezzo A, et al.: Ketoconazole prevents acute respiratory failure in critically ill surgical patients. *J Trauma* 1988; 28:648–654.

69. Leeman M, Boeynaems J, Degaute J, et al.: Administration of dazoxiben, a selective thromboxane synthetase inhibitor in the adult respiratory distress syndrome. *Chest* 1985; 87:726–730.

70. Yu M, Tomasa G: A double-blind, prospective, randomized trial of ketoconazole, a thromboxane synthetase inhibitor, in the prophylaxis of the adult respiratory distress syndrome. *Crit Care Med* 1993; 21:1635–1642.

71. Holcroft JW, Vassar MJ, Weber CJ: Prostaglandin E1 in patients with the adult respiratory distress syndrome. *Chest* 1989; 96:114–119.

72. Bone RC, Slotman G, Maunder R, et al.: Randomized double-blind, multicenter study of prostaglandin E1 in patients with the adult respiratory distress syndrome. *Chest* 1989; 96:114–119.

73. Melot C, Lejeune P, Leeman M, et al.: Prostaglandin E1 in patients with the adult respiratory distress syndrome. *Chest* 1989; 96:114–119.

74. Hallman M, Spragg R, Harrell JH, et al.: Evidence of lung surfactant abnormality in respiratory failure. *J Clin Invest* 1982; 70:673:683.

75. Petty TL, Silver GW, Paul GW, et al.: Abnormalities in lung elastic properties and surfactant function in adult respiratory distress syndrome. *Chest* 1979; 75:571–574.

76. Jobe A, Ikegami M: Surfactant for the treatment of respiratory distress syndrome. *Am Rev Respir Dis* 1987; 136:1256–1275.

77. Merritt TA, Hallman M, Bloom BT, et al.: Prophylactic treatment of very premature infants with human surfactant. *N Engl J Med* 1986; 315:785–790.

78. Horbar JD, Soll RF, Sutherland JM, et al.: A multicenter, randomized, placebo-controlled trial of surfactant therapy for respiratory distress syndrome. *N Engl J Med* 1989; 320:959–965.

79. Cooke R: The current use of exogenous surfactants in the newborn. *Brit J Obstet Gynaecol* 1995; 102:679–91.

80. Enhorning G: Surfactant replacement in adult respiratory distress syndrome. *Am Rev Respir Dis* 1989; 140:281–283.

81. Anzeuto A, Baughman R, Guntupalli K, et al.: An international, randomized, placebo-controlled trial evaluating the safety and efficacy of aerosolized surfactant in patients with sepsis-induced ARDS (abstract). *Am J Respir Crit Care Med* 1994; 149:A567.

82. Frostell CG, Blomqvist H, Hedenstierna G, et al.: Inhaled nitric oxide selectively reverses human hypoxic pulmonary vasoconstriction without causing systemic vasodilation. *Anesthesiology* 1993; 78:427–35.

83. Rossaint R, Falke KJ, Lopez F, et al.: Inhaled nitric oxide for the adult respiratory distress syndrome. *N Engl J Med* 1993; 328:399–405.

PHYSIOLOGIC THERAPEUTIC INTERVENTIONS

JESSE HALL AND GREGORY A. SCHMIDT

Physiologic Interventions in ARDS

It is hoped that further explication of mechanisms of injury (see Chaps. 100 and 101) eventually will lead to innovative pharmacologic therapies. At present management of these patients relies on meticulous supportive therapy, while underlying diseases are diagnosed and treated. Even if new pharmacologic agents become available, the same supportive therapy will be necessary to maintain a viable patient to benefit from treatment.

OXYGEN THERAPY

Upon presentation, the patient with acute respiratory distress syndrome (ARDS) should receive supplemental oxygen provided by high flow or rebreather mask. Tracheal Fi_{O_2} rarely exceeds 0.60 in the typical dyspneic, tachypneic patient, regardless of the type of mask system used.[1] Nonetheless, the initial administration of an $Fi_{O_2} > 50$ percent serves both diagnostic and therapeutic purposes. A large intrapulmonary shunt is suggested by a minimal increase in Pa_{O_2} (< 100 mmHg). If the response to oxygen is better than this, etiologies of respiratory distress and radiologic infiltrates lacking large intrapulmonary shunts should be considered (e.g., pleural effusions, pulmonary emboli). Even when arterial Pa_{O_2} increases minimally, oxygen delivery to peripheral tissues may increase significantly, due to the steep slope of the oxyhemoglobin dissociation curve in the range of these abnormal values (see Fig. 102-1).

AIRWAY MANAGEMENT AND INITIAL USE OF MUSCLE RELAXATION AND SEDATION

Intubation should be performed early and electively in most patients. Noninvasive mask ventilation has been used successfully in patients with pulmonary edema complicating left ventricular failure and with patients with exacerbations of chronic obstructive pulmonary disease, but is rarely indicated in patients with ARDS.[2]

If hypoperfusion is present, as in the patient with hypotension, cardiovascular instability, or the hyperdynamic circulation of sepsis, oxygen delivery may be compromised not only by hypoxemia but by an inadequate cardiac output as well. In this circumstance, sedation and muscle relaxation should be instituted immediately, as a means to diminish the oxygen requirement of the skeletal muscles. Patients with extreme hypoxemia despite ventilator management (as described below) should be treated in a similar fashion. Finally, muscle relaxation will also allow cooling of the febrile patient without shivering, an important consideration in this group of individuals with borderline oxygen delivery.

VENTILATOR PARAMETERS

Initial ventilator settings are selected to provide adequate oxygenation and ventilation, with a minimal risk of barotrauma. This is accomplished best with an Fi_{O_2} of 1.0, tidal volume of 6 to 8 mL/kg and respiratory rate of 25. Patients may be permitted to initiate breaths with an assist control or

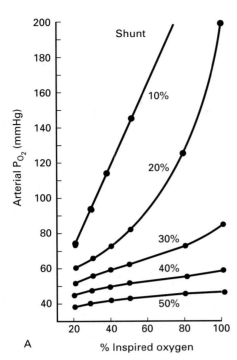

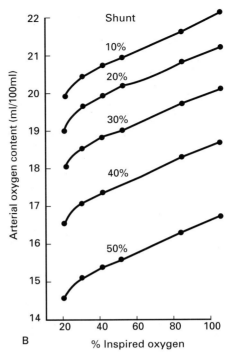

FIGURE 102-1 The effect of intrapulmonary shunt on gas exchange and oxygen delivery. In *panel A*, Pa_{O_2} is plotted against Fi_{O_2} for varying shunt fractions. Note that for higher shunt fractions (> 30 percent), Pa_{O_2} increases minimally with increase in Fi_{O_2}. For this reason, ARDS and other disease processes with large shunts are termed oxygen *refractory*. Nonetheless, as shown in *panel B*, even small changes in Pa_{O_2} are associated with relatively large changes in arterial oxygen content and, hence, oxygen delivery. This is so because these small increments in Pa_{O_2} occur on the steep portion of the oxyhemoglobin dissociation curve, and, hence, hemoglobin saturation increases significantly. Thus, high concentrations of oxygen are the appropriate initial management for patients with ARDS. (*Reproduced with permission from Dantzker RM: Gas exchange in the adult respiratory distress syndrome. Clin Chest Med 1982; 3:57–67.*)

synchronized intermittent mandatory ventilation mode with minimal sensitivity ($-$ 2 cmH_2O).

As noted above, patients who have shock complicating ARDS or who cannot be adequately oxygenated may require early muscle relaxation. The goal of low tidal volume use is to maintain peak airway pressures < 40 cmH_2O, which usually can be achieved with the strategy described despite marked reductions in lung compliance. Such low tidal volume ventilation is appropriate to the reduced functional residual capacity (FRC) in edematous lungs and has been shown to be safe in a diverse population of patients.[3] This may avoid lung injury and capillary leak associated with larger tidal volumes and larger pressure excursions[4–6] (Fig. 102-2) and facilitates the use of greater positive end-expiratory pressure (PEEP) to reduce shunt without excessive end-inspiratory pressures. As illustrated in Figure 102-3, the pressure-volume curve in ARDS has a sigmoidal shape, with a lower and an upper inflection point (LIP and UIP). The UIP, usually seen at a pressure between 20 to 35 cmH_2O, indicates that further increases in pressure result in less volume change, presumably because some alveoli are maximally stretched. When patients were ventilated to keep the peak airway pressure < 40 cmH_2O (tidal volume less than 6 mL/kg), gas exchange, lung mechanics, and weaning rate were improved compared to randomized controls.[7] Several

studies have suggested that low tidal volume ventilation also confers improved circulatory function on patients with ARDS.[7,8]

Low tidal volume ventilation may result in hypercapnea. Rather than reverting to larger tidal volumes, many authors now recommend permissive hypercapnea in patients with severe ARDS.[9–11] This is generally well tolerated if carbon dioxide levels are allowed to increase slowly. The benefit of correction of acid-base state with bicarbonate infusion is unclear. Permissive hypercapnea to a Pa_{CO_2} causing arterial blood pH of 7.2 to 7.3 may be used if necessary to achieve peak airway pressures ≤ 40 cmH_2O. However, this ventilator strategy still requires further assessment in prospective trials. For such significant levels of hypercapnea, sedation and muscle relaxation may be necessary to overcome the patient's drive to breathe.

Intermittent positive-pressure ventilation with high concentrations of oxygen will achieve an acceptable Pa_{O_2} (≥ 50 mmHg) and O_2 saturation (Sa_{O_2} ≥ 90 percent) in many patients; unfortunately, continuous administration of such high concentrations of oxygen may cause further lung injury. Clinically, it is often difficult to distinguish the sequelae of acute lung injury from the complications of the therapy it requires.[12] Nonetheless, there also are limits on the degree of hypoxemia that may be tolerated, and an Sa_{O_2} approaching

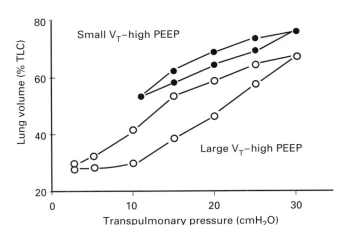

FIGURE 102-2 Comparison of pulmonary pressure-volume rela-tionships during canine acid aspiration pneumonitis between two groups: open circles denote large tidal volume–low PEEP (3 cmH$_2$O); closed circles denote small tidal volume–high PEEP (13 cmH$_2$O). Note that increasing PEEP by 10 cmH$_2$O caused a large increase in end-expired lung volume such that tidal volume was halved to maintain end-inspired lung volume and transpul-monary pressure. This ventilatory pattern reduced the edema by 50 percent compared with the large tidal volume–low PEEP pat-tern. (*Reproduced and adapted with permission from Corbridge TC, Wood LDH, Crawford GP, et al.: Adverse effects of large tidal volume and low PEEP in canine acid aspiration. Am Rev Respir Dis 1990; 142:311–315.*)

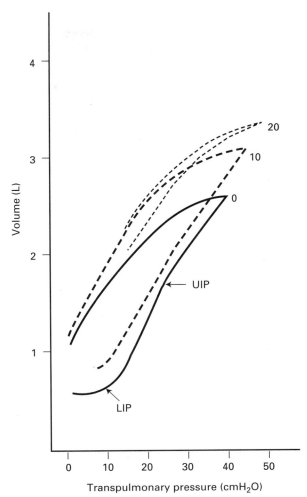

FIGURE 102-3 Static pressure-volume curve is shown for a patient with early ARDS at various levels of PEEP. Without PEEP, the curve demonstrates marked hysteresis and an inflection point on the inflation limb. At 20 cmH$_2$O PEEP, the lower inflec-tion point is lost, and the inflation-deflation curves are more nearly superimposable with an increased slope, indicating improved compliance associated with alveolar recruitment. Patients not exhibiting such inflection points prior to application of PEEP are less likely to exhibit alveolar recruitment with improvement in gas exchange. (*Modified and reproduced with permission from Benito S, LeMaire F: Pulmonary pressure-volume relationship in acute respiratory distress syndrome in adults: role of positive end-expiratory pressure. J Crit Care 1990; 5:27–34.*)

75 percent may result in global myocardial hypoxia and acute dilated cardiomyopathy, which progresses rapidly to cardiac arrest.[13] Positive end-expiratory pressure is utilized in this setting to provide adequate oxygenation without incurring oxygen toxicity.

Preventing alveolar and airway pressure from falling to atmospheric by application of a retard valve on the ventila-tor (PEEP) or providing a positive pressure by mask throughout the respiratory cycle (CPAP) exploits the hys-teresis of the inflation and deflation limbs of each breath. Over the course of five to eight breaths, the increased end-expired pressure increases end-inspired volume to achieve alveolar recruitment by expansion of collapsed units and translocation of fluid from flooded units to the interstitial space; PEEP then prevents the derecruitment of these units at end-expiration.[7,14] The resulting increase in FRC is indi-cated by an increase in lung compliance and is associated with an improvement in gas exchange caused by perfusion of recruited air space. Interestingly, lung liquid is not decreased by PEEP[14] but merely redistributed. Recent evi-dence suggests that a level of PEEP should be chosen that is sufficient (usually 10 to 15 cmH$_2$O) to prevent excessive derecruitment at end-expiration to protect the lung from the shear forces associated with repeated recruitment and col-lapse. This approach to PEEP, along with the aforementioned low tidal volume strategy which attempts to maintain peak airway pressure < 40 cmH$_2$O, is termed the "open lung" approach, and has been validated in critically ill patients.[7] Alveolar recruitment may not occur in advanced prolifera-tive-phase ARDS because edema contributes less to shunt

while alveolar obliteration with fibrosis unresponsive to PEEP contributes more.

Positive end-expiratory pressure should be titrated to achieve an Fi$_{O_2}$ of ≤ 0.60 and should be added in increments of 3 to 5 cmH$_2$O. With each increment in PEEP, alveolar recruitment and lung mechanical changes tend to be com-plete and stable after five to eight breaths, and improvement in arterial saturation follows within minutes. Accordingly, improvement in respiratory system compliance and oxy-genation can be rapidly determined during this time, just as the potential for PEEP to decrease venous return can be detected rapidly by hypotension. This allows a rapid achievement of the level of PEEP that improves oxygenation without decreasing cardiac output and oxygen delivery, as opposed to the hours of assessment that might occur if many serial blood gas and cardiac output determinations were performed. Some data suggest that a subset of patients with ARDS do not exhibit lung mechanics as described above.[15] Specifically, their inflation volume-pressure curve is convex upward, and lung compliance measurements do not correlate well with alveolar recruitment (Fig. 102-3). To the extent this is true, the thoracic gas volume increment occurring with PEEP might correlate better with alveolar recruitment.[15]

If PEEP levels beyond those associated with ongoing alveolar recruitment are applied, lung hyperexpansion may result, risking barotrauma without benefit to gas exchange. Such excessive PEEP levels are recognized by cardiovascular effects of lung hyperinflation—hypotension and tachycardia. Patients receiving drugs that diminish tone in the peripheral circulation (e.g., nitrates or narcotics) or who have a component of hypovolemia are particularly prone to these adverse cardiovascular effects of PEEP.[16] Both diminished vascular tone and hypovolemia diminish mean systemic pressure, which in turn causes a decrease in venous return and cardiac output. Furthermore, PEEP actually may increase resistance to venous return so that cardiac output is reduced by PEEP even when mean systemic pressure increases just as much as right atrial pressure;[17] accordingly, PEEP-induced hypotension needs to be treated by temporary reduction in the PEEP and then by expansion of the circulating volume. Vasoactive drugs that increase vascular tone may be useful in this setting as well.

While PEEP constitutes standard supportive therapy for patients with ARDS, there is no evidence that PEEP prevents patients with predisposing conditions from progressing to ARDS. Accordingly, PEEP should not be used unless lung oxygen exchange is severely impaired.[18] Titration of PEEP therapy is often associated with an apparent improvement in the chest radiograph, but this is the result of an increase in gas volume and not a decrease in lung edema, which tends to remain the same or increase with application of PEEP.[14]

While PEEP is used in the majority of patients with acute respiratory failure and severe hypoxemia, PEEP may be deleterious in instances of focal lung injury such as lobar pneumonia.[9,19] In patients with focal disease, PEEP may not recruit the consolidated lung but rather hyperinflate normal lung, and, at high levels, cause an increase in intrapulmonary shunt. Nonetheless, a trial of PEEP is warranted in most patients since varying degrees of lung edema may be present in regions distant from the radiologically apparent pneumonia.

In extremely hypoxemic patients, an incremental application of PEEP may not be desirable. Immediately applying 15 to 20 cmH_2O PEEP (provided the tidal volume is 5 to 7 ml/kg) may improve oxygen saturation if it does not reduce blood pressure to an unacceptable level. Positive end-expiratory pressure then can be titrated down from the initial level after reducing Fi_{O_2} until Sa_{O_2} decreases to about 90 percent.

Rarely, even a PEEP level of 20 cmH_2O does not achieve 90 percent saturation of arterial hemoglobin with an Fi_{O_2} of 1.0. In this circumstance, tidal volume may be reduced further (and permissive hypercapnea undertaken) and PEEP levels of 20 to 30 cmH_2O may be applied. Such severe lung injury coupled with high PEEP levels is associated with a very high incidence of barotrauma, and it is advisable to have chest tubes available at the bedside for a rapid response to pneumothorax.[20]

This approach to PEEP almost will invariably permit reduction of Fi_{O_2} to ≤ 0.60 within the early hours of stabilization of the patient on a ventilator. Positive end-expiratory pressure should not be used, however, to minimize intrapulmonary shunt or administration of oxygen, but rather the least amount of PEEP that achieves > 90 percent saturation or arterial hemoglobin on an Fi_{O_2} of 0.60 should be used. It is important that arterial oxygen content—and hence oxygen delivery to peripheral tissues—be maintained at a high level in these patients by transfusion to a hemoglobin level of > 13 to 14 g/dL.

Reduction of PEEP levels, even for short periods of time, is often associated with alveolar derecruitment and, hence, rapid arterial hemoglobin desaturation. Thus, once endotracheal tube suctioning has been accomplished for diagnostic purposes, nursing and respiratory therapy staff should be instructed to keep times for airway disconnections to a minimum, or to use an in-line suctioning system that maintains sterility and positive pressure. This is accomplished with a suctioning catheter residing in a sterile sheath and entering the endotracheal tube through a tight-sealing diaphragm. These suctioning systems generally are effective for lesser levels of PEEP (< 15 cmH_2O) but often leak if greater levels are attempted.

CIRCULATORY MANAGEMENT OF ARDS

While PEEP is employed widely to support gas exchange during mechanical ventilatory support, there are no data indicating that its use has improved survival. This may relate to the fact that it is purely supportive management and does not improve underlying lung damage and its associated pulmonary edema and may itself cause further lung injury. Conceivably measures that reduce edemagenesis in ARDS could diminish the duration of potentially dangerous ventilator, PEEP, and oxygen therapy thereby improving outcome. Most patients with ARDS do not die during the early phase of disease as a consequence of severe hypoxemia, but rather over days to weeks, frequently with evidence of hypermetabolism, nosocomial infection, and multiple system organ failure.[21] Some have argued that an approach to patients with ARDS that maximizes oxygen delivery to peripheral tissues will avoid these late complications of acute lung injury and its associated conditions.[22] One such method of increasing oxygen delivery is to administer fluids aggressively in hope of increasing cardiac output. This position is advocated as well to address the finding in some clinical investigations that an oxygen extraction or utilization defect may exist in patients with sepsis and ARDS,[23,24] although recent studies have called the existence

TABLE 102-1   Studies Relating Oxygen Consumption ($\dot{V}_{O_2}$) to Delivery (Q_{O_2})

Ref. No.	Number of Patients	Disease	$Q_{O_2}\Delta$ by	If $\dot{V}_{O_2}$ Independently Measured by Expired Gas	If $\dot{V}_{O_2}$ Measured by Fick Determination
25	12	Septic shock	PEEP	No	Yes
26	14	Septic shock	Dobutamine	No	Yes
27	17	ARDS	Transfusion	No	Yes
28	16	Sepsis	Time	No	Yes
29	8	ARDS	PEEP/volume	No	NR
30	9	ARDS	PEEP	No	Yes
31	10	Septic shock	Dobutamine	No	Yes

of this purported abnormality into question, at least as being clinically relevant.[25–32] The consequence of an approach of maximizing oxygen delivery could be escalating requirements for mechanical ventilation, oxygen, and PEEP, and to the extent that intensity and duration of supportive therapy were greater determinants of complications and organ dysfunctions, the net result could be detrimental. A diametrically opposed approach, which explores an aggressive but cautious reduction in ventricular preload without decreasing cardiac output early in the course of ARDS, could result in a reduction in edemagenesis and, hence, its treatment. The justification for this approach derives from both animal models[32–37] and clinical data.

Several retrospective studies have reported a correlation between survival and net diuresis or reduction in pulmonary capillary wedge pressure in patients with ARDS.[38–40] Prospective data collection also has demonstrated that titration of therapy to minimize extravascular lung water results in decreased ventilator and ICU days.[41]

While fluid restriction and judicious volume reduction may improve lung function, many clinicians are concerned that excessive application of such measures could result in hypoperfusion and organ failure. This concern has been heightened by a notion that patients with sepsis and other conditions predisposing to ARDS exhibit an oxygen extraction defect in peripheral tissues, and hence require supranormal levels of oxygen delivery to avoid tissue hypoxia and dysfunction. Much of this speculation has been fueled by studies in patients with sepsis and ARDS who exhibited an increase in oxygen consumption when oxygen delivery was altered by manipulations of PEEP, vasoactive drugs, or fluid and blood administration.[23,24,42] In these early clinical studies, oxygen consumption ($\dot{V}_{O_2}$) and oxygen delivery (Q_{O_2}) were measured by data collected during right heart catheterization. Since oxygen consumption was measured by Fick determination, there was a shared variable (cardiac output) in the measurements of Q_{O_2} and $\dot{V}_{O_2}$. This raised the possibility of mathematical coupling of data and a spurious relationship between $\dot{V}_{O_2}$ and Q_{O_2} being seen during the various manipulations directed at changing oxygen delivery. In fact, when studies measuring $\dot{V}_{O_2}$ independently (at the mouth by metabolic cart) were performed, similar patient groups with sepsis and ARDS did not exhibit this dependence of $\dot{V}_{O_2}$ on Q_{O_2} (see Table 102-1).

Table 102-1 summarizes studies examining whether oxygen consumption ($\dot{V}_{O_2}$) is dependent on oxygen delivery (Q_{O_2}) in patients with sepsis and ARDS. When $\dot{V}_{O_2}$ is measured independently of Q_{O_2} by metabolic cart, no dependence was observed. When $\dot{V}_{O_2}$ is measured by Fick determination at the time of right heart catheterization, a spurious correlation was observed. Accordingly, the implication that greater oxygen deliveries are appropriate for these patients does not appear warranted.

A number of studies have been conducted attempting to evaluate prospectively the benefit of increasing Q_{O_2} in critically ill patients. In two studies, no benefit was seen, and in one, a significantly greater mortality was observed in patients taken to a high cardiac output with the use of vasoactive drugs.[43–45] Accordingly, fluid restriction in patients with ARDS as well as attempts to diurese the patient within the limits of an adequate cardiac output is advocated as the best course. Monitoring the pulmonary capillary wedge pressure (Pcwp) can be useful in this setting, and a reduction of Pcwp can be accomplished safely in most patients.[39] Rather than striving for a specific "optimal" oxygen delivery, treatment should be guided by the usual parameters of organ perfusion and function that are routinely followed in all critically ill patients—mental status, urine output and concentration, circulatory adequacy, and metabolic evidence of anaerobic metabolism.

MONITORING THE PATIENT WITH ARDS

Changes in intrapulmonary shunt, oxygen consumption, or perfusion are frequent and relatively sudden in patients with ARDS; all influence arterial hemoglobin saturation. Pulse oximetry is thus useful as a continuous measure of the adequacy of blood oxygen levels, at least in patients with a stable circulation. It is still advisable to obtain frequent arterial blood gases in the first day of management to correlate to pulse oximetry readings and to avoid mismeasurement of arterial hemoglobin saturation in the patients with various degrees of hypoperfusion.

CIRCULATORY MANAGEMENT OF ARDS

As mentioned above, right heart catheterization is useful in many patients, although debate continues over whether invasive measurements confer true benefit as regards morbidity and mortality. The measurement of the pulmonary capillary wedge pressure will on occasion identify patients with "clear-cut" ARDS who prove to have significant left ventricular dysfunction and hydrostatic edema. The benefit of identifying such patients is clear. There are other means of determining the cause of pulmonary edema when the clinical setting and findings are not definitive. The protein content of edema fluid in ARDS is 70 percent to 90 percent of the plasma concentration.[46,47] By contrast, cardiogenic edema is transudative in nature, with a protein content less than 50 percent of that of the patient's plasma. Thus, simply sampling edema fluid in the intubated patient and performing a simple protein analysis can be extremely useful. This analysis has no diagnostic value unless performed early in the course of edemagenesis, since there is active clearance of crystalloid from alveolar liquid, which results in an increase in the ratio of pulmonary edema to plasma protein ratio in recovering heart failure patients. Failure to concentrate alveolar protein signals persistent leak and a poorer prognosis.[47]

Invasive hemodynamic monitoring also is useful in patients with sepsis as an antecedent to ARDS. Many of these patients are hypovolemic, likely related to intravascular volume lost through their diffuse capillary leak and sequestration of circulating volume in the venous capacitance vessels. Volume resuscitation is appropriate to the extent that hypovolemia is the cause of hypoperfusion superimposed on their hypoxemia, but excessive volume administration may cause worsening pulmonary edema. Measurements of pulmonary capillary wedge pressure and cardiac output help avoid excessive fluid administration.

Since the greatest uncertainty regarding specifics of cardiopulmonary function and dysfunction exists early in the course of acute lung injury, we advocate early use of right-heart catheterization followed by a daily approach of questioning the ongoing need for an indwelling invasive device is advised.

INNOVATIVE SUPPORTIVE INTERVENTIONS

INVERSE RATIO VENTILATION

Inverse ratio ventilation (IRV) involves prolongation of inspiratory time so that the inspiratory to expiratory time ratio (I:E) exceeds 1, as opposed to the usual ratios of 1:2 or 1:3 employed during conventional ventilation. The purported benefits of this ventilatory strategy are more optimal distribution of ventilation and alveolar recruitment at lower airway inflating pressures.[38–51] A number of studies have indicated that intrapulmonary shunt can be reduced substantially with IRV, and some authors have suggested it be used as a "salvage" strategy for patients who cannot be adequately treated with conventional ventilation and PEEP.[50,52,53]

In the absence of prospective trials comparing IRV to routine mechanical ventilation strategies (including low tidal volume ventilation and permissive hypercapnea), it is most appropriate to consider IRV as innovative and, at best, a salvage strategy for patients failing routine therapy. One possi-

ble effect of shortened expiratory time is dynamic hyperinflation with intrinsic PEEP ($PEEP_i$). Thus, the use of IRV could result in higher levels of PEEP than were initially abandoned in the pursuit of routine mechanical ventilation of a given patient with ARDS. Were this the sole mechanism of improved alveolar recruitment and diminished intrapulmonary shunt, IRV should not be used. However, at least some anecdotal reports have suggested that oxygenation is improved through alternative mechanisms with this ventilatory strategy.[54]

It is important to note that all patients will require heavy sedation, and many will require paralysis to tolerate IRV. Since many patients managed with prolonged muscle relaxation have exhibited protracted syndromes of neuromuscular weakness during their recovery from critical illness, this is a potential weakness of this ventilatory strategy.[55,56] When IRV is contemplated, an initial database should be collected including minute ventilation, tidal volume, mean airway pressure (MAP), $PEEP_i$, arterial blood gases, and hemodynamics. I:E ratios should then be altered gradually (e.g., 1:3, 1:2, 1:1, 2:1, 2.5:1, 3:1) with recollection of data with each incremental change. A diminished intrapulmonary shunt at a $PEEP_i$ and MAP less than the prior settings on routine mechanical ventilation would indicate a successful intervention.

HIGH-FREQUENCY AND CONSTANT FLOW VENTILATION

A natural extension of the notion of use of low tidal volume ventilation to minimize lung injury is use of extremely low tidal volumes and high rates (e.g., tidal volume in the range 1 to 5 mL/kg and rates of 60 to 3000). The widest clinical application has been high-frequency jet ventilation (HFJV). A number of crossover and prospective randomized trials comparing HFJV to conventional ventilation have been reported.[57–62] While this ventilatory mode appears to be safe in the hands of investigators reporting these results, it did not cause reduced incidence of barotrauma, improved gas exchange, or better outcome. In many patients with high minute ventilation requirements or greatly deranged lung mechanics, CO_2 elimination may not be possible.[57]

Constant flow ventilation (CFV) is yet another alternative mode of ventilation. This approach relies less on bulk flow and completely on intrapulmonary momentum exchange to effect alveolar ventilation,[63] but requires careful placement of the inflow gas jets to bypass the bottleneck of facilitated diffusion in the proximal airways.[64] This technique and the related use of tracheal gas insufflation[65,66] may find application in the future but should be viewed as experimental modes at the present time.

PATIENT POSITIONING

Side-to-side positioning of the patient is well described as improving gas exchange in the patient with asymmetric alveolar filling disease. Similar reduction of intrapulmonary shunt and improved oxygenation has been described in patients with ARDS shifted to a prone position.[67,68] These observations are consistent with positional changes in ARDS patients exploiting the gravitational distribution of blood flow to reduce shunt. This strategy is best reserved for patients who cannot be managed adequately in the supine position.

EXTRACORPOREAL MEMBRANE OXYGENATION

Use of an extracorporeal device to achieve gas exchange provides the theoretical benefit of lung "rest" until recovery is well established. The earliest large multicenter trial of this therapy, using venoarterial extracorporeal membrane oxygenation (ECMO), was reported in 1979.[69] In this study, patients with advanced ARDS requiring toxic concentrations of oxygen were enrolled, and survival was not improved with ECMO. After this report, interest waned in the use of this technology in ARDS. Over the next decade, however, increased survival was demonstrated in neonates with respiratory distress syndrome (RDS) and recent studies have suggested that it may be beneficial in this form of respiratory failure. A number of European and American investigators now have returned to various ECMO strategies. Most popular is use of veno-venous bypass to achieve extracorporeal carbon dioxide removal ($ECCO_2R$) with only a fraction of oxygenation provided by the extracorporeal circuit; further blood oxygenation is achieved by apneic ventilation in the paralyzed patient by continuous flow provided by a cannula placed in the trachea, along with low-frequency positive-pressure ventilation.[70,71] Interestingly, reported survival is improved from earlier reports of ECMO in ARDS, but clear differences in survival between this approach and conventional ventilator strategies have not been demonstrated. Final results of the single large American study are not yet available. At present, this therapy is best considered experimental and should be restricted to large centers with both experience in and resources for this intensive therapy.

MANAGEMENT DURING RECOVERY FROM THE EXUDATIVE PHASE OF ARDS

Rapid recovery from ARDS, generally within 2 to 3 days, is encountered and is likely determined by resolution of the predisposing cause and arguably by appropriate cardiovascular interventions. Such recovery is heralded by diminished shunt, increased lung compliance, and diminishing oxygen requirements. When Fi_{O_2} can be reduced to 0.40 to 0.50, consideration can be given to cautious reduction in PEEP. On occasion, however, even small decrements in PEEP will be associated with sudden arterial desaturation, perhaps related to alveolar flooding or collapse related to surfactant deficiency or dysfunction. When this occurs, PEEP levels often must be increased above the former level for alveolar recruitment. PEEP should be reduced in small decrements (2 to 3 cmH_2O), with several hours of observation between adjustments.

When the patient has achieved an Fi_{O_2} of 0.40 and PEEP < 10 cmH_2O, evaluation for spontaneous ventilation can be undertaken. If central nervous system depression, muscle weakness, or new lung insults have not occurred during the course of acute illness, rapid progression to CPAP is appropriate, with prompt extubation. In anticipation of these events, sedation and muscle relaxation should be discontinued as soon as edema resolves.

MANAGEMENT OF THE PATIENT IN PROLIFERATIVE-PHASE ARDS

Unfortunately, many patients with ARDS will progress over the first week of mechanical ventilation to disordered healing and severe lung fibrosis. This is usually characterized by increasing airway pressures, diminished lung compliance, a "honey-comb" appearance on the chest radiograph, progressive pulmonary hypertension, and extremely high minute ventilation requirements (> 20 L/min). Barotrauma is a prominent feature of their course and multiple organ failures often accrue.

Many of the specifics and goals of therapy delineated above for management of exudative-phase ARDS require modification if this disease progression occurs. Since patients with proliferative-phase ARDS often have lessened vascular permeability and pulmonary edema, strategies to reduce lung water (e.g., fluid restriction and diuresis) are often of little benefit. Since alveolar pressures are particularly high in these patients, attempts to reduce pulmonary vascular pressure may cause increased dead space and hypoperfusion. Thus, earlier strategies to reduce Pcwp may have to be aborted and fluid liberalization undertaken.

Day-to-day management of these patients is dominated by attention to the many complications arising during prolonged mechanical ventilatory support. Nosocomial infections are common, and complicating gram-negative pneumonia is particularly problematic. Nutritional support is crucial and should be instituted if recovery is not likely to be complete within the first several days of management. The role of corticosteroids in the treatment of lung inflammation and disordered healing is discussed in Chap. 10; at present, this must be considered an untested therapy.

Conclusion

While a large number of clinical conditions can result in acute lung injury and ARDS, a relatively small number of entities (sepsis, acid aspiration, trauma) account for the vast majority of patients. As the understanding of the factors that take patients from "at risk" to actual pulmonary capillary leak grows, more specific pharmacologic interventions will be identified and evaluated. Promising avenues include antioxidants, antilipids, and possibly biologics. It is likely that any effective therapy will require early identification of patients at risk and early administration.

Regardless of the progress of pharmacotherapy, appropriate supportive therapy is necessary to stabilize the patient and provide a window for treatment of underlying processes. Ventilator management of patients with the early, exudative phase of ARDS should begin with an Fi_{O_2} of 1.0, tidal volume 6 to 7 mL/kg, and respiratory rate of 20 to 28. During initial stabilization on the ventilator, sedation and, on occasion, muscle relaxation are warranted to minimize oxygen consumption and airway pressures. Subsequent goals of supportive therapy include the least PEEP that achieves a 90 percent saturation of an adequate circulating hemoglobin (> 13 g/dL) on a nontoxic Fi_{O_2} (< 0.60).

While controversial, a circulatory management that is directed at reduction of lung microvascular pressures and, thereby, limits edemagenesis is worth considering. This goal can be achieved with an approach of reduction of pulmonary capillary wedge pressure within the limits of an adequate cardiac output. At present, clinical data do not support an approach of maximizing oxygen delivery by maximizing cardiac output. Rather, the adequacy of cardiac output should be determined by classic measures of adequate organ perfusion.

Proliferative, late-phase ARDS is signaled by a large dead-space fraction (and, hence, high minute ventilation requirement), high airway pressures (reflecting further reductions in lung compliance), and varying degrees of pulmonary hypertension. The chest radiograph often demonstrates a "honeycomb" appearance. In this phase of ARDS, hypovolemia is poorly tolerated, since it may further increase dead space and have adverse effects on venous return. The use of corticosteroids in this setting requires further confirmation by clinical studies and must be weighed against the risks related to nosocomial superinfection.

References

1. Gibson RL, Comer PB, Beckham RW, et al.: Actual tracheal oxygen concentrations with commonly used oxygen equipment. *Anesthesiology* 1976; 44(1):71.

2. Meyer TJ, Hill NS: Noninvasive positive pressure ventilation to treat respiratory failure. *Ann Int Med* 1994; 120:760–770.

3. Lee PC, Helsmoortel CM, Cohn SM, et al.: Are low tidal volumes safe? *Chest* 1990; 97:425–29.

4. Bshouty Z, Ali J, Younes M: Effect of tidal volume and PEEP on rate of edema formation in in situ perfused canine lobes. *J Appl Physiol* 1988; 64:1900–1902.

5. Corbridge TC, Wood LDH, Crawford GP, et al.: Adverse effects of large tidal volume and low PEEP in canine acid aspiration. *Am Rev Respir Dis* 1990; 142:311–315.

6. Marini JJ: Lung mechanics in the adult respiratory distress syndrome: recent conceptual advances and implications for management. *Clin Chest Med* 1990; 11(4):673–90.

7. Amato MBP, Barbas CSV, Medieros DM, et al.: Beneficial effects of the "open lung approach" with low distending pressures in acute respirtory distress syndrome. *Am J Respir Crit Care Med* 1995; 152:1835–46.

8. Kiiski R, Takala J, Kari A, et al.: Effect of tidal volume on gas exchange and oxygen transport in the adult respiratory distress syndrome. *Am Rev Respir Dis* 1992; 146:1131–5.

9. Hall JB, Schmidt GA, Wood LDH. Acute hypoxemic respiratory failure, in Murray JF, Nadel JA (eds): *Textbook of Respiratory Medicine*. WB Saunders, Philadelphia, 1994:2589–2613.

10. Kollef MH, Schuster DP: The acute respiratory distress syndrome. *N Engl J Med* 1995; 332:27–38.

11. Hickling KG, Henderson SJ, Jackson R: Low mortality associated with low volume pressure limited ventilation with permissive hypercapnia in severe adult respiratory distress syndrome. *Intensive Care Med* 1990; 16:372–7.

12. Tierney DF, Ayers L, Kasuyama RS.: Altered sensitivity to oxygen toxicity. *Am Rev Respir Dis* 1977; 115(suppl):59–65.

13. Walley KR, Becker CJ, Hogan RA, et al.: Progressive hypoxemia limits left ventricular oxygen consumption and contractility. *Circ Res* 1988; 63:849–859.

14. Pare PD, Warriner E, Baile M, et al.: Redistribution of pulmonary extravascular water with positive end-expiratory pressure in canine pulmonary edema. *Am Rev Respir Dis* 1983; 127:590–593.

15. Ranieri VM, Eissa NT, Corbeil C, et al.: Effects of positive end-expiratory pressure on alveolar recruitment and gas exchange in patients with the adult respiratory distress syndrome. *Am Rev Respir Dis* 1991; 144:544–551.

16. Goldberg H, Rabson J: Control of cardiac output by systemic vessels: circulatory adjustments to acute and chronic respiratory failure and the effect of therapeutic interventions. *Am J Cardiol* 1981; 47:696–702.

17. Fessler HE Brower RG, Wise RA, et al.: Effects of positive end-expiratory pressure on the gradient for venous return. *Am Rev Respir Dis* 1991; 143:19–24.

18. Pepe PE, Hudson LD, Carrico CJ: Early application of positive end-expiratory pressure in patients at risk for the adult respiratory-distress syndrome. *N Engl J Med* 1984; 311:281–286.

19. Hall JB, Wood LDH. Acute hypoxemic respiratory failure, in Hall JB, Schmidt GA, Wood LDH (eds): *Principles of Critical Care*. New York, McGraw-Hill, 1992:1634–1658.

20. Kirby RR, Downs JB, Civetta JM, et al.: High level positive and expiratory pressure (PEEP) in acute respiratory insufficiency. *Chest* 1975; 67:156–163.

21. Bone RC, Balk R, Slotman G, et al.: Adult respiratory distress syndrome: sequence and importance of development of multiple organ failure. *Chest* 1992; 101:320–26.

22. Shoemaker WE, Appel PL, Kram HB, et al.: Prospective trial of supranormal values of survivors as therapeutic goals in high-risk surgical patients. *Chest* 1988; 94:1176–86.

23. Haupt MT, Gilbert EM, Carlson RW: Fluid loading increases oxygen consumption in septic patients with lactic acidosis. *Am Rev Respir Dis* 1985; 131:912.

24. Schumacker PT, Cain SM: The concept of a critical oxygen delivery. *Intensive Care Med* 1987; 13:223.

25. Wysocki M, Besbes M, Roupie E, et al.: Modification of oxygen extraction ratio by change in oxygen transport in septic shock. *Chest* 1992; 102:221–226.

26. Ronco JJ, Phang PT, Walley KR, et al.: Oxygen consumption is independent of changes in oxygen delivery in severe adult respiratory distress syndrome. *Am Rev Respir Dis* 1991; 143:1267–1273.

27. Ronco JJ, Fenwick JC, Wiggs BR, et al.: Oxygen consumption is independent of increases in oxygen delivery by dobutamine in septic patients who have normal or increased plasma lactate. *Am Rev Resp Dis* 1993; 147:25–31.

28. Vermeij CG, Feenstra BWA, Adrichem WJ, et al.: Independent oxygen uptake and oxygen delivery in septic and postoperative patients. *Chest* 1991; 99:1438–1443.

29. Annat G, Viale JP, Percival C, et al.: Oxygen delivery and oxygen uptake in adult respiratory distress syndrome. Lack of relationship when measured independently in patients with normal blood lactate concentrations. *Am Rev Respir Dis* 1986; 133:999–1001.

30. Carlile PV, Gray BA: Effect of opposite changes in cardiac output and arterial P_{O_2} in relationship between mixed venous P_{O_2} and oxygen transport. *Am Rev Respir Dis* 1989; 140:891–898.

31. Manthous CA, Schumacker PT, Pohlman A: Absence of supply dependence of oxygen consumption in patients with septic shock. *J Crit Care* 1993; 8:203–211.

32. Prewitt RM, McCarthy J, Wood LDH: Treatment of acute low pressure edema in dogs: relative effects of hydrostatic and oncotic pressure, nitroprusside, and positive end expiratory pressure. *J Clin Invest* 1981; 67:409–417.

33. Long GR, Breen PH, Mayers I, Wood LDH: Treatment of canine aspiration pneumonitis: fluid volume reduction vs. fluid volume expansion. *J Appl Physiol* 1988; 65:1736–1744.

34. Sznajder JI, Zucker AR, Wood LDH, Long GR: Effects of plasmapheresis and hemofiltration on acid aspiration pulmonary edema. *Am Rev Respir Dis* 1986; 134:222–228.

35. Zucker AR, Becker CJ, Berger S, et al.: Pathophysiology of treatment of canine kerosene pulmonary injury: the effects of plasmapheresis and positive end-expiratory pressure on canine kerosene pulmonary injury. *J Crit Care* 1989; 4:184–193.

36. Zucker AR, Wood LDH, Curet-Scott M, et al.: Partial lung bypass reduces kerosene lung injury in dogs. *J Crit Care* 1991;

37. Wood LDH, Prewitt RM: Cardiovascular management in acute hypoxemic respiratory failure. *Am J Cardiol* 1981; 47:963–972.

38. Simons RS, Berdine GG, Seidenfeld JJ, et al.: Fluid balance and the adult respiratory distress syndrome. *Am Rev Respir Dis* 1987; 135:924–29.

39. Humphrey H, Hall J, Sznajder I, et al.: Improved survival in ARDS patients associated with a reduction in pulmonary capillary wedge pressure. *Chest* 1990; 97:1176–80.

40. Mitchel JP, Schuller D, Calandrino FS, et al.: Improved outcome based on fluid management in critically ill patients requiring pulmonary artery catheterization. *Am Rev Respir Dis* 1992; 145:990–998.

41. Eisenberg PR, Hansrough JR, Anderson D, Schuster DP: A prospective study of lung water measurements during patient management in an intensive care unit. *Am Rev Respir Dis* 1987; 136:662–68.

42. Hudson LD: Fluid management strategy in acute lung injury. *Am Rev Respir Dis* 1992; 145:988–989.

43. Tuchschmidt J, Fried J, Astiz M, Rackow E: Elevation of cardiac output and oxygen delivery improves outcome in septic shock. *Chest* 1992; 102:216–20.

44. Yu M, Levy MM, Smith P, et al.: Effect of maximizing oxygen delivery on morbidity and mortality rates in critically ill patients: a prospective, randomized, controlled study. *Crit Care Med* 1993; 21(6):830–838.

45. Hayes MA, Timmins AC, Yau EH, et al.: Elevation of systemic oxygen delivery in the treatment of critically ill patients. *N Engl J Med* 1994; 330:1717–22.

46. Fein A, Grossman RF, Jones JG, et al.: The value of edema fluid protein measurement in patients with pulmonary edema. *Am J Med* 1979; 67:32.

47. Matthay MA, Wiener-Kronish JP: Intact epithelial barrier function is critical for the resolution of alveolar edema in humans. *Am Rev Respir Dis* 1990; 142:1250.

48. Abraham E, Yoshihara G: Cardiorespiratory effects of pressure controlled inverse ratio ventilation in severe respiratory failure. *Chest* 1989; 96:1356–1359.

49. Gurevitch MJ, Van Dyke J, Young ES, et al.: Improved oxygenation and lower peak airway pressure in severe adult respiratory distress syndrome: treatment with inverse ratio ventilation. *Chest* 1986; 89:211–213.

50. March TW, Marini JJ: Inverse ratio ventilation in ARDS: rationale and implementation. *Chest* 1991; 100:494–504.

51. Ravizza AF, Carugo D, Cerchiari EL, et al.: Inversed ratio and conventional ventilations: comparison of the respiratory effects (abstract). *Anesthesiology* 1983; 59:A523.

52. Tharratt RS, Allen RP, Albertson TE: Pressure controlled inverse ratio ventilation in severe adult respiratory failure. *Chest* 1988; 94:755–762.

53. Cole AGH, Weller SF, Sykes MK: Inverse ratio ventilation compared with PEEP in adult respiratory failure. *Intensive Care Med* 1984; 10:227–232.

54. Manthous CA, Schmidt GA: IRV in ARDS: improved oxygenation without autoPEEP. *Chest* 1993; 103:953–54.

55. Shapiro JM, Condos R, Cole RP: Myopathy in status asthmaticus: relation to neuromuscular blockade and corticosteroid administration. *J Int Care Med* 1993; 8:144–152.

56. Douglass JA, Tuxen D, Horne M, et al.: Myopathy in severe asthma. *Am Rev Respir Dis* 1992; 146:517–19.

57. MacIntyre NR, Follett JV, Dietz JL, et al.: Jet ventilation at 100 breaths per minute in adult respiratory failure. *Am Rev Respir Dis* 1986; 134:897–901.

58. Borg UR, Stoklosa JC, Siegel JH, et al.: Prospective evaluation of combined high-frequency ventilation in post-traumatic patients with adult respiratory distress syndrome refractory to optimized conventional ventilatory management. *Crit Care Med* 1989; 17:1129–1141.

59. Schuster DP, Klain M, Snyder JV: Comparison of high frequency jet ventilation to conventional ventilation during severe acute respiratory failure in humans. *Crit Care Med* 1982; 10:625–630.

60. Holzapfel L, Robert D, Perrin F, et al.: Comparison of high frequency jet ventilation to conventional ventilation in adults with respiratory distress syndrome. *Intensive Care Med* 1987; 13:100–5.

61. Carlon GC, Howland WS, Ray C, et al.: High-frequency jet ventilation: a prospective randomized evaluation. *Chest* 1983; 84:551–9.

62. Carlon GC, Howland WS, Groeger JS, et al.: Role of high-frequency jet ventilation in the management of respiratory failure. *Crit Care Med* 1984; 12:777–779.

63. Schumacker PT, Sznajder I, Nahum A, Wood LDH: Ventilation-perfusion inequality during constant flow ventilation. *J Appl Physiol* 1987; 62(3):1255–1263.

64. Breen PH, Sznajder JI, Morrison P, et al.: Constant flow ventilation in anesthetized patients: efficacy and safety. *Anesth Analg* 1986; 65:1161–1169.

65. Marini JJ: Tracheal gas insufflation: a useful adjunct to ventilation? *Thorax* 1994; 49(8):735–7.

66. Nahum A, Ravenscraft SA, Nakos G, et al.: Effect of catheter flow direction on CO_2 removal during tracheal gas insufflation in dogs. *J Appl Phys* 1993; 75(3):1238–46.

67. Piehl M, Brown R: Use of extreme position changes in acute respiratory failure. *Crit Care Med* 1976; 4:13–14.

68. Langer M, Mascheroni D, Marcolin R, et al.: The prone position in ARDS patients. *Chest* 1988; 94:103–107.

69. Zapol WM, Snider MT, Hill JD, et al.: Extracorporeal membrane oxygenation in severe acute respiratory failure. *JAMA* 1979; 242:2193–2196.

70. Morris AH, Wallace CJ, Clemmer TP, et al.: Extracorporeal CO_2 removal therapy for adult respiratory distress syndrome patients. *Respir Care* 1990; 35:224–231.

71. Gattinoni L, Presenti A, Mascheroni D, et al.: Low frequency positive-pressure ventilation with extracorporeal CO_2 removal in severe acute respiratory failure. *JAMA* 1986; 256:881–886.

PHARMACOLOGY OF SYSTEMIC CRITICAL ILLNESS

Chapter 103

PULMONARY DEFENSE AGAINST INFECTION AND THE SYSTEMIC INFLAMMATORY RESPONSE: SEPSIS AND MULTISYSTEM ORGAN DYSFUNCTION

THEODORE LEWIS, JR., AND PATRICK MURRAY

Normal Lung Defenses

The advent of the human immunodeficiency virus (HIV) and acquired immunodeficiency syndrome (AIDS) and the dramatic growth of organ transplantation have had major impacts on the study of infectious diseases of the lung. Research driven by the clinical importance of these conditions and their associated immunocompromised states has enhanced the understanding of lung defenses and how those defenses can fail. It is now necessary to be familiar with many pathogens previously considered rare, to expand the diagnostic arsenal, and utilize many new therapies. An equally rapid change in the systemic manifestations of infec-

tion has demonstrated that many complications of infection result from interactions between microbe and host defenses.[1] This information is well incorporated into an understanding of lung defenses. Several excellent reviews of lung defenses are available, and only a brief review is offered below.[2–4]

The defenses of the lung may be considered anatomically and functionally. Anatomically, the lung is defended by upper airway defenses and alveolar defenses. Functionally, these defenses include structural, cellular, and humoral mechanisms. In the upper airway, structural defenses are very important. Particulate matter is trapped in mucus and transported out of the airway by ciliary motion. The extensive branching of the airway facilitates this process by increasing the likelihood of particulate impact on the airway mucosa. Immunoglobulin secreted into the mucous, largely IgA, also enhances particulate capture.[5] Cellular immunity also may be stimulated by antigenic presentation in the upper airway by lymphoid follicles adjacent to the airway mucosa. Substances secreted in the mucus such as lysozyme or lactoferrin are toxic to the microbe or inhibit growth.[6,7]

CELLULAR DEFENSES

In the alveolus, cellular and humoral defenses predominate. Structural defenses are less important, though surfactant may play a role in promoting uptake of antigen by resident cellular defenses.[8] The macrophage plays several critical roles. Macrophages reside within the alveolar space, the interstitium, and the pleural space. They are capable of phagocytosing particulate matter and microbes. This uptake largely is mediated by receptors for complement or the Fc region of IgG.[9] Opsonization of particulates or microbes with complement or immunoglobulin facilitates macrophage uptake of pathogens. Receptors for specific microbial components also exist.[10] Binding of macrophage surface receptors is a powerful stimulus for macrophage activation, enhancing macrophage killing.[11]

The alveolar macrophage kills microbes by a number of mechanisms (see Chap 33). During phagocytosis the macrophage releases oxygen radicals (in particular hypochlorous acid and hydroxyl radicals) into phagosomes and the surrounding environment.[8] Proteases, collagenases, and lyzozyme are also released into phagosomes and play a role in microbe killing.[8] Macrophage antimicrobial activity is upregulated by cytokines, in particular interferon γ, but also tumor necrosis factor alpha, TNF α, and granulocyte-monocyte colony stimulating factor (GM CSF).[12–14] Macrophage activity may be diminished by IL-4, IL-10, transforming growth factor β, (TGF β) and macrophage deactivating factor.[15,16]

The macrophage also recruits other cellular defenses into areas of inflammation. Cytokines, chemoattractants, and leukotrienes are released, inducing migration of polymorphonuclear leukocytes (PMN) into the area of infection. PMN migration is a complex process of adherance to vascular endothelium, diapedisis through the vascular wall, and pulmonary interstitium. Several substances produced by alveolar macrophages facilitate this process, including leukotriene B$_4$, platelet activating factor, IL-8, IL-1, and others.[8] Leukocyte recruitment also is augmented by cytokines released by other cells resident in the lungs (fibroblast and endothelial cells) in response to TNF or IL-1 released by alveolar macrophages.[17,18] Leukocyte migration also may occur in response to complement fragments or bacterial products themselves. Upon arriving in an area of inflammation, PMNs recognize and phagocytose microbes. This process again is greatly facilitated by complement and antibody bound to the microbe.[19,20] Fusion of phagosome with lysosome results in microbial killing. Killing may occur through oxidative mechanisms, enzymatic mechanisms, or nonenzymatic methods, such as defensins or bactericidal-permeability increasing protein.[21,22] Lysosomal activity of the PMN is increased by activation. Several substances activate PMNs

including IL-1, TNF α, and granulocyte-monocyte colony stimulating factor.[8] Release of lysosomal contents from PMN can occur without phagocytosis, resulting in the discharge of free radicals and enzymes into the immediate local environment.[23] These contents, in particular nitric oxide (NO) may decrease PMN activation locally.

Lymphocyte recruitment into infected regions allows presentation of antigens to lymphocytes. Presentation probably occurs at dendritic cells as well as alveolar macrophages.[3] Antigen presentation requires processing of the microbial protein into antigen (often peptide fragments) and its association with proteins of either class I or class II major histocompatibility complex (MHC). Interaction with T cells through the T-cell receptor then allows T-lymphocyte recognition and activation. The subsequent proliferation of either cytotoxic or helper T cells is dependent on the antigen presenting cell and the MHC with which the antigen is associated. Presentation of antigen with MHC class I molecules, T-cell binding, and local cytokine release results in the proliferation of cytotoxic T cells (CD8+). These are capable of the destruction of cells that present microbial antigens, thus serving to eradicate infected cells.[24] Presentation of antigen with MHC class II molecules results in the development of helper T lymphocytes (CD4+).[25] These cells release products such as interferon γ, resulting in the above-noted augmentation of macrophage bacterial killing. Helper T cells are also important in clonal proliferation of B lymphocytes, through direct cell-to-cell interactions and the release of IL-2, IL-4, and IL-5, and stimulation of antibody production, resulting in the development of specific humoral immunity.[26] The type of response generated by CD4+ cells may reflect further differentiation of these cells into subtypes. In mice, these subtypes (Th1 and Th2) produce varying cytokines,[27] and such subtypes appear to be present in humans.[28]

HUMORAL DEFENSES

Humoral mechanisms play an important role in alveolar defenses. Specific antibodies (IgA and IgG) in the alveolar fluid serve as powerful opsonins, allowing better uptake of pathogens by macrophages and PMNs. IgM and IgG antibodies activate the complement cascade through the classic pathway. Binding of C3 to microbial surfaces in the presence of factors B and D and properdin also activates the complement cascade (alternative pathway). Both pathways result in the eventual generation of the membrane attack complex (C5b-8,9). The membrane attack complex is bound to the microbial cell surface, forming pores in the cell membrane. These pores allow the egress of water, ions, and soluble molecules, eventually causing cell death.[29] Complement fragments also serve as opsonins and chemoattractants for PMNs (see above).

It is apparent from the previous discussion that there are multiple positive feedback loops between cellular and humoral components. Regulatory mechanisms are necessary to prevent an excessive inflammatory response and inappropriate tissue injury. Several such mechanisms appear to be important. It already has been noted that some cytokines (IL-4, IL-10) and TGF β downregulate cellular components of the inflammatory response.[30] Other factors directly antagonize the effects of inflammatory mediators. Soluble receptors to TNF have been identified.[31] These receptors bind to TNF and prevent its binding to cellular receptors, blocking the action of the cytokine.[31] A naturally occurring receptor antagonist of IL-1 also has been noted.[32] It blocks the effect of IL-1 at its target receptors. The role these agents play in pulmonary defenses remains to be elucidated. The balance that results between enhancers and suppressors of inflammation determines the effectiveness with which infection is controlled and the extent of tissue injury.

SPECIFIC PATHOGENS

Within this framework of lung defenses the response to particular types of pathogens may be examined. Extracellular bacteria, bacteria that replicate in the extracellular spaces (*Streptococcus pneumoniae*, *Haemophilus influenzae*, and some gram-negative organisms), are eradicated by several mechanisms. They may be phagocytosed by macrophages, a process that is expedited by complement and specific IgG antibodies. Antibody and complement also may be directly bactericidal, as noted above. Extracellular bacteria are phagocytosed and destroyed by PMNs. Organisms that are capable of reproducing within cells (*Mycrobacterium tuberculosis*, *Legionella pneumophilia*, *Listeria monocytogenes*) are protected against extracellular defenses. Killing of these organisms depends on cellular immune defenses. Activation of alveolar macrophages by interferon produced by helper CD4+ cells allows killing of intracellular organisms. T-cell-mediated defenses are also important in the defense against viruses such as cytomegalovirus and herpes viruses, where cellular expression of viral antigen causes activation of CD8+ cells, which then lyse the infected cell. Defense against fungal infections such as *Cryptococcus neoformans*, *Histoplasma capsulatum*, or *Coccidioides immitis* requires both CD4+ and CD8+ T cells. Other fungal infections, in particular *Aspergillus fumigatus*, require intact polymorphonuclear leukocyte function to eradicate. *Pneumocytis carinii* is attacked by both humoral and cellular mechanisms.

Infectious pneumonia results when there is an imbalance between the infecting agent and the defense mechanisms discussed. Such an imbalance occurs when there is a large innoculum of an infectious agent delivered to the lower airway, which overwhelms the defense systems, or when a virulent organism is capable of avoiding resident defenses. Clinical pneumonia, manifested by local effects on lung structure and gas exchange, and systemic inflammation (fever, shock, organ dysfunction), are the result of interactions between the infecting agent, toxins it may produce, and the host defenses. These relationships are discussed in the following section. Abnormalities in host defenses increase susceptibility to infection and alter the normal host response. Pulmonary infections in the setting of compromised host defenses are discussed in Chaps. 103 and 104.

Systemic Inflammatory Responses

The complex interactions of structural, cellular, and humoral components of pulmonary defenses serve as a useful framework to consider the systemic effects of infection and host response. It should be noted that systemic inflammation is a common consequence of infection elsewhere in the body and of noninfectious inflammatory states such as pancreatitis or the adult respiratory distress syndrome. Nevertheless the same cellular constituents (macrophage-monocytes, polymorphonuclear leukocytes and lymphocytes) and humoral constituents (cytokines, antibody, complement) are important in systemic inflammation.[1] Furthermore, pulmonary infection may initiate the systemic inflammatory process in the absence of systemic infection.[33,34]

The clinical manifestations of ongoing systemic inflammation span a continuum that ranges from simple fever to shock and death. A systematic classification of these clinical signs been has proposed to allow assessment of severity of illness and comparison of patients receiving therapy.[35] *The systemic inflammatory response syndrome* (SIRS) is defined by disordered temperature regulation, tachycardia, hyperventilation, and/or changes in white blood cell count or differential. *Sepsis* describes the SIRS when there is clear evidence of infection. *Severe sepsis* reflects the signs of systemic inflammation and infection with organ system dysfunction or hypotension responsive to therapy. *Septic shock* is defined as sepsis with hypotension refractory to volume therapy and evidence of end-organ dysfunction. The SIRS may be complicated by the development of *multiple organ dysfunction syndrome (MODS)*, defined as altered organ dysfunction in an acutely ill patient that requires intervention to maintain homeostasis. These definitions may appear artificial, but they allow comparison of patients with different primary disease states complicated by systemic inflammation.

Comparisons among large numbers of patients further are facilitated by the use of physiologic scoring systems, which allow grouping according to severity of illness. The Acute Physiology and Chronic Health Evaluation (APACHE) and Simplified Acute Physiology Score (SAPS) are two examples of such systems.[36,37] These systems are not examined in detail, but the standardization of severity of illness is critical in the assessment of efficacy of therapy in the SIRS.

PATHOPHYSIOLOGY OF SYSTEMIC INFLAMMATION

The interactions between microbes and host cells can induce many changes in the host defense network. These responses may be caused by products released by the microbe (exotoxins) or by structural components within the microbe released during cell destruction. Toxic shock syndrome toxin-1 (TSST-1) and *Pseudomonas* toxin A are examples of exotoxins.[38] The cell wall lipopolysaccharides (LPS) of gram-negative organisms are referred to as endotoxins.[38] Gram-negative infections are common among causes of SIRS and have been studied extensively in animals and humans.[1] This paradigm will be utilized to examine mechanisms of systemic inflammation.

ENDOTOXIN

Gram-negative endotoxins are structures composed of a variety of sugars attached to a lipid A moeity.[39,40] The saccharide component of the molecule varies widely across species, but the lipid A component appears to be preserved.[41,42] Endotoxin has been demonstrated in the serum of patients with sepsis.[43,44] The degree of endotoxemia may correlate with survival.[45] Infusions of endotoxin in animals and humans duplicate many of the phenomena seen in sepsis and septic shock. In humans, infusion of LPS causes a flu-like illness characterized by headache, myalgias, and fever. Hypotension associated with systemic vasodilation also is noted.[46] In animal models, infusion of antibodies against LPS protects against the adverse effects of infusion of bacteria.[47]

Endotoxin is bound by a soluble lipopolysaccharide binding protein (LBP). Binding of LPS to LBP enhances macrophage response to LPS.[48] This complex then binds to monocytes at the CD14 receptor and initiates the cytokine inflammatory process.[49] Endotoxin also causes the release of platelet-activating factor (PAF).[50,51] In some animal models the release of PAF occurs prior to the release of TNF.[52] Endotoxin administration provokes the synthesis and release of IL-1 and IL-8 by monocyte-macrophages.[53]

PLATELET-ACTIVATING FACTOR

Increased PAF activity has been reported in patients with sepsis.[54] Infusion of PAF in some animal species (pigs in particular) causes many of the changes seen in septic shock, with a mortality approaching 50 percent.[55] Doses of PAF required to cause shock were substantially less than doses of endotoxin required to achieve the same effect.[56] Hypotension induced by PAF infusion is blocked by the administration of NG-nitro-L-arginine, an inhibitor of nitric oxide synthetase.[57] Antagonists of PAF have been demonstrated to protect against the development of disseminated intravascular coagulation in rats treated with endotoxin.[58] Platelet-activating factor also contributes to the cytokine cascade by stimulating production of IL-1 and IL-2.[59] Agents that block PAF activity have had variable activity on release of TNF during endotoxin infusion (55, 57).

TUMOR NECROSIS FACTOR

Increases in TNF concentrations have been documented in patients with gram-negative septic shock,[60] though variability is reported. Infusion of TNF in animals also causes systemic changes that mimic those of septic shock or LPS infusion, including death.[61] Increases in TNF concentration precede the adverse hemodynamic and systemic manifestations of endotoxemia. Treatment with antibodies directed against TNF allows survival to animals given lethal doses of LPS or bacteria.[62,63] Tumor necrosis factor is released by macrophages in response to other infectious stimuli including TSST-1 and fungal organisms.[64,65] Unlike LPS, TSST-1 requires the presence of T lymphocytes to induce expression of TNF.[65]

Release of TNF from monocytes has several effects on the inflammatory process and end organs. In a mouse model of endotoxemia, these effects appear to be mediated in large part by interaction with one (TNF R-1) of two distinct membrane-associated receptors (TNF R-1 and TNF R-2).[66] TNF stimulates the release of other cytokines. Following LPS administration there is an increase in circulating IL-1 concentrations, followed by an increase in concentrations of IL-6 and IL-8. These increases are attenuated by the administration of antibodies to TNF.[67] TNF also causes the release of GM-CSF.[68]

Tumor necrosis factor causes prostaglandin synthesis in the hypothalamus leading to hyperthermia.[69] Tumor necrosis factor induces production of nitric oxide synthetase in vascular smooth muscle, which causes increase in nitric oxide and resultant relaxation.[70] In isolated vessels, this smooth-muscle relaxation is not attenuated by vasoconstrictors or sympathetic stimulation.[71,72] Disordered production of ni-tric oxide may occur in the myocardium as well.[73] Administration of TNF also has effects (either direct or indirect) on the endothelium. Infusion of TNF increases pulmonary capillary permeability.[74] Tumor necrosis factor promotes the expression of tissue factor, a potent procoagulant, on endothelial cells.[75]

INTERLEUKIN-1

Concentrations of IL-1 have been reported to be increased in sepsis, though this finding, as with TNF, is not uniform.[45,76] The infusion of IL-1, like PAF and TNF, causes many of the changes associated with septic shock, including fever, hypotension, and changes in white blood cell counts.[77] Blockade of IL-1 by antibody or infusion of antagonist attenuates the effects of bacterial or LPS infusion.[78,79]

Interleukin 1 shares many effects with TNF. It causes the release of IL-6 and IL-8.[80,81] It causes increased vascular permeability.[82] It also causes increases in prostaglandins in the hypothalamus, causing fever.[69] One of the more important effects of IL-1 may be its amplification of the effects of TNF.[83] Low doses of TNFα, when given to rabbits alone, caused little change in the animals. When the same dose of TNFα was given in conjunction with IL-1 it caused extensive tissue damage.

OTHER CYTOKINES

Both IL-6 and IL-8 are increased in patients with sepsis.[84,85] They may be better predictors of outcome in sepsis than other cytokines, in that increases in each have been correlated with severity of illness.[85,86] However, unlike TNF or IL-1, infusions of IL-6 or IL-8 do not cause the hemodynamic changes typical of sepsis.[87,88] Even though they cannot be responsible for all the manifestations of sepsis, each of these cytokines has important effects in the inflammatory process. Interleukin-6 may have several roles in the inflammatory process. Infusion of endotoxin activates the coagulation cascade in chimpanzees. This process is attenuated by monoclonal antibodies directed against IL-6.[89] Activation of the clotting cascade may be mediated by IL-6 induced expression of tissue factor from endothelial cells.[90] Interleukin-6 also may modulate the inflammatory response by the synthesis of IL-1 receptor antagonist (IL-1ra) or release of soluable TNF receptors (TNF sRp55).[91] Interleukin-8 has important effects on the interaction between PMNs and the endothelium. Incubation of PMNs with IL-8 caused increased expression of the PMN adhesion-promoting receptor CD11/CD18.[92] Local administration of IL-8 in rabbits results in PMN accumulation and plasma leakage.[93] In baboons IL-8 administration results in margination of PMNs.[88]

ARACHIDONIC ACID METABOLITES

Metabolites of arachidonic acid (eicosonoids) are extensively reviewed in Chaps. 12 and 13. Products of both cyclooxygenase and lipoxygenase pathways have been reported to be increased in systemic inflammatory states. Thromboxane B_2 and 6-keto-prostaglandin $F_{1\alpha}$ are increased in patients with gram-negative sepsis.[94,95] Leukotrienes are increased in patients with the adult respiratory distress syndrome, a frequent complication of systemic inflammatory states.[96] Both thromboxanes and leukotrienes have been shown to increase vascular permeability.[97] Inhibitors of cyclooyenase attenuate the effects of endotoxin in animal models.[98]

THE INFLAMMATORY NETWORK

The preceding discussion represents an overview of the complex interactions of the components of the inflammatory response. The release of various cytokines and mediators has potent effects on "downstream" effectors, but also upregulates and downregulates "upstream" effectors. Indeed, the image of an inflammatory cascade probably is misleading, as it suggests unidirectional flow through the system. Several authors have likened the system to a network.[99,100] It also should be noted that cells involved in the inflammatory response may release mediators that act in predominantly autocrine and paracrine fashion, achieving important effects without detectable circulating levels. It is, as noted, the effects of the primary insult and the sum of these complex local and distant interactions that determine the clinical manifestations of SIRS.

CLINICAL MANIFESTATIONS OF SYSTEMIC INFLAMMMATION

Disordered thermal regulation is a hallmark of the SIRS. Fever, the most common manifestation, results from the effects of TNF and IL-1 on prostaglandin synthesis in the hypothalamus.[69] Hyperventilation may be a secondary effect of temperature on the hypothalamus or carotid body.[101] Alternatively, a mechanism similar to the effect of cytokines on hypothalamic temperature regulation might result in a direct stimulatory effect of cytokines on the hypothalamus or medullary respiratory center.[102] Changes in white blood cell count reflect the effects of PAF, IL-8, and GM-CSF on peripheral neutrophils. The hypotension that frequently complicates sepsis results from several effects. Primary among these are profound vasodilation (both venous and arterial), intravascular volume depletion, and cardiac dysfunction. Vasodilation probably is caused by mediators such as leukotrienes and nitric oxide. The latter may occur in vascular smooth muscle as the result of upregulation of both constitutive and inducible nitric oxide synthetase by PAF, TNF and IL-1.[103] Peripheral venodilation results in pooling of blood in capacitance beds, with a consequent decrease in the mean systemic pressure.[104] This decrease in venous pressure is compounded further by volume reduction caused by the fluid leak that results from the effect of eicosonoids and PMNs on capillaries.[97] Volume infusion increases mean systemic pressure and unmasks arteriolar vasodilatation. This arteriolar vasodilatation is manifest as the high cardiac output hypotension typical of septic shock.[105] Hypotension is responsible for half of the deaths associated with SIRS.[106,107]

Despite the profound vasodilatation and increased cardiac output associated with sepsis, there is often myocardial dysfunction.[108] Ejection fraction of both ventricles usually is depressed and associated with biventricular dilation (increased end-diastolic volume, EDV). Development and early reversal of this acute dilated cardiomyopathy are positive prognostic markers in canine and human septic shock.[107–110] There are several potential etiologies of this myocardial depression including myocardial hyporesponsiveness to catecholamines[111] and a circulating myocardial depressant factor.[112] The impaired myocardial function may be reproduced by the infusion of endotoxin or TNFα. Recently myocardial NO synthesis has been suggested as an etiology for impaired myocardial performance.[113–115] Coronary hypoperfusion does not appear to be a significant factor.[116,117]

Endothelial injury and organ dysfunction also are expected complications of activation of the cytokine network. Activation of the clotting cascade by IL-6 or PAF-induced expression of tissue factor may precipitate microthrombus formation and disseminated intravascular coagulation (DIC). Similarly PMN sequestration may cause local microvascular injury. Leukocyte-induced injury may result in complement activation and further inflammation. Microcirculatory manifestations of sepsis are more difficult to quantify, but regional vasoconstriction is known to occur in septic shock, masked clinically by overall decreased SVR. Early effects of sepsis in various animals include pulmonary arterial vasoconstriction, impaired mesenteric arterial relaxation[118,119] with reduced intestinal capillary density,[120] and hepatic vein sphincter constriction (another cause of splanchnic blood pooling in septic canines).[39] Diminished endothelium-dependent relaxation is found in ex vivo animal models of sepsis.[121–123]

This impaired vascular function may affect oxygen utilization during sepsis. Oxygen consumption is increased in sepsis, but tissue oxygen extraction defects have been found in whole-body and regional[124] animal models of sepsis. Proposed causes of this oxygen extraction defect include a direct cellular (e.g., mitochondrial) effect and mismatch of tissue blood supply and demand caused by microvascular (endothelial and vascular smooth muscle) dysfunction and thrombosis.[125] Studies have not confirmed the existence of an oxygen extraction defect in septic humans, despite contrary clinical evidence (elevated mixed venous oxygen saturation and narrow arteriovenous oxygen content difference during lactic acidemia).[126,127] In fact, there is an alternative (nonischemic) explanation for sepsis-associated lactic acidemia,[128,129] and experimental data refute the presence of tissue hypoxia in this population.[130–132]

Whatever the mechanism, the clinical ramifications of this ongoing endothelial injury include pulmonary capillary leak with resultant ARDS, renal failure, hepatic failure and DIC. It is this spectrum of complications of systemic complications that constitutes the multiple organ dysfunction syndrome.

Multiple organ dysfunction syndrome (MODS) is defined by evidence of dysfunction in three or more organ systems. It is responsible for death in close to 50 percent of those patients who die of sepsis.[133] When present for a period of >72 h following admission to an intensive care unit, MODS is associated with a very poor prognosis.[134]

Therapy of Sepsis

PRIMARY THERAPY

The therapy of systemic inflammation, in particular that of sepsis and septic shock, may be viewed as primary and supportive. Primary therapy is directed at removing the inflammatory stimulus. In sepsis, this requires a thorough search for the source of infection and the application of appropriate antibiotics. The use of appropriate antibiotics has been shown to have a significant impact on mortality in sepsis.[45] Recognition of conditions that are refractory to antimicrobial therapy such as abscess and noninfectious causes of SIRS such as pancreatitis and salicylate intoxication[135] are also critically important.

SUPPORTIVE THERAPY

MONITORING AND THERAPEUTIC GOALS
Patients manifesting features diagnostic of sepsis syndrome require careful monitoring and an aggressive diagnostic and therapeutic approach. Admission to an intensive care unit permits vigilant monitoring and manipulation of hemodynamic parameters and end-organ functions. If refractory hypotension and/or end-organ dysfunction develop, a rapidly escalating course of therapy is required to avoid death from cardiovascular collapse and/or subsequent multiple systems organ failure. Hemodynamic therapeutic endpoints in septic shock are difficult to firmly define. Simple goals are an adequate mean arterial blood pressure (MAP) (usually >70 mmHg) and oxygen delivery that allows reversal of clinically detectable end-organ dysfunction (confusion, oliguria) or clear-cut tissue hypoperfusion (peripheral capillary refill, decrease mixed venous oxygen concentration (Mv_{O_2}), large arteriovenous difference in oxygen content $D(A-V)_{O_2}$). Difficulties in further assessment of adequacy of tissue perfusion have led to the practice of attempting to augment oxygen delivery until resolution of lactic acidemia. This presumes that this reflects tissue anaerobic metabolism, which may not always be the case (see above). More recently, gastric mucosal pH has been used as a marker of tissue hypoxia.[136]

Further increase in oxygen delivery, once the above goals are achieved, is advocated by those who believe that septic patients manifest a tissue oxygen extraction defect of sufficient severity to develop pathologic supply dependence (PSD) of oxygen consumption ($\dot{V}_{O_2}$) on oxygen delivery (Q_{O_2}). This phenomenon has been demonstrated convincingly in septic laboratory animals.[124] Human studies in sepsis and ARDS have not found pathological supply dependence of O_2 when methodological flaws have been eliminated.[126,127,137,138] Studies demonstrating improved outcomes with deliberate supranormal oxygen delivery in high-risk surgical patients[139] and other critically ill patients[140] have been criticized for randomization deficiencies[139] or analytical deficiencies.[140] Other positive outcomes with this approach may be explained on the basis of selective improvements in splanchnic perfusion,[141,142] particularly in view of the negative,[143] and even harmful,[144] outcomes of other studies. It should be noted that maximizing oxygen delivery does have potential harmful sequelae, including exacerbation of ARDS (fluid loading increases lung water); catecholamine-induced arrhythmia, myocardial ischemia, and increased tissue oxygen consumption; and the uncertain effects of erythrocyte transfusion (see below). It therefore seems prudent at the present time to titrate hemodynamic management of septic shock to clinically definable parameters[127] of adequate tissue perfusion, rather than to attempt to correct a presumed occult tissue oxygen debt.[145]

FLUID THERAPY
For the reasons noted above, aggressive volume administration is the mainstay of septic shock resuscitation. Frequently many liters of fluid must be administered through multiple large-bore intravenous accesses to achieve timely and adequate resuscitation. Progressive diffuse capillary leak necessitates continued large fluid requirements even after stabilization. Complications of fluid resuscitation include precipitation or aggravation of acute hypoxemic respiratory failure (particularly when pulmonary capillary leak is prominent), peripheral edema formation (which may impair wound healing), and gut mucosal edema. Aggressive volume resuscitation should therefore be titrated to appropriate endpoints.

FLUID CHOICE
Considerable controversy exists regarding the choice of resuscitation fluid-crystalloid (isotonic saline or Ringer's lactate solution; hypertonic saline is also sometimes used) versus colloid [albumin, dextrans, hyoxyethyl starch (Hetastarch)] in septic patients and others. Initial resuscitation with colloid is achieved more rapidly, requires less total volume (1 to 2 L colloid versus 4 to 8 L crystalloid), and better preserves plasma colloid osmotic pressure, with variable effects on pulmonary or peripheral edemagenesis.[146,147] Despite these apparent advantages, however, studies in septic shock[148] and other populations with diffuse capillary leak[149] have not documented improved outcome with respect to morbidity (including pulmonary edemagenesis) or mortality with colloid resuscitation. Cost, anaphylactic reactions, and infection risk argue against routine use of particular colloids. Crystalloid resuscitation is adequate in many cases.

BLOOD
The optimal target hematocrit in septic patients is another controversial issue. Unlike hypovolemic-hemorrhagic shock,[150] improved oxygen-carrying capacity at "normal" hematocrits may not translate into improved tissue oxygen delivery in septic patients,[151] possibly because of the rheologic effects altered erythrocyte deformability and microvas-

cular dysregulation and thrombosis-stasis in sepsis.[151,152] The risk of transfusion-borne infection is another concern. Indications to transfuse for correction of inadequate oxygen delivery must be evaluated on a case-by-case basis at this point.

INOTROPIC AGENTS

Inotropic agents and vasopressors frequently are necessary to maintain adequate blood pressure despite massive fluid resuscitation.

DOPAMINE

Dopamine (DA) is administered widely at low "renal" doses in patients with shock and oliguria, particularly when azotemia develops. DA at doses of 0.5 to 2.0 μg/kg/min increases renal blood flow (RBF) and mesenteric BFR, along with a lesser increase in glomerular filtration rate (GFR) and increased UOP, which results in large part from antagonism of tubular sodium reabsorption. These effects are less well documented in septic patients; two recent studies found no increase in GFR,[153,154] or gastric pH (an index of splanchnic perfusion) at approximately 3 μg/kg/min in this population, despite increased UOP. Data suggesting that α-adrenergic effects (splanchnic vasoconstriction) may develop in some individuals at doses as low as 5.0 μg/kg/min also cause concern.[155] No study has demonstrated improved outcomes (renal function, mortality) in septic patients treated with DA, although low-dose (0 to 2 μg/kg/min) therapy seems unlikely to have harmful effects. DA at >2 to 4 μg/kg/min has positive inotropic (β-adrenergic) effects, superior to NE in this regard in recent dog[156] and human[157] studies. In addition, DA at 2 to 6 μg/kg/min has a venoconstrictor effect. During septic shock resuscitation, vigorous fluid administration initially may be accompanied by temporizing use of the venoconstrictor, inotropic, and vasopressor effects of DA. Following successful fluid resuscitation, DA should be tapered (if possible) to at most 2 μg/kg/min.

DOBUTAMINE

Dobutamine (DB) is an effective inotropic agent in septic shock. Even in those without marked left ventricle (LV) dysfunction, DB allows maintenance of adequate cardiac output-oxygen delivery at lower levels of left ventricular end-diastolic pressure and volume (LVEDP and LVEDV) than dopamine.[158,159] This is crucial in those patients who develop ARDS and are therefore prone to exacerbation of pulmonary edema at "normal" LV-filling pressures-volumes. Some also utilize DB to maximize oxygen delivery in this setting.[160] Increased mesenteric blood flow may be another salutary (β_2-adrenergic) effect of DB. Unlike DA, DB has no direct renal vasodilator or renal tubular effect. (See Chap. 23). Complications from DB therapy in septic shock include arrhythmogenesis, intolerance of peripheral vasodilator (β_2-adrenergic) effect with aggravation of hypotension, and potential provocation of LV diastolic dysfunction when LVEDV is inadequate. Regardless of the indication for its use, invasive hemodynamic monitoring is recommended to guide DB use in this setting.

DOPEXAMINE

Dopexamine (DX) is not currently in widespread use in the United States, but offers renal and mesenteric vasodilator effects and a positive inotropic effect, without the potential for α-adrenergic receptor stimulation and vasoconstriction. Interesting clinical data suggest a protective effect in high-risk surgical patients,[141] possibly through selective splanchnic vasodilation.[160]

VASOPRESSOR AGENTS

Vasopressor agents may be necessary to support blood pressure when profound vasodilatation results in severe hypotension refractory to volume loading and inotropic agents.

NOREPINEPHRINE

In patients with hypotension refractory to fluid resuscitation and DA at 20 to 25 μg/kg/min, the more potent α-adrenergic effect of this compound (along with a myocardial β-adrenergic effect) has been repeatedly demonstrated to attain satisfactory MAP values,[161] although the adequacy of prior volume resuscitation in such studies is sometimes questionable.[162–164] This effect is mostly due to an increase in systemic vascular resistance, with little or no change in cardiac output.[156,157,165] This may be particularly important in patients with significant pulmonary hypertension, in whom right ventricular coronary perfusion is critically dependent on adequate systemic (and thus coronary) arterial pressure; this effect may, however, be counterbalanced by increased (α-adrenergically stimulated) pulmonary vascular resistance and RV afterload with this agent.[165,166] Although renal function clearly benefits from adequate perfusion pressure (autoregulation of RBF and GFR dramatically decline at MAP <85 mmHg), in nonseptic animal studies,[167] norepinephrine (NE) also causes renal arterial vasoconstriction, which may be blunted by concomitant low-dose DA therapy.[168] Renal oxygen consumption is directly proportional to tubular reabsorptive work, decreasing with RBF and GFR, so relative renal hypoperfusion may be better tolerated than in other organs.[169] The balance of potential beneficial and harmful renal effects of NE therapy on renal function and viability in septic shock are not discernible based on available data.[170] There are inconclusive data regarding the effect of NE therapy on mesenteric perfusion adequacy in septic shock. Augmented tissue perfusion pressure may not achieve adequate mesenteric oxygen delivery because of vasoconstriction and potentially catecholamine-induced increased demand.[157,171,172] If hemodynamically tolerated, the addition of inotropes and mesenteric vasodilators (DB, DX) to adequate volume resuscitation seems the preferable approach to septic shock management.

PHENYLEPHRINE

This is a pure α-adrenergic agonist, so that it lacks the β-adrenergically mediated tachycardic and arrhythmogenic effects of NE. Phenylephrine (PE) has been used successfully to increase blood pressure (again, increasing SVR without inotropic effect), urine output, and oxygen delivery in patients with septic shock refractory to fluid and inotropic support.[173]

EPINEPHRINE

At low doses, this catecholamine has strong inotropic (β-adrenergic) and vasoconstrictor (α-adrenergic) effects at high doses. Epinephrine has been studied in the therapy of septic shock refractory to fluid loading[174] or fluids and DA.[166] Cardiac output increased in all studies, and SVR increased in some.[175] Despite improved oxygen delivery, there is evidence (increased lactate with increased lactate/pyruvate ratio) that epinephrine simultaneously induces or aggravates anaerobic metabolism in such patients.[176,177] Arrhythmia is less frequent than might be expected with epinephrine therapy in septic patients. Considering the available data, epinephrine is used as an agent of last resort in hemodynamic management of septic adults.

EXPERIMENTAL THERAPY

The therapy outlined above still results in a significant mortality in patients with severe sepsis and septic shock. Frustration with standard therapy along with a growing understanding of the roles of exogenous and endogenous inflammatory mediators in the SIRS has prompted extensive research in modulating the inflammatory response. Initial efforts utilized nonspecific immunosuppressive agents, but have progressed to include immunotherapy directed at bacterial products or the use of endogenous specific regulators of the inflammatory network. Substances that block secondary mediators or end-organ effects of the inflammation also are being examined. To date, this therapy has been exciting in the laboratory and disappointing in patient care, but as understanding of the complexity of the inflammatory response grows, it is hoped that these innovative therapies will be implemented better.

CORTICOSTEROIDS

Initial attempts to modulate the inflammatory network relied on nonspecific immunosuppression, in particular the use of corticosteroids. Rat models of bactermic shock demonstrated a protective effect of dexamethasone.[178] Some clinical studies suggested efficacy as well, but two large randomized clinical trials demonstrated no overall benefit to the administration of corticosteroids to patients with septic shock.[179,180]

ANTIBODIES AGAINST ENDOTOXIN

Recognition that LPS plays a major role in the pathogenesis of gram-negative sepsis leads to attempts to neutralize the substance by passive immunization. Initial efforts utilized antiserum against the J5 mutant of *Escherichia coli*, a mutant whose LPS consisted of lipid A and a short side chain. Animals immunized with the J5 antiserum were protected against typically lethal bacteremia.[181] A trial of the J5 human antiserum administered to humans with sepsis resulted in a significant reduction in mortality in patients with bacteremia.[182] However a subsequent study utilizing anti-*E. coli* J5 IgG demonstrated no benefit.[183]

Monoclonal antibodies to LPS were developed to provide a more specific therapy and reduce the risk of transmission of infection. Two monoclonal antibodies against the lipid A moiety of LPS have been tested extensively. Both HA-1A, a human IgM, and E5, a murine IgM, have been demonstrated to protect animals against bacteremia,[184,185] although efficacy in animals has been questioned.[186] Initial reports of use of HA-1A suggested improved survival in a subgroup of study patients with gram-negative bacteremia.[187] Subsequent review of the analysis of the data suggested that this conclusion was not supported.[186] A second, larger randomized trial examined the effect of HA-1A on patients with gram-negative septic shock.[188] There was no effect of the administration of HA-1A on mortality in patients with gram-negative bacteremia and shock. Therapy with E5 monoclonal antibodies also has had little clinical success. The initial clinical trial demonstrated no overall benefit in mortality, though a retrospective subgroup analysis suggested benefit in patients with gram-negative bacteremia without shock.[189] A second randomized trial has been presented in abstract form.[190] No overall survival benefit was demonstrated, though a subgroup analysis suggested improved survival in patients with organ failure without refractory shock. Thus, at the present time, the use of antibody therapy directed against endotoxin cannot be supported.

Other agents that neutralize LPS have been considered in the therapy of gram-negative sepsis. Bactericidal permeability-increasing protein is a neutrophilic granular protein which binds LPS with greater affinity than LBP.[191] Bactericidal permeability-increasing protein also has bactericidal properties, making it an attractive agent in the therapy of sepsis.[192] In a mouse model administration of BPI protected against *E. coli* sepsis.[193] Clinical trials utilizing BPI are in process. Other inhibitors of LPS include other naturally occurring LPS binding proteins and analogues of lipid A.[194]

ANTIBODIES AGAINST INFLAMMATORY MEDIATORS

The demonstration of increases in levels of endogenous anti-inflammatory mediators has prompted the attempts to inhibit them with passive immunization. Inhibition of endogenous inflammatory mediators is appealing, because it could allow attenuation of the inflammatory response to other pathogens such as gram-positive bacteria or fungi. Monoclonal antibodies against TNF and IL-1 have been developed and tested in animal models, and antibodies against TNF have undergone clinical testing.

Primate models of bacteremic septic shock have suggested anti-TNF antibodies were protective. When administered prior to or soon after exposure to *E. coli* or *S. aureus*, anti-TNF antibodies improved survival.[67,195] When administered later, the effect was lost.[67] It should also be noted that some animal models suggest that anti-TNF antibodies are detrimental in some intracellular infections such as *Listeria monocytogenes*.[196] Clinical studies of anti-TNF antibodies have to date been disappointing. A large randomized study of monoclonal antibodies to TNF α in patients with sepsis syndrome found a reduction in mortality at 3 days following therapy in both low- and high-dose treatment groups, but these differences were no longer significant at 28 days.[197] At the present time, therapy with monoclonal antibodies to TNF is not supported.

Monoclonal antibodies directed against IL-1 also have been developed. In mouse models, these antibodies appear to protect against endotoxemia.[198] However, because of the availability of naturally occurring immodulators against IL-1, these monoclonal antibodies have not been developed extensively.

NATURAL IMMUNOMODULATORS

Several substances have been isolated from animals and humans that appear to limit the effect of mediators of the inflammatory network. Two of these substances have been studied extensively—soluble TNF receptors and IL-1 receptor antagonists.

Soluble receptors to TNF (sTNFR) have been identified in humans given endotoxin and patients with sepsis syndrome.[199,200] In primate models, administration of sTNFR attenuates the hemodynamic response to bacteremia.[199] Unfortunately, preliminary data from clinical trials with sTNFR, in particular the 75-kDa form of the receptor attached to the Fc fragment of human IgG, have been reported to suggest higher mortality among treated patients.[194] Further studies with the 55-kDa form of sTNFR are expected.

Antagonists to the IL-1 receptor (IL-1ra) have been identified in humans.[32] Administration of IL-1ra to animals reduced mortality following lethal endotoxin dosage.[201] Protection against hypotension was also afforded rabbits given *S. epidermidis*.[202] Initial clinical trials with IL-1ra also were promising.[203] However, a larger clinical study demonstrated no difference in survival time between placebo and higher dose IL-1ra.[204] A retrospective analysis of the study suggested improved survival time in patients with a predicted mortality of ≥24 percent. Prospective studies will be needed to better test the use of IL-1ra in this high-risk population. To date neither sTNFR nor IL-1ra can be recommended for therapy of SIRS.

PLATELET-ACTIVATING-FACTOR ANTAGONISTS

The prominent role PAF plays in animal models of sepsis has led to trials of antagonists of PAF in sepsis and septic shock. In a mouse model of endotoxemia, the PAF antagonist CL 184,005 normalized blood pressure when administered to hypotensive animals following endotoxin challenge.[205] In a canine model, the PAF antagonist TCV-309 attenuated hypotension and increased effective vascular compliance and cardiac output.[100] A clinical trial of the PAF antagonist PN 52021 did not demonstrate a survival benefit in patients with sepsis syndrome.[206] Further analysis of the study demonstrated improved survival in patients with sepsis syndrome caused by gram-negative organisms and patients with septic shock from gram-negative organisms. Additional studies will be necessary to confirm this finding in a prospective fashion.

EICOSONOID MODULATORS

Because of the adverse effects associated with thromboxane and leukotrienes in inflammatory states, modulators of arachidonic acid metabolism have been utilized in animal models of sepsis. Administration of ibuprofen, a cyclooxygenase inhibitor attenuated the hypotension associated with endotoxin in dogs.[104] This effect occurred despite an increase in concentration of cytokines.[207] In humans given endotoxin, ibuprofen prevented fever but did not alter production of TNFα.[208] In one small clinical trial administration of ibuprofen to patients with the sepsis syndrome resulted in a reduction of urinary metabolites of thromboxane and 6-keto-prostaglandin $F_{1\alpha}$ and a trend toward reversal of shock that did not reach statistical significance.[209]

The inhibitor of thromboxane synthetase ketoconazole has been tested in patients with the sepsis syndrome.[210] Treatment with 400 mg of ketoconazole within 24 h of admission with sepsis resulted in a significant reduction in the incidence of ARDS. Mortality also was reduced. Animal evidence argues that this effect may be independent of thromboxane synthetase inhibition.[211]

END ORGAN INTERVENTIONS

In addition to efforts to alter the inflammatory network, there has been increasing focus on blunting the end-organ effects of the SIRS. Two important areas of experimental therapy include inhibitors of nitric oxide synthetase and antioxidant therapy.

INHIBITION OF NITRIC OXIDE

The well documented effects of unregulated nitric oxide (NO) production by inducible NO synthase (iNOS) in septic shock[212,213] and cytokine-induced hypotension[214] include vasopressor-refractory relaxation of vascular smooth muscle and probably myocardial depression (see above). Experimental data demonstrate reversal of septic hypotension[213] and restoration of vasopressor-responsiveness[215] by inhibition of NO synthesis. Myocardial depression is reversed only partially by NOS inhibition[216] without evidence for the potential confounding effect of coronary vasoconstriction.[217] Recent data suggest a synergistic effect of NOS inhibition and dobutamine in reversing canine septic shock.[218] Although universally increasing blood pressure in animals with septic shock, outcomes with respect to organ function and mortality frequently have been negative. NOS inhibition in this setting has been associated with increased renal vascular resistance, decreased renal blood flow,[219,220] intestinal ischemia and increased capillary leak,[221] worsening myocardial function[222] and oxygen delivery,[223,224] hepatic dysfunction,[224] and increased mortality.[224,225] One of these studies found that *partial* NOS inhibition improved survival in septic rats.[225] Whether improved vasopressor responsiveness translates into decreased morbidity and mortality in human septic shock is unproven. Inhibition of NOS in small numbers of humans with septic shock[226–228] and a similar syndrome induced by IL-2 therapy[229] had peripheral vascular and myocardial effects similar to those seen in animals, without detectable effects on end-organ function and mortality.

One explanation for the mixed results of NOS inhibition in septic shock concerns the physiologic role of NO (produced constitutively by eNOS) in the regulation of organ and tissue perfusion. For example, NOS inhibition decreases renal medullary blood flow and oxygenation[230] and increases systemic blood pressure. Downregulation of eNOS production[231] may explain the endothelium-dependent vasodilator hyporesponsiveness (see above) and examples of focal vasoconstriction (see above) in septic shock. Inhibition of NOS appears to reduce splanchnic perfusion[232] and does not improve impaired intestinal or systemic oxygen extraction despite increasing blood pressure in animals with septic shock.[233] Indeed, administration of a nitric oxide donor increased splanchnic blood flow in endotoxemic dogs.[234]

The potential utility of selective iNOS inhibition with preserved eNOS activity is obvious. Lower doses or particular forms of nitrogen-substituted L-arginine derivatives may achieve this goal in septic shock therapy. Other agents are more selective in inhibiting the iNOS isozyme. For example, L-canavanine (a selective iNOS inhibitor) augments contraction of aortas from endotoxemic rats ex vivo[235] and increases blood pressure in endotoxemic rats but not controls.[236] The therapeutic utility of any NOS inhibitor may also be confounded by beneficial effects of NO in sepsis. NO has antimicrobial-immunomodulating[224] and antithrombotic[237] effects and may have organ-specific protective effects in sepsis.[13]

Alternatively, manipulation of other signal transduction pathways, which seem to play a role in sepsis-induced vascular smooth-muscle hypocontractility, may confer a selectively beneficial vasopressor effect in septic shock. Inhibition of guanylyl cyclase is one potential option.[238,239] Reversal of blunted intracellular calcium mobilization is another.[240] The contribution of excessive NO production caused by NOS to sepsis-induced vascular dysfunction varies according to the caliber of vessel[113] and species[233] studied, so that other sepsis-induced vascular effects may have important therapeutic implications.

Thus, manipulation of the NOS system offers the possibility of important hemodynamic benefits in patients with septic shock, but with potential detriment to microcirculatory regulation and tissue perfusion. Currently, studied agents cannot be recommended until their impact on end-organ function is better delineated.

ANTIOXIDANT THERAPY

Because many pathways of inflammation end with activation of leukocytes and release of free radicals, it has been argued that antioxidant therapy would be useful in sepsis. Infusion of superoxide dismutase in mice protects against the effects of endotoxin.[241] Administration of N-acetylcysteine to dogs prior to a bolus of endotoxin resulted in a higher extraction ratio of oxygen consumption to oxygen delivery, lower levels of lactic acid, and lower levels of tumor necrosis factor.[242] There was no difference in hemodynamics. Another class of antioxidants, lazaroids, has been tested in a canine model of endotoxemia. Pretreatment with U-74389G reduced intrapulmonary shunt in dogs given endotoxin.[243] There was no difference in hemodynamics. Finally, administration of N-acetylcysteine to patients with septic shock resulted in increased oxygen consumption[244] in the treated group. A retrospective grouping of patients into those who "responded" to N-acetylcysteine found a higher survival in

that group. Further studies are clearly necessary to assess the efficacy of antioxidant therapy in the SIRS.

Prognosis

The prognosis in patients with ongoing systemic inflammation is obviously dependent on the extent of that inflammation and the extent of end-organ injury. A recent prospective evaluation of the SIRS confirmed that the extent of inflammation, as quantified by number of criteria met by which the syndrome is diagnosed, correlated well with mortality.[245] More than 3700 patients on general medicine wards or in critical care units were surveyed, and 68 percent met criteria for the SIRS. Patients who did not meet criteria for SIRS had a mortality of 3 percent. Those patients who met two criteria for SIRS had a mortality of 6 percent, those who met three criteria 9 percent, and those with four criteria 18 percent. Patients who had culture-positive sepsis had an overall mortality of 16 percent compared with 10 percent in those with sepsis but without positive cultures. Mortality was greater still in those with severe sepsis and worse in those with positive cultures (20 percent in the culture-positive severe sepsis group, 16 percent in the culture-negative severe sepsis group). Mortality in those who developed septic shock was 46 percent, and there was no difference between those with and those without positive cultures. These figures are supported in recent clinical trials in sepsis. The mortality for patients treated with placebo in the IL1-ra study noted above was 34 percent (80 percent of those patients were in shock upon presentation).[204] Similarly mortality for placebo-treated patients in the HA-1A trial cited above was 32 percent (septic shock was part of the entry criteria for the study).[188]

These mortality rates are in the lower range of rates previously reported for sepsis and septic shock.[109] It is likely that, while there have been no dramatic breakthroughs in the therapy of SIRS, familiarity with sepsis and its complications has refined supportive therapy. A similar phenomenon has been described in ARDS and was particularly pronounced in patients with ARDS-complicating sepsis.[246] It does not seem overly optimistic to hope that supportive care will continue to be refined and better understanding of the inflammatory network and its actions will allow judicious utilization of immunomodulatory and end-organ therapy to improve further prognosis in the SIRS and MODS.

References

1 Bone R: The pathogenesis of sepsis. *Ann Intern Med* 1991; 115:457.

2. Skerrett S: Host defenses against respiratory infection. *Med Clin North Am* 1994; 78:941.

3. Toews G: Pulmonary defense mechanisms. *Sem Resp Inf* 1993; 8:160.

4. Rose R: The host defense network of the lungs: An overview, Niederman M, Sarosi G, Glassroth J (eds): in *Respiratory Infections. A Scientific Basis for Management*. Philadelphia, WB Saunders, 1994.

5. Danielle R: Immunoglobulin secretion in the airways. *Ann Rev Physiol* 1990; 52:177.

6. Konstan M, Chen P, Sherman J, et al.: Human lung lysozyme: Sources and properties. *Am Rev Resp Dis* 1981; 131:120.

7. Halliwell B, Gutteridge J: Oxygen free radicals and iron in relation to biology and medicine: Some problems and concepts. *Arch Biochem Biophys* 1986; 246:501.

8. Sibille Y, Reynolds H: Macrophages and polymorphonuclear neutrophils in lung defense and injury. *Am Rev Respir Dis* 1990; 141:471.

9. Wright S, Detmers P: Receptor mediated phagocytosis, Crystal R, West J (eds): in *The Lung: Scientific Foundations*. New York, Raven, 1991.

10. Stahl P: The macrophage mannose receptor: Current status. *Am Rev Respir Cell Mol Biol* 1990; 2:317.

11. Kaltreider H: Macrophages, lymphocytes and anti-body and cell-mediated immunity, Murray J, Nadel J (eds): in *Textbook of Respiratory Medicine*. Philadelphia, WB Saunders, 1994.

12. Murray H: Interferon gamma, the activated macrophage, and host defense against microbial challenge. *Ann Intern Med* 1988; 108:595.

13. Harbrecht BG, Billiar TR, Stadler J, et al.: Nitric oxide synthesis serves to reduce hepatic damage during acute murine endotoxemia. *Crit Care Med* 1992; 20:1568.

14. Ganz T: Macrophage function. *New Horizons* 1993; 1:23.

15. Moore K, O'Garra A, Malefty W, et al.: Interleukin-10. *Ann Rev Immunol* 1993; 11:165.

16. Palladino M, Morris R, Starnes H, Levinson A: The transforming growth factor-betas. A new family of immunoregulatory molecules. *Ann New York Acad Sci* 1990; 593:181.

17. Rolfe M, Kunkel S, Standiford T, et al.: Pulmonary fibroblast expression of interleukin-8: A model for alveolar macrophage-derived cytokine networking. *Am J Respir Cell Molec Biol* 1991; 5:493.

18. Strieter R, Kunkel S, Showell H, et al.: Endothelial cell gene expression of a neutrophil chemotactic factor by TNF-alpha, LPS and IL-1 beta. *Science* 1989; 243:1467.

19. Ravetch J, Kinet J: Fc receptors. *Ann Rev Immunol* 1991; 9:457.

20. Wilson J, Andriopoulous N, Fearon D: CR1 and the cell membrane proteins that bind C3 and C4. A basic and clinical review. *Immunol Res* 19XX; 6:192.

21. Elsbach P, Weiss J: Bactericidal/permeability increasing protein and host defense against gram-negative bacteria and endotoxin. *Curr Opin Immunol* 1993; 5:103.

22. Ganz T, Selsted M, Lehrer R: Defensins. *Eur J Haematol* 1990; 44:1.

23. Goldstein I, Shak S: Host defenses in the lung: Neutrophils, complement and other humoral mediators, in Murray J, Nadel J (eds): *Textbook of Respiratory Medicine*. Philadelphia, WB Saunders, 1994.

24. Abbas A, Lichtman A, Pober J: Immunity to microbes, in Abbas A, Lichtman A, Pober J (eds): *Cellular and Molecular Immunology*. Philadelphia, WB Saunders, 1994.

25. Abbas A, Lichtman A, Pober J: Molecular basis of T cell antigen recognition and activation, in Abbas A, Lichtman A, Pober J (eds): *Cellular and Molecular Immunology*. Philadelphia, WB Saunders, 1994.

26. Abbas A, Lichtman A, Pober J: B cell activation and antibody production, in Abbas A, Lichtman A, Pober J (eds): *Cellular and Molecular Immunology*. Philadelphia, WB Saunders, 1994.

27. Mosmann T, Coffman R: Th1 and Th2 cells: Different patterns of lymphokine secretion lead to different functional properties. *Ann Rev Immunol* 1989; 7:145.

28. Romagnani S: Th1 and Th2 subsets: Doubt no more. *Immunol Today* 1991; 12:256.

29. Abbas A, Lichtman A, Pober J: The complement system, in Abbas A, Lichtman A, Pober J (eds): *Cellular and Molecular Immunology*. Philadelphia, WB Saunders, 1994.

30. Dinarello C: Interleukin-1 and interleukin-1 antagonism. *Blood* 1991; 77:1627.

31. Van Zee K, Kohno T, Fischer E, et al.: Tumor necrosis factor soluble receptor circulate during experimental and clinical inflammation and can protect against excessive tumor necrosis factor a in vitro and in vivo. *Proc Nat Acad Sci* 1992; 89:4845.

32. Arend W: Interleukin-1 receptor antagonist: A new member of the interleukin-1 family. *J Clin Invest* 1991; 88:1445.

33. Parker M, Ognibene F, Rogers P, et al.: Severe *Pneumocystis carinii* pneumonia produces a hyperdynamic profile similar to bacterial pneumonia with sepsis. *Crit Care Med* 1994; 22:50.

34. Fukushima R, Alexander J, Gianotti L, Ogle C: Isolated pulmonary infection acts as a source of systemic tumor necrosis factor. *Crit Care Med* 1994; 22:114.

35. Bone R, et al.: American College of Chest Physicians/Society of Critical Care Medicine Consensus Conference Committee: Definitions for sepsis and organ failure and guidelines for the use of innovative therapies in sepsis. *Crit Care Med* 1992; 20:864.

36. Knauss W, Draper E, Wagner D, et al.: APACHE II: A severity of disease classification system. *Crit Care Med* 1985; 13:818.

37. Le Gall J, Loirat P, Alperovitch A, et al.: A simplified acute physiology score for ICU patients. *Crit Care Med* 1984; 12:975.

38. Hewlett, E: Toxins and other virulence factors, in Mandel G, Bennett J, Dolin R (eds): *Principles and Practice of Infectious Diseases*. New York, Churchill-Livingstone, 1995.

39. Manthous C, Hall J, Samsel R: Endotoxin in human disease. Part 1: Biochemistry, assay and possible role in diverse disease states. *Chest* 1993; 104:1572.

40. Manthous CA, Hall JB, Samsel RW: Endotoxin in human disease (Part 2). *Chest* 1993; 104:1872.

41. Westphal O, Hann K, Himmelspach K: Chemistry and immunochemistry of bacterial lipopolysaccharide as cell wall antigens and endotoxins. *Prog Allergy* 33.

42. Brade H, Brade L, Schade U, et al.: Structure, endotoxicity, immunogenicity and antigenicity of bacterial lipopolysaccharides. *Prog Clin Biol Res* 1988; 272:17.

43. Danner R, Elin R, Hosseini J, et al.: Endotoxemia in human septic shock. *Chest* 1990; 99:169.

44. Behre G, Schedel I, Nentwig B, et al.: Endotoxin concentration in neutropenic patients with suspected Gram-negative sepsis: Correlation with clinical outcome and determination of antiendotoxin care antibodies during therapy with polyclonal immunoglobulin-M-enriched immunoglobulins. *Antimicrob Agents Chemother* 1992; 36:2139.

45. Barriere S, Lowry S: An overview of mortality risk prediction in sepsis. *Crit Care Med* 1995; 23:376.

46. Suffredini A, Fromm R, Parker M, et al.: The cardiovascular response of normal humans to administration of endotoxin. *N Eng J Med* 1989; 321:280.

47. Teng H, Kaplan H, Herbert J, et al.: Protection against gram-negative bacteremia and endotoxemia with monoclonal IgM antibody. *Proc Natl Acad Sci* 1985; 82:1790.

48. Schumann R, Leong S, Flaggs G, et al.: Structure and function of lipopolysaccharide binding protein. *Science* 249:1429.

49. Wright S, Ramos R, Tobias P, et al.: CD14, a receptor for complexes of lipopolysaccharide (LPS) and LPS binding protein. *Science* 1990; 249:1431.

50. Koltai M, Hosford D, Guinot P, et al.: Platelet-activating factor (PAF): A review of its effects, antagonists and possible future clinical applications. *Drugs* 1991; 42:9.

51. Koltai M, Hosford D, Guinot P, et al.: Platelet-activating factor (PAF): A review of its effects, antagonists and possible future clinical applications. *Drugs* 1991; 42:174.

52. Klosterhalfen B, Horstmann-Jungemann K, Vogel P, et al.: Time course of various inflammatory mediators during recurrent endotoxemia. *Biochem Pharmacol* 1992; 43:2103.

53. Ulich T, Watson L, Songmei Y, et al.: The intratracheal administration of endotoxin and cytokines: I. Characterization of LPS-induced IL-1 and TNF mRNA expression and LPS-, IL-1-, and TNF-induced inflammatory infiltrate. *Am J Pathol* 1991; 138:1485.

54. Heuer H, Darius H, Lohmann H, et al.: Platelet-activating factor type activity in plasma from patients with septicemia and other diseases. *Lipids* 1991; 26:1381.

55. Mozes T, Zijlstra F, Heiligers J: Sequential release of tumour necrosis factor, platelet-activating factor and eicosonoids during endotoxic shock in anesthetized pigs: Protective effects of indomethacin. *Br J Pharmacol* 1991; 104:691.

56. Koltai M, Hosford D, Braquet P: Platelet-activating factor in septic shock. *New Horizons* 1993; 1:87.

57. Szabo C, Wu C, Mitchell J, et al.: Platelet-activating factor contributes to the induction of nitric oxide synthase by bacterial lipopolysaccharide. *Circ Res* 1993; 73:991.

58. Yokota Y, Inamura N, Asano M, et al.: Effect of FR128998, a novel PAF antagonist, on endotoxin-induced disseminated intravascular coagulation. *Eur J Pharmacol* 1994; 258:239.

59. Pignol B, Henane S, Sorlin B, et al.: Effect of long-term treatment of platelet-activating factor on IL-1 and IL-2 production by rat spleen cells. *J Immunol* 1990; 145:980.

60. Groote M, Martin M, Densen P, et al.: Plasma tumor necrosis factor levels in patients with presumed sepsis: Results in those treated with antilipid A antibody vs placebo. *J Am Med Assoc* 1989; 262:249.

61. Tracey K, Beutler B, Lowry S, et al.: Shock and tissue injury induced by recombinant human cachectin. *Science* 1986; 234:470.

62. Beutler BM, Cerami A: Passive immunization against cachectin/tumor necrosis factor protects mice from lethal effect of endotoxin. *Science* 1995; 229:869.

63. Tracey K, Fong J, Hesse D, et al.: Anti-TNF a monoclonal antibodies prevent septic shock during lethal bacteremia. *Nature* 1987; 330:662.

64. Dooley D, Cox R, Hestilow K, et al.: Cytokine induction in human coccidioidomycosis. *Infection Immun* 1994; 62:3980.

65. Kum W, Laupland K, See R, Chow A: Improved purification and biologic activities of staphylococcal toxic shock syndrome toxin 1. *J Clin Micro* 1993; 31:2654.

66. Pfeffer K, Matsuyama T, Kundig T, et al.: Mice deficient for the 55 kd tumor necrosis factor receptor are resistant to endotoxic shock, yet succumb to L. monocytogenes infection. *Cell* 1993; 73:457.

67. Fong Y, Tracey K, Moldawer L, et al.: Antibodies to cachectin/TNF reduce interleukin-1-β and interleukin-6 appearance during lethal bacteremia. *J Exp Med* 1989; 170:1627.

68. Koeffler H, Gasson J, Ranyard J: Recombinant human TNF α stimulates production of G-CSF. *Blood* 1987; 70:55.

69. Saper C, Breder C: The neurologic basis of fever. *N Eng J Med* 1994; 330:1880.

70. Moncada S, Palmer R, Higgs E: Nitric oxide: Physiology, pathophysiology and pharmacology. *Pharmacol Rev* 1991; 43:109.

71. Julou-Schaeffer F, Gray G, Fleming I, et al.: Loss of vascular responsiveness induced by endotoxin involves the L-arginine pathway. *Am J Physiol* 1990; 259:H1038.

72. Gonzalez C, Fernandez A, Martin C, et al.: Nitric oxide from endothelium and smooth muscle modulates responses to sympathetic nerve stimulation: Implications for endotoxin shock. *Biochem Biophys Res Commun* 1992; 186:150.

73. Schulz R, Nava E, Moncada S: Induction and potential biological relevance of a Ca^{2+}-independent nitric oxide synthase in the myocardium. *Br J Pharmacol* 1992; 105:575.

74. Stephens K, Ishizaka A, Larrick J, Raffin T: Tumor necrosis factor causes increased pulmonary capillary permeability and edema: Comparison to septic acute lung injury. *Am Rev Resp Dis* 1988; 137:1364.

75. Taylor F, Chang A, Morrissey L, et al.: Lethal *E. coli* sepsis is prevented by blocking tissue factor with monoclonal antibody. *Circ Shock* 1991; 33:127.

76. Girardin E, Grau G, Dayer J: Tumor necrosis factor and interleukin-1 in the serum of children with severe infectious purpura. *N Eng J Med* 1988; 319:397.

77. Smith J, Urba W, Curtis B, et al.: The toxic and hematologic effects of interleukin-1 alpha administered in a phase I trial to patients with advanced malignancies. *J Clin Oncol* 1992; 10:1141.

78. Lemay L, Otterness I, Vander M, Kluger M: In vivo evidence that the rise in plasma IL-6 following injection of a fever-inducing dose of LPS is mediated by IL-1β. *Cytokine* 1990; 2:199.

79. Wakabayashi G, Gelfand J, Burke J, et al.: A specific receptor antagonist for interleukin-1 prevents *Esherichia coli*-induced shock in rabbits. *FASEB J* 1991; 5:338.

80. Wong G, Clark S: Multiple actions of interleukin-6 within a cytokine network. *Immunol Today* 1988; 9:137.

81. Strieter M, Chensue S, Basha M, et al.: Human alveolar macrophage gene expression of interleukin-8 by tumor necrosis factor α, lipopolysaccharide, and interleukin 1β. *Am J Respir Cell Mol Biol* 1990; 2:321.

82. Royall J, Berkow R, Beckman J, et al.: Tumor necrosis factor and interleukin-1 increase vascular endothelial permeability. *Am J Physiol* 1989; 257:L399.

83. Okusawa S, Gelfand J, Ikejima T, et al.: Interleukin 1 induces a shock-like state in rabbits: Synergism with tumor necrosis factor and the effect of cyclooxygenase inhibition. *J Clin Invest* 81:1162.

84. Waage A, Brandtzaeg P, Halstensen A, et al.: The complex pattern of cytokines in serum from patients with meningococcal septic shock: Association between interleukin 6, interleukin 1, and fatal outcome. *J Exp Med* 1989; 169:333.

85. Hack C, Hart M, van Schijndel R, et al.: Interleukin-8 in sepsis: Relation to shock and inflammatory mediators. *Infect Immun* 1992; 60:2835.

86. Hack C, DeGroot E, Felt-bersma R, et al.: Increased plasma levels of interleukin-6 in sepsis. *Blood* 1989; 74:1704.

87. van Gameren M, Willemse P, Mulder N, et al.: Effects of recombinant human interleukin-6 in cancer patients: A phase I-II study. *Blood* 1994; 84:1434.

88. Van Zee K, Fischer E, Hawes A, et al.: Effects of intravenous IL-8 administration in non-human primates. *J Immunol* 1992; 148:1746.

89. van der Poll T, Levi M, Hack C, et al.: Elimination of interleukin 6 attenuates coagulation activation in experimental endotoxemia in chimpanzees. *J Exp Med* 1994; 179:1253.

90. Nawroth P, Stern D: Modulation of endothelial cell hemostatic properties by tumor necrosis factor. *J Exp Med* 1986; 163:740.

91. Tilg H, Trehu E, Atkins M, et al.: Interleukin-6 (IL-6) as an anti-inflammatory cytokine: induction of circulating IL-1 receptor antagonist and soluble tumor necrosis factor receptor p55. *Blood* 1994; 83:113.

92. Detmars P, Powell D, Walz A, et al.: Differential effects of neutrophil-activating peptide 1/IL-8 and its homologues on leukocyte adhesion and phagocytosis. *J Immunol* 1991; 147:4211.

93. Colditz I: Effect of exogenous prostaglandin E2 and actinomycin D on plasma leakage induced by neutrophil-activating peptide-1/interleukin-8. *Immunol Cell Biol* 1990; 68:397.

94. Halushka P, Reines H, Barrow S, et al.: Elevated plasma 6-keto-prostaglandin $F_{1-\alpha}$ in patients with septic shock. *Crit Care Med* 1985; 13:451.

95. Reines H, Cook J, Halushka P: Plasma thromboxane concentrations are raised in patients dying with septic shock. *Lancet* 1982; 1:174.

96. Bernard G, Korley V, Chee P, et al.: Persistent generation of peptido leukotrienes in patients with the adult respiratory distress syndrome. *Am Rev Resp Dis* 1991; 144:263.

97. Bone R: Phospholipids and their inhibitors: A critical evaluation of their role in the treatment of sepsis. *Crit Care Med* 1992; 20:884.

98. Balk R, Jacobs R, Tryka A, et al.: Low dose ibuprofen reverses the hemodynamic alterations of canine endotoxin shock. *Crit Care Med* 1988; 16:1128.

99. Elias J, Freundlich B, Kern J, Rosenbloom J: Cytokine networks in the regulation of inflammation and fibrosis in the lung. *Chest* 1990; 97:1439.

100. Balkwill F, Burke F: The cytokine network. *Immunol Today* 1989; 10:299.

101. Slutsky A, Phillipson E: Hyperventilation syndromes, in Murray J, Nadel J (eds): *Textbook of Respiratory Medicine.* Philadelphia, WB Saunders, 1994.

102. Breder C, Tsujimoto M, Terano Y, et al.: Distribution and characterization of tumor necrosis factor-alpha-like immunoreactivity in the murine central nervous system. *J Comp Neurol* 1993; 337:543.

103. Szabo C: Alterations in nitric oxide production in various forms of circulatory shock. *New Horizons* 1995; 3:2.

104. Yamanaka S, Iwao H, Yukimura T, et al.: Effect of the platelet-activating factor antagonist, TCV-309, and the cyclo-oxygenase inhibitor, ibuprofen, on the haemodynamic changes in canine experimental endotoxic shock. *Br J Pharmacol* 1993; 110:1501.

105. Winslow E, Loeb H, Rahimtoola S, et al.: Hemodynamic studies and results of therapy in 50 patients with bacteremic shock. *Am J Med* 1973; 54:421.

106. Ruokenen E, Takala J, Kari A, Alhava E: Septic shock and multiple organ failure. *Crit Care Med* 1991; 19(9):1146.

107. Parrillo JE: Pathogenetic mechanisms of septic shock. *N Engl J Med* 1993; 328:1471.

108. Parker MM, Parillo JE: Myocardial function in septic shock. *J Crit Care* 1990; 5:47.

109. Parrillo JE (moderator): Septic shock in humans: Advances in the understanding of pathogenesis, cardiovascular dysfunction, and therapy. *Ann Intern Med* 1990; 113:227.

110. Parker MM, Shelhammer JH, Natanson C, et al.: Serial cardiovascular variables in survivors and nonsurvivors of human septic shock: Heart rate as an early predictor of prognosis. *Crit Care Med* 1987; 15:923.

111. Bersten AD, Sibbald WJ, Hersch M, et al.: Interaction of sepsis and sepsis plus sympathomimetics on myocardial oxygen availability. *Am J Physiol* 1992; 262(4 Pt 2):H1164.

112. Silverman HJ, Penaranda R, Orens B, Lee NH: Impaired beta-adrenergic receptor stimulation of cyclic adenosine monophosphate in human septic shock: Association with myocardial hyporesponsiveness to catecholamines. *Crit Care Med* 1993; 21(1):31.

113. Schulz R, Nava E, Moncada S: Induction and potential relevance of Ca^{2+} independent nitric oxide synthase in the myocardium. *Br J Pharmacol* 1992; 105:575.

114. Finkel MS, Oddis CV, Jacob TD, et al.: Negative inotropic effects of cytokines on the heart mediated by nitric oxide. *Science* 1992; 257:387.

115. Brady AJB, Poole-Wilson PA, Harding SE, et al.: Nitric oxide production within cardiac myocytes reduces their contractility in endotoxemia. *Am J Physiol* 1992; 263:H1963.

116. Parrillo JE, Burch C, Shelhammer JH, et al.: A circulating myocardial depressant substance in humans with septic shock. *J Clin Invest* 1985; 76:1539.

117. Solomon MA, Correa R, Alexander HR, et al.: Myocardial energy metabolism and morphology in a canine model of sepsis. *Am J Physiol* 1994; 266(2 Pt 2):H757.

118. Zweifach BW, Nagler AL, Thomas L: The role of epinephrine in the reactions produced by endotoxins of gram negative bacteria. *J Exp Med* 1956; 103:865.

119. Rubinstein I, Gao X-p: Regulation of arteriolar diameter in the peripheral microcirculation during acute exposure lipopolysaccharide. *Clin Res* 1994; 42(3):350A.

120. Drazenovic R, Samsel RW, Wylam ME, et al.: Regulation of perfused capillary density in canine intestinal mucosa during endotoxemia. *Am J Physiol* 1992; 72(1):259.

121. Altura BM, Gebrewold A, Burton RW: Failure of microscopic metarterioles to elicit vasodilator responses to acetylcholine, bradykinin, histamine, and substance P after ischemic shock, endotoxemia, and trauma. *Microcirc Endothel Lymphat* 1985; 2:121.

122. Umans JG, Wylam ME, Samsel RW, et al.: Effects of endotoxin in vivo on endothelial and smooth muscle function in rabbit and rat aorta. *Am Rev Respir Dis* 1993; 148:1638.

123. Wylam ME, Samsel RW, Umans JG, et al.: Endotoxin in vivo impairs endothelium-dependent relaxation of canine arteries in vitro. *Am Rev Respir Dis* 1990; 142:1263.

124. Nelson DP, Beyer C, Samsel RW, et al.: Pathological supply dependence of O_2 uptake during bacteremia in dogs. *Am J Physiol* 1987; 63(4):1487.

125. Schumacker PT, Samsel RW: Oxygen delivery and uptake by peripheral tissues: Physiology and pathophysiology. *Crit Care Clin* 1989; 5(2):255.

126. Manthous CA, Schumacker PT, Pohlman A, et al.: Absence of supply dependence of oxygen consumption in patients with septic shock. *J Crit Care* 1993; 8:1.

127. Russell JA, Phang TP: The oxygen delivery/consumption controversy. *Am J Respir Crit Care Med* 1994; 149:533.

128. Curtis SE, Cain SM: Regional and systemic oxygen delivery/uptake relations and lactate flux in hyperdynamic, endotoxin-treated dogs. *Am Rev Respir Dis* 1992; 145:348.

129. Siegel JH, Cerra FB, Coleman B, et al.: Physiological and metabolic correlations in human sepsis. *Surgery* 1979; 886:163.

130. Hotchkiss RS, Rust RS, Dence CS, et al.: Evaluation of the role of cellular hypoxia in sepsis by the hypoxic marker [^{18}F]fluoromisonidazole. *Am J Physiol* 1991; 261:R965.

131. Hotchkiss RS, Karl IE: Reevaluation of the role of cellular hypoxia and bioenergetic failure in sepsis. *J Am Med Assoc* 1992; 267:1503.

132. Solomon MA, Alexander HR, Balaban RS, et al.: Myocardial cytosolic phosphorylation potential in a canine sepsis model. *Clin Res* 1991; 39:164A.

133. Bone RC: Sepsis and its complications: The clinical problem. *Crit Care Med* 1994; 22:S8.

134. Knaus W, Wagner D: Multiple systems organ failure: Epidemiology and prognosis. *Crit Care Clin* 1989; 5:221.

135. Leatherman J, Schmitz P: Fever, hyperdynamic shock, and multiple-system organ failure. A pseudo-sepsis syndrome associated with chronic salicylate intoxication *Chest* 1991; 100:1391.

136. Gutierrez G, Palizas F, Doglio G, et al.: Gastric intramucosal pH as a therapeutic index of tissue oxygenation in critically ill patients. *Lancet* 1992; 339:195.

137. Ronco JJ, Fenwick JC, Tweeddale MG, et al.: Identification of the critical oxygen delivery for anaerobic metabolism in critically ill septic and nonseptic humans. *J Am Med Assoc* 1993; 270(14):1724.

138. Wysocki M, Besbes M, Roupie E, Brun-Buisson C: Modification of oxygen extraction ratio by change in oxygen transport in septic shock. *Chest* 1992; 102:221.

139. Shoemaker WC, Appel PL, Kram HB, et al.: Prospective trial of supranormal values of survivors as therapeutic goals in high-risk surgical patients. *Chest* 1988; 94:1176.

140. Tuchschmidt J, Fried J, Astiz M, Rackow E: Elevation of cardiac output and oxygen delivery improves outcome in septic shock. *Chest* 1992; 102:216.

141. Boyd O, Grounds RM, Bennett ED: A randomized clinical trial of the effect of deliberate perioperative increase of oxygen delivery on mortality in high-risk surgical patients. *J Am Med Assoc* 1993; 270:2699.

142. Smithies M, Yee TH, Jackson L, et al.: Protecting the gut and liver in the critically ill: Effects of dopexamine. *Crit Care Med* 1994; 22:789.

143. Yu M, Levy MM, Smith P, et al.: Effect of maximizing oxygen delivery on morbidity and mortality rates in critically ill patients: A prospective, randomized, controlled study. *Crit Care Med* 1993; 21:830.

144. Hayes MA, Timmins AC, Yau EHS, et al.: Elevation of systemic oxygen delivery in the treatment of critically ill patients. *N Engl J Med* 1994; 330:1717.

145. Shoemaker WC, Appel PL, Kram HB: Role of oxygen debt in the development of organ failure, sepsis, and death in high-risk surgical patients. *Chest* 1992; 102:208.

146. Astiz ME, Galera-Santiago A, Rackow EC: Intravascular volume and fluid therapy for severe sepsis. *New Horizons* 1993; 1:127.

147. Rackow EC, Falk JL, Fein A, et al.: Fluid resuscitation in circulatory shock: A comparison of the cardiorespiratory effects of albumin, hetastarch, and saline solutions in patients with hypovolemic and septic shock. *Crit Care Med* 1983; 11:839.

148. Rackow EC, Mecher C, Astiz ME, et al.: Effect of pentastarch and albumin infusion on cardiorespiratory function and coagulation in patients with severe sepsis and systemic hypoperfusion. *Crit Care Med* 1989; 17:394.

149. Pockaj BA, Yang JC, Lotze MT, et al.: A prospective randomized trial evaluating colloid versus crystalloid resuscitation in the treatment of the vascular leak syndrome associated with interleukin-2 therapy. *J Immunother* 1994; 15(1):22.

150. Fortune JB, Feustel PJ, Saifi J, et al.: Influence of hematocrit on cardiopulmonary function after acute hemorrhage. *J Trauma* 1987; 27:243.

151. Rogers F, Dunn R, Barrett T, et al.: Alteration of capillary flow during sepsis. *Circ Shock* 1985; 15:105.

152. Voerman H, Fonk T, Thijs L: Changes in hemorheology in patients with sepsis or septic shock. *Circ Shock* 1989; 29:219.

153. Duke GJ, Briedis JH, Weaver RA: Renal support in critically ill patients: Low-dose dopamine or low-dose dobutamine? *Crit Care Med* 1994; 22:1919.

154. Olson D, Pohlman A, Lavoie A, et al.: Effects of dopamine on regional blood flow in the sepsis syndrome. *Am J Respir Crit Care Med* 1995; 151(4):A446.

155. D'Orio V, El Allaf D, Juchmes J, Marcelle R: The use of low doses of dopamine in intensive care medicine. *Arch Int Physiol Biochem* 1984; 92:S11.

156. Karzai W, Reilly JM, Hoffman WD, et al.: Hemodynamic effects of dopamine, norepinephrine, and fluids in a dog model of sepsis. *Am J Physiol* 268:H692.

157. Marik PE, Mohedin M: The contrasting effects of dopamine and norepinephrine on systemic and splanchnic oxygen utilization during hyperdynamic sepsis. *J Am Med Assoc* 1994; 272(7):1354.

158. Vincent JL, Roman A, Kahn RJ: Dobutamine administration in

159. Vincent JL, Van Der Linden P, Domb M, et al.: Dopamine compared with dobutamine in experimental septic shock: Relevance to fluid administration. *Anesth Analg* 1987; 66:565.

160. Shoemaker WC, Appel PL, Kram HB: Hemodynamic and oxygen transport effects of dobutamine in critically ill general surgical patients. *Crit Care Med* 1986; 14:1032.

161. Martin C, Papazian L, Perrin G, et al.: Norepinephrine or dopamine for the treatment of hyperdynamic septic shock? *Chest* 1993; 103:1826.

162. Vincent JL, Preiser JC: Inotropic agents. *New Horizons* 1993; 1:137.

163. Desjars P, Pinaud M, Potel G, et al.: A reappraisal of norepinephrine therapy in human septic shock. *Crit Care Med* 1987; 15:134.

164. Desjars P, Pinaud M, Bugnon D, et al.: Norepinephrine therapy has no deleterious effects in human septic shock. *Crit Care Med* 1989; 17:426.

165. Schrueder WO, Schneider AJ, Groeneveld J, Thijs LG: Effect of dopamine vs norepinephrine on hemodynamics in septic shock. *Chest* 1989; 95:1282.

166. Martin C, Perrin G, Saux P, et al.: Effects of norepinephrine on right ventricular function in septic shock patients. *Intensive Care Med* 1994; 20(6):444.

167. Vander AJ: Renal blood flow and glomerular filtration, in Vander AJ (ed): *Renal Physiology*, 5th ed. New York, McGraw-Hill, 1995:24–50.

168. Schaer GL, Fink MP, Parrillo JE: Norepinephrine alone versus norepinephrine plus low-dose dopamine: Enhanced renal blood flow with combination pressor therapy. *Crit Care Med* 1985; 13:492.

169. Brezis M, Rosen S: Hypoxia of the renal medulla—its implications for disease. *N Engl J Med* 1995; 332:647.

170. Redl-Wenzl EM, Armbruster C, Edelmann G, et al.: The effects of norepinephrine on hemodynamics and renal function in severe septic shock states. *Intensive Care Med* 1993; 19(3):151.

171. Ruokonen E, Takala J, Kari A, et al.: Regional blood flow and oxygen transport in septic shock. *Crit Care Med* 1993; 21:1296.

172. Hansen PD, Coffey SC, Lewis FR Jr: Changes in oxygen consumption relative to oxygen delivery in endotoxemic dogs given adrenergic agents. *J Surg Res* 1994; 57(1):156.

173. Gregory JS, Bonfiglio MF, Dasta JF, et al.: Experience with phenylephrine as a component of the pharmacologic support of septic shock. *Crit Care Med* 1991; 19(11):1395.

174. Moran JL, O'Fathartaigh MS, Peisach AR, et al.: Epinephrine as an inotropic agent in septic shock: a dose-profile analysis. *Crit Care Med* 1993; 21(1):70.

175. Bollaert PE, Bauer P, Audibert G, et al.: Effects of epinephrine on hemodynamics and oxygen metabolism in dopamine-resistant septic shock. *Chest* 1990; 98:949.

176. Wilson W, Lipman J, Scribante J, et al.: Septic shock: Does adrenaline have a role as a first-line inotropic agent? *Anaesth Intens Care* 1992; 20(4):470.

177. Levy B, Bollaert PE, Nace L, et al.: Epinephrine or norepinephrine-dobutamine for dopamine resistant septic shock. *Am J Respir Crit Care Med* 1995; 151:A447.

178. Pitcairn M, Schuler J, Erve P, et al.: Glucocorticoid and antibiotic effect on experimental gram-negative bacteremic shock. *Arch Surgery* 1975; 110:1012.

179. Sprung C, Panagiota C, Marcial R, et al.: The effects of high-dose corticosteroids in patients with septic shock: a prospective, controlled study. *N Eng J Med* 1984; 311:1137.

180. Bone R, Fischer C, Clemmer T, et al.: A controlled trial of high-

dose methylprednisolone in the treatment of severe sepsis and septic shock. *N Eng J Med* 1987; 317:653.

181. Ziegler E, McCutchan J, Douglas H, et al.: Prevention of lethal pseudomonas bacteremia with epimerase-deficient *E. coli* antiserum. *Trans Assoc Am Physicians* 1975; 88:101.

182. Ziegler E, McCutchan A, Fierer J, et al.: Treatment of bacteremia and shock with human antiserum to a mutant *Escherichia coli. N Eng J Med* 1982; 307:1225.

183. Calandra T, Glauser M, Schellekens J, et al.: Treatment of gram-negative septic shock with human IgG antibody to *Escherichia coli* J5: A prospective, double blinded, randomized study. *J Infect Dis* 1988; 158:312.

184. Teng N, Kaplan H, Hebert J, et al.: Protection against gram-negative bacteremia and endotoxemia with human monoclonal IgM antibodies. *Proc Natl Acad Sci* 1985; 82:1790.

185. Young L, Gascon R, Alam S, Bermudez L: Monoclonal antibodies for treatment of gram-negative infections. *Rev Infect Dis* 1989; 11:S1564.

186. Warren H, Danner R, Munford R: Sounding board: Anti-endotoxin monoclonal antibodies. *N Eng J Med* 1992; 326:1153.

187. Ziegler E, Fischer C, Sprung C, et al.: Treatment of gram-negative bacteremia and shock with HA-1A human monoclonal antibody against endotoxin: A randomized, double blind, placebo controlled trial. *N Eng J Med* 1991; 324:429.

188. McCloskey R, Straube R, Sanders C, et al.: Treatment of septic shock with human monoclonal antibody HA-1A: A randomized, double blind, placebo controlled trial. *Ann Intern Med* 1994; 121:1.

189. Greenman R, Schein R, Martin M, et al.: A controlled trial of E5 murine monoclonal IgM antibody to endotoxin in the treatment of gram-negative sepsis. The XOMA Sepsis Study Group. *J Am Med Assoc* 1991; 266:1097.

190. Wenzel R, Bone R, Fein A, et al.: Results of a second double-blind, randomized, controlled trial of anti-endotoxin antibody E5 in gram-negative sepsis [Abstract]. Program and Abstracts of the Thirty First Interscience Conference of Antimicrobial Agents and Chemotherapy: 294, 1991.

191. Heumann D, Gallay P, Betz-Corradin S, et al.: Competition between bactericidal/permeability-increasing protein and lipopolysaccharide binding protein for lipopolysaccharide binding to monocytes. *J Infect Dis* 1993; 167:1351.

192. Weiss J, Elsbach P, Shu C, et al.: Human bactericidal/permeability increasing protein and a recombinant NH2-fragment terminal cause killing of serum resistant gram-negative bacteria in whole blood and inhibit tumor necrosis factor release induced by bacteria. *J Clin Invest* 1992; 90:1122.

193. Evans T, Carpenter A, Martin R, Cohen J: Protective effect of bactericidal/permeability increasing protein (BPI) in experimental gram-negative sepsis with a rough organism [abstract]. Program and Abstracts of the Thirty Third Interscience Conference of Antimicrobial Agents and Chemotherapy: 378, 1993.

194. Lynn W, Cohen J, Adjunctive therapy for septic shock: A review of experimental approaches. *Clin Infect Dis* 1995; 20:143.

195. Hinshaw L, Emerson T, Taylor F, et al.: Lethal *Staphylococcus aureus*-induced shock in primates: Prevention of death with anti-TNF antibody. *J Trauma* 1992; 33:568.

196. Nakane A, Minagawa T, Kato K: Endogenous tumor necrosis factor (cachectin) is essential to host resistance against *Listeria monocytogenes* infection. *Infect Immunol* 1988; 56:2563.

197. Abraham E, Wunderlink R, Silverman H, et al.: Efficacy and safety of monoclonal antibody to human tumor necrosis factor α in patients with sepsis syndrome: A randomized, controlled, double-blind, multicenter clinical trial. *J Am Med Assoc* 1995; 273:934.

198. McNamara M, Norton J, Nauta R, Alexander H: Interleukin-1 receptor antibody (IL-1rab) protection and treatment against lethal endotoxemia in mice. *J Surg Res* 1993; 54:316.

199. van Zee K, Kohno T, Fischer E, et al.: Tumor necrosis factor soluble receptors circulate during experimental and clinical inflammation and can protect against excessive tumor necrosis factor a in vitro and in vivo. *Proc Natl Acad Sci* 1992; 89:4845.

200. Froon A, Bemelmans M, Greve J, et al.: Increased plasma concentrations of soluble tumor necrosis factor receptors in sepsis syndrome: Correlation with plasma creatinine values. *Crit Care Med* 1994; 22:803.

201. Alexander H, Doherty G, Buresh C, et al.: A recombinant human receptor antagonist to interleukin-1 improves survival after lethal endotoxemia in mice. *J Exp Med* 1991; 173:1029.

202. Aiura K, Gelfand J, Burke J, et al.: Interleukin-1 (IL-1) receptor antagonist prevents *Staphylococcus epidermidis*-induced hypotension and reduces circulating levels of tumor necrosis factor and IL-1β in rabbits. *Infect Immun* 1993; 61:3342.

203. Fisher C, Slotman G, Opal S, et al.: Initial evaluation of human recombinant interleukin-1 receptor antagonist in the treatment of sepsis syndrome: A randomized, open label, placebo-controlled multicenter trial. *Crit Care Med* 1994; 22:12.

204. Fisher C, Dhainaut J, Opal S, et al.: Recombinant human interleukin 1 receptor antagonist in the treatment of patients with sepsis syndrome: Results from randomized, double-blind, placebo-controlled trial. *J Am Med Assoc* 1994; 271:1836.

205. Torley L, Pickett W, Carroll M, et al.: Studies of the effect of a platelet-activating factor antagonist, CL 184,005, in animal models of gram-negative bacterial sepsis. *Antimicrob Agents Chemother* 1992; 36:1971.

206. Dhainaut J, Tenaillon A, Tulzo Y, et al.: Platelet activating factor receptor antagonist BN 52021 in the treatment of severe sepsis: A randomized, double blind, placebo controlled, multicenter clinical trial. *Crit Care Med* 1994; 22:1720.

207. Coran A, Drongowski R, Paik J, Remick D: Ibuprofen intervention in canine septic shock: Reduction of pathophysiology without decreased cytokines. *J Surg Res* 1992; 53:272.

208. Michie H, Manogue K, Spriggs D, et al.: Detection of circulating tumor necrosis factor after endotoxin administration. *N Eng J Med* 1988; 318:1481.

209. Bernard G, Reines H, Halushka P, et al.: Prostacyclin and thromboxane A2 formation is increased in human sepsis syndrome. Effects of cyclooxygenase inhibition. *Am Rev Resp Dis* 1991; 144:1095.

210. Yu M, Tomasa G: A double blind, prospective, randomized trial of ketoconazole, a thromboxane synthetase inhibitor, in the prophylaxis of the adult respiratory distress syndrome. *Crit Care Med* 1993; 21:1635.

211. Williams J, Maier R: Ketoconazole inhibits alveolar macrophage production of inflammatory mediators involved in acute lung injury (adult respiratory distress syndrome). *Surgery* 1992; 112:270.

212. Kilbourn RG, Jubran A, Gross SS, et al.: Reversal of endotoxin-mediated shock by N^G-methyl-L-arginine, an inhibitor of nitric oxide synthesis. *Biochem Biophys Res Comm* 1990; 172(3):1132.

213. Vallance P, Moncada S: Role of endogenous nitric oxide in septic shock. *New Horizons* 1993; 1(1):77.

214. Hibbs JB, Westenfelder C, Taintor R, et al.: Evidence for cytokine-inducible nitric oxide synthesis from L-arginine in patients receiving interleukin-2 therapy. *J Clin Invest* 1992; 89:867.

215. Landin L, Lorente JA, Renes E, et al.: Inhibition of nitric oxide synthesis improves the vasoconstrictive effect of noradrenaline in sepsis. *Chest* 1994; 106:250.

216. Herbertson MJ, Werner HA, Handel J, Walley KR: L-Nitro argi-

nine partially reverses decreased myocardial contractility in endotoxemia. *Am J Respir Crit Care Med* 1995; 151(4):A15.

217. Cohen R, Huberfeld S, Genovese J, et al.: Coronary blood flow and myocardial function after nitric oxide synthetase inhibition in endotoxemic dogs. *Am J Respir Crit Care Med* 1995; 151(4):A16.

218. Kilbourn RG, Cromeens DM, Chelly FD, Griffith OW: N^G-methyl-L-arginine, an inhibitor of nitric oxide formation, acts synergistically with dobutamine to improve cardiovascular performance in endotoxemic dogs. *Crit Care Med* 1994; 22:1835.

219. Tolins JP, Raij L: Modulation of systemic blood pressure and renal hemodynamic responses by endothelium-derived relaxing factor (nitric oxide), in Moncada S, Higgs EA (eds): *Nitric oxide from L-arginine.* New York, Elsevier Science, 1990:463–473.

220. Walder CE, Thiemermann C, Vane JR: The involvement of endothelium-derived relaxing factor in the regulation of renal cortical blood flow in the rat. *Br J Pharmacol* 1991; 102:967.

221. Hutcheson IR, Whittle BR, Boughton-Smith NK: Role of nitric oxide in maintaining vascular integrity in endotoxin-induced acute intestinal damage in the rat. *Br J Pharmacol* 1990; 101:815.

222. Klabunde RE, Ritger RC: N^G-monomethyl-L-arginine (NMA) restores arterial blood pressure but reduces cardiac output in a canine model of endotoxin shock. *Biochem Biophys Res Commun* 1991; 178:1135.

223. Cobb JP, Natanson C, Banks SM, et al.: N^ω-Amino-L-arginine, an inhibitor of nitric oxide synthase, raises vascular resistance but increases mortality rates in awake canines challenged with endotoxin. *J Exp Med* 1992; 176:1175.

224. Danner RL: Nitric oxide: A therapeutic target in sepsis, pp778–780, in Natanson C (moderator): Selected treatment strategies for septic shock based on proposed mechanisms of pathogenesis. *Ann Intern Med* 1994; 120:771.

225. Nava E, Palmer RM, Moncada S: The role of nitric oxide in endotoxin shock: Effects of N^ω-monomethyl-L-arginine.

226. Petros A, Bennett D, Vallance P: Effect on nitric oxide synthase inhibitors on hypotension in patients with septic shock. *Lancet* 1991; 338:1557.

227. Schilling J, Cakmaci M, Battig U, et al.: A new approach to treatment of hypotension in human septic shock by N^G-monomethyl-L-arginine, an inhibitor of nitric oxide synthetase. *Intens Care Med* 1993; 19:227.

228. Petros A, Lamb G, Leone A, et al.: Effects of a nitric oxide synthase inhibitor in humans with septic shock. *Cardiovasc Res* 1994; 28:34.

229. Kilbourn RG, Logothetis CJ, Striegel A, et al.: N^G-monomethyl-L-arginine (NMA), an inhibitor of nitric oxide (NO) production reverses interleukin-2 mediated hypotension in humans. *Endothelium* 1993; 1:S14.

230. Brezis M, Heyman SN, Dinour D, et al.: The role of nitric oxide in renal medullary oxygenation. Studies in isolated and intact rat kidneys. *J Clin Invest* 1991; 88(2):390.

231. Liu SF, Adcock IM, Barnes PJ, Evans TW: Differential regulation of the constitutive and inducible NO synthase by endotoxin in vivo in the rat. *Am J Respir Crit Care Med* 1995; 151:A15.

232. Mulder MF, Van Lambalgen AA, Huisman E, et al.: Protective role of NO in the regional hemodynamic changes during acute endotoxemia in rats. *Am J Physiol* 1994; 266:H1558.

233. Schumacker PT, Kazaglis J, Connolly H, et al.: Systemic and gut O_2 extraction during endotoxemia. Role of nitric oxide synthesis. *Am J Respir Crit Care Med* 1995; 151:107.

234. Zhang H, Rogiers P, Spapen H, et al.: NO donor SIN-1 can increase splanchnic blood flow during endotoxic shock. *Am J Respir Crit Care Med* 1995; 151:A16.

235. Umans JG, Samsel RW: L-Canavanine selectively augments contraction in aortas from endotoxemic rats. *Eur J Pharmacol* 1992; 210:343.

236. Liaudet L, Feihl F, Hurni JM, Perret C: L-Canavanine selectively inhibits inducible NO synthase in endotoxemia. *Am J Respir Crit Care Med* 1995; 151:A16.

237. Schultz PJ, Raij L: Endogenously synthesized nitric oxide prevents endotoxin-induced glomerular thrombosis. *J Clin Invest* 1992; 90:1718.

238. Keaney JF, Puyana JC, Francis S, et al.: Methylene blue reverses endotoxin-induced hypotension. *Circ Res* 1994; 74:1121.

239. Schneider F, Lutun P, Hasselman M, et al.: Methylene blue increases systemic vascular resistance in human septic shock. Preliminary observations. *Intens Care Med* 1992; 18(5):309.

240. Preiser JC, Moulart D, Cosyns B, Vincent JL: Administration of the calcium agonist BAY K 8644 in endotoxic shock. *Circ Shock* 1991; 35(4):199.

241. Broner C, Shenep J, Stidham G, et al.: Effect of scavengers of oxygen-derived free radicals on mortality in endotoxin-challenged mice. *Crit Care Med* 1988; 16:848.

242. Bakker J, Zhang H, Depierreux M, et al.: Effects of N-acetylcysteine in endotoxic shock. *J Crit Care* 1994; 9:236.

243. Johnson D, Hurst T, Prasad K, et al.: Lazaroid pretreatment preserves gas exchange in endotoxin-treated dogs. *J Crit Care* 1994; 9:213.

244. Spies C, Reinhart K, Witt I, et al.: Influence of N-acetylcysteine on indirect indicators of tissue oxygenation in septic shock patients: Results of a prospective, randomized, double blind study. *Crit Care Med* 1994; 22:1738.

245. Rangel-Frausto M, Pittet D, Costigan M, et al.: The natural history of the systemic inflammatory response syndrome: A prospective study. *J Am Med Assoc* 1995; 273:117.

246. Milberg J, Davis D, Steinburg K, Hudson L: Improved survival of patients with acute respiratory distress syndrome (ARDS): 1983–1993. *J Am Med Assoc* 1995; 273:306.

Chapter 104

PULMONARY INFECTIONS IN PATIENTS RECEIVING IMMUNE SUPPRESSIVE THERAPY

THEODORE H. LEWIS, JR.

The expanding use of chemotherapy for malignancy and inflammatory diseases and bone marrow and solid organ transplantation has led to an increasingly large population of patients at risk for pulmonary infection. These patients are at risk for other pulmonary complications as well. Pulmonary involvement of the malignancy, inflammatory disease, drug toxicity, radiation toxicity, and volume overload (or congestive heart failure) all may cause pulmonary disease in this patient population. Infection, however, is the predominant concern. Understanding these infectious complications of immunosuppressive therapy requires an understanding of pulmonary defense mechanisms and the impact of the treatment (as well as the underlying disease) upon those defenses. Immunosuppressive therapies result in either cytopenias (in particular, neutropenia) or impaired T-cell–mediated immunity. Patients receiving cytotoxic chemotherapy typically develop neutropenia, while patients who have undergone organ transplantation have impaired T-cell–mediated immunity. Patients who have received bone marrow transplants (particularly allogeneic transplants) suffer from both types of immunosuppression. Indeed, many patients develop both cytopenia and impaired T-cell function. (Lymphoma patients treated with cytotoxic therapy and corticosteroids are one example.) High dose cytotoxic therapy also may result in impaired macrophage and lymphocyte function.[1] Nevertheless, it is useful to consider infections associated with these isolated defects in pulmonary defenses, recognizing that many patients may fall into both categories.

Pulmonary Infections in Neutropenic Patients

Neutropenia is a common complication of hematologic malignancies and chemotherapy. It also may complicate other conditions, such as human immunodeficiency virus (HIV) infection and its therapies.[2] The risk of infection increases with the severity of neutropenia and its duration.[3] More aggressive chemotherapeutic regimens may result in profound neutropenia. Growth factor therapy has been effective in speeding marrow recovery and reducing infectious complications[4,5] but is not always effective, nor can it be universally applied; thus, neutropenia remains a significant problem. Neutrophils are critically important in the defense against bacteria and opportunistic fungi.[6,7] Thus, patients with neutropenia are at increased risk for bacterial and fungal infection.

In patients with neutropenic infections, the lung is a common site of infection. Unfortunately, while a definitive diagnosis may be established, fever and/or pulmonary infiltrates in neutropenic patients often cannot be attributed to a specific organism. Aggressive empiric therapy and a careful diagnostic approach offer the best chance of supporting patients until their neutropenia resolves.

BACTERIAL INFECTIONS

Bacterial infections are the most common cause of infection in neutropenic host. The lungs are the portal of entry for 25 percent of bacteremic episodes.[7] The spectrum of pathogens responsible for bacteremic infections in neutropenic host is changing. Gram-positive bacteremias are more common, while gram-negative infections are less frequently identified.[8] In one recent study, the incidence of gram-negative organisms in bacteremia was 16 percent.[9] This shift in the type of microbes responsible for infection is caused by increased use of long-term indwelling venous access devices, increased use of prophylactic antibiotics (such as trimethoprim-sulfamethoxazole or quinolones), and/or increased mucositis complicating high-dose chemotherapy. Gram-negative infections remain a concern, however, because of the rapidity with which they can progress to shock and death.

GRAM-NEGATIVE INFECTION

The gram-negative organisms that cause disease in the neutropenic host are those that cause noscocomial infections in the general hospitalized population, enteric organisms, e.g., *Pseudomonas aeruginosa*, *Escherichia coli*, and *Klebsiella pneumoniae*.[10] *Pseudomonas* is of particular concern because of its extreme pathogenicity. *Pseudomonas* releases exotoxins and proteases, causing significant pulmonary parenchymal destruction.[11] This can result in life-threatening pulmonary hemorrhage in thrombocytopenic patients (Fig. 104-1). *Pseudomonas* can also cause activation of the systemic inflammatory network through endotoxins present in the cell wall.

GRAM-POSITIVE INFECTION

Gram-positive organisms that cause infection in neutropenic patients are those associated with skin, such as *Staphylococcus aureus* and *Staphylococcus epidermidis*, or the oral cavity, such as viridans group streptococci. In general, these organisms are less virulent than gram-negative infections.[12] However, increasing experience with viridans group streptococci suggests that bacteremia with these organisms, and *Streptococcus mitus* in particular, is associated with significant morbidity and mortality.[9] A syndrome of rash, palmar desquamation, hypotension, adult respiratory distress syndrome, and death has been described in neutropenic patients infected with these organisms.[9]

The incidence of specific etiologic organisms in bacterial pneumonia in the neutropenic patient has been less well studied than bacteremia. One study utilizing bronchoscopy with bronchoalveolar lavage (BAL) and protected brush to evaluate infiltrates in immunocompromised hosts found that 22 percent of infiltrates were attributable to bacterial pneumonia,[13] of which 80 percent were gram-negative organisms. However, this patient population was a heterogeneous group, which included patients positive for human immunodeficiency virus (HIV) and transplant patients as

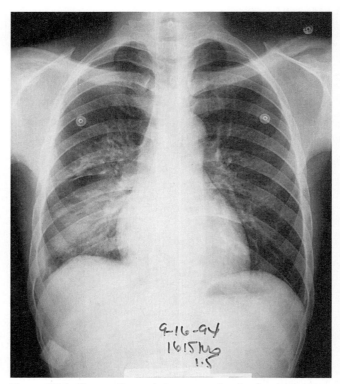

Figure 104-1   Chest radiograph demonstrating focal pulmonary hemorrhage in a young woman with *Pseudomonas aeruginosa* pneumonia and sepsis complicating chemotherapy-induced neutropenia.

well as neutropenic patients. Unfortunately, other bronchoscopy studies have had similarly mixed populations.[14]

Unusual bacterial organisms may cause pneumonia in neutropenic hosts. *Legionella pneumophila* (and other *Legionella* species) and *Nocardia asteroides* have been reported to cause pneumonia in neutropenic hosts, though an associated cell-mediated immune defect is usually present.[7] *Mycobacterium tuberculosis* may also complicate neutropenia,[7] although it is an unusual pathogen in this population. Atypical mycobacteria are unusual pathogens in the neutropenic host except in chronic lymphocytic leukemia and hairy-cell leukemia.[15]

CLINICAL PRESENTATION

The clinical presentation of pulmonary infection in neutropenic patients differs from that in nonneutropenic patients. Cough and sputum production appear to be less frequent symptoms.[16] Physical examination may be unrevealing. Chest radiography usually demonstrates an abnormality, but findings may be subtle and CT scanning may increase the sensitivity of radiographic assessment.[17]

DIAGNOSIS

The diagnosis of bacterial pneumonia in neutropenia patients is problematic, because patients may often be treated with broad-spectrum empiric antibiotics prior to the development of radiographic abnormalities. This reduces the likelihood of an accurate microbiologic diagnosis of a bacterial pneumonia by blood culture or bronchoscopy.[18] Because of this, many patients are treated empirically for common bacterial organisms (see below). Failure to respond to empiric therapy mandates bronchoscopy in pursuit of less common pathogens.

TREATMENT

The therapy of bacterial pneumonia in neutropenic patients is directed at the organisms common to these patients and modified by the results of diagnostic testing. Most authorities believe empiric therapy with a β-lactam antibiotic (ceftazidime or imipenem) is effective in the majority of cases.[19] The need for an aminoglycoside at the outset is determined in part by the severity of neutropenia and the susceptibilities of gram-negative organisms within a given institution.[10] The increasing incidence of severe gram-positive infections suggests that the addition of vancomycin to this empiric regimen may be indicated, but present recommendations argue for waiting until a gram-positive pathogen is identified.[10,19] Lack of improvement with such a regimen should prompt bronchoscopy if a diagnosis has not been made with blood cultures. Identification of *Legionella* species would necessitate the addition of erythromycin (4 g intravenously daily). Nocardia requires therapy with trimethoprim/sulfamethoxazole (TMP/SMX) (15 mg/kg/day of TMP, 75 mg/kg/day of SMX).

Patients with *S. mitis* bacteremia have a high incidence of adult respiratory distress syndrome. There has been some early evidence to support the use of corticosteroid administration in this very specific group of patients,[105] though the study cited was historically controlled.

FUNGAL INFECTIONS

Fungal infections are a common, devastating problem in neutropenic hosts. The fungi that typically cause disease in neutropenia are opportunistic rather than pathogenic fungi, in particular *Aspergillus* and *Candida* species.[7,20] Other fungal infections, such as mucormycosis, are observed occasionally.[21]

ASPERGILLOSIS

Aspergillus species usually cause pulmonary disease, though dissemination may occur. There are many *Aspergillus* species, but disease typically is associated with *A. fumigatus* and *A. flavus*.[22] *Aspergillus* species are not part of the normal host flora but are ubiquitous in the environment. Inhalation of spores by immunocompromised patients results in infection. Outbreaks of *Aspergillus* infection have been associated with construction or renovation within or adjacent to hospitals.[23]

Invasive aspergillosis presents a major diagnostic and therapeutic problem in neutropenic patients. *Aspergillus* infections cause about 8 percent of febrile episodes in neutropenic patients.[24] Duration of neutropenia is an important factor in *Aspergillus* infection. In one study, the risk of developing invasive aspergillosis during neutropenia was initially 1 percent per day but increased to > 4 percent per day after day 20.[25] Recent series have noted much lower attack rates.[26] The incidence of invasive aspergillosis is very high in patients with a prior episode of aspergillosis and neutropenia. In one study, 75 percent of patients with acute nonlymphocytic leukemia and fungal infection developed a second invasive fungal infection during subsequent episodes of neutropenia, and 52 percent of episodes of neutropenia were complicated by fungal infection.[27] The majority of these invasive infections were due to *Aspergillus* species.

CLINICAL PRESENTATION

The clinical presentation of invasive aspergillosis is nonspecific. Fever, chest pain, cough and hemoptysis all may be presenting symptoms. The radiographic presentation is also nonspecific, ranging from "normal" chest radiograph to dense focal infiltrates to diffuse patchy infiltrates (Fig. 104-2).[28,29] While the routine chest radiographic findings in invasive aspergillosis are nonspecific, chest computed tomography (CT) may offer a more specific pattern. The appearance of an area of low attenuation around a pulmonary mass has been reported to be an early manifestation of invasive aspergillosis in neutropenic patients (Fig. 104-3).[30] This "halo sign" has, however, been reported in other pulmonary infections associated with cavitary infiltrates. The sensitivity of CT in the diagnosis of invasive aspergillosis is variable.[16,30]

DIAGNOSIS

The diagnosis of invasive *Aspergillus* infection in neutropenic patients is often difficult. Sputum cultures or cultures of nasal swabs may demonstrate *Aspergillus* species. When sputum cultures were positive in nonsmoking neutropenic patients, they had a very high correlation with invasive pulmonary aspergillosis.[31] While the significance of a positive sputum may be debated,[32] most authors would consider a culture positive for *Aspergillus* from the respiratory tract very suggestive of invasive disease in a neutropenic patient with fevers.[10,16]

Bronchoscopy often is utilized to diagnose aspergillosis in neutropenic patients. Unfortunately, the sensitivity of bronchoscopy for establishing a diagnosis is poor. Bronchoalveolar lavage has the best sensitivity of bronchoscopic techniques—about 53 percent.[33] Transbronchial biopsy appears to add little to washings.[33,34] Bronchoscopy had a 75 percent positive predictive value.[33]

Open lung biopsy is the other diagnostic modality utilized in invasive pulmonary aspergillosis. Unlike sputum culture or bronchoalveolar lavage, open lung biopsy demonstrates tissue invasion. Unfortunately, its sensitivity is also poor. Two series of patients (one in acute leukemia, the other in bone marrow transplants) noted cases of invasive pulmonary fungal disease discovered at autopsy that were not detected at open biopsy.[35,36] Nevertheless, because of the toxicities of high-dose amphotericin, open lung biopsy usually is recommended when invasive aspergillosis is suspected in a neutropenic patient and cannot be diagnosed by less invasive studies.[32]

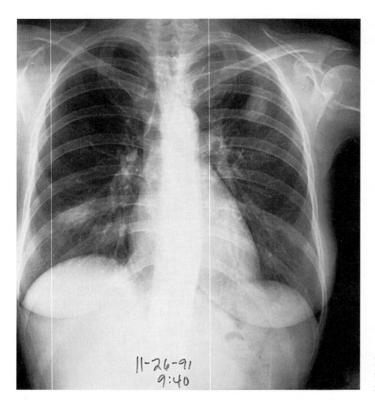

FIGURE 104-2 Chest radiograph demonstrating patchy infiltrates (one with cavitation) due to *Aspergillus fumigatus* in a neutropenic bone marrow transplant recipient.

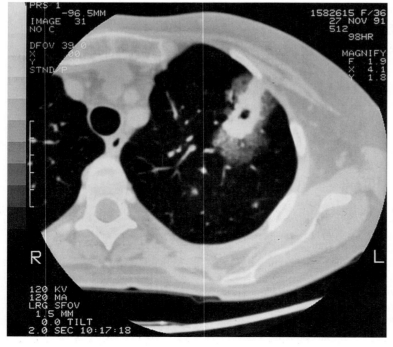

FIGURE 104-3 Chest CT demonstrating dense, high-attenuation infiltrate surrounded by area of lower attenuation. This is the "halo sign." Cavitation is also noted in the infiltrate. The infiltrate is due to *Aspergillus fumigatus.*

THERAPY

The therapy of invasive aspergillosis is evolving. The disease has been felt to have a dismal prognosis in patients with neutropenia, with mortality rates of 95 percent.[37] However, several factors may have a positive influence on outcome. These include early diagnosis, aggressive antifungal therapy, and control of the underlying malignancy.[38,39]

Amphotericin B remains the drug of choice for invasive aspergillosis. In one group of neutropenic patients treated with high-dose (1.0 to 1.5 mg/kg/day) amphotericin, 13 of 14 patients survived.[38] Lower doses of amphotericin (0.5 mg/kg/day), used empirically, have been associated with the development of invasive aspergillosis.[38,40] Amphotericin has been utilized as primary (inhaled and intranasal) and secondary (intravenous) prophylaxis against Aspergillus in patients undergoing multiple courses of cytotoxic chemotherapy.[41,42] The development of liposomal preparations of amphotericin may allow the administration of higher doses with less toxicity.[43]

Itraconazole is another antifungal agent with significant activity against Aspergillus.[44] It has been utilized in patients with invasive aspergillosis[45] and in those with neutropenia and invasive aspergillosis.[45,46] In neutropenic patients with invasive aspergillosis treated with itraconazole (400 mg/day), response rates of 66 to 75 percent are reported. Itraconazole currently is available only as an oral medication, which may limit its use in patients with chemotherapy-induced mucositis. Randomized trials of itraconazole versus high-dose amphotericin in neutropenic patients are necessary to determine which regimen has greater efficacy and tolerability and less toxicity. It also should be noted that itraconazole use has been implicated in the development of resistance to amphotericin B.[7] The significance of this phenomenon will have to be explored further. Itraconazole also has been used as part of a primary prophylaxis regimen. In a historically controlled study of patients with hematologic malignancies, itraconazole (200 mg/day) combined with nasal amphotericin significantly reduced the risk of Aspergillus infection.[47]

CANDIDIASIS

Invasive Candida infections are common in neutropenic patients, but Candida pneumonia is unusual.[48] Isolated Candida pneumonia was noted in less than 5 percent of autopsies at a cancer hospital.[49] The spectrum of Candida species causing disease in neutropenic patients is changing[16]; C. krusei and C. tropicalis are becoming more frequent causes of infections. The clinical presentation of pulmonary candidiasis is nonspecific. Patients typically present with fever. Physical examination is often unrevealing. Radiographic manifestations include patchy peripheral infiltrates, but the chest radiograph may be normal.[49] Patients who have Candida species recovered from pulmonary sources (sputum, bronchoscopic specimens) should be evaluated for disseminated candidiasis, but documentation of tissue invasion or fungemia is appropriate before instituting antifungal therapy. Disseminated candidiasis is more likely in patients with Candida found in multiple sites (multicolonized).[50]

The therapy of Candida infections also is changing. Amphotericin B remains the primary therapy, but, increasingly, fluconazole is being utilized. In neutropenic patients with acute disseminated candidiasis, fluconazole therapy (400 mg/day for 3 days followed by 200 mg/day) resulted in a clinical response in 67 percent of patients.[51] Comparison with amphotericin in a large series has not yet been done. Fluconazole has been utilized as primary prophylaxis for invasive fungal infections.[52] Deep fungal infections were reduced, though breakthrough was seen by fluconazole-resistant species such as C. krusei or Aspergillus species. Amphotericin (0.5 to 0.7 mg/kg/day) has been utilized as prophylaxis in neutropenic patients who remain febrile despite broad-spectrum antibacterials.[53] The incidence of fungal infections was reduced. However, breakthrough infections with Aspergillus species have been reported at these lower doses of amphotericin.[38]

VIRAL INFECTIONS

Viral pneumonias occasionally may complicate neutropenia, but they are seen much more frequently in the setting of marrow transplantation.[16] Herpesviruses (HSV) cause most infections in neutropenic patients, and (in nontransplant patients) herpes simplex infections are the most common. Pneumonia secondary to HSV is rare. In one series of 20 patients with HSV pneumonia, only two were neutropenic with hematologic malignancies without marrow transplant.[54] Nevertheless, when HSV is recovered from neutropenic patients with lung lesions, antiviral therapy is indicated, but an aggressive search for other pathogens should be carried out, as co-infection is common.[54] The clinical presentation is one of fever, cough, and dyspnea.[54] Chest radiographs may demonstrate focal, multifocal, or diffuse infiltrates.[54] Therapy for HSV pneumonia is acyclovir (30 mg/kg/day in three divided intravenous doses, adjusted for renal function).

Varicella zoster virus also may cause pneumonia in neutropenic patients.[16] In adults, reactivation and dissemination is the more common cause of pneumonia, but primary infection may occur. Vesicles typically are present, though they may be subtle or absent. Chest radiography usually demonstrates a diffuse nodular or interstitial diffuse infiltrate.[55] Acyclovir (15 to 30 mg/kg/day in three divided intravenous doses, adjusted for renal function) is the appropriate therapy for varicella zoster pneumonia.

APPROACH TO PNEUMONIA IN THE NEUTROPENIC HOST

Investigators at the National Institutes of Health, National Cancer Institutes, and elsewhere have developed an approach to fevers and pulmonary infiltrates that is accepted widely.[56] Focal pulmonary infiltrates are classified as early, refractory, or late. Neutropenic patients who develop fevers and infiltrates simultaneously are considered to have "early" infiltrates and have a high likelihood of having a bacterial infection. Broad-spectrum antibacterial antibiotics should be administered. Examination of sputum and blood cultures is mandated. Some authors would also argue that bronchoscopy should be considered.[32] Failure of the patient to respond to therapy (continued fever, progressing infiltrates) leads to classification of the infiltrate as "refractory." Unusual organisms such as *Legionella* species, *Nocardia*, *Actinomycetes*, or fungi become more likely etiologic agents. Aggressive diagnostic procedures such as bronchoscopy are indicated. If no etiology is found, open lung biopsy should be considered.[57] Neutropenic patients who develop pulmonary infiltrates after having received antibacterials for several days are considered to have "late" infiltrates. Like refractory infiltrates, the etiologic agents that typically cause late infiltrates are fungal organisms or unusual bacteria, and aggressive diagnostic measures are indicated. Such measures also are indicated for diffuse lung lesions, which are unlikely to be due to typical bacterial infections. Viral infections, *Legionella* infection, *Mycoplasma pneumoniae* infection and noninfectious processes may all cause diffuse lung lesions.

Finally, it is important to note that many neutropenic patients also have defects of cellular or humoral defenses. Some chemotherapies are associated with impaired cell-mediated immunity,[58] and some diseases (lymphoma, chronic lymphocytic leukemia) may impair cell-mediated immunity. Consequently, the patient with neutropenia may also be at risk for pathogens typically associated with altered cellular immunity (see below).

Pulmonary Infections in Solid-Organ Transplant Recipients

The complex immune responses to allogeneic tissue grafts require aggressive suppression of the host's (or, in the case of an allogeneic bone marrow transplant, the graft's) cellular immunity if the graft is to survive. This suppression places the host at risk for many infections, and pulmonary infections are a large portion of these infections. The pulmonary complications of organ transplantation have been well reviewed; only brief discussion follows.[59–61]

PATHOPHYSIOLOGY

The recognition of alloantigen and components of a foreign major histocompatibility complex (MHC or human leukocyte antigens) on either lymphocytes or antigen-presenting cells in the allograft elicits a complex response that depends upon the cell recognizing the foreign material and the class of MHC that differs from the host. Class I MHC alloantigens are recognized by CD8+ lymphocytes and result in the generation of cytotoxic T lymphocytes (CTL); class II MHC alloantigenic differences result in the stimulation of CD4+ lymphocytes.[62] These differences are not absolute.[62] The growth and differentiation of CD8+ CTL is largely dependent upon activation of CD4+ lymphocytes.[62]

Activation of CD4+ lymphocytes occurs when activation of the T-cell receptor–CD3 (TCR) complex leads to increases in intracellular calcium, activating, in turn, calcineurin. Calcineurin results in dephosphorylation of a cytoplasmic component called the nuclear factor of activated T cells

(NFATc), allowing its migration into the T-cell nucleus. Coincident with this dephosphorylation, protein kinase C– and tyrosine kinase–mediated promoters such as AP-1 and NF-κB are increased in the T-cell nucleus. Interaction of NFAT with AP-1 results in binding of the complex to the IL-2 promoter and upregulation of IL-2 production.[63] The transcription of IL-2 may be upregulated by CD28-mediated pathways as well as TCR-mediated pathways that utilize non-calcium-dependent mechanisms.[63] Increases in IL-2 causes increases in other components of the cytokine network as well as proliferation of lymphocytes and activation of CTLs and other effector cells such as macrophages.[64] Proliferation and activation of these cells results in graft rejection.

Graft survival thus requires the modulation of the immune response to alloantigen. Several methods of reducing the T-cell–mediated response are utilized in organ transplant recipients. Corticosteroids reduce the immune response through a number of mechanisms, including reduction of IL-2 production by T cells[65] and IL-1, IL-2, INF-γ, and TNF-α production by macrophages.[64] Modulators of calcineurin block its phosphatase activity, ultimately inhibiting transcription of the IL-2 gene. Two such agents are currently utilized, cyclosporin A and tacrolimus (FK506). Each binds with a specific binding protein(s) (cyclophilin and FK-binding proteins).[66] The drug-binding protein complex inhibits calcineurin phophorylation of NFATc, blocking its entry into the nucleus.[66] Rapamycin, an experimental agent, acts to inhibit lymphocyte proliferation responding to a number of stimuli, including IL-2, IL-3, IL-4, stimulation of the TCR, and stimulation of CD28.[64] Other agents, e.g., azathiaprine, reduce the number of lymphocytes by inhibiting proliferation; still others directly reduce numbers of lymphocytes, e.g., corticosteroids or monoclonal antibodies against T cell surface receptors (OKT3, antithymocyte globulin).

The remarkable success that has been achieved at impairing the cellular immune response to allografts, improving graft survival, also reduces the ability of the host to utilize the cellular defense against infection. Infections by agents that are normally handled by cellular defenses are common in transplant recipients. The likelihood of infection is influenced by the type of organ transplant and the duration and degree of immunosuppression.[67]

The type of transplant a patient receives has an important impact on the infections that may complicate the procedure (Table 104-1). Infections were more common in liver, heart, and heart-lung transplants than in renal transplants.[68] Furthermore, the types of infections varied with the type of transplant.[68] Nevertheless, the lung is a frequent source of infection in transplant patients, and infectious pneumonitis contributes substantially to mortality in transplants.[69]

The type of infection also varies with the time from transplantation (Fig. 104-4). Bacterial infections are common soon after transplantation, but pneumonia caused by encapsulated organisms may occur remote from the transplant. Infection from HSV and *Candida* may also occur in the first month following transplant. Cytomegalovirus, other fungal infections, and infection with *Pneumocystis carinii* tend to occur after the first month.[69,70]

TABLE 104-1   Infection and Morbidity Due to Cytomegalovirus (CMV) Infection among Different Transplant Groups[a]

Type of Transplant	Total No. Patients	No. of Patients with Infections, Percent of Total	NO. OF SYMPTOMATIC PATIENTS		NO. OF PATIENTS WITH CMV PNEUMONIA	
			Infected, %	Total, %	Infected, %	Total, %
Kidney	131	79/131 (60)	13	8	4	2
Liver	93	55/93 (59)	49	29	5	3
Heart	48	44/48 (92)	27	25	9	8
Heart-lung	31	22/31 (71)	55	39	45	32

[a] Reflecting the University of Pittsburgh transplant experience.
SOURCE: From HO and Dummer,[68] with permission.

Viral Infections

Infection with herpesviruses is common in transplant recipients. Cytomegalovirus (CMV), HSV, and varicella virus are major pathogens. Infection with CMV occurs in many transplant recipients, with infection rates of 50 to 70 percent in patients who were seronegative prior to transplant and received a CMV-positive organ (D+/R-).[71] Seronegative patients who receive seronegative organs are virtually free of CMV infection assuming that CMV-negative blood products are utilized.

Pneumonitis is the most common severe complication of CMV infection. In some series, CMV pneumonia complicates close to 30 percent of transplants.[69] It may occur as early as the second week following transplantation, though onset prior to the fourth week is unusual.[69] Peak incidence is 8 to 12 weeks posttransplant.[70,72] Increases in immunosuppression (treatment of graft rejection) may be associated with CMV infection over a greater period of time.

CLINICAL MANIFESTATIONS

Cytomegalovirus pneumonitis typically presents with non-specific systemic symptoms such as fever, malaise, and myalgias. Cough and dyspnea are common chest symptoms.[73] Abnormal laboratory values include increased liver function enzymes, leukopenia, and thrombocytopenia.[73] Radiographic manifestations range from normal chest films to diffuse interstitial infiltrates. Nodules and focal infiltrates also may be seen.[73] The spectrum of disease associated with CMV ranges from mild respiratory symptoms to respiratory failure and death. In lung and heart-lung transplants, the

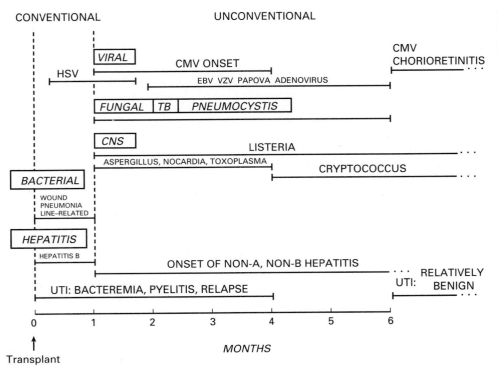

FIGURE 104-4 Varying infections over time in renal transplant recipients. (*From Rubin et al.,*[71] *with permission.*)

severity of illness correlates with the serologic status of the recipient. Seronegative recipients of seropositive organs are at greatest risk for symptomatic disease and mortality.[71]

DIAGNOSIS

The diagnosis of CMV pneumonitis may be problematic, because many asymptomatic patients shed virus in respiratory secretions, blood, and urine.[5] Bronchoscopy with BAL and transbronchial biopsy is an important tool in the diagnosis of CMV pneumonitis. Bronchoalveolar lavage has a sensitivity of > 80 percent for CMV pneumonitis, but is not specific.[75] Many investigators argue that tissue, transbronchial biopsy or open lung biopsy confirmation is necessary before a diagnosis of CMV pneumonia can be made.[76] This is particularly true in lung transplant patients, where CMV growth from BAL does not correlate with pneumonitis on pathology.[77] In recipients of other organ transplants the presence of CMV in bronchoalveolar lavage in the clinical setting of pneumonitis warrants careful consideration of therapy.

THERAPY

Ganciclovir is the therapy of choice for CMV pneumonitis. The use of ganciclovir has reduced the mortality of CMV pneumonitis from 75 percent in untreated patients to 13 percent in heart transplant recipients.[78] The use of adjunctive immunoglobulin therapy is being studied.

The efficacy of prophylactic therapy for CMV pneumonia is controversial. Some measures are clearly efficacious. If a recipient is seronegative for CMV, use of a seronegative organ is preferable, and any blood products utilized should be seronegative. The rate of CMV infection and disease in seronegative recipients of seronegative organs is very low.[71] Unfortunately, the use of seronegative organs is not always possible when the patient is critically ill or organs are in short supply.[71]

Several forms of medical prophylaxis have been attempted in solid-organ transplants to decrease the incidence and severity of CMV pneumonitis. High-dose oral acyclovir has been utilized with conflicting results.[79,80] Ganciclovir has also been utilized as a prophylactic agent. In cardiac transplant patients, ganciclovir reduced the incidence of CMV disease.[81] However, ganciclovir prophylaxis in lung transplant patients did not provide a benefit for D+/R- transplants, i.e., those patients with the greatest likelihood of developing severe disease.[82] A recent study compared acyclovir with ganciclovir for chemoprophylaxis of CMV infection in lung transplant recipients.[83] It was noted that during the early part of the study, the incidence of CMV infection and pneumonitis was reduced in those patients who received ganciclovir. However, this benefit had been lost at 2 years posttransplant, suggesting that longer-term prophylaxis might be necessary. Thus, the role of chemoprophylaxis in CMV pneumonia remains to be defined.

Bacterial Infections

Bacterial infections cause significant pulmonary disease in transplant recipients. Bacterial pneumonia is particularly common in lung transplant recipients, accounting for 50 percent of infections.[84] Gram-negative bacteria and staphylococcal infections occur early. Infection with encapsulated organisms occurs months or years after transplantation.[70] *Legionella* species also may cause pneumonia in transplant recipients.[85] Patients with prior tuberculosis infection may suffer reactivation.

CLINICAL PRESENTATION

The presentation of bacterial pneumonia in transplant recipients is similar to that of nonimmunocompromised hosts.[85] Rapid onset of cough, dyspnea, and hyperpyrexia is typical. Radiographically, bacterial pneumonias usually present with focal infiltrates, although *Legionella* may present as a diffuse interstitial lung lesion.[86]

DIAGNOSIS

The diagnosis of bacterial pneumonia in transplant recipients is made as in other hosts. Blood cultures remain the standard, and bronchoscopic techniques are used to obtain specimens for bacteriology. The specificity and sensitivity of BAL and protected brush specimens for the diagnosis of bacterial pneumonia in the transplant population remains to be defined fully.[76] Interpretation of the results of bronchoscopy is often complicated by prior administration of antibiotics.

THERAPY

The therapy of bacterial pneumonia in transplant recipients is determined optimally by microbiologic data. However, empiric therapy is often necessary while sputum, bronchoscopic specimens, and blood cultures are being analyzed. Empiric antibacterial therapy should be broad-spectrum, covering enteric gram-negative organisms and *Staphylococcus* species. In patients with diffuse lung lesions, strong consideration of therapy against *Legionella* species is warranted.

Prophylactic therapy against bacterial pneumonia has been utilized in lung transplant patients.[84] A regimen using ceftazidime and clindamycin has been shown to reduce the incidence of pneumonia from 48 to 9 percent.[84]

PROGNOSIS

The response of pneumonia in transplant patients to antibacterial therapy is variable, depending upon the organism causing pneumonia. In one series, the development of gram-negative pneumonia (often as a superinfection) was associated with a high mortality.[86]

Pneumocystis Carinii Pneumonia

The significant cell-mediated immune defect associated with transplantation readily explains the increased incidence of *Pneumocystis carinii* pneumonia (PCP) in transplant recipients. Previously, PCP was seen in 8 to 11 percent of transplant recipients.[88] However, the widespread use of prophylaxis against PCP has reduced dramatically this incidence.

CLINICAL PRESENTATION

Transplant recipients who develop PCP typically do so 3 to 4 months following transplant, although PCP has been reported years after transplantation. The presentation of PCP in transplant recipients differs from that in patients with HIV infection. The duration of symptoms is usually days to weeks,[88] as opposed to weeks to months in HIV-infected patients.[89] Common symptoms include fever, nonproductive cough, and dyspnea.

Physical examination findings are often subtle. Radiographic manifestations include the typical diffuse interstitial infiltrates but also focal infiltrates, masses, and pleural effusions.[88]

DIAGNOSIS

The diagnosis of PCP in transplant recipients may be made by examination of induced sputum, BAL, or biopsy specimens. The sensitivity of sputum induction for the detection has been reported to be as high as 64 percent in non-HIV-infected patients.[90] Bronchoalveolar lavage has a high sensitivity,[88] although probably not equal to its sensitivity in HIV-infected patients.

THERAPY

The treatment of PCP in transplant recipients is similar to its treatment in HIV-infected patients. The drug of choice for treatment is TMP/SMX (15 mg/kg/day of TMP and 75 mg/kg/day of SMX in three to four divided doses). Patients who have allergies to sulfa preparations should be treated with pentamidine (4 mg/kg/day). Treatment response rates in PCP pneumonia complicating organ transplantation are variable. Survival rates of 8 to 38 percent are reported, depending in part upon the transplanted organ.[61,88]

The role of corticosteroids in the treatment of established PCP with significant hypoxemia has not been well studied. Most transplant recipients, unlike HIV-infected patients, are receiving treatment with corticosteroids at the time of development of PCP. Consequently, most patients receive higher doses of steroids in response to the "stress" of pneumonia. Firm guidelines for indications, dose and duration of steroid therapy in the posttransplant setting have not been delineated.

Primary prophylaxis against PCP in transplant recipients has had a dramatic impact on the incidence of the disease. Most authors feel that low-dose TMP/SMZ approaches 100 percent in efficacy.[69,91] Three double-strength tablets weekly may be sufficient.[68]

Fungal Infections

The T-cell dysfunction associated with transplant immunosuppression, in combination with the suppressive effects of corticosteroids on polymorphonuclear leukocytes puts transplant recipients at increased risk of fungal infections.

Transplant recipients, like HIV-infected patients, are at risk for reactivation or new infection with pathogenic fungi such as *Cryptococcus neoformans*, *Histoplasma capsulatum*, and *Coccidioides immitis*. They are also at risk for infection with *Aspergillus fumigatus* and *Candida* species. Fungi caused 26 percent of pneumonias in one series of renal transplant recipients.[87]

The epidemiology and pathogenesis of endemic fungal infections is discussed in Chap. X. There are many similarities between fungal infection in HIV-infected patients and transplant patients. Only a brief overview follows.

HISTOPLASMOSIS

Histoplasmosis is rare outside of the midwestern river valleys. It may complicate transplantation as reactivation of prior infection or occur as a new infection.[92] In endemic regions, histoplasmosis may complicate 0.5 to 2.1 percent of transplants (the latter figure associated with an outbreak of the disease).[92,93]

The incidence of dissemination during histoplasmosis is much greater in transplant recipients than in normal hosts (77 percent in one series).[92] Clinical manifestations are usually those of disseminated disease; fever is the most common presenting symptom.[92] Physical findings are often nonspecific. The chest radiograph may be normal in approximately 50 percent of patients.[94] Diagnosis may be established by examination of blood, bone marrow, lung, and liver. Histoplasma antigen may prove useful. Therapy with amphotericin is currently the standard management. The role of azole antifungal agents remains to be fully delineated.

COCCIDIOIDOMYCOSIS

Infection with *C. immitis* is a significant problem in endemic regions of the southwest. One series of renal transplant recipients noted a 7 percent rate of infection.[95] Dissemination is much more frequent than in normal host. Pulmonary symptoms are common. Chest radiographs typically demonstrate bilateral miliary or interstitial infiltrates.[94] Diagnosis may be established by bronchoscopy. Bronchoalveolar lavage has been shown to identify *C. immitis* in 31 percent of non-HIV-infected individuals subsequently shown to have coccidioidomycosis.[96] Culture of BAL was positive in all cases. Transbronchial biopsies were positive in the 8 subjects in whom they were performed. Amphotericin remains the therapy of choice, though experience with itraconazole and fluconazole is growing.

ASPERGILLOSIS

Invasive aspergillosis complicates 1.5 to 5 percent of liver transplants.[97,98] The incidence of aspergillosis appears to be higher in liver transplant patients than in renal transplant recipients.[99] The clinical presentation is nonspecific. Cough, chest pain and hemoptysis may occur. Chest radiographs may demonstrate peripheral wedge-shaped infiltrates.[94] Diagnosis has previously required tissue documentation of hyphal invasion,[94] but because of its lethality, some authors have suggested that the presence of the organism in sputum should be regarded as significant.[97] Amphotericin remains the mainstay of therapy, but experience with itraconazole is growing.

CANDIDIASIS

Candidal pneumonia is unusual in organ transplant recipients. It is typically a manifestation of disseminated candidiasis.[94] Clinical manifestations are nonspecific. Chest radiography demonstrates similarly nonspecific patchy bilateral infiltrates. Diagnosis requires documentation of *Candida* species in blood or tissue invasion, as sputum cultures frequently reflect colonization. Therapy of deep *Candida* infections initially should be amphotericin until the organism is speciated. Some *Candida* species may be treated with fluconazole, though invasive *Candida* infections should be treated with amphotericin.

Pulmonary Infections in Recipients of Bone Marrow Transplant

The infectious pulmonary complications of bone marrow transplantation encompass the pulmonary infections discussed in the two preceding sections. Patients who have undergone bone marrow transplantation are subject to a prolonged period of neutropenia followed by impaired cellular and humoral immune function. Those patients who have undergone allogeneic bone marrow transplantation (ALBMT) also require further immunosuppression to prevent or ameliorate graft-versus-host disease (GVHD). This immunosuppression usually utilizes cyclosporine and corticosteroids. Thus, patients who have received an ALBMT suffer impairment of neutrophil, T-cell, and B-cell function.[1] The differences in immune impairment between ALBMT and autologous bone marrow transplants (ABMT) result in a difference between the incidence of pneumonia and pneumonitis (25.3 versus 4.1 percent)[101] and causes of pneumonia (37 percent viral pneumonias versus no viral pneumonias). It should be noted that the incidence of pulmonary complications in this study was much less than that of other experiences.[102] Nevertheless, the incidence of CMV pneumonia is much less in ABMT patients.[103] The time-course of pulmonary complications following bone marrow transplantation involves three discrete stages (see Fig. 104-5).[1] The first stage begins with the onset of neutropenia and lasts approximately 30 to 40 days, ending with engraftment. Prolongation of the first stage due to delayed engraftment or failure to engraft places the patient at risk for invasive fungal infection (see "Approach to Pneumonia in the Neutropenic Host," above). The second stage reflects return of immune function. This phase generally lasts 90 to 120 days.[1] Viral infections (particularly CMV infection in allogeneic transplant patients) are important complications during the second phase following transplant. Acute GVHD may complicate allogeneic transplants during this period and prolong it by preventing immune recovery.[100] The third phase following transplant consists of eventual return to normal immune function. This may occur 1 to 2 years fol-

lowing transplantation. Reactivation with varicella zoster may occur during this phase.[1] Infection with encapsulated bacterial organisms may also occur during this period because of persistent B-cell dysfunction. Chronic GVHD may also be present during the third phase of transplantation, contributing to immunosuppression and possibly causing lung disease.

BACTERIAL PNEUMONIA

The spectrum of bacterial infections seen in bone marrow transplant patients during the initial or aplastic period is similar to that seen in other neutropenic patients. The incidence of bacterial pneumonia reported varies greatly from one series to another, reflecting perhaps differing diagnostic criteria, ranging from only 2 percent in autopsy series to 50 percent in clinical series.[105,106] Gram-positive organisms are increasingly common causes of infection.[8] Clinical presentation is similar to that of other neutropenic hosts. Diagnosis continues to rest upon blood cultures, while the role of bronchoscopy is evolving. Empiric therapy with broad-spectrum antibiotics remains important in treating febrile episodes in neutropenic hosts.[19] It should be noted that these patients are also susceptible to infection with *Legionella* species.[105,107] In regions or institutions where *Legionella* is endemic consideration of empiric therapy directed against the organism is appropriate in marrow recipients with pneumonia.

In the later stages of transplantation pneumonia due to *S. pneumonia* and *H. influenzae* may result in overwhelming infection.[105] This susceptibility to bacterial pneumonia late in marrow transplantation is in part due to diminished levels of anti-polysaccharide antibodies.[108] The clinical presentation may be that of lobar pneumonia or overwhelming sepsis.[105] Antibacterial therapy is typically broad in its coverage to treat the possibility of *H. influenzae* as well as other gram-negative organisms. Prophylactic measures that may be useful include oral penicillin or TMP/SMZ and intravenous immune globulin infusion.[109,110]

FUNGAL PNEUMONIA

Fungal infections in marrow transplant recipients present a major diagnostic and therapeutic challenge. *Candida* and *Aspergillus* species are the predominant cause of fungal infections in marrow recipients, but infection with pathogenic fungi has also been reported.[111] Risk factors for deep fungal infection include prolonged neutropenia, allogeneic bone marrow transplant, and the development of severe GVHD.[112]

Aspergillus infection is common in bone marrow transplant recipients. It may account for one-third of nosocomial pneumonias in such patients.[113] *Aspergillus* infection usually occurs during the initial aplastic phase of transplantation but may be seen in the second and third phases as well, particularly in patients with GVHD. The clinical presentation is that seen in other neutropenic hosts: fever, cough, occasionally pleuritic chest pain, and hemoptysis. The chest radiograph may demonstrate focal infiltrates and nodules or may be normal.[28,29] The role of CT has been discussed above.

Diagnosis of invasive aspergillosis is difficult in marrow transplant recipients, as in other hosts. Sputum cultures or cultures of nasal swabs may demonstrate *Aspergillus* species. As noted above, positive sputum cultures in neutropenic nonsmokers had a very high correlation with invasive pulmonary aspergillosis.[31] Bronchoscopy often is utilized in an attempt to diagnose aspergillosis in bone marrow patients. Bronchoalveolar lavage has the best sensitivity of bronchoscopic techniques, with a reported sensitivity of 53 percent.[33] Transbronchial biopsy appears to add little to washings.[33,34] Bronchoscopy had a 75 percent positive predictive value.[33] A recent study in marrow recipients noted a similar overall sensitivity for BAL in detecting *Aspergillus* but also noted that, in patients with diffuse lung lesions due to aspergillosis, the sensitivity was 100 percent.[114] Open lung biopsy also is used to diagnose aspergillosis when other modalities fail, and it allows demonstration of tissue invasion. However, in one series of bone marrow transplant patients who underwent open lung biopsy, several cases of pulmonary aspergillosis were noted at autopsy that had not been diagnosed at open lung biopsy within the preceding 10 days.[36] The used of CT scanning with open biopsy (or video-assisted biopsy) may improve sensitivity for diagnosing pulmonary aspergillosis.

The standard therapy of invasive aspergillosis remains high-dose amphotericin B. As noted above, 13 of 14 neutropenic patients treated with high-dose (1.0 to 1.5 mg/kg/day) amphotericin survived.[38] Side effects are common. Liposomal preparations of amphotericin may allow the administration of higher doses with less toxicity.[43] Itraconazole also has been utilized in a marrow transplant recipient with invasive aspergillosis.[115] Both amphotericin and itraconazole have been utilized as prophylaxis against *Aspergillus* in patients undergoing cytotoxic chemotherapy.[41,42,47]

Candida infection is the other common fungal infection in marrow transplant recipients. *Candida* pneumonia is usually a manifestation of disseminated candidiasis; as many as 50 percent of patients who die of disseminated candidiasis have pulmonary involvement.[112] Diagnosis of *Candida* pneumonia requires documentation of tissue invasion. Demonstration of *Candida* in respiratory secretions should prompt a search for fungemia or other evidence of dissemination.

The therapy of *Candida* infection in marrow recipients is currently amphotericin B. Empiric antifungal therapy is typically initiated in marrow recipients who remain febrile despite broad-spectrum antibacterial antibiotics during the aplastic phase. Fluconazole may also be used to treat some *Candida* infections. In a recent trial noted above, there was a 67 percent response rate in marrow recipients with disseminated candidiasis treated with fluconazole.[51] Fluconazole has also been used for prophylaxis against candidal infections in bone marrow transplant recipients.[52] Fluconazole does not treat infection with *C. kruzei*, and there may be an increase in infections with this organism in patients treated with prophylactic fluconazole.[52]

VIRAL PNEUMONIA

Viral pneumonias continue to pose a major problem for bone marrow transplant recipients. Cytomegalovirus (CMV), varicella-zoster virus (VZV), and herpes simplex virus (HSV) may cause infection in marrow recipients, as may other respiratory viruses. Pneumonia caused by HSV is unusual,[109] and mucocutaneous involvement is almost always present. Pneumonia due to VZV is typically associated with disseminated infection following reactivation.[109] Rarely, VZV infection occurs in the absence of cutaneous lesions. Human herpesvirus type 6 and respiratory syncytial virus also have been reported as associated with pneumonitis in transplant recipients.[127,128]

Cytomegalovirus infection occurs in about 50 percent of allogeneic bone marrow transplant patients.[109] It is more frequent and severe in patients who are seropositive prior to transplant.[109] One-third of patients who develop CMV infection (or about 15 percent of all transplant patients) develop CMV pneumonitis.[116] Pneumonitis usually occurs during transplantation but may occur later if GVHD has caused continued immunosuppression. Pneumonitis due to CMV is rare in ABMT patients,[101,117] despite similar rates of infection.

The clinical presentation of CMV pneumonitis is one of dyspnea and non-productive cough. Fever and crackles on chest auscultation are common exam findings. Chest radiographs usually demonstrate an interstitial infiltrate.[118] Diagnosis may be made by demonstration of cytopathologic changes in the lung. Documentation of CMV in bronchoalveolar lavage of an allogeneic marrow transplant recipient with interstitial pneumonia should prompt therapy.

Treatment of CMV infection in bone marrow transplant recipients has been disappointing. While ganciclovir has had a significant impact upon survival in CMV pneumonia in solid-organ transplant patients, survival among ALBMT patients with CMV pneumonia has been < 50 percent when they were treated with ganciclovir alone.[119,120] The addition of high-titer CMV-specific immune globulin to ganciclovir has improved the survival of transplant recipients with CMV pneumonitis to 52 to 70 percent.[121,122]

Prophylaxis against CMV infection has been attempted with ganciclovir and CMV-specific immune globulin. Administration of ganciclovir to CMV-seropositive ALBMT recipients reduced the incidence of CMV infection from 56 to 20 percent.[123] There appeared to be less CMV disease as well. Neutropenia complicated the therapy, and there was no difference in overall survival between groups. Similar results were noted in another study that utilized ganciclovir as primary prophylaxis in conjunction with CMV hyperimmune globulin.[124] Ganciclovir has also been used as prophylaxis against CMV pneumonitis, utilizing routine BAL to identify patients shedding CMV in the lungs.[125] Patients with positive BAL cultures were treated with either ganciclovir or placebo. The mortality from CMV pneumonitis was reduced from 70 percent in the control group to 25 percent in the treatment group. The administration of CMV-specific immune globulin has resulted in reduction in viremia but does not appear to reduce the incidence of pneumonitis.[126]

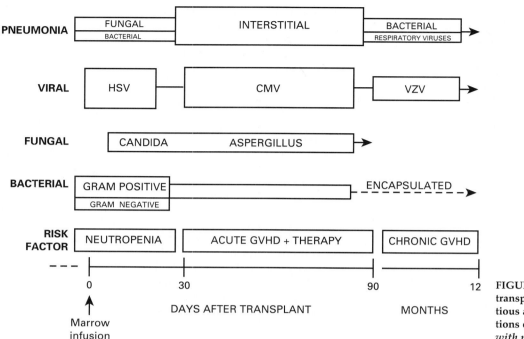

FIGURE 104-5 Stages of marrow transplantation and typical infectious and noninfectious complications over time. (*From Winston,*[110] *with permission.*)

PNEUMOCYSTIS CARINII PNEUMONIA

Infection with PCP has become rare among bone marrow transplant recipients. Effective prophylaxis with TMP/SMZ has virtually eliminated the disease in compliant patients.[135] In patients unable or unwilling to take TMP/SMZ, PCP still occurs.[101] In patients unable to take TMP/SMZ, aerosolized pentamidine is an effective alternative.

NONINFECTIOUS PULMONARY DISEASE

There are several life-threatening, noninfectious pulmonary complications of bone marrow transplantation. Alveolar hemorrhage and idiopathic pneumonia syndrome are seen in both ABMT and ALBMT.[103,129] Bronchiolitis obliterans is an important late complication of ALBMT.[130] The former complications may be mistaken for infectious processes. Bronchiolitis obliterans tends to present later in the course of transplantation and is usually readily diagnosed by pulmonary function testing and chest radiography.

ALVEOLAR HEMORRHAGE

Diffuse alveolar hemorrhage (DAH) complicating bone marrow transplant was initially described in autologous marrow recipients, occurring in 21 percent of the patients.[129] Subsequently, the incidence has been noted to range from 1 to 10 percent, and it has been described in allogeneic transplant recipients.[131,132] The onset of alveolar hemorrhage ranged from 7 to 40 days following transplant, with the median at 12 days.[129] The clinical presentation is one of dyspnea or cough, but hemoptysis was not reported. Fever is a common clinical finding. Chest radiography demonstrates bilateral infiltrates. The diagnosis of alveolar hemorrhage may be made by assessment of lack of clearing of blood in

serial aliquots of BAL fluid or by quantitation of hemosiderin in alveolar macrophages.[129,133]

Initial reports of DAH noted mortality rates that approached 100 percent.[129,102] Subsequently two historically controlled studies demonstrated a significant improvement in survival when high-dose corticosteroids were given.[132,134] Survival to discharge in the larger of the two studies was 9.1 percent among patients who received supportive therapy and 33 percent among those treated with high-dose steroids.[132]

IDIOPATHIC PNEUMONIA SYNDROME

The incidence of interstitial pneumonia of unknown etiology varies from series to series but may approach 40 percent of transplant recipients.[102,109] It appears in both ALBMT and ABMT patients, though it seems to be more frequent in the latter.[103] The syndrome typically manifests itself 40 to 50 days following transplant, but there is an earlier peak in the first 14 days.[103] Clinical manifestations are largely progressive dyspnea and cough. Chest radiograph usually demonstrates a diffuse interstitial lung lesion. Diagnosis requires demonstration of alveolar damage, interstitial infiltration, or fibrosis in the absence of infectious organisms.

Idiopathic pneumonia syndrome is associated with a mortality of 71 percent, though only 32 percent of patients died of progressive respiratory failure.[103] Infection complicating the course of the idiopathic lung lesion was common. Some patients appeared to benefit from corticosteroids, though the response rate is yet to be fully defined.

DIAGNOSTIC APPROACH

The broad spectrum of pulmonary pathology that complicates bone marrow transplantation mandates an aggressive diagnostic strategy. Because alveolar hemorrhage may appear to mimic infectious pneumonias and probably benefits from radically different therapy (corticosteroids versus antibiotics), early bronchoscopy is appropriate to establish or exclude DAH. If the patient fails to respond to broad-spectrum antimicrobials and no diagnosis is established on bronchoscopy, then either repeat bronchoscopy or open lung biopsy should be strongly considered. Focal infiltrates that remain undiagnosed should raise concern about aspergillosis, as the diagnosis may be missed even with open biopsy.

Summary

Infectious pulmonary complications are common in immunosuppressed hosts. While many pathogens occur in all immunocompromised groups, each immunologic defect is marked by the prevalence of particular agents. It is important to note that many patients have defects of neutrophil and lymphocyte function, predisposing them to a broader range of infections. Finally, our understanding of immune defects and their complications has allowed the institution of effective prophylaxis against a number of infectious agents. Continued research is necessary to refine these prophylactic regimens. It is also important to utilize the lessons learned in neutropenic patients and organ transplant recipients as aggressive immunomodulatory therapy is used in other diseases.

References

1. Hiemenz J, Greene J: Special considerations for the patient undergoing allogeneic or autologous bone marrow transplantation. *Hematol Oncol Clin North Am* 1993; 7:961–1002.
2. Scadden D, Zon L, Groopman J: Pathophysiology and management of HIV-associated hematologic disorders. *Blood* 1989; 74:1455–1465.
3. Bodey G, Buckley M, Sathe Y, et al.: Quantitative relationships between circulating leukocytes and infection in patients with acute leukemia. *Ann Intern Med* 1966; 64:328–340.
4. Antman K, Griffin J, Elias A: Effect of recombinant human granulocyte-macrophage colony-stimulating factor on chemotherapy-induced myelosuppression. *N Engl J Med* 1988; 319:593–598.
5. Crawford J, Ozer H, Stoller R: Reduction by granulocyte colony stimulating factor of fever and neutropenia induced by chemotherapy in patients with small-cell lung cancer. *N Engl J Med* 1991; 325:164–170.
6. Sibille Y, Reynolds H: Macrophages and polymorphonuclear neutrophils in lung defense and injury. *Am Rev Respir Dis* 1990; 141:471–501.
7. Schaffner A, Davis D, Schaffner T, et al.: In vitro susceptibility of fungi to killing by neutrophil granulocytes discriminates between primary pathogenicity and opportunism. *J Clin Invest* 1986; 78:511–524.
7. Lee J, Pizzo P: Management of the cancer patient with fever and prolonged neutropenia. *Hematol Oncol Clin North Am* 1993; 7:937–960.
8. Bochud P, Calandra T, Francioli P: Bacteremia due to *viridans* streptococci in neutropenic patients: A review. *Am J Med* 1994; 97:256–264.
9. Bochud P, Eggiman P, Calandra T, et al.: Bacteremia due to *viridans* streptococcus in neutropenic patients with cancer: Clinical spectrum and risk factors. *Clin Infect Dis* 1994; 18:25–31.
10. Schimpff S: Infections in the cancer patient-diagnosis, prevention and treatment, in Mandell G, Bennett J, Dolin R (eds): *Principles and Practice of Infectious Diseases*. New York, Churchill-Livingstone, 1995.
11. Wiener-Kronish J, Tsutomo S, Ichidai K, et al.: Alveolar epithelial injury and pleural empyema in acute *P. aeurginosa* pneumonia in anesthetized rabbits. *J Appl Phys* 1993; 75:1661–1669.
12. Rubin M, Hawthorn J, Marshall D, et al.: Gram-positive infections and the use of vancomycin in 550 episodes of fever and neutropenia. *Ann Intern Med* 1988; 108:30–35.
13. Xaubet A, Torres A, Marco F, et al.: Pulmonary infiltrates in immunocompromised patients: Diagnostic value of telescoping plugged catheter and bronchoalveolar lavage. *Chest* 1989; 95: 130–135.
14. Meduri G, Stover D, Greeno R, et al.: Bilateral bronchoalveolar lavage in the diagnosis of opportunistic pulmonary infections. *Chest* 1991; 100:1272–1276.
15. Bennet C, Vardiman J, Golumb H: Disseminated atypical mycobacterial infection in patients with hairy cell leukemia. *Am J Med* 1986; 80:891–896.
16. Rivera M, Jules-Elysee K, Stover D: Nontransplant chemotherapy immunosuppression, in Niderman M, Sarosi G, Glassroth J, (eds): *Respiratory Infections: A Scientific Basis for Management*. Philadelphia, Saunders, 1994.
17. Barloon T, Galvin J, Mori M, et al.: High-resolution ultrafast chest CT in the clinical management of the febrile bone marrow transplant patients with normal or nonspecific chest roentgenograms. *Chest* 1991; 99:928–933.
18. Chastre J, Viau F, Brun P, et al.: Prospective evaluation of the protected specimen brush for the diagnosis of pulmonary infections in ventilated patients. *Am Rev Respir Dis* 1984; 130: 924–929.
19. Pizzo P: Management of fever in patients with cancer and treatment-induced neutropenia. *N Engl J Med* 1993; 328:1323–1332.
20. DeGregorio M, Lee W, Linker C, et al.: Fungal infections in patients with acute leukemia. *Am J Med* 1982; 73:543–548.
21. Sugar A: Mucormycosis. *Clin Infect Dis* 1992; 14:S126–129.
22. Young R, Jennings A, Bennett J: Species identification of invasive aspergillosis in man. *Am J Clin Pathol* 1972; 58:554–557.
23. Walsh T, Dixon D: Nosocomial aspergillosis: Environmental microbiology, hospital epidemiology, diagnosis, and treatment. *Eur J Epidemiol* 1989; 5:131–142.
24. Davies S: Fungal pneumonia. *Med Clin North Am* 1994; 78:1049–1065.
25. Gerson S, Talbot G, Hurwitz S, et al.: Prolonged granulocytopenia: The major risk factor for invasive pulmonary aspergillosis in patients with acute leukemia. *Ann Intern Med* 1984; 100:345–351.
26. McWhinney P, Kibbler C, Hamon M: Progress in the diagnosis and management of aspergillosis in bone marrow transplantation: 13 years experience. *Clin Infect Dis* 1993; 17:397–404.
27. Robertson M, Larson R: Recurrent fungal pneumonias in patients with acute nonlymphocytic leukemia undergoing multiple courses of intensive chemotherapy.
28. Sinclair A, Rossof A, Coltman C: Recognition and successful management in pulmonary aspergillosis in leukemia. *Cancer* 1978; 42:2019–2024.
29. Pennington J: Aspergillosis pneumonia in hematologic malignancy: Improvements in diagnosis and therapy. *Arch Intern Med* 1977; 137:769.
30. Kuhlman J, Fishman E, Burch P, et al.: Invasive pulmonary aspergillosis in acute leukemia: The contribution of CT to early diagnosis and aggressive management. *Chest* 1987; 92:95–99.

31. Yu V, Muder R, Poorsattar A: Significance of isolation of *Aspergillus* from the respiratory tract in diagnosis of invasive pulmonary aspergillosis. *Am J Med* 1986; 81:249–254.

32. Suffredini A: Diagnosis of infection: Noninvasive and invasive procedures, in Shelhamer J (moderator): Respiratory disease in the immunocompromised patient. *Ann Intern Med* 1992; 117:415–431.

33. Kahn F, Jones J, England D: The role of bronchoalveolar lavage in the diagnosis of invasive pulmonary aspergillosis. *Am J Clin Pathol* 1986; 86:518–523.

34. Albeda S, Talbot, Gerson S: Role of fiberoptic bronchoscopy in the diagnosis of invasive pulmonary aspergillosis in patients with acute leukemia. *Am J Med* 1984; 76:1027–1033.

35. McCabe R, Brooks R, Mark J, Remington J: Open lung biopsy in patients with acute leukemia. *Am J Med* 1985; 78:609–616.

36. Crawford S, Hackman R, Clark J: Open lung biopsy diagnosis of diffuse pulmonary infiltrates after marrow transplantation. *Chest* 1988; 94:949–953.

37. Walsh T: Management of immunocompromised patients with evidence of an invasive mycosis. *Hematol Oncol Clin North Am* 1993; 7:1003–1026.

38. Burch P, Karp J, Merz W, et al.: Favorable outcome of invasive aspergillosis in patients with acute leukemia. *J Clin Oncol* 1987; 5:1985–1993.

39. Ribrag V, Dreyfus F, Venot A: Prognostic factors of invasive pulmonary aspergillosis in leukemic patients. *Leuk Lymph* 1993; 10:317–321.

40. Pizzo P: Empirical therapy and prevention in the immunocompromised host, in Mandell G, Bennett J, Dolin R (eds): *Principles and Practice of Infectious Disease*. New York, Churchill-Livingstone, 1995.

41. Meyers J, Spencer H, Watts J, et al.: Cytomegalovirus pneumonia after human marrow transplantation. *Ann Intern Med* 1975; 82:181–188.

42. Karp J, Burch P, Merz W: An approach to intensive antileukemia therapy in patients with previous invasive aspergillosis. *Am J Med* 1988; 85:203–206.

43. Mills W, Chopra R, Linch D, Goldstone A: Liposomal amphotericin B in the treatment of fungal infections in neutropenic patients: A single-centre experience of 133 episodes in 116 patients. *Br J Haematol* 1994; 86:754–760.

44. Graybill J: Future directions of antifungal chemotherapy. *Clin Infect Dis* 1992; 14:(S1):S170–S181.

45. Denning D, Lee J, Hostetler J, et al.: NIAID Mycoses Study Group multicenter trial of oral itraconazole therapy for invasive aspergillosis. *Am J Med* 1994; 97:135–144.

46. van't Wout J: Itraconazole in neutropenic patients. *Chemotherapy* 1992; 38:(S1):S23–S26.

47. Todeschini G, Murari C, Bonesi R, et al.: Oral itraconazole plus nasal amphotericin B for prophylaxis of invasive aspergillosis in patients with hematological malignancies. *Eur J Clin Microbiol Infect Dis* 1993; 12:614–618.

48. Sobel J, Vazquez J: Candidemia and systemic candidiasis. *Semin Respir Infect* 1990; 5:1123–1137.

49. Dubois P, Myerowitz R, Allen C: Pathological correlation of pulmonary candidiasis in immunosuppressed patients. *Cancer* 1977; 40:1026–1036.

50. Martino P, Girmena C, Micozzi A, et al.: Prospective study of *Candida* colonization, use of amphotericin B and development of invasive mycosis in neutropenic patients. *Eur J Clin Microbiol Infect Dis* 1994; 13:797–804.

51. de Pauw B, Raemaekers J, Donnelly J, et al.: An open study on the safety and efficacy of fluconazole in the treatment of disseminated *Candida* infections in patients treated for hematological malignancies. *Ann Hematol* 1995; 70:83–87.

52. Goodwin J, Winston D, Greenfield R, et al.: A controlled trial of fluconazole to prevent fungal infections in patients undergoing bone marrow transplant. *N Engl J Med* 1992; 326:845–851.

53. EORTC International Antimicrobial Therapy Cooperative Group: Empiric antifungal therapy in febrile granulocytic patients. *Am J Med* 1989; 86:668–672.

54. Ramsey P, Fife K, Hackman R, et al.: Herpes simplex pneumonia: Clinical, virologic and pathologic features in 20 patients. *Ann Intern Med* 1982; 97:813–820.

55. Cate T: Viral pneumonia in immunocompetent adults, in Niederman M, Sarosi G, Glassroth J (eds): *Respiratory Infections: A Scientific Basis for Management*. Philadelphia, Saunders, 1994.

56. Walsh T, Rubin M, Pizzo P: Respiratory diseases in patients with malignant neoplasms, in Shelhamer J, Pizzo, Parillo J, Masur H (eds): *Respiratory Disease in the Immunocompromised Host*. Philadelphia, Lippincott, 1991.

57. Dichter J, Levine S, Shelhamer J: Approach to the immunocompromised host with pulmonary symptoms. *Hematol Oncol Clin North Am* 1993; 7:887–912.

58. Balow J: Cyclophosphamide suppression of established cell-mediated immunity. *J Clin Invest* 1975; 56:65070.

59. Rubin R, Johnson P (eds): Pulmonary infection in solid organ transplant recipients. *Semin Respir Infect* 1990; 5.

60. Ettinger N, Trulock E: Pulmonary considerations of organ transplantation (Parts I,II,III). *Am Rev Respir Dis* 1991; 143:1386–1405, 144:213–223, 433–451.

61. Trulock E (ed): Infectious complications of organ transplantation. *Semin Respir Infect* 1993; 8.

62. Abbas A, Lichtman A, Pober J: Immune responses to tissue transplant, in Abbas A, Lichtman A, Pober J (eds): *Cellular and Molecular Immunology*. Philadelphia, Saunders, 1994.

63. Abbas A, Lichtman A, Pober J: Molecular basis of T cell antigen recognition and activation, in Abbas A, Lichtman A, Pober J (eds): *Cellular and Molecular Immunology*. Philadelphia, Saunders, 1994.

64. Superdock K, Helderman J: Immunosuppressive drugs and their effects. *Semin Respir Infect* 1993; 8:152–159.

65. Boumpas D, Anastassiou E, Older S, et al.: Dexamethasone inhibits human interleukin 2 but not interleukin 2 receptor gene expression in vitro at the level of nuclear transcription. *J Clin Invest* 1991; 87:1739–1747.

66. Schreiber S, Crabtree G: The mechanism of action of cyclosporin A and FK506. *Immunol Today* 1992; 13:136–142.

67. Ho M, Dummer J: Infections in transplant recipients, in Mandell G, Bennett J, Dolin R (eds): *Principles and Practice of Infectious Diseases*. New York, Churchill Livingstone, 1995.

68. Dummer S, Ho M, Simmons R: Infections in solid organ transplant recipients, in Mandell G, Bennett J, Dolin R (eds): *Principles and Practice of Infectious Diseases*. New York, Churchill Livingstone, 1995.

69. Dummer S, Kusen S: Liver transplantation and related infections. *Semin Respir Infect* 1993; 8:191–198.

70. Rubin R, Wolfson J, Cosimi A, Tolkoff-Rubin N: Infection in the renal transplant recipient. *Am J Med* 1981; 70:405–411.

71. Bailey T: Prevention of cytomegalovirus disease. *Semin Respir Infect* 1993; 8:225–232.

72. Dummer J, White L, Ho M, et al.: Morbidity of cytomegalovirus infection in recipients of heart or lung transplants. *J Infect Dis* 1985; 152:1182–1191.

73. Anderson D, Jordan M: Viral pneumonia in recipients of solid organ transplants. *Semin Respir Infect* 1990; 5:38–49.

74. Ho M, Cytomegalovirus, in Mandell G, Bennett J, Dolin R (eds): *Principles and Practice of Infectious Diseases*. New York, Churchill Livingstone, 1995.

75. Stover D, Zaman M, Hajdu S, et al.: Bronchoalveolar lavage in the diagnosis of diffuse pulmonary infiltrates in the immunocompromised host. *Ann Intern Med* 1984; 101:1–7.

76. Ettinger N: Invasive diagnostic approach to pulmonary infiltrates. *Semin Resp Infect* 1993; 8:168–176.

77. Ettinger N, Bailey T, Trulock E, et al.: Cytomegalovirus infection and pneumonitis: Impact after isolated lung transplantation. Washington University Lung Transplant Group. *Am Rev Respir Dis* 1993; 147:1017–1023.

78. Kirklin J, Naftel D, Levine T, et al.: Cytomegalovirus infection after heart transplantation: Risk factors for infection and death: A multi-institutional study. The Cardiac Transplant Research Database Group. *J Heart Lung Transplant* 1994; 13:394–404.

79. Balfour H, Chace B, Stapleton J, et al.: A randomized, placebo controlled trial of oral acyclovir for the prevention of cytomegalovirus disease in recipients of renal allografts. *N Engl J Med* 1989; 320:1381–1387.

80. Bailey T, Ettinger N, Storch G, et al.: Failure of high-dose oral acyclovir with or without immune globulin to prevent primary CMV disease in solid organ transplant recipients. *Am J Med* 1993; 95:273–278.

81. Merigan T, Renlund D, Keay S, et al.: A controlled trial of ganciclovir to prevent cytomegalovirus disease after heart transplantation. *N Engl J Med* 1992; 326:1182–1186.

82. Bailey T, Trulock E, Ettinger N, et al.: Failure of prophylactic ganciclovir to prevent cytomegalovirus disease in recipients of lung transplants. *J Infect Dis* 1992; 165:548–552.

83. Duncan S, Grgurich W, Iacono A: A comparison of ganciclovir and acyclovir to prevent cytomegalovirus after lung transplantation. *Am J Respir Crit Care Med* 1994; 150:146–152.

84. Paradis I, Williams P: Infection after lung transplantation. *Semin Respir Dis* 1993; 8:207–215.

85. Mermel L, Maki D: Bacterial pneumonia in solid organ transplantation. *Semin Respir Med* 1990; 5:10–29.

86. Ampel N, Wing E: *Legionella* infection in transplant patients. *Semin Respir Infect* 1990; 5:30–37.

87. Ramsey P, Rubin R, Tolkoff-Rubin N, et al.: The renal transplant with fever and pulmonary infiltrates: Etiology, clinical manifestations and management. *Medicine* 1980; 59:205–222.

88. Dummer J: *Pneumocystis carinii* infections in transplant recipients. *Semin Respir Med* 1990; 5:50–57.

89. Kovacs J, Hiemenz J, Macher A, et al.: *Pneumocystis carinii* pneumonia: A comparison between patients with the acquired immunodeficiency syndrome and patients with other immunodeficiencies. *Ann Intern Med* 1984; 100;663–671.

90. Godwin C, Brown D, Masur H, et al.: Sputum induction: A quick and sensitive technique for diagnosing *Pneumocystis carinii* pneumonia in immunosuppressed patients. *Respir Care* 1991; 36:33–39.

91. Rubin R: Infectious disease complications of renal transplantation. *Kidney Int* 1993; 44:221–236.

92. Wheat L, Smith E, Sathapatayavongs B, et al.: Histoplasmosis in renal allograft recipients: Two large urban outbreaks. *Arch Intern Med* 1983; 143:703–707.

93. Davies S, Sarosi G, Peterson P, et al.: Disseminated histoplasmosis in renal transplant recipients. *Am J Surg* 1979; 137:686–691.

94. Zeluff B: Fungal pneumonia in transplant recipients. *Semin Respir Infect* 1990; 5:80–89.

95. Cohen I, Galgiani J, Potter D, Ogden D: Coccidioidomycosis in renal replacement therapy. *Arch Intern Med* 1982; 142:489–494.

96. DiTommasso J, Ampel N, Sobonya R, Bloom J: Bronchoscopic diagnosis of pulmonary coccidioidomycosis: Comparison of cytology, culture, and transbronchial biopsy. *Diagn Microbiol Infect Dis* 1994; 18:83–87.

97. Kusne S, Torres-Cisneros J, Manez R, et al.: Factors associated with invasive lung aspergillosis and significance of positive *Aspergillus* culture after liver transplantation. *J Infect Dis* 1992; 166:1379–1383.

98. Singh N, Mieles L, Yu V, Gayowski T: Invasive aspergillosis in liver transplant patients with candidemia and consumption coagulopathy and failure of prophylaxis with low-dose amphotericin B. *Clin Infect Dis* 1993; 17:906–908.

99. Boon A, O'Brien D, Adams D: 10-year review of invasive aspergillosis detected at necropsy. *J Clin Pathol* 1991; 44:452–454.

100. Paulin T, Ringden O, Nilsson B: Immunological recovery after bone marrow transplantation: Role of age, graft versus host disease, prednisolone treatment and infections. *Bone Marrow Transplant* 1986; 1:317–328.

101. Gentile G, Micozzi A, Girmenia C, et al.: Pneumonia in allogeneic and autologous bone marrow recipients: A retrospective study. *Chest* 1993; 104:371–375.

102. Jules-Elysee K, Stover D, Yahalom J, et al.: Pulmonary complications in lymphoma patients treated with high-dose chemotherapy and autologous bone marrow transplantation. *Am Rev Respir Dis* 1992; 146:485–491.

103. Clark J, Hansen J, Hertz M, et al.: Idiopathic pneumonia syndrome after bone marrow transplantation. *Am Rev Respir Dis* 1993; 147:1601–1606.

104. Dompeling E, Donnelly J, Raemaekers J, DePauw B: Pre-emptive administration of corticosteroids prevents the development of ARDS associated *Streptococcus mitis* bacteremia following chemotherapy with high-dose cytarabine. *Ann Hematol* 1994; 69–71.

105. Crawford S: Bone-marrow transplantation and related infections. *Semin Respir Infect* 1993; 8:183–190.

106. Krowka M, Rosenow E, Hoagland H: Pulmonary complications of bone marrow transplantation. *Chest* 1985; 87:237–246.

107. Benz-Lemione E, Dewail V, Castel O, et al.: Nosocomial legionnaire's disease in a marrow transplant unit. *Bone Marrow Transplant* 1991; 7:61–63.

108. Lum L: Immune recovery after bone marrow transplantation. *Hematol Oncol Clin North Am* 1990; 4:659–675.

109. Winston D: Infections in bone marrow transplant recipients, in Mandell G, Bennett J, Dolin R (eds): *Principles and Practice of Infectious Diseases*. New York, Churchill Livingstone, 1995.

110. Sullivan K, Kopecky K, Jacom J, et al.: Immunomodulatory and antimicrobial efficacy of intravenous immunoglobulin in bone marrow transplantation. *N Engl J Med* 1990; 323:705–712.

111. Riley D, Galgiani J, O'Donnell M, et al.: Coccidioidomycosis in bone marrow recipients. *Transplantation* 1993; 45:1531–1533.

112. Goodrich J, Reed E, Mori M, et al.: Clinical features and analysis of risk factors for invasive candidal infection after marrow transplantation. *J Infect Dis* 1991; 164:731–740.

113. Pannuti C, Gingrich R, Pfaller M, et al.: Nosocomial pneumonia in adult patients undergoing bone marrow transplantation: A 9-year study. *Bone Marrow Transplant* 1991; 9:77–84.

114. McWhinney P, Kibbler C, Hamon M, et al.: Progress in the diagnosis and management of aspergillosis in bone marrow transplantation: 13 years' experience. *Clin Infect Dis* 1993; 17:397–404.

115. Denning D, Stepan D, Blume K, Steven D: Control of invasive pulmonary aspergillosis with oral itraconazole in a bone marrow transplant patient. *J Infect* 1992; 24:73–79.

116. Meyers J, Flournoy N, Thomas E: Risk factors for cytomegalovirus infection after human marrow transplantation. *J Infect Dis* 1986; 153:478–488.

117. Ljungman P, Biron P, Bosi A, et al.: Cytomegalovirus interstitial pneumonia in autologous bone marrow transplant recipient. Infectious Disease Working Party of European Group for Bone Marrow Transplantation. *Bone Marrow Transplant* 1994; 13: 209–212.

118. Meyers J, Spencer H, Watts J, et al.: Cytomegalovirus pneumonia after human marrow transplantation. *Ann Intern Med* 1975; 82:181–188.

119. Ettinger N, Selby P, Powles R, et al.: Cytomegalovirus pneumo-

nia: The use of ganciclovir in marrow transplant recipients. *J Antimicrob Chemother* 1989; 24:53–62.

120. Crumpacker C, Marlowe S, Zhang J, et al.: Treatment of cytomegalovirus pneumonia. *Rev Infect Dis* 1988; 10:538S-546S.

121. Emanuel D, Cunningham I, Jules-Elysee K, et al.: Cytomegalovirus pneumonia after bone marrow transplantation successfully treated with the combination of ganciclovir and high dose intravenous immune globulin. *Ann Intern Med* 109:777–782.

122. Reed E, Bowden R, Dandliker P, et al.: Treatment of cytomegalovirus pneumonia with ganciclovir and intravenous cytomegalovirus immunoglobulin in patients with bone marrow transplants. *Ann Intern Med* 1988; 109:783–788.

123. Winston D, Ho W, Bartoni K, et al.: Ganciclovir prophylaxis of cytomegalovirus infection and disease in allogeneic bone marrow transplant recipients: Results of a placebo-controlled, double-blind trial. *Ann Intern Med* 1993; 118:179–184.

124. von Bueltzingsloewen A, Bordigoni P, Witz F, et al.: Prophylactic use of ganciclovir for allogeneic bone marrow transplant recipients. *Bone Marrow Transplant* 1993; 12:197–202.

125. Schmidt G, Horak D, Niland J, et al.: A randomized, controlled trial of prophylactic ganciclovir for cytomegalovirus pulmonary infection in recipients of allogeneic bone marrow transplants; The City of Hope-Stanford-Syntex CMV Study Group. *N Engl J Med* 1991; 324:1005–1011.

126. Bowden R, Risher L, Rogers K, et al.: Cytomegalovirus (CMV)-specific intravenous immunoglobulin for the prevention of primary CMV infection and disease after marrow transplant. *J Infect Dis* 1991; 164:483–487.

127. Pitalia A, Liu-yin J, Freemont A, et al.: Immunohistological detection of human herpes virus 6 in formalin-fixed, paraffin-embedded lung tissues. *J Med Virol* 1993; 41:103–107.

128. Englund J, Sullivan C, Jordan C, et al.: Respiratory syncytial virus infection in immunocompromised adults. *Ann Intern Med* 1988; 109:203–208.

129. Robbins R, Linder J, Stahl M, et al.: Diffuse alveolar hemorrhage in autologous bone marrow transplant recipients. *Am J Med* 1989; 87:511–518.

130. Ralph D, Springmeyer S, Sullivan K, et al.: Rapidly progressive air-flow obstruction in marrow transplant recipients: Possible association between obliterative bronchiolitis and chronic graft-versus-host disease. *Am Rev Respir Dis* 1984; 129:641–644.

131. Mulder P, Meinesz A, de Vries E, Mulder N: Diffuse alveolar hemorrhage in autologous bone marrow transplant recipients (letter). *Am J Med* 1991; 90:278–280.

132. Metcalf J, Rennard S, Reed E, et al.: Corticosteroids as adjunctive therapy for diffuse alveolar hemorrhage associated with bone marrow transplantation. *Am J Med* 1994; 96:327–333.

133. Kahn F, Jones J, England D: Diagnosis of pulmonary hemorrhage in the immunocompromised host. *Am Rev Respir Dis* 1987; 136:155–160.

134. Chao N, Duncan S, Long G, et al.: Corticosteroid therapy for diffuse alveolar hemorrhage in autologous bone marrow transplant recipients. *Ann Intern Med* 1991; 114:145–146.

135. Winston D: Prophylaxis and treatment of infection in the bone marrow transplant recipient. *Curr Clin Top Infect Dis* 1993; 13:293–321.

Chapter 105 _____
PULMONARY INFECTIONS IN HIV-INFECTED INDIVIDUALS

THEODORE H. LEWIS, JR.

Impact of HIV Infection on Pulmonary Defenses

It is estimated that 10 million people worldwide and approximately 1 million people in the United States are infected with the human immunodeficiency virus (HIV). The immunocompromised state of patients infected with this virus is unique in many ways. It affects virtually all facets of pulmonary defense, leading to many different pulmonary infections. The lungs are the most frequent site of infectious complications in HIV infection.[1] The degree of immunosuppression increases over the course of the disease, changing the infections to which the patient is susceptible. This immunosuppression and its progression results from a decline in the number of circulating CD4+ helper lymphocytes. HIV infects cells that express the CD4 receptor, including CD4+ lymphocytes and alveolar macrophages, as well as colonic epithelium, central nervous system glial cells, and others. Alveolar macrophages are able to survive infection and may act as a reservoir of virus. There is some evidence that the function of HIV-infected macrophages is impaired. Some authors have noted that objective measures of phagocytosis are unchanged during HIV infection,[2] whereas others have noted decreased recognition and binding.[3] Measures of cell killing also appear to be reduced.[3,4] Lymphocytes infected by HIV are often destroyed by cytotoxic T cells as they express viral antigen; others fall victim to apoptosis.[5] The result is a progressive decline in total number of helper T cells. Lymphocyte function is also impaired following infection with HIV. Lymphocyte proliferation is a response to soluble antigens in HIV-infected men with normal numbers of CD4+ T cells.[5] T lymphocyte production of interferon-γ in response to IL-2 stimulation is reduced in patients with advanced HIV infection.[6] This decline in number and function of CD4+ lymphocytes impairs both cellular and humoral immunity through loss of the mechanisms described in the preceding chapter. The absolute number of circulating CD4+ lymphocytes correlates well with the degree of immune impairment and the type of infections for which the patient is at risk[7] (Fig. 105-1). Pulmonary pathogens that possess a high degree of virulence tend to occur early in the course of HIV infection. Pathogens that are easily handled by normal pulmonary defenses occur later in the course of HIV infection.

Tuberculosis and HIV Infection

One pathogen that is capable of causing disease in normal hosts is *Mycobacterium tuberculosis*. Tuberculosis infects one-third of the world's population, 10 million people in the United States. It is estimated that 40 percent of HIV-infected individuals are infected with *M. tuberculosis* worldwide, and close to one-half of HIV-infected individuals in Africa are believed to be infected with tuberculosis.[8] In the United States these percentages are far less, but certain groups in

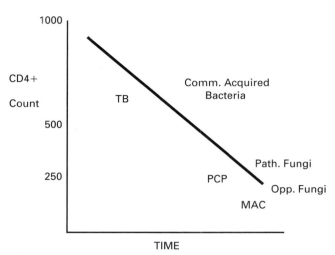

FIGURE 105-1 Progressive fall in CD4+ lymphocyte count associated with opportunistic infections. (*From Long et al.,*[17] *with permission.*)

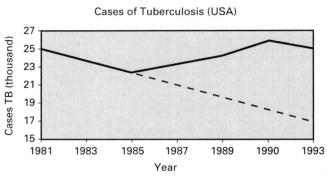

FIGURE 105-2 Cases of tuberculosis reported in the United States 1981–1993 (*solid line*) compared with the expected decline in tuberculosis (*dotted line*).

high-risk areas may have rates of coinfection in excess of 40 percent.[9]

PATHOPHYSIOLOGY

Mycobacterium tuberculosis generally enters the body by inhalation of droplet nuclei generated by the cough of a patient with active pulmonary tuberculosis. Bacilli are phagocytosed initially by alveolar macrophages. The tuberculosis bacillus is capable of avoiding destruction by the alveolar macrophage, possibly by disruption of phagosome-lysosome fusion.[10] It then replicates within the macrophage. Tuberculosis bacilli may travel through lymphatics or the blood to lymph nodes or other regions of the body. Approximately 6 to 8 weeks following infection cell-mediated immunity develops and there is an influx of monocytes and CD4+ lymphocytes into areas where the tuberculosis bacillus has proliferated, forming collections of these cells known as granulomas. Lymphokines and cytokines released by these cells cause activation of macrophages, leading to the death of the organism. The infection is usually contained by these defenses, and only 10 percent of patients infected with tuberculosis will develop active (uncontrolled) disease over their lifetime, about 5 percent in the first 2 years following infection. Organisms may persist within granulomata without causing clinical disease, but serving as a nidus for reactivation in the event that the cell-mediated immunity against *M. tuberculosis* should wane.

EPIDEMIOLOGY

The impairment of cell-mediated immunity that occurs during HIV infection probably increases susceptibility to *M. tuberculosis*. In the United States the incidence of tuberculosis had declined steadily from the 1950s until 1984, when the trend reversed and the incidence increased (Fig. 105-2). There is substantial evidence that this increase in the number of cases of tuberculosis is in large part due to the increase in

HIV infection. Tuberculosis infection increased disproportionately in young minority patients—the same patient group with rapidly increasing rates of HIV infection.[9] Coinfection with tuberculosis is extremely common in HIV-infected patients in Africa, approaching 50 percent.[8] Infection following exposure to tuberculosis appears to be increased in patients with HIV infection. At least 50 percent of HIV-infected patients exposed to a single case of active tuberculosis developed evidence of infection with *M. tuberculosis*.[11] Infection following exposure in non-HIV-infected patients is approximately 30 percent.[12]

Several other factors probably contribute to the increase in tuberculosis cases in the United States. Tuberculosis has been reported in homeless patients, a group with a high incidence of HIV infection. These patients have poor access to health care and often live in shelters with crowded conditions and inadequate ventilation. Tuberculosis is also common among immigrants to the United States.

NATURAL HISTORY

The natural history of tuberculosis infection is altered in patients with HIV infection. In the above-noted outbreak of tuberculosis, active disease developed in 37 percent of cases *exposed* within 15 weeks of exposure.[11] This contrasts with normal rates of active disease of 3 to 5 percent of *infected* cases within the first year following infection. Patients with preexisting infection with *M. tuberculosis* who become infected with HIV have reactivation of tuberculosis at rates of 5 to 7 percent per year,[13] contrasting with lifetime activation rates of 6 to 10 percent in non-HIV-infected individuals. Unfortunately infection with *M. tuberculosis* may increase the progression of HIV infection,[14] probably because the cytokines released in response to *M. tuberculosis* upregulate viral replication.

CLINICAL PRESENTATION

The clinical manifestations of tuberculosis are protean and depend on the site of active disease. In HIV-infected patients, pulmonary disease is very common, but as many as 70 percent of patients may have extrapulmonary disease.[15] Symptoms of tuberculosis in HIV-infected patients are very nonspecific. They include systemic symptoms such as weight loss, night sweats, and chills; pulmonary symptoms such as cough, chest pain, or hemoptysis; and extrapulmonary symptoms such as headache, abdominal pain, and/or bone pain. Physical signs are equally nonspecific, including adenopathy, cachexia, fever, pulmonary signs of consolidation, and extrapulmonary signs which vary with the involved organ system.

The radiographic manifestations of pulmonary tuberculosis are also dramatically affected by HIV infection. The classic signs of upper lobe infiltrates with cavitation are much less common in patients with HIV infection when compared with immunocompetent hosts. Features often thought of as radiographic signs of primary tuberculous infection such as adenopathy and lower lobe infiltrates are frequently seen in HIV infection. Normal radiographs may also be noted, even when *M. tuberculosis* is found in the sputum. These variable radiographic presentations are to some extent dependent on the stage of HIV infection and corresponding immunosuppression. Radiographic features of "typical" tuberculous pulmonary disease are seen early in HIV infection, whereas those features considered "atypical" are seen late in the course of the disease (Table 105-1,[17] Figs. 105-3 and 105-4). It has become increasingly important to recognize the variable radiographic presentations of pulmonary tuberculosis, because misdiagnosis is common.[16] Misdiagnosis results in delay in the institution of therapy and failure to isolate infectious patients. This in turn poses a risk to other patients and health care workers.

DIAGNOSIS

Because HIV-infected patients lack specific symptoms, signs, or radiographic findings of tuberculosis, the disease should be suspected in any HIV-infected patient who presents with pulmonary disease. The diagnosis of tuberculosis is suggested by demonstration of pathologic changes consistent with tuberculous infection or evidence of cell-mediated immunity against the organism. It is confirmed by the demonstration of organisms in bodily fluids or tissue. Confirmation of infection is increasingly important to document sensitivity of the organism to antituberculosis therapy.

TUBERCULIN SKIN TESTING
Reactivity to tuberculin-purified protein derivative is the benchmark of cell-mediated immunity against *M. tuberculosis*. HIV infection, presumably because of its effect on cell-

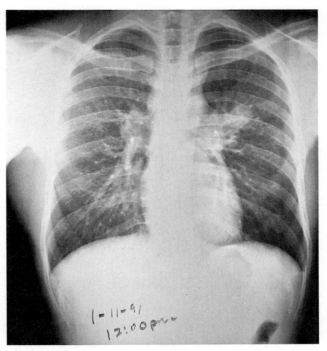

FIGURE 105-3 Chest radiograph of HIV positive individual with fevers and weight loss. Note mediastinal and hilar adenopathy. Mediastinoscopy demonstrated poorly formed granulomas which grew *M. tuberculosis*.

mediated immunity, has been shown to decrease the sensitivity of reaction to tuberculin purified protein derivative (PPD) as an indicator of infection. Anergy and negative PPDs are more common in advanced HIV infection as CD4+ lymphocyte counts decrease.[18] Anergy also appears to be a marker for severity of immunosuppression. Failure to respond to delayed-type hypersensitivity skin testing predicted the development of AIDS-defining infections.[19]

The incidence of active tuberculosis in HIV-infected patients with a positive reaction to tuberculin skin testing has been reported to be between 7.9 and 10.4 cases per 100 patient-years.[13,20] A negative reaction to tuberculin associated with cutaneous anergy also defined a group of patients at high risk for developing active tuberculosis, 12.4 cases per 100 patient-years.[20] The incidence of active tuberculosis was substantially less in patients who failed to react to tuberculin but did react to other delayed-type hypersensitivity (DTH) skin testing.[20] Even lower rates of active pulmonary tuberculosis may occur in HIV-infected tuberculin-negative patients, with a case attack rate of 0.3 cases per 100 patient-years noted.[13] This discrepancy between attack rates in HIV-infected tuberculin-skin-test-negative patients may be due to differing endemnicities of tuberculosis in the communities studied.

Current recommendations suggest that all HIV-infected patients be tested for reactivity to tuberculin. They should also be tested for cutaneous anergy. Because of the diminished response to tuberculin PPD, a reaction is considered positive when there is 5 mm of induration.[21] Testing should be done soon after the diagnosis of HIV infection in an effort to establish baseline markers of infection.

TABLE 105-1   Radiographic Presentations of Tuberculosis in HIV Infected Patients[a]

	% of infiltrates	
Normal	Early 5	Late 20
Adenopathy (without infiltrate)	Early 7	Late 20
Infiltrates	Early 88	Late 60
Cavitary	Early 76	Late 33
Adenopathy	Early 39	Late 80

[a] Adapted from Ref. 17.

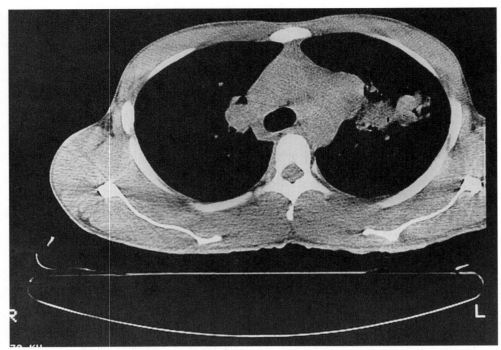

FIGURE 105-4 Computed axial tomography of chest demonstrating mediastinal and hilar adenopathy noted on chest film in Fig. 105-3.

SPUTUM EXAMINATION

Detection of acid-fast bacilli in smears of sputum is very specific for *M. tuberculosis*, with specificities of 98 to 99 percent reported.[22,23] Unfortunately sputum smears are not very sensitive, with sensitivities ranging from 45 to 55 percent.[22,23] In HIV-infected patients with advanced disease, the sensitivity of sputum smears may be less because of fewer cases of cavitary disease.[24]

Sputum mycobacterial cultures are both sensitive and specific. In the above-noted study the sensitivity of sputum cultures was 81.5 percent.[22] Recent studies of patients with HIV infection undergoing bronchoscopy noted "prebronchoscopy" sputum cultures were positive in 89 percent of patients eventually found to have tuberculosis.[25] Unfortunately sputum cultures may take weeks to demonstrate growth of *M. tuberculosis*. The time needed for *M. tuberculosis* to grow from culture may be substantially shortened by the use of the Bactec system, which utilizes uptake and release of radio-labeled carbon by the organism to signal growth. Polymerase chain reaction may also hasten identification of organisms grown in culture. Nevertheless diagnosis by sputum culture still requires weeks.

BLOOD CULTURES

In tuberculosis patients not infected with HIV mycobacterial bacteremia is very rare. In HIV-infected patients the incidence of mycobacteremia is much more common. Typically, the organism found is *M. avium*, but in a substantial number of patients *M. tuberculosis* is found. The likelihood of finding *M. tuberculosis* in the blood of HIV-infected patients with active tuberculosis depends on the severity of CD4+ lymphocyte depletion.[26] In those patients with severely reduced CD4+ lymphocyte counts (<100 cells per milliliter) the incidence of mycobacteremia of active tuberculosis was 49 percent, while no patients in whom the CD4+ lymphocyte count was greater than 300 cells per milliliter were found to have mycobacteremia.

BRONCHOSCOPY

Bronchoscopy is an important tool in evaluating pulmonary processes in HIV-infected patients. Its primary role in the diagnosis of pulmonary tuberculosis is largely expediting the process, allowing an earlier diagnosis in 33 percent of HIV-infected patients.[25] Samples obtained at bronchoscopy include bronchoalveolar lavage and transbronchial biopsies. Bronchoalveolar lavage typically is done with 120 ml of normal saline, often lavaging both lungs.[27] The lavage should be performed on lobes that are most affected radiographically. Bronchial alveolar lavage (BAL) is less sensitive than sputum smears in HIV-infected patients, with 23 percent of patients found to have acid-fast organisms on smears of the BAL and 62 percent having cultures positive for *M. tuberculosis*.[25] In the same study transbronchial biopsy was shown to demonstrate granulomata in only 19 percent of HIV-infected patients who underwent biopsy. Despite the lack of sensitivity of transbronchial biopsy, it was the sole early diagnostic test that suggested a diagnosis of tuberculosis.

OTHER TESTS

The diagnosis of tuberculosis may be made by growth of *M. tuberculosis* from other tissues, such as bone marrow aspirates or lymph node biopsies. Tuberculosis may also be found in urine culture.

THERAPY

The therapy of tuberculosis in HIV-infected patients is similar to therapy in normal hosts. Antituberculosis therapy is utilized with two specific goals: prevention of active disease in previously infected patients and treatment of active disease.

Therapy of active tuberculosis in HIV-infected patients relies on the same principles of drug use as therapy in non-HIV-infected patients. Specifically therapy with at least two bactericidal agents to which the organism is susceptible must be administered for at least 9 months to prevent the development of drug resistance. Isoniazid (INH) and rifampin are two highly effective bactericidal agents that are well tolerated. The addition of pyrazinamide for the initial 2 months allows the duration of therapy to be reduced to 6 months in normal hosts. Because of the high incidence of INH and multiple-drug-resistant isolates, four agents should be used initially (see below) unless the incidence of INH resistance in the community is less than 4 percent.[28] Currently the American Thoracic Society recommends INH (3 to 5 mg/kg per day), rifampin (10 mg/kg per day), pyrazinamide (15 to 30 mg/kg per day) and ethambutol (15 to 25 mg/kg per day) for 2 months, followed by 4 months of INH and rifampin if the organisms isolated are susceptible to these agents.[28] (Ethambutol is continued until sensitivities are determined or if resistance is documented.) Several studies have examined the efficacy of both 6- and 9-month therapy in HIV-infected patients.[29,30] These studies noted an excellent response to antituberculosis therapy, with 96 percent of treated patients in whom repeat smears were obtained demonstrating conversion to negative smears.[30] Unfortunately mortality ranged from 45 to 77 percent in treated patients, though tuberculosis was thought to play a role in only 6 to 8 percent of these deaths. A recent study from Zaire compared 6 months with 12 months of therapy.[31] Relapse was more common in patients treated for 6 months (9 percent) than in patients treated for 12 months (1.9 percent). Mortality in this study was 31 percent at 24 months; mortality due to tuberculosis accounted for 20 (8 percent) of deaths.

DRUG RESISTANCE

Resistance to INH or multiple antituberculosis therapies has been noted worldwide. Multi-drug-resistant (MDR) tuberculosis has been reported in several instances in the United States, particularly in HIV-infected patients.[32,33] Nosocomial outbreaks of MDR tuberculosis have been reported in the last several years.[34,35] The impact of infection with MDR tuberculosis in HIV-infected patients has been profound. AIDS patients infected with MDR tuberculosis were found to have a 90 percent mortality from tuberculosis.[36] In those patients who received two or more drugs to which the organism was susceptible there was still a 32 percent mortality. Median survival in patients with MDR tuberculosis was 12 months less than that in patients infected with susceptible or single-drug-resistant organisms.

TOXICITY

In the two series of HIV-infected patients for tuberculosis noted above the incidence of toxicity requiring change of therapy ranged from 6 to 18 percent.[29,30] Toxicities included hepatitis, anorexia, and rash.

PROPHYLAXIS

It was noted earlier that patients with previous infection with *M. tuberculosis* have a very high rate of reactivation. Because of this, a positive PPD in an HIV-infected patient always warrants therapy, regardless of age or duration of positive PPD. Current CDC guidelines for prophylaxis recommend isoniazid, 5 mg/kg per day or alternative thrice weekly regimens, for 1 year. There have been no prospective trials of isoniazid prophylaxis in HIV-infected patients, but it has been noted in studies of PPD-positive HIV-infected patients that previous INH therapy protected against the development of active tuberculosis.[13]

A more complex question arises in HIV-infected patients who are anergic. These patients develop active tuberculosis at a rate equal to that of patients who are PPD positive. Because of this high rate of active disease among anergic HIV-infected patients, some authors have argued for isoniazid prophylaxis in this patient population as well.[20] It should be noted that this study was done in a population with a high incidence of tuberculosis. Whether prophylactic antituberculosis therapy should be used in anergic HIV-infected patients in all regions of the world remains unstudied. HIV-infected patients who are exposed to tuberculosis should receive prophylactic therapy regardless of their PPD status because of the high incidence of primary infection and progression to active disease.[37]

PROGNOSIS

The overall prognosis for tuberculosis in HIV-infected patients is poor. The prognosis of untreated disease is difficult to discern, but given the fact that "missed diagnoses" are usually found at autopsy, it is likely very poor. Those patients with tuberculosis who have sensitive organisms have an excellent response to therapy, but also have a poor prognosis because of co-morbid HIV-related illnesses.[29-31] Finally, patients with tuberculosis caused by MDR *M. tuberculosis* also have a poor prognosis, because of failure to control the infection.[36]

Bacterial Pneumonia in HIV Infection

Bacterial infections of the respiratory system have been increasingly recognized as a cause of morbidity and mortality in HIV-infected patients.[38] In a recent study of respiratory infections in HIV-infected patients, the overall incidence of bacterial pneumonia exceeded the incidence of *Pneumocystis carinii* pneumonia.[39] Recurrent bacterial pneumonias is an AIDS-defining condition, according to the Centers for Disease Control.[40]

PATHOPHYSIOLOGY

Bacterial infection of the lung typically occurs with inhalation or aspiration of organisms, though hematogenous spread may also occur. Opsonization of encapsulated extracellular bacteria by macrophages and polymorphonuclear leukocytes occurs with destruction of the organism. HIV infection could adversely affect this process at a number of steps. HIV infection causes a nonspecific polyclonal gammopathy, but production of specific antibody (particularly IgG$_2$) in response to challenge with pneumococcal polysaccharide.[41] Clearance of opsonized particles by alveolar macrophages may be reduced, as evidenced by impaired clearance of complement opsonized particles by the reticuloendothelial system in HIV-infected patients.[42] Defects in reticuloendothelial cell ability to phagocytose opsonized particles also results in a greater incidence of bacteremia in infections with encapsulated organisms such as *Streptococcus pneumoniae*.[43]

The organisms causing bacterial pneumonia in HIV-infected patients, as with normal hosts, vary depending on the location in which the infection was acquired. Community acquired organisms are similar to those which cause community acquired pneumonia (CAP) in the normal host. *Streptococcus pneumoniae* is the most common cause of bacterial CAP in HIV-infected patients, accounting for between 30 and 70 percent of cases. *Haemophilus influenzae* is another common etiologic agent, causing pneumonia much more often in HIV-infected patients (3 to 40 percent of cases) than in non-HIV-infected patients (<10 percent of cases).[44,45] *Staphylococcus aureus* often is noted as a cause of bacterial pneumonia in HIV-infected patients.[38,39] This may be due to the high incidence of intravenous drug use.[46] Enteric gram-negative organisms may cause pneumonia in hospitalized patients or patients with neutropenia. *Rhodo-coccus equi* has been identified as the cause of bacterial pneumonia in a surprising number of HIV-infected patients.[47]

EPIDEMIOLOGY

Bacterial pneumonia occurs with greater frequency in intravenous drug abusing patients with HIV infection.[39] Inner city minority patients with HIV infection have a greater incidence of bacterial pneumonia than homosexual or bisexual patients.[44]

Bacterial pneumonia may occur early in the course of HIV infection, before the advent of opportunistic infections. This is not surprising, given the virulence of the organisms. Nevertheless infection occurs more often in patients with reduced numbers of CD4+ lymphocytes. In a recent prospective study of respiratory infections in HIV-infected patients, the incidence of bacterial pneumonia was three times greater in HIV-positive individuals with CD4+ counts <250 cells per cubic millimeter than patients whose CD4+ count was >250 cells per cubic millimeter.[39]

CLINICAL MANIFESTATIONS

The clinical presentation of pneumonia in HIV-infected patients differs little from that seen in non-HIV-infected patients. Most patients with bacterial pneumonia have fever, cough, and sputum production.[48] Purulent sputum argues against a diagnosis of *Pneumocystis carinii*. Dyspnea and chest pain also are common. The tempo with which symptoms develop may help differentiate bacterial pneumonia from opportunistic pneumonias such as *Pneumocystis carinii*. Symptoms associated with bacterial pneumonia usually are present for hours to days, while those associated with *Pneumocystis pneumoniae* may be present for weeks to months.[49,50] Physical examination is not mentioned frequently in the literature and is probably not specific. Laboratory data may demonstrate an elevated white blood cell count, though rarely >15,000 cells per milliliter.[49] Immature leukocytes often are present even in the setting of neutropenia.[49]

Radiography of the chest in HIV-infected patients with bacterial pneumonia may demonstrate focal consolidation or a diffuse reticular pattern. Focal consolidation (segmental, lobar, or multilobar) occurs in 45 to 70 percent of patients[48,49] (Fig. 105-5). Patients with bacterial pneumonia and a diffuse reticular pattern on chest radiograph are often infected with *H. influenzae*. Infection with *Pseudomonas* species may be associated with cavitary nodules on chest radiograph.[51]

DIAGNOSIS

The diagnosis of bacterial pneumonia is a controversial area in non-HIV-infected hosts.[52] These controversies are probably equally applicable in HIV-infected patients. Varying diagnostic methods have been used in studies of bacterial pneumonia in HIV-infected patients.[53,54]

Examination of expectorated sputum may suggest the diagnosis of bacterial pneumonia.[52] A sample with >25

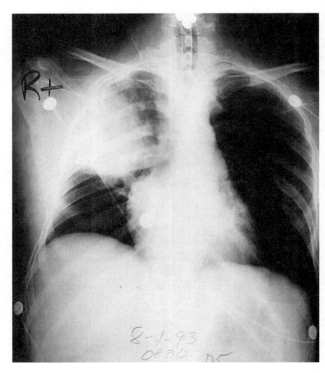

FIGURE 105-5 Chest radiograph of HIV-positive drug abuser with severe pneumococcal pneumonia.

polymorphonuclear cells with < five squamous cells may be helpful if a predominant organism is noted. Many clinicians, however, would not alter therapy based on results of sputum Gram stains. Routine bacterial cultures of sputum specimens are probably not useful.

Bronchoscopy is utilized extensively in the diagnosis of pulmonary infiltrates in HIV-infected patients. Quantitative culture of bronchoalveolar lavage and bronchial brushings, have been studied extensively in non-HIV-infected patients.[55] In one study of HIV-infected patients, bronchoalveolar lavage with quantitative culture was said to be 62 percent "sensitive" in diagnosing bacterial pneumonia, though a definitive diagnosis was based on response to antibacterial antibiotics.[53] Bronchoscopy with protective brushing and quantitative culture was said to be 53 percent sensitive and 75 percent specific.[56]

Blood cultures are positive in many HIV-infected patients with bacterial pneumonia, particularly those with pneumococcal pneumonia.[57] Positive blood cultures have been reported in 25 to 75 percent of patients with pneumococcal pneumonia.[58] Bacteremia appears to be less frequent in *H. influenzae* pneumonia, occurring in 12 to 25 percent of cases.[44,53]

THERAPY

HIV-infected patients with documented or suspected bacterial pneumonia should be treated with therapy aimed at common organisms, in particular *S. pneumoniae* and *H. influenzae*. Penicillin or erythromycin usually are appropriate to treat *S. pneumoniae*; however, the incidence of resistance to penicillin and cephalosporins is increasing[59] and has been reported in HIV-infected patients.[60] A third-generation cephalosporin will cover *H. influenzae*. In patients in whom *Pnuemocystis carinii* is suspected, trimethoprim-sulfamethoxazole is active against common bacterial pathogens as well. Patients who are hospitalized or are neutropenic should be treated for enteric gram negatives such as *Pseudomonas aeriginosa*. *Rhodococcus equi* is susceptible to erythromycin, vancomycin, flouroquinolones, and aminoglycoside.[61] Patients who fail to respond to antibacterial therapy should be evaluated for coincident infections.[49]

PROPHYLAXIS

Because of the frequency of bacterial pneumonias in HIV-infected patients, prophylaxis against these infections is appropriate. Vaccines against *S. pneumoniae* and *H. influenzae* are available. The utility of pneumococcal vaccine has been studied extensively in non-HIV-infected patients.[62] Its efficacy has not been extensively tested in HIV-infected patients, though in one series of patients with pneumococcal pneumonia, most were infected with serotypes included in the 23-valent vaccine. Unfortunately, there have been several reports of subprotective antibody responses to vaccination in patients with HIV infection.[63] Current CDC guidelines recommend pneumococcal vaccine for patients >2 years of age having HIV infection.[64]

Antibacterial prophylaxis may also have some role in prevention of bacterial pneumonia. Trimethoprim-sulfamethoxazole is active against *S. pneumoniae* and *H. influenzae*. It is recommended for prophylaxis against *Pneumocystis carinii* and may have some efficacy in prevention of bacterial infection. Penicillin prophylaxis might be warranted for patients with recurrent pneumococcal disease.[46]

PROGNOSIS

Despite the high incidence of bacteremia, mortality from bacterial pneumonia in HIV-infected patients generally is uncommon. In one series of 18 patients with bacterial pneumonia, 16 responded to antibacterial antibiotics and two died.[53] Patients with pneumococcal pneumonia have mortality rates around 10 percent,[46,48] less than that typically reported for pneumococcal pneumonia in non-HIV-infected patients.[65] However, not all reports are so optimistic. In one series of 14 AIDS patients with bacteremic pneumococcal pneumonia, eight patients died.[66] In the same report there was only one death in 12 cases of bacteremic pneumoccal pneumonia in HIV-infected patients who did not meet CDC criteria for AIDS.

Prognosis appears worse in other bacterial infections. *Pseudomonas* infection has been associated with mortalities of 33 to 37 percent.[51,67] Infection with *R. equi* is associated with a 60 percent mortality.[68]

Pneumocystis carinii Pneumonia in HIV Infection

Pneumocystis carinii pneumonia (PCP) has been the predominant respiratory complication of HIV infection in developed nations.[1] Before the advent of primary prophylaxis against PCP, it was the AIDS-defining illness in >60 percent of HIV-infected individuals who progressed to AIDS.[69] In a comparison of HIV-infected men receiving primary prophylaxis against PCP with those who did not, 60 percent of those not taking prophylaxis developed *Pneumocystis* pneumonia during the course of their illness, and in 46 percent it was the AIDS-defining illness.[70] Importantly, in those patients taking PCP prophylaxis, the incidence of PCP decreased 28 percent; in 14 percent, it was the AIDS-defining illness. Thus PCP is an extremely important pulmonary pathogen in HIV-infected patients and one that is treatable and preventable.

PATHOPHYSIOLOGY

Pneumocystis carinii resembles a fungus more than a protozoa, based on ribosomal RNA analysis. It is carried in the alveoli of many species, including humans. Infection with *Pneumocystis carinii* probably occurs in childhood for most individuals. Over 66 percent of children demonstrate serologic evidence of infection by age 4 years.[71] In animal models PCP occurs during immunosuppression by reactivation of latent infection,[72] but new infection cannot be excluded as a cause of disease in immunocompromised hosts.[73]

The development of active pneumonia with *P. carinii* is very unusual in normal hosts. Both cellular and humoral defenses appear to play a role in controlling infection.[74] Animal studies using mice with severe combined immunodeficiency (SCID) demonstrate the importance of CD4+ T lymphocytes.[75] In humans infection is most often seen in patients with impaired CD4+ T-cell function or reduced numbers of these cells. When there is impaired T-helper-cell response to *P. carinii*, the organism was attached to type I epithelial cells, resulting in destruction of these cells.[76] Subsequently, the alveolar spaces are filled by an eosinophilic, amorphous material composed of degenerating organisms, host cells, and lipoprotein-like material.[77] Disease progression is marked by mononuclear cell infiltration of the interstitium. Progression to respiratory failure may occur from filling of alveolar spaces by the eosinophilic debris or polymorphonuclear-leukocyte-mediated alveolar damage.

EPIDEMIOLOGY

Pneumocystis carinii pneumonia affects all risk groups patients for HIV infection. It is interesting to note that it appears to be much less common in Africa than in the developed nations. A recent study from Rwanda noted that of 47 patients with HIV infection and AIDS with pulmonary disease, 5 cases of PCP were diagnosed.[78]

CLINICAL MANIFESTATIONS

Cough and dyspnea are the symptoms that are most common in HIV-infected patients with PCP. The time course of symptoms has been mentioned, with PCP in HIV-infected patients often causing symptoms for weeks prior to diagnosis.[50] Physical examination reveals fever. Chest examination is often normal,[50] though crackles or wheezes may be heard. Extrapulmonary involvement with PCP may occur, though physical examination findings are nonspecific.[79]

Pneumocystis carinii pneumonia typically presents with a diffuse reticular or interstitial pattern on chest radiograph (Fig. 105-6), but patients may present with normal chest radiographs.[80] Apical infiltrates may occur in HIV patients with PCP, usually in patients receiving aerosolized pentamidine[81] (Fig. 105-7). Apical infiltrates have been reported in HIV-infected patients with PCP not receiving inhaled pentamidine.[82] Spontaneous pneumothorax also occurs (Fig. 105-8).

DIAGNOSIS

Because of the nonspecific presentation of PCP, diagnosis requires demonstration of the organism in sputum or pathologic specimens.

NONSPECIFIC MARKERS

There are some diagnostic studies which, while not specific for PCP, are very sensitive to the presence of infection. Serum lactate dehydrogenase is increased in >90 percent of HIV-infected patients with PCP.[83] Serum lactate dehydrogenase (LDH) also predicts severity of disease.[83,84] Unfortunately, LDH may be increased in a number of disease states, including other lung diseases, liver disease, muscle injury, and hemolysis. Galium 67 scanning also is a sensitive test of pulmonary infection with PCP[85] (Fig. 105-9). Galium uptake in the lung that is greater than uptake in the liver was found in

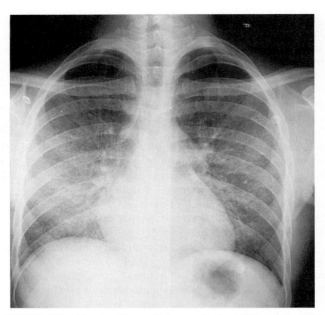

FIGURE 105-6 Chest radiograph demonstrating diffuse intestitial infiltrate in an HIV-infected patient with PCP.

90 percent of patients with PCP. Pulmonary function testing also may be abnormal in the presence of PCP. The diffusing capacity for carbon monoxide and the partial pressure of oxygen in arterial blood during exercise are decreased with PCP.[86]

FIGURE 105-7 Chest radiograph demonstrating upper lobe predominant interstitial infiltrate in patient with PCP that developed while being treated with inhaled pentamidine.

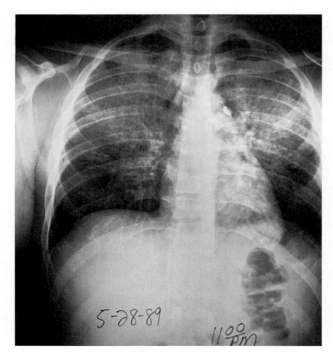

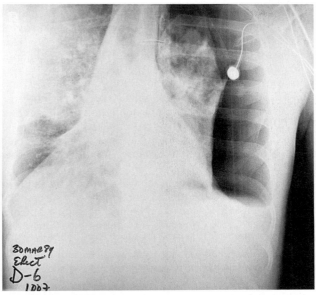

FIGURE 105-8 Chest radiograph demonstrating spontaneous pneumothorax in an HIV-infected patient with PCP.

SPUTUM EXAMINATION

Demonstration of *P. carinii* in sputum and in pathologic specimens remains the standard by which infection is diagnosed. The ability to diagnose PCP by examination of expectorated sputum has reduced greatly the need for invasive diagnostic procedures in centers where the technique has been developed. Several studies have demonstrated sensitivities that range from 45 to 75 percent.[87] Sputum production is induced by inhalation of aerosolized hypertonic saline. Sputum then may be stained with conventional stains such as methenamine silver, Giemsa, or monoclonal antibody stains against *P. carinii* itself. The highest reported sensitivities are obtained using monoclonal antibody staining, but specificity is reduced when compared with conventional stains.[88]

BRONCHOSCOPY

Fiberoptic bronchoscopy has been the primary tool for diagnosing PCP. Organisms may be identified in bronchoalveolar lavage fluid or in transbronchial biopsy. Bronchoalveolar lavage has been shown to have a sensitivity of 89 percent in diagnosing PCP in HIV-infected patients.[89] Bilateral lavage may increase the sensitivity of bronchoalveolar lavage by a small amount.[27]

Transbronchial biopsy also may be utilized to diagnose PCP. Transbronchial biopsy alone has a sensitivity of 91 percent for the diagnosis of PCP in HIV-infected patients.[89] Others have reported that transbronchial biopsy actually is less sensitive than bronchoalveolar lavage.[90] Because of the risk of pneumothorax and bleeding, transbronchial biopsy has been reserved for those patients in whom sputum and bronchoalveolar lavage do not yield a diagnosis or patients in whom there is a strong suspicion of another infection or pulmonary process.

It should be noted that some authors have argued that bronchoscopy is unnecessary in patients with known HIV

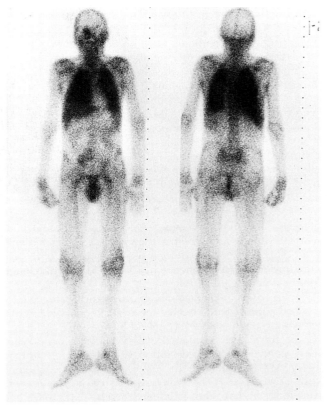

FIGURE 105-9 Ga[67] scan demonstrating pulmonary uptake in a patient with PCP.

infection and a clinical picture consistent with PCP.[91] A decision analysis utilizing a patient not on prophylactic therapy with a typical clinical presentation suggested there was no significant difference in outcome with reduced cost.[92] However, as primary and secondary prophylaxis against PCP are utilized increasingly, it has become less common,[70] making confirmation of the diagnosis more important.

THERAPY

There are several agents that are effective against *Pneumocystis carinii*. Trimethoprim-sulfamethoxazole (TMP/SMZ) and pentamidine remain mainstays of therapy. Atovaquone, dapsone, trimetrexate, and clindamycin and primaquine have been utilized as alternatives.

TREATMENT

The treatment of acute PCP in HIV-infected patients is initiated with TMP/SMZ, unless there is a known allergy to sulfur-containing medications. The dosage of TMP/SMZ is 15 mg/kg per day of trimethoprim and 75 mg/kg per day of sulfamethoxazole in three to four divided doses. Intravenous and oral administration appear to be equally efficacious (in those patients who are well enough to tolerate oral medications). Treatment should continue for 3 weeks.

Utilizing this regimen, survival rates of 60 to 90 percent are reported.[93–95] Unfortunately, the incidence of toxicity with TMP/SMZ is exceedingly high, in some series reaching 90 percent. Toxicities requiring alternative therapy occur in 35 to 50 percent.[93,94] Toxicities include rash, bone marrow suppression, and hyperkalemia.[95,96]

In those patients with moderate to severe cases of PCP who cannot tolerate TMP/SMZ, pentamidine remains the second-line therapy. Pentamidine is dosed 4 mg/kg per day in a single dose intravenously over 1 h. Several studies have compared pentamidine to TMP/SMZ.[93–95] In two of the studies cited, the two drugs were equally efficacious; in the third, TMP/SMZ was found to have greater efficacy (86 versus 60 percent survival). Pentamidine also has a significant incidence of drug toxicities, including hypotension, hyperglycemia and hypoglycemia, renal dysfunction, and bone marrow suppression. Because the toxicities associated with TMP/SMZ are less severe than those associated with pentamidine and it may be more efficacious, TMP/SMZ remains first-line therapy for PCP.

Because of the high incidence of drug toxicity among HIV-infected patients being treated for PCP, alternative therapies have been sought actively. Dapsone, atovaquone, and trimetrexate have been compared with TMP/SMZ.[97–99] When used alone, each has been found to be less effective than TMP/SMZ, though toxicities were less than those associated with TMP/SMZ. The combination of dapsone with trimethoprim has been compared with TMP/SMZ and found to have equal efficacy in mild to moderate PCP.[100] Similarly, the combination of clindamycin and primaquine has been compared with TMP/SMZ in a small trial and was found to have equal efficacy.[101]

It became clear early in the HIV epidemic that HIV-infected patients with PCP often worsened after the initiation of therapy. This prompted several investigators to administer corticosteroids to patients with severe PCP. Controlled trials of the administration of corticosteroids to patients with severe PCP demonstrated that corticosteroids substantially reduced the incidence of respiratory failure or death.[102,103] A consensus panel from the National Institute of Health and University of California recommended that patients with PCP and arterial hypoxemia Pa_{O_2} <70 mmHg breathing room air or an alveolar arterial gradient [$(A-a)D_{O_2}$] of 35 mmHG, receive 80 mg of prednisone (or its equivalent) daily with initiation of therapy for PCP.[104]

PROPHYLAXIS

In the absence of prophylaxis, PCP is the most common respiratory complication of HIV infection. Patients with PCP have very high relapse rates following apparently successful therapy. Because of the high incidence of infection and recurrence, primary and secondary prophylaxis has been initiated. Both TMP/SMZ and inhaled pentamidine have been shown to reduce the incidence of primary PCP.[105,106] When directly compared, TMP/SMZ has been shown to be more effective than inhaled pentamidine for secondary prophylaxis.[107] In the study of HIV-infected patients with CD4 lymphocyte counts <200 cells per milliliter, there were no episodes of PCP in patients taking TMP/SMZ (80 mg of

trimethoprim per 400 mg of sulfamethoxazole daily or 160 mg of trimethoprim per 800 mg of sulfamethoxazole daily) over a period of 250 days. There was an 11 percent incidence of PCP in patients taking inhaled pentamidine (300 mg by nebulizer monthly). Unfortunately, adverse reactions were much more common in the TMP/SMZ groups (21 and 26 percent) than the inhaled pentamidine group (none). Subsequent studies have suggested that lower-dose TMP/SMZ regimens such as 160 mg of trimethoprim per 800 mg of sulfamethoxazole three times weekly is equally effective with a lower incidence of adverse reactions (9 percent).[108]

Dapsone has also been studied as primary prophylaxis. When compared with inhaled pentamidine, dapsone (100 mg twice weekly) was found to be effective, with a 3 percent incidence of PCP.[109] Comparison of dapsone (100 mg daily) with TMP/SMZ (160 mg of trimethoprim per 800 mg of sulfamethoxazole) found the two regimens had equal efficacy.[110] The incidence of adverse effects was also the same, with a very large number of patients developing limiting toxicity.

Secondary prophylaxis also has been documented to be effective.[111,112] Once again, TMP/SMZ was more effective than pentamidine, though both were less effective when utilized as secondary prophylaxis than when used for primary prophylaxis. The incidence of recrudescent PCP was 11 percent in 17 months of observation in patients treated with TMP/SMZ compared with 27 percent in patients treated with inhaled pentamidine.[112] Adverse reactions were more common in the TMP/SMZ-treated patients. It also was noted that the incidence of bacterial infections was reduced in patients treated with TMP/SMZ.[112]

In conclusion, therapy for primary or secondary prophylaxis against PCP in HIV-infected patients should be initiated with TMP/SMZ (160 mg of trimethoprim per 800 mg of sulfamethoxazole) three times weekly in those patients without prior severe reaction to the drug. If the patient is intolerant of TMP/SMZ, then inhaled pentamidine (300 mg monthly) or dapsone (50 to 100 mg daily) may be utilized. The addition of pyrimethamine (50 mg weekly) to dapsone provides effective prophylaxis against *Toxoplasma gondii*.[113]

PROGNOSIS

The response of HIV-infected patients to therapy for PCP has been described. Survival ranges from 65 to 90 percent. In those patients with PCP that is severe enough to warrant mechanical ventilation, the survival is much worse.[114] Current reports suggest that mortality of HIV-infected patients with PCP who require mechanical ventilation is 76 to 91 percent.[114,115] Factors that correlate with decreased likelihood of survival include lower CD4+ lymphocyte counts, pneumothorax, and duration of therapy prior to respiratory failure.[115,116]

Fungal Pneumonia in HIV Infection

Fungal infections are common in HIV-infected patients. More than 20 percent of AIDS-defining illnesses are due to fungal infection.[117] In some areas, the incidence of fungal infection is higher. Several fungal species have been reported to cause infection in HIV-infected patients, but three soil-dwelling fungi predominate. *Cryptococcus neoformans* is ubiquitous, causing disease worldwide.[78] *Coccidioides immitis* and *Histoplasma capsulatum* are common causes of disease in regions in which they are endemic. Finally, infections with *Aspergillus* species appears to be increasing in frequency in HIV-infected patients.

PATHOPHYSIOLOGY

Fungal infections have been classified into infections by primary pathogens and opportunists.[118] Primary pathogens (*C. neoformans, C. immitis, H. capsulatum,* and *Blastomyces dermatitidis*) are capable of surviving the defenses of naive phagocytes. Activation of macrophages by T cells is necessary for containment of the infection. Opportunists (*Aspergillus, Mucorales*) are killed by the polymorphonuclear leukocytes.[118] Infection with *Candida* species defies this classification, as impairment of T-cell-dependent mechanisms results in mucosal overgrowth but rarely deep tissue invasion. Tissue invasion occurs in the setting of phagocyte impairment.[118] Impairment of T-cell-dependent macrophage activation makes infection with primary pathogenic fungi an expected complication of HIV infection. Much as with tuberculosis, patients with HIV infection who have been previously infected with a fungus may suffer reactivation of that organism, or new infection may occur.[119]

Several generalizations may be made about infection with endemic fungi in HIV-infected patients. First, fungal infections occur in all HIV risk groups. Second, fungal infection is often a systemic disease[120–122] with a nonspecific presentation. Pulmonary disease often is present but may be asymptomatic. Third, response to therapy occurs in the majority of patients, but without maintenance therapy relapse is the rule. Beyond these generalizations each of the major fungal infections affecting HIV-infected patients is briefly discussed.

CRYPTOCOCCUS NEOFORMANS

EPIDEMIOLOGY

Cryptococcus neoformans is the most common cause of deep tissue fungal infection in HIV-infected patients.[117] It occurs worldwide and is a common cause of lung disease in parts of Africa.[78] The fungus is found in soil, particularly in soil enriched with bird or bat excrement. Both homosexuality and IV drug abuse have been reported as the predominant risk factor for HIV infection in patients with cryptococcosis,[121,123] suggesting there is no specific risk group association.

CLINICAL MANIFESTATIONS

The clinical manifestations of cryptococcal infection in HIV-infected individuals reflect the systemic nature of the infection. Most patients present with fevers and malaise.[121] Meningitis is the most common presentation, and >70 percent of patients presented with headache. Cough was pre-

sent in 31 percent. Physical examination is often unrevealing. Meningismus was found in only 24 percent.[121]

Pulmonary involvement in patients with cryptococcosis is common, though isolated pulmonary involvement is thought to be unusual.[123] However, a recent African study reported 37 patients with pulmonary cryptococcosis, of whom 29 had "primary" pulmonary cryptococcosis.[124] Almost all these patients presented with cough, whereas 51 percent had fever and 46 percent had dyspnea.

The radiographic presentation of cryptococcosis also is variable. Normal chest radiographs have been reported in one-third of patients with positive respiratory cultures. A diffuse interstitial abnormality usually is cited as the most common radiographic abnormality,[117,123] though focal infiltrates (Fig. 105-10), adenopathy, and cavitation have been reported.

DIAGNOSIS

The diagnosis of cryptococcosis is facilitated by the ability to detect fungal antigen (CRAG) in blood and cerebrospinal fluid (CSF). CRAG is positive in the CSF in 91 percent of patients with meningitis, and in the serum in 98 percent.[120] Serum CRAG was found to be positive in all patients tested with documented pulmonary cryptococcosis. This finding was not demonstrated in the Rwandan study, where CRAG was not found in patients with isolated pulmonary cryptococcosis.[124] The discrepancy between this and previous studies is not readily explained, although earlier detection of cryptococcal infection may have allowed diagnosis prior to

FIGURE 105-10 Chest radiograph demonstrating a focal infiltrate in an HIV-positive hemophiliac found to be positive for *C. neoformans* on BAL and transbronchial biopsy.

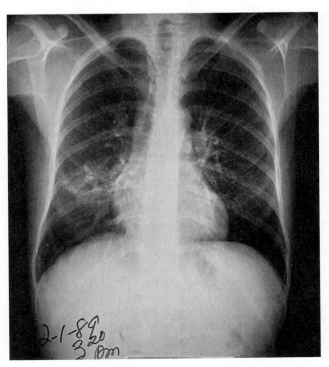

dissemination. Alternatively, technical differences between CRAG testing may have played a role.

Isolation of *C. neoformans* from bronchoalveolar lavage is common in pulmonary cryptococcosis. Several series have documented isolation of the fungus in more than 80 percent of the patients sampled.[121,123] Organisms also may be demonstrated in pathologic material obtained in transbronchial biopsy.

THERAPY

Amphotericin B has been the mainstay of treatment of active cryptococcosis in HIV-infected individuals.[117,121] In a comparative study of amphotericin and fluconazole in HIV-infected patients with cryptococcal meningitis, amphotericin (0.4 mg/kg) resulted in a complete resolution of evidence of cryptococcal infection in 40 percent.[124] A positive response to therapy was seen in 67 percent of patients.

Several studies have documented some efficacy of the oral azoles, fluconazole and itraconazole, in cryptococcal meningitis.[124–126] In these studies, fluconazole (200 mg per day) was successful in the treatment of 34 percent of patients, and a positive response was obtained in 60 percent.[121] A retrospective review of fluconazole (400 mg per day) in cryptococcosis demonstrated that of 30 patients, none died within the first 30 days even though several patients had high titers of CRAG and altered mental status.[126] Treatment with itraconazole in African patients with pulmonary cryptococcosis prevented the development of disseminated cryptococcosis.[78] Seventy percent of those patients with pulmonary disease who did not receive anticryptococcal therapy developed disseminated disease. Thus, the role of oral azoles in the induction therapy of HIV-associated cryptococcal disease is evolving. Currently fluconazole (and perhaps itraconazole) is appropriate for isolated pulmonary cryptococcosis. Severe pulmonary disease or meningitis probably should be treated with high dose amphotericin.

Life-long secondary prophylaxis (maintenance therapy) is required in HIV-infected patients with cryptococcosis. Amphotericin B is effective at preventing recurrent disease,[121] but its requirement for intravenous administration and renal toxicities make long-term usage difficult. Both fluconazole and itraconazole have been evaluated as maintenance therapy. Fluconazole (200 mg per day) was associated with only a 3 percent relapse rate of cryptococcal infection in HIV-infected patients with meningitis whose CSF cultures had been sterilized after amphotericin therapy.[127] Itraconazole, as noted earlier, prevented dissemination in HIV-infected patients with pulmonary cryptococcosis.[124]

HISTOPLASMA CAPSULATUM

EPIDEMIOLOGY

Infection with *Histoplasma capsulatum* is common among HIV-infected patients who live in, or have lived in, areas in which the fungus is endemic. These regions include the valleys of the Mississippi, Ohio, and St. Lawrence rivers and the Carribean islands. Histoplasmosis is reported in 2 to 5 percent of patients with AIDS in these regions.[128] Active disease

is probably the result of both new infection and reactivation.[120]

CLINICAL MANIFESTATIONS

Histoplasmosis in HIV-infected patients typically presents with fever and wasting.[129] However, respiratory complaints may predominate.[120] Physical examination may demonstrate hepatomegaly or splenomegaly.[120,129] A small number of patients (10 to 12 percent) present with a sepsis-like syndrome.[129] This syndrome proved rapidly fatal in 44 percent of these patients.[120] Chest radiography typically demonstrates a diffuse lung lesion[120,129] (Fig. 105-11), but 25 to 43 percent of HIV-infected patients with histoplasmosis may have normal chest radiographs. Anemia, thrombocytopenia, and leukopenia are common.[117,129]

DIAGNOSIS

Diagnosis of histoplasmosis requires demonstration of the organism. *Histoplasma capsulatum* may be identified in the blood by buffy coat stain or in bone marrow.[129] Bronchoscopy also may demonstrate the organism in 75 to 85 percent of patients.[120] *Histoplasma capsulatum* polysaccharide antigen may be detected in 95 percent of cases of disseminated histoplasmosis.[120]

THERAPY

Induction therapy of histoplasmosis may be accomplished with amphotericin or itraconazole. Amphotericin remains the mainstay of initial therapy. Improvement has been reported in 77 to 87 percent of patients treated with amphotericin.[120,130] Itraconazole also has been utilized as initial

FIGURE 105-11 Chest radiograph demonstrating diffuse, nodular interstitial infiltrate in HIV-positive patient with disseminated histoplasmosis.

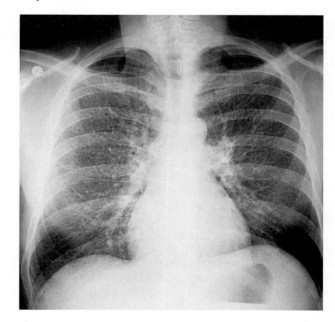

therapy. Nine of 12 HIV-infected patients with histoplasmosis treated with itraconazole (400 mg per day) demonstrated improvement, and seven achieved a remission of their disease.[131] In the same study, 10 patients were treated with fluconazole (100 to 800 mg per day); four patients had improvement or remission.[131] Another study of HIV-infected patients with disseminated histoplasmosis without meningitis or shock treated with itraconazole (600 mg per day, followed by 400 mg per day) found that 85 percent responded to therapy.[132] In patients with severe disseminated disease (meningitis, shock), amphotericin remains the agent of choice for induction of therapy.

Maintenance therapy of histoplasmosis in HIV-infected patients has been achieved with amphotericin and itraconazole.[130,133] Once again, ease of administration and complications associated with amphotericin diminish its role as a maintenance therapy. Itraconazole prevented recurrence of histoplasmosis in 95 percent of HIV-infected patients with *H. capsulatum* infection.[133] Fluconazole also has been used as maintenance therapy, though with less efficacy than itraconazole, and provides an alternative for patients who cannot tolerate itraconazole.[134] *Histoplasma capsulatum* var. capsulatum antigen may be followed as a means of early diagnosis of recurrence.[120]

PROGNOSIS

The prognosis of HIV-infected patients with disseminated histoplasmosis has improved with maintenance therapy. Median survival in the patients treated with itraconazole following amphotericin induction was 98 weeks.[133] Death was often the result of progressive HIV infection or other opportunistic infections.

COCCIDIOIDES IMMITIS

EPIDEMIOLOGY

Like infection with *H. capsulatum*, infection with *Coccidioides immitis* is common in individuals who live in areas in which the fungus is endemic. As many as 30 percent of individuals in Tuscon, Arizona, demonstrate infection with *C. immitis* when skin tested, and it is estimated that the incidence of new infection is 3 percent per year.[134] In a recent prospective cohort analysis of HIV-infected patients in an area endemic for *C. immitis*, the estimated cumulative incidence of active coccidioidomycosis for 41 months was 25 percent.[135] Risk for the development of active coccidioidomycosis among this group of patients correlated with CD4 lymphocyte counts <250 cells per milliliter and a diagnosis of AIDS.[136] It is interesting to note that evidence of prior infection with *C. immitis* was not associated with increased risk of infection. Coccidioidomycosis has been noted in all groups at risk for HIV infection.[121]

CLINICAL MANIFESTATIONS

The clinical manifestations of coccidioidomycosis are similar to those of other fungal infections in HIV-infected patients. Prolonged fever and wasting are typical. Pulmonary symptoms are common.[117] Physical examination findings may reflect pulmonary disease or cutaneous involvement. Chest radiography was abnormal in 75 percent of patients in one of the largest series reported.[36] Both focal and diffuse pulmonary infiltrates were reported. Large nodules have been reported as a common radiographic manifestation.[119]

DIAGNOSIS

The diagnosis of coccdioidomycosis requires the demonstration of *C. immitis* by staining or in culture. Serologies are often positive in HIV-infected patients with coccidioidomycosis, but may be negative in patients with severe immunocompromise or overwhelming infection.[122] The diagnosis may be made readily in patients with pulmonary involvement. In one large study of coccidioidomycosis in HIV-infected patients, 51 patients had pulmonary involvement. A diagnosis was made by examination of sputum or bronchoscopically obtained material in 32 patients.[122] An interesting study of bronchoalveolar lavage done in the same highly endemic region found only one case of coccidioidomycosis in 36 bronchoalveolar lavage specimens from HIV-infected patients.[137] In addition to bronchoalveolar lavage, bronchoscopic inspection may suggest the diagnosis of coccidioidal infection if large endobronchial ulcers are noted.[119] It should be noted that there is a high incidence of coexisting opportunistic infections in HIV-infected patients presenting with coccidioidomycosis.[122,138] Specimens should be examined closely for multiple pathogens. Specimens from patients suspected of having coccidioidomycosis should be processed by expert laboratories, as there is a significant risk of infection of laboratory personnel.[119]

THERAPY

The therapy of coccidioidomycosis in HIV-infected patients is evolving. Amphotericin has been the standard of care.[117] In the large review cited, the mortality in all patients given amphotericin was 42 percent.[122] Fluconazole has been studied in the treatment of coccidioidal meningitis and pulmonary coccidioidomycosis in HIV-infected and non-HIV-infected patients and found to have varying efficacy.[139,140] No direct comparisons with amphotericin have been performed.

PROGNOSIS

Like other disseminated fungal infections in HIV-infected patients, coccidioidomycosis is a progressive disease if untreated. Survival is dependent on the severity of the disease at presentation and the underlying HIV-related illness.

OTHER FUNGAL INFECTIONS

Two other fungal infections have been reported with increasing frequency in the HIV-infected population—*Aspergillus* infections and blastomycosis.

Invasive infection with *Aspergillus* has been reported in patients late in the course of HIV-infection. Many HIV-infected patients with invasive aspergillosis have CD4+ counts of <100 cells per milliliter.[141,142] In addition, many patients are neutropenic (absolute neutrophil count <1000 cells per milliliter).[141,142] The lungs are the most common site of infection.[142] Clinical manifestations including fever, cough, and dyspnea are the most common symptoms, although chest pain and hemoptysis also occur.[142] Chest radiograph may demonstrate focal infiltrates, nodules, or diffuse infiltrates.[142] Cavitation also may be seen on chest film.[142] The diagnosis of invasive aspergillosis is a difficult one to establish. In one large series, *Aspergillus* species were cultured from the respiratory tract of 4 percent of patients with AIDS.[141] *Aspergillus* was believed to be invasive in only 11 percent of these patients. Therefore culture of *Aspergillus* from sputum or bronchoalveolar lavage is not diagnostic. Transbronchial biopsy or transthoracic needle biopsy may establish the diagnosis. Endobronchial ulceration and pseudomembranes have also been described.[143] Therapy for invasive *Aspergillus* infection typically requires amphotericin B, though itraconazole also holds promise in those patients able to take oral medications.[144] The overall response rate and survival are poor.[142]

Infection with *Blastomyces dermatitidis* recently has been reported with increasing frequency in HIV-infected individuals.[145,146] Blastomycosis appears to be a late complication, with more than 85 percent of cases with CD4+ counts of <200 cells per milliliter. Dissemination occurred with equal frequency when compared with non-HIV-infected patients, but meningeal disease was more common.[146] Pulmonary disease was present in 80 percent of patients.[145] Radiographic abnormalities were noted in 73 percent of patients, and diffuse lung lesions were the most common abnormality.[145] Diagnosis requires demonstration of typical histologic appearance in sputum, BAL, or other pathologic specimens or growth in culture. The latter often requires 2 to 4 weeks. Response to therapy has been poor, with a mortality of 54 percent.[146] Amphotericin is still the drug of choice, because of the high incidence of central nervous system infection.[145]

PRIMARY FUNGAL PROPHYLAXIS

Fungal infections remain a cause of significant morbidity and mortality in HIV-infected patients. Because of the success of prophylaxis against *P. carinii*, other infections, such as fungal infections, may become more common. To date, this has not been reported.[70] Nevertheless, interest in primary prophylaxis against fungal infections seems appropriate. A large trial was recently completed, which examined the effects of fluconazole in the prevention of fungal infections in patients with advanced HIV. Fluconazole clearly protected against the development of cryptococcosis and candidiasis. There was no protective effect against aspergillosis or histoplasmosis, though the numbers of these infections were small. Overall survival was not different between those receiving fluconazole and those treated with clotrimazole troches (the control group). At the present time, primary prophylaxis against fungal infection in HIV-infected patients remains an area of investigation.

Other Pulmonary Infections

There are many other pulmonary infections which complicate HIV infection. Two of these infections, warrant specific mention. They are atypical mycobacterial infection and cytomegalovirus infection.

Infection with atypical mycobacteria, in particular with *M. avium* complex (MAC), has been recognized as a common infectious complication which occurs late in the course of HIV infection. Patients typically present with fevers and wasting and often have adenopathy. Isolated pulmonary disease is unusual in MAC infection,[147] and isolation of the organism usually represents colonization. However, pulmonary disease can occur, and both parenchymal and endobronchial disease have been described.[148,149] Furthermore, isolation of MAC from the respiratory tract portends disseminated disease in many patients.[150] If there is evidence of localized pulmonary or disseminated MAC, therapy should be instituted. Therapy should include a macrolide antibiotic such as clarithromycin or azithromycin, ethambutol, and possibly a quinolone antibiotic like ciprofloxacin or ofloxacin.[150] Pulmonary disease in HIV-infected patients caused by *M. kansasii* has also been reported.[151]

Cytomegalovirus (CMV) is the cause of several different clinical syndromes in HIV-infected patients, including retinitis, colitis, esophagitis, and adrenalitis.[152] Nevertheless, its role as a pulmonary pathogen appears to be limited. Early reports suggested that CMV pneumonitis was a common cause of pulmonary pathology in patients with AIDS.[153] However, subsequent studies demonstrated no adverse effects associated with CMV cultured from bronchoalveolar lavage fluid.[154] In fact, detection of CMV in BAL was associated with a better outcome from PCP and was not associated with subsequent disseminated CMV disease. Thus, therapy of CMV in HIV-infected patients is warranted only if there is CMV disease outside the lungs, or if there is no other cause of pulmonary disease and cytopathologic changes of CMV are documented in the lungs.

Noninfectious Pulmonary Disease

Noninfectious diseases can also cause pulmonary complications in HIV-infected patients. Malignancies associated with HIV infection, Kaposi's sarcoma in particular, can involve the lungs. Two pneumonitides also may affect HIV-infected patients: nonspecific pneumonitis and lymphocytic pneumonitis.

KAPOSI'S SARCOMA

Kaposi's sarcoma (KS) is the most common HIV-associated malignancy. It may cause pulmonary involvement, which can be fatal. Pulmonary disease is common at autopsy in HIV-infected patients with KS, approaching 20 percent of those with cutaneous lesions.[155] Isolated pulmonary disease is unusual, but certainly described.[156]

PATHOGENESIS
The understanding of the origins of KS in HIV-infected patients is evolving. Increased expression of cytokines by HIV-infected lymphocytes, in conjunction with the HIV-1 Tat protein, may drive the proliferation of vascular endothelium and smooth muscle that characterizes KS.[157] The increased

prevalence of KS in homosexual populations suggested that a sexually transmitted agent might be causative.[158] Recently nonhuman, herpes virus-like DNA has been indentified in KS, suggesting a possible viral etiology of the malignancy.[159] Similar DNA sequences have been detected in non-HIV-infected patients with KS.[160]

EPIDEMIOLOGY

Kaposi's sarcoma has been a frequent complication of HIV infection among homosexuals, but is much less common among other HIV risk groups.[161] Within the homosexual population, the occurrence of KS is associated with certain sexual practices.[162] It is interesting to note that the incidence of KS, even among high-risk groups, has declined in the United States.[163]

CLINICAL PRESENTATION

The clinical presentation of KS is similar to that of many infectious pulmonary complications of HIV infection. Patients often present with fever, cough, and dyspnea.[156] Hemoptysis and hoarseness may also be presenting symptoms.[164] Physical examination is equally nonspecific, although the presence of cutaneous KS should heighten suspicion of pulmonary involvement. Radiographic appearance is typically that of diffuse coarse nodular or interstitial infiltrates.[165] Pleural effusions are common (Fig. 105-12). Hilar adenopathy may be noted, but is not typical.[164]

DIAGNOSIS

The definitive diagnosis of KS requires histologic examination of involved tissue. Unfortunately, in the case of pulmonary KS this often requires open lung biopsy.[156] The yield

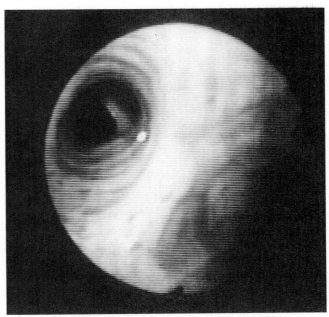

FIGURE 105-13 Endobronchial lesions of Kaposi's sarcoma.

from bronchoscopic biopsies, both endobronchial and transbronchial, is variable.[166–168] Excessive bleeding has been reported with bronchoscopic biopsies,[169] though others have commented on the safety of the procedure.[156] Because of the low yield and reported risk of bronchoscopic biopsies, many authors argue that the distinctive appearance of endobronchial KS is adequate to establish the diagnosis of pulmonary KS,[169,170] particularly when cutaneous disease (Figs. 105-13 and 14) is present. Thoracentesis and pleural biopsy have also been similarly unrewarding methods to obtain a

FIGURE 105-12 Chest radiograph of HIV-positive patient with pulmonary Kaposi's sarcoma.

FIGURE 105-14 Endobronchial lesions of Kaposi's sarcoma.

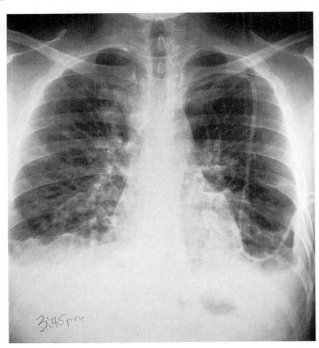

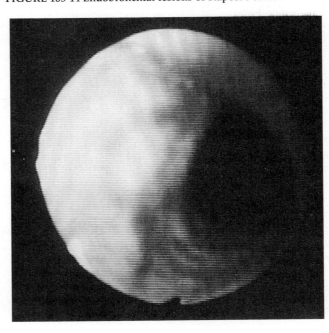

tissue diagnosis.[166] Open-lung biopsy remains the most assured means of obtaining a tissue diagnosis, but its use in HIV-related lung lesions is restricted to unusual cases,[171] for example, an HIV-infected patient with progressive pulmonary disease, negative bronchoalveolar lavage, and transbronchial biopsy and no other signs of KS.

THERAPY

Combined modality chemotherapy has been utilized to treat pulmonary KS. A regimen consisting of doxorubicin, bleomycin, and vincristine has had a 60 percent response rate in pulmonary KS.[172] Radiation therapy has been used for palliation of localized lesions and diffuse disease.[173]

PROGNOSIS

The prognosis of HIV-infected patients with pulmonary KS is poor. In the above-noted chemotherapy study, median survival of responders was 10 months.

LYMPHOMA

Lymphoma is the second most common malignancy to complicate HIV infection. Lymphoma may complicate the course of up to 25 percent of HIV-infected patients[164] and may soon account for > 25 percent of all non-Hodgkin's lymphoma.[174] Pulmonary involvement is seen in 25 percent of cases, and <10 percent of patients in two series.[175,176] Symptoms typically are the result of extrapulmonary manifestations of the lymphoma. Radiographic findings range from adenopathy to parenchymal infiltrates.[177] Diagnosis is usually made from sites outside the chest (bone marrow biopsy, lymph node biopsy). In those unusual individuals with primary intrathoracic lymphoma diagnosis may require open biopsy. Therapy requires combined modality chemotherapy.[178]

INTERSTITIAL PNEUMONITIS

Nonspecific interstitial pneumonitis (NIP) and lymphocytic interstitial pneumonitis (LIP) are two "noninfectious" complications of HIV infection. They are reported with varying frequency in series of pulmonary complications of HIV infection, ranging from uncommon to > 30 percent of cases of pneumonitis.[179,180] In several series, NIP has been much more common than LIP in adults.[180,181] In children, LIP is a common complication of HIV infection, often associated with pulmonary lymphoid hyperplasia.[182]

PATHOGENESIS

The pathologic changes of NIP and LIP are similar, in that both demonstrate lymphocytic and plasma cell infiltration.[181] The degree of cellularity appears greater in patients with LIP, and cellular infiltration occurs in the alveolar septae. The cellularity in NIP is localized to peribronchial, perivascular, and paraseptal regions.[181] Alveolar damage is more extensive in LIP[181]; extrathoracic lymphocytic proliferation is much more common in LIP.[183] Because of the similarities of pathology between these two entities, the possibility of a common etiologic agent has been considered. Recent evidence suggests that HIV itself may be responsible.[181,184] Epstein-Barr virus (EBV) has also been implicated in LIP,[185] though the above-noted study found little evidence for EBV infection in patients with nonspecific interstitial pneumonitis.[181]

CLINICAL MANIFESTATIONS

Patients presenting with interstitial pneumonitis typically have pulmonary symptoms, usually cough[180]; fever is also common.[180] It should be noted, however, that in one series of HIV-infected patients without symptoms or plain chest radiographic abnormalities, 48 percent had pathologic changes consistent with NIP.[186] Physical examination and chest radiography were indistinguishable from opportunistic infection.[180]

DIAGNOSIS

The diagnosis of LIP or NIP is made by documentation of absence of opportunistic infection with histology consistent with interstitial pneumonitis. In children, a clinical picture consistent with LIP and absence of opportunistic infection by BAL may be considered adequate to establish the diagnosis[182]; however, many pediatricians would confirm the diagnosis with open biopsy prior to treatment.

TREATMENT

In many patients, NIP and LIP are minimally symptomatic and observation alone is appropriate.[180,186] In those patients with LIP and progressive symptoms, corticosteroids have been shown to improve symptoms and physiologic parameters in both children and adults.[187,188]

PROGNOSIS

The prognosis of NIP and LIP in HIV-infected patients is, in general, good.[180,186] Response to therapy for LIP with corticosteroids is frequent in those patients with progressive symptoms. Major morbidity and mortality are primarily due to coincident opportunistic infections.

References

1. Murray J, Mills J: Pulmonary infectious complications of human immunodeficiency virus infection. *Am Rev Respir Dis*, 1990; 141:1356, 1582.
2. Washburn R, Tuazon C, Bennett J: Phagocytic and fungicidal activity of monocytes from patients with acquired immunodeficiency syndrome. *J Infect Dis* 1985; 151:565.
3. Chaturvedi S, Frame P, Newman S: Macrophages from human immunodeficiency virus positive persons are defective in host defense against Histoplasma capsulatum. *J Infect Dis* 1995; 171:320.
4. Smith P, et al.: Monocyte function in the acquired immune deficiency syndrome. *J Clin Invest* 1984; 74:2121.
5. Fauci A: Immunopathogenic mechanisms in human immunodeficiency virus (HIV) infection. *Ann Intern Med* 1991; 114:678.
6. Murray H, Scavuzzo D, Kelly C, et al.: T4+ cell production of interferon gamma and the clinical spectrum of patients at risk for and with the acquired immunodeficiency syndrome. *Arch Intern Med* 1988; 148:1613.
7. Masur H, et al.: CD4 counts as predictors of opportunistic pneumonias in human immunodeficiency virus (HIV) infection. *Ann Intern Med* 1989; 111:223.

8. Sundre P, ten Dam G, Kochi A: Tuberculosis: a global overview of the situation today. *Bull WHO* 1992; 70:149.

9. Centers for Disease Control: Prevention and control of tuberculosis in U.S. communities with at-risk minority populations, and prevention and control of tuberculosis among homeless persons: Recommendations of the Advisory Council for the Elimination of Tuberculosis. *MMWR* 1992; 41:1.

10. Armstrong J, Hart P: Response of cultured macrophages to *Mycobacterium tuberculosis*, with observations on fusion of lysosomes and phagosomes. *J Exp Med* 1971; 134:713.

11. Daley C, Small P, Schecter G, et al.: An outbreak of tuberculosis with accelerated progression among persons infected with the human immunodeficiency virus. An analysis using restriction length polymorphisms. *N Eng J Med* 1992; 326:231.

12. Bloch A, Rieder H, Kelly G, et al.: The epidemiology of tuberculosis in the United States. *Sem Resp Infect* 1989; 4:157.

13. Selwyn P, Hartel D, Lewis V, et al.: A prospective study of the risk of tuberculosis among intravenous drug users with human immunodeficiency virus infection. *N Engl J Med* 1989; 320:545.

14. Whalen C, Horsburgh C, Hom D, et al.: Accelerated course of human immunodeficiency virus infection after tuberculosis. *Am J Resp Crit Care Med* 1995; 151:129.

15. Pitchenik AE, Burr J, Suarez M, et al.: Human T-cell lymphotropic virus-III (HTLV-III) seropositivity and related disease among 71 consecutive patients in whom tuberculosis was diagnosed. *Am Rev Respir Dis* 1987; 135:875.

16. Flora G, Modilevsky T, Antoniskis D, Barnes P: Undiagnosed tuberculosis in patients with human immunodeficiency virus infection. *Chest* 1990; 98:1056.

17. Long R, et al.: The chest roentgenogram in pulmonary tuberculosis patients seropositive for human immunodeficiency virus type 1. *Chest* 1991; 99:123.

18. Markowitz N, Hansen N, Wilcosky T, et al.: Tuberculin and anergy testing in HIV-seropositive and HIV-seronegative persons. *Ann Intern Med* 1993; 119:185.

19. Blatt S, Hendrix C, Butzin C, et al.: Delayed type hypersensitivity skin testing predicts progression to AIDS in HIV-infected patients. *Ann Intern Med* 1993; 119:177.

20. Moreno S, Baraia-Etxaburu J, Bouza E, et al.: Risk for developing tuberculosis among anergic patients infected with HIV. *Ann Intern Med* 1993; 119:194.

21. CDC: Purified protein derivative (PPD)-tuberculin anergy and HIV infection: Guidelines for anergy testing and management of anergic persons at risk of tuberculosis. *MMWR* 1991; 40:27.

22. Levy H, Feldman C, Sacho H, et al.: A reevaluation of sputum microscopy and culture in the diagnosis of pulmonary tuberculosis. *Chest* 1989; 95:1193.

23. Gordin F, Slutkin G: The validity of acid-fast smears in the diagnosis of pulmonary tuberculosis. *Arch Pathol Lab Med* 1990; 114:1025.

24. Klein N, Duncanson F, Lenox T, et al.: Use of mycobacterial smears in the diagnosis of pulmonary tuberculosis in AIDS/ARC patients. *Chest* 1989; 95:1190.

25. Kennedy DJ, Lewis WP, Barnes PF: Yield of bronchoscopy for the diagnosis of tuberculosis in patients with human immunodeficiency virus infection. *Chest* 1992; 102:1040.

26. Jones BE, Young SM, Antoniskis D, et al.: Relationship of the manifestations to tuberculosis to CD4 cell counts in patients with human immunodeficiency virus infection. *Am Rev Respir Dis* 1993; 148:1292.

27. Meduri G, Stover D, Greeno R, et al.: Bilateral bronchoalveolar lavage in the diagnosis of opportunistic pulmonary infections. *Chest* 1991; 100:1272.

28. American Thoracic Society: Treatment of tuberculosis and tuberculosis infection in adults and children. *Am J Resp Crit Care Med* 1994; 149:1359.

29. Small P, et al.: Treatment of tuberculosis in patients with advanced human immunodeficiency virus infection. *N Eng J Med* 1991; 324:289.

30. Jones B, Otaya M, Antoniskis D, et al.: A prospective evaluation of antituberculosis therapy in patients with human immunodeficiency virus infection. *Am J Resp Crit Care Med* 1994; 150:1499.

31. Perriens J, St Louis M, Muhadi Y, et al.: Pulmonary tuberculosis in HIV infected patients in Zaire. A controlled trial for either 6 or 12 months. *N Eng J Med* 1995; 332:779.

32. Fischl MA, Uttamchandani RB, Daikos GL, et al.: An outbreak of tuberculosis caused by multiple-drug resistant tubercle bacilli among patients with HIV infection. *Ann Intern Med* 1992; 117:177.

33. Nosocomial transmission of multi-drug resistant tuberculosis among HIV-infected persons—Florida and New York, 1988–1991. *MMWR* 1991; 40:585.

34. Edlin B, Tokars J, Grieco M, et al.: An outbreak of multi-drug resistant tuberculosis among hospitalized patients with the acquired immunodeficiency syndrome. *N Eng J Med* 1992; 326:1514.

35. Beck-Sague C, Dooley S, Hutton M, et al.: Hospital outbreak of multi-drug resistant *Mycobacterium tuberculosis* infection. *J Am Med Assoc* 1992; 268:1280.

36. Fischl MA, Daikos GL, Uttamchandani RB, et al.: Clinical presentation and outcome of patients with HIV infection and tuberculosis caused by multiple-drug resistant bacilli. *Ann Intern Med* 1992; 117:184.

37. Centers for Disease Control: The use of preventive therapy for tuberculosis infection in the United States. Recommendations of the advisory committee for elimination of tuberculosis. *MMWR* 1990; 39:9.

38. Rosen M: Pneumonia in patients with HIV infection. *Med Clin NA* 1994; 78:1067.

39. Wallace J, Rao V, Glassroth J, et al.: Respiratory illness in persons with human immunodeficiency virus infection. *Am Rev Resp Dis* 1993; 148:1523.

40. Centers for Disease Control: 1993 revised classification system for HIV infection and expanded surveillance case definitions for AIDS among adolescents and adults. *MMWR* 1992; 41:1.

41. Parkin J et al.: Immunoglobulin G subclass deficiency and susceptibility to pyogenic infections in patients with AIDS related complex and AIDS. *AIDS* 1989; 3:37.

42. Bender B, Bohnsack J, Sourlis S, et al.: Demonstration of defective C3-receptor-mediated clearance by the reticuloendothelial system in patients with acquired immunodeficiency syndrome. *J Clin Invest* 1987; 79:715.

43. Simberkoff M, El-Sadr W, Schiffman G, Rahal J: *Streptococcus pneumoniae* infections and bacteremia in patients with acquired immunodeficiency syndrome, with a report of pneumococcal vaccine failure. *Am Rev Resp Dis* 1984; 130:1174.

44. Schlamm H, Yancovitz S: *Haemophilus influenzae* pneumonia in young adults with AIDS, ARC, or risk of AIDS. *Am J Med* 1989; 86:11.

45. Caiaffa WT, Graham NMH, Vlahov D: Bacterial pneumonia in adult populations with human immunodeficiency virus (HIV) infection. *Am J Epidemiol* 1993; 138(11):909.

46. Daley C: Bacterial pneumonia in HIV-infected patients. *Sem Resp Infect* 1993; 8:104.

47. Weingarten J, Huang D, Jackman J: *Rhodococcus equi* pneumonia. *Chest* 1988; 94:195.

48. Krumholz H, Sande M, Lo B: Community-acquired bacteremia in patients with acquired immunodeficiency: Clinical presentation, bacteriology and outcome. *Am J Med* 1989; 86:776.

49. Janoff EN, Breiman RF, Daley CL, et al.: Pneumococcal disease during HIV infection. Epidemiologic, clinical, and immunologic perspectives. *Ann Intern Med* 1992; 117:314.

50. Kovacs J, et al.: *Pneumocystis carinii* pneumonia: A comparison between patients with acquired immunodeficiency syndrome and patients with other immunodeficiencies. *Ann Intern Med* 1984; 100:663.

51. Franzetti M, Cernuschi M, Esposito R, et al.: Pseudomonas infections in patients with AIDS and AIDS-related complex. *J Intern Med* 1992; 231:437.

52. Niederman M, Bass J, Campbell G, et al.: Guidelines for the initial management of adults with community acquired pneumonia: Diagnosis, assessment of severity, and initial antimicrobial therapy. American Thoracic Society. *Am Rev Resp Dis* 1993; 148:1418.

53. Magnenat J, et al.: Mode of presentation and diagnosis of bacterial pneumonia in human immunodeficiency virus infected patients. *Am Rev Respir Dis* 1991; 144:917.

54. Polsky B, Gold J, Wimberly E, et al.: Bacterial pneumonia in patients with the acquired immunodeficiency syndrome. *Ann Intern Med* 1986; 104:38.

55. Baselski V, Wunderink R: Bronchoscopic diagnosis of pneumonia. [Review] *Clin Microbiol Rev* 1994; 7:533.

56. Ferrer M, Torres A, Xaubet A, et al.: Diagnostic value of telescoping plugged catheters in HIV-infected patients with pulmonary infiltrates. *Chest* 1992; 102:76.

57. Janoff EN, O'Brien J, Thompson P, et al.: *Streptococcus pneumoniae* colonization, bacteremia, and immune response among persons with human immunodeficiency virus infection. *J Infect Dis* 1993; 167:49.

58. Cohn, D: Bacterial pneumonia in the HIV-infected patient. [Review] *Infect Dis Clin North Am* 1991; 5:485.

59. Friedland I, McCracken G: Management of infections caused by antibiotic-resistant *Streptococcus pneumoniae*. *N Eng J Med* 1994; 331:377.

60. Penicillin-resistant pneumococcal meningitis in an HIV-infected man. *N Eng J Med* 1991; 325:1047.

61. Nordmann P, Ronco E: In vitro antimicrobial susceptibility of *Rhodococcus equi*. *J Antimicrob Chemo* 1992; 29:383.

62. Shapiro E, Berg T, Austrian R, et al.: The protective efficacy of polyvalent pneumococcal polysaccharide vaccine. *N Eng J Med* 1991; 325:1453.

63. Ballet JJ, Sulcebe G, Coudere LJ, et al.: Impaired antipneumococcal antibody response in patients with AIDS-related persistent generalized lymphadenopathy. *Clin Exp Immunol* 1987; 68:479.

64. Centers for Disease Control: Immunziation practices advisory committee. Pneumococcal polysaccharide vaccine. *MMWR* 1988; 40:64.

65. Davies S: Pneumococcal pneumonia, in Niederman M, Sarosi G, Glassroth J (eds): *Respiratory Infections. A scientific basis for management*. Philadelphia, WB Saunders, 1994.

66. Pesola GR, Charles A: Pneumococcal bacteremia with pneumonia. *Chest* 1992; 101:150.

67. Nelson MR, Shanson DC, Barter GJ, et al.: *Pseudomonas* septicaemia associated with HIV. *AIDS* 1991; 5:761.

68. Drancourt M, Bonnet E, Gallais H, et al.: *Rhodococcus equi* infection in patients with AIDS. *J Infect* 1992; 24:123.

69. Hopewell P: *Pneumocystis carinii* pneumonia: Diagnosis. *J Infect Dis* 1988; 157:1115.

70. Hoover D, Saah AJ, Bacellar H, et al.: Clinical manifestations of AIDS in the era of pneumocystis prophylaxis. *N Engl J Med* 1992; 329:1922.

71. Pifer L, Hughes W, Stagno S, Woods D: *Pneumocystis carinii* infection: evidence for high prevalence in normal and immunosuppressed children. *Pediatrics* 1978; 61:35.

72. Frenkel J, Good J, Schultz J: Latent *Pneumocystis* infection in rats, relapse and chemotherapy. *Lab Invest* 1966; 15:1559.

73. Walzer P, Kim C, Linke M, et al.: Outbreaks of *Pneumocystis carinii* pneumonia in colonies of immunodeficient mice. *Infect Immunol* 1989; 57:62.

74. Su T, Martin W: Pathogenesis and host response in *Pneumocystis carinii* pneumonia. *Ann Rev Med* 1994; 45:261.

75. Harmsen A, Stankiewicz M: T cells are not sufficient for resistance to *Pneumocystis carinii* pneumonia in mice. *J Protozool* 1991; 38:44S.

76. Yoneda K, Walzer P: Interaction of *Pneumocystis carinii* with host lungs: An ultrastructural study. *Infect Immun* 1980; 29:692.

77. Zimmerman P, Martin J: in Niederman M, Sarosi G, Glassroth J (eds): *Pneumocystis carinii in Respiratory Infections: A Scientific Basis for Management*. Philadelphia, WB Saunders, 1994.

78. Batungwanayo J, Taelman H, Lucas S, et al.: Pulmonary disease associated with the human immunodeficiency virus in Kigali, Rwanda. A fiberoptic bronchoscopic study of 111 cases of undetermined etiology. *Am J Resp Crit Care Med* 1994:149:1591.

79. Northfelt D, Clement M, Safrin S: Extrapulmonary pneumocystosis: Clinical features in human immunodeficiency virus infection. *Medicine* 1990; 69:392.

80. Levine S, White D: *Pneumocystis carinii*. *Clin Chest Med* 1988; 9:395.

81. Jules-Elysee K, Stover D, Zaman M, et al.: Aerosolized pentamidine: Effect on diagnosis and presentation of *Pneumocystis carinii* pneumonia. *Ann Intern Med* 1990; 112:750.

82. Shin M, Veal C, Jessup J, et al.: Apical *Pneumocystis carinii* pneumonia in AIDS patients not receiving inhaled pentamidine prophylaxis. *Chest* 1991; 100:1462.

83. Zaman M, White D: Serum lactate dehydrogenase levels and *Pneumocystis carinii* pneumonia. *Am Rev Respir Dis* 1988; 137:796.

84. Lipman M, Goldstein E: Serum lactate dehydrogenase predicts mortality in patients with AIDS and *Pneumocystis* pneumonia. *West J Med* 1988; 149:486.

85. Tuazon L, et al.: Sensitivity of gallium[67] scintigraphy and bronchial washings in the diagnosis and treatment of *Pneumocystis carinii* pneumonia in patients with the acquired immune deficiency syndrome. *Am Rev Respir Dis* 1985; 132:1087.

86. Hopewell P, Luce J: Pulmonary involvement in the acquired immunodeficiency syndrome. *Chest* 1985; 84:104.

87. Digby T, et al.: Usefulness of induced sputum in the diagnosis of *Pneumocystis carinii* pneumonia in patients with the acquired immunodeficiency syndrome. *Am Rev Respir Dis* 1986; 133:515.

88. Kovacs J, Ng V, Masur H, et al.: Diagnosis of *Pneumocystis carinii* pneumonia: Improved detection in sputum with use of monoclonal antibodies. *N Eng J Med* 1988; 318:589.

89. Broaddus C, Dake MD, Stulbarg MS, et al.: Bronchoalveolar lavage and transbronchial biopsy for the diagnosis of pulmonary infections in the acquired immunodeficiency syndrome. *Ann Intern Med* 1985; 102:747.

90. Weldon-Linne C, Rhone D, Bourassa R: Bronchoscopy specimens in adults with AIDS. Comparative yields of cytology, histology and culture for diagnosis of infectious agents. *Chest* 1990; 98:24.

91. Luce J, Stover D: Controversies in pulmonary medicine: Presumed *Pneumocystis carinii* pneumonia should be treated empirically in a patient with the acquired immunodeficiency syndrome. *Am Rev Resp Dis* 1988; 138:1076.

92. Tu JV, Biem HJ, Detsky AL: Bronchoscopy vs. empirical therapy in HIV-infected patients with presumptive *Pneumocystis carinii* pneumonia. *Am Rev Respir Dis* 1993; 148:370.

93. Wharton JM, Coleman DL, Wofsy CB, et al.: Trimethoprim-sulfamethoxazole or pentamidine for *Pneumocystis carinii* pneumonia in the acquired immunodeficiency syndrome. A prospective randomized trial. *Ann Intern Med* 1986; 105:37.

94. Klein NC, Duncanson FP, Lenox TH, et al.: Trimethoprim-sulfamethoxazole versus pentamidine for *Pneumocystis carinii* pneumonia in AIDS patients: Results of a large prospective randomized treatment trial. *AIDS* 1992; 6:301.

95. Sattler FR, Cowan R, Nielson DM, et al.: Trimethoprim-sulfamethoxazole compared with pentamidine for treatment of *Pneumocystis carinii* pneumonia in the acquired immunodeficiency syndrome. A prospective, noncrossover study. *Ann Int Med* 1988; 109:280.

96. Greenberg S, Reiser I, Shyan-Yih C, Porush J: Trimethoprim-sulfamethoxazole induces reversible hyperkalemia. *Ann Intern Med* 1993; 119:291.

97. Safrin S, Sattler F, Lee B, et al.: Dapsone as a single agent is suboptimal therapy for *Pneumocystis carinii* pneumonia. *J Acquired Immune Defic Synd* 1991; 4:244.

98. Hughes W, Leoung G, Kramer F, et al.: Comparison of atovaquone (566C80) with trimethoprim sulfamethoxazole to treat *Pneumocystis carinii* pneumonia in patients with AIDS. *N Engl J Med* 1993; 328:1521.

99. Sattler F, Frame P, Davis R, et al.: Trimetrexate with leucovorin versus trimethoprim-sulfamethoxazole for moderate to severe episodes of *Pneumocystis carinii* pneumonia in patients with AIDS: A prospective, controlled multicenter investigation of the AIDS Clinical Trials Group Protocol 029/031. *J Infect Dis* 1994; 170:165.

100. Medina I, Mills J, Leoung G, et al.: Oral therapy for *Pneumocystis carinii* pneumonia in the acquired immunodeficiency syndrome: A controlled trial of trimethoprim-sulfamethoxazole versus trimethoprim-dapsone. *N Eng J Med* 1990; 323:776.

101. Toma E, Fournier S, Dumont M, et al.: Clindamycin/primaquine versus trimethoprim-sulfamethoxazole as primary therapy for *Pneumocystis carinii* pneumonia in AIDS: A randomized, double-blind pilot trial. *Clin Infect Dis* 1993; 17:178.

102. Bozette S, et al.: A controlled trial of early adjunctive treatment with corticosteroids for *Pneumocystis carinii* pneumonia in the acquired immunodeficiency syndrome. *N Engl J Med* 1990; 323:1451.

103. Gagnon S, et al.: Corticosteroids as adjunctive therapy for severe *Pneumocystis carinii* pneumonia in the acquired immunodeficiency syndrome. *N Engl J Med* 1990; 323:1444.

104. Consensus statement on the use of corticosteroids as adjunctive therapy for *Pneumocystis* pneumonia in the acquired immunodeficiency syndrome. *N Engl J Med* 1990; 323:1500.

105. Fischl M, Dickinson G, LaVoie L: Safety and efficacy of sulfamethoxazole and trimethoprim chemoprophylaxis for *Pneumocystis carinii* pneumonia in AIDS. *J Am Med Assoc* 1988; 259:1185.

106. Hirschel B, Lazzarin A, Chopard P, et al.: A controlled trial of inhaled pentamidine for primary prevention of *Pneumocystis carinii* pneumonia. *N Engl J Med* 1991; 324:1079.

107. Schneider ME, Hoepelman AIM, Schattenkerk JK, et al.: A controlled trial of aerosolized pentamidine or trimethoprim-sulfamethoxazole as primary prophylaxis against *Pneumocystis carinii* pneumonia in patients with human immunodeficiency virus infection. *N Engl J Med* 1992; 327:1836.

108. Stein D, Stevens R, Terry C, et al.: Use of low-dose trimethoprim-sulfamethoxazole thrice weekly for primary and secondary prophylaxis of *Pneumocystis carinii* pneumonia in human immunodeficiency virus-infected patients. *Antimicrob Agents Chemo* 1991; 35:1705.

109. Torres R, Barr M, Thorn M, et al.: Randomized trial of dapsone and aerosolized pentamidine for the prophylaxis of *Pneumocystis carinii* pneumonia and Toxoplasmic encephalitis. *Am J Med* 1993; 95:573.

110. Blum R, Miller L, Gaggini L, Cohn D: Comparative trial of dapsone versus trimethoprim/sulfamethoxazole for primary prophylaxis of *Pneumocystis carinii* pneumonia. *J Acquired Immune Defic Synd* 1992; 5:341.

111. Leoung G, et al.: Aerosolized pentamidine for prophylaxis against *Pneumocystis carinii* pneumonia. The San Francisco community prophylaxis trial. *N Engl J Med* 1992; 323:769.

112. Hardy W, Feinberg J, Finkelstein D, et al.: A controlled trial of trimethoprim-sulfamethoxazole or aerosolized pentamidine for secondary prophylaxis of *Pneumocystis carinii* pneumonia in patients with the acquired immunodeficiency syndrome. *N Engl J Med* 1992; 327:1842.

113. Girard P, Landman R, Gaudebout C, et al.: Dapsone-pyrimethamine compared with aerosolized pentamidine as primary prophylaxis against *Pneumocystis carinii* pneumonia and toxoplasmosis HIV infection. *N Eng J Med* 1993; 328:1514.

114. Hawley P, Ronco J, Guillemi S, et al.: Decreasing frequency but worsening mortality of acute respiratory failure secondary to AIDS-related *Pneumocystis carinii* pneumonia *Chest* 1994; 106:1456.

115. Staikowsky F, Lafon B, Guidet B, et al.: Mechanical ventilation for *Pneumocystis carinii* pneumonia in patients with the acquired immunodeficiency syndrome. Is the prognosis really improved? *Chest* 1993; 104:756.

116. Wachter R, Luce J, Safrin S, Berrios D, et al.: Cost and outcome of intensive care for patients with AIDS, *Pneumocystis carinii* pneumonia, and severe respiratory failure. *J Am Med Assoc* 1995; 273:230.

117. Stansell JD; Pulmonary fungal infections in HIV-infected persons. *Sem Resp Inf* 1993; 8:116.

118. Schaffner A, Davis D, Schaffner T, et al.: In vitro susceptibility of fungi to killing by neutrophil granulocytes discriminates between primary pathogenicity and opportunism. *J Clin Invest* 1986; 78:511.

119. Davies S: Fungal pneumonia. *Med Clin North Am* 1994; 78:1049.

120. Wheat L, et al.: Disseminated histoplasmosis in the acquired immune deficiency syndrome: Clinical findings, diagnosis and treatment, and review of the literature. *Medicine* 1990; 69:361.

121. Chuck S, Sande M: Infections with *Cryptococcus neoformans* in the acquired immunodeficiency syndrome. *N Eng J Med* 1989; 321:794.

122. Fish D, Ampel N, Galgiani J, et al.: Coccidioidomycosis during human immunodeficiency virus infection. A review of 77 patients. *Medicine* 1990; 69:384.

123. Chechani V, Kamholz S: Pulmonary manifestations of disseminated cryptococcosis in patients with AIDS. *Chest* 1990; 98:1060.

124. Batungwanayo J, Taelman H, Bogaerts J, et al.: Pulmonary cryptococcosis associated with HIV-1 infection in Rwanda: A retrospective study of 37 cases. *AIDS* 1994; 8:1271.

125. Saag M, Powderly W, Cloud G, et al.: Comparison of amphotericin B with fluconazole in the treatment of acute AIDS-associated cryptococcal meningitis. *N Eng J Med* 1992; 326:83.

126. Nightingale S: Initial therapy for acquired immunodeficiency syndrome-associated cryptococcus with fluconazole. *Arch Inter Med* 1995; 155:538.

127. Bozzette S, Larsen P, Chiu J, et al.: A placebo controlled trial of maintenance therapy of cryptococcal meningitis in the acquired immuno deficiency syndrome. California Collaborative Treatment Group. *N Engl J Med* 1992; 324:580.

128. Wheat L: Histoplasmosis in AIDS. *AIDS Clin Care* 1992; 4:1.

129. Sarosi G, Johnson P: Progressive disseminated histoplasmosis in the acquired immunodeficiency syndrome: A model for disseminated disease. *Sem Resp Inf* 1990; 5:146.

130. McKinsey D, Gupta M, Riddler S, et al.: Long-term amphotericin B therapy for disseminated histoplasmosis in patients

with the acquired immunodeficiency syndrome (AIDS). *Ann Intern Med* 1989; 111:655.

131. Sharkey-Mathis P, Velez J, Fetchick R, Graybill J: Histoplasmosis in the acquired immunodeficiency syndrome (AIDS): Treatment with itraconazole and fluconazole. *J Acquired Immune Defic Synd* 1993; 6:809.

132. Wheat J, Hafner R, Korzun A, et al.: Itraconazole treatment of disseminated histoplasmosis in patients with the acquired immunodeficiency syndrome. *Am J Med* 1995; 98:336.

133. Wheat J, Hafner R, Wulfsohn M, et al.: Prevention of relapse of histoplasmosis with itraconazole in patients with the acquired immunodeficiency syndrome. *Ann Intern Med* 1993; 118:610.

134. Norris S, Wheat J, McKinsey D, et al.: Prevention of relapse of histoplasmosis with fluconazole in patients with the acquired immunodeficiency syndrome. *Am J Med* 1994; 96:504.

135. Ampel N, Dols C, Galgiani J: Coccidioidomycosis during human immunodeficiency virus infection: Results of a prospective study of coccidioidal endemic area. *Am J Med* 1993; 94:235.

136. Dodge R, Lebowitz M, Barbee R, et al.: Estimates of *C. immitis* infection by skin test reactivity in an endemic community. *Am J Pub Health* 1985; 75:863.

137. Sobonya R, Barbee R, Wiens J, Trego D: Detection of fungi and other pathogens in immunocomprised patients by bronchoalveolar lavage in an area endemic for coccidioidomycosis. *Chest* 1990; 97:1349.

138. Mahaffey K, Hippenmeyer C, Mandel R, Ampel N: Unrecognized coccidioidomycosis complicating *Pneumocystic carinii* pneumonia in patients with the human immunodeficiency virus and treated with corticosteroids: A report of two cases. *Arch Intern Med* 1993; 153:1496.

139. Galgiani J, Catanzaro A, Cloud G, et al.: Fluconazole therapy for coccidioidal meningitis. The NIAID-Mycoses Study Group. *Ann Intern Med* 1993; 119:28.

140. Catanzaro A, Galgiani J, Levine B, et al.: Fluconazole in the treatment of chronic pulmonary and non-meningeal disseminated coccidioidomycosis. The NIAID Mycoses Study Group. *Am J Med* 1995; 98:249.

141. Purcell K, Telzak E, Armstrong D: *Aspergillus* species colonization and invasive disease in patients with AIDS. *Clin Infect Dis* 1992; 14:141.

142. Khoo S, Denning D: Invasive aspergillosis in patients with AIDS. *Clin Infect Dis* 1994; 19:S41.

143. Denning D, Follansbee S, Scolaro M, et al.: Pulmonary aspergillosis in the acquired immunodeficiency syndrome. *N Eng J Med* 1991; 324:654.

144. Denning D, Lee J, Hostetler J, et al.: NIAID Mycoses Study Group multicenter trial of oral itraconazole therapy for invasive aspergillosis.

145. Pappas P, Pottage J, Powderly W, et al.: Blastomycosis in patients with the acquired immunodeficiency syndrome. *Ann Intern Med* 1992; 116:847.

146. Witzig R, Hoadley D, Greer D, et al.: Blastomycosis and human immunodeficiency virus; three new cases and review. *Southern Med J* 0000; 87:0000.

147. Tenholder M, Moser R, Tellis C: Mycobacteria other than tuberculosis. Pulmonary involvement in patients with acquired immunodeficiency syndrome. *Arch Intern Med* 1988; 148:953.

148. Packer S, Cesario T, Williams J: *Mycobacterium avium-intracellulare* complex infection presenting as endobronchial lesions in immunosuppressed patients. *Ann Intern Med* 1988; 109:389.

149. Kalayjian R, Toosi Z, Tomashefski J, et al.: Pulmonary infections due to infection by *Mycobacterium avium* complex in patients with AIDS. *Clin Infect Dis* 1994; 20:1186.

150. Chin DP: *Mycobacterium avium* complex and other nontuberculous mycobacterial infections in patients with HIV. *Sem Resp Inf* 1993; 8(2):124.

151. Levine B, Chaisson RE: *Mycobacterium kansasii*: A cause of treatable pulmonary disease associated with advanced human immunodeficiency virus (HIV) infection. *Ann Intern Med* 1991; 114:861.

152. Chaisson R, Volberding P: Clinical manifestations of HIV infection, in Mandell G, Bennett J, Dolin R (eds): *Principles and Practice of Infectious Diseases.* New York, Churchill-Livingstone, 1995.

153. Jacobson M, Mills J: Cytomegalovirus infection. *Clin Chest Med* 1988; 9:443.

154. Bozzette S, Arcia J, Bartok A, et al.: Impact of *Pneumocystis carinii* and cytomegalovirus on the course and outcome of atypical pneumonia in advanced human immunodeficiency virus disease. *J Infect Dis* 1992; 165:93.

155. Ognibene F, Shelhamer J: Kaposi's sarcoma. *Clin Chest Med* 1988; 9:459.

156. Ognibene F, Steis R, Macher A, et al.: Kaposi's sarcoma causing pulmonary infiltrates and respiratory failure in the acquired immunodeficiency syndrome. *Ann Intern Med* 1985; 102:472.

157. Ensoli B, Barillari G, Gallo R: Cytokines and growth factors in the pathogenesis of AIDS-associated Kaposi's sarcoma. *Immunol Rev* 1992; 127:147.

158. Miles S: Pathogenesis of HIV-related Kaposi's sarcoma. *Curr Opin Oncol* 1994; 6:497.

159. Chang Y, Cesarman E, Pessin M, et al.: Identification of herpesviruslike DNA sequences in AIDS-associated Kaposi's sarcoma. *Science* 1994; 266:1865.

160. Moore P, Chang Y: Detection of herpesvirus-like DNA sequences in Kaposi's sarcoma in patients with and without HIV infection. *N Eng J Med* 1995; 332:1181.

161. Haverkos H, Drotman D: Prevalence of Kaposi's sarcoma among patients with AIDS. *N Eng J Med* 1985; 312:1518.

162. Beral V, Bull D, Jaffe H, et al.: Risk of Kaposi's sarcoma and sexual practices associated with faecal contact in homosexual or bisexual men with AIDS. *Lancet* 1992; 339:632.

163. Des Jarlais D, Stoneburner R, Thomas P, Friedman S: Declines in proportion of Kaposi's sarcoma among cases of AIDS in multiple risk groups in New York City. *Lancet* 1987; 2(8566):1024.

164. Irwin D, Kaplan L: Pulmonary manifestations of acquired immunodeficiency syndrome-associated malignancies. *Sem Resp Inf* 1993; 8:139.

165. Davis S, Henschke C, Chamides B, et al.: Intrathoracic Kaposi's sarcoma in AIDS patients: Radiographic-pathologic correlation. *Radiology* 1987; 163:495.

166. Meduri G, Stover D, Lee M, et al.: Pulmonary Kaposi's sarcoma in the acquired immune deficiency syndrome. Clinical, radiographic, and pathologic manifestations. *Am J Med* 1986; 81:11.

167. Garay S, Belenko M, Fazzini E, Schinella R: Pulmonary manifestations of Kaposi's sarcoma. *Chest* 1987; 91:39.

168. Hamm P, Judson M, Aranda C: Diagnosis of pulmonary Kaposi's sarcoma with fiberoptic bronchoscopy and endobronchial biopsy. A report of five cases. *Cancer* 1987; 59:807.

169. Pitchenik A, Fischl M, Saldana M: Kaposi's sarcoma of the tracheobronchial tree. Clinical, bronchoscopic, and pathologic features. *Chest* 1985; 87:122.

170. Wallace J: Mimics of infectious pneumonia in persons infected with human immunodeficiency virus, in Niederman M, Sarosi G, Glassroth J (eds): *Respiratory Infections.* Philadelphia, WB Saunders.

171. Stulbarg M, Golden J: Open lung biopsy in the acquired immunodeficiency syndrome (AIDS) (editorial). *Chest* 1987; 91:639.

172. Gill P, Akil B, Colletti P, et al.: Pulmonary Kaposi's sarcoma: Clinical findings and results of therapy. *Am J Med* 1989; 87:57.

173. Nobler M: Pulmonary irradiation for Kaposi's sarcoma in AIDS. *Am J Clin Oncol* 1985; 8:441.

174. Gail M, Pluda J, Rabkin C, et al.: Projections of the incidence of non-Hodgkin's lymphoma related to acquired immunodeficiency syndrome. *J Nat Cancer Inst* 1991; 83:695.

175. Zeigler J, Beckstead J, Voberding P, et al.: Non-Hodgkin's lymphoma in 90 homosexual men related to generalized lymphadenopathy and the acquired immunodeficiency syndrome. *N Eng J Med* 1984; 311:565.

176. Kaplan L, Abrams D, Feigal E, et al.: AIDS-associated non-Hodgkin's lymphoma in San Francisco. *J Am Med Assoc* 1989; 261:719.

177. Sider L, Weiss A, Smith M, et al.: Varied appearance of AIDS related lymphomas in the chest. *Radiology* 1989; 1712:629.

178. Gill P, Levine A, Krailo M, et al.: AIDS related malignant lymphoma: Results of prospective treatment trials. *J Clin Oncol* 1987; 5:1322.

179. Stover D, White D, Romano P, et al.: Spectrum of pulmonary diseases associated with the acquired immunodeficiency syndrome. *Am J Med* 1985; 78:429.

180. Suffredini A, Ognibene F, Lack E, et al.: Nonspecific interstitial pneumonitis: A common cause of pulmonary disease in the acquired immunodeficiency syndrome. *Ann Intern Med* 1987; 107:7.

181. Travis W, Fox C, Devaney K, et al.: Lymphoid pneumonitis in 50 adult patients infected with the human immunodeficiency virus: Lymphocytic interstitial pneumonitis versus nonspecific interstitial pneumonitis. *Hum Pathol* 1992; 23:529.

182. Rubenstein A, Morecki R, Silverman B, et al.: Pulmonary disease in children with acquired immune deficiency syndrome and AIDS related complex. *J Pediatr* 1986; 108:498.

183. Itescu S, Brancato L, Buxbaum J, et al.: A diffuse infiltrative CD8 lymphocytosis syndrome in human immunodeficiency virus (HIV) infection: A host immune response associated with HLA-DR5. *Ann Intern Med* 1990; 112:3.

184. Resnick L, Pitchenik A, Fisher E, et al.: Detection of HTLV III/LAV-specific IgG and antigen in bronchoalveolar lavage fluid from two patients with lymphocytic interstitial pneumonitis associated with AIDS-related complex. *Am J Med* 1987; 82:553.

185. Andiman W, Eastmann R, Martin R, et al.: Opportunistic lymphoproliferation associated with Epstein-Barr viral DNA in infants and children with AIDS. *Lancet* 1985; 2:1390.

186. Ognibene F, Masur H, Rogers P, et al.: Nonspecific interstitial pneumonitis in asymptomatic patients infected with human immunodeficiency virus (HIV). *Ann Intern Med* 1988; 109:874.

187. Rubenstein A, Bernstein L, Charytan M, et al.: Corticosteroid treatment for pulmonary lymphoid hyperplasia in children with the acquired immune deficiency syndrome. *Pediatr Pulmonol* 1988; 4:13.

188. Morris J, Rosen M, Marchevsky A, Teirstein A: Lymphocytic interstitial pneumonia in patients at risk for the acquired immune deficiency syndrome. *Chest* 1987; 91:63.

PHARMACOLOGY OF CRITICAL CARE ILLNESS IN INFANTS AND CHILDREN

MARC B. HERSHENSON

This chapter focuses on the pharmacology of life-threatening pediatric respiratory illnesses. In addition, because of the complex nature of respiratory disease in critically ill children, related topics such as cardiopulmonary resuscitation, hemodynamic support, sedation, and muscle relaxation also are discussed. Though differences in drug disposition between children and adults are cited when necessary, the interested reader is encouraged to study one of the excellent reviews of pediatric critical care pharmacology.[1,2] Only a few general comments on pediatric pharmacodynamics are offered here.

BIOAVAILABILITY

Bioavailability is defined as the rate and extent of drug absorption. In the intensive care unit, most drugs are administered intravenously, thereby obviating most problems associated with drug absorption. However, even intravenous administration may be problematic in the treatment of small infants. For example, significant errors may result when small dosage volumes are required. The lack of small, accurate syringes with minimal dead space makes injection of small volumes difficult, and errors in the dilution of drugs may lead to either under- or overdosage. In addition, the low intravenous infusion rates required for small infants can lead to significant delays in the initiation or termination of drug treatments, as the medication slowly travels from the injection port or burette to the actual intravenous site. Knowledge of the intravenous system employed minimizes problems of this nature.

On occasion, intraosseous delivery is required for the emergency administration of resuscitative fluids and drugs.[3] This method has been shown to be significantly more effective than endotracheal drug administration, the other alternative to intravenous drug delivery.[4] Saline, colloids, bicarbonate, calcium, catecholamines, and even muscle relaxants have been demonstrated to be effectively and rapidly delivered by this route of administration.[5] Issues of bioavailability also arise when β_2-adrenergic agonists are administered in the treatment of asthma. These concerns are addressed below.

DISTRIBUTION

The distribution of a drug depends on its water- or fat-solubility, polarity, pH, and molecular weight as well as the patient's body composition and cardiac output. These chemical factors, in turn, determine whether the drug will be tightly protein-bound or whether it will penetrate the extravascular space, intracellular compartment, or central nervous system. Many drugs, such as theophylline, are less avidly bound to plasma proteins in the neonate and infant than in the older patient. This causes an increase in the apparent volume of distribution and a decrease in the plasma drug concentration obtained following a standard dosage.

Highly lipid-soluble drugs may accumulate in the tissues and produce a reservoir of drug that can prolong drug action. This is a critical point when administering sedatives in the critical care unit. For example, administration of the first dose of thiopental leads to rapid onset and termination of anesthesia, as the drug redistributes from the highly perfused brain to other tissues such as fat and muscle. With subsequent doses, however, the accumulation of thiopental in these tissue stores reduces the concentration gradient between these compartments and the central nervous system, prolonging the duration of action. Eventually, the tissue storage sites become completely saturated, causing the duration of action of thiopental to be dependent on its biotransformation and elimination by the liver (elimination half-life, 5 to 12 h). Although thiopental now is rarely administered in the pediatric critical care unit, concern for prolonged sedation also holds true for other lipid-soluble drugs such as diazepam, which is often given in repeated doses for the treatment of status epilepticus.

ELIMINATION

After biotransformation—whereby the drug is altered by oxidation, reduction, hydrolysis, or conjugation—elimination occurs, predominantly through the bile and/or urine. Biotransformation, which takes place primarily in the hepatic microsomes, generally transforms drugs into more polar compounds, enhancing their elimination. Many drug metabolites retain activity. The benzodiazepines are especially notable in this regard.

Pharmacology of Specific Disease Entities and Clinical Situations

STATUS ASTHMATICUS AND SEVERE ASTHMA

It has been suggested that wheezing infants fail to respond to bronchodilators because of a deficiency in airway smooth muscle.[6] It is now clear, however, that normal infants may exhibit greater airway cholinergic responsiveness than adults,[7] consistent with the notion that asthma may occur early in life. The pharmacologic treatment of acute asthma in children, as in adults, primarily consists of β_2-adrenergic agonists, corticosteroids, and aminophylline (Table 106-1).

β_2-ADRENERGIC AGONISTS

In severe asthma or status asthmaticus, β_2-adrenergic agonists are best delivered in the form of continuous nebulized albuterol. Continuous therapy does not cause cardiotoxicity in children[8] and is more effective than intermittent nebulized albuterol in this patient population.[9]

Selective β_2-adrenoceptor agonists, such as albuterol and terbutaline, have been administered safely by continuous intravenous infusion.[10,11] A comparison of the bronchodilating effects of terbutaline given either intravenously or by

TABLE 106-1   Pharmacologic Treatment of Acute Asthma in Children

Agent	Dose
Albuterol	0.1–0.3 mg/kg/h by nebulizer (max, 10 mg/h)
Terbutaline	10 µg/kg IV over 30 min, followed by 0.1 µg/kg/min infusion; max, 4 µg/kg/min
Methylprednisolone	2 mg/kg IV followed by 0.5–1 mg/kg every 6 h
Aminophylline	6 mg/kg IV over 20–30 min, followed by 1.0 mg/kg/h infusion; titrate to serum level
Ipratropium bromide	250 µg by nebulizer every 3–6 h

metered-dose inhaler (MDI) showed that intravenous administration produced no greater bronchodilation than did aerosol delivery; furthermore, intravenous administration increased heart rate and tremor.[12] Although this study was conducted in adults with asthma, it appears that maximal β_2-selective stimulation in the lung can be achieved by the inhaled route. Nevertheless, the use of intravenous terbutaline may be warranted in patients with impending respiratory failure. Isoproterenol should not be used because of its nonselective cardiac effects.[13]

β_2-adrenergic agonists also can be delivered by MDI and a spacer device. Although this method of administration can be as effective in the treatment of acute asthma in children as use of the nebulized drug,[14] the efficacy of this method in endotracheally intubated pediatric patients has not been tested. However, it has recently been demonstrated that the delivery of β_2-adrenergic agonists by MDI has no effect whatsoever on resistive pressure in mechanically ventilated adults.[15] These data suggest that drug deposition along the endotracheal tube makes delivery by MDI untenable in endotracheally intubated patients.

CORTICOSTEROIDS

It is now generally agreed that suppression of airway inflammation with corticosteroids should be the mainstay of pharmacologic therapy for chronic asthma. The utility of corticosteroids in the treatment of acute childhood asthma has been well demonstrated.[16–18]

AMINOPHYLLINE

Intravenously administered aminophylline when given with corticosteroids and β_2-adrenergic agonists has been shown in three recent studies to be of no additional benefit in the treatment of acute asthma in children.[19–21] Thus, aminophylline treatment no longer should be included in the routine treatment of status asthmaticus. The use of aminophylline in the treatment of children with impending respiratory failure may still be warranted, however, as these patients were excluded from the above studies.

OTHER AGENTS

The efficacy of anticholinergic agents, disodium cromoglycate, or nedocromil in the treatment of critically ill children with asthma has not been investigated. The addition of ipratropium bromide solution to nebulized albuterol has been noted to improve pulmonary function in children with acute asthma presenting to an emergency room.[22] Untested treatments such as inhalational anesthesia, magnesium sulfate, or ketamine are discussed elsewhere in this book.

BRONCHIOLITIS

Bronchodilators, corticosteroids, and ribavirin have all been employed in the treatment of viral bronchiolitis in infants, all with questionable benefit. Research examining the efficacy of these agents in the treatment of bronchiolitis has been hampered by the use of clinical scoring systems as well as by difficulty in distinguishing acute bronchiolitis from an acute exacerbation of asthma.

β_2-ADRENERGIC AGONISTS

Of the six studies that have examined the effects of bronchodilators on airflow in patients with bronchiolitis,[23-28] three show improvement following treatment with β_2-adrenergic agonists. In one instance, 13 of 14 mechanically ventilated infants exhibited a 30 percent increase in expiratory flow after treatment.[23] On the other hand, one study showed a reduction of airflow following salbutamol treatment, probably secondary to airway collapse.[26] Another study demonstrated a salutary effect of racemic epinephrine but not salbutamol, suggesting that α-adrenergic stimulation may be helpful in this disease, possibly by reducing airway microvascular leak.[27]

CORTICOSTEROIDS

Systemic administration during the acute phase of bronchiolitis does not appear to improve pulmonary function.[29] On the other hand, administration of nebulized beclomethasone has been shown to improve airflow in infants suffering from persistent wheezing 6 to 28 weeks following acute bronchiolitis.[30]

RIBAVIRIN

Despite initial enthusiasm for its use,[31] the efficacy of ribavirin in the treatment of bronchiolitis caused by respiratory syncytial virus (RSV) has not been proven. Recent studies indicate that ribavirin fails to improve either pulmonary function in previously healthy infants with RSV bronchiolitis[32] or clinical outcome in mechanically ventilated patients with RSV lower respiratory tract disease.[33] Nevertheless, it appears from the latter study that ribavirin can be administered safely to mechanically ventilated infants if desired.

BRONCHOPULMONARY DYSPLASIA

The pharmacologic treatment of infants with acute "exacerbations" of bronchopulmonary dysplasia (BPD) largely consists of measures employed in the treatment of acute asthma (see above). Corticosteroids have been shown to improve pulmonary function[34-36] and speed extubation[34,37-41] in patients with BPD, though data demonstrating a beneficial effect on the natural history of the disease are disappointing.[38-41] Infants with BPD exhibit airway hyperresponsive-

ness and appear to benefit from both β_2-adrenergic agonists[42-45] and ipratropium.[46] Diuretics are also widely employed in the treatment of BPD, though their effect on pulmonary function has been proven only in the subacute setting.[47,48]

CARDIOPULMONARY RESUSCITATION

For a complete review of pediatric advanced life support, the reader is referred to the latest American Heart Association guidelines for cardiopulmonary resuscitation.[4] Unlike that in adults, cardiac arrest in infants and children is almost always the culmination of a progressive deterioration in respiratory and subsequently circulatory function. Accordingly, early evidence of respiratory and circulatory failure must be promptly detected and treated, great care must be taken to assure adequate oxygenation and ventilation during resuscitative efforts, and it must be realized that the outcome of out-of-hospital cardiopulmonary resuscitation in children is universally poor.[49,50]

The most common rhythm disturbances associated with cardiovascular collapse in children are asystole and idioventricular bradycardia. As in adults, epinephrine, a potent α- and β-adrenergic agonist, is the most effective drug for the treatment of asystole. A recent study suggesting that high-dose epinephrine improves the neurologic outcome of children with asystole[51] has led workers to recommend a 10-fold greater dose (0.1 mg/kg) for second and subsequent doses of epinephrine in the treatment of unresponsive asystole. Calcium and bicarbonate are of uncertain efficacy and are recommended only for documented hypocalcemia and prolonged cardiac arrest, respectively. The efficacy of atropine in the treatment of asystole is also unproven. Atropine is effective in the treatment of vagally mediated bradycardia following intubation attempts, but it is not as effective as epinephrine in the treatment of bradycardia associated with low cardiac output.

CIRCULATORY SHOCK/MYOCARDIAL DYSFUNCTION

DOPAMINE

Dopamine and dobutamine remain the agents most commonly employed in the treatment of myocardial dysfunction in infants and children. Early studies suggested that, on average, infants and young children required greater dopamine infusion rates to produce the hemodynamic effects observed in adults.[52] However, other reports demonstrated significant increments in stroke volume and shortening fraction with dopamine infusion rates as low as 2 μg/kg/min.[53,54] Although higher clearance rates[55] and maturational differences in ventricular compliance, innervation, and receptor density[56] increase required dopamine infusion rates in young infants, the pharmacokinetics of dopamine are highly variable, even in hemodynamically stable children.[57] The hemodynamic response to dopamine infusion may be influenced by such factors as hepatic and renal function, endogenous epinephrine stores and release, serum protein concentration, adrenal function, concurrent analgesic administration, and other factors.[55-57] Thus, infusions must be titrated individually to measured changes in the patient's hemodynamic response. A final point: there are data to indicate that relatively high infusion rates of dopamine do not adversely affect renal function in infants,[58,59] as they do in adults.

DOBUTAMINE

The pharmacokinetics of dobutamine in infants and children are comparable to those of dopamine. Wide variability of hemodynamic responses and clearance kinetics has been noted, indicating that dobutamine infusions must be titrated individually. Infusion rates $\leq$ 0.5 to 1.0 μg/kg/min have been demonstrated to increase cardiac index in some patients.[60,61] One study has suggested that patients 1 year of age or younger have an attenuated response to dobutamine.[62] As in adults, the drug appears to be a relatively selective inotropic agent with lesser chronotropic effects, though this finding is not universal.[60,61,63] Finally, systemic hypotension in response to dobutamine has occasionally been noted in children.[62]

AMRINONE

The hemodynamic effects of amrinone, a bipyridine derivative with inotropic and vasodilator actions, have been studied in children with congenital heart disease. In the earliest study, amrinone failed to increase significantly cardiac index, while systemic vascular resistance decreased substantially.[64] A second study, in which preload was kept constant by colloid infusion, noted significant increases in cardiac output with amrinone, though dopamine was required to maintain arterial pressure in some patients.[65] Interestingly, the sole child with pulmonary hypertension in the latter study showed a beneficial reduction in pulmonary artery pressure during amrinone infusion. Similarly, infants and children with cardiac left-to-right shunts and pulmonary artery hypertension demonstrated selective reductions in pulmonary vascular resistance during amrinone infusion.[66] Thus, amrinone may have a role in the treatment of patients with pulmonary hypertension.

CARDIAC ARRHYTHMIAS

A complete discussion of cardiac arrhythmias and their treatment is beyond the scope of this chapter. Cardiac arrhythmias due to primary cardiac disease are rare in children; the most common arrhythmias, asystole and idioventricular bradycardia, occur as a result of hypoxemia, acidosis, or hypotension.

Supraventricular tachycardia (SVT) is the most common arrhythmia causing circulatory compromise in infants. It may occur in infants with underlying structural malformations, Wolff-Parkinson-White syndrome, or those with no apparent cardiac disease; SVT is also an infrequent complication of bronchiolitis[67] and asthma.[68] Although vagal maneuvers are often successful in temporarily interrupting SVT,[69] the purine nucleotide adenosine can be most useful in the diagnosis and treatment of SVT in infants and children. Termination of SVT by adenosine—which induces transient atrioventricular (AV) conduction delay and block (the half-life of adenosine is < 10 s)—is diagnostic of arrhythmias

requiring AV or AV nodal reentry for the tachycardia circuit.[70] These arrhythmias constitute the majority of supraventricular tachycardias in children. On the other hand, supraventricular arrhythmias not dependent on AV conduction for the tachycardia circuit (such as ectopic atrial tachycardia or atrial flutter) will respond by transient loss of the ventricular complex on the electrocardiogram, with persistence of the atrial tachycardia. Ventricular arrhythmias should not be affected by adenosine treatment. (Thus, wide QRS tachycardias that respond to adenosine are supraventricular in origin.)

Other treatments for SVT in infants and children include transesophageal atrial pacing, electrical cardioversion, verapamil, beta-adrenoceptor blockade, and phenylephrine (Table 106-2). However, verapamil has been associated with cardiovascular collapse in young infants[69,71]; for this reason, it should not be used for babies with SVT. Significant hypotension also may occur in infants receiving beta-blocking drugs for SVT. Finally, digoxin may be used to reduce ventricular rate in patients with SVT.

ANESTHETICS AND MUSCLE RELAXANTS FOR ENDOTRACHEAL INTUBATION

It generally is accepted by most pediatric intensivists that infants and children should be deeply sedated prior to endotracheal intubation. The only exceptions to this rule are moribund patients requiring cardiopulmonary resuscitation and possibly patients with upper airway obstruction in whom endotracheal intubation may be difficult to accomplish. (These patients generally can be anesthetized safely using inhalational anesthesia.) Of course, the severity of cardiac and pulmonary dysfunction in critically ill children makes anesthetic induction challenging, primarily by limiting the choice of anesthetic agents available. For example, thiopental, a useful drug for the anesthetic induction of previously healthy infants and children, often results in profound hemodynamic compromise when administered in full dosage to critically ill patients. Such consequences may not be limited to patients with obvious cardiac disease. For example, administration of thiopental to asthmatic patients, in combination with the change from negative- to positive-pressure ventilation, may precipitate severe hypotension and cardiac arrest, especially in the presence of hypovolemia. Another point to remember is that, while it is tempting to administer lower doses of anesthetic agents to

TABLE 106-2   Pharmacologic Treatment of SVT in Infants and Children

Agent	Dose
Adenosine	0.1 mg/kg rapid IV; may increase dose 0.05 mg/kg every 2 min to max of 0.25 mg/kg or 12 mg
Esmolol	0.1–0.5 mg/kg IV over 1 min
Verapamil	0.1–0.3 mg/kg IV over 2–3 min; maximum, 5 mg; should not be given to infants <1 year of age
Phenylephrine	5–10 μg/kg over 20–30 s

TABLE 106-3   Anesthetic Agents Employed for Endotracheal Intubation

Agent	Dose	Comments
Thiopental	3–5 mg/kg	May cause profound hemodynamic instability
Midazolam	0.1–0.3 mg/kg	Supplementation with fentanyl often required
Fentanyl	3–5 μg/kg	Supplementation with midazolam often required
Ketamine	1–3 mg/kg	Requires coadministration of muscle relaxant

critically ill children (in the mistaken belief that this approach will minimize side effects), partial sedation often results in an uncooperative patient with inadequate airway reflexes, making pulmonary aspiration more likely and endotracheal intubation more difficult. Finally, because of the intense vagal stimulation provoked by endotracheal intubation in infants and children, atropine should be administered prior to laryngoscopy.

Anesthetic agents employed for endotracheal intubation include thiopental, midazolam, fentanyl, ketamine, and propofol (Table 106-3).

THIOPENTAL

As mentioned above, there are few indications for thiopental in the pediatric intensive care unit, owing to its depressant effects on venous tone and myocardial function. Perhaps one exception is the older child with closed head injury and increased intracranial pressure. Thiopental is rapid-acting (loss of consciousness in 10 to 15 s; duration 10 to 15 min) and reduces intracranial pressure by its depressant effect on cerebral metabolic rate and blood flow. Thus, it is an excellent choice for the rapid-sequence intubation of patients with normal cardiovascular systems and increased intracranial pressure. The safety of thiopental administration may be enhanced by volume leading prior to induction. As discussed previously, the rapid action of thiopental is a function of high cerebral blood flow and rapid redistribution to tissue stores. Repeated doses will lead to an increased duration of action, which will ultimately depend on hepatic elimination (half-time: 5 to 12 h).

MIDAZOLAM

Since the mid-1980s, the benzodiazepine midazolam has been used for the endotracheal intubation of infants and children with hemodynamic instability. Unlike diazepam, midazolam exerts central nervous system effects rapidly and may therefore be used as an induction agent. Maximal depression occurs at 1 to 5 min after intravenous administration (slightly slower than thiopental), and its duration of action is approximately 15 min. Greater doses (up to 0.3 mg/kg) are often necessary for the adequate sedation of infants and children during endotracheal intubation, and supplementation with a narcotic (fentanyl) also may be required. Unlike thiopental, midazolam has relatively small effects on the normal cardiovascular system and is therefore a safer choice in hemodynamically unstable patients. Like

barbiturates, benzodiazepines have a salutary effect on intracranial pressure.

FENTANYL

The short-acting narcotic fentanyl has also been used for the deep sedation of infants and children prior to endotracheal intubation, especially those with cardiac disease. Although fentanyl alone may not abate all airway reflexes, administration in higher doses (up to 5 μg/kg) and/or supplementation with midazolam (0.1 mg/kg) will allow endotracheal intubation without hemodynamic compromise. Unlike morphine, fentanyl does not cause histamine release; thus, fentanyl rarely decreases blood pressure, even in patients with poor left ventricular function.

KETAMINE

Ketamine is a dissociative anesthetic that actually stimulates the central nervous system. Aside from being an excellent analgesic, ketamine has been used for the endotracheal intubation of critically ill infants and children (intravenous dose, 1 to 2 mg/kg). Ketamine exerts its central nervous system effects rapidly (slightly more slowly than thiopental), with consciousness returning in 10 to 15 min (though full recovery may take longer). Ketamine actually increases blood pressure and heart rate except in patients in whom the autonomic nervous system is blocked, in which case ketamine causes direct myocardial depression. Ventilation also is maintained, and bronchial smooth muscle tone is relaxed. Ketamine therefore is preferred for the deep sedation and endotracheal intubation of young patients with heart disease and asthma. However, there are several disadvantages. Ketamine increases airway reflexes, leading to increased secretions, coughing, and occasionally, laryngospasm. These factors, combined with the increase in skeletal muscle tone following ketamine administration, require that the drug be given with a vagolytic agent and muscle relaxant. Ketamine also increases intracranial pressure and may cause dysphoria, especially in older children.

PROPOFOL

Propofol, a hindered phenolic compound, recently has been used for the anesthetic induction of infants and children.[72] The main advantage of propofol is its high lipid solubility, leading to a large volume of distribution (the tissues cannot be saturated) and rapid onset and offset. However, propofol may reduce significantly systemic vascular resistance and blood pressure.[73] Profound hemodynamic compromise has also been associated with prolonged propofol administration.[74] Therefore the role of propofol in the pediatric intensive care unit remains to be defined.

MUSCLE RELAXANTS

Muscle relaxants often are administered concurrently with anesthetics to prevent movement and aid visualization during endotracheal intubation. In critically ill infants and children, a rapid-sequence or modified rapid-sequence technique is often required, necessitating the use of relatively rapidly acting muscle relaxants, including succinylcholine, mivacurium, atracurium, and vecuronium (Table 106-4). Succinylcholine, a depolarizing muscle relaxant, has

TABLE 106-4   Muscle Relaxants

	Priming Dose[a]	Intubation Dose	Time to Complete Block (min)	Maintenance Infusion
Depolarizing				
Succinylcholine	—	1–2 mg/kg	1.0	—
Nondepolarizing				
Mivacurium	—	0.2 mg/kg	1.5	5–30 µg/kg/min
Atracurium	0.06 mg/kg	0.6 mg/kg	1.5	0.4–0.8 mg/kg/h
Vecuronium	0.01 mg/kg	0.1 mg/kg	1.5	0.075 mg/kg/h
Pancuronium	0.01 mg/kg	0.1 mg/kg	2.5	—

[a] Addition of a priming dose, given 3–6 min before intubation, will accelerate the onset of block.

the advantage of rapid action (30 to 60 s), which reduces the risk of hypoxia or aspiration of gastric contents. However, succinylcholine administration holds many disadvantages, including (1) muscle depolarization, with consequent increments in serum potassium concentration; (2) stimulation of cardiac muscarinic receptors, which can result in bradycardia and cardiac arrest, especially after the second dose (atropine should always be given prior to succinylcholine administration in children); and (3) increased risk of malignant hyperthermia. Succinylcholine is contraindicated after traumatic and burn injuries: because of increased muscarinic receptor density, which occurs 6 days to 6 months after injury, succinylcholine may cause massive depolarization and life-threatening hyperkalemia. Neuromuscular disease, which also increases the number of muscarinic receptors susceptible to depolarization, and renal failure with hyperkalemia are also contraindications to the use of succinylcholine. Succinylcholine-induced fasciculations also may increase intracranial pressure, though fasciculations often do not occur in infants and increments in intracranial pressure may be prevented by concurrent use of thiopental. In light of these problems and the fact that critically ill infants often must be hand-ventilated prior to intubation, even if succinylcholine is given, many practitioners are turning to alternative, nondepolarizing muscle relaxants (Table 106-4). In a preliminary study of infants < 1 year of age, mivacurium, a new agent with a short duration of action,[75]

induced complete neuromuscular blockade of the thumb in approximately 30 s, though at that time intubating conditions were suboptimal relative to succinylcholine.[76] Atracurium and vecuronium produce adequate muscle relaxation for endotracheal intubation within approximately 90 s. Both mivacurium and atracurium induce histamine release, whereas vecuronium does not.

PROLONGED SEDATION AND ANALGESIA

A wide range of sedatives and analgesics are available for the treatment of critically ill infants and children (Table 106-5). The use of these agents for endotracheal intubation has been discussed previously. In selecting the right agent(s) for other tasks, one must consider carefully the desired effect(s) of treatment. Too often, for example, patients are sedated for nonpainful procedures with narcotics, or, conversely, anesthetized for painful procedures with benzodiazepines or chloral hydrate. Consideration of the exact intent of therapy, along with attention to potential side effects and duration of action, generally leads to the correct regimen.

BENZODIAZEPINES
Benzodiazepines provide superior sedation and amnesia but little analgesia; they often are combined with a narcotic for this reason. Like thiopental, the benzodiazepines have relatively long elimination half-lives but short durations of

TABLE 106-5   Sedatives and Analgesics for the Treatment of Critically Ill Infants and Children

	Single Dose	Duration of Action	Infusion
Benzodiazepines			
Midazolam	0.1 mg/kg IV	15 min	0.025–0.100 mg/kg/h
Diazepam	0.1–0.2 mg/kg IV	20–60 min	—
Lorazepam	0.05 mg/kg IV	2–6 h	—
Narcotics			
Morphine	0.1–0.3 mg/kg IV	2–4 h	10–30 µg/kg/h
Fentanyl	1–5 µg/kg IV	30 min	2–5 µg/kg/h after loading dose
Methadone	0.1–0.2 mg/kg IV	6–12 h	—
Other agents			
Ketamine	1–3 mg/kg	1 h	0.5–2 mg/kg/h
Chloral hydrate	30–75 mg/kg	4–6 h	—
Propofol	0.2–2.5 mg/kg	5 min	0.5–3.0 mg/kg/h

action, due to high fat solubility and subsequent redistribution from the central nervous system. If the interval between succeeding doses is less than the time required for elimination (or if the drug is given as a continuous infusion), the concentration gradient driving redistribution will diminish, increasing the duration of action. After initial administration, midazolam has a rapid onset and offset and therefore is a poor (i.e., inconvenient) choice for prolonged sedation when given in bolus form. For prolonged sedation, midazolam may be used as constant infusion. However, one should be aware that for reasons described above, continuous administration of midazolam may result in prolonged sedation even after the infusion is discontinued. Furthermore, reversible neurologic symptoms such as dystonia and choreoathetosis have been reported after midazolam infusion[77] and may represent benzodiazepine withdrawal, persistent effects of the drug, or the combined effects of multiple pharmacologic agents.

Diazepam, like midazolam, rapidly affects the central nervous system. Its duration of action is slightly longer than midazolam (20 to 60 min). Therefore, the administration of diazepam as an intermittent bolus (for example, every 2 to 4 h) often fails to provide adequate sedation. Somewhat fortuitously, the long elimination half-life of the drug (20 to 40 h) often leads to an "enhanced" sedative effect after repeated doses. Lorazepam is a less lipid-soluble, longer-acting benzodiazepine (peak effect 45 to 50 min; duration of effect, 2 to 6 h). The longer central nervous system effects but shorter elimination half-life (10 to 20 h) of lorazepam makes it superior to diazepam for prolonged sedation.

NARCOTICS

Narcotics are the most commonly used class of drugs for analgesia in the pediatric intensive care unit. In addition to their analgesic properties, narcotics induce decreased responsiveness to external stimulation and a reduction in the level of consciousness. Nevertheless, the sedative properties of narcotics are inferior to those of the benzodiazepines. Amnesia following narcotic administration is incomplete even at high doses. For this reason, narcotics often are combined with a benzodiazepine for added sedation and amnesia.

Morphine has a duration of action of 2 to 5 h, depending on route of administration. Although intramuscular administration gives less dramatic peak effects and a longer duration of action, it is so unpleasant that pediatric patients will deny pain in order to avoid injections; therefore, the intravenous route is preferred. Morphine may also be given as a constant infusion. Due to histamine release, hypotension frequently occurs with morphine administration. The most common indication for morphine in the pediatric intensive care unit is therefore routine analgesia and sedation in patients without serious hemodynamic instability.

Fentanyl, unlike morphine, rarely decreases blood pressure, even in patients with poor cardiac function. Thus, fentanyl is commonly used for the analgesia and sedation of patients with hemodynamic instability. The duration of fentanyl's effect is 20 to 30 min; like midazolam, fentanyl is an inconvenient choice for prolonged use when given in bolus form. Fentanyl may also be given as a continuous infusion;

however, potential problems include tolerance, narcotic withdrawal, and neurologic toxicity. For example, in a study of newborn infants, each receiving a continuous infusion of fentanyl, increasingly higher plasma fentanyl concentrations were required to maintain the same degree of sedation.[78] In a prospective study examining the occurrence of opioid withdrawal in the pediatric intensive care unit, all infants receiving fentanyl for a period of greater than or equal to 9 days (57 percent of the total) exhibited withdrawal symptoms.[79] Finally, movement disorders have been noted following cessation of fentanyl infusions in infants and young children.[77,80]

Meperidine offers no advantage to morphine with regard to hemodynamic or respiratory effects. Indeed, meperidine causes significant histamine release and direct myocardial depression. Potential advantages include less biliary tract spasm and the oral route of administration.

Methadone has recently been advocated as a narcotic and sedative in the pediatric critical care unit,[81] mainly because of its long duration of action. (Often 8- to 12-h dosing becomes adequate.) Methadone may be given intravenously or by mouth. Because of its duration of action, methadone is an excellent choice for busy nursing units.

When narcotics are administered on an "as needed" basis, the patient inevitably suffers from severe pain prior to the next dose (a pain cycle). For morphine, intravenous boluses must be given at intervals of no more than 2 to 4 h so as to avoid a pain cycle. Such frequent administration may be difficult or impossible for busy nursing units. In such cases, intermittent methadone, a continuous infusion of morphine or fentanyl, or patient-controlled anesthesia (PCA) may be preferable. The last of these, PCA, has been used with excellent results in adolescents and children as young as 6 years of age.[82] With this technique, patients self-administer small boluses of morphine every 6 to 15 min using a computer-controlled infusion pump (the specific time period of "lockout" is selected by the physician, as is the maximum cumulative dose). Contraindications include severe pain, inability to push the button or understand the concept of PCA, or uncooperativeness.

OTHER SEDATIVE AGENTS

The physiologic effects of ketamine are described above. Ketamine is an excellent sedative and analgesic, which may be given as a bolus or by continuous infusion. The effects of ketamine on blood pressure and heart rate make it an excellent choice for patients with cardiovascular heart disease. However, increased secretions, airway reflexes, skeletal muscle tone, and dysphoria accompany ketamine use, often necessitating the coadministration of vagolytics, muscle relaxants, and benzodiazepines.

Chloral hydrate has been used for years to sedate infants and children. It may be given enterally or rectally and has an onset of effect of 15 to 30 min; the duration of effect is 4 to 6 h. As with other lipophilic anesthetics (barbiturates, benzodiazepines), the duration of effect is shorter than the elimination half-life (4 to 12 h). Thus, administration of multiple doses leads to a prolonged duration of central nervous system effects. There is little or no depression of central respiratory drive, though chloral hydrate may preferentially reduce upper airway muscle activity,[83] leading to an inability to clear the airway. Chloral hydrate has minimal analgesic activity. The most common use of chloral hydrate is the sedation of nonintubated patients for noninvasive procedures.

As described above, propofol has recently been approved for use in the intensive care unit. Propofol is a good sedative and amnestic but a poor analgesic. The main advantage of propofol is its rapid offset. Although propofol may be given as a constant infusion, prolonged infusions may increase risk of infection (due to its emulsion vehicle) and have been associated with myocardial depression and seizures.[74,84] Thus, the role of propofol in the pediatric intensive care unit has not been established.

PROLONGED MUSCLE RELAXATION

The potential advantages of succinylcholine for endotracheal intubation are discussed above. For prolonged muscle relaxation, however, the nondepolarizing agents are administered, either by bolus or continuous infusion (Table 106-4). Pancuronium is the most commonly used agent and has a duration of action of 45 to 60 min. Some 60 to 80 percent of the drug is excreted by the kidney; the remainder is eliminated through the hepatobiliary tract. Pancuronium blocks cardiac muscarinic receptors weakly, causing tachycardia; there is no histamine release. Thus, for infants, in whom cardiac output is relatively heart rate–dependent, pancuronium is an excellent choice for routine paralysis in the intensive care unit.

Atracurium is a moderately short-acting nondepolarizing muscle relaxant, whose chief attributes are its relatively short time of onset and metabolism in the serum by Hoffmann degradation and ester hydrolysis. Thus, atracurium may be given to patients with renal or hepatic failure. For prolonged muscle relaxation, the short duration of action of atracurium makes administration by intermittent injection impractical; constant infusion is preferable. Finally, atracurium causes slight histamine release and may therefore cause hypotension when given as a bolus.

Vecuronium is another moderately short-acting muscle relaxant. It is metabolized almost completely by the liver (renal metabolism is 10 to 20 percent). Like atracurium, vecuronium is more conveniently administered as a constant infusion. Cardiac muscarinic receptors are not blocked and histamine is not released; thus, of all the muscle relaxants, this drug has the fewest cardiovascular effects.

Mivacurium, an agent with a short duration of action, recently has been introduced and may be used by constant infusion. Like atracurium, mivacurium induces histamine release.

Continuous infusions of pancuronium and vecuronium have been associated with residual weakness, which may persist ≥ 6 months.[85–88] Most of these cases have occurred in asthmatic patients concurrently receiving corticosteroids. The etiology of this generalized myopathy is unclear but may stem from the above aminosteroid structure of the drug; when these agents are combined with corticosteroids, an accelerated steroid myopathy may result. Continuous administration of atracurium, a quarternary ammonium compound, has not as yet been associated with myopathy,

TABLE 106-6   Drugs Employed to Treat Hypertensive Emergencies

Agent	Dose
Nitroprusside	1–5 μg/kg/min
Labetalol	0.25 mg/kg over 2 min; 0.4–1.0 mg/kg/h
Nifedipine	0.25–0.5 mg/kg, up to 10 mg

though experience with this drug is limited. Aside from structural differences, the lack of side effects following atracurium administration may result from its metabolism in the serum (see above). Whatever the cause, continuous administration of muscle relaxants should be limited whenever possible, and overdosing should be avoided by periodically allowing the partial return of muscle function or by monitoring neuromuscular blockade using a peripheral nerve stimulator.

HYPERTENSION

The list of drugs employed to treat hypertensive emergencies in the pediatric critical care unit is a short one (Table 106-6). Continuous infusions of nitroprusside and labetalol are most commonly used; sublingual nifedipine is also effective. Although there is a risk of both cyanide and thiocyanate overdose with nitroprusside administration, clinical toxicity is rare. Labetalol, a nonselective β-adrenergic blocking drug with some α-adrenergic blocking activity, should be avoided in patients with bronchospasm or heart failure. Though nifedipine may be given sublingually, it should not be administered without establishing intravenous access appropriate for critically ill children with severe hypertension.

RENAL FAILURE

Renal disease may reduce or prevent the elimination of drugs administered in the pediatric intensive care unit. Accurate assessment of renal function, frequent determination of plasma drug concentrations, and periodic readjustment of drug dosages are all required to prevent drug overdosage. For a review of the adjustments in drug therapy that are required for renal failure, the reader is referred to an excellent review of the subject.[89]

SEIZURES

The treatment of status epilepticus (Table 106-7) may be partitioned into two phases: (1) an early phase, in which seizures are abolished by treatment with short-acting benzodiazepines (lorazepam or diazepam), and (2) a late phase in which an additional agent (phenytoin or phenobarbital) is given to prevent recurrence. Phenytoin is preferred over phenobarbital because it does not cause sedation, which may interfere with the neurologic exam. Pentobarbital, general anesthesia, and midazolam by continuous infusion[90] have each been used successfully for the treatment of seizures unresponsive to the above medications or for those lasting

TABLE 106-7 Treatment of Status Epilepticus

Agent	Dose
Early phase	
Lorazepam	0.03–0.05 mg/kg IV in up to three repeated doses every 5–10 min
Diazepam	0.2–0.5 mg/kg IV in up to three repeated doses every 5–10 min
Late phase	
Phenytoin	15–20 mg/kg IV, rate no greater than 1 mg/kg/min
Phenobarbital	15–20 mg/kg IV, rate no greater than 30 mg/min
Persistent seizures	
Midazolam	0.15 mg/kg IV followed by continuous infusion of 1 µg/kg/min, or
Pentobarbital	5 mg/kg IV

1 h or more. One should not forget that electrolyte abnormalities are important causes of seizures in infants; a bedside determination of blood glucose should be obtained immediately and glucose administered if needed. Other electrolyte abnormalities should also be considered.

References

1. Notterman DA: Pediatric pharmacotherapy, in Chernow B (ed): *The Pharmacologic Approach to the Critically Ill Patient*, 3d ed. Baltimore: Williams & Wilkins, 1994:139–145.
2. Susia GM, Dionne RE: Pharmacokinetics–pharmacodynamics: Drug delivery and therapeutic monitoring, in Holbrook PR (ed): *Textbook of Pediatric Critical Care*. Philadelphia: Saunders, 1993.
3. Guy J, Haley K, Zuspan SJ: Use of intraosseous infusion in the pediatric trauma patient. *J Pediatr Surg* 1993; 28:158.
4. Emergency Cardiac Care Committee and Subcommittees, American Heart Association: Guidelines for cardiopulmonary resuscitation and emergency cardiac care: Part VI. Pediatric advanced life support. *JAMA* 1992; 268:2262.
5. Tobias JD, Nichols DG: Intraosseous succinylcholine for orotracheal intubation. *Pediatr Emerg Care* 1990; 6:108.
6. Lenney W, Milner AD: At what age do bronchodilators work? *Arch Dis Child* 1978; 53:532.
7. Tepper RS: Airway reactivity in infants: A positive response to methacholine and metaproterenol. *J Appl Physiol* 1987; 62:1155.
8. Katz RW, Kelly HM, Crowley MR, et al.: Safety of continuous nebulized albuterol for bronchospasm in infants and children. *Pediatrics* 1993; 92:666.
9. Papo MC, Frank J, Thompson AE: A prospective, randomized study of continuous versus intermittent nebulized albuterol for severe status asthmaticus in children. *Crit Care Med* 1993; 21:1479.
10. Bohn D, Kalloghlian A, Jenkins J, et al.: Intravenous salbutamol in the treatment of status asthmaticus in children. *Crit Care Med* 1984; 12:892.
11. Fuglsang G, Pedersen S, Borgstrom L: Dose-response relationships of intravenously administered terbutaline in children with asthma. *J Pediatr* 1989; 114L:315.
12. Thiringer G, Svedmyr N: Comparison of infused and inhaled terbutaline in patients with asthma. *Scand J Respir Dis* 1976; 57:17.
13. Kerem E, Levison H, Schuh S, et al.: Efficacy of albuterol administered by nebulizer versus spacer device in children with acute asthma. *J Pediatr* 1993; 123:313.
14. Maguire JF, O'Rourke PP, Colan SD, et al.: Cardiotoxicity during treatment of severe childhood asthma. *Pediatrics* 1991; 88:1180.
15. Manthous CA, Hall JB, Schmidt GA, Wood LD: Metered-dose inhaler versus nebulized albuterol in mechanically ventilated patients. *Am Rev Respir Dis* 1993; 148:1567.
16. Tal A, Levy N, Bearman JE: Methylprednisone therapy for acute asthma in infants and toddlers: A controlled clinical trial. *Pediatrics* 1990; 86:350.
17. Gleeson JG, Loftus BG, Price JF: Placebo controlled trial of systemic corticosteroids in acute childhood asthma. *Acta Paediatr Scand* 1992; 79:1052.
18. Scarfone RJ, Fuchs SM, Nager AL, Shane SA: Controlled trial of oral prednisone in the emergency department treatment of children with acute asthma. *Pediatrics* 1993; 92:513.
19. DiGiulio GA, Kercsmar CM, Krug SE, et al.: Hospital treatment of asthma: Lack of benefit from theophylline given in addition to nebulized albuterol and intravenously administered corticosteroid. *J Pediatr* 1993; 122:464.
20. Carter E, Cruz M, Chesrown S, et al.: Efficacy of intravenously administered theophylline in children hospitalized with severe asthma. *J Pediatr* 1993; 122:470.
21. Strauss RE, Wertheim DL, Bonagura VR, Valacer DJ: Aminophylline therapy does not improve outcome and increases adverse effects in children hospitalized with acute asthmatic exacerbations. *Pediatrics* 1994; 93:205.
22. Reisman J, Galdes-Sebalt M, Kazim F, et al.: Frequent administration by inhalation of salbutamol and ipratropium bromide in the initial management of severe acute asthma in children. *J Allergy Clin Immunol* 1988; 81:16.
23. Mallory GB, Motoyama EK, Koumbourlis AC, et al.: Bronchial reactivity in infants in acute respiratory failure with viral bronchiolitis. *Pediatr Pulmonol* 1989; 6:253.
24. Tepper RS, Rosenberg D, Eigen H, Reister T: Bronchodilator responsiveness in infants with bronchiolitis. *Pediatr Pulmonol* 1994; 17:81.
25. Soto ME, Sly PD, Uren E, et al.: Bronchodilator response during acute viral bronchiolitis in infancy. *Pediatr Pulmonol* 1985; 2:85.
26. Hughes DM, Lesouëf PN, Landau LI: Effect of salbutamol on respiratory mechanics in bronchiolitis. *Pediatr Res* 1987; 22:83.
27. Sanchez I, De Koster J, Powell RE, et al.: Effect of racemic epinephrine and salbutamol on clinical score and pulmonary mechanics in infants with bronchiolitis. *J Pediatr* 1993; 122:145.
28. Sly PD, Lanteri CJ, Raven JM: Do wheezy infants recovering from bronchiolitis respond to inhaled salbutamol? *Pediatr Pulmonol* 1991; 10:36.
29. Springer C, Bar-Vishay E, Uwayyed K, et al.: Corticosteroids do not affect the clinical or physiological status of infants with bronchiolitis. *Pediatr Pulmonol* 1990; 9:181.
30. Maayan C, Itzhaki T, Bar-Vishay E, et al.: The functional response of infants with persistent wheezing to nebulized beclomethasone dipropionate. *Pediatr Pulmonol* 1986; 2:9.
31. Smith DW, Frankel LR, Mathers LH, et al.: A controlled trial of aerosolized ribavirin in infants receiving mechanical ventilation for severe respiratory syncytial virus infection. *N Engl J Med* 1991; 325:24.
32. Janai HK, Stutman HR, Zaleska M, et al.: Ribavirin effect on pulmonary function in young infants with respiratory syncytial virus bronchiolitis. *Pediatr Infect Dis J* 1993; 12:214.
33. Meert KL, Sarnaik AP, Gelmini MJ, Lieh-Lai MW: Aerosolized ribavirin in mechanically-ventilated children with respiratory syncytial virus lower respiratory tract disease: A prospective, double-blind, randomized trial. *Crit Care Med* 1994; 22:566.
34. Avery GB, Fletcher AB, Kaplan M, Brudno DS: Controlled trial of

dexamethasone in respirator-dependent infants with bronchopulmonary dysplasia. *Pediatrics* 1985; 75:106.

35. Yeh TF, Torre JA, Rastogi A, et al.: Early postnatal dexamethasone therapy in premature infants with severe respiratory distress syndrome: A double-blind, controlled study. *J Pediatr* 1990; 117:273.

36. LaForce WR, Brudno DS: Controlled trial of beclomethasone propionate by nebulization in oxygen- and ventilator-dependent infants. *J Pediatr* 1993; 122:285.

37. Mammel MC, Green TP, Johnson DE, Thompson TR: Controlled trial of dexamethasone therapy in infants with bronchopulmonary dysplasia. *Lancet* 1983; 1:1356.

38. Cummings JJ, D'Eugenio DB, Gross SJ: A controlled trial of dexamethasone in preterm infants at high risk for bronchopulmonary dysplasia. *N Engl J Med* 1989; 320:1505.

39. Harkavy KL, Scanlon JW, Chowdry PK, Grylack LJ: Dexamethasone therapy for chronic lung disease in ventilator- and oxygen-dependent infants: A controlled trial. *J Pediatr* 1989; 115:979.

40. Kazzi NJ, Brans YW, Poland RL: Dexamethasone affects the hospital course of infants with bronchopulmonary dysplasia who are dependent on artificial ventilation. *Pediatrics* 1990; 86:722.

41. Collaborative Dexamethasone Trial Group: Dexamethasone therapy in neonatal chronic lung disease: An international placebo-controlled trial. *Pediatrics* 1991; 88:421.

42. Motoyama EK, Fort MD, Klesh KW, et al.: Early onset of airway reactivity in premature infants with bronchopulmonary dysplasia. *Am Rev Respir Dis* 1987; 136:50.

43. Northway WH Jr, Moss RB, Carlisle KB, et al.: Late pulmonary sequelae of bronchopulmonary dysplasia. *N Engl J Med* 1990; 323:1793.

44. de Kleine MJ, Roos CM, Voorn WJ, et al.: Lung function 8–18 years after intermittent positive pressure ventilation for hyaline membrane disease. *Thorax* 1990; 45:941.

45. Denjean A, Guimaraes H, Migdal M, et al.: Dose-related bronchodilator response to aerosolized salbutamol (albuterol) in ventilator-dependent infants. *J Pediatr* 1992; 120:974.

46. Brundage KL, Mohsini KG, Froese AB, Fisher JT: Bronchodilator response to ipratropium bromide in infants with bronchopulmonary dysplasia. *Am Rev Respir Dis* 1990; 142:1137.

47. Rush MG, Engelhardt B, Parker RA, Hazinski TA: Double-blind, placebo-controlled trial of alternate-day furosemide therapy in infants with bronchopulmonary dysplasia. *J Pediatr* 1990; 117:112.

48. Kao LC, Durant DJ, McCrea RC, et al.: Randomized trial of long-term diuretic therapy for infants with oxygen-dependent bronchopulmonary dysplasia. *J Pediatr* 1994; 124:772.

49. O'Rourke PP: Outcome of children who are apneic and pulseless in the emergency room. *Crit Care Med* 1986; 14:466.

50. Biggart MJ, Bohn DJ: Effect of hypothermia and cardiac arrest on outcome of near-drowning accidents in children. *J Pediatr* 1990; 117:179.

51. Goetting MG, Paradis MA: High-dose epinephrine improves outcome from pediatric cardiac arrest. *Ann Emerg Med* 1991; 20:22.

52. Lang P, Williams RG, Norwood WI, Casteneda AR: The hemodynamic effects of dopamine in infants after corrective cardiac surgery. *J Pediatr* 1980; 96:630.

53. Driscoll DJ, Gillette PC, Duff DF, McNamara DG: The hemodynamic effect of dopamine in children. *J Thorac Cardiovasc Surg* 1979; 78:765.

54. Disessa TG, Leitner M, Ti CC, et al.: The cardiovascular effects of dopamine in the severely asphyxiated neonate. *J Pediatr* 1981; 99:772.

55. Notterman DA, Greenwald BM, Moran F, et al.: Dopamine clearance in critically ill infants and children: Effect of age and organ system dysfunction. *Clin Pharm Ther* 1990; 48:138.

56. Zaritsky A, Chernow B: Use of catecholamines in pediatrics. *J Pediatr* 1984; 105:341.

57. Eldadah MK, Schwartz PH, Harrison R, Newth CJL: Pharmacokinetics of dopamine in infants and children. *Crit Care Med* 1991; 19:1008.

58. Perez CA, Reimer JM, Schreiber MD, et al.: Effect of high-dose dopamine on urine output in newborn infants. *Crit Care Med* 1986; 14:1045.

59. Outwater KM, Treves ST, Lang P, et al.: Renal and hemodynamic effects of dopamine in infants following cardiac surgery. *J Clin Anesth* 1990; 2:253.

60. Habib DM, Padbury JF, Anas NG, et al.: Dobutamine pharmacokinetics and pharmacodynamics in pediatric intensive care patients. *Crit Care Med* 1992; 20:601.

61. Berg RA, Donnerstein RL, Padbury JF: Dobutamine infusions in stable, critically ill children: Pharmacokinetics and hemodynamic actions. *Crit Care Med* 1993; 21:678.

62. Perkin RM, Levin DL, Webb R, et al.: Dobutamine: A hemodynamic evaluation in children with shock. *J Pediatr* 1982; 100:977.

63. Bohn DJ, Poirer CS, Edmonds JF, Barker GA: Hemodynamic effects of dobutamine after cardiopulmonary bypass in children. *Crit Care Med* 1980; 8:367.

64. Berner M, Jaccard C, Oberhansli I, et al.: Hemodynamic effects of amrinone in children after cardiac surgery. *Int Care Med* 1990; 16:85.

65. Lynn AM, Sorensen GK, Williams GD, et al.: Hemodynamic effects of amrinone and colloid administration in children following cardiac surgery. *J Cardiothorac Vasc Anesth* 1993; 7:560.

66. Robinson BW, Gelband H, Mas MS: Selective pulmonary and systemic vasodilator effects of amrinone in children: New therapeutic implications. *J Am Coll Cardiol* 1993; 21:1461.

67. Donnerstein RL, Berg RA, Shehab Z, Ovadia M: Complex atrial tachycardias and respiratory syncytial virus infections in infants. *J Pediatr* 1994; 125:23.

68. Cook P, Scarfone RJ, Cook RT: Adenosine in the termination of albuterol-induced supraventricular tachycardia. *Ann Emerg Med* 1994; 24:316.

69. Sreeram N, Wren C: Supraventricular tachycardia in infants: response to initial treatment. *Arch Dis Child* 1990; 65:127.

70. Ralston MA, Knilans TK, Hannon DW, Daniels SR: Use of adenosine for diagnosis and treatment of tachyarrhythmias in pediatric patients. *J Pediatr* 1994; 124:139.

71. Epstein ML, Kiel EA, Victorica BE: Cardiac decompensation following verapamil therapy in infants with supraventricular tachycardia. *Pediatrics* 1985; 75:737.

72. Hannallah RS, Baker SB, Casey W, et al.: Propofol: Effective dose and induction characteristics in unpremedicated children. *Anesthesiology* 1991; 74:217.

73. Short SM, Aun CS: Haemodynamic effects of propofol in children. *Anaesthesia* 1991; 46:783.

74. Parke TJ, Stevens JE, Rice AS, et al.: Metabolic acidosis and fatal myocardial failure after propofol infusion in children: Five case reports. *Br Med J* 1992; 305:613.

75. Woelfel SK, Brandom BW, McGowan FX Jr, Cook DR: Clinical pharmacology of mivacurium in pediatric patients less than two years old during nitric oxide-halothane anesthesia. *Anesth Analg* 1993; 77:713.

76. Gronert B, Woelfel S, Cook DR: Comparison of equipotent intubating doses of mivacurium and succinylcholine in infants 2–12 months old. (abstr) *Anesthesiology* 1993; 79:A932.

77. Bergman I, Steeves M, Burckart G, Thompson A: Reversible neurologic abnormalities associated with prolonged intravenous midazolam and fentanyl administration. *J Pediatr* 1991; 119:644.

78. Arnold JH, Truog RD, Scavone JM, Fenton T: Changes in the pharmacodynamic response to fentanyl in neonates during continuous infusion. *J Pediatr* 1991; 119:639.

79. Katz R, Kelly HW, Hsi A: Prospective study on the occurrence of withdrawal in critically ill children who receive fentanyl by continuous infusion. *Crit Care Med* 1994; 22:763.

80. Lane JC, Tennison ST, Lawless ST, et al.: Movement disorder after withdrawal of fentanyl infusion. *J Pediatr* 1991; 119:649.

81. Berde CB, Beyer JE, Bournaki M-C, et al.: Comparison of morphine and methadone for prevention of postoperative pain in 3- to 7-year old children. *J Pediatr* 1991; 119:136.

82. Berde CB, Lehn BM, Yee JD, et al.: Patient-controlled analgesia in children and adolescents: A randomized, prospective comparison with intramuscular administration of morphine for postoperative analgesia. *J Pediatr* 1991; 118:460.

83. Hershenson MB, Brouillette RT, Olsen E, Hunt CE: The effect of chloral hydrate on genioglossus and diaphragmatic activity. *Pediatr Res* 1984; 18:516.

84. DeFries CB, Wong HC: Seizures and opisthotonos after propofol anesthesia. *Anesth Analg* 1992; 75:630.

85. Segredo V, Caldwell JE, Matthay MA, et al.: Persistent paralysis in critically ill patients after long-term administration of vecuronium. *N Engl J Med* 1992; 327:524.

86. Douglass JA, Tuxen DV, Horne M, et al.: Myopathy in severe asthma. *Am Rev Respir Dis* 1992; 146:517.

87. Kupfer Y, Namba T, Kaldawi E, Tessler S: Prolonged weakness after long-term infusion of vecuronium bromide. *Ann Intern Med* 1992; 117:484.

88. Hansen-Flaschen J, Cowen J, Raps EC: Neuromuscular blockade in the intensive care unit: More than we bargained for. *Am Rev Respir Dis* 1993; 147:234.

89. St Peter WL, Halstenson CE: Pharmacologic approach in patients with renal failure: Treatment, in Chernow B (ed): *The Pharmacologic Approach to the Critically Ill Patient,* 3d ed. Baltimore: Williams & Wilkins, 1994:41–79.

90. Rivera R, Segnini M, Baltodano A, Perez V: Midazolam in the treatment of status epilepticus in children. *Crit Care Med* 1993; 21:991.

TREATMENT OF DISORDERED BREATHING

Chapter 107

EFFECTS OF COPD ON SLEEP

MELVIN LOPATA

Along with the many studies that have defined the nature and extent of primary sleep disorders resulting in impaired breathing, there has been increased recognition of sleep-induced respiratory dysfunction in primary pulmonary disorders, mainly chronic obstructive pulmonary disease (COPD). This chapter reviews the effects of COPD on nocturnal (sleep-related) respiration, the marked impairment of ventilation and gas exchange that occurs during sleep in some patients with COPD, as well as its causes, consequences, and treatment.

Sleep has a primary effect on respiratory control that can result in significant alterations of respiratory drive and respiratory mechanics. These sleep-related changes in respiration have little functional influence on ventilation and gas exchange in healthy adults but can have profound impact on patients with respiratory disease.

The most apparent change in respiratory mechanics associated with non–rapid-eye-movement (NREM) sleep pertains to the upper airway. Pharyngeal resistance increases more than twice that during waking, probably owing to a decrease in activity of the upper airway dilating muscles, whose function it is to maintain the integrity and patency of the upper airway during inspiration.[1,2] In contrast, during NREM sleep, respiratory muscle activity either does not change (diaphragm)[3,4] or is increased (inspiratory intercostals and diaphragm).[3,5,6]

Rapid eye movement (REM) sleep is inherently an unsteady state characterized by bursts of phasic eye movements (REMs) and skeletal muscle twitching, along with loss of tone of the postural muscles.[7] During REM sleep, breathing is also unsteady or irregular.[8] In contrast to the relatively regular irregularity—that is, periodic breathing at sleep onset—respiration during REM sleep is usually irregularly irregular with sudden changes, especially shallow, rapid respirations, associated with bursts of REMs,[4,9] though periodic breathing can occur as well.[8] Apneas may also appear at this time.[10] As in NREM sleep, upper airway muscle activity is diminished, especially with REMs, and pharyngeal resistance increases in REM sleep as well.[1,11] In contrast to NREM sleep, inspiratory intercostal muscle activity is inhibited during REM sleep, resulting in diminished displacements of the rib cage or even in paradoxical movement of the chest wall (abdomen out and rib cage in) during inspiration. Thus, REM sleep represents a precarious period for respiration, which can become critical in patients with respiratory disease.

The effects of sleep on ventilation and oxygenation in patients with COPD have been the subject of investigation for many years. Although early studies demonstrated that arterial oxygen tension or saturation decreased and CO_2 tension increased in patients with COPD during sleep,[2,12–16] the reported degree of blood gas worsening was variable and not even considered by some investigators to be greater than normal.[13–15] Not until continuous monitoring of arterial oxygen saturation (Sa_{O_2}) was possible did the extent of sleep-induced impairment of oxygenation become known.[17,18] From the works of Flick and Block and Douglas and colleagues,[17,18] it was demonstrated clearly in these patients that oxygen desaturation during sleep could be severe and prolonged and that REM sleep was the state typically associated with such desaturation (Fig. 107-1).

Although almost all patients studied and reported have severe airway obstruction (i.e., $FEV_1 < 1$ L), the degree of nocturnal hypoxemia as well as CO_2 retention was quite variable.[2,12–14,16,18,19,22] The decrease in Sa_{O_2} and Pa_{O_2} varies from 4 to 70 percent and 5 to 35 mmHg, respectively, whereas the increase in Pa_{CO_2} ranges from 5 to 15 mmHg.[12–14,17,18] Three distinct patterns of oxygen desaturation related to different sleep stages and incurring different degrees and durations of hypoxemia have been recognized.

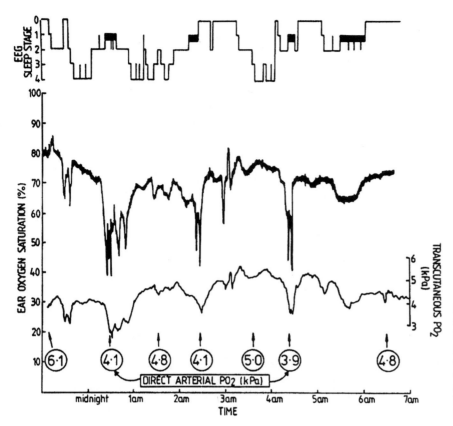

FIGURE 107-1 Continuous oxygen saturation, transcutaneous PO_2, and sleep state [closed bars = rapid eye movement (REM) sleep] in a patient with severe airway obstruction and daytime hypoxemia and hypercapnia. Note decrease in baseline saturation at sleep onset and episodic desaturation, the most severe being in REM sleep (1 pka = 7.5 mmHg). (*From Flenly,*[66] *with permission.*)

The first occurs at sleep onset and is evident by a mild to moderate decrease of the waking baseline oxygen saturation, or tension, which persists throughout sleep.[13,18] Superimposed on this baseline shift are two types of episodic desaturations; one occurs in stages I and II NREM sleep and REM sleep and is associated with the periodic breathing evident in these sleep states.[8,9] This disordered breathing is manifest as periodic hypopneas or apneas, often due to upper airway obstruction; hence it is similar to the disordered breathing of sleep apnea. The degree of associated desaturation is usually mild to moderate and of relatively brief duration (< 30 s)[19,22] (see Fig. 108-1, Chap. 108). The second pattern of episodic desaturation occurs essentially during REM sleep and may account for > 50 percent of the transient desaturations and usually the great majority of severe desaturations.[22] These desaturations usually are associated with some decrease in respiratory effort evident by decreased chest wall or pleural pressure excursions.[17,19,22,23] There also may be no obvious change in the ventilatory pattern.[22] These episodes of desaturation can be the most severe and prolonged, lasting from 5 to over 30 min[17,19,22] (see Fig. 108-2).

What is the prevalence of sleep-associated hypoxemia in patients with COPD and which patients are at risk for developing significant oxygen desaturation during sleep? Studies reporting on sleep effects in COPD usually have included relatively few patients who were selected for their severe airway obstruction.[12–22,24,25] Most, if not all, patients in this group experience nocturnal decreases in Pa_{O_2} and, depending on the baseline Pa_{O_2}, many show oxygen desaturation.

However, the degree of desaturation is quite variable.

Patients classified as "blue bloaters" have been shown to be at risk for severe nocturnal desaturation. These patients have severe hypoxemia, hypercapnia, and cor pulmonale and are often obese, as opposed to the thin, mildly hypoxemic, normocapneic "pink puffers." The former group has been shown to have severe and prolonged oxygen desaturation during sleep compared with the mild impairment of oxygenation seen in the latter.[17,19–21,25,26] The degree of airway obstruction does not distinguish between those patients who experience desaturation.[13–17]

The most apparent reason for the susceptibility of the blue bloater to nocturnal desaturation is the presence of a low waking Pa_{O_2} and thereby a low baseline oxygen saturation. By being on the steep part of the oxygen dissociation curve, changes in Pa_{O_2} can result in profound changes in saturation and could explain the differences between the blue bloater and pink puffer.[25] Thus, the true risk factor may be the waking Pa_{O_2} or saturation. Baseline Pa_{O_2} above 60 mmHg and saturation > 90 percent would not be associated with nocturnal deterioration of oxygenation, whereas lesser values would be a harbinger of sleep-induced hypoxia. Indeed, a number of studies have shown a significant relationship between the degree of nocturnal hypoxemia or desaturation and the baseline or waking Pa_{O_2} or Sa_{O_2},[13,15,24,25,27–29] such that the lower the baseline value, the greater the nocturnal deterioration. Daytime hypoxemia has been found to account for three-fourths of the variation in nocturnal hypoxemia.[25] Thus, waking Pa_{O_2} is probably the best predictor of nocturnal desaturation, but patients with reasonable

$Pa_{O_2} > 60$ mmHg can experience significant desaturation.[19,20,22] However, one study has shown that the great majority of such patients do not develop severe nocturnal hypoxia.[30]

The impairment of oxygenation during sleep can result in physiologic dysfunction due to tissue hypoxia. Episodes of oxygen desaturation, whether associated with hypopneas and apneas or REMs, uniformly result in increased pulmonary artery pressure (PAP).[12,17,31,32] Although most of the patients studied have waking pulmonary hypertension, which worsens during sleep,[12,22,32] patients with normal baseline pulmonary pressures also can show increases in PAP associated with oxygen desaturation.[7] The degree of PAP elevation is inversely proportional to the degree of desaturation. The mechanism mediating the pulmonary hypertension is probably pulmonary vasoconstriction induced by hypoxia or possibly acidosis secondary to acute hypoventilation occurring with the desaturation episode.[31,32] The fact that pulmonary vascular resistance increases with the PAP elevation[32] and that oxygen administration, which eliminates the desaturation, eliminates the increase in PAP during sleep supports the role of hypoxia as the main culprit.[31,32] Based on the relationship between hypoxia and pulmonary hypertension[33] and the known effects on pulmonary pressure of sleep-induced hypoxemia in the sleep apnea syndrome,[34,35] the occurrence of sleep-related pulmonary hypertension in COPD is certainly not unexpected. However, the importance of this process relates to the premise that episodes of transient increase in PAP during sleep can lead to sustained pulmonary hypertension.[36,37] This contention implicates sleep-related desaturation in the natural history and daytime morbidity of COPD and presupposes the use of nocturnal oxygen therapy to prevent hypoxemia and its pulmonary vascular sequelae.

Interestingly, left ventricular function apparently is not impaired during the desaturation episodes because pulmonary capillary wedge pressure is not increased during these periods[31,32]; however, it has been calculated that during sleep in those patients who desaturate, there is an increased demand for myocardial blood flow equivalent to that of maximal exercise.[32]

Patients with severe COPD are at risk for sudden death, presumably because of arrhythmias,[38–40] probably occurring during sleep.[41,42] At least three studies have documented electrocardiographic (ECG) changes and multiple arrhythmias at night in these patients,[43–45] though sleep was not documented electroencephalographically in two.[43,45] Premature ventricular contractions, often frequent and multifocal, unsustained ventricular tachycardia, and idioventricular rhythm have been shown to occur during sleep,[43–45] especially at the nadir of a severe episode of desaturation.[44]

Electrocardiographic abnormalities—such as ST-T depression, right bundle branch block, and prolonged QT interval—have also been associated with sleep.[45] The patients at greatest risk are those who experience desaturation the most during sleep[44]–those with low baseline Pa_{O_2} or Sa_{O_2}. Elimination of nocturnal desaturation with oxygen decreases the number of premature ventricular contractions (PVCs) and may eliminate the occurrence of arrhythmias,

such as ventricular tachycardia and idioventricular rhythm, as well as the described ECG abnormalities.[43,45] The potential efficacy of oxygen to reduce the risk of sleep-induced arrhythmia and sudden death implies the benefits of nocturnal oxygen therapy.

Sleep is disturbed in patients with severe COPD.[12,22] When sought, complaints are common, including sleeping difficulty with repeated awakenings and daytime somnolence.[19,27] Monitoring of sleep architecture confirms disturbed sleep, and findings from multiple studies are fairly consistent. Generally, total sleep time is decreased and there may be an increase in sleep latency.[12,46] The decreased time in sleep is due to multiple arousals resulting in more time spent in wakening.[12,14,27,46–48] The effects of this fractionated sleep on specific sleep states are not clear. Although there is some evidence for reduction in REM and slow-wave sleep,[14,22,24] the changes in these sleep states are quite variable and may not be different from those of a healthy population of the same age. Though the number of arousals has been shown to be related to the severity of oxygen desaturation (i.e., patients with the lowest Sa_{O_2} had the greatest number of arousals or awakenings[27]), only half of arousals are associated with episodes of desaturation, and there is no relationship between the number of arousals and the number of desaturation episodes per hour of sleep.[27,47] One study has shown that pink puffers with less severe daytime hypoxemia and nocturnal desaturation had more disturbed sleep than blue bloaters.[46] These data indicate that poor oxygenation is not the sole cause of arousal and disturbed sleep—that other factors, such as nocturnal dyspnea, retained secretions, and cough must be important as well. The multifactorial mechanisms for causing sleep disruption are supported by the variable effects of nocturnal oxygen on this pattern of disturbed sleep. Preventing desaturation by administering oxygen via a nasal cannula has not been shown to improve sleep dramatically, although there are reports of improved sleep efficiency with oxygen administration.[14,48] Other studies have shown no improvement[24,36] or only an insignificant trend toward improvement.[49]

The mechanisms of sleep-induced hypoxemia in COPD must be understood in the context of the three patterns of oxygen desaturation. The decrease in baseline Sa_{O_2} at sleep onset, the desaturation associated with periodic breathing during mostly light NREM sleep, and the prolonged REM desaturations are all abnormalities based on disease-exaggerated sleep state and stage effects on respiratory control, ventilation, and respiratory mechanics. The sleep-induced hypoventilation at sleep onset, resulting in minimal changes in Pa_{O_2} in healthy individuals, results in significant desaturation in hypoxemic patients on the steep part of their O_2-dissociation curve. Middle-aged to elderly men with COPD, especially if plagued by the common afflictions of obesity and snoring, experience periodic breathing and associated apneas and hypopneas during early sleep, as do their non-smoking counterparts, and even without meeting criteria for sleep apnea, these men will experience significant desaturation due to their abnormal baseline blood gases. Patients with COPD may also have true sleep apnea, which is discussed elsewhere (see Chap. 108). The striking effect of REM sleep on respiratory function and chest wall mechanics in healthy individuals becomes profound in patients with COPD and results in far more severe oxygen desaturation than that occurring in the other stages.

The mechanism of REM-induced blood gas abnormalities has been studied in a number of laboratories and is reasonably well understood. Both hypoventilation and gas-exchange abnormalities have been implicated as the cause of hypoxemia. Hypoventilation, as denoted by an increase in Pa_{CO_2}, does occur[12–14,18,50] and is associated with decreased ventilation[1,50] and respiratory effort, as indicated by decreased chest wall displacement and inspiratory pressure generation.[1,19,50,51] The decrease in ventilation is mainly due to tidal volume reduction,[1,50] and thoracic displacement is diminished more than that of the abdomen.[1,51] The cause of this impaired ventilation is in large part due to REM-induced inhibition of intercostal/accessory muscles whose activity is necessary to compensate for impaired diaphragmatic function in patients with chronic airway obstruction.[18,41] A decrease or loss of phasic and tonic inspiratory intercostal/accessory activity as well as expiratory activity results in chest wall distortion and reduced functional residual capacity.[26,51,52] As a result, both hypoventilation and impaired gas exchange occur, though the relative contribution of both of these pathophysiologic components to REM-induced hypoxemia is not really known.[53,54] Also contributing to the impaired ventilation in these patients is sleep, and especially REM-induced increases in upper airway resistance.[55]

The rise in Pa_{CO_2} indicative of hypoventilation, which occurs during these episodes, is rather modest compared with the fall in Pa_{O_2}, likely due to the large body stores of CO_2 compared with those of oxygen.[50] Though this hypoventilation is probably mostly due to REM inhibition of postural muscles, which include the intercostal/accessory muscles, the detection of diminished diaphragmatic electromyogram (EMG), and mouth occlusion pressure as well as decreased oxygen utilization during REM desaturations suggest that a more global component of hypoventilation also occurs.[1,55,56]

However, centrally mediated impairment of respiratory drive does not appear to contribute greatly to REM hypoventilation, because almitrine and progesterone (peripheral and central respiratory stimulants, respectively), when tested in patients with COPD, result in less overall nocturnal desaturation due to increase in waking Pa_{O_2} but do not really eliminate or alter the nocturnal episodes that cause desaturation.[57–63]

It is not clear whether there should be specific treatment for sleep-associated oxygen desaturation in COPD. Certainly, nocturnal desaturation can be prevented by administering oxygen, which can also prevent nocturnal exacerbation of pulmonary hypertension and arrhythmias and may improve sleep quality.[14,24,31,32,46,48,49] As noted, intermittent yet chronic pulmonary hypertension and sleep disruption have been proposed to contribute to the sequelae of COPD by leading to sustained pulmonary hypertension or by contributing to the development of CO_2 retention. However, even if this contention were true, no evidence exists that treatment with nocturnal oxygen would prevent

the sequelae or alter the natural course of the disease. In this regard the inability of 12-h nocturnal oxygen administration to improve survival in patients with severe COPD certainly does not support nocturnal oxygenation only.[64] However, since the Nocturnal Oxygen Therapy Trial study did not investigate sleep behavior, the results do not definitively negate such use of oxygen.

The consideration of nocturnal oxygen in patients who demonstrate sleep-induced hypoxemia is rather moot because the majority of patients who significantly desaturate are severely hypoxemic and generally already meet the criteria for continuous oxygen therapy.[64] The real consideration for nocturnal therapy is in those patients whose waking Pa_{O_2} is above 60 mmHg. About one-quarter of these patients will experience REM desaturation, but usually not to a severe degree, and there is no way to predict who is at risk.[30] However, a recent multicenter but retrospective study has shown that in selected COPD patients with a daytime Pa_{O_2} of > 60 mmHg and followed for up to 7½ years, those with nocturnal oxygen desaturation had a shorter survival than those without nocturnal desaturation.[65] Patients with desaturation treated with oxygen tended to survive longer than those not treated with O_2, but the differences did not achieve significance.

Thus current data, though emphasizing the need for prospective studies, do not justify the use of supplemental oxygen to correct nocturnal O_2 desaturation. A sleep study may be warranted in patients with a Pa_{O_2} of > 60 mmHg if they have sleep-related complaints or pulmonary hypertension or hypercapnia. If REM desaturations are present, nocturnal or continuous oxygen may be warranted. Therapy with oxygen should result in amelioration of the sleep complaint or the pulmonary vasculature and blood gas abnormalities to justify its long-term use. However, it also is likely that patients with these clinical features may have sleep apnea. Proving the efficacy of nocturnal oxygen in this clinical context requires extensive longitudinal studies that are yet to be performed.

Another therapeutic approach to prevent nocturnal oxygen desaturation is using drugs that stimulate ventilation (see Chap. 67). Both almitrine and progesterone have been studied and have generally been found to improve nocturnal oxygenation without affecting the REM events that cause the desaturation.[57–63] This improvement is due to the ability of these drugs to increase waking Pa_{O_2}.[57–62] As with oxygen therapy, which is more effective than drugs in improving oxygenation, the efficacy and cost-effectiveness of drug therapy is not known and the routine use of drugs cannot be justified at this time.

References

1. Hudgel DW, Martin RJ, Johnson B, Hill P: Mechanics of the respiratory system and breathing pattern during sleep in normal humans. *J Appl Physiol* 1984; 56:133–137.
2. Robin ED: Some interrelations between sleep and disease. *Ann Intern Med* 1958; 102:669–675.
3. Lopes JM, Tabachnik E, Muller NL, et al.: Total airway resistance and respiratory muscle activity during sleep. *J Appl Physiol* 1983; 54:773–777.

4. Tusiewicz K, Moldafsky H, Brian SC, Bryan AC: Mechanics of the rib cage and diaphragm during sleep. *J Appl Physiol* 1977; 43:600–602.

5. Tabachnik E, Muller NL, Bryan C, Levison H: Changes in ventilation and chest wall mechanics during sleep in normal adolescents. *J Appl Physiol* 1987; 51:557–564.

6. Warner G, Skatrud JB, Dempsey JA: Effect of hypoxia-induced periodic breathing on upper airway obstruction during sleep. *J Appl Physiol* 1987; 62:2201–2211.

7. Aseunsky E, Kleetman N: Regularly occurring periods of eye mobility and concomitant phenomena during sleep. *Science* 1953; 118:273–274.

8. Webb P: Periodic breathing during sleep. *J Appl Physiol* 1974; 37:899–909.

9. Bulow K: Respiration and wakefulness in man. *Acta Physiol Scand* 1963; 59:1–110.

10. Krieger J, Turlot JC, Mangin P, Kurtz D: Breathing during sleep in normal young and elderly subjects: Hypopneas, apneas and correlated factors. *Sleep* 1983; 6:108–120.

11. Önal E, Lopata M: Periodic breathing and the pathogenesis of occlusive sleep apneas. *Am Rev Respir Dis* 1982; 126:676–680.

12. Coccagna G, Lugaresa E: Arterial blood gases and pulmonary and systemic arterial pressure during sleep in chronic obstructive pulmonary disease. *Sleep* 1978; 1:117–124.

13. Koo KW, Sax DS, Snider GL: Arterial blood gases and pH during sleep in chronic obstructive pulmonary disease. *Am J Med* 1975; 58:663–670.

14. Leitch AG, Clancy LJ, Leggett RJE, et al.: Arterial blood gas tensions, hydrogen ion, and electroencephalogram during sleep in patients with chronic ventilatory failure. *Thorax* 1976; 31:730–735.

15. Pierce AK, Jarrett CE, Werkle G, Miller WF: Respiratory function during sleep in patients with chronic obstructive lung disease. *J Clin Invest* 1966; 45:631–636.

16. Trask CH, Cree EM: Oximeter studies on patients with chronic obstructive emphysema, awake and during sleep. *N Engl J Med* 1962; 266:639–642.

17. Douglas NJ, Calverley PMA, Leggett RJE, Brash HM: Transient hypoxemia during sleep in chronic bronchitis and emphysema. *Lancet* 1979; 1:1–4.

18. Flick MR, Block AJ: Continuous in vivo monitoring of arterial oxygenation in chronic obstructive lung disease. *Ann Intern Med* 1977; 36:725–730.

19. Arand DL, McGinty DJ, Littner MR: Respiratory patterns associated with hemoglobin desaturation during sleep in chronic obstructive pulmonary disease. *Chest* 1981; 80:183–190.

20. DeMarco FJ, Wynne JW, Block AJ: Oxygen desaturation during sleep as a determinant of the "blue and bloated" syndrome. *Chest* 1981; 79:621–625.

21. Gimeno F, van Veenen R, Steenhuis EJ: Ear oximetry studies during sleep in patients with severe chronic obstructive pulmonary disease in a stable state. *Ann Allergy* 1986; 56:142–144.

22. Wynne JW, Block AJ, Hemenway J, et al.: Disordered breathing and oxygen desaturation during sleep in patients with chronic obstructive lung disease (COLD). *Am J Med* 1979; 66:573–579.

23. Hudgel DW, Martin RJ, Capehart M, et al.: Contribution of hypoventilation to sleep oxygen desaturation in chronic obstructive pulmonary disease. *J Appl Physiol* 1983; 55:669–677.

24. Fleetham J, Mezon B, West P, et al.: Sleep, arousals, and oxygen desaturation in chronic obstructive pulmonary disease. *Am Rev Respir Dis* 1982; 126:429–433.

25. Stradling JR, Lane DJ: Nocturnal hypoxemia in chronic obstructive pulmonary disease. *Clin Sci* 1983; 64:213–222.

26. Catterall JR, Douglas NJ, Calverley PMA, et al.: Transient hypoxemia during sleep in chronic obstructive pulmonary disease is not a sleep apnea syndrome. *Am Rev Respir Dis* 1983; 128:24–29.

27. Cormick W, Olson L. Hensley JM, Saunders NA: Nocturnal hypoxemia and quality of sleep in patients with chronic obstructive lung diseases. *Thorax* 1986; 41:846–854.

28. Fleetham JA, Mezon B, West P: Chemical control of ventilation and sleep arterial oxygen desaturation in patients with COPD. *Am Rev Respir Dis* 1980; 122:583–589.

29. Tatsumi K, Kimura H, Kunitomo F, et al.: Sleep arterial oxygen desaturation and chemical control of breathing during wakefulness in COPD. *Chest* 1986; 90:6–73.

30. Fletcher EC, Miller J, Divine GW, et al.: Nocturnal oxyhemoglobin desaturation in COPD patients with arterial oxygen tensions above 60 mmHg. *Chest* 1987; 92:604–608.

31. Boysen PG, Block AJ, Wynne JW, et al.: Nocturnal pulmonary hypertension in patients with chronic obstructive pulmonary disease. *Chest* 1979; 76:536–542.

32. Fletcher EC, Levin DC: Cardiopulmonary hemodynamics during sleep in subjects with chronic obstructive pulmonary disease: The effect of short and long-term oxygen. *Chest* 1984; 85:6–14.

33. Abraham AS, Kay JM, Cole RB, Pincock AC: Hemodynamic and pathologic study of the effect of chronic hypoxia and subsequent recovery on the heart and pulmonary vasculature of the rat. *Cardiovasc Res* 1971; 5:95–102.

34. Coccagna G, Mantovani M, Brignani F, et al.: Continuous recording of the pulmonary and systemic arterial pressure during sleep in syndromes of hypersomnia with periodic breathing. *Bull Physiopathol Respir* 1972; 8:1159–1172.

35. Tilkian AG, Guilleminault C, Schroeder JS, et al.: Hemodynamics in sleep induced apnea. *Ann Intern Med* 1976; 85:714–719.

36. Nattie EE, Bartlett D, Johnson K: Pulmonary hypertension and right ventricular hypertrophy caused by intermittent hypoxia and hypercapnia in the rat. *Am Rev Respir Dis* 1978; 118:653–658.

37. Ressl J, Urbanova D, Widimsky J, et al.: Reversibility of pulmonary hypertension and right ventricular hypertrophy induced by intermittent high altitude hypoxia in rats. *Respiration* 1974; 31:38–46.

38. Burrows B, Earle RH: Course and prognosis of chronic obstructive lung disease. *N Engl J Med* 1969; 280:397–404.

39. Diener CV, Burrows B: Further observations on the course and prognosis of chronic obstructive lung disease. *Am Rev Respir Dis* 1976; 111:719–724.

40. Holford FD, Mithoefer JC: Cardiac arrhythmias in hospitalized patients with COPD. *Am Rev Respir Dis* 1973; 108:879–895.

41. Hudson LD, Kurt TL, Petty TL, Genton E: Arrhythmias associated with acute respiratory failure in patients with chronic airway obstruction. *Chest* 1973; 63:661–665.

42. Smolensky M, Halberg F, Sargent F II: Chronobiology of the life sequence, in Itoh S, Ogata K, Hoshimure H (eds): *Advances in Climatic Physiology*. Tokyo: Igaku Shoin, 1972: 281–318.

43. Flick MR, Block AJ: Nocturnal vs diurnal cardiac arrhythmias in patients with chronic obstructive pulmonary disease. *Chest* 1979; 75:8–11.

44. Shepard JW, Garrison MW, Grither DA, et al.: Relationship of ventricular ectopy to nocturnal oxygen desaturation in patients with chronic obstructive pulmonary disease. *Am J Med* 1985; 78:28–34.

45. Tirlapur VG, Mir MA: Nocturnal hypoxemia and associated electrocardiographic changes in patients with chronic obstructive airways disease. *N Engl J Med* 1982; 306:125–130.

46. Calverley PMA, Brezinova V, Douglas NJ, et al.: The effect of oxygenation on sleep quality in chronic bronchitis and emphysema. *Am Rev Respir Dis* 1982; 126:206–210.

47. Brezinova V, Catterall JR, Douglas NJ, et al.: Night sleep of patients with chronic ventilatory failure and age matched controls: Number and duration of the EEG episodes of intervening wakefulness and drowsiness. *Sleep* 1982; 5:123–130.

48. Kearley R, Wynne JW, Block AJ, et al.: The effect of low flow oxygen on sleep-disordered breathing and oxygen desaturation: A

study of patients with chronic obstructive lung disease. *Chest* 1980; 78:682–685.

49. Goldstein RS, Ramcharan V, Bowes G, et al.: Effect of supplemental nocturnal oxygen on gas exchange in patients with severe obstructive lung disease. *N Engl J Med* 1984; 310:425–429.

50. Catterall JR, Calverley PMA, MacNee W, et al.: Mechanism of transient nocturnal hypoxemia in hypoxic chronic bronchitis and emphysema. *J Appl Physiol* 1985; 59:1698–1703.

51. Johnson MW, Remmers JE: Accessory muscle activity during sleep in chronic obstructive pulmonary disease. *J Appl Physiol* 1984; 57:1011–1017.

52. Muller NL, Francis PW, Gurwitz D, et al.: Mechanism of hemoglobin desaturation during rapid-eye movement sleep in normal subjects and in patients with cystic fibrosis. *Am Rev Respir Dis* 1980; 121:463–469.

53. Findley LJ, Ries AL, Lisi GM, Wagner PD: Hypoxemia during apnea in normal subjects: Mechanisms and impact of lung volume. *J Appl Physiol* 1983; 55:1777–1783.

54. Hudgel DW, Devadatta P: Decrease in functional residual capacity during sleep in normal humans. *J Appl Physiol* 1984; 57:1319–1322.

55. Ballard RD, Clover CW, Suh BY: Influence of sleep on respiratory function in emphysema. *Am J Respir Crit Care Med* (In press).

56. Fletcher EC, Gray BA, Levin DC: Nonapneic mechanisms of arterial oxygen desaturation during rapid-eye movement sleep. *J Appl Physiol* 1983; 54:632–639.

57. Connaughton JJ, Douglas NJ, Morgan AD, et al.: Almitrine improves oxygenation when both awake and asleep in patients with hypoxia and carbon dioxide retention caused by chronic bronchitis and emphysema. *Am Rev Respir Dis* 195; 132:206–210.

58. Daskalopoulou E, Patakas D, Tsara V, et al.: Almitrine effect on nocturnal hypoxemia in patients with chronic obstructive pulmonary disease (COPD). *Bull Clin Respir Physiol* 1987; 23(suppl):185s–190s.

59. Dolly FR, Block AJ: Medroxyprogesterone acetate and COPD: Effect on breathing and oxygenation in sleeping and awake patients. *Chest* 1983; 84:394–398.

60. Marrone O, Milone F, Coppola P, et al.: Effects of almitrine bismesylate on nocturnal hypoxemia in patients with chronic bronchitis and obesity. *Eur J Respir Dis* 1986; 69(suppl 146):641–648.

61. Racineux JL, Meslier N, Hubert P: The effect of long-term almitrine therapy on sleep hypoxemia in patients with chronic airways obstruction. *Bull Clin Resp Physiol* 1987; 23(suppl):183s.

62. Skatrud JB, Dempsey JA, Iber C, Berssenbrugge A: Correction of CO_2 retention during sleep in patients with chronic obstructive pulmonary diseases. *Am Rev Respir Dis* 1981; 124:260–268.

63. Tatsumi K, Kimura H, Kunitomo F, et al.: Effect of chlormadinone acetate on sleep arterial oxygen desaturation in patients with chronic obstructive pulmonary disease. *Chest* 1987; 91:688–692.

64. Nocturnal Oxygen Therapy Trial Group: Continuous or nocturnal oxygen therapy in hypoxemic chronic obstructive lung disease. *Ann Intern Med* 1980; 93:391–398.

65. Fletcher EC, Donner CF, Midgram B, et al.: Survival in COPD patients with a daytime $PaO_2 > 60$ mmHg with and without nocturnal oxyhemoglobin desaturation. *Chest* 1992; 101:649–655.

66. Flenly DC: Sleep in chronic obstructive lung disease. *Clin Chest Med* 1985; 6:651–661.

Chapter 108 _____
CLINICAL EVALUATION OF HYPOVENTILATION SYNDROMES: AN OVERVIEW

MELVIN LOPATA

Pathogenesis: Differential Diagnosis

Laboratory Evaluation

Neuromuscular Disease

Primary Alveolar Hypoventilation

Therapeutics

Epilogue

Patients with unexplained chronic or acute-on-chronic CO_2 retention present a challenge to the clinician. Sorting out the cause or disease entity is often an unstructured, confusing process, and until recently, therapeutic options were limited and less than efficacious. The goal of this chapter is to put the problem of disorders of respiratory control into perspective to explain the nature and pathophysiology of impaired control of ventilation, and to provide a logical and practical scheme for evaluating such patients and instituting proper therapy.

Though the focus of this text is from a pharmacologic perspective, drug therapy for most if not all of the causes of hypoventilation syndrome has not been shown to be effective. Thus, the emphasis of this chapter includes nonpharmacologic treatment modalities. The scope of the clinical problem is demonstrated by presenting brief vignettes of two actual patients. The outcomes are given at the end of the chapter.

Patient 1: A 51-year-old male with a 3-month history of progressive exertional dyspnea, orthopnea, and daytime somnolence. Arterial blood gases: Pa_{O_2}, 53 mmHg; Pa_{CO_2}, 59 mmHg; pH, 7.34. Pulmonary function tests: FVC, 2.5 L; FEV_1, 2.0 L.

Patient 2: A 46-year-old male, 50-pack per year cigarette smoker, presents with chronic cough, effort dyspnea, peripheral edema, and fatigue. Arterial blood gases: Pa_{O_2}, 52 mmHg; Pa_{CO_2}, 55 mmHg; pH, 7.36. Pulmonary function tests: FVC, 2.4 L; FEV_1, 1.4 L.

These two patients have quite different primary diseases that share a common end result—that is, hypercapnic respiratory failure, a term that can be used interchangeably with alveolar hypoventilation and CO_2 retention. Though the primary pathology in these diseases is different, there is a commonality of pathophysiology. By virtue of the presence of CO_2 retention, these diseases are disorders of respiratory control. By various mechanisms, the many disorders of respiratory control all affect the respiratory control system and impair the function of the complex regulatory process that normally maintains a narrow range of Pa_{CO_2}.

Pathogenesis: Differential Diagnosis

The diseases associated with alveolar hypoventilation are shown in Table 108-1. To understand how a given disease may cause CO_2 retention, one must understand the organization of the respiratory control system, which is made up of the central and peripheral nervous systems, respiratory muscles, and bellows (lungs and chest wall) components that in concert serve to control ventilation.[2] Thus the primary drive to breathe is initiated in the brainstem and transmitted to the spinal cord and the respiratory motor neurons of the peripheral nerves, which carry the impulses to the respiratory muscles whose contraction powers the bellows to effect ventilation. Alveolar ventilation primarily serves to regulate alveolar and, thereby, arterial Pa_{CO_2}. Through the peripheral and central chemoreceptors and by way of reflexes generated in the airways, lung parenchyma, and chest wall, various feedback processes fine-tune the control system. Under varied metabolic, environmental, and even disease states, a narrow range of Pa_{CO_2} is maintained to optimize the Pa_{O_2}.[2] By functionally interrupting the control system anywhere along the control arc from the CNS to the bellows, disease processes may impair the ability of the

TABLE 108-1 Causes of Hypoventilation

Central (CNS)
    Idiopathic (primary)
    CVA, tumor, infection
    Syringobulbia
    Trauma
    Metabolic, hypothyroidism, metabolic alkalosis
Neuromuscular
    Anterior horn cells
        Poliomyelitis
        Amyotrophic lateral sclerosis
        Syringomyelia
    Peripheral nerves
        Polyneuropathy (Guillain-Barré syndrome)
        Phrenic nerve injury (secondary to cardiac hypothermia)
        Multiple sclerosis
        Postpolio syndrome
    Motor end plate
        Myasthenia gravis
        Lambert-Eaton syndrome
        Botulism
    Muscle
        Dystrophies
        Myopathies
            Hereditary (acid maltase deficiency)
            Inflammatory
            Metabolic
Bellows (lung/chest wall)
    COPD
    Kyphoscoliosis
    Obesity

system to regulate ventilation normally, causing inappropriately decreased alveolar ventilation and CO_2 retention.[1] This implies that CO_2 retention is essentially caused by a respiratory neuromechanical defect. However, this is not entirely correct, since gas exchange abnormalities caused by ventilation-perfusion mismatching can also impair CO_2 elimination and cause CO_2 retention.[3] However, in the presence of a normal control system, disease-associated hyperventilation should serve to maintain the Pa_{CO_2} in the normal or hypocapnic range. Even with impaired gas exchange, CO_2 retention probably occurs only when some component of the control system is impaired functionally.

It is informative to categorize diseases causing alveolar hypoventilation according to the component of the control system affected by the disease. Table 108-1 categorizes these diseases automatically as central, neuromuscular (subdivided into anterior motor horn cell, peripheral nerves, motor end plate, muscle), and bellows (lung/chest wall). In considering the differential diagnosis of a patient with a hypoventilation syndrome, rather than evoking the extensive list in Table 108-1, it is convenient to consider the differential diagnosis in light of a limited but very practical set of categories: bellows dysfunction, neuromuscular disease, primary (idiopathic) alveolar hypoventilation, and sleep apnea syndrome. In such a sequence, diseases affecting the bellows (lung/chest wall) first must be considered—mainly chronic obstructive pulmonary disease (COPD), since it is the most

common disease causing hypoventilation. Once bellows dysfunction as the primary cause is ruled out, the broad category of neuromuscular disease must be considered. In spite of the many diseases in this class, a generic approach to the evaluation can result in the exclusion or inclusion of this category before other diagnostic methods are used to isolate the particular disease. If neuromuscular disease is excluded, primary alveolar hypoventilation (PAH) as a diagnosis of exclusion now must be considered. However, at this point a sleep study would be done, in part to establish or exclude the presence of sleep apnea—namely, obstructive sleep apnea. As noted above, this diagnostic sequence is largely conceptual; one may have considered sleep apnea earlier in the evaluation, but the sequence emphasizes that at some point most, if not all, patients with hypoventilation (excluding COPD) should undergo a sleep study.

The evaluation of hypoventilation, as with any clinical disorder, starts with the history. With the above disease categories in mind, it is clear that inquiries regarding a past medical history of pulmonary, neurologic, chest wall, and metabolic disease as well as prescription drug usage (i.e., diuretics) must be made. A history of recent open-heart surgery (i.e., coronary artery bypass) or a more likely scenario of a difficult-to-wean postoperative coronary surgery patient should suggest immediately phrenic nerve injury due to cardiac hypothermia.[4] Eliciting a careful family history can be quite important in directing the evaluation toward genetic neuromuscular diseases.

There is a spectrum of symptoms offered by patients with chronic hypoventilation syndromes that are nonspecific or common to many of the causative diseases. Complaints of fatigability, daytime somnolence, disturbed sleep, and morning headaches can be elicited from most such patients and point to the detrimental effects that all these diseases have on sleep. Disabling hypersomnolence coupled with disturbing snoring, especially in an obese patient, certainly suggests sleep apnea, but even in the disease the symptoms may not be dramatic.

Specific symptoms such as effort dyspnea or cough with sputum production, especially in a smoker, mandate evaluation of the severity of obstructive lung disease. Patients with neuromuscular disease variably complain of dyspnea in the upright position but often not to a severe degree, while patients with PAH may not be dyspneic at all.[5,6] An important variant of the complaint of shortness of breath is that of worsening dyspnea in the supine position. This symptom, which should be elicited from all these patients, characteristically suggests neuromuscular disease with diaphragmatic paralysis as the causative disease process.[6,7]

In the physical examination, the following abnormalities must be evaluated: evidence of airway obstruction (wheezing, rhonchi, prolonged expiration), kyphoscoliosis, obesity, muscular weakness, neurologic deficits (sensory and motor), and signs of cor pulmonale and congestive heart failure. The latter cardiac findings are not specific for any disease entity, but their presence is evidence of severe sequelae of the disease process. Complementing supine dyspnea as a symptom of diaphragmatic dysfunction is the physical sign of paradoxical chest wall movement caused by assuming the supine position. In this circumstance, the rib cage and abdomen do not move synchronously or in and out together but rather paradoxically—i.e., during inspiration the rib cage moves outward and the abdomen inward, with this pattern reversing during expiration.[7]

Laboratory Evaluation

The laboratory examination supplements the investigative process and narrows the etiologic choices for definitive diagnosis. To start, basic blood studies should be performed. Serum electrolytes and biochemistry, along with arterial blood gases, enable the identification of metabolic abnormalities that either cause or contribute to hypoventilation, such as metabolic alkalosis, hypokalemia, hypophosphatemia, hypomagnesemia, and hypothyroidism.[8–12]

The next step in the evaluation involves the pulmonary function laboratory and is directed at establishing the presence of bellows dysfunction (see Table 108-1) and its causative role in the hypoventilation process. Since COPD is the most common cause of CO_2 retention, the question to be asked is: Does the patient have airway obstruction, and if so, is it severe enough to cause alveolar hypoventilation? In patients with COPD, the level of Pa_{CO_2} is hyperbolically related to the degree of airway obstruction as reflected by the FEV_1. The Pa_{CO_2} is maintained at eucapnic or hypocapnic levels as the FEV_1 declines with progressive disease until a critical level of obstruction at an FEV_1 of 1 to 1.3 L is reached, after which CO_2 retention tends to occur.[5] Thus hypoventilation caused by COPD occurs in the face of severe airway obstruction typically at an FEV_1 of <1 L. As such, in the presence of obstructive lung disease, an FEV_1 of >1 to 1.3 L, suggests that a process other than COPD is causing or contributing to the CO_2 retention.

Similarly, patients with kyphoscoliosis typically hypoventilate only when a severe degree of chest wall distortion and functional impairment is reached. Thus, most such patients will have severe lateral scoliosis with a Cobb's angle of more than 120° and a vital capacity of <1 L.[13]

Another relatively simple test to assess mechanical limitation to ventilation is to determine the effects of voluntary hyperventilation on the Pa_{CO_2}. Normal individuals or patients with central and often neuromuscular causes of hypoventilation will be able to decrease the Pa_{CO_2} > 20 mmHg; a patient with bellows dysfunction severe enough to cause hypoventilation will be able to reduce the Pa_{CO_2} ≤ 10 mmHg.[5] Thus, at this point in the evaluation, the next question is: Can the patient decrease his or her Pa_{CO_2} with voluntary hyperventilation? A 20 mmHg decrease in Pa_{CO_2} makes mechanical impairment of the bellows unlikely as a major cause of CO_2 retention. The ability to hyperventilate adequately is consistent with the presence of PAH and OHS but does not exclude neuromuscular disease.[6]

Neuromuscular Disease

If the above procedures exclude bellows dysfunction as a cause of CO_2 retention, the evaluation proceeds to neuromuscular disease as the causative process. Certainly patients may have diseases that are quite evident or easily diagnosed, especially if the process is diffuse or systemic with neural or muscle group involvement other than that of the respiratory system. However in many diseases the respiratory motor neurons, nerves, or muscles may be the first, only, or major components involved, resulting in significant diaphragmatic dysfunction or paralysis.[6] These patients may present with CO_2 retention without obvious neurologic deficits, and the effects of diaphragm paralysis may be quite subtle and therefore overlooked.[6,14]

An approach to the evaluation of neuromuscular disease is first to demonstrate the presence of diaphragm paralysis and thereby establish its role in the hypoventilation state. Subsequently (or concurrently), the diagnosis of the specific disease entity must be determined. Respiratory muscle function and to some extent the function of the diaphragm can be assessed utilizing the pulmonary function laboratory and radiologic techniques.

There are no specific effects of diaphragm paralysis on pulmonary function tests, but characteristic changes do occur; when present, they support the presence of neuromuscular disease. A decrease of the forced vital capacity (FVC) of 50 percent or more in the supine position suggests the possible presence of bilateral diaphragmatic weakness or paralysis[6,14,15] and points to the importance of performing upright and supine spirometry. A nonconcentric restrictive process occurs quite typically in patients with neuromuscular disease and diaphragmatic paralysis. In such instances, the resting lung volume is relatively well preserved but the inspiratory capacity is markedly impaired, resulting in a normal or slightly reduced functional residual capacity (FRC) and a markedly reduced vital capacity (VC) and total lung capacity (TLC).[16]

The measurement of respiratory pressures developed by maximum isometric contraction of the inspiratory and expiratory muscles is another sensitive way to screen for and document quantitatively the presence of respiratory muscle weakness.[17,18] Mouth pressure can be measured very easily and noninvasively while the patient inspires maximally or expires against a closed airway. The ability to generate maximum mouth pressure is diminished in patients with respiratory muscular dysfunction, and both inspiratory and expiratory pressures can be diminished, though not necessarily to an equal degree.[18,19] Similar results are evident when pleural or transdiaphragmatic pressures are recorded.[7,19,20] Impaired pressure generation, especially when patient cooperation and optimal effort is assured, provides strong support for neuromuscular disease as the culprit in the hypoventilation workup. Normal pressures[17] do not rule out this category of disease but do make it unlikely.

Fluoroscopy is the time-honored method for detecting diaphragmatic dysfunction or paralysis. The lack of diaphragmatic movement or, more specifically, paradoxical, upward movement during a brief inspiratory effort has been regarded as the classic sign of diaphragmatic paralysis. Unfortunately, this technique, the results of which are often difficult to interpret, can provide misleading, false-negative data.[7] This occurs because patients, especially early in the course of their disease, often manifest predominantly inspiratory muscle dysfunction, and the preservation of expiratory abdominal muscle function permits the patient to compensate for his or her diaphragmatic paralysis. Compensation occurs with the development of a strategy of breathing that utilizes the functioning abdominal muscles to support the action of the nonfunctioning diaphragm.[6,7] This involuntary strategy entails contracting the abdominal muscles during expiration, forcing the diaphragm upward or cephalad, such that during the subsequent inspiration gravity and passive recoil of the thorax cause the diaphragm to descend and thus effect inspiration. This action of the expiratory muscles promotes and assists inspiration and allows the patient to compensate for the lack of diaphragmatic function. If one were viewing diaphragmatic movement by fluoroscopy in a patient effecting these maneuvers, the diaphragm would be seen to descend during inspiration; hence, the false-negative result.[7]

This successful strategy of breathing depends in large part on gravity and the upright position. When the patient assumes the supine position, neither gravity nor thoracic recoil assists inspiratory movement of the diaphragm and compensation is lost, resulting in the classic symptom of supine dyspnea.

Normally, the rib cage and abdomen move synchronously with respiration, outward with inspiration and inward with expiration. This synchrony occurs because diaphragmatic contraction results in descent of the diaphragm, which increases abdominal pressure moving the abdominal wall outward. Concurrently, diaphragmatic action elevates the lower rib cage, moving it outward, and any intercostal recruitment will expand and displace outward the upper rib cage. All these actions cause outward synchrony during inspiration, which reverses during expiration.[7] With diaphragmatic paralysis, the intact inspiratory intercostal and accessory muscles elevate and move the rib cage outward, increasing thoracic volume and decreasing intrathoracic pressure, thus pulling the diaphragm cephalad along with the abdominal contents, and the abdominal wall moves inward; the rib cage and abdomen now move paradoxically.[6,7] As discussed above, expiratory recruitment of the abdominal muscles can elicit compensation to prevent such paradoxical movement, but only in the upright position; thus, the classical sign of supine paradoxical movement of the rib cage and abdomen results. Through simple observation or by recording rib cage and abdominal motion with specific sensing devices, one can document supine paradoxical movement, supporting the diagnosis of dia-phragmatic paralysis.

If these physiologic tests support the presence of neuromuscular disease as the cause of the hypoventilation syndrome, a vigorous neurologic evaluation must ensue. This should include nerve conduction studies and electromyography to detect generalized neurologic involvement and to distinguish between neuropathic and myopathic disease. In the latter case a muscle biopsy will probably be indicated.

Primary Alveolar Hypoventilation

If respiratory muscle function is intact and no neurologic deficits are evident, PAH must be considered.[21–23] Since there is no specific test for this disease, it essentially becomes a diagnosis of exclusion. Therefore, one can entertain a diagnosis of PAH when chronic hypercapnic respiratory failure occurs in the absence of pulmonary disease, chest wall disease, neuromuscular disease, and obstructive sleep apnea. Characteristically, because of the so-called impairment of automatic brainstem respiratory function, there is a diminished or absent ventilatory response to CO_2 and hypoxic stimulation as well as to exercise.[21–23]

At this point, even if one is secure in a diagnosis, there is one more test that must be part of any evaluation of hypoventilation, i.e., a nocturnal polysomnogram. A sleep study may already have been considered or indicated because of a high suspicion of sleep apnea, yet symptoms of obstructive sleep apnea (OSA) may be subtle or mild and may overlap with those of the other diseases, especially PAH, such that OSA may be missed. Thus, there are two reasons to perform a sleep study on these patients: (1) to determine the presence or absence of OSA, a treatable disease, and (2) to determine the degree of arterial oxygen desaturation and CO_2 elevation during sleep in patients with kyphoscoliosis, neuromuscular disease, and PAH and to assess their response to assisted ventilation.[6,24–26] This latter justification is based on data clearly showing that patients in these categories will demonstrate significant worsening of their hypoxemia, hypercapnia, and acidosis during sleep, especially REM sleep. This nocturnal deterioration of ventilation and gas exchange creates a vicious cycle that promotes progression of the hypoventilation state and it sequelae—i.e., cor pulmonae and right heart failure.[6,27] Breaking this cycle with nocturnal ventilatory assist provides a therapeutic modality for these patients (a topic reviewed in detail later in the chapter).

Nocturnal polysomnography, the monitoring of multiple physiologic parameters during sleep, will detect the presence of sleep-disordered breathing, which will be different in patients with OSA than in those in the other disease categories. Patients with OSA will demonstrate periodic, usually repetitive apneas (cessation of airflow at nose and mouth), during which there is continuing evidence of respiratory muscle activity—i.e., chest wall movement[28] (Fig. 108-1). In patients with kyphoscoliosis, neuromuscular disease, and PAH, there may be irregular breathing, short central apneas, or diminished tidal volume and chest wall excursions, or there may be little overt evidence of disordered breathing; however, all of these are associated with prolonged oxygen desaturation or worsening of the arterial blood gases, this being especially severe during REM sleep[27] (Fig. 108-2).

Once a diagnosis is secure and the status of sleep-disordered breathing is known, the next step is to consider therapeutic alternatives for the chronic disease state. There are principles of therapy generic to most patients with chronic hypoventilation as well as therapeutic interventions specific to certain diseases. Neurologic diseases that can be specifically treated are myasthenia gravis and, debatably, multiple sclerosis, though the latter rarely is associated with respiratory failure. Hypothyroidism is treatable and electrolyte imbalance—whether it be metabolic alkalosis, hypophosphatemia, hypomagnesemia, or hypokalemia—usually is reversible.

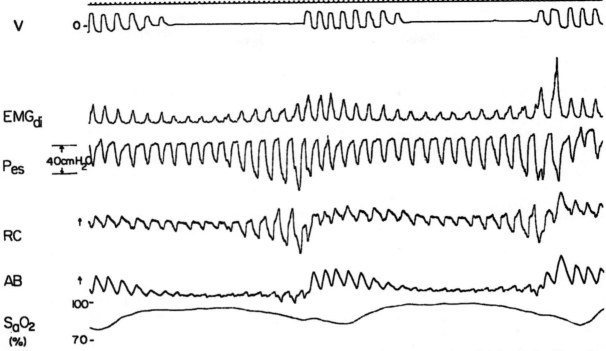

FIGURE 108-1 Obstructive sleep apnea. Continuous recording of flow (V), diaphragmatic EMG (EMGdi), esophageal pressure (Pes), rib cage (RC) and abdominal (AB) motion, and oxygen saturation (Sa$_{O_2}$) in a patient with sleep apnea. Note the occurrence of two apneas (cessation of airflow) but with continued and even increasing respiratory effort evident by EMGdi, Pes, RC, and AB tracings. Each apnea is associated with periodic oxygen desaturation. P$_{es}$: esophageal pressure; RC: rib cage; AB: abdomen.

FIGURE 108-2 Oxygen desaturation induced by REM in a patient with neuromuscular disease. Continuous recording of right and left electrooculogram (LEOG and REOG), submental electromyogram (EMG), electroencephalogram (EEG), electrocardiogram (ECG), airflow, esophageal pressure, and oxygen saturation. Note conjugate eye movements (REMs), diminution of airflow, and decline in pleural pressure with progressive and prolonged oxygen desaturation to 50 percent. (*From Arand et al.,*[71] *with permission.*)

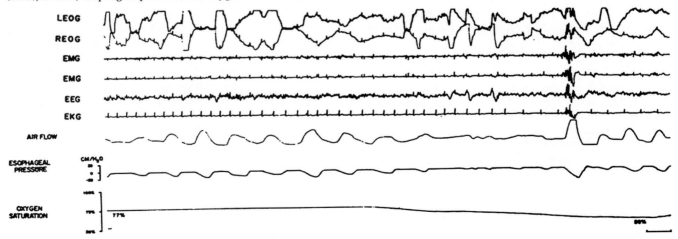

Therapeutics

The course or manifestations of most hyperventilation disorders have not been shown to be influenced or improved by pharmacologic therapy. In patients with COPD, a number of drugs directed at the hypoventilating state have been studied. Almitrane, a piperazine derivative that stimulates the peripheral chemoreceptors, has been shown in patients with COPD and CO_2 retention to increase minute ventilation, slightly reduce Pa_{CO_2}, and increase Pa_{O_2}, the latter mostly through improvement in lung ventilation:perfusion matching.[29] Medroxyprogesterone, another ventilatory stimulant, possibly via brainstem respiratory neurons,[30] and protriptyline, a tricyclic antidepressant that suppresses REM sleep, may also increase ventilation and somewhat decrease Pa_{CO_2} in hypoventilating patients with COPD.[31–33] However, any positive effects of these drugs in these types of patients have not been sufficiently great or consistent to warrant the consideration of these drugs as therapeutic options. Other agents, such as theophylline and acetezolamide have been studied and shown not to have any benefit.[32,34] The other disease under this purview that has been subjected to pharmacologic intervention is PAH. Many respiratory stimulants including theophylline, progesterone, and acetezolamide have not been shown to consistently reduce Pa_{CO_2} in PAH patients.[35] Intravenous doxapram may be effective in improving ventilation and gas exchange, but this therapeutic modality does not offer an efficacious or practical option for chronic therapy.[36]

Two common diseases associated with alveolar hypoventilation, COPD and sleep apnea, can be singled out for the specific approach to their treatment.

Patients with severe irreversible airway obstruction typically receive an intensive regimen of bronchodilators, including inhaled beta agonists and anticholinergics, theophylline, and probably corticosteroids. The efficacy of these drugs is variable, but even when there is significant improvement of airway obstruction and symptoms, it is unlikely that respiratory failure will be reversed in COPD patients. Since these patients also manifest severe hypoxemia, they are invariably candidates for chronic domiciliary oxygen therapy. Indeed, this is the one therapeutic regimen that can result in improved survival in this patient group, and it should be the mainstay of treatment.[37,38]

If one assumes that respiratory failure in COPD is dependent on the development of diaphragmatic fatigue,[39,40] then the use of methods to rest the respiratory muscles—inspiratory muscle rest (IMR)—is a logical extension of this assumption. Unfortunately, there are no hard data to support the premise that patients with severe COPD develop inspiratory muscle fatigue. It has been shown in patients with COPD that ventilatory support with negative- or positive-pressure ventilation can unload and "rest" the diaphragm, and there have been a number of clinical trials testing the efficacy of intermittent assisted ventilation in such patients.[41–45] The studies have generally been unrandomized and uncontrolled, have had a variable time of ventilator use, and did not necessarily demonstrate that the method of ventilation suppressed spontaneous diaphragmatic activity.

Again, the results have not been uniform, some studies demonstrating improvement in the clinical status and arterial blood gases of the treated patients and others demonstrating no effect. Of importance, the best designed trial thus far carried out, with patients randomized to either daytime negative-pressure ventilation or sham ventilation, failed to show any benefit of IMR.[46] Current data thus do not support IMR as an effective form of therapy in hypoventilating patients with COPD. However, recent trials using positive-pressure ventilation via a nasal mask have been promising results.[47–50] These results, coupled with the relative ease and comfort of using this form of ventilatory assist, especially during sleeping hours, should stimulate large and properly designed trials to test this methodology. Because of the relatively high prevalence of this disorder and the great expense of home ventilatory therapy, definitive data confirming the efficacy of IMR are mandatory before it can be accepted as a therapeutic option in these patients.

The association of obesity with cardiorespiratory failure was recognized early in this century and was codified in the medical literature as the Pickwickian syndrome.[51] It is now clear that most Pickwickians or—stated more appropriately—patients with obesity-hypoventilation syndrome, have obstructive sleep apnea. Hypoventilation, usually associated with cor pulmonale, is a serious sequela of the sleep apnea syndrome, which, along with these complications, is eminently treatable. The therapeutic options for sleep apnea are relatively broad, including surgical measures (uvulpalatopharyngoplasty, or UPPP, and mandibular advancement), dental appliances, and pharmacologic, positional, and dietary approaches.[52–56] However, in hypoventilating patients with significant morbidity and probably increased mortality,[57] only two forms of therapy should be considered initially: tracheostomy and nasal continuous positive airway pressure (NCPAP).[58,59] The former will clearly cure obstructive apnea and result in dramatic clinical and blood gas improvement, but the latter may be just as effective yet is noninvasive and relatively free of complications and side effects.[58,59] Administered by means of a high-flow air compressor via a tight-fitting nose mask to achieve pressure levels of 5 to 15 cmH_2O, NCPAP essentially results in splinting the upper airway and preventing the passive collapse which causes obstructive apnea.[59] If NCPAP is found to be effective in preventing obstructive apnea and reversing the sleep disruption and oxygen desaturation evident in the baseline polysomnograph and if it is tolerated and accepted by the patient, it is the preferable method of treatment.[60] Failing those criteria, tracheostomy becomes the treatment of choice. Patients treated with NCPAP must be carefully followed to assure compliance with therapy.[61] Effective therapy should result in improvement and likely resolution of the CO_2 retention.[62,63] This response along with the expected dramatic clinical improvement is most gratifying and stresses the importance of recognizing and diagnosing this disease so that it can be so treated.

The two diseases just discussed, COPD and sleep apnea, are both rather prevalent and can coexist in the same patient. This overlap of two highly morbid diseases probably results in additive effects of both disease processes on the sleep-induced blood gas impairment and on daytime respiratory dysfunction as well. The presence of the mechanical and gas exchange abnormalities of airway obstruction in patients with sleep apnea as the predominant complaint may well contribute to the development of hypercapnia and pulmonary hypertension in these patients.[64–66] On the other hand, the presence of sleep apnea in patients with chronic airway obstruction can result in hypercapnia and pulmonary hypertension that may be attributed to the COPD because the presence of sleep apnea may not be recognized. Such recognition is critical for proper management, since sleep apnea is treatable and its complications are reversible, in contrast to COPD.[67–69] Patients with COPD who have sleep apnea usually demonstrate obesity, daytime somnolence, and snoring.[68] One must be especially aware of the COPD patient with CO_2 retention who does not manifest the severe degree of airway obstruction that is characteristically associated with hypercapnia (see above). An FEV_1 of greater than 1 to 1.3 L in such a clinical setting should arouse suspicion of disease in addition to COPD, mainly sleep apnea, and warrants the appropriate evaluation. The remarkable clinical benefit from treating sleep apnea should not be missed by failing to consider this diagnosis in certain patients with chronic airway obstruction.

Common to most patients with hypoventilation is the risk of experiencing sleep-disordered breathing, which is associated with nocturnal worsening of the already impaired arterial blood gases. Especially vulnerable during REM sleep, these patients as a rule manifest sleep-induced hypoxemia, hypercapnia, and respiratory acidosis.[25,26,70–73] Except for sleep apnea, where sleep is associated with repetitive upper airway occlusions, the mechanism of sleep-disordered breathing is not well understood. Sleep, especially during REM, may result in further central depression of ventilatory drive or selective inhibition of intercostal/accessory muscle activity.[74,75] Either perturbation can result in worsening hypoventilation and the above noted changes in blood gases as well as sleep disruption and fragmentation. The common daytime symptoms of fatigue and somnolence may be a product of this secondary sleep disorder.

Sleep-induced hypoventilation can be prevented by instituting ventilatory support during sleep. This can be accomplished by a number of methods of assisted ventilation, including the rocking bed as well as negative- and positive-pressure ventilation.[27,76] The rocking bed, a classic but time-worn method, is rather inefficient, and its use has generally been supplanted by newer technology. Negative-pressure ventilation (NPV) classically was effected by means of the iron lung, but these days is more likely to be administered via the cuirass ventilator or the pneumowrap (poncho).[76] It can be quite effective in ventilating hypoventilating patients, even those with kyphoscoliotic chest wall deformity.[77–81] How-ever, it is often difficult to capture the patient who tends to breathe around or through the negative pressure cycles, and when successful, NPV has one significant drawback; the generated negative airway pressure may result in passive collapse of the upper airway and intermittent upper airway obstruction—that is, obstructive sleep apnea—with the same consequence to gas exchange and sleep architecture as found in primary sleep apena.[82] Under these circumstances, continued efficacious use of NPV necessitates treatment of sleep apnea, either NCPAP or tracheostomy. This course makes NPV a less than desirable treatment option.

Positive-pressure ventilation (PPV) obviates the upper airway problems of NPV. Also, when the assist/control mode of a volume-cycled ventilator is utilized, PPV allows for easier capture of the patient's ventilatory cycle than with NPV. The drawback of PPV has been that its use necessitated a tracheostomy for access to the airway for the ventilator.[83] This problem has recently been obviated by the demonstrated ability to effect PPV via the nose by means of a tight-fitting nose mask.[84,85] Nasally applied PPV (NPPV) is convenient and can be effected easily. It has been shown to inhibit spontaneous respiratory muscle activity in normal subjects and hypoventilation patients, so that ventilation can be controlled or assisted.[50] Though this is a relatively new method of providing assisted ventilation, there is accumulating evidence of the short- and long-term efficacy of NPPV and the relatively high rate of patient acceptance and compliance with its use.[86–91] The described side effects of NPPV (e.g., gastric distention, nasal bridge abrasion, and mask leak) have been mild and infrequent.[42,81,84] At the present time, NPPV is probably the preferred choice for instituting nocturnal ventilatory assist in these patients.

It must be emphasized that most patients with hypoventilation syndromes, though manifesting chronic respiratory failure, are not ventilator-dependent and can sustain adequate ventilatory function during waking hours. It is nocturnally, during sleep, that ventilatory assistance is required to prevent the disease-related deterioration of respiratory control and its sequelae. It is also apparent that the effects of this sleep-disordered breathing are causally related to the progression of daytime respiratory failure and the downhill course of the hypoventilation process. Nocturnal support of ventilation, whether by NPV or PPV, can effect marked clinical improvement (decreased fatigue, somnolence, dyspnea, sleep disruption, and improvement of cor pulmonale with resolution of congestive heart failure) and, most important, improvement of the arterial blood gases—even normalization of the Pa_{CO_2}.[81,84–91] It is important to emphasize that resolution of alveolar hypoventilation with successful nocturnal ventilation clearly denotes the critical importance of the sleep disorder in the pathophysiology of the disease process. Although the underlying processes themselves may not be treatable, the sleep-disordered breathing can well be controlled and its effects reversed.

Prior to initiating chronic assisted ventilation, the degree of sleep-disordered breathing must be determined by baseline nocturnal polysomnography. There are no tested criteria for instituting nocturnal ventilation, but the presence of sleep-, especially REM-, induced hypoventilation (or apnea) with O_2 desaturation in patients with chronic hypercapnia certainly warrants therapy. Subsequently, the prevention of documented sleep-induced dysfunction by the chosen form of ventilation must be verified.

The reason for the ability of nocturnal therapy to effect global improvement of chronic hypoventilation without affecting the primary elements of the disease process is unknown. As in sleep apnea, the effects of the nighttime perturbation of the central nervous system may result in further impairment of respiratory control, this being prevented and possibly reversed by the use of nocturnal ventilation. One also may speculate that assisted ventilation results in resting the stressed, functionally remaining respiratory muscles, so that their overall function is improved.[50] These are interesting ideas and are the subject of further investigation.

Nocturnal assisted ventilation must be considered lifelong therapy. Patients with nonprogressive disease—that is, PAH, some neuromuscular disorders, and possibly kyphoscoliosis—can do well and remain stable for an indefinite period.[84–91] Patients with progressive neuromuscular disease or those with a superimposed respiratory infection may not be able to sustain adequate ventilation even during waking hours and require ventilatory support either continuously or for a major part of the day. Noninvasive NPPV can be effective in these patients, but if such daytime ventilatory needs are long-term, PPV via a tracheostomy or NPV may be more efficacious than NPPV.[81] The need for chronic, continuous ventilatory support at home or in an institution will depend on the nature of the primary disease and its natural history.

Epilogue

Patient 1: The patient's dyspnea limited him to walking one block; also, he could not lie supine and slept almost upright. Physical examination revealed paradoxical chest wall motion while supine and he had mild upper extremity weakness. Laboratory findings: a decrease in FVC from 2.5 L upright to 1.5 L supine, a nonconcentric restrictive defect (TLC, 65 percent; FRC, 99 percent; RV, 107 percent), and myopathic motor unit potentials on electromyography of the upper extremity. Muscle biopsy (deltoid) revealed acid maltase deficiency. A nocturnal polysomnogram demonstrated episodes of hypopnea and O_2 desaturation, which were pronounced in REM sleep (O_2 saturation, 50%); this was reversed with NPPV. Six months after nightly therapy with NPPV, arterial blood gases were as follows: Pa_{O_2}, 78 mmHg; Pa_{CO_2}, 44 mmHg; pH, 7.40.

Patient 2: The patient's hypoventilation had been attributed to COPD, but his relatively well-preserved FEV_1 and a subsequently elicited history of daytime somnolence and snoring led to the ordering of a nocturnal polysomnogram. This showed severe obstructive sleep apnea (apnea index, 60/h; minimum O_2 saturation, 40%), which was completely reversed with NCPAP at 10 cmH_2O. After 3 months of nightly NCPAP, the patient's arterial blood gases were as follows: Pa_{O_2}, 70 mmHg; Pa_{CO_2}, 42 mmHg; pH, 7.42.

References

1. Lopata M, Lourenço RV: Evaluation of respiratory control. *Clin Chest Med* 1980; 1:33.
2. Irsigler GB, Severinghaus JW: Clinical problems of ventilatory control. *Annu Rev Med* 1980; 31:1009.
3. West JB: Causes of carbon dioxide retention in lung disease. *N Engl J Med* 1971; 284:1232.
4. Kohorst WR, Schonfeld SA, Altman M: Bilateral diaphragmatic paralysis following topical cardiac hypothermia. *Chest* 1984; 85:65.
5. Rhoads GG, Brody JS: Idiopathic alveolar hypoventilation: Clinical spectrum. *Ann Intern Med* 1969; 71:271.
6. Newsom-Davis J, Goldman M, Loh L, Casson M: Diaphragm function and alveolar hypoventilation. *Quarterly J Med* 1976; 45:87.
7. Loh L, Goldman M, Newsom-Davis J: The assessment of diaphragm function. *Medicine* 1977; 56:165.
8. Weiner M, Chausow A, Szidon P: Reversible respiratory muscle weakness and hypothyroidism. *Br J Dis Chest* 1986; 80:391.
9. Zwillich CW, Pierson DJ, Hofeldt FD, et al.: Ventilatory control in myxedema and hypothyroidism. *N Engl J Med* 1976; 292:662.
10. Javaheri S, Kazemi H: Metabolic alkalosis and hypoventilation in humans. *Am Rev Respir Dis* 1987; 36:1011.
11. Newman JH, Neff TA, Ziporin P: Acute respiratory failure associated with hypophosphatemia. *N Engl J Med* 1977; 296:1101.
12. Dhingra S, Solven F, Wilson A, McCarthy DS: Hypomagnesia and respiratory muscle power. *Am Rev Respir Dis* 1984; 129:497.
13. Bergofsky E: Respiratory failure disorders of the thoracic cage. *Am Rev Respir Dis* 1979; 119:643.
14. Sivak ED, Ahmad M, Hanson MR, Wilbourn AJ: Respiratory insufficiency in adult-onset acid maltase deficiency. *South Med J* 1987; 80:205.
15. Sivak ED, Streib EW: Management of hypoventilation in motor neuron disease presenting with respiratory insufficiency. *Ann Neurol* 1980; 7:188.
16. Rideau Y, Jankowski LW, Grellet J: Respiratory function in the muscular dystrophies. *Muscle Nerve* 1981; 4:155.
17. Black LF, Hyatt RE: Maximal respiratory pressures: Normal values and relationship to age and sex. *Am Rev Respir Dis* 1969; 99:696.
18. Black LF, Hyaff RE: Maximal static respiratory pressures in generalized neuromuscular disease. *Am Rev Respir Dis* 1971; 103:641.
19. Demedts M, Beckers J, Rochette F, Bulcke J: Pulmonary function in moderate neuromuscular disease without respiratory complaints. *Eur J Respir Dis* 1982; 63:62.
20. Gibson GJ, Pride NB, Newsom-Davis J, Loh L: Pulmonary mechanics in patients with respiratory muscle weakness. *Am Rev Respir Dis* 1977; 115:389.
21. Richter T, West JR, Fishman AP: The syndrome of alveolar hypoventilation and diminished sensitivity of the respiratory center. *N Engl J Med* 1957; 256:1165.
22. Fishman AP, Goldring RM, Turino GM: General alveolar hypoventilation: A syndrome of respiratory and cardiac failure in patients with normal lungs. *Quarterly J Med* 1966; 35:261.
23. Mellins RB, Balfour HH, Trino GM, Winters RW: Failure of automatic control of ventilation (Ondine's curse). *Medicine* 1970; 49:487.
24. Braun NMT, Arora NS, Rochester DF: Respiratory muscle and pulmonary function in polymyositis and other proximal myopathies. *Thorax* 1983; 38:616.
25. Mezon BL, West P, Isreal J, Kryger M: Sleep breathing abnormalities in kyphoscoliosis. *Am Rev Respir Dis* 1982; 122:617.
26. Guilleminault C, Kurlame G, Winkle R, Miles LE: Severe kyphoscoliosis, breathing and sleep. *Chest* 1982; 79:626.
27. Hill NS: Noninvasive ventilation. Does it work, for whom, and how? *Am Rev Respir Dis* 1993; 147:1050.
28. Orr WC: Utilization of polysomnography in the assessment of sleep disorders. *Med Clin North Am* 1985; 69:1153.
29. Stradling JR, Nicholl CG, Coever D, et al.: The effects of oral almitrane on pattern of breathing and gas exchange in patients with chronic obstructive pulmonary diseases. *Clin Sci* 1984; 66:435.
30. Skatrud JB, Dempsey JA, Kaiser DG: Ventilatory response to

medroxyprogesterone acetate in normal subjects: Time course and mechanism. *J Appl Physical* 1978; 44:939.

31. Skatrud JB, Dempsey JA, Bhansali P, et al.: Determinants of chronic carbon dioxide retention and correction in humans. *J Clin Invest* 1980; 65:13.

32. Skatrud JB, Dempsey JA: Relative effectiveness of acetazolamide versus medroxyprogesterone acetate in correction of carbon dioxide retention. *Am Rev Respir Dis* 1983; 127:405.

33. Series F, Comier Y: Effects of protriptyline on diurnal and nocturnal oxygenation in patients with chronic obstructive pulmonary disease. *Ann Intern Med* 1990; 113:507.

34. Ebden P, Vathenen AS: Does aminophylline improve nocturnal hypoxia in patients with chronic airflow obstruction? *Eur J Respir Dis* 1987; 71:334.

35. Altose MD, Hudgel DW: The pharmacology of respiratory depressants and stimulants. *Clin Chest Med* 1986; 7:481.

36. Lugliani R, Whipp BJ, Wasserman K: Doxapram hydrochloride: A respiratory stimulant for patients with alveolar hyperventilation. *Chest* 1979; 76:414.

37. Nocturnal Oxygen Therapy Trial Group: Continuous or nocturnal oxygen therapy in hypoxemic chronic obstructive lung disease. *Ann Intern Med* 1980; 93:391.

38. The Medical Research Council Working Party: Long-term domiciliary oxygen therapy in chronic hypoxic cor pulmonale complicating chronic bronchitis and emphysema. *Lancet* 1981; i:681.

39. Macklem PT, Roussos C: Respiratory muscle fatigue: A cause of respiratory failure. *Clin Sci* 1977; 53:419.

40. Kongragunta VR, Druz WS, Sharp JT: Dyspnea and diaphragmatic fatigue in patients with chronic obstructive pulmonary disease: Responses to theophylline. *Am Rev Respir Dis* 1988; 137:662.

41. Braun N, Marino WD: Effect of daily intermittent rest of respiratory muscles in patients with severe chronic airflow limitation (abstr). *Chest* 1984; 85:595S.

42. Van Weerden GJ: Preliminary results of periodic ambulant ventilatory treatment in patients suffering from severe chronic nonspecific respiratory disease. *Folia Med Neder* 1966; 9:125.

43. Cropp A, DiMarco AF: Effects of intermittent negative pressure ventilation in respiratory muscle function in patients with severe chronic obstructive pulmonary disease. *Am Rev Respir Dis* 1987; 135:1056.

44. Gutierrez M, et al.: Weekly cuirass ventilation improves blood gases and inspiratory muscle strength in patients with chronic airflow limitation and hypercarbia. *Am Rev Respir Dis* 1988; 138:616.

45. Zibrak JD, et al.: Evaluation of intermittent long-term negative pressure ventilation in patients with severe chronic obstructive pulmonary disease. *Am Rev Respir Dis* 1988; 138:1515.

46. Martin JG: Clinical intervention in chronic respiratory failure. *Chest* 1990; 97:105.

47. Laier-Groenveld G, Huttemann U, Criee CP: Noninvasive nasal ventilation in acute and chronic ventilatory respiratory failure. *Chest* 1990; 97:A237.

48. Waldhorn RE: Nocturnal nasal intermittent positive pressure ventilation with bi-level positive airway pressure (BIPAP) in respiratory failure. *Chest* 1992; 101:516.

49. Meduri GU, Abou-Shala N, Fox RC, et al.: Noninvasive face mask mechanical ventilation in patients with acute hypercapnic respiratory failure. *Chest* 1991; 100:445.

50. Carrey Z, Gottfried SB, Levy RD: Ventilatory muscle support in respiratory failure with nasal positive pressure ventilation. *Chest* 1990; 97:150.

51. Burwell C, Rabin E, Whaley R, Bilkman A: Extreme obesity associated with alveolar hypoventilation: A Pickwickian syndrome. *Am J Med* 1956; 21:811.

52. Fujita S, Conway W, Zorick F, Roth T: Surgical correction of anatomic abnormalities in obstructive sleep apnea syndrome: Uvulopalatopharyngoplasty. *Otolaryngol Head Neck Surg* 1981; 89:923.

53. Powell NB, Guilleminault C, Riley RW, Smith L: Mandibular advancement and obstructive sleep apnea syndrome. *Bull Eur Physiopathol Respir* 1983; 19:607.

54. Strohl KP, et al.: Progesterone administration and progressive sleep apneas. *JAMA* 1980; 245:1230.

55. Braunell LG, West P, Sweatman P, et al.: Protriptyline in obstructive sleep apnea. *N Engl J Med* 1982; 307:1037.

56. Smith PL: Weight loss in mildly to moderately obese patients with obstructive sleep apnea. *Ann Intern Med* 1985; 103:850.

57. Ke J, Roth T: Mortality and apnea index in obstructive sleep apnea: Experience in 385 male patients. *Chest* 1988; 94:9.

58. Guilleminault C, et al.: Obstructive sleep apnea and tracheostomy: Long-term follow-up experience. *Arch Intern Med* 1981; 141:985.

59. Sullivan CE, Issa FG, Berthon-Jones M, Eves L: Reversal of obstructive sleep apnea by continuous positive airway pressure applied through the nares. *Lancet* 1981; i:62.

60. Popkin J, Rutherford R, Lue F, et al.: A one-year randomized trial of nasal CPAP versus protryptyline in the management of obstructive sleep apnea. *Sleep Res* 1988; 17:237.

61. Grunstein RR, Dood MJ, Costas L, Sullivan CE: Home nasal CPAP for sleep apnea—Acceptance of home therapy and its usefulness. *Aust NZ J Med* 1986; 16:635.

62. Rapoport DM, Sorkin B, Garay SM, Goldring RM: Reversal of the "Pickwickian syndrome" by long-term use of nocturnal nasal airway pressure. *N Engl J Med* 1982; 307:931.

63. Firth RW, Cont BR: Severe obstructive sleep apnea treated with long-term nasal positive airway pressure. *Thorax* 1985; 40:45.

64. Lopata M, Önal E: Mass loading, sleep apnea and the pathogenesis of obesity hypoventilation. *Am Rev Respir Dis* 1982; 126:640.

65. Bradley TD, et al.: Role of diffuse airway obstruction in the hypercapnia of obstructive sleep apnea. *Am Rev Respir Dis* 1986; 134:920.

66. Leech JA, Önal E, Bahr P, Lopata M: Determinants of hypercapnia in patients with sleep apnea syndrome. *Chest* 1987; 92:807.

67. Guilleminault C, Cummiskey J, Motta J: Chronic obstructive airflow disease and sleep studies. *Am Rev Respir Dis* 1980; 122:397.

68. Flenley DC: Sleep in chronic obstructive lung disease. *Clin Chest Med* 1985; 6:651.

69. Fletcher EC, Schaaf JW, Miller J, Fletcher JG: Long-term cardiopulmonary sequelae in patients with sleep apnea and chronic lung disease. *Am Rev Respir Dis* 1987; 135:525.

70. Wynne JW, et al.: Disordered breathing and oxygen desaturation during sleep in patients with chronic obstructive lung disease (COLD). *Am J Med* 1979; 66:537.

71. Arand DL, McGinty DJ, Littner MR: Respiratory patterns associated with hemoglobin desaturation during sleep in chronic obstructive pulmonary disease. *Chest* 1981; 80:183.

72. Skatrud J, Iber H, McHugh W, et al.: Determinants of hypoventilation during wakefulness and sleep in diaphragmatic paralysis. *Am Rev Respir Dis* 1980; 121:587.

73. Smith REM, Calverly PMA, Edwards RHT: Hypoxemia during sleep in Duchenne muscular dystrophy. *Am Rev Respir Dis* 1988; 137:884.

74. Muller NL, Francis PW, Gurwitz N, et al.: Mechanism of hemoglobin desaturation during REM sleep in normal subjects and in patients with cystic fibrosis. *Am Rev Respir Dis* 1980; 121:463.

75. Johnson MW, Remmers JE: Accessory muscle activity during sleep in chronic obstructive pulmonary disease. *J Appl Physiol* 1984; 57:1011.

76. Hill NS: Clinical applications of body ventilators. *Chest* 1986; 90:897.

77. Holtackers TR, Loosbrock LM, Gracey DR: The use of the chest cuirass in respiratory failure of neurologic origin. *Respir Care* 1982; 27:271.

78. Goldstein RS, Gee JBL, Cole DR, et al.: Reversal of sleep-induced hypoventilation and chronic respiratory failure by nocturnal negative pressure ventilation in patients with restrictive ventilatory impairment. *Am Rev Respir Dis* 1987; 135:1049.

79. Driver AG, Blackburn BB, Marcuard SP, Austin EH: Bilateral diaphragm paralysis treated with cuirass ventilation. *Chest* 1987; 136:1276.

80. Celli BR, Rassulo J, Corral R: Ventilatory muscle dysfunction in patients with bilateral idiopathic diaphragmatic paralysis: Reversal by intermittent external negative pressure ventilation. *Am Rev Respir Dis* 1987; 136:1276.

81. Mohn CH, Hill NS: Long-term follow up of nocturnal ventilatory assistance in patients with respiratory failure due to Duchenne-type muscular dystrophy. *Chest* 1990; 97:91.

82. Glenn WW, et al.: Combined central alveolar hypoventilation and upper airway obstruction: Treatment by tracheostomy and diaphragm pacing. *Am J Med* 1978; 64:50.

83. Hoeppner VH, Cockcroft DW, Dosman JA, Cotton DJ: Nighttime ventilation improves respiratory failure in secondary kyphoscoliosis. *Am Rev Respir Dis* 1984; 129:240.

84. Kirby GR, Mayer LS, Pingleton SK: Nocturnal positive pressure ventilation via nasal mask. *Am Rev Respir Dis* 1987; 135:738.

85. Leger P, Jennequin J, Gerard M, Robert D: Home positive pressure ventilation via nasal mask for patients with neuromuscular weakness or restrictive lung or chest-wall disease. *Respir Care* 1989; 34:73.

86. Ellis ER, Bye PT, Bruderer JW, Sullivan CE: Treatment of respiratory failure during sleep in patients with neuromuscular disease: Positive-pressure ventilation through a nose mask. *Am Rev Respir Dis* 1987; 135:148.

87. DiMaco AF, Connors AF, Altose MD: Management of chronic alveolar hypoventilation with nasal positive pressure breathing. *Chest* 1987; 92:952.

88. Ellis ER, et al.: Noninvasive ventilatory support during sleep improves respiratory failure in kyphoscoliosis. *Chest* 1988; 94:811.

89. Bach JR, Alba AS: Management of chronic alveolar hypoventilation by nasal ventilation. *Chest* 1990; 97:52.

90. Heckmatt JZ, Loh L, Dubowitz V: Night-time nasal ventilation in neuromuscular disease. *Lancet* 1990; 10:579.

91. Goldstein RS: Hypoventilation: Neuromuscular and chest wall disorders. *Clin Chest Med* 1992; 13:507.

Chapter 109 _____

TREATMENT OF OBSTRUCTIVE SLEEP APNEA

ROBERT C. BASNER

Obstructive Sleep Apnea
  Etiologies
  Specific therapies

Periodic Breathing and Central Sleep Apnea
  Etiologies
  Specific therapies

Obstructive Sleep Apnea

ETIOLOGIES

Obstructive sleep apnea (OSA) may be defined as a disorder in which during sleep, repetitive episodes of total cessation of airflow at the nose and mouth occur for at least 10 s in the presence of continued respiratory effort (obstructive apnea), or there are decreases in airflow that are disproportionate to any decreases in respiratory effort (hypopnea). (See Fig. 108-2.) Both species of obstructive respiratory events are manifestations of partial or complete paroxysmal closure of the pharyngeal airway, typically at the level of the soft palate (velopharynx) and/or tongue (oro/hypopharynx).[1,2] A characteristic pathophysiologic sequence occurs during and following obstructive events, including repeated inspiratory effort against the obstruction, cortical arousal, and release of the obstruction followed by resumption of ventilation. Obstructive events thus are, virtually by definition, associated with transient arousals, though not necessarily awakenings, from sleep, and significant decreases in oxygen saturation of hemoglobin. Both the acute and long-term consequences of OSA can be understood in the context of this pathophysiology. The syndrome of OSA is defined as the presence of five or more obstructive apneas and hypopneas per hour of sleep,[3] in the setting of signs or symptoms of sequelae of these events. Excessive daytime sleepiness (EDS) is the most characteristic of these sequelae. Snoring, obesity, and systemic hypertension are common but not essential correlates of the syndrome. Obstructive sleep apnea is a prevalent condition in adults,[4,5] with peak prevalence reported in the sixth decade.[6]

From a practical perspective, respiratory effort is often difficult to measure and may be physiologically irregular or periodic in certain sleep stages, such that the differentiation among obstructive respiratory events, exaggerated respiratory periodicity, central apneas, alveolar hypoventilation, and sleep exacerbation of ventilation-perfusion mismatching is often not readily apparent.

Along with the difficulties involved in accurately diagnosing OSA,[7] the clinician is faced with two surprising dilemmas regarding treatment: no consensus currently exists as to which patients with uncomplicated OSA need treatment, and treatment modalities continue to be less than ideally effective.[8,9] The repetitive asphyxia of OSA, with its attendant chemical and mechanical perturbations, would be expected to predispose to acute and chronic cardiovascular and cerebrovascular derangements, particularly among susceptible populations[10-14]; abrupt and repetitive arousals might similarly endanger cardiovascular homeostasis during sleep[15-18] while also leading to sleep fragmentation and EDS.[8,19]

In contrast to the pathophysiologic concerns noted above, the association between OSA and long-term cardiovascular and cerebovascular sequelae has not been well established. Studies that have investigated such an association tend to be retrospective, with small numbers, and many do not explicitly account for the many variables present in these populations.[20-26] Further, for acute cardiovascular events as well as sudden unexplained nocturnal death, it is not clear to what extent OSA plans an independent or additive role as opposed to effects of sleep and different sleep stages and circadian variation in neural, endocrine, and hemostatic functions.[25,26] Nevertheless, such data as are available suggest that cardiovascular mortality is increased in patients with untreated OSA[23,27]; this excess mortality appears to increase with increasing severity of the OSA,[27] correlating with an apnea index of greater than 20 events per hour.[27] Data suggesting that successful treatment of OSA may ameliorate some of the associated adverse cardiovascular conditions[11,13,14,23] provide a further link between OSA and cardiovascular dysfunction while also highlighting the importance of accurate diagnosis and treatment of OSA.

1053

Numerous studies support the impression that OSA patients may be objectively sleepy during the day,[5,8,30] as measured by multiple sleep latency testing (MSLT).[31] Severely decreased latencies to sleep during such testing have been correlated with decrements in vigilance and performance; thus the MSLT represents an objective and standardized means of measuring physiologically significant EDS.[31] Data suggest that patients with more than mild OSA carry a relatively high risk of being involved in a motor vehicle accident due to excessive sleepiness; some of these accidents can involve fatalities.[28–30] At the same time, it should be pointed out that the degree of sleepiness on MSLT does not necessarily correlate with the frequency of motor vehicle accidents on OSA patients.[28,30] Any patient who is known to have fallen asleep while driving is dangerously sleepy and should be removed from driving as well as from any and all activities in which falling asleep unexpectedly would endanger the patient or others—pending successful diagnosis and treatment.[28,29]

Patients with more than mild OSA have increased mortality rates if untreated. The cardiovascular and neurocognitive morbidity, including loss of productivity and disrupted family and social function, must also be taken into account. With these considerations in mind, treatment of the patient with OSA should be individualized to the greatest extent possible. Because the asphyxia, arousal, and efforts against upper airway obstruction of OSA[32,33] have all been associated with adverse cardiovascular effects and/or daytime morbidity and mortality, these are the endpoints that must be followed in treating OSA. The success of treatment is measured both clinically and by polysomnography. The following discussion of specific treatment modalities should be considered with these issues in mind.

SPECIFIC THERAPIES

NASAL POSITIVE AIRWAY PRESSURE

Nasal positive airway pressure (NPAP) is the treatment of choice of most adult patients with OSA. Other modalities, which aim to treat OSA definitively, should be considered only when a patient cannot or will not be successfully treated with NPAP. Nasal positive airway pressure involves the use of a tight-fitting nasal mask, secured by soft headgear and attached to an electrically driven unit that delivers pressurized air up to 20 cmH_2O, which is maintained throughout the respiratory cycle (continuous positive airway pressure, or CPAP) or adjusted to deliver an inspiratory pressure higher than the expiratory pressure (bilevel PAP). Current devices are equipped with internal flow transducers, which allow for detection of total flow rates with continuous adjustment for transient air leaks and pressure changes. Some data suggest that less positive pressure is necessary to overcome airway resistance in expiration versus inspiration,[34] and this is the rationale for the use of bilevel PAP, which theoretically can avoid subjecting the patient to greater than necessary expiratory pressures (as may be the case with CPAP). Extensive documentation of the ability of CPAP to achieve improved respiratory and sleep parameters[35–37] and preliminary data indicating similar compliance rates with CPAP and bilevel PAP[38] suggest that in most cases, CPAP, rather than bilevel PAP, may be prescribed. However, objective and subjective measures of long-term compliance with CPAP have shown surprisingly low rates, despite the apparent success of CPAP titration in the laboratory.[8] Newer strategies of NPAP, aimed at self-adjusting airway pressures throughout the respiratory cycle, are evolving, which would have the theoretical advantages of more accurate breath-to-breath pressure delivery, improved patient compliance, and decreased need for laboratory titration. It is not known whether such devices will prove to be practical or to be more effective in OSA than current devices.

The current widespread lack of systematic diagnostic and therapeutic polysomnography and follow-up have added to the relatively disappointing success rates with CPAP. Routine use of two separate sessions of laboratory polysomnography—the first diagnostic and the second therapeutic—is essential. Teaching, including mask-fitting and exposure to CPAP, should be provided prior to attempting titration. The titration itself is done under strict guidelines with continuous assessment and teaching regarding the technician's technique. Clearly, the sleep clinician's prior and meaningful knowledge of the patient's history, exam, and pertinent cardiorespiratory lab data will allow for the greatest possible planning for such titration, which may ideally involve CPAP, bilevel PAP, nasal intermittent positive pressure ventilation, or oxygen alone or in combination with positive airway pressure[39–41] based on the expectations and expertise of the sleep clinician, and the evolving polysomnogram. There are times when such a titration is clearly not optimal within a single session, and the decision regarding a second titration session must be considered.

In all cases, patients require routine follow-up at 2 weeks and at intervals thereafter, including at 1 year. This strategy is more cost- and labor-intensive than may have been formerly thought necessary and seemingly opposes the tide of current health-care policy. However, other therapies, as outlined below, offer less chance of success, with perhaps more cost and risk to the patient than the approach for using NPAP.

PHARMACOLOGIC THERAPY

Pharmacologic therapy has little if any usefulness in the contemporary management of OSA. Stimulants, such as methylphenidate and pemoline, have not been shown to benefit the cardiorespiratory perturbations of OSA, nor indeed in a systematic fashion to benefit the EDS of OSA syndrome. Such therapy is not recommended for the treatment of OSA, and failure to achieve amelioration of EDS from standard therapy should alert the clinician to the possibility of a problem with the chosen therapy or an inaccurate or possibly an additional diagnosis.[7,42] The tricyclic antidepressants, particularly the more alerting agents of this class, have been used to treat OSA. The rationale for such treatment has been twofold: (1) these medications potently suppress REM sleep, the sleep stage commonly associated with worsened sleep-disordered breathing and oxygen desaturation of hemoglobin,[43] and (2) at least one of these agents has been associated with preferentially increased upper airway nerve activity in decerebrate cats.[44] These medications have not generally been shown to be effective in patients with OSA[45,46] and can be associated with significant side effects at the dosages that might be clinically useful. Such side effects—which may include urinary hesitancy, impotence, postural hypotension, sedation, and cardiac arrhythmia—may be particularly problematic in just those groups of patients most likely to have OSA. Medroxyprogesterone has been found to be of benefit as a respiratory stimulant in patients with hypoventilation syndromes other than OSA (see Chap. 108); it does not have an established role in the treatment of OSA, particularly in the absence of diurnal hypoventilation.[47] Other respiratory stimulants, including theophylline and acetazolamide, have not been shown to be effective in OSA, although they may be tried in other sleep-related respiratory disorders (see below).

Probably most pertinent to the discussion of pharmacologic agents in OSA is mention of those agents with potential adverse effects on the syndrome, particularly since many patients with OSA will be found to be using such agents chronically. Ethanol is acutely and chronically sleep disruptive, appears to inhibit upper airway dilator muscle activity preferentially,[48] and has been shown to worsen sleep-disordered breathing in snorers and patients with OSA.[49,50] Other sedative hypnotics, including certain benzodiazepines and barbiturates, are also potentially sleep-disruptive, may also preferentially inhibit upper airway muscle activity, and may also worsen sleep-disordered breathing in OSA.[44,51] Newer hypnotics, such as the imidazopyridines, have not been studied in patients with OSA. The decision to allow the use of any sedative-hypnotic agent in patients diagnosed with or suspected of having OSA should ideally be made with objective evidence of the patient's sleep and respiration on pharmacoactive levels of the medication. Many other medications that the patient with OSA may be taking can be sleep-disruptive; an exhaustive discussion of such medications is beyond the scope of this chapter.[7]

SURGICAL APPROACHES

Certain functional or anatomic abnormalities are sometimes present in adult patients with OSA; such abnormalities include nasal septal deviation, adenotonsillar hypertrophy, nasopharyngeal tumor, rhinitis, macroglossia, micro- and retrognathia, and vocal cord dysfunction.[52] Identification and treatment of such specific defects can be of obvious importance to the patient's well-being aside from possibly ameliorating sleep-disordered breathing or allowing improved compliance with NPAP. In our experience, however, it is not common for a specific abnormality amenable to surgical intervention to be found in adults,[52] or for surgical therapy for a specific anatomic defect to be successful in eliminating adult OSA. Numerous nonspecific pharyngeal surgical procedures designed to widen the pharyngeal air space have been used to attempt to treat OSA definitively. Uvulopalatopharyngoplasty (UPPP) is the most commonly performed and well-documented of these procedures. UPPP alone does not consistently achieve physiologically acceptable amelioration of sleep-disordered breathing, although subjective improvement is common.[52a] Even in those patients who are "preselected" for UPPP by cephalometry, fiberoptic endoscopy with Mueller maneuver, and segmental upper airway pressure measurements to define the site of anatomic or functional narrowing, few with significant OSA prior to surgery are left without significant OSA, and it is difficult to predict from current data which site of pharyngeal narrowing actually predicts a better UPPP outcome.[9,53,54] Perioperative and early and late postoperative complications must also be considered.[55] Diverse methods of maxillomandibular advancement as well as numerous other soft tissue resections—including midline partial glossectomy and resection of redundant aryepiglottic folds—have also been used to widen the pharyngeal airway in patients with OSA.[52] Two points concerning all of these procedures require emphasis. First, these procedures should be offered only to those patients who cannot or will not successfully use NPAP and in whom surgery can be safely performed. Only a small minority of OSA patients will, with careful and knowledgeable management, meet these criteria. Second, objective documentation of the results of such surgery should be obtained. In this setting, if significant OSA remains and NPAP continues to be unsuccessful or unacceptable, permanent tracheostomy should be considered.[56] Laser-assisted uvulopalatoplasty, a procedure developed for the treatment of snoring,[57] has recently begun to be performed in some centers as an outpatient procedure for the treatment of OSA. It is mentioned here only to point out that to date there are no controlled data justifying the use of this procedure for such treatment.

NASAL AND ORAL DEVICES

The use of numerous devices for internally or externally dilating the nasopharyngeal[58] and oropharyngeal[59,60] airway has been attempted to definitively treat OSA. As with surgical therapies, such devices have been shown to have limited effectiveness overall in patients with OSA, particularly more severe OSA, where definitive therapy appears most important.

WEIGHT LOSS AND POSITIONAL THERAPY

Weight loss, when applicable, has been found to be of benefit in reducing the severity of sleep-disordered breathing in some[61] but not all[62] studies of patients with OSA. Weight loss should be considered an adjunctive rather than a definitive treatment approach in all but the mildest cases of OSA. In our experience, advising the patient to lose weight at the time of assessment and diagnosis is rarely successful without specific nutritional counseling and supportive therapy. Further, the motivation for losing weight is more likely to be present after successful treatment has been initiated, when the burden of excessive sleepiness and neurocognitive deficits has been relieved.

In some patients with OSA, there is a striking increase in obstructive events in the supine versus the lateral decubitus position. This appears to be particularly true in those patients with lesser degrees of apnea frequency.[63] Such a positional effect should be known from the polysomnography results, and, if present, may be addressed by using a foam wedge to keep the patient in the lateral position, or by sewing a tennis ball into the back of his or her nightshirt. Such therapy itself may interfere with sleep, and the patient should be monitored clinically as well as with objective measures of gas exchange and daytime sleepiness.

Periodic Breathing and Central Sleep Apnea

ETIOLOGIES

Respiratory periodicity is a physiologic occurrence at sleep onset, as awake and behavioral drive is withdrawn and metabolic regulation predominates.[64] Relatively lower chemoresponsiveness at this time results in hypoventilation, followed by hyperventilation, until a stable metabolic set point is reached. The transient arousals that may accompany the fluctuations in mechanical and chemical stimuli at sleep onset may exaggerate the hyperventilatory response to the preceding hypoventilation and propagate the periodicity until sleep consolidation is established. Conditions in which relative hypocapnia is present, as with hypoxemia from any cause (a classic example being high altitude) or in which chemoreception is impaired (as from neurologic disease or circulatory perturbations in congestive heart failure), may allow exaggeration of the metabolic respiratory response. Such situations can result in Cheyne-Stokes breathing and outright central apneas at the nadir of the ventilatory cycle. Repetitive arousals may thus result from and lead to instability of respiratory drive and thus create a syndrome of gas-exchange abnormality and sleep disruption.

Central sleep apnea, defined as a transient and repetitive cessation of respiratory effort during sleep, is much less prevalent as a syndrome than OSA.[65] It may be present in association with chronic centrally mediated alveolar hypoventilation syndromes and with hypoventilation resulting from neuromuscular disorders.[66] It should be noted that a strict separation between central and obstructive sleep apnea may be misleading physiologically: OSA is also typically associated with periodicity of respiratory effort, with occlusion of the upper airway generally occurring at the nadir of the respiratory effort.[67] Such a pattern of apnea, with occluded efforts early and late in the event, has been shown in patients with Cheyne-Stokes respiration associated with congestive heart failure.[68] Upper-airway occlusion may itself promote ventilatory instability, either reflexively[69] or by exaggerating chemical stimuli changes, further propagating the periodicity of ventilatory and upper-airway muscle neural output, and arousal. The efficacy of NPAP in the treatment of periodic breathing[70] and central apneas during sleep[71] highlights the similarities in underlying respiratory instability of the two conditions.

SPECIFIC THERAPIES

Because the syndrome of central apnea during sleep tends to be a sleep-related exaggeration of underlying cardiorespiratory insufficiency or secondary to neurologic defect, as discussed above, treatment of the underlying condition should be the primary goal of therapy. When such treatment has been optimized and sleep fragmentation and gas-exchange abnormalities continue to be physiologically or symptomatically significant, treatment aimed specifically at the sleep-induced perturbation is warranted. Administration of supplemental oxygen under controlled conditions is a rational approach to such patients, in whom hypoxemia with relative hypocapnia underlies the respiratory instability. In most other patients with central sleep apnea, who tend to have chronic hypoventilation, treatment during sleep is essentially the same as that for other patients with chronic alveolar hypoventilation (see Chap. 108). Respiratory stimulants have been tried in patients with hypercapnic central sleep apnea[66] with variable success; part of the difficulty with these medications is their stimulant effect on sleep itself. For most patients, some form of noninvasive nocturnal ventilation will have the greatest chance at reversal of nocturnal and diurnal gas exchange perturbations and restoration (or preservation) of sleep consolidation. Such patients should be titrated polysomnographically, preferably with measurement of gas exchange rather than oxygen saturation of hemoglobin alone. A tight-fitting nasal mask may be used to deliver the appropriate regimen of positive pressure, be it continuous PAP,[66,71] bilevel PAP, or intermittent positive-pressure ventilation.[72]

References

1. Shepard JJ Jr, Thawley SE: Localization of upper airway collapse during sleep in patients with obstructive sleep apnea. *Am Rev Respir Dis* 1990; 141:1350.
2. Hudgel DW, Harasick R, Katz RL, et al.: Uvulopalatopharyngoplasty in obstructive apnea: Value of preoperative localization of site of upper airway narrowing during sleep. *Am Rev Respir Dis* 1991; 143:942.
3. Guilleminault C: Sleep and breathing, in Guilleminault C (ed): *Sleeping and Waking Disorders: Indications and Techniques.* Menlo Park, CA: Addison Wesley, 1982:155–182.
4. Young T, Palta M, Dempsey J, et al.: Occurrence of sleep disordered breathing among middle-aged adults. *N Engl J Med* 1993; 328:1230.
5. Lavie P: Incidence of sleep apnea in a presumably healthy working population: A significant relationship with excessive daytime sleepiness. *Sleep* 1983; 6:312.
6. Gislason T, Almqvist M, Eriksson G, et al.: Prevalance of sleep apnea syndrome among Swedish men: An epidemiological study. *J Clin Epidemiol* 1988; 41:571.
7. Basner RC, Önal E: Dealing with the differential diagnosis of obstructive sleep apnea syndrome. *Comp Ther* 1994; 20:273.
8. Kribbs NB, Pack AI, Kline LR, et al.: Objective measurement of patterns of nasal CPAP use by patients with obstructive sleep apnea. *Am Rev Respir Dis* 1993; 147:887.
9. Sher AE, Thorpy MJ, Shprintzen RJ, et al.: Predictive value of Mueller's maneuver in selection of patients for uvulopalatopharyngoplasty. *Laryngoscope* 1985; 95:1483.
10. Tilkian AG, Guilleminault C, Schroeder JS, et al.: Hemodynamics in sleep-induced apnea. *Ann Intern Med* 1976; 85:714.
11. Guilleminault C, Connolly SJ, Winkle RA: Cardiac arrhythmia and conduction disturbances during sleep in 400 patients with sleep apnea syndrome. *Am J Cardiol* 1983; 52:490.
12. Shepard JW Jr: Gas exchange and hemodynamics during sleep. *Med Clin North Am* 1985; 69:1243.
13. Fletcher EC, Miller J, Schaaf JW, et al.: Urinary catecholamines before and after tracheostomy in patients with obstructive sleep apnea and hypertension. *Sleep* 1987; 10:35.
14. Jennum P, Wildschiodtz G, Christensen NJ, et al.: Blood pressure, catecholamines, and pancreatic polypeptide in obstructive

sleep apnea with and without nasal continuous positive airway pressure (nCPAP) treatment. *Am J Hypertens* 1989; 2:847.

15. Hedner J, Ejnell H, Sellgren J, et al.: Is high and fluctuating muscle nerve sympathetic in the sleep apnoea syndrome of pathogenetic importance for the development of hypertension? *J Hypertens* 1988; 6:529.

16. Ringler J, Basner RC, Shannon R, et al.: Hypoxemia alone does not explain blood pressure elevations after obstructive apneas. *J Appl Physiol* 1990; 69:2143.

17. Davies RJO, Belt PJ, Roberts SJ, et al.: Arterial blood pressure responses to graded transient arousal from sleep in normal humans. *Am Rev Respir Dis* 1993; 74:1123.

18. Somers VK, Dyken ME, Mark AL, Abboud FM: Sympathetic activity during sleep in normal subjects. *N Engl J Med* 1993; 328:303.

19. Philip P, Stoohs R, Guilleminault C: Sleep fragmentation in normals: A model for sleepiness associated with upper airway resistance syndrome. *Sleep* 1994; 17:242.

20. Williams AJ, Houston D, Finberg S, et al.: Sleep apnea syndrome and essential hypertension. *Am J Cardiol* 1985; 55:1019.

21. Fletcher EC, DeBehnke RD, Lovoi MS, et al.: Undiagnosed sleep apnea in patients with essential hypertension. *Ann Intern Med* 1985; 103:190.

22. Warley ARH, Mitchell JH, Stradling JR: Prevalence of nocturnal hypoxaemia amongst men with mild to moderate hypertension. *Q J Med* 1988; 256:637.

23. Partinen M, Jamieson A, Guilleminault C: Long-term outcome for obstructive sleep apnea syndrome patients: Mortality. *Chest* 1988; 94:1200.

24. Millman RP, Redline S, Carlisle CC, et al.: Daytime hypertension in obstructive sleep apnea: Prevalence and contributing risk factors. *Chest* 1991; 99:861.

25. Harrison MJG, Pollock S, Kendall BE, et al.: Effect of haematocrit on carotid stenosis and cerebral infarction. *Lancet* 1981; ii:114.

26. Tofler GH, Brezinski D, Schafer AI, et al.: Concurrent morning increase in platelet aggregability and the risk of myocardial infarction and sudden cardiac death. *N Engl J Med* 1987; 316:1514.

27. He J, Kryger MH, Zorick FJ, et al.: Mortality and apnea index in obstructive sleep apnea: Experience in 385 male patients. *Chest* 1988; 94:9.

28. Findley LJ, Levinson MP, Bonnie RJ: Driving performance and automobile accidents in patients with sleep apnea. *Clin Chest Med* 1992; 13:427.

29. Dement WC (chair): *Wake Up America: A National Sleep Alert*: vol I. Executive summary and report of the National Commission on Sleep Disorders Research, U.S. Department of Health and Human Services, Washington, D.C. 1993.

30. Aldrich MS: Automobile accidents in patients with sleep disorders. *Sleep* 1989; 12:487.

31. Carskadon MA (chair): Guidelines for the multiple sleep latency test (MSLT): A standard measure of sleepiness. *Sleep* 1986; 9:519.

32. Scharf SM, Bianco JA, Tow DE, et al.: The effect of large negative intrathoracic pressure on left ventricular function in patients with coronary artery disease. *Circulation* 1981; 63:871.

33. Tolle FA, Judy WV, Yu PI, et al.: Reduced stroke volume related to pleural pressure in obstructive sleep apnea. *J Appl Physiol* 1983; 55:1718.

34. Sanders MH, Moore SE: Inspiratory and expiratory partitioning of airway resistance during sleep in patients with sleep apnea. *Am Rev Respir Dis* 1983; 127:554.

35. Sullivan CE, Issa FG, Berthon-Jones M, et al.: Home treatment of obstructive sleep apnea with continuous positive airway pressure applied through a nose mask. *Bull Eur Physiopathol Respir* 1984; 20:49.

36. Rajagopal KR, Bennett LL, Dillard TA, et al.: Overnight nasal CPAP improves hypersomnolence in sleep apnea. *Chest* 1986; 90:172.

37. Kribbs NB, Pack AI, Kline LR, et al.: Effects of one night without nasal CPAP treatment on sleep and sleepiness in patients with obstructive sleep apnea. *Am Rev Respir Dis* 1993; 147:1162.

38. Reeves-Hoche MK, Hudgel D, Meck R, et al.: Continuous versus bilevel positive airway pressure for obstructive sleep apnea. *Am J Respir Crit Care Med* 1995; 151:443.

39. Motta J, Guilleminault C: Effects of oxygen administration in sleep-induced apneas, in Guilleminault C (ed): *Sleep Apnea Syndromes*: vol II. New York: Liss, 1978:137–144.

40. Martin RJ, Sanders MH, Gray BA, Pennock BE: Acute and long term ventilatory effects of hyperoxia in the adult sleep apnea syndrome. *Am Rev Respir Dis* 1982; 125:175.

41. Smith PL, Haponik EF, Bleecker ER: The effects of oxygen in patients with sleep apnea. *Am Rev Respir Dis* 1984; 130:958.

42. *International Classification of Sleep Disorders: Diagnostic and Coding Manual*. Lawrence, KS: Allen Press, 1990.

43. Smith PL, Haponik EF, Allen RP, Bleecker ER: The effects of protriptyline in sleep disordered breathing. *Am Rev Respir Dis* 1983; 127:8.

44. Bonora M, St John WM, Bledsoe TA: Differential elevation by protriptyline and depression by diazepam of upper airway respiratory motor activity. *Am Rev Respir Dis* 1985; 13:41.

45. Hanzell DA, Proia NG, Hudgel DW: Response of obstructive sleep apnea to fluoxetine and protriptyline. *Chest* 1983; 100:416.

46. Brownell LG, Perez-Padilla R, West P, Kryger MH: The role of protriptyline in obstructive sleep apnea. *Bull Eur Physiopathol Respir* 1983; 19:621.

47. Cook WR, Benich J, Wooten SA: Indices of severity of obstructive sleep apnea syndrome do not change during medroxyprogesterone therapy. *Chest* 1989; 96:262.

48. Krol RC, Knuth SL, Bartlett D: Selective reduction of genioglossal muscle activity by alcohol in normal human subjects. *Am Rev Respir Dis* 1984; 129:247.

49. Issa FG, Sullivan CE: Alcohol, snoring, and sleep apnea. *Neurol Neurosurg Psychiatry* 1982; 45:353.

50. Scrima L, Broudy M, Nay K, et al.: Increased severity of obstructive sleep apnea after bedtime alcohol ingestion: Diagnostic potential and proposed mechanisms of actions. *Sleep* 1982; 5:318.

51. Hishikawa Y, Furuya E, Wakamatsu H: Hypersomnia and periodic respiration-presentation of two cases and comment on the physiopathogenesis of the Pickwickian syndrome. *Folia Psychiatr Neurol Jpn* 1970; 24:163.

52. Sher AE: The upper airway in obstructive sleep apnea syndrome: Pathology and surgical management, in Thorpy MJ (ed): *Handbook of Sleep Disorders*. New York: Marcel Dekker, 1990:311–335.

52a. Miljekig H, Mateika S, Haight JS, et al.: Subjective and objective assessment of uvulopalatopharyngoplasty for treatment of snoring and obstructive sleep apnea. *Am J Respir Crit Care Med* 1994; 150:1286.

53. Ryan CF, Dickson RI, Lowe AA, et al.: Upper airway measurements predict response to uvulopalatopharyngoplasty in obstructive sleep apnea. *Laryngoscope* 1990; 100:248.

54. Rojewski TE, Schuller DE, Clark RW, et al.: Videoendoscopic determination of the mechanism of obstruction in obstructive sleep apnea. *Otolaryngol Head Neck Surg* 1984; 92:127.

55. Fairbanks DN: UPPP complications and avoidance strategies. *Otolaryngol Head Neck Surg* 1990; 102:239.

56. Fairbanks DNF: Tracheostomy for obstructive sleep apnea:

Indications and techniques, in Fairbanks DNF, Fujita S (eds): *Snoring and Obstructive Sleep Apnea*. New York: Raven Press, 1994:169–177.

57. Kamami YV: Laser CO_2 for snoring: Preliminary results. *Acta Otorhinolaryngol Belg* 1990; 44:451.

58. Nahmias JS, Karetzky MS: Treatment of the sleep apnea syndrome using a nasopharyngeal tube. *Chest* 1988; 94:1142.

59. Schmidt-Nowara WW, Meade TE, Hays MB: Treatment of snoring and obstructive sleep apnea with a dental orthosis. *Chest* 1991; 99:1378.

60. Eveloff SE, Rosenberg CL, Carlisle CC, Millman RP: Determinants of efficacy of a mandibular advancement device for the treatment of OSA (abstr). *Am Rev Respir Dis* 1993; 147:252.

61. Smith PL, Gold AR, Meyers DA, et al.: Weight loss in mildly to moderately obese patients with obstructive sleep apnea. *Ann Intern Med* 1985; 103:850.

62. Guilleminault C, Eldridge FL, Tilkian A, et al.: Sleep apnea due to upper airway obstruction. *Arch Intern Med* 1977; 137:296.

63. Cartwright RD: Effect of position on sleep apnea therapy. *Sleep* 1984; 110:7.

64. Phillipson EA: Control of breathing during sleep. *Am Rev Respir Dis* 1978; 118:909.

65. Guilleminault C, Tilkian A, Dement WC: The sleep apnea syndromes. *Annu Rev Med* 1976; 27:475.

66. Bradley TD, Phillipson EA: Central sleep apnea. *Clin Chest Med* 1992; 13:493.

67. Önal E, Lopata M: Periodic breathing and the pathogenesis of occlusive sleep apneas. *Am Rev Respir Dis* 1982; 126:676.

68. Alex CG, Önal E, Lopata M: Upper airway occlusion during sleep in patients with Cheyne-Stokes respiration. *Am Rev Respir Dis* 1986; 133:42.

69. Sullivan CE, Murphy E, Kozar LF, et al.: Waking and ventilatory responses to laryngeal stimulation in sleeping dogs. *J Appl Physiol* 1978; 45:681.

70. Takasaki Y, Orr D, Popkin J, et al.: Effect of nasal continuous positive airway pressure on sleep apnea in congestive heart failure. *Am Rev Respir Dis* 1989; 140:1578.

71. Hoffstein V, Slutsky AS: Central sleep apnea reversed by continuous positive airway pressure. *Am Rev Respir Dis* 1987; 135:1210.

72. Ellis ER, Bye PTP, Bruderer JW, et al.: Treatment of respiratory failure during sleep in patients with neuromuscular disease. *Am Rev Respir Dis* 1987; 135:148.

PART 6

TREATMENT OF IDIOPATHIC LUNG DISEASES

IDIOPATHIC PARENCHYMAL LUNG DISEASES

Chapter 110

IDIOPATHIC PULMONARY FIBROSIS

EUGENE J. SULLIVAN AND TALMADGE E. KING, Jr.

Introduction

Idiopathic pulmonary fibrosis (IPF) is an intraalveolar and interstitial disease of uncertain etiology. The estimated prevalence is 5 to 29 individuals per 100,000 population.[1–3] Patients generally present in the fifth or sixth decade of life. Although the process is chronic, the pathogenesis appears to follow injury to the alveolar wall leading to an influx of inflammatory and immune effector cells, i.e., "alveolitis." It is the presence of this ongoing alveolitis that causes the derangement of the alveolar and interstitial architecture. The ensuing fibrosis results in loss of alveolar gas exchanging units. Because patients frequently present at mid-to-late stages of the disease successful management of the disease is difficult. The average length of survival after presentation is 3 to 5 years, with 50% of patients dying of progressive disease within 5 years. Few controlled clinical trials have been performed, and none have included sufficient numbers of patients to provide data to support a specific treatment approach. Consequently, treatment is largely empirical.

Diagnosis

CLINICAL FEATURES

A key to the diagnosis of IPF is to exclude carefully other causes of diffuse parenchymal lung disease.[4] Often this can be done by taking a careful history but not infrequently lung tissue examination is necessary to confirm or establish a specific diagnosis. Important categories of diseases or processes to consider include: connective tissue diseases, diseases associated with occupational and environmental exposures, drug-induced diseases (particularly chemotherapeutic agents), and several idiopathic syndromes with similar clinical, radiographic, or histopathologic features to IPF (for example respiratory bronchiolitis associated interstitial lung disease or stage III sarcoidosis). Review of the environment (home and work), especially as it relates to pets (particularly birds), air conditioners, humidifiers, hot tubs, saunas, evaporative cooling systems (e.g., swamp coolers), damp basements, etc., is extremely valuable.

Common presenting symptoms are progressive breathlessness with exertion and persistent nonproductive cough. Physical examination reveals tachypnea and bibasilar end-inspiratory dry rales. Clubbing of the digits is found in some patients, usually late in the course of the disease. Signs of pulmonary hypertension and cor pulmonale are generally secondary manifestations of advanced pulmonary fibrosis.

DIAGNOSTIC STUDIES

LUNG IMAGING STUDIES

The chest roentgenogram is frequently the first study to suggest the presence of diffuse parenchymal lung disease. The most common radiographic abnormality is a reticular or reticulonodular pattern, although mixed patterns of alveolar filling and increased interstitial markings may be seen. The chest roentgenogram may be normal in documented cases of diffuse parenchymal lung disease, particularly hypersensitivity pneumonitis and sarcoidosis but is very rarely normal in IPF. The physician should not ignore or incompletely evaluate an asymptomatic patient with an abnormal chest radiograph or a mildly symptomatic patient with a normal chest radiograph. These stages of disease may represent early and potentially reversible phases of the disease with a more likely positive response to therapy.

High-resolution computed tomography (HRCT) scanning is more sensitive and specific for the detection of ILD than chest radiograph. HRCT is especially helpful in detecting the presence of disease in symptomatic patients with a normal chest radiograph. Furthermore, HRCT identifies disease progression better than does routine chest x-ray. However, a normal HRCT does not rule out the presence of interstitial lung disease in all cases.[5] A typical HRCT appearance in the proper clinical setting is pathognomonic of IPF. The "proper clinical setting" is difficult to define: a middle-aged or elderly patient with diffuse parenchymal lung disease, symptoms of cough or dyspnea of greater than one year's duration, crackles on chest examination, and progressive disease as measured by physiologic testing (restrictive ventilatory defect with reduced diffusing capacity). These manifestations of the disease are generally present in mid-to-late stages and frequently identify the patient at a point when treatment is less likely to be of help in improving symptoms or altering the outcome. In addition, the conditions that are most important to distinguish from IPF, because they tend to be more treatable, are confused with it (e.g., hypersensitivity pneumonitis, sarcoidosis, cryptogenic organizing pneumonia, and eosinophilic pneumonia).[6]

HRCT findings in IPF include a marked peripheral and subpleural distribution of the interstitial densities. The involvement is patchy with areas of reticulation intermingled with areas of normal tissue, and this type of involvement is often associated with cystic spaces 2 to 4 mm in diameter. Correlation of the HRCT findings with the histopathological manifestations in IPF is incomplete. "Hazy" or "ground-glass" increase in lung density (that is, an increase in CT lung density that does not obscure the underlying lung parenchyma) or consolidation (a marked increase in attenuation with obliteration of underlying

anatomic features) is thought to correlate with early disease histopathologically, signifying alveolitis and potential therapeutic responsiveness.[7–9] In IPF, there is often little correlation between the grade of increase in attenuation and disease activity as assessed by the pathologic evaluation.[10]

In more "advanced" disease, there is a lower lung zone predominant reticular pattern, consisting largely of thickened interlobular septa and intralobular lines, often associated with honeycombing, traction bronchiectasis and subpleural fibrosis. In addition, parenchymal opacification may represent end-stage fibrosis rather than alveolitis in some cases.[11] The nearby presence of other indications of fibrosis (traction bronchiectasis or bronchiolectasis, anatomic distortion, and discernible cysts) can be helpful in resolving the distinction between alveolitis and fibrosis.[10,12,13]

The predictive value of HRCT in determining the response to treatment and prognosis in IPF is unclear.[4] A better response to therapy[7,14] and higher actuarial survival[14] is observed in IPF patients with a predominantly ground-glass pattern than with a mixed or predominantly reticular appearance. Although the ground glass opacities in IPF is sometime reversible,[7–9] more commonly it precedes the development of lung fibrosis.[7–9,15] Only a minority of patients with a predominant reticular pattern show a response to therapy. Serial HRCTs in treated patients showed that while an initial ground glass pattern may regress towards normal (or progress to a reticular pattern in a minority of unresponsive patients), a reticular pattern failed to regress in any patient and in most instances progressed in patients with IPF.[15,16] Also, the HRCT pattern appear to be independent of most physiologic measures of lung function (particularly, FVC, or DLCO).[14]

PULMONARY FUNCTION TESTS

Unless complicated by another pulmonary process, for example emphysema, most patients with IPF have a restrictive defect with reduced TLC, FRC, and RV. Flow rates appear decreased (FEV_1 and FVC) but this is related to the decreased lung volumes. The FEV_1/FVC ratio is usually normal and often increased. Smoking history must be considered when interpreting the functional studies. The finding of a restrictive pattern and an obstructive airflow limitation may occur in patients with IPF and previously existing COPD. Reduction in lung compliance is also common.

A decrease in the diffusing capacity for CO (DL_{CO}) is common and is due in part to effacement of the alveolar capillary units but more importantly to the extent of mismatching of ventilation and perfusion of the alveoli. Lung regions with reduced compliance due either to fibrosis or excessive cellularity may be ventilated poorly, but still be well perfused. A frequent mistake is to equate the extent of severity of the DCO reduction with disease stage. In some cases of IPF there can be considerable reduction in lung volumes and/or severe hypoxemia but normal or only slightly reduced DLCO. The DLCO also is not a useful method to follow the course of patients with IPF.

The resting arterial blood gas may be normal or reveal hypoxemia and respiratory alkalosis. Importantly, a normal resting PaO_2 does not rule out significant hypoxemia during exercise or sleep. Because undetected exercise-induced hypoxemia likely accelerates the development of pulmonary hypertension and cor pulmonale, it is important to perform exercise testing with arterial blood gases so that appropriate oxygen supplementation can be instituted.

Unfortunately, physiologic tests are not sensitive nor specific for the presence of inflammation in the lung parenchyma. In fact, in patients with early disease, the routine pulmonary function tests may be normal. Reductions in the VC do correlate with the degree of fibrosis present, and show a relationship with the overall histologic derangements. A marked reduction in the VC (< 50 percent of predicted), is associated with pulmonary hypertension and a reduced 2 year survival. Reduction of the TLC correlates with neither the histopathologic finding[17] nor prognosis and survival.[18] The compliance, maximum transpulmonary pressure, and coefficient of elastic retraction of the lung correlate well with the degree of fibrosis, but do not exclude the presence of cellularity.[17] The D_LCO has no correlation with the histologic stage of the disease. Patients with a normal D_LCO usually do not have significant gas exchange abnormalities, whereas patients with values <70 percent of predicted frequently have such changes at rest or with exercise. Survival is longer in patients with a more normal D_LCO (> 45 percent of predicted values).[19] A marked reduction of the D_LCO and resting hypoxemia is associated with pulmonary hypertension and decreased survival. Patients with a predominantly fibrotic process have greater abnormalities of the $P(A-a)O_2$ when compared to those with more cellular changes. Alterations in exercise gas exchange when compared to other indices of lung function correlate best with histopathologic findings.[17,20] We believe serial measurements of exercise gas exchange is the most sensitive physiologic indicator of the clinical course of IPF and appear to be the best predictors of responsiveness to treatment.

BRONCHOALVEOLAR LAVAGE

The value of subsegmental bronchoalveolar lavage (BAL) in the clinical staging and management of IPF patients remains to be established.[21] BAL lymphocytosis (>15%) tends to identify patients with a predominant inflammatory component histopathologically and a greater likelihood of response to corticosteroid therapy. On the other hand, neutrophilia and/or eosinophilia (>5%) appears to identify a more fibrotic stage of the disease and lack of response to corticosteroid therapy.

LUNG BIOPSY

Tissue examination is the most definitive method to diagnose and stage the disease so that appropriate prognostic and therapeutic decisions can be made. The major histopathologic features of IPF are: **1.** accumulation of alveolar macrophages and lymphocytes in the alveolar spaces with relatively intact alveolar walls; **2.** thickened, edematous alveolar walls with fibrinous exudate, mononuclear cell infiltration, and fibroblast proliferation; and **3.** aberrant extracellular matrix deposition with prominent accumulation of collagen and elastin resulting in broad bands of fibrosis and cystic spaces ("honeycombing"). All of the above pathologic patterns are frequently seen in adjacent sections of lung tissue from the same patient.

Treatment of IPF

INDICATIONS FOR THERAPY

IPF patients generally experience a relentless progression to endstage lung disease and death. Consequently, we believe that early and aggressive treatment directed at general suppression of this "immune-inflammatory process" should be tried in most patients. The two major approaches to drug therapy used to date have been corticosteroids and cytotoxic medications.[22,23] The concensus is that these drugs have broad anti-inflammatory and/or antifibrotic properties but the specific mechanism of their action in the lung is poorly understood.[23] The treatment period should be not less than three to six months regardless of the agent used. This period of time is required to determine the efficacy of the therapy.

DETERMINING THERAPEUTIC RESPONSIVENESS AND PROGNOSIS

Only limited data exists regarding the determinants of responsiveness to treatment in IPF. Favorable indicators of survival include: cellular histology at diagnosis, younger age, female gender, earlier stage of disease (less dyspnea, more normal lung function, less parenchymal disease on chest radiograph, elevated circulating immune complexes), increased lymphocytes in BAL, and a beneficial response to corticosteroid therapy.[24–26] Patients with IPF can be placed into lower and higher risk categories based on clinical symptoms (dyspnea, the more severe, the greater the risk of progression), smoking history (more pack-years, the worse the prognosis), severity of the initial lung function (worse the DLCO and gas exchange with exercise, the worse the prognosis), BAL cellular content (neutrophilia or eosinophilia suggest advanced disease with poorer prognosis), and need for immunosuppressive therapy.[21,27]

In addition to close monitoring for drug side effects and complications, patients should have a thorough evaluation at 3, 6, 12 months and annually after drug therapy has been initiated. This assessment should include careful history and examination, chest radiograph, pulmonary function testing to include lung volumes and diffusing capacity, and resting and exercise gas exchange.

In general, the "responsive" patient will report a decrease in symptoms. Radiographic improvement may occur but is not a usual finding even when the patients has considerable symptomatic improvement. Physiologic improvement, i.e., increase TLC, D_LCO or have an improvement in the exercise—induced oxygen desaturation can be seen and is important to determine. It is important to recognize that *no further decline* in lung function or other parameter of disease activity is a positive outcome given the almost invariable progressive nature of IPF. However, most patients with IPF experience episodes of increased dyspnea, decreased exercise capacity, or other declines in their functional status during the course of their illness. Clinical deterioration is due most frequently to disease progression but also may be caused by disease-associated complications and adverse effects of therapy.[28] These complications include heart failure, bronchogenic carcinoma, pulmonary infections, thromboembolism, pneumothorax, and corticosteroid-induced metabolic side effects and myopathy. Identifying the cause of the clinical deterioration is very important since it will determine the therapeutic intervention required and will influence the patient's prognosis and length of survival.

THERAPEUTIC ALTERNATIVES

CORTICOSTEROIDS
Corticosteroids are used in the initial treatment of most patients with IPF. Stabilization or improvement occurs in 20 to 40 percent of patients.

Mechanism(s) of action
Corticosteroids modify inflammatory and immune processes by effects on leukocyte function and leukocyte traffic and alteration in humoral processes. The ability of corticosteroids to inhibit recruitment of neutrophils and monocyte-macrophages to an inflammatory site may be the most pertinent mechanism of action against the perpetuation of inflammation in the lung injury process.

Dose and Route of Administration
The proper dose for the initiation of corticosteroid therapy is unknown. High dose corticosteroid therapy should be used to treat IPF, 1 to 1.5 mg per kilogram per day (using ideal body weight) not to exceed 100 mg per day. Prednisone is given as a single oral dose in the morning and may be maintained at this dose for 12 weeks. If the patient is stable or improved, the prednisone dose is gradually tapered over 4 to 5 weeks to 0.5 mg per kilogram per day (using ideal body weight) and maintained at this lower dose for the next 12 weeks. After 6 months, if the patient remains stable or improved, the prednisone gradually is tapered to 0.25 mg per kilogram per day (using ideal body weight) and maintained at that level until one year after the initiation of corticosteroid therapy. If the patient has deteriorated despite the corticosteroid therapy, a cytotoxic agent is considered while generally maintaining corticosteroid therapy at a reduced dose, usually 0.25 mg/kg/day as tolerated.

High-dose parenteral corticosteroid therapy (methylprednisolone 250 mg every 6 hours intravenously) has been recommended as the initial treatment in patients with rapidly progressive IPF.[22] This treatment may be given for 3 to 5 days to see if it initiates a response, primarily a reduction in symptoms and improvement in gas exchange. Improvements in chest radiographs generally are appreciated only if there was a significant component of alveolar infiltrate suggestive of acute/subacute alveolitis. No controlled clinical trials exist to support this recommendation and personal experience of success with this regimen exists in only a few cases.

Side Effects/Complications
Although therapy with corticosteroids usually is tolerated by patients, side effects are common and potentially disabling.[22] Some patients develop side effects of corticosteroids more readily than others at equivalent doses. Peptic ulcer disease, posterior capsular cataracts, increased intraocular pressure, hypertension, endocrine and metabolic alterations (deposition and redistribution of fatty tissue with truncal obesity, moon facies, menstrual irregularities, impotence, hyperglycemia, hypokalemia, metabolic alkalosis, and secondary adrenal insufficiency) may occur. Potential musculoskeletal complications are osteoporosis, vertebral compression fractures, aseptic necrosis of femoral and humeral heads, and myopathy. The latter may impair diaphragmatic and intercostal muscle strength and endurance, and these changes may complicate the assessment of therapeutic efficacy. Psychologic effects including euphoria, depression, or psychosis may also be encountered, especially in elderly patients.[29] Corticosteroid therapy may suppress the immune response to skin tests; therefore, when possible, tuberculin skin testing is advisable prior to the initiation of corticosteroid therapy. Routine isoniazid prophylaxis for corticosteroid-treated patients, even those with positive tuberculin skin tests results, is not indicated in most cases. Methods to reduce the risk of corticosteroid-induced osteoporosis should be instituted, especially in postmenopausal women, since even short term therapy (3 to 6 months) may cause reductions in bone mass. Unfortunately, the success of such regimens remains to be determined.

CYCLOPHOSPHAMIDE
Cyclophosphamide (Cytoxan) has been demonstrated to be effective in the treatment of pulmonary fibrosis in a few small clinical trials.[30–37]

Mechanism of Action
Cyclophosphamide is an alkylating agent of the nitrogen mustard group that is an inactive drug that is metabolized in vivo by the cytochrome P-450 mixed function oxidase system to its active metabolites which are responsible for the clinical actions and adverse effects of cyclophosphamide.[22] Hence, the activity of the hepatic microsomal enzymes is very important in determining the ultimate effect of this agent. Lymphoid tissues appear to be particularly sensitive to treatment with alkylating agents with decreases in both T cells and B cells, although the lymphocytic populations are probably not equally affected. The specific functional significance of these alterations in cell populations is yet unclear. In addition to its immunological effects, the alkylating agents exert anti-inflammatory actions.

Dose and Route of Administration
Cyclophosphamide usually is administered in a daily oral dose. The recommended dose is approximately 2 mg per kilogram per day, although the optimal dose in IPF is unknown. Exceeding 200 mg per day is not recommended, and most of patients at National Jewish Center for Immunology and Respiratory Disease take doses of 100 to 150 mg/day. Therapy usually is initiated at 50 mg/day of cyclophosphamide orally, for 1 week. Thereafter, the dose is increased each 7 to 10 days by 25 mg until a maximum dose of 100 to 150 mg per day is reached. The white blood cell count should be monitored each week for the first 4 to 6 weeks or until 2 weeks after a stable dose is achieved. It sometimes can be monitored every 2 or 3 weeks thereafter as long as the white blood cell count is > 4000. In the event leukopenia (WBC < 3000) occurs the cyclophosphamide

should be discontinued for several days (usually 5 to 7 days) until the white blood cell count recovers to a level > 4000. Then the drug is reintroduced at a lower dose to maintain this WBC level. Urinalysis should be performed every 6 to 8 weeks to monitor for signs of bladder irritation, i.e. occult hematuria. Increased fluid intake, 8 glasses of water or more per day, and frequent bladder emptying are recommended to pre-vent hemorrhagic cystitis. A trial of at least 3 to 6 months is needed to ensure an adequate opportunity for clinical response.

Periodic parenteral pulse therapy with cyclophosphamide has not been sufficiently assessed in IPF, although it has been efficacious in some other clinical processes with immune-inflammatory mechanisms such as systemic lupus erythematosis.[30] Parenteral cyclophosphamide therapy has been given in combination with parenteral corticosteroids as the initial treatment in patients with rapidly progressive and severe courses of IPF.[22] A single daily dose of approximately 2 mg per kilogram (based on ideal body weight) is administered intravenously over 30 to 60 minutes, with a 250 to 500 ml fluid bolus. As in parenteral methylprednisolone therapy, we recommend that this treatment be given for 3 to 5 days to see if it initiates a reduction in symptoms and improvement in gas exchange. Although no controlled clinical trials of parenteral cyclophosphamide or methylprednisolone for IPF exist, this approach is suggested in the subset of IPF patients with rapidly progressive and severe disease since survival in this group of patients is short unless the deterioration can be halted.

Side Effects/Complications[22]
Hematologic alterations are common and frequently require dose adjustment. Leukopenia, anemia and thrombocytopenia are the most commonly reported hematologic toxicities. In some cases, the hematologic effects of cyclophosphamide may persist for several months despite discontinuance of the drug. In pulse therapy with cyclophosphamide the nadir for leukocyte counts usually occurs 8 to 12 days after dosing and returns to normal in 2 to 3 weeks. Bacterial and opportunistic infections can occur during treatment, and while often these infectious complications are associated with leukopenia, they can occur in the absence of peripheral blood abnormalities. Herpes zoster is also frequently reported during cyclophosphamide therapy. Urologic complications of hemorrhagic cystitis and carcinoma of the bladder are known, although these are thought to be less common in the dose range utilized in IPF as compared to the higher dosages recommended in chemotherapeutic regimens. Infertility in males may occur and is potentially irreversible. Ovarian failure and amenorrhea is a well-documented complication of cyclophosphamide with ovarian fibrosis and follicular destruction. Because of potential teratogenic effects, all possible efforts should be made to avoid conception in a woman receiving cyclophosphamide. Gastrointestinal symptoms of stomatitis, nausea, and diarrhea may occur. Hepatotoxicity with cholestasis is a rare complication. Several of our patients have complained of extreme fatigue while taking cyclophosphamide, sometimes requiring withdrawal of the drug. Therapy with cyclophosphamide is reported to increase the risk of subsequent malignancy. Several reports

suggest that both total dose and duration of treatment likely impact on the risk of malignancy. Side effects and complications have prompted permanent discontinuance of cyclophosphamide in very few of our patients.

AZATHIOPRINE
Azathioprine (Imuran) has been used to treat pulmonary fibrosis with limited effectiveness (most often used in combination with low dose corticosteroids).[37–42]

Mechanism of Action
Azathioprine has cytotoxic effects and has also been reported to suppress natural killer cell activity, antibody production, and antibody-dependent cellular cytotoxicity.

Dose and Route of Administration
The recommended dose for azathioprine in IPF is 1 to 2 mg per kilogram, although the optimal dose for treatment of IPF is as yet undetermined. The authors generally do not recommend exceeding 200 mg per day. As in cyclophosphamide therapy, we recommend a trial of at least 3 to 6 months duration to ensure an adequate opportunity for clinical response.

Side Effects/Complications
It is estimated that significant adverse drug reactions resulting in discontinuance of azathioprine occur in 20 to 30 percent of patients. Gastrointestinal complaints are the most frequent side effects including nausea and vomiting, and less commonly peptic ulcer disease and diarrhea. Hematologic adverse effects include leukopenia, anemia, thrombocytopenia, pure red cell aplasia, and pancytopenia. Mild elevation of hepatic enzymes has been described in approximately 5 percent of patients treated with azathioprine, although reports of severe hepatitis, progressive hepatic cirrhosis, and cholestasis are rare. Although normal births have been reported in patients having received azathioprine during pregnancy, there are also reports of significant neonatal complications and chromosomal damage in the offspring of patients treated with azathioprine during pregnancy. There is conflicting data regarding the carcinogenic potential of azathioprine. The risk of malignancy is increased in renal transplant patients treated with azathioprine and corticosteroids.

COLCHICINE
Known as a poison for centuries, the extract of *Colchicum autumnale* has been used in the treatment of gout since the 1700s. The alkaloid, colchicine, was first isolated from colchicum in 1820 and has established itself as a mainstay in the treatment of gout.

Mechanism(s) of Action
By binding to the microtubular protein tubulin, colchicine interferes with the function of the cell's mitotic spindles, leading to arrest of cell division. Colchicine has also been shown to inhibit granulocyte migration and to inhibit the release of several proteins from cells. In addition, it may also interfere with the synthesis and secretion of collagen from fibroblasts and may increase collagen degradation by enhancing the action of collagenase.

The possibility that colchicine may be of therapeutic use in IPF has been suggested by several *in vitro* and animal studies. In 1977, Chuensumran and colleagues[43] reported that colchicine reduced pulmonary protein metabolism and probably reduced collagen synthesis in a paraquat induced model of chronic pneumonitis in the mouse. Dubrawksy and colleagues[44] found that colchicine reduced collagen deposition and improve pressure volume characteristics in rat lung following irradiation. Using a rat bleomycin lung injury model, Zhang and coworkers,[45] found that colchicine administration resulted in decreased fiber deposition and total lung hydroxyproline content. In addition, histopathologic proliferation of fibroblasts were said to have "dropped slightly". Rennard and coworkers[46] demonstrated that colchicine blocked the *in vitro* release of fibronectin and alveolar macrophage derived growth factor (AMDGF) from cultured alveolar macrophages harvested from patients with IPF. Fibronectin and AMDGF are felt to be important modulators of fibroblast proliferation. Colchicine treatment resulted in decreased fibronectin production and increased IL-1 production from alveolar macrophages which were cultured from patients with interstitial lung disease associated with collagen vascular disease.[47]

There has been limited clinical experience with colchicine that might be relevant regarding its potential use in IPF. Colchicine is used in Familial Mediterranean Fever where it prevents acute attacks of fever and polyserositis and the development of amyloidosis.[48] One study also has suggested that colchicine may halt the progression of disease in patients with progressive systemic sclerosis.[49] Colchicine also may be beneficial in reducing mortality in hepatic cirrhosis of various etiologies.[50] Finally, colchicine is known to decrease secretion of neutrophil elastase in vitro and has been shown to result in reduced bronchoalveolar lavage neutrophil elastase concentration in former smokers with COPD.[51] While none of these diseases bear a striking resemblance to IPF, the beneficial effects of colchicine in disorders characterized by inflammation and progressive scarring is perhaps relevant.

The only report on the clinical use of colchicine in patients with IPF was a retrospective case series.[52] There were considerable flaws in the study design (for example, 12 of the 35 subjects were excluded from the study because of lack of follow-up data, the diagnosis of IPF was not confirmed by tissue examination in a substantial proportion of patients, and the patients received multiple treatment regimens). Improved outcome, defined as a decrease in symptoms and a 15 percent increase in vital capacity or diffusing capacity for carbon monoxide, was reported in 5 (20 percent) patients. Three of these received colchicine as sole therapy. Nine patients (40 percent) were regarded as stable, and 9 patients (40 percent) were felt to be worse. One patient was felt to have improvement in her chest X-ray. She had received colchicine as sole therapy. During the follow-up period 6 of the 23 patients died, two of metastatic carcinoma and 4 of progressive respiratory failure. Thus, although the in vitro actions of colchicine suggest that it might be useful in idiopathic pulmonary fibrosis, convincing clinical data are lacking.

Dose and Route of Administration
The authors have used an oral dose of 0.6 mg once or twice daily or a single dose of 1.2 mg daily depending on patient tolerance.

Side Effects/Complications
Few side effects have been encountered in the IPF patients we have treated with colchicine. The most common are usually gastrointestinal and consist of abdominal pain, nausea, vomiting or diarrhea. Prolonged administration may have the potential to cause bone marrow suppression with agranulocytosis, thrombocytopenia, and aplastic anemia. Other reported adverse reactions include peripheral neuritis and myopathy. The possibility of increased colchicine toxicity in the presence of renal or hepatic dysfunction should be considered.

METHOTREXATE
The established clinical use of methotrexate can be divided into two categories: antineoplastic (acute lymphoblastic leukemia in children, trophoblastic tumors in women, osteosarcoma, mycosis fungoides, etc.), and immunosuppressive (rheumatoid arthritis, refractory psoriasis, possibly asthma). There are few published data on the use of methotrexate for interstitial lung disease.[53–57] Scott and Bacon[54] pub-lished an anecdotal report of 3 patients with a clinical diagnosis of fibrosing alveolitis associated with connective tissue disease who were treated with methotrexate. All patients demonstrated improvement in symptoms, two patients had radiologic improvement, and one had improvement in pulmonary function.

Mechanism(s) of Action
Methotrexate is a folic acid analog that inhibits the enzyme dihydrofolate reductase, blocking thymidylate and purine synthesis. Like most antimetabolites methotrexate is particularly toxic for rapidly dividing cells. Its immunosuppressive properties can likely be attributed to inhibition of replication and function of T lymphocytes and possibly B lymphocytes. It may also interfere with neutrophil chemotaxis.

Dose and Route of Administration
Methotrexate often is administered orally or intramuscularly at doses of 15 to 30 mg per week. Oral therapy has been given in the treatment of sarcoidosis (10 mg once a week).[56] We recommend an initial dose of 7.5 mg once weekly, with increments by 2.5 mg every 2 weeks until a maximal dose of 15 mg is achieved, for a 4 to 6 months trial. Serial white blood counts and liver function studies should be obtained at least monthly to monitor for bone marrow suppression and liver toxicity. Liver biopsy has been advocated, even in the absence of liver function abnormalities, when the dose exceeds 1 gram or after 18 months to 2 years of continuous treatment to detect subclinical hepatotoxicity.

Side Effects/Complications
The side effects of methotrexate differ depending on whether it is used in high doses as an antineoplastic or in

lower doses over longer term as an immunosuppressive agent. In lower doses the most serious toxicities are hepatic fibrosis (in up to 10 percent of cases when the dose exceeds 5 g) and interstitial pneumonitis leading to pulmonary fibrosis (in 5 percent of cases). Obviously, this last toxicity can be problematic when treating patients for IPF whose condition worsens. Other toxicities include bone marrow suppression, gastrointestinal distress (nausea), alopecia and skin rash. Methotrexate is markedly teratogenic and may transiently suppress gonadal function. The oncogenic potential of methotrexate remains controversial.

PENICILLAMINE

Penicillamine first was isolated in 1953 from the urine of patients with liver disease who were receiving penicillin. The *D* isomer is used clinically. Several animal studies suggest a possible role for penicillamine in treatment of fibrotic lung disorders.[58–61] Penicillamine improves the degree of cutaneous fibrosis in patients with systemic sclerosis. Its effect on the pulmonary interstitial fibrosis associated with connective tissue disease is unclear. Two retrospective studies compared the outcomes of patients with scleroderma who received penicillamine with those who did not.[62,63] Both studies reported that penicillamine therapy was associated with improvement in DLCO but not in other PFT parameters. In an open trial of penicillamine (750 mg daily) plus prednisone (60 mg daily for 1 month followed by a 6 month taper) in 7 patients with rheumatoid arthritis and interstitial lung disease, there was a significant improvement in vital capacity after one month with no deterioration after a mean follow-up of 48 months.[64] There was also an improvement in CO diffusion. Little information regarding patient characteristics, previous therapy or other measures of disease severity is stated in this report.

The experience with penicillamine in patients with IPF is limited.[65–68] Penicillamine plus prednisolone was superior to prednisolone alone and prednisolone plus azathioprine, based upon improvements in vital capacity and rest and exercise oxygenation.[65] Based upon a report in four patients, it appeared that the addition of azathioprine enhanced the effectiveness of the penicillamine/prednisolone regimen. A pilot study[69] of 18 patients with interstitial lung disease who had failed to respond to high dose corticosteroids or immunosuppressives demonstrated clinical improvement in dyspnea in 5 patients, two remained unchanged, and eleven continued to deteriorate. One patient had improved spirometry. Two patients suffered important side effects (reversible proteinuria and skin rash). Nine patients died during the follow-up period which ranged from 39 to 61 months. Of the nine patients who died, only one had associated connective tissue disease. The median survival of the entire group was 55 months. This compared favorably with that of historical controls (17 months). Chapela and colleagues[70] described their findings in 12 patients with fibrotic lung disease (11 IPF, 1 HSP) who received penicillamine. All were considered "end stage" and were on oxygen therapy. Seven of the twelve had received corticosteroids in the past without improvement. Penicillamine was administered at 300 mg/day for 3 weeks, followed by 600 mg/day. They report that all patients improved clinically and functionally during the first year of treatment. There was moderate improvement in vital capacity and total lung capacity with no change in compliance. In addition there was an increase in Pa_{O_2} at rest and a lesser decrease during exercise. After 2 to 5 year follow-up, 8 patients had died (7 of progressive cardiopulmonary insufficiency and 1 of spontaneous pneumothorax) and 4 continued to improve. Survival rates were improved significantly compared to historic controls with end stage disease. No side effects were noted. Because of the potential side effect, especially nephrotoxicity, temper the use of colchicine in IPF; however, the development of novel lysyl oxidase inhibitors may be an important advance in the management of pulmonary fibrosis.

Mechanism(s) of Action

Penicillamine is a chelator of copper, mercury, zinc and lead, and promotes excretion of these metals in the urine. It is this property that explains its clinical utility in Wilson's disease and heavy metal poisoning. It also is used in patients with cysteinuria because it binds to cysteine, decreasing the formation of cysteine stones. Another established clinical use for penicillamine is in patients with rheumatoid arthritis. The mechanism of action in these patients is unclear. Postulated mechanisms include the inhibition of collagen synthesis by interfering with collagen crosslinking by inhibition of lysyl oxidase, suppression of T-cell function, and reduction in the concentrations of IgM rheumatoid factor.

Dose and Route of Administration

The dosage regimen recommended is that used for the management of rheumatoid arthritis. Treatment is initiated at a single oral dose of 125 mg to 250 mg daily (given 1 to 2 hours apart from food, milk or other medicines) for 4 to 8 weeks. The dose was escalated on a weekly basis to a final dose of 500 mg daily. Higher doses (up to 1000 mg per day) can be tried if well-tolerated by the patient. The medication must be given for a prolonged period before its effectiveness can be determined (4 to 6 months).

Side Effects/Complications

Reported side effects include: nausea, vomiting, diarrhea, dyspepsia, anorexia, transient loss of taste for sweet and salt, cutaneous lesions, hematologic toxicity (leukopenia, aplastic anemia, agranulocytopenia), renal toxicity (reversible proteinuria and hematuria, nephrotic syndrome), myasthenia gravis and bronchoalveolitis. In the past, preparations of penicillamine contained trace amounts of penicillin. While this is no longer the case, some of the reactions which occur may be explained by cross-reactivity with penicillin. Most side effects are experienced during the first 18 months of therapy. Concomitant drug therapy should be closely monitored since adverse reactions may occur.

CYCLOSPORINE

In addition to its use in the prevention of allograft rejection, cyclosporine has been demonstrated to be effective in a variety of T cell mediated disorders, such as uveitis, psoriasis, rheumatoid arthritis, primary biliary cirrhosis. It also has been tried in other fibrotic conditions, for example scleroderma, sarcoidosis.[71–74] Few studies have evaluated the efficacy of cyclosporine in IPF and the results have not been impressive.[73,75,76] A possible benefit from the use of cyclosporine is in IPF patients who are awaiting lung transplantation has been suggested.[75,76] High dose corticosteroid is a relative contraindication to lung transplantation, because of the many associated side effects and the potential for impaired healing of the surgical anastimosis. Unfortunately, in these patients it often is difficult to decrease the dose of corticosteroids to an acceptable level without precipitating a clinical deterioration. The addition of cyclosporine may allow the reduction of corticosteroid without a worsening of the underlying disease.[76]

Mechanism(s) of Action

Cyclosporine exerts an inhibitory effect on T cells. It is known to suppress antibody response to T cell dependent antigens, delayed type hypersensitivity, and allograft rejection. There is apparently no myelotoxicity associated with the therapeutic use of cyclosporine.

Dose and Route of Administration

The optimal dose for cyclosporine is unknown and largely depends upon how well it is tolerated. Oral cyclosporine is usually given at 10 mg per kg per day, lower maintenance doses may be indicated (5 to 8 mg/kg/day). Blood levels are closely monitored in most instances where this drug is used (aim is to achieve specific whole blood 24-hour trough levels of 100 to 200 ng/mL).

Side Effects/Complications

The major adverse reactions are renal dysfunction (which limits it usefulness most frequently), tremor, hirsutism, hypertension, and gum hyperplasia.

POTENTIAL FUTURE THERAPIES FOR PULMONARY FIBROSIS

Antioxidants

It has been suggested that epithelial cell injury in IPF may be caused by oxygen radicals derived from alveolar macrophages and neutrophils.[77–79] Patients with IPF have reduced epithelial lining fluid glutathione levels when compared with normal controls.[80] Glutathione is an effective scavenger of toxic oxidants and suppresses lung fibroblast proliferation in response to mitogens. It also has been shown that increased serum concentrations of the antioxidant enzyme Cu/Zn superoxide dismutase occur in IPF and correlates with disease activity and neutrophil degranulation.[81] Thus, these finding suggest that there may be an oxidant-antioxidant imbalance in the lower respiratory tract of patients with IPF.[78] Taurine (a natural free-amino acid) and niacin also inhibit the development of fibrosis (better than either agent alone) in an animal model.[82] There is little experience with pharmacologic manipulation of the oxidant-antioxidant balance in patients with IPF, but this may be an important direction of future research.[23,83,84]

Cytokine and Growth Factor Inhibitors

The retention of leukocytes in the lung and the generation of fibrogenic cytokines likely play an important role in the ongoing inflammatory and fibrotic process. Recently, reports describe the use of antibodies to interrupt these processes in animal models of lung fibrosis.[85,86] CD-11*a* and CD-11*b* are leukocyte integrins that are involved in leukocyte trafficking and retention in the lung. Piguet and coworkers,[85] reported that anti-CD-11 antibodies prevented collagen deposition in mice treated with intratracheal bleomycin. These antibodies were effective when given on days 20 and 25 after instillation of bleomycin, a time when fibrosis has already become established.

Increased concentrations of interleukin-1 beta (IL-1β) and tumor necrosis factor-alpha (TNF-α) have been identified in lungs of patients with IPF.[87–89] Thus it has been postulated that administration of inhibitors of these mediators may prevent the development or progression of fibrosis and there is some evidence from animal models to support this hypothesis.[90–92] Granulocyte macrophage colony stimulating factor (GM-CSF) increases the production of IL-1 and TNF-α and induces alveolar macrophages to produce increased amounts of IL-1ra (the inhibitor of IL-1).[93] Interestingly, GM-CSF appears to have anti-fibrotic properties. The administration of GM-CSF decreased the amount of fibrosis whereas anti-GMCSF antibodies increased the amount of fibrosis in an animal model of pulmonary fibrosis.[94] Unfortunately, an elegant study demonstrated that fibroblast proliferation and induction of myofibroblast-like cells occurred when low levels of GM-CSF was subcutaneously administered to rats.[95] Interestingly, similar myofibroblast-like cells are found in the lungs of patients with IPF.[96,97]

Transforming growth factor beta (TGF-β) is a cytokine, which is known to induce the proliferation of fibroblasts and stimulate the synthesis of collagen and fibronectin by fibroblasts. TGF-β expression is increased in the lungs of patients with IPF (98–100). Consequently, there is a lot of interest in the potential anti-fibrotic role of anti-TGF-β antibodies. Giri and colleagues[86] demonstrated that antibodies to TGF-β$_1$ and TGF-β$_2$ significantly reduced the accumulation of collagen induced by bleomycin in the lungs of mice. Unfortunately, several problems appear to hamper the possible usefulness of anti-TGF-β antibodies in the treatment of lung fibrosis, for example, all fibrotic processes do not appear to involve TGF-β,[101] and depletion of TGF-β may cause other inflammatory processes.[102]

Other antifibrotic agents are being developed for the treatment of lung fibrosis, for example, Pirfenidone and gamma interferon inducers. Gamma interferon decreases collagen production by fibroblasts in vitro and it has been suggested that its administration or induction may influence collagen production in lung fibrosis.[103,104] Production of gamma interferon is reduced in patient with IPF.[105] However, systemic toxicity appears to limit its potential usefulness.

Angiotensin-Converting Enzyme Inhibitors

It has been demonstrated in a number of animal models that angiotensin-converting enzyme Inhibitors ameliorated the anatomic and biochemical manifestations of lung injury in these models.[106–108] The antifibrotic effect of these compounds is likely unrelated to their ACE inhibitory action. It appears that it is the presence of a thiol group which confers antifibrotic activity as the non-thiol ACE inhibitor CG13945 did not protect from hydroxyproline accumulation.[109] Nguyen and coworkers[110] demonstrated that captopril inhibits the proliferation of human lung fibroblasts in vitro. This inhibitory effect was particularly evident in fibroblasts which had been stimulated with basic fibroblast growth factor (bFGF). As in the radiation studies, it seems to be the thiol group and not the ACE inhibition which inhibits proliferation. Penicillamine and glutathion mimic the effects of captopril but lisinopril, a non-thiol ACE inhibitor, does not. Also, addition of exogenous Angiotensin 2 did not inhibit the captopril effect.[110]

Overall, these findings are intriguing and raise the possibility that new therapies will be developed that will prove beneficial in the therapy of IPF. In particular, aerosolized preparations may avoid some of the systemic problems encountered with the use of current agents.

NONPHARMACOLOGIC THERAPIES

The care of patients with IPF should encompass both pharmacologic and nonpharmacologic approaches. Oxygen supplementation, occupational and physical therapy, and psychosocial support all contribute to the patient's overall functional status and quality of life. Although there are no randomized trials to demonstrate the benefits of supplemental oxygen therapy in patients with IPF we feel that it is reasonable to extrapolate from the proven benefits in hypoxic patients with chronic obstructive pulmonary disease. We use the standard established criteria to determine when to begin patients on supplemental oxygen. Physical and occupational therapy helps to teach patients oxygen conservation strategies, thus allowing them to accomplish more of their activities of daily living with the limited pulmonary function that they have. These patients need encouragement to gradually develop a routine conditioning program to improve muscle strength and cardiovascular efficiency. Daily walks and stationary bicycling can assist in weight control and improve the patient's sense of well-being. Finally, consultation with a mental health care provider may prove beneficial. Many patients with IPF have difficulty dealing with the severity of their illness and the lifestyle changes which become necessary. Anxiety and depression are relatively common in these patients and they may benefit from supportive psychotherapy, relaxation training and/or psychopharmacotherapy.

INDICATIONS FOR LUNG TRANSPLANTATION

Lung transplantation is an important management option for patients with IPF < age 60 (some transplant groups require age < 55), who have experienced progressive phys-iologic deterioration despite the above outlined approaches to drug management.[111] While lung transplant programs vary as to their specific criteria for appropriate patient selection, the following need to be considered: life expectancy, cardiac status, previous chest surgeries, general fitness and nutritional status, other organ disease, immuno-competency, psychologic status, and familial support system. If this option is being considered, the patient should be referred for further evaluation and counseling at a nearby lung transplant center. Early referral (for example when supplemental oxygen at rest or with exercise is required) is important since most patients with IPF die waiting to receive a transplant.

References

1. Crystal RG, Bitterman PB, Rennard SI, Hance AJ, Keogh BA: Interstitial lung diseases of unknown cause. Disorders characterized by chronic inflammation of the lower respiratory tract. *N Engl J Med* 1984; 310:154.
2. Scott J, Johnston I, Britton J: What causes cryptogenic fibrosing alveolitis? A case-control study of environmental exposure to dust. *Br Med J* 1990; 301:1015.
3. Coultas DB, Zumwalt RE, Black WC, Sobonya RE: The epidemiology of interstitial lung disease. *Am J Respir Crit Care Med* 1994; 150:967.
4. Raghu G: Interstitial lung disease: a diagnostic approach. Are CT scan and lung biopsy indicated in every patient? *Am J Respir Crit Care Med* 1995; 151:909.
5. Lynch DA, Rose C, Way DE, King TE Jr: Hypersensitivity pneumonitis: sensitivity of high resolution CT in a population-based study. *Am J Roentgenol* 1992; 159:469.
6. Tung KT, Wells AU, Rubens MB, Kirk JM, du Bois RM, Hansell DM: Accuracy of the typical computed tomographic appearances of fibrosing alveolitis. *Thorax* 1993; 48:334.
7. Lee JS, Im JG, Ahn JM, Kim YM, Han MC: Fibrosing alveolitis: prognostic implication of ground-glass attenuation at high-resolution CT. *Radiology* 1992; 184:451.
8. Terriff BA, Kwan SY, Chan-Yeung MM, Muller NL: Fibrosing alveolitis: chest radiology and CT as predictors of clinical and functional impairment at follow-up in 26 patients. *Radiology* 1992; 184:445.
9. Bessis L, Callard P, Gotheil C, Biaggi A, Grenier P: High-resolution CT of parenchymal lung disease: precise correlation with histologic findings. *Radiographics* 1992; 12:45.
10. Leung AN, Miller RR, Muller NL: Parenchymal opacification in chronic infiltrative lung disease: CT-pathologic correlation. *Radiology* 1993; 188:209.
11. Remy-Jardin M, Remy J, Wallaert B, Bataille D, Hatron PY: Pulmonary involvement in progressive systemic sclerosis: sequential evaluation with CT, pulmonary function tests, and bronchoalveolar lavage. *Radiology* 1993; 188:499.
12. Nishimura K, Kitaichi M, Izumi T, Nagai S, Kanaoka M, Itoh H: Usual interstitial pneumonia: histologic correlation with high-resolution CT. *Radiology* 1992; 182:337.
13. Remy-Jardin M, Giraud F, Remy J, Copin MC, Gosselin B, Duhamel A: Importance of ground-glass attenuation in chronic diffuse infiltrative lung disease: pathologic-CT correlation. *Radiology* 1993; 189:693.
14. Wells AU, Hansell DM, Rubens MB, Cullinan P, Black CM, du Bois RM: The predictive value of appearances on thin-section computed tomography in fibrosing alveolitis. *Am Rev Respir Dis* 1993; 148:1076.

15. Akira M, Sakatani M, Ueda E: Idiopathic pulmonary fibrosis: progression of honeycombing at thin-section CT. *Radiology* 1993; 189:687.

16. Wells AU, Rubens MB, du Bois RM, Hansell DM: Serial CT in fibrosing alveolitis: prognostic significance of the initial pattern. *AJR* 1993; 161:1159.

17. Fulmer JD, Roberts WC, von Gal ER, Crystal RG: Morphologic-physiologic correlates of the severity of fibrosis and degree of cellularity in idiopathic pulmonary fibrosis. *J Clin Invest* 1979; 63:665.

18. Turner-Warwick M, Burrows B, Johnson A: Cryptogenic fibrosing alveolitis: clinical features and their influence on survival. *Thorax* 1980; 35:171.

19. Tukiaininen P, Taskinen E, Holsti P, Korhola O, Valle M: Prognosis of cryptogenic fibrosing alveolitis. *Thorax* 1983; 38:349.

20. Newman SL, Michel RP, Wang NS: Lingular lung biopsy: is it representative? *Am Rev Respir Dis* 1985; 132:1084.

21. Watters LC, Schwarz MI, Cherniack RM, Waldron JA, Dunn TL, Stanford RE, King TE Jr: Idiopathic pulmonary fibrosis: Pretreatment bronchoalveolar lavage cellular constituents and their relationships with lung histopathology and clinical response to therapy. *Am Rev Respir Dis* 1987; 135:696.

22. Mortenson RL, King TE Jr: Idiopathic pulmonary fibrosis, in Lichtenstein, LM, Fauci AS (eds): *Current Therapy in Allergy, Immunology, and Rheumatology,* St. Louis, B.C. Decker, Inc., 1992; pp 233.

23. Hunninghake GW, Kalica AR: Approaches to the treatment of pulmonary fibrosis. *Am J Respir Crit Care Med* 1995; 151:915.

24. Schwartz DA, Helmers RA, Galvin JR, Van Fossen DS, Frees KL, Dayton CS, Burmeister LF, Hunninkhake GW: Determinants of survival in idiopathic pulmonary fibrosis. *Am J Respir Crit Care Med* 1994; 149:450.

25. van Oortegem K, Wallaert B, Marquette CH, Ramon P, Perez T, Lafitte JJ, Tonnel AB: Determinants of response to immunosuppressive therapy in idiopathic pulmonary fibrosis. *Eur Respir J* 1994; 7:1950.

26. Agusti C, Xaubet A, Agusti AGN, Roca J, Ramirez J, Rodriguez-Roisin R: Clinical and functional assessment of patients with idiopathic pulmonary fibrosis: results of a 3 year follow-up. *Eur Respir J* 1994; 7:643.

27. Schwartz, DA, Van Fossen DS, Davis CS, Helmers RA, Dayton CS, Burmeister LF, Hunninkhake GW: Determinants of progression in idiopathic pulmonary fibrosis. *Am J Respir Crit Care Med* 1994; 149:444.

28. Panos RJ, Mortenson R, Niccoli SA, King TE Jr: Clinical deterioration in patients with idiopathic pulmonary fibrosis. Causes and assessment. *Am J Med* 1990; 88:396.

29. Schreiner R, Mortenson RL, Ikle D, King TE Jr: Interstitial Lung Disease in the Elderly, in Mahler D (eds): *Pulmonary Disease in the Elderly,* New York, Marcel Dekker, Inc, 1993; pp 339. (Lenfant C, ed. Lung Biology in Health and Disease).

30. Baughman RP, Lower EE: Use of intermittent, intravenous cyclophosphamide for idiopathic pulmonary fibrosis. *Chest* 1992; 102:1090.

31. Fort JG, Scovern H, Abruzzo JL: Intravenous cyclophosphamide and methylprednisolone for the treatment of bronchiolitis obliterans and interstitial fibrosis associated with crysotherapy. *J Rheumatol* 1988; 15:850.

32. Johnson MA, Kwan S, Snell NJC, Nunn AJ, Darbyshire JH, Turner-Warwick M: Randomized controlled trial comparing prednisolone alone with cyclophosphamide and low dose prednisolone in combination in cryptogenic fibrosing alveolitis. *Thorax* 1989; 44:280.

33. Meuret G, Fueter R, Gloor F: Early stage of fulminant idiopathic pulmonary fibrosis cured by intense combination therapy using cyclophosphamide, vincristine, and prednisone. *Respiration* 1978; 36:228.

34. Patel AR, Shah PC, Rhee HZ, Sassoun H: Cyclophosphamide therapy and interstitial pulmonary fibrosis. *Cancer* 1976; 38:1542.

35. Silver RM, Warrick JH, Kinsella MB, Staudt LS, Bauman MH, Strange C: Cyclophosphamide and low-dose prednisone therapy in patients with systemic sclerosis (scleroderma) with interstitial lung disease. *J Rheumatol* 1993; 20:838.

36. van de Laar MA, Westerman CJ, Wagenaar SS, Dinant HJ: Beneficial effect of intravenous cyclophosphamide and oral prednisone on D-penicillamine-associated bronchiolitis obliterans. *Arthritis Rheum* 1985; 28:93.

37. Weese WC, Levine BW, Kazemi H: Interstitial lung disease resistant to corticosteroid therapy Report of three cases treated with azathioprine or cyclophosphamide. *Chest* 1975; 67:57.

38. Matthay RA, Hudson LD, Petty TL: Acute lupus oneumonitis: response to azathioprine therapy. *Chest* 1973; 69:117.

39. Cegla UH, Kroidl RF, Meier-Sydow J, Thiel C, Czarnecki GV: Therapy of the idiopathic fibrosis of the lung. Experiences with three therapeutic principles corticosteroids in combination with azathioprine, D-penicillamine, and para-amino-benzoate. *Pneumonologie* 1975; 152:75.

40. Winterbauer RH, Hammar SP, Hallman KO, Hays JE, Pardee NE, Morgan EH, Allen JD, Moores KD, Bush W, Walker JH: Diffuse interstitial pneumonitis Clinicopathologic correlations in 20 patients treated with prednizone/azathioprine. *Am J Med* 1978; 65:661.

41. Rowen AJ, Reichel J: Dermatomyositis with lung involvement, successfully treated with azathioprine. *Respiration* 1983; 44:143.

42. Raghu G, Depaso WJ, Cain K, Hammar SP, Wetzel CE, Dreis DF, Hutchinson J, Pardee NE, Winterbauer RH: Azathioprine combined with prednisone in the treatment of idiopathic pulmonary fibrosis: a prospective, double-blind randomized, placebo-controlled clinical trial. *Am Rev Respir Dis* 1991; 144:291.

43. Chuensumran O, Khurana ML, Varshney S, Niden AH: Effect of colchicine on pulmonary collagen cynthesis In vivo. *Am Rev Respir Dis* 1977; 115:315.

44. Dubrawsky C, Dubravsky NB, Withers HR: The effect of colchicine on the Accumulation of Hydroxyproline and on lung compliance after irradiation. *Rad Res* 1978; 73:111.

45. Zhang L, Zhu Y, Luo W: The protective effect of colchicine on bleomycin-induced pulmonary fibrosis in rats. *Chin Med Sci J* 1992; 7:58.

46. Rennard SI, Bitterman PB, Ozaki T, Rom WN, Crystal RG: Colchicine suppresses the release of fibroblast growth factors from alveolar macrophages in vitro The basis of a possible therapeutic approach to the fibrotic disorders. *Am Rev Respir Dis* 1988; 137:181.

47. Saito Y: The effects of various drugs and immune complexes on the function of alveolar macrophages from patients with collagen-vascular diseases with interstitial pneumonia. *Arerugi* 1990; 39:532.

48. Zemer D, Pras M, Sohar E, Modan M, Cabili S, Gafni J: Colchicine in the prevention and treatment of the amyloidosis of familial Mediterranean fever. *N Engl J Med* 1986; 314:1001.

49. Alarcon-Segovia D, Ramos-Niembro F, Ibanez de Kasep G, Alcocer J, Tamayo RP: Long-term evaluation of colchicine in the treatment of scleroderma. *J Rheumatol* 1979; 6:705.

50. Kershenobich D, Vargas F, Garcia-Tsao G, Perez Tamayo R, Gent M, M. R.: Colchicine in the treatment of cirrhosis of the liver. *N Engl J Med* 1988; 318:1709.

51. Cohen AB, Girard W, Mclarty J, Starcher B, Davis D, Stevens M, Rosenbloom J, Kucich U: A controlled trial of colchicine to reduce the elastase load in the lungs of ex-cigarette smokers

with chronic obstructive pulmonary disease. *Am Rev Respir Dis* 1991; 143:1038.

52. Peters SG, McDougall JC, Douglas WW, Coles DT, DeRemee RA: Colchicine in the treatment of pulmonary fibrosis. *Chest* 1993; 103:101.

53. Lacher MJ: Spontaneous remission response to methotrexate in sarcoidosis. *Ann Intern Med* 1968; 69:1247.

54. Scott DGI, Bacon PA: Response to methotrexate in fibrosing alveolitis associated with connective tissue disease. *Thorax* 1980; 35:725.

55. Lower EE, Baughman RP: The use of low dose methotrexate in refractory sarcoidosis. *Am J Med Sci* 1990; 299:153.

56. Baughman RP, Lower EE: The effect of corticosteroid or methotrexate on lung lymphocytes and macrophages in sarcoidosis. *Am Rev Respir Dis* 1990; 142:1268.

57. Lower EE, Baughman RP, Winget D: The long term use of methotrexate in patients with chronic symptomatic sarcoidosis. *Sarcoidosis* 1992; 9:465.

58. Ward WF, Shih-Heollwarth A, Tuttle RD: Collagen Accumulation in Irradiated Rat Lung: Modification by D-Penicillamine. *Radiology* 1983; 146:533.

59. Ekimoto H, Aikawa M, Ohnuki T: Immunological Involvement in Pulmonary Fibrosis Induced by Peplomycin. *Jour Antibio* 1985; 38:94.

60. Molteni A, Ward WF, Ts'ao C: Monocrotaline-Induced Pulmonary Fibrosis in Rats: Amelioration by Captotril and Penicillamine. *Proc Soc Exper Bio & Med* 1985; 180:112.

61. Geismar LS, Hennessey SH, Reiser KM, Last JA: D-Penicillamine prevents collagen accumulation in lungs of rats given bleomycin. *Chest* 1986; 89:153.

62. Steen VD, Owens GR, Redmond C, Rodnan GP, Medsger TAJ: The effect of D-penicillamine on pulmonary findings in systemic sclerosis. *Arthritis Rheum* 1985; 28:882.

63. DeClerk LS, Dequeker J, Francx L, Demedts M: D-Penicillamine Therapy and Interstitial Lung Disease in Scleroderma: A Long-Term Followup Study. *Arth & Rheum* 1987; 30:643.

64. van der Schee AC, Dinkla BA, Festen JJM: Penicillamine for Interstitial Lung Disease in Rheumatoid Arthritis. 1989; 56:134.

65. Cegla UH: Treatment of idiopathic fibrosing alveolitis. Therapeutic experiences with azathioprine-prednisolone and D-Penicillamine-prednisolone combination therapy. *Schw Med Woch* 1977; 107:184.

66. Goodman M, Turner-Warwick M: Pilot study of penicillamine therapy in corticosteroid failure patients with widespread pulmonary fibrosis. *Chest* 1978; 74:338.

67. Meier-Sydow J, Rust M, Kronenberger H, Thiel C, Amthor M, Riemann H: Long-term follow-up of lung function parameters in patients with idiopathic pulmonary fibrosis treated with prednisone and azathioprine or D-penicillamine. *Prax Pneumol* 1979; 33:680.

68. Liebetrau G, Pielesch W, Ganguin HG, Jung A, Jung H: Therapy of pulmonary fibrosis with D-penicillamine. *Z Gesamte Inn Med* 1982; 37:263.

69. Goodman M, Knight RK, Turner-Warwick M: Modulation of autoimmunity and disease. *Prague Praeger* 1981; 1981:291.

70. Chapela R, Zuniga G, Selman M: D-Penicillamine in the therapy of fibrotic lung diseases. *Int Jour Clin Pharm Ther Tox* 1986; 24:16.

71. Worle B, Hein R, Krieg T, Meurer M: Cyclosporin in localized and systematic scleroderma. A clinical study. *Dermatologica* 1990; 181:215.

72. Alegre J, Teran J, Alvarez B, Viejo JL: Successful use of cyclosporine for the treatment of aggressive pulmonary fibrosis in a patient with rheumatoid arthritis. *Arth & Rheum* 1990; 33:1594.

73. Moolman JA, Bardin PG, Rossouw DJ, Joubert JR: Cyclosporin as a treatment for interstitial lung disease of unknown aetiology. *Thorax* 1991; 46:592.

74. Baughman RP, Lower EE, Lynch JP III: Treatment modalities for sarcoidosis. *Clin Pulm Med* 1994; 1:223.

75. Alton EW, Johnson M, Turner-Warwick M: Advanced cryptogenic fibrosing alveolitis: preliminary report on treatment with cyclosporin A. *Respir Med* 1989; 83:277.

76. Venuta F, Rendina EA, Ciriaco P, De Giacomo T, Pompeo E, Bachetoni A, Ricci C: Efficacy of cyclosporin to reduce steroids in patients with idiopathic pulmonary fibrosis before lung transplantation. *J Heart Lung Transplant* 1993; 12:909.

77. Cantin AM, North SL, Fells GA, Hubbard RC, Crystal RG: Oxidant-mediated epithelial cell injury in idiopathic pulmonary fibrosis. *J Clin Invest* 1987; 79:1665.

78. Cantin AM, Larivee P, Begin RO: Extracellular glutathione suppresses human lung fibroblast proliferation. *Am Jour Resp Cell & Molec Bio* 1990; 3:79.

79. McLaughlin GE, Frank L: Effects of the 21-aminosteroid, U74389F, on Bleomycin-induced Pulmonary Fibrosis in Rats. *Crit Care Med* 1994; 22:313.

80. Cantin AM, Hubbard RC, Crystal RG: Glutathione deficiency in the epithelial lining fluid of the lower respiratory tract in idiopathic pulmonary fibrosis. *Am Rev Respir Dis* 1989; 139:370.

81. Borzi RM, Grigolo B, Meliconi R, Fasano L, Sturani C, Fabbri M, Porstmann T, Facchini A: Elevated serum superoxide dismutase levels correlate with disease severity and neutrophil degranulation in idiopathic pulmonary fibrosis. *Clinical Sci* 1993; 85:353.

82. Wang QJ, Giri SN, Hyde DM, Li C: Amelioration of bleomycin-induced pulmonary fibrosis in hamsters by combined treatment with taurine and niacin. *Biochem Pharmacol* 1991; 42:1115.

83. Borok Z, Buhl R, Grimes GJ, Bokser AD, Hubbard RC, Holroyd KJ, Roum JH, Czerski DB, Cantin AM, Crystal RG: Effect of glutathione aerosol on oxidant-antioxidant imbalance in idiopathic pulmonary fibrosis. *Lancet* 1991; 338:215.

84. Meyer A, Buhl R, Magnussen H: The effect of oral N-acetylcysteine on lung glutathione levels in idiopathic pulmonary fibrosis. *Eur Respir J* 1994; 7:431.

85. Piguet PF, Rosen H, Vesin C, Grau GE: Effective treatment of the pulmonary fibrosis elicited in mice by bleomycin or silica with anti-CD 11 antibiotics. *Am Rev Resp Dis* 1993; 147:435.

86. Giri SN, Hyde DM, Hollinger MA: Effect of antibody to transforming growth factor beta on bleomycin induced accumulation of lung collagen in mice. *Thorax* 1993; 48:959.

87. Zhang Y, Lee TC, Guillemin B, Yu MC, Rom WN: Enhanced IL-1 beta and tumor necrosis factor-alpha release and messenger RNA expression in macrophages from idiopathic pulmonary fibrosis or after asbestos exposure. *J Immunol* 1993; 150:4188.

88. Piguet PF, Ribaux C, Karpuz V, Grau GE, Kapanci Y: Expression and localization of tumor necrosis factor-alpha and its mRNA in idiopathic pulmonary fibrosis. *Am J Pathol* 1993; 143:651.

89. Nash JR, McLaughlin PJ, Butcher D, Corrin B: Expression of tumour necrosis factor-alpha in cryptogenic fibrosing alveolitis. *Histopathology* 1993; 22:343.

90. Piguet PF, Collart MA, Grau GE, Sappino AP, Vassalli P: Requirement of tumor necrosis factor for the development of silica-induced pulmonary fibrosis. *Nature* 1990; 344:245.

91. Piguet PF, Vesin C, Grau GE, Thompson RC: Interleukin 1 receptor antagonist (IL-1ra) prevents or cures pulmonary fibrosis elicited in mice by bleomycin or silica. *Cytokine* 1993; 5:57.

92. Piguet PF, Vesin C: Treatment by human recombinant soluble TNF receptor of pulmonary fibrosis induced by bleomycin or silica in mice. *Eur Respir J* 1994; 7:515.

93. Janson RW, King TE Jr, Hance KR, Arend WP: Enhanced production of IL-1 receptor antagonist by alveolar macrophages

from patients with interstitial lung disease. *Am Rev Respir Dis* 1993; 148:495.

94. Piguet PF, Grau GE, de Kossodo S: Role of granulocyte-macrophage colony-stimulating factor in pulmonary fibrosis induced in mice by bleomycin. *Exp Lung Res* 1993; 19:579.

95. Rubbia-Brandt L, Sappino AP, Gabbiani G: Locally applied GM-CSF induces the accumulation of alpha-smooth muscle actin containing myofibroblasts. *Virchows Arch B Cell Pathol Incl Mol Pathol* 1991; 60:73.

96. Leslie KO, King TE Jr, Low RB: Smooth muscle actin is expressed by airspace fibroblast-like cells in idiopathic pulmonary fibrosis and hypersensitivity pneumonitis. *Chest* 1991; 99:47.

97. Ohta K, Mortenson RL, Clark RAF, Hirose N, King TE Jr: Immunohistochemical identification and characterization of smooth muscle cells in idiopathic pulmonary fibrosis. *Am J Respir Crit Care Med* 1995; 152:1659.

98. Khalil N, Bereznay O, Sporn M, Greenburg AH: Macrophage production of transforming growth factor β and fibroblast collagen synthesis in chronic pulmonary inflammation. *J Exp Med* 1989; 70:727.

99. Broekelmann TJ, Limper AH, Colby TV, McDonald JA: Transforming growth factor beta 1 is present at sites of extracellular matrix gene expression in human pulmonary fibrosis. *Proc Natl Acad Sci USA* 1991; 88:6642.

100. Khalil N, O'Connor RN, Unruh HW, Warren PW, Flanders KC, Kemp A, Bereznay OH, Greenburg AH: Increased production and immunohistochemical localization of transforming growth factor-beta in idiopathic pulmonary fibrosis. *Am J Respir Cell Mol Biol* 1991; 5:155.

101. Moreland LW, Goldsmith KT, Russell WJ, Young KR Jr, Garver RI Jr: Transforming growth factor beta within fibrotic scleroderma lungs. *Am J Med* 1992; 93:628.

102. Shull MM, Ormsby I, Kier AB, Pawlowski S, Diebold RJ, Yin M, Allen R, Sidman C, Proetzel G, Calvin D, et al.: Targeted disruption of the mouse transforming growth factor-beta 1 gene results in multifocal inflammatory disease. *Nature* 1992; 359:693.

103. Okada T, Sugie I, Aisaka K: Effects of gamma-interferon on collagen and histamine content in bleomycin-induced lung fibrosis in rats. *Lymphokine Cytokine Res* 1993; 12:87.

104. Zia S, Hyde DM, Giri SN: Effects of an interferon inducer bropirimine on bleomycin-induced lung fibrosis in hamsters. *Pharmacol Toxicol* 1992; 71:11.

105. Prior C, Haslam PL: In vivo levels and in vitro production of interferon-gamma in fibrosing interstitial lung diseases. *Clin Exp Immunol* 1992; 88:280.

106. Molteni A, Ward WF, Ts'ao C, Solliday NH: Moncrotaline-induced cardiopulmonary damage in rats: amelioration by the angiotensin-converting enzyme inhibitor CL242817 (42370). *Proc Soc Exper Bio & Med* 1986; 182:483.

107 Ward WF, Molteni A, Ts'ao C: Radiation-induced endothelial dysfunction and fibrosis in rat lung: modification by the angiotensin coverting enzyme inhibitor CS 242817. *Rad Res* 1989; 117:342.

108. Ward WF, Molteni A, Ts'ao C, Hinz JM: Captopril Reduces Collagen and Mast Cell Accumulation in Irradiated Rat Lung. *Int Jour Rad Onc Bio Phys* 1990; 19:1405.

109. Ward WF, Molteni A, Ts'ao C, Hinz JM: Radiation Pneumotoxicity in Rats: Modification by Inhibitors of Angiotensin Converting Enzyme. *Int Jour Rad Onc Bio Phys* 1992; 22:623.

110. Nguyen L, Ward WF, Ts'ao C, Molteni A: Captopril inhibits proliferation of human lung fibroblasts in culture: a potential antifibrotic mechanism. *Proc Soc Exper Bio & Med* 1994; 205:80.

111. Kaiser LR, Cooper JD: The current status of lung transplantation. *Advances in Surgery* 1992; 25:259.

Chapter 111, Part 1

CONNECTIVE TISSUE DISORDERS INVOLVING THE LUNG–ETIOLOGY, PATHOGENESIS, AND DIAGNOSIS

REBECCA L. MORTENSON AND THOMAS CORBRIDGE

Rheumatoid Arthritis

Systemic Lupus Erythematosus

Progressive Systemic Sclerosis

Polymyositis/Dermatomyositis

Sjogren's Syndrome

Mixed Connective Tissue Disease

Ankylosing Spondylitis

Psoriatic Arthritis

Behcet's Disease

Relapsing Polychondritis

The connective tissue disorders are a heterogeneous group of diseases characterized by immune-inflammatory-mediated aberrancies of multiple organ systems. These disorders frequently exhibit pulmonary manifestations, which may specifically involve airways, vasculature, alveoli, interstitium, or pleura.

Rheumatoid Arthritis

Rheumatoid arthritis (RA) is a systemic disease characterized by an inflammatory destructive synovitis of disarthrodial joints. A subpopulation of rheumatoid patients, including those of the male sex, and those with severe destructive arthritis, highly increased rheumatoid factors, subcutaneous nodules or other extra-articular rheumatoid manifestations, is at greater risk of lung involvement. The pleuropulmonary manifestations of RA are many and complex, involving multiple sites within the chest: lung parenchyma, tracheobronchial tree, pleura, pulmonary vasculature, and larynx. Drug treatment of RA also may induce lung disease that is difficult to distinguish from the underlying disorder itself. Unlike many of the other connective tissue diseases involving the lung, the pleuropulmonary

manifestations of RA have been relatively well-defined (Table 111-1).

INTERSTITIAL LUNG DISEASE

The observed frequency of interstitial lung disease in RA ranges from 20 percent to 40 percent. The wide variability in this range relates to differences in selected methods of detection (clinical, physiologic, radiologic, or histopathologic). Furthermore, many studies have not controlled for the potential impact of drug and occupational exposures. The prevalence of interstitial lung disease correlates with increased titers of rheumatoid factor, the presence of other extra-pulmonary manifestations of disease, and the severity and duration of arthritis. Pulmonary fibrosis precedes the onset of arthritis in 10% to 15% of cases. Interstitial fibrosis occurs more commonly in men despite the known predilection of RA for women.

Dry cough or dyspnea on exertion are the most common presenting symptoms, although immobility of patients from joint involvement often delays patient awareness of the latter. Physical signs of interstitial lung disease usually are limited to tachypnea and bibasilar inspiratory crackles. In some cases, physical signs may be quite subtle or absent. With

TABLE 111B-1 Pleuropulmonary Manifestations of Connective Tissue Disorders. RA, rheumatoid arthritis; SLE, systemic lupus erythematosus; PSS, progressive systemic sclerosis; PM-DM, polymyositis-dermatomyositis; SS, Sjogren's syndrome; MCTD, mixed connective tissue disease; AS, ankylosing spondylitis; PA, psoriatic arthritis; RP, relapsing polychondritis. UIP, usual interstitial pneumonitis; LIP, lymphocyte interstitial pneumonitis; BOOP, bronchiolitis obliterans organizing pneumonia; DAD, diffuse alveolar damage; AIP, acute interstitial pneumonitis; PAH, primary arterial hypertension; Dz, disease.

	RA	SLE	PSS	PM-DM	SS
ILD/Intra-alveolar Dz					
UIP	++	Rare (chronic interstitial pneumonitis)	+++	++	++
LIP					+
BOOP	+			+	+
DAD				+	+
AIP		+			
Alveolar Hemorrhage	Rare	+	Rare		
Pleural Dz	++	++	+	+	+
Airways Dz					
Upper Airways Dz	++	+			
Bronchitis	++				+++
Bronchiectasis	Rare				Rare
Bronchiolitis Obliterans	+	? (one case report)			+
Follicular Bronchiolitis	+				+++
Pulmonary Vascular Dz					
Vasculitis	Rare	+	Rare	Rare	Rare
PAH	+	Rare	++	Rare	Rare
Aspiration			++ (esophageal dysfunction)	++ (pharyngeal dysfunction)	
Respiratory Muscle Dysfunction		++ Diaphragm dysfunction; atelectasis		+++	
Malignancy			+ (lung Ca)	++	+ (lymphoreticular malignancies)
Other	Apical fibrobullous disease (rare)			Pulmonary alveolar proteinosis (rare)	

	MCTD	AS	PA	Behcets	RP
ILD/Intraalveolar Dz					
UIP	++				
LIP					
BOOP					
DAD					
AIP					
Alveolar Hemorrhage	Rare				
Pleural Dz	+	+			
Airways Dz					
Upper Airways Dz		+			++ (Laryngotracheal chondritis)
Bronchitis					++ (Bronchial chondritis & stenosis)
Bronchectasis					
Pulmonary Vascular Dz				+ (venous thrombosis; aneurysms)	
Vasculitis	+			+	
PAH	++				
Aspiration	++				
Respiratory Muscle Dysfunction	+ (Diaphragm dysfunction)				
Malignancy					
Other		Rare Apical fibrobullous dz; atypical mycobacterial infection; Aspergillomas	Apical fibrobullous dz		

more advanced pulmonary fibrosis, cyanosis, and signs of pulmonary hypertension may be present. Clubbing occurs in up to 75 percent of patients. Pulmonary function testing reveals a restrictive ventilatory defect with reduction in diffusing capacity. As in idiopathic pulmonary fibrosis, chest roentgenograms generally reveal peripheral and lower zone reticular or reticulonodular opacities, sometimes with superimposed areas of hazy, alveolar opacities. Honeycombing often is seen with disease progression. Pleural disease is a frequently associated finding, occurring in approximately 20 percent of patients with pulmonary fibrosis. Histopathologically, the interstitial lung disease seen in association with RA generally is indistinguishable from usual interstitial pneumonitis, unless there are detectable features of lymphocytic infiltration with lymphoid germinal follicles surrounding bronchovascular bundles ("follicular bronchiolitis"), pleural fibrosis, or rheumatoid nodules.

The pathogenesis of pulmonary fibrosis in RA remains unclear, but numerous immune and cellular events have been clarified in recent investigations.[1,2] Activated macrophages elaborating superoxide anion, neutrophil chemotactic factor, fibronectin, as well as increased concentration of neutrophils have been confirmed in bronchoalveolar lavage fluid of patients with RA-associated pulmonary fibrosis, but not in patients with RA alone.[3] Proteinases, such as neutrophil collagenase, are increased in BAL fluid in patients with pulmonary fibrosis. This, combined with the known high incidence of nonhomozygous M_1 alpha$_1$ antiprotease phenotypes in patients with RA and pulmonary fibrosis[4,5] suggests that protease and antiprotease imbalance are important in the development or perpetuation of lung injury and subsequent fibrosis. Other mediators of the inflammatory response such as interleukin-1, interferon-alpha, interferon-gamma, and macrophage derived growth factor have also been implicated in the development if the fibrotic response in RA.[6]

The presence of pulmonary fibrosis in RA contributes to a poorer prognosis with increased morbidity and mortality. Although the course of the disease is often variable, the majority of patients experience slow progression. A small, but definite, subpopulation exhibits fulminant progression.

BRONCHIOLITIS OBLITERANS ORGANIZING PNEUMONITIS

Bronchiolitis obliterans organizing pneumonitis (BOOP) is a well documented complication of RA. In a recent study of histopathology in RA-associated interstitial lung disease, the prevalence of BOOP was slightly greater than that of fibrosing alveolitis (usual interstitial pneumonitis).[7,8,9] Patients typically present with a subacute, flu-like illness characterized by increasing shortness of breath, cough, malaise, and fever. Physical exam findings include crackles and rarely wheezes on lung auscultation. The chest radiograph often reveals bilateral diffuse alveolar opacities (classically in with a peripheral distribution). Migrating infiltrates have also been described.[9] The clinical presentation is frequently misdiagnosed as infectious pneumonia, for which antibiotic therapy is prescribed without benefit for variable periods of time before a definitive tissue diagnosis is obtained. While

there is evidence that BOOP associated with connective tissue disorders has a poorer prognosis than idiopathic BOOP (better termed cryptogenic organizing pneumonitis), the large majority of patients respond well to corticosteroid therapy. This suggests that early determination of the specific histologic findings in patients with RA-associated interstitial lung disease may better determine prognosis and management.

AIRWAY DISEASE

Several studies have indicated a high prevalence of obstructive lung disease in patients with RA (ranging from 20 to 40 percent of patients).[10,11] Although the spectrum of histopathologic lesions underlying airflow obstruction has not been described fully, it generally is accepted that patients with RA are at greater risk for the development of bronchiolitis obliterans and bronchiectasis.

Bronchiolitis obliterans (or constrictive bronchiolitis) leading to progressive obstructive airflow limitation and hypoxemia is an unusual but devastating occurrence in RA. Reports have suggested an association with the use of D-penicillamine.[12] Symptoms include worsening dyspnea and dry cough. Lung ausculatory findings include inspiratory crackles or a mid-inspiratory squeak. Chest roentgenograms and CT scans are usually normal, although they may demonstrate lung hyperinflation. Lung biopsy usually confirms the diagnosis, revealing lymphoplasmocytic infiltration of bronchiolar walls with associated granulation tissue leading to constriction and obliteration of airway lumens. Unfortunately, bronchodilator and immunosuppressive treatment generally is ineffective, and prognosis is poor with death ensuing within months to a few years after recognition of the diagnosis.

Respiratory tract infection is common in patients with RA, contributing to morbidity and the cause of death in 15 to 19 percent of patients.[13] The reasons underlying increased risk of infection are not known. Bronchiectasis occurs infrequently in patients with RA. Whether it occurs as a primary manifestation of RA, or rather as a result of recurrent infections, is unclear. When present, bronchiectasis usually is found in patients with severe, long-standing disease, although there are rare reports of bronchiectasis predating the onset of arthritis. Rarely recurrent pulmonary infections lead to chronic respiratory failure. Traction bronchiectasis occurs as a secondary phenomenon of end-stage fibrosis, and is due to the tethering effect of the surrounding scarred lung parenchyma on the airways. However, bronchiectasis occurs in patients independent of fibrotic lung disease.

PLEURAL DISEASE

Twenty percent of patients develop symptomatic pleural disease, the majority of which have mild pleurisy.[14] Only about 5 percent develop pleural effusions during the course of their disease.[15] Men in their fourth and fifth decades are at greatest risk.[15] Effusions generally are small, unilateral, and nearly always exudative as defined by protein and lactate dehydrogenase concentrations. Markedly decreased pleural glucose concentrations are characteristic with 75% of patients demonstrating a glucose level of less than 50 mg/dl.[16] Defective transport of glucose from blood to the pleural space has been implicated as the cause of this finding.[17] Pleural fluid pH of < 7.2 is common. Rheumatoid factor and RA cells (granulocytes containing rheumatoid factor complex) may be present, but are nonspecific, also occurring in effusions associated with SLE, pneumonia, tuberculosis, and malignancy.

RHEUMATOID NODULES

Pulmonary necrobiotic nodules are rare, but like rheumatoid pleural effusions, are more common in men than women[15] and generally cause no symptoms. Nodules vary in size from 0.5 to 7.0 cm and generally occur peripherally with an upper and mid lung zone predominance. They are usually non-calcified, and ≤ 50 percent cavitate.[15] The pathogenesis of rheumatoid nodules is unknown, but possible mechanisms include vasculitis and immune complex deposition. There also may be an association with cigarette smoking.[18] No radiographic features can differentiate rheumatoid nodules from lung carcinomas, and hence invasive testing for tissue diagnosis often is indicated. The presence of rheumatoid nodules in patients with pneumoconiosis is referred to as "Caplan's syndrome".

PULMONARY VASCULAR DISEASE

Pulmonary vascular involvement in RA (other than that associated with pulmonary fibrosis) is uncommon. Primary vascular involvement possibly results from immune complex deposition and complement activation leading to necrotizing arteritis, although pulmonary vasculitis with fibrinoid necrosis of vessel walls was not seen in a study of lung biopsies in RA.[7] Pulmonary arterial hypertension with medial hypertrophy and intimal fibrosis has been described.[19]

FIBROBULLOUS DISEASE

Although usually associated with ankylosing spondylitis and the HLA-B27 histocompatibility antigen, apical fibrobullous pulmonary parenchymal disease has been reported uncommonly in seropositive RA in the absence of HLA-B27.[20] Rarely, this finding may precede signs of arthritis.[21]

CRICOARYTENOID ARTHRITIS

Cricoarytenoid arthritis is an inflammatory arthritis with synovial proliferation in the cricoarytenoid joint, which may result in intermittent sore throat, hoarseness, gagging, or difficulty with inspiration. Laryngoscopic examination reveals limitation of vocal cord abduction during respiration due to fixation of the cricoarytenoid joint,[22,23] and there may be flattening of the inspiratory component of the flow-volume loop consistent with extrathoracic obstruction. Occasionally, life-threatening obstruction occurs.[24] Upper airway obstruction also occurs from rheumatoid nodules involving the larynx, or rarely from arteritis of the vasa nervorum of laryngeal nerves.[22] The prevalence of upper airway disease is not known, but it may be as great as 50 percent if CT scanning is used as the diagnostic tool.[22]

Systemic Lupus Erythematosus

Systemic lupus erythematosus (SLE) is defined both by its clinical features and by the presence of antibodies in the blood directed against component(s) of cell nuclei. Antinuclear antibodies have not been shown to be directly involved in the pathogenesis of the disease, and patients with SLE often have other circulating antibodies that react with cell membranes or serum components. Some antibodies may be directly responsible for disease manifestations, while others may play a role in the immune dysregulation that underlies the disease. The development of multiple antibodies in patients with SLE may be a sequela of polyclonal B-cell activation. Alternatively, the immune response in SLE may be stimulated specifically by antigens. Evidence of a genetic factor in the pathogenesis of SLE in humans suggests a gene or genes linked to the HLA-DR and DQ loci in the class II immune-response complex. Genetic predisposition could depend on multiple variables, including the determination of antigens for which tolerance fails, the characteristics of autoantibodies that are formed, and immune-complex clearing mechanisms.

Pleuropulmonary manifestations of SLE occur frequently and contribute significantly to morbidity and mortality. Multiple tissue sites can be affected, including lung parenchyma, pleura, pulmonary vasculature, respiratory muscles, and airways. There appears to be little correlation between pulmonary complications and general activity or duration of disease, positive serology, immune complexes in skin or renal biopsies, or the presence of circulating immune complexes.

ACUTE INTERSTITIAL PNEUMONITIS

The onset of abrupt cough, fever, and dyspnea with patchy alveolar opacities on chest radiograph in the patient with SLE can signify infection, alveolar hemorrhage, or acute lupus pneumonitis. Infection is the cause in up to 70 percent of cases in this setting, mandating that infection be considered first and foremost in patients with compatible clinical features.[18,25] Alveolar hemorrhage is reasonably likely if bronchoalveolar lavage fluid is bloody and does not clear with sequential lavages (see below). Once infection and alveolar hemorrhage have been excluded, acute interstitial pneumonitis becomes a clinical diagnosis of exclusion. A high index of suspicion is warranted in the postpartum period, during which the risk of acute lupus pneumonitis is increased for unknown reasons.[26] Laboratory studies are helpful, since 81 percent to 83 percent of patients with SLE-associated interstitial pneumonitis have anti-SS-A antibodies.[27,28] However, open lung biopsy frequently is required to establish a definitive diagnosis, and in some cases, even large tissue samples do not provide specific findings. Histology generally reveals nonspecific findings of diffuse alveolar damage (DAD), alveolar septal inflammation, hyaline membrane formation, mononuclear cell infiltration, and edema.[29] Biopsies are quite useful in ruling out other etiologies of lung disease, and therefore contribute to formulating more reliable management plans.

PULMONARY HEMORRHAGE

Alveolar hemorrhage in SLE varies from a mild, chronic form (which may remain subclinical), to an acute and massive alveolar filling process. Fortunately, massive bleeding occurs in only 1 to 2 percent of cases.[9] Alveolar hemorrhage may be a variant of acute lupus pneumonitis, given the similarity of histologic findings in both conditions. In both conditions, there may be a component of DAD along with alveoli filled with blood. Patients with alveolar hemorrhage frequently have hemosiderin laden macrophages and, in patients with recurrent hemorrhage, there may be a component of alveolar septal fibrosis as well. Vasculitis is unusual, although recent studies have better described a distinctive small vessel vasculitis ("capillaritis") in some of these patients.[30]

Detecting alveolar hemorrhage can be difficult even in cases of massive bleeding. This is particularly true in patients without apparent hemoptysis. A significant decrease in hematocrit over 12 to 24 hours should raise suspicion. An increase in diffusing capacity for carbon monoxide also is suggestive, however, measuring diffusing capacity is difficult in severely ill patients. Moreover, the diffusing capacity may not be increased in patients with transient bleeding, and a normal or low diffusing capacity does not reliably rule out the presence of alveolar blood. Bronchoalveolar lavage demonstrating a bloody return that does not clear with repeated washing or lung biopsy usually are required to establish a more definitive diagnosis.

CHRONIC INTERSTITIAL PNEUMONITIS

Chronic interstitial pneumonitis is an exceedingly rare manifestation of SLE characterized by progressive dyspnea, cough, bibasilar crackles, and diffuse interstitial opacities on chest radiograph.[31] Most investigators believe that chronic diffuse interstitial disease is the end result of recurrent episodes of acute lupus pneumonitis. Histologically, the interstitial process in chronic disease is far more cellular than fibrotic, even in autopsy studies. The low incidence of chronic interstitial pneumonitis may relate to the poor survival of patients with acute interstitial pneumonitis (which may be associated with a 50 percent mortality rate),[25] or to complete recovery between episodes of acute pneumonitis in some cases. Chronic interstitial lung disease can significantly impact on activities of daily living, but is rarely the sole cause of death in patients with SLE.

PLEURAL DISEASE

Clinical manifestations of pleural disease are common in patients with SLE. At autopsy, evidence of pleuritis, pleural thickening or pleural effusions is reported in 47 to 83 percent of patients.[29,32,33,34] Pleural effusions generally are small, bilateral, and exudative. They are characterized by the following: 1) clear serous or serosanguinous fluid (grossly bloody effusions are rare); 2) normal glucose (low in rare cases); 3) variable white blood cell counts and differential blood cell counts; 4) LE cells, immune complexes, and reduced complement components; and 5) a ratio of ANA in the pleural fluid to that in the serum of greater than or equal to 1 (the presence of ANA in the pleural fluid is not specific for SLE).[35,36]

PULMONARY VASCULAR DISEASE

Although clinically important pulmonary hypertension is seldom seen in patients with SLE, histopathologic abnormalities of the pulmonary vasculature are common. Various lesions have been described including vasculitis, thrombosis, medial hypertrophy and intimal fibrosis, and a condition very similar to what is seen in patients with primary pulmonary hypertension.[36] Changes have been seen in arterioles, muscular and elastic arteries, and pulmonary veins.[37]

DIAPHRAGMATIC DYSFUNCTION

Elevated hemidiaphragms are a frequent finding in patients with SLE. In some cases, this is the result of decreases in lung parenchymal volume caused by atelectasis or fibrosis. In other cases, there is no intrinsic parenchymal disease to explain this finding. In some cases, transdiaphragmatic pressures are decreased while innervation of the diaphragm remains intact, suggesting the presence of a primary myopathy of the diaphragm. Progressive diaphragmatic dysfunction (colorfully referred to as the "shrinking lung syndrome") manifests clinically as dyspnea and radiographically by a poorly moving and elevated diaphragm.[38] Pulmonary function tests demonstrate a restrictive pattern that is often difficult to distinguish from a lung parenchymal abnormality. Longitudinal studies of some of these patients show that it is sometimes a reversible condition.[39]

ATELECTASIS

Atelectasis frequently is described in pathologic, radiologic, and clinical studies of pulmonary aspects of SLE. Basilar, linear atelectatic opacities above the diaphragms often are noted on chest radiographs.[40] Although the mechanisms responsible for this finding have not been completely elucidated, it is likely that diaphragmatic dysfunction and the lack of a vigorous breath is the cause in some cases. Restrictive ventilatory defects usually are present, and there may be a decrease in static lung compliance that reverses after delivery of a mechanically delivered positive pressure breath.[39] Although most patients with atelectasis on chest radiograph report dyspnea, it is unclear whether atelectasis contributes meaningfully to this symptom or whether both dyspnea and atelectasis are caused by other pathological processes, such as diaphragmatic dysfunction. It also is unclear whether atelectasis predisposes to the increased incidence of respiratory tract infections seen in these patients.

UPPER AIRWAY DISEASE

Upper airway obstruction resulting from laryngeal inflammation and laryngospasm has been reported in patients with SLE. Epiglottitis, cricoarytenoid arthritis and necrotizing tracheitis also have been recognized.[9,36,41] However, clinically significant hypopharyngeal or laryngeal involvement is quite rare.

OBSTRUCTIVE LUNG DISEASE

Physiologic evidence of obstructive airflow limitation is found in very few nonsmoking patients with SLE.[42] Rare patients have been described with significant airflow obstruction.[43,44] Bronchodilator responsiveness has not been demonstrated. In other cases, inflammation of the airways has been found coincident with other pathologic processes involving the lung parenchyma.[32]

Progressive Systemic Sclerosis

Progressive systemic sclerosis (scleroderma) is a connective tissue disorder of variable course and unknown cause that can involve skin, lungs, gastrointestinal tract, kidneys, and heart. Lung involvement is common and is a chief contributor to morbidity and mortality in many patients.[45] As in RA and SLE, epidemiological studies have shown that progressive systemic sclerosis (PSS) occurs more often in adult females and in nonwhites. Similarly, mortality from PSS is greater in females than in males, and in nonwhites.

Studies attempting to address the etiology of PSS have focused on families, genetic markers of disease (e.g., human leucocyte antigen types), immunological and endocrine-metabolic factors, as well as toxic exposures. Family studies suggest an increased risk among first-degree relatives, especially those with shared HLA phenotypes. Reports of HLA class I, class II and III associations suggest that several MHC genes may influence susceptibility to and progression of PSS in some ethnic groups. A few reports exist of one family member having PSS and another member having another connective tissue disease, suggesting a common genetic risk may exist for PSS and other like diseases. Increased chromosomal breakage and sister chromatid exchanges have also been found in patients with PSS compared to controls. Serologic investigations in PSS offer promise epidemiologically with antibody markers potentially aiding in patient classification and prognosis determination. The relationship of cellular immune mechanisms to collagen and the immunopathology of PSS has been an area of intense investigation, although thus far, these processes can not confidently be implicated in the pathogenesis of PSS. Microvascular abnormalities are prominent in pathogenesis of PSS. Repeated episodes of endothelial injury may result in inadequate tissue perfusion, platelet aggregation and mediator release, which ultimately may lead to connective tissue deposition.[46] A serum cytotoxic factor causing endothelial injury also has been suspected in PSS.[47]

Various chemical agents have been associated with scleroderma-like conditions, such as vinyl chloride, organic solvents, trichlorethylene, aniline-denatured rapeseed oil, L-hydroxytryptophan, carbidopa therapy, pentazocine, and silicone or paraffin implantation. The incidence and mechanism of sclerodermatous changes associated with these agents are not well understood.

INTERSTITIAL LUNG DISEASE

Diffuse interstitial fibrosis occurs in the majority of patients with PSS, although it varies widely with regard to extent and severity of disease. At autopsy, interstitial lung disease (ILD) has been reported in 60 to 100 percent of cases, although ILD was not necessarily the cause attributed to death.[48,49] Patients generally present with dyspnea on exertion and cough with advancing disease, although they frequently are asymptomatic during the early phases of disease. Often, a sedentary lifestyle resulting from limitation of physical activity masks progressive lung involvement. Early in ILD, chest roentgenograms reveal increased linear or reticular opacities in the periphery of the lower zones, which then progress to more diffuse and prominent reticulonodular opacities with honeycombing.[50,51,52] Occasionally, areas of alveolar hazy opacities can be detected as well. Pulmonary physiological studies may be normal or reveal a restrictive defect, evidence of small airways disease, or a reduced diffusing capacity.[53] A reduction in respiratory muscle strength also is common. Bronchoalveolar lavage studies have demonstrated increased inflammatory cells in patients with PSS with and without ILD in variable patterns, making this procedure of uncertain clinical utility.[9] Histopathologic examination of lung tissue reveals fibrosis of alveolar septa with variable degrees of inflammatory infiltration.[54] Ultrastructural studies reveal endothelial and epithelial injury associated with alveolar septal edema and excess collagen deposition. Progressive architectural distortion generally occurs at variable rates, leading to coalescence of alveolar spaces to form "honeycomb" cysts. Clinical series studying the natural history of scleroderma ILD by physiologic measures suggest an overall indolent progression of disease, although there is substantial individual variability.

PLEURAL DISEASE

Signs and symptoms of pleural disease are uncommon in patients with PSS. However, autopsy series have clearly demonstrated evidence of pleural adhesions in a large number of cases, suggesting that subclinical or occult pleural inflammation is common.[55]

PULMONARY HYPERTENSION

Pulmonary hypertension can develop from progressive pulmonary fibrosis, or it can occur in isolation. The latter occurs more commonly in patients with the CREST variant of systemic sclerosis.[56] Pathologically, muscular hypertrophy of the media and circumferential deposition of collagen in the intima narrows the lumen of arterioles to increase pulmonary vascular resistance. Because the lung parenchyma may be normal, pulmonary function tests may reveal normal lung volumes and airflows with an isolated decrease in diffusing capacity. Although not invariably the case, isolated pulmonary arterial hypertension usually progresses, resulting in significant dyspnea on exertion, right heart strain, and even death.

ASPIRATION PNEUMONITIS

Aspiration pneumonitis is a potential sequela of gastroesophageal reflux and esophageal dysmotility. Esophageal dysfunction has been reported to occur in up to 87% of patients with PSS,[57] placing patients at great risk of oropharyngeal and reflux aspiration. Recurrent aspiration always should be in the differential diagnosis of patients with abnormal chest radiographs, particularly if abnormalities are present in dependent lung zones. The actual frequency and extent of aspiration in this patient population is not known. Twelve out of 13 patients with PSS studied for the presence of gastroesophageal reflux and occult aspiration were found to have laryngeal changes suggestive of aspiration.[58] Current methods of detection do not study patients over prolonged periods of time (and are therefore not optimal to quantify episodic events). This likely results in a substantial incidence of false negative studies.

BRONCHOGENIC CARCINOMA

There appears to be an association between PSS with pulmonary fibrosis and the development of bronchogenic carcinoma that is not explained by cigarette smoking. Several cases of adenocarcinoma and squamous cell carcinoma in PSS have been reported in the literature.[59] The relative risk of developing lung cancer in patients with scleroderma may be as high as 17,[60] which is similar to the reported increased relative risk in patients with idiopathic pulmonary fibrosis.[61] Carcinoma is thought to arise from the intense epithelial hyperplasia that accompanies the fibrotic process.[45]

Polymyositis-Dermatomyositis

Polymyositis-dermatomyositis (PM-DM) is an idiopathic inflammatory disease of muscle and skin mediated by autoimmune and cellular events that usually cause proximal muscle weakness. Although PM and DM are considered to be the same disease, muscle or skin manifestations may predominate in some patients.[62] PM-DM has been associated with malignancies in patients > 50 years of age.[63] Malignancy can precede or follow the development of clinical signs of PM-DM. PM-DM also may occur in patients with well established RA, SLE, or scleroderma.

INTERSTITIAL/INTRAALVEOLAR LUNG DISEASE

The reported incidence of ILD in PM-DM is variable ranging from 5% in those studies using radiographic criteria alone, to 40% in those investigations utilizing physiologic criteria for diagnosis.[62,64] Interestingly, a much greater incidence has been reported in Japan.[65] Clinical, radiographic, and physiologic features of ILD in this group of patients are similar to those seen in other connective tissue disorders. There has been no consistent relationship between the level of serum muscle enzymes and the development of ILD. However, there is a higher incidence of ILD in patients with anti-Jo-1 antibodies than in patients without anti-Jo-1 antibodies. Histopathological patterns of usual interstitial pneumonitis, BOOP, and diffuse alveolar damage (DAD), have all been clearly demonstrated in PM-DM.[62,66] Of these, BOOP has the most favorable prognosis. Patients with DAD have a uniformly poor outcome, often dying within weeks of diagnosis. Patients with usual interstitial pneumonitis typically demonstrate progressive disease, although the clinical course is often variable.

ASPIRATION PNEUMONITIS

Aspiration pneumonitis appears to be a common consequence of impaired hypopharyngeal muscle function and failure to protect the airway.[67] Diffuse myopathy with muscle bundle atrophy, termed cricopharyngeal achalasia, predisposes to massive aspiration pneumonitis.

RESPIRATORY FAILURE SECONDARY TO RESPIRATORY MUSCLE DYSFUNCTION

Respiratory muscle weakness decreases total lung capacity, interferes with the cough mechanism, and predisposes to mucus plugging and atelectasis. Rarely, severe muscle weakness results in life-threatening hypercapneic respiratory failure.[67] Although not common, respiratory muscle weakness may occur before peripheral muscle weakness, thereby masking the underlying cause of ventilatory failure.[68]

PULMONARY HYPERTENSION

Pulmonary arterial hypertension can occur secondary to 1) vascular destruction associated with ILD; 2) chronic hypoxemia associated with respiratory muscle dysfunction or ILD; or 3) congestive heart failure/cardiomyopathy.[62] Primary pulmonary arterial hypertension also can occur as a result of a primary fibroproliferative process involving the walls of arterioles of the lung leading to lumenal obliteration and significant increases in pulmonary vascular resistance. This form of pulmonary hypertension is unresponsive to treatment and invariably portends a poor outcome.[69]

Sjogren's Syndrome

Sjogren's syndrome (SS) classically presents with keratoconjunctivitis sicca, xerostomia, and polyarthritis. It may occur alone (primary SS) or in association with another connective tissue disease (secondary SS). Sjogren's syndrome is characterized by lymphocytic infiltration and destruction of exocrine glands. The actual mechanism of destruction of salivary and lacrimal glands is unclear, but the aggressive lymphocytic infiltration likely contributes directly or indirectly to signaling for cell-mediated tissue destruction. Local immunoglobulin synthesis propagates immune complex formation which contributes to chronic stimulation of B cells and the resultant hypergammaglobulinemia, and increase autoantibodies seen in these patients. Antibodies to extractable nuclear antigens (anti-Ro or anti-SSA and anti-La or anti-SSB) are relatively sensitive and specific for Sjogren's syndrome. Up to 90 percent of patients are rheumatoid factor positive, and up to 80 percent have positive antinuclear antibodies.[70]

DESICCATION OF THE TRACHEOBRONCHIAL TREE

Involvement of nasopharnygeal mucosa can lead to abnormalities of smell and taste. Chronic hoarseness often results from dryness of the hypopharyngeal mucosa. Xerotrachea leads to persistent dry cough in up to 25 percent of patients and predisposes to inspissated secretions, mucus plugging, airflow obstruction, recurrent atelectasis, pneumonia, and bronchiectasis.[71,72] Bronchoscopic examination generally reveals dry, erythematous bronchial mucosa.

INTERSTITIAL/INTRAALVEOLAR LUNG DISEASE

Diffuse interstitial lung disease occurs more commonly in patients with secondary SS (perhaps affecting as many as 50 percent of patients) than in patients with primary disease.[70] Signs and symptoms are as described in previous sections related to ILD. Chest radiographs can be normal, but more often show bilateral reticulonodular opacities. Importantly, the spectrum of pathologic findings differs somewhat from other connective tissue diseases. In addition to previously described histologic patterns of usual interstitial pneumonitis and bronchiolitis obliterans organizing pneumonitis, lymphocytic interstitial pneumonitis (LIP) is a well established complication of Sjogren's syndrome. LIP is a benign, polyclonal lymphoproliferation in the lung, frequently with germinal centers and noncaseating granulomas. The latter finding has occasionally been confused with hypersensitivity pneumonitis and sarcoidosis, particularly since hilar and mediastinal adenopathy are occasionally present. Rarely, LIP evolves into lymphoma. There have been several cases of lymphoma presenting as diffuse reticular pulmonary infiltrates without nodular masses or lymphadenopathy.[73] This highlights the importance of lung biopsy in SS-associated ILD.

DIFFUSE OR FOCAL NODULAR PARENCHYMAL DISEASE

Lymphoid parenchymal lung disease is a relatively unique feature of SS and ranges from benign bronchial submucosal lymphocytic infiltration to LIP, pseudolymphoma, and uncommonly malignant lymphoreticular neoplasm. Pseudolymphoma in SS is characterized by tumor-like proliferation of lymphocytes without histologic evidence of malignancy in extrasalivary sites such as the lungs, reticuloendothelial system, and kidneys.[74] Lymphoid architecture usually is preserved. In contrast, lymphomas are characterized by imma-

ture lymphocytes, monoclonal gammopathy, and loss of normal lymph node architecture.[75] Most of the lymphomas are of B cell origin (including well-differentiated lymphocytic lymphoma, mixed small cell and large cell lymphoma, lymphomatoid granulomatomatosis, Waldenstrom's macroglobulinemia, and sarcoma) occur in < 5 percent of patients with SS.[70]

PLEURAL DISEASE

Pleurisy and exudative pleural effusions occur in SS. Since SS frequently is associated with other connective disorders, it has been difficult to determine whether pleural disease is the result of SS or the associated disorder.

Mixed Connective Tissue Disease

Mixed connective tissue disease (MCTD) is characterized by the presence of high titer anti-RNP (ribonuclear protein) in patients with features of SLE, PSS, and PM-DM. The majority of patients with MCTD suffer pulmonary complications.

INTERSTITIAL LUNG DISEASE

Clinical, radiographic, and physiologic features of ILD in MCTD are similar to those previously described in association with other connective tissue disorders. However, histologic features are somewhat unique. The primary lesion appears to be a proliferative vasculopathy with intimal thickening and medial muscular hypertrophy of pulmonary arteries and arterioles that is more prominent than interstitial fibrosis.[9,76]

PLEURAL DISEASE

Pleuritis and pleuritic chest pain occur in more than one-third of patients, although findings of pleural thickening or effusion on chest radiographs are unusual.[76]

PULMONARY VASCULAR DISEASE

Pulmonary arterial hypertension is a major cause of clinical demise in patients with MCTD. It can occur as a secondary event in patients with severe interstitial pulmonary fibrosis or in patients with recurrent thromboembolic events; or it can be the result of primary plexogenic arteriopathy with or without associated vasculitis.[77] Thromboembolic disease should be suspected in patients with pulmonary hypertension and predominant clinical features of SLE. These patients should be tested for the presence of antiphospholipid antibody (and in the usual ways for the presence of thromboembolic disease).

ASPIRATION PNEUMONITIS
As in patients with PSS and PS-DM, patients with MCTD commonly develop esophageal dysmotility, placing them at increased risk of recurrent aspiration.[76]

PULMONARY HEMORRHAGE

Alveolar hemorrhage has been reported in patients with MCTD and SLE-like features.[78] The risk of hemorrhage may be increased in patients with concurrent renal failure.

DIAPHRAGMATIC DYSFUNCTION

Given that patients with MCTD have features of both SLE and PM-DM, it is not surprising that diaphragmatic dysfunction with ventilatory failure is a potential complication of this disease.[76]

Ankylosing Spondylitis

Ankylosing spondylitis (AS) is one of the seronegative spondyloarthropathies, in which inflammation occurs at the attachment of ligaments and joint capsule to bone. Fibrosis and ossification result in syndesmophyte formation, squaring of the vertebral bodies, ankylosis of the joints, and calcification of spinal ligaments and intervertebral discs.[70] More than 90 percent of patients with AS are HLA-B27 positive, but only about 20 percent of HLA-B27 positive patients develop AS.[9] Commonly, patients with AS present with sacro-illiac joint involvement, back pain, early morning stiffness, and restriction of spinal movement. Constitutional symptoms may occur. Extraarticular manifestations include the development of iritis and uveitis, and aortic valve insufficiency. Pleuropulmonary complications are often asymptomatic, and generally do not occur until late in the course of the disease.[79]

CHEST WALL ABNORMALITIES

Ankylosis of the costovertebral junctions and thoracic spine leads to fixation of the thoracic cage around a fairly normal resting lung volume. Total lung capacity is often low and residual volume high reflecting limitation of chest wall excursion with deep breaths.[9,80] Maintenance of resting lung volume likely protects against the development of severe hypoventilation and cor pulmonale (such as is seen in patients with severe kyphoscoliosis).[9] Restricted chest wall movement may, however, interfere with cough and mucus clearance and may predispose patients to pulmonary infection. It is not clear, however, that bacterial infection is more common in this patient group.

UPPER LOBE FIBROBULLOUS DISEASE

Upper lobe fibrotic or fibrobullous changes have been clearly described in AS.[79] While this finding has been noted late in the course of disease, it does not seem to correlate with the severity of ankylosis.[81] Patients are generally free of respiratory symptoms, unless fibrobullous changes are complicated by secondary infection. There has been concern that apical fibrosis is a risk factor for the development of "scar carcinoma."[82]

INFECTIOUS COMPLICATIONS

It is not clear that AS predisposes to common bacterial infections. The reported association with tuberculosis is suspect given upper lobe changes may be due solely to the underlying disease, and many patients thought to have tuberculosis did not have positive sputum cultures or respond to antimycobacterial therapy.[9] Still, the presence of apical fibrobullous disease does increase the risk developing atypical mycobacterial infection,[83] and the risk of colonization with aspergillus species and formation of aspergilloma.[79]

CRICOARYTENOID ARTHRITIS

As in RA, cricoarytenoid arthritis has been recognized in AS. It can complicate upper airway endoscopy and intubation, and rarely cause acute respiratory failure and cor pulmonale.[84]

PLEURAL DISEASE

Apical pleural thickening may be seen early in the course of this disease, often in conjunction with apical fibrobullous changes. Otherwise, pleural disease is unusual.

Psoriatic Arthritis

Psoriatic arthritis is a distinct inflammatory arthritis involving the proximal interphalangeal and distal interphalangeal joints. Patients may also demonstrate spondyloarthritis, sacroiliitis and/or ankylosing spondylitis with or without associated arthritis of the hands and feet. Similar to AS, upper zone pulmonary fibrosis has been recognized in patients psoriatic spondylitis.[85]

Behcet's Disease

Behcet's disease is thought to be an immune-mediated disease, although little is understood regarding its pathogenesis. Diagnosis is based on the presence of three of the following features: 1) recurrent ulcers of the mouth, 2) recurrent genital ulcers, 3) uvetis, 4) cutaneous vasculitis, 5) synovitis, and 6) meningoencephalitis.[9] Pulmonary manifestations are uncommon. They include lymphocytic, necrotizing vasculitis involving pulmonary arteries, veins, and capillaries with associated venous thrombosis and pulmonary aneurysms.[86] Pleuritis also occurs with symptoms of cough, dyspnea, pleuritic chest pain, and hemoptysis. Chest radiographs may reveal fleeting bilateral alveolar opacities and occasionally evidence of pulmonary arterial aneurysms. Pulmonary angiograms better define vascular involvement.

Relapsing Polychondritis

Relapsing polychondritis is a rare disease characterized by inflammatory destruction of cartilaginous structures throughout the body. Clinical features include auricular chondritis, nonerosive inflammatory polyarthritis, nasal chondritis, ocular inflammation, chondritis of the laryngotracheobronchial structures, and cochlear or vestibular damage.[70] Biopsy of an involved cartilaginous structure demonstrating histologic features of chondritis confirms the diagnosis, but is not mandatory.

LARYNGOTRACHEAL AND BRONCHIAL CHONDRITIS

Laryngotracheal and bronchial chondritis may lead to airway collapse or airway stenosis.[87] Airflow obstruction may predispose to respiratory tract infection. Clinical studies that help characterize the type and location of airway obstruction include the flow-volume loop, tracheal tomography or CT scanning, and bronchoscopy.

RESPIRATORY INFECTIONS

The increased occurrence of respiratory infection likely results from insufficient clearance of respiratory secretions, a direct complication of airway stenosis or ineffective cough secondary to dynamic airway collapse.

References

1. Weiland JE, Garcia JG, Davis WV, Gadlek JE: Neutrophil collagenase in rheumatoid interstitial lung disease. *J Appl Physiol* 62:628–33, 1987.
2. DeHoratius RJ, Abruzzo JL, Williams RC Jr: Immunofluorescent and immunologic studies of rheumatoid lung. *Arch Intern Med* 129:441–46, 1972.
3. Cervantes-Perez P, Toro-Perez AH, Rodriguez-Juardo P: Pulmonary involvement in rheumatoid arthritis. *JAMA* 17:1715–19, 1980.
4. Geddes DM, Webley M, Brewerton DA, et al.: Alpha-1 antitrypsin phenotypes in pulmonary fibrosis and rheumatoid arthritis. *Lancet* 2:1049–50, 1977.
5. Michalski JP, McCombs CC, Scopelitis E: Alpha-1 antitrypsin phenotypes including M subtypes in pulmonary disease associated with rheumatoid arthritis and systemic sclerosis. *Arthritis Rheum* 29:586–91, 1986.
6. Shannon TM, Gale ME: Noncardiac manifestations of rheumatoid arthritis in the thorax. *J Thoracic Imaging* 7:19–30, 1992.
7. Yousem SA, Colby TV, Carrington CB: Lung biopsy in rheumatoid arthritis. *Am Rev Respir Dis* 131:770–77, 1985.
8. King TE JR: Bronchiolitis, in King TE, Schwarz MI (eds): *Interstitial Lung Disease*, 2d ed. St. Louis, Mosby–Year Book, pp 463–95, 1993.
9. King TE Jr: Connective tissue disease, in King TE, Schwarz MI (eds): *Interstitial Lung Disease*, 2d ed. St. Louis, Mosby–Year Book, pp 308, 1993.
10. Geddes DM, Webley M, Emerson PA: Airways obstruction in rheumatoid arthritis. *Ann Rheum Dis* 38:222–25, 1979.
11. Sassoon CS, McAlpine SW, Taskin DP, et al.: Small airways function in nonsmokers with rheumatoid arthritis. *Arthritis Rheum* 27:1218–26, 1984.
12. Epler GR, Snider GL, Gaensler EA, et al.: Bronchiolitis and bronchitis in connective tissue disease: a possible relationship to the use of D-penicillamine. *JAMA* 242:528–32, 1979.
13. Koota K, Isomaki H, Mutru O: Death rate and causes of death in RA patients during a period of five years. *Scand J Rheumatol* 6:241–44, 1977.
14. MacFarlane JD, Dieppe PA, Rigden BG, et al.: Pulmonary and pleural lesions in rheumatoid disease. *Br J Dis Chest* 72:288–300, 1978.
15. Walker WC, Wright V: Pulmonary lesions and rheumatoid arthritis. *Medicine* 47:501–20, 1968.
16. Lillington GA, Carr DT, Mayne JG: Rheumatoid pleurisy with effusion. *Arch Intern Med* 128:764–68, 1971.
17. Dodson WH, Hollingsworth JW: Pleural effusions in rheumatoid arthritis. Impaired transport of glucose. *N Engl J Med* 276:1337–41, 1966.
18. Hunninghake GK, Fauci AS: Pulmonary involvement in the collagen vascular diseases. *Am Rev Respir Dis* 119:471–503, 1979.
19. Kay JM, Banik S: Unexplained pulmonary hypertension with pulmonary arteritis in rheumatoid disease. *Chest* 75:739–41, 1979.
20. Petrie GR, Bloomfield P, Grant IWB, Crompton GK: Upper lobe fibrosis and cavitation in rheumatoid disease. *Br J Dis Chest* 74:263–67, 1980.
21. Strohl KP, Feldman NT, Ingram RH: Apical fibrobullous disease with rheumatoid disease. *Chest* 75:739–41, 1979.
22. Lawry GV, Finnerman ML, Hanafee WN, et al.: Laryngeal involvement in rheumatoid arthritis. *Arthritis Rheum* 27:873–82, 1984.
23. Lavoy MR, Hughes GRV: Laryngeal obstruction and rheumatoid arthritis: a case report. *J Rheumatol* 7:759–60, 1980.
24. Gereud A, Ejnell H, Mansoon I, et al.: Severe airway obstruction caused by laryngeal rheumatoid arthritis. *J Rheumatol* 13:948–51, 1986.
25. Matthay RA, Schwartz MI, Petty TL, et al.: Pulmonary manifestations of systemic lupus erythematosus: review of twelve cases of acute lupus pneumonitis. *Medicine* 54:397–409, 1975.
26. Leikin JB, Arof HM, Pearlman LM: Acute lupus pneumonitis in the postpartum period: a case history and review of the literature. *Obstet Gynecol* 68:29S–31S, 1986.
27. Boulware DW, Hedgpeth MT: Lupus pneumonitis anti-SSA (Ro) antibodies. *J Rheumatol* 16:479–81, 1989.
28. Hedgpeth MT, Boulware DW: Interstitial pneumonitis in antinuclear antibody negative systemic lupus erythematosus: a new clinical manifestation and possible association with anti-Ro (SSA) antibodies. *Arthritis Rheum* 31:345, 1988.
29. Haupt HM, Moore GM, Hutchins GM: The lung in systemic lupus erythematosus: analysis of the pathologic changes in 120 patients. *Am J Med* 72:791–98, 1981.
30. Myers JL, Katzenstein AL: Microangiitis in lupus induced pulmonary hemorrhage. *Am J Clin Pathol* 85:522–56, 1986.
31. Eisenberg H, Dubois EL, Sherwin RP, et al.: Diffuse interstitial lung disease in systemic lupus erythematosus. *Ann Intern Med* 79:37–45, 1973.
32. Purnell DC, Baggenstoss AH, Olsen AM: Pulmonary lesions in disseminated lupus erythematosus. *Ann Intern Med* 42:619–28, 1955.
33. Alarcon-Segovia D, Alarcon-Segovia DG: Pleuropulmonary manifestations of systemic lupus erythematosus. *Dis Chest* 39:7–17, 1961.
34. Gross M, Esterly JR, Earle RH: Pulmonary alterations in systemic lupus erythematosus. *Am Rev Respir Dis* 105:572–77, 1972.
35. Good JT, King TE, Antony VB, et al.: Lupus pleuritis: clinical factors and pleural fluid characteristics with special reference to pleural fluid and antinuclear antibodies. *Chest* 84:714–718, 1983.
36. Wiedemann HP, Matthay RA: Pulmonary manifestations of systemic lupus erythematosus. *J Thorax Imaging* 7:1–18, 1992.
37. Fayemi AO: Pulmonary vascular disease in systemic lupus erythematosus. *Am J Clin Pathol* 65:284–90, 1976.

38. Thompson PJ, Dhillon DP, Ledingham J, et al.: Shrinking lungs, diaphragmatic dysfunction, and systemic lupus erythematosus. *Am Rev Respir Dis* 132:926–28, 1985.

39. Martens J, Demedts M, Vanmeenen MT, et al.: Respiratory muscle dysfunction in systemic lupus erythemtosus. *Chest* 84:170–75, 1983.

40. Levin DC: Proper interpretation of pulmonary roentgen changes in systemic lupus erythematosus. *AJR* 3:510–17, 1971.

41. Kovarsky J: Otorhinolaryngologic complications of rheumatic diseases. *Semin Arthritis Rheum* 14:141–50, 1984.

42. Andonopoulos AP, Constantopoulos SH, Galanopoulou V, et al.: Pulmonary function of nonsmoking patients with systemic lupus erythematosus. *Arthritis Rheum* 17:1–10, 1974.

43. Kallenbach J, Zwi S, Goldman HI: Airways obstruction in a case of disseminated lupus erythematosus. *Thorax* 33:814–15, 1978.

44. Kinney WW, Angelillo VA: Bronchiolitis in systemic lupus erythematosus. *Chest* 82:646–49, 1982.

45. Arroliga AC, Podell DN, Matthay RA: Pulmonary manifestations of scleroderma. *J Thorax Imaging* 7:30–45, 1992.

46. LeRoy EC: Scleroderma (systemic sclerosis), in Kelley WN, Harris ED Jr, Ruddy S, Sledge CB (eds): *Textbook of Rheumatology*, Philadelphia, WB Saunders, p 1183, 1985.

47. Cohen S, Johnson AR, Hurd E: Cytotoxicity of sera from patients with scleroderma: effects on human endothelial cells and fibroblasts in culture. *Arthritis Rheum* 26:170–78, 1982.

48. Weaver AL, Divertie MB, Titus JL: Pulmonary scleroderma. *Dis Chest* 54:490–98, 1968.

49. Young RH, Mark GJ: Pulmonary vascular changes in scleroderma. *Am J Med* 64:998–1003, 1978.

50. Schurawitzki H, Stiglbauer R, Graninger W, et al.: Interstitial lung disease in progressive systemic sclerosis: high resolution CT versus radiography. *Radiology* 176:755–59, 1990.

51. Boyd JA, Patrick SL, Reeves RJ: Roentgen changes observed in generalized scleroderma. *Arch Intern Med* 94:248–58, 1954.

52. Weaver AL, Divertie MB, Titus JL: The lung in scleroderma. *Mayo Clin Proc* 42:754–66, 1967.

53. McCarthy DS, Baragar FD, Dhingra S, et al.: The lung in systemic sclerosis (scleroderma): a review and new information. *Seminin Arthritis Rheum* 17:271–83, 1988.

54. Flint A, Colby TV: Connective tissue disorders and disease, in Flint A, Colby TV (eds): *Surgical Pathology of Diffuse Infiltrative Lung Disease*. Orlando, Florida, Grune and Stratton, 1987.

55. D'Angelo WA, Fries JF; Masi AT, et al.: Pathologic observations in systemic sclerosis (scleroderma). *Am J Med* 46:428–40, 1969.

56. Stupi AM, Steen VD, Owens GR, et al.: Pulmonary hypertension in the CREST syndrome variant of systemic sclerosis. *Arthritis Rheum* 29:515–24, 1986.

57. Geppert T: Clinical features, pathogenic mechanisms, and new developments in the treatment of systemic sclerosis. *Am J Med Sci* 299:193–209, 1990.

58. Johnson DA, Drane WE, Curran J, et al.: Pulmonary disease in progressive systemic sclerosis: a complication of gastroesophageal reflux and occult aspiration? *Arch Intern Med* 149:589–93, 1989.

59. Talbott JH, Barrocas M: Carcinoma of the lung in systemic sclerosis: a tabular review of the literature and a detailed report of the roentgenographic changes in two cases. *Semin Arthritis Rheum* 9:191–217, 1980.

60. Peters-Golden M, Wise RA, Hochberg M, et al.: Incidence of lung cancer in systemic sclerosis. *J Rheumatol* 12:1136–39, 1985.

61. Turner-Warwick M, Lebowitz M, Burrows B, et al.: Cryptogenic fibrosing alveolitis and lung cancer. *Thorax* 35:496–99, 1980.

62. Schwarz MI: Pulmonary and cardiac manifestations of polymyositis-dermatomyositis. *J Thorax Imaging* 7:46–54, 1992.

63. Mancul LA, Jin A, Pritchard KI, et al.: The frequency of malignant neoplasms in patients with polymyositis-dermatomyositis: a controlled study. *Arch Intern Med* 145:1835–39, 1985.

64. Lakhanpal S, Lie JT, Conn DL, et al.: Pulmonary disease in polymyositis/dermatomyositis: a clinicopathological analysis of 65 autopsy cases. *Ann Rheum Dis* 46:23–29, 1987.

65. Takizawa H, Shiga J, Moroi Y, et al.: Interstitial lung disease in dermatomyositis: clinicopathologic study. *J Rheumatol* 14:102–07, 1987.

66. Tazelaar HD, Viggiano RW, Pickersgill J, et al.: Interstitial lung disease in polymyositis and dermatomyositis: clinical features and prognosis is correlated with histological finding. *Am Rev Resp Dis* 141:727–33, 1990.

67. Dickey BF, Myers AR: Pulmonary disease in polymyositis/dermatomyositis. *Semin Arthrit Rheum* 14:60–76, 1984.

68. Blumberg PE, Byrne H, Kakulas BA: Polymyositis presenting with respiratory failure. *J Neurol Sci* 65:221–29, 1989.

69. Bunch TW, Tancredii RC, Lie JT: Pulmonary hypertension in polymyositis. *Chest* 79:105–07, 1981.

70. Tanoue LT: Pulmonary involvement in collagen vascular disease: a review of the pulmonary manifestations of the Marfan syndrome, ankylosing spondylitis, Sjogren's syndrome, and relapsing polychondritis. *J Thorax Imaging* 7:62–77, 1992.

71. Constantopoulus SH, Drosos AA, Maddison PJ, et al.: Xerotrachea and interstitial lung disease in primary Sjogren's syndrome. *Respiration* 46:310–14, 1984.

72. Strimlan CV, Rosenow EC III, Divertie MB, et al.: Pulmonary manifestations of Sjogren's syndrome. *Chest* 70:354–61, 1976.

73. Hansen LA, Prakash UBS, Colby TV: *Pulmonary lymphoma in Sjogren's syndrome.* Mayo Clin Proc 64:920–31, 1989.

74. Talal N, Sokoloff L, Barth WF: Extrasalivary lymphoid abnormalities in Sjogren's syndrome (reticulum cell sarcoma, "pseudolymphoma", macroglobulinemia). *Am J Med* 43:50–65, 1967.

75. Kennedy JL, Nathwani BN, Burke JS, et al.: Pulmonary lymphoma and other pulmonary lymphoid lesions. *Cancer* 56: 539–52, 1985.

76. Sullivan WD, Hurst DJ, Harmon CE, et al.: A prospective evaluation emphasizing pulmonary involvement in patients with mixed connective tissue disease. *Medicine* 63:92–107, 1984.

77. Hosada Y, Suzuki Y, Takano M, et al.: Mixed connective tissue disease with pulmonary hypertension: a clinical and pathological study. *J Rheumatol* 14:826–30, 1987.

78. Prakash UBS: Lungs in mixed connective tissue disease. *J Thorax Imaging* 7:55–61, 1992.

79. Rosenow EC, Strimlan CV, Muhrn JR, et al.: *Pleuropulmonary manifestations of ankylosing spondylitis*, Mayo Clin Proc 52:641–49, 1977.

80. Sharp JT, Sweany SK, Henry JP, et al.: Lung and thoracic compliances in ankylosing spondylitis. *J Lab Clin Med* 63:254–63, 1964.

81. Hillerdal G: Ankylosing spondylitis lung disease. An underdiagnosed entity? *Eur J Respir Dis* 64:437–41, 1983.

82. Ahern MJ, Maddison P, Mann S, et al.: Ankylosing spondylitis and adenocarcinoma of the lung. *Ann Rheum Dis* 41:292–94, 1982.

83. Gacad G, Massaro D: Pulmonary fibrosis and group IV mycobacterial infection of the lung in ankylosing spondylitis. *Am Rev Respir Dis* 109:274–78, 1974.

84. Libby DM, Schley WC, Smith JP: Cricoarytenoid arthritis in ankylosing spondylitis. A cause of respiratory failure and cor pulmonale. *Chest* 80:641–42, 1981.

85. Guzman LR, Gall EP, Pitt M, et al.: Psoriatic spondylitis: association with advanced nongranulomatous upper lobe pulmonary fibrosis. *JAMA* 239:1416–17, 1978.

86. Efthimiou J, Johnston C, Spiro SG, et al.: Pulmonary disease in Bechet's syndrome. *QJ Med* 58:259–80, 1986.

87. Michet CJ, McKenna CH, Luthra HS, et al.: Relapsing polychondritis. *Ann Intern Med* 104:74–78, 1986.

Chapter 111, Part 2

CONNECTIVE TISSUE DISORDERS INVOLVING THE LUNG–TREATMENT

REBECCA L. MORTENSON AND THOMAS CORBRIDGE

Interstitial/Intraalveolar Disease
  Usual interstitial pneumonitis
  Lymphocytic interstitial pneumonitis
  Bronchiolitis obliterans organizing pneumonia
  Diffuse alveolar damage
  Acute interstitial pneumonitis
  Alveolar hemorrhage

Airways Disease
  Upper airway obstruction
  Bronchitis and bronchiectasis
  Bronchiolitis obliterans

Pulmonary Vascular Disease
  Vasculitis
  Pulmonary arterial hypertension

Aspiration

Respiratory Muscle Dysfunction

Pleural Disease

The pleuropulmonary manifestations of the connective tissue disorders are many and complex, requiring a multidisciplinary approach to patient care, including patient education, careful attention to general medical needs (e.g., birth control measures and vaccinations), psychosocial support, close surveillance of pulmonary disease activity, and skillful prescription and monitoring of pharmacologic therapy (Table 111-1). The principal therapeutic strategy in these diseases is to maintain adequate disease suppression without accumulating unacceptable medication side effects and to protect the patient from additional insults such as aspiration and pulmonary infection. This can be a formidable task.

Interstitial and Intraalveolar Lung Disease

Determination of optimal treatment of interstitial lung disease (ILD) associated with the connective tissue disorders is clouded by the heterogeneity of these pathologic processes and limited data regarding specific treatment regimens. Even though the medical treatment of choice may be immunosuppressive therapy for all of the interstitial diseases, it is important to differentiate between the histologic patterns of usual interstitial pneumonitis (UIP), lymphocytic interstitial pneumonitis (LIP), bronchiolitis obliterans organizing pneumonia (BOOP), diffuse alveolar damage (DAD), acute interstitial pneumonitis (AIP), and alveolar hemorrhage, each of which may demonstrate variable rates of progression and each of which may respond differently to pharmacologic therapy. Accordingly, decisions regarding when to treat, with what to treat, and how long to treat may vary significantly.

USUAL INTERSTITIAL PNEUMONITIS

In general, survival of patients with connective tissue disorder–associated UIP is decreased compared to that of those without pulmonary fibrosis. However, prolonged and relatively stable disease occurs in many patients; overall, this group of patients seems to survive longer than those with idiopathic pulmonary fibrosis.[1] This is not to say that cases of rapidly progressive ILD of the Hammon-Rich variety do not occur.[2] Clinical outcome in response to treatment is difficult to assess due to insufficient numbers of patients in clinical studies, the lack of tissue confirmation of UIP in many cases, variability in modes of treatment, and the lack of studies controlled for the natural history of the disease.

There are patients with UIP associated with rheumatoid arthritis (RA), progressive systemic sclerosis (PSS),

TABLE 111-1 General Measures in the Management of Connective Tissue Disease–Associated Interstitial Lung Disease

Patient education	Directed at the disease process, medications, and medication side effects
Regular interval monitoring	Assessment of PFTs, gas exchange, CXR, and review of medications every 3 to 6 months depending on disease activity; surveillance labs if on immunosuppressive therapy: CBC, LFTs, potassium, and urinalysis
Surveillance for infection if on immunosuppressive therapy	Patient education regarding symptoms/signs of infection
Birth control	Pregnancy should be avoided during heightened disease activity and cytotoxic therapy
Immunizations	Annual influenza vaccine, and pneumococcal vaccine
Psychological support	Directed at coping with chronic disease

ABBREVIATIONS: PFT = pulmonary function test; CXR = chest radiograph; CBC = complete blood count; LFT = liver function test.

polymyositis-dermatomyositis (PM-DM), and mixed connective tissue disease (MCTD) who have improved symptomatically and physiologically from the use of corticosteroid therapy. General guidelines for the use of corticosteroids are given in Table 111-2. Walker and Wright noted short-lived objective improvement in 44 percent of 25 patients with ILD and RA.[3] Turner-Warwick and Evans noted improved exercise tolerance in 43 percent and improved chest radiographs in 22 percent of 23 patients given corticosteroids for RA-associated ILD.[4] It is possible that patients with a high degree of lung tissue cellularity respond better to corticosteroid administration than patients with a predominantly fibrotic pattern.[5] In systemic lupus erythematosus (SLE), little is known regarding the responsiveness of chronic interstitial disease to pharmacologic treatment, but it is probably not very good.[6,7] In PSS, case reports have demonstrated objective improvement in symptoms, pulmonary function tests, and bronchoalveolar lavage (BAL) findings, although to date there are no controlled trials demonstrating a long-term benefit to corticosteroid therapy.[1,8,9] Corticosteroids are probably of benefit in up to 40 percent of patients with PM-DM.[1,10–12] In MCTD, early reports suggested a significant benefit to the use of corticosteroids. Harmon and coworkers noted that 12 of 14 patients with symptomatic lung disease and MCTD demonstrated objective improvement following administration of corticosteroids.[13] However, Wiener-Kronish and colleagues followed five patients with MCTD and rapidly progressive pulmonary disease secondary to either ILD or pulmonary arterial hypertension (PAH).[14]

Corticosteroid therapy proved ineffective in all cases. In Sullivan's et al.,[15] about half of patients followed with serial pulmonary function tests demonstrated improvement in diffusing capacity following corticosteroids, and about one-third of corticosteroid nonresponders improved on cyclophosphamide. As in the other connective tissue disorders, there are no controlled trials of corticosteroids or other cytotoxic agents in MCTD-associated lung disease from which to draw strong conclusions regarding the efficacy of therapy.

Azathioprine, methotrexate, D-penicillamine, and cyclophosphamide have all been used alone or in combination with corticosteroids for the treatment of connective tissue disorder–associated UIP. However, experience with these agents for the treatment of parenchymal lung disease in these disorders is quite limited, and their use in this setting should still be regarded as experimental. Potential complications of these agents are given in Table 111-3. Azathioprine and methotrexate have both been used successfully to treat patients with PM-DM and may allow for a decrease in corticosteroid dose in some cases.[16–18] It should be kept in mind that patients on methotrexate can develop methotrexate lung toxicity, which can be confused with progression of the underlying disorder. D-penicillamine is an anti-inflammatory/immunosuppressive drug that inhibits intra- and intermolecular cross-linking of collagen. Steen and colleagues[19] reviewed serial pulmonary functions in PSS patients receiving D-penicillamine. They found a significant increase in diffusing capacity and forced vital capacity in treated versus

TABLE 111-2 General Guidelines for Corticosteroid Treatment in Connective Tissue Disorder–Associated Interstitial Lung Disease

- Initiating dose: Prednisone (or its equivalent) 1.0 mg/kg ideal body weight/day in a single dose. Attempt to sustain 1.0 mg/kg (ideal body weight)/day for 6 to 12 weeks before tapering.
- Duration of therapy: Patients with BOOP or LIP can often be tapered from prednisone over 3 to 6 months. Patients with UIP generally require a slower taper: e.g., to a prednisone dose of 0.25 mg/kg (ideal body weight)/day over 3 to 6 months. Further taper or cessation in UIP is guided by disease activity.
- Intravenous pulse methylprednisolone: Utilized in some cases of fulminant (Hamman-Rich variant) ILD, DAD, or BOOP. A common dose is 1 g over 30 min q 24 h for 3 to 5 consecutive days.

TABLE 111-3   Potential Complications of Corticosteroids, Cyclophosphamide, Azathioprine, D-Penicillamine, and Methotrexate

Drugs	Selected potential complications	Clinical surveillance schemes
Prednisone	Posterior subcapsular cataracts; increased intraocular pressure	Baseline eye examination; annual examinations thereafter or sooner if symptoms occur
	Hyperglycemia, hypokalemia, metabolic alkalosis	Blood glucose, electrolytes at 2 weeks and every 3 months thereafter
	Osteoporosis; vertebral compression fractures, aseptic necrosis	24-h urine collection for calcium and creatinine; spinal bone densitometry analysis; serum osteocalcin level; careful serial measurement of height; physical conditioning program; calcium and vitamin D supplements; calcitonin or etidronate in severe cases
	Systemic hypertension	Serial blood pressure measurements, manage appropriately
	Peptic ulcer disease	Surveillance, manage appropriately
	Infection	Surveillance, manage appropriately
	Secondary adrenal insufficiency	Measure serum cortisol, cosyntropin stimulation test, treat appropriately
	Menstrual irregularity; impotence	Usually improves after drug withdrawal
	Proximal myopathy including diaphragmatic dysfunction	Regular exercise program; may require drug withdrawal
	Euphoria, depression, psychosis	Psychological evaluation and medical management if necessary
Cyclophosphamide	Hematologic abnormalities: leukopenia, anemia thrombocytopenia (rare), hematologic malignancies (rare)	CBC weekly during the first 6 to 8 weeks of induction therapy (until a given dose maintains WBC of 3000–6000); then once every 5 to 6 weeks
	Nausea, diarrhea	Often can avoid by introducing at 50 mg daily, then adjust dose upward during induction
	Hemorrhagic cystitis, carcinoma of bladder	UA once monthly; maintain adequate hydration; stop therapy temporarily for microhematuria, permanently for gross hematuria
	Potential teratogenic effects; infertility, ovarian failure, amenorrhea	Avoid use in circumstances of potential pregnancy
	Infection	Close surveillance, manage appropriately
Azathioprine	Leukopenia, anemia thrombocytopenia	CBC weekly during the first 6 to 8 weeks of induction therapy (until a given dose maintains WBC of 3000–6000); then once every 5 to 6 weeks
	Nausea, diarrhea	May minimize by starting at low doses (e.g., 50 mg/day)
	Hepatic enzyme elevation	Avoid use in patients with underlying liver disease. LFTs every 6 to 8 weeks
	Potential teratogenic effects; infertility, ovarian failure, amenorrhea	Avoid use in circumstances of potential pregnancy
	Infection	Close surveillance, manage appropriately
D-penicillamine	*Early* (first few months) dermatitis, altered taste pemphigus, itching, drug fever	CBC, UA monthly, surveillance and appropriate management
	Late (1–2 years) stomatitis, nausea, leukopenia, thrombocytopenia, protienuria, autoimmune disease	
Methotrexate	Leukopenia, anemia thrombcytopenia	CBC every 6 to 8 weeks
	Hepatic enzyme elevation, chronic liver fibrosis and cirrhosis	Avoid use in patients with underlying liver disease. LFTs every 6 to 8 weeks, consider liver biopsy after total dose of 1.5 g
	Infection	Close surveillance, manage appropriately
	Drug-induced lung disease	High index of suspicion when there is progressive pulmonary disease during treatment
	Drug accumulation	Use with care in patients with third-space compartments such as pleural effusions and ascites
	Nausea, diarrhea	May be less common at lower doses
	Nephropathy	Follow electrolytes, BUN, creatinine and UA every 6 to 8 weeks

ABBREVIATIONS: WBC = white blood cell count; UA = urinalysis; See also Table 111-1.
SOURCE: Modified from Mortensen and King[60] with permission.

untreated patients. In addition, a significantly greater number of untreated patients demonstrated progression of dyspnea, crackles, and radiographic evidence of lung fibrosis. Silver and coworkers[20] reported a small number of patients with PSS in whom treatment with the combination of low-dose prednisone (10 mg or less per day) and oral cyclophosphamide (1 to 1.5 mg/kg/day) improved the rate of decline in pulmonary function and the degree of dyspnea.

Until more clinical treatment trial data become available, three general guidelines merit consideration in the determination of when to treat, how aggressively to treat, and how long to treat: (1) the rate of physiologic deterioration, (2) the histologic cellularity of the lung tissue, and (3) the overall functional status of the patient with consideration of the level of risk that immunosuppressive therapy will present to the individual patient. First line therapy should consist of corticosteroids (see Table 111-2 for dosing guidelines). Other immunosuppressive agents should be reserved for corticosteroid nonresponders, patients who develop severe corticosteroid side effects, and, perhaps patients with fulminant disease.

In rare patients with severe progressive UIP, lung transplantation may be an option. Many patients are excluded from this consideration because of the involvement of multiple organ systems with connective tissue disorder or because of severe functional limitation and deconditioning.

LYMPHOCYTIC INTERSTITIAL PNEUMONITIS

Lymphocytic interstitial pneumonitis is usually found in association with Sjogren's syndrome (SS). Although controlled trials are lacking, LIP may be more responsive to corticosteroids and thus has a better prognosis than UIP. There is less experience with the use of nonsteroidal immunosuppressive therapies. As in UIP, these agents are generally reserved for patients who progress despite corticosteroid use or who develop severe corticosteroid side effects; thus, they should still be considered experimental. Patients with LIP merit surveillance for the possibility of evolution into lymphoma.

BRONCHIOLITIS OBLITERANS ORGANIZING PNEUMONITIS

Patients with BOOP in the setting of a connective tissue disorder tend to be less responsive to treatment than patients with idiopathic BOOP (cryptogenic organizing pneumonitis). Still, this histologic lesion and the accompanying clinical syndrome is, in most cases, quite corticosteroid-responsive and certainly predicts a better prognosis than UIP. A small number of patients with BOOP and a connective tissue disorder have a fulminant course unresponsive to corticosteroid therapy. Few data are available regarding the use of other cytotoxic agents in this disease; as in UIP and LIP, these agents are reserved for patients unresponsive to or intolerant of corticosteroid treatment.

DIFFUSE ALVEOLAR DAMAGE

The histologic pattern of DAD has been well described in a population of patients with PM-DM, but it probably occurs in other connective tissue disorders as well. Tazelaar and colleagues[21] carefully reviewed lung biopsies from a series of patients with PM-DM–associated diffuse parenchymal disease and demonstrated that nearly one-quarter of these patients had damaged alveolar lining cells, hyaline membranes, intraalveolar edema, and focal hemorrhage consistent with DAD. In this study, patients uniformly experienced respiratory failure and death within weeks despite therapy with corticosteroids. Given the cellular nature and high mortality associated with this condition, patients with histopathologic features of DAD probably merit aggressive immunosuppressive therapy with high-dose corticosteroids and possibly the addition of a second immunosuppressive agent. Importantly, serious infection should be excluded before embarking on such therapy.

ACUTE INTERSTITIAL PNEUMONITIS

Acute interstitial pneumonitis (AIP) has most often been described in SLE, although cases have been reported in other connective tissue disorders with SLE-like features. Fortunately, AIP is rare, but it is associated with mortality rates in the range of 50 percent.[22] Corticosteroid treatment is reported to be effective in some cases, but clinical deterioration on corticosteroids also occurs.[22] The addition of cyclophosphamide or azathioprine to corticosteroid therapy is reasonable in the critically ill patient who is unresponsive to corticosteroids alone,[23] although there are no controlled trials demonstrating the efficacy or safety of this approach. As stated previously, exclusion of an acute infectious etiology (often requiring lung biopsy) is important prior to initiation of aggressive immunosuppressive therapy. Limited data are available regarding the benefits of plasmapheresis in SLE-associated AIP.[24]

ALVEOLAR HEMORRHAGE

There are marked histologic and clinical similarities between alveolar hemorrhage and AIP in the setting of a connective tissue disorder (usually SLE). Corticosteroids have been reported to be of benefit,[1] but there are no controlled studies demonstrating efficacy and safety in alveolar hemorrhage. For patients who do not respond initially to corticosteroids, cyclophosphamide or azathioprine have been tried,[25] but again data regarding efficacy and safety are not available. Cyclophosphamide may help to suppress "rebound" antibody production in patients receiving plasmapheresis as a part of their treatment regimen.[26]

Airways Disease

UPPER AIRWAY OBSTRUCTION

Management of cricoarytenoid arthritis depends on the severity of related symptoms and activity of the underlying disease. Treatment options include prednisone 20 mg daily plus aspirin or a nonsteroidal anti-inflammatory agent for 2 to 3 weeks.[27] Symptomatic relief of hoarseness sometimes can be achieved with benzonatate, throat lozenges and frequent sips of water. Surgical lateralization of the vocal cords or tracheostomy may be necessary in severe cases.

BRONCHITIS AND BRONCHIECTASIS

Bronchitis and bronchiectasis occur most often in patients with RA and SS. Treatment is similar to that in patients with large airway disease secondary to other conditions. There are no good data demonstrating that treatment of the underlying connective tissue disorder affects large airway function, although systemic corticosteroids given to patients with relapsing polychondritis and laryngotracheal and bronchial chondritis may improve airflow obstruction.[28] Airway hyperreactivity as assessed by methacholine challenge has not been well studied in this patient population, and a bronchodilator response appears to be a variable finding. If there is demonstration of response to inhaled bronchodilators or airway hyperreactivity during pulmonary function tests, inhaled bronchodilators and inhaled corticosteroids may be beneficial. In patients with significant amounts of excess mucus, inhaled bronchodilators and theophylline may aid in mucus clearance. In patients with thick secretions, mucolytic agents such as guiafenesin and maintenance of adequate hydration are of limited benefit. In patients with desiccation of the tracheobronchial tree, maintaining a humidified environment and the addition of an inhaled corticosteroid (which theoretically may decrease lymphocytic infiltration of the bronchial mucosa) may help. Physical maneuvers including aerobic exercise, chest percussion and postural drainage, and use of expiratory resistance valves aids in mucus clearance in some patients. Broad-spectrum antibiotics are indicated when there is an increase in the volume of mucus or in purulence.

BRONCHIOLITIS OBLITERANS

Bronchiolitis obliterans (or constrictive bronchiolitis) is a rare manifestation of RA and SS.[1] In RA, bronchiolitis obliterans has been associated with the use of D-penicillamine[29,30] and gold.[31,32] Treatment of this cause of progressive airflow obstruction is generally ineffective. Geddes and colleagues[33] reported six patients (five of whom had RA) with rapidly fatal disease unresponsive to inhaled bronchodilators or corticosteroids. Since then, patients have been described with variable clinical courses. Penny and coworkers[34] reported two patients with RA who developed obliterative bronchiolitis while taking D-penicillamine. One patient died of respiratory failure soon after diagnosis; the other stabilized on a combination of prednisone and azathioprine. Van de Laar and coworkers[35] reported one patient with bronchiolitis obliterans in the setting of D-penicillamine in whom the combination of intravenous cyclophosphamide and prednisone was thought to be of benefit.

Until further data are available, patients with bronchiolitis obliterans should be treated first with corticosteroids, reserving other immunosuppressive agents for corticosteroid nonresponders, corticosteroid-intolerant patients, and patients with fulminant disease. Although a definitive association between D-penicillamine or gold and bronchiolitis obliterans in RA has yet to be proved, the available literature supports stopping these drugs in patients with clinical or pathologic features consistent with bronchiolitis obliterans as a part of the overall treatment strategy.

Pulmonary Vascular Disease

VASCULITIS

Pulmonary vasculitis is uncommon in the connective tissue disorders but causes significant morbidity and mortality. Because of its low incidence, there are no clinical therapeutic trials confined to connective tissue disorders on which to base standard recommendations for treatment. In general, if the vasculitis is damaging a vital organ system, aggressive therapeutic intervention with corticosteroid therapy and other toxic agents such as cyclophosphamide is warranted to avoid serious organ dysfunction and irreversible damage. In some cases with apparently milder organ involvement, it may be clinically desirable to attempt treatment with corticosteroids alone to avoid a more toxic regimen. When the more conservative treatment approach of corticosteroids alone is selected, close clinical follow-up is essential to monitor for disease progression. These patients may initially respond to corticosteroids but subsequently experience progressive lung parenchymal damage as well as other organ system damage, particularly affecting the kidneys and gastrointestinal tract. Any evidence of progressive organ dysfunction in the setting of corticosteroid therapy alone is an indication for the addition of a second immunosuppressive agent. The combination of chronic low-dose cyclophosphamide and prednisone is effective in inducing remission in a number of the systemic vasculitic syndromes including Wegener's granulomatosis, corticosteroid-resistant systemic vasculitis of the polyarteritis nodosa group, corticosteroid-resistant Takayasu's arteritis, and corticosteroid-resistant angiitis of the central nervous system. Lacking specific treatment data in the connective tissue disorders with associated pulmonary vasculitis, this treatment combination appears to be the most reasonable approach. An alternative of intravenous pulse cyclophosphamide administered at 0.5 to 7.5 mg/m^2 body surface area has been used successfully to treat nephritis, cerebritis, and thrombocytopenia in SLE.[36,37] However, the efficacy of pulse cyclophosphamide has not been established in systemic vasculitis. In fact, the protocol of monthly pulses of cyclophosphamide is significantly less effective in inducing sustained remissions in Wegener's granulomatosis than in the low-dose daily protocol.[38–41] Suggested treatment guidelines for combination oral cyclophosphamide and prednisone are included in Table 111-4.

PULMONARY ARTERIAL HYPERTENSION

Although reversible vasospasm has been postulated as one mechanism in the pathogenesis of pulmonary arterial hypertension in the connective tissue disorders, most evidence suggests that the vascular defect becomes fixed and nonreactive relatively early in the course of disease. Vasodilator therapy has had little impact on decreasing pulmonary artery pressures or pulmonary vascular resistance, nor has it

TABLE 111-4   General Guidelines for Corticosteroid-Cyclophosphamide Treatment in Connective Tissue Disease-Associated Systemic Vasculitis

Corticosteroids
- Initiate prednisone therapy at 1 mg/kg/day in divided doses (every 6 to 8 h) for the first week.
- Consolidate the dose of prednisone to a single daily dose over the ensuing 2 to 3 weeks.
- After 1 month of prednisone therapy, initiate a gradual taper to alternate-day schedule over a 2-month period.
- The alternate-day dose should gradually be tapered during the treatment period. Total duration of treatment should be determined by the clinical circumstances.

Cyclophosphamide
- Therapy should be initiated at 2 mg/kg/day in a single daily dose.
- In fulminant cases, a dose of 4 mg/kg/day can be given every 24 h for 2 to 3 days, followed by 2 mg/kg/day (note that dosage reduction is appropriate in significant renal insufficiency).
- Thereafter, the dose should be adjusted to maintain a peripheral leukocyte count of 3000 to 6,000 cells/mm^3. The dose of cyclophosphamide required to maintain the leukocyte count in the recommended range tends to decrease as steroids are tapered and must be monitored closely.
- The duration of therapy in severe, fulminant cases of vasculitis should be approximately 1 year after induction of disease remission.

affected clinical outcome.[42–47] Resting and exercise gas exchange should be assessed, and supplemental oxygen should be supplied to maintain an arterial P_{O_2} of 60 mmHg.

In SLE or MCTD with associated antiphospholipid syndrome, pulmonary hypertension can result from recurrent pulmonary embolism. Treatment regimens for the antiphospholipid syndrome are still in evolution, but data thus far suggest that corticosteroids and immunosuppressive agents probably are not effective in reducing antibody titers.[48] Long-term anticoagulation with heparin and/or warfarin may reduce thrombosis in some patients.

Aspiration

Patients with PSS, PM-DM, and MCTD are at particular risk for the development of aspiration pneumonitis. This may be due to esophageal dysfunction (as in PSS),[49,50] hypopharyngeal dysfunction (as in PM-DM),[51] gastroesophageal reflux, or a combination of all three. A high index of suspicion for oropharyngeal and reflux aspiration is warranted in this patient population, particularly if there are complaints of difficulty initiating the swallow, dysphagia, cough after swallowing, or symptoms of gastroesophageal reflux disease (including its possible contribution to nocturnal respiratory events). Recurrent aspiration should be in the differential diagnosis of an abnormal chest radiograph, particularly if changes are present in dependent lung zones. In selected cases, fluoroscopic evaluation of the swallowing mechanism, esophogram, a nuclear medicine reflux aspiration scan, 24-h monitoring of esophageal pH, or esophageal motility studies may aid in diagnosis.

Treatment of dysphagia starts with safe swallowing techniques. Rarely, bypassing the esophagus with a gastric or jejunal feeding tube is required. Treatment of gastroesophageal reflux consists of elevation of the head of the bed with bed blocks (or the use of a wedge-shaped pillow), avoidance of large and late meals, weight loss, dietary mod-

ification, avoidance of alcohol and smoking, and pharmacologic manipulation.[52,53] Medications that decrease lower esophageal sphincter pressure (e.g., theophylline, oral beta-agonists, anticholinergics, and calcium channel blockers) should be discontinued if possible. The addition of an H_2-receptor antagonist, such as ranitidine or famotidine, decreases esophageal exposure to acid by decreasing gastric acidity and volume. In severe cases, the use of a proton pump inhibitor (such as omeprazole) or the addition of a prokinetic agent (such as metaclopramide hydrochloride or cisapride) to improve gastric and esophageal emptying and increase lower esophageal sphincter tone may be beneficial.

Respiratory Muscle Dysfunction

Respiratory muscle weakness is most often seen in PM-DM. It interferes with cough, predisposes to mucous plugging and atelectasis, and rarely results in hypercapneic respiratory failure.[51] Although not common, respiratory muscle weakness may occur before peripheral muscle weakness.[54] Treatment of the underlying connective tissue disorder with corticosteroids is the mainstay of therapy. Noninvasive facemask ventilation may also be of benefit in this clinical setting.

Pleural Disease

Few data are available regarding the efficacy of therapy in connective tissue pleural disease. In the setting of RA pleuritis, Light recommends initial treatment with nonsteroidal anti-inflammatory agents followed by oral corticosteroids in nonresponsive patients.[55] Some patients seemingly respond to corticosteroids[56] while others do not.[57] Decortication may be necessary in nonresponsive patients at risk for forming a fibrous pleural peel. Patients with RA-associated pleural effusion are at increased risk of developing an infected parapneumonic effusion, which is managed the usual way. In contrast to RA, SLE pleuritis appears to respond quite well to corticosteroid therapy. Hunder and colleagues[58] reported rapid improvement in 5 out of 6 patients with SLE pleural effusions after initiation of corticosteroids. Winslow and colleagues[59] reported rapid clearance in 10 out of 11 patients treated with corticosteroids, compared with 10 of 16 in patients who were not treated.

References

1. King TE Jr: Connective tissue disease, in King TE, Schwarz MI (eds): *Interstitial Lung Disease*, 2d ed. St. Louis: Mosby Year Book 1993: 308.
2. Dixon AS, Dixon J, Ball J: Honeycomb lung and chronic rheumatoid arthritis. *Ann Rheum Dis* 1957; 16:241–245.
3. Walker WC, Wright V: Pulmonary lesions and rheumatoid arthritis. *Medicine* 1968; 48:501–520.
4. Turner-Warwick M, Evans RC: Pulmonary manifestations of rheumatoid disease. *Clin Rheum Dis* 1977; 3:549–564.
5. Doctor L, Snider GL: Diffuse interstitial pulmonary fibrosis associated with arthritis. *Am Rev Respir Dis* 1962; 85:413–422.
6. Holden M: Massive pulmonary fibrosis due to systemic lupus erythematosus. *NY State J Med* 1973; 73:462–465.
7. Holgate ST, Galss DN, Haslam P, et al.: Respiratory involvement in systemic lupus erythematosus: A clinical and immunological study. *Clin Exp Immunol* 1976; 24:385–395.
8. Kallenberg CGM, Jansen HM, Elema JD, et al.: Steroid-responsive interstitial pulmonary disease in systemic sclerosis: Monitoring by bronchoalveolar lavage. *Chest* 1984; 86:489–492.
9. Salomon A, Appel B, Dougherty EF, et al.: Scleroderma: Pulmonary and skin studies before and after treatment with cortisone. *Arch Intern Med* 1955; 95:103–111.
10. Henriksson KG, Sandstedt P: Polymyositis treatment and prognosis: A study of 107 patients. *Acta Neurol Scand* 1982; 65:280–300.
11. Vihino M, Arahi S, Voshida O, et al.: High single dose alternate day therapy regimens in treatment of polymyositis. *J Neurol* 1985; 232:175–178.
12. Yanagisawa T, Sueishi M, Nawata Y, et al.: Methylprednisolone pulse therapy in dermatomyositis. *Dermatologica* 1983; 167:47–51.
13. Harmon C, Wolfe JF, Lillard S, et al.: Pulmonary involvement in mixed connective tissue disease (MCTD). *Arthritis Rheum* 1976; 19:801.
14. Wiener-Kronish JP, Solinger AM, Warnock ML, et al.: Severe pulmonary involvement in mixed connective tissue disease. *Am Rev Respir Dis* 1981; 124:499–503.
15. Sullivan WD, Hurst DJ, Harmon CE, et al.: A prospective evaluation emphasizing pulmonary involvement in patients with mixed connective tissue disease. *Medicine* 1984; 63:92–107.
16. Bunch TW: Prednisone and azathioprine for polymyositis: Long-term follow up. *Arthritis Rheum* 1981; 24:45–48.
17. Bunch TW, Worthington, JW. Combs JJ, et al.: Azathioprine with prednisone for polymyositis: A controlled clinical trial. *Ann Intern Med* 1980; 92:365–369.
18. Metzger AL, Bohan A, Goldberg LS, et al.: Polymyositis and dermatomyositis: Combined methotrexate and corticosteroid therapy. *Ann Intern Med* 1978; 81:182–89.
19. Steen VD, Owens GR, Redmond C, et al.: The effect of D-penicillamine on pulmonary findings in systemic sclerosis. *Arthritis Rheum* 1985; 28:882–888.
20. Silver RM, Miller KS, Kinsella MB, et al.: Evaluation and management of scleroderma lung disease using bronchoalveolar lavage. *Am J Med* 1990; 88:470–476.
21. Tazelaar HD, Viggiano RW, Pickersgill J, et al.: Interstitial lung disease in polymyositis and dermatomyositis: Clinical features and prognosis correlated with histological finding. *Am Rev Respir Dis* 1990; 141:727–733.
22. Matthay RA, Schwarz MI, Petty TL, et al.: Pulmonary manifestations of systemic lupus erythematosus: Review of twelve cases of acute lupus pneumonitis. *Medicine* 1975; 54:397–409.
23. Matthay RA, Hudson LD, Petty TL: Acute lupus pneumonitis: Response to azathioprine therapy. *Chest* 1973; 69:117–120.
24. Ibister JP, Ralston M, Hayes JM, et al.: Fulminant lupus pneumonitis with acute renal failure and RBC aplasia: Successful management with plasmapheresis and immunosuppression. *Arch Intern Med* 1981; 141:1081–1083.
25. Eagen JW, Memoli VA, Roberts JL, et al.: Pulmonary hemorrhage in systemic lupus erythematosus. *Medicine* 1978; 57:545–560.
26. Millman RP, Cohen TB, Levinson AI, et al.: Systemic lupus erythematosus complicated by acute pulmonary hemorrhage: Recovery following plasmapheresis and cytotoxic therapy. *J Rheumatol* 1981; 8:1021–1023.
27. Lavoy MR, Hughes GRV: Laryngeal obstruction and rheumatoid arthritis: A case report. *J Rheum* 1980; 7:759–760.
28. Stokes LT, Turner-Warwick M: Lungs and connective tissue disorders, in Murray JF, Nadel JA (eds): *Textbook of Respiratory Medicine*. Philadelphia, Saunders, 1988: 1462–1485.
29. Epler GR, Snider GL, Gaensler EA, et al.: Bronchiolitis and bronchitis in connective tissue disease: A possible relationship to the use of D-penicillamine. *JAMA* 1979; 242:528–532.
30. Wolfe F, Schurle DR, Lin JJ, et al.: Upper and lower airways disease in penicillamine treated patients with rheumatoid arthritis. *J Rheum* 1983; 10:406–410.
31. O'Duffy JD, Luthra HS, Unni KK, et al.: Bronchiolitis in a rheumatoid arthritis patient receiving aurafin. *Arthritis Rheum* 1986; 29:556–559.
32. Holness L, Tennenbaum J, Cooter NBE, et al.: Fatal bronchiolitis obliterans associated with chrysotherapy. *Ann Rheum Dis* 1983; 42:593–596.
33. Geddes DM, Corrin B, Brewerton DA, et al.: Progressive airway obliteration in adults and its association with rheumatoid disease. *Q J Med* 1977; 184:427–444.
34. Penny WJ, Knight RK, Rees AM, et al.: Obliterative bronchiolitis in rheumatoid arthritis. *Ann Rheum Dis* 1982; 41:469–472.
35. van de Laar MAFJ, Westermann CJJ, Wagenaar SS, et al.: Beneficial effect of intravenous cyclophosphamide and oral prednisone on D-penicillamine-associated bronchiolitis obliterans. *Arthritis Rheum* 1985; 28:93–97.
36. Boumpas DT, Austin HA III, Vaughn EM, et al.: Controlled trial of pulse methylprednisolone versus 2 regimens of pulse cyclophosphamide in severe lupus nephritis. *Lancet* 1992; 340:741–745.
37. Steinberg AD, Steinberg SC: Long-term preservation of renal function in patients with lupus nephritis receiving treatment that includes cyclophosphamide versus those treated with prednisone only. *Arthritis Rheum* 1991; 34:945–950.
38. Cupps TR, Fauci AS: The vasculiditis, in Smith LH Jr (ed): *Major Problems in Internal Medicine*. Philadelphia, Saunders, 1981: 1.
39. Fauci AS, Dale DC, Balow JE: Glucocorticosteroid therapy: Mechanism of action and clinical consideration. *Ann Intern Med* 1976; 84:304.
40. Fauci AS, Haynes BF, Katz P, et al.: Wegener's granulomatosis: Prospective clinical and therapeutic experience with 85 patients for 21 years. *Ann Intern Med* 1983; 98:76.
41. Fauci AS: Cytotoxic and other immunoregulatory agents, in Kelly WN, Harris ED Jr, Ruddy S, Sledge CB (eds): *Textbook of Rheumatology*. Philadelphia, Saunders, 1985: 833.
42. Ungerer RG, Tashkin DP, Furst D, et al.: Prevalence and clinical

coorelates of pulmonary arterial hypertension in progressive systemic sclerosis. *Am J Med* 1983; 75:65–74.

43. Demedts M: Pulmonary hypertension in connective tissue disease. *Clin Rheum* 1990; 1:20–21.

44. Kasukawa R, Nishimaki T, Takagi T, et al.: Pulmonary hypertension in connective tissue diseases: Clinical analysis of sixty patients in a multi-institutional study. *Clin Rheumatol* 1990; 9:56–62.

45. Young ID, Ford SE, Ford TM: The association of pulmonary hypertension with rheumatoid arthritis. *J Rheum* 1989; 9: 1266–1269.

46. Sharma S, Vaccharajani A, Mandke J: Severe pulmonary hypertension in rheumatoid arthritis. *Int J Cardiol* 1990; 2:220–222.

47. Mahowald ML, Weir EK, Ridley DJ, et al.: Pulmonary hypertension in systemic lupus erythematosus: Effect of vasodilators on pulmonary hemodynamics. *J Rheum* 1985; 12:773–777.

48. Howe HS, Boey ML, Fong KY, et al.: Pulmonary hemorrhage, pulmonary infarction and the lupus anticoagulant. *Ann Rheum Dis* 1988; 47:869–872.

49. Geppert T: Clinical features, pathogenic mechanisms, and new developments in the treatment of systemic sclerosis. *Am J Med Sci* 1990; 299:193–209.

50. Johnson DA, Drane WE, Curran J, et al.: Pulmonary disease in progressive systemic sclerosis: A complication of gastroesophageal reflux and occult aspiration? *Arch Intern Med* 1989; 149:589–593.

51. Dickey BF, Myers AR: Pulmonary disease in polymyositis/dermatomyositis. *Semin Arthritis Rheum* 1984; 14:60–76.

52. Hixson LJ, Kelley CL, Jones WN, et al.: Current trends in the pharmacotherapy for gastroesophageal reflux disease. *Arch Intern Med* 1992; 152:717–723.

53. Kitchin LI, Castell DO: Rationale and efficacy of conservative therapy for gastroesophageal reflux disease. *Arch Intern Med* 1991; 151:448–454.

54. Blumberg PE, Byrne E, Kakulas BA: Polymyositis presenting with respiratory failure. *J Neurol Sci* 1989; 65:221–229.

55. Light RW: Pleural disease due to collagen vascular diseases, in Light RW (ed): *Pleural Diseases*. Philadelphia, Lea & Febiger, 1983; 163–171.

56. Walker WC, Wright V: Rheumatoid pleuritis. *Ann Rheum Dis* 1967; 26:467–474.

57. Mays EE: Rheumatoid pleuritis: Observations in eight cases and suggestions for making the diagnosis in patients without the "typical" findings. *Dis Chest* 1968; 53:202–214.

58. Hunder GG, McDuffie FC, Hepper NGG: Pleural fluid complement in systemic lupus erythematosus and rheumatoid arthritis. *Ann Intern Med* 1972; 76:357–362.

59. Winslow WA, Ploss LN, Loitman B: Pleuritis in systemic lupus erythematosus: Its importance as an early manifestation in diagnosis. *Ann Intern Med* 1958; 49:70–88.

60. Mortenson RL, King TE: Idiopathic pulmonary fibrosis, in Lichtenstein LM, Fauci AS (eds): *Current Therapy in Allergy, Immunology and Rheumatology*. St Louis, Mosby-Year Book, 1992: 233–241.

Chapter 112

SARCOIDOSIS
RICHARD H. WINTERBAUER

Initial Laboratory Evaluation
 Selecting the patient who may benefit from therapy

Treatment
 Effect of corticosteroids

Alternative Therapies
 Nonsteroidal anti-inflammatory agents
 Chloroquine
 Methotrexate
 Inhaled corticosteroids

The diagnostic criteria for sarcoidosis are (1) a compatible clinical picture; (2) histologic demonstration of noncaseating granuloma; and (3) exclusion of other diseases capable of producing a similar histologic or clinical picture. Since the clinical picture is variable and the histologic changes are nonspecific, sarcoidosis for the major part is a diagnosis of exclusion. Multiple diseases—including tuberculosis, fungal infections, and lymphoma—may mimic either the clinical or histologic features of sarcoidosis. Virtually every organ is at risk for involvement with sarcoidosis. Pulmonary disease is almost universal and serves as a common denominator of the illness. An abnormal chest roentgenogram is present in 95 percent of patients with sarcoidosis.

 Pulmonary sarcoidosis has been grouped into three stages by plain chest roentgenographic pattern. The stages parallel the natural progression of the disease and relate to overall prognosis. Stage I is defined as bilateral hilar lymphadenopathy (BHL) with or without right paratracheal adenopathy and normal pulmonary parenchyma. The combination of BHL on roentgenogram, no symptoms, and a negative physical examination has proved to be highly specific for sarcoidosis. Stage II roentgenograms show BHL and parenchymal disease. Stage III roentgenograms demonstrate parenchymal disease in the absence of hilar adenopathy. Approximately 50 percent of sarcoid patients present in stage I, and they are often asymptomatic. Some 25 percent of patients present with stage II and 20 percent with stage III disease.[1]

Initial Laboratory Evaluation

A recommended initial laboratory evaluation of patients with sarcoidosis is listed in Table 112-1. The white blood count, hematocrit, and platelet count are measured because granulomatous involvement creates marked splenomegaly in 2 to 3 percent of patients with associated hypersplenism,

TABLE 112-1   Recommended Initial Laboratory Evaluation of Patients with Sarcoidosis

1. Peripheral blood counts	3. Urinalysis
White blood cells	4. Intermediate-strength PPD
Hematocrit	(anergic controls are unnecessary)
Platelets	5. Pulmonary function tests
2. Serum chemistries	Forced vital capacity
Calcium	$DL_{CO_{SB}}$
Alkaline phosphatase	
Glucose	

anemia, and thrombocytopenia.[2] In addition, there is an association between sarcoidosis and autoimmune thrombocytopenia in rare individuals. Approximately 2 percent of sarcoid patients will have hypercalcemia with an attendant risk of nephrocalcinosis and stones.[3] Although hypercalciuria occurs in normocalcemic patients with sarcoidosis, urinary calcium exertion need not be measured in the absence of stone or nephrocalcinosis. At necropsy, 70 percent of sarcoid patients have hepatic granulomata and 25 percent have hepatomegaly during life.[4] The alkaline phosphatase is typically the only measurable abnormality and gives some estimate of the patient's granuloma burden. The incidence of tuberculosis has decreased in more recent series as the disease has become less prevalent. Nevertheless, patients with a positive purified protein derivative (PPD) who are to receive corticosteroid therapy should be given 300 mg of isoniazid for 6 months as prophylaxis.

 Pulmonary function tests have a poor correlation with histologic severity of disease but, in general, tend to sort the extremes in separating mild from severe illness.[5] A restrictive ventilatory defect is the typical finding in pulmonary sarcoidosis. At present, there is no conclusive evidence that measurements of arterial blood gas tensions, pulmonary compliance, or pulmonary exercise testing add significantly to the sensitivity and specificity of the vital capacity and dif-

TABLE 112-2   Guidelines for the Use of CT and HRCT in the Diagnosis and Management of Pulmonary Sarcoidosis

1. Neither CT nor HRCT findings should be considered diagnostic of sarcoidosis. Certain patterns are compatible with sarcoidosis but require diagnostic confirmation.
2. Neither CT nor HRCT images accurately predict the natural history or therapeutic outcome of sarcoidosis.
3. Neither CT nor HRCT offers an advantage over the combination of history of symptoms, chest roentgenogram, and FVC in assessing the need for therapy, response to therapy, or progression of disease in patients with sarcoidosis.
4. There is no evidence that HRCT increases the diagnostic yield of TBBX in sarcoidosis.
5. In patients with illnesses clinically compatible with sarcoidosis (central nervous system disease, hypercalcemia, ocular disease), normal chest roentgenograms, and no readily available biopsy site, a CT scan to demonstrate occult intrathoracic adenopathy may point to fiberoptic bronchoscopy with TBBX and/or mediastinoscopy as the next diagnostic step.
6. Only rare patients with sarcoidosis will benefit from lung CT or HRCT in the diagnosis and management of their disease.

ABBREVIATIONS: CT = computed tomography; HRCT = high-resolution computed tomography; FVC = forced vital capacity; TBBX = transbronchial biopsy.

fusing capacity for carbon monoxide in detecting the presence of parenchymal sarcoidosis, assessing the extent of disease, or measuring changes in the disease course.[5]

Conventional computed tomography (CT) or high-resolution computed tomography (HRCT) has been proposed as helpful in the diagnosis and management of sarcoidosis.[6–8] Suggested guidelines for the use of CT and HRCT in pulmonary sarcoidosis are listed in Table 112-2.

SELECTING THE PATIENT WHO MAY BENEFIT FROM THERAPY

The initial therapeutic decision in the patient with sarcoid is whether to treat or not. The decision process begins by recognizing subgroups with different patterns of disease progression.[9] Approximately 75 percent of patients with sarcoidosis will have spontaneous remission or mild, stable disease not requiring steroid therapy.[9] Indications for treatment in 10 percent will be involvement of a critical extrapulmonary organ such as the eye, brain, or heart, while only 15 percent will require treatment for progressive pulmonary disease. Recognition of the latter subgroup is important, for clinicians can then avoid giving corticosteroids to a patient who ultimately would have spontaneous resolution and can provide early therapy for those patients destined to have progressive pulmonary disease. Roentgenographic patterns, sequential pulmonary function testing, and clinical patterns of disease have all been used to predict the outcome of sarcoidosis. Although loose correlations exist, none of these techniques has been reliable enough to become clinical dogma. For example, patients with stage I roentgenographic disease have an 80 percent frequency of spontaneous remission within 2 years of onset; stage II disease has a 65 percent chance of spontaneous remission; and stage III, a 30 percent chance.[10] Erythema nodosum and acute arthritis indicate an

excellent prognosis with an approximate 85 percent frequency of spontaneous remission. At the opposite extreme, patients with hepatomegaly, central nervous system involvement, upper airway disease, lupus pernio, bone lesions, nephrocalcinosis, or cor pulmonale all have less than a 25 percent chance of remission within 2 years, either with or without therapy.[11] Severely symptomatic patients are more likely to have persistent disease. Persistence of symptoms for more than 2 years markedly reduces the chance of spontaneous remission. Racial factors are important, as black patients are more likely to develop chronic, progressive disease. While admittedly imperfect, these clinical criteria are still the best data on which to base treatment decisions. Laboratory tests such as serum angiotensin-converting enzyme, bronchoalveolar lavage (BAL) cell populations, and gallium 67 scans have not proved to add significantly to treatment decisions.[9]

Since clinical patterns, roentgenographic appearance, and serologic measures are imperfect in predicting the natural course of sarcoidosis, decisions regarding whom to treat remain murky. Suggested guidelines for initiation of treatment in pulmonary sarcoidosis are listed in Table 112-3. These suggestions are based on personal experience and offered as a general guide to patient management. The recommendations are largely based on patient symptoms. Until therapy becomes available that results in cure, elimination of symptoms is a reasonable therapeutic goal. The treatment of chest x-ray or pulmonary function abnormalities alone in the absence of symptoms should be discouraged.

Treatment

EFFECT OF CORTICOSTEROIDS

The majority of sarcoid patients receiving corticosteroids show a beneficial response, but this represents disease suppression and not cure. For example, Harkleroad and colleagues studied 25 patients randomized to treatment and control groups that were similar in sex, age, race, degrees of pulmonary dysfunction, chest x-ray stage, and duration of disease.[12] The patients were evaluated initially and at 6 months, 1 to 2 years, and 10 to 15 years with complete spirometric studies, single-breath DL_{CO}, and arterial blood

TABLE 112-3   Guidelines for Initiation of Treatment in Patients with Pulmonary Sarcoidosis

1. Asymptomatic patients with pulmonary sarcoidosis should not receive corticosteroids.
2. Patients with significant respiratory symptoms, abnormal pulmonary function tests, and a diffuse abnormality on chest x-ray should receive treatment.
3. Patients with minimal symptoms might best be managed by serial evaluations at 2 to 3 month intervals and with treatment reserved until there is evidence of disease progression.
4. Patients with disease of greater than 2 years duration with deterioration in pulmonary function (FVC decrease $\geq 10\%$, DL_{CO} decrease $\geq 20\%$, increase in D[A-a] $O_2 \geq 5$ mmHg) over time are candidates for steroid therapy.

gases. Prednisone was given in a dose of 15 mg daily for 6 to 24 months. There was no difference between the two groups in radiologic staging and pulmonary function tests after follow-up of ≥10 years.[12] Israel and colleagues conducted a controlled, double-blinded, randomized trial of prednisone 15 mg daily for 3 months versus placebo in the treatment of pulmonary sarcoidosis.[13] Epidemiologic and clinical characteristics of the treatment and control groups were similar. Outcome was evaluated by radiographic evolution of disease, vital capacity, and clinical symptoms. In 46 patients with pulmonary parenchymal sarcoidosis, significant improvement was evident at the end of the treatment period, but no difference between treated patients and controls was demonstrable after a mean interval of 5.4 years.[13] Johns and colleagues studied a large group of patients with a longer duration of treatment (1 year).[14] Over 90 percent of patients treated for symptomatic pulmonary sarcoidosis showed improvement in symptoms, chest roentgenogram, and pulmonary function tests. Only one-third remained improved after therapy was discontinued at 1 year.

The optimal dose and duration of steroid therapy for sarcoidosis has never been scientifically defined. Generally, an initial dose of 30 mg of prednisone daily is adequate. Larger doses are rarely required. Symptomatic improvement is rapid, with maximum improvement frequently present at 2 weeks. Failure to improve after a month of treatment defines a steroid-resistant illness and longer trials rarely, if ever, are successful. Patients with disease of less than 6 months duration show the greatest therapeutic benefit. Improvement more often is reflected by an increase in vital capacity than changes in the diffusing capacity. A course of 6 to 12 months generally is recommended, but it must be realized that, even with prolonged treatment, a large percentage of patients will relapse when therapy is stopped.

Alternate-day therapy can be very effective in maintaining improvement and may decrease side effects. Spratling and colleagues evaluated the effectiveness of alternate-day corticosteroids by randomizing patients with stage II disease to receive 6 months of either daily or alternate-day prednisone.[15] Total dosage was equivalent. Both groups showed statistically significant improvement in pulmonary function (TLC, FVC, FEV_1, DL_{CO}) at 3 and 6 months, and there were no significant differences between the two groups. Roentgenographic improvement was also the same in both groups.

The treated patient is at risk for numerous complications of corticosteroid therapy. Some of the undesirable effects of steroids can be obviated through careful education of the patient. For instance, patients must be warned of increase in appetite and possible weight gain; attention to caloric restriction should begin on the first day of treatment. Similarly, patients should be warned of the potential for water retention and instructed in the reduction of dietary salt. Patients should be urged to exercise as much as they can; thus the myopathy and osteoporosis associated with corticosteroids can be at least partially offset. In addition, other side effects—such as mood changes including euphoria, sleep deprivation, epigastric distress, and the elevation of blood sugar with polyuria and polydypsia—should be explained in detail to the patient.

Alternative Therapies

There are only four alternative treatments for systemic disease that we consider adequately substantiated to incorporate into current clinical practice. These are nonsteroidal anti-inflammatory drugs (NSAIDs) for the treatment of acute arthritis and/or erythema nodosum; chloroquine, which has been especially effective in the treatment of skin disease; oral methotrexate for multisystem sarcoidosis; and inhaled budesonide for pulmonary sarcoidosis. Budesonide is not yet available in the United States but it has a substantial experience in Europe and Canada. Other therapies that have been tried include chlorambucil, cyclosporine, azathioprine, cyclophosphamide, and ketoconazole. Support for use of these is exclusively anecdotal. Reference 16 provides a detailed review of their use in sarcoidosis.

NONSTEROIDAL ANTI-INFLAMMATORY AGENTS

The NSAIDs (indomethacin, ibuprofen, salicylates) may control the acute inflammatory symptoms of sarcoidosis presenting with arthritis and/or erythema nodosum. Anti-inflammatory agents are effective in approximately one-third of cases of acute sarcoid arthritis. Therapy can start with indomethacin, 25 to 50 mg three times a day. If symptomatic relief does not occur within 7 days, systemic corticosteroids should be given. Since acute arthritis and erythema nodosum from sarcoidosis usually remit by 3 months, corticosteroid treatment for these symptoms should be limited to 3 months.

CHLOROQUINE

In 1953, Schaffer and colleagues published the first report of a patient with sarcoidosis who responded to an oral antimalarial agent.[17] Since then, 25 investigations of the efficacy of chloroquine, hydroxychloroquine, and quinacrine have been found in the English medical literature. Most studies have involved patients with cutaneous sarcoidosis or combined cutaneous and pulmonary lesions. Many of these studies involve patients who had previously failed a trial of corticosteroids. All but one of the studies showed at least temporary improvement in cutaneous lesions. Pulmonary lesions have shown less consistent improvement.

The first prospective study was performed by Morse and coworkers in 1961.[18] After 6 months of therapy with chloroquine at a daily dose of 500 mg, the skin lesions in all seven patients improved. Four of the seven patients suffered a relapse after discontinuation of therapy but responded well after drug therapy was resumed.[18] Relapse after cessation of drug treatment has been seen in multiple studies, confirming that chloroquine suppresses but does not cure the cutaneous lesions.

The only randomized, double-blind clinical trial was reported by the British Tuberculosis Association in 1967.[19] Fifty-seven patients received either chloroquine therapy or placebo for 4 months. Chest roentgenographic assessment showed substantial improvement in the chloroquine group at 4 and 6 months but no difference between the two groups at 12 months (8 months after stopping therapy).[19] The most recent clinical trial used hydroxychloroquine in patients with cutaneous sarcoidosis and produced regression of the skin disease in 12 of 17 patients within 4 to 12 weeks.[20] In two of eight patients with pulmonary sarcoidosis, roentgenographic improvement was seen. No ocular toxicity was noted.

The effectiveness of chloroquine in the treatment of hypercalcemia also has been demonstrated, as initially reported in 1963. Most recently, Adams and colleagues have studied this phenomenon.[21] They found that chloroquine inhibited the overproduction of 1,25-dihydroxyvitamin D within days, a finding contrary to previous suggestions that oral chloroquine regimens of longer duration were required. The investigators studied the pulmonary alveolar macrophages from their patients in vitro by exposing them to a chloroquine concentration that was an order of magnitude lower than the serum concentration achieved in patients receiving such therapy. Chloroquine completely inhibited the 25-OH-D$_3$-1 hydroxylation reaction within hours.[21] The exact mechanism by which chloroquine inhibits the pulmonary macrophage 1,25-dihydroxyvitamin D synthesis in sarcoidosis is not known.

Chloroquine therapy has not enjoyed wide popularity, partly because of the concern over retinal toxicity.[22] However, in comparison with corticosteroids, the side effect profile of chloroquine may be preferable. Complications of chloroquine therapy occur relatively infrequently, and most are transient and reversible with discontinuation of therapy. In patients with rheumatoid arthritis, chloroquine side effects occur in 3 to 7 percent of patients. The most common complaints are nausea and diarrhea. The most common ocular changes associated with chloroquine therapy are corneal deposition and retinopathy.[22] Corneal deposits occur in about 95 percent of patients receiving long-term therapy with 250 mg/day of chloroquine, but over 90 percent of these patients are asymptomatic.[22] Corneal deposition has no direct relationship to the development of retinopathy and is entirely reversible, disappearing within 6 to 8 weeks after discontinuation of therapy. Chloroquine-induced retinopathy was first recorded by Hobbs and colleagues in 1958.[23] The overall incidence of retinopathy in patients receiving chloroquine therapy is estimated to be 0.45 to 2 percent.[22] The size of the daily dose rather than total drug exposure correlates with the development of eye disease. Based upon more than 6000 patient-years of drug exposure in patients with rheumatoid arthritis, MacKenzie found no detectable eye disease in patients receiving less than 4 mg/kg/day of chloroquine or less than 5.6 mg/kg/day of hydroxychloroquine.[24] Daily dose must be calculated based on ideal body weight, not the actual weight of the patient.[24] Reports in which chloroquine-induced retinopathy has occurred in patients receiving 250 mg/day or less of chloroquine usually have exceeded 4 mg/kg/day. The fear of late-onset chloroquine-induced retinopathy is now questioned by many investigators and is not felt to be a major concern. Although correlating drug dose to the weight of the patient has been shown to decrease the risk of retinopathy, it is more important to have regular ocular examinations and frequent screenings to detect and prevent retinal toxicity. Ophthalmologic examination should be performed before therapy is initiated in all patients and repeated approximately every 6 months during therapy.

Antimalarial agents have a strong record of success in the treatment of disfiguring sarcoidosis skin lesions such as lupus pernio, plaques, and nodules. Intralesional steroid injections and topical corticosteroids are much less effective. Although corticosteroids remain the therapy of choice for progressive cutaneous sarcoidosis, chloroquine is a viable alternative in patients who cannot tolerate corticosteroid therapy or as adjunctive therapy in patients with poorly controlled disease. An initial 14-day course of 500 mg/day of chloroquine phosphate followed by the smaller of either 250 mg/day or 4 mg/kg/day of ideal body weight as maintenance therapy is recommended. Chloroquine and hydroxychloroquine may be considered in the treatment of sarcoidosis-associated hypercalcemia in patients who cannot tolerate corticosteroids. Prior to therapy, baseline liver function tests are recommended to ensure adequate liver function for normal metabolism and excretion of chloroquine. Acute toxic hepatitis can occur in patients with porphyria cutanea tarda who receive high doses of chloroquine.

METHOTREXATE

The most promising alternative to corticosteroids in the treatment of pulmonary sarcoidosis is low-dose methotrexate. Methotrexate is a commonly used antimetabolite in cancer chemotherapy that is becoming increasingly popular in the treatment of various nonmalignant diseases such as rheumatoid arthritis, inflammatory bowel disease, asthma, graft-versus-host disease, psoriasis, and Reiter's syndrome. Although its exact mechanism of action is unclear, it is unlikely that the beneficial effects of low dose methotrexate are related to its immunosuppressive effects, as these effects are subtle at best when compared to those of cyclosporine, cyclophosphamide, or azathioprine. It has been postulated that the effects of methotrexate are related to alterations in the local inflammatory response, as methotrexate is known to inhibit macrophage function and chemotaxis. Methotrexate diminishes peripheral blood B-lymphocyte and monocyte activity but has little affect on T lymphocytes.

Lower and Baughman studied the effects of low-dose methotrexate therapy in 15 sarcoidosis patients with either progressive disease or severe side effects from prednisone.[25] Patients received 10 mg of methotrexate weekly given as a single oral dose. All patients had previously been treated with prednisone, although not all patients were on prednisone at the time of the study. Disease duration ranged from 1 to 23 years; only one patient had disease for less than 2 years. All patients had lung involvement; however, in several patients, multiorgan disease was present. All patients received methotrexate for a minimum of 6 months. After 8 months of treatment, 13 of 14 patients were subjectively improved, while objective improvement was noted in 12 patients. Objective improvement was defined as greater than 15 percent improvement in vital capacity (5 patients), improvement in chest roentgenogram (6 patients), and greater than 50 percent reduction in skin lesions (4 patients) or liver function abnormalities (2 patients). Disease relapsed in 5 patients as methotrexate was being withdrawn. A single case of drug-related leukopenia occurred. Of the 11 patients who were concurrently receiving prednisone therapy, 6 were able to have their corticosteroids discontinued, while prednisone requirements decreased in 3 patients.

In a second study, Baughman and Lower studied the effect of methotrexate therapy on BAL lymphocytes and macrophages.[26] Patients were treated for at least 6 months with either 10 mg of methotrexate per week or a tapering dose of prednisone. Both groups showed significant improvement in vital capacity with therapy. In addition, the percentage of lymphocytes in BAL fell significantly for both the prednisone and methotrexate groups. The authors also noted that the amount of hydrogen peroxide and tumor necrosis factor released by the alveolar macrophages was significantly reduced after both therapies.

It appears that the risk-benefit ratio of methotrexate is low in comparison to that of prednisone. Liver disease, including cirrhosis, can be seen with methotrexate but the incidence is low and dose-related. Concern has been voiced over the potential for malignancy associated with long-term use of methotrexate; however, several studies have shown no increased risk in patients followed for more than 7 years after completion of methotrexate treatment.[27,28] Unfortunately, the drug has the potential to induce an allergic pneumonitis that may complicate its use in sarcoidosis. This reaction is characterized by dyspnea, nonproductive cough, fever, and hypoxemia in association with diffuse pulmonary infiltrates. Hilar adenopathy and pleural effusions may be seen. Most patients recover with discontinuation of the drug.

INHALED CORTICOSTEROIDS

Inhaled corticosteroids became available in 1978 for the treatment of patients with bronchial asthma. Early attempts to use inhaled beclomethasone dipropionate (BPT) for the treatment of pulmonary sarcoidosis were not successful. However, budesonide, available since 1982 for asthma, is part of a newer generation of more potent inhaled corticosteroids. These new agents have revived the enthusiasm for aerosolized corticosteroid therapy in pulmonary sarcoidosis. A number of studies have now looked at both the in vitro and in vivo effects of inhaled budesonide. Animal studies have shown that local instillation of inhaled steroids into the bronchial tree has resulted in higher tissue concentrations than systemic administration.[29] These studies were confirmed in humans who were undergoing thoracic surgery for localized lesions.[30] Patients were given inhaled budesonide 1600 μg as a single dose immediately before general anesthesia. Lung tissue samples obtained from the periphery of the lung showed tissue concentrations of budesonide high enough to cause receptor binding and exert local anti-inflammatory effect. Since budesonide is rapidly inactivated in the liver after systemic absorption, systemic bioavailability is low and high doses can be used by inhalation with a low risk of systemic side effects.

In the first clinical trials with inhaled budesonide for sarcoidosis, Selroos treated 20 patients with biopsy-proven disease.[29,30] All patients had chest roentgenographic stage II or III disease. Of the 20 patients, 9 had been treated earlier with oral corticosteroids but not within the 6 months preceding the study. Patients were initially given 800 μg of budesonide twice daily for 3 to 6 months; the dosage was then reduced to 800 μg per day. Sixteen patients demonstrated roentgenographic improvement, with three completely normalizing. The vital capacity improved in some patients but the change for the whole group was not statistically significant. Spiteri and colleagues compared 4 months of inhaled budesonide with placebo in a small group of patients with grade III abnormalities on their chest roentgenograms.[31] Distribution studies showed that 10 percent of the inhaled drug was deposited in the alveolar region. All 10 treated sarcoid patients had symptomatic relief with no adverse effects. Of the 10 patients, 3 showed significant resolution on chest roentgenogram. No significant difference in pulmonary function was noted. At the cellular level, a significant decrease in BAL lymphocytosis was seen after 16 weeks. No similar change was observed in the placebo group. During therapy, a change in the phenotype and functional characteristics of the alveolar macrophage population was noted; alveolar macrophages became better stimulators of autologous peripheral blood mononuclear cells. These data suggest that inhaled budesonide can modulate immunologic reactions in the lung in pulmonary sarcoidosis while also producing symptomatic relief with minimal side effects.

Studies have indicated that patients initially treated with oral glucocorticosteroids who have relapsed after stopping treatment could be successfully treated with inhaled budesonide alone at a dose of 1200 to 1600 μg daily, and budesonide has a systemic steroid-sparing capability in patients who require long-term maintenance therapy.[32,33]

The results with budesonide have been mixed, however. For example, Erkkilä and colleagues randomized 19 patients with newly detected pulmonary sarcoidosis (10 with stage I and 9 with stage II disease) between inhaled budesonide at 1600 μg/day and placebo for 8 to 10 weeks.[34] At the end of the trial period, no significant changes were noted in chest radiographs or lung function tests. However, decreases in serum angiotensin-converting enzyme (SACE) and β_2-microglobulin as well as BAL-hyaluronan levels were found in the budesonide-treated patients without similar changes in the placebo group. In addition, a significant decrease in the percentage of BAL T lymphocytes and a drop in the CD4/CD8 ratio was found in the treated group.

The major advantage of inhaled corticosteroids is safety, and their role will most likely be as systemic steroid-sparing agents in patients with symptomatic pulmonary sarcoidosis. The improvement with aerosolized therapy is slow compared to that seen with systemic steroids. Maximum improvement typically occurs within 2 to 3 weeks in patients receiving systemic steroids but may take 2 months or longer with inhaled steroids. The best therapy may be a combination of systemic and inhaled corticosteroids for rapid initial improvement and then maintenance therapy with inhaled corticosteroids to minimize or eliminate long-term oral corticosteroids.

References

1. Sharma OP: Sarcoidosis. *Disease-a-Month* 1990; 36:469–535.

2. Fordice J, Katras T, Jackson RE, et al.: Massive splenomegaly in sarcoidosis. *South Med J* 1992; 85:775–778.

3. Cuppage FE, Emmott DF, Duncan KA: Renal failure secondary to sarcoidosis. *Am J Kidney Dis* 1988; 11:519–520.

4. Cunningham D, Mills PR, Quigley EM, et al.: Hepatic granulomas: Experience over a 10-year period in the West of Scotland. *Q J Med* 1982; 51:162–170.

5. Winterbauer RH, Hutchinson JF: Clinical significance of pulmonary function tests. *Chest* 1980; 78:640–647.

6. Dawson WB, Müller NL: High resolution computed tomography in pulmonary sarcoidosis. *Semin Ultrasound CT MR* 1990; 11:423–429.

7. Kuhlman JE, Fishman EK, Hamper UM, et al.: The computed tomographic spectrum of thoracic sarcoidosis. *Radiographics* 1989; 9:449–466.

8. Sider L, Horton ES Jr: Hilar and mediastinal adenopathy in sarcoidosis as detected by computed tomography. *J Thorac Imaging* 1990; 5:77–80.

9. Winterbauer RH, Hammar SP: Sarcoidosis and idiopathic pulmonary fibrosis: A review of recent events, in Simmons DH (ed): *Current Pulmonology*, vol 7. Chicago, Year Book, 1986: 117–164.

10. Hillerdal G, Osterman NK, Schmekel B: Sarcoidosis: Epidemiology and diagnosis: A 15 year European study. *Am Rev Respir Dis* 1984; 130:29–32.

11. Neville E, Walker AN, James DG: Prognostic factors predicting the outcome of sarcoidosis: An analysis of 818 patients. *Q J Med* 1983; 52:525–533.

12. Harkleroad LE, Young RL, Savage PJ, et al.: Pulmonary sarcoidosis: Long-term follow-up of the effects of steroid therapy. *Chest* 1982; 82:84–87.

13. Israel HL, Fouts DW, Beggs RA: A controlled trial of prednisone treatment of sarcoidosis. *Am Rev Resp Dis* 1973; 107:609–614.

14. Johns CJ, Schonfeld SA, Scott PP, et al.: Longitudinal study of chronic sarcoidosis with low-dose maintenance corticosteroid therapy. *Ann NY Acad Sci* 1986; 465:702–712.

15. Spratling L, Tenholder MF, Underwood GH, et al.: Daily vs alternate day prednisone therapy for stage II sarcoidosis. *Chest* 1985; 88:687–690.

16. Kirtland SH, Winterbauer RH: Selected aspects of sarcoidosis, in Tierney D (ed): *Current Pulmonology*, vol 15, Chicago, Year Book, 1994: 399–439.

17. Schaffer B, Cahn MM, Levy EJ: Sarcoidosis apparently cured by quinacrine (Atabrine) hydrochloride. *Arch Dermatol* 1953; 67: 640–641, .

18. Morse SI, Cohn ZA, Hirsch JG, et al.: The treatment of sarcoidosis with chloroquine. *Am J Med* 1961; 30:779–784.

19. Research Committee of the British Tuberculosis Association: Chloroquine in the treatment of sarcoidosis: A report from the Research Committee of the British Tuberculosis Association. *Tubercle* 1967; 148:257–272.

20. Jones E, Callen JP: Hydroxychloroquine is effective therapy for control of cutaneous sarcoidal granulomas. *J Am Acad Dermatol* 1990; 23:487–489.

21. Adams JS, Diz MM, Sharma OP: Effective reduction in the serum 1,25-dihydroxyvitamin D and calcium concentration in sarcoidosis-associated hypercalcemia with short-course chloroquine therapy. *Ann Intern Med* 1989; 111:437–438.

22. Easterbrook M: Ocular effects and safety of antimalarial agents. *Am J Med* 1988; 85:23–29.

23. Hobbs HE, Sorsby A, Friedman A: Retinopathy following chloroquine therapy. *Lancet* 1958; ii:478–480.

24. MacKenzie AH: Dose refinements in long-term therapy of rheumatoid arthritis with antimalarials. *Am J Med* 1983; 75:40–45.

25. Lower EE, Baughman RP: The use of low dose methotrexate in refractory sarcoidosis. *Am J Med Sci* 1990; 299:153–157.

26. Baughman RP, Lower EE: The effect of corticosteroid or methotrexate therapy on lung lymphocytes and macrophages in sarcoidosis. *Am Rev Respir Dis* 1990; 142:1268–1271.

27. Toews GB, Lynch JP III: Methotrexate in sarcoidosis. *Am J Med Sci* 1990; 300:33–36.

28. Tugwell P, Bennett K, Bell M, et al.: Methotrexate in rheumatoid arthritis: Feedback on American College of Physicians Guidelines. *Ann Intern Med* 1989; 110:581–583.

29. Selroos O: Inhaled corticosteroids and pulmonary sarcoidosis. *Sarcoidosis* 1988; 5:104–105.

30. Selroos OB: Use of budesonide in the treatment of pulmonary sarcoidosis. *Ann NY Acad Sci* 1986; 465:713–721.

31. Spiteri MA, Newman SP, Clark SW, et al.: Inhaled corticosteroids can modulate the immunopathogenesis of pulmonary sarcoidosis. *Eur Respir J* 1989; 2:218–224.

32. Morgan AD, Johnson MA, Kerr I, et al.: The action of an inhaled corticosteroid as a steroid sparing agent in chronic pulmonary sarcoidosis. *Am Rev Respir Dis* 1987; 135:A349.

33. Gupta SK: Treatment of sarcoidosis patients by steroid aerosol: A ten-year prospective study from Eastern India. *Sarcoidosis* 1989; 6:51–54.

34. Erkkilä S, Fröseth B, Helström PE, et al.: Inhaled budesonide influences cellular and biochemical abnormalities in pulmonary sarcoidosis. *Sarcoidosis* 1988; 5:106–110.

Chapter 113

TREATMENT OF PULMONARY HYPERTENSION

HAROLD I. PALEVSKY

The Pulmonary Circulation

The pulmonary circulation is unique among the organ vascular beds in that it accommodates the entire cardiac output. Through vascular recruitment and distention, this high-capacitance, low-resistance circuit can normally accommodate several multiples of resting cardiac output with only slight increments in pulmonary arterial pressure.[1] The normal low pulsatile pulmonary arterial pressure is sufficient to overcome pulmonary vascular resistance and to keep pulmonary blood flow equal to systemic blood flow. This is accomplished with an average pressure decrease (in mean pressure) of only 5 to 10 mmHg between the pulmonary artery and left atrium. In normal subjects under age 40, even during exertion, the upper limit of mean pulmonary arterial pressure at sea level is 30 mmHg; in trained athletes achieving cardiac outputs greater than 20 L/min, mean pulmonary arterial pressures may be greater.[2]

Because of the effect of hypoxemia on resting pulmonary arterial tone, the criteria for defining pulmonary hypertension depends on altitude; while at sea level, a resting mean pulmonary arterial pressure > 20 mmHg is considered abnormal; at an altitude of 15,000 ft, the normal range for resting mean pulmonary arterial pressure extends to 25 mmHg. Resting pulmonary hypertension at sea level, even if only mild, generally signifies a limitation of the pulmonary vascular tree and/or an elevated pulmonary blood flow. The abnormal pulmonary arterial pressures increase significantly when either vascular tone or blood flow increases (e.g., during acute hypoxia or exertion). In all pulmonary hypertensive states, the pressures are important only in terms of the strain imposed on the right ventricle, with intermittent increases in right ventricular afterload of lesser significance than sustained increases. However, over time, even intermittent strain on the right ventricle results in muscular hypertrophy and may possibly cause heart failure.

Pulmonary hypertension is frequently not diagnosed until right ventricular hypertrophy or rightsided heart failure is detected. The normal right ventricle can generate systolic pressures up to approximately 50 mmHg in response to an acute increase in afterload (i.e., acute pulmonary embolism). If the afterload has developed gradually so that the right ventricle has had time to hypertrophy, it can generate substantially higher pressures, even up to systemic arterial pressure levels. However, if the increased afterload is maintained, it is likely that the ventricle will dilate and ultimately fail.

The pulmonary vascular bed is frequently described by an equation relating inflow and outflow pressures to the pulmonary blood flow (cardiac output), which equation is analogous to Ohm's law:

$$\text{Pulmonary vascular resistance} = \frac{\begin{array}{c}\text{mean pulmonary} \\ \text{arterial pressure} \\ \text{(mmHg)}\end{array} - \begin{array}{c}\text{mean pulmonary} \\ \text{arterial wedge} \\ \text{pressure (mmHg)}\end{array}}{\text{pulmonary blood flow (L/min)}}$$

Expressed this way, the normal pulmonary vascular resistance is approximately 1 U. Resistance also may be expressed in dyne·s·cm^{-5} by multiplying the numerator of this equation by 79.9; expressed in this manner, the normal pulmonary vascular resistance is approximately 50 to 100 dyne·s·cm^{-5}.

This resistance equation, adapted from Poiseuille's law, is based on the laminar flow of a Newtonian fluid through rigid tubes and does not readily apply to the pulmonary circulation. The normal pulmonary vascular bed is composed of elastic, distensible vessels, not rigid tubes; they change in diameter with changes in pulmonary blood volume, flow, and pressure. Pulmonary blood flow is pulsatile and turbulent rather than laminar. The pulmonary blood volume is altered by changes in blood flow, transthoracic pressures, and the gravitational effects of posture. Blood is a non-Newtonian fluid; its apparent viscosity changes with different flow velocities. Thus, the resistance equation may not accurately describe the highly distensible, normal pulmonary circulation; it may be more relevant to the abnormal pulmonary circulation in which vessel walls are thickened and have become more rigid.

Because the relationship between pressure and flow in the normal pulmonary circulation is not linear, resistance is not a constant but varies with the flow through the system, with the pressure drop across the pulmonary circulation, and with the other factors noted above. This complicates interpretation of calculated values for pulmonary vascular resistance, especially in evaluating the effect of a therapeutic intervention on the pulmonary circulation. The substitution of mean pulmonary arterial pressure for the pressure decrease between the pulmonary artery and the left atrium in the numerator of the resistance equation further deprives the calculation of any physiologic meaning.

Pathogenesis of Pulmonary Hypertension

The major causative factor in the development of pulmonary hypertension is an increase in the pulmonary vascular resistance, which is localized primarily to the precapillary arteries and arterioles.[3] This increase in vascular resistance may be anatomic or vasoconstrictive in origin. Often—particularly in long-standing pulmonary vascular processes—both mechanisms are involved.[4,5] Regardless of cause, when the pulmonary vascular reserve is compromised by a progressive reduction in the extent and/or the distensibility of the pulmonary vascular bed, increases in cardiac output result in elevation of pulmonary arterial pressures. Over time, lesser increments in pulmonary blood flow (cardiac output) are required to generate pulmonary hypertension. Eventually, even the resting cardiac output results in increased pulmonary arterial pressures.

OXYGEN TENSIONS

The most potent stimulus for pulmonary vasoconstriction is alveolar hypoxia acting on the adjacent small pulmonary arteries and arterioles. Systemic arterial hypoxemia augments the local effects of alveolar hypoxia indirectly through sympathetic neural reflexes.[6] In chronic hypoxemia, the effects of these pulmonary vasoconstrictor stimuli often are augmented by increased blood viscosity caused by sec-

ondary polycythemia. Episodic exacerbations of hypoxemia result in progressive pulmonary vascular impairment and may lead to development of sustained pulmonary hypertension, even though recovery from early episodes is frequently associated with the return of pulmonary arterial pressures to normal levels.[7]

ACID-BASE STATUS

Acidosis (pH < 7.2) also elicits pulmonary vasoconstriction. In humans, acidosis acts synergistically with hypoxia, whereas alkalosis diminishes the vasoconstrictive response to hypoxia.[1]

CARBON DIOXIDE

Carbon dioxide contributes to pulmonary hypertension predominantly by causing respiratory acidosis rather than by direct vasoconstriction.[1] Metabolic alkalosis induced by sodium bicarbonate administration can overcome the pressor effects of respiratory acidosis induced by acute hypercapnia.[8] In chronic lung diseases, carbon dioxide retention may be self-perpetuating; hypercapnia blunts the responsiveness of respiratory centers to carbon dioxide and promotes retention of bicarbonate by the kidney.[9] Not only the hypercapnia resulting from disorders to the lungs or ventilation, but also that seen in response to metabolic alkalosis, results in ventilatory depression, with consequent progressive hypercapnia, hypoxia, and pulmonary vasoconstriction.

MEDIATORS OF VASCULAR TONE

Investigations into the mechanisms by which vascular smooth muscle tone is regulated have placed renewed emphasis on the role of the pulmonary endothelium in the uptake and metabolism of vasoactive compounds and have led to the description of potent mediators of both vasodilation and vasoconstriction.

Among the compounds described, prostacyclin (prostaglandin I_2), the predominant metabolite of arachidonic acid, appears to play an important role in the local modulation of vascular tone.[10] Endothelium-derived relaxing factor (EDRF) is a product of the intact vascular endothelium and acts on adjacent vascular smooth muscle. After intensive efforts to characterize EDRF, it appears that it may be the short-lived, diffusible, free radical nitroxide (NO·), which acts by stimulating guanylate cyclase in the smooth muscle to increase cyclic guanosine monophosphate levels.[11,12] Both of these mediators have been introduced into clinical trials in the treatment of pulmonary hypertension (see "Treatment of Pulmonary Hypertension," below).

Endothelins, a family of 21-amino-acid peptides, are circulating hormones with potent smooth muscle constrictive effects.[13] These compounds are produced by both pulmonary vascular endothelial cells and bronchiolar respiratory epithelial cells and, in experimental preparations, can cause both significant pulmonary vasoconstriction and airways smooth muscle constriction. There is speculation that one or more of the endothelins may be the mediator of hypoxic pulmonary vasoconstriction.[14,15]

Additional mediators of vascular tone will be identified in the future, and modification of the balance between the mediators of vasodilation and vasoconstriction will be of clinical relevance in the management of pulmonary vascular disease states.

Treatment of Pulmonary Hypertension

At present, the treatment of pulmonary hypertension is directed toward any reversible component of the underlying pathogenetic process while relieving any hypoxemia, hypercapnia, or acidosis that might be contributing to right-sided heart strain. In addition to specific measures, several categories of treatment may be helpful in patients with pulmonary hypertension regardless of cause (Table 113-1).

OXYGEN SUPPLEMENTATION

In patients demonstrating any arterial hypoxemia—resting, exertional, or nocturnal—there is a role for oxygen supplementation in treating hypoxic vasoconstriction. The objective is to reduce the afterload on the right ventricle, while also reducing any contribution of the hypoxemia to arrhythmogenesis. Consideration should be given to performing a sleep study in the evaluation of unexplained pulmonary hypertension. Exertional arterial desaturation should be considered in all patients with a decreased diffusing capacity (e.g., < 60 percent of predicted value)[16,17]; these patients should be exercised to tolerance while arterial oxygen saturation is monitored with pulse oximetry. Although oxygen administration entails some risk in patients with obstructive pulmonary disease by decreasing respiratory drive and alveolar ventilation and thereby worsening respiratory acidosis, oxygen supplementation to maintain an arterial oxygen tension of > 60 mmHg, or an arterial oxygen saturation of > 90 percent, has been shown to reduce the mortality of cor pulmonale and improve cognitive function and quality of life in patients with advanced obstructive pulmonary disease.[9,18–21] Although the best data are available for COPD, it is likely that oxygen supplementation is of similar benefit in other advanced pulmonary conditions resulting in pulmonary hypertension. In primary pulmonary hypertension, a Mayo Clinic study has shown that decreased systemic arterial oxygen saturation (Sa_{O_2} was the single factor most predictive of patient survival).[22] In this and other studies, decreased Sa_{O_2} was associated with a high incidence of sudden death.

TABLE 113-1   Pulmonary Hypertension: Pharmacologic Therapy

Treat any underlying disorders that can be treated
Oxygen supplementation
Treatment of right heart failure
  low salt diet
  diuretics
  digitalis
  phlebotomy
Anticoagulation or antiplatelet agents
Vasodilators

TREATMENT OF RIGHT HEART FAILURE

Right-sided heart failure in pulmonary hypertension and cor pulmonale may be transient if the exacerbating factors can be controlled. The usual therapies for heart failure are used: low-salt diet and administration of digitalis and diuretics.[1,23] Phlebotomy to decrease the circulating blood volume (and hematocrit) may be of benefit in patients with secondary polycythemia; repeated phlebotomies may be needed to maintain the benefit.[24]

DIGITALIS

The use of digitalis in right ventricular dysfunction and failure remains controversial; it has been shown to improve right ventricular function only when left heart dysfunction also is present.[25] Digitalis directly increases pulmonary vascular resistance and has a high incidence of toxicity in patients with cor pulmonale.[23,26] Despite this, digitalis is used routinely in patients receiving calcium channel blockers as vasodilating agents (see "Vasodilators," below). In this situation, the concurrent administration of digitalis may serve to offset the negative inotropic effects of calcium channel blockade on cardiac function.

DIURETICS

Diuretics have a long-standing role in the treatment of symptomatic consequences of right heart failure such as peripheral edema, systemic venous congestion, and hepatic distention. They also can provide symptomatic relief of dyspnea and orthopnea in chronic cor pulmonale.[27] In these patients, left ventricular function is thought to be compromised by right ventricular hypertrophy and dilatation and by alterations in the geometry and function of the intraventricular septum. Diuretics should be given with care, particularly in patients with abnormalities of ventilatory control, because metabolic alkalosis may complicate their use; alkalosis, in turn, contributes to ventilatory insufficiency by depressing the ventilatory response to carbon dioxide. Moreover, diuresis may increase blood viscosity by increasing the hematocrit. In patients with right heart failure, excessive diuresis results further may in inadequate filling of the right side of the heart and compromise cardiac output and arterial oxygenation.

ANTICOAGULATION

In situ thrombosis as a consequence of endothelial injury and abnormal blood flow has been observed to occur in the pulmonary microvasculature in all forms of pulmonary hypertension.[28–32] It is likely that this process further compromises the cross-sectional area of the pulmonary circulation, causing progressive increase in pulmonary vascular resistance and contributing to the deteriorating course observed in most patients with pulmonary hypertension. Moreover, once the patient progresses to right heart failure, peripheral venous thrombosis and pulmonary embolism occurs as consequences of venous dilation and stasis and decreased physical activity. Both retrospective[22] and, more recently, prospective data on the survival of patients with primary pulmonary hypertension (PPH) have shown that anticoagulation (usually with warfarin) provides a survival benefit.[33] While not a universal finding, some studies have found elevated concentrations of fibrinopeptide A (indicative of ongoing thrombosis)[34,35] and increased urinary excretion of metabolites of thromboxane A$_2$ (indicative of platelet activation)[36,37] in patients with PPH and other types of pulmonary vascular disease. Based on these hypotheses and observations, anticoagulation with warfarin or adjusted dose subcutaneous heparin or treatment with antiplatelet agents (aspirin, possibly in combination with dipyridamole) is recommended for patients with pulmonary hypertension. Caution is indicated in patients with pulmonary hypertension who manifest syncope (up to 55 percent of patients with PPH).[38,39] Routine prophylaxis with subcutaneous heparin is advisable during all periods of hospitalization or prolonged immobility.

The occurrence of in situ thrombosis in patients with PPH raises speculation that the improved outcomes that have been reported with long-term prostacyclin infusions, even in patients who do not exhibit substantial acute hemodynamic effects (see below), may be caused by the potent effect of prostacyclin on inhibiting platelet aggregation.[40] Similarly, there is a theoretical basis to suspect that heparin administered subcutaneously may be preferable to warfarin in the long-term management of pulmonary hypertension because of its inhibitory effects on smooth-muscle (and endothelial) cell proliferation.[41]

VASODILATORS

Pulmonary vasodilator therapy is based on the premise that pulmonary vasoconstriction is an important component of pulmonary hypertension.[3,4] This vasoconstriction may be the primary cause of increased pulmonary vascular resistance or it may be secondary to the distension of pulmonary blood vessels by increased intraluminal pressures.[5] The goal has been to decrease right ventricular afterload and to arrest and reverse obliterative changes in the pulmonary vascular bed. While vasodilators have been most extensively studied in primary pulmonary hypertension, the general principles and findings are likely applicable to other pulmonary hypertensive conditions.

VASODILATOR RESPONSES

The optimal response to the acute administration of a vasodilator agent in pulmonary hypertension would be a reduction in pulmonary arterial pressure (unaccompanied by any change in pulmonary wedge pressure) accompanied by an increase in cardiac output, resulting in a decrease in pulmonary vascular resistance; the systemic arterial blood pressure and oxygenation should be little affected. Unfortunately, this pattern of response is seen in only approximately 15 percent to 25 percent of patients.[42] In primary pulmonary hypertension, the most frequent response to vasodilation is an increase in cardiac output without much change in either pulmonary arterial (or wedge) pressure or arterial oxygen tension (up to one-half of patients).[42,43] This response pattern also results in a decrease in the calculated pulmonary vascular resistance, but without a decrease in the hemodynamic load of the right ventricle

and may be accompanied by an improved sense of well-being and an improved exercise tolerance. However, despite the increase in cardiac output and the decrease in calculated pulmonary vascular resistance, clinical improvement may be short-lived unless the pulmonary arterial pressure (and right ventricular work) also decreases. Occasionally, the improvements in exercise hemodynamics are of greater magnitude than the changes in resting values; this may account for clinical improvement beyond that anticipated by the resting vasodilator responses.

Unfortunately, vasodilating agents often affect the systemic vascular bed more than they do the pulmonary vascular bed. If systemic vasodilation predominates and cardiac output increases in response to this, the increase in blood flow (cardiac output) through a restricted pulmonary vascular bed will cause pulmonary arterial pressure (and right ventricular work) to increase (despite a decrease in calculated pulmonary vascular resistance). If systemic vasodilation predominates and the cardiac output fails to increase, systemic hypotension will result. This hypotension may be difficult to treat, even after vasodilator administration is discontinued. Volume administration often is unsuccessful, and vasopressors administered to cause systemic vasoconstriction may worsen the pulmonary hypertension, acutely increasing the right ventricular afterload. Systemic hypotension may cause decreasing coronary arterial perfusion and myocardial ischemia (particularly in the right ventricle), which can precipitate or worsen cardiac function and, in particular, ventricular failure. The possible serious adverse consequences of administering vasodilating agents make it essential that "trials" be performed by experienced personnel in a hospital setting where continuous monitoring of pulmonary and systemic hemodynamics, as well as arterial oxygenation, is possible (Table 113-2).

DEFINING FAVORABLE VASODILATOR RESPONSIVENESS

Various criteria have been proposed for defining a "positive" or favorable response to the acute administration of vasodilator agents.[43,44] These criteria usually involve some combination of a reduction in pulmonary vascular resistance with a decrement in pulmonary arterial pressure. If sustained, the combination of a decrease in pulmonary arterial pressure and a decrease in pulmonary vascular resistance can be expected to be of clinical benefit by decreasing the work of the right ventricle.

More important than just evoking in acute vasodilator response is establishing criteria that predict long-term clinical vasodilator responses and/or patient survival. Reeves

---

TABLE 113-2   Monitoring during Vasodilator Administration

Systemic arterial blood pressure
Electrocardiogram
Arterial oxygen saturation
Pulmonary arterial pressures
   systolic, diastolic, and mean
Pulmonary artery occlusion (wedge) pressure
Cardiac output

and co-workers have shown that patients who had a reduction in pulmonary vascular resistance > 30 percent during an acute vasodilator trial were more likely to demonstrate sustained clinical improvement than patients who did not have acute responses of this magnitude; 33 of 53 responders were improved, while only 4 of 64 nonresponders were improved.[45] Supporting this observation are studies using high doses of calcium channel antagonists (see below)[33]; these also suggest that, the greater the magnitude of the resistance change to acute vasodilator administration, the more likely there is to be long-term clinical and hemodynamic benefit. This is particularly true when the decrease in calculated pulmonary vascular resistance is associated with a decrease in pulmonary arterial pressure.

SCREENING FOR VASODILATOR RESPONSIVENESS

The administration of vasodilators in evaluating for pulmonary vascular responsiveness poses a dilemma; although many patients with PPH who respond favorably to the acute administration of a vasodilator agent benefit from long-term vasodilator therapy, the acute administration of vasodilators, particularly long-acting agents, can be dangerous. This has encouraged the search for potent, short-acting pulmonary vasodilating agents that can be administered safely for the assessment of pulmonary vasoreactivity. An ideal screening agent for acute pulmonary vascular responsiveness should have the following properties: (1) it should be an agent that elicits pulmonary vasodilation at a dose that has little or no effect on the systemic circulation; (2) it should be short-acting and should be cleared rapidly from the body, so that baseline hemodynamic state is rapidly reestablished once administration is discontinued; (3) it should be easy to administer accurately in an incremental dosing regimen; (4) the hemodynamic and side effects of the screening agent should predict effects that longer-acting agents will elicit; that is, it should identify those patients who will respond to longer-acting vasodilators as well as those who will experience adverse events; and (5) it should identify those patients who will not respond to pulmonary vasodilator therapy. Thus, use of an ideal screening agent should expedite the identification of patients in whom the risk-benefit profile warrants a search for the optimal, longer-acting vasodilator agent and the elimination from further studies of those patients who either cannot respond or who would experience adverse consequences of the drug therapy.

Of the short-acting, intravenously administered agents listed in Table 113-3, four have been used as potential screening agents for assessing acute pulmonary vasodilator responsiveness: prostacyclin and its analog iloprost, acetylcholine, and adenosine.

Prostacyclin

Prostacyclin has been the most intensively studied of these agents.[46] It is a potent pulmonary vasodilator and inhibitor of platelet aggregation normally produced by vascular endothelial cells. According to the criteria above, it is an excellent screening agent for accessing pulmonary vasodilator responsiveness. It has a short half-life (less than 5 minutes), its hemodynamics effects resolve rapidly and incremental intravenous dosing can be used to assess pul-

TABLE 113-3   Potential Screening Agents for the Assessment of Pulmonary Vascular Responsiveness

Acetylcholine
Adenosine
Amrinone
Nitric oxide
Nitroglycerin
Prostacyclin (PGI_2) and analogs
Prostaglandin E_1
Sodium nitroprusside

monary arterial vasodilator responses without undo effect on the systemic circulation. Acute prostacyclin administration has been well tolerated by patients with PPH and has been shown to predict pulmonary vasodilator responses to standard vasodilator agents.[47–51] Prostacyclin also appears to identify those patients with PPH who will not respond to administration of more traditional, standard vasodilators. Prostacyclin has recently been approved by the Food and Drug Administration for continuous intravenous infusion for the long-term treatment of primary pulmonary hypertension, see below. Continuous intravenous infusion is required since no long acting analogs of prostacyclin are available.

Iloprost

Iloprost is a short-acting, stable carbacyclin derivative of prostacyclin that has similar pharmacologic effects on the pulmonary circulation in patients with PPH.[52,53] However, iloprost is somewhat more stable than prostacyclin, with a half-life > 10 min, and can be stored at room temperature. Iloprost is currently an investigational agent with very limited availability and for which no long-acting analogs are available.

Acetylcholine

Acetylcholine is another drug suitable as a screening agent for pulmonary vasodilating capacity; it has a short pharmacologic half-life and is well-tolerated by patients. Acetylcholine was used to test for vasodilation in patients with PPH in the 1950s; however, it was abandoned when orally administered vasodilators became available. Acetylcholine has been compared with prostacyclin as screening agents for pulmonary vasodilator potential in PPH.[50] Both agents were successful in identifying patients with PPH whose conditions responded to standard vasodilator agents, although the magnitude of the responses to prostacyclin tended to be greater. This suggests that acetylcholine may be useful in screening to identify those patients with PPH who are likely to respond to treatment with standard vasodilators.

Adenosine

Adenosine, a purine nucleoside with a very short pharmacologic half-life (< 10 s), recently has been shown to be a potent pulmonary vasodilator in vitro.[54] In initial trials in patients with PPH, adenosine has demonstrated pulmonary vasodilating properties without significant systemic side effects in dosages up to 300 μg/kg per min.[55,56]

A recent comparison of the acute hemodynamic effects of adenosine and prostacyclin infusions in PPH found that at maximal tolerated dosing adenosine (200 ± 53 ng/kg per min) caused a 33 ± 18 percent decrease in pulmonary vascular resistance, a 52 ± 25 percent increase in cardiac output, and no effect on pulmonary or systemic arterial pressures.[51] Prostacyclin (8 ± 4 ng/kg per min) produced a 22 ± 18 percent decrease in pulmonary vascular resistance, a 25 ± 26 percent increase in cardiac output in association with a 14 ± 6 percent decrease in systemic arterial pressure, and no change in pulmonary arterial pressure. Adenosine is readily available (although not approved for use as a pulmonary vasodilator) and appears to be effective, safe, and relatively inexpensive for use in screening for pulmonary vascular responsiveness.

STANDARD VASODILATOR THERAPY

Most attempts to vasodilate the pulmonary circulation have involved the use of longer-acting agents, familiar as systemic vasodilators, that can be administered orally. These agents have not been uniform or consistent in their pulmonary vasodilator capabilities, and all have elicited adverse as well as desirable beneficial responses.[43] A wide range of different pharmacologic classes is represented by the available agents (Table 113-4): α-adrenergic antagonists, β-adrenergic agonists, calcium channel–blocking agents, inhibitors of angiotensin-converting enzyme, nitrates, and "direct-acting" vasodilator agents.[42,57–62] In patients who demonstrate vasodilator responsiveness to administration of a screening agent, it may be necessary to test multiple agents of different pharmacologic classes, since striking variability in responses to different agents is a common finding. Some investigators have proposed that since the long-term effects of high-dose calcium channel antagonists are more consistent than those obtained with other agents, only this class of agents need be tested. This certainly shortens the drug trials but may miss a favorable response to another agent, a circumstance that would be anticipated to occur in a minority of instances.

After identifying an agent that can elicit acute vasodilation, it is uncertain how the response will change over time. Some patients with PPH clearly maintain their vasodilator responsiveness and appear to benefit from long-term therapy. Other patients with PPH respond well initially to the administration of a vasodilator agent but lose responsiveness over time.[43,44,62,63] In these individuals it is difficult to distinguish the mechanisms responsible for this change in drug effect; that is, tachyphylaxis or progression of the underlying pathologic process.

It also is uncertain whether the lack of an acute vasodilator response signifies that no benefit can be expected from long-term vasodilator therapy. Patients often report an improved sense of well-being when being treated, despite often only exhibiting minimal hemodynamic improvement. Since some of the newer pulmonary vasodilator agents (in particular, the calcium channel-blocking agents) usually are well-tolerated by patients, many patients are tried on long-term treatment, even though no significant acute vasodilator response was elicited during short-term drug trials. Chronic intravenous prostacyclin therapy has been shown to be of long-term benefit in patients who did not respond to acute infusion with pulmonary vasodilation.

PULMONARY VASODILATING AGENTS

The classes of agents used as pulmonary vasodilators are presented in Table 113-4. Many of these agents have been used less frequently in the treatment of chronic pulmonary hypertension (i.e., PPH) since the introduction of high-dose calcium channel blockade and continuous intravenous prostacyclin therapy. However, in other situations, such as acute pulmonary hypertension after cardiac surgery, various of the listed agents continue to be used.

Sodium Nitroprusside

Sodium nitroprusside, a very short-acting agent available only for intravenous administration, has relatively balanced vasodilating effects on arterial and venous resistance vessels. In some individuals with primary pulmonary hypertension, acute administration of nitroprusside-elicited pulmonary vasodilation.[64] This agent still is used in evaluating the reversibility of pulmonary hypertension caused by left heart disease during heart transplant evaluations and after cardiac surgery. For sustained vasodilation, a combination of hydralazine and a nitrate may reproduce the response to nitroprusside.

Nitroglycerin and Long-Acting Nitrates

Nitroglycerin and nitrates induce smooth muscle relaxation by a mechanism that entails the release of nitric oxide (NO) (see "Nitric Oxide," below). In an animal model of pulmonary hypertension, nitroglycerin increased cardiac output and decreased pulmonary arterial pressures.[65] In humans, nitroglycerin and long-acting nitrates have sometimes reduced pulmonary arterial pressure and pulmonary vascular resistance without eliciting much systemic arterial vasodilation.[66] The availability of topical, sublingual, and oral preparations for long-term therapy has simplified the use of nitroglycerin for the chronic management of the few patients with pulmonary hypertension who respond by pulmonary vasodilation during acute testing with this agent.

β-Adrenergic Agonists

Isoproterenol has been used as a pulmonary vasodilator since the early 1960s. A powerful sympathomimetic amine

---

TABLE 113-4   **Agents Used As Pulmonary Vasodilator Agents (Short- and Long-Term Administration)**

Acetylcholine
Adenosine
α-Adrenergic antagonists
Angiotensin-converting enzyme inhibitors
β-Adrenergic agonists
Calcium channel blockers
E-series prostaglandins
Nitrates
Nitric oxide
Nonspecific antihypertensive agents (sodium nitroprusside, hydralazine, diazoxide)
Prostacyclin (PGI$_2$) and analogs
Serotonin (S$_2$) receptor blockers

that acts on β-adrenergic receptors throughout the body, isoproterenol leaves α-adrenergic receptors unaffected. It increases the cardiac output through its chronotropic and inotropic effects in addition to increasing venous return by evoking peripheral vasodilation. When administered intravenously or sublingually, pulmonary arterial pressure either remains unchanged or occasionally increases; calculated pulmonary vascular resistance usually decreases.[67] In a few patients, pulmonary arterial pressures and pulmonary vascular resistance decreased after isoproterenol and, in some, symptomatic and hemodynamic improvement were sustained by the chronic administration of isoproterenol sublingually.[68] Other β-adrenergic agonists (e.g., terbutaline) may be of benefit for those patients who demonstrated pulmonary vasodilation to isoproterenol.[69]

α-Adrenergic Antagonists

Several α-adrenergic antagonists are available for use in pulmonary hypertension. Tolazoline hydrochloride was the first oral agent used as a pulmonary vasodilator. It was effective when given intravenously but not orally; it is of historical interest only because equally effective α-adrenergic antagonists, with fewer side effects, currently are available for oral administration.

Phentolamine is a potent α-adrenergic antagonist that exerts its effects at both the pre- and postsynaptic receptors. It blocks the reuptake of norepinephrine, thereby increasing sympathetic tone and exerting chronotropic and inotropic effects on the heart. In a few PPH patients, particularly those with the veno-occlusive histology, α-adrenergic blockade using phentolamine produced a favorable hemodynamic response.[70,71] Experience with other α-adrenergic blocking agents (e.g., prazosin and phenoxybenzamine) is much more limited. Nonetheless, in a few patients, these agents also have been shown to cause pulmonary vasodilation.[71,72] Prazosin, which only blocks the postsynaptic (α_1) α-adrenergic receptor sites, has not been used widely because of its reputation for inducing tachyphylaxis. However, loss of effect may be caused by progression of the underlying disease. Phentolamine is no longer marketed for oral use, although a limited supply may be available for those patients who are refractory to other pulmonary vasodilators. The unavailability and uncertainty that handicaps the use of the α-adrenergic blockers seems destined to decrease their use in the treatment of pulmonary hypertension.

Hydralazine

Hydralazine, a direct acting vasodilator, has undergone extensive studies as a systemic antihypertensive agent where its primary effect is to dilate precapillary resistance vessels; it also has a lesser effect on venous beds. Hydralazine also increases cardiac output, both by a positive inotropic effect and by evoking tachycardia; the latter seems to be a central nervous system reflex response to the drug-induced drop in systemic vascular resistance.

Hydralazine was used extensively in primary pulmonary hypertension after a 1980 report that, when taken orally, it affected both acute and chronic reductions in pulmonary vascular resistance at rest and during exercise.[73] However, initial enthusiasm was tempered by subsequent reports

describing the serious complications of hydralazine usage.[74] Many of the complications are shared with other vasodilators, notably systemic arterial hypotension.[75] Prediction of responders is unreliable. One study found that patients with lesser degrees of pulmonary hypertension respond better to hydralazine as a pulmonary vasodilator than do those with higher pressures.[76] This result is not unexpected since, with time and prolonged elevation of pulmonary artery pressures, patients tend to develop a fixed and unresponsive vasculature, possibly because of increasing fibrosis in the pulmonary vascular lesions.

Angiotensin-Converting Enzyme Inhibitors

Attempts to use angiotensin-converting enzyme inhibitors (e.g., captopril) in patients with primary pulmonary hypertension have met with varying degrees of success. Unfortunately, although a few dramatic instances of pulmonary vasodilation are reported, as a rule this class of agents has not been useful.[77,78]

Calcium Channel Blockers

Nifedipine, verapamil, and diltiazem are the calcium "channel blockers" (calcium channel antagonists) that have had the greatest use in the treatment of primary pulmonary hypertension. They are all believed to act primarily by inhibiting the influx of calcium into pulmonary vascular smooth muscle cells, thus inhibiting muscular contraction and resulting in vasodilation. In experimental studies in animals, nifedipine proved to be the most potent pulmonary vasodilator of the three[79]; verapamil had the greatest (undesirable) negative inotropic effects.[80] In some patients, acute administration of these agents elicited the desirable responses of reducing pulmonary arterial pressures and pulmonary vascular resistance. At present, nifedipine is the most frequently used calcium channel blocker for primary pulmonary hypertension although some patients who have systemic side effects to nifedipine can better tolerate diltiazem. Unfortunately, not all patients respond well to calcium blockers, and not all who respond acutely sustain improvement on chronic therapy.

Adverse responses to calcium channel antagonists are relatively infrequent. In a few patients, cardiac output increases while pulmonary vascular tone appears to be unaffected. This leads to increased pulmonary arterial pressures. In others, the negative inotropic effects of calcium blockade result in fatigue and signs of right ventricular failure during chronic maintenance therapy. To offset this, it has become standard to place patients receiving calcium channel antagonists on digitalis (see "Digitalis," above).

Approximately 10 years ago, Rich and Brundage began studying the role of high-dose calcium channel–blocking agents in the treatment of primary pulmonary hypertension.[81] This was based on the observation that there was not a linear dose-response and that some patients required substantial doses of nifedipine or diltiazem before decreasing pulmonary vascular resistance. In their initial study of 13 PPH patients who did not respond to conventional doses of calcium channel antagonists, they observed substantial responses to high doses of calcium channel antagonists in 8 patients. Four of 5 patients restudied after 1 year of therapy exhibited sustained vasodilator responsiveness and demonstrated regression of right ventricular hypertrophy.

In a subsequent study of 64 PPH patients, Rich and colleagues found that 17 (26 percent) responded to high-dose calcium channel antagonists with a > 20 percent decrease in both pulmonary artery pressure and pulmonary vascular resistance.[33] In this group, 5-year survival was 94 percent, as compared to 55 percent in the group of nonresponders (a majority of whom were anticoagulated). In comparison, the 5-year survival of patients in the NIH-PPH registry was only 38 percent.[38]

Prostaglandins

The lung, and in particular the pulmonary vascular endothelium, is one of the major sites of prostaglandin synthesis and inactivation.[82] Prostaglandin and leukotriene precursors, intermediates, and metabolites contribute importantly to normal pulmonary vascular tone. In particular, prosta-glandin $F_{2\alpha}$ and thromboxane A_2 are potent vasoconstrictors (and platelet aggregators), where prostaglandins E_1 and I_2 (prostacyclin) are potent vasodilators (and inhibitors of platelet aggregation). It has been suggested that derangements in the prostaglandin systems may be involved in the pathogenesis of both primary and secondary pulmonary hypertension, and that many of the vasodilators listed above may work, in part, by modulating prostaglandin balance.[36,37,83]

Initial attempts to influence the prostaglandin systems directly in primary pulmonary hypertension involved trials of cyclooxygenase inhibitors administered orally. Although occasional case reports suggest that indomethacin may play a role in the treatment of primary pulmonary hypertension, this experience has rarely been confirmed.[84]

Prostaglandin E_1 is available for intravenous infusion to maintain the patency of the ductus arteriosus in newborns with congenital heart disease, and to try and decrease pulmonary vascular resistance in neonates with persistent pulmonary hypertension of the newborn. There is only limited experience using this agent in other pulmonary hypertensive conditions.[85]

Prostacyclin (PGI_2) is a potent pulmonary vasodilator and inhibitor of platelet aggregation. Currently, only available for intravenous infusion, as noted above, prostacyclin has been advocated as a screening agent to test the ability of the pulmonary vascular bed to dilate.[48,50] More recently, studies have been undertaken on the role of continuous intravenous infusion of prostacyclin in the management of PPH patients who have failed all other therapies. Initially this approach was thought to be best-suited for supporting severely ill patients with PPH who were awaiting heart-lung or lung transplantation (e.g., a bridge to transplantation). However, in patients who exhibit pronounced response to PGI_2 infusion, the infusion is being maintained long-term (> 5 years) with consideration of transplantation only if symptoms recur or if complications ensue.[40,86,87] The delivery system requires a portable infusion pump and a Hickman type central venous catheter; frequent dosing increments are required to maintain responses and complications (including death) have occurred as a consequence of thrombosis or infection of the indwelling catheter, or interruptions of drug delivery caused by pump malfunction or other reasons. Despite these problems, data from a 12-week long prospective randomized trial comparing conventional therapy with continuous intravenous prostacyclin infusion in severe primary pulmonary hypertension found that prostacyclin produced symptomatic and hemodynamic improvement, as well as improved survival.[87A] Data from a long-term follow-up study showed three years survival on continuous intravenous prostacyclin therapy to be 63.3 percent as compared to 40.6 percent in the historical control group.[87] Patient exercise capacity and functional status also were substantially improved. Prostacyclin has recently been approved by the US Food and Drug Administration for continuous intravenous therapy of severe primary pulmonary hypertension (New York Heart Association Class III and Class IV patients).

Nitric Oxide

Nitric oxide was identified as endothelial-derived relaxing factor (EDRF) in 1987.[88,89] One of the most important products of endothelial cells, nitric oxide acts through cyclic guanosine 5' monophosphate (cyclic GMP) to cause smooth muscle cell vasodilation; it also has inhibitory effects on platelet aggregation and antimitogenic activity. In conditions that result in endothelial cell dysfunction, such as hypoxia, increased shear stress, and the toxic effects of fibrin and its degradation products, EDRF release is inhibited, contributing to the development of increased pulmonary vascular resistance and pulmonary hypertension.[90]

Efforts to treat a spectrum of different pulmonary hypertensive states with nitric oxide are increasingly being undertaken.[91–95] Nitric oxide is a gas, administered by inhalation at a concentration of up to 80 ppm. Nitric oxide is very short-acting, being inactivated almost immediately by hemoglobin through generation of methemoglobin. Because NO is only delivered to ventilated lung units, and is rapidly bound, the pulmonary vasodilation it produces does not increase V/Q mismatch nor does it cause systemic vasodilation or hypotension.

Nitric oxide is as effective a pulmonary vasodilator as prostacyclin in patients with PPH and persistent pulmonary hypertension of the newborn (PPHN).[96–98] Similar observations have been made in the treatment of acute respiratory distress syndrome (ARDS), where NO has been found to produce selective pulmonary vasodilation and improved gas exchange. This is in contrast to prostacyclin or PGE_1, which in ARDS causes decrease in lower pulmonary arterial pressures but increase in shunt fraction and decreased systemic pressure.[92,93]

Nitric oxide administration currently is most practical for those patients requiring mechanical ventilation (i.e., ARDS and PPHN). Nitric oxide and NO_2 analyzers must be part of the inhalation circuit, and NO and NO_2 scrubbers should be part of the exhalation circuit. Long-term therapy appears possible; in the studies of ARDS, a patient received NO at concentrations up to 80 ppm for 52 days without apparent complications (i.e., lung injury or the development of methemoglobinemia).[92] Initial trials of chronic NO administration through transtracheal catheters or nasal cannula in other pulmonary vascular disease states are now under way.[99,100]

The Future

There has been considerable progress in the treatment of pulmonary hypertension since pharmacologic therapy was first undertaken 40 years ago. The prognosis for patients is much better now than it was even 10 years ago. Further advances in the understanding of the processes taking place at the endothelial and smooth muscle cell level, as well as new pharmacologic options and advances in delivery systems, should further improve the therapeutic options and approaches to this difficult group of disorders.

References

1. Fishman AP: Pulmonary circulation, in Fishman AP (ed): *Handbook of Physiology*, Section III, vol. I. Bethesda, American Physiological Society, 1985:93.
2. Palevsky HI: Exercise and the pulmonary circulation, in Leff A (ed): *Cardiopulmonary Exercise Testing*. Orlando, FL, Grune & Stratton, 1986:89.
3. Wagenvoort CA, Wagenvoort N: *Pathology of Pulmonary Hypertension*. New York, Wiley, 1977.
4. Fishman AP, Pietra GG: Primary pulmonary hypertension. *Ann Rev Med* 1980; 31:421.
5. Hyman AL: Pulmonary vaso-constriction due to non-occlusive distention of large pulmonary arteries in the dog. *Circ Res* 1986; 23:401.
6. Archer SL, McMurtry IF, Weir EK: Mechanisms of acute hypoxic and hyperoxic changes in pulmonary vascular reactivity, in Weir EK, Reeves JT (eds): *Pulmonary Vascular Physiology and Pathophysiology*. New York, Marcel Dekker, 1989:241.
7. Unger M, Atkins M, Briscoe WA, et al: Potentiation of pulmonary vasoconstriction with intermittent repeated hypoxia. *J Appl Physiol* 1977; 43:662.
8. Chang AC, Zucker HA, Hickey PR, Wessel DL: Pulmonary vascular resistance in infants after cardiac surgery: role of carbon dioxide and hydrogen ion. *Crit Care Med* 1995; 23:568.
9. Derenne J-P, Fluery B, Pariente R: Acute respiratory failure of chronic obstructive lung disease. *Am Rev Respir Dis* 1988; 138:1006.
10. Van Grondelle A, Worthen GS, Ellis D, et al.: Altering hydrodynamic variables influences PGI_2 production by isolated lung and endothelial cells. *J Appl Physiol* 1984; 57:388.
11. Peach MJ, Johs RA, Rose Jr CE: The potential role of interactions between endothelium and smooth muscle in pulmonary vascular physiology and pathophysiology, in Weir EK, Reeves JT (eds): *Pulmonary Vascular Physiology and Pathophysiology*. New York, Marcel Dekker, 1989:643.
12. Cremona G, Dinh-Xuan AT, Higenbottam TW: Endothelium-derived relaxing factor and the pulmonary circulation. *Lung* 1991; 169:185.
13. Lerman A, Hildebrand Jr FL, Margulies KB, et al.: Endothelin: a new cardiovascular regulatory peptide. *Mayo Clin Proc* 1990; 64:1441.
14. Vanhoutte PG: Endothelium and control of vascular function. State of the art. *Hypertension* 1989; 13:658.
15. Steward DJ, Levy RD, Cernacek P, et al.: Increased plasma endothelin-1 in pulmonary hypertension: marker or mediator of disease? *Ann Intern Med* 1991; 114:464.
16. Owens GR, Rogers RM, Pennock BE, et al.: The diffusing capacity as a predictor of arterial oxygen desaturation during exercise in patients with chronic obstructive pulmonary disease. *N Engl J Med* 1984; 310:1218.
17. Kelley MA, Panettieri Jr RA, Krupinski AV: Resting single-breath diffusing capacity as a screening test for exercise induced hypoxemia. *Am J Med* 1986; 80:807.
18. Flenley DC: Long-term home oxygen therapy. *Chest* 1985; 89:99.
19. Timms RM, Khaja RU, Williams GW: The nocturnal oxygen therapy trial. Hemodynamic response to oxygen therapy in chronic obstructive pulmonary disease. *Ann Intern Med* 1985; 102:29.
20. Cooper CB, Waterhouse J, Howard P: Twelve year clinical study of patients with hypoxic cor pulmonale given long-term domiciliary oxygen therapy. *Thorax* 1987; 42:105.
21. Ferguson GT, Cherniack RM: Management of chronic obstructive pulmonary disease. *N Engl J Med* 1993; 328:1017.
22. Fuster V, Steele PM, Edwards WD, et al.: Primary pulmonary hypertension: natural history and the importance of thrombosis. *Circulation* 1984; 70:580.
23. Rubin LJ, Peter RH: Therapy of pulmonary heart disease, in Rubin LJ (ed): *Pulmonary Heart Disease*. Boston, Martinus Nijhoff Publishing, 1984:325.
24. McGrath RC, Weil JV: Adverse effects of normovolemic polycythemia and hypoxia on hemodynamics in the dog. *Circ Res* 1978; 43:793.
25. Mathur PN, Powles RCP, Pugsley SO, et al.: Effects of digoxin on right ventricular function in severe chronic airflow obstruction. *Ann Intern Med* 1981; 92:283.
26. Coates AL, Desmond K, Asher MI, et al.: The effect of digoxin on exercise capacity and exercising cardiac function in cystic fibrosis. *Chest* 1982; 82:543.
27. Fishman AP: Chronic cor pulmonale. *Am Rev Respir Dis* 1976; 114:775.
28. Weir EK, Archer SL, Edwards JE: Chronic primary and secondary thromboembolic pulmonary hypertension. *Chest* 1988; 93:149S.
29. Voelkel NF, Weir EK: Etiologic mechanisms in primary pulmonary hypertension, in Weir EK, Reeves JT (eds): *Pulmonary Vascular Physiology and Pathophysiology*. New York, Marcel Dekker, 1989:513.
30. Rich S, Brundage BH: Pulmonary hypertension: A cellular basis for understanding the pathophysiology and treatment. *J Am Coll Cardiol* 1990; 14:545.
31. Cohen M, Fuster V, Williams WD: Anticoagulation in the treatment of pulmonary hypertension, in Fishman AP (ed): *The Pulmonary Circulation: Normal and Abnormal Mechanisms, Management, and the National Registry*. Philadelphia, PA, University of Pennsylvania Press, 1990:501.
32. Rich S: The role of thrombosis in pulmonary hypertension. *Chest* 1993; 103:660.
33. Rich S, Kaufmann E, Levy PS: The effect of high doses of calcium-channel blockers on survival in primary pulmonary hypertension. *N Engl J Med* 1992; 327:76.
34. Eisenberg PR, Lucore C, Kaufman L, et al.: Fibrinopeptide A levels indicative of pulmonary vascular thrombosis in patients with primary pulmonary hypertension. *Circulation* 1990; 82:841.
35. Schulman LL, Grossman BA, Owen J: Platelet activation and fibrinopeptide formation in pulmonary hypertension. *Chest* 1993; 104:1690.
36. Christman BW, McPherson CD, Newman JH, et al.: An imbalance between the excretion of thromboxane and prostacyclin metabolites in pulmonary hypertension. *N Engl J Med* 1992; 327:70.
37. Adatia I, Barrow SE, Stratton PD, et al.: Thromboxane A_2 and prostacyclin biosynthesis in children and adolescents with pulmonary vascular disease. *Circulation* 1993; 88:2117.
38. Rich S, Dantzker DR, Ayres SM, et al.: Primary pulmonary hypertension: A national prospective study. *Ann Intern Med* 1987; 107:216.

39. Hughes JD, Rubin LJ: Primary pulmonary hypertension: an analysis of 28 cases and a review of the literature. *Medicine (Baltimore)* 1986; 65:56.

40. Higenbottam TW, Spiegelhalter D, Scott JP, et al.: Prostacyclin (epoprostenol) and heart-lung transplantation as treatments for severe pulmonary hypertension. *Br Heart J* 1993; 70:366.

41. Hirsh J: Heparin. *N Engl J Med* 1991; 324:1565.

42. Rubin LJ (chairman). Primary pulmonary hypertension: an ACCP consensus statement. *Chest* 1993; 104:236.

43. Weir EK, Rubin LJ, Ayres SM, et al.: The acute administration of vasodilators in primary pulmonary hypertension: experience from the National Institutes of Health registry on primary pulmonary hypertension. *Am Rev Respir Dis* 1989; 140:1623.

44. Palevsky HI, Schloo BL, Pietra GG, et al.: Primary pulmonary hypertension: vascular structure, morphometry and responsiveness to vasodilator agents. *Circulation* 1989; 80:1207.

45. Reeves JT, Groves BM, Turkevich D: The case for treatment of selected patients with primary pulmonary hypertension. *Am Rev Respir Dis* 1986; 134:342.

46. Bonow RO, Galie N, Gheorghiade M, Magnani B: Prostacyclin: basic principles and clinical application in congestive heart failure and primary pulmonary hypertension. *Am J Cardiol* 1995; 75:1A.

47. Rubin LJ, Groves BM, Reeves JT, et al.: Prostacyclin-induced acute pulmonary vasodilation in primary pulmonary hypertension. *Circulation* 1982; 66:334.

48. Long W, Barst R, Fishman AP, et al.: Acute hemodynamic effects of prostacyclin in 65 primary pulmonary hypertension patients. *J Crit Care* 1986; 1:127.

49. Barst RJ, Hall JC, Stalcup SA: Response to prostacyclin predicts response to subsequent vasodilator therapy in children and young adults with primary pulmonary hypertension, in Doyle EF, Engle MA (eds): *Cardiology*. New York, Springer-Verlag, 1986:952.

50. Palevsky HI, Long W, Crow J, Fishman AP: Prostacyclin and acetylcholine as screening agents for acute pulmonary vasodilator responsiveness in primary pulmonary hypertension. *Circulation* 1990; 82:2018.

51. Nootens M, Schrader B, Kaufmann E, et al.: Comparative acute effects of adenosine and prostacyclin in primary pulmonary hypertension. *Chest* 1995; 107:54.

52. Scott JP, Higenbottam TW, Wallwork J: The acute effect of the synthetic prostacyclin analogue iloprost in primary pulmonary hypertension. *Br J Clin Pharmacol* 1990; 6:231.

53. Dinh-Xuan AT, Higgenbottam TW, Scott JP, et al.: Effects of long-term treatment with iloprost, a prostacyclin analogue, on exercise tolerance in patients with primary pulmonary hypertension. *Am Rev Respir Dis* 1990; 141:A889.

54. McCormack DG, Clarke B, Carnes PJ: Characterization of adenosine receptors in human pulmonary arteries. *Am J Physiol* 1989; 256:H41.

55. Evans TW, McCormack DG, Morgan JM, et al.: Adenosine as a vasodilator in primary pulmonary hypertension. *Am Rev Respir Dis* 1990; 141:A665.

56. Inbar S, Schrader BJ, Kaufmann E, et al.: Effects of adenosine in combination with calcium channel blockers in patients with primary pulmonary hypertension. *J Am Coll Cardiol* 1993; 2:413.

57. Peter RH, Rubin L: The pharmacologic control of the pulmonary circulation in pulmonary hypertension. *Adv Intern Med* 1984; 29:494.

58. McGoon MD, Vliestra RE: Vasodilator therapy for primary pulmonary hypertension. *Mayo Clin Proc* 1984; 59:672.

59. McLeod AA, Jewitt DE: Drug treatment of primary pulmonary hypertension. *Drugs* 1986; 31:177.

60. Weir EK: Acute vasodilator testing and pharmacological treatment of primary pulmonary hypertension, in Fishman AP (ed): *The Pulmonary Circulation: Normal and Abnormal: Mechanisms, Management and the National Registry*. Philadelphia, PA, University of Pennsylvania Press, 1990:485.

61. Eysmann SB, Palevsky HI, Reichek N, et al.: Echo/Doppler and hemodynamic correlates of vasodilator responsiveness in primary pulmonary hypertension. *Chest* 1991; 99:1066.

62. Weir EK: The United States experience with the acute and chronic treatment of primary pulmonary hypertension. *Eur Heart J* 1988; 9(suppl):33.

63. Dantzker DR, D'Alonzo GE, Gianotti L, et al.: Vasodilators and primary pulmonary hypertension: variability of long-term response. *Chest* 1989; 95:1185.

64. Fuleihan DS, Mookherjee S, Potts J, et al.: Sodium nitroprusside: a new role as a pulmonary vasodilator. *Am J Cardiol* 1979; 43:405.

65. Pearl RG, Rosenthal MH, Ashton JPA: Pulmonary vasodilator effects of nitroglycerin and sodium nitroprusside in canine oleic acid induced pulmonary hypertension. *Anesthesiology* 1983; 58:514.

66. Pearl RG, Rosenthal MH, Schroeder JS, Ashton JPA: Acute hemodynamic effects of nitroglycerin in pulmonary hypertension. *Ann Intern Med* 1983; 99:9.

67. Lupi-Herrera E, Bialostozky D, Sobrino A: The role of isoproterenol in pulmonary artery hypertension of unknown etiology (primary). *Chest* 1981; 79:292.

68. Pietro DA, LaBresh KA, Shulman RM, et al.: Sustained improvement in primary pulmonary hypertension during six years of treatment with sublingual isoproterenol. *N Engl J Med* 1984; 310:1032.

69. Person B, Proctor RJ: Primary pulmonary hypertension: response to indomethacin, terbutaline and isoproterenol. *Chest* 1979; 76:601.

70. Ruskin JN, Hutter AM: Primary pulmonary hypertension treated with oral phentolamine. *Ann Intern Med* 1979; 90:772.

71. Palevsky H, Pietra GG, Fishman AP: Pulmonary veno-occlusive disease and its response to vasodilator agents. *Am Rev Respir Dis* 1990; 142:426.

72. Coma-Canella I, Lopez-Sendon J: Hemodynamic effects of nifedipine, nitroglycerin and prazosin in pulmonary hypertension following ingestion of toxic oil. *Eur Heart J* 1983; 4:566.

73. Rubin LJ, Peter RH: Oral hydralazine therapy for primary pulmonary hypertension. *N Engl J Med* 1980; 302:69.

74. Packer M, Greenberg B, Masore B, Dash H: Deleterious effects of hydralazine in patients with pulmonary hypertension. *N Engl J Med* 1982; 306:1326.

75. Packer M: Vasodilator therapy for primary pulmonary hypertension: limitations and hazards. *Ann Intern Med* 1985; 103:258.

76. Lupi-Herrera E, Sandoval J, Seoane M, Bialastozky D: The role of hydralazine therapy for pulmonary arterial hypertension of unknown cause. *Circulation* 1982; 65:645.

77. Rich S, Martinez J, Lam W, Rosen KM: Captopril as treatment for patients with pulmonary hypertension. *Br Heart J* 1982; 48:272.

78. Leier CV, Bambach D, Nelson S, et al.: Captopril in primary pulmonary hypertension. *Circulation* 1983; 67:155.

79. Young TE, Lundquist LJ, Chesler E, Weir EK: Comparative effects of nifedipine, verapamil and diltiazem on experimental pulmonary hypertension. *Am J Cardiol* 1983; 51:195.

80. Henry PD: Comparative pharmacology of calcium antagonists: nifedipine, verapamil and diltiazem. *Am J Cardiol* 1980; 46:1047.

81. Rich S, Brundage BH: High-dose calcium channel blocking therapy for primary pulmonary hypertension: Evidence for long-term reduction in pulmonary arterial pressure and regression of right ventricular hypertrophy. *Circulation* 1987; 76:134.

82. Dusting GJ, Moncada S, Vane JR: Prostaglandins, their intermediates and precursors: cardiovascular actions and regulatory roles in normal and abnormal circulatory systems. *Prog Cardiovasc Dis* 1979; 6:405.

83. Das UK: Prostaglandins and pulmonary hypertension: further evidence. *Med Hypothesis* 1981; 7:621.

84. Hermiller JB, Bambach D, Thompson MJ, et al.: Vasodilators and prostaglandin inhibitors in primary pulmonary hypertension. *Ann Intern Med* 1982; 97:480.

85. Long WA, Rubin LJ: Prostacyclin and PGE$_1$ treatment of pulmonary hypertension. *Am Rev Respir Dis* 1987; 136:773.

86. Rubin LJ, Mendoza J, Hood M, et al.: Treatment of primary pulmonary hypertension with continuous intravenous prostacyclin (epoprostenol). *Ann Intern Med* 1990; 112:485.

87. Barst RJ, Rubin LJ, McGoon MD, et al.: Survival in primary pulmonary hypertension with long-term continuous intravenous prostacyclin. *Ann Intern Med* 1994; 121:409.

87a. Barst, R. J., Rubin, L. J., Long, W. A., et al.: A comparison of continuous intravenous epoprostenol (prostacyclin) with conventional therapy for primary pulmonary hypertension. *N Engl J Med* 1996; 334:296.

88. Ignarro LJ, Buga GM, Wood KS, et al.: EDRF produced and released from artery and vein is nitric oxide. *Proc Natl Acad Sci USA* 1987; 84:9265.

89. Palmer RMJ, Ferrige AG, Moncada S: Nitric oxide release accounts for the biological activity of EDRF. *Nature* 1987; 327:524.

90. Dinh-Xuan AT, Higenbottam TW, Clelland CA, et al.: Impairment of endothelium-dependent pulmonary artery relaxation in chronic obstructive lung disease. *N Engl J Med* 1991; 324:1539.

91. Higenbottam T: Inhaled nitric oxide: A magic bullet? *Quart J Med* 1993; 86:555.

92. Rossaint R, Flake KJ, Lopez F, et al.: Inhaled nitric oxide for the adult respiratory distress syndrome. *N Engl J Med* 1993; 328:399.

93. Zapol WM, Rimar S, Gillis N, et al.: Nitric oxide and the lung: an NHLBI workshop summary. *Am J Respir Crit Care Med* 1994; 149:1375.

94. Rossaint R, Pison U, Gerlach H, Falke KJ: Inhaled nitric oxide: its effects on pulmonary circulation and airway smooth muscle cells. *Eur Heart J* 1993; 14(suppl I):133.

95. Fink MP (ed): Nitric oxide. *New Horizons* 1995; 3:1.

96. Pepke-Zaba J, Higenbottam TW, Dinh-Xuan AT, et al.: Inhaled nitric oxide as a cause of selective pulmonary vasodilation in pulmonary hypertension. *Lancet* 1991; 338:1173.

97. Roberts JD, Polaner DM, Lang P, et al.: Inhaled nitric oxide in persistent pulmonary hypertension of the newborn. *Lancet* 1992; 340:818.

98. Kinsella JP, Neish SR, Shaffer E, et al.: Low dose inhalational nitric oxide in persistent pulmonary hypertension of the newborn. *Lancet* 1992; 340:819.

99. Snell GI, Salamonsen RF, Bergin P, et al.: Inhaled nitric oxide used as a bridge to heart-lung transplantation in a patient with end-stage pulmonary hypertension. *Am J Respir Crit Care Med* 1995; 151:1263.

100. Hess D, Kacmarek R, Imanaka H, et al.: Administration of inhaled nitric oxide by nasal cannula. *Am J Respir Crit Care Med* 1995; 151:A44.

Chapter 114 _____
PULMONARY HEMOSIDEROSIS
LEWIS W. NEESE
EDWARD C. ROSENOW, III
AND JEFFREY L. MYERS

Epidemiology

Pathology

Pathogenesis

Clinical Features
    Signs and symptoms
    Laboratory findings
    Roentgenographic features
    Pulmonary function testing

Diagnosis

Treatment
    Corticosteroids
    Azathioprine
    Other therapies

Prognosis

Pulmonary hemosiderosis is a term that has been used in the past to describe all causes of pulmonary hemorrhage. This term is somewhat confusing, as the primary problem is one of hemorrhage, and the hemosiderosis represents a secondary reaction to blood in the lung. These various syndromes are now classified as diffuse alveolar hemorrhage (DAH).[1] Idiopathic pulmonary hemosiderosis (IPH) describes those cases occurring in children or, less frequently, in adults that are considered idiopathic in regard to etiology. Some would question whether this represents a distinct clinical entity. Many of the cases reported in the literature occurred prior to the advent of electron microscopy and immunofluorescence techniques. It is possible that some of the cases may actually have been DAH associated with systemic or extrapulmonary disorders and therefore not truly "idiopathic." Also, many recent cases in the literature have not been followed extensively to exclude other causes of DAH that may become evident with time. However, many patients have been thoroughly evaluated without an apparent cause found to explain pulmonary hemorrhage, suggesting that this may indeed be a distinct entity. Much attention has focused on the search for the cause of this disease; however, little is known about the true pathogenesis.

Idiopathic pulmonary hemosiderosis is an uncommon cause of DAH. Clinically it is manifest by recurrent hemoptysis, iron-deficiency anemia, and migratory pulmonary infiltrates. The usual natural history is characterized by frequent exacerbations and remissions. This natural history makes evaluation of therapeutic programs difficult.

Although typically a disease of children, as many as 15 percent of cases occur in adults.[2] Idiopathic pulmonary hemosiderosis is a diagnosis of exclusion, with other causes of DAH excluded. Therapeutic options are limited in IPH and the overall prognosis remains poor.

Epidemiology

The epidemiologic data concerning IPA are limited because this is such an uncommon disease. Most reports document small series of patients or isolated cases. Few large series have been reported in the literature describing long-term follow-up of these patients. As noted above, IPH is predominantly a disease of young children, occurring in infants as young as 4 months old.[2] The sex distribution in children is almost equal.[2,3] Adults, usually below age 30, do constitute a significant proportion of patients. Among adults, males predominate two to one.[2] The disease in adults tends to be milder than it is in children.[4] Familial occurrences have been reported in siblings and offspring, although no pattern of inheritance has been established.[5–8]

Pathology

The histologic findings in IPH are nonspecific and vary depending on the chronicity of the disease. The lungs at autopsy following acute episodes of bleeding are usually bulky and heavy and show evidence of acute hemorrhage.[9]

Erythrocytes and hemosiderin-laden macrophages are seen filling the alveolar spaces in this setting. (Fig. 114-1). Hyperplasia, degeneration, and shedding of alveolar epithelial cells with marked alveolar capillary dilatation and tortuousity has been described as a common finding in most patients regardless of their clinical state. Though nonspecific, these findings do suggest a form of alveolar injury. Other findings, although not invariably present, are also seen. Various stages of interstitial fibrosis and hemosiderosis are present in chronic cases. The absence of significant pulmonary fibrosis in some cases of long duration suggests that the degree of fibrosis cannot be predicted by the duration of the disease. Degeneration of the elastic fiber network is also frequently seen, occurring in pulmonary vessels as well as the interstitium. Bronchial and mediastinal lymph nodes are frequently enlarged and hemosiderotic.[9] Taken together, these findings are nonspecific and can be seen in a variety of disorders.

Ultrastructural studies by electron microscopy also reveal evidence of nonspecific lung injury. Some studies have demonstrated no abnormalities of the alveolar capillary

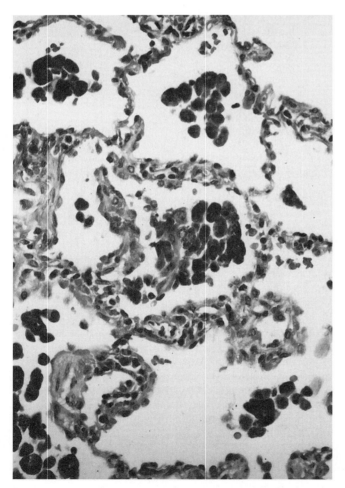

FIGURE 114-1 Light microscopy from a patient with idiopathic pulmonary hemosiderosis. The most prominent feature is the numerous hemosiderin-laden macrophages seen filling the alveoli. Mild alveolar septal thickening is present secondary to infiltration by inflammatory cells.

endothelium or basement membranes,[10] whereas others have documented breaks in the continuity,[11] thickening or concentric layering,[12–14] or splitting of the alveolar capillary basement membrane with deposition of amorphous material and fibrils.[15] These findings suggest an injury at the level of the alveolar capillary membrane by an as yet unidentified agent. Degeneration of type I pneumocytes, which occurs in many types of lung injury, results in small portions of exposed basement membrane. Increased numbers of type II pneumocytes are also seen, which is felt to indicate a state of lung repair.[10] Immunofluorescent studies have failed to demonstrate deposition of immunoglobins, complement, or immune complexes.[10,11,15]

Pathogenesis

The syndrome of IPH was first described by Virchow over a century ago. Despite the passing of one hundred years, the etiology of IPH remains a mystery to this day. Many theories have been put forth through the years, although none have been conclusively proven. The natural history of the disease—with frequent remissions—and its low incidence makes it difficult to perform detailed clinical, pathologic, and epidemiologic studies.

Initial theories concerning the pathogenesis of IPH included speculation that there were developmental defects of the pulmonary elastic fibers. It was felt that these defects could result in fragility of the alveolar capillary walls, with a resulting predisposition to bleeding. Histologic studies have demonstrated degeneration of these fibers within the interstitium and pulmonary vessels of patients with IPH. However, these fibers have also been shown to be normal in many cases of IPH, especially those of short duration. It has been shown that similar alterations occur in other conditions, such as long-standing cases of left ventricular failure. Most investigators believe that the elastic fiber abnormalities represent a secondary phenomenon related to the development of interstitial hemosiderosis.[9] Probst speculated that the pulmonary elastic fibers contained an abnormal mucopolysaccharide with an affinity for inorganic iron.[16] He theorized that these fibers accumulated iron, which decreased the strength of the fibers and predisposed them to breakage, resulting in rupture of small alveolar vessels. These observations were not confirmed by other investigators.[9]

Severe mitral stenosis was once a very common cause of DAH secondary to markedly elevated pulmonary venous pressures. Early investigators speculated that in IPH there might be a defect in vasomotor control within the pulmonary circulation that led to transient increases in pulmonary venous pressure with subsequent hemorrhage. This theory was felt to explain the reports of exacerbations of IPH during pregnancy. The disorder has been noted in some patients during the seventh month of pregnancy, a time when the increase in plasma volume is at its maximum.[17] Right heart catheterization studies have failed to support this theory.

Soergel and Sommers reported histologic findings from tissue obtained by open lung biopsies and autopsy specimens from 18 patients with IPH.[2,9] Striking degeneration, hyperplasia, and shedding of alveolar epithelial cells was described. The investigators suggested that the primary pathogenic mechanism was an abnormality of alveolar epithelial growth and function. This abnormality of epithelial cells ultimately affected the mechanical stability of the alveolar capillaries, resulting in widespread hemorrhages. It was also speculated that a nonspecific injury, such as a viral infection or inhalation of an irritating or allergenic substance, might be responsible for the alveolar injury. Other investigators have also theorized that environmental exposures may play a role. An epidemiologic study from Greece demonstrated a clustering of cases in rural areas where chronic exposure to insecticides was felt to play a potential role.[7] There has also been a report of a young patient with numerous exacerbations of his disease presumably secondary to the effects of cigarette smoking.[18]

Much of the attention concerning the pathogenesis of IPH has focused upon immunologic mechanisms. Although never proven, this theory remains attractive for several reasons: (1) the histologic findings of alveolar damage are similar to those seen in immune-mediated diseases such as systemic lupus erythematosus and Goodpasture's syndrome[1]; (2) there is an association between IPH and other immune-mediated diseases such as cow's milk sensitivity,[19–23] celiac disease,[24–28] autoimmune thyrotoxicosis,[29] autoimmune hemolytic anemia,[30] and IgA monoclonal gammopathy[31]; (3) some patients have been noted to have nonspecific increases in serum IgA[32]; and (4) there are reported cases of response to immunosuppressive therapy.

Cow's milk allergy has been proposed as a possible mechanism to explain some cases of IPH occurring in small children. Cow's milk sensitivity in children typically presents with malabsorption, protein-losing enteropathy, chronic rhinitis, and enterocolitis. Many of these patients have persistent pulmonary disease. Heiner and associates described a series of 7 patients with hypersensitivity to cow's milk and prominent respiratory complications including cough, dyspnea, and migratory pulmonary infiltrates on chest x-ray.[19] All of the patients had iron-deficiency anemia at initial presentation and four patients gave a history of hemoptysis. All of the patients were found to have antibodies to milk constituents, including lactalbumin and casein. Of the total, 6 patients had resolution of their pulmonary symptoms after removal of cow's milk from their diet. Similar results were noted by other investigators.[20–23] These children appear to lose their sensitivity to milk with time. The significance of these findings is unclear, as many normal infants may also have antibodies to cow's milk. It has been speculated that immune complex deposition or an Arthus-like reaction may be responsible for the pulmonary hemorrhage seen in some of these patients.

An association with celiac disease has been described in several adult patients with IPH. Wright and colleagues studies seven patients with presumed IPH and minimal if any gastrointestinal symptoms; subsequently jejunal biopsies were performed to evaluate the presence of celiac disease.[24] Three of the patients had villous atrophy on biopsy consistent with celiac disease. Other investigators reported similar findings.[26,27] Respiratory symptoms improved in some of these patients after a gluten-free diet was instituted.

Clinical Features

SIGNS AND SYMPTOMS

Presenting symptoms can vary greatly. The typical presentation consists of recurrent hemoptysis, iron-deficiency anemia, and transient pulmonary infiltrates. The hemoptysis may consist of recurrent episodes of massive, life-threatening bleeding or intermittent episodes of blood-streaked sputum. Young children frequently present with chronic cough, dyspnea, and an abnormal chest x-ray without significant hemoptysis, as they may be unable to expectorate the blood and therefore swallow it.[33] Fever is frequently present and is felt to represent a systemic response to blood within the alveoli or interstitium. Pallor, failure to thrive, and tachypnea are frequent presenting manifestations in children. In approximately 20 percent of cases generalized lymphadenopathy and hepatosplenomegaly are found.[2]

Recurrent episodes of bleeding may eventually lead to pulmonary fibrosis with resultant increasing dyspnea, bibasilar crackles on auscultation of the lungs, and digital clubbing. The degree of pulmonary fibrosis is not felt to be predictable from the number of episodes of significant bleeding or the duration of the disease.[2] With progression of the pulmonary fibrosis, cor pulmonale may become a prominent clinical feature, although it is reported in a small minority of patients.[2–4]

LABORATORY FINDINGS

The laboratory findings in IPH are nonspecific. The most striking abnormality is the hypochromic microcytic anemia. This is typically seen in all patients except those with long-standing inactive disease and occurs even in the absence of hemoptysis.[2] The degree of anemia can be marked. The severity of the anemia is frequently out of proportion to the amount of reported hemoptysis and the chest radiographic findings.[4] Serum iron concentrations usually are decreased, with an increased total iron binding capacity consistent with iron deficiency. Bone marrow aspirates reveal an absence of stainable iron and erythroid hyperplasia. The reticulocyte count may be elevated, which in the setting of anemia may suggest hemolysis.[5] Iron deficiency develops despite normal or increased levels of total body iron because the erythron is unable to mobilize iron stored as hemosiderin within alveolar macrophages.[5,11] Mild eosinophilia has been reported in several patients.[2,11] Serum bilirubin levels may be elevated during acute bleeding episodes, presumably secondary to breakdown of intraalveolar blood.[2] Tests for fecal occult blood are frequently positive in young children.[2,11]

Hemosiderin-laden alveolar macrophages are a common, although nonspecific, finding in IPH. They can be found in sputum, tracheal aspirates, bronchoalveolar lavage, and gastric aspirates in patients with DAH from any cause. They may not be present during acute episodes of hemorrhage. They typically are seen 48 h after the initial bleeding episode and are usually cleared from the lung within 2 weeks. The absence of hemosiderin-laden macrophages does not exclude the possibility of a recent or remote episode of bleeding.[34]

ROENTGENOGRAPHIC FEATURES

The chest radiograph typically demonstrates bilateral alveolar infiltrates during acute episodes. The apices and costophrenic angles are usually spared.[35] These findings are nonspecific and can mimic pneumonia or congestive heart failure. Following acute episodes, chest roentgenograms may revert to normal within 1 to 2 weeks.[2,4,34] Many patients are left with a residual diffuse reticulonodular infiltrate on chest radiograph that may persist, depending on the chronicity of the disease. (Fig. 114-2). Enlarged hilar lymph nodes are frequently seen during acute episodes.[35] With time and repeated episodes of hemorrhage, pulmonary fibrosis may become prominent. Progressive massive fibrosis has also been reported in one patient.[36]

Computed tomography (CT) of the chest will frequently reveal abnormalities in patients who are considered to have normal chest x-rays.[35] Areas of increased density are noted on CT scans, corresponding to alveolar hemorrhage or accumulation of hemosiderin-laden macrophages. Fine thickening of interlobular septa is seen in patients with repeated episodes of hemorrhage. In patients with long-standing disease, evidence of pulmonary fibrosis and subpleural honeycombing is frequently seen.[37] Magnetic resonance imaging of the pulmonary parenchyma reveals a decreased signal on T2-weighted images secondary to the paramagnetic effect of ferric iron.[38]

PULMONARY FUNCTION TESTING

Pulmonary function testing is nonspecific but may be of value in assessing the course of the disease. Tests may be normal during initial episodes. With acute alveolar hemorrhage the diffusing capacity (DL_{CO}) may be increased due to increased uptake of carbon monoxide by free hemoglobin within the alveoli.[4] As the disease progresses and pulmonary fibrosis intervenes, a restrictive ventilatory defect with decreased total lung capacity, vital capacity, and lung compliance becomes prominent. The DL_{CO} and oxygen saturation gradually decline as the degree of pulmonary fibrosis increases.[39,40]

Diagnosis

The clinical diagnosis of IPH can be difficult. The hemoptysis itself may not always be a prominent clinical feature. The amount of hemoptysis may be small and out of proportion to objective findings on chest x-ray.[4] The hemorrhagic episodes in small children may go unnoticed, as they will frequently swallow the blood. Many of these patients will have positive tests for occult fecal hemoglobin and gastric aspirates containing hemosiderin-laden macrophages. These patients may present with anemia and undergo extensive gastrointestinal evaluations to discover a source of the bleeding. Other patients may present with scanty hemoptysis, mild anemia, and minimal chest x-ray findings, which may be overlooked.

Idiopathic pulmonary hemosiderosis is a diagnosis of exclusion. It is therefore important to rule out other systemic and extrapulmonary causes of DAH and to perform frequent monitoring of patients. There are reports of patients initially diagnosed as IPH who were later found to have other causes for their pulmonary hemorrhage, such as Goodpasture's syndrome or connective tissue diseases.[41–43] The presence of hemosiderin-laden macrophages in pulmonary or gastric secretions suggests recent alveolar hemorrhage, but this is a nonspecific finding. A careful family history may reveal other family members with a history of recurrent hemoptysis and anemia suggestive of IPH. A urinalysis and serum creatinine are essential to evaluate renal function and the possibility of a coexisting glomerulonephritis. Antineutrophil cytoplasmic antibodies (ANCA) should be checked to rule out the possibility of Wegener's granulomatosis or nonWegener's capillaritis. Antiglomerular membrane antibodies should also be evaluated, as well as immunofluorescent studies of available lung and renal tissue to exclude Goodpasture's syndrome. The presence of connective tissue diseases should be explored by serologic testing and a thorough physical examination. Severe mitral stenosis and left atrial myxoma are uncommon causes of DAH.[44] Echocardiography is an important diagnostic tool necessary to evaluate the possibility of these rare conditions.

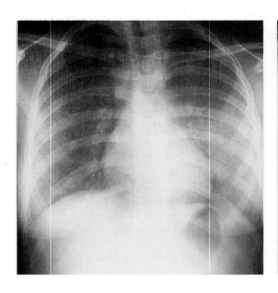
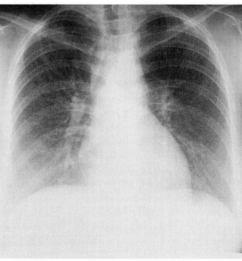

FIGURE 114-2 *A.* Chest radiograph from a young patient with idiopathic pulmonary hemosiderosis following an episode of acute hemoptysis. Diffuse alveolar infiltrates are noted, greater in the left mid-lung. *B.* Chest radiograph from the same patient 12 years later demonstrates a diffuse reticulonodular pattern suggesting pulmonary fibrosis.

Coagulation studies will rule out significant coagulopathies predisposing patients to bleeding. In small children with IPH, cow's milk sensitivity may be present. The presence of antibodies to cow's milk products can provide additional clues to this uncommon entity. The presence of celiac disease in adults should be explored. Gastrointestinal symptoms, if present, should prompt a jejunal biopsy. Most patients will require a tissue biopsy of the lung to confirm the diagnosis.

Treatment

The therapy for IPH has, overall, been unsatisfactory. No controlled, perspective studies have been performed to evaluate any therapeutic program. Because many patients experience spontaneous remissions of their disease, such studies would be difficult to perform and evaluate. Much of the attention has focused on immunosuppressive treatment, with varying degrees of success. There is hope that a better understanding of the pathogenesis of this uncommon entity will lead to improved treatments.

Acute exacerbations of IPH are typically treated symptomatically. Blood transfusions are often required in severe cases with prominent anemia. Most patients with iron-deficiency anemia will require iron replacement therapy, as the body is unable to utilize the iron that is stored within macrophages as hemosiderin. Oxygen therapy frequently is required in severe exacerbations associated with hypoxemia and also chronic cases with significant pulmonary fibrosis.

One of the first therapies for IPH was splenectomy. Some investigators theorized that IPH was an immunohematologic problem and that therefore splenectomy might improve the clinical course. Many patients with severe, relapsing disease have undergone this procedure on an elective basis. The survival and course of these patients appeared to be no better than those of other patients with IPH.[2,40]

Young children with IPH should be evaluated for cow's milk sensitivity. A trial of a milk-free diet would appear to be warranted in children, given the innocuous nature of this therapy. Because of the possibility of coexisting celiac disease in adults, a trial of a gluten-free diet may also be indicated.

CORTICOSTEROIDS

The role of corticosteroids in IPH remains unclear. Most patients with acute exacerbations do appear to improve following initiation of steroid therapy. Corticosteroids appear to improve the immediate prognosis and also possibly speed recovery.[2,3] These observations must be considered with caution, given the fact that many patients appear to improve without any therapy. How corticosteroids provide a beneficial effect remains unknown. Some would argue that this improvement supports the theory that IPH is primarily an immunologic disease, although this has not been substantiated. Alternatively, corticosteroids may exert a positive effect through their membrane-stabilizing properties and reduction of capillary leak.[45] It does appear that a trial of corticosteroids is warranted in acute episodes.

The data concerning the use of corticosteroids in chronic cases are less convincing. It appears that long-term steroid therapy does not alter the disease's course or prognosis.[2,3] Corticosteroid treatment should be individualized in these patients depending on their clinical course. Other factors also have to be considered, including the risk of infection and, in children, growth retardation associated with chronic steroid use.

AZATHIOPRINE

Azathioprine is an immunosuppressive antimetabolite with profound effects on cellular immunity. Either alone or in combination with corticosteroids, azathioprine has shown some potential benefit in acute exacerbations and presention of relapses.[15,46,47] These findings are difficult to interpret with such small numbers of patients reported. Azathioprine must be used cautiously in patients with IPH because of the known associated risks, including reversible bone marrow suppression, hepatotoxicity,[48] and increased risks for infection.

OTHER THERAPIES

There are case reports in the literature of successful treatment of IPH with other agents. Cyclophosphamide was used successfully to treat a 5-year-old child with significant hemoptysis that was refractory to prednisone and azathioprine.[49] The complications of cyclophosphamide use are numerous and include infection, bladder toxicity, malignancies, and gonadal failure.[48] Given the frequency and severity of side effects associated with the use of cyclophosphamide, use of this therapy for IPH would appear to be too great a risk without more supportive data concerning its efficacy.

Chloroquine has been shown to be beneficial in two patients with IPH.[50] Unfortunately, treatment was limited in one patient by retinal changes associated with chloroquine. Again, with such small numbers and a disease known for spontaneous remissions, these data are difficult to interpret. There has been a report of one patient who responded to plasmapheresis.[51] One patient with IPH has successfully undergone lung transplant.

Prognosis

The overall prognosis for patients with IPH remains poor. The average survival following the onset of symptoms is 2½ years.[2] Various clinical outcomes have been noted. Many patients have severe, unremitting disease characterized by repeated episodes of hemoptysis and early death. Some patients become symptom-free after initial episodes. Other patients have recurring bouts of hemoptysis manifest by chronic dyspnea and persistent anemia with eventual progression to pulmonary fibrosis. Certain factors do appear to have prognostic significance. Adults tend to have a milder, more chronic form of the disease.[4] The severity of the disease at its onset does not affect overall survival. Overall survival in children appears to be better in females than males. Also, the earlier the patient's age at onset, generally the less favorable the prognosis.[3]

References

1. Murray JF, Nadel JA: *Textbook of Respiratory Medicine*, 2d ed. Philadelphia, Saunders, 1994.
2. Soergel KH, Sommers SC: Idiopathic pulmonary hemosiderosis and related syndromes. *Am J Med* 1962; 32:499.
3. Chryssanthopoulos C, Cassimos C, Panagiotidou C: Prognostic criteria in idiopathic pulmonary hemosiderosis in children. *Eur J Pediatr* 1983; 140:123.
4. Morgan PGM, Turner-Warwick M: Pulmonary hemosiderosis and pulmonary hemorrhage. *Br J Dis Chest* 1981; 75:225.
5. Thaell JF, Greipp PR, Stubbs SE, Siegal GP: Idiopathic pulmonary hemosiderosis: Two cases in a family. *Mayo Clin Proc* 1978; 53:113.
6. Beckerman RC, Taussig LM, Pinnas JL: Familial idiopathic pulmonary hemosiderosis. *Am J Dis Child* 1979; 133:609.
7. Cassimos CD, Chryssanthopoulos C, Panagiotidou C: Epidemiologic observations in idiopathic pulmonary hemosiderosis. *J Pediatr* 1983; 102:698.
8. Breckenridge RL, Ross JS: Idiopathic pulmonary hemosiderosis: A report of familial occurrence. *Chest* 1979; 75:636.
9. Soergel KH, Sommers SC: The alveolar epithelial lesion of idiopathic pulmonary hemosiderosis. *Am Rev Respir Dis* 1962; 85:540.
10. Irwin RS, Cottrell TS, Hsu KC, et al.: Idiopathic pulmonary hemosiderosis: An electron microscopy and immunofluorescent study. *Chest* 1974; 65:41.
11. Hyatt RW, Adelstein ER, Halazun JF, Lukens JN: Ultrastructure of the lung in idiopathic pulmonary hemosiderosis. *Am J Med* 1972; 52:822.
12. Gonzalez-Crussi F, Hull MT, Grosfeld JL: Idiopathic pulmonary hemosiderosis: Evidence of capillary basement membrane abnormality. *Am Rev Respir Dis* 1976; 114:689.
13. Cutz E: Idiopathic pulmonary hemosiderosis and related disorders in infancy and childhood. *Perspect Pediatr Pathol* 1987; 11:47.
14. Corrin B, Jagusch M, Dewar A, et al.: Fine structural changes in idiopathic pulmonary hemosiderosis. *J Pathol* 1987; 153:249.
15. Yeager H, Powell D, Weinberg RM, et al.: Idiopathic pulmonary hemosiderosis: Ultrastructural studies and response to azathioprine. *Arch Intern Med* 1976; 136:1145.
16. Probst A: Morphologie and Pathogenese der essentiellen Lungenhaemosiderose. *Virchows Arch Pathol Anat* 1955; 326:633.
17. Gurewich V, Thomas MA: Idiopathic pulmonary hemosiderosis in pregnancy. *N Engl J Med* 1959; 261:1154.
18. Lowry R, Buick B, Riley M: Idiopathic pulmonary hemosiderosis and smoking. *Ulster Med J* 1993; 62:116.
19. Heiner DC, Sears JW, Kniker WT: Multiple precipitins to cow's milk in chronic respiratory disease. *Am J Dis Child* 1962; 103:634.
20. Williams S, Craver RD: Cow's milk–induced pulmonary hemosiderosis. *J LA St Med Soc* 1989; 141:19.
21. Boat TF, Polmar SH, Whitman V, et al.: Hyperreactivity to cow milk in young children with pulmonary hemosiderosis and cor pulmonale secondary to nasopharyngeal obstruction. *J Pediatr* 1975; 87:23.
22. Lee SK, Kniker WT, Cook CD, Heiner DC: Cow's milk-induced pulmonary disease in children. *Adv Pediatr* 1978; 25:39.
23. Galant S, Nussbaum E, Wittner R, Et al: Increased IgD milk antibody responses in a patient with Down's syndrome, pulmonary hemosiderosis, and cor pulmonale. *Ann Allergy* 1983; 51:446.
24. Wright PH, Menzies IS, Pounder RE, Keeling PWN: Adult idiopathic pulmonary hemosiderosis and celiac disease. *QJ Med* 1981; 197:95.
25. Mah MW, Priel IE, Humen DP, et al.: Idiopathic pulmonary hemosiderosis, complete heart block and celiac disease. *Can J Cardiol* 1989; 5:191.
26. Pacheco A, Casanova C, Fogue L, Sueiro A: Long-term clinical follow-up of adult idiopathic pulmonary hemosiderosis and celiac disease. *Chest* 1991; 99:1525.
27. Reading R, Watson JG, Platt JW, Bird AG: Pulmonary hemosiderosis and gluten. *Arch Dis Child* 1987; 62:513.
28. Wright PH, Buxton-Thomas M, Keeling PWN, Kreel L: Adult idiopathic hemosiderosis: A comparison of lung function changes and the distribution of pulmonary disease in patients with and without celiac disease. *Br J Dis Chest* 1983; 77:282.
29. Bain SC, Bryan RL, Hawkins JB: Idiopathic pulmonary hemosiderosis and autoimmune thyrotoxicosis. *Respir Med* 1989; 83:447.
30. Rafferty JR, Cook MK: Idiopathic pulmonary hemosiderosis with autoimmune hemolytic anemia. *Br J Dis Chest* 1984; 78:282.
31. Nomura S, Kanoh T: Association of idiopathic pulmonary hemosiderosis with IgA monoclonal gammopathy. *Thorax* 1987; 42:696.
32. Valassi-Adam H, Rouska A, Karpouzas J, Matsaniotis N: Raised IgA in idiopathic pulmonary hemosiderosis. *Arch Dis Child* 1976; 50:320.
33. Matsaniotis N, Karpuozas K, Apostolopouloc E, Messaritakis J: Idiopathic pulmonary hemosiderosis in children. *Arch Dis Child* 1968; 43:307.
34. Sherman JM, Winnie G, Thomassen MJ, et al.: Time course of hemosiderin production and clearance by human pulmonary macrophages. *Chest* 1984; 86:409.
35. Akyar S, Ozbek SS: Computed tomography findings in idiopathic pulmonary hemosiderosis. *Respiration* 1993; 60:63.
36. Buschman DL, Ballard R: Progressive massive fibrosis associated with idiopathic pulmonary hemosiderosis. *Chest* 1993; 104:293.
37. Lynch DA, Brasch RC, Hardy KA, Webb WR: Pediatric pulmonary disease: Assessment with high-resolution ultrafast CT. *Radiology* 1990; 176:243.
38. Rubin GD, Edwards DK, Reicher MA, et al.: Diagnosis of pulmonary hemosiderosis by MR imaging. *AJR* 1989: 152:573.
39. Allue X, Wise MB, Beaudry PH: Pulmonary function studies in idiopathic pulmonary hemosiderosis in children. *Am Rev Respir Dis* 1973; 107:410.
40. Repetto G, Lisboa C, Empiranza E, et al.: Idiopathic pulmonary hemosiderosis: Clinical, radiological, and respiratory function studies. *Pediatrics* 1967; 40:24.
41. Lemley DE, Katz P: Rheumatoid-like arthritis presenting as idiopathic pulmonary hemosiderosis: A report and review of the literature. *J Rheum* 1986; 13:854.
42. Katz SM, Foster E, Miller AS, et al.: Goodpasture's syndrome mimicking idiopathic pulmonary hemosiderosis. *Ann Clin Lab Sci* 1989; 19:280.
43. Case Records of the Massachusetts General Hospital: Case#16-1993. *N Engl J Med* 1993; 328:1183.
44. Chaudhry AA, Dobson CM, Simpson FG: Pulmonary hemosiderosis associated with left atrial myxoma. *Thorax* 1991; 46:539.
45. Boumpas DT, Chrousos GP, Wilder RL, et al.: Glucocorticoid therapy for immune-mediated diseases: basic and clinical correlates. *Ann Intern Med* 1993; 119:1198.
46. Rossi GA, Balzano E, Battistini E, et al.: Long-term prednisone and azathioprine treatment of a patient with idiopathic pulmonary hemosiderosis. *Pediatr Pulmonol* 1992; 13:176.
47. Byrd RB, Gracey DR: Immunosuppressive treatment of idiopathic pulmonary hemosiderosis. *JAMA* 1973; 226:458.
48. Luqmani RA, Palmer RG, Bacon PA: Azathioprine, cyclophosphamide, and chlorambucil. *Bailliére's Clin Rheum* 1990; 4:595.
49. Colombo JL, Stolz SM: Treatment of life-threatening primary pulmonary hemosiderosis with cyclophosphamide. *Chest* 1992; 102:959.
50. Bush A, Sheppard MN, Warner JO: Chloroquine in idiopathic pulmonary hemosiderosis. *Arch Dis Child* 1992; 67:625.
51. Pozo-Rodriguez F, Freire-Campo JM, Gutierrez-Millet V, et al.: Idiopathic pulmonary hemosiderosis treated with plasmapheresis. *Thorax* 1980; 35:399.

Chapter 115

GOODPASTURE'S SYNDROME

EUGENE F. GEPPERT

Etiology and Pathogenesis

Signs, Symptoms, and Laboratory Abnormalities

Diagnosis

Treatment
    Plasmapheresis
    Corticosteroids
    Cyclophosphamide
    Respiratory support
    The results of treatment

Summary

Goodpasture's syndrome is a rare disease whose prognosis has been improved substantially by the development of drug therapy. The major components of the classic form of the disease are rapidly progressive glomerulonephritis and pulmonary hemorrhage together with the production of antiglomerular basement membrane (anti-GBM) antibodies. As such, Goodpasture's syndrome is considered to be one of the pulmonary-renal syndromes in a group that also includes Wegener's granulomatosis, pulmonary hemorrhage with microscopic polyangiitis, systemic lupus erythematosus, mixed cryoglobulinemia, Henoch-Schönlein purpura, and others. Goodpasture's syndrome stands out from the other diseases because the anti-GBM antibody contributes so much to the correct diagnosis. Indeed, some authorities prefer to define a disease called anti-GBM antibody–mediated disease to refer to all the patients who have this laboratory abnormality, no matter what variation of signs and symptoms they have at presentation. According to this view, a patient with an abnormal level of anti-GBM antibody might lack one of the cardinal features of Goodpasture's syndrome, such as renal insufficiency or hemoptysis, and yet would be considered to belong to the group of patients with anti-GBM antibody disease. This chapter considers Goodpasture's syndrome as the classic triad of glomerulonephritis, lung hemorrhage, and anti-GBM antibodies, but the guidelines for therapy also cover the clinical situations in which one of the elements of the syndrome is missing.

Much has been learned during the past 30 years about the pathophysiology, diagnosis, and treatment of Goodpasture's syndrome, and these advances in knowledge have benefited patients in the form of a decreasing morbidity and mortality from the disease.

Etiology and Pathogenesis

Goodpasture's syndrome is a classic example of an autoimmune disorder because the patient produces antibodies directed against one of the body components—in this case, against a membrane protein present in the glomerular and alveolar basement membranes. It is unclear, however, why affected patients produce the antibodies. The answer seems to lie in a combination of heredity and environment. A genetic predisposition to this disorder is suggested by a number of observations. Familial clusterings of the disease have been the subject of a number of reports.[1–6] In addition, an association has been found between the syndrome and the major histocompatibility complex.[7–9] These studies show that two-thirds of patients who are positive for anti-GBM antibody have the human leukocyte antigen HLA DR2, as do one-quarter of controls. Furthermore, genetics seems to play a role in the type of antibodies produced by these patients. Rees and coworkers[3,10] have shown that the susceptibility to anti-GBM disease depends on the inheritance of certain "GM allotypes" of immunoglobulin heavy chains. Certain of these are increased in patients with anti-GBM disease. It may be that the inheritance of these traits predisposes some patients to the possible development of Goodpasture's syndrome under the right environmental conditions. Such conditions might, for example, include an infection or toxin exposure that damages the basement membrane and thereby exposes one of its antigenic components. If the patient responds by developing antibodies to this antigen, the clinical disease might result.[11]

Biochemists have made considerable progress in identifying the "Goodpasture antigen," that is, the membrane component to which the anti-GBM antibodies are directed.[12] It is one of the regions in the type IV collagen molecule that forms the backbone of the basement membrane. For reasons not yet totally clear, the basement membranes of the alveolar wall and the renal glomerulus seem to bind the antibodies better than basement membranes at other sites.[13]

What sorts of environmental conditions might expose the basement membrane and set up the conditions for the patient to begin making antibodies against basement membrane collagen? This is an area of speculation, but the case records of patients with Goodpasture's syndrome contain possible clues. Patients have developed the disease after influenza,[14–18] and patients have had rehemorrhages after infections, fluid overload, or oxygen exposure.[19,20] Exposure to the fumes of hydrocarbon solvents has also been found in the histories of a number of patients, although only in a small percentage.[6,11,21–24] Finally, cigarette smoking has a strong association with pulmonary hemorrhage in anti-GBM disease. Donaghy and Rees[25] found that of 37 of their patients with anti-GBM disease who smoked, all had pulmonary hemorrhage, whereas only 20 percent of the non-smokers in their series had this finding. They conjectured that smoking might increase lung permeability and in that way predispose to the formation of anti-GBM antibodies. Other reports support the association with smoking.[10,11]

In summary, Goodpasture's syndrome is a disease in which a genetically predisposed subject suffers an injury to basement membrane that exposes type IV collagen molecules and results in the formation of antibodies, which, in turn, combine with basement membranes in the glomerulus of the kidney and the alveolar wall to incite an additional injury, resulting in alveolar hemorrhage and renal failure.

Signs, Symptoms, and Laboratory Abnormalities

There is a great deal of variation in the pattern of appearance of the symptoms of Goodpasture's syndrome. Kelly and Haponik[11] have carefully reviewed the literature and concluded that hemoptysis is the most common presenting symptom. In the majority of cases, hemoptysis comes before renal failure, generally by an interval of 8 to 12 months. Hemoptysis can be mild or severe; indeed, patients with severe disease continue to die today of hemoptysis in spite of appropriate drug therapy. During the period of acute pulmonary hemorrhage, systemic symptoms are common, including fever, chills, and sweats. Fatigue and weakness generally correlate with the degree of anemia.[15] Chest pain is seen in some patients, probably caused by coughing. Other symptoms include gross hematuria and weight loss in some patients. Pallor is the most common sign of anti-GBM disease. Crackles are also common. Less common signs include heart murmur, hepatomegaly, edema, hypertension, and fundoscopic changes.

The most striking laboratory abnormality is anemia, but Kelly and Haponik[11] found that microcytic indices were uncommon, suggesting that factors other than blood loss were contributing. White blood counts are increased in up to one-half of patients, often with increased immature forms.[16,24] Urinalysis is abnormal and often shows microscopic or gross hematuria, proteinuria, and red blood cell casts.

The chest roentgenogram in Goodpasture's syndrome usually shows diffuse consolidation, often with sparing of the apices and bases.[26]

One laboratory test that can be useful in monitoring pulmonary hemorrhage in Goodpasture's syndrome is the diffusing capacity of carbon monoxide (DL_{CO}) measured in the pulmonary function laboratory.[27] Since this test measures intravascular and extravascular blood in the lung, DL_{CO} may be increased dramatically after alveolar hemorrhage has taken place.

Diagnosis

When a patient presents with the new onset of a pulmonary-renal syndrome, time is critical. If treatment is delayed, the patient may suffer progressive loss of renal function by the hour, and, at any moment, a fatal pulmonary hemorrhage may supervene. The diagnostic workup should include blood samples for the following: (1) anti-GBM antibody assay; (2) antineutrophil cytoplasmic antibody assay (positive in Wegener's granulomatosis, systemic necrotizing vasculitis, pauci-immune glomerulonephritis, and Henoch-Schönlein purpura); and (3) antinuclear antibody (positive in connective tissue diseases such as systemic lupus erythematosus). In many cases, it is also highly desirable to obtain a biopsy for speedy diagnosis. A biopsy of the kidney is often the first choice, since glomerular lesions can be immediately diagnostic or at least can limit the differential diagnosis in such a way that, together with clinical and serologic findings, a diagnosis can be made.[28] The characteristic renal lesion of Goodpasture's syndrome is linear immunofluorescent staining of the GBM with IgG, often together with crescentic glomerulonephritis. When a lung biopsy is chosen over kidney biopsy, the best technique is thoracoscopic biopsy. This method allows large biopsies to be taken and causes significantly less trauma to the patient than full thoracotomy techniques. Lung tissue obtained at biopsy should be processed immediately to look for linear fluorescence of IgG along the alveolar basement membrane. Alveolar hemorrhage itself is nonspecific.

Treatment

Advances in treatment have decreased the mortality of Goodpasture's syndrome from almost 90 percent to $\leq$ 25 percent.[11,29] Current treatment is a combination of plasmapheresis and drug therapy, which together are designed to decrease the concentration of circulating anti-GBM antibodies in the patient's blood.

PLASMAPHERESIS

In treatment by plasma exchange, whole blood is removed from the patient so that cells can be separated from the antibody-rich proteins. Cells are reinfused with donor plasma,

plasma protein, or albumin in saline. As reported by Lockwood and colleagues,[30] this therapy helps to improve the creatinine clearance of patients who still have some residual renal function, and it rapidly controls pulmonary hemorrhage. Plasmapheresis is used at the beginning of the patient's therapy, and it can be reinstituted later if the patient has a relapse of alveolar hemorrhage. Kelly and Haponik[11] recommend as a guideline that 4-L exchanges should be carried out every 1 to 3 days for 14 days, or until anti-GBM antibody titer is normal. If the patients still has alveolar hemorrhages at that point, the plasmapheresis should be continued. Drug therapy should be given concomitantly. In addition, patients with a significant degree of renal failure will require hemodialysis.

CORTICOSTEROIDS

When the patient's degree of alveolar hemorrhage is not considered to be life-threatening, Kelly and Haponik[11] recommend prednisone at a dose of 1 to 2 mg/kg/day for 8 to 12 weeks.

When the patient's degree of alveolar hemorrhage is life-threatening, they recommend methylprednisolone at a dose of 5 to 15 mg/kg/day for 1 to 3 days, after which prednisone can be substituted as above.

CYCLOPHOSPHAMIDE

Kelly and Haponik[11] recommend a dose of 2 to 3 mg/kg/day for 8 to 12 weeks given either orally or intravenously, but this dose should be adjusted for leukopenia ($<4000/mm^3$) and thrombocytopenia ($<100,000/mm^3$).

RESPIRATORY SUPPORT

Patients with respiratory failure need endotracheal intubation, mechanical ventilation, oxygen, and positive end-expiratory pressure.

THE RESULTS OF TREATMENT

With aggressive treatment, it is now possible to save the lives of approximately 80 percent of patients with Goodpasture's syndrome, although many will complete treatment with a significant degree of chronic renal failure that may require maintenance dialysis. Treatment is often given for up to 12 weeks and then discontinued. Relapse is seen in some cases if the treatment is tapered at a time when the patient is still producing anti-GBM antibodies.[15] Recurrence following remission is rare.[11] The many patients who achieve remission are capable of returning to work without the need for chronic drug therapy.

Summary

Goodpasture's syndrome is a rare disease in which proper pharmacotherapy together with plasmapheresis plays a lifesaving role. By decreasing the production of the auto-antibodies that are the root cause of the disease, cyclophos-phamide and corticosteroids together with plasmapheresis and hemodialysis allow many patients to recover residual glomerular function and to survive acute pulmonary hemorrhage.

References

1. D'Apice AJF, Kincaid-Smith P, Becker GJ, et al.: Goodpasture's syndrome in identical twins. *Ann Intern Med* 1978; 88:61.
2. Gossain VV, Gerstein AR, Janes AW: Goodpasture's syndrome: A familial occurrence. *Am Rev Respir Dis* 1972; 105:621.
3. Rees AJ, Demaine AG, Welsh KI: Association of immunoglobulin Gm allotypes with anti-glomerular basement membrane antibodies and their titers. *Hum Immunol* 1984; 10:213.
4. Stanton MC, Tange JD: Goodpasture's syndrome: Pulmonary hemorrhage associated with glomerluonephritis. *Australas Ann Med* 1958; 7:132.
5. Maddock RK, Stevens LE, Reemtsma K, Bloomer HA: Goodpasture's syndrome: Cessation of pulmonary hemorrhage after bilateral nephrectomy. *Ann Intern Med* 1967; 67:1258.
6. Savage COS, Pusey CD, Bowman C, et al.: Anti-glomerular basement membrane antibody mediated disease in the British Isles 1980–1984. *Br Med J* 1986; 292:301.
7. Perl SI, Pussel BA, Charlesworth JA, et al.: Goodpasture's (Anti-GBM) disease and HLA-DRW2. *N Engl J Med* 1981; 305:463.
8. Rees AJ, Peters DK, Compston DAS, Batchelor JR: Strong association between HLA-DRW2 and antibody-mediated Goodpasture's syndrome. *Lancet* 1978; 1:966.
9. Dunkley H, Chapman JR, Burke J, et al.: HLA-DR and -DQ in Anti-GBM disease. *Dis Markers* 1991; 9:249.
10. Rees AJ, Lockwood CM: Anti-glomerular basement membrane antibody-mediated nephritis, in Schrier RW, Gottschalk CW (eds): *Disease of the Kidney*. Boston: Little Brown, 1988: 2091–2126.
11. Kelly PT, Haponik EF: Goodpasture syndrome: Molecular and clinical advances. *Medicine* 1994; 73:171.
12. Wieslander J, Barr JF, Butowski RJ, et al.: Goodpasture antigen of the glomerular basement membrane: Localization to noncollagenous regions of type IV collagen. *Proc Natl Acad Sci USA* 1984; 81:3838.
13. Weber M, Pullig O: Different immunologic properties of the globular NC1 domain of collagen type IV isolated from various human basement membranes. *Eur J Clin Invest* 1992; 22:138.
14. Wilson CB, Dixon FJ: Anti-glomerular basement membrane antibody-induced glomerulonephritis. *Kindey Int* 1973; 3:74.
15. Benoit FL, Rulon CB, Theil GB, et al.: Goodpasture's syndrome: A clinicopathologic entity. *Am J Med* 1964; 37:424.
16. Proskey AJ, Weatherbee L, Easterling RE, et al.: Goodpasture's syndrome: A report of five cases and review of the literature. *Am J Med* 1970; 48:162.
17. Wilson CB, Smith RC: Goodpasture's syndrome associated with influenza A2 virus infection. *Ann Intern Med* 1972; 76:91.
18. Perez GO, Bjornsson S, Ross AH, et al.: A mini-epidemic of Goodpasture's syndrome. *Nephron* 1974; 13:161.
19. Bowley NB, Steiner RE, Chin WS: The chest x-ray in anti-glomerular antibody disease (Goodpasture's syndrome). *Clin Radiol* 1979; 30:419.
20. Rees AJ, Lockwood CM, Peters DK: Enhanced allergic tissue injury in Goodpasture's syndrome by intercurrent bacterial infection. *Br Med J* 1977; 2:723.
21. Heale WF, Mathiesson AM, Niall JF: Lung hemorrhage and nephritis. *Med J Aust* 1969; 2:355.
22. Beirne GJ, Brennan JT: Glomerulonephritis associated with hydrocarbon solvents. *Arch Environ Health* 1972; 25:365.
23. Briggs WA, Johnson JP, Teichman S, et al.: Antiglomerular base-

ment membrane antibody–mediated glomerulonephritis and Goodpasture's syndrome. *Medicine (Baltimore)* 1979; 58:348.

24. Teague CA, Doak PB, Simpson IJ, et al.: Goodpasture's syndrome: An analysis of 29 cases. *Kidney Int* 1978; 13:492.

25. Donaghy M, Rees AJ: Cigarette smoking and lung hemorrhage in glomerulonephritis caused by autoantibodies to glomerular basement membrane. *Lancet* 1983; 2:1390.

26. Müller NL, Miller RR: Diffuse pulmonary hemorrhage. *Radiol Clin North Am* 1991; 29:965.

27. Addleman M, Logan AS, Grossman RF: Monitoring intrapulmonary hemorrhage in Goodpasture's syndrome. *Chest* 1985; 87:119.

28. Travis WD, Colby TV, Lombard C, Carpenter AH: A clinicopathologic study of 34 cases of diffuse pulmonary hemorrhage with lung biopsy confirmation. *Am J Surg Pathol* 1990; 14:1112.

29. Rosenblatt SG, Knight W, Bannayan GA, et al.: Treatment of Goodpasture's syndrome with plasmapheresis. *Am J Med* 1979; 66:698.

30. Lockwood CM, Rees AJ, Pearson TA, et al.: Immunosuppression and plasma-exchange in the treatment of Goodpasture's syndrome. *Lancet* 1976; 1:711.

Chapter 116

WEGENER'S GRANULOMATOSIS

EUGENE F. GEPPERT

Wegener's granulomatosis is a rare disease characterized by granulomatous inflammation of the respiratory tract and necrotizing vasculitis affecting small to medium-sized vessels (e.g., capillaries, venules, arterioles, and arteries). Necrotizing glomerulonephritis is common, and this disease is strongly associated with antineutrophil cytoplasmic antibodies in the patient's blood.[1] During the past 35 years, pharmacotherapy has greatly improved for patients with this previously fatal illness.[2]

Pathogenesis

The etiology of Wegener's granulomatosis is still unknown. One hypothesis that has been considered is that this disease might result from an infection. It is common for physicians initially to misdiagnose pulmonary Wegener's granulomatosis as a subacute pneumonia. The illness is often characterized by fever, leukocytosis, and sputum production together with findings of consolidation on the chest roentgenogram. In addition, scattered case reports have even suggested the possibility that antimicrobial drugs might at times provide a partial treatment,[3–5] although these observations have not translated into consistent benefit for most patients in one careful study.[6] Since conventional methods of culture of lung tissue had never revealed an infecting microbe, Hoffman and associates[7] decided to search for a pathogen by using the techniques of in situ hybridization on specimens obtained at open lung biopsy from patients with Wegener's granulomatosis. They found no nucleic-acid sequences homologous to adenovirus, cytomegalovirus, enterovirus, herpes simplex virus, varicella zoster virus, influenza, parainfluenza, rhinovirus, or respiratory syncytial virus. These investigators

did document that neutrophils were present in the bronchoalveolar lavage fluid of patients with active disease. In addition, the lavage fluid contained an increased concentration of IgG c-ANCA (an antineutrophil cytoplasmic antibody) in patients whose disease was active, but this increased concentration was not found during remission from the disease. Thus, although no evidence has been found for an infectious etiology, neutrophils were present in the lungs at the time when Wegener's granulomatosis was advancing.

A contemporary hypothesis concerning the etiology of Wegener's granulomatosis considers the possibility that the serum antibody that is viewed as a laboratory test for the disease in most cases—the antineutrophil cytoplasmic antibody—might also play a central role in pathogenesis of the disease.[8] To explain this hypothesis, it is first necessary to review what is known about the biochemistry of antineutrophil cytoplasmic antibodies and the proteins with which they combine.

A number of different antineutrophil cytoplasmic antibodies are associated with such diseases as Wegener's granulomatosis, microscopic polyangiitis, segmental necrotizing glomerulonephritis, and others. As explained in the review of Galperin and Hoffman,[8] an understanding of the antineutrophil cytoplasmic antibody starts with an understanding of the biochemical composition of the human neutrophil. These cells have primary cytoplasmic granules that contain the proteins myeloperoxidase, proteinase 3, and many other proteins. The antineutrophil cytoplasmic antibodies, or ANCAs, react to proteins within neutrophil granules. In 1985, van der Woude and coworkers discovered that ANCA was present in 25 of 27 patients with active Wegener's granulomatosis.[9] Since this initial discovery, there have been large changes in the method used to perform the assay, and a great deal more has been learned about the specific antigens within neutrophils that elicit the antibody formation in various diseases. The initial assay was the indirect immunofluorescent technique. By this method, isolated normal human neutrophils are cytocentrifuged onto slides, fixed in ethanol, incubated with the patient's serum, and finally stained with fluoresceinated secondary antihuman immunoglobulin antibodies. The slides are examined on a fluorescent microscope and, when ANCAs are present, two patterns of fluorescence are noted. One is labeled "c-ANCA," in which the fluorescence is seen over the neutrophil's cytoplasm. The other was labeled "p-ANCA" in which the fluorescence is seen in a perinuclear position. Both antibodies are directed against proteins in the cytoplasmic primary granules. The apparent perinuclear location of p-ANCA is an artifact relating to the method of cell fixation.

Currently, attempts are being made to refine the assay by converting it from indirect fluorescence using cells to an enzyme-linked immunosorbent assay (ELISA) that uses purified antigens. Research biochemists have shown that the antigen responsible for the c-ANCA pattern is a 29-kDa serine proteinase called proteinase 3.[10–12] The antigen that is most commonly found in patients who are positive for p-ANCA is myeloperoxidase. The new ELISA assays use one of several techniques to determine seropositivity for the ANCAs.[8] In the direct ELISA, purified proteinase 3 or myeloperoxidase is bound to wells and incubated with the patient's serum. If ANCA is present, it will bind to the fixed protein. As a last step, the serum is washed away and labeled antihuman immunoglobulin reacts with the complex. Bound antibody is detected by means of the labeled second antibody.

Recent studies that have used an ELISA method have shown that a majority of c-ANCA-positive sera react with proteinase 3.[13,14] Since the correlation is not perfect, there may be antibodies directed against antigens other than proteinase 3. Similarly, the correlation between p-ANCA and myeloperoxidase is not perfect. At the present time, it is not clear whether ELISA techniques will replace indirect immunofluorescence. Nevertheless, it is possible to say that most patient sera that show the c-ANCA pattern are detecting antibodies to proteinase 3 and that very many of the sera that show the p-ANCA pattern are detecting antibodies to myeloperoxidase.

According to the hypothesis that ANCA might play a central role in the pathogenesis of Wegener's granulomatosis, circulating ANCAs might enhance the activation of neutrophils and monocytes, cause them to adhere to the walls of blood vessels, and finally injure them.[8] For this pathogenic sequence to happen, three events must take place.[15] First, the ANCA must interact with viable leukocytes in the blood. Second, ANCAs must be capable of activating the neutrophil. Last, the combination of the ANCA and the activated neutrophil must cause injury to the blood vessel. There is now enough in vitro evidence that it will be possible to pursue this hypothesis further (summarized in Ref. 8).

Evidence collected so far does not support a genetic predisposition to Wegener's granulomatosis. A recent study of HLA alleles in 83 patients did not show any genetic type to be unusually common in patients with this disease (Hoffman, unpublished data, cited in Ref. 8).

Signs and Symptoms

The signs and symptoms of Wegener's granulomatosis at the time of presentation are extremely variable. Systemic symptoms include fever and weight loss. Often, patients with fever and respiratory symptoms are initially thought to have pneumonia and are treated with antimicrobials on an empiric basis. In the series of Hoffman and associates, 23 percent of the patients had fever at presentation and half had fever at some time during the course of their illness. Weight loss of more than 10 percent of usual body weight was seen in 15 percent of patients at presentation and 35 percent of the patients overall, and patients were often thought to have an occult malignancy. Most patients first sought medical care because of symptoms referable to the upper airway or the respiratory tract.

Oral ulcers are common and may be either painful or painless. Purulent or bloody nasal discharge is also seen frequently. If the earliest manifestations of Wegener's involvement of the upper respiratory tract do not lead to diagnosis, more advanced manifestations such as recurrent epistaxis, mucosal ulcerations, nasal septal perforation, and nasal deformity ("saddle nose") may supervene. The common symptoms of lower respiratory tract involvement by Wegener's granulomatosis include cough, hemoptysis, and pleuritic pain. Eye symptoms are quite frequent during the course of the disease. Especially characteristic signs are proptosis and loss of conjugate gaze due to the buildup of retroorbital inflammatory tissue. The majority of patients have musculoskeletal symptoms such as arthralgias and myalgias. A variety of skin rashes are seen: palpable purpura, ulcers, vesicles, papules, and subcutaneous nodules. Both the central and peripheral nervous system may be involved, although rarely at presentation. Mononeuritis multiplex is seen in about one-sixth of the patients; the central nervous system (CNS) abnormalities that are seen include stroke and cranial nerve abnormalities. The most common cardiac abnormality is pericarditis, sometimes manifest by chest pain. In rare instances, the inflammation of Wegener's granulomatosis can involve almost any system of the body or tissue.

Diagnosis

Wegener's granulomatosis is a clinicopathologic diagnosis. This means that the diagnosis requires a characteristic tissue biopsy together with a compatible set of signs and symptoms. Laboratory testing can add important support to a clinicopathologic diagnosis that is borderline or tentative. The most important criterion for diagnosis is the presence of granulomatous vasculitis on biopsy of the lung. Supporting data come from the clinical laboratory, the pulmonary function laboratory, and radiologic studies.

CLINICAL LABORATORY DATA

The sera of most patients who have Wegener's granulomatosis is positive for c-ANCA, the cytoplasmic antineutrophil cytoplasmic antibody, which in most cases really represents IgG antibody to proteinase 3. A minority of patients with Wegener's granulomatosis are positive for p-ANCA or are not positive to either c-ANCA or p-ANCA. The value of a positive c-ANCA test in a patient with signs and symptoms compatible with Wegener's granulomatosis is that it provides substantial support for the diagnosis. In itself, the c-ANCA test is not absolutely diagnostic of Wegener's granulomatosis. The sensitivity and specificity of the c-ANCA test (indirect immunofluorescence) vary according to how controls are chosen. One widely quoted figure is at least 80 percent for sensitivity and up to 97 percent for specificity.[8] In a study in which cases and controls came from the medical practices of pulmonologists, the sensitivity was 65 percent and the specificity only 77 percent.[16] It is very likely that these statistics will change along with important changes in the method of the assay in the near future.

Since ANCA is not absolutely specific for Wegener's granulomatosis, what are some of the other diseases associated with a positive test? One of the ANCA-positive diseases is microscopic polyangiitis. This disease is a systemic nongranulomatous vasculitis of small vessels (arterioles, capillaries, venules) that sometimes also involves larger vessels. It often causes a segmental necrotizing glomerulonephritis and sometimes causes diffuse alveolar hemorrhage. This disease is usually positive for the p-ANCA but occasionally the c-ANCA may be positive. Other diseases associated with a positive ANCA test include Churg-Strauss syndrome and polyarteritis nodosa. The specificity of the ANCA will likely change as the assay is improved with the use of molecular techniques.

In the late 1980s, articles appeared supporting the idea that the degree of positivity of the ANCA test might correlate with the clinical activity of Wegener's granulomatosis. Unfortunately, the correlation is not so good that it can take the place of the physician's clinical judgment. Currently, therefore, decisions about whether the disease is active or in remission or relapse cannot depend only on the changes in the titer of the ANCA test in an individual patient.

The clinical laboratory can also contribute helpful information about patients with Wegener's granulomatosis when the complete blood count and erythrocyte sedimentation rate are measured. Patients with Wegener's granulomatosis often have an elevated white blood count with a mean value in one series[6] of $10,500/mm^3$. Anemia is found in about three-quarters of patients and thrombocytosis is seen in two-thirds. The erythrocyte sedimentation rate is elevated in the majority with a mean value of 71 mm/h and a range from 17 to 140 mm/h.[6]

PULMONARY FUNCTION TESTS

The abnormalities measured in the pulmonary function tests of patients with Wegener's granulomatosis vary strikingly according to whether the pattern of disease involves the bronchial airways or only the alveolar parenchyma.[6] A restrictive pattern is seen in patients who have suffered extensive parenchymal infiltrates or major alveolar hemorrhage. In some cases, drug-induced pneumonitis caused by the patient's treatment with cyclophosphamide may contribute to the restrictive defect. Active endobronchial disease is common in Wegener's granulomatosis and, even with treatment, the endobronchial disease may regress but leave significant endobronchial scars that limit expiratory airflow. This group of patients will have obstructive abnormalities on spirometry and the flow volume loop. Patients with tracheal stenosis will show a pattern of upper airway obstruction on the flow volume loop with a visible plateau in inspiratory and expiratory flows. Patients with Wegener's who have pulmonary function testing during periods of diffuse alveolar hemorrhage will have increased diffusing capacity for carbon monoxide (DL_{CO}) due to the uptake of carbon monoxide by intraalveolar blood.

RADIOLOGIC STUDIES

A number of studies have contributed to our knowledge of patterns of abnormality in the chest roentgenograms and CT scans of patients with Wegener's granulomatosis.[6,17–19]

At the time of diagnosis, many patients with pulmonary Wegener's granulomatosis have either bilateral patchy pulmonary infiltrates or nodules, often with central cavitation. Pleural effusions are occasionally present. In patients who have bronchial obstruction, atelectasis may be seen. Patients who present with diffuse alveolar hemorrhage have dense bilateral infiltrates reminiscent of pulmonary edema. Occasional patients are found to have hilar and mediastinal lymph node enlargement. Recent articles have contributed new patterns to the spectrum of roentgenographic abnormalities. Aberle and associates[18] commented on the occasional patient whose chest roentgenogram shows a pattern of prominent bronchovascular markings. Papiris and associates[19] have reported patients with cuffing around the bronchovascular bundles on CT scans. No roentgenographic pattern is specific for Wegener's granulomatosis, but the most characteristic pattern is bilateral multiple cavities.

THE SURGICAL PATHOLOGY OF BIOPSIES

Although it is possible to make a diagnosis of Wegener's granulomatosis from biopsies from various tissues, lung tissue is preferred. Although tissues from the head and neck are more accessible than those of the lung, experience has shown that a diagnosis of Wegener's granulomatosis can only be made about 23 percent of the time on nasal or other head/neck tissues.[20] Kidney biopsies from patients with Wegener's granulomatosis typically show segmental necrotizing glomerulonephritis, but this same renal pattern of abnormality is shared by other diseases in the family of systemic vasculitides. Although the pathologist will search the renal biopsy for vasculitis, this finding is present in only about 8 percent of biopsies.[6] Thus, the kidney does not typically show the granulomatous vasculitis that is necessary to give strong support to a diagnosis of Wegener's granulomatosis. Skin biopsies have the same problem; the skin typically shows a leukocytoclastic angiitis in patients with Wegener's granulomatosis, not a granulomatous reaction.

Lung tissue obtained by fiberoptic bronchoscopy with transbronchial biopsy[21] sometimes contains enough tissue to make a diagnosis of Wegener's granulomatosis. More commonly, a large biopsy of lung obtained by thoracoscopy or open lung biopsy is required to show the pattern of abnormalities that allows confident diagnosis.[22–24] The appearance of the biopsies differs according to the patient's pulmonary presentation.

In patients with diffuse alveolar hemorrhage, lung tissue is submitted for immunofluorescent staining and for standard histopathologic stains. In Wegener's granulomatosis, immunofluorescent staining is completely negative or shows only sparse granular IgG. This pattern of staining is sometimes referred to as "pauci-immune" and indicates that neither complexes nor antibasement membrane antibodies are present. In routine stains, intraalveolar red blood cells are seen together with hemosiderin deposition within alveolar macrophages in some cases. Neutrophilic capillaritis is also seen in the majority of cases. In some patients with the acute alveolar hemorrhage of Wegener's granulomatosis, typical granulomatous inflammation is seen as well, but not all cases have this feature. Indeed, a type of acute alveolar hemorrhage has recently been described in which there is no granulomatous inflammation in the lung and the patients are positive for ANCA that is antimyeloperoxidase.[25] This disease, called isolated pulmonary hemorrhage, is one of a series of diseases that must be considered along with Wegener's granulomatosis in the differential diagnosis of diffuse alveolar hemorrhage. Clinical laboratory data help to make the distinctions among these diseases: systemic lupus erythematosus (with anti-double-stranded DNA antibodies), Goodpasture's syndrome (with antiglomerular basement membrane antibodies), rheumatoid arthritis (with rheumatoid factors), and IgA nephropathy (with immunofluorescence on skin biopsy). In patients who have diffuse alveolar hemorrhage secondary to Wegener's granulomatosis, the patient should be started on emergency treatment as soon as the lung biopsy and ANCA results are obtained, since any delay in therapy could result in death or irreversible renal failure.

In patients with possible Wegener's granulomatosis who do not present with acute alveolar hemorrhage, lung biopsies should be obtained from multiple sites and examined for the characteristic changes. The three types of changes sought include vasculitis, necrosis, and granulomatous inflammation.

The vasculitis seen in lung biopsies of patients with Wegener's granulomatosis varies from none at all to extensive involvement of arteries, veins, and capillaries. The earliest visible lesion in the lung[22] is a small focus of necrosis of collagen. The pathologic lesion that then follows is the formation of palisading granulomas and micronecrosis. At a later stage, macronecrosis is seen, and it may form "geographic" shapes. Fibrosis appears as a reparative process. Mark and associates[22] found that when lung biopsies from patients with Wegener's granulomatosis were compared with biopsies from patients with diseases that could be confused with Wegener's, the major discriminating features were palisading granulomas or palisading histiocytes in vascular walls and in extravascular tissue, microabscesses or fibrinoid necrosis in vascular walls, leukocytoclastic capillaritis, diffuse granulomatous tissue, and granulomatous bronchiolitis. The main diseases in the histopathologic differential diagnosis are tuberculosis and fungal lung diseases that sometimes show similar types of necrosis.

The granulomatous inflammation often seen in lung biopsies is one of the most important criteria for the diagnosis of Wegener's granulomatosis. These granulomatous inflammatory lesions are somewhat diffuse, not tightly packed, like the granulomas of sarcoidosis. Scattered giant cells are often seen.

In addition to vasculitis, necrosis, and granulomatous inflammation, many other histopathologic lesions are seen in the biopsies of patients with Wegener's granulomatosis. It is worth noting that in many cases, major histopathologic hallmarks of the disease may not be seen; it is especially in these cases that data other than the lung biopsy may allow the diagnosis to be made. Features such as concomitant sinus disease, hemoptysis, a renal biopsy showing segmental necrotizing glomerulonephritis, and a positive c-ANCA test can provide the support necessary to make a confident diagnosis in these difficult cases.

Drug Therapy

During the last 40 years, the introduction of pharmacotherapy for patients with Wegener's granulomatosis has made an enormous difference in prognosis.[2] Before drug therapy, Wegener's granulomatosis was uniformly fatal within about 5 months. The introduction of glucocorticoid therapy made only a small difference; as a result, patients lived up to 1 year. The major breakthrough came in 1973, when Fauci and Wolff showed that a combination of glucocorticoids with cyclophosphamide could induce a remission in many patients.[26] Although this represents a very great achievement in drug therapy, long-term evaluation of the patients treated with this drug regimen has revealed many forms of drug toxicity; for this reason, the search for better regimens continues.

Wegener's granulomatosis is a chronic disease. Current therapy can induce remissions, but relapses are common, even after many years. The general strategy is first to stabilize the patient, then induce a remission, and finally continue treatment for a reasonable time interval before withdrawing therapy gradually and watching the patient closely for any signs of a relapse.

At the time of the initial diagnosis, some patients with Wegener's granulomatosis are desperately ill. The current recommended drug regimen for these patients[27] is to give a daily oral dose of cyclophosphamide (up to 4 mg/kg) and methylprednisolone (1 g) for about 3 days. After that, the doses are reduced to the more conventional range, as detailed in the following paragraph.

Patients who are not desperately ill at presentation with Wegener's granulomatosis are treated with daily oral therapy with cyclophosphamide (2 mg/kg) and prednisone (1 mg/kg) for 1 month. If the patient improves substantially—as shown by suppression of clinical signs of disease, stabilization of the creatinine clearance, and at least partial resolution of lung consolidation on roentgenograms—the prednisone dose is tapered to an every-other-day regimen during the next 2 months. Cyclophosphamide is continued for at least 1 year after the patient has a complete remission and is then tapered by decrements of 25 mg every 2 to 3 months until the drug is discontinued or the patient suffers a relapse that requires augmentation of therapy. If the patient suffers a relapse, the standard protocol is begun anew with cyclophosphamide (2 mg/kg) and prednisone (1 mg/kg).

The standard protocol detailed above induces remission in about three-quarters of the patients with Wegener's granulomatosis, and the typical time to remission is 1 to 3 months. An unfortunate subgroup of patients show refractoriness to therapy and may go for many years without entering a remission. Since the drugs used to induce a remission are toxic, it is not surprising that many patients experience significant morbidity from treatment. Hoffman[27] has listed the morbidities of cyclophosphamide as follows: cystitis (43 percent), pulmonary insufficiency (17 percent), bladder cancer (2.8 to 4.2 percent), and infections requiring a stay in the hospital for intravenous antimicrobials (46 percent). Chronic therapy with glucocorticoids also is associated with significant side effects.

In the search for alternative drug regimens that will give relief to patients with Wegener's granulomatosis, trials of pulse therapy with cyclophosphamide were carried out. This therapy has had some success in treating patients with lupus nephritis. Unfortunately this strategy did not work, since an unacceptably high percentage of patients suffered relapse of Wegener's granulomatosis after an initial induction of remission.[28–30]

Since some patients with Wegener's granulomatosis cannot tolerate cyclophosphamide, it would be very useful to have an alternative regimen. Preliminary work has shown promise for methotrexate combined with glucocorticoids.[31] More studies are needed to evaluate this therapy, but the results of weekly administration of methotrexate at a mean stable dose of 20 mg resulted in good improvement in three-quarters of the 29 patients who took this experimental therapy.

Other forms of experimental therapy are in the early stages of evaluation. Although there has been mention in the literature of cases of Wegener's granulomatosis that seemed to respond to trimethoprim-sulfamethoxazole, the initial results of an open prospective study with this drug were not encouraging.[6] If this antimicrobial has a role in the treatment of Wegener's granulomatosis, it is not yet well defined.

In summary, the most effective drug yet found in the treatment of Wegener's granulomatosis is cyclophosphamide. A possible alternative drug that looks promising is methotrexate. Both these drugs are administered along with glucocorticoids in most cases. The goal of therapy is to induce a remission of the disease so that the patient can enjoy a prolonged interval free of its manifestations.

Clinical Outcome and Morbidity

The outcome of treatment of Wegener's granulomatosis has been best studied by the group at the U.S. National Institutes of Health and reported in 1992 by Hoffman and associates.[6] This group treated 158 patients with Wegener's granulomatosis using standard therapy of glucocorticoid and cyclophosphamide, as outlined above. Three-quarters of the patients achieved a complete remission. One of the best indicators that the regimen is working is the rate at which glucocorticoid can be withdrawn. Among the patients of Hoffman and coworkers who achieved remission on standard therapy, conversion from daily to alternate-day prednisone occurred within a median of 3.2 months. The median time to complete discontinuation of glucocorticoids was 12 months. One year was also the median time required to achieve a complete remission. About 1 out of 12 patients was refractory to the regimen, but even these often had a remission after continuing the regimen for 4 to 6 years. Half of the patients who had a remission later suffered a relapse. A total of 46 percent of all the patients' time was spent in remission.

The morbidity suffered by patients on standard therapy for Wegener's granulomatosis included morbidity from the disease and its treatment and from the treatment alone. Renal insufficiency in Wegener's granulomatosis is often severe, and many patients required dialysis or transplantation. Other occasional morbidities seen included hearing loss, nasal deformity, visual loss, chronic sinus dysfunction and pulmonary insufficiency. Morbidities related to cyclophosphamide included ovarian failure and an increased incidence of bladder cancer and lymphoma. Infectious morbidities were also common, and included pneumonias, sinus infections, and herpes zoster infections.

Summary

Wegener's granulomatosis is a chronic systemic disease with prominent pulmonary manifestations in many patients. Modern standard drug therapy with glucocorticoids and cyclophosphamide has greatly extended the life span of patients with this disease and has undoubtedly lessened the renal, pulmonary, and upper airway morbidity. The challenge for the future will be to develop alternative therapies that are less toxic than current therapy.

References

1. Jennette CJ, Falk RJ, Adrassy K, et al.: Nomenclature of systemic vasculitides: Proposal of an International Consensus Conference. *Arthritis Rheum* 1994; 37:187.
2. Hoffman GS: Wegener's granulomatosis: Changing perceptions of a once-fatal disease. *Clev Clin J Med* 1994; 61:412.
3. Israel HL: Sulfamethoxazole-trimethoprim therapy for Wegener's granulomatosis. *Arch Intern Med* 1988; 143:2293.

4. West BC, Todd JR, King JW: Wegener granulomatosis and trimethoprim-sulfamethoxazole: Complete remission after a twenty-year course. *Ann Intern Med* 1987; 106:840.

5. Puolijoki H, Liippo K, Raitio M, Tala E: Wegener's granulomatosis: Treatment under revision? *Respiration* 1992; 59:116.

6. Hoffman GS, Kerr GS, Leavitt RY, et al.: Wegener granulomatosis: An analysis of 158 patients. *Ann Intern Med* 1992; 116:488.

7. Hoffman GS, Sechler JMG, Gallin JI, et al.: Bronchoalveolar lavage analysis in Wegener's granulomatosis. *Am Rev Respir Dis* 1991; 143:401.

8. Galperin C, Hoffman GS: Antineutrophil cytoplasmic antibodies in Wegener's granulomatosis and other diseases: Clinical issues. *Clev Clin J Med* 1994; 61:416.

9. van der Woude FJ, Lobatto S, Permin H, et al.: Autoantibodies against neutrophils and monocytes: Tool for diagnosis and marker for disease activity in Wegener's granulomatosis. *Lancet* 1985; 1:425.

10. Lüdemann J, Utecht B, Gross WL: Anti-neutrophil cytoplasmic antibodies in Wegener's granulomatosis recognize an elastinolitic enzyme. *J Exp Med* 1990; 171:357.

11. Niles JL, McCluskey RT, Ahmad MF, Arnaout MA: Wegener's granulomatosis autoantigen is a novel serine proteinase. *Blood* 1989; 74:1888.

12. Goldschmeding R, van der Schoot CE, ten Bokkel Huinink D, et al.: Wegener's granulomatosis antibodies identify a novel diisopropilfluorophosphate-binding protein in the lysosomes of normal human neutrophils. *J Clin Invest* 1989; 84:1577.

13. Nölle B, Specks U, Lüdemann J, et al.: Anticytoplasmic antibodies: Their immunodiagnostic value in Wegener's granulomatosis. *Ann Intern Med* 1989; 111:28.

14. Cohen Tervaert JW, Goldschmeding R, Elema JD, et al.: Autoantibodies against myeloid lysosomal enzymes in crescentic glomerulonephritis. *Kidney Int* 1990; 37:799.

15. Jennette JC, Ewert BH, Falk RJ: Do antineutrophil cytoplasmic autoantibodies cause Wegener's granulomatosis and other forms of necrotizing vasculitis? *Rheum Dis Clin North Am* 1993; 19:1.

16. Davenport A, Lock RJ, Wallington TB: Clinical relevance of testing for antineutrophil cytoplasm antibodies (ANCA) with a standard indirect immunofluorescence ANCA test in patients with upper or lower respiratory tract symptoms. *Thorax* 1994; 49:213.

17. Cordier JF, Valeyre D, Guillevin L, et al.: Pulmonary Wegener's granulomatosis: A clinical and imaging study of 77 cases. *Chest* 1990; 97:906.

18. Aberle DR, Gamsu G, Lynch D: Thoracic manifestations of Wegener granulomatosis: Diagnosis and course. *Radiology* 1990; 174:703.

19. Papiris SA, Manoussakis MN, Drosos AA, et al.: Imaging of thoracic Wegener's granulomatosis: The computed tomographic appearance. *Am J Med* 1992; 93:530.

20. Devaney KO, Travis WD, Hoffman GS, et al.: Interpretation of head and neck biopsies in Wegener's granulomatosis: A pathologic study of 126 biopsies in 70 patients. *Am J Surg Pathol* 1990; 14:555.

21. Lombard CM, Duncan SR, Rizk NW, Colby TV: The diagnosis of Wegener's granulomatosis from transbronchial biopsy specimens. *Hum Pathol* 1990; 21:838.

22. Mark EJ, Matsubara O, Tan-Liu NS, Fienberg R: The pulmonary biopsy in the early diagnosis of Wegener (pathergic) granulomatosis: A study based on 35 open lung biopsies. *Hum Pathol* 1988; 19:1065.

23. Travis WD, Colby TV, Lombard C, Carpenter HA: A clinicopathologic study of 34 cases of diffuse pulmonary hemorrhage with lung biopsy confirmation. *Am J Surg Pathol* 1990; 14:1112.

24. Travis WD, Hoffman GS, Leavitt RY, et al.: Surgical pathology of the lung in Wegener's granulomatosis. *Am J Surg Pathol* 1991; 15:315.

25. Bosch X, Font J, Mirapeix E, et al.: Antimyeloperoxidase autoantibody-associated necrotizing alveolar capillaritis. *Am Rev Respir Dis* 1992; 146:1326.

26. Fauci AS, Wolff SM: Wegener's granulomatosis: Studies in eighteen patients and a review of the literature. *Medicine* 1973; 52:535.

27. Hoffman GS: Treating Wegener's granulomatosis: How far have we come? *Clev Clin J Med* 1994; 61:414.

28. Hoffman GS, Leavitt RY, Fleisher TA, et al.: Treatment of Wegener's granulomatosis with intermittent high-dose intravenous cyclophosphamide. *Am J Med* 1990; 89:403.

29. Drosos AA, Sakkas LI, Soussia A, et al.: Pulse cyclophosphamide therapy in Wegener's granulomatosis: A pilot study. *J Intern Med* 1992; 232:279.

30. Reinhold-Keller E, Kekow J, Schnabel A, et al.: Influence of disease manifestation and antineutrophil cytoplasmic antibody titer on the response to pulse cyclophosphamide therapy in patients with Wegener's granulomatosis. *Arthritis Rheum* 1994; 6:919.

31. Hoffman GS, Leavitt RY, Kerr GS, Fauci AS: The treatment of Wegener's granulomatosis with glucocorticoids and methotrexate. *Arthritis Rheum* 1992; 35:1322.

PART 7

SPECIAL TREATMENT MODALITIES

AEROSOL THERAPY
JONATHAN S. ILOWITE AND ALAN M. FEIN

Fundamentals of Aerosol Therapy

Types of Aerosol Delivery Devices

Delivery of Aerosolized Medications to Mechanically Ventilated Patients

Inhaled Antibiotics
Prevention of pneumonia
Treatment of infection in cystic fibrosis
Treatment of *pneumocystis carinii* pneumonia

Novel Agents Administered by Aerosol Therapy
Recombinant human DNase
Aerosolized amiloride, gene therapy in cystic fibrosis
Surfactant replacement therapy in acute lung injury
Other therapies

Conclusions

Aerosol therapy has undergone a major resurgence of interest for a number of reasons. Potential advantages of administering pharmaceuticals directly to the lung include the following:

1. Potential for a quicker, more potent effect
2. Potential avoidance of systemic side effects
3. Avoidance of the gastrointestinal tract and subsequent degradation of drug

However, the delivery of drugs by aerosol can be difficult. Some potential disadvantages of aerosol therapy include the following:

1. Difficulty determining dose of drug actually delivered to the lung
2. Difficulty in formulation and manufacturing of drugs for aerosol delivery
3. Ineffective patient technique in using the delivery device
4. Poor patient compliance with aerosol therapy

This chapter reviews the science of aerosol therapy and uses these principles to help practitioners maximize the advantages of aerosol therapy.

Fundamentals of Aerosol Therapy

An aerosol is a suspension of liquid droplets of particles in the air. Aerosols are characterized by average size and by the variability in size. Most often, particles are characterized by their mass median aerodynamic diameter (MMAD), which describes the diameter of a particle (usually in microns) around which the suspension is equally divided by mass (i.e., half of the total mass of the particles is greater than the MMAD and half is less). The variability of the particles around the mean is usually described by the geometric standard deviation (GSD), which is computed by plotting the distribution of particle sizes on log normal paper. Aerosols with GSDs < 1.2 are considered to be *monodisperse*. Monodisperse aerosols technically are difficult to manufacture, and their use has been confined to research purposes. Most aerosols used in clinical medicine have GSDs > 2 and are termed *heterodisperse*.

Particles will deposit in the respiratory tract by three major mechanisms: impaction, sedimentation, and diffusion.[1] *Impaction* refers to the momentum of a particle that will carry the particle into a bifurcation of an airway while the airstream in which it was suspended makes the turn (Fig. 117-1). This is the major mechanism that accounts for deposition of particles in the nasopharynx and oropharynx, and it is a useful defense mechanism for the lung to keep particles out of the lower respiratory tract. In general, particles with a MMAD > 6 to 8 μ are deposited in the oropharynx by impaction. Furthermore, since momentum is also a function of velocity, the greater the inhalation flow rate, the more likely that particles will be deposited by impaction. Particles that penetrate deeper into the lungs, i.e., the small airways and alveoli, will be deposited mainly by sedimentation. *Sedimentation* refers to the deposition of particles by gravitational forces. Sedimentation occurs as a function of the MMAD and residence time. Larger particles settle out faster, and the more time the suspension is in the respiratory tract, the greater the fraction of the suspension that settles out and

THREE MECHANISMS OF AEROSOL DEPOSITION

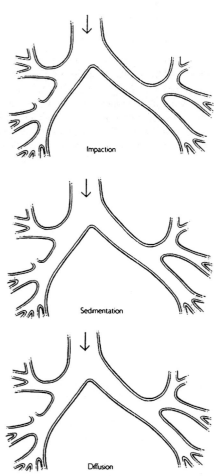

FIGURE 117-1 Mechanisms of deposition of aerosol. Impaction occurs when the momentum of a particle is too great to allow it to remain suspended as the airstream changes direction in the oropharynx or airway bifurcation. Sedimentation occurs when the airstream slows sufficiently to allow particles to settle out by force of gravity. Diffusion occurs by Brownian motion of small particles striking the epithelial surface. (*From Ilowite,*[67] *with permission.*)

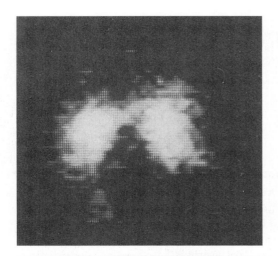

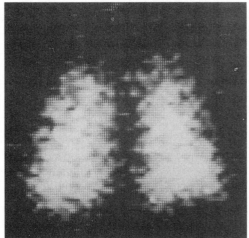

FIGURE 117-2 Effect of inspiratory flow rate. Gamma camera images of a radiolabeled aerosol are shown. The image at left was made with a fast inspiratory flow and demonstrates a more proximal airway deposition than the image at right, where the aerosol was inhaled more slowly. Note that the image at left also shows aerosol in the stomach, which represents aerosol swallowed after orpharyngeal impaction. (*From Ilowite,*[67] *with permission.*)

is deposited on the airway surface. In general, particles of 1 to 5 μ are deposited chiefly by sedimentation, and it is this range of particles that is ideal for aerosol delivery systems. Particles smaller than 1 μ tend to be too light to be influenced by gravitational forces; they are deposited only if random (Brownian) motion puts them in contact with the epithelium—i.e., by diffusion. This process is relatively inefficient, and many submicronic particles will be exhaled; hence, the deposition fraction is small.

Other factors influence the regional distribution of aerosol in the lung besides particle size. Inspiratory flow has already been mentioned, and high flows favor impaction in the proximal airways and oropharynx (Fig. 117-2). In addition, disease may alter the normal distribution of aerosol in the lung. In particular, chronic obstructive lung disease (COPD),[2] cystic fibrosis,[3] and asthma are associated with a more hetero-

geneous distribution of aerosol than that found in normal subjects.[4] This is probably secondary to the alteration of normal airway geometry as well as an altera-tion in the normal distribution and velocity of airflow in obstructed airways. A typical distribution pattern of aerosol in a normal subject is compared to one in a patient with obstructive lung disease in Fig. 117-3.

Types of Aerosol Delivery Devices

Four types of aerosol delivery devices have been developed for use in the clinical setting: the small-volume nebulizer (SVN), the metered-dose inhaler (MDI), the dry powder inhaler (DPI), and the ultrasonic nebulizer (UN). The SVN uses a source of compressed air to force a stream of liquid

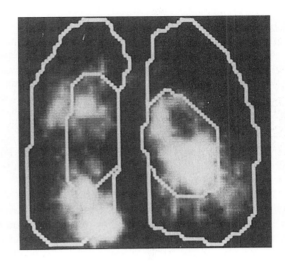

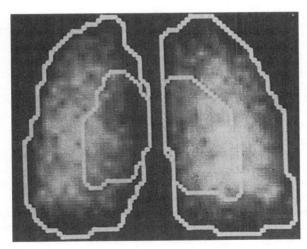

Figure 117-3 The effects of pulmonary disease. The distribution of aerosol is markedly more heterogeneous in the patient with cystic fibrosis and severe airway obstruction (*left*) than it is in the patient with mild cystic fibrosis and normal pulmonary function (*right*) breathing the same radiolabeled aerosol. (*From Ilowite,*[67] *with permission.*)

into a narrow opening, where it is exploded by the jet stream into a cloud of aerosol droplets. This cloud of droplets is usually too large and heterodisperse to be of clinical use. The nebulizer also has baffles and valves that trap the larger particles and allow only the smaller particles to pass through to the inhalation end.

Unfortunately, drug delivery by SVN is not a very efficient process.[5] A number of technical factors determine the actual amount of drug delivered by a SVN. Efficiency varies substantially by brand, and, sometimes, lot numbers of the same device.[6] The flow of gas through the nebulizer affects performance. In general, higher flow rates will produce smaller particles and increase the efficiency of the product; it generally is recommended that most nebulizers be operated with ≥ 6 L/min flow of driving gas.[7] Even when run to "dry-

ness," approximately 50 percent of the medication remains in the nebulizer. This results from evaporation of the eluent during nebulization and adherence of the liquid to the walls and tubing of the nebulizer.[8] This "dead volume" can be decreased by diluting the medication in a larger volume in the nebulizer; a volume of ≥ 4 ml has been recommended by some authors.[9] However, it may be impractical to adjust the volume when administering "unit dose" medications. Patient compliance may decrease with use of larger volumes, because it will take a longer time to complete the nebulization. Similarly, efficiency can be increased by using a trigger that allows only the driving gas into the nebulizer during inspiration.[10] This will decrease the aerosol, which normally is formed during the expiratory phase and is wasted. However, use of this system greatly increases the time for nebulization and may decrease compliance. Breathing pattern should be slow, relaxed tidal breathing. Even using optimal technique, the amount of drug that is deposited in the patient's lungs is only about 5 to 10 percent of the dose administered in the nebulizer. A summary of technique for using an SVN is shown in Table 117-1.

Ultrasonic nebulizers (USNs) use a special type of crystal (pizo-electric) that is sensitive to electric current. The crystal transforms the electric current to mechanical oscillations, which, in turn, are transmitted to the liquid to be nebulized. This mechanical disturbance causes an aerosol to form at the liquid-air interface, which can be inhaled directly or, with some devices, blown by a small fan. The particles size varies among USN, depending on the frequency response of the pizo-electric crystals.[11] The major advantage of USNs is their efficiency (as great as 27 percent for some models[12]). However, disadvantages—including expense, the need for electricity to operate them, the lack of disposability, and the concern that the heat generated during nebulization might denature some pharmaceuticals—have greatly limited their use up to the present time.

A MDI contains medication either suspended or dissolves in a propellant mixture. The propellant contains a mixture of chlorofluorocarbons (CFCs) and surfactants and other solvents. When the MDI is actuated, the aerosol suspension is released from the tip of the canister at a high velocity (60 mph)[13] and the particle size is exceedingly large (greater than 30 μ).[14] Fortunately, the aerosol volume slows down rapidly and the propellant evaporates, leaving an aerosol that is usually the correct size for lung deposition, around 3 to 4 μ.

Using a MDI correctly is not an easy task. A summary of recommended instructions is shown in Table 117-2.[15] Many patients are unable to perform the maneuver correctly.[16]

TABLE 117-1   Use of a Small Volume Nebulizer

Place drug in nebulizer.
Dilute drug with proper eluent if necessary.
Set driving gas flow at 6–10 L/min.
Connect patient to SVN with mouthpiece.
Have patient inhale slowly and deeply.
Continue treatment until no aerosol is produced (nebulizer can be tapped gently near the end of treatment to facilitate complete emptying).

TABLE 117-2   Use of a Metered-Dose Inhaler

1. Remove the cap and hold inhaler upright.
2. Shake the inhaler.
3. Tilt head back slightly and breathe out.
4. Position the inhaler either in the mouth or 1–2 in away from open mouth.
5. Press down on inhaler to release medication at the onset of a slow inspiration.
6. Breathe in slowly (3–5 s).
7. Hold breath for 10 s.
8. Repeat puffs as directed. Wait 1 min in between puffs.

Common mistakes include inhaling too rapidly and failure to synchronize inhalation with activation of the MDI. Both errors result in an exceedingly large oropharyngeal deposition with little deposition in the lung. A table of common errors in technique is shown in Table 117-3. A source of controversy is whether it is preferable to put the MDI directly in the mouth with lips closed around the mouthpiece or to hold the MDI 1 to 2 in away from the mouth.[17,18] The latter has the theoretical advantage of allowing more time for the aerosol plume to evaporate and slow down, thus enhancing efficiency. However, careful aim of the MDI is necessary with this method, or the aerosol will not be delivered into the mouth at all. The authors prefer the closed-mouth technique, especially with older or less reliable patients.

Even when technique is optimal, only 10 to 15 percent of the aerosol will be delivered into the respiratory tract.[19] The distribution differs from that of the SVN, however, with almost all wasted aerosol due to oropharyngeal impaction. A number of devices have been invented to attempt to decrease oropharyngeal deposition. These devices are collectively termed "spacers," as all are placed between the MDI and the patient's mouth. While they differ in size, shape, and operating features, all use the same general principle; i.e., because there is now a space between the patient and the MDI, the aerosol slows down and evaporates, thereby decreasing oropharyngeal deposition.[20] Another advantage of spacer devices is a decreased requirement for exact timing of inspiration and MDI actuation. Thus, even if actuation precedes inspiration by a few seconds, enough aerosol will remain suspended in the spacer device to ensure adequate delivery to the respiratory tract. The spacer device also decreases the tendency for patients to stop inhaling when they feel the "jolt" of aerosol released from an MDI. By

TABLE 117-3   Common Errors in MDI Use

1. Failure to coordinate inspiration with actuation of the canister
2. Failure to breathe in slowly and deeply.
3. Failure to remove the cap of the inhaler.
4. Incorrect positioning of the inhaler
5. Failure to hold breath
6. Failure to tilt head back
7. Failure to exhale completely before beginning maneuver
8. Failure to wait between puffs.

reducing oropharyngeal deposition, spacer devices also reduce the common side effects of aerosolized steroids, such as dysphonia and thrush. The major disadvantage of spacers is the added bulk of the device, which decreases the easy portability of the MDI.

An MDI has been developed that automatically actuates upon inspiration. Thus, the most common error in MDI use is eliminated while compactness and portability are maintained.[21] However, patients still must be trained carefully in its use, and the device does not prevent the patient from stopping inhalation when the aerosol is released. Furthermore, oropharyngeal deposition is not reduced with this device.

The future of MDIs is in doubt, because they use CFCs as propellant. Chlorofluorocarbons have clearly been shown to be an environmental hazard, leading to ozone depletion in the upper atmosphere and global warming.[22,23] An international consensus leading to the phaseout of CFCs has been achieved. Twenty-seven nations signed this Montreal protocol[24] in 1987, which originally agreed to decrease production of CFCs by 50 percent by 1999. More recently, the parties agreed to terminate production of CFCs completely by the year 2000. Although an exemption has been granted to medical devices that use CFCs, it is doubtful that, as production ceases, MDI manufacturers will be able to procure adequate supplies of CFCs at a reasonable price. Thus, MDI manufacturers will be forced to find substitutes for existing CFCs. Such research is already under way; however, it is unknown at this time whether all the manufacturing, testing, and regulatory steps will be in place soon enough to avoid a shortage of MDIs in the near future.[25]

Dry-powder inhalers (DPI) are devices in which the medication is administered to the patient in powder form. The medication must be loaded individually (SDIs) or multiple doses may be preloaded in certain devices (MDIs). The DPIs have many of the same advantages as MDIs—i.e., they are portable, require no external air source or electricity, and are quick and easy to use. They even have an advantage over MDIs in that they are breath-actuated. Furthermore, they do not use CFCs as a propellant and thus are potential substitutes for MDIs if the latter become unavailable in the future. The single-dose devices (Rotohaler and Spinhaler) are cumbersome in that each time the DPI is used, a small gelatin capsule containing the medicine must be inserted into the device. Newer MDIs (Diskhaler and Turbohaler) have eliminated this problem by loading multiple doses (8 and 200, respectively) onto the device itself. These newer devices are not yet available in the United States.[26]

The deposition efficiency, regional distribution, and clinical effect is similar for DPIs and MDIs in stable patients. This, coupled with their ease of use (especially the multidose models), have made DPIs a useful alternative to MDIs in these patients. One drawback to these devices, however, is the need for rapid inspiratory flow rates to actuate them and to disperse the agglomerates of particles into a respirable size. There is the concern that in patients with severe obstruction or in young children, inadequate flow rate will be obtained to facilitate adequate deposition.[27,28] This concern requires further study before DPIs are recommended in these situations. Another concern is that the devices will lead

TABLE 117-4   **Comparison of Aerosol Devices**

	Nebulizer	MDI	MDI and spacer	Powder inhaler
Ease of use	Yes	No	Yes	+/-
Speed of use	Slow	Fast	Fast	Fast
Use of CFCs	No	Yes	Yes	No
Fast inspiratory flow necessary	No	No	No	Yes
Compact	No	Yes	No	Yes
Need for compressed gas source	Yes	No	No	No
Oropharyngeal deposition	Low	High	Low	High
Suitable for mechanical ventilation	Yes	+/-	Yes	No
Multidose	No	Yes	Yes	Yes, but not in the United States

to more side effects when used with corticosteroid medications, since, with high inspiratory flows, more of the medication will be deposited in the oropharynx and larynx. Another less important consideration is that not all drugs can be manufactured in powder form.

Thus, no "perfect" aerosol device exists at the current time. Each type of device has its particular advantages and disadvantages. These are summarized in Table 117-4.

Delivery of Aerosolized Medications to Mechanically Ventilated Patients

Most studies of aerosol therapy have focused on nonintubated, stable patients. However, aerosol therapy frequently is employed in the intensive care unit to deliver a variety of medications to intubated patients. Aerosol delivery may be affected adversely by a number of conditions. For one, the endotracheal tube and ventilator tubing may trap aerosolized medication, preventing the medication from reaching the airways at all. Second, the high humidity in the endotracheal tube and ventilator tubing may cause hygroscopic growth of the aerosol particle, which may result in a less than optimal particle size for delivery into the respiratory tract. Third, the type of ventilator, the ventilator settings, and the interface between the nebulizer and the ventilator all may have profound effects on the efficiency of delivery.[29] Finally, the state of the patient's illness may affect drug delivery, drug distribution, and the pharmacokinetics of inhaled medication.

Small-volume nebulizers are the most common method of delivering medication to intubated patients. In older ventilators, this was accomplished by attaching a continuous nebulizer system to the inspiratory limb of the ventilator tubing. However, this required careful readjustment of the ventilator settings to compensate for the added inspiratory flow of gas from the nebulizer system. Newer ventilators now have settings that allow nebulization to occur using the ventilator as the source of compressed gas. Aerosols usually are delivered only during the inspiratory cycle, which allows the clinician to keep the ventilator settings and monitoring capabilities intact during nebulization. Most studies have found that aerosol delivery by SVN is very inefficient, with many stud-

ies showing delivery of about 3 to 5 percent of the dose in the nebulizer.[30,31] Most studies have shown that delivery can be improved by using higher-volume fills, lower inspiratory flows and respiratory rates, greater endotracheal tube sizes, and less humidification of the inspired gas.[32,33]

Delivery of aerosol by MDI connected to the ventilator circuit has undergone renewed interest in view of the poor delivery of medication by SVN. Various adapters have been developed to interface between the MDI and the ventilator circuit. Two types of adapters are available commercially; one type is an adapter that allows the MDI to be released directly into the ventilator tubing, and the other type is a spacer device similar to that used with conventional MDI therapy. In general, studies have shown that spacer devices perform better than the other adapters in delivering medication to the respiratory tract.[34,35] Studies attempting to quantitate delivery of medication have produced widely varying results. Delivery through conventional adapters has been estimated at around 5 percent, whereas studies using spacer devices have shown delivery varying from 6 to 30 percent. More recently, investigators have examined delivery by MDI through catheters placed directly into the endotracheal tube. These studies are promising, showing 30 to 100 percent delivery.[36,37]

Bronchodilator effect has also varied widely among studies, which have examined the in vivo effect of bronchodilators on obstructed, intubated patients. Measurement of bronchodilator effect is difficult in uncooperative intubated patients; investigators have examined peak airway pressure, peak and static airway pressure, airway resistance, and expiratory resistance by the "interrupter" technique as an index of bronchodilator response. Most studies have used a "unit dose" of albuterol by SVN, whereas puffs from the MDI has varied from 2 to 10. Most investigators (with some exceptions) have concluded that both methods were equally effective in achieving bronchodilation.[38,39,40]

It is difficult to recommend a specific algorithm for administration of bronchilators to intubated patients. Dosage will vary widely, based on the nebulizer or MDI used, the adapter interface to the patient, and the ventilator and tubing used. Even if we had a better understanding of these factors, which would allow us to estimate dosage delivered, patient response to the same dosage of medication also varies widely. Furthermore, patient response is difficult to assess. In view of the quicker inhalation time and the ease of administration, we favor delivery of bronchodilators by MDI for most patients. The medications should be delivered by a spacer device, not a conventional adapter. In addition, an attempt to gauge the results of therapy on lung mechanics should help determine efficacy of dosage in the individual patient.

Inhaled Antibiotics

PREVENTION OF PNEUMONIA

Aerosol therapy for lung infection is an appealing concept. Antibiotic delivery by aerosol can achieve high sputum levels of antibiotic while avoiding systemic toxicity and poor penetration of antibiotics. However, early studies in the intensive care unit (ICU) were disappointing. Studies were aimed at reducing the high level of nosocomial pneumonia in intubated patients in the ICU. Early studies using polymyxin B showed that one could reduce the rate of gram-negative colonization in intubated patients.[41] In particular, few patients developed colonization with *Pseudomonas aeruginosa* during treatment with aerosolized polymyxin B.[42] However, when this drug was given on a long-term basis to all patients in the ICU, unusual organisms emerged and caused a high mortality in the treated patients, leading to the abandonment of this form of therapy.[43] In evaluating these early studies, however, certain flaws are apparent. Little attention was given to the nebulizer, particle size, dosage, etc., in these studies. It is likely that very minute quantities of aerosol were actually deposited in the respiratory tract and that most of the medication was deposited in the oropharynx and endotracheal tube. Perhaps if these studies were repeated using methods to bypass the oropharynx, prevention of pneumonia could be achieved without alteration of the orpharyngeal flora or the emergence of resistant organisms.

TREATMENT OF INFECTION IN CYSTIC FIBROSIS

Recurrent, chronic, and progressive endobronchial infections are the hallmark of patients with cystic fibrosis (CF) and a major cause of morbidity and mortality; *P. aeruginosa* is the principal pathogen (see also Chap. 93).[44] Much attention has been focused on the use of inhaled aminoglycosides in this disease, in view of the activity of these agents against *P. aeruginosa*, the systemic toxicity, and the poor bronchial penetration of these agents when given systemically. Early studies showed that inhaled aminoglycosides could reduce the need for hospitalization, improve pulmonary function, and improve weight gain and growth in these patients with virtually none of the systemic side effects of the aminoglycosides.[45,46] Recently, higher doses of aminoglycosides have been administered, serum concentrations reaching the therapeutic range. Nevertheless, no systemic oto- or nephrotoxicity was seen in this study. However, a high incidence of resistant *P. aeruginosa* emerged during therapy.[47] Most recently, a double-blind crossover study has confirmed the value of inhaled tobramycin in the treatment of CF patients chronically infected with *P. aeroginosa*. Improvements in pulmonary function were seen during the treatment period, as well as a substantial decrease in the density of *P. aeroginosa* in the sputum.[48]

TREATMENT OF *PNEUMOCYSTIS CARINII* PNEUMONIA

Pneumocystis carinii pneumonia (PCP) is the most common opportunistic infection in patients with acquired immunodeficiency syndrome (AIDS); this infection has a high morbidity and mortality (see also Chap. 105).[49] Systemic therapy is associated with significant side effects, frequently resulting in a need to change therapy. Attention has focused on aerosol therapy as an alternative to treat this disease and a way of preventing infection. Initial studies in animals showed that pentamidine had unique characteristics ideally suited for aerosol delivery. Aerosol studies showed that very high concentrations could be obtained in the lung with virtually no systemic absorption or toxicity.[50] Since PCP pneumonia is an alveolar disease, attention focused on the design of a nebulizer that would maximize alveolar absorption.[51]

Two nebulizers have gained widespread use for delivery of aerosolized pentamidine. The Respirgard II nebulizer (Marquest, Englewood, CO) has a particle size of around 1 μ, which is suited ideally for the delivery of medication to the alveolar region. However, it delivers < 5 percent of the total dose to the patient.[52] Nevertheless, it has been studied in a large number of patients and has been found to be an effective agent in the prevention of PCP in AIDS patients, both as secondary prophylaxis for patients who have already had PCP and for primary prophylaxis in high-risk patients.[53] The recommended dose of pentamidine is 300 mg every 4 weeks, although greater doses have not been evaluated. The Fisoneb nebulizer (Fisons Corp., Rochester, NY) also has been found to be effective in clinical studies. This is an ultrasonic nebulizer, and the efficiency of delivery is greater, probably as high as 25 percent.[52] However, because of the larger particle size, approximately 3 to 4 μ, the regional distribution of the aerosol is not ideal, and tracheobronchial deposition may lead to more frequent side effects, such as cough and bronchospasm. Direct studies comparing the effectiveness of the two apparatuses have not been done.

A recent study compared the effectiveness of aerosolized pentamidine versus oral bactrim for prophylaxis of PCP. Oral bactrim was a superior agent; thus, aerosolized pentamidine should be reserved for patients who are intolerant of oral bactrim.[54] Reports of transmission of tuberculosis by aerosol therapy have also diminished the initial enthusiasm for this form of therapy. Tuberculosis precautions should be used by all caregivers who administer aerosolized pentamidine for prophylaxis.

Aerosolized pentamidine has also been used for treatment of mild to moderate PCP.[55] It has not been found to be as effective as oral or intravenous therapy. Further research using higher doses of medication or more efficient delivery systems before use of aerosolized pentamidine for treatment of PCP can be recommended.

Novel Agents Administered by Aerosol Therapy

RECOMBINANT HUMAN DNASE

Accumulations and persistence of viscous secretions in human airways has been a particular problem in a number of respiratory diseases, including CF (see Chaps. 91 to 95), bronchiectases, chronic bronchitis, pneumonia, and exacerbations of chronic obstructive pulmonary disease. Conventional mucolytics, such as acetylcysteine, have little if any benefit in these conditions. The viscosity of the sputum results primarily from the large amount of native DNA released by inflammatory cells into the airways.[56] Recently, a human form of recombinant human DNase (rhDNAse, Genentech) has been developed (see Chap. 69). Early studies showed that rhDNAse effectively decreased the viscosity of CF sputum.[57] Clinical studies in patients with CF have shown an improvement in lung function and a reduction in the relative risk of respiratory tract infection with continuous treatment using rhDNase.[58] Patients had an improved sense of well-being and spent less time in the hospital than the placebo group. Further studies are in progress to determine optimal dose and duration of treatment. A preliminary phase II study has suggested that the medication also may have benefit in reducing mortality in patients with purulent infectious exacerbation of chronic obstructive pulmonary disease.

AEROSOLIZED AMILORIDE, GENE THERAPY IN CYSTIC FIBROSIS

Another approach to CF patients has been the use of aerosolized amiloride (see also Chap. 92). Amiloride is a sodium channel blocker that inhibits the absorption of sodium when applied to the airway epithelial cells of CF patients. This might result in mucus that is less viscous and easier to clear. Pilot studies in CF patients showed a reduction in the loss of lung function after treatment with aerosolized amiloride.[59] Further studies are presently under way.

An even more novel approach to CF patients is gene therapy (see also Chap 95). Laboratory studies have been performed to evaluate the transfer of vectors encoding the replacement gene for the protein responsible for the ion transport defect in CF airways.[60] Studies have shown that the gene can be bound effectively to liposomes, which are phospholipid vesicles suitable for aerosolization. These liposome-DNA complexes can be aerosolized and deposited onto the surface of the CF airway, where they can enter the cell and the gene can be incorporated into the nucleus of the airway epithelial cell. Efficient liposome-mediated gene transfer to respiratory epithelium has been reported.[61]

SURFACTANT REPLACEMENT THERAPY IN ACUTE LUNG INJURY

Among the most important advances in the management of neonatal respiratory distress syndrome has been the incorporation of surfactant replacement into the standard of care for this condition. Since the primary pathophysiologic determinant of infantile acute lung injury is immaturity of surfactant production, replacement has resulted in dramatic acute improvements in gas exchange, pulmonary mechanics, and ventilatory requirements as well as a reduction in barotrauma. Most importantly, survival has improved significantly (35 to 50 percent), with concomitant reduction in the frequency of bronchopulmonary dysplasia resulting from prolonged mechanical ventilation.[62] Surfactant replacement has been applied both to rescue in patients with established disease and for prophylaxis of premature infants at high risk for developing ARDS. Surfactant in neonates is usually administered by bolus through the endotracheal tube, although recent investigations have suggested more efficient delivery by aerosol. The types of surfactant available include synthetic, animal-derived, and recombinant, all of which have been utilized clinically.

Quantitative and qualitative surfactant deficiencies have been described in both early and late phases of ARDS.[63] Lack of effective surface-active material is believed to result from damage to surfactant-producing type II pneumocytes, inhibition by protein-rich edema fluid, and proteolytic damage. This lack of effective surfactant accounts in part for the atelectasis, shunt, and reduced compliance that characterize ARDS in adults. In addition, surfactant apoproteins have been recognized as important in enhancing host defense against bacterial and fungal pathogens; therefore, deficiency may account for the high-risk incidence of ventilator-associated pneumonia described in ARDS.

There is, therefore, strong support for the hypothesis that exogenous surfactant replacement might have similar if not greater benefit than that observed in neonatal lung injury. Alternative methods for delivery of surfactant in ARDS may be by boluses through the endotracheal tube, directed bronchoscopically throughout the lung. Spragg and colleagues reported that relatively small doses of porcine surfactant could be given safely. These investigators decided that transiently improved gas exchange overcame surfactant inhibition of plasma.[64] A recent phase II trial in 59 patients suggested that survival might be improved utilizing bronchoscopically instilled repetitive doses of bovine surfactant.[65] Concern over the cost and safety of delivering large boluses of surface-active material into an adult airway has resulted in trials of aerosolized surfactant. However, the only randomized controlled trial published to date has not demonstrated either physiologic or survival advantage in ARDS due to severe sepsis.[66] Failure to improve outcome has been attributed to several factors, including the use of a relatively inactive synthetic surfactant. Therapy aimed at improving pulmonary physiologic homeostasis may not be able to affect a fundamentally systemic disease (sepsis) or diseases in which there is limited nebulizer efficiency. At present, there remains limited evidence supporting exogenous surfactant administration as of more than theoretical benefit in ARDS. The uncertainties surrounding surfactant replacement in ARDS include the following:

1. Composition of surfactant, including both phospholipid and apoprotein.

2. Timing of therapy: At which stage in ARDS should surfactant be administered?
3. Type and pattern of mechanical ventilation to promote optimal distribution of surfactant.
4. Dose: Balancing cost against sufficient quantities to overcome inhibition of the alveolar level.
5. Delivery system: Bolus, nebulization, or nebulizer. Significant focus on improving efficiency of delivery by nebulization has the potential to significantly reduce dose and therefore cost of therapy.

OTHER THERAPIES

This review is not intended to provide an exhaustive list of all potential uses for aerosol therapy. Investigators are presently evaluating aerosolized cyclosporine for lung transplant patients and other diseases. Aerosolized amphotericin is being evaluated for the prevention and treatment of fungal infection of the lung in immunocompromised patients. Aerosolized insulin and growth hormone are being evaluated for replacement therapy in these endocrinopathies. Aerosolized α_1-antiprotease replacement therapy as well as synthetic antiprotease therapy are being evaluated in deficiency states and in CF.

Conclusions

Aerosol therapy has a growing importance in pulmonary pharmacology. Careful attention to the scientific principles of aerosol delivery has greatly increased the use of aerosols in the treatment of lung disease. The future of aerosol therapy is very exciting, and many new agents and improved delivery systems will be arriving soon.

References

1. Dolovich MB: Clinical aspects of aerosol physics. *Respir Care* 3G:931–938, 1991.
2. Dolovich MB, Sanchis J, Rossman C, Newhouse MT: Aerosol penetrance: A sensitive index of peripheral airway obstmetioll. *J Appl Physiol* 40:468–471, 1976.
3. Ilowite JS, Gorvoy JD, Smaldone GC: Quantitative deposition of aerosolized gentamicin in cystic fibrosis. *Am Rev Respir Dis* 136:1445–1449, 1987.
4. Newman SP: Delivery of therapeutic aerosols, in Witek TJ, Schachter EN (eds): *Advances in Respiratory Care Pharmacology.* Philadelphia, Lippincott, 1988, 53–82.
5. Mercer TT: Production of therapeutic aerosol: Principles and techniques. *Chest* 80:813–817, 1981.
6. Alvine GF, Rodgers P, Fitzsimmons KM, Ahrens RC: Disposable jet nebulizers: How reliable are they? *Chest* 101:316–319, 1992.
7. Kacmarek RM, Hess D: The interface between patient and aerosol generator. *Respir Care* 36:952–976, 1991.
8. Mercer TT: Production of therapeutic aerosols: Principles and techniques. *Chest* 80:813–817, 1981.
9. Newman SP: Aerosol deposition considerations in inhalation therapy. *Chest* 88(suppl):152S–160S, 1985.
10. Kradjan WA, Lakshminarayan S: Efficacy of air compressor-driven nebulizers. *Chest* 87:512–516, 1985.
11. Phipps PR, Gonda T: Droplets produced by medical nebulizers: Some factors affecting their size and solute concentration. *Chest* 97:1327–1332, 1990.
12. Ilowite JS, Baskin MI, Sheetz MS, Abd AG: Delivered dose and regional distribution of aerosolized pentamidine using different delivery systems. *Chest* 99:1139–1144, 1991.
13. Pederson S, Mortensen S: Use of different inhalation devices in children. *Lung* 168(suppl):653–657, 1990.
14. Moren F, Andersen J: Fraction of the dose exhaled after the administration of pressurized inhalation aerosols. *Int J Pharm* 6:295–300, 1980.
15. Newman SP, Pavia D, Clarke SW: Simple instructions for using pressurized aerosol bronchodilators. *J R Soc Med* 73:776–779, 1980.
16. Orehek J, Gayrard P, Grimand CH, Charpin J: Patient error in the use of bronchodilator metered aerosols. *Br Med J* 1:76–77, 1976.
17. Dolovich M, Ruffin RE, Roberts R, Newhouse MT: Optimal delivery of aerosols from metered dose inhalers. *Chest* 80(suppl):911S–915S, 1981.
18. Lawford P, McKenzie D: Pressurized bronchodilator aerosol technique: Influence of breath-holding time and relationship of inhaler to the mouth. *Br J Dis Chest* 76:229–233, 1982.
19. Newman SP, Pavia D, Moren F, et al: Deposition of pressurized aerosols in the human respiratory tract. *Thorax* 36:52–55, 1981.
20. Konig P: Spacer devices used with metered-dose inhalers: Breakthrough or gimmick? *Chest* 88:276–284, 1985.
21. Newman SP, Weisz AWB, Talaeen N, Clarke SW: Improvement of drug delivery with a breath actuated pressurized aerosol for patients with poor inhaler technique. *Thorax* 46:712–716, 1991.
22. Fisher DA, Hales CH, Wang WC, et al.: Model calculations of the relative effects of CFCs and their replacements on global warming. *Nature* 344:513–516, 1990.
23. Molina MJ, Rowland F: Stratospheric risk for chlorofluoromethanes: Chlorine atom–catalysed destruction of ozone. *Nature* 249:815–812, 1974.
24. Technology Review Panel Technical Options Committee on Aerosols, Sterilants and Miscellaneous Uses: *Aerosols, Sterilants, and Miscellaneous Uses of CFCs* (pursuant to the Montreal Protocol). Nairobi, Kenya: United Nations Environment Programme, 1989.
25. Balmes JR: Propellant gases in metered dose inhalers: Their impact on the global environment. *Respir Care* 36:1037–1044, 1991.
26. Persson G, Cruvstad E, Stahl E: A new multiple dose powdered inhaler (Turbohaler), compared with a pressurized inhaler: A study of terbutaline in asthmatics. *Eur Respir J* 1:681–684, 1988.
27. Pedersen S, Hansen OR, Fugisang G: Influence of inspiratory flow rate upon the effect of a Turbohaler. *Arch Dis Child* 65:308–319, 1990.
28. Engel T, Heinig JM, Medsen F, Nikander K: Peak inspiratory flowrate and inspiratory vital capacity of patients with asthma measured with and without a new dry powder inhaler device (Turbohaler). *Eur Respir J* 3:1037–1041, 1990.
29. Hess D: How should bronchodilators be administered to patients on ventilators? *Respir Care* 36:377–394, 1991.
30. MacIntyre NR, Silver RM, Miller CW, et al.: Aerosol delivery in intubated, mechanically ventilated patients. *Crit Care Med* 13:81–84, 1985.
31. O'Doherty MJ, Thomas SHL, Page CG, et al.: Delivery of a nebulized aerosol to a lung model during mechanical ventilation. *Am Rev Respir Dis* 146:383–388, 1992.
32. O'Riordan TG, Green MJ, Perry RJ, Smaldone GC: Nebulizer

function during mechanical ventilation. *Am Rev Respir Dis* 145:1117–1122, 1992.

33. Fuller HD, Dolovich MB, Posmituck G, et al.: Pressurized aerosol versus jet aerosol delivery to mechanically ventilated patients. *Am Rev Respir Dis* 141:440–444, 1990.

34. Bishop MJ, Larson RP, Buschman DL: Metered dose inhaler aerosol characteristics are affected by the endotracheal tube actuator/adapter used. *Anesthesiology* 73:1263–1265, 1990.

35. Rau JL, Harwood RJ, Gruff JL: Evaluation of a reservoir device for metered-dose bronchodilator delivery to intubated adults. *Chest* 102:924–930, 1992.

36. Taylor REI, Lerman J, Chambers C, Dolovich M: Dosing efficiency and particle size characteristics of pressurized metered-dose inhaler aerosols in narrow catheters. *Chest* 103:920–924, 1993.

37. Niven RW, Kacmarek RM, Brain JD, Peterfreulld RA. Small bore nozzle extensions to improve the delivery efficiency of drugs from metered dose inhalers: Laboratory evaluation. *Am Rev Respir Dis* 147:1590–1594, 1993.

38. Guitierrez CJ, Nelson R: Short-term bronchodilation in mechanically ventilated patients receiving metaproterenol via small volume nebulizer (SVN) or metered-dose inhaler (MDI). *Respir Care* 33:910–913, 1988.

39. Bakow ED, Galgon P, Bachman V, Lucke J: Beta-agonist delivery in-line with a ventilator circuit by either metered dose inhaler or updraft nobulizer in a distal or proximal position. *Respir Care* 34:1027–1029, 1989.

40. Manthous CA, Schmidt GA, Hall JB, Wood DH: Metered dose inhaler versus nebulized albuterol for the treatment of bronchospasm in mechanically ventilated patients. *Am Rev Respir Dis* 148:1567–1571, 1993.

41. Greenfield S, Teres D, Bushnell LS, et al.: Prevention of gram-negative bacillary pneumonia using aerosol polymyxin as prophylaxis: I. Effect on colonization pattern of the upper respiratory tract of seriously ill patients. *J Clin Invest* 52:2935–2940, 1973.

42. Klick JM, DuMoulin GC, Hedley-Whyte J, et al.: Prevention of gram-negative bacillary pneumonia using polymyxin aerosol as prophylaxis: II. Effect on the incidence of pneumonia in seriously ill patients. *J Clin Invest* 55:514–519, 1975.

43. Feeley TW, DuMoulin GC, Hedley-Whyte J, et al.: Aerosol polymyxin and pneumonia in seriously ill patients. *N Engl J Med* 293:471–475, 1975.

44. Marks MI: The pathogenesis and treatment of pulmonary infections in patients with cystic fibrosis. *J Pediatr* 98:173–179, 1981.

45. Kun P, Landau LI, Phelan PD: Nebulized gentamicin in children and adolescents with cystic fibrosis. *Austr Paediatr J* 20:43–45, 1984.

46. Hodson ME, Penketh ARL, Batten JC: Aerosol carbenicillin and gentamicin treatment of *Pseudomonas aeruginosa* infection in patients with cystic fibrosis. *Lancet* 2:1137–1139, 1981.

47. Smith AL, Ramsey BW, Hedges DL, et al.: Safety of aerosol tobramycin administration for 3 months to patients with cystic fibrosis. *Pediatr Pulmonol* 7:265–271, 1989.

48. Ramsey BW, Darkin HL, Eisenberg JD, et al.: Efficacy of aerosolized tobramycin in patients with cystic fibrosis. *N Engl J Med* 328:1740–1746, 1993.

49. Devita VT, Broder S, Fauci AS: Developmental therapeutics and the acquired immunodeficiency syndrome. *Ann Intern Med* 106:568–581, 1987.

50. Debs RJ, Straubinger RMW, Brunette EN: Selective enhancement of pentamidine uptake in the lung by aerosolization and delivery in liposomes. *Am Rev Respir Dis* 135:731–737, 1987.

51. Montgomery AB, Debs RJ, Luce JM: Selective delivery of pentamidine to the lung by aerosol. *Am Rev Respir Dis* 137:477–478, 1988.

52. Ilowite JS, Baskin MI, Sheetz MS, Abd AG: Delivered dose and regional distribution of aerosolized pentamidine using different delivery systems. *Chest* 99:1139–1144, 1991.

53. Leoung GS, Feigal DW Jr, Montgomery AB, et al.: Aerosolized pentamidine prophylaxis following *Pneumocystis carinii* pneumonia in AIDS patients: The San Francisco Community Prophylaxis trial. *N Engl J Med* 323:769, 1990.

54. Hardy WD, Feinberg J, Finkelstein DM, et al.: A controlled trial of trimethoprim-sulfamethoxazole or aerosolized pentamidine for secondary prophylaxis of *Pneumocystis carinii* pneumonia in patients with acquired immunodeficiency syndrome. *N Engl J Med* 327:1842, 1992.

55. Montgomery AB, Debs RJ, Luce JM: Aerosolized pentamidine as sole therapy for *Pneumocystis carinii* pneumonia in patients with acquired immunodeficiency syndrome. *Lancet* 2:480–483, 1987.

56. Potter JL, Spector S, Matthews LW, Lenin J: Studies on pulmonary secretions: 3. The nucleic acids in whole pulmonary secretions from patients with cystic fibrosis, bronchiectasis, and laryngectomy. *Am Rev Respir Dis* 99:909–916, 1969.

57. Shak S, Capon DJ, Hellmiss R, et al.: Recombinant human DNase reduced the viscosity of cystic fibrosis sputum. *Proc Natl Acad Sci USA* 87:9188–9192, 1990.

58. Hubbard RC, McElvaney NG, Birrer P, et al.: A preliminary study of aerosolized recombinant human deoxyribonuclease I in the treatment of cystic fibrosis. *N Engl J Med* 326:812–815, 1992.

59. Knowles MR, Church NL, Waltner WE, et al.: A pilot study of aerosolized amiloride for the treatment of cystic fibrosis lung disease. *N Engl J Med* 322:1189–1194, 1990.

60. Hyde SC, Gill DR, Higgins CF, et al.: Correction of the ion transport defect in cystic fibrosis transgenic mice by gene therapy. *Nature* 362:250–255, 1993.

61. Alton EWFW, Middleton PG, Caplen NJ, et al.: Non-invasive liposome-mediated gene delivery can correct the ion transport defect in cystic fibrosis mutant mice. *Nature Genet* 5:135–142, 1993.

62. Enhoring G, Shennan AT: Surfactant supplementation in the neonatal period, in Fishman AP (ed): *Update: Pulmonary Diseases and Disorders.* New York: McGraw-Hill, 1992:213–223.

63. Pison U, Obertacke U, Brand M, et al.: Altered pulmonary surfactant in uncomplicated and septicemia-complicated courses of acute respiratory failure. *J Trauma* 30:19–26, 1990.

64. Spragg RG, Gilliard N, Richman P, et al.: Acute effects of a single dose of porcine surfactant on patients with the adult respiratory distress syndrome. *Chest* 105:195–202, 1994.

65. Gregory TJ, Longmore WJ, Moxley MA, et al.: Surfactant repletion following survanta supplementation in patients with acute respiratory distress syndrome (ARDS). *Am J Respir Crit Care Med* 149:(4):A124, 1994.

66. Anzueto A, Baughman R, Guntupalli K, et al.: An international, randomized placebo-controlled trial evaluating the safety and efficacy of aerosolized surfactant in patients with sepsis-induced ARDS. *Am J Respir Crit Care Med* 149:A567, 1994.

67. Ilowite J: Techniques of aerosol therapy. *Emerg Med* April 1991, p. 69.

Chapter 118

LUNG TRANSPLANT PHARMACOLOGY

ALBERTO DE HOYOS
RONALD F. GROSSMAN

Transplantation of the kidney, liver, and heart are well-established therapeutic modalities for individuals with irreversible failure of these organs. By contrast, lung and heart-lung transplants have been feasible therapeutic strategies for patients with end-stage parenchymal and vascular disease for just over a decade.[1,2] As recently as 1985, fewer than 10 people had received successful isolated lung transplants worldwide. Since 1987, the number of transplants has rapidly increased so that by April 1994, more than 2780 isolated lung transplants had been performed. The current level of success of lung transplantation is critically dependent on the availability of effective immunosuppressive drugs. It was not until the introduction of cyclosporin A into clinical practice that lung transplantation became a clinical reality.[3,4] As experience accumulates, survival rates continue to improve. This improvement is due in part to better donor and recipient selection, improved organ preservation, better perioperative care, innovative surgical techniques, and, most of all, to new immunosuppressive regimens. Morbidity and mortality have shifted from surgical-related complications (dehiscence of the airway anastomosis) in the early experience, to infection and chronic rejection in long-term survivors. This chapter outlines the evolving indications for transplantation, mechanisms of rejection, the most commonly used antirejection agents, and the current management of common medical problems in lung transplant recipients.

Indications for Lung Transplantation

The indication for lung transplantation is irreversible, progressively disabling end-stage pulmonary disease.[5] Pathophysiologically this can be parenchymal (restrictive, obstructive, infective) or vascular. Three procedures are available: single, bilateral, and heart-lung transplantation. The indications for each type have evolved with the clinical experience accumulated and are listed in Table 118–1. Choice of a particular type of transplant depends not only on the underlying disease but also on the local expertise of the operating team and the availability of donor organs.

SINGLE LUNG TRANSPLANT

Single lung transplantation was performed initially in patients with end-stage fibrotic lung disease.[2] The poor compliance and increased vascular resistance of the native lung ensure that both ventilation and perfusion are preferentially diverted to the transplanted lung.[2] Single lung transplantation also can be successfully performed in patients with obstructive lung disease and in patients with primary or secondary pulmonary hypertension.[6,7] Advantages of single lung transplantation include improved utilization of scarce donor organs, increased likelihood of transplantation (since a single lung donor is more frequent than a double or heart-lung donor), avoidance of removal of a normally functioning heart, and simpler technical operation.

DOUBLE LUNG TRANSPLANT

The major indication for double lung transplantation is bilateral pulmonary sepsis. The presence of sepsis in the remaining native lung precludes single lung transplant because the native lung would be a continuous source of infection in a chronically immunosuppressed host. Bilateral lung transplantation also has been used in patients with pulmonary hypertension and obstructive lung disease.[8]

TABLE 118-1   Lung Transplant Indications

Single Lung Transplant
  Idiopathic pulmonary fibrosis
  Hypersensitivity pneumonitis
  Sarcoidosis
  Pneumoconiosis
  Drug-induced lung disease
  Collagen vascular disease limited to lung
  Pulmonary vascular disease
  Chronic obstructive lung disease
Double or Bilateral Lung Transplant
  Chronic obstructive lung disease
    Emphysema
    α1-antitrypsin deficiency
    Bronchiolitis obliterans
  Chronic pulmonary infection
    Bronchiectasis
    Cystic fibrosis
  Pulmonary vascular disease
  Other
Heart-Lung Transplant
  Pulmonary vascular disease
    Eisenmenger syndrome
  Chronic pulmonary infection
  Parenchymal lung disease with nonrecoverable heart disease
  Parenchymal lung disease with unrelated severe cardiac
  dysfunction

HEART-LUNG TRANSPLANT

Combined heart-lung transplant is offered in most centers, to patients with parenchymal or vascular disease with coexisting cardiac dysfunction (primary and secondary pulmonary hypertension with irreversible heart failure, or lung disease with intrinsic heart disease) and, in some centers, to patients with cystic fibrosis as part of the "domino procedure."[9]

Overview of Transplant Immunology

Most human transplants are allografts in which the donor and recipient are homologous; that is, of the same species but genetically nonidentical. The recipient's immune system can identify the donor organ as being "non self." Allogenic responses exhibit extraordinary strength (10 to 100 times stronger than that of nominal antigens), and can be stimulated by two different sets of antigen-presenting cells from the donor or the recipient.

MECHANISMS OF T-CELL RECOGNITION OF ALLOANTIGEN

The recipient's immune system recognizes proteins encoded by the major histocompatibility complex (MHC) of the donor's genes as non-self.[10] The principal targets of the immune response to allografts are the MHC molecules themselves, and T-cell recognition of allo-MHC is the primary and central event that initiates allograft rejection.

Allorecognition involves a tripartite structure consisting of T cells (recipient), antigen-presenting cells (recipient or donor), and a peptide bound in the groove of the MHC molecule of antigen-presenting cells. T cells recognize allogenic MHC molecules and other antigens through the T-cell receptor, a complex transmembrane glycoprotein associated with at least four other peptides comprising the CD3 molecule.[11] T cells recognize intact allo-MHC molecules on the surface of donor or stimulator cells in the so-called *direct pathway*. This form of antigen recognition is responsible for the strong proliferative response to alloantigens and the events leading to the early acute rejection of allografts.[12] In the so-called *indirect pathway*, T cells recognize processed allogenic MHC molecules in the context of self antigen-presenting cells.[13] In general, peptides presented in association with MHC class I molecules are processed through the endogenous pathway, and those presented by the MHC class II molecules are processed through the exogenous pathway. T cells primed by the direct pathway play a dominant role in acute or early allograft rejection, whereas T cells primed by the indirect pathway play the dominant role in chronic rejection.

T-CELL COLLABORATION IN ALLOGRAFT RESPONSES

Human T cells are segregated into CD4+ and CD8+ cells according to their cell-surface markers and their MHC recognition pattern (CD4/MHC II; CD8/MHC I).[14] Functionally, however, there is no strict dichotomy between these two subsets. Whereas the CD4+ T cell generally is considered to be a cytokine-producing helper cell, CD4+ cells also exert effector functions such as cytotoxic activity, allograft rejection, and graft-versus-host disease. Conversely, CD8+ T cells, considered to be cytolytic cells, also can proliferate autonomously to allogenic stimuli and release a number of cytokines.

ACCESSORY AND ADHESION MOLECULES AND ALLOGRAFT REJECTION

The accessory molecules CD4 and CD8 determine the interaction of the T-cell receptor and the MHC products presenting the antigen (class II and class I, respectively).[15] For T cells to become activated, two signals are required: (1) antigen recognition and engagement by the T-cell receptor–CD3 complex, and (2) costimulation by signals provided by antigen-presenting cells. During the initial events of the inflammatory response, circulating leukocytes contact an unknown or recognized antigen on graft vascular endothelium or enter a site of inflammation, then recirculate to host lymph nodes to disseminate widely their information to other as yet uncommitted cells. Such cell movement entails a complex series of events involving activation of accessory adhesion molecules. When endothelial cells lining the vessels of a transplanted organ become activated, they may produce or express a number of cytokines, such as tumor necrosis factor (TNF) or interferon-γ (IFN-γ), or upregulate their adhesion molecules, particularly selectins. As a result, leukocytes begin to slow and stick via upregulated selectin receptors on their surfaces. Because binding to selectins is relatively weak, the leukocytes are pushed aside by the force of flow, only to interact with the next selectin on the same or adjacent endothelial cell (rolling). The presence of cytokines in this microenvironment and the binding to selectins result in a conformational shift of integrin receptors on the leukocytes from low to high avidity. The upregulated β2-integrin receptors (particularly leukocyte function associated antigen-1; LFA-1) then adhere "secondarily" to other molecules appearing on endothelial cells, such as intercellular adhesion molecule-1 (ICAM-1), causing permanent binding of the host cell to graft vasculature, activating the leukocytes further, and initiating changing patterns of cell migration.[16]

THE REJECTION PROCESS

The immune response to an allograft can be divided into two limbs: (1) the afferent limb, which involves the engagement and recognition of foreign antigens on the transplanted organ; and (2) the efferent limb, which comprises the clonal proliferation of alloantigen-stimulated cytotoxic lymphocytes, generation of inflammatory cytokines, and destruction of the transplanted organ.

THE AFFERENT LIMB
Alloantigens shed from the transplanted organ gain access and reach the regional lymph nodes where they are encountered by recipient T lymphocytes. Graft antigens are recognized either directly or indirectly in association with major histocompatibility complex molecules on the surface of donor or recipient antigen-presenting cells, respectively. The recognition of antigen in combination with costimulatory membrane and soluble signals results in T-cell activation.

THE EFFERENT LIMB
Once alloantigens have been presented to T cells and transcription of specific genes has occurred, an amplification process is initiated resulting in clonal proliferation of cytotoxic T lymphocytes with ensuing damage to the transplanted organ.[17] One of the earliest events of T-cell activation involves the synthesis and release of interleukin-2 (IL-2) and synthesis and expression of IL-2 receptors.[18] Interleukin-2 causes proliferation of T cells bearing IL-2 receptors, as well as inducing synthesis of other cytokines such as interferon-γ, tumor necrosis factor, and B-cell growth and differentiation factors (IL-4, IL-5, and IL-6). Interferon-γ induces expression of MHC class II molecules on cells of the transplanted organ and triggers or activates macrophage function. Interleukin-4 (IL-4), IL-5, and IL-6 induce clonal expansion of B cells. Under the influence of the cytokines in the microenvironment, the dividing T cells assume more specific functions such as cytotoxicity; macrophages become activated and release their lysosome contents; B cells differentiate to plasma cells and produce immunoglobulins; and cells bearing Fc receptors (NK cells, macrophages) participate in antibody-dependent cellular cytotoxicity (ADCC). The result of this cascade of events is inexorable and progressive graft destruction.[19]

Immunosuppression

Available immunosuppressive agents and their mechanisms of action are outlined in Fig. 118-1 and Table 118-2. No immunosuppressive drug or regimen can be considered ideal; all have side effects and potential adverse consequences, and none uniquely inhibits lymphocytes activated by and directed against donor-specific alloantigens.

TECHNIQUES OF IMMUNOSUPPRESSION

Modulation of the normal immune response is the major challenge for successful lung transplantation. Immunosuppression therapy for organ transplantation uses combinations of cyclosporin A, prednisone, and azathioprine with or without a polyclonal or monoclonal antilymphocyte agent for induction therapy. These strategies stem from the principle that lower doses of multiple agents can be administered with greater efficacy and diminished toxicity as compared with individual agents alone. There are 3 immunosuppressive strategies: (1) prophylaxis against early acute rejection; (2) long-term maintenance prophylaxis; and (3) treatment of acute and chronic rejection. The goal of therapy is to provide sufficient immunosuppression to retard or attenuate rejection without causing undesirable toxicity or side effects such as infection and neoplasms.

EARLY REJECTION PROPHYLAXIS
Early rejection prophylaxis uses intensive immunosuppressive regimens that are designed to minimize the possibility of rejection during the fragile postoperative stage of transplantation. During this initial phase, the objectives are (1) to prevent or delay rejection during the recovery phase after transplant, minimizing the early use of corticosteroids; (2) to avoid complications; and (3) to inhibit the immune response in the critical "priming" period, possibly setting the stage for better long-term reduced rejection and need for enhanced immunosuppression.

MAINTENANCE IMMUNOSUPPRESSION
Long-term prophylaxis attempts to create a balance between prevention of rejection and side effects. Doses of immunosuppressive drugs are titrated on the basis of drug levels, biopsy evidence of rejection, prior rejection history, and evidence of side effects. The standard regimen is based on triple-drug therapy; namely, cyclosporin A, azathioprine, and prednisone. Two-pronged regimes omit the prednisone but are not used commonly because of fears that such patients may be more susceptible to chronic rejection.

TREATMENT OF ACUTE REJECTION
Treatment for episodes of acute rejection depends on the severity of rejection, previously administered immunosuppressive agents, and the presence of preformed antibodies. Agents employed include methylprednisolone and polyclonal or monoclonal antilymphocyte preparations. Minimal (grade I) rejection does not usually prompt augmentation in immunosuppression; rather, biopsy frequency is increased.

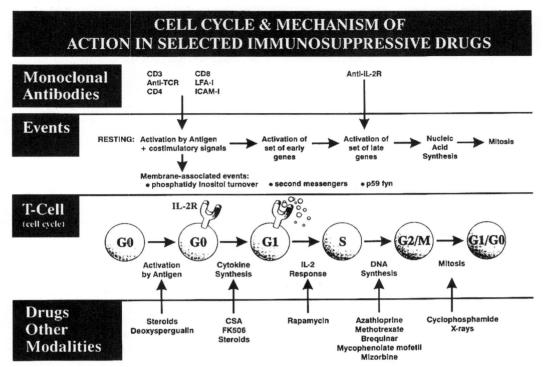

FIGURE 118-1 The cell cycle is demonstrated. The site of action of various immunosuppressive drugs is shown.

TABLE 118-2

	Azathioprine	Cyclosporine	Methyl-prednisolone (MP) Prednisone (P)	ATG
Initial	4 mg/kg preop 1–3 mg/kg/d	10 mg/kg/d	MP: 500 mg IV intraop 125 mg IV x 3 days P: 1 mg/kg/d	10–20 mg/kg x 3–5 days T cells: 10–20%
Maintenance	1.5–2 mg/kg/d	↓ gradually to 6 mg/kg/d	P: 1 mg/kg/d	
Rejection acute or early	No change	No change	MP: 1 g IV/d x 2–3 days P: 1 mg/kg/d ↓ gradually to maintenance dose	10–20 mg/kg x 3–5 days
Rejection chronic or late	No change	No change	MP: 1 g IV/d x 2–3 days if recurrent P: 1 mg/kg/d ↓ gradually to maintenance dose	10–20 mg/kg x 3–5 days

Mild, moderate, or severe rejection (grade II or greater) almost always mandates increased immunosuppression with methylprednisolone given intravenously. This is followed by transient increase in the orally administered corticosteroid and tapering doses during the subsequent 4 to 6 weeks. Rejection episodes refractory to high doses of corticosteroids warrant lympholytic therapy.

TREATMENT OF CHRONIC REJECTION

Chronic rejection is manifested clinically as a bronchiolitis obliterans syndrome. Although in many instances its course is progressive, augmented immunosuppression usually is indicated. Newly diagnosed chronic rejection is treated with methylprednisolone 1 g daily intravenously for three consecutive days followed by boost and taper of prednisone. Failure to improve or recurrent disease warrants a trial of cytolytic therapy with antilymphocyte globulin or OKT3.

Immunosuppressive Drugs

Immunosuppressive drugs are classified according to their mechanism of action (Fig. 118-1).

CALCINEURIN INHIBITORS

CYCLOSPORIN A

Cyclosporin A is currently the mainstay of immunosuppressive therapy.

Structure and Source

Cyclosporin A, a fungal antibiotic, is a neutral, lipophilic, cyclic undecapeptide extracted from *Tolypocladium inflatum Gams*. For clinical use, cyclosporin is stabilized with castor oil (cremophor) and olive oil for intravenous and oral administration, respectively. The relative bioequivalence of oral to intravenous doses is 1:3.

Mechanism of Action

Cyclosporin readily and passively diffuses into the cytoplasm of T cells, inhibiting T-cell function in the G_0 phase of the cell cycle.[20] Activation of T cells through the T-cell receptor results in activation of early genes encoding lymphokines, growth factors, and their receptors. Upon activation, intracytosolic Ca^{2+} increases. Cytosolic Ca^{2+} binds to calmodulin, which, in turn, binds to the calmodulin-dependent phosphatase calcineurin; activated calcineurin dephosphorylates the cytoplasmic subunit of nuclear factor of activated T cells (NF-AT$_c$), resulting in its translocation from the cytoplasm into the nucleus to form a competent transcriptional activator, initiating transcription of mRNA for a variety of cytokines including IL-2. Cyclosporin A prevents the initiation of transcription of mRNA encoding a variety of cytokines including interleukin-2, interferon-γ, and tumor necrosis factor. Decreased expression of these cytokines results in impaired proliferation and differentiation of helper T cells and cytotoxic T-cell development, B-cell activation, and differentiation of macrophages.

The subcellular mechanism of action of cyclosporin has been linked to the high-affinity binding protein cyclophilin (CyP).[21] Collectively, cyclophylin and the FK-506 binding protein (FKBP) are termed *immunophilins*. They share the ability to catalyze the *cis-trans* intraconversion of peptidyl-prolyl bonds, a property known as rotamase or isomerase activity. Rotamase activity may serve to promote protein folding in cells. The complex of immunosuppressive drugs and their corresponding binding protein (cyclosporine-cyclophiline and FK-506-FKBP), but not the drugs alone, then home in on calcineurin (an enzyme with phosphatase activity) and prevents it from activating (dephosphorylating) the cytosolic component of the nuclear factor of activated T cells (NF-AT).[22] Calcineurin and the immunophilins block the assembly of a functional transcription factor, thereby inhibiting the activation of early genes on which T cell activation and proliferation are crucially dependent.

Absorption

Cyclosporin absorption in the gastrointestinal tract is highly variable and incomplete; bioavailability is about 30 percent (range 5 percent to 70 percent) but may increase with increasing dosage and duration of treatment.[23] Interpatient variation in bioavailability (ninefold) may be due to differences in gastric emptying rate, bile acid levels, gastrointestinal motility, and/or metabolism by enzymes in gastrointestinal mucosa.[24] Following absorption, cyclosporin is distributed initially within the blood, where 60 percent to 70 percent is taken up by blood cells, mostly erythrocytes (41 percent to 58 percent), and the remainder is bound to plasma lipoproteins, mostly high-density lipoproteins (18 percent to 22 percent).[25]

Protein Binding

In plasma, >80 percent of cyclosporin binds avidly to lipoproteins. The major fractions involved are high (HDL) and low (LDL) density lipoproteins.

Half-life

The half-life of cyclosporin is 19 h, ranging from 10 to 27 h.

Time to Peak Plasma or Blood Concentration

The time to peak plasma level after oral administration of cyclosporin is 3.5 h. Whole blood concentrations may be two to nine times plasma concentration. Distribution in blood is concentration- and temperature-dependent.[26]

Metabolism and Elimination

Cyclosporin is metabolized by the cytochrome P-450 IIIA enzyme system, resulting in demethylation, hydroxylation, and cyclization, but with preservation of the cyclic structure.[27] Metabolism occurs primarily in the liver but some prehepatic, presystemic metabolism by cytochrome P-450 IIIA enzymes present in the gastrointestinal mucosa also occurs following oral administration. There is no single major metabolic pathway, and more than 30 metabolites have been observed. The most active metabolites show 10 percent to 20 percent of the immunosuppressant activity of the parent compound. Clearance of cyclosporin shows wide interindividual variability (sixfold). Clearance is greater in children and decreased in patients with hepatic impairment, reduced serum low-density lipoprotein levels, and in the elderly. More than 90 percent of cyclosporin is excreted in bile with <1 percent excreted as unchanged cyclosporin. Only 6 percent is eliminated in the urine (0.1 percent unchanged).

Drug Interactions

Interactions between cyclosporin and other drugs include those that influence the metabolism of cyclosporin and interactions that potentiate the drug's nephrotoxicity. Table 118-3 summarizes the drug interactions involving cyclosporin.

Side/Adverse Effects

NEPHROTOXICITY Nephrotoxicity is the major adverse effect of cyclosporin and occurs in approximately one-third of all patients. Acute nephrotoxicity is related to drug-plasma concentrations and usually is reversible on reduction of the dose, although prolonged administration has been associated with progressive and irreversible renal dysfunction. In the early stages of the disorder, renal dysfunction is likely due to vasoconstriction of the afferent glomerular arteriole secondary to a cyclosporin-induced imbalance in the concentrations of the vasodilator prostacyclin and its vasoconstrictor antagonist thromboxane A_2.[28] Thromboxane A_2 induces arterial vasoconstriction and proliferation and migration of vascular smooth muscle cells into the vascular intima.[29,30] Another potential mechanism is inhibition of regulators of the production of the potent vasoconstrictor endothelin. During later stages of nephrotoxicity, chronic vasculointerstitial changes occur with cell damage, glomerulopathy, arteriolopathy and interstitial fibrosis. This form of

nephrotoxicity appears after months of therapy and usually is irreversible.

HYPERTENSION Hypertension is usually moderate to severe and dose-related. A variety of mechanisms may contribute to its pathogenesis including impaired sodium excretion, enhanced sympathetic nervous activity, effects on renal prostaglandin metabolism, and direct injury to endothelial cells with release to endothelin.[31] Hypertension may occur independently of nephrotoxicity and may be difficult to treat.

HEPATOTOXICITY Although rare, cyclosporin may induce centrilobular fatty changes and hepatocyte necrosis.[32] This results in cholestasis with hyperbilirubinemia and elevation of serum levels of aminotransferases. Chronic cyclosporin-induced hepatic dysfunction is associated with an increased incidence of cholelithiasis presumably because of altered lithogenicity of the bile.

NEUROTOXICITY Even though cyclosporin is not believed to cross the intact blood-brain barrier, neurologic side effects occur in approximately 20 percent of recipients of renal and liver transplants.[33,34] Symptoms include tremor, ataxia, confusion, agitation, depression, sleep disturbances, headaches, lethargy or coma, convulsions, cortical blindness, and burning palmar and plantar paresthesias. The mechanism of neurotoxicity is unknown, but disturbances of the blood-brain barrier or cyclosporin metabolites may be related.

MALIGNANCIES Malignancies in cyclosporin-treated patients show a disproportionate high incidence of lymphomas (27 percent versus 11 percent) and Kaposi sarcoma (8 percent versus 3 percent) when compared with patients receiving azathioprine plus prednisone.[35] Lymphomas in cyclosporin-treated patients usually occur earlier (15 versus 48 months posttransplant). They frequently involve lymph nodes (39 percent versus 23 percent) and less frequently the central nervous system (15 percent versus 38 percent).[36]

Dose

Cyclosporin is administered initially at 2 to 3 mg/kg per day intravenously over 2 to 6 h and converted to an oral regimen of 7 to 15 mg/kg per day in divided doses as soon as feasible. Dosage may be subsequently reduced gradually to a maintenance dose of 3 to 8 mg/kg per day to achieve desired target trough levels.

Monitoring

Two methods are available for specific assay of the cyclosporin parent compound: radioimmunoassay (RIA) and high-performance liquid chromatography (HPLC). The specific antibody against cyclosporin gives a selective measure of the parent compound without interference from drug metabolites (30 metabolites identified). Therefore, 12 h trough levels of the cyclosporin parent compound should be measured routinely by RIA. Whole blood is the matrix of choice to determine cyclosporin levels. If plasma or serum are used, a standard protocol with respect to time and temperature should be used. Target blood concentrations during

Table 118-3 Drug Interactions with Cyclosporin

Drug Class	Known Interaction	Suspected/Possible Interaction
Increased trough blood level		
Antimicrobials	Erythromycin Josmycin Ketoconazole	Amikacin Fluconazole Intraconazole Metronidazole Norfloxacin
Ca^{++}Channel Antagonists	Diltiazem Nicardipine Verapamil	
H2-Receptor Antagonists		Cimetidine Ranitidine
Oral Anticoagulants		Warfarin
Decreased trough blood level		
Anticonvulsants	Carbamazepine Phenobarbital Phenytoin	Primidone
Antimicrobials	Rifampicin	Pyrazinamide Sulphadiazine

the first three months are 250 to 340 ng/ml; the dose is titrated to achieve trough concentrations of 200 to 250 ng/ml by 6 months and 150 to 200 ng/ml by 12 months posttransplant. Blood pressure and serum creatinine concentrations are monitored every 2 weeks during the first 3 months of therapy and then every 2 months. Cyclosporin dosage should be reduced by 25 percent to 50 percent if serum creatinine increases by more than 30 percent above baseline, even if values remain within the normal range. Addition of diltiazem may prove beneficial in achieving a reduction in the dose and in attenuating the nephrotoxicity.[37]

TACROLIMUS

Tacrolimus, formerly known as FK-506, is a macrolide antibiotic with similar but more potent (10 to 100 times) immunosuppressant properties than cyclosporin, inhibiting cell-mediated and humoral immune responses. At present, it continues under intensive clinical investigation, but published peer-reviewed publications are few.

Structure and Source

Tacrolimus, a hydrophobic macrocyclic lactone, was first isolated in 1985 from the fermentation broth of *Streptomyces tsukubaensis*, a soil microorganism found in northern Japan.[38]

Mechanism of Action

As for cyclosporin, tacrolimus binds with high affinity to a family of immunosuppressant binding proteins (immunophilins). The main FK-506 binding protein is a 12-kDa molecule, FKBP12. FKBP12 is a peptidyl-propyl *cis-trans* isomerase (rotamase), which catalyzes proline peptide bond isomerization, a rate-limiting step in protein folding.[39,40] Although cyclosporin and tacrolimus are potent inhibitors of rotamase activity, it is unlikely that this effect is implicated in the immunosuppressant action of the drugs. Instead, the immunophilin-drug complex, the active moiety, binds to and inhibits calcineurin, a calmodulin- and calcium-dependent serine/threonine phosphatase involved in signal transduction.[41]

Absorption

Tacrolimus is poorly and erratically absorbed after oral administration.[42] The absolute oral bioavailability ranges from 5 percent to 67 percent (mean 27 percent). The presence of food may decrease its absorption.

Tissue Distribution

Tacrolimus is highly lipophilic and undergoes extensive tissue distribution.[42] Drug concentrations in the lung, spleen, heart, kidney, and pancreas exceed those in plasma. In the vascular compartment, erythrocytes sequester tacrolimus, binding 75 percent to 80 percent of the drug, with the result that whole blood concentrations are approximately 10 to 30 times greater than plasma concentrations.[43]

Protein Binding

Tacrolimus binds avidly (88 percent) to plasma proteins, predominantly the nonlipoprotein fraction containing albumin and α1 acid glycoprotein.[44]

Half-life

Plasma half-life of tacrolimus ranges from 5.5. to 16.6 h (mean 8.7 h).[42]

Time to Peak Plasma or Blood Concentration

Peak plasma concentration after a single oral dose of tacrolimus occurs at 0.5 to 8 h.

Metabolism and Elimination

Tacrolimus is metabolized almost completely by the liver; <1 percent of the parent drug is excreted unchanged in the bile, urine, and feces.[42] Hepatic metabolism occurs primarily through the cytochrome P-450 subtypes Ia and IIIa, with demethylation and hydroxylation representing the main metabolic pathways.[45] Two of the nine metabolites identified exhibit immunosuppressant activity in vitro. Hepatic dysfunction is associated with increased plasma concentrations, prolonged half-life, and reduce clearance, whereas pharmacokinetics are not modified with renal impairment.[46]

Drug Interactions

Tacrolimus is a potent inhibitor of cytochrome P-450–dependent drug metabolism.[47] This enzyme system is responsible for oxidation of calcium channel blocking agents, corticosteroids, cyclosporin, macrolide antibiotics, and other drugs. Since tacrolimus and cyclosporin are both substrates for cytochrome P-450, each drug can act as a competitive inhibitor of the other's metabolism.[48] Increased plasma concentrations of tacrolimus have been associated with coadministration of cytochrome P-450 inhibitors such as ketoconazole, fluconazole, itraconazole, trimethoprim/sulfamethoxazole, diltiazem, and erythromycin.

Side/Adverse Effects

The principal adverse effects of tacrolimus are nephrotoxicity, infectious and malignant complications, neurotoxicity, and diabetogenic effects, all of which also have been associated with conventional immunosuppressive therapies, including cyclosporin.[49,50] Gingival hyperplasia, hirsutism, and hypercholesterolemia do not appear to be significant side effects.

Dosage

Following transplantation, tacrolimus is administered by intravenous infusion until oral therapy is feasible. A dose of 0.05 to 0.1 mg/kg is given over 24 h. Oral therapy usually is started with 0.15 mg/kg twice daily. The optimum dosage regimen for tacrolimus continues to be refined.

Monitoring

Recommended trough concentrationss of tacrolimus in plasma and in whole blood are 0.5 to 2 μg/L and 15 to 20 μg/L, respectively. Measurement in whole blood is the method of choice.

PURINE SYNTHESIS INHIBITORS

AZATHIOPRINE

Azathioprine {6-[(1-methyl-4-nitro-1H-imidazol-5-yl)thio]-1H-purine} a synthetic imidazolyl derivative of 6-mercaptopurine, is a purine analogue that inhibits cell-mediated and humoral immunity. It is widely used as an immunosuppressant in organ transplantation.

Structure and Source

Azathioprine and its related compound 6-mercaptopurine are purine analogues that interfere with DNA synthesis.

Mechanism of Action

Azathioprine itself is not an active compound. In the liver and erythrocytes, it is metabolized to 6-mercaptopurine, the active molecule.[51] Hypoxanthine phosphoribosyl transferase metabolizes 6-mercaptopurine to 6-thioinosinic acid, a competitive inhibitor of inosine monophosphate dehydrogenase (IMD); inhibition of this enzyme suppresses several steps in the synthesis of adenine and guanine by preventing interconversion of purine bases, especially inosinic and guanylic acid.[52] The end result is inhibition of the synthesis of DNA, RNA, and proteins necessary for cell differentiation and function.

Absorption

Azathioprine is well-absorbed after oral administration.

Protein Binding

Approximately 30 percent of circulating azathioprine is protein bound.

Half-life

The half-life of azathioprine is 3 to 5 h, with clearance from the blood resulting from uptake by cells, renal excretion, and metabolic degradation.

Time to Peak Plasma Concentration

Maximum serum concentration occurs at 1 to 2 h after oral administration of azathioprine. Blood concentrations have little predictive value for therapy since the magnitude and duration of clinical effects correlate with thiopurine nucleotide concentrationsin tissues rather than with plasma drug concentrations.

Metabolism and Elimination

Azathioprine and 6-mercaptopurine ultimately are oxidized in the liver by xanthine oxidase to the inactive molecule 6-thiouric acid. About one-half of an oral dose is found excreted in the urine within the first 24 h.[53] Although hepatic metabolism is important, the effects of liver disease on azathioprine metabolism remain unclear. The half-life of azathioprine may increase in renal failure, although this effect is generally not clinically significant. Two to 10 percent of the oral dose is excreted unchanged in the urine.[54]

Drug Interactions

Allopurinol, by blocking xanthine oxidase, reduces the metabolism of azathioprine, resulting in accumulation of azathioprine and its metabolites. When azathioprine and allopurinol are to be used concurrently, the dose of azathioprine must be reduced by 75 percent and close monitoring

performed to avoid toxicity, usually in the form of leukopenia.[52]

Side/Adverse Effects

The primary clinical concern is bone marrow suppression, with leukopenia rather than thrombocytopenia and anemia being the major manifestations.[55,56] This is usually dose-dependent and may occur late in the course of therapy. Dose reduction or temporary withdrawal allow reversal of these manifestations. Predisposition to infection may occur due to leukopenia or functional impairment of lymphocyte and macrophage function. Dosage should be adjusted to maintain the leukocyte count at 3500 to 4000/mm. Other side effects include gastrointestinal manifestations, liver and lung injury, predisposition to malignancy, and teratogenic effects.

Dosage

Azathioprine usually is started intravenously in doses of 1 to 2.5 mg/kg and converted to oral therapy when feasible. The dose is adjusted to maintain the leukocyte count above 3500/mm.

CORTICOSTEROIDS

Corticosteroids (prednisone, prednisolone, and methylprednisolone) have been used for prophylaxis and treatment of rejection since the beginning of clinical organ transplantation in the 1950s. Corticosteroids inhibit the cellular cascade of the inflammatory and immune response at virtually all levels, including neutrophil and monocyte migration into inflammatory sites, macrophage antigen presentation to lymphocytes, lymphocyte proliferation and differentiation into effector cell, and cytokine production. They suppress macrophage generation and release of arachidonic acid-derived proinflammatory prostaglandins and leukotrienes. Corticosteroids also induce lympholysis through *apoptosis*, a specific form of hormone-stimulated programmed cell death.

Structure and Source

Corticosteroids are 21-carbon steroid molecules whose biologic activity requires the presence of a hydroxyl group at carbon 11 (C-11), a ketone oxygen at C-3, an unsaturated bond between C-4 and C-5, and a ketone oxygen at C-20. The synthetic corticosteroids were developed to enhance anti-inflammatory activity and reduce mineralocorticoid activity.

Mechanism of Action

Glucocorticoids diffuse through the cell membranes and bind to cytoplasmic glucocorticoid receptors (GRs), a member of the superfamily of receptors derived from genes with homology to the oncogene *erbA*.[57] (See also Chaps. 3 and 55). The hormone-binding region of the glucocorticoid receptor usually is occupied by a 90-kDa heat-shock protein (HSP-90).[58] Glucocorticoid binding displaces HSP-90 and induces an allosteric change in the glucocorticoid receptor, allowing the receptor-hormone complex to translocate to the nucleus where it binds to target glucocorticoids response elements

(GREs) in the DNA through the DNA-binding region of the glucocorticoid receptor. This results either in inhibition (nGRE) or stimulation (+GRE) of transcription in steroid-responsive target genes. Corticosteroids inhibit the transcription of several cytokines including IL-1, TNF-α, GM-CSF, IL-3, IL-4, IL-5, IL-6, and IL-8.[59] By contrast, synthesis of lipocortin-1, β adrenoreceptors, and endonucleases is stimulated by binding of glucocorticoid receptors to +glucocorticoid response elements. Lipocortin-1 inhibits phospholipase A_2 activity, resulting in inhibition of synthesis of prostaglandins, leukotrienes, and platelet-activating factor, all of which have proinflammatory properties.

Absorption
Prednisone is 80 percent to 90 percent absorbed after oral administration and is not influenced by food intake.

Time to Peak Plasma Concentration
Prednisone is biologically inactive and must be converted to prednisolone. Peak prednisolone concentration is reached in 1 to 2 h. Concentrations of prednisolone achieved after oral prednisone are only slightly less than after the same dose of prednisolone given intravenously. Prednisone conversion is depressed in patients with severe liver disease, but it is doubtful that this factor is clinically significant.

Protein Binding
In plasma, glucocorticoids are bound to plasma proteins. Corticosteroid-binding globulin (CBG; transcortin), an α-globulin synthesized by the liver, binds 75 percent of the circulating hormone. The remainder is bound loosely to albumin (15 percent) or free (10 percent) and is available to exert its effect on target cells. When plasma cortisol concentrations exceed 20 to 30 μg/dl, CBG is saturated, and the concentration of free hormone rises rapidly.

Half-life
The half-life of cortisol in the circulation ranges from 80 to 115 min; half-life for other glucocorticoids is as follows: prednisone 3.4 to 3.8 h; prednisolone 2.1 to 3.5 h; methylprednisolone 1.3 to 3.1 h; dexamethasone 1.8 to 4.7 h. The relative potency of glucocorticoids correlates more with their affinity for the cytoplasmic glucocorticoid receptor than with their half-life.

Metabolism and Elimination
Elimination is primarily by biotransformation to inactive compounds. Only a small fraction of the parent biologically active compound is excreted through the kidney. Hepatic conjugation generates water-soluble sulfate esters of glucuronide which are excreted through the bile and urine as 11-oxy-17-ketosteroids.

Drug Interactions
Drugs that induce hepatic microsomal enzymes may alter corticosteroid elimination. Barbiturates, phenytoin, rifampin, carbamazepine, and ephedrine all increase elimination. This effect is much greater on methylprednisolone than

on prednisone. Oral contraceptives impair elimination by increasing the cortisol and prednisolone-binding protein transcortin.

Side/Adverse Effects
The physiologic and pharmacologic effects of corticosteroids are not distinct, but are on a continuum dependent on the concentration, duration of exposure, and a multitude of cell and tissue variables. Among common adverse effects are hypertension, negative balance of calcium and nitrogen, truncal obesity, moon facies, facial erythema, thin and fragile skin, acne, suppression of growth in children, hyperglycemia, hyperlipoproteinemia, atherosclerosis, sodium retention, hypokalemia, secondary adrenal insufficiency, myopathy, osteoporosis, osteonecrosis, alterations in mood, susceptibility to infections and posterior subcapsular cataracts. Uncommon adverse effects include metabolic alkalosis, hyperosmolar nonketotic diabetic coma, "silent" intestinal perforation, glaucoma, benign intracranial hypertension, spontaneous fractures, and psychosis. Rare side effects include congestive heart failure, hirsutism, secondary amenorrhea, fatty liver, pancreatitis, convulsions, exophthalmos, and allergy to synthetic corticosteroids resulting in angioedema.

Dosage
Recent clinical and experimental evidence support a beneficial role for corticosteroids in the healing of the airway anastomosis. Most transplant centers initiate immunosuppression with corticosteroids during the operative procedure. Typically, methylprednisolone 500 mg is administered intravenously just prior to perfusion of the graft. This is followed by 1.5 to 2 mg/kg daily for 3 days and converted to oral prednisone when the patient is able to tolerate this route. Prednisone usually is started at a dose of 0.5 to 1 mg/kg per day and gradually tapered to a maintenance dose of 0.1 to 0.2 mg/kg per day over several months.

Acute episodes of allograft rejection are treated with methylprednisolone 1 g intravenously daily for 3 days, followed by oral prednisone 1 mg/kg per day and gradually tapered to the maintenance dose during the ensuing 3 to 4 weeks. Although episodes of chronic rejection in the form of bronchiolitis obliterans are treated with the same initial pulse therapy with methylprednisolone, a more gradual taper is advised to stabilize or prevent further deterioration of lung function. This approach has not been validated.

CYTOLYTIC AGENTS

ANTILYMPHOCYTE GLOBULINS
Antilymphocyte globulins are powerful immunosuppressant agents used for prophylaxis and treatment of severe or corticosteroid-resistant episodes of allograft rejection. When used prophylactically, they significantly reduce the frequency and intensity of rejection and have corticosteroid-sparing effects. However, they may increase the incidence and severity of infections and predispose to malignancies.

Structure and Source

Antithymocyte, antilymphocyte, or antilymphoblast globulins are polyclonal antisera prepared by repeated sensitization of an animal with parenteral injection of human thymocytes, lymphocytes, or lymphoblasts.[60] The serum is purified by exchange chromatography and double precipitation to obtain the active fraction containing the relevant IgGs.

Mechanism of Action

Antilymphocyte globulins contain antibodies of defined specificity against membrane-bound molecules on T cells such as CD2, CD4, CD8, CD18, MHC class II, and CD3. They cause lymphocyte depletion by complement-dependent lysis, and opsonization and destruction by the reticuloendothelial system through the interaction of IgG with the Fc receptor of macrophages.

Drug Interaction

Patients who have developed hypersensitivity to heterologous proteins may show signs of cross-intolerance to the antilymphocyte globulin.

Side/Adverse Effects

Side effects include fever, shivering, arthralgias, skin rashes, and, much less frequently, anaphylactoid reactions (hypotension, respiratory distress, urticaria, purpura). Intense T-cell inhibition increases the incidence of viral infections and lymphomas.[61]

Dosage

The dose varies according to the source and strength of the commercial product. Recommended doses for prophylaxis vary from 1.25 to 2.5 mg/kg per day to 10 to 15 mg/kg per day intravenously. In all cases, the dose is adjusted to maintain the lymphocyte count between 100 and 200 cells/ml and/or the E rosette lymphocytes between 5 percent and 10 percent. Usual treatment is 1 to 2 weeks, either simultaneously or sequentially with cyclosporin A–based regimens. Treatment should be stopped if anaphylaxis, neutropenia of <2,000 cells/ml, or thrombocytopenia of <50,000/ml develops. Neutropenia and thrombocytopenia result from contamination with antineutrophil and antiplatelet antibodies.

OKT3

OKT3 is a mouse antihuman antibody specifically directed against the CD3 component of the T-cell receptor complex of T cells. OKT3 has been extensively used in renal transplantation but its use in lung transplantation has been reserved for steroid-resistant acute or chronic rejection. It is considered the most potent antirejection therapy currently available.

Structure and Source

OKT3 is a murine monoclonal IgG2a antibody obtained from a hybridoma cell line.[62] The hybridoma is injected into the peritoneal cavity of mice and the antibody obtained by harvesting the ascitic fluid.

Mechanism of Action

OKT3 binds to the epsilon moiety of the CD3 molecule, opsonizing circulating lymphocytes and facilitating their removal by the reticuloendothelial system. Additionally, by binding to the CD3 molecule OKT3 may modulate the T-cell receptor complex, rendering T cells inactive and unable to recognize alloantigen.[63]

Side/Adverse Effects

Side effects include fever, chills, headache, rigors, myalgia, nausea, vomiting, diarrhea, thrombocytopenia, leukopenia, arthritis, pruritus, rash, tachycardia, hypertension, hypotension, angina, and an aseptic meningitis syndrome. The initial few doses of OKT3 often are accompanied by systemic release of lymphokines which, in turn, enhance synthesis of inflammatory mediators resulting in a systemic inflammation response.[64] Other rare, but potentially serious, manifestations of the CRS are pulmonary edema, which tends to occur in patients who already are fluid-overloaded, myocardial depression, neurotoxicity (seizures, encephalitis), thrombosis, and an anaphylactoid response in previously sensitized patients. Isotypic and idiotypic antibodies against OKT3 develop in 30 percent of patients; these may diminish the efficacy of OKT3 and preclude subsequent administration of other mouse monoclonal antibodies.

Dosage

OKT3 usually is given in doses of 2.5 to 5 mg intravenously daily for 10 to 21 days. For the first 3 days, recommended premedication includes methylprednisolone 1 mg/kg, acetaminophen 650 mg orally or indomethacin 50 to 100 mg per rectum, diphenhydramine hydrochloride 50 mg intravenously, and ranitidine hydrochloride 50 mg intravenously. Conventional concomitant immunosuppression usually is decreased during OKT3 therapy. Circulating lymphocyte count returns to pretreatment levels in 1 to 2 days after discontinuation of treatment.

Antiviral Agents

ACYCLOVIR

Acyclovir {9-[(2-hydroxyethoxy)methyl]guanine} is a synthetic antiviral drug with activity limited to herpesviruses. It is more active against herpes simplex virus types 1 and 2 and varicella zoster virus; infections caused by cytomegalovirus and Epstein-Barr virus do not respond.

Structure and Source

Acyclovir is an acyclic analogue of guanosine developed during efforts to prepare synthetic nucleoside analogues, substituting the normal cyclic carbohydrate ring with an acyclic side chain, with retention of substrate activity.

Mechanism of Action

Acyclovir is a prodrug. After uptake by an infected cell, acyclovir is phosphorylated to an inactive monophosphate form by a virus-specific thymidine kinase and then is phosphorylated to diphosphate and triphosphate forms by cellular guanylate kinases.[65] Acyclovir triphosphate, the active form, inhibits viral DNA polymerase and competes with deoxyguanosine triphosphate to act as a terminator of biosynthesis of the viral DNA strand.[66] Viral DNA that has been chain-terminated by acyclovir becomes irreversibly damaged. Uptake and activation of the drug by cells expressing a viral thymidine kinase is the most important explanation for the selective antiviral activity of acyclovir compared with its effects on uninfected cells. Because cytomegalovirus (CMV) lacks a thymidine kinase, acyclovir has limited activity against this virus.[67]

Absorption

After oral administration, acyclovir is absorbed slowly and incompletely with a bioavailability of 15 percent to 30 percent. Gastrointestinal absorption is not significantly affected by food.

Protein Binding

Protein binding of acyclovir is low in the range of 10 percent to 30 percent.

Half-life

Half-life of acyclovir after oral and intravenous administration is 3.3 and 3.9 h, respectively. Half-life increases with decreased creatinine clearance.

Time to Peak Serum Concentration

The time to peak serum concentration is 1.7 h after oral administration.

Metabolism and Elimination

Acyclovir trapped and phosphorylated by the herpesvirus thymidine kinase in infected cells intracellularly persists well after the clearance of acyclovir from the plasma. The metabolic fate of acyclovir involves hydroxylation and oxidation and urinary excretion as inactive metabolites. Renal excretion is by both glomerular filtration and tubular secretion. Fecal elimination is insignificant (<2 percent). Patients with acute or chronic renal impairment require a reduction in the dose. Removal of acyclovir is accelerated fourfold during hemodialysis.

Drug Interactions

Probenecid significantly reduces tubular secretion, increasing the plasma half-life by 20 percent and serum concentrations by 50 percent, thus enhancing the potential for nephrotoxicity. Nephrotoxicity is also enhanced by other concomitantly administered nephrotoxic drugs.

Side/Adverse Effects

Reversible renal toxicity occurs in 5 percent to 10 percent of patients and is more common after rapid intravenous bolus administration, with high doses, concurrent dehydration, and preexisting renal impairment.[68] Renal toxicity is caused by tubular crystallization and precipitation of the drug causing a crystalline nephropathy. Other adverse effects include neuropsychiatric disturbances such as confusion, delirium,

lethargy, tremors, and seizures. Renal and neurologic side effects correlate with the serum concentration of the drug and occur most commonly when it exceeds 25 μg/ml.[69]

Dosage

For prophylaxis, acyclovir is given 400 mg three times daily for the first three months posttransplantation. Treatment for Herpes zoster requires 800 mg fives times daily for 7 to 10 days. Although acyclovir does not reduce the frequency of cytomegalovirus infection in transplant patients, it reduces the severity of the disease. Patients with acute or chronic renal impairment require a reduction in dose or increase in interval of administration.

GANCICLOVIR

Ganciclovir {9-[(1,3-dihydroxy-2-propoxy)methyl]guanine} (DHPG), an acyclic nucleoside analogue of guanine, inhibits the replication of all human herpesviruses, including cytomegalovirus.

Structure and Source

As a derivative of acyclovir, ganciclovir also is an acyclic analogue of guanosine.

Mechanism of Action

Ganciclovir is a prodrug. In cytomegalovirus-infected cells, ganciclovir is phosphorylated to the 3'-ganciclovir monophosphate by a cellular deoxyguanosine kinase.[70] Further phosphorylation occurs by several cellular kinases to produce ganciclovir triphosphate. In cytomegalovirus-infected cells, there is approximately a 10-fold increased concentration of both cellular kinases and ganciclovir triphosphate than in noninfected cells. It inhibits viral DNA synthesis by two mechanisms: (1) by competitive inhibition of deoxyguanosine incorporation into DNA by DNA polymerase, and (2) by incorporating itself into viral DNA, causing subsequent termination or very limited elongation of viral DNA.[71]

Absorption

After oral administration, ganciclovir is absorbed poorly with a bioavailability of approximately 3 percent to 4.6 percent.[72] Therefore, ganciclovir is only available for intravenous infusion.

Protein Binding

Protein binding of ganciclovir is low, in the range of 1 percent to 2 percent.

Half-life

In patients with normal renal function, the plasma half-life after 1-h intravenous infusion is approximately 2.9 h.

Time to Peak Plasma Concentration

The time to peak plasma concentration is the time to reach the end of the intravenous infusion (approximately 1 h).

Metabolism and Elimination

In virus-infected cells, ganciclovir triphosphate is metabolized slowly, with 60 percent to 70 percent remaining intracellularly 18 h after removal of ganciclovir from the extracellular fluid. More than 90 percent of the drug is excreted unchanged in the urine by glomerular filtration, and a much smaller amount possibly by tubular secretion. There are no known metabolites of ganciclovir.

Drug Interactions

Probenecid may reduce the renal clearance of ganciclovir by reducing tubular secretion. Concurrent use with zidovudine may result in increased myelosuppression by additive effect rather than by pharmacokinetic interaction.

Side/Adverse Effects

The most common adverse effects are neutropenia and thrombocytopenia.[73] Overall, neutropenia (< 1000 cells/ml) occurs in 38 percent and severe neutropenia (< 500 cells/ml) in 16 percent of patients. Neutropenia tends to occur during the second week of therapy and is usually reversible after discontinuation or reduction of the drug. Other adverse effects include fever, rash, anemia, nausea, vomiting, and mild elevations in creatinine and liver function tests values.

Dosage

For prophylaxis against cytomegalovirus, the usual dose of 5 mg/kg twice daily for 14 days, followed by 5 mg/kg three times weekly for three months. Substantial reductions in the dose and dosing intervals are necessary in patients with renal insufficiency. Hemodialysis efficiently reduces concentrations of ganciclovir in plasma by approximately 50 percent, and it is recommended to administer this drug after dialysis.

CMV IMMUNE GLOBULIN

Monoclonal anti-CMV antibodies, unselected immunoglobulins (hyperimmune plasma), or CMV immune globulin have been used in the attempt to prevent CMV disease. Although there have been no direct clinical comparisons between CMV immune globulin and the other preparations, there are several theoretical reasons why CMV immune globulin may be preferable and is the product most widely used.

Structure and Source

CMV immune globulin is produced from plasma obtained from normal volunteer blood donors. An enzyme-linked immunosorbent assay (ELISA) for antibody to CMV is used to screen donor blood and ensure high antibody titers. After suitable screening, about 4 percent to 9 percent of the donor population is selected for contribution to a plasma pool. Usually more than 2000 donors contribute to a single plasma pool.[74] Compared with unselected globulin, CMV immune globulin is five- to eightfold richer in specific anti-CMV antibody. CMV immune globulin is manufactured by using the classic Cohn-Oncley fractionation method, with a terminal ultrafiltration step to modify it for intravenous administra-

tion. The preparation contains primarily immunoglobulin IgG comprising all four subclasses and trace amounts of IgA and IgM.

Mechanism of Action

The mechanism of action of anti-CMV immune globulin is unknown. The antibody may neutralize directly CMV antigen, block cytotoxic T-cell recognition of virus-infected cells, or enhance antibody-dependent cell-mediated cytotoxicity against the virus.

Adverse/Side Effects

Adverse or side effects are observed in approximately 5 percent of the infusions. Chest tightness, muscle cramps, back pain, flushing, chills, and wheezing are the most common. Persons with selective IgA deficiency have the potential for developing antibodies to IgA and could have anaphylactic reactions to subsequent administration of blood products that contain IgA.

Dosage

The optimal dose, duration, and timing of CMV immune globulin remain to be established. While passive immunization with this product does not prevent infection (seroconversion), it does prevent the emergence of serious symptomatic disease. CMV immune globulin is indicated for prophylaxis against primary CMV disease in CMV seronegative recipients of allografts from CMV seropositive donors and has been extended to include all seropositive lung transplant recipients as well. CMV immune globulin plus ganciclovir may be beneficial in the treatment of established CMV disease. The recommended dosage of CMV immune globulin is 150 mg/kg intravenously within 72 h of transplantation. The same dose is repeated two weeks later and then followed by 100 mg/kg every two weeks for 6 additional doses.

Prophylaxis of Infection

Infection remains a major cause of morbidity and the major cause of mortality after lung transplantation.[75] Most infections occur during the first few months after transplantation, and the lung itself is frequently the target of infection. The risk of infection during maintenance immunosuppression is low in the absence of augmented immunosuppression. Many common infections can be prevented with the use of appropriate prophylactic regimens. In the first postoperative month, the major causes of infection are bacterial, and usually involve the wound, the lung, the pleural space, or, rarely, the mediastinum and the urinary tract. These infections are readily treated with antibiotics. Between 1 to 6 months after transplant immunosuppression reaches its peak, cytomegalovirus and Herpes simplex virus infections appear, and opportunistic infections become more common. In the late posttransplant period (after 6 months), the incidence and types of infection in transplant recipients are similar to those in the general population. Bacterial bronchitis and recurrent pneumonias are common in patients who develop chronic rejection in the form of bronchiolitis obliterans.

Prevention of infection begins with a comprehensive medical assessment including a detailed history of past or recurrent infections, immunization and travel history, and screening for the presence of active indolent infection. Serologic testing to detect antibodies against herpes simplex virus, Epstein-Barr virus, cytomegalovirus, varicella zoster virus, hepatitis B virus, and hepatitis C virus complements this assessment. Potential lung donors seropositive for human immunodeficiency virus (HIV) or hepatitis virus B or C are excluded from consideration. A detailed bronchoscopic examination is performed to detect evidence of gross infection and to obtain samples for bacteriology.[76]

BACTERIAL

Antibacterial prophylaxis for patients with underlying septic lung disease (cystic fibrosis, bronchiectasis) is targeted against the microorganisms responsible for the most recent exacerbation. Since *Pseudomonas* species are the most common microorganisms isolated, a third-generation cephalosporine (ceftazidime 2 g IV three times daily) plus an aminoglycoside (tobramycin 100 to 160 mg IV three times daily) is administered for 7 to 10 days. For patients without septic lung disease, antibacterial prophylaxis is initiated with ceftazidime (1 g IV three times daily) plus clindamycin (600 mg IV three times daily) and adjusted according to results of cultures from donor and recipient. This regimen is continued for 2 days after transplantation.

CYTOMEGALOVIRUS

Prevention of primary CMV infection, the most common viral infection following lung transplantation, is accomplished best by avoiding exposure to the virus.[77] A policy of transplanting only lungs from seronegative donors to seronegative recipients would be ideal; however, with the prevalence of seropositive individuals ranging from 45 percent to 79 percent, and, given the scarcity of donors, this is not always feasible. All CMV positive and seromismatched recipients receive prophylaxis with CMV hyperimmune globulin and ganciclovir. Reinstitution of ganciclovir during intense antirejection therapy may be a vital component of the prophylactic strategy, and it probably should be given to all patients receiving courses of antilymphocyte globulin or OKT3 to treat acute or chronic rejection. Seronegative recipients of seronegative donors do not receive ganciclovir or hyperimmune globulin but do receive acyclovir prophylaxis for herpes simplex virus infection. They also should receive only blood products from seronegative donors.

PNEUMOCYSTIS CARINII

Since the institution of prophylactic regimens, infection with this microorganism has been almost eradicated.[78] Various regimens including trimethoprim/sulfamethoxazole (one double-strength tablet twice daily every other day, or twice daily three times per week) have been highly effective in preventing infection and are continued indefinitely. Patients who have a history of serious reactions to sulfa drugs may receive aerosol pentamidine 300 mg every month or the combination of dapsone plus trimethoprim, 100 mg daily three times per week and 200 mg twice daily three times per week, respectively.

FUNGI

Infections with *Aspergillus* and *Candida* have been reported in 5 percent to 14 percent of lung transplant recipients. *Candida* has been identified as a cause of urinary tract infection, pleural infection, and candidemia. *Aspergillus* species are ubiquitous organisms in the environment, and the respiratory tract of patients with end-stage parenchymal lung disease may easily become colonized. No standard practice exists to prevent infection by these microorganisms. Commonly employed strategies include low-dose intravenous amphotericin B or itraconazole. Patients whose sputum reveals *Aspergillus* species preoperatively should receive itraconazole 200 mg orally daily for two months. All other patients routinely receive mycostatin 100,000 U swish-and-swallow four times daily for two months.

Complications

REJECTION

Hyperacute rejection is caused by preexisting antibodies in the recipient's circulation that bind to the vascular endothelium of the graft. This form of rejection has been virtually eliminated by preoperative cross-matching of donor and recipient. Acute rejection is the result of a complex cellular immune response directed against specific antigenic determinants in donor cells. Histologically acute rejection is characterized by necrosis of parenchymal cells and perivascular mononuclear infiltrates with or without lymphocytic bronchiolitis or alveolitis. Chronic lung rejection is characterized by obliterative fibrosis of the small peripheral airways.[79] The lesion progresses from an inflammatory nonocclusive bronchiolitis to partial or complete obliteration of bronchioles by fibro-cellular tissue plugs (Masson's bodies). It also may present as proliferation of intimal smooth muscle cells in the walls of the pulmonary arteries in the form of accelerated atherosclerosis. Chronic rejection is now recognized as the most important cause of late graft failure and death.

ACUTE REJECTION

Episodes of acute rejection are almost universal among lung transplant recipients. The first episode commonly occurs at the end of the first week or ten days following transplant, but may occur as early as 48 h. Rejection episodes decrease in frequency after the first three months. Mild cases are usually asymptomatic, and the condition is suspected because of widening of the alveolar-arterial oxygen gradient, leukocytosis, or reticular or acinar lung infiltrates. In more severe cases, clinical manifestations may include nonproductive cough, persistent fever, dyspnea, tightness of the chest, and decreased exercise tolerance, often accompanied by hypoxemia, crackles, deterioration in pulmonary function tests, and progressive roentgenographic infiltrates. Separating rejection from infection is often not possible, and confirmation of the diagnosis requires tissue obtained from transbronchial lung biopsy for histopathology. Treatment is with pulsed methylprednisolone therapy, 1 g IV daily for three consecutive days, followed by a temporary increase in the oral prednisone dose with tapering over the subsequent 4 to 6 weeks.[80] The vast majority of cases respond rapidly. If symptoms and findings persist a second course of methylprednisolone or antilymphocyte globulin is usually effective. Persistent ongoing rejection may require the addition of OKT3 or rescue therapy with tacrolimus.

CHRONIC REJECTION

Bronchiolitis obliterans appears to be an immune-mediated phenomenon targeted against the epithelial component of small airways and affecting up to 50 percent of long-term survivors of lung and heart-lung transplantation.[81] It may develop as early as 2 months or more than 4 years after transplant; most cases appear by the end of the first year. Most often it has an insidious onset with gradual development of dyspnea on exertion, malaise, and productive or nonproductive cough, but, occasionally, a more rapid and fulminant course can be seen. The diagnosis is confirmed by finding an obstructive or mixed obstructive-restrictive pattern on pulmonary function testing and/or demonstrating obstructive endobronchial plugs in small airways. The earliest physiologic abnormality is usually a decline in the airflow rate in the midvital capacity range.[82] The chest roentgenogram may be normal in early stages, but patchy interstitial-acinar infiltrates with or without pleural thickening and hyperinflation may be observed later. Colonization with *Staphylococcus aureus* or *Pseudomonas* species occurs commonly, and recurrent episodes of bronchitis and pneumonitis eventually develop. With early diagnosis, it can be reversed or arrested in some patients by enhancing the level of immunosuppression, usually with pulse methylprednisolone or with polyclonal antilymphocyte globulin.[83] Temporarily increasing the dose of prednisone and pushing azathioprine to tolerance may be helpful adjunctive steps. Relapses of bronchiolitis obliterans usually are treated with another course of antilymphocyte serum. About two-thirds of patients have a clearcut clinical response with improvement in symptoms and in lung function. Only in about one-third to one-half of these is the response sustained. Another less fortunate group of patients fail to respond to any form of therapy, experience a gradual decline in lung function, and eventually become fully disabled or die. For some, retransplantation has been performed successfully.

BRONCHIOLITIS OBLITERANS ORGANIZING PNEUMONIA

It is characterized by acute or subacute onset of dyspnea, tachypnea, hypoxemia, and focal or diffuse alveolar pulmonary infiltrates and a restrictive pattern on pulmonary function testing. Pathologically, the most striking abnormality is the filling of terminal and respiratory bronchioles, alveolar ducts, and alveolar spaces with plugs of loose granulation and connective tissue. Occasionally lipid-laden macrophages are seen, but active lymphocytic infiltrates are rare. Treatment with high-dose methylprednisolone followed by boost and taper doses of prednisone (as in acute rejection) results in resolution of symptoms and radiologic abnormalities.

INFECTIOUS COMPLICATIONS

Lung transplants have the highest rate of infection of all solid organ transplants, with an incidence around 65 percent, about double that of heart transplants, and far greater than the 5 percent to 10 percent incidence seen in kidney transplants.[84]

BACTERIAL

The clinical presentation of bacterial pneumonia may be fulminant with the sudden onset of symptoms over 12 to 24 h. Bacterial bronchitis, wound infections, mediastinitis, empyema, and occasionally sepsis, account for most of the remaining bacterial infections. Cystic fibrosis patients are particularly prone to develop serious infections by *Pseudomonas* species. The diagnosis of bacterial pneumonia is made by the usual criteria of a pulmonary infiltrate, fever, and isolation of a pathogen from a lower respiratory tract specimen. Although fever, dyspnea, leukocytosis, crackles, and pulmonary infiltrates in the early postoperative period are highly suggestive of pneumonia, acute allograft rejection cannot be excluded clinically and invasive procedures usually are required. Expectorated sputum or suctioned secretions in intubated patients provide an adequate specimen for Gram stain and culture. If not, samples can be obtained bronchoscopically. Quantitative culture of bronchoalveolar lavage fluid and protected brush specimens has not been validated in lung transplant recipients, and the preadministration of antibiotics, a rather common circumstance, complicates the interpretation of the data. Gram-negative microorganisms, especially *Pseudomonas* species, are responsible for about 75 percent of all bacteria pneumonias.[85] Other commonly isolated microorganisms are *Haemophilus* influenzae, *Enterobacter* species, *Escherichia coli*, *Staphylococcus aureus*, and oral bacteria. Less commonly, *Serratia marcescens*, *Acinetobacter*, and *Legionella pneumophila* are isolated. A commonly used empiric regimen includes an aminoglycoside plus a third-generation cephalosporin or an antipseudomonal penicillin. Once the sensitivities of the microorganisms are determined, appropriate antibiotics are selected and administered for 10 to 14 days. Occasionally, patients with unresolved lung abscess may benefit from lung resection.

VIRAL

Cytomegalovirus infection is defined as isolation or identification of cytomegalovirus from any site (blood, urine, sputum, stool) or positive seroconversion (presence of cytomegalovirus IgM or fourfold increase in IgG titers) in the absence of clinical symptoms. By contrast, cytomegalovirus disease is defined as invasive or symptomatic cytomegalovirus infection with histologic evidence of viral cytopathic effects or a positive cytomegalovirus culture from a deep tissue specimen in the setting of suggestive clinical manifestations. Infection with cytomegalovirus has a peak incidence between the end of the first and fourth month posttransplant, the period of most intense immunosuppression.[86] The rate of infection varies according to the preoperative serologic status of the donor and recipient and the degree of immunosuppression. All serologic combinations, except donor-negative/recipient-negative, are at high risk of developing symptomatic infection. The prevalence of cytomegalovirus infection in seronegative recipients of seropositive donors has been in the 67 percent to 100 percent range, similar to other organ transplant recipients. By contrast, the prevalence of infection in seronegative recipients of seronegative donors (who also receive only blood products from seronegative donors) is <10 percent.[87] Primary infection occurs when a seronegative recipient is infected with latent virus from a seropositive donor (graft or blood transfusions). Reactivation infection occurs when endogenous latent virus is reactivated under the influence of immunosuppression in a seropositive recipient. Superinfection is characterized by infection of a seropositive recipient with a different strain of cytomegalovirus acquired from a seropositive donor. Clinically, infection develops more commonly in recipients at risk for primary infection (60 percent) than in those at risk for reactivation (20 percent) or superinfection (20 percent to 40 percent).[88] Furthermore, primary cytomegalovirus disease is often more severe and tends to present earlier than that observed in superinfection or reactivation infection. Polyclonal or monoclonal antilymphocyte preparations are the most potent reactivators of active cytomegalovirus infection.[89] Cyclosporin A and tacrolimus are poor reactivators of cytomegalovirus, but once the virus is activated, cyclosporin and tacrolimus effectively block the cytotoxic T-cell response against cytomegalovirus and thereby increase viral replication.[90] Cytomegalovirus itself may cause leukopenia, inversion of T-helper/T-suppressor cell ratios, and depression of cell-mediated immunity and alveolar macrophage function. Patients with cytomegalovirus infection are at greater risk for superinfection from gram-negative bacilli and opportunistic pathogens. Cytomegalovirus may interact with the allograft to induce dysfunction or provoke rejection.[91] Although the exact sequence of events is still controversial, most data suggest that allograft rejection precedes active cytomegalovirus infection. An increase in the level of immunosuppression during rejection may be responsible for the occurrence of cytomegalovirus infection. Conversely, cytomegalovirus induces MHC class I and II antigen expression through release of interferons, which may further contribute to/or precipitate allograft rejection. Augmentation of immunosuppression to treat rejection further promotes viral replication.

Cytomegalovirus causes a wide range of clinical manifestations and infection as with the other herpes viruses, is lifelong, and is incurable. Syndromes of moderate intensity include a flu-like illness, persistent fever, atypical lymphocytosis, chemical hepatitis, leukopenia, and myalgias and arthralgias. Severe syndromes include interstitial pneumonitis, hepatitis, gastrointestinal hemorrhage and ulceration, retinitis, and disseminated disease. Frequently, the target of disease is the organ that is transplanted. More hepatitis occurs in liver transplants and more pneumonitis occurs in lung transplants. Furthermore, the incidence of symptomatic cytomegalo-virus disease is significantly greater among lung transplant recipients than in renal transplants. In lung transplant recipients, the respiratory and gastrointestinal tracts are affected most commonly. Clinical features of cytomegalovirus pneumonitis include a subacute onset, dry cough, tachypnea, dyspnea, hypoxemia, and roentgenographic infiltrates that range from a subtle micronodular appearance to a diffuse bilateral whiteout.[92] Gastrointestinal involvement is signalled by symptoms such as abdominal pain, nausea, vomiting, weight loss, dysphagia, bleeding or ulceration, or, rarely, perforation of any part of the gut. Rare manifestations of cytomegalovirus in transplant patients include retinitis, myocarditis, pancreatitis, acalculous cholecystitis, encephalitis, and adrenalitis.

Isolation of virus from blood (viremia) provides definitive evidence of active cytomegalovirus infection and correlates closely with disease. Employing monoclonal antibodies against the 71-kDa immediate, early antigen of cytomegalovirus incubated on fibroblast monolayers has decreased the incubation time from several weeks to 16 to 24 h.[93] Similarly, the cytomegalovirus antigenemia assay, which detects cytomegalovirus antigen on circulating leukocytes by immunoperoxidase, is a marker of active infection as antigenemia does not occur in healthy cytomegalovirus seropositive individuals. More recently the polymerase chain reaction technique has been used to detect target DNA sequences of cytomegalovirus in circulating leukocytes or plasma. The presence of actively replicating virus in the blood, as indicated by the presence of mRNA for late viral antigens, might be a better marker for cytomegalovirus disease than the presence of cytomegalovirus DNA per se as it detects only actively replicating virus. While these tests are of interest, the diagnosis of cytomegalovirus pneumonitis requires cytologic or histologic confirmation. Standard cytologic examination of bronchoalveolar fluid for cells with viral inclusions has a low sensitivity (21 percent) but a high specificity (98 percent).[84] Bronchoalveolar lavage cells also can be stained directly for the presence of viral antigen. A sensitivity of 86 percent, a specificity of 84 percent, and a negative predictive value of 96 percent for cytomegalovirus pneumonitis has been reported with this technique. The sensitivity of transbronchial biopsies for the diagnosis of cytomegalovirus pneumonia in lung transplant recipients has not been determined. Cytomegalovirus can be recognized in tissue by the characteristic "owl's eye" inclusion bodies. These diagnostic Cowdry type A intranuclear inclusions indicate tissue-invasive infection. In the appropriate clinical setting, presumptive evidence of cytomegalovirus infection is considered adequate for initiation of antiviral therapy with ganciclovir in combination with CMV immune globulin for two to three weeks. Most centers recommend a short, intensive induction treatment followed by a longer period of lower doses. Moderate reduction in the immunosuppressive regimen is usually necessary and well-tolerated.

OTHER VIRAL INFECTIONS

In the absence of acyclovir prophylaxis, infection with Herpes simplex virus usually occurs during the first three weeks posttransplant.[94] The majority of infections represent viral reactivation and involve the oropharyngeal mucosa. Herpes simplex virus pneumonitis is rare and can present in two forms: focal or multifocal pulmonary involvement arising from direct contiguous spread from the oropharynx, or diffuse pulmonary involvement arising from hematogenous dissemination. The clinical features are nonspecific and include fever, cough, dyspnea, and hypoxemia. The diagnosis requires tissue confirmation with immunofluorescent staining. Intravenous acyclovir 10 mg/kg every 8 h for 10 to 14 days is highly effective therapy for infections with these viruses.

Infection with Varicella zoster virus presents with mucocutaneous involvement causing oropharyngeal ulcers and cutaneous eruptions; infection also may present asymptomatically with viral shedding as the sole manifestation. Most infections represent recrudescence of previous infection although primary infections also may occur. The presence of prolonged fever or continued formation of new crops of skin lesions is a useful clue for the presence of infection. The diagnosis is usually made clinically by the appearance of the skin lesions and is supported by the demonstration of multinucleated giant cells on a Tzanck smear of a vesicular lesion. Zoster is diagnosed clinically by the presence of pain and skin lesions along dermatomes.

Clinical manifestations of Epstein-Barr virus infection usually occur during the first three months posttransplant and resemble a mononucleosis-type syndrome with fever, malaise, pharyngitis, adenopathy, and atypical lymphocytosis. Its most ominous significance, however, is its association with posttransplant lymphoproliferative disorders. No effective therapy exists for infection with Epstein-Barr virus.

The respiratory syncytial virus is an uncommon cause of interstitial pneumonitis in lung transplant recipients. Clinical manifestations include fever, cough, and ear or sinus involvement. Wheezing may be a prominent physical finding. The seasonal nature of the infection (winter and spring) and the high frequency of upper respiratory tract symptoms and signs should suggest the possibility of infection with this virus. Infection with respiratory syncytial virus is treated with aerosolized ribavirin (6 g reconstituted in 300 ml of sterile water to a final concentration of 20 mg/ml and administered 12 to 18 h per day for 3 to 7 days), although no clinical trials have been conducted in this patient population.

FUNGAL

Invasive fungal infections are the most lethal of all infections in transplant recipients. They occur relatively infrequently and mostly in patients who have other complications or are treated frequently for episodes of rejection. Fungal infections can be considered in two categories: (1) those mycoses with geographic distribution such as histoplasmosis, coccidiomycosis, and blastomycosis; and (2) the ubiquitous mycoses such as aspergillosis, candidiosis, and mucormycosis, which tend to cause potentially lethal disease in immunocompromised hosts.

The clinical presentation of invasive pulmonary aspergillosis includes nonspecific symptoms such as fever, dyspnea, dry cough, and pleuritic chest pain or hemoptysis. Wheezing is particularly prominent in patients with tracheobronchial involvement, and bronchoscopic examination may reveal pseudomembranes that cover the bronchial mucosa, often extending to subsegmental orifices.[95] The radiographic features are variable with focal, nodular, or diffuse infiltrates. Some patients demonstrate peripheral triangular infiltrates that arise as a result of vascular invasion and infarction. Because colonization is common among transplant recipients, the diagnosis of tissue-invasive aspergillosis requires biopsy of infected tissues. Transbronchial biopsies, however, may be unrewarding even in the setting of tissue invasion. Multiple positive cultures from respiratory secretions in patients on high-dose corticosteroids or receiving antilymphocyte products is disturbing as it may signal invasive pulmonary infection.

Candidiasis is the most common fungal infection reported in liver and heart-lung transplant recipients. Although isolation of *Candida* from respiratory secretions is not unusual, candida pneumonitis occurs infrequently. Mucocutaneous involvement is most common but other presentations include mediastinitis, colonization and infection of intravascular catheters, mycotic aneurysms of vascular anastomosis, and disseminated infection.

Amphotericin B still is regarded as the treatment of choice for infections with *Aspergillus* and *Candida*. However, because of the additive nephrotoxicity with cyclosporin, itraconazole and fluconazole may be acceptable alternatives for *Aspergillus* and *Candida*, respectively. Response to either form of treatment, however, is disappointing once deep-seated infections are diagnosed.

PARASITIC

Pneumocystis carinii has been eradicated almost completely from the lung transplant population since the routine use of trimethoprim/sulfamethoxazole as prophylaxis. The diagnosis usually is made on expectorated or induced sputum, or in bronchoalveolar lavage fluid. First-line drugs for treatment include trimethoprim/sulfamethoxazole, pentamidine, and the combination of clindamycin plus primaquine.

MYCOBACTERIAL INFECTIONS

Infections with *Mycobacterium* occur infrequently. The onset of infection is usually late, with the majority of patients developing the disease after six months to a year after transplant. Respiratory symptoms may be minimal and prolonged fever or persistent pulmonary infiltrates may be the only manifestations. The majority of infections are caused by reactivation of tuberculous mycobacteria in the recipient; however, infections with mycobacteria other than tuberculosis or reactivation of previously undetected disease in the transplanted allograft also can occur. The diagnosis is suspected by identification of acid-fast bacilli on pulmonary secretions or tissue specimens and is confirmed by culture and isolation of the microorganisms. Tuberculin skin testing is not helpful because of the high incidence of cutaneous anergy while on immunosuppression. Mycobacterial disease in transplant recipients usually responds to standard antituberculous therapy. Short-course therapy with three drugs is usually effective, but some authors recommend 18-month regimens with two or three drugs. The possibility of drug interactions and toxicities must be taken into account and doses of immunosuppressants adjusted accordingly. The incidence of reactivation of tuberculosis is low even among transplant recipients who are tuberculin positive before transplant and isoniazid prophylaxis is not routinely recommended in most centers.

NEOPLASIA

Malignancies that show a disproportionate increase in transplant recipients include those in which viral infections, particularly those of the herpesvirus group, are thought to play a part. These include non-Hodgkin lymphoma, Kaposi sarcoma, cancer of the vulva and vagina, hepatocarcinoma, carcinoma of the pharynx and esophagus, leukemia, and invasive cancer of the cervix. In 1993 the Transplant Tumor Registry reported 7248 types of cancer in 6798 transplant recipients.[35] Most have developed in kidney (5912) or heart (527) transplant recipients, while only 44 cancers have been reported in lung transplant or heart-lung transplant recipients, this reflecting the greater number and longer follow-up of kidney transplant recipients. Data from several large kidney and heart transplant programs show an overall incidence of cancer ranging from 3 percent to 9 percent, with a mean of 6 percent.

Transplant recipients develop a variety of malignancies that are uncommon in the general population: lymphomas (23 percent versus 5 percent), lip cancer (7 percent versus 0.3 percent), Kaposi sarcoma (6 percent versus a negligible incidence), hypernephroma (5 percent versus 2 percent), and carcinomas of the vulva and perineum (4 percent versus 0.5 percent). The most common tumors reported to the Transplant Tumor Registry are carcinomas of the skin and lips (37 percent). While in the general population basal cell carcinoma outnumbers squamous cell carcinoma (5 to 1), the reverse is true in transplant patients (1 to 1.8). Squamous cell cancers in the transplant population also appear at an earlier age, more often are multiple, and are more aggressive than in the general population.

POSTTRANSPLANT LYMPHOPROLIFERATIVE DISORDERS

The great majority of lymphomas after transplantation are non-Hodgkins lymphomas, which make up 94 percent of the total (65 percent in the general population) while only 2 percent to 5 percent are cases of Hodgkin disease (14 percent in the general population). Two large epidemiologic studies in renal transplant recipients showed a 28- to 49-fold increase in frequency of lymphomas compared with age-matched controls.[96] A predisposition to posttransplant lymphoproliferative disorders has been noted in organ transplant recipients since 1968, long before the advent of cyclosporin. The spectrum of lymphoproliferative disorders ranges from a slow-growing polyclonal proliferation of lymphocytes to a very aggressive monoclonal malignancy that is rapidly fatal. Almost all of these tumors are of the B-cell type and are associated with the presence of Epstein-Barr virus (EBV) infection.[97] Posttransplant lymphomas differ from their counterpart in the general population in that extranodal involvement is more common (69 percent versus 24 percent to 48 percent), central nervous system involvement is more common (28 percent versus 1 percent), and isolated CNS involvement is common in transplant patients but rare in the general population.

Epstein-Barr–related lymphoma and lower-grade lymphoproliferative disorders are reported in 2 percent to 10 percent of lung transplant recipients.[98] The major predisposing factors appear to be the intensity and duration of immunosuppression and the use of anti–T cell antibodies. Clinical presentation of these disorders may be as innocuous as an incidental finding on a chest roentgenogram. More often, however, patients complain of fatigue, low-grade fever, adenopathy, or gastrointestinal symptoms. Most of these neoplasms occur during the first year posttransplant and have an unusual propensity to involve the transplanted lung. The cornerstone of therapy appears to be reduction of immunosuppression. Adjunctive measures such as chemotherapy and acyclovir also have been tried with some success in polyclonal proliferations. In cases of truly localized disease, complete resection appears to be curative. Long-term prognosis remains unclear. Prognosis for patients with aggressive disease is dismal regardless of therapy.

HYPERTENSION

Hypertension may occur independently of cyclosporin-induced renal toxicity and may require treatment with antihypertensives. β-adrenoceptor blocking agents are not recommended due to their potential role in increasing serum cholesterol levels. Withdrawal of corticosteroids in renal transplant patients results in significant reductions in blood pressure and in the number of antihypertensive agents required by patients maintained on cyclosporin. First-line therapy relies on calcium channel antagonists, particularly nifedipine, which does not compete with cyclosporin for cytochrome P-450 IIIA metabolism.[99] For patients with persistent edema or hyperkalemia, loop diuretics might be combined with sodium restriction. Angiotensin-converting enzyme in-hibitors may exacerbate glomerular hypovascularity and renal function by unloading the efferent arteriole, and, therefore, are not commonly recommended. Diltiazem is an attractive therapy because of its renal protective effect.

HYPERLIPIDEMIA

Patients on cyclosporin and/or prednisone tend to have hyperlipidemia with elevations in all fractions.[100] Corticosteroids appear to be the single most important contributing factor for hypercholesterolemia after transplant. Plasma levels appear to peak in the first three to six months posttransplant, the time during which most episodes of rejection are usually treated. The contribution of cyclosporin to posttransplant hypercholesterolemia is more difficult to discern. The mechanism may involve cyclosporin-induced enzymatic inhibition of oxidation of bile acid intermediates in the liver, with resultant increase in intracellular cholesterol and downregulation of LDL receptor synthesis. Withdrawal of corticosteroids in cyclosporin-treated transplant recipients decreases total serum cholesterol levels by 13 percent to 18 percent, but the total to high-density lipoprotein ratios remain unchanged. Optimization of immunosuppression and maintenance of body weight are important factors in limiting the severity of posttransplant hyperlipidemia. The greatest benefit derives from the avoidance of unnecessary treatment of rejection with corticosteroids. Bile acid binding resins such as cholestyramine have been used to reduce serum cholesterol levels. Since these agents can decrease micelle formation and fat absorption, care must be used to avoid interfering with cyclosporin absorption. Gemfibrozil reduces hepatic triglyceride and very-low-density lipoprotein synthesis and production; however, it does not lower cholesterol. Since both gemfibrozil and cyclosporin have been associated with increased gallstone formation, patients should be monitored for this complication. 3-hydroxy-3-methylglutaryl-coenzyme A (HMG CoA) reductase inhibitors such as mevalamic acid (lovastatin) lower total serum cholesterol and low-density lipoprotein levels in cyclosporin-treated cardiac transplant recipients. However, this drug has been associated with rhabdomyolysis and acute renal failure when used in conjunction with cyclosporin. Lower doses can lower cholesterol with fewer complications. Provastatin successfully lowers serum cholesterol in cyclosporin-treated renal transplant recipients and may have fewer side effects.

NEPHROTOXICITY

Cyclosporin nephrotoxicity is characterized by fluid retention, increased serum creatinine and urea concentration, a fall in glomerular filtration rate, decreased sodium and potassium excretion, and high blood pressure. Risk factors include trough whole blood levels of cyclosporin greater than 400 ng/ml, preexisting renal damage, hypertension, and use of other nephrotoxic drugs. Acute nephrotoxicity begins during the first 7 days of therapy, a subacute form most frequently but not extensively between 7 and 60 days, and a chronic form as early as 30 days. Acute nephrotoxicity is manifested by increases in creatinine and urea nitrogen with preserved urine volumes and sodium excretion. When cyclosporin doses are reduced, renal function usually improves completely. Subacute nephrotoxicity also is manifested by increases in creatinine and urea nitrogen. As in acute toxicity, this form also is reversible upon reduction in cyclosporin dosages. Chronic nephrotoxicity is characterized by significant reductions in glomerular filtration rate and increases in creatinine and urea nitrogen usually during the first six months of therapy, which worsens over three to four years. Thereafter, in most patients, the renal deterioration appears to stabilize. At this point, however, significant increases in creatinine and urea nitrogen are almost universal. Because the great majority of lung transplant recipients are not yet at the five-year survival mark, the extent of this complication may not be realized fully. The most common pharmacologic approach to decrease nephrotoxicity is the use of calcium channel antagonists to counteract the cyclosporin-induced vasoconstriction and mesangial cell calcium uptake. Calcium channel antagonists improve the early and long-term renal function of kidney transplant recipients. A second strategy employs agents that alter the prostacyclin/thromboxane balance. Results with iloprost (prostacyclin analogue), enisoprost (prostaglandin E1 analogue), fish oils

(thromboxane antagonists), and picotamide (inhibitor of thromboxane synthesis and receptor function) are equivocal. A third approach is the administration of cytochrome P-450 IIIA system inhibitors such as ketoconazole, diltiazem, or verapamil to reduce cyclosporin doses and to block the generation of putative, but yet unknown, nephrotoxic metabolites. A fourth strategy is the administration of pentoxifylline, a cytokine inhibitor that has been shown to mitigate renal dysfunction in transplant recipients. Careful control of trough concentrations and combination immunosuppression can, by using significantly lower doses of each agent, reduce renal toxicity.

The clinical presentation and morphology of tacrolimus nephrotoxicity is identical to those of cyclosporin, and the incidence of this adverse effect is broadly similar for patients treated with either drug. The incidence of nephrotoxicity necessitating withdrawal from therapy in renal transplant recipients is similar for tacrolimus and cyclosporin. Chronic nephrotoxicity occurs in 30 percent to 50 percent of liver transplants treated with tacrolimus.

References

1. Jamieson SW, Reitz BA, Oyer PE, et al.: Combined heart and lung transplantation. *Lancet* 1983; i:1130.
2. Toronto Lung Transplant Group: Unilateral lung transplantation for pulmonary fibrosis. *N Engl J Med* 1986; 314:1140.
3. Macoviak JA: Four year experience with cyclosporine for heart and heart-lung transplantation. *Transplant Proc* 1985; 17(suppl 2):97.
4. Borel J, Feurer C, Gubler HB, Stahelin H: Biologic effects of cyclosporine A: a new antilymphocytic agent. *Agents Actions* 1976; 6:465.
5. Marshall SE, Kramer MR, Lewiston NJ, et al.: Selection and evaluation of recipients for heart-lung and lung transplantation. *Chest* 1990; 98:1488.
6. Mal H, Andreassian B, Pamela F, et al.: Unilateral lung transplantation in end-stage pulmonary emphysema. *Am Rev Respir Dis* 1989; 140:797.
7. Maurer JR, Winton TL, Patterson GA, Williams TR: Single-lung transplantation for pulmonary vascular disease. *Transplant Proc* 1991; 23:1211.
8. Cooper JD, Patterson GA, Grossman R, et al.: Double-lung transplant for advanced chronic obstructive lung disease. *Am Rev Respir Dis* 1989; 139:303.
9. Yacoub MH, Banner NR, Khaghani A, et al.: Heart-lung transplantation for cystic fibrosis and subsequent domino heart transplantation. *J Heart Transplant* 1990; 9:459.
10. Mason DW, Morris PJ: Effector mechanisms in allograft rejection. *Annu Rev Immunol* 1986; 4:119.
11. Borst J, Alexander S, Elder J, Terhorst C: The T3 complex on human T lymphocytes in-volves four structurally distinct glycoproteins. *J Biol Chem* 1983; 258:5135.
12. Sayegh M, Watschinger B, Carpenter CB: Mechanisms of T cell recognition of alloantigen. The role of peptides. *Transplantation* 1994; 57:1295.
13. Shoskes D: Indirect presentation of MHC antigens in transplantation. *Immunol Today* 1994; 15:32.
14. Swain SL: T cell subsets and the recognition of MHC class. *Immunol Rev* 1983; 74:129.
15. Neefjes J, Momburg F: Cell biology of antigen presentation. *Curr Opin Immunol* 1993; 5:27.

16. Gorski A: The role of cell adhesion molecules in immunopathology. *Immunol Today* 1994; 15:252.

17. Heemann UW, Tullius SG, Azuma H, et al.: Adhesion molecules and transplantation. *Ann Surg* 1994; 219:4.

18. Hayry P: Intragraft events in allograft destruction. *Transplantation* 1985; 38:1–4.

19. Aschner N: Cellular events within the rejecting allograft. *Transplantation* 1984; 35:193.

20. Borel JF, Feurer C, Magnee C, Stahelin H: Effects of the new anti-lymphocyte peptide cyclosporine A in animals. *Immunology* 1977; 32:1017.

21. Handschumacher RE, Harding MW, Rice J, Drugge RJ: Cyclophilin: a specific cytosolic binding protein for cyclosporine A. *Science* 1984; 226:544.

22. Liu J, Farmer JD Jr, Lane WS, et al.: Calcineurin is a common target of cyclophilin-cyclosporin A and FKBP-FK506 complexes. *Cell* 1991; 66:807.

23. Kahan BD, Van Buren CT, Lin SN, et al.: Immunopharmacological monitoring of cyclosporin A–treated patients. *Transplantation* 1982; 34:36.

24. Wood AJ, Maurer G, Niederberger W, Beveridge T: Cyclosporine: pharmacokinetics, metabolism and drug interactions. *Transplant Proc* 1983; 15:2409.

25. Niederberger W, Lemaire M, Maurer G, et al.: Distribution and binding of cyclosporine in blood and tissues. *Transplant Proc* 1983; 15(suppl 1):203.

26. Atkinson K, Boland J, Britton K, Biggs J: Blood and tissue distribution of cyclosporine in humans and mice. *Transplant Proc* 1983; 15(suppl 1):214.

27. Maurer G, Loosli HR, Schrier E, Keller B: Disposition of cyclosporine in several animal species and man. 1. Structural elucidation of its metabolites. *Drug Metab Dispos* 1984; 12:120.

28. Weir MR, Klassen DK, Shen SY, et al.: Acute effects of IV cyclosporine on renal function in healthy humans. *Transplant Proc* 1989; 21:915.

29. Kawaguchi A, Goldman MN, Shapiro R, et al.: Increase in urinary thromboxane B_2 in rats caused by cyclosporine. *Transplantation* 1985; 40:214.

30. Hoover EL, Harrison BS, Williams WW, et al.: Decrease in cyclosporin mediated prostacyclin production in renal versus carotid arteries. A mechanism for cyclosporine-induced hypertension. *J Surg Res* 1990; 48:481.

31. Curtis JJ, Luke RG, Jones P, Diethelm AG: Hypertension in cyclosporin-treated renal transplant recipients is sodium dependent. *Am J Med* 1988; 85:134.

32. Vine W, Billiar T, Simmons R, Bowers LD: Cyclosporine-induced hepatotoxicity: a microassay by hepatocytes in tissue culture. *Transplant Proc* 1988; 29(suppl 3):859.

33. De Groen PC, Aksamit AJ, Rakela J, et al.: Central nervous system toxicity after liver transplantation. The role of cyclosporine and cholesterol. *N Engl J Med* 1987; 317:861.

34. Adams DH, Ponsford S, Gunson B, et al.: Neurological complications following liver transplantation. *Lancet* 1987; i:949.

35. Penn I: Incidence and treatment of neoplasia after transplantation. *J Heart Lung Transplant* 1993; 12:S328.

36. Penn I: The changing pattern of posttransplant malignancies. *Transplant Proc* 1991; 23:1101.

37. Weir MR: Therapeutic benefits of calcium channel blockers in cyclosporine-treated organ transplant recipients: blood pressure control and immunosuppression. *Am J Med* 1991; 90(5A):32S.

38. Kino T, Hatanaka H, Miyata S, et al.: FK-506, a novel immunosuppressant isolated from a Streptomyces. II. Immunosuppressive effect of FK-506 in vitro. *J Antibiot* 1987; 40:1256.

39. Siekierka JJ, Hung SHY, Poe M, et al.: A cytosolic binding protein for the immunosuppressant FK-506 has peptidyl-prolyl isomerase activity but is distinct from cyclophilin. *Nature* 1989; 341:755.

40. Harding MW, Galat A, Uehling DE, Schreiber SL: A receptor for the immunosuppressant FK-506 is a *cis-trans* peptidyl-prolyl isomerase. *Nature* 1989; 341:758.

41. Kay JE, Benzie CR, Goddier MR, et al.: Inhibition of T-lymphocyte activation by the immunosuppressive drug FK-506. *Immunology* 1989; 67:473.

42. Venkataramanan R, Jain A, Cadoff E, et al.: Pharmacokinetics of FK 506: preclinical and clinical studies. *Transplant Proc* 1990; 22(suppl 1):52.

43. Jusko WJ, D'Ambrosio RD: Monitoring FK 506 concentrations in plasma and whole blood. *Transplant Proc* 1991; 23:2732.

44. Habucky K, Flowers J, Warty VJ, et al.: Blood protein binding (BPB) of FK-506 (F) in various species. Abs. Pharmaceutical Research 1992; 9(suppl):S-334.

45. Sattler M, Guengerich FP, Yun CH, et al.: Cytochrome P-450 3A enzymes are responsible for biotransformation of FK 506 and rapamycin in man and rat. *Drug Metab Dispos* 1992; 20:753.

46. Jain AB, Abu-Elmagd K, Abdallah H, et al.: Pharmacokinetics of FK 506 in liver transplant recipients after continuous intravenous infusion. *J Clin Pharmacol* 1993; 33:606.

47. Ali Shah I, Whiting PH, Omar G, et al.: Effects of FK 506 on human hepatic microsomal cytochrome P450–dependent drug metabolism in vitro. *Transplant Proc* 1991; 23:2783.

48. Omar G, Shah A, Thompson AW, et al.: FK 506 inhibition of cyclosporine metabolism by human liver microsomes. *Transplant Proc* 1991; 23:934.

49. McCauley J: The nephrotoxicity of FK 506 as compared to cyclosporine. *Current Opinion in Nephrology and Hypertension* 1993; 2:662.

50. Tabasco-Minguillan J, Mieles L, Caroll P, et al.: Long-term insulin requirement after liver transplantation with FK 506 in american veterans. *Transplant Proc* 1993; 25:677.

51. Clements PJ, Davis J: Cytotoxic drugs: their clinical application to the rheumatic diseases. *Semin Arthritis Rheum* 1986; 15:231.

52. Bertino JR: Chemical action and pharmacology of methotrexate, azathioprine and cyclophosphamide in man. *Arthritis Rheum* 1973; 16:79.

53. Bach JF, Dardenne M: The metabolism of azathioprine in renal failure. *Transplantation* 1971; 12:253.

54. Huskisson EC: Azathioprine. *Clin Rheum Dis* 1984; 10:325.

55. Lorenzen I, Videbaek A: Treatment of collagen diseases with cytostatics. *Lancet* 1965; ii:558.

56. Berry H, Liyanage SP, Durance RA, et al.: Azathioprine and penicillamine in treatment of rheumatoid arthritis. *Br Med J* 1976; 1:1052.

57. Hollenberg SM, Giguere V, Segui P, Evans RM: Colocalization of DNA-binding and transcriptional activation functions in the human glucocorticoid receptor. *Cell* 1987; 49:39.

58. Miyata Y, Yahara I: Cytoplasmic 8 S glucocorticoid receptor binds to actin filaments through the 90-kDa heat shock protein moiety. *J Biol Chem* 1991; 266:8779.

59. Knudsen PJ, Dinarello CA, Strom TB: Glucocorticoids inhibit transcriptional and post-transcriptional expression of interleukin 1 in U937 cells. *J Immunol* 1987; 139:4129.

60. Starzl TE, Marchioro TL, Porter KA, et al.: The use of heterologous antilymphoid agents in canine renal and liver homotransplantation and in human renal homotransplantation. *Surg Gynecol Obstet* 1967; 124:301.

61. Kahan BD: Timeline of immunosuppression. *Transplant Proc* 1993; 25(suppl 3): 1.

62. Kung PC, Goldstein G, Reinherz EL, Schlossman SF: Monoclonal antibodies defining distinctive human T cell surface antigens. *Science* 1979; 206:347.

63. Reinherz EL, Meuer S, Fitzgerald KA, et al.: Antigen recognition

by human T lymphocytes is linked to surface expression of the T3 molecular complex. *Cell* 1982; 30:735.

64. Ortho Multicenter Transplant Study Group: A randomized clinical trial of OKT3 monoclonal antibody for acute rejection of cadaveric renal transplants. *N Engl J Med* 1985; 313:337.

65. Dorsky DI, Crumpacker CS: Drugs five years later: acyclovir. *Ann Intern Med* 1987; 107:859.

66. St. Clair MH, Furman PA, Lubbers CM, Elion GB: Inhibition of cellular α and virally induced deoxyribonucleic acid polymerases by the triphosphate of acyclovir. *Antimicrob Agents Chemother* 1980; 18:741.

67. Wade JC, Hintz M, McGuffin RW, et al.: Treatment of cytomegalovirus pneumonia with high-dose acyclovir. *Am J Med* 1982; 73(suppl):249.

68. Keeney RE, Kirk LE, Brigden D: Acyclovir tolerance in humans. *Am J Med* 1982; 73(suppl):176.

69. Bean B, Aeppli D: Adverse effects of high-dose intravenous acyclovir in ambulatory patients with acute herpes zoster. *J Infect Dis* 1985; 151:362.

70. Cheng YC, Grill SP, Dutschman GE, et al.: Effect of 9-(1,3-dihydroxy-2-propoxymethyl)guanine, a new anti-herpes compound, on synthesis of macromolecules in herpes simplex virus-infected cells. *Antimicrob Agents Chemother* 1984; 26:283.

71. Tyms AS, Davis JM, Clarke JR, Jeffries DJ: Synthesis of cytomegalovirus DNA is an antiviral target late in virus growth. *J Gen Virol* 1987; 68:1563.

72. Jacobson MA, De Miranda P, Cederberg DM, et al.: Human pharmacokinetics and tolerance of oral ganciclovir. *Antimicrob Agents Chemother* 1987; 31:1251.

73. Harbison MA, De Girolami PC, Jenkins JL, Hammer SM: Gancyclovir therapy of severe cytomegalovirus infections in solid-organ transplant recipients. *Transplantation* 1988; 46:82.

74. Snydman DR: Prevention of cytomegalovirus-associated diseases with immunoglobulin. *Transplant Proc* 1991; 23(suppl 3): 131.

75. Maurer JR, Tullis DE, Grossman RF, et al.: Infectious complications following isolated lung transplantation. *Chest* 1992; 101:1056.

76. Todd TRJ: Early postoperative management following lung transplantation. *Clin Chest Med* 1990; 11:259.

77. Ettinger NA, Bailey TC, Trulock EP, et al.: Cytomegalovirus infection and pneumonitis. Impact after isolated lung transplantation. *Am Rev Respir Dis* 1993; 147:1017.

78. Gryzan S, Paradis IL, Zeevi A, et al.: Unexpectedly high incidence of *Pneumocystis carinii* infection after lung-heart transplantation. *Am Rev Respir Dis* 1988; 137:1268.

79. Yousem SA, Berry GJ, Brunt EM, et al.: A working formulation for the standardization of nomenclature in the diagnosis of heart and lung rejection. *J Heart Lung Transplant* 1990; 9:593.

80. Reitz BA, Gaudiani VA, Hunt SA, et al.: Diagnosis and treatment of allograft rejection in heart-lung transplant recipients. *J Thorac Cardiovasc Surg* 1983; 85:354.

81. Burke CM, Theodore J, Baldwin JC, et al.: Twenty-eight cases of human heart-lung transplantation. *Lancet* 1986; i:517.

82. Otulana BA, Higenbottam T, Scott J, et al.: Lung function associated with histologically diagnosed acute lung rejection and pulmonary infection in heart-lung transplant patients. *Am Rev Respir Dis* 1990; 142:329.

83. Glanville A, Baldwin J, Burke C, et al.: Obliterative bronchiolitis after heart-lung transplantation: apparent arrest by augmented immunosuppression. *Ann Intern Med* 1987; 107:300.

84. Ettinger NA, Trulock EP: Pulmonary considerations or organ transplantation. Part 3. *Am Rev Respir Dis* 1991; 144:433.

85. Dauber JH, Paradis IL, Dummer JS: Infectious complications in pulmonary allograft recipients. *Clin Chest Med* 1990; 11:291.

86. The TH, van den Berg AP, van Son WJ, et al.: Monitoring for cytomegalovirus after organ transplantation: a clinical perspective. *Transplant Proc* 1993; 25(suppl 4):5.

87. Farrugia E, Schwab TR: Management and prevention of cytomegalovirus infection after renal transplantation. *Mayo Clin Proc* 1992; 67:879.

88. Ho M: Cytomegalovirus infection and indirect sequelae in the immunocompromised transplant patient. *Transplant Proc* 1991; 23(suppl 1):2.

89. Rubin RH, Tolkoff-Rubin NE, Oliver D, et al.: Multicenter seroepidemiologic study of the impact of cytomegalovirus infection on renal transplantation. *Transplantation* 1985; 40:243.

90. Rubin RH, Tolkoff-Rubin NE: The impact of infection on the outcome of transplantation. *Transplant Proc* 1991; 23:2068.

91. Schrier RD, Rice GPA, Oldstone MBA: Suppression of natural killer cell activity and T cell proliferation by fresh isolates of human cytomegalovirus. *J Infect Dis* 1986; 153:1084.

92. Glenn J: Cytomegalovirus infections following renal transplantation. *Rev Infect Dis* 1981; 3:1151.

93. Paya CV, Wold AD, Smith TF: Detection of cytomegalovirus infections in specimens other than urine by the shell vial assay and conventional tube cell cultures. *J Clin Microbiol* 1987; 25:755.

94. Smyth RL, Higenbottam TW, Scott JP, et al.: Herpes simplex virus infection in heart-lung transplant recipients. *Transplantation* 1990; 49:735.

95. Kramer MR, Denning DW, Marshall SE, et al.: Ulcerative tracheobronchitis after lung transplantation. A new form of invasive aspergillosis. *Am Rev Respir Dis* 1991; 144:552.

96. Kinlen LJ: Incidence of cancer in rheumatoid arthritis and other disorders after immunosuppressive treatment. *Am J Med* 1985; 78(suppl 1A):44.

97. Nalesnik MA, Makowka L, Starzl TE: The diagnosis and treatment of posttransplant lymphoproliferative disorders. *Curr Probl Surg* 1988; 25:371.

98. Randhawa PS, Yousem SA, Paradis IL, et al.: The clinical spectrum, pathology and clonal analysis of Epstein-Barr virus–associated lymphoproliferative disorders in heart-lung transplant recipients. *Am J Clin Pathol* 1989; 92:177.

99. Morales JM, Andres A, Prieto C, et al.: Calcium antagonist treatment of recipients minimises early cyclosporine nephrotoxicity in renal transplantation: a prospective randomized trial. *Transplant Proc* 1989; 21:137.

100. de Hoyos A, Maurer JR: Complications following lung transplantation. *Sem Thorac Cardiovasc Surg* 1992; 4:132.

Chapter 119 _____

PHARMACOLOGIC MANAGEMENT OF AIRWAY CALIBER DURING SURGICAL ANESTHESIA

CAROL A. HIRSHMAN

Inhalation Anesthetics

Induction Agents
  Barbiturates
  Ketamine
  Propofol

Neuromuscular Blocking Drugs

Local Anesthetics

Conclusions

Smooth-muscle contraction largely is responsible for the rapid decrease in airway caliber seen during anesthesia and provoked by the presence of irritating substances in the airway. Parasympathetic nervous system stimulation plays a major role. The local anesthetics affect airway caliber by blocking airway reflexes, whereas inhalational anesthetics, induction agents, and neuromuscular blocking drugs modulate smooth muscle tone by direct effects on airway smooth muscle, as well as by indirect effects on nerves.[1] The mechanisms by which these four classes of drugs alter airway tone are a topic of considerable clinical interest, particularly in patients with asthma in whom airway constriction easily is precipitated. The opioids and benzodiazepines have little effect on airway tone and reactivity and is not discussed.

Inhalational Anesthetics

The potent inhalational anesthetics historically fall into two groups: those available prior to 1956 and those available after that date. The anesthetics available prior to 1956 include ether, cyclopropane, and chloroform, which are no longer used. In 1956, they were replaced by halothane, followed by enflurane, isoflurane and, more recently, desflurane, and in some countries sevoflurane. The clinical popularity of the potent inhalational anesthetics is based largely on their lack of flammability, ease with which depth of anesthesia is changed, rapid awakening, and low incidence of toxicity. A common way of comparing potencies of different inhalational anesthetics is the minimal alveolar

concentration (MAC). A dose of 1 MAC is defined as the end-tidal anesthetic concentration that will prevent movement in response to surgical incision in 50 percent of patients. In individual patients, adequate anesthesia is provided by doses ranging from 0.2 to 2 MAC.

Potent inhalational anesthetics such as halothane prevent and reverse bronchoconstriction by: (1) blocking airway neural reflexes, (2) directly relaxing airway smooth muscle, and (3) inhibiting mediator release. The action of potent inhalational anesthetics on airway reflexes has been studied for decades, and the ability of halothane, cyclopropane, ether, and enflurane to block a wide variety of airway reflexes has been well established. Reflex airway stimulation involves afferent receptors, afferent neural pathways, central synapses, efferent pre- and postganglionic nerves, and the ganglia. Inhalational anesthetics may block at any of those sites, but the precise site of action of inhalational anesthetics in the reflex pathway is not known. It is likely that the actions of inhalational anesthetics on this reflex are complex and that inhibition occurs at more than one site.[2] Inhalational anesthetics bronchodilate unconstricted[3] as well as constricted airways, since airways of many species, including the human, have resting vagal tone.

At high clinical concentrations, all the commonly used inhalational anesthetics studied (halothane, isoflurane, enflurane, and sevoflurane) are equally effective at preventing and reversing bronchoconstriction when airway changes are assessed by conventional means.[3] However, recent studies from Brown et al.[4], using high-resolution computed tomography, a more sensitive technique, confirmed a long-

supplied as a 1% emulsion. Injection of 2 mg/kg induces anesthesia within 10 to 20 s, like thiopental, but the emergence from anesthesia is more rapid. Data on airway tone and responsiveness with this agent are only starting to emerge. A recent report in patients with chronic obstructive pulmonary disease who required mechanical ventilation noted decreases in airway resistance after administration of propofol. In asymptomatic patients with asthma and in nonasthmatic patients, there is a significantly lower incidence of wheezing after tracheal intubation when propofol, rather than a barbiturate, was used to induce anesthesia.[6] These studies suggest that propofol may be a useful alternative for rapid induction of anesthesia in patients at risk for the development of bronchospasm. However, the mechanisms by which propofol acts on airways are not known.

Neuromuscular Blocking Drugs

Although neuromuscular blocking drugs are not anesthetics, they are used to facilitate tracheal intubation to provide muscle relaxation intraoperatively. Two main classes are available: the depolarizing and nondepolarizing blocking agents. Succinylcholine is the major nondepolarizing neuromuscular blocker used today to facilitate intubation. A dose of 0.5 to 1 mg/kg first induces muscle fasciculations, then paralysis within 60 to 90 s that becomes maximal at 2 min. The drug is metabolized rapidly by plasma pseudocholinesterases, and its effects are gone in 3 to 5 min. There are many nondepolarizing neuromuscular blockers currently available with differing onsets of action of duration, including d-tubocurarine, gallamine, pancuronium, vecuronium, atracurium, and more recently mivicurium, pipecuronium, rocuronium, and doxacurium. The oldest drug of this class, d-tubocurarine, is rarely used today.

There are few controlled studies regarding the effects of neuromuscular blocking drugs on airway tone in humans. One study found little effect in normal subjects, while another study found that pulmonary resistance was greater in subjects with pulmonary disease who were paralyzed with d-tubocurarine than in comparable subjects paralyzed with pancuronium.[9]

Neuromuscular blocking agents possess two characteristics that theoretically can alter airway tone and reactivity. To interact with nicotinic cholinergic receptors at the neuromuscular junction of skeletal muscle, these agents must resemble acetylcholine structurally. Thus, it is likely that these agents also will bind to muscarinic receptors located on ganglia, nerve endings, and airway smooth muscle and interact with tissue cholinesterases, altering neurally mediated control of airway tone. Moreover, many, but not all, of these agents are capable of inducing histamine release from mast cells lining the blood vessels into which they are injected.[9]

Gallamine no longer is administered clinically to induce muscle paralysis because its use was associated with tachycardia. This is caused by blockade of the cardiac M_2-muscarinic receptors. M_2-muscarinic receptors also are located presynaptically on parasympathetic postganglionic nerves. Activation of these M_2-muscarinic receptors limits the release of acetylcholine from the nerves. Thus, blockade of neuronal M_2-muscarinic receptors potentiates vagally induced bronchoconstriction. Conversely, blockade of M_3-muscarinic receptors on the airway smooth muscle inhibits vagally mediated bronchoconstriction. Therefore, agents that have only M_3- or both M_2- and M_3-muscarinic antagonist activity should not increase airway tone. Pancuronium and pipecuronium have both M_2- and M_3-antagonist activity. Mivicurium blocks M_3-receptors, whereas doxacurium and vecuronium are antagonists with neither M_2- nor M_3-muscarinic receptor antagonist activity.

The administration of d-tubocurarine and atracurium to healthy subjects is associated with increases in plasma histamine concentration and significant hypotension, but wheezing has generally not been reported. A study by Mehr and associates[10] in this laboratory showed that atracurium constricted peripheral airways in dogs at doses that produced significant cardiovascular effects. The airway constriction, however, was short-lived and was totally prevented by H_1-histamine receptor antagonist pretreatment.

Since chemists are now able to synthesize neuromuscular blocking drugs that avoid most of the unwanted side effects, it seems reasonable to select agents that lack M_2-muscarinic receptor blocking activity or histamine releasing properties, particularly in patients at risk for developing bronchospasm.

Cholinesterase inhibitors such as neostigmine, physostigmine, and edrophonium are used to reverse neuromuscular blockade caused by nondepolarizing neuromuscular blockers. These agents inhibit the destruction of endogenously released acetylcholine at the motor end plate. This allows the concentrations of acetylcholine to increase to the point where the neuromuscular block is overcome. Similar effects can occur at parasympathetic efferent nerve terminals, provoking airway constriction by activation of M_3-muscarinic receptors on airway smooth muscle. However, these effects can readily be prevented and reversed by muscarinic antagonists such as atropine and glycopyrrolate.

Local Anesthetics

Local anesthetics prevent the generation and conduction of nerve impulses in any part of the nervous system and in any type of fiber, including the nerves in the lung that modulate airway tone. Their main site of action is the cell membrane, where they inhibit voltage-sensitive sodium channels, thereby preventing the transient increase in permeability to sodium ions required for an action potential.

Local anesthetics are characterized in two major groups on the basis of their metabolism: esters and amides. Esters, such as tetracaine and procaine, are metabolized by plasma esterases. Amides, such as lidocaine and bupivacaine, are degraded by the liver. Local anesthetics, administered by the intravenous or the aerosol route, have been used to prevent bronchospasm for many years. They are particularly effective at preventing airway constriction provoked by airway irritation. The mechanisms involved include interruption of irritant reflex arcs, direct relaxation of airway smooth muscle, and inhibition of mediator release from mast cells.

Lidocaine is the most widely used of the local anesthetics, and most of the research related to airways involved this agent. Local anesthetics such as lidocaine directly relax airway smooth muscle. This relaxation is associated with decreases in concentrations of intracellular calcium. Lidocaine also inhibits release of histamine from mast cells. However, the drug concentrations required for these effects are about 100 times greater than can be administered safely to humans.

Lidocaine is extremely effective at preventing irritant-induced bronchoconstriction in humans, but is ineffective against agonists that constrict directly airway smooth muscle.[11] Effective plasma concentrations range from 2 to 4 µg/mL. Aerosol administration offers no advantage over the intravenous route and may even provoke bronchoconstriction in patients with hyperreactive airways. Procaine, hexylcaine, and bupivacaine offer no advantage over lidocaine in this regard and in some instances are less effective. Lidocaine, in a dose of 1.5 to 2 mg/kg, is widely used to attenuate the reflex bronchoconstriction induced by tracheal intubation. The protective effect is typically gone in 5 min. An infusion of 1 to 3 mg/min produces a more prolonged effect.

Brown and colleagues[12] demonstrated that an orally active local anesthetic, mexiletine, was as effective as intravenous lidocaine at preventing the reflex component of histamine-induced bronchoconstriction in dogs.[12] This occurred at therapeutic plasma levels with a prolonged duration of action. These studies must be repeated in humans, but they suggest that orally active local anesthetics may be useful in the prevention of irritant-induced bronchoconstriction in humans.

Conclusions

Many anesthetics or anesthetic adjuncts can theoretically alter airway tone and reactivity. These include ultra-short-acting induction agents, inhalational and local anesthetics, and neuromuscular blockers. The effects of thiobarbiturates on airways are controversial. A new agent, propofol, appears promising as an induction agent that prevents bronchoconstriction, but its mechanism of action on airways is unknown. The effects of the commonly used neuromuscular blockers are probably minimal. By contrast, inhalational anesthetics and local anesthetics are extremely effective at inhibiting airway reflexes. Inhalational anesthetics also directly relax the airway smooth muscle at greater, but still clinically relevant, concentrations, making these agents potent bronchodilators. The application of patch clamp techniques and fluorescent dyes to measure intracellular calcium ion concentrations in airway smooth muscle and nerves is now increasing understanding of the cellular mechanisms involved.

References

1. Hirshman CA, Bergman NA: Factors influencing intrapulmonary airway calibre during anaesthesia. *Br J Anaesth* 1990; 65:30.
2. Warner DO, Vetterman J, Brichant JF, Rehder K: Direct and neurally mediated effects of halothane on pulmonary resistance in vivo. *Anesthesiology* 1990; 72:1057.
3. Jones RM: Clinical comparison of inhalational anaesthetic agents. *Br J Anaesth* 1984; 56:57S.
4. Brown RH, Zerhouni EA, Hirshman CA: Comparison of low concentrations of halothane and isoflurane as bronchodilators. *Anesthesiology* 1993; 78:1097.
5. Yamakage M, Hirshman CA: Volatile anesthetics and airway smooth muscle function. *Curr Opin Anesth* 1994; 7:531.
6. Pizov R, Brown RH, Weiss YS, et al.: Wheezing during induction of general anesthesia in patients with and without asthma: a randomized blinded trial. *Anesthesiology* 1995; 82:1111.
7. Hirshman CA, Downes H, Farbood A, Bergman NA: Ketamine block of bronchospasm in experimental canine asthma. *Br J Anaesth* 1979; 51:713.
8. Wilson LE, Hatch DJ, Rehder K: Mechanisms of the relaxant action of ketamine on isolated porcine trachealis muscle. *Br J Anaesth* 1993; 71:544.
9. Bowman WC: Non-relaxant properties of neuromuscular blocking drugs. *Br J Anaesth* 1982; 54:147.
10. Mehr E, Hirshman CA, Lindeman KS: Mechanism of action of atracurium on airways. *Anesthesiology* 1992; 76:448.
11. Downes H, Gerber N, Hirshman CA: IV Lignocaine in reflex and allergic bronchoconstriction. *Br J Anaesth* 1980; 52:873.
12. Brown RH, Robbins W, Staats P, Hirshman CA: Prevention of bronchoconstriction by an orally active local anesthetic. *Am J Respir Crit Care Med* 1995; 151:1239.

INDEX

INDEX

The letter *f* or *t* following a page number indicates that either a figure or a table is being referenced.

ISBN 0-07-037096-6

90000>